Oxford Textbook of

Obstetric Anaesthesia

Oxford Textbooks in Anaesthesia

Oxford Textbook of Anaesthesia for the Elderly Patient
Edited by Chris Dodds, Chandra M. Kumar, and Bernadette Th.Veering

Oxford Textbook of Anaesthesia for Oral and Maxillofacial Surgery
Edited by Ian Shaw, Chandra M. Kumar, and Chris Dodds

Principles and Practice of Regional Anaesthesia, Fourth Edition
Edited by Graeme McLeod, Colin McCartney, and Tony Wildsmith

Oxford Textbook of Cardiothoracic Anaesthesia
Edited by R. Peter Alston, Paul S. Myles, and Marco Ranucci

Oxford Textbook of Transplant Anaesthesia and Critical Care
Edited by Ernesto A. Pretto, Jr., Gianni Biancofiore, Andre De Wolf, John R. Klinck, Claus Niemann, Andrew Watts, and Peter D. Slinger

Oxford Textbook of Obstetric Anaesthesia
Edited by Vicki Clark, Marc Van de Velde, and Roshan Fernando

Oxford Textbook of

Obstetric Anaesthesia

Edited by

Dr Vicki Clark, MB. ChB., FRCA

Consultant Anaesthetist
Simpson Centre for Reproductive Health
Royal Infirmary
Edinburgh, UK

Professor Marc Van de Velde, MD, PhD, EDRA

Professor of Anesthesiology
Department of Cardiovascular Sciences
KU Leuven
Chair
Department of Anesthesiology
UZ Leuven
Leuven, Belgium

Dr Roshan Fernando, MB. ChB., FRCA

Consultant Anaesthetist and Honorary Senior Lecturer
Department of Anaesthesia
University College London Hospitals NHS Foundation Trust
London, UK

OXFORD
UNIVERSITY PRESS

OXFORD
UNIVERSITY PRESS

Great Clarendon Street, Oxford, OX2 6DP,
United Kingdom

Oxford University Press is a department of the University of Oxford. It furthers the University's objective of excellence in research, scholarship, and education by publishing worldwide. Oxford is a registered trade mark of Oxford University Press in the UK and in certain other countries

First Edition published in 2016

Published in the United States of America by Oxford University Press
198 Madison Avenue, New York, NY 10016, United States of America

British Library Cataloguing in Publication Data
Data available

Library of Congress Control Number: 2016938518

ISBN 978–0–19–871333–3

Dedications

Vicki Clark

To Richard and my parents, colleagues, and patients, all of whom in their different ways, helped to make this textbook possible. Their contributions, known and unknown, small or large, have all been invaluable and my thanks go to them.

Roshan Fernando

To all my family who have supported me throughout my career and especially to my wife Anelia and our little girl Nia for making it special.

Marc Van de Velde

To my parents, Karel and Vera, for their everlasting love and support.

To my loving wife Eva, for making my life complete.

To Juliette, Ella, Bas, Michiel, and Sofie for bringing joy, laughter and warmth into my life. I couldn't dream of better kids.

Preface

Providing obstetric anaesthesia in the delivery suite and maternity theatre presents a challenge to every practising anaesthetist. Not only are there two patients to consider, often with opposing needs, but the physiology and anatomy of the pregnant woman varies significantly from her non-pregnant counterpart. Furthermore, many procedures are done as emergencies with additional risk factors. And in recent years, the complexity of care of the pregnant population has been increased by factors such as rising maternal age and co-morbidities which in the past may have precluded pregnancy. There is therefore a need for a comprehensive, up-to-date textbook covering all aspects of care for parturients including recent approaches to neuraxial anaesthesia, new technologies, drugs, protocols, and guidelines.

This textbook brings together international contributors who are experts in their fields and who have provided in-depth, evidence-based chapters on obstetric anaesthesia with practical information and guidance that we hope will be of value for those working in the maternity environment wherever they happen to practise.

Contents

Abbreviations

5-HT	5-hydroxytryptamine (serotonin)
AAGBI	Association of Anaesthetists of Great Britain and Ireland
AAP	American Association of Pediatrics
ACOG	American College of Obstetricians and Gynecologists
ACTH	adrenocorticotropic hormone
AD	autosomal dominant
ADE	absorption, distribution, metabolism, and elimination
AED	antiepileptic drug
AFE	amniotic fluid embolism
AFLP	acute fatty liver of pregnancy
AHD	acquired heart disease
AIH	autoimmune hepatitis
AKI	acute kidney injury
ALP	alkaline phosphatase
ALT	alanine transaminase
ANA	antinuclear antibody
AP	alkaline phosphatase
APACHE	Acute Physiology and Chronic Health Evaluation
APH	antepartum haemorrhage
APS	antiphospholipid syndrome
aPTT	activated partial thromboplastin time
AR	autosomal recessive
ARDS	acute respiratory distress syndrome
AROM	artificial rupture of the membranes
ART	assisted reproductive technology
ASA	American Society of Anesthesiologists
ASD	atrial septal defect
ASM	airway smooth muscle
AST	aspartate transaminase
ATP	Adenosine triphosphate
AUROC	area under the receiver operating characteristic curve
AV	atrioventricular
AVM	arteriovenous malformation
BMI	body mass index
bpm	beats per minute
BPP	biophysical profile score
cAMP	cyclic adenosine monophosphate
CBG	corticosteroid-binding globulin
CD	Caesarean Delivery
CDC	Centers for Disease Control and Prevention
CEI	continuous epidural infusion
CEMACH	Confidential Enquiry into Maternal and Child Health
CEMD	Confidential Enquiry into Maternal Deaths
CF	cystic fibrosis
CGRP	calcitonin gene-related peptide
CHD	congenital heart disease
CI	confidence interval
CIPCEA	computer-integrated patient-controlled epidural analgesia
CK	creatine kinase
CKD	chronic kidney disease
CMACE	Centre for Maternal and Child Enquiries
CMV	cytomegalovirus
CNB	central neuraxial blockade
CNS	central nervous system
CO	cardiac output
CO_2	carbon dioxide
COX	cyclooxygenase
CPAP	continuous positive airway pressure
CPR	cardiopulmonary resuscitation
CRH	corticotropin-releasing hormone
CS	Cushing's syndrome
CSA	Continuous Spinal Anaesthesia
CSE	combined spinal–epidural
CSF	cerebrospinal fluid
CSH	cranial subdural haematoma
CTG	cardiotocography
CTPA	computed tomography pulmonary angiography
CVA	cerebrovascular accident
CVC	central venous catheter
CVS	cardiovascular system
CXR	chest X-ray
CYP	cytochrome p450
DAS	Difficult Airway Society
DCM	dilated cardiomyopathy
DDI	decision to delivery interval
DHPR	dihydropyridine
DIC	disseminated intravascular coagulation
DKA	diabetic ketoacidosis
DM	diabetes mellitus
DMARD	Disease modifying anti-rheumatic drugs

DPG	diphosphoglycerate
DVT	deep vein thrombosis
EA	epidural anaesthesia
EC_{50}	median effective concentration
ECC	excitation–contraction coupling
ECG	electrocardiogram
ED	Ehlers–Danlos
ED_{50}	effective dose in 50% of subjects
ED_{95}	effective dose in 95% of subjects
EFM	electronic fetal monitoring
EP	ectopic pregnancy
EPAU	early pregnancy assessment unit
EREM	extended-release epidural morphine
ERPHD	European Registry on Pregnancy and Heart Disease
ESBL	extended-spectrum beta-lactamase
ESC	European Society of Cardiology
ESRD	end-stage renal disease
ETT	endotracheal tube
EUA	examination under anaesthetic
FAS	fetal alcohol syndrome
FBC	full blood count
FBS	fetal blood sampling
FDA	Food and Drug Administration
FER	frozen embryo replacement
FET	frozen embryo transfer
FEV_1	forced expiratory volume in 1 second
FFN	fetal fibronectin
FHR	fetal heart rate
FIGO	Federation Internationale des Gynécologues et des Obstétriciens
FLF	fetal lung fluid
FPG	fasting plasma glucose
FRC	functional residual capacity
FSH	follicle-stimulating hormone
FVC	forced vital capacity
GA	general anaesthesia
GABA	gamma-aminobutyric acid
GBS	Guillain–Barré syndrome
GDM	gestational diabetes mellitus
GFR	glomerular filtration rate
GGT	gamma-glutamyl transferase
GH	gestational hypertension or growth hormone
GI	gastrointestinal
GMC	General Medical Council
GnRH	gonadotropin-releasing hormone
GOR	gastro-oesophageal reflux
GP	general practitioner
hCG	human chorionic gonadotropin
HCM	hypertrophic cardiomyopathy
HDU	high dependency unit
HELLP	haemolysis, elevated liver enzyme levels, and low platelet count
HIT	heparin-induced thrombocytopenia
HLHS	hypoplastic left heart syndrome
HPA	hypothalamic–pituitary–adrenal
HR	heart rate
HSV	herpes simplex virus
HUS	haemolytic uraemic syndrome
ICD-10	International Classification of Diseases, tenth revision
ICNARC	Intensive Care National Audit and Research Centre
ICP	intracranial pressure
ICS	inhaled corticosteroid
ICSI	intracytoplasmic sperm injection
ICU	intensive care unit
IE	infective endocarditis
IHD	ischaemic heart disease
IIH	Idiopathic intracranial hypertension
ILCOR	International Liaison Committee on Resuscitation
IM	intramuscular
INR	international normalized ratio
IR	interventional radiology
ITP	idiopathic thrombocytopenic purpura
ITU	intensive therapy unit
IUGR	intrauterine growth restriction
IV	intravenous
IVC	inferior vena cava
IVF	in vitro fertilization
LA	local anaesthetic
LABA	long-acting beta-2-agonist
LAST	local anaesthetic systemic toxicity
LBP	low back pain
LDH	lactate dehydrogenase
LFT	liver function test
LH	luteinizing hormone
LMA	laryngeal mask airway
LMN	Lower Motor Neuron
LMWH	low-molecular-weight heparin
LOR	loss of resistance
LOS	lower oesophageal sphincter
LRTA	leukotriene-receptor antagonist
LSB	lumbar sympathetic block
LUD	left uterine displacement
MAC	minimum alveolar concentration
MAHA	microangiopathic haemolytic anaemia
MBRRACE-UK	Mothers and Babies: Reducing Risk through Audits and Confidential Enquiries across the United Kingdom
MCA	middle cerebral artery
MCV	mean cell volume
MDE	Maternal Death Enquiry
MELD	Model of End Stage Liver Disease
MEWS	Modified Early Warning Score
MFS	Marfan syndrome
MG	myasthenia gravis
MH	malignant hyperthermia
MHRA	Medicines & Healthcare products Regulatory Agency
MHS	malignant hyperthermia-susceptible
MI	myocardial infarction
MLAC	minimum local analgesic concentration
MLAD	minimum local analgesic dose
MMR	maternal mortality ratio
MPM	Mortality Probability Model
MRI	Magnetic Resonance Imaging

MRSA meticillin-resistant *Staphylococcus aureus*
NA neuraxial anaesthesia
NAFLD non-alcoholic fatty liver disease
NAP National Audit Project
NICE National Institute of Health and Care Excellence
NMB neuromuscular blockade
NMDA N-methyl-D-aspartate
NO nitric oxide
NSAID non-steroidal anti-inflammatory drug
NT nuchal translucency
NYHA New York Heart Association
O_2 oxygen
OAA Obstetric Anaesthetists' Association
ODP operating department practitioner
OGTT oral glucose tolerance test
OHSS ovarian hyperstimulation syndrome
OR odds ratio/Operating Room
PAC pulmonary artery catheter
$PaCO_2$ arterial partial pressure of carbon dioxide
PAI plasminogen activator inhibitor
PAPP-A pregnancy-associated plasma protein-A
PB pudendal block
PCA patient-controlled analgesia
PCB paracervical block
PCEA patient-controlled epidural analgesia
PCO_2 partial pressure of carbon dioxide
PCR polymerase chain reaction
PD pharmacodynamics
PDPH postdural puncture headache
PDPM postdural puncture meningitis
PEEP positive end-expiratory pressure
PEF peak expiratory flow
PEFR peak expiratory flow rate
PG prostaglandin
PIP positive inspiratory pressure
PK pharmacokinetics
PND paroxysmal nocturnal dyspnoea
PPCM peripartum cardiomyopathy
PPH postpartum haemorrhage
PPROM preterm premature rupture of membranes
PPSP persistent postsurgical pain
PRB pregnancy-related backache
PROM premature rupture of membranes
PSO paramedian sagittal oblique
PT prothrombin time
PTE pulmonary thromboembolism
PVB paravertebral block
RA rheumatoid arthritis
RBC red blood cell
RBF renal blood flow
RCOG Royal College of Obstetricians and Gynaecologists
RCT randomized controlled trial
REM rapid eye movement
RHD rheumatic heart disease
RR relative risk
RSI rapid sequence induction
RYR1 ryanodine
SA spinal anaesthesia
SABA short-acting beta-2-agonist
SAD supraglottic airway device
SaO_2 arterial oxygen saturation
SAPS Simplified Acute Physiology Score
SCASMM Scottish Confidential Audit of Severe Maternal Morbidity
SCI spinal cord injury
SGA small for gestational age
SH spinal haematoma
SIGN Scottish Intercollegiate Guidelines Network
SLE systemic lupus erythematosus
SNP single nucleotide polymorphism
SSRI selective serotonin reuptake inhibitor
SSS single-shot spinal
SV stroke volume
SVR systemic vascular resistance
SVT supraventricular tachycardia
T1D type 1 diabetes
T2D type 2 diabetes
T_3 triiodothyronine
T_4 thyroxine
TAP transversus abdominis plane
TB tuberculosis
TBG thyroxine-binding globulin
TCPC total cavopulmonary connection
TENS transcutaneous electrical nerve stimulator
TM transverse median
TSH thyroid-stimulating hormone
TT thrombin time
TTP thrombotic thrombocytopenic purpura
TTTS twin-to-twin transfusion syndrome
TV tidal volume
UDCA ursodeoxycholic acid
UFH unfractionated heparin
UKHCDO United Kingdom Haemophilia Centre Doctors' Organisation
UKOSS UK Obstetric Surveillance System
ULN upper limit of normal
UMN Upper Motor Neuron
V/Q ventilation/perfusion
VAPS visual analogue pain scale
VAS visual analogue scale
VBAC vaginal birth after caesarean
VD vaginal delivery
VRS verbal rating score
VSD ventricular septal defect
VT ventricular tachycardia
VTE venous thromboembolism
vWD von Willebrand disease
vWF von Willebrand factor
WFSA World Federation of Societies of Anaesthesiologists
WHO World Health Organization

Contributors

Colleen D. Acosta, Researcher, National Perinatal Epidemiology Unit, Nuffield Department of Population Health, University of Oxford, Oxford, UK

Karel Allegaert, Department of Development and Regeneration, KU Leuven, Belgium; Intensive Care and Department of Surgery, Erasmus MC-Sophia Children's Hospital, Rotterdam, the Netherlands

John A. Anderson, Consultant in Obstetrics and Gynaecology, Bradford Royal Infirmary, Bradford, UK

Michelle J. Arcache, Specialist Anaesthesiologist, Department of Anaesthesia, University of Cape Town, Cape Town, South Africa

Sarah L. Armstrong, Consultant Anaesthetist, Frimley Health NHS Foundation Trust, Frimley, Surrey, UK

Salma Ballal, Liverpool Women's NHS Foundation Trust, Liverpool, UK

Philip Barclay, Consultant Anaesthetist, West Middlesex University Hospital, Chelsea and Westminster NHS Foundation Trust, London, UK

Jessica Bauerle, Department of Anesthesiology, Perioperative and Pain Medicine, Brigham and Women's Hospital, Boston, MA, USA

Julie-Clare Becher, Department of Neonatology, Simpson Centre for Reproductive Health, Royal Infirmary of Edinburgh, Edinburgh, UK

Marie-Pierre Bonnet, Anesthesia and Critical Care Department, Hôpital Cochin, Hôpitaux Universitaires Paris Centre, Assistance Publique-Hôpitaux de Paris, Paris; INSERM UMR1153, Obstetrical, Perinatal and Paediatric Epidemiology Research Team (Epopé), Center for Epidemiology and Statistics Sorbonne Paris Cité, Paris France

Kate Bramham, Clinical Research Fellow, Women's Health Academic Centre, King's Health Partners, King's College London, London, UK

James P. R. Brown, Consultant Anesthesiologist, Department of Anesthesiology, BC Women's Hospital, Vancouver, Canada; Clinical Assistant Professor, University of British Columbia, Vancouver, Canada

Roch Cantwell, Consultant Perinatal Psychiatrist, NHS Greater Glasgow and Clyde; Honorary Clinical Senior Lecturer, University of Glasgow, Glasgow, UK

Giorgio Capogna, Head of Department, Department of Anaesthesiology Città di Roma Hospital, Rome; Director, European School of Obstetric Anesthesia, Rome, Italy

David Cassiman, Professor of Medicine, Division of Gastroenterology and Hepatology, University Hospital Gasthuisberg, University of Leuven, Belgium

Susan Catling, Consultant Anaesthetist, Department of Anaesthesia, Singleton Hospital, Swansea, UK

Anne Alice Chantry, INSERM UMR1153, Obstetrical, Perinatal and Paediatric Epidemiology Research Team (Epopé), Center for Epidemiology and Statistics Sorbonne Paris Cité, Paris France; Baudelocque Midwives School, Paris Descartes University (Paris 5), Paris, France

Katherine Cheesman, Consultant Anaesthetist, Guy's & St Thomas NHS Trust, London, UK

Vicki Clark, Consultant Anaesthetist, Simpson Centre for Reproductive Health, Royal Infirmary, Edinburgh, UK

Elizabeth Combeer, Consultant Anaesthetist, Frimley Health NHS Foundation Trust, Frimley, Surrey, UK

E. Sarah Cooper, Consultant Obstetrician, Simpson Centre for Reproductive Health, Royal Infirmary of Edinburgh, Edinburgh, UK

Catherine Cromey, Consultant Anaesthetist, Department of Anaesthesia, Morriston Hospital, Swansea, UK

Vegard Dahl, Professor, Head of Department of Anaesthesia and Intensive Care, Akershus University Hospital, Loerenskog, Norway

Diane De Neubourg, Leuven University Fertility Centre, Department of Obstetrics and Gynaecology, University Hospitals Leuven, Leuven, Belgium

Fiona C. Denison, Reader in Maternal and Fetal Health and Consultant Obstetrician, MRC Centre for Reproductive Health, University of Edinburgh, Queen's Medical Research Institute, Edinburgh, UK

Jan Deprest, Department of Obstetrics and Gynecology, Fetal Medicine Unit, University Hospitals Leuven, Leuven, Belgium

Roland Devlieger, Department of Obstetrics and Gynaecology, University Hospitals Leuven, Leuven, Belgium

Sarah Devroe, Department of Anaesthesiology, University Hospitals Leuven, Leuven; Department of Cardiovascular Sciences, Section Anesthesiology, Obstetric Anesthesia, KU Leuven and UZ Leuven, Leuven, Belgium

Daryl P. Dob, Consultant Anaesthetist, Magill Department of Anaesthesia, Chelsea and Westminster Hospital, London, UK

M. Joanne Douglas, Professor Emeritus, Department of Anesthesiology, Pharmacology and Therapeutics, University of British Columbia and BC Women's Hospital, Vancouver, Canada

Timothy J. Draycott, Professor, Department of Women's Health, Southmead Hospital, Bristol

Kate Drummond, Department of Neurosurgery, The Royal Melbourne Hospital; Department of Surgery, University of Melbourne; Melbourne Brain Centre at The Royal Melbourne Hospital, Melbourne, Australia

W. Colin Duncan, Senior Lecturer in Reproductive Medicine, University of Edinburgh; Consultant Gynaecologist, Simpson Centre for Reproductive Health, Royal Infirmary, Edinburgh, UK

Robert A. Dyer, Professor and Second Chair, Department of Anaesthesia, University of Cape Town, Cape Town, South Africa

Thomas Erb, Professor of Anaesthesia, Departement of Anaesthesia, University Children's Hospital beider Basel, Basel, Switzerland

Roshan Fernando, Consultant Anaesthetist and Honorary Senior Lecturer, Department of Anaesthesia, University College London Hospitals NHS Foundation Trust, London, UK

Timothée Fraisse, Pharmaceutical Medicine Specialist, MFGI, Lyon, France

Miguel Garcia, Specialist Registrar in Anaesthesia, Department of Anaesthesia, University Hospitals Bristol, Bristol, UK

Michael A. Gatzoulis, Professor of Cardiology, Department of Cardiology, Royal Brompton Hospital and National Heart and Lung Institute, Imperial College, London, UK

Thierry Girard, Professor of Anaesthesia, Department of Anesthesiology, Operative Intensive Care, Preclinical Emergency Medicine and Pain Management, University Hospital Basel, Basel, Switzerland

Ian A. Greer, Vice-President, The University of Manchester; Dean, Faculty of Medical and Human Sciences, The University of Manchester; Director, Manchester Academic Health Science Centre (MAHSC), Manchester, UK

James Griffiths, Department of Anaesthesia, Royal Women's Hospital, Melbourne; Department of Pharmacology and Therapeutics, University of Melbourne, Melbourne, Australia

Suni Halder, Consultant Anaesthetist, Nuffield Department of Anaesthesia, John Radcliffe Hospital, Oxford University NHS Foundation Trust Hospitals, Oxford, UK

Rachel Hignett, Consultant Anaesthetist, Simpson Centre for Reproductive Health, Royal Infirmary of Edinburgh, Edinburgh, UK

David Hill, Consultant Anaesthetist, Ulster Hospital, Belfast, UK

Beverley J. Hunt, Professor of Thrombosis & Haemostasis, Kings College and Consultant in Departments of Haematology, Pathology and Rheumatology, Guy's & St Thomas' NHS Foundation Trust, London, UK

Tauqeer Husain, Consultant Anaesthetist, Department of Anaesthesia & Perioperative Medicine, University College Hospital, London, UK

Sudhir Immani, Consultant Anaesthetist, Obstetric Anaesthesia Clinical lead, University Hospital Waterford, Republic of Ireland

Rehana Iqbal, Consultant Anaesthetist, Lecturer in Medical Ethics & Law, St. George's University Hospitals NHS Foundation Trust, London, UK

Yves Jacquemyn, Gynaecologist, Antwerp University Hospital, Belgium

Ewen D. Johnston, Department of Neonatology, Simpson Centre for Reproductive Health, Royal Infirmary of Edinburgh, Edinburgh, UK

Ross Junkin, Consultant Anaesthetist, Department of Anaesthesia, University Hospital Crosshouse, Kilmarnock, UK

Oonagh Keag, Registrar in Obstetrics & Gynaecology, Simpson Centre for Reproductive Health, Royal Infirmary of Edinburgh

Mirjana Kendrisic, Department of Anaesthesia and Intensive Therapy, General Hospital Sremska Mitrovica, Sremska Mitrovica, Serbia

Marian Knight, Research Professor in Public Health, National Perinatal Epidemiology Unit, Nuffield Department of Population Health, University of Oxford, Oxford, UK

Oliver Kraemer, Obstetrics and Gynaecology, Clinica Santa Chiara, Locarno, Switzerland

Anneke Kwee, Gynaecologist, University Medical Center Utrecht, The Netherlands

Sapna Ladani, Specialist Training Registrar in Haematology and Honorary Clinical Lecturer, University Hospitals of Leicester, Leicester, UK

Pierre-Antoine Laloë, Consultant in Anaesthetics, Calderdale Royal Hospital, Halifax, UK

Ruth Landau, Professor of Anesthesiology, Associate Director of Obstetric Anesthesia, Columbia University Medical Center; Director of the Center for Precision Medicine, Department of Anesthesiology, Columbia University College of Physicians & Surgeons, New York, USA

Eldrid Langesaeter, Department of Anesthesiology, Division of Emergencies and Critical Care, and National Resource Centre for Women's Health, Oslo University Hospital, Oslo, Norway

Patricia Lavand'homme, Department of Anaesthesiology, St Luc Hospital University Catholic of Louvain Medical School, Brussels, Belgium

Serene Leo, Consultant, KK Women's and Children's Hospital, Singapore

David M. Levy, Consultant Anaesthetist, Nottingham University Hospitals NHS Trust, Nottingham, UK

York-Mui Liu, Research Fellow in Obstetric Anaesthesia, Department of Anaesthesia, University College London Hospital, London, UK

John Loughrey, Consultant Anaesthetist, The Rotunda Hospital, Dublin, Ireland

Nuala Lucas, Consultant Anaesthetist, Northwick Park Hospital, Harrow, Middlesex, UK

Ioanna Mavridou, Consultant Anaesthetist, Department of Anaesthesia, University College London Hospital, London, UK

Grace McClune, Consultant Anaesthetist, Royal Infirmary, Little France, Edinburgh, UK

Elizabeth M. McGrady, Consultant Anaesthetist, Department of Anaesthesia, Glasgow Royal Infirmary and Princess Royal Maternity Unit

Alistair G. McKenzie, Consultant Anaesthetist, Simpson Centre for Reproductive Health, Royal Infirmary of Edinburgh, Edinburgh, UK

Simon Millar, Consultant Anaesthetist, Department of Anaesthesia, Royal Alexandra Hospital, Paisley, UK

Alistair Milne, Consultant Anaesthetist, Department of Anaesthesia, Royal Infirmary, Little France, Edinburgh, UK

Vibeke Moen, Consultant Anaesthetist, Department of Anaesthesia and Intensive Care, Kalmar County Hospital, Kalmar, Sweden

Wint Mon, Research Fellow in Obstetric Anaesthesia, Department of Anaesthesia, University College London Hospital, London, UK

Neil A. Muchatuta, Consultant Anaesthetist, Department of Anaesthesia, St Michael's Hospital, University Hospitals Bristol, Bristol, UK

Mary C. Mushambi, Consultant Anaesthetist, Leicester Royal Infirmary, Leicester, UK

Catherine Nelson-Piercy, Professor of Obstetric Medicine, Women's Health Academic Centre, King's Health Partners, London; Consultant Obstetric Physician, Guys and St. Thomas' NHS Foundation Trust and Imperial College Healthcare NHS Trust, London, UK

Patchareya Nivatpumin, Assistant Professor, Department of Anesthesiology, Faculty of Medicine Siriraj Hospital, Mahidol University, Bangkok, Thailand

Jane E. Norman, Professor of Maternal and Fetal Health, University of Edinburgh; Director of the Tommy's Centre for Maternal and Fetal Health, Edinburgh, UK

Geraldine O'Sullivan,[†] Previously Consultant Anaesthetist, Guy's & St. Thomas NHS Trust Hospital, London, UK

Clemens Ortner, Assistant Professor, Department of Anesthesiology and Pain Medicine, University of Washington Medical Center, Seattle, WA, USA

Michael J. Paech, Winthrop Professor and Chair of Obstetric Anaesthesia Pharmacology, Pharmacy and Anaesthesiology Unit, School of Medicine and Pharmacology, The University of Western Australia, Perth, Australia

Outi Palomäki, Senior Consultant in Obstetrics and Gynaecology, Tampere University Hospital, Finland

Rajesh Pandey, Consultant Anaesthetist, Leicester General Hospital, Leicester, UK

Sue Pavord, Consultant Haematologist and Senior Lecturer in Medical Education, University Hospitals of Leicester, Leicester, UK

Linzi Peacock, Consultant Anaesthetist, Simpson Centre for Reproductive Health, Royal Infirmary of Edinburgh, Edinburgh, UK

Elspeth E. Pickering, Consultant Anaesthetist, Magill Department of Anaesthesia, Chelsea and Westminster Hospital, London, UK

Borislava Pujic, Department of Anaesthesia, Gynaecology & Obstetrics, University Hospital, Clinical Centre of Vojvodina, Novi Sad, Serbia

Fabienne Roelants, Department of Anaesthesiology, St Luc Hospital University Catholic of Louvain Medical School, Brussels, Belgium

Eva Roofthooft, Department of Anesthesiology, ZNA Middelheim and Paola Children's Hospital, Ziekenhuis Netwerk Antwerpen, Antwerp, Belgium

Francesca Russo, Department of Obstetrics and Gynecology, Fetal Medicine Unit, University Hospitals Leuven, Leuven, Belgium

Ieva Saule, Anaesthetist, East Midlands School of Anaesthesia, Nottingham, UK

Helen Scholefield, Consultant Obstetrician, Liverpool Women's NHS Foundation Trust, Liverpool, UK

Alex Tiong Heng Sia, Professor and Chairman of Medical Board, KK Women's and Children's Hospital and Duke-NUS Graduate Medical School, Singapore

Maria-Elisabeth Smet, Department of Obstetrics and Gynaecology, University Hospitals Leuven, Leuven, Belgium

Ban Leong Sng, Adjunct Assistant Professor and Senior Consultant, KK Women's and Children's Hospital and Duke-NUS Graduate Medical School, Singapore

Mieke A. Soens, Department of Anesthesiology, Perioperative and Pain Medicine, Brigham and Women's Hospital, Boston, MA, USA

Ulrich J. Spreng, Head of Department of Anaesthesia and Intensive Care, Baerum Hospital, Vestre Viken HT, Baerum, Norway

Gary M. Stocks, Consultant Anaesthetist, Queen Charlotte's Hospital, Du Cane Road, London, UK

Wendy H. L. Teoh, Adjunct Assistant Professor, Duke-NUS Graduate Medical School Singapore; Senior Consultant, Department of Women's Anesthesia, KK Women's & Children's Hospital, Singapore

Roulhac D. Toledano, Assistant Clinical Professor of Anaesthesiology, SUNY Downstate Medical Center; Director of Obstetric Anesthesia, NYU Lutheran, Brooklyn, NY, USA

Derek J. Tuffnell, Consultant in Obstetrics and Gynaecology, Bradford Royal Infirmary, Bradford, UK

Kristel Van Calsteren, Department of Development and Regeneration, KU Leuven; Obstetrics and Gynecology, University Hospitals Leuven, Leuven, Belgium

Marc Van de Velde, Professor of Anesthesiology, Department of Cardiovascular Sciences, KU Leuven; Chair, Department of Anesthesiology, UZ Leuven, Leuven, Belgium

Tim Van Mieghem, Consultant in Obstetrics and Gynecology, Department of Obstetrics and Gynecology, Fetal Medicine Unit, University Hospitals Leuven, Leuven, Belgium

Johan Verhaeghe, Professor of Medicine, Department of Maternal Care, University Hospital Gasthuisberg, Leuven, Belgium

Chris Verslype, Professor of Medicine, Department of Hepatology, University Hospital Gasthuisberg, Leuven, Belgium

Petri Volmanen, Chief Physician, Programme for Patient safety, Institute of Health and Welfare, Helsinki, Finland

Michelle Walters, Consultant Anaesthetist, William Harvey Hospital, East Kent Hospitals University Foundation NHS Trust, Ashford, UK

Mark Wigginton, Consultant Paediatric Anaesthetist, Leeds Children's Hospital, Leeds Teaching Hospitals NHS Trust, Leeds, UK

Kate Wiles, NIHR Doctoral Research Fellow in Obstetric Nephrology, King's College, London, UK; Guys and St. Thomas' NHS Foundation Trust, London, UK

Steve Yentis, Consultant Anaesthetist, Chelsea and Westminster Hospital, London; Honorary Reader, Imperial College London, London, UK

Gordon Yuill, Consultant Obstetric Anaesthetist, Department of Anaesthesia, Stepping Hill Hospital, Stockport, UK

PART 1

History of obstetric anaesthesia

CHAPTER 1

Historic timeline of obstetric anaesthesia

Alistair G. McKenzie

Events up to 1950

Antiquity to the 1840s

The severity of the pain of labour has been recognized for millennia, featuring in many books of the Old Testament of the Bible.[1] It was widely believed inappropriate to interfere with this 'women's heritage'—pain was considered to have a dual role: punishment and redemption.[2] Indeed, in 1591, Eufame MacCalyean was executed in Edinburgh, Scotland, having been found guilty of many charges, including requesting a witch to relieve the pains of childbirth.[3] In 1777, Anton Mesmer introduced mesmerism and by 1836, French physician Dr Grubert of Lyons suggested applying this to provide pain relief in labour—but held back, not wishing to defy the book of Genesis.[4] Within a decade, attitudes changed and mesmerism was used to alleviate labour pains: in January 1844 by JP Lynell of Manchester, United Kingdom,[5] and in March 1846 by WB Fahnestock of Lancaster, Pennsylvania, United States.[6] In the early 1840s, James Young Simpson, Professor of Midwifery in Edinburgh, United Kingdom, was using a large dose of laudanum (tincture of opium) to facilitate turning the fetus in labour.[7] Soon after the introduction of general anaesthesia (GA; ether) by William Morton on 16 October 1846, it was James Young Simpson who would revolutionize obstetrics by adopting ether to facilitate delivery.

General anaesthesia, analgesia, and amnesia

Introduction of inhalation anaesthesia in obstetrics

1847 (19 January)

James Young Simpson (Edinburgh) (Figure 1.1) was the first in the world to administer ether (by inhalation) in obstetrics.[8] He then searched for an anaesthetic agent more suitable for use in obstetrics.

1847 (25 January)

First ether anaesthesia for caesarean section was administered by SJ Tracey at St Bartholomew's Hospital, London. This was reported in the *London Medical Gazette* with the comment that 'prolonged exhibition of ether was not allowed lest it might interfere with the contraction of the uterus'.[9]

1847 (February)

Adam Hammer was the first in Germany to use ether for pain relief in labour.[10]

1847 (March)

James Young Simpson wrote: 'it will be necessary to ascertain anaesthesia's precise effects, both upon the action of the uterus and on the assistant abdominal muscles; its influence, if any, upon the child; whether it has a tendency to haemorrhage or other complications.'[8] Unfortunately this was not followed up for nearly a century.

1847 (April)

The first obstetric anaesthetic in the United States was by Dr Nathan Cooley Keep, who administered ether for relief of labour pain to Fanny Longfellow, wife of the poet Henry Wadsworth Longfellow (who also participated in the administration).[11]

1847 (May)

NI Pirogoff in Russia expounded on the rectal route for administration of ether in obstetrics.[12]

1847 (8 November)

James Young Simpson was the first to use chloroform in obstetrics. A week later he published the second edition of a pamphlet describing the inhalation of chloroform in 50 cases. Thereafter, for the rest of his life, he promoted chloroform.[13]

1847 (December)

James Young Simpson published *Answer to the Religious Objections*,[14] a pamphlet in which he rather exaggerated potential religious objections to anaesthesia/analgesia for childbirth—to get the public on his side.[15]

1853

John Snow smelled ether on the breath of neonates delivered from mothers who had received ether, surmising placental transmission.[16]

1853 (April)

John Snow administered chloroform to Queen Victoria during the birth of her eighth child, Prince Leopold.

1857 (April)

Queen Victoria again received chloroform from John Snow for the birth of her ninth child (Princess Beatrice). Many authors have declared that this *narcose à la reine* set the seal of respectability on obstetric analgesia; however this may be mythical: the chloroformings of the Queen were not well publicized,[17] excepting

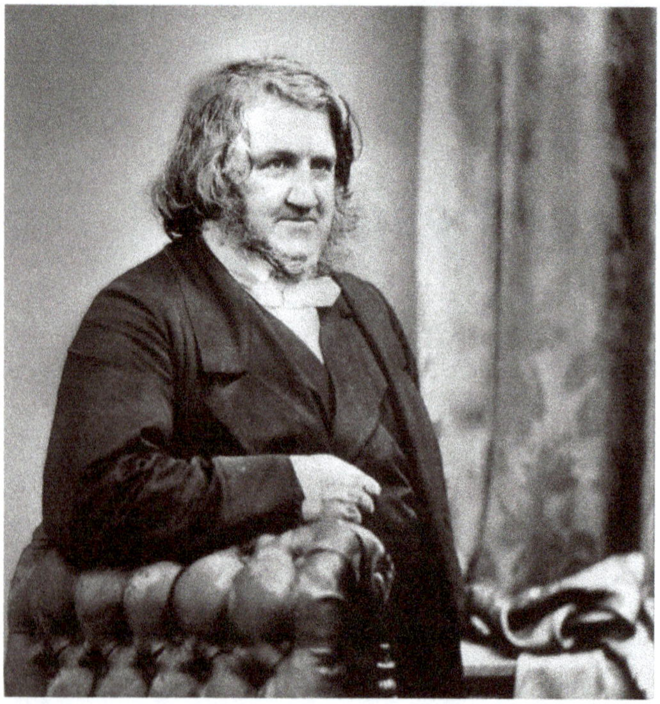

Figure 1.1 James Young Simpson (1811–1870) in 1850. He was first to use ether in obstetrics in January 1847, introduced chloroform in November 1847, and championed analgesia in childbirth.
Image courtesy of the Royal College of Physicians of Edinburgh.

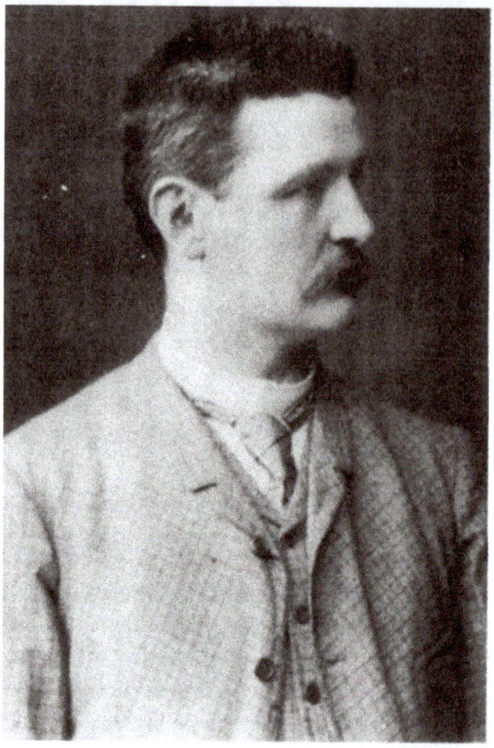

Figure 1.2 Stanislav Sigismund Klikovich (1853–1910)—the first (1880) to use nitrous oxide in obstetrics.
Reproduced from *Materials for the history of scientific and applied activities in Russia in the realms of zoology and allied branches of knowledge during the last 35 years 1850–90* by A. Bogdanov, Moscow, 1892.

London's social elite.[18] Anaesthesia for childbirth progressively became commonplace through public acclaim.

1858

John Snow noted that Dr EW Murphy and Dr E Rigby pioneered relief from pain by inhalation in obstetric cases without loss of consciousness—though this condition was not called 'analgesia' at that time.[19]

1866

Robert Ellis, Obstetric Surgeon to the Chelsea, Brompton and Belgrave Dispensaries in London, described his alcohol-ether-chloroform apparatus for use in obstetrics.[20]

1874

Swiss obstetrician (in Basel), Paul Zweifel, deduced placental transfer by demonstrating that chloroform was present in the umbilical blood of neonates born to chloroformed mothers.[21] He wondered whether this could be a factor in neonatal jaundice, but this was never found to be so.

1880

Stanislav Sigismund Klikovich (Figure 1.2), a doctor in St Petersburg, Russia, was the first to use nitrous oxide in obstetrics—he administered it with oxygen.[22]

1928–32

National Birthday Fund for Maternity Services was inaugurated in London with an address by Lucy Baldwin (the Prime Minister's wife). In 1930, this became the National Birthday Trust Fund, which proceeded to organize supply of chloroform in glass capsules (brisettes) for analgesia in labour, including administration by supervised midwives. Within 10 years these were withdrawn because of high mortality. An alternative was the Mennell chloroform inhaler (modified Junker bottle).[25]

1933

RJ Minnitt in Liverpool, United Kingdom, modified the McKesson oxygen therapy apparatus for self-administration of nitrous oxide with air in labour.[26]

1934–35

Wesley Bourne (Canada) used cyclopropane[27] and also divinyl ether in obstetrics.[28]

1936

Minnitt produced the 'Queen Charlotte' model of his gas-air analgesia apparatus,[29] which was approved by the Central Midwives Board for use by midwives.

1937

Professor Chassar Moir designed an attachment for the above-mentioned apparatus, which allowed a limited amount of pure nitrous oxide to be inhaled before continuing with the mixture.[30] (This invalidated the endorsement for use by midwives.)

1943

Inhalation of Trilene® was found to be a useful method of analgesia in labour. In **1949**, the 'Emotril' draw-over inhaler was designed.[31]

Parenteral amnesia—The Vogue for 'Twilight Sleep'

1902

'Dammerschlaf' (twilight sleep), a technique of initial injection of morphine with hyoscine (scopolamine) and repeat doses of the latter, was used for labour by von Steinbuchel of Graz, Austria.[11]

1906

Carl J Gauss of Freiburg, Germany, popularized twilight sleep, reporting 1000 cases.[11] The injections were subcutaneous or intramuscular. Media coverage led women in Europe and the United States to demand twilight sleep from their obstetricians. Of course there was a depressant effect on the newborns.[11]

Rectal agents including Avertin® for pain relief in labour

1926

Rectal tribromoethanol (Avertin®) was introduced for basal narcosis and was soon adopted to provide amnesia in childbirth. Problems encountered were prolongation of labour and respiratory depression in the neonate. By the 1950s, it was usually reserved for treatment of eclampsia.[35,36]

1930

Gwathmey (New York) introduced a rectal mixture of ether with quinine, alcohol, and olive oil. This was given in combination with hypodermic morphine and intramuscular (IM) magnesium sulphate.[37]

1935

Rosenfield and Davidoff (Boston) used rectal paraldehyde for amnesia, in combination with oral Nembutal®.[38]

1939

McCormick (Indiana) modified Gwathmey's technique for rectal ether mixture (having devised apparatus for administration) by omitting quinine, and giving oral pentobarbitone sodium (Nembutal®) instead of IM magnesium sulphate.[39]

Obstetric flying squad

1929

Professor E Farquhar Murray (Newcastle-upon-Tyne, United Kingdom), addressing the Edinburgh Obstetric Society, conceived the idea of an obstetric flying squad—for domiciliary treatment of obstetric emergencies.[40]

1932

The first operational squad began at Bellshill (near Glasgow), Scotland—called the 'Special Outdoor Treatment Unit'.[40]

1935

The Bellshill unit comprised two doctors and two nurses, who travelled by automobile with apparatus for blood transfusion or intravenous (IV) saline; they had access to 25 universal blood donors.[41]

1948

Obstetric flying squads had been established in many centres in the United Kingdom.[42]

1940–50

In the Bellshill unit, most anaesthetics were administered by junior doctors: Pentothal® (79%), chloroform (12%).[43]

From 'Twilight Sleep' to IV barbiturates

1934

Katherine Lloyd-Williams (Royal Free Hospital, London) published her book *Anaesthesia and Analgesia in Labour* which included the barbiturates sodium amytal, Nembutal®, pernocton, and sodium evipan (hexobarbitone).[44]

1934

Irving et al. at the Boston Lying-in Hospital, United States, researched the effects of popular methods of analgesia, and recommended oral Nembutal® (pentobarbitone sodium) combined with hypodermic scopolamine. There some practitioners began to avoid morphine because it induced neonatal respiratory depression.[38]

1940

The synthetic opioid pethidine (meperidine, Demerol®) was first used in labour by Benthin in Germany.

1943

Gilbert and Dixon (Baltimore) were first in the United States to use Demerol in obstetrics.[45]

1944

Spitzer was the first to use pethidine for obstetric analgesia in Britain.[46]

Figure 1.3 Anaesthesia timeline 1900–1983.

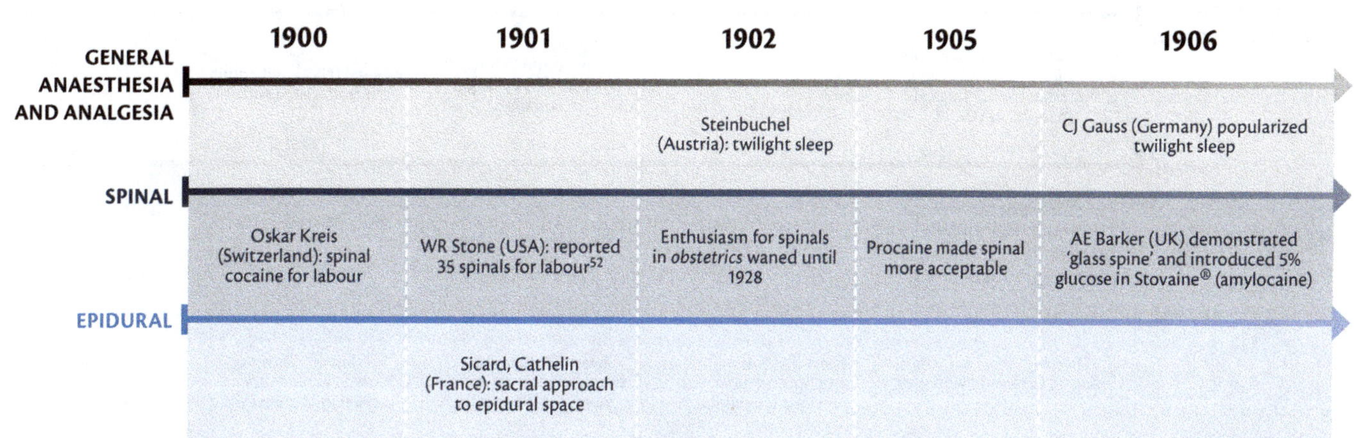

1945

IV pentothal began to be advocated, particularly for caesarean delivery.[47]

Resuscitation of the newborn

1934

Resuscitation of the newborn was often the task of the attending anaesthetist. Instruction in Katherine Lloyd-Williams' book included: clearing the airway, administration of carbon dioxide and oxygen, hypodermic Lobeline, and gentle compression of the chest (no mention of intubation); other stimulant drugs were camphor, Coramine®, and Cardiazol®.[44]

Acid aspiration syndrome

1946

Curtis L Mendelson (Figure 1.4), obstetrician at the New York Lying-in Hospital, reported 66 cases of aspiration of gastric contents during obstetric anaesthesia. Five of the patients aspirated solid material and two of these died of asphyxia. The patients who aspirated liquid (none of whom died) had a different clinical picture: respiratory distress and chest X-ray appearance of soft mottled densities which cleared in 7–10 days. Mendelson showed that instillation of dilute acid into the lungs of anaesthetized rabbits produced a similar syndrome.[49]

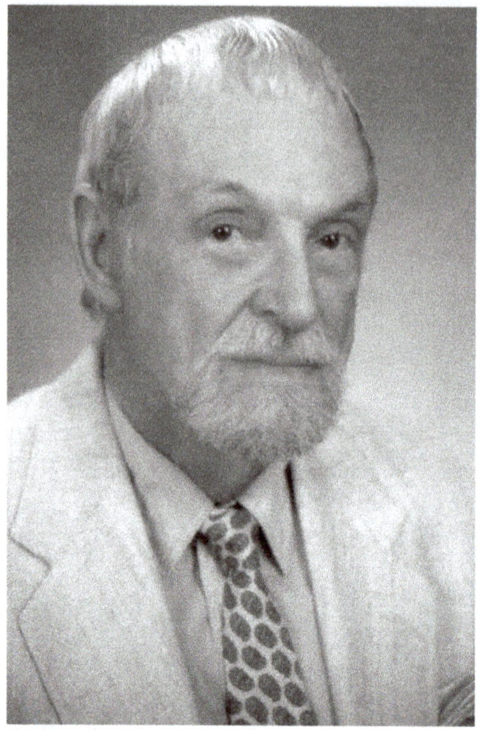

Figure 1.4 Curtis L Mendelson (1913–2002) described the acid aspiration syndrome of pregnancy in 1945.
Image courtesy of Professor J Roger Maltby, author of *Notable Names in Anaesthesia*, London, 2002.

Concept and introduction of regional anaesthesia in obstetrics

1848

James Young Simpson introduced the *concept* of chemical local anaesthesia (LA), experimenting with the application of chloroform and other substances to animals and humans.[50] Unfortunately Simpson lacked both LA agent (cocaine introduced 1884) and the means to inject it (hypodermic needle and syringe introduced by Alexander Wood 1853). If these had been available to him, he would almost certainly have introduced LA in obstetrics.

1900

Sixteen years after Carl Koller introduced the use of cocaine for LA (1884) and 2 years after August Bier performed the first deliberate spinal, Oskar Kreis in Basel, Switzerland, was the first to try intradural spinal block using cocaine for analgesia in labour.[51] Enthusiasm for spinal block waned until after 1905 (see later).

1908

Pudendal block was described by WB Muller in Germany.[53]

1909

Uptake of caudal analgesia (sacral epidural) in obstetrics (see later).

1926

Paracervical block was described by Gellert in Germany.[54]

	1907	1909	1910	1911	1921
GENERAL ANAESTHESIA AND ANALGESIA	Hewitt's textbook: chloroform choice for analgesia in labour, but ether for full surgical anaesthesia (UK)[23]		Papaveretum first used in obstetrics by Jaeger (Germany)[34]	Guedel (USA): self-admin of nitrous oxide with air	
SPINAL	Hewitt's textbook: spinal not even mentioned (UK) Dean described continuous spinal—not accepted (UK)				
EPIDURAL	Hewitt's textbook: sacral epidural not even mentioned (UK)	Stoeckel (Germany) attempted caudal with procaine for childbirth	Läwen (Germany) used caudal with procaine for operative obstetrics	Schlimpert (Germany) used caudal for pain relief in obstetrics[68]	F Pagés Miravé (Spain) introduced lumbar approach

Spinal anaesthesia

Uptake of spinal anaesthesia … and decline by 1948

1905

Popularization of procaine facilitated uptake of spinal anaesthesia as it caused less irritation of meninges; concurrent factors in the United States were availability of finer needles which reduced spinal headache, and rubber gloves (introduced by WS Halsted in 1890) and development of aseptic technique.[55]

1906–07

AE Barker in the United Kingdom demonstrated the 'glass spine', showing the importance of curves and gravity, and introduced 'heavy' Stovaine® (amylocaine) made hyperbaric by the addition of glucose.[56]

1907

Henry P Dean described 'continuous spinal anaesthesia', but this was not accepted at the time.[57]

1912

Babcock (Philadelphia) rendered Stovaine® hypobaric by addition of 10% alcohol.[55] It was not known then that 10% alcohol is potentially neurotoxic.

1927

George Pitkin (New Jersey) introduced hypobaric spinocaine (procaine + alcohol).[55]

Ephedrine was first used to restore blood pressure (BP) during spinal anaesthesia.[58]

1928

George Pitkin also rendered procaine hyperbaric, and was the first to use this for delivery: his so-called controllable spinal anaesthesia.[59]

1940

Walter Lemmon (Philadelphia) revived 'continuous spinal anaesthesia' using novocaine (procaine) with a malleable needle and special rubber tubing attached to the hub.[63]

1944

EB Tuohy described alternative technique: passing a size 4 ureteral catheter *through* a 15-gauge spinal needle.[64]

1948

An article by Bourne and Williams drew attention to serious problems of spinal anaesthesia in obstetrics: maternal collapse, headache, and neurological complications.[67]

Epidural analgesia

Uptake of epidural analgesia

1901

In Paris, J Sicard (neurologist) and F Cathelin (urologist) independently used the sacral approach to the epidural space.[68]

1909

Though initially sceptical, German obstetrician and gynaecologist Walter Stoeckel in Marburg noted Cathelin's publication, and attempted to use 'sacral anaesthesia' with procaine to achieve painless child birth.[69]

1910

Arthur Läwen in Leipzig, Germany, also used the sacral approach to inject procaine in operative obstetrics. He favoured the sitting position and used sodium bicarbonate to alkalinize novocaine chloride, which increased rate, onset, and duration; this had a high success rate and he renamed the method 'extradural anaesthesia'.[68]

1921

The lumbar approach was introduced by Fidel Pagés Miravé in Madrid, Spain, who published *Metameric Anaesthesia*. He died on active service soon after and the method was temporarily forgotten.[68]

1928

Pickles and Jones (Providence, Rhode Island) reported 28 deliveries under single-shot procaine injected into the sacral hiatus.[70]

1930

Eugan Bogdan Aburel (Figure 1.5), a Romanian doctor working in Paris, published five papers on the afferent innervation of the uterus.[71]

1931

Aburel presented a paper on continuous caudal and lumbo-aortic plexus block for pain relief in childbirth.[71]

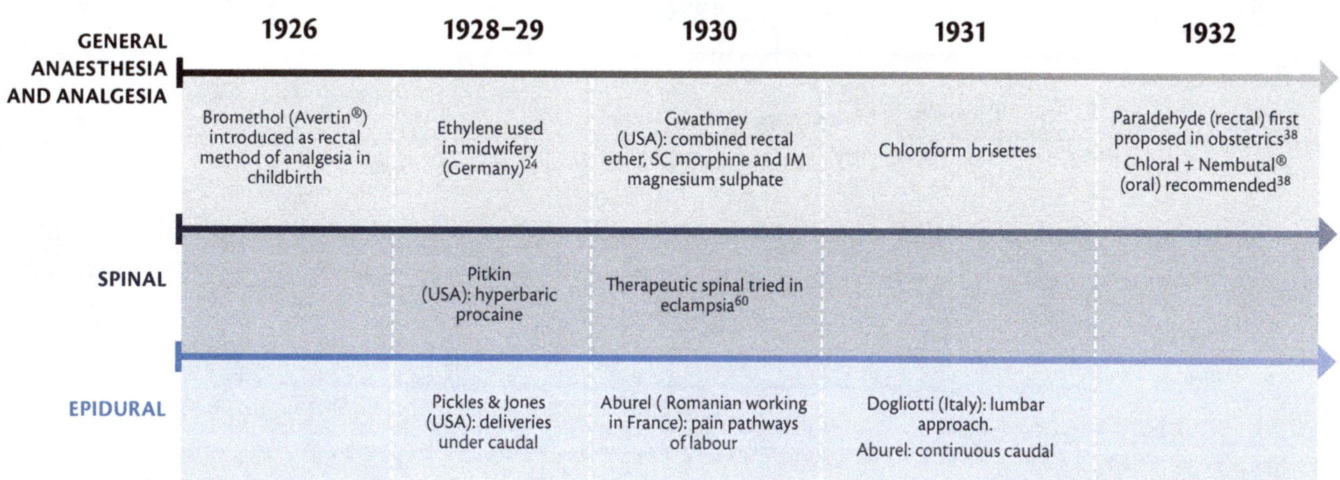

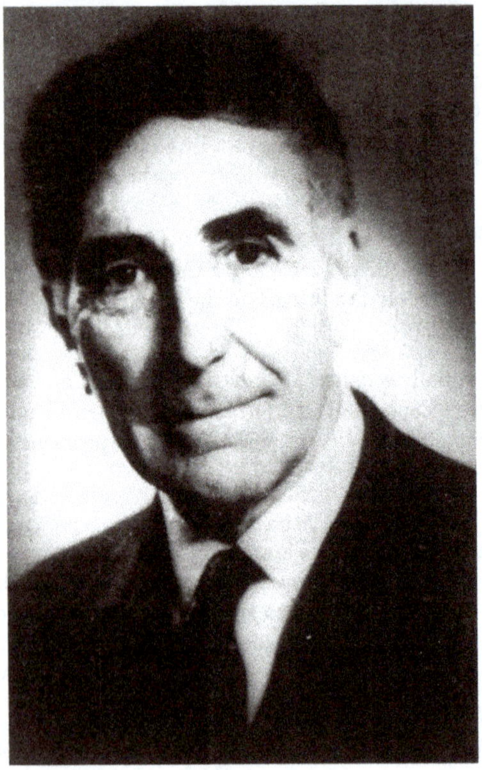

Figure 1.5 Eugen Bogdan Aburel (1899–1975) described the pain pathways of labour in 1930 and continuous caudal analgesia in 1931.
Reproduced with permission from I Curelaru and L Sandu, 'Eugen Bogdan Aburel (1899–1975)', *Anaesthesia*, Volume 37, p. 663, Copyright © 1982 John Wiley & Sons.

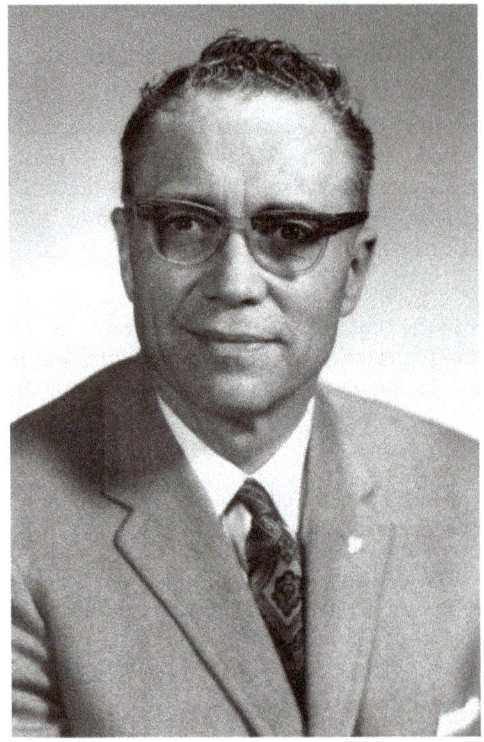

Figure 1.6 Robert A Hingson (1913–1996) popularized continuous caudal analgesia in 1942, introducing plastic catheters and malleable steel needles.
Image courtesy of the Wood Library-Museum of Anesthesiology, Schaumburg, Illinois.

1931

Turin surgeon, Achille Maurio Dogliotti, unaware of Pagés Miravé's work, published a paper on the lumbar approach in *Societa Piemontese di Chirurgia*, and popularized the technique.[68]

1933

John GP Cleland (Oregon City, Oregon), unaware of Aburel's work, researched the afferent innervation of the uterus and published on the use of paravertebral blocks for painless childbirth, and *caudal catheter* for analgesia in the second stage of labour.[72]

1938

Graffagnino and Seyler of New Orleans were the first to use epidural lumbar block in labour (single shot).[73]

1942

Robert Hingson (Philadelphia) (Figure 1.6) and Waldo Edwards (Staten Island, New York) popularized continuous caudal analgesia.[74]

1945

Edward Boyce Tuohy at the Mayo Clinic described a 15-gauge needle with a Huber point (tip designed by Ralph Huber) and a stilette, manufactured by Becton Dickenson.[77] The Huber-tip

	1933	1934	1935	1936	1937
GENERAL ANAESTHESIA AND ANALGESIA	Minnitt (UK): modified McKesson apparatus for self-administration of nitrous oxide with air	Barbiturates for labour—Irving (USA), K Lloyd-Williams (UK). Cyclopropane used by Bourne (Canada)	Rosenfield & Davidoff (USA): rectal paraldehyde. Divinyl ether used by Bourne (Canada)	Minnitt (UK): Queen Charlotte model for nitrous oxide with air	Chassar Moir (UK) attachment for 100% nitrous oxide
SPINAL		K Lloyd-Williams in her book + Franken & O'Connor described spinal for caesarean delivery[47]			Fairfield (UK): high mortality if caesarean delivery done under spinal[61]
EPIDURAL	Cleland (USA): paravertebral block and caudal catheter	Per K Lloyd-Williams: sacral anaesthesia *not* commonly used in the UK			

prevented plugging with tissue and enabled choice of direction of a catheter through the needle.

1949

Manual Martinez Curbelo in Havana, Cuba, described use of the above-described Tuohy needle for continuous epidural injection of procaine via silk catheter (lumbar or low thoracic levels) in 59 surgical cases (including gynaecology).[78]

1949

C Flowers, obstetrician at Baltimore (independently) used the Tuohy needle with the first plastic catheter (polyethylene) in obstetrics.[79]

1949

Torsten Gordh (Karolinska Hospital, Stockholm) published the first clinical account of lidocaine, an amide-type LA with more penetrative power and less toxicity than all previous LAs (esters).[80] This major advance would have a profound influence on events from the 1950s onwards.

Events from 1950 onwards

Non-pharmacological methods of analgesia

1950

Although Grantly Dick Read (general practitioner in England) first published *Revelation of Childbirth* in 1942, it was from about 1950 that his method of education and relaxation really became popular.[81]

1950

Velvosky and Nicolaiev in the Soviet Union employed a method of psychological preparation with hypnosis and oxygen.[11]

1952

Fernand Lamaze, Director of the Metal-Workers Lying-in Hospital in Paris, introduced the Lamaze Method of psychoprophylaxis, which became popular throughout France and was also popularized in the United States.[11]

1954

Grantly Dick Read republished his book under the title *Childbirth Without Fear.*[81]

1965

Publication of the gate control theory of pain by Melzack and Wall instigated interest in transcutaneous electrical nerve stimulation (TENS).

1975

Leonid Persianinov in Russia claimed good analgesia in labour by electroanalgesia—the application of low-intensity current to the forehead and mastoid processes.[82]

1980

TENS was reported as a safe and useful analgesia method in labour. Two pairs of electrodes were placed on the lower back and low intensity background current applied, with controls to increase the amplitude for contractions.[83] This method has remained quite popular for early labour in the United Kingdom.

Resuscitation of the newborn

1953

Virginia Apgar, anaesthetist (Professor) at Columbia Presbyterian Hospital, New York, described a simple, reliable system for evaluating newborns: the Apgar score.[84] In time, this was adopted worldwide.

1957

Bingham (Northern Ireland), reported on current practice: 'gastric oxygen' was used pending availability of a person competent to perform tracheo-bronchial toilet and intubation.[85]

Demission of anaesthetists from neonatal resuscitation

Although Moir and Thorburn's textbook of 1986[119] still had a chapter on neonatal resuscitation, this was gradually eschewed by obstetric anaesthetists, whose full attention was required for the mother. This was borne out by a case in the Confidential Enquiry into Maternal Deaths (CEMD) in the United Kingdom 1997–99 where the anaesthetist was distracted by resuscitating the baby.[209]

General anaesthesia and analgesia

Developments in use of inhalation anaesthetic agents

1953

The problem of delayed chloroform poisoning was noted.[86]

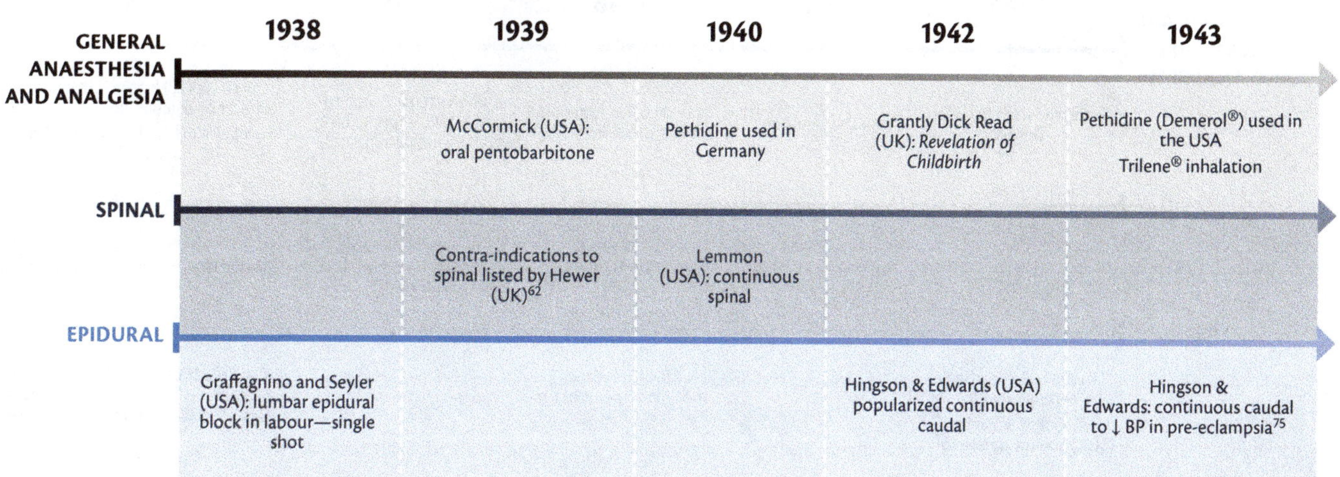

1956

Halothane was introduced and soon was embraced for GA in obstetric practice.

1962–85

Methoxyflurane was tried for labour analgesia in North America in 1962 and in the United Kingdom in 1966.[87] In 1970, it was approved for obstetric analgesia in the United Kingdom at a concentration of 0.35% in air via a Cardiff inhaler. Owing to concerns about renal impairment, it was withdrawn around 1985.

1990s

Isoflurane superseded halothane.

2000

Sevoflurane became commonly used.

The response to Mendelson's paper

1951

Morton and Wylie noted the difficulties of thorough gastric emptying by means of a stomach tube.[89]

1956

JM Holmes advocated induction of vomiting with apomorphine to empty the stomach as an alternative to passing a wide-bore stomach tube.[92]

1957

Bingham reported on 'balanced anaesthesia' for caesarean delivery in 614 cases between 1948 and 1956. Initially reserved for cases of vomiting during surgery, intubation was then adopted routinely. About half the patients received thiopentone, suxamethonium, pethidine, nitrous oxide, and oxygen with no added volatile anaesthetic agent. Cyclopropane was used in 246, gallamine in 368, and gallamine or d-tubocurarine in 132 cases.[85]

1957

Dinnick, concurring with Mendelson, suggested that prophylactic antacids could prevent the acid-aspiration syndrome.[93]

1959

Hamer-Hodges et al. published a series of 2000 patients of whom 1529 had an operative delivery, describing the use of thiopentone, suxamethonium, and intubation for caesarean delivery, which was safe for both mother and baby. This technique was developed for fetal interests rather than protection of the mother from aspiration. Further details were atropine (vagolytic essential with light GA), no pre-oxygenation, and 60% nitrous oxide with oxygen.[94]

1961

Brian Sellick (Middlesex Hospital, London) described his manoeuvre of cricoid pressure to hold back stomach contents during induction of anaesthesia.[95] This was gradually adopted in British practice.

1962

Bannister and Sattilaro suggested that a pH below 2.5 was critical for aspirate to cause severe lung reaction.[96]

1965

Selwyn Crawford (Birmingham, United Kingdom) provided guidelines for fasting in labour.[98,101]

1966

Taylor and Pryse-Davies (Queen Charlotte's Maternity Hospital, London) repeated some of Mendelson's work and recommended routine administration of antacids before anaesthesia: magnesium trisilicate mixture.[100]

1974

Roberts and Shirley reported that (in addition to pH < 2.5) the volume of gastric aspirate (>25 mL) was critical to development of severe lung damage.[102]

1974

Gertie F Marx (Figure 1.7) and Girvice W Archer (New York) demonstrated the marked desaturation of pregnant women within 60 seconds of apnoea (compared with non-pregnant controls), thereby emphasizing the importance of preoxygenation at induction of GA and prompt re-oxygenation following endotracheal intubation.[103]

1978

Wilson in Edinburgh demonstrated that the main determinant of delayed gastric emptying in labour is the administration of narcotic analgesics, whereas epidural analgesia has little or no effect on gastric emptying.[104]

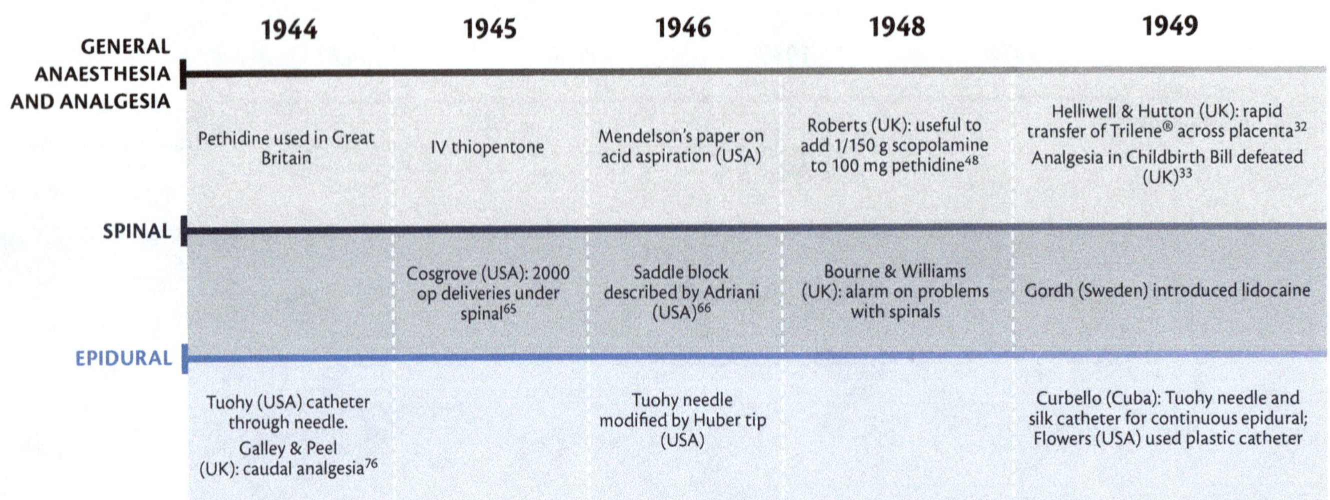

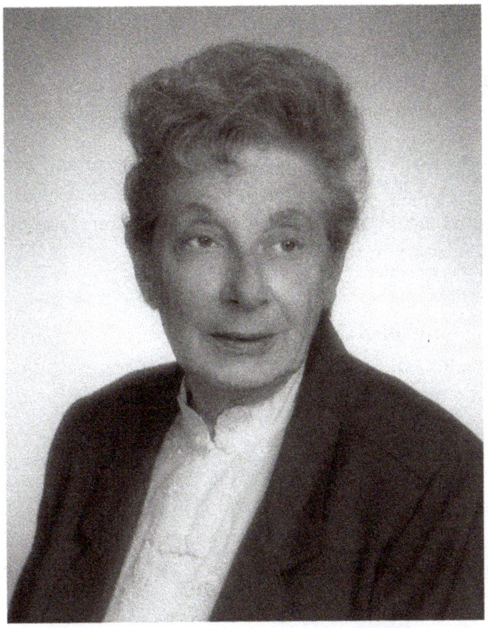

Figure 1.7 Gertie Florentine Marx (1912–2004) practised and taught epidural analgesia in obstetrics from 1945 over five decades in New York. She published prolifically and became known as 'the mother of obstetric anaesthesia'. She was the second woman (the first was Virginia Apgar) to receive the Distinguished Service Award of the American Society of Anesthesiologists, and a long spinal needle was named in her honour.
Image courtesy of the Wood Library-Museum of Anesthesiology, Schaumburg, Illinois.

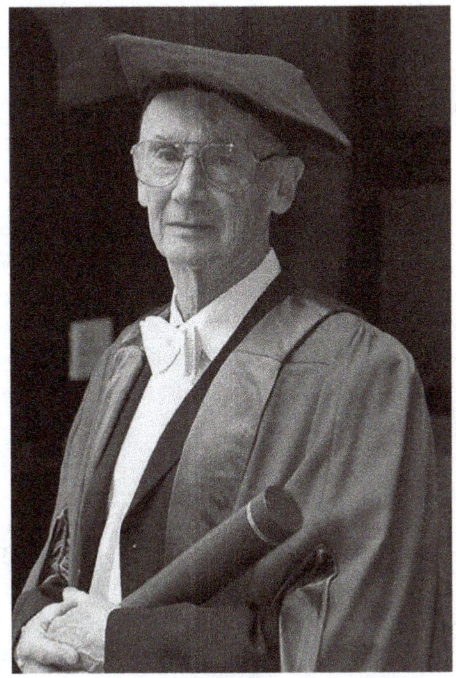

Figure 1.8 Michael E. Tunstall (1928–2011) introduced Entonox in 1961, described a 'failed intubation drill' in 1976, and advocated use of an 'isolated forearm technique' to avoid awareness under general anaesthesia for obstetrics in 1977.
Image courtesy of Mrs A Tunstall, Aberdeen, UK

1979

Gibbs et al. (Florida) reported that aspiration of particulate antacid produced severe lung pathology,[105] and went on to state that non-particulate antacid (0.3 M sodium citrate) was preferable.[106]

Entonox®

1961

Work by Michael E Tunstall (Portsmouth, England) (Figure 1.8) in conjunction with British Oxygen Company produced a pre-mix of nitrous oxide and oxygen in equal proportions (Entonox®), which was rapidly adopted for inhalation analgesia in labour.[108]

1962

Cole and Nainby-Luxmore drew attention to possible fetal compromise due to low maternal oxygen levels with 'gas and air'.[109]

1963

Nevertheless, nitrous oxide with as low as 20% oxygen, continued to be self-administered in obstetrics, using the new 'Lucy Baldwin' machine.[110]

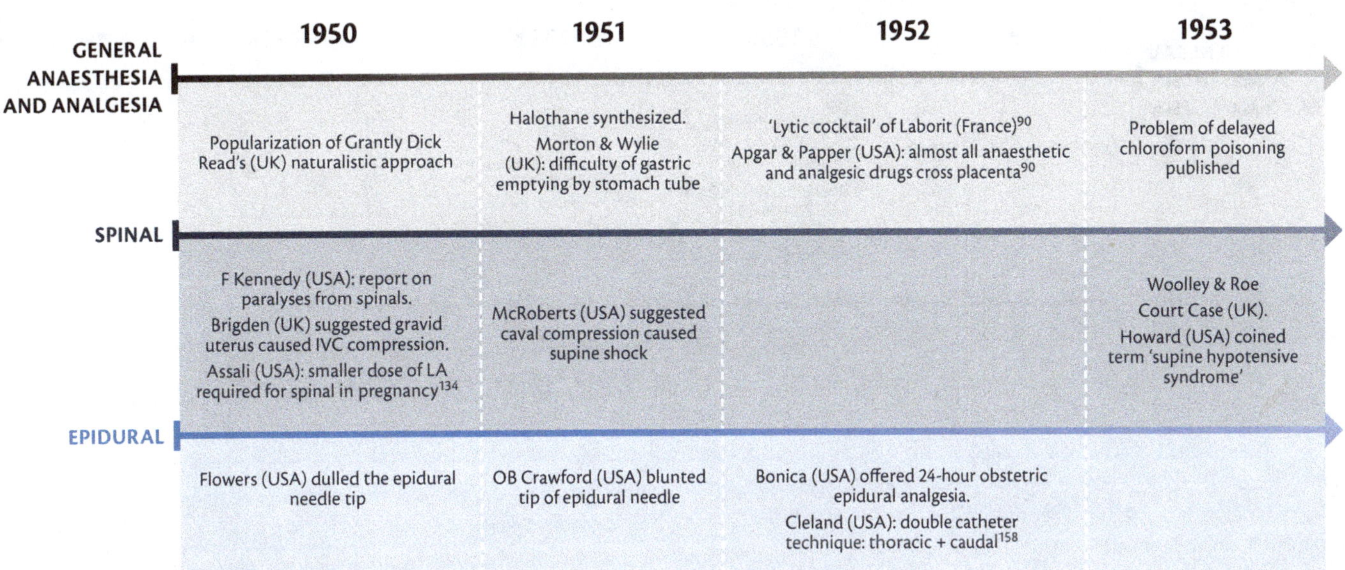

1970

Approval for 'gas and air' was withdrawn in the United Kingdom.

Awareness

1969

Wilson and Turner in Edinburgh published a seminal paper on awareness during caesarean delivery under GA. At that time the usual GA for caesarean delivery was based on the original 'Liverpool technique' of ventilation with nitrous oxide and oxygen *only*—at least until after delivery. In their series of 150 patients they reported unpleasant recall in 17.5% of cases.[111] By appearing in the *BMJ* this paper reached a wide general readership, and was instrumental in the decline of the original 'Liverpool technique'.

1970

Moir (Glasgow) recommended 0.5% halothane with 50% each of nitrous oxide and oxygen, plus a muscle relaxant as a suitable general anaesthetic for caesarean delivery: this provided safety, no increase in haemorrhage, minimal neonatal depression, and a much lower incidence of awareness.[112]

1977

Tunstall advocated use of an isolated forearm (IFA) technique to avoid awareness under GA for obstetrics.[113]

The obstetric flying squad

1957

Stabler enunciated the principles for obstetric flying squads.[114]

1960

Adamson et al. described results for 138 GAs given by the Edinburgh squad—in the majority, open chloroform was used. He suggested use of a specialist anaesthetist.[114]

1951–61

In 305 anaesthetics given by the Bellshill squad, the usual method was thiopentone (98%); gastric lavage was carried out before induction. The equipment carried by the team included an oxygen cylinder, Ambu respirator, laryngoscope, and endotracheal tubes, but apparently intubation was infrequent.[43]

1961

Argent and Evans described use of thiopentone and suxamethonium followed by intubation, and maintenance of anaesthesia with nitrous oxide, oxygen, and ether, but spontaneous ventilation. The equipment was bulky.[114]

1967

Dallas recommended thiopentone, suxamethonium, endotracheal intubation, and intermittent positive pressure respiration with air from an Ambu bag, thus using light equipment.[114]

1969

Davies (Cambridge, United Kingdom) described portable equipment aiming for pre-oxygenation, IV barbiturate, suxamethonium, endotracheal intubation, and positive pressure respiration with nitrous oxide and oxygen, using intermittent suxamethonium.[114]

1970s–1980s

By 1976, improvements in UK provision of antenatal care and obstetric management and decline in home deliveries (<4%) called into question the justification for continuing the flying squads.[40]

In 1980, a survey found that over half the squads answered ten or fewer calls per annum—most were subsequently disbanded.[115]

Advances in airway management and prevention of Mendelson's syndrome

1980s

Tunstall's failed intubation drill (first described in 1976) was widely adopted.[116]

1984

Cormack and Lehane provided a laryngoscopy grading system.[117]

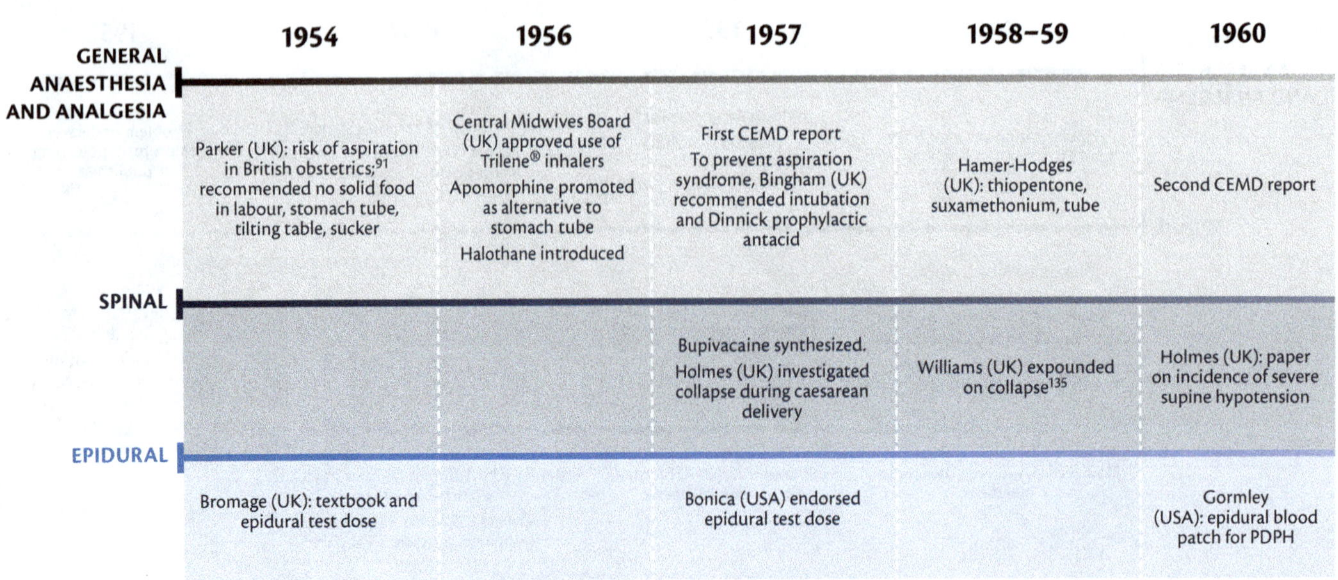

1986

Modern 'rapid sequence induction' (RSI) had developed piecemeal through successive CEMD reports and was described in standard textbooks.[119]

1986

Laryngeal mask airway (LMA) introduced.

1989

The CEMD report for 1982–84 suggested use of H_2-receptor antagonists and ranitidine became standard practice.[121]

1990

It was suggested that the LMA should be considered for rescuing the airway in cases of difficult intubation.[122]

Reduction of deaths from pulmonary aspiration

By **1994** the reduction in deaths from pulmonary aspiration was attributed to prophylaxis with H_2 receptor antagonists.[124] By the **late 1990s**, there had been a dramatic swing to spinal anaesthesia instead of GA for operative obstetrics in the United Kingdom, Germany, France, and the United States, which probably contributed even more to the continued decline in such deaths.

Cricoid pressure revisited

2003

A magnetic resonance imaging study by KJ Smith et al. (Hamilton, Ontario) revealed the alignment of the oesophagus to be lateral to the cricoid cartilage in more than 50% and application of cricoid pressure increased this lateral displacement to 90%.[127]

This has called into question the use of cricoid pressure in RSI.

Remifentanil

2004

A case series of remifentanil technique in GA for caesarean delivery was published.[128] Since then remifentanil infusion has become recognized as useful for the following indications: intraoperative analgesia, avoidance of hypertensive response to intubation, avoidance of neuromuscular blocking agents, intraoperative control of BP in pre-eclampsia, AND reducing volatile requirements.

Box 1.1 The Foster Kennedy report

- In 1950, Foster Kennedy, a neurologist trained at The National Hospital for Neurology and Neurosurgery, London, but working in New York, published a review entitled 'The grave spinal cord spinal paralyses caused by spinal anaesthesia'.
- This described a collection of catastrophic sequelae following spinal anaesthesia, with detailed neurological but little anaesthetic information.
- Published in *Surgery, Gynecology and Obstetrics*, the paper was widely read by surgeons, and led to some decline in spinal anaesthesia in the United States.
- It fuelled a far greater decline in spinal anaesthesia in the United Kingdom, where concern was further generated by the publicity about the Woolley and Roe case (Box 1.2).

Data from Kennedy F, Effron AS, Perry G, The grave spinal cord paralyses caused by spinal anaesthesia, Surgery, *Gynecology and Obstetrics*, 1950; 91: 385–98.

Spinal anaesthesia

Near demise of spinal anaesthesia in the United Kingdom

The concern generated by Bourne and Williams' paper (1948) was cemented by two other (non-obstetric) events:

1950

The Foster Kennedy report—see Box 1.1.[131]

1953

The Woolley and Roe case—see Box 1.2.[132]

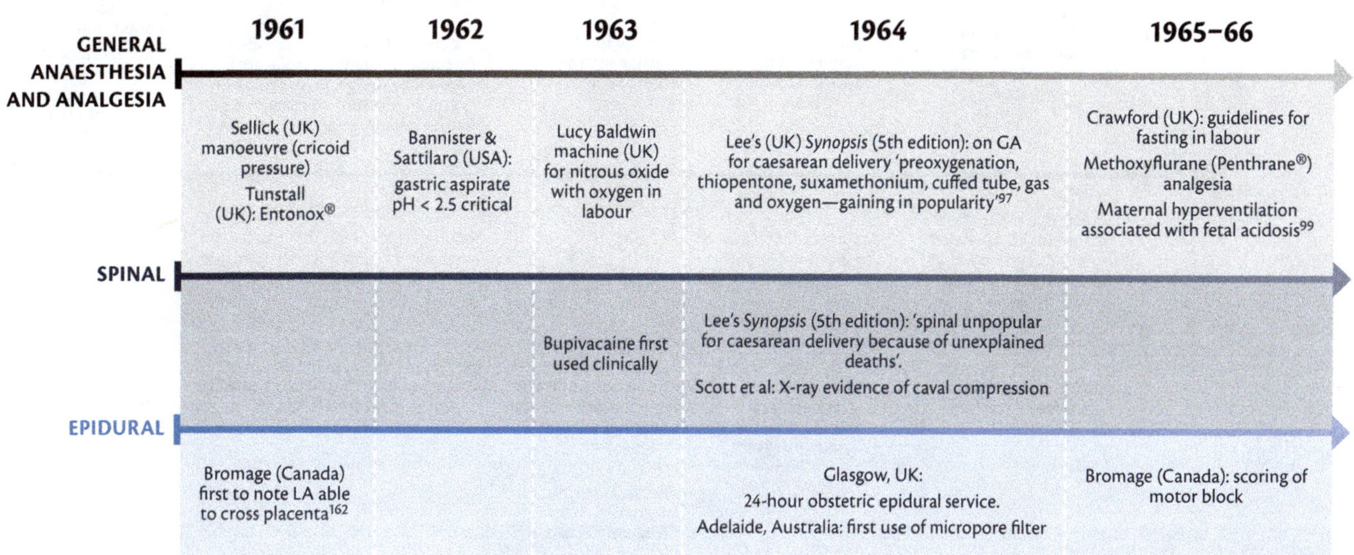

Box 1.2 The Woolley and Roe case

- In October 1947 at Chesterfield Hospital in England, Albert Woolley underwent a semilunar cartilage removal and Cecil Roe had a hydrocele repaired, both under spinal anaesthesia on the same operating list, by the same anaesthetist.
- By the next day both men developed lower limb paralysis and incontinence, which progressed to permanent paraparesis.
- They sued the Ministry of Health, the case coming to court in October 1953.
- The judge ruled that inadvertent contamination of the LA had occurred, with no negligence.
- The plaintiffs received no compensation.
- Following the case there was a profound decline in spinal anaesthesia in the United Kingdom.

Data from Cope RW, The Woolley and Roe Case; Woolley and Roe versus Ministry of Health and Others, *Anaesthesia*, 1954; 9: 249–70.

Spinal anaesthesia went into decline in the UK for nearly 30 years (though it remained in favour for obstetric use in the United States).

Elucidation of the supine hypotensive syndrome of pregnancy

1950

Brigden, Howarth, and Sharpey-Schafer at St Thomas' Hospital, London, suggested that in the supine position the gravid uterus could cause obstruction to flow in the great veins of the abdomen.[133]

1951

McRoberts in Houston, Texas, suggested caval compression as the cause of supine shock in pregnancy.[133]

1953

Howard in Dallas, Texas, concurred with McRoberts, coining the term 'supine hypotensive syndrome'.[133]

1957

Anaesthetist Frank Holmes in Edinburgh suggested that caval compression was compounded by vasodilatation due to spinal block to cause sudden circulatory collapse during caesarean delivery under spinal anaesthesia.[133]

1960

Holmes published on the incidence of severe supine hypotension in advanced pregnancy (8.2%) and on management by turning the patient semi-lateral.[133]

1963

Anaesthetist Bruce Scott (Figure 1.9) and obstetrician Melville Kerr (Simpson Memorial Maternity Pavilion, Edinburgh) concluded from inferior vena cava (IVC) pressure measurements that in the supine position the gravid uterus occluded the IVC, but there was also collateral flow, which was adequate in most cases.[133]

1964

Scott, Kerr, and radiologist Samuel in Edinburgh produced the first X-ray evidence of caval compression in late pregnancy.[133]

1967

Lees, Scott, Kerr and Taylor in Edinburgh used invasive monitoring to demonstrate that most pregnant women could compensate for IVC compression by increase in SVR (vasoconstriction).[133] This mechanism was disabled by spinal anaesthesia.

1968

Bieniarz, working with R Caldeyro-Barcia in Montevideo, Uruguay, reported that the gravid uterus also compressed the abdominal aorta.[133]

	1967	1968–69	1970	1972	1973–74
GENERAL ANAESTHESIA AND ANALGESIA	Beazley (UK): parenteral & inhalation methods gave only 60% adequate analgesia in labour	Wilson (UK): awareness under GA for caesarean delivery 17.5%	Approval for nitrous oxide with air withdrawn in the UK	CEMD: deaths due to anaesthesia unchanged for 20 years. Crawford (UK) recommended preop magnesium trisilicate, followed by wedge, preoxygenation, cricoid pressure, thiopentone, suxamethonium, endotracheal tube[101]	Electro-analgesia popular in Russia. Roberts & Shirley (USA): gastric aspirate volume > 25 mL critical
SPINAL	Edinburgh group: most parturients compensated for caval compression by vasoconstriction—disabled by spinal!	Argument for return to spinal use in the UK obstetrics		Crawford (UK) pointed out two main drawbacks of spinal: hypotension and PDPH	
EPIDURAL	Lumbar approach became preferred method	Moir & Willocks (UK): epidural reduced need for caesarean delivery	British workers: efficacy of epidural dependent on experience of operator[171] Midwives topping-up epidurals as permitted by (UK) Central Midwives Board	Lumbar epidural described in detail by Crawford (UK)	Pearson & Davies (UK): use of epidural reduced fetal distress

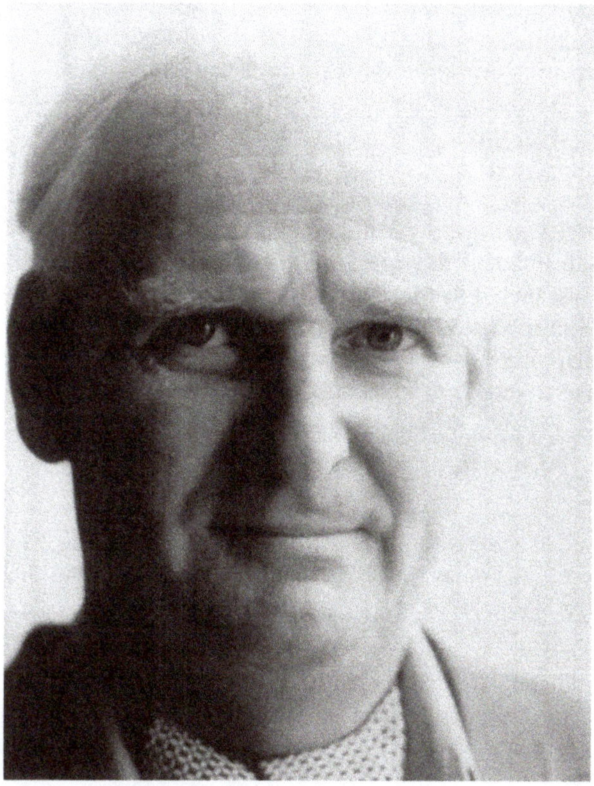

Figure 1.9 D Bruce Scott (1926–1998) played a key role in elucidation of the supine hypotensive syndrome of late pregnancy (1960s), developed knowledge about the circulatory effects of epidural anaesthesia, studied local anaesthetic toxicity, and was renowned as a teacher. He was the second President of the Obstetric Anesthetists' Association.

Photograph in Department of Anaesthesia, Critical Care & Pain Medicine, Royal Infirmary of Edinburgh.

1969

By this time it was clear that supine hypotension could be avoided by lateral tilt, and there was some argument for a return to spinal subarachnoid block in obstetrics.[136]

1972

Selwyn Crawford in Birmingham, United Kingdom, conducted a trial of tilt versus non-tilt of patients undergoing caesarean delivery under GA; the status of the neonates revealed the importance of tilt for fetal welfare—Crawford recommended a tilt angle of 15°.[133]

The resurgence of spinal anaesthesia in the United Kingdom

1980s

In the United Kingdom, spinal anaesthesia for obstetrics (although popular in some countries) was considered too problematic: 64% incidence of hypotension,[139] 24% incidence of headache,[139] and unpredictability of spread of plain (isobaric) 0.5% bupivacaine.[140] Hypotension could be managed with vasopressors and the spread controlled by use of hyperbaric solutions and positioning to enhance thoracic curvature. But, owing to the high incidence of postdural puncture headache (PDPH) in the obstetric population, the epidural remained the usual form of neuraxial anaesthesia for caesarean delivery until the availability of reliable pencil point needles.

Early 1990s

Although designs of pencil-point spinal needles had been published by Whitacre[141] (USA) in 1951 and Sprotte[142] (Germany) in 1987, it was not until the 1990s that these became widely used in obstetric anaesthesia practice.

1992

A study at the University of Natal, South Africa showed that rapid crystalloid preload caused unacceptable increases in central venous pressure (CVP) yet did not prevent spinal-induced hypotension at caesarean delivery.[143]

1995

Obstetric anaesthetists in Glasgow confirmed that preloading was not required to prevent spinal-induced hypotension at caesarean delivery—vasopressor use was more effective.[145]

1995

I Russell in Hull, United Kingdom, began to add diamorphine to intrathecal hyperbaric 0.5% bupivacaine to improve

	1976–77	1978–79	1980	1981	1983
GENERAL ANAESTHESIA AND ANALGESIA	Tunstall (UK): failed intubation drill; IFA technique to avoid awareness	Gibbs (USA) recommended 0.3M sodium citrate rather than 'mag trisil'	TENS reported as safe & useful analgesia method in labour	Enflurane reported as satisfactory analgesia in labour[88]	Crawford (UK) reported normal labour does *not* retard gastric emptying time[107]
SPINAL		Crawford called for spinal to be used more widely in the UK[137]	Moir called for spinal to be used more widely in the UK[138]	Brownridge (Australia): combined spinal–epidural (CSE)	
EPIDURAL	Carrie (UK): paramedian approach[174]	Bromage (USA) book *Epidural Analgesia*: spread determined by dose[176] Use of epidural morphine published (Israel)	FDA banned use of 0.75% bupivacaine in obstetrics[178]	Moore (USA) recommended epidural test dose include epinephrine. Thorburn & Moir (UK): 0.5% bupivacaine associated with motor block and intervention	Preload of 2 L recommended for caesarean delivery Disapproval of stopping epidural for second stage of labour

postoperative analgesia following spinal anaesthesia for caesarean delivery.[146]

1998

A study in Belfast, United Kingdom, found that addition of intrathecal diamorphine also improved intraoperative analgesia during spinal anaesthesia for caesarean delivery (reduced need for intraoperative analgesic supplementation.[147] The technique was adopted widely in the United Kingdom, becoming established practice.

1999

In the United Kingdom, to manage spinal-induced hypotension at caesarean delivery, 95% of obstetric anaesthetists used boluses of ephedrine as the sole vasopressor.[148]

2003

A study in Leeds, United Kingdom, found that the optimum dose of intrathecal diamorphine to prevent intraoperative supplementation of spinal anaesthesia for caesarean delivery was 0.4 mg.[149]

2004

Ngan Kee (Hong Kong) showed that during spinal anaesthesia for elective caesarean delivery, phenylephrine infusion to maintain BP at 100% of baseline conferred the best outcome for both mother (less nausea) and baby (highest umbilical artery pH).[150]

2006

In the United Kingdom, use of phenylephrine as first-line vasopressor by obstetric anaesthetists had increased to 51%.[148]

2010

A study in the United Kingdom found that for high-risk caesarean deliveries, choice of phenylephrine versus ephedrine made no difference to fetal acidosis.[148]

Epidural analgesia

Advances in epidural analgesia

1952

John Bonica at Tacoma, Washington was one of the first to offer a 24-hour obstetric anaesthesia service with emphasis on continuous caudal or epidural analgesia.[157]

1954

Philip Bromage (then in England) (Figure 1.10) published the first edition of his textbook on epidural analgesia, in which he described a test dose to safeguard against 'total spinal' and systemic toxicity.[159]

1957

Bonica et al. opined that the test dose manoeuvre was extremely valuable, though not an absolute safeguard.[160]

1957

New LAs became available, synthesized by Bo Af Ekenstam (laboratories of Bofors Nebel-Pharma): mepivacaine (1956), bupivacaine, and ropivacaine (1957).

1960

The 'blood patch' method of treating PDPH was introduced by Gormley of Pennsylvania.[161] In time, this would become the gold standard of treatment.

1963

Bupivacaine was first used clinically, but did not become commonly used in obstetrics until the 1970s.

1964

Probably the first 24-hour epidural service in the United Kingdom was established at the Queen Mother's Hospital, Glasgow, by Donald D Moir: this utilized intermittent top-ups with lignocaine.

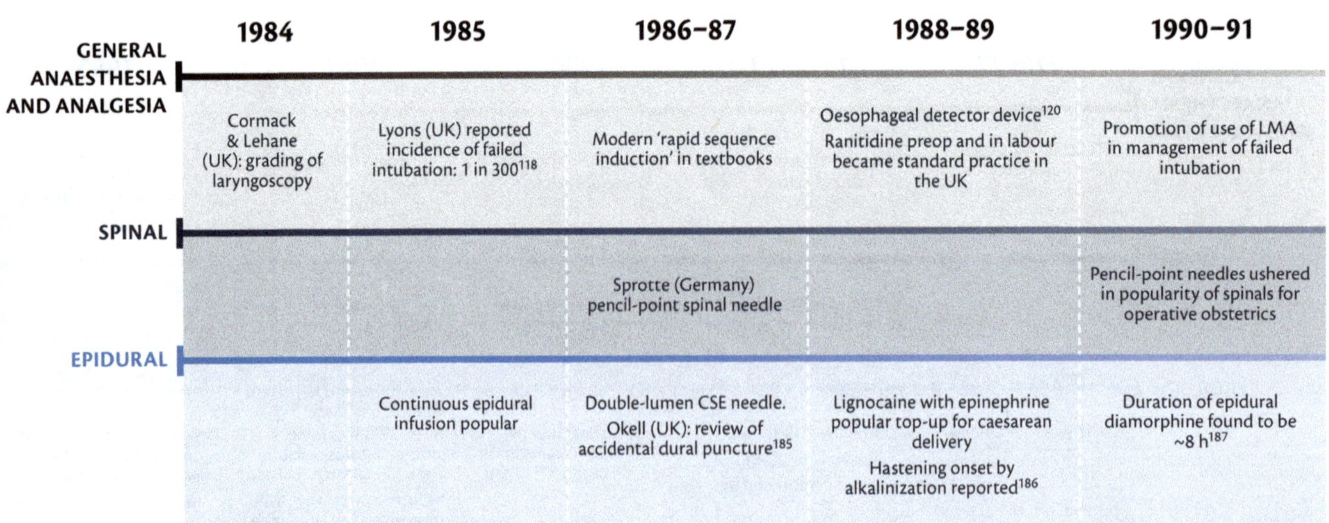

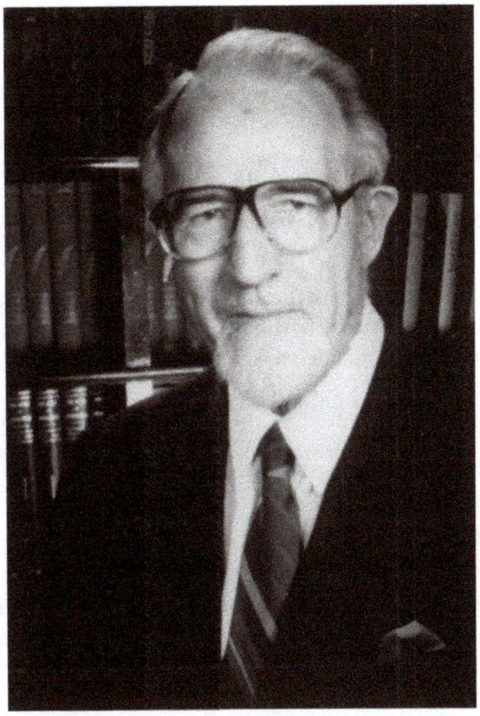

Figure 1.10 Philip Raikes Bromage (1920–2013) published a textbook on epidural anaesthesia in 1954 and introduced a scoring system for motor block in 1965.
Portrait photograph reproduced with kind permission from McGill Department of Anesthesia, Montreal, Canada.

1965

Bromage (then Professor at McGill University, Montreal) introduced a scoring system for motor block.[163]

1967

The lumbar approach to the epidural space became preferred to caudal.

1968

Moir and Willocks reported on 300 continuous and 62 single-shot epidural blocks (using lignocaine with epinephrine) administered during labour at the Queen Mother's Hospital, Glasgow.[164] Besides analgesia, indications for the continuous method included incoordinate uterine action, severe pre-eclampsia, and selected cases of cardiac and respiratory disease. The single-shot method was found to be excellent for forceps delivery where it also reduced blood loss.

Advances in epidural needles and catheters

1950–1970s

In the United States, R Hustead and OB Crawford blunted the Tuohy needle, while J Weiss added wings.[165] In 1960, in the United Kingdom, J Alfred Lee (author of *A Synopsis of Anaesthesia*), added 1 cm-wide alternate black and metallic markings to the shaft of the epidural needle[166]—this reduced the incidence of dural puncture. DB Scott in 1964 described prolonging the hub to prevent kinking of the catheter.[167]

Regarding the epidural catheter, Lee in 1962 described a nylon catheter with a non-patent tip, lateral eye, and length calibrations.[168]

From the above, there developed the modern epidural needle and catheter.

Adoption of micropore filters for epidural catheters

1964–1970s

1961–64 saw the need for scrub-up before each epidural top-up to maintain sterility: this was frequent owing to the short duration of lidocaine. Various mechanical schemes were designed to avoid touching syringe/catheter; these were cumbersome.

Developments in the plastics industry combined with increased demand for micropore filters in microbiology led to mass production.

1964 James Saunders (Adelaide, Australia) was the first to use in obstetrics.

	1992	1994	1995–96	1998	1999
GENERAL ANAESTHESIA AND ANALGESIA	Gastric emptying by orogastric tube done before emergency caesarean delivery by 62% in Denmark[123]	Fall in deaths from pulmonary aspiration attributed to H_2 antagonist and rise in neuraxial anaesthesia	Consensus: nil advantage in propofol over thiopentone for caesarean delivery[125]	Muscle relaxants reviewed[126]	Role of anaesthetist in management of pre-eclampsia and eclampsia recognized
SPINAL	Rout et al. (South Africa): preload not efficacious at caesarean delivery in preventing hypotension FDA withdrew microcatheters (<24 gauge) for CSA[64]	Risk recognized of 'high spinal or total spinal' when spinal performed for caesarean delivery in presence of epidural block[144]	Glasgow (UK) group confirmed preload not required to prevent hypotension at caesarean delivery	Call for reappraisal of spinal anaesthesia in severe pre-eclampsia[226]	Edinburgh (UK) group showed spinal as safe as epidural in severe pre-eclampsia
EPIDURAL	Comparison of top-ups, infusion, and PCEA: little difference	Increasing acceptance of low-dose bupivacaine with fentanyl mixtures	'Walking' epidural popularized (CSE) Ropivacaine marketed	Use of 0.1% bupivacaine with fentanyl 2 mcg/mL: less instrumental deliveries than with 0.25% bupivacaine	Attention to neurological complications of obstetric neuraxial anaesthesia[191]

1965 Bruce Scott (Edinburgh) attached 0.2 μm millipore filters to epidural catheters.

1972 J Desmond was probably first to use the filters in North America.

1975 J Selwyn Crawford (Birmingham, United Kingdom) recommended the filters.

1977 E Abouleish in the United States disputed the need.

From the late 1970s the filter became a standard component of the epidural pack.[169]

1970s

Bupivacaine top-ups superseded lidocaine.

Labour analgesia: parenteral/inhalational versus epidural

Reasons advanced for resistance to epidurals included:

- parenteral/inhalation methods adequate
- concerns that epidural was detrimental to fetus.

1967

Beazley et al. found that only 60% of women had adequate analgesia from parenteral and inhalation methods in labour.[170]

1968

Moir and Willocks found that epidural analgesia reduced the need for caesarean delivery for maternal distress.[164]

1974

Pearson and Davies found that epidural analgesia avoided fetal depressant effects of potent opioid and sedative drugs.[172]

1974

Crawford reported that epidural analgesia did not reduce uterine tone.[173]

1978

Jouppila demonstrated that epidural analgesia did not diminish measured placental blood flow (radioactive clearance method).[175]

Epidural anaesthesia for caesarean delivery

Late 1970s

There was an upsurge of interest in epidural analgesia for caesarean delivery in the United Kingdom.[177]

1980s

Epidural anaesthesia was commonly used for caesarean delivery in the United Kingdom. By 1983, a preload of 2 L of Hartmann's solution was recommended to protect against hypotension.[179]

Further advances in epidural analgesia

1979

Publication of the use of epidural morphine at the Hadassah Hospital, Jerusalem, captured the interest of all anaesthetists, including those in obstetrics.[180]

1981

Moore and Batra recommended that the test dose include epinephrine 15 mcg to diagnose inadvertent IV injection (this dose of epinephrine consistently raised heart rate during the first minute after injection).[181]

1980s

Continuous epidural infusion for pain relief in labour became popular. There were many papers on epidural infusion versus top-ups.

Infusion advantages:

- Maintenance of stable level of analgesia[182,184]
- More stable heart rate and BP[183]

	2000–01	2002–03	2004	2007	2008
GENERAL ANAESTHESIA AND ANALGESIA	Remifentanil PCA	Cricoid pressure revisited	Chronic pain after caesarean delivery: incidence higher if GA than neuraxial anaesthesia CEMACH report: need for anaesthetic antenatal clinic for high risk cases	Anaesthetic antenatal assessment of obese women common. CEMACH report urged use of obstet. early warning system (EWS)	TAP blocks after caesarean delivery Cell salvage (blood conservation) promoted in obstetric haemorrhage
SPINAL		Optimum dose of intrathecal diamorphine found 0.4 mg. Supplemental oxygen no longer recommended for elective caesarean delivery[151]	Assessing spinal block level: cold, pinprick and touch compared[152] Ngan Kee (Hong Kong): phenylephrine infusion to maintain BP	Use of alcohol swab and filter straw recommended for adding non-sterile wrapped opioid to LA injectate[153]	Van de Velde (Belgium) found inserting epidural catheter intrathecally in cases of accidental dural puncture did not reduce PDPH[195]
EPIDURAL	Epidural with 0.125% bupivacaine shown *not* a cause of increased operative deliveries Levobupivacaine introduced COMET study	Postpartum backache reviewed: found *not* increased by epidural for delivery[192]	RCoA *Good Practice with Epidural Analgesia in Hospital Setting*[193] Spinal epidural abscess found to be a *rare* complication[194]	NPSA *Safer Practice with Epidural Injections and Infusions* AAGBI guidelines on treating severe LA toxicity[212]	NICE recommend that ultrasound may be effective in achieving correct placement of epidural catheters[196]

- Less frequent need for bolus.[182,184]

Infusion disadvantages:

- Increased total dose of LA[184]
- Potential for increased motor block.[182]

Early 1990s

Low-concentration bupivacaine with fentanyl solutions were popularized (the addition of fentanyl was synergistic and could reduce the amount of bupivacaine).[188]

Mid 1990s

Patient-controlled epidural analgesia (PCEA) in labour was popularized.[189]

1996

Having been first used clinically in 1993, ropivacaine was marketed in the United Kingdom.[190] Promoters suggested it would reduce undesirable motor block. However, it was not commercially competitive against racemic bupivacaine, as by this time excellent results were being obtained with low-concentration bupivacaine/fentanyl mixtures.

Combined spinal–epidural techniques

1981

P Brownridge (Adelaide) described CSE technique for caesarean delivery.[198]

1986

Following publication on CSE by the Romanian, Ioan Curelaru, in 1979, Karl Wiegand in Germany worked on a double-lumen CSE needle for which a patent was granted.[68]

1995

'Walking' epidural in labour concept was popularized by BM Morgan (Queen Charlotte's & Chelsea Hospital, London) and advanced the usage of CSE.[199]

Audits of maternal mortality and morbidity

The confidential enquiries into maternal deaths for England and Wales

1957

The first report of the CEMD in England and Wales for the triennium 1952–54 was published. Anaesthetists were involved from the start. Initially there were 44 maternal deaths for every 1000 deliveries. Notable details in the first report[200] included:

- a total of 49 deaths attributable to anaesthesia
- 32 deaths following inhalation of stomach contents
- six deaths under chloroform
- two cases in which the obstetrician 'managed' anaesthesia and delivery single-handed
- in addition to the 49 deaths ascribed to anaesthesia, at least 20 more were identified where anaesthesia was contributory.

Haemorrhage was the second commonest direct cause of death—in the years following 1957 it became appreciated that the anaesthetist could play a major role in management of haemorrhage.

1960

In the report for 1955–57, endotracheal intubation was advised for patients with full stomach and for forceps in the lithotomy position.[201]

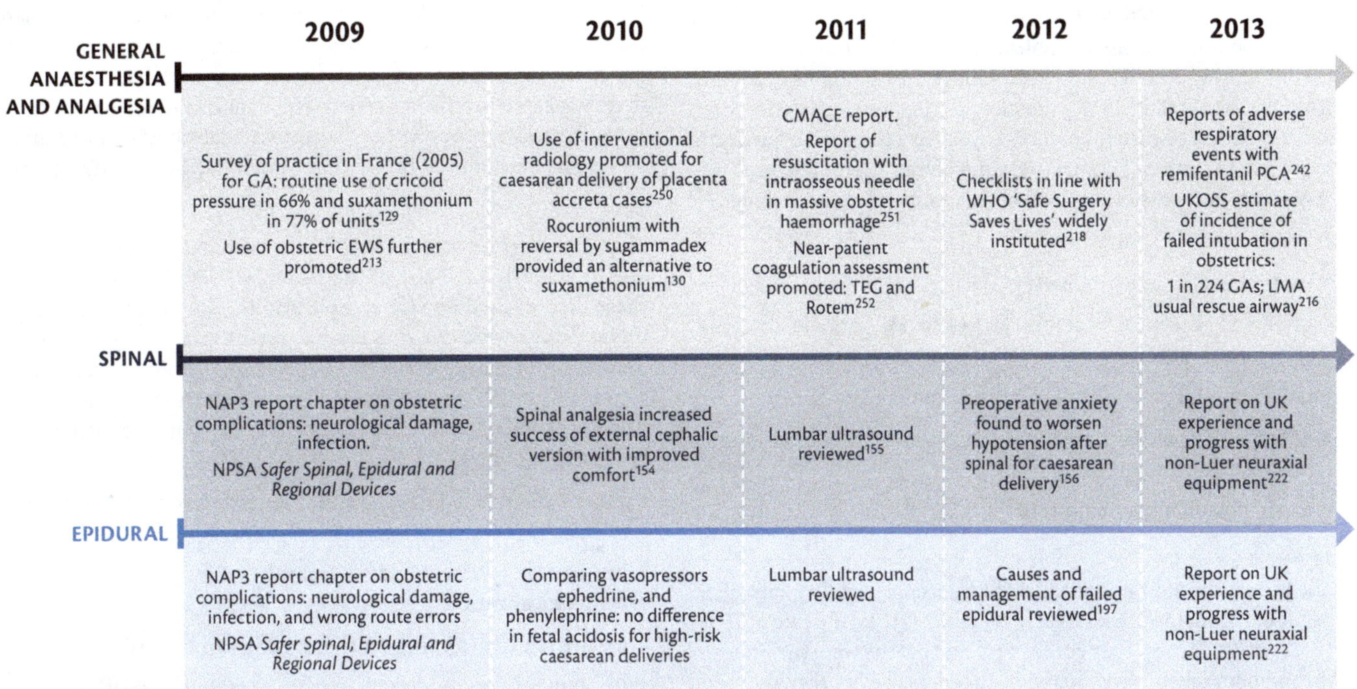

1972

By this time it was evident that the number of deaths due to anaesthetic complications had remained unchanged for nearly 20 years.[202] This stimulated interest in neuraxial analgesia as an alternative method.

1979

The report for 1973–75 included 13 deaths from inhalation of gastric contents despite antacids—in 12, cricoid pressure was not properly applied. There were two deaths from 'total spinal' complication of epidural analgesia. The report emphasized the need for experienced anaesthetists (rather than unsupervised trainees) and for monitoring the patients.[203]

1986

The report for 1979–81 showed that anaesthesia was the third commonest cause of maternal death. Causes again included inhalation of stomach contents (eight) and difficulty with endotracheal intubation (eight cases—four oesophageal intubations). There were three deaths from haemorrhage with poor anaesthetic management; three patients with severe kyphoscoliosis died from respiratory problems. The authors recommended a drill for management of bleeding and early multidisciplinary consultation for patients with kyphoscoliosis.[204]

The confidential enquiries into maternal deaths in the United Kingdom

1991

The first UK report (for 1985–87) revealed six deaths due to problems with tracheal intubation, one death due to inhalation of gastric contents, and one death (patient with severe congenital heart disease) due to cardiovascular collapse under epidural anaesthesia. The authors commented that a failed intubation drill should be agreed and practised; extra anaesthetic apparatus for a difficult intubation was suggested.[205]

1994

In the report for 1988–90 there were five deaths due to anaesthesia, with the following causes: problems with tracheal tube (one), hypotension during spinal anaesthesia followed by pulmonary oedema from excess IV fluid (one), substandard postoperative care (one), and aspiration of gastric contents (two). Also there were ten deaths to which anaesthesia contributed, involving haemorrhage, bronchospasm, and possible aspiration. Recommendations included:[124]

- provision of CO_2-analyser
- monitoring by pulse oximetry
- giving H_2-receptor blocking drugs to all patients who may require anaesthesia
- emptying the stomach before extubation
- adequate IV access and provision of blood products for suspected haemorrhage cases
- use of postoperative pain relief service.

1996

The report for 1991–93 revealed a maternal mortality rate of six per 100,000 maternities—nearly 12-fold less than the rate of 70 for 1952–54.[206] The top four causes of direct deaths were thrombosis/thromboembolism, hypertensive disorders, early pregnancy, and haemorrhage—anaesthesia was ranked eighth. There were eight deaths directly attributable to anaesthesia (substandard care in seven); causes included hypoxia and airway obstruction (five), acute respiratory distress syndrome (two), and failure of tissue perfusion (one). All the direct deaths associated with anaesthesia for caesarean delivery involved the use of GA.

Morbidity audit

1998

Noting the falling numbers of maternal deaths in the United Kingdom (revealed by the CEMD report for 1991–93), Mantel et al. in South Africa proposed that more useful information might be obtained from audit of severe acute maternal morbidity or 'near miss'.[207]

2000

Scottish Assessors for the CEMD began a series of pilot exercises, which led to collection of data on defined categories of severe maternal morbidity in all consultant-led maternity units in Scotland: the *Scottish Confidential Audit of Severe Maternal Morbidity* (SCASMM), which has produced nine reports funded by NHS Quality Improvement Scotland—the latest in March 2013.[208]

2001

The Report on CEMD in the United Kingdom for 1997–99[209] (and subsequent reports) included information on 'near misses' and severe maternal morbidity based on the Scottish audit of these outcomes.

Confidential Enquiry into Maternal and Child Health (CEMACH)

2004

The report on CEMD in the United Kingdom for 2000–02 came for the first time under the auspices of CEMACH and marked 50 years of this audit.[210]

There were six direct deaths due to anaesthesia—all associated with GA, that is, nil attributable to neuraxial anaesthesia. Of these, three were due to difficult intubation, two resulted from hypoventilation in isolated sites, one from anaphylaxis. In addition there were 20 deaths in which perioperative anaesthetic management contributed (five cases of substandard perioperative care and five cases of substandard management of haemorrhage; in addition there were two deaths in women who declined blood products).

Nevertheless, the report revealed that anaesthesia for caesarean section had become 30 times safer than it had been in the 1960s.

2007

The CEMACH report for 2003–05 again included six direct deaths due to anaesthesia. Four of the patients were obese and three of these died of fatal airway complications. The other three anaesthetic deaths were due to a cardiac arrest in a septic patient, LA toxicity from a drug error (IV bupivacaine), and a haemothorax secondary to CVP line insertion. For the first time the report identified a top ten of recommendations, the following being most relevant to anaesthetists: [211]

- in pre-eclampsia, treat systolic hypertension of 160 mmHg or more
- any patient with a previous caesarean delivery should have placental localization
- ensure regular training (obstetric 'skills and drills')
- implement a modified early obstetric warning score (MEOWS) system

- urgent guidelines for obesity, sepsis, and pain/bleeding in early pregnancy.

Centre for Maternal and Child Enquiries (CMACE)

2011

The triennial review on maternal deaths in the United Kingdom for 2006–08 was published by CMACE,[214] the new name adopted by CEMACH on becoming an independent charity in 2009. The report revealed that sepsis had become the leading cause of direct maternal death, with a reduction in deaths due to thromboembolism and haemorrhage. There were seven direct deaths due to anaesthesia: four from postoperative complications, two from failure to ventilate, and one from leucoencephalitis. Again the report listed a top ten of recommendations, notably:

- treat systolic hypertension above 150 mmHg
- address clinical skills and training: 'Back to Basics'
- routine use of MEOWS chart
- communication and early referral of high-risk cases to specialists
- appropriate multidisciplinary specialist care for serious medical conditions
- serious incident reporting.

UK Obstetric Surveillance System (UKOSS)

2005

A joint initiative began between the Royal College of Obstetricians and Gynaecologists and the National Perinatal Epidemiology Unit (United Kingdom). Surveys of rare disorders have been conducted through a monthly card mailing to nominated obstetricians, midwives, and anaesthetists in each hospital in the United Kingdom with a consultant obstetric unit.[215]

Mothers and babies: reducing the risk through audits and confidential enquiries across the UK (MBRRACE-UK)

2010

Competitive tender was invited for the UK Confidential Enquiries into Maternal Deaths, and this was won by MBRRACE-UK.[217]

Audit of complications of central neuraxial block and efforts to improve safety

Systemic toxicity

2001

Levobupivacaine introduced.

Wrong route of drug administration:

- 2007 National Patient Safety Agency (NPSA) in England—Patient Safety Alert 21: safer practice with epidural injections and infusions[219]
- 2009 NPSA Patient Safety Alert—Safer Spinal (intrathecal), Epidural and Regional Devices.[220]

Neurological sequelae

2008

National Institute for Health and Clinical Excellence (NICE) in England and Wales—suggested making use of ultrasound for guiding catheterization of epidural space.[196]

2009

The Report of the Third National Audit Project of the Royal College of Anaesthetists—*Major Complications of Central Neuraxial Block in the United Kingdom* (NAP3)—included a chapter on obstetric practice.[221]

Epidural haematoma and infection

2009

The NAP3 Report included incidence and pointed out how to deal with coagulopathy and use of anticoagulants, and provided guidelines for avoiding infection including epidural abscess.[221]

Role of the anaesthetist in the management of pre-eclampsia and eclampsia

1980s

Pre-eclampsia was recognized as one of the main indications for epidural analgesia in labour (provided coagulation profile satisfactory).[119]

For caesarean delivery, epidural anaesthesia was recommended with the proviso that any tendency to hypotension must be carefully controlled;[223] spinal anaesthesia was often discouraged because of a presumed risk of severe hypotension.

1992

A study by Hood challenged the view that spinal anaesthesia was unsafe in severe pre-eclampsia.[224]

1995

Wallace et al. at the Parkland Hospital (Dallas, Texas) compared three methods of anaesthesia for caesarean delivery of severe pre-eclamptics: general, epidural, and CSE—they found no severe hypotension in the spinal group and all methods acceptable.[225]

1999

Obstetric anaesthetists in Edinburgh confirmed that spinal was as safe as epidural anaesthesia in severe pre-eclampsia; indeed they suggested spinal to be preferable on grounds of better intraoperative analgesia.[227]

2005

The Edinburgh group further found that severe pre-eclampsia conferred an ability to sustain arterial pressure after spinal block for caesarean delivery, as these patients required less vasopressor compared with normotensive parturients.[228]

Progress in eclampsia 2002–04

The Magpie Trial (2002) revealed that magnesium sulphate halves the risk of eclampsia.[229]

It was recognized that the obstetric anaesthetist has a key role in the emergency management of imminent and manifested eclamptic seizures—airway management and prompt commencement of magnesium sulphate infusion—team performance improvable by simulation drills.[230]

Role of the anaesthetist in the management of labour and postoperative pain

1980s

The few contraindications to epidural analgesia were enumerated. It was recognized that the offer of epidural analgesia would often persuade a parturient to accept augmentation with oxytocin; and (besides pain relief) there were many other indications for epidural analgesia in labour: pre-eclampsia, multiple pregnancy, and cardiac and respiratory disease.[119]

Thorburn and Moir pointed out that repeated boluses of 0.5% bupivacaine for epidural analgesia in labour was associated with profound motor block and increased intervention. In this group, spontaneous deliveries were reduced to 31%, compared with 53% for 0.25% bupivacaine.[231]

For the second stage of labour it was noted that allowing epidural analgesia to wear off increased maternal distress without improving outcome—and that such practice should be discouraged.[232]

1990s

Use of 0.1% bupivacaine with fentanyl 2 mcg/mL for epidural analgesia (compared with 0.25% bupivacaine) was shown to reduce instrumental deliveries.[233]

Comparison of intermittent top-ups, infusions, and PCEA found little difference in delivery outcome.[234]

Use of the 'walking' epidural, although enabling mobilizing, did not appear to confer any change in delivery outcome compared with the above.[235]

A study on mobilizing found that this made no difference to duration of labour or delivery outcome.[236]

While recognizing that fluid preload was not required for epidural analgesia using dilute bupivacaine, it was also noted that preloading may temporarily decrease uterine activity.[237]

The minimum local analgesic concentration (MLAC) of epidural bupivacaine was shown to increase with progression of labour.[238]

2000

Loughnan et al. (London) in a randomized study found that epidural analgesia with 0.125% bupivacaine was not associated with increases in either instrumental or operative deliveries.[239]

2001

Comparative Obstetric Mobile Epidural Trial (COMET) study in the United Kingdom found a reduced *instrumental* vaginal delivery rate with CSE and low-dose infusion techniques compared with traditional epidural.[240]

2001

Remifentanil patient-controlled anaesthesia (PCA) was introduced as alternative analgesia in labour, especially where epidural not an option.[241]

2004

A study in Denmark found that chronic pain after caesarean delivery was higher with GA compared to neuraxial anaesthesia.[243]

2008

McDonnell in Galway, Ireland introduced transversus abdominis plane (TAP) block for analgesia after caesarean delivery.[244]

Advances in management of major obstetric haemorrhage—role of the anaesthetist

1950s

Although David Massa (Anaesthesia Resident) at the Mayo Clinic introduced the plastic 'Rochester' cannula,[245] metal needles (e.g. Mitchell) were still commonly used for IV access.

1964

Deseret introduced the Angiocath, a PVC, hypodermic-style needle with flash-back chamber and flow control plug.[245]

1970s

Glass bottles as containers for IV fluids and blood were superseded by plastic bags. These both reduced risk of air embolism and permitted pressurization for rapid infusion.

1980s

The Report on CEMD for 1976–78 emphasized the need for a simple protocol for anticipation and treatment of postpartum haemorrhage.[246] This was re-emphasized in the report for 1979–81, which recommended a drill for management of bleeding.[204]

1990s

Rapid infusers with blood warming capability were improved (e.g. the 'Level 1' series) and recommended.[247]

Autologous blood transfusion (cell salvage) was promoted[248] and developed.

2000 onwards

Novel medical, surgical, radiological, and haematological interventions were developed, with anaesthetists establishing a key role in management.[249] Also multidisciplinary working practices were encouraged and national guidelines implemented.[250]

Professional organizations and associations

1968

An informal group of interested anaesthetists met in Liverpool, United Kingdom, at the invitation of Dr THL Bryson (Liverpool) and Dr M Lewis (Belfast)—and hatched the idea of the Obstetric Anaesthetists' Association (OAA).

1969

The OAA was constituted at a spring meeting in Glasgow hosted by Dr DD Moir—the inaugural elected president was Dr JS Crawford (Birmingham) (Figure 1.11).

At a meeting in Kansas City, Missouri, the initial plans for a parallel organization were made.

1970

At Nashville, Tennessee, the Society for Obstetric Anesthesia and Perinatology (SOAP) was founded—the first president was Robert F Hustead, MD.

1987

Responding to the Report on CEMD in England and Wales for 1979–81, the OAA in conjunction with AAGBI published a report outlining far-sighted proposals for improving the quality and safety of obstetric anaesthesia in the United Kingdom.[253]

1992

The OAA launched its official journal: the *International Journal of Obstetric Anesthesia*.

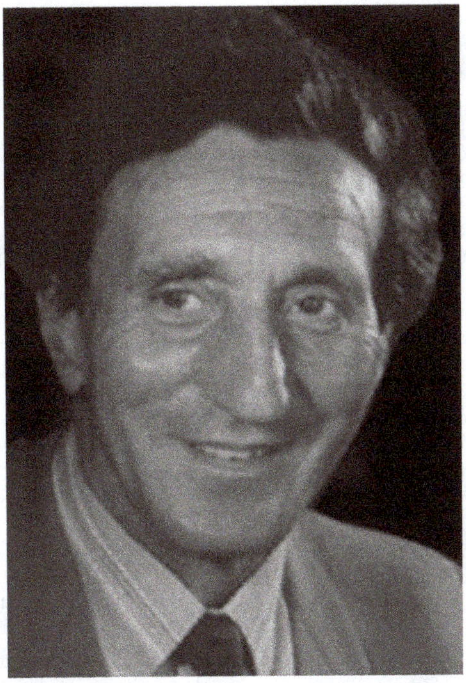

Figure 1.11 Jeff Selwyn Crawford (1922–1988) published the first edition of *Principles & Practice of Obstetric Anaesthesia* in 1959, provided guidelines for fasting in labour (1965), designed a wedge to provide lateral tilt of the pregnant woman placed supine (1972), and was inaugural President of the Obstetric Anesthetists' Association.

Image courtesy of the Obstetric Anaesthetists' Association.

References

1. Lull CB, Hingson RA. *Control of Pain in Childbirth* (2nd ed). Philadelphia, PA: Lippincott Co.; 1945:121–2.
2. Caton D. The secularisation of pain. *Anesthesiology* 1985; 62:493–501.
3. Davison MHA. *The Evolution of Anaesthesia*. Altrincham: John Sherratt & Son; 1965:212–15.
4. Scheff R (trans). *Henri Chapelain Archives* [English translation of the Chapelain archives from original documents in French.] Park Ridge. IL: Wood Library-Museum Archives Collection; 1988:176–7.
5. Lynell JP. Labour in mesmeric state. *ZOIST II* 1844; 5:120–23.
6. Lee CA. Artificial somnambulism in Pennsylvania. *Boston Med J* 1846; 35:194.
7. Zuck D. Simpson as a teacher—a student's notebook. *Br J Anaesth* 1976; 48:1103–11.
8. Simpson JY. On the inhalation of sulphuric ether in the practice of midwifery. *Edin Monthly J Med Sci* 1847; 3:721–32.
9. [Report] St. Bartholomew's Hospital. Caesarean operation, performed by Mr. Skey at St. Bartholomew's Hospital. *London Med Gaz* 1847; 48:212–13.
10. Goerig M, Streckfess W. Adam Hammer (1818–1878)—remarks on a forgotten pioneer of ether anaesthesia in obstetrics. *Anasthesiol Intensivmed Notfallmed Schmerzther* 2004; 39:265–75.
11. Clark RB, Pitcock CD. From Fanny to Fernand—consumerism in pain control during the birth process. In Fink BR, Morris LE, Stephen CR (eds) *Proceedings of Third International Symposium on the History of Anesthesia*. Park Ridge, IL: Wood Library-Museum; 1992:106–10.
12. Secher O. Nikolai Ivanovich Pirogoff. *Anaesthesia* 1986; 41:829–37.
13. Simpson JY. *Account of a New Anaesthetic Agent, as a Substitute for Sulphuric Ether in Surgery and Midwifery*. Edinburgh: Sutherland & Knox; 1847.
14. Simpson JY. *Answer to the Religious Objections Advanced Against the Employment of Anaesthetic Agents in Midwifery and Surgery*. Edinburgh: Sutherland & Knox; 1847.
15. Farr AD. Religious opposition to obstetric anaesthesia: a myth? *Anna Sci* 1983; 40:159–77.
16. Snow J. On the administration of chloroform during parturition. *Assoc Med J* 1853; 1:500–2.
17. Connor H, Connor T. Did the use of chloroform by Queen Victoria influence its acceptance in obstetric practice? *Anaesthesia*1996; 51:955–7.
18. Caton D. John Snow's Practice of Obstetric Anesthesia. Anesthesiology 2000; 92: 247–52.
19. Snow J. *On Chloroform and Other Anaesthetics*. London: John Churchill; 1858:318.
20. Ellis R. *Safe Abolition of Pain in Labour and Surgical Operations by Anaesthesia with Mixed Vapours*. London: Robert Hardwicke; 1866.
21. Caton D. Paul Zweifel—an early contributor to obstetric anesthesia. In Fink BR, Morris LE, Stephen CR (eds) *Proceedings of Third International Symposium on the History of Anesthesia*. Park Ridge, IL: Wood Library-Museum; 1992:103–5.
22. Richards W, Parbrook GD, Wilson J. Stanislav Klikovich (1853–1910)—pioneer of nitrous oxide and oxygen analgesia. *Anaesthesia* 1976; 31:933–40.
23. Hewitt FW. *Anaesthetics and their Administration* (3rd ed). London: Macmillan & Co.; 1907.
24. Hewer CL. *Recent Advances in Anaesthesia and Analgesia* (1st ed). London: J&A Churchill; 1932:51.
25. Drury PME. The National Birthday Trust Fund. *History Anaesth Soc Proc* 1999; 26:23–7.
26. Minnitt RJ. A new technique for the self-administration of gas-air analgesia in labour. *Lancet* 1934; i:1278.
27. Bourne W. Cyclopropane anaesthesia in obstetrics. *Lancet* 1934; 2:20–1.
28. Bourne W. Vinyl ether obstetrical anaesthesia for general practice. *Can Med Assoc J* 1935; 33:629–32.
29. Minnitt RJ. The history and progress of gas and air analgesia for midwifery. *Proc Roy Soc Med* 1944; 37:45.
30. Moir C. Nitrous oxide analgesia in obstetrics—a new type of machine for self-administration of gas. *Lancet* 1937; i:615–18.
31. Epstein HG, Macintosh RR. Analgesia inhaler for trichlorethylene. *Br Med J* 1949; 2:1092–4.
32. Helliwell PJ, Hutton AM. Analgesia in obstetrics. *Anaesthesia* 1949; 4:18–21.
33. Barnett R. "The future of the midwife depends on her power to relieve pain". The rise and fall of the Analgesia in Childbirth Bill (1949). *Int J Obstet Anesth* 2007; 16:35–39.
34. Jaeger W. Versuche zur herabsetzung des wehenschmerzes bei der geburt. *Zentralblatt für Gynäkologie* 1910; 46.
35. Hewer CL. *Recent Advances in Anaesthesia and Analgesia* (3rd ed). London: J&A Churchill; 1939:287.
36. Goodman LS, Gilman A. *The Pharmacological Basis of Therapeutics* (2nd ed). New York: Macmillan; 1955:93–97.
37. Gwathmey JT. Obstetrical analgesia: a further study based on more than twenty thousand cases. *Surg Gynec Obstet* 1930; 51:190–5.
38. Hewer CL. *Recent Advances in Anaesthesia and Analgesia* (3rd ed). London: J&A Churchill; 1939:285–6.
39. Lull CB, Hingson RA. *Control of Pain in Childbirth* (2nd ed). Philadelphia, PA: Lippincott Co.; 1945:156–65.
40. Fergusson ILC, Watson JM. Assessment of the obstetric flying squad in an urban area. *Br Med J* 1976; 1:446–8.
41. Thomson HJ. Maternity emergency service. *Br Med J* 1936; I:235.
42. Lloyd HN. Discussion on emergency obstetrical service (the flying squad)—its use and abuse. *Proc Roy Soc Med* 1949; 42:1–10.
43. Liang DYS. The emergency obstetric service—Bellshill Maternity Hospital, 1933–1961. *J Obstet Gynaecol Br Emp* 1963; 70:83–93.
44. Lloyd-Williams KG. *Anaesthesia and Analgesia in Labour*. London: Edward Arnold & Co.; 1934.

45. Gilbert G, Dixon AB. Observations on demerol as an obstetric analgesic. *Am J Obstet Gynecol* 1943; 45:320.
46. Spitzer W. Obstetric analgesia with pethidine. *Br Med J* 1944; 1:179–81.
47. Lull CB, Hingson RA. *Control of Pain in Childbirth* (2nd ed). Philadelphia, PA: Lippincott Co.; 1945:165–7, 203.
48. Roberts H. Pethidine and scopolamine in labour. *Br Med J* 1948; 2:590–3.
49. Mendelson CL. The aspiration of stomach contents into the lungs during obstetric anesthesia. *Am J Obstet Gynecol*1946; 52:191–205.
50. Simpson JY. Local anaesthesia: notes on its artificial production by chloroform, etc, in the lower animals, and in man. *Prov Med Surg J* 1848; S1–12:365–71.
51. Kreis O. Über Medullarnarkose bei Gabärenden. *Centralblatt für Gynäkologie* 1900; 28:724 (translated as 'On spinal narcosis during labour'. *Int J Obstet Anesth* 2000; 9:174–8).
52. Stone WR. Cocainization of the spinal cord by means of lumbar puncture during labor. *Am J Obstet Gynecology* 1901; 63:145–55.
53. Muller WB. *Narkologie. Ein Handbuch der Wissenschaft über allgemeine u. locale Schmerzbetäubung* (2nd ed). Berlin: R. Trenkel; 1908.
54. Gellert PH. Aufhebung der Wehenschmerzen und Wehenüberdruck. *Monatschr Geburtsh Gynäk* 1926; 73:143.
55. Winnie AP. The early history of regional anaesthesia in the United States. In Scott DB, McClure J, Wildsmith JAW (eds) *Regional Anaesthesia 1884–1984*. Södertälje: ICM AB; 1984:35–8.
56. Lee JA. Arthur Edward James Barker 1850–1916: British pioneer of regional analgesia. *Anaesthesia* 1979; 34:885–91.
57. Akhtar M. Henry Percy Dean: an early British pioneer of spinal analgesia. *Anaesthesia* 1972; 27:330–3.
58. Ockerblad NF, Dillon TG. The use of ephedrine in spinal anesthesia (preliminary report). *JAMA* 1927; 88:1135–6.
59. Pitkin G. Controllable spinal anesthesia. *Am J Surg* 1928; 5:537–53.
60. Paramour RH. A case of eclampsia treated with spinal anaesthesia. *Br Med J* 1930; I:15.
61. Fairfield L. Maternity work in L.C.C. hospitals, 1931–1936. *Proc Roy Soc Med* 1938; 31:237–50.
62. Hewer CL. *Recent Advances in Anaesthesia and Analgesia* (3rd ed). London: J&A Churchill; 1939:187–8.
63. Lemmon WT. A method for continuous spinal anaesthesia. *Ann Surg* 1940; 111:144.
64. Denny NM, Selander DE. Continuous spinal anaesthesia. *Br J Anaesth* 1998; 81:590–7.
65. Lull CB, Hingson RA. *Control of Pain in Childbirth* (2nd ed). Philadelphia, PA: Lippincott Co.; 1945:129.
66. Adriani J, Roma-Vega D. Saddle block anesthesia. *Am J Surg* 1946; 71:12–18.
67. Bourne AW, Williams LH. *Recent Advances in Obstetrics and Gynecology* (7th ed). London: Churchill; 1948:114–18.
68. Goerig M, Freitag M, Standl T. One hundred years of epidural anaesthesia—the men behind the technical developments. In Diz JC, Franco A, Bacon DR, *et al.* (eds) *The History of Anaesthesia*. International Congress Series No. 1242. Amsterdam: Elsevier Science; 2002:203–12.
69. Doughty A. Walter Stoeckel (1871–1961); a pioneer of regional analgesia in obstetrics. *Anaesthesia* 1990; 45:468–71.
70. Pickles W, Jones SS. Regional anesthesia in obstetrics, with a report of 28 deliveries under epidural block. *N Engl J Med* 1928; 199:988–94.
71. Curelaru I, Sandu L. Eugan Bogdan Aburel (1899–1975): the pioneer of regional analgesia for pain relief in childbirth. *Anaesthesia* 1982; 37:663–9.
72. Cleland JGP. Paravertebral anesthesia in obstetrics. *Surg Gynecol Obstet* 1933; 57:51–62.
73. Graffagnino P, Seyler LW. Epidural anesthesia in obstetrics. *Am J Obstet Gynecol* 1938; 35:597.
74. Hingson RA, Edwards WB. Continuous caudal anesthesia. *Curr Res Anesth Analg* 1942; 21:301–11.
75. Hingson RA, Edwards WB. Continuous caudal analgesia: an analysis of the first 10000 confinements thus managed with the report of the authors' first 1000 cases. *JAMA* 1943; 123:538–46.
76. Galley AH, Peel JH. Continuous caudal analgesia in obstetrics. *Proc Roy Soc Med* 1944; 37:680–4.
77. Maltby JR. *Notable Names in Anaesthesia*. London: Royal Society of Medicine Press; 2002:216–18.
78. Curbelo MM. Continuous peridural segmental anesthesia by means of a ureteral catheter. *Anesth* Analg 1949; 28:13–23.
79. Flowers C. Continuous peridural anesthesia and analgesia for labor, delivery and caesarean section. *Anesth* Analg 1949; 28:181–9.
80. Gordh T. Xylocain—a new local analgesic. *Anaesthesia* 1949; 4:4–9.
81. Read GD. *Childbirth Without Fear* (2nd ed). London: William Heinemann; 1953.
82. Persianinov LS. The use of electro-analgesia in obstetrics and gynecology. *Acta Obstet Gynecol Scand* 1975; 54:373–84.
83. Miller Jones CMH. Transcutaneous nerve stimulation in labour. *Anaesthesia* 1980; 35:372–5.
84. Apgar V. A proposal for a new method of evaluation of the newborn infant. *Anesth Analg* 1953; 32:260–7.
85. Bingham W. Balanced anaesthesia for Caesarean section. *Anaesthesia* 1957; 12:435–52.
86. Lunt RL. Delayed chloroform poisoning in obstetric practice. *Br Med J* 1953; 1:489–90.
87. Major V, Rosen M, Mushin WW. Methoxyflurane as an obstetric analgesic: a comparison with trichloroethylene. *Br Med J* 1966; 2:1554–61.
88. Abboud TK, Shnider SM, Wright RG, *et al.* Enflurane analgesia in obstetrics. *Anesth Analg Curr Res* 1981; 60:133.
89. Morton HJV, Wylie WD. Anaesthetic deaths due to regurgitation or vomiting. *Anaesthesia* 1951; 6:190.
90. Roberts H. The trend in obstetric analgesia and anaesthesia. In Evans FT, Gray TC (eds.) *Modern Trends in Anaesthesia*. London: Butterworth & Co.; 1958:196–205.
91. Parker RB. Risk from the aspiration of vomit during obstetric anaesthesia. *Br Med J* 1954; 2:65–9.
92. Holmes JM. The prevention of inhaled vomit during obstetric anaesthesia. *J Obstet Gynaecol Br Emp* 1956; 63:239.
93. Dinnick OP. Discussion on anaesthesia for obstetrics: an evaluation of general and regional methods. *Proc Roy Soc Med* 1957; 50:547–56.
94. Hamer Hodges RJ, Bennett JR, Tunstall ME, *et al.* General anaesthesia for operative obstetrics. *Br J Anaesth* 1959; 31:152–63.
95. Sellick BA. Cricoid pressure to control regurgitation of stomach contents during induction of anaesthesia. *Lancet* 1961; 2:404–6.
96. Bannister WK, Sattilaro AJ. Vomiting and aspiration during anaesthesia *Anesthesiology* 1962; 23:251–64.
97. Lee JA, Atkinson RA. *A Synopsis of Anaesthesia* (5th ed). Bristol: John Wright & Sons Ltd.; 1964.
98. Crawford JS. *Principles and Practice of Obstetric Anaesthesia* (2nd ed). Oxford: Blackwell; 1965.
99. Moya F, Morishima H, Shnider SM, *et al.* Influence of maternal hyperventilation on the newborn infant. *Am J Obstet Gynecol* 1965; 91:76–84.
100. Taylor G, Pryse-Davies J. The prophylactic use of antacids in the prevention of acid pulmonary aspiration syndrome. *Lancet* 1966; 1:288–91.
101. Crawford JS. *Principles and Practice of Obstetric Anaesthesia* (3rd ed.). Oxford: Blackwell Scientific Publications; 1972.
102. Roberts RB, Shirley MA. Reducing the risk of acid aspiration during caesarean section. *Anesth Analg* 1974; 53:859–68.
103. Archer GW, Marx GF. Arterial oxygen tension during apnoea in parturient women. *Br J Anaesth* 1974; 46:358–60.
104. Wilson J. Gastric emptying in labour: some recent findings and their clinical significance. *J Int Med Res* 1978 Suppl. 1:54–62.

105. Gibbs CP, Schwartz DJ, Wynne JW, *et al.* Antacid pulmonary aspiration in the dog. *Anesthesiology* 1979; 51:380.
106. Gibbs CP, Wynne JW. Maternal mortality and anaesthesia. *Br J Anaesth* 1980; 52:842.
107. Crawford JS. The stages and phases of labour: an outworn nomenclature that invites hazard. *Lancet* 1983; 2:271–2.
108. Tunstall ME. Obstetric analgesia: the use of a fixed nitrous oxide and oxygen mixture from one cylinder. *Lancet* 1961; 2:964.
109. Cole PV, Nainby-Luxmore RC. The hazards of gas and air in obstetrics. *Anaesthesia* 1962; 17:505–18.
110. McAneny TM, Doughty AG. Self-administered nitrous oxide/oxygen analgesia in obstetrics. *Anaesthesia* 1963; 18:488–97.
111. Wilson J, Turner DJ. Awareness during caesarean section under general anaesthesia. *Br Med J* 1969; 1:280–3.
112. Moir D. Anaesthesia for Caesarean section. An evaluation of a method using low concentrations of halothane and 50 per cent oxygen. *Br J Anaesth* 1970; 42:136–42.
113. Tunstall ME. Detecting wakefulness during general anaesthesia for caesarean section. *Br Med J* 1977; 1:1321.
114. Davies CK. Anaesthesia for an obstetric flying squad. *Br J Anaesth* 1969; 41:545–50.
115. Royal College of Obstetricians and Gynaecologists. *Survey of Obstetric Flying Squads.* London: RCOG Press; 1980.
116. Tunstall ME. Failed intubation drill (News & Notices: The OAA). *Anaesthesia* 1976; 31:850.
117. Cormack RS, Lehane J. Difficult intubation in obstetrics. *Anaesthesia* 1984; 39:1105–11.
118. Lyons G. Failed intubation—six years experience in a teaching maternity unit. *Anaesthesia* 1985; 40:759–62.
119. Moir DD, Thorburn J. *Obstetric Anaesthesia and Analgesia* (3rd ed). London: Bailliere-Tindall; 1986.
120. Wee MYK. The oesophageal detector device. Assessment of a new method to distinguish oesophageal from tracheal intubation. *Anaesthesia* 1988; 43:27–9.
121. Department of Health. *Report on Confidential Enquiries into Maternal Deaths in England and Wales 1982–84.* London: HMSO; 1989.
122. McClune S, Regan M, Moore J. Laryngeal mask for Caesarean section. *Anaesthesia* 1990; 45:227–8.
123. Helbo-Hansen HS, Bang U. Current Danish practice for aspiration prophylaxis in obstetric anaesthesia: a survey. *Int J Obstet Anesth* 1993; 2:233–5.
124. Department of Health, Welsh Office, Scottish Office Home & Health Department, *et al. Report on CEMD in the United Kingdom 1988–90.* London: HMSO; 1994.
125. Lyons G. Anaesthesia and analgesia for caesarean section. In Adams AP, Cashman JN (eds) *Recent Advances in Anaesthesia and Analgesia 19.* Edinburgh: Churchill Livingstone; 1995:55–70.
126. Ward SJ, Rocke DA. Neuromuscular blocking drugs in pregnancy and the puerperium. *Int J Obstet Anesth* 1998; 7:251–60.
127. Smith KJ, Dobranowski J, Yip G, *et al.* Cricoid pressure displaces the esophagus: an observational study using magnetic resonance imaging. *Anesthesiology* 2003; 99:60–4.
128. Van de Velde M, Teunkens A, Kuypers M, *et al.* General anaesthesia with target controlled infusion of propofol for planned caesarean section: maternal and neonatal effects of a remifentanil-based technique. *Int J Obstet Anesth* 2004; 13:153–8.
129. Benhamou D, Bouaziz H, Chassard D, *et al.* Anaesthetic practices for scheduled caesarean delivery: a 2005 French national survey. *Eur J Anaesthesiol* 2009; 26:694–700.
130. Pühringer FK, Kristen P, Rex C. Sugammadex reversal of rocuronium-induced neuromuscular block in Caesarean section patients: a series of seven cases. *Br J Anaesth* 2010; 105:657–60.
131. Kennedy F, Effron AS, Perry G. The grave spinal cord paralyses caused by spinal anaesthesia. *Surg Gynecol Obstet* 1950; 91:385–98.
132. Cope RW. The Woolley and Roe Case; Woolley and Roe versus Ministry of Health and Others. *Anaesthesia* 1954; 9:249–70.
133. Mckenzie AG. Researches on supine hypotension in pregnancy. In Diz JC, Franco A, Bacon DR, *et al.* (eds) *The History of Anaesthesia.* International Congress Series No. 1242. Amsterdam: Elsevier Science; 2002:597–601.
134. Assali NS, Prystowski H. Studies on autonomic blockade. Comparison between the effects of tetraethylammonium chloride (TEAC) and high selective spinal anaesthesia on the blood pressure of normal and toxaemic pregnancy. *J Clin Invest* 1950; 29:1354–60.
135. Williams B. Collapse from spinal analgesia in pregnancy. *Anaesthesia* 1958; 13:448–53.
136. Williams B. The present place of spinal subarachnoid analgesia in obstetrics. *Br J Anaesth* 1969; 41:628–34.
137. Crawford JS. Experience with spinal analgesia in a British obstetric unit. *Br J Anaesth* 1979; 51:531.
138. Moir DD. *Obstetric Anaesthesia and Analgesia* (2nd ed). London: Bailliere Tindall; 1980.
139. Russell IF. Spinal anaesthesia for caesarean section; the use of 0.5% bupivacaine. *Br J Anaesth* 1983; 55:309–13.
140. Russell IF. Inadvertent total spinal for caesarean section. *Anaesthesia* 1985; 40:199–200.
141. Hart JR, Whitacre RJ. Pencil-point needle in prevention of postspinal headache. *JAMA* 1951; 147:657–8.
142. Sprotte G, Schedel R, Pajunk H. Eine atraumatische universalkanule fur einzeitige regional-regionanasthesien. *Anaesthesie* 1987; 10:104–8.
143. Rout CC, Akoojee SS, Rocke DA, *et al.* Rapid administration of crystalloid preload does not decrease the incidence of hypotension after spinal anaesthesia for elective caesarean section. *Br J Anaesth* 1992; 68:394–7.
144. Gupta A, Enlund G, Bengtsson M, *et al.* Spinal anaesthesia for caesarean section following epidural analgesia in labour. *Int J Obstet Anesth* 1994; 3:153–6.
145. Jackson R, Reid JA, Thorburn J. Volume preloading is not essential to prevent spinal-induced hypotension at Caesarean section. *Br J Anaesth* 1995; 75:262–5.
146. Graham D, Russell I. Double-blind study to assess the analgesic sparing effect of 0.3 mg diamorphine given intrathecally at elective Caesarean section. *Int J Obstet Anesth* 1995; 4:179–80.
147. Kelly MC, Carabine UA, Mirakhur RK. Intrathecal diamorphine for analgesia after Caesarean section. *Anaesthesia* 1998; 53:231–7.
148. Cooper DW, Sharma S, Orakkan P, *et al.* Retrospective study of association between choice of vasopressor given during spinal anaesthesia for high-risk caesarean delivery and fetal pH. *Int J Obstet Anesth* 2010; 19:44–49.
149. Saravanan S, Robinson APC, Qayoum Dar A, *et al.* Minimum dose of intrathecal diamorphine to prevent intraoperative supplementation of spinal anaesthesia for Caesarean section. *Br J Anaesth* 2003; 91:368–72.
150. Ngan Kee WD, Khaw KS, Ng FF. Comparison of phenylephrine infusion regimens for maintaining maternal blood pressure during spinal anaesthesia for Caesarean section. *Br J Anaesth* 2004; 92:469–74.
151. Khaw KS, Wang CC, Ngan Kee WD, *et al.* Effects of high inspired oxygen fraction during elective caesarean section under spinal anaesthesia on maternal and fetal oxygenation and lipid peroxidation. *Br J Anaesth* 2002; 88:18–23.
152. Russell IF. A comparison of cold, pinprick and touch for assessing the level of spinal block at caesarean section. *Int J Obstet Anesth* 2004; 13:146–52.
153. Hemmingway CJ, Malhotra S, Almeida M, *et al.* The effect of alcohol swabs and filter straws on reducing contamination of glass ampoules used for neuraxial injections. *Anaesthesia* 2007; 62:286–8.
154. Weiniger CF, Ginosar Y, Elchalal U, *et al.* Randomized controlled trial of external cephalic version in term multiparae with or without spinal analgesia. *Br J Anaesth* 2010; 104:613–18.
155. Gambling DR. Lumbar ultrasound: useful gadget or time-consuming gimmick? *Int J Obstet Anesth* 2011; 20:318–20.

156. Orbach-Zinger S, Ginosar Y, Elliston J, *et al.* Influence of preoperative anxiety on hypotension after spinal anaesthesia in women undergoing Caesarean delivery. *Br J Anaesth* 2012; 109:144–54.
157. Maltby JR. *Op. cit.*; 22–4.
158. Cleland JGP. Continuous epidural and caudal block in obstetrics and surgery with postoperative analgesia. *Anesth Analg Curr Res* 1952; 31:289–300.
159. Bromage PR. *Spinal Epidural Anaesthesia.* Edinburgh: E&S Livingstone; 1954.
160. Bonica JJ, Backup PH, Anderson CE, *et al.* Peridural block: analysis of 3637 cases and a review. *Anesthesiology* 1957; 18:723–84.
161. Cullen SC. Treatment of postspinal headache. *Anesthesiology* 1960; 21:565–6.
162. Bromage PR, Robson JG. Concentrations of lignocaine in the blood after intravenous, intramuscular, epidural and endotracheal administration. *Anaesthesia* 1961; 16:461–78.
163. Bromage PR. A comparison of the hydrochloride and carbon dioxide salts of lidocaine and prilocaine in epidural analgesia. *Acta Anaes Scand* 1965; Suppl. XVI:55–69.
164. Moir DD, Willocks J. Epidural analgesia in British obstetrics. *Br J Anaesth* 1968; 40:129–38.
165. Frölich MA, Caton D. Pioneers in epidural needle design. *Anesth Analg* 2001; 93:215–20.
166. Lee JA. Specially marked needle to facilitate extradural block. *Anaesthesia* 1960; 15:186.
167. Scott DB. A modified Tuohy needle. *Br J Anaesth* 1964; 36:816.
168. Lee JA. A new catheter for continuous extradural analgesia. *Anaesthesia* 1962; 17:248–50.
169. McKenzie AG. The introduction of micropore filters for epidural catheters. *Int J Obstet Anesth* 2001; 10:248.
170. Beazley JM, Leaver EP, Morewood JHM, *et al.* Relief of pain in labour. *Lancet* 1967; 1:1033–5.
171. Doughty A. Epidural analgesia in labour: the past, the present and the future. *J Roy Soc Med* 1978; 71:879–84.
172. Pearson JF, Davies P. The effect of continuous lumbar epidural analgesia upon fetal acid-base status during the first stage of labour. *J Obstet Gynaecol Br Commonw* 1974; 81:971–9.
173. Crawford JS. An appraisal of lumbar epidural blockade in patients with a singleton fetus presenting by the breech. *J Obstet Gynaecol Br Commonw* 1974; 81:867–72.
174. Carrie LES. The paramedian approach to the epidural space. *Anaesthesia* 1977; 32:670.
175. Jouppila R, Jouppila P, Hollmen A, *et al.* Effect of segmental extradural analgesia on placental blood flow during normal labour. *Br J Anaesth* 1978; 50:563–6.
176. Bromage PR. *Epidural Analgesia.* Philadelphia, PA: WB Saunders; 1978.
177. Moir DD. (Editorial) Extradural analgesia for Caesarean section. *Br J Anaesth* 1979; 51:79–80.
178. Birnbach DJ. Obstetric anesthesiology in the new millennium. *Anesth Analg* 2000; 90:1241–3.
179. Lewis M, Thomas P, Wilkes RG. Hypotension during epidural analgesia for Caesarean section. *Anaesthesia* 1983; 38:250–3.
180. Behar M, Magora F, Olshwang D, *et al.* Epidural morphine in treatment of pain. *Lancet* 1979; 1:527–9.
181. Moore DC, Batra MS. The components of an effective test dose prior to epidural block. *Anesthesiology* 1981; 55:693–6.
182. Hicks JA, Jenkins JG, Newton MC, *et al.* Continuous epidural infusion of 0.075% bupivacaine for pain relief in labour. *Anaesthesia* 1988; 43:289–92.
183. Lamont RF, Pinney D, Rodgers P, *et al.* Continuous versus intermittent epidural analgesia: a randomised trial to observe obstetric outcome. *Anaesthesia* 1989; 44:893–6.
184. Li DF, Rees GAD, Rosen M. Continuous epidural infusion of 0.0625% or 0.125% bupivacaine for pain relief in primigravid labour. *Br J Anaesth* 1985; 57:264–70.
185. Okell RW, Sprigge JS. Unintentional dural puncture. A survey of recognition and management. *Anaesthesia* 1987; 42:1110–13.
186. Sweeney N, Denson D, Juneja MM, *et al.* The effect of pH on the onset and duration of epidural lidocaine in the parturient. *Reg Anesth* 1989; 14 Suppl:16.
187. Patrick J. A comparison of epidural diamorphine with intramuscular papaveretum following caesarean section. *Int J Obstet Anesth* 1991; 1:25–8.
188. Stoddart AP, Nicholson KEA, Popham PA. Low dose bupivacaine/fentanyl epidural infusions in labour and mode of delivery. *Anaesthesia* 1994; 49:1087–90.
189. Gambling DR, Bogod D. Epidural infusions in labour should be abandoned in favour of patient-controlled epidural analgesia (Controversy). *Int J Obstet Anesth* 1996; 5:59–63.
190. McClure JH. Ropivacaine. *Br J Anaesth* 1996; 76:300–7.
191. Loo CC, Dahlgren G, Irestedt L. Neurological complications in obstetric regional anaesthesia. *Int J Obstet Anesth* 2000; 9:99–124.
192. Howell CJ, Dean T, Lucking L, *et al.* Randomised study of long term outcome after epidural versus non-epidural analgesia during labour. *Br Med J* 2002; 325:357–9.
193. Royal College of Anaesthetists, Royal College of Nursing, Association of Anaesthetists of Great Britain and Ireland, *et al. Good Practice in the Management of Continuous Epidural Analgesia in the Hospital Setting.* London: Royal College of Anaesthetists; 2004.
194. Schroeder TH, Krueger WA, Neeser E, *et al.* Spinal epidural abscess—a rare complication after epidural analgesia for labour and delivery. *Br J Anaesth* 2004; 92:896–8.
195. Van de Velde M, Schepers R, Berends N, *et al.* Ten years of experience with accidental dural puncture and post-dural puncture headache in a tertiary obstetric anaesthesia department. *Int J Obstet Anesth* 2008; 17:329–35.
196. National Institute for Health and Clinical Excellence. *Ultrasound Guided Catheterisation of the Epidural Space: Understanding NICE Guidance.* London: NICE; 2008.
197. Hermanides J, Hollmann MW, Stevens MF, *et al.* Failed epidural: causes and management. *Br J Anaesth* 2012; 109:144–54.
198. Brownridge P. Epidural and subarachnoid analgesia for elective Caesarean section. *Anaesthesia* 1981; 36:70.
199. Morgan BM. 'Walking' epidurals in labour. *Anaesthesia* 1995; 50:839–40.
200. Walker AL, Wrigley AJ, Marston AD, *et al. Report on CEMD in England and Wales 1952–54.* London: Ministry of Health; 1957.
201. Walker AL, Wrigley AJ, Marston AD, *et al. Report on CEMD in England and Wales 1955–57.* London: Ministry of Health; 1960.
202. Arthure H, Tomkinson J, Organe G, *et al. Report on CEMD in England and Wales 1967–69.* London: DHSS; 1972.
203. Tomkinson J, Turnbull A, Robson G, *et al. Report on CEMD in England and Wales 1973–75.* London: DHSS; 1979
204. Turnbull AC, Tindall VR, Robson G, *et al. Report on CEMD in England and Wales 1979–81.* London: DHSS; 1986.
205. Department of Health, Welsh Office, Scottish Office Home & Health Department, *et al. Report on CEMD in the United Kingdom 1985–87.* London: HMSO; 1991.
206. Department of Health, Welsh Office, Scottish Office Home & Health Department, *et al. Report on CEMD in the United Kingdom 1991–93.* London: HMSO; 1996.
207. Mantel GD, Buchmann E, Rees H, *et al.* Severe acute maternal morbidity: a pilot study of a definition for a near-miss. *Br J Obstet Gynaecol* 1998; 105:985–90.
208. NHS Quality Improvement Scotland. *Scottish Confidential Audit of Severe Maternal Morbidity (SCASMM).* http://www.healthcareimprovementscotland.org/our_work/reproductive,_maternal__child/reproductive_health.aspx
209. Department of Health, Scottish Executive Health Department, Department of Health, Social Services and Public Safety, Northern Ireland. *Why Mothers Die. Fifth Report on Confidential Enquiries into Maternal Deaths in the United Kingdom, 1997–1999.* London: RCOG Press; 2001.

210. Department of Health, Scottish Executive Health Department, Department of Health, Social Services and Public Safety, Northern Ireland. *Why Mothers Die. Sixth Report on Confidential Enquiries into Maternal Deaths in the United Kingdom, 2000–2002.* London: RCOG Press; 2004.
211. Lewis G (ed). *The Confidential Enquiry into Maternal and Child Health (CEMACH). Saving Mothers' Lives: Reviewing Maternal Deaths to Make Motherhood Safer—2003–2005.* London: CEMACH; 2007. http://www.cemach.org.uk
212. Association of Anaesthetists of Great Britain & Ireland. *Guidelines for the Management of Severe Local Anaesthetic Toxicity.* London: AAGBI, 2007.
213. Swanton RDJ, Al-Rawi S, Wee MYK. A national survey of obstetric early warning systems in the United Kingdom. *Int J Obstet Anesth* 2009; 18:253–7.
214. CMACE. Saving Mothers' Lives: reviewing maternal deaths to make motherhood safer: 2006–08. The Eighth Report on Confidential Enquiries into Maternal Deaths in the United Kingdom. *Br J Obstet Gynaecol* 2011; 118 Suppl 1:1–203.
215. National Perinatal Epidemiology Unit. *UK Obstetric Surveillance System (UKOSS).* University of Oxford. http://www.npeu.ox.ac.uk/ukoss
216. Quinn AC, Milne D, Columb M, *et al.* Failed tracheal intubation in obstetric anaesthesia: a 2 yr national case-control study in the UK. *Br J Anaesth* 2013; 110:74–80.
217. National Perinatal Epidemiology Unit. *MBRRACE-UK: Mothers and Babies: Reducing Risk through Audits and Confidential Enquiries across the UK.* University of Oxford. https://www.npeu.ox.ac.uk/mbrrace-uk
218. Toledo P. What's new in obstetric anesthesia: the 2011 Gerard W. Ostheimer lecture. *Int J Obstet Anesth* 2012; 21:68–74.
219. National Patient Safety Agency. Patient Safety Alert 21: *Safer Practice with Epidural Injections and Infusions.* NPSA; 2007. www.saferhealthcare.org.uk
220. National Patient Safety Agency. Patient Safety Alert: *Safer Spinal, Epidural and Regional Anaesthesia Devices*—Part A. NPSA; 2009. http://www.nrls.npsa.nhs.uk/resources/patient-safety-topics/medical-device-equipment/?entryid45=94529
221. Royal College of Anaesthetists. *Report and Findings of the Third National Audit Project: Major Complications of Central Neuraxial Block in the United Kingdom.* London: Royal College of Anaesthetists, 2009. http://www.rcoa.ac.uk/nap3
222. Kinsella SM. The shock of the 'Nuer': the UK experience with new non-Luer neuraxial equipment and implications for obstetric anaesthesia. *Int J Obstet Anesth* 2013; 22:1–5.
223. Hodgkinson R, Husain FJ, Hayashi RH. Systemic and pulmonary blood pressure during caesarean section in parturients with gestational hypertension. *Can Anaesth Soc J* 1980; 27:389–94.
224. Hood DD, Boese PA. Epidural and spinal anaesthesia for caesarean section in severely pre-eclamptic patients (abstract). *Reg Anesth* 1992; 17:35.
225. Wallace DH, Leveno KL, Cunningham FG *et al.* Randomized comparison of general and regional anesthesia for caesarean delivery in pregnancies complicated by severe preeclampsia. *Obstet Gynaecol* 1995; 86:193–9.
226. Howell P. Spinal anaesthesia in severe preeclampsia: time for reappraisal, or time for caution? *Int J Obstet Anesth* 1998; 7:251–60.
227. Sharwood-Smith G, Clark VA, Watson E. Regional anaesthesia for caesarean section in severe preeclampsia: spinal anaesthesia is the preferred choice. *Int J Obstet Anesth* 1999; 8:85–9.
228. Clark VA, Sharwood-Smith G, Stewart AVG. Ephedrine requirements are reduced during spinal anaesthesia for caesarean section in preeclampsia. *Int J Obstet Anesth* 2005; 14:9–13.
229. The Magpie Trial Collaborative Group. Do women with pre-eclampsia, and their babies, benefit from magnesium sulphate? The Magpie Trial: a randomised placebo-controlled trial. *Lancet* 2002; 359:1877–90.
230. Thompson S, Neal S, Clark VA. Clinical risk management in obstetrics: eclampsia drills. *Br Med J* 2004; 328:269–71.
231. Thorburn J, Moir DD. Extradural analgesia: the influence of volume and concentration of bupivacaine on the mode of delivery, analgesic efficacy and motor block. *Br J Anaesth* 1981; 53:933–9.
232. Phillips KC, Thomas TA. Second stage of labour with or without extradural analgesia. *Anaesthesia* 1983; 38:972–6.
233. James KS, McGrady E, Quasim I, *et al.* Comparison of epidural bolus administration of 0.25% bupivacaine and 0.1% bupivacaine with 0.0002% fentanyl for analgesia during labour. *Br J Anaesth* 1998; 81:507–10.
234. Purdie J, Reid J, Thorburn J, *et al.* Continuous extradural analgesia: comparison of midwife top-ups, continuous infusions and patient controlled administration. *Br J Anaesth* 1992; 68:580–4.
235. Collis RE, Davies DWL, Aveling W. Randomised comparison of combined spinal-epidural and standard epidural analgesia in labour. *Lancet* 1995; 345:1413–16.
236. Collis RE, Harding SA, Morgan BM. Effect of maternal ambulation on labour with low-dose combined spinal-epidural analgesia. *Anaesthesia* 1999; 54:535–9.
237. Cheek TG, Samuels P, Miller F, *et al.* Normal saline i.v. fluid load decreases uterine activity in active labour. *Br J Anaesth* 1996; 77:632–5.
238. Capogna G, Celleno D, Lyons G, *et al.* Minimum local analgesic concentration of extradural bupivacaine increases with progression of labour. *Br J Anaesth* 1998; 80:11–13.
239. Loughnan BA, Carli F, Romney M, *et al.* Randomized controlled comparison of epidural bupivacaine *versus* pethidine for analgesia in labour. *Br J Anaesth* 2000; 84:715–19.
240. Comparative Obstetric Mobile Epidural Trial (COMET) Study Group UK. Effect of low-dose mobile versus traditional techniques on mode of delivery. *Lancet* 2001; 358:19–23.
241. Blair JM, Hill DA, Fee JPH. Patient-controlled analgesia for labour using remifentanil: a feasibility study. *Br J Anaesth* 2001; 87:415–20.
242. Muchatuta NA, Kinsella SM. Remifentanil for labour analgesia: time to draw breath? *Anaesthesia* 2013; 68:231–5.
243. Nikolajsen L, Sorensen HC, Jensen TS, *et al.* Chronic pain following caesarean section. *Acta Anaesthesiol Scand* 2004; 48:111–16.
244. McDonnell JG, Curley G, Carney J, *et al.* The analgesic efficacy of transversus abdominis plane block after caesarean delivery: a randomized controlled trial. *Anesth Analg* 2008; 106:186–91.
245. Rivera AM, Strauss KW, van Zundert A, *et al.* The history of peripheral intravenous catheters: how little plastic tubes revolutionized medicine. *Acta Anaesth Belg* 2005; 56:271–82.
246. Department of Health and Social Security. *Report on Confidential Enquiries into Maternal Deaths in England and Wales 1976–78.* London: HMSO; 1982.
247. Browne DA, De Boeck R, Morgan M. An evaluation of the Level 1 blood warmer series. *Anaesthesia* 1990; 45:960–3.
248. Turner DAB. Blood conservation (Editorial). *Br J Anaesth* 1991; 66:281–4.
249. Walfish M, Neuman A, Wlody D. Maternal haemorrhage. *Br J Anaesth* 2009; 103 Supplement 1:i47–i56.
250. Association of Anaesthetists of Great Britain and Ireland, Thomas D, Wee M, *et al.* Blood transfusion and the anaesthetist: management of massive haemorrhage. *Anaesthesia* 2010; 65:1153–61.
251. Chatterjee DJ, Bukunola B, Samuels TL, *et al.* Resuscitation in massive obstetric haemorrhage using an interosseous needle. *Anaesthesia* 2011; 66:306–10.
252. Stocks G. Monitoring transfusion requirements in major obstetric haemorrhage: out with the old and in with the new? *Int J Obstet Anesth* 2011; 20:275–8.
253. Association of Anaesthetists of Great Britain & Ireland and Obstetric Anaesthetists' Association. Anaesthetic Services for Obstetrics—a Plan for the Future. London, 1987.

PART 2

Maternal and fetal physiology

CHAPTER 2

Physiological changes associated with pregnancy

Roulhac D. Toledano

Introduction

Pregnancy triggers significant systemic and organ-specific changes that start soon after conception, become more marked as gestation advances and during labour and delivery, and, most commonly, resolve in the early postpartum period. These physiological alterations, which serve to accommodate the developing fetus and the increased metabolic demands of pregnancy, as well as to prepare the parturient for blood loss at delivery, are generally tolerated well in healthy females. However, they may compromise the parturient with pre-existing or pregnancy-related disease, unmask and/or worsen previously unidentified disease, and complicate the anaesthetic management of pregnant patients presenting for obstetric or non-obstetric surgery. They may also alter diagnostic and laboratory criteria and limit the management and treatment options available to obstetric patients. As a result, an understanding of the anatomical, functional, and biochemical adaptations to pregnancy is essential for health care providers. This chapter reviews the organ-specific and systemic changes associated with pregnancy, with emphasis, when applicable, on how they affect anaesthetic management.

The central nervous system

The central nervous system (CNS) undergoes significant changes during pregnancy (see Table 2.1). Pregnant women experience slight changes in pain perception and pain threshold (see Chapter 15), decreases in anaesthetic requirements, problems with attention, concentration, and memory,[1] disruptions in sleep patterns, increased dependence on the sympathetic nervous system, and, possibly, an increase in cerebral blood flow,[2] without detectable changes in cerebrovascular autoregulation.[3] The clinical implications and mechanism of many of these changes remain unclear or difficult to quantify.

Anaesthetic requirements

The minimum alveolar concentration (MAC) of volatile agents during general anaesthesia is reduced in pregnancy. In an early study, Palahniuk and colleagues found that the MAC for halothane and isoflurane was 25% and 40% lower, respectively, in pregnant ewes compared to non-pregnant controls.[4] A subsequent study in rabbits by Datta et al. proposed that the MAC of halothane correlated inversely with progesterone levels.[5] Other investigators postulated that increased concentrations of endorphins and dynorphins may increase the pain threshold and affect anaesthetic requirements.[6] Studies of human subjects by Chan and colleagues found similar decreased MAC requirements starting early in pregnancy, reporting the MAC of isoflurane to be reduced by 28% at 8–12 weeks' gestation.[7] In another study of females undergoing elective termination of pregnancy, investigators determined median decreases in the MAC of halothane and enflurane of 27% and 30%, respectively, at 8–13 weeks' gestation.[6] Labour appears to decrease the MAC of volatile agents even further.[8] Chan and other investigators determined that the MAC of isoflurane remained decreased (by roughly one-third) for 24–36 hours postpartum and returned to non-pregnant values by 72 hours.[9]

Although it is difficult to extrapolate these findings to other gestational stages of pregnancy and to all volatile agents, it appears that maternal anaesthetic requirements for volatile agents are reduced early in pregnancy and return to normal levels by postpartum day 3. As a result, it has become standard over the past several decades to administer less than 1 MAC of volatile agent (0.5–0.75%), with or without nitrous oxide, during caesarean delivery under general anaesthesia. The reduced MAC has been considered adequate to anaesthetize the mother, with minimal tocolytic and neonatal depressant effects. A target 0.5 MAC of sevoflurane and up to 1 MAC of desflurane also appears not to inhibit the frequency and amplitude of myometrial contractions induced by exogenously administered oxytocin.[10]

The routine use of low concentrations of volatile agents for caesarean delivery under general anaesthesia has contributed to a higher incidence of intraoperative awareness and subsequent recall among parturients. Indeed, investigators have begun to question whether a decreased MAC during pregnancy correlates with

Table 2.1 Central nervous system changes of pregnancy

Parameter	Change
Pain threshold	Increased
MAC of volatile agents	Decreased
Local anaesthetic requirements	Decreased
Cerebrovascular autoregulation	No change
Cerebrovascular blood flow	+/–*
Dependence on the sympathetic nervous system	Increased

*Data are conflicting.

enhanced brain sensitivity to volatile anaesthetic effects; if not, pregnant and non-pregnant patients may require similar doses of anaesthetics to prevent intraoperative awareness.[11] Although the incidence of intraoperative awareness during caesarean delivery has declined to an estimated 0.26%, prevention of this untoward complication remains a challenge for obstetric anaesthetists balancing concerns for uterine tone, maternal anaesthetic depth, and fetal well-being.[12] In the absence of a definitive monitor and reproducible clinical signs to assess anaesthetic depth, investigators have recently advocated a target of 0.7 MAC, which corresponds to a bispectral index value below 60 yet does not appear to increase the incidence of uterine atony and neonatal depression, during caesarean delivery under general anaesthesia.[12] Supplemental nitrous oxide, particularly in emergency caesarean deliveries, may further minimize the risk of awareness. Other investigators concur that a target of less than 0.8–1.0 MAC will provide sufficient maternal unconsciousness without affecting neonatal outcomes, blood loss, or uterine contraction in response to oxytocin.[13] Despite notable progress, intraoperative awareness remains a highly undesirable outcome with the potential for long-term sequelae, such as post-traumatic stress disorder, in a small subset of patients. Intraoperative awareness may also present a medicolegal challenge for anaesthetists.

Local anaesthetic requirements

Local anaesthetic requirements for both peripheral and neuraxial anaesthetic procedures appear to be reduced in obstetric patients, most likely as a collective result of anatomical, mechanical, and biochemical changes. Neuraxial local anaesthetic requirements are reduced early in pregnancy, presumably due to chronic exposure to progesterone, and reach 40% of non-pregnant requirements by term gestation. An increase in epidural fat content during pregnancy and the distension of the epidural venous plexus by the enlarging uterus contribute to this dose reduction by decreasing both the volume of the epidural space and of cerebrospinal fluid (CSF) per spinal segment. Decreases in the specific gravity and pH of CSF during pregnancy may also contribute to the observed decreased requirements of spinally administered local anaesthetics. These dose requirements return to baseline within 24 hours postpartum.[14]

The autonomic nervous system

Pregnant patients develop increasing reliance on the sympathetic nervous system throughout pregnancy. This phenomenon, which peaks at term and returns to baseline within 2 days postpartum, accounts in part for the occasional severe haemodynamic derangements associated with the sympathectomy of neuraxial blockade, as well as the relatively high pressor requirements that otherwise healthy parturients experience during spinal anaesthesia.[15] The downregulation of the parasympathetic nervous system towards term gestation, in turn, may have a sparing effect, preventing more frequent episodes of severe bradycardia in the setting of high sympathectomies.

The cardiovascular system

The cardiovascular system undergoes several changes during pregnancy, including increases in plasma volume, red blood cell (RBC) mass, and cardiac output (CO) and decreases in blood pressure and systemic vascular resistance (SVR) (see Table 2.2).

Table 2.2 Cardiovascular changes of pregnancy

Parameter	Change
Plasma volume	Increased
RBC mass	Increased
Cardiac output	Increased
Blood pressure	Decreased
Systemic vascular resistance	Decreased
Myocardial contractility	No change/increase*

*Data are inconclusive.

Although myocardial contractility remains unchanged, or is, possibly, slightly increased, the increased CO may unmask underlying or pregnancy-related heart conditions or precipitate acute deterioration in patients with previously asymptomatic heart disease. Aortocaval compression, neuraxial procedures, and general anaesthetics may further contribute to maternal cardiac decompensation and fetal compromise.

Cardiac output

An increase in CO begins as early as 5 weeks' gestation and continues throughout pregnancy, peaking at 28–34 weeks' gestation and, again, during the second stage of labour. At its height during pregnancy, CO reaches 50% above baseline. It increases an additional 15–25% during early labour and the active phase of labour, and reaches 50% above term pregnancy values during the second stage of labour. The highest CO, however, is in the immediate postpartum period, when it reaches 80% above prelabour values. Uterine involution and the resultant autotransfusion, which outpaces blood loss at delivery, accounts in part for the postpartum increase in CO. Cardiac patients are at particular risk during this period.

Both an increased stroke volume (SV) and heart rate (HR) contribute to the increased CO of pregnancy, but the former contributes to a greater degree (see Figure 2.1). SV increases early in pregnancy and declines very slightly at term. The maternal HR increases as early as 5 weeks' gestation and reaches 15–20 beats/min above baseline by 32 weeks' gestation.[16] At term, sustained maternal tachycardia is primarily responsible for the high CO.

Aortocaval compression

Maternal positioning influences the pregnancy-induced increase in CO. Sharp reductions in CO are seen in some women in the supine position as early as 18–20 weeks' gestation, if not earlier, when the enlarging uterus begins to compress the inferior vena cava (IVC) and, less often, the aorta. The IVC may become partially or completely occluded, resulting in dramatically decreased venous return to the right atrium and a related decrease in CO. Collateral circulation through the paravertebral and azygos veins only partially compensates for the decreased venous return. At term, aortocaval compression in the supine position may reduce CO by as much as 30%, and up to 15% of parturients experience signs and symptoms of the supine hypotensive syndrome, including hypotension, sweating, bradycardia, syncope, nausea and vomiting, and mental status changes.[17] Uteroplacental perfusion also decreases as a result of decreased uterine blood flow and increased uterine venous pressure, compromising fetal well-being.

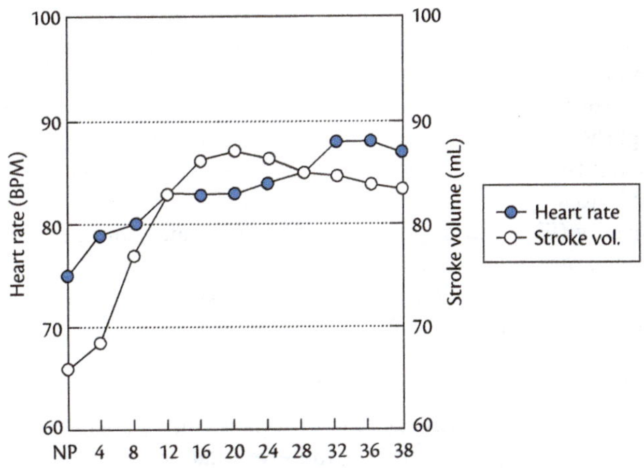

Figure 2.1 This figure was published in *Creasy & Resnik's Maternal-Fetal Medicine: Principles and Practice*, RK Creasy, R Resnik, JD Iams, *et al* (eds), Maternal Cardiovascular, Respiratory, and Renal Adaptation to Pregnancy, p.102–9, Copyright Elsevier (2009). Adapted from *Americal Journal of Physiology – Heart and Circulatory Physiology*, Robson SC, Hunter S, Boys RJ, *et al.* Serial Study of Factors Influencing Changes in Cardiac Output during Human Pregnancy, 256, 4, 1989, p. H1060, ©The American Physiological Society (APS).

General and neuraxial anaesthesia impair sympathetic tone and compromise the normal physiological response to aortocaval compression, exacerbating maternal hypotension and further reducing cardiac preload and output. Although data are inconclusive, left uterine displacement (LUD) with either a wedge placed under the patient's right side or a 15–20° tilt of the operating table should be maintained during all procedures involving pregnant women after mid-gestation. During caesarean deliveries, LUD should be maintained until the baby is delivered; studies have demonstrated improved Apgar scores and reduced neonatal depression in the setting of LUD.[18] Employing LUD is also an essential, initial component of successful cardiopulmonary resuscitation of pregnant patients in cardiac arrest, as the obstructive effects of the gravid uterus on the great vessels attenuate the efficacy of compressions. Occasionally, manual displacement of the uterus to the left, for example, during an acute episode of fetal hypoxia, right uterine displacement, or additional LUD of up to a 30° tilt may be required to relieve IVC compression and maintain maternal and fetal well-being. Assuming the lateral recumbent position or a knee-chest position may also help to maintain CO during procedures, such as spinal or epidural placement.

Blood pressure and systemic vascular resistance

In general, both arterial blood pressure and SVR decrease during pregnancy, although several factors affect blood pressure measurements, including maternal age, positioning, gestational age, comorbidities, and parity. The systolic and diastolic blood pressures begin to drop at 7 weeks' gestation, but the diastolic pressure decreases to a greater extent, reaching 10 mmHg (1.33 kPa) below baseline at 24–32 weeks. This discrepancy accounts for the slight increase in pulse pressure in the early third trimester. Thereafter, both the systolic and diastolic pressures rise slowly towards prepregnant values, although they increase above baseline during labour. The magnitude of this increase is dependent on the patient's position and the degree of pain she experiences during labour, as well as the intensity of uterine contractions.

SVR begins to decrease as early as 5 weeks' gestation as a result of the potent vasodilating effects of progesterone and prostacyclin and, as pregnancy progresses, the low-resistance uteroplacental circulation. Endothelium-derived factors such as nitric oxide may also initiate vasodilation early in pregnancy. The decrease in SVR rises progressively after 14–24 weeks' gestation, and represents a 21% decrease from baseline by term.

Blood volume

Cardiovascular changes of pregnancy can be attributed in part to several haematological changes. Plasma volume expands gradually throughout pregnancy, starting as early as 6 weeks' gestation and peaking at 32–34 weeks. Sodium and water retention contribute to an average gain in plasma volume of 1200–1600 mL by the third trimester, which represents roughly a 45% increase above non-pregnant values.[19] A portion of this retained fluid is transferred into the interstitial space as a result of low colloid oncotic pressure during pregnancy. The RBC mass increases also, beginning at 8–10 weeks' gestation, but a disproportionate increase in plasma volume contributes to a relative anaemia of pregnancy. Despite increased erythropoiesis, haemoglobin, haematocrit, and blood viscosity decrease during pregnancy.

Cardiac evaluation

Cardiovascular changes during pregnancy affect the physical findings on cardiac examination, as well as cardiac diagnostic test results (see Table 2.3). The enlarging uterus shifts the heart to the left, slightly anterior, and in a transverse direction, resulting in a cephalad and lateral shift of the maximal cardiac impulse. The leftward shift also contributes to an enlarged cardiac silhouette on chest radiograph and, as pregnancy progresses, a left axis deviation on electrocardiogram (ECG). Additional changes that may be detected on ECG include sinus tachycardia, premature atrial and ventricular contractions, periods of supraventricular tachycardia and ventricular extrasystoles, shortened PR and uncorrected QT intervals, fleeting ST segment and T wave changes, inverted T waves in leads V1, V2, and, less commonly, V3, an attenuated Q wave in lead aVF, and a Q wave and inverted T waves in lead III. The increased incidence of cardiac arrhythmias during pregnancy is attributed in part to a stretching of the cardiac conduction pathways related to the increased SV and resultant cardiac chamber enlargement, as well as to hormonal and autonomic changes. Pregnant women in their late thirties and forties are more likely to have comorbidities that predispose them to arrhythmias. Women who were successfully treated for heart disease as infants and have

Table 2.3 Changes detected on cardiac evaluation during pregnancy

Left axis deviation by 3rd trimester	Tachycardia, other arrhythmias
Left ventricular enlargement	Audible splitting of S1
Prominent jugular venous pulsation	Tricuspid, pulmonic regurgitation
Detectable venous hum	Audible 3rd heart sound
Audible systolic ejection murmur	Premature atrial contractions
Leftward point of maximal impulse	Premature ventricular contractions

now reached childbearing age may also have arrhythmias and residual cardiac anomalies.

Several additional changes can be detected on cardiovascular examination. The left and right ventricles may be palpable as a result of the hyperdynamic circulation, although palpation becomes more difficult as the breasts and abdomen continue to enlarge. Prominent jugular venous pulsations, basal crepitations due to atelectasis from compression by the gravid uterus, and lower extremity oedema may be among the physical findings during normal pregnancy. Heart murmurs and heart sounds that are difficult to hear in non-pregnant individuals become more audible during pregnancy. A grade II systolic ejection murmur is commonly auscultated over the pulmonary and tricuspid areas, and a third heart sound is often present late in pregnancy. There is an audible splitting of S1 and, in the third trimester, S2, and the venous hum is common in pregnancy. Tricuspid and pulmonary regurgitation occurs in the majority of pregnant patients at term, while mitral valve regurgitation occurs in roughly one-third of patients. Diastolic murmurs may uncommonly be detected as a result of the increased blood flow, but more likely represent pathological conditions that warrant further investigation.

On echocardiogram the left ventricle is enlarged as a result of a 50% increase in mass at term. The eccentric hypertrophy is a result of an increase in the size rather than number of cardiomyocytes. Right-sided regurgitation is commonly detected, and may persist until the early postpartum period. Valvular annular dilatation and, less commonly, a small pericardial effusion of no known clinical significance may also be visualized.

The respiratory system

The respiratory system undergoes profound hormonal, circulatory, and mechanical alterations during pregnancy. Pregnant women may experience shortness of breath, nasal congestion, tachypnoea, epistaxis, sleep-disordered breathing, snoring, and voice changes, among other signs and symptoms that often worsen as gestation advances. Pregnancy is also accompanied by increased pulmonary blood flow, structural changes to the thoracic and rib cages, a 4 cm elevation of the diaphragm, and alterations in the balance of bronchoconstrictor and bronchodilator prostanoids. Of particular clinical relevance, pregnancy is marked by airway changes that may contribute to difficult and failed intubations, as well as changes in lung function and oxygen consumption that lead to prompt desaturation during periods of apnoea. Maternal weight gain, breast enlargement, predisposition to gastro-oesophageal disorders, and comorbidities, such as obesity and pre-eclampsia, as well as the occasional emergent nature of obstetric cases, compound these challenges.

Lung volumes and capacities

Alterations in respiratory function during pregnancy can be attributed to anatomical and hormonal changes, as well as to changing metabolic demands. With upward uterine displacement of the diaphragm and a related 35–45% decrease in chest wall compliance, expiratory reserve volume and residual volume fall by 25% and 15%, respectively.[20] As a result, functional residual capacity (FRC) drops markedly after 5 months' gestation, reaching 80% of prepregnancy values by term. Supine positioning, obesity, and the induction of general anaesthesia exacerbate this decrease. Tidal volume (TV) increases by 45% early in pregnancy, primarily as a result of the respiratory stimulant effects of increased serum progesterone levels, while inspiratory reserve volume increases very slightly. Vital capacity and total lung capacity show little to no change (see Figure 2.2). Airflow mechanics, as measured by forced expiratory volume in 1 second (FEV_1) and the FEV_1/forced vital capacity (FVC) ratio, peak expiratory flow rates, and the shape of the flow–volume curve are also unchanged during pregnancy. These changes in lung volumes, capacities, and airflow mechanics are summarized in Table 2.4.

Ventilation and arterial blood gases

There are several clinical implications of the changes in lung function during pregnancy. Minute ventilation increases up to 45% above baseline, primarily as a result of the increase in TV from roughly 500 to 700 mL per breath. The increase in minute ventilation, which starts during the first trimester and remains constant or increases slightly towards term, overcompensates for the increased carbon dioxide production during pregnancy and contributes to a decrease in the arterial partial pressure of carbon dioxide ($PaCO_2$), which reaches approximately 30 mmHg (4.0 kPa) already early in pregnancy. An increase in renal excretion of plasma bicarbonate partially compensates for this respiratory alkalosis, but the pH remains slightly more alkalotic than the normal state (see Table 2.5). Respiratory alkalosis results in a leftward shift in the oxyhaemoglobin dissociation curve, increasing the affinity of maternal haemoglobin for oxygen. An increase in erythrocyte 2,3-diphosphoglycerate during pregnancy, though, shifts the curve to the right, favouring oxygen transfer to the fetus (see Figure 2.3). Although alkalosis in the CSF and blood normally suppress hypoxic drive, women experience a twofold increase in the hypoxic ventilatory response during pregnancy.[21]

Pregnancy-induced hyperpnoea also contributes to a change in arterial oxygenation tension. The arterial partial pressure of oxygen (PaO_2) increases slightly during pregnancy, ranging from 107 mmHg (14.3 kPa) in the first trimester to 103 mmHg (13.7 kPa) in the third trimester, a process that may facilitate oxygen transfer across the placenta. However, increased oxygen consumption, which reaches up to 60% above baseline at term, may account for a PaO_2 of less than 100 mmHg (13.3 kPa) in many pregnant patients by mid-gestation. A lower PaO_2 may also result from small airway closure and the related ventilation/perfusion (V/Q) mismatch that occurs when closing capacity exceeds FRC. A reduced CO, as seen when parturients assume the supine position, may further reduce the PaO_2.

Apnoeic hypoxaemia

Decreased FRC, coupled with increased oxygen consumption, results in rapid oxygen desaturation during periods of apnoea in pregnant patients. Labouring, obese, and septic obstetric patients, and, in particular, obese labouring patients, appear to be at greatest risk for developing hypoxaemia rapidly during even short periods of apnoea, such as upon induction of general anaesthesia for caesarean delivery or during eclamptic seizures.[22] Oxygen consumption increases throughout pregnancy and reaches its peak at term, when it averages 331 mL/min at rest and 1167 mL/min with exercise.[23] It increases an additional 40–75% during labour, and even more in obese pregnant women in labour, although these

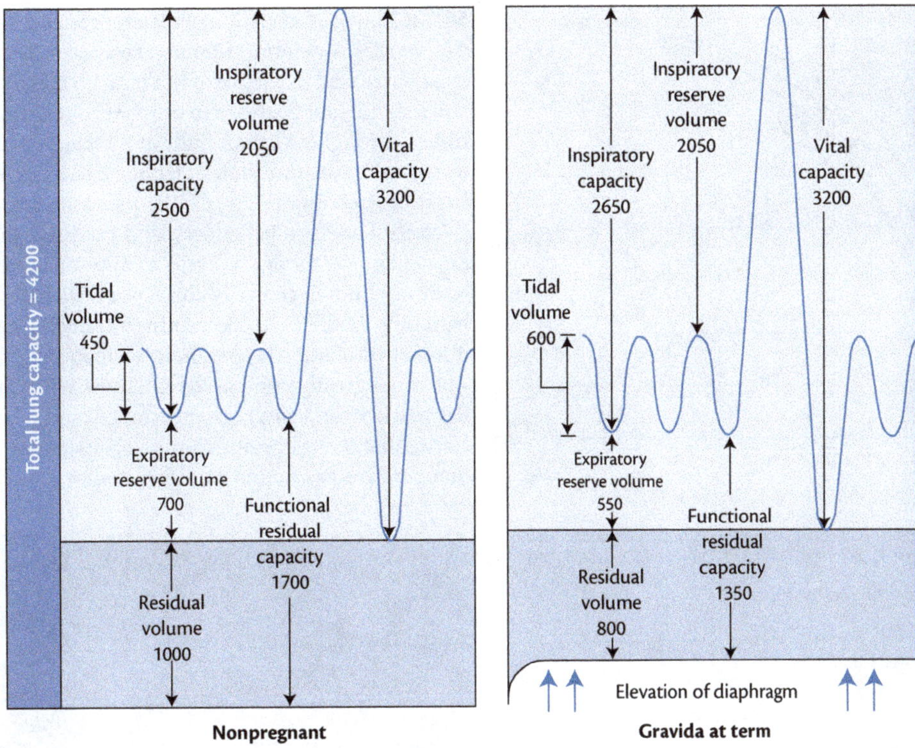

Figure 2.2 Changes in lung volumes during pregnancy.

Reproduced with permission from MS Suresh, BS Segal, RL Preston, *et al., Shnider and Levinson's Anesthesia for Obstetrics*, Fifth Edition, Baltimore, MA: Lippincott Williams & Wilkins, 1–17. Copyright © 2013. This figure was originally in Bonica JJ (ed) *Principles and Practice of Obstetric Analgesia and Anesthesia*. Philadelphia, PA: Davis, 1967:24, © F.A. Davis.

increased metabolic requirements can be mitigated by effective analgesia, such as epidural blockade.[24] Simultaneously, parturients have reduced oxygen storage in a smaller FRC. The net effect is a reduced apnoea tolerance in pregnancy and in conditions that contribute to additional imbalances between oxygen consumption and FRC.

Studies have demonstrated that oxygen desaturation occurs more rapidly during periods of apnoea in pregnancy. McClelland and colleagues found that the median time required for arterial oxygen saturation (SaO_2) to fall below 90% after complete denitrogenation was 4 min 52 s in pregnant subjects, compared to 7 min 25 s in non-pregnant subjects.[25] All subjects in this simulation study desaturated to an SaO_2 below 40% in less time than deemed necessary to resume spontaneous ventilation after the administration of 1 mg/kg intravenous succinylcholine.[26] The study also found that, across all subjects that were preoxygenated, the pregnant subjects desaturated from 90% to 40% SaO_2 in 35 s, compared to 45 s in non-pregnant subjects. The labouring patient with a body mass index (BMI) of 50 kg/m^2 exhibited the fastest arterial desaturation, falling below 90% in 98 s, compared to 292 s in a standard pregnant patient.[22] These findings highlight the importance of limiting the number and duration of attempts at laryngoscopy and of re-establishing ventilation promptly after unsuccessful intubation. Finally, McClelland et al. demonstrated an almost directly proportional relationship between apnoea tolerance and preoxygenation status, although a plateau was reached in which increasing time spent preoxygenating resulted

Table 2.4 Respiratory changes during pregnancy

Lung volumes, capacities, and airflow mechanics	Change
Tidal volume	+33–45%
Expiratory reserve volume	−20–25%
Inspiratory reserve volume	+5%
Residual volume	−15–20%
Total lung capacity	−5%
Vital capacity	No change
Inspiratory capacity	+6–15%
Functional residual capacity	−20%
FEV_1	No change
FEV_1/FVC	No change
Peak expiratory flow	No change
Flow–volume loop	No change

Table 2.5 Arterial blood gas measurements during pregnancy

Parameter	Non-pregnant	Pregnant
pH	7.4	7.4–7.44
PaO_2 (mmHg)	100	103–107[a]
$PaCO_2$ (mmHg)	40	30
HCO_3 (mEq/L)	24	20

[a]Note that the PaO_2 may vary in each trimester.

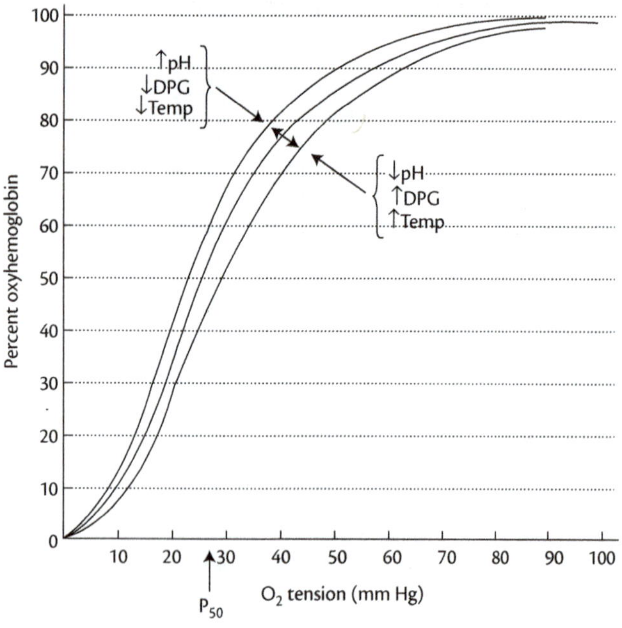

Figure 2.3 Oxyhaemoglobin dissociation curve.
This figure was published in *Creasy & Resnik's Maternal-Fetal Medicine: Principles and Practice*, RK Creasy, R Resnik, JD Iams, *et al.* (eds), Respiratory Diseases in Pregnancy, p. 928, Copyright Elsevier (2009).

in gradually less benefit to apnoea tolerance. Two minutes of complete denitrogenation by tidal breathing of 100% oxygen with a tight-fitting facemask, a process that is accelerated by the reduced FRC and increased minute ventilation of pregnancy, provided roughly 3.5–6 min before the SaO_2 fell below 90% in normal, healthy parturients at term.[27]

Airway changes during pregnancy and labour and delivery

Airway changes during pregnancy and over the course of labour and delivery complicate the perioperative management of parturients. Swelling of the oropharyngeal tissue, a decrease in the size of the glottic aperture, and mucosal friability are present from early gestation until several days postpartum, but are most pronounced near term and during labour and delivery. Fat deposition related to maternal weight gain, increased tongue size, an increase in airway connective tissue, fluid retention, capillary engorgement, and decreased soft tissue mobility contribute to these changes. Full dentition in the majority of women of childbearing age, enlarged breasts, inappropriately applied cricoid pressure during attempts at tracheal intubation, and the fact that parturients undergoing emergency caesarean delivery during general anaesthesia are rarely fasted compound concerns about the obstetric airway, particularly for anaesthetists and trainees with little experience administering general anaesthetics to this patient population.

Although recent data suggest that the incidence of difficult or failed intubations in obstetric patients is decreasing, whether or not the maternal airway is more difficult anatomically is still debated in the literature.[28] Using standardized photography, Pilkington and colleagues documented an incidence of 36% and 42% of Mallampati class 3 and class 4, respectively, in obstetric patients at 12 weeks' gestation; the respective rates were 29% and 56% at 38 weeks' gestation, which represent a 34% increase in class 4 airways.[29] A deterioration in airway classification, as manifested by an increased incidence of Mallampati class 3 and class 4 airways and a significant decrease in oropharyngeal area and volume, continues throughout labor, and, in a recent study, was found to be unrelated to the duration of labour and intravenous fluid administration (see Figure 2.4).[30] The presence of comorbidities, such as obesity and pre-eclampsia, and excessive fluid administration may magnify these changes. While an increasing Mallampati score does not necessarily correspond with difficult tracheal intubation,[31] Rocke et al. determined that the relative risk (RR) of difficult intubation in pregnant women with class 3 airways was 7.58 times greater compared with those with class 1 airways.[32] The RR reached 11.3 in pregnant women with class 4 airways, indicating that using various combinations of risk factors may enable preoperative prediction of difficult airway encounters.[32] Because

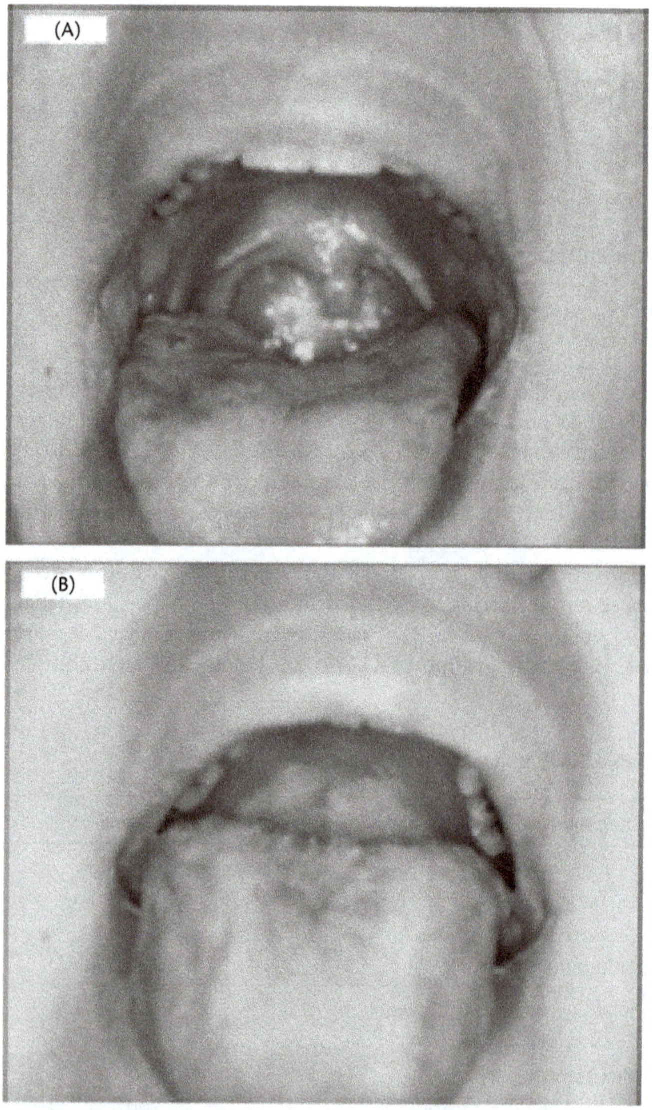

Figure 2.4 Airway changes during labour and delivery. (A) Prelabour (B) Postlabour.
Reproduced with permission from Kodali, BS, Chandrasekhar, S, Bulich, LN, *et al.*, Airway Changes during Labor and Delivery, *Obstetric Anesthesia Digest*, Volume 28, Issue 3, pp. 357–362, Copyright © 2008 Wolters Kluwer Health, Inc.

labour and delivery is associated with additional airway changes, it is essential to reassess the Mallampati classification and other aspects of the airway in labouring women who present for caesarean delivery prior to initiation of an anaesthetic.

Although anaesthesia-related maternal mortality is rare, airway catastrophes remain the leading cause of death from general anaesthesia in the obstetric population.[33] As a result, maintaining constant vigilance and pursuing strategies to manage the obstetric airway are paramount. Access to video laryngoscopes and other airway adjuvants, availability of a short-handle laryngoscope, optimization of maternal positioning and preoxygenation, familiarity with the emergency airway algorithm for obstetric patients, immediate availability of experienced anaesthesia providers, and early initiation of neuraxial blockade in patients with known or suspected difficult airways may help minimize or avoid airway complications in obstetric patients. Avoidance of nasal intubation and nasal suctioning, preparedness to use a smaller endotracheal tube (6.0 or 6.5 mm), and limiting the number and duration of attempts at intubation are essential measures to decrease complications associated with excessive bleeding and airway oedema. Early identification of patients at risk for emergency operations, such as those with dysfunctional labour, ongoing communication with the obstetrics team, and continued vigilance during emergence and recovery, when complications arise with equal or greater frequency,[34] may help to avoid difficulties in the airway management of individual patients. While aspiration prophylaxis, restriction of oral intake of solids, and rapid sequence induction (RSI) with cricoid pressure have never been proven to reduce maternal morbidity,[35] they are still considered by most practitioners to be standards of care.

Haematology and immunology of pregnancy

Pregnancy is marked by significant changes in plasma volume, RBC mass, and leucocyte number and function, as well as in the delicate balance between clot formation and thrombosis prevention. Notable changes in platelet count and function also affect a small percentage of both healthy pregnant women and those with coexisting disease. Many of these haematological and immunological adaptations to pregnancy prepare the mother for blood loss at delivery and optimize maternal–fetal immunologic interactions. However, they may also predispose the parturient to venous thromboembolism (VTE) during pregnancy and to haemorrhagic complications in the peripartum period. This section reviews the haemostatic system, common platelet disorders, and changes in the immunologic system during pregnancy.

Haemostasis

The haemostatic system, which establishes a delicate balance between clot formation and prevention of thrombosis, undergoes profound local and systemic changes during pregnancy (see Table 2.6). Broadly speaking, pregnancy is a prothrombotic state associated with increased clotting capacity and decreased anticoagulant and fibrinolytic activity. Concentrations of von Willebrand factor (vWF) and factors VII, VIII, IX, X, and XII increase to varying degrees (see Table 2.7). Fibrinogen (factor I) levels also increase, reaching a mean value of 450 mg/dL during pregnancy.[36] Levels of factors II and V, however, remain stable, and the concentration of factor XI decreases slightly. The activity of anticoagulant protein S declines to roughly one-third of normal during the second and third trimesters, decreasing even further in the setting of caesarean delivery or infection.[37] A related increased resistance to activated protein C contributes to the observed increase in thrombin formation during pregnancy. With regard to proteins that inhibit clot lysis, plasminogen activator inhibitor (PAI) types 1 and 2, triple, if not quadruple, during pregnancy, and peak at term. This increase is attributed to rich sources of PAI-1 in the uterine decidua and to placental production of PAI-2.[38] Venous stasis resulting from compression of the IVC and adjacent vessels by the enlarged uterus further increases the risk of VTE, which may be sixfold higher during pregnancy.[39]

While pregnancy is a prothrombotic state, obstetric complications associated with impaired decidualization or haemorrhage into the decidua may result in massive haemorrhage and disseminated intravascular coagulation (DIC) more swiftly than anticipated. Under normal conditions, a progesterone-mediated increase in tissue factor (TF) and, secondarily, PAI-1 in the uterine decidua serves to mediate haemostasis during the third stage

Table 2.6 Haematological parameters

Parameter	Non-pregnant adult	Term parturient	General trend
Erythropoietin (U/L)	4–27	14–222	Increased
Haemoglobin (g/dL)	12–15.8	9.5–15	Decreased
Haematocrit (g/dL)	35.4–44.4	28–40	Decreased
Mean corpuscular haemoglobin (pg/cell)	27–32	29–32	No change
Mean corpuscular volume (m^3)	79–93	81–99	No change
Platelet (10^9/L)	165–415	146–429	Decreased
RBC count (10^6/mm^3)	4–5	2.7–4.4	Decreased
White blood cell count (10^3/mm^3)	3.5–9.1	5.9–16.9	Increased

Table 2.7 Changes in coagulation and fibrinolytic parameters during pregnancy

Parameter	Change
Factor I (fibrinogen)	Increased
Factor VII (proconvertin)	Increased
Factor VIII (antihaemophilic factor)	Increased
Factor IX (Christmas factor)	Increased
Factor X (Stuart–Prower factor)	Increased
Factor XII (Hageman factor)	Increased
vWF (von Willebrand factor)	Increased
PAI-1, PAI-2	Increased
Factor II (prothrombin)	No change
Factor V (proaccelerin)	No change
Factor XI (plasma thromboplastin antecedent)	Decreased
Protein S	Decreased

of labour, protecting the mother from haemorrhagic complications.[40] However, the principal role of decidual TF in maintaining haemostasis is jeopardized in conditions of impaired decidualization, such as placenta accreta, ectopic pregnancy, and placenta praevia. Decidual TF also appears to play a central role in haemorrhagic complications associated with placenta abruption; high levels of TF in the setting of inadequate haemostasis lead to excessive thrombin formation, exhaustion of clotting factors, hypofibrinogenaemia, and, possibly, DIC.[41] Massive haemorrhage from any of several other obstetric complications, including uterine atony, retained products of conception, amniotic fluid embolism, uterine inversion, and birth trauma, as well as from trauma, sepsis, and large-volume blood transfusions may also rapidly evolve into DIC in obstetric patients.

Physiological anaemia of pregnancy

A disproportionate expansion of maternal plasma volume relative to the increase in RBC mass during pregnancy results in physiological anaemia. Beginning as early as 6 weeks' gestation, plasma volume progressively expands until it reaches 45% above baseline by 32–34 weeks. This increase appears to be mediated by enhanced aldosterone activity, an oestrogen- and nitric oxide-mediated increase in plasma renin activity early in pregnancy, and the reduced plasma osmolality at which vasopressin is secreted during pregnancy, and correlates with the observed increase in plasma-mature adrenomedullin.[42] RBC volume, on the other hand, declines early in pregnancy, reaches prepregnancy values by 16 weeks' gestation, and peaks at term. The ultimate rise in RBC mass to 17–30% above baseline is due to an increase in erythropoietin activity, but does not match the plasma expansion during earlier gestation. Haemodilution results in characteristically lower RBC, haemoglobin, and haematocrit counts, but does not alter the mean corpuscular volume or the mean corpuscular haemoglobin concentration during pregnancy (see Table 2.6). The average haemoglobin concentration of parturients at term is 12.5 g/dL, somewhat above the World Health Organization's cut-off of 11 g/dL for anaemia of pregnancy.[43] Failure to meet the increasing iron, vitamin B_{12}, and folate requirements during pregnancy can lead to further declines in haemoglobin and haematocrit concentrations and result in pathological anaemia. Overall, the disproportionate increase in plasma volume and RBC mass observed in normal pregnancy results in decreased blood viscosity, which reduces resistance to blood flow through the uteroplacental circulation, and sufficient hypervolaemia to ensure delivery of vital nutrients to the fetus, maintain maternal blood pressure in the setting of decreased vascular tone, and prepare the mother for blood loss at delivery.

Platelet number and function

The platelet count falls by an estimated 10% during normal pregnancy, with the greatest drop occurring in the third trimester.[44] However, roughly 8% of pregnant women have or develop some form of more severe thrombocytopaenia, as defined by a platelet count below 150×10^9/L.[45] Incidental thrombocytopaenia of pregnancy, also known as gestational thrombocytopaenia, affects up to 5% of these patients,[46] and accounts for an estimated 75% of all cases of thrombocytopaenia during pregnancy.[47] This benign condition, which usually presents in the third trimester and resolves within 7 days postpartum, is due primarily to haemodilution that results from the increase in plasma volume during pregnancy.[48] Although the literature is inconclusive, a mild intravascular coagulation within the uteroplacental circulation that leads to increased platelet destruction and that is compensated for by increased, albeit inadequate, platelet production may also play a role in the pathogenesis of gestational thrombocytopaenia.[49] Increased platelet aggregation in response to epinephrine and arachidonic acid, among other things, and an immune-mediated component may further contribute. In general, patients with gestational thrombocytopaenia have no prior history of thrombocytopaenia in the non-gravid state, remain asymptomatic throughout pregnancy, and do not require any medical therapy. Up to one-fifth of these patients may experience a recurrence in subsequent pregnancies, and there is little to no known risk of neonatal thrombocytopaenia in infants born to these mothers. In the absence of a coexisting platelet disorder, patients with gestational thrombocytopaenia usually maintain platelets counts greater than 70×10^9/L. If platelets fall below this cut-off or if the patient experiences any clinically significant bleeding, other sources of thrombocytopaenia must be considered.

An estimated 25% of the cases of significant thrombocytopaenia during pregnancy are due to disease processes that may lead to bleeding complications in the peripartum period or that may indicate a more complex underlying disorder.[50] Of these, the majority is related to hypertensive disorders of pregnancy, and a small portion is secondary to immune processes, such as idiopathic thrombocytopenic purpura (ITP). ITP, which affects an estimated 2 per 1000 pregnant[51] women, must be distinguished from gestational thrombocytopaenia because of potential, albeit uncommon, bleeding complications for both mother and neonate. Patients with ITP have a history of bleeding in the non-pregnant state, may have platelet counts below 70×10^9/L, although the median range in one large study was 85×10^9/L,[52] present with low platelet counts early in pregnancy, and may not experience resolution of the disease after delivery. A mild, progressive decline in count may be observed as gestation advances. Treatment with corticosteroids, intravenous immunoglobulin, immunosuppressive agents, and, in refractory cases, splenectomy, most often in the second trimester, may be necessary, although conservative management of this autoimmune disorder is increasingly common.[53] Because ITP is a quantitative, rather than qualitative platelet disorder, routine management also appears to be appropriate prior to initiation of neuraxial blockade, provided platelet count remains above a certain, practitioner-specific or institutional-specific range. Neonates of mothers with ITP are at risk of thrombocytopaenia; parturients with ITP are at increased risk of peripartum haemorrhage.

The immune system

The blood leucocyte count rises steadily as gestation advances and during the puerperium, while chemotaxis and adherence functions of some polymorphonuclear leucocytes decrease, starting at the second trimester and continuing until term. Markers of inflammation, such as C-reactive protein, the erythrocyte sedimentation rate, and complement factors C3 and C4, are also elevated to varying degrees at different gestational ages. In general, normal leucocyte counts during gestation range from 5000 to 12,000/μL and average 14,000–16,000/μL during labour and in the early postpartum period. The aetiology of this increase has not been elucidated, but may be related to a reappearance of leucocytes that had been previously sequestered. The distribution of cell types also changes during pregnancy, as manifested by a significant increase in granulocytes and CD8 T lymphocytes and a sharp reduction in CD4 T lymphocytes and monocytes during the third trimester.[54] Overall, depressed leucocyte function appears to be of little clinical significance, but may account in part for pregnancy-related remission of some autoimmune disorders, as well as the mildly increased susceptibility of pregnant women to certain infections.

The immunology of pregnancy is complex and has not yet been fully elaborated, although several theories have been proposed. Briefly, one long-standing theory regarding how the fetus evades maternal rejection proposes that the placenta serves as a mechanical barrier, barring interaction between fetal antigens and the maternal immune system. However, more recent evidence suggests that the trophoblast–decidual interface is not impermeable, as evidenced by the fact that fetal cells circulate in the maternal blood long after delivery.[55] Another theory proposes that pregnancy is a state of systemic immune suppression, which permits the mother to tolerate the foreign fetus and partially explains the improvement in some autoimmune diseases often observed during pregnancy. However, critics of this theory challenge that an intact maternal immune system appears to evade infection despite chronic exposure to pathogens. Additional theories propose deletion of immune cells that recognize paternal alloantigens from the maternal immune system, a state of localized immune suppression, and a lack of placental expression of certain human leucocyte antigens, among others, and are beyond the scope of this chapter.[56]

The gastrointestinal system

The gastrointestinal (GI) system undergoes several changes during pregnancy, many of which have been attributed to changes in the hormonal milieu. In general, pregnant women are prone to develop disorders of the oropharynx, ranging from benign changes in taste perception[57] and salivary composition[58] to gingival bleeding associated with periodontal disease; of the stomach, oesophagus, and intestines, such as gastro-oesophageal reflux (GOR), hyperemesis gravidarum, and constipation and bloating; and of the anorectum, including haemorrhoids, anal fissures, proctitis, and faecal incontinence.[59] Mechanical and, primarily, hormonal changes in the GI system that may predispose pregnant women to pulmonary aspiration are of particular clinical relevance to anaesthesia providers.

Gastro-oesophageal reflux

GOR affects an estimated 30–50% of pregnant women at some stage during pregnancy, although the true incidence may be as high as 80% in some patient populations.[60] While it occasionally represents an exacerbation of pre-existing disease, it most often develops *de novo* during pregnancy, presenting late in the first trimester, worsening as gestation advances, and resolving soon after delivery.[61] Heartburn is a common symptom of reflux, but a small percentage of patients remain asymptomatic throughout pregnancy. Risk factors for symptomatic disease appear to be advancing gestational age, pre-existing GOR, and multiparity, although the data are conflicting.[62]

The pathogenesis of reflux during pregnancy has not been fully elucidated in the literature, but progesterone-induced changes in the lower oesophageal sphincter (LOS) tone are believed to play a primary role. Briefly, in the first trimester of pregnancy the LOS decreases its responsiveness to stimuli that normally serve to increase pressure and minimize reflux. Thereafter, LOS pressure falls progressively until it reaches 30–50% of prepregnancy values by 36 weeks' gestation, and gradually rebounds over the course of 1–4 weeks postpartum.[63] Mechanical displacement of the stomach upward and laterally by the enlarging uterus, most commonly in the second half of gestation, appears to play a secondary role.

The clinical implications of the high incidence of GOR among parturients remain unresolved in the literature. Recent data suggest that reflux is unlikely to be a significant risk factor for pulmonary aspiration, particularly in the setting of normal gastric emptying (see 'Gastrointestinal Motility and Acidity').[64] Indeed, anaesthesia providers routinely anesthetize patients with GOR without using full stomach precautions. In the obstetric population, recent studies have reported the successful performance of caesarean deliveries in healthy term parturients using laryngeal mask airways[65] in lieu of tracheal intubation, as well as the provision of labour analgesia with subanaesthetic concentrations of volatile agents via facemask without adverse sequelae.[66] Increased awareness of nil per os (NPO) guidelines, routine use of aspiration prophylaxis, and the broadening indications for regional anaesthesia in the obstetric population have contributed to a marked decline in the incidence of pulmonary aspiration.

Gastrointestinal motility and acidity

Recent studies have cast doubt on the traditional dogma that pregnant women have increased gastric acidity, increased gastric volume, and decreased gastric motility, prompting a more liberal approach to full stomach precautions in pregnancy.[67] Historically, pregnancy has been associated with delayed gastric emptying has been attributed to all obstetric patients, presumably due primarily to hormonally induced changes in gastric motility. However, studies that measure gastric transit time by the absorption of orally administered acetaminophen[68] and ultrasound,[69] among other methods, have determined that there is no change in gastric emptying during pregnancy.

Gastric acid production also appears to be either unchanged or decreased during pregnancy. Van Thiel et al.'s early study evaluating gastric pH in pregnant volunteers at 12, 24, and 36 weeks' gestation and at 1 and 4 weeks postpartum found no difference in basal gastric pH or in peak acid output during pregnancy compared with postpartum values.[70] Similarly, a non-invasive radiotelemetry study used to assess gastric acidity and the effects of antacids in term parturients and non-pregnant women found no significant difference in basal gastric acidity between the two subject groups.[71] A study comparing gastric pH in pregnant women scheduled for caesarean delivery and in non-pregnant patients undergoing elective surgery, however, found a slight difference in pH (2.4 ± 1.4 vs 3.0 ± 1.9, $P < 0.05$), but no difference in serum gastrin levels.[72] The lower pH among the pregnant patients may be attributable to their higher level of preoperative anxiety. The finding that the frequency and severity of peptic ulcer disease decreases during pregnancy may reflect decreased acid production, although it may be related to diet and other factors.[73]

In contrast to the findings that pregnant women have normal gastric emptying and unchanged or reduced gastric acid production, labouring pregnant women and women who have received systemic[74] or neuraxial opioids[75] have delayed gastric emptying and may be at increased risk for pulmonary aspiration. Carp and colleagues performed ultrasound examinations of the stomach contents in 39 parturients in active labour and found that up to two-thirds of labouring women had evidence of solid food particles, independent of the interval between the last oral intake and the ultrasound scan.[76] Investigators also performed ultrasound examination of stomach contents in postpartum women and non-pregnant volunteers and found that 19 of 20 postpartum patients had food particles in their stomachs 4 hours after a standardized meal compared with 4 of 21 in the non-pregnant group.[77] Gastric emptying returns to prepregnancy measurements within 24 hours after delivery.[78] Gastric pH, which may decrease during labour, has also been found to be similar to that of non-pregnant, fasting individuals scheduled for elective surgery by 18 hours postpartum.[79]

Aspiration precautions

Many of the traditional pulmonary aspiration precautions have not been proven to reduce the frequency or severity of aspiration, yet there is sufficient evidence that such precautions are reasonable and, in most cases, unlikely to cause harm. Preoperative fasting, pharmacological prophylaxis, and careful patient positioning, among other things, play an important role for anaesthetists caring for pregnant patients who may present at any gestational age for obstetric or non-obstetric surgery under regional or general anaesthesia. Current American Society of Anesthesiologists (ASA) guidelines permit clear liquids during labour, clear liquids up to 2 hours prior to scheduled caesarean delivery, and fatty solids up to 8 hours prior to scheduled surgery. Other national organizations have similar recommendations (see Obstetric Anaesthetists Association guidelines in Appendix 1). In practice, labouring women may be required to refrain from oral intake, although this trend appears to be changing towards a more liberal approach. The ASA Task Force on Obstetric Anesthesia has supplemented these recommendations with an additional aspiration prophylaxis regimen of timely administered non-particulate antacids, H_2 receptor antagonists, and/or metoclopramide.[80] A recent review supports the use of H_2 receptor antagonists and non-particulate antacids, but found that neither proton pump inhibitors nor metoclopramide was effective, although this observation is not consistent.[81] RSI and maintenance of cricoid pressure until proper endotracheal tube placement is confirmed also remain standards of practice for emergency obstetric surgery and, in most cases, for elective caesarean delivery under general anaesthesia, although inappropriately applied cricoid pressure may cause more harm than benefit and neither practice has been proven to decrease the incidence of aspiration. Other manoeuvers that appear to minimize the risk of aspiration and improve maternal and fetal safety include maintenance of LUD until the baby has been delivered, use of a ramp (such as the Troop Elevation Pillow®) to elevate the patient's shoulders and achieve the sniffing position, and, possibly, positioning the patient in a 20–30° head-up position to lengthen the apnoeic time before hypoxaemia develops.[82] Continued vigilance during extubation, emergence, and recovery is also required.

Hepatic and biliary function

Hepatic function changes during pregnancy, although hepatic blood flow remains unchanged. The gallbladder also undergoes characteristic changes during pregnancy, many of which predispose pregnant patients to obstetric cholestasis.

The liver

The liver is displaced in a posterosuperior direction by the gravid uterus, but does not change in size or volume. Hepatic blood flow also remains unchanged during pregnancy, at roughly 25–35% of CO. Hepatic function, however, undergoes significant changes, many of which are reflected in liver function test results (see Table 2.8). Alkaline phosphatase levels increase up to fourfold, primarily due to placental production, and return to normal within 3–6 weeks after delivery. Plasma cholesterol and triglyceride levels also increase from baseline. In contrast, liver transaminases (alanine transaminase and aspartate transaminase) and gamma-glutamyl transferase decline during pregnancy, but may peak in the first several days to a week postpartum, most commonly in response to obstetric interventions, such as caesarean delivery. Serum albumin levels also decline, primarily as a result of increased plasma, contributing to a dramatic decrease in colloid oncotic pressure and predisposing pregnant women to oedema formation. Maternal bilirubin levels remain unchanged during pregnancy, despite transfer of small volumes of fetal bilirubin into the maternal circulation.

Several other changes in liver function are also attributed to increased levels of oestrogen and progesterone. Stigmata associated with advanced liver disease, such as spider naevi and palmar erythema, may be detected in normal, healthy pregnant patients and have no clinical significance in this context.[83] Oestrogen is also believed to accelerate the production of fibrinogen and several other coagulation factors, while progesterone plays a role in the increase in cytochrome P450 isoenzyme levels. Coagulation abnormalities that increase bleeding tendency, though, are not normal in pregnancy and point to underlying disease or the exogenous administration of anticoagulants. Finally, production of specific binding proteins, including thyroxine-binding globulin (TBG) and corticosteroid-binding globulin (CBG), increases during pregnancy, decreasing the free portion of certain hormones.

The gallbladder

Changes in gallbladder function during pregnancy are attributed largely to elevated levels of reproductive hormones, which

Table 2.8 Liver function tests during pregnancy

Test	Result
Alkaline phosphatase	2- to 4-fold increase by term
Liver transaminases (ALT, AST)	Decrease by term
Cholesterol	Increase
Gamma-glutamate transaminase	No change to slight decrease
Triglycerides	2- to 3-fold increase

contribute to biliary stasis, prolonged intestinal transit, and increased levels of cholesterol in the bile and predispose pregnant and postpartum patients to gallstone formation. A genetic component may render some pregnant women particularly susceptible to the cholestatic effects of reproductive hormones, contributing to the elevated incidence of obstetric cholestasis among certain patient populations, such as women of South Asian and South American descent. Multiparity, advancing gestation, history of cholestasis, twin gestation, and an elevated prepregnancy BMI[84] appear to be additional risk factors for intrahepatic cholestasis of pregnancy.

Parturients with gallbladder disease are more likely than healthy pregnant counterparts to have peripartum complications, such as fetal arrhythmias, meconium-stained amniotic fluid, intrauterine demise, and spontaneous preterm labour, which are thought to be related to elevated maternal and/or fetal serum bile acids.[85] They are also more likely to present to the delivery suite for early induction of labour, most often at 37 weeks' gestation, and to the main operating theatre for cholecystectomy, one of the most common non-obstetric surgeries during pregnancy. During the first year postpartum, gallbladder disease is among the most common non-obstetric cause of maternal hospital admission.[86]

The genitourinary system

Changes in kidney function and in uterine anatomy and blood flow present early in pregnancy and have profound clinical implications, particularly as gestation advances.

The upper and lower urinary tracts

Kidney, ureteral, and bladder changes accompany different stages of pregnancy. Anatomically, the kidneys elongate by 1–1.5 cm and increase in volume by 30%, partly in response to a 50–85% increase in renal blood flow (RBF) that starts early in the first trimester, peaks at 26 weeks, and declines slightly at term.[87] Relaxin, a hormone secreted by the corpus luteum, the decidua, and the placenta appears to play a role in the initiation and modulation of augmented renal hemodynamics.[88] Nitric oxide may also play a role, contributing to renal vasodilation and increased renal plasma flow and glomerular filtration rate (GFR). The renal pelvices, calyces, and ureters begin to dilate as early as 7 weeks' gestation due to both the vasodilating effects of progesterone and, later, the mechanical compression of the ureters at the pelvic brim. A protective effect of the sigmoid colon on the left, dextrorotation of the uterus, and positional compression by the right ovarian vein contribute to more marked ureteral dilation on the right. Hormonal changes also affect the bladder and urethral mucosa, which becomes more hyperaemic and congested. Although data are conflicting, the bladder develops an increased capacity and becomes displaced upwards and anteriorly by the gravid uterus; by the third trimester, it protrudes markedly into the abdomen and undergoes additional anatomical distortions. The net result of many of these anatomical changes is an increased incidence of ascending urinary tract infections (UTIs), hydronephrosis, and symptomatic urolithiasis during pregnancy. Indeed, urological emergencies account for a small percentage of the estimated 1–2% of non-obstetric operations among pregnant women reported annually in the United States.

Increased RBF and decreased renal vascular resistance contribute to changes in kidney function during pregnancy. The GFR begins to increase soon after conception, reaches a 40–65% increase above prepregnant levels by the beginning of the second trimester, and tapers, if not decreases, towards term.[89] This increase in GFR, from roughly 100 mL/min to 150 mL/min, leads to a decrease in serum creatinine, urea, and uric acid concentrations and an increase in the urinary excretion of albumin, low-molecular-weight proteins, amino acids, water-soluble vitamins, and glucose. Additional changes in kidney function during pregnancy include alterations in osmoregulation, manifested by decreased serum osmolality, and an increased urinary excretion of bicarbonate, which serves to compensate for the respiratory alkalosis of pregnancy. The decrease in serum bicarbonate that accompanies increased urinary bicarbonate excretion may diminish the buffering capacity of blood. Changes in the renin–angiotensin–aldosterone system contribute to a dramatic plasma volume expansion during pregnancy, and elevated levels of erythropoietin contribute to the expansion in RBC mass that peaks at term.

These changes in renal function result in characteristic clinical and laboratory findings that must be distinguished from pathological states (see Table 2.9). Mild glucosuria is a normal finding during pregnancy and is not diagnostic of diabetes mellitus (DM); by the third trimester, glucose excretion increases significantly in healthy pregnant individuals and may reach three times higher than non-pregnant values. If DM is suspected, a glucose challenge test must be performed. Mild proteinuria below 300 mg/24 h is also common during pregnancy, although further investigation may be warranted to rule out UTIs or previously undetected kidney disorders. Significant proteinuria in the setting of new onset hypertension, however, is highly suggestive of pre-eclampsia. During normal pregnancy, serum albumin decreases in association with plasma volume expansion and increased urinary excretion. An abnormally high urinary excretion of albumin occurs in patients with pre-eclampsia and contributes to more significant intravascular contraction. Serum creatinine and urea levels decrease to 0.5–0.6 mg/dL and 9 mg/dL, respectively, during pregnancy; higher values may suggest underlying renal disease, although they are within normal limits for non-pregnant patients. Sodium retention, which results in part from stimulation of the renin–aldosterone system, contributes to increased total body water and plasma volume. As a result, a mild hyponatraemia develops during pregnancy, and thirst and water retention occur at a different, lower plasma

Table 2.9 Kidney function during pregnancy compared with the non-pregnant state

Test	Pregnancy	Non-pregnant
Plasma blood urea nitrogen	9–12 mg/dL	11–20 mg/dL
Plasma Cr	<1.0 mg/dL	<1.3 mg/dL
Plasma Na	130–140 mEq/L	135–145 mEq/L
Plasma HCO_3	18–20 mEq/L	22–28 mEq/L
Urinary protein excretion	<300 mg/24 h	<150 mg/24 h
Plasma albumin	2.5–3.2 g/dL	3.5–4.5 g/dL

sodium concentration in pregnant compared with non-pregnant patients.[90] Serum uric acid, which is expected to decrease by roughly 25–30% by mid-gestation, reaches non-pregnant levels by term. Elevated serum uric acid levels may indicate poor kidney function and be suggestive of pre-eclampsia in the setting of new onset hypertension. Tests that are commonly used to evaluate kidney function, such as the Cockroft–Gault formula and the estimated GFR from the Modification of Diet in Renal Disease formula, may not reflect the true GFR during pregnancy.[91] A 24-hour urine collection for creatinine clearance is a cumbersome test of debatable accuracy during pregnancy;[92] if used to assess renal function during pregnancy, a 30% increase above the prepregnancy value should be expected. Finally, the increased GRF may also alter clearance of medications that are excreted through the kidney.

The uterus

The uterus, normally pear-shaped, expands more in length than width and exits the pelvis by 12 weeks' gestation. Thereafter, it displaces the intestines laterally and superiorly and ultimately rotates rightward in the abdominal cavity, impeded by the rectosigmoid on the left. The term uterus pushes the liver in a posterosuperior direction, forces the diaphragm upward roughly 4 cm, and shifts the heart leftward. When the parturient is erect, the abdominal wall supports the enlarging uterus; in the supine position, the uterus rests on the vertebral column and the great vessels.

Uteroplacental blood flow, derived primarily from the uterine and ovarian arteries, increases from roughly 50 mL/min at 10 weeks' gestation to 450–700 mL/min, or greater, near term. Hormonal-induced increases in arterial diameter and decreases in vascular resistance as gestation advances contribute to this increase. Uterine venous drainage also increases during pregnancy, a process facilitated by changes in venous calibre and distensibility. Uterine blood flow, which is not autoregulated, declines in the presence of factors that increase uterine vascular resistance or decrease perfusion pressure. For example, it decreases during contractions, particularly during prolonged periods of hypertonus, and during episodes of acute or chronic maternal hypertension and hypotension. It also diminishes in response to certain exogenously administered α-adrenergic agonists, including epinephrine used to evaluate intravascular epidural cannulation. Ephedrine is an exception to this generalization on account of its primary β-adrenergic effect.[93]

Modern obstetric anaesthesia practice has changed with the better understanding of factors that affect uterine blood flow. The efficacy of the traditional epidural 'test dose' with an epinephrine-containing local anaesthetic has been challenged in part due to concerns that decreased uteroplacental blood flow may accompany a positive test result. Additionally, concerns about the adverse effects of high levels of circulating maternal catecholamines related to stress or anxiety have led some practitioners to reassess the wisdom of withholding premedications from parturients in certain clinical scenarios. For example, the administration of a single dose of intravenous anxiolytic medication, such as midazolam, during epidural placement for labour analgesia, for pregnant women undergoing non-obstetric surgery, and for patients scheduled for caesarean delivery may be appropriate for individual patients. One double-blinded, randomized, placebo-controlled trial of 60 parturients undergoing caesarean delivery who received either 1 mcg/kg of fentanyl and 0.02 mg/kg of midazolam or placebo immediately prior to spinal anaesthesia found no difference between groups in neonatal outcomes (Apgar score, continuous oxygen saturation, neurobehavioral scores) or maternal recall of the birth.[94] Finally, maternal hypotension related to neuraxial procedures, hypovolaemia, supine hypotensive syndrome, or haemorrhage, among other things, is an important cause of suboptimal uterine blood flow and warrants immediate correction, including maintenance of LUD, appropriately timed intravenous administration of crystalloid or colloid fluids, and appropriate use of vasopressors, to optimize maternal and fetal well-being. It is also important to bear in mind that the increased uterine blood flow at term, which accounts for at least 10% of maternal CO, places patients with obstetric complications at risk for significant haemorrhage. Additional factors that affect uteroplacental blood flow are covered in greater detail in Chapter 3.

Endocrinology

Pregnant women experience profound changes in glucose metabolism, as well as in thyroid, pituitary, and adrenal gland function. Some of these changes may predispose pregnant patients to disease states, such as ketosis, hypothyroidism, and hyperthyroidism, particularly in the absence of strict glycaemic control and nutritional supplements. They may also adversely affect fetal growth and development.

Glucose metabolism

Profound changes in maternal metabolism during pregnancy serve to accommodate increased maternal energy needs and fetal growth requirements. In general, pregnant patients experience increased insulin secretion in conjunction with a progressive insulin resistance, as well as fasting hypoglycaemia and postprandial hyperglycaemia. Increased levels of growth hormone (GH), cortisol, and human placental lactogen (HPL), among other diabetogenic hormones, account for the progressive insulin resistance of pregnancy, although the precise mechanism has not been elucidated. Broadly speaking, insulin resistance permits preferential use of fatty acids, triglycerides, and ketone bodies for maternal fuel sources, while preserving glucose and amino acids for the fetus. Fetal glucose levels are maintained at roughly 80% of maternal serum levels by facilitated diffusion across the placenta down a concentration gradient. Amino acids are actively transported across the placenta.

Several factors contribute to decreased maternal fasting glucose, including increased plasma volume, reduced hepatic glycogen stores, and the increasing demands of the fetoplacental unit as gestation advances. The increased fetal needs and accelerated maternal metabolic rate, coupled with relative insulin deficiency and reduced glycogen stores, place the mother at risk for ketosis, particularly during the second and third trimesters. Without adequate oral or intravenous nutrients, the mother may swiftly deplete glycogen stores and resort to lipolysis and ketone body production, a process frequently referred to as 'accelerated starvation of pregnancy'.[95] Changes in postprandial glucose levels, on the other hand, are mild in healthy pregnant women, but may be exaggerated in obese women who exhibit more insulin resistance than non-obese counterparts.

Pregnancy in diabetic patients may be complicated by congenital malformations, prematurity of the newborn, fetal hypoglycaemia, fetal macrosomia, birth related injuries, an increased risk of perinatal mortality,[96] maternal diabetic ketoacidosis (DKA), and an increased incidence of maternal comorbidities, such as chronic hypertension, pregnancy-induced hypertension, and diabetic nephropathy. The likelihood of caesarean delivery and neonatal admission to the intensive care unit is also higher in diabetic parturients compared with healthy counterparts. DKA during pregnancy is associated with a high morbidity and mortality for both mother and fetus, although advances in management have vastly reduced the risk of mortality. As in the non-pregnant population, DKA occurs in the setting of insulin deficiency (relative or absolute) with a concurrent increase in glucagon. Increased glucose production, decreased glucose utilization in the peripheral tissues, and lipolysis with ketone body formation ensue. Sequelae include osmotic diuresis and maternal dehydration, with associated water and electrolyte disturbances, as well as a decrease in maternal pH from ketone body accumulation. If fluid loss is severe, cardiovascular collapse and shock may result. The fetus commonly develops a non-reassuring heart rate pattern, which most often resolves once maternal fluid and electrolyte imbalances are corrected.

Given the sharp worldwide rise in maternal obesity in recent decades, it is likely that obstetric anaesthesia providers will be caring for diabetic pregnant patients both on the labour and delivery unit and in the main operating suites with increasing frequency. It is essential that the anaesthetist bear in mind the type of maternal DM and the nature and extent of end-organ involvement, as well as the patient's medical regimen and most recent glucose level. Management involves balancing insulin therapy in patients with type 1 diabetes to prevent both DKA and hypoglycaemic episodes. For patients with type 2 diabetes, avoiding hyperglycaemic, hyperosmolar syndromes that can lead to dehydration, decreased uterine perfusion, and electrolyte imbalances is essential.[97] Of note, general anaesthesia may mask the signs and symptoms of hypoglycaemia, and patients with autonomic dysfunction related to DM, as well as patients in DKA, may exhibit profound haemodynamic instability following neuraxial anaesthesia. Finally, as the incidence of obesity and type 2 diabetes rises in the obstetric population, anaesthesiologists may encounter additional, related challenges, such as difficulties with the maternal airway, intravenous access, monitoring, positioning, transport, and neuraxial anatomy.

Thyroid function

Several biochemical changes in thyroid function, many of which are of minor consequence in conditions of iodine sufficiency, occur at different stages of pregnancy (see Figure 2.5).[98] During the first trimester, human chorionic gonadotropin (hCG), which shares structural similarities with thyroid stimulating hormone (TSH, thyrotropin), stimulates TSH receptors in thyroid tissue, leading to a transient increase in free thyroxine (T_4). Through a feedback loop, increased levels of thyroid hormones suppress TSH. As a result, between 8 and 14 weeks' gestation, relatively low TSH with mildly elevated free T_4 is not uncommon and of little clinical significance. However, certain conditions that are associated with increased levels of hCG, such as molar pregnancy or hyperemesis gravidarum, may cause a prolonged or exaggerated increase in T_4 and lead to transient thyrotoxicosis.

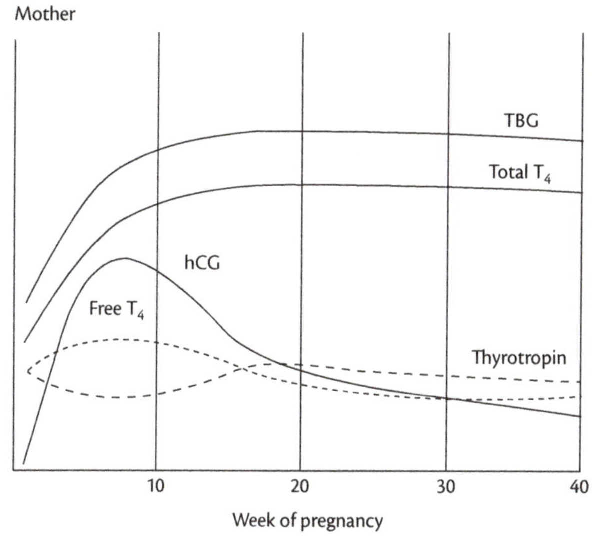

Figure 2.5 Relative changes in maternal and fetal thyroid function during pregnancy.

From *The New England Journal of Medicine*, Burrow GN, Fisher DA, Larsen PR, Maternal and fetal thyroid function, 331, 16. Copyright © 1994 Massachusetts Medical Society.

Additional changes in thyroid function are related to either rising oestrogen levels or to modifications in the peripheral metabolism of thyroid hormones.[99] Elevated circulating oestrogen promotes increased production of binding proteins, such as TBG, from the liver. The two- to threefold increase in basal TBG leads to a reduction in the free, active thyroid hormones, T_4 and triiodothyronine (T_3), and, in turn, stimulation of the hypothalamic–pituitary–thyroid axis. Slightly elevated TSH levels are common during this stage of pregnancy, after the first trimester and continuing to term, but generally remain within the reference range. When dietary iodine is plentiful, there is only a mild change in free hormone levels, but several complications related to low T_3 and T_4 may occur in iodine-deficient states. Of note, total (free and bound) T_4 and T_3 levels are increased during this stage as a result of the increased production of TBG and reduced clearance induced by the hyperoestrogenic state; it is important to distinguish between free and total thyroid hormone levels and to bear in mind the trimester-specific normative data when interpreting laboratory values.[100] Another change in thyroid activity, most commonly during the second half of pregnancy, is related to the activity of three enzymes that catalyse the deiodination of thyroid hormones. Briefly, two of these enzymes are abundant in the placenta and may alter thyroid hormone levels (low T_3 and high reverse T_3).

The pathological states that result from iodine-deficient hypothyroidism or from hyperthyroidism, which has multiple possible aetiologies, are of particular clinical relevance to anaesthesia providers. The increase in renal clearance of iodine during pregnancy, in conjunction with increased sequestration of iodine by the fetoplacental unit, contributes to iodine deficiency in the absence of nutritional supplements. Reduced dietary iodine results in chronic thyroid stimulation, which manifests with increased TSH, increased thyroglobulin levels in the thyroid gland, and goitrogenesis. In the absence of iodine deficiency, the differential diagnosis of goitre during pregnancy includes Graves' disease, excess iodine intake, Hashimoto's thyroiditis, lymphoma, and thyroid cancer, among others.

Graves' disease is by far the most common cause of hyperthyroidism during pregnancy, although other aetiologies, such as toxic multinodular goitre, hyperemesis gravidarum, and gestational trophoblastic disease, should be considered in the differential diagnosis.[101] Of these, management of hydatidiform mole poses a particular challenge, as evacuation of molar pregnancy may be accompanied by thyroid storm, trophoblastic emboli, severe haemorrhage, DIC, and cardiopulmonary arrest, among other things.[102] Adequate intravenous access, invasive haemodynamic monitors, immediate availability of blood products, and premedication with antithyroid drugs and beta-adrenergic blockers may be required prior to surgical treatment of a hydatidiform mole.[103]

Thyroid storm, a life-threatening exacerbation of thyrotoxicosis, is rare during pregnancy, but may also be precipitated by labour, caesarean delivery, infection, and pre-eclampsia.[104] Signs and symptoms of hyperthyroidism and this rare complication may be incorrectly attributed to the hypermetabolic state of pregnancy. Sustained tachycardia, weight loss, goitre, ophthalmopathy, GI symptoms, elevated free T_3 and T_4 with suppressed TSH, and, in the case of thyroid storm, thermoregulatory dysfunction and CNS changes, including delirium and agitation, may be suggestive of active, and possibly life-threatening, thyroid dysfunction. Treatment of pregnant women in crisis is similar to that of non-pregnant patients, and includes propylthiouracil, iodine, dexamethasone, beta-adrenergic blockers, such as propranolol, labetalol, or esmolol, fluid hydration, and nutritional support.[105] Of note, fetal bradycardia, hypoglycaemia, and intrauterine growth restriction are associated with prolonged beta-adrenergic therapy. Successful use of esmolol in a parturient in an acute situation without adverse sequelae to the mother or fetus has been reported.[106]

The pituitary gland

The pituitary gland enlarges during pregnancy, reaching its peak size in the immediate postpartum period and returning to normal dimensions within 6 months of delivery.[107] Clinically, this oestrogen-mediated hyperplasia results most notably in rising levels of prolactin (PRL) throughout gestation, which may adversely affect pregnant women with pre-existing prolactinomas. In contrast to PRL, GH secretion from the pituitary decreases, starting in the second half of pregnancy when the placenta increases production of a GH variant.[108] Pregnant women with acromegaly, though, will experience an increase in both pituitary and placental GH secretion. Adrenocorticotropic hormone levels increase progressively later in pregnancy, most likely as a result of placental production and despite elevated levels of bound and free cortisol.[109] Other anterior pituitary hormones experience fluctuating levels during pregnancy: TSH levels decline early in pregnancy, but return to the normal range as gestation advances, and luteinizing hormone and follicle-stimulating hormone levels decrease during the first trimester in response to placental sex steroid production.[110] With regard to the posterior pituitary, oxytocin levels increase throughout pregnancy, rising further at term and peaking during the second stage of labour. Arginine vasopressin is released at a lower plasma osmolality and is metabolized more rapidly in pregnant patients compared with non-pregnant counterparts.

Anaesthetic implications of an enlarged pituitary gland, placental production of pituitary hormones, and changes in the hypothalamic–pituitary axis are rare. However, pituitary enlargement may predispose parturients to Sheehan's syndrome, an uncommon hypopituitarism specific to parous women caused by anterior pituitary lobe necrosis in the setting of obstetric haemorrhage.[111] Pregnant patients with acromegaly may experience any of the complications normally associated with the disease, including soft tissue changes, carbohydrate intolerance, overt diabetes, hypertension, and cardiac disease. The soft tissue changes do not appear to affect the genital tract or otherwise complicate vaginal delivery. Pregnancy-related insulin resistance is an additive risk among acromegalic obstetric patients.

The adrenal glands

The adrenal glands, which are responsible for the production of mineralocorticoids, glucocorticoids, and sex steroids, undergo several changes during pregnancy. Bound and free, metabolically active cortisol levels increase progressively during pregnancy due to a combination of factors, including increased production, an oestrogen-mediated increase in CBG in the liver, and a decrease in metabolic clearance. Urinary free cortisol levels are elevated in parturients due to the two- to threefold rise in cortisol levels by term.[112] Renin activity peaks early in pregnancy and declines in the third trimester, coinciding with a rise in angiotensin II.[113] The net result is that plasma aldosterone levels increase roughly 20 times above non-pregnant levels by late gestation. This increase correlates with other physiological changes of pregnancy, including the increase in GFR and the sharp rise in progesterone, which competitively inhibits both aldosterone-mediated sodium retention and sodium-potassium exchange.[114] Overall, the activation of the renin–angiotensin–aldosterone system during pregnancy appears to result from the decreased vascular responsiveness to angiotensin II, despite elevated levels, and to the related fall in blood pressure.[115] It also contributes to the increase in plasma volume. With regard to sex steroids, testosterone levels are low to normal until late second trimester, but increase thereafter and may exceed non-pregnant values at term.

Of the many physiological and potential pathological changes of the adrenal glands during pregnancy, phaeochromocytomas, which occur in roughly 1 per 50,000 pregnancies, pose particular diagnostic and therapeutic challenges.[116] The typical presenting symptoms, including heart palpitations, headaches, sweating, episodic elevations in blood pressure, nausea, vomiting, and visual changes, may be misdiagnosed as pre-eclampsia/eclampsia or attributed to exacerbations of the normal physiological changes of pregnancy. Plasma catecholamine levels or 24-hour urine testing for catecholamines and their metabolites should be evaluated in all pregnant patients who present with any combination of these signs and symptoms, particularly before 20 weeks' gestation. Magnetic resonance is the imaging test of choice for localization of the tumour, and is considered safe in pregnancy. Ultrasonography, also safe during pregnancy, is not sensitive in identifying extra-adrenal phaeochromocytomas, which comprise roughly 10% of these neuroendocrine tumours. Computed tomography is not recommended due to fetal exposure to ionizing radiation.

The musculoskeletal system

Pregnant women commonly experience changes in the musculoskeletal system that contribute to a high incidence of low back pain (LBP), distort the anatomical landmarks that are traditionally used to identify the L3–4 interspace, and complicate neuraxial procedures. Hormonal changes are thought to contribute to both LBP and to changes in the perivertebral ligamentous structures. The ligamentum flavum, for example, becomes softer and more difficult to distinguish from other structures during epidural needle advancement. Weight gain during pregnancy, which often exceeds the recommended 12.5 kg, and the progressive accentuation of lumbar lordosis as gestation advances make it difficult for term parturients to attain appropriate positioning during neuraxial procedures and most likely contribute to the perception of narrow interspaces during attempts to initiate epidural placement using the midline approach. The accumulation of adipose tissue in the epidural space may increase the posterior epidural space depth in parturients, as well as alter local anaesthetic dose requirements and spread. Maternal obesity also contributes to an increase in the skin to epidural space distance and presents additional challenges for obstetric anaesthesia providers.

Maternal obesity

Maternal obesity poses several challenges to obstetric anaesthesia providers. Obese parturients are a high-risk group for perioperative airway catastrophe, often have unidentifiable anatomical landmarks for initiation of neuraxial procedures, and have a higher risk of anaesthesia-related mortality than non-obese pregnant counterparts.[117] Several factors contribute to difficult airway management in this patient population, including a high prevalence of obstructive sleep apnoea, a vastly reduced FRC, increased baseline oxygen consumption, and a predisposition to develop pronounced narrowing of the pharyngeal airway during pregnancy.[118] In addition, maternal obesity is associated with an increased risk of thromboembolism, cardiovascular disorders, hypertensive disorders of pregnancy, and gestational diabetes, as well as a higher risk of emergency caesarean delivery[119] and surgery for postpartum haemorrhage.[120] These and other complications associated with maternal obesity are covered in detail in Chapter 39.

Low back pain

Back pain may affect over 70% of women at some point during their pregnancy and, based on findings from several randomized controlled trials and prospective cohort studies, appears unrelated to the type of analgesia, if any, received by the parturient.[121] LBP presents in a small percentage of patients towards the end of the first trimester. However, the incidence increases dramatically as gestation advances.[122] Although the severity of LBP improves for the majority of patients after delivery, up to 40% of patients report ongoing musculoskeletal pain during the first 18 months postpartum and up to one-fifth of these women experience severe ongoing LBP.[123] Unfortunately, a large percentage of patients who experience LBP in their first pregnancy will have recurrent symptoms in subsequent pregnancies, and up to 19% of women who experience LBP in an initial pregnancy report avoidance of future pregnancies for fear of recurrent musculoskeletal pain.[124]

The aetiology of LBP during pregnancy is multifactorial, although hormonal and mechanical factors predominate. Relaxin, a hormone known to be involved in pelvic connective tissue remodelling in several mammalian species, appears to contribute, although its role has not been confirmed.[125] The increasing lumbar lordosis as gestation advances, which places additional strain on the lower back and alters the centre of gravity, the increased spinal load related to fetal weight, weight gain during pregnancy, the decreased stability of the pelvic girdle, muscular dysfunction, pre-existing LBP, and maternal age also play a role. Whether mode of delivery affects the incidence of LBP is debated in the literature. However, epidural analgesia does not appear to independently affect the incidence.[126] Regardless of the aetiology, LBP during pregnancy rarely requires medical intervention and responds to postural changes, exercises, and activity. Patient education is another cornerstone in the management of LBP during pregnancy.

Key points

- The MAC of volatile agents is reduced during pregnancy; the routine administration of <1 MAC, however, may contribute to a higher incidence of intraoperative awareness and postoperative recall among pregnant women.
- Volatile agents contribute to a reduction in both myometrial contractility and myometrial response to oxytocin in a dose-dependent fashion.
- Both plasma volume and RBC mass increase during pregnancy, but the former increases to a greater extent, resulting in a physiological anaemia.
- Airway changes resulting in worsening airway classification have been observed over the course of pregnancy and during labour and delivery. Worsening airway classification appears to correspond with difficult tracheal intubation in pregnant women undergoing caesarean delivery during general anaesthesia.
- Thrombocytopaenia is the most common coagulation disorder during pregnancy. Most pregnant women experience a 10% drop in platelet count. Up to 5% experience gestational thrombocytopaenia, a benign condition that does not require medical therapy or cause clinically significant bleeding.
- Gastric pH and gastric emptying time do not differ significantly between pregnant and non-pregnant patients, but heartburn is relatively common in parturients and may predispose parturients to GOR.
- Uterine blood flow increases to a maximum of 700 mL/min at term, which represents 10% of CO.
- GFR increases by up to 65% above baseline during pregnancy, resulting in serum creatinine and urea levels of 0.5 mg/dL and 9 mg/dL respectively.
- Both decreased FRC and increased oxygen consumption contribute to rapid oxygen desaturation during periods of apnoea during pregnancy.
- CO increases throughout pregnancy, reaching its peak at 80% above prelabour values immediately postpartum as a result of the autotransfusion associated with uterine involution.

- Although blood flow to the liver remains at its prepregnant range of 25% of CO, hepatic function changes dramatically during pregnancy.
- Pregnancy is marked by an increased coagulation activity and decreased anticoagulation and fibrinolytic activity.
- LBP affects an estimated 80% of pregnant patients at some point during pregnancy.
- Obesity, a growing problem among industrial countries, is associated with a higher risk of emergency caesarean deliveries, maternal airway catastrophes, difficult initiation of neuraxial blockade, and maternal mortality.

References

1. Keenan PA, Yaldoo DT, Stress ME, *et al.* Explicit memory in pregnant women. *Am J Obstet Gynecol* 1998; 179:731–7.
2. Nevo O, Soustiel JF, Thaler I. Maternal cerebral blood flow during normal pregnancy: a cross-sectional study. *Am J Obstet Gynecol* 2010; 203:475.e1–6.
3. Bergersen TK, Hartgill TW, Pirhonen J. Cerebrovascular response to normal pregnancy: a longitudinal study. *Am J Physiol Heart Circ Physiol* 2006; 290:H1856–61.
4. Palahniuk RJ, Shnider SM, Eger EI. Pregnancy decreases the requirements for inhaled anesthetic agents. *Anesthesiology* 1974; 41:82–3.
5. Datta S, Migliozzi RP, Flanagan HL, *et al.* Chronically administered progesterone decreases halothane requirements in rabbits. *Anesth Analg* 1989; 68:46–50.
6. Chan MT, Mainland P, Gin T. Minimum alveolar concentration of halothane and enflurane are decreased in early pregnancy. *Anesthesiology* 1996; 85:782–6.
7. Gin T, Chan MT. Decreased minimum alveolar concentration of isoflurane in pregnant humans. *Anesthesiology* 1994; 81:829–32.
8. Erden V, Erkalp K, Yangin Z, *et al.* The effect of labor on sevoflurane requirements during cesarean delivery. *Int J Obstet Anesth* 2011; 20:17–21.
9. Chan MT, Gin T. Postpartum changes in the minimum alveolar concentration of isoflurane. *Anesthesiology* 1995; 82:1360–3.
10. Yildiz K, Dogru K, Dalgic H, *et al.* Inhibitory effects of desflurane and sevoflurane on oxytocin-induced contractions of isolated pregnant human myometrium. *Acta Anaesthesiol Scand* 2005; 49:1355–9.
11. Ueyama H, Hagihira S, Takashina M, *et al.* Pregnancy does not enhance volatile anesthetic sensitivity on the brain: an electroencephalographic analysis study. *Anesthesiology* 2010; 113:577–84.
12. Robins K, Lyons G. Intraoperative awareness during general anesthesia for cesarean delivery. *Anesth Analg* 2009; 109:886–90.
13. Chin KJ, Yeo SW. Bispectral index values at sevoflurane concentrations of 1% and 1.5% in lower segment cesarean delivery. *Anesth Analg* 2004; 98:1140–4.
14. Abouleish EI. Postpartum tubal ligation requires more bupivacaine for spinal anesthesia than does cesarean delivery. *Anesth Analg* 1986; 65:897–900.
15. Assali NS, Prystowsky H. Studies on autonomic blockade. I. comparison between the effects of tetraethylammonium chloride (TEAC) and high selective spinal anesthesia on blood pressure of normal and toxemic pregnancy, *J Clin Invest* 1950; 29:1354–66.
16. Robson SC, Hunter S, Boys RJ, *et al.* Serial study of factors influencing changes in cardiac output during human pregnancy. *Am J Physiol* 1989; 256:H1060–5.
17. Bucklin BA, Fuller AJ. Physiologic changes of pregnancy. In Suresh MS, Segal BS, Preston RL, *et al.* (eds), *Shnider and Levinson's Anesthesia for Obstetrics.* Baltimore, MD: Lippincott Williams & Wilkins; 2013:1–17.
18. Crawford JS, Burton M, Davies P. Anaesthesia for section: further refinements of a technique. *Br J Anaesth* 1973; 45:726–32.
19. Monga M. Maternal cardiovascular, respiratory, and renal adaptation to pregnancy. In Creasy RK, Resnik R, Iams JD, *et al.* (eds) *Creasy & Resnik's Maternal-Fetal Medicine: Principles and Practice.* Philadelphia, PA: Saunders Elsevier; 2009:101–9.
20. Wise RA, Polito AJ, Krishnan V. Respiratory physiologic changes in pregnancy. *Immunol Allergy Clin North Am* 2006; 26:1–12.
21. Moore LG, McCullough RE, Weil JV. Increased HVR in pregnancy: relationship to hormonal and metabolic changes, *J Appl Physiol* 1987; 62:158–63.
22. McClelland SH, Bogod DG, Hardman JG. Pre-oxygenation and apnoea in pregnancy: changes during labour and with obstetric morbidity in a computational simulation, *Anaesthesia* 2009; 64:371–7.
23. Pernoll ML, Metcalfe J, Kovach PA, *et al.* Ventilation during rest and exercise in pregnancy and postpartum. *Respir Physiol* 1975; 25:295–310.
24. Pearson JF, Davies P. The effect of continuous lumbar epidural analgesia on the acid-base status of arterial blood during the first stage of labour. *J Obstet Gynaecol Br Commonw* 1973; 80:218–24.
25. McClelland SH, Bogod DG, Hardman JG. Apnoea in pregnancy: an investigation using physiological modelling. *Anaesthesia* 2008; 63:264–9.
26. Benumof JL, Dagg R, Benumof R. Critical hemoglobin desaturation will occur before return to an unparalyzed state following 1 mg/kg intravenous succinylcholine. *Anesthesiology* 1997; 87:979–82.
27. McClelland SH, Bogod DG, Hardman JG. Pre-oxygenation in pregnancy: an investigation using physiological modelling. *Anaesthesia* 2008; 63:259–63.
28. Goldszmidt E. Is there a difference between the obstetric and non-obstetric airway? In Halpern SH, Douglas MJ (eds) *Evidence-Based Obstetric Anesthesia.* Malden, MA: Blackwell Publishing; 2005:225–36.
29. Pilkington S, Carli F, Dakin MY, *et al.* Increase in Mallampati score during pregnancy, *Br J Anaesth* 1995; 74:638–42.
30. Kodali BS, Chandrasekhar S, Bulich LN, *et al.* Airway changes during labor and delivery. *Anesthesiology* 2008; 108:357–62.
31. Isono S. Mallampati classification, an estimate of upper airway anatomical balance, can change rapidly during labor. *Anesthesiology* 2008; 108:347–9.
32. Rocke DA, Murray WB, Rout CC, *et al.* Relative risk analysis of factors associated with difficult intubation in obstetric anesthesia. *Anesthesiology* 1992; 77:67–73.
33. Mhyre JM. Maternal mortality. *Curr Opin Anaesthesiol* 2012; 25:277–85.
34. Mhyre JM, Riesner MN, Polley LS, *et al.* A series of anesthesia-related maternal deaths in Michigan, 1985–2003. *Anesthesiology* 2007; 106:1096–104.
35. Goldszmidt E. Principles and practices of obstetric airway management. *Anesthesiol Clin* 2008; 26:109–25.
36. Abbassi-Ghanavati M, Greer LG, Cunningham FG. Pregnancy and laboratory studies: a reference table for clinicians. *Obstet Gynecol* 2009; 114:326–31.
37. Lockwood CJ and Silver RM. Coagulation disorders in pregnancy. In Creasy RK, Resnik R, Iams JD, *et al.* (eds) *Creasy & Resnik's Maternal-Fetal Medicine: Principles and Practice.* Philadelphia, PA: Saunders Elsevier; 2009:825–54.
38. Bremme KA. Haemostatic changes in pregnancy. *Best Pract Res Clin Haematol* 2003; 16:153–68.
39. Lockwood CJ. Thromboembolic disease in pregnancy. In Creasy RK, Resnik R, Iams JD, *et al.* (eds) *Creasy & Resnik's Maternal-Fetal Medicine: Principles and Practice.* Philadelphia, PA: Saunders Elsevier; 2009:855–68.
40. Erlich J, Parry GC, Fearns C, *et al.* Tissue factor is required for uterine hemostasis and maintenance of the placental labyrinth during gestation. *Proc Natl Acad Sci USA* 1999; 96:8138–43.

41. Mackenzie AP, Schatz F, Krikum G, *et al.* Mechanisms of abruption-induced premature rupture of the fetal membranes: thrombin enhanced decidual matrix metalloproteinase-3 (stromelysin-1) expression. *Am J Obstet Gynecol* 2004; 191:1996–2001.
42. Hayashi Y, Ueyama H, Mashimato T, *et al.* Circulating mature adrenomedullin is related to blood volume in full-term pregnancy. *Anesth Analg* 2005; 101:1816–20.
43. McLintock C, Repke JT, Bucklin B. Hematologic disease in pregnancy. In Powrie RO, Greene MF, Camann W (eds) *de Swiet's Medical Disorders in Obstetric Practice*. Hoboken, NJ: Wiley-Blackwell; 2010:48–81.
44. Kelton JG. Idiopathic thrombocytopenia purpura complicating pregnancy. *Blood Reviews* 2002; 16:43–6.
45. Verdy E, Bessous V, Dreyfus M, *et al.* Longitudinal analysis of platelet count and volume in normal pregnancy. *Thromb Haemost* 1997; 77:806–7.
46. Burrows RF, Kelton JG. Incidentally detected thrombocytopenia in healthy mothers and their infants. *N Engl J Med* 1988; 319:142–5.
47. Myers B. Diagnosis and management of maternal thrombocytopenia in pregnancy. *Br J Haematol* 2012; 158:3–15.
48. Burrows RF, Kelton JG. Thrombocytopenia at delivery: a prospective survey of 6715 deliveries. *Am J Obstet Gynecol* 1990; 162:731–4.
49. Bremme KA. Haemostatic changes in pregnancy. *Best Pract Res Clin Haematol* 2003; 16:153–68.
50. Bockenstedt PL. Thrombocytopenia in pregnancy. *Hematol Oncol Clin North Am* 2011; 25:293–310.
51. Gernsheimer TB. Thrombocytopenia in pregnancy: is this immune thrombocytopenia or ...?. *Hematology Am Soc Hematol Educ Program* 2012; 2012:198–202.
52. Webert KE, Mittal R, Sigouin C, *et al.* A retrospective 11-year analysis of obstetric patients with idiopathic thrombocytopenic purpura. *Blood* 2003; 102:4306–11.
53. Kelton JG. Idiopathic thrombocytopenic purpura complicating pregnancy. *Blood Rev* 2002; 16:43–6.
54. Cunningham FG, Leveno KJ, Bloom SL, *et al.* Maternal physiology. In Cunningham FG, Leveno KJ, Bloom SL, *et al.* (eds), *Williams Obstetrics* (23rd ed). New York: McGraw Hill; 2010:107–35.
55. Bianchi DW, Zickwolf GK, Weil GJ, *et al.* Male fetal progenitor cells persist in maternal blood for as long as 27 years postpartum. *Proc Natl Acad Sci USA* 1996; 93:705–8.
56. Mor G, Abrahams VM. The immunology of pregnancy. In Creasy RK, Resnick R, Iams JD, *et al.* (eds), *Creasy & Resnik's Maternal-Fetal Medicine: Principles and Practice*, Philadelphia, PA: Saunders Elsevier; 2009:87–99.
57. Kölble N, Hummel T, von Mering R, *et al.* Gustatory and olfactory function in the first trimester of pregnancy. *Eur J Obstet Gynecol Reprod Biol* 2001; 99:179–83.
58. Laine MA. Effect of pregnancy on periodontal and dental health. *Acta Odontol Scand* 2002; 60:257–64.
59. Chaliha C, Sultan AH, Bland JM, *et al.* Anal function: effect of pregnancy and delivery. *Am J Obstet Gynecol* 2001; 185:427–32.
60. Richter JE. Gastroesophageal reflux disease during pregnancy. *Gastroenterol Clin North Am* 2003; 32: 235–61.
61. Richter,JE. Review article: The management of heartburn in pregnancy. *Aliment Pharmacol Ther* 2005; 22:749–57.
62. Marrero JM, Goggin PM, de Caestecker JS, *et al.* Determinants of pregnancy heartburn. *Br J Obstet Gynaecol* 1992; 99:731–4.
63. Van Thiel DH, Gavaler JS, Joshi SN, *et al.* Heartburn of pregnancy. *Gastroenterology* 1977; 72:666–8.
64. Hardy JF, Lepage Y, Bonneville-Chouinard N. Occurrence of gastroesophageal reflux on induction of anaesthesia does not correlate with the volume of gastric contents. *Can J Anaesth* 1990; 37:502–8.
65. Han TH, Brimacombe J, Lee EJ, *et al.* The laryngeal mask airway is effective (and probably safe) in selected healthy parturients for elective cesarean section: a prospective study of 1067 cases. *Can J Anaesth* 2001; 48:1117–21.
66. Klomp T, van Poppel M, Jones L, *et al.* Inhaled analgesia for pain management in labour. *Cochrane Database Syst Rev* 2012; 9:CD009351.
67. de Souza DG, Doar LH, Mehta SH, *et al.* Aspiration prophylaxis and rapid sequence induction for elective cesarean delivery: time to reassess old dogma? *Anesth Analg* 2010; 110:1503–5.
68. Macfie AG, Magides AD, Richmond MN, *et al.* Gastric emptying in pregnancy. *Br J Anaesth* 1991; 67:54–7.
69. Wong CA, McCarthy RJ, Fitzgerald PC, *et al.* Gastric emptying of water in obese pregnant women at term. *Anesth Analg* 2007; 105:751–5.
70. Van Thiel DH, Gavaler JS, Joshi SN, *et al.* Heartburn of pregnancy. *Gastroenterology* 1977; 72:666–8.
71. O'Sullivan GM, Bullingham RE. The assessment of gastric acidity and antacid effect in pregnant women by a non-invasive radiotelemetry technique. *Br J Obstet Gynaecol* 1984; 91:973–8.
72. Hong JY, Park JW, Oh JI. Comparison of preoperative gastric contents and serum gastrin concentrations in pregnant and nonpregnant women. *J Clin Anesth* 2005; 17:451–5.
73. Cappell MS. Gastric and duodenal ulcers during pregnancy. *Gastroenterol Clin North Am* 2003; 32:263–308.
74. Nimmo WS, Wilson J, Prescott LF. Narcotic analgesics and delayed gastric emptying during labor. *Lancet* 1975; 1:890–3.
75. Kelly MC, Carabine UA, Hill DA, *et al.* A comparison of the effect of intrathecal and extradural fentanyl on gastric emptying in laboring women. *Anesth Analg* 1997; 85:834–8.
76. Carp H, Jayaram A, Stoll M. Ultrasound examination of the stomach contents of parturients. *Anesth Analg* 1992; 74:683–7.
77. Jayaram A, Bowen MP, Deshpande S, *et al.* Ultrasound examination of the stomach contents of women in the postpartum period. *Anesth Analg* 1997; 84:522–6.
78. Gin T, Cho AM, Lew JK, *et al.* Gastric emptying in the postpartum period. *Anaesth Intensive Care* 1991; 19:521–4.
79. Gaiser R. Physiologic changes of pregnancy. In Chestnut DH, Polley LS, Tsen LC, *et al.* (eds) *Chestnut's Obstetric Anesthesia*. Philadelphia, PA: Mosby Elsevier; 2009:15–36.
80. American Society of Anesthesiologists Task Force on Obstetric Anesthesia. Practice guidelines for obstetric anesthesia: an updated report by the American Society of Anesthesiologists Task Force on Obstetric Anesthesia. *Anesthesiology* 2007; 106:843–63.
81. Paranjothy S, Griffiths JD, Broughton HK, *et al.* Interventions at caesarean section for reducing the risk of aspiration pneumonitis. *Int J Obstet Anesth* 2011; 20:142–8.
82. O'Sullivan G, Segal S. NPO controversies—pulmonary aspiration: risks and management. In Suresh MS, Segal BS, Preston RL, *et al.* (eds) *Shnider and Levinson's Anesthesia for Obstetrics*. Baltimore, MD: Lippincott Williams & Wilkins; 2013:403–11.
83. Kumar S, Balki M, Williamson C, *et al.* Disorders of the liver, biliary system and exocrine pancreas in pregnancy. In Powrie RO, Greene MF, Camann W (eds) *de Swiet's Medical Disorders in Obstetric Practice*. Hoboken, NJ: Wiley-Blackwell; 2010:223–55.
84. Ko CW, Beresford SA, Schulte SJ, *et al.* Incidence, natural history, and risk factors for biliary sludge and stones during pregnancy. *Hepatology* 2005; 41:359–65.
85. Glantz A, Marschall HU, Mattsson LA. Intrahepatic cholestasis of pregnancy: relationships between bile acid levels and fetal complication rates. *Hepatology* 2004; 40:467–74.
86. Lydon-Rochelle M, Holt VL, Martin DP, *et al.* Association between method of delivery and maternal rehospitalization. *JAMA* 2000; 283:2411–16.
87. Toledano RD. Urologic emergencies and nonobstetric surgery during pregnancy. In Gainsburg D, Bryson E, Frost E (eds), *Anesthesia in Urologic Surgery*. New York: Springer Science and Business Media; 2014:215–42.
88. Smith MC, Murdoch AP, Danielson LA, *et al.* Relaxin has a role in establishing a renal response in pregnancy. *Fertil Steril* 2006; 86:253–5.

89. Jeyabalan A, Conrad KP. Renal function during normal pregnancy and preeclampsia. *Front Biosci* 2007; 12:2425–37.
90. Brown MA, Mangos GJ, Peek M, *et al.* Renal disease in pregnancy. In Powrie RO, Greene MF, Camann W (eds) *de Swiet's Medical Disorders in Obstetric Practice.* Hoboken, NJ: Wiley-Blackwell; 2010:182–208.
91. Williams DJ, Davidson JM. Renal disorders. In Creasy RK, Resnik R, Iams JD, *et al.* (eds) *Creasy & Resnik's Maternal-Fetal Medicine: Principles and Practice*, Philadelphia, PA: Saunders Elsevier; 2009:905–25.
92. Côté AM, Firoz T, Mattman A, *et al.* The 24-hour urine collection: gold standard or historical practice? *Am J Obstet Gynecol* 2008; 199:625.e1–6.
93. Zakowski MI, Ramanathan S. Uteroplacental circulation and respiratory gas exchange. In Suresh MS, Segal BS, Preston RL, *et al.* (eds) *Shnider and Levinson's Anesthesia for Obstetrics.* Philadelphia, PA: Lippincott Williams & Wilkins; 2013:18–45.
94. Frölich MA, Burchfield DJ, Euliano TY, *et al.* A single dose of fentanyl and midazolam prior to Cesarean section have no adverse neonatal effects. *Can J Anaesth* 2006; 53:79–85.
95. Kamalakannan D, Baskar V, Barton DM, *et al.* Diabetic ketoacidosis in pregnancy. *Postgrad Med J* 2003; 79:454–7.
96. Yang J, Cummings EA, O'Connell C, *et al.* Fetal and neonatal outcomes of diabetic pregnancies. *Obstet Gynecol* 2006; 108:644–50.
97. Greene MF, Solomon CG, Lee SL, *et al.* Diabetes mellitus in pregnancy. In Powrie RO, Greene MF, Camann W (eds) *de Swiet's Medical Disorders in Obstetric Practice*, Hoboken, NJ: Wiley-Blackwell; 2010:293–321.
98. Glinoer D. What happens to the normal thyroid during pregnancy? *Thyroid* 1999; 9: 631–5.
99. Burrow GN, Fisher DA, Larsen PR. Maternal and fetal thyroid function. *N Engl J Med* 1994; 331:1072–8.
100. Ain KB, Mori Y, Refetoff F. Reduced clearance rate of thyroxine-binding globulin (TBG) with increased sialylation: a mechanism for estrogen-induced elevation of serum TBG concentration. *J Clin Endocrinol Metab* 1987; 65:689–96.
101. Nader S. Thyroid disease and pregnancy. In Creasy RK, Resnik R, Iams JD, *et al.* (eds) *Creasy & Resnik's Maternal-Fetal Medicine: Principles and Practice.* Philadelphia, PA: Saunders Elsevier; 2009:995–1014.
102. Celeski D, Micho J, Walters L. Anesthetic implications of a partial molar pregnancy and associated complications. *AANA J* 2001; 69:49–53.
103. Morgan LS. Hormonally active gynecologic tumors. *Semin Surg Oncol* 1990; 6:83–90.
104. Burch HB, Wartofsky L. Life threatening thyrotoxicosis. Thyroid storm. *Endocrinol Metab Clin North Am* 1993; 22:263–77.
105. Casey BM, Leveno KJ. Thyroid disease in pregnancy. *Obstet Gynecol* 2006; 108:1283–92.
106. Isley WL, Dahl S, Gibbs H. Use of esmolol in managing a thyrotoxic patient needing emergency surgery. *Am J Med* 1990; 89:122–3.
107. Gonzalez JG, Elizondo G, Saldivar D, *et al.* Pituitary gland growth during normal pregnancy: an in vivo study using magnetic resonance imaging, *Am J Med* 1988; 85:217–20.
108. Frankenne F, Closset J, Gomez F, *et al.* The physiology of growth hormones (GHs) in pregnant women and partial characterization of the placental GH variant. *J Clin Endocrinol Metab* 1988; 66:1171–80.
109. Sasaki A, Shinkawa O, Yoshinaga K. Placental corticotropin-releasing hormone may be a stimulator of maternal pituitary adrenocorticotropic hormone secretion in humans, *J Clin Invest* 1989; 84:1997–2001.
110. Molitch ME, Peaceman A. Pituitary and adrenal disease in pregnancy. In Powrie RO, Greene MR, Camann W (eds) *de Swiet's Medical Disorders in Obstetric Practice.* Hoboken, NJ: Wiley-Blackwell; 2010:335–51.
111. Feinberg EC, Molitch ME, Endres LK, *et al.* The incidence of Sheehan's syndrome after obstetric hemorrhage. *Fertil Steril* 2005; 84:975–9.
112. Nolten WE, Lindheimer MD, Rueckert PA, *et al.* Diurnal patterns and regulation of cortisol secretion in pregnancy. *J Clin Endocrinol Metab* 1980; 51:466–72.
113. Wilson M, Morganti AA, Zervoudakis I, *et al.* Blood pressure, the renin-aldosterone system and sex steroids throughout normal pregnancy. *Am J Med* 1980; 68:97–104.
114. Ehrlich EN, Lindheimer MD. Effect of administered mineralocorticoids or ACTH in pregnant women. Attenuation of kaliuretic influence of mineralocorticoids during pregnancy. *J Clin Invest* 1972; 51:1301–9.
115. Nader S. Other endocrine disorders of pregnancy. In Creasy RK, Resnik R, Iams JD, *et al.* (eds) *Creasy & Resnik's Maternal-Fetal Medicine: Principles and Practice.* Philadelphia, PA: Saunders Elsevier; 2009:1015–40.
116. Martin FM, Rowland RG. Urologic malignancies in pregnancy. *Urol Clin North Am* 2007; 34:53–9.
117. Kayem G, Kurinczuk J, Lewis G, *et al.* Risk factors for progression from severe maternal morbidity to death: a national cohort study, *PLoS One* 2011; 6:e29077.
118. Tagaito Y, Isono S, Remmers JE, *et al.* Lung volume and collapsibility of the passive pharynx in patients with sleep-disordered breathing. *J Appl Physiol* 2007; 103:1379–85.
119. Doherty DA, Magann EF, Francis J, *et al.* Pre-pregnancy body mass index and pregnancy outcomes. *Int J Gynaecol Obstet* 2006; 95:242–7.
120. Hood DD, Dewan DM. Anesthetic and obstetric outcome in morbidly obese parturients. *Anesthesiology* 1993; 79:1210–18.
121. Breen TW. Epidural analgesia and back pain. In Halpern SH, Douglas MJ (eds) *Evidence-Based Obstetric Anesthesia.* Malden, MA: Blackwell Publishing; 2005;208–16.
122. Kristiansson P, Svardsudd K, von Schoultz B. Back pain during pregnancy: a prospective study. *Spine* 1996; 21:702–9.
123. George JW, Skaggs CD, Thompson PA, *et al.* A randomized controlled trial comparing a multimodal intervention and standard obstetrics care for low back and pelvic pain in pregnancy. *Am J Obstet Gynecol* 2013;208:295.e1–7.
124. Brynhildsen J, Hansson A, Persson A, *et al.* Follow-up of patients with low back pain during pregnancy. *Obstet Gynecol* 1998; 91:182–6.
125. Kristiansson P, Svärdsudd K, von Schoultz B. Serum relaxin, symphyseal pain, and back pain during pregnancy. *Am J Obstet Gynecol* 1996; 175:1342–7.
126. Breen TW, Ransil B, Groves P, *et al.* Factors associated with back pain after childbirth. *Anesthesiology* 1994; 81:29–34.

CHAPTER 3

Placenta and uteroplacental perfusion

Marie-Pierre Bonnet and Anne Alice Chantry

Introduction

The placenta is a dynamic organ from fetal origin with specific characteristics. Its anatomy changes throughout the pregnancy. The placenta has three main functions that are all necessary for adequate embryonic and fetal development: fetal protection and nutrition, and hormonal secretion. The chorionic villus, located in the intervillous space, is the main placental unit implicated in the exchanges between mother and fetus.

Any change in placental development and function can have a negative effect on fetal well-being. Uteroplacental perfusion is the major determinant of fetal oxygenation and nutrient delivery, but due to its limited autoregulation, it is particularly dependent on maternal haemodynamics. Consequently, any significant decrease in maternal blood pressure or cardiac output can affect uteroplacental perfusion and hence can impact on the fetus, with potential lethal consequences for the fetus.

Most anaesthetic drugs, except for neuromuscular blocking agents, can cross the placental barrier and directly affect the fetus. Indirectly, the anaesthetic technique can affect the fetus by disturbing uteroplacental perfusion. As such, anaesthetists caring for pregnant women should have excellent knowledge of the placenta, its function, and the determinants of uteroplacental perfusion.

Placental development, anatomy, and uteroplacental perfusion

Early development of the placenta

After being fertilized in the external third of the Fallopian tube, the egg moves towards the uterine cavity. During its progression, the fertilized egg is subject to some intrinsic modifications, the first divisions leading to the blastocyst stage at day 5. The blastocyst corresponds to the primitive stage of the fetus and the placenta, with on one hand, the trophoblast (future placenta and membranes) and on the other hand, the endoderm (corresponding to the future fetus).

Six days after fertilization, the blastocyst joins the uterine epithelium. At that stage, the trophoblast differentiates into an inner layer, the cytotrophoblast, and an outer layer, the syncytiotrophoblast. This syncytiotrophoblast proliferates and penetrates the external third of the endometrium, and then extends to create a sea of circulating maternal blood (lacunar network), establishing the uteroplacental circulation. This process constitutes the beginning of implantation. About 10 days after fertilization, implantation into the endometrium is complete and the syncytiotrophoblast develops all around the egg (Figure 3.1).[1,2]

From day 13, the extravillous cytotrophoblast cells invade the syncytiotrophoblast and are responsible for endometrial spiral uterine artery remodelling. This represents the primary development of the chorionic villi, which constitute the functional units of the human placenta in its definitive structure from 3 weeks of gestation. During the following weeks, part of the modified endometrium, called the basili decidua, forms some incomplete divisions, the septa. A cotyledon is composed of several chorionic villi included between two septa. As the pregnancy goes on, the fetus grows and is progressively exteriorized with its membranes out of the endometrium, while the placenta partly implanted in the endometrium constitutes the functional interface between mother and fetus.

Excessive trophoblastic invasion can be responsible for pathological presentations, such as choriocarcinoma, a malignant trophoblastic cancer deriving from the placenta, or placenta accreta, which is a pathological invasion by the chorionic villi of the superficial myometrium leading to an abnormally deep attachment of the placenta to the uterus.

Embryology of the uteroplacental perfusion

During the first trimester, placental development occurs in specific and optimum conditions for angiogenesis and vasculogenesis: low oxygen concentrations and anaerobic metabolism.[3,4] From the second week of gestation, clusters of extravillous cytotrophoblastic cells obstruct the diameter of uterine spiral arteries to limit diffusion of nutrients and oxygen towards the developing fetus and to activate remodelling of the endothelium of uterine spiral arteries. This remodelling deeply modifies the structure of the endothelium: cells of the smooth uterine muscle are replaced by cytotrophoblasts and spiral arteries become dilated, inelastic, and non-contractile, resulting in a low-resistance, poorly regulated uteroplacental perfusion. After 3 weeks of gestation, the chorionic villi have their definitive structure (Figure 3.2). The syncytiotrophoblast borders the intervillous space and is directly in contact with maternal blood.

After 10 weeks of gestation, clusters of cytotrophoblasts that were obstructing the spiral arteries progressively disappear and arterial maternal blood fills the intervillous space without resistance. Consequently, the oxygen tension in the intervillous space

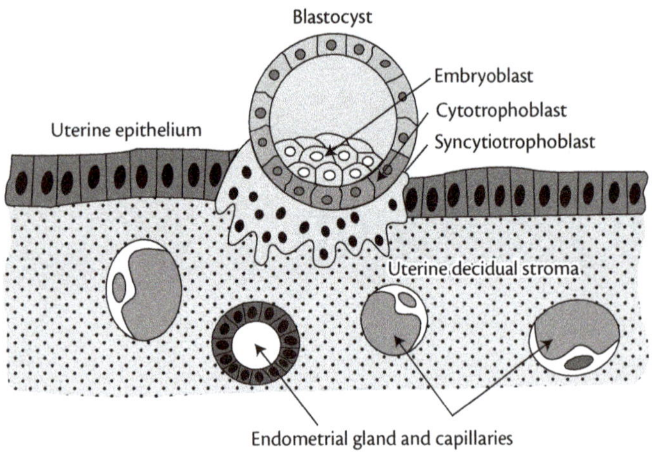

Figure 3.1 During implantation of the blastocyst, trophoblast cells in direct contact with maternal tissues syncytially fuse and give rise to the syncytiotrophoblast. Only this multinucleated tissue is able to penetrate the uterine epithelium and to implant the developing embryo.

increases throughout the first trimester of pregnancy from 2.7 to 8.0 kPa (20 mmHg to 60 mmHg).[5] Maternal placental circulation is fully established at the end of the first trimester of pregnancy. Thereafter, the placental structure remains stable. However until the end of pregnancy, chorionic villi continue to grow, divide, and become more numerous, parallel to the increasing needs of nutrient, exchange, and endocrine functions of the placenta.

Abnormal trophoblastic invasion of the endometrium could have different consequences. Insufficient trophoblastic invasion induces abnormal remodelling of the uterine spiral arteries and generates low placental perfusion and placental hypoxia. This phenomenon not only impacts on fetal development, with an increased risk of fetal growth restriction, but it can also be responsible for maternal endothelium dysfunction leading to pre-eclampsia.[6,7] Pregnancy hypertensive disorders appearing before 34 weeks of gestation are related to an abnormal trophoblastic invasion,[8] whereas pre-eclampsia occurring after 34 weeks of gestation seem to be associated with normal trophoblastic invasion in the first weeks, but with late atherosclerotic changes in spiral arterioles.[9,10]

Macroscopic anatomy of the placenta

The placenta constitutes the interface between the fetus and the endometrium. Placentation can take place anywhere in the uterine

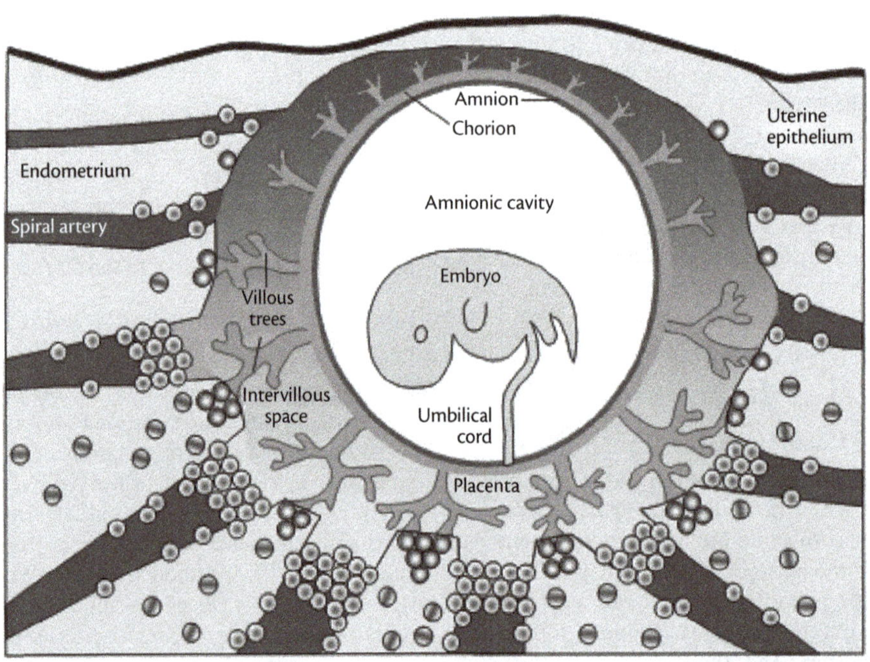

Figure 3.2 Schematic representation of the developing embryo and its surrounding tissues at about 8–10 weeks of pregnancy. The amnionic cavity with the embryo inside is marked off by the amnion that has already contacted the chorion. From the chorion, villous trees protrude into the intervillous space where some villi have direct contact with the basal plate (anchoring villi). At these sites, trophoblastic cell columns are the source for all extravillous trophoblast cells invading maternal tissues. Interstitial trophoblast cells derived from these columns invade endometrium and myometrium, while a subset of these cells penetrates the spiral arteries first as intramural and then as endovascular trophoblast cells. Onset of maternal blood flow into the placenta starts in the upper regions of placenta (the abembryonic pole) where development is slightly delayed. The local high concentrations of oxygen contribute to the regression of villi at the abembryonic pole. This in turn leads to the formation of the smooth chorion, the fetal membranes.

cavity, but is generally located on the upper third of the cavity and extends towards the uterine fundus. In case of placenta praevia, the placenta is implanted in the lower segment of the uterus (0.3–3% of pregnancies), and induces a risk for severe obstetric haemorrhage. This pathological placental localization can also be responsible for fetal malposition and fetal growth restriction, due to the low vascularization of this uterine area.

The human placenta is haemochorial, meaning that maternal blood directly bathes fetal tissues. Until 9–10 weeks of gestation, its structure is very thin. From 12 weeks of gestation, it grows dramatically, reaching at that time 18–20 cm in diameter and being 3 cm thick. At term, its weight is normally equivalent to a sixth of the fetal weight, from 400 to 600 g. But the placental weight/fetal weight ratio changes throughout pregnancy: during the first trimester, the placenta weighs more than the fetus; then from 14–16 weeks of gestation the placental weight/fetal weight ratio is around 1; and afterwards, the fetus becomes heavier than the placenta. This ratio reflects fetal well-being and is an indicator of an ongoing healthy pregnancy.

The mature placenta has two different faces. The chorionic face is the smooth fetal face, which is composed of two membranes: the amnion and the chorion. Made up of different layers, the amnion is the thin inner membrane (0.02–0.5 mm),[11] directly in contact with the amniotic fluid and covering the umbilical cord. It delimits the amniotic cavity. The outer membrane in contact with the endometrium becomes the chorial plate of the placenta. On the fetal side of the placenta, fetal vessels deriving from the umbilical vessels can be observed. These vessels also vascularize the chorion and transfer nutrients by diffusion to the amnion. The Benckiser syndrome is a fetal haemorrhage, often severe, resulting from the rupture of one or more velamentous praevia fetal vessels.

On the other placental side, called the maternal side or basal plate, cotyledons can be seen. These cotyledons result from the pooling of numerous villous trees tightly packed together. The basal plate is composed of modified endometrium and is in contact with the myometrium during the whole pregnancy. After birth, as a result of uterine contractions, the basili decidua (modified endometrium) separates from the myometrium for placental delivery.

The intervillous space, the place where maternofetal exchange occurs, is exactly localized between the chorial plate and the basal plate.

Anatomy of uteroplacental perfusion

Fetal–maternal exchange occurs in the intervillous space containing the chorionic villi. Its overall surface is estimated at 12 m^2 at term, whereas the functional surface of exchange is estimated at 1.8 m^2. The intervillous space overall contains a total volume of 150 mL of maternal blood, renewed three or four times per minute. The intervillous space is perfused by the uteroplacental arteries, derived from the remodelling of the uterine spiral arteries, which are themselves branches of the hypogastric arteries. Ovarian arteries also contribute for a small proportion to uteroplacental perfusion (10–20%). Uterine blood flow represents 3.5% of cardiac output in early pregnancy and 15–20% at term.

Oxygenated maternal blood comes from the uterine spiral arteries into the intervillous space, exchanges occurring at the level of the chorionic villi. Nutrients and oxygen enter the embryonal circulation by allantoidal vessels, future umbilical vessels (one vein, two arteries) coming from the terminal portion of the abdominal aorta or primitive arteries of the fetus. In the fetal vascular system, the umbilical vein transports the oxygenated blood and the umbilical arteries drain the fetal blood poorly concentrated in oxygen. This blood goes back to the basal plate through the intervillous space and is drained by uteroplacental veins located in the endometrium, and then by the uterine veins.

Regulation and measurement of uteroplacental perfusion

To maintain normal oxygen and nutrient delivery to the fetoplacental unit, the uteroplacental perfusion increases 15–20-fold during pregnancy. At term, it represents 15–20% of cardiac output. Due to the trophoblastic endothelial invasion and functional denervation of the spiral arteries, the uteroplacental circulation is usually considered as maximally vasodilated, with little or no ability for autoregulation. As a consequence, the uteroplacental perfusion mainly depends on maternal blood flow, and a decrease in uteroplacental perfusion can be observed in different circumstances (Table 3.1):

- Any significant maternal hypotension (i.e. in case of maternal hypovolaemia, sympathetic blockade in the context of neuraxial anaesthesia or analgesia, use of vasodilatory drugs, or aortocaval compression syndrome).
- Excessive vasoconstriction of the uterine arteries secondary to maternal hypertension, use of vasopressors, or catecholamines. Changes in PO_2 and PCO_2 can also have an impact on spiral artery tone: chronic hyperoxia and hypocapnia induce a decrease in uteroplacental perfusion.
- Frequent and prolonged uterine contractions and uterine hypertonus decrease uterine venous return and can also reduce uteroplacental perfusion.

Any change in uterine circulation directly impacts on the intervillous circulation. But even if the uteroplacental circulation is a widely dilated low-resistance system with a perfusion that is largely pressure dependent, there is still a place for moderate regulation. Prostacyclin and nitric oxide, by maintaining vasodilatation and inducing refractoriness to vasoconstrictor substances

Table 3.1 Causes of decreased uteroplacental perfusion

Decrease in maternal arterial blood pressure	Aortocaval compression syndrome Sympathetic blockade (neuraxial anaesthesia) Vasodilatory drugs Hypovolaemia
Excessive vasoconstriction of the uterine arteries	Maternal arterial hypertension Vasopressors Catecholamines Secondary to changes in PO_2 and PCO_2: Chronic hyperoxia Chronic hypercapnia
Increased uterine venous pressure	Frequent and prolonged uterine contractions/uterine hypertonus During uterine contractions

such as angiotensin II,[12] seem to play a major role in the control of the fetoplacental circulation. Prostacyclin is a prostaglandin I_2 usually produced by the vascular endothelium. During pregnancy, production of prostacyclin increases because of uterine vascular production.[13] Similarly, the endothelial synthesis of nitric oxide by the uterine arteries increases during pregnancy secondary to a greater nitric oxide synthase activity.[14]

Uteroplacental perfusion can be evaluated by various methods. The most common one is Doppler ultrasonography.[15] Measurement of red blood cell velocity of blood flowing through the uterine arteries allows estimation of uteroplacental blood flow. Moreover, several indices of vascular impedances can be calculated by using the arterial velocity waveform: the Pulsatility Index (PI), calculated as the difference between the peak systolic and the end diastolic flow velocity, divided by the mean flow velocity, and the Resistance Index (RI), estimated by comparing systolic and diastolic waveforms. Normally, the uterine vascular bed is a low-resistance circuit and flow continues throughout diastole. As resistance increases, diastolic velocity decreases in relation to systolic flow and the RI increases. Finally, Doppler ultrasonography is a non-invasive method that gives rapid results but with some limitations: the reproducibility of the measurement greatly depends on the examination of the same portion of uterine artery, precise measurements are also required otherwise inducing large errors in blood flow estimation. These limitations should be kept in mind when interpreting uteroplacental blood flow by Doppler ultrasonography.

Placental physiology

Placental functions differ with species, and results from animal studies should be interpreted with caution. The human placenta has multiple functions: it acts as a barrier, and an endocrine organ, and it is responsible for transfer of respiratory gases and nutrients to the fetus.

Transport mechanisms through the placenta

Substances are transported through the placenta by different mechanisms:

Passive diffusion

Passive diffusion is mainly driven by the concentration gradient across the membrane, without expenditure of cellular energy. It includes molecules of low molecular weight and not linked to proteins. Most drugs are transferred by this mechanism.

Facilitated diffusion

As for passive diffusion, the concentration gradient is responsible for the transfer through the membrane but with a maximum rate (saturation), determined by the number of membranous carrier protein complexes ('facilitators') and by the interaction between the carrier and the substance being transported. This is the main transportation route of relatively lipid-insoluble molecules. Some other substances can also be transported linked to another molecule, mostly sodium, whose concentration gradient facilitates the transfer of the first substance (secondary active transport or co-transport), and without cellular energy expenditure.

Active transport

Active transport involves the transport of a substance across cell membranes needing a protein membrane carrier, and requiring cellular energy. Usually, it occurs against a concentration, electrical, or pressure gradient. These protein carriers protect the fetus against foreign and potentially teratogenic compounds.

Pinocytosis

In pinocytosis, molecules are surrounded by the cell membrane, and can cross the cytoplasm to fuse with the other side of the cell. This process requires energy and concerns large molecules.

Several factors impact on the transplacental transfer of a substance and can affect maternal–fetal exchange (Table 3.2):

- Molecular weight and lipophilic quality of the substance: provided the molecular weight is lower than 1000 Da, the lower the molecular weight, the greater the diffusion; highly lipid-soluble drugs penetrate the cell membrane easily, but can also lead to trapping of drugs within placental tissue.
- Maternal and fetal plasma pH changes the ionization of drugs according to their pKa. Fetal pH is lower than maternal pH. Weak bases are more ionized and accumulate in the fetus. Fetal acidosis greatly enhances maternal-to-fetal transfer of basic drugs, such as local anaesthetics and opioids ('ion trapping').[16]
- Protein binding: only the free part of the drug diffuses through the placenta, in particular for non-lipophilic or ionized molecules. Plasma protein concentrations and in particular albumin and alpha-1-glycoprotein concentrations in the mother and the fetus influence the placental transfer of the drug. Typically, albumin concentration is higher in fetal plasma than in maternal plasma. Consequently the fetal concentration of a substance with strong binding to albumin will be higher than its concentration in maternal blood. Fetal blood typically contains 40% of the alpha-1-glycoprotein maternal concentrations.
- Maternal plasma concentration of the substance, and the kinetics of its concentration (depending on the dose, and on the mode of administration). Both define for a substance a fetal exposition time.

Table 3.2 Major maternal factors modifying transplacental transfer of a substance

Factor	Increased transplacental transfer	Decreased transplacental transfer
Molecular weight	<1000 Da	>1000 Da
Lipid solubility	Lipophilic	Hydrophilic
pH vs pKa determining the amount of ionized drug	High proportion of un-ionized drug Fetal acidosis	High proportion of ionized drug
Protein binding	High unbound fraction Alpha-1-glycoprotein binding	Low unbound fraction Albumin binding
Maternal plasma concentration	High	Low
Uteroplacental blood flow	High	Low
Placental fixation and metabolism	Low	High

- Uteroplacental perfusion, directly influencing the transfer of lipophilic substances, but with a weak impact on low lipophilic and ionized substances.
- Surface and thickness of the exchange zone, particularly in the context of vasculoplacental pathology (pre-eclampsia).
- Placental fixation or metabolism of drugs (e.g. corticosteroids).

Protective functions of the placenta

The placenta is an imperfect protective barrier for the fetus against substances circulating in the maternal blood: many small xenobiotics cross the placenta by simple diffusion, and some bigger ones can be transported by specific systems. However, several protective mechanisms also take place in the placenta, reducing the transfer of some potentially toxic substances. One of these protective systems is the production of cytochrome P450 isoenzymes, metabolizing certain drugs and xenobiotics.[17] There are also export pumps on the maternally facing membrane of the syncytiotrophoblast, such as multidrug resistance proteins, placenta-specific ATP-binding cassette proteins, breast cancer resistance protein, and mitoxantrone resistance-associated protein.[18] These pumps remove toxic substances from the fetal circulation.

Most proteins cannot cross the placenta barrier. But maternal antibodies, mainly immunoglobulins G, are transported through the placenta by pinocytosis and provide passive immunity to the fetus. However, some virus, such as *Cytomegalovirus*, rubella, varicella, polio, coxsackie viruses, and, in a minority of cases, HIV (1.5–2% of pregnancies in HIV-positive mothers[19]), can infect the fetus. Generally, bacteria and parasites do not cross the placenta. Only *Toxoplasma gondii* and *Treponema pallidum* can be transmitted to the fetus through the placenta.

Thus, the protective role of the placenta is not perfect, and the best protection against maternal–fetal transmission of infection is primary prevention.

Placental endocrine functions

The placenta has polyvalent endocrine functions. It produces peptide and steroid hormones (Table 3.3), essential for pregnancy, and some placental proteins, whose role is still not well defined.

From a very early stage in pregnancy, the placenta produces progesterone and oestrogens by converting steroid precursors with placental enzymes. Then, it releases them into both maternal and fetal circulations. The corpus luteum also produces progesterone, but by the ninth week of gestation, it atrophies and the placenta becomes the main producer of circulating progesterone and oestrogens. Peptide hormones, close to the hypothalamic and hypophyseal hormones, are also secreted by the placenta, such as placental growth hormone (GH), human chorionic gonadotropin (hCG), human placental lactogen, and a number of growth factors (endocrine gland-derived vascular endothelial growth factor, epidermal growth factor, insulin-like growth factors, and platelet-derived growth factor). All of these factors play a key role in embryonic and fetal growth and allow the placenta to influence and control the fetal environment.[20]

Progesterone inhibits uterine contractions. Oestrogens act as specialized growth hormones for the mother's reproductive organs.[21] hCG helps prolong the life of the corpus luteum in early pregnancy. With oestradiol and glucocorticoids, it also stimulates the cytotrophoblast cell fusion and the functional differentiation of the villous trophoblast.[22] Human placental lactogen modulates embryonic development and stimulates the production of insulin-like growth factors, insulin, adrenocortical hormones, and pulmonary surfactant.[23] It may also play a role in angiogenesis.[24] Placental GH may be involved in maternal adjustment to pregnancy and in placental development via an autocrine or paracrine mechanism.[25]

Table 3.3 Main endocrine functions of the placenta

Hormones	Functions
Steroids	
Progesterone	Inhibition of uterine contractions
Oestrogens (oestrone, oestradiol, oestriol)	Growth hormone for the mother's reproductive organs (breasts, uterus, cervix and vagina) Stimulation of the cytotrophoblast cell fusion and of functional differentiation of the villous trophoblast
Peptide hormones	
Placental growth hormone (GH)	Maternal adjustment to pregnancy Placental development Stimulation of the production of insulin-like growth factors
Human chorionic gonadotropin (hCG)	Prolongation of the life of the corpus luteum Stimulation of cytotrophoblast cell fusion and of functional differentiation of the villous trophoblast
Human placental lactogen	Modulation of embryonic development Stimulation of the production of insulin-like growth factors, insulin, adrenocortical hormones and pulmonary surfactant Angiogenesis
Growth factors	
Endocrine gland-derived vascular endothelial growth factor (EG-VEGF) Epidermal growth factor (EGF) Insulin-like growth factor (IGF) Platelet-derived growth factor (PGF)	Role in fetal-placental growth throughout gestation

Metabolic functions of the placenta

Apart from its protective and endocrine functions, the placenta is responsible for all exchanges between the mother and the fetus. This organ provides oxygen, water, carbohydrates, fatty acids, amino acids, vitamins, minerals and other nutrients to the fetus from the maternal circulation. Simultaneously, it removes carbon dioxide and other waste products from the fetal circulation. The placenta also requires oxygen and nutrients for itself, and removes its own metabolites.

Transfer of respiratory gases

The respiratory function of the placenta is five times less efficient than the lung for oxygen transfer, but the large surface of exchange partly compensates for this. Oxygen diffusion through the placenta is poor, and oxygen transfer mainly depends on oxygen partial pressure gradient between maternal blood in the spiral arteries (13.3 kPa) and fetal blood (2.2–3.7 kPa). Despite low oxygen partial pressures in the intervillous space, the fetal oxygen blood content is high enough (23 mL per 100 mL of blood) to provide aerobic metabolism. Indeed, the oxygen affinity is higher for fetal haemoglobin than for maternal haemoglobin, and the fetal haemoglobin concentration is between 17 and 20 g/dL. In case of maternal anaemia, a 50% or more decrease in haemoglobin maternal level is needed to impact on fetal oxygen transfer. Oxygen transfer from the mother to the fetus is about 80 mL/min, for a fetal oxygen consumption of 8 mL/kg fetal body weight.[26] A rate-limiting factor for oxygen transfer is the uteroplacental perfusion. Fetal hypoxia is observed in case of a 50% or more decrease in uteroplacental blood flow. Conversely, carbon dioxide is 20 times more diffusible than oxygen and haemoglobin affinity for carbon dioxide is lower for fetal haemoglobin than for maternal haemoglobin.

Transport and metabolism of carbohydrates

For the fetus, the main source of energy is glucose. As fetal gluconeogenesis is very poor, fetal glucose mainly comes from the maternal circulation. Glucose transfer occurs via facilitated diffusion with a number of glucose transporters (GLUTs) involved, located both at the maternal blood-facing and the fetal capillary-facing membranes of placental tissues. Cellular distribution of GLUTs changes during pregnancy, suggesting modifications in their functions between early and late pregnancy.[27] Only 28% of the absorbed glucose is transferred to the fetus, due to placental glucose consumption.[28]

Transport and metabolism of amino acids

Amino acids are needed for fetal protein synthesis and metabolism. As amino acid concentration is higher in the umbilical venous blood than in the maternal blood, transport of amino acids from the mother to the fetus is active, involving amino acid transporters that require energy coming from the large sodium gradient generated by Na,K-ATPase pumps.[29]

Transport and metabolism of lipids

As they are lipophilic, the large majority of free fatty acids cross the placental membrane through a simple passive diffusion mode, except arachidonic acid, which is actively transported.[30]

Transplacental transfer of anaesthetic drugs

The study of placental drug transfer encounters several methodological limitations: first, wide interspecies variation in placental anatomy and physiology limit the extension of results from animal to human studies;[31] second, experimental studies on drug transport performed on human placental slices or isolated villi, membrane vesicles, homogenates, or tissue culture cells do not take into account the dual perfusion (maternal and fetal) of the placenta *in situ*; finally, due to ethical concerns for maternal and fetal safety, clinical studies are rarely performed. Most of the time, data on the placental transfer of anaesthetic agents have been extrapolated from measurements of drug concentrations in the maternal and umbilical cord blood at the time of delivery allowing the calculation of the ratio of umbilical vein/maternal artery or vein concentrations. This ratio, called the fetal/maternal (F/M) ratio, is used as a surrogate of drug transplacental transfer, the umbilical vein blood concentration representing the fetal blood concentration of the drug. For a given drug, a high F/M ratio suggests a high placenta transfer. Large inter- and intra-individual variations of these ratios reported across studies highlight the fact that maternal and fetal concentrations are also influenced by maternal drug metabolism, the placenta, the fetus, and by intrapartum changes. Consequently, these kinds of studies need large numbers of study subjects. *In vitro* models of dual-perfused human placenta have also been developed and are now validated for the study of maternal–fetal transport. Placental transfer can also be reported as a ratio referred to as the index transfer. This is defined as the ratio of the drug clearance/reference compound clearance (i.e. creatinine, or tritiated water) and allows interplacental comparisons. Transplacental transfer of the main anaesthetic drugs has been studied using these types of methods.

With the exception of neuromuscular blocking agents, all anaesthetic drugs are lipophilic and consequently migrate through the placental barrier. However, the placenta itself may take up highly lipophilic drugs, creating a placental drug depot that limits placental transfer of these drugs. Major characteristics of drug transfer for anaesthetic drugs are listed in Table 3.4.

Hypnotic drugs

The high lipophilic properties of induction agents enhance their transfer across the placenta.

Thiopental is the most widely studied anaesthetic drug. The thiopental F/M ratio is between 0.43 and 0.96, 1–3 minutes after its intravenous administration.[32] Thiopental is a highly protein-bound drug. Consequently, its transplacental transfer is strongly affected by maternal and fetal protein concentrations, with a greater free fraction in fetal blood (33). Thiopental transplacental transfer is higher than for midazolam (F/M ratio = 0.66) (34). However, due to its possible negative effect on the fetus, administration of midazolam to the mother is not recommended.[35]

For etomidate, the F/M ratio is 0.5, 6–10 minutes after injection,[36] but the use of etomidate for induction of anaesthesia is not recommended, as it has been associated with fetal transient hypocorticoid syndrome.[37]

Propofol F/M ratios between 0.2 and 0.8 have been reported 4–10 minutes after its intravenous administration.[38–40] The transplacental transfer of propofol is strongly influenced by maternal and fetal protein concentrations, placental clearance of propofol increasing with increasing fetal albumin concentrations. The free propofol concentration remains unchanged, indicating that the pharmacological effects of propofol on the fetus can be expected to be fairly constant and predictable based on maternal propofol concentrations.[41]

Inhalation anaesthetic agents

Due to their high liposolubility and low molecular weight, inhaled anaesthetic agents cross the placenta very easily. In case of caesarean delivery under general anaesthesia, a prolonged induction–delivery time interval may induce neonatal general

Table 3.4 Placental transfer of anaesthetic drugs

Drug	Molecular weight (Da)	pKa	Lipid solubility	% protein binding	F/M ratio
Thiopental	132	7.6	580	75	0.4–0.9
Propofol	178	11	4700	98	0.5–0.8
Morphine	285	7.9	1.4	30	0.61
Fentanyl	336	8.4	816	84	0.37–0.57
Sufentanil	386	8.0	1727	93	0.81
Remifentanil	376	7.1	50	70	0.55–0.88
Suxamethonium	399	–	–	–	0.02
Rocuronium	530	–	–	30	0.16
Atracurium	145	–	–	80	0.07
Cisatracurium	929	–	–	–	–
Vecuronium	558	8.9	16	90	0.11
2-Chloroprocaine	271	8.9	0.14	–	–
Lidocaine	234	7.9	2.9	64	0.5–0.7
Bupivacaine	288	8.2	28	96	0.2–0.4
Levobupivacaine	288	8.1	28	97	0.3
Ropivacaine	274	8.0	3	90–95	0.2

anaesthesia. The transplacental transfer of nitrous oxide is very rapid, with an F/M ratio of 0.8 within 3 minutes of continuous inhalation.[42] There is no available data on the F/M ratio of desflurane and sevoflurane.

Opioids

Transplacental transfer of lipophilic opioids mostly depends on the fetal pH and protein concentrations; it increases in case of fetal acidosis.

Sufentanil is the most lipophilic opioid currently used. An F/M ratio of 0.81 has been reported. Its transplacental diffusion is limited by linking with alpha-1-glycoprotein and its placental capture.[43]

Fentanyl is a highly lipid-soluble drug with high albumin binding. After maternal epidural administration, the F/M ratios reported are between 0.37 and 0.57,[44] but compared to sufentanil, fentanyl has lower lipophilic solubility. Consequently, in case of epidural or intrathecal administration, there is less binding of fentanyl onto the spinal cord, resulting in a higher systemic concentration and hence increased fetal fentanyl exposure.[44]

For remifentanil, the F/M ratio is around 0.55 when administered as patient-controlled analgesia for labour,[45] and 0.88 when it is given as a continuous intravenous infusion before or during caesarean delivery. It is rapidly metabolized by fetal esterases or redistributed, hence limiting its effects on the neonate.[46]

Morphine is a hydrophilic compound that exhibits membrane-limited transfer, with low placental tissue content and a fast washout. An F/M ratio of 0.61 has been reported 30 minutes after its intravenous administration.[47] Following morphine intrathecal administration, the Umbilical artery/maternal artery ratio is around 0.92, but the absolute fetal morphine concentrations are lower than those inducing neonatal side effects. The placental transfer of morphine is apparently not affected by the administration of naloxone.[47]

Muscle relaxants

As muscle relaxants are fully ionized components, their transplacental transfer is very low. For succinylcholine, the F/M ratio is of 0.02. Succinylcholine is not detected in the umbilical venous blood after a single injection with a dose lower than 300 mg.[48] Concerning non-depolarized muscle relaxants, the F/M ratios are also very low, between 0.07 (atracurium) and 0.11 (vecuronium), but the fetal blood concentration increases over time.[49] No data are available on placental transfer of rocuronium. Maternal administration of muscle relaxants has no impact on neonatal well-being.

Local anaesthetics

Local anaesthetics readily cross the placenta by simple diffusion. Even if there are differences in structure and lipid solubility between ropivacaine and bupivacaine, their placental transfer is comparable.[50] After epidural administration of bupivacaine, the F/M ratio is 0.31.[51] After intrathecal administration, this ratio is 0.34. Plasma umbilical venous bupivacaine concentration after intrathecal anaesthesia is 7% of that found after epidural anaesthesia.[52]

Lidocaine is bound to alpha-1-glycoprotein that decreases during pregnancy, leading to a higher free fraction of lidocaine in pregnant women than in non-pregnant controls.[53] In the acidotic fetus, 'ion trapping' phenomenon of local anaesthetic drugs is observed: as their pK is close to the physiologic pH, decreases in fetal pH increase the proportion of ionized local anaesthetic drugs, resulting in a large amount of local anaesthetic in fetal plasma. This phenomenon is classically described with all local anaesthetics and in particular with lidocaine.[16,54] For chloroprocaine as for lidocaine and bupivacaine, placental transfer increases linearly as the fetal pH decreases. But conversely to these two local anaesthetics, clearance of chloroprocaine does not return to baseline when fetal pH is restored to 7.4. Maternal protein binding limits placental transfer of lidocaine and bupivacaine, but not of chloroprocaine.[16]

Conclusion

The placenta is a dynamic organ with a complex structure constituting the anatomical and functional connection between the mother and the fetus. The main functional units of the placenta are the chorionic villi located in the intervillous space. The placenta helps to protect the fetus against some xenobiotics and infectious agents. Moreover, it releases many hormones involved in the development of pregnancy. Finally, the placenta provides oxygen and nutrients to the fetus while removing carbon dioxide and other waste products to ensure fetal growth.

As autoregulation of the placental circulation is limited, maternal haemodynamic status and uteroplacental perfusion should be kept stable to avoid any impact on fetal well-being, in particular while performing general or neuraxial anaesthesia.

With the exception of muscle relaxants, all anaesthetics drugs easily cross the placenta, and anaesthetists should be aware of their potential complications for the fetus and neonates.

References

1. Bernischke K, Kaufmann P. *Pathology of the Human Placenta.* Berlin: Springer; 2000.
2. Pidoux G, Gerbaud P, Cocquebert M, *et al.* Review: Human trophoblast fusion and differentiation: lessons from trisomy 21 placenta. *Placenta* 2012; 33 Suppl:S81–6.
3. Genbacev O, Zhou Y, Ludlow JW, *et al.* Regulation of human placental development by oxygen tension. *Science* 1997; 277(5332):1669–72.
4. Jauniaux E, Watson AL, Hempstock J, *et al.* Onset of maternal arterial blood flow and placental oxidative stress. A possible factor in human early pregnancy failure. *Am J Pathol* 2000; 157(6):2111–22.
5. Jauniaux E, Watson A, Burton G. Evaluation of respiratory gases and acid-base gradients in human fetal fluids and uteroplacental tissue between 7 and 16 weeks' gestation. *Am J Obstet Gynecol* 2001; 184(5):998–1003.
6. Malassine A, Frendo JL, Evain-Brion D. Trisomy 21- affected placentas highlight prerequisite factors for human trophoblast fusion and differentiation. *Int J Dev Biol* 2010; 54(2-3):475–82.
7. Redman CW, Sargent IL. Latest advances in understanding preeclampsia. *Science* 2005; 308(5728):1592–4.
8. Moldenhauer JS, Stanek J, Warshak C, *et al.* The frequency and severity of placental findings in women with preeclampsia are gestational age dependent. *Am J Obstet Gynecol* 2003; 189(4):1173–7.
9. Ness RB, Roberts JM. Heterogeneous causes constituting the single syndrome of preeclampsia: a hypothesis and its implications. *Am J Obstet Gynecol* 1996; 175(5):1365–70.
10. Redman CW, Sargent IL. Placental debris, oxidative stress and pre-eclampsia. *Placenta* 2000; 21(7):597–602.
11. Mamede AC, Carvalho MJ, Abrantes AM, *et al.* Amniotic membrane: from structure and functions to clinical applications. *Cell Tissue Res* 2012; 349(2):447–58.
12. Rosenfeld CR. Mechanisms regulating angiotensin II responsiveness by the uteroplacental circulation. *Am J Physiol Regul Integr Comp Physiol* 2001; 281(4):R1025–40.
13. Magness RR, Rosenfeld CR, Hassan A, *et al.* Endothelial vasodilator production by uterine and systemic arteries. I. Effects of ANG II on PGI2 and NO in pregnancy. *Am J Physiol* 1996; 270(6 Pt 2):H1914–23.
14. Sladek SM, Magness RR, Conrad KP. Nitric oxide and pregnancy. *Am J Physiol* 1997; 272(2 Pt 2):R441–63.
15. Urban G, Vergani P, Ghidini A, *et al.* State of the art: non-invasive ultrasound assessment of the uteroplacental circulation. *Semin Perinatol* 2007; 31(4):232–9.
16. Johnson RF, Herman NL, Johnson HV, *et al.* Effects of fetal pH on local anesthetic transfer across the human placenta. *Anesthesiology* 1996; 85(3):608–15.
17. Pasanen M. The expression and regulation of drug metabolism in human placenta. *Adv Drug Deliv Rev* 1999; 38(1):81–97.
18. Marin JJ, Macias RI, Serrano MA. The hepatobiliary-like excretory function of the placenta. A review. *Placenta* 2003; 24(5):431–8.
19. Soilleux EJ, Coleman N. Transplacental transmission of HIV: a potential role for HIV binding lectins. *Int J Biochem Cell Biol* 2003; 35(3):283–7.
20. Siler-Khodr T. Endocrine and paracrine function of the human placenta. In Polin RA Fox WW (eds) *Fetal and Neonatal Physiology* (2nd ed). Philadelphia, PA: WB Saunders; 1998:89–102.
21. Page K. *The Physiology of the Human Placenta.* London: University College; 1993.
22. Malassine A, Cronier L. Hormones and human trophoblast differentiation: a review. *Endocrine* 2002; 19(1):3–11.
23. Handwerger S, Freemark M. The roles of placental growth hormone and placental lactogen in the regulation of human fetal growth and development. *J Pediatr Endocrinol Metab* 2000; 13(4):343–56.
24. Corbacho AM, Martinez De La Escalera G, Clapp C. Roles of prolactin and related members of the prolactin/growth hormone/placental lactogen family in angiogenesis. *J Endocrinol* 2002; 173(2):219–38.
25. Lacroix MC, Guibourdenche J, Frendo JL, *et al.* Human placental growth hormone—a review. *Placenta* 2002; 23 Suppl A:S87–94.
26. Longo L. Respiration in the fetal-placental unit. In Cowett RM (ed) *Principles of Perinatal-neonatal Metabolism.* New York: Springer-Verlag; 1991:304–15.
27. Baumann MU, Deborde S, Illsley NP. Placental glucose transfer and fetal growth. *Endocrine* 2002; 19(1):13–22.
28. Morriss FJ. Placental transport. In Knobil E, Neill JD (eds) *The Physiology of Reproduction.* New York: Raven Press; 1994:813–61.
29. Yudilevich DL, Sweiry JH. Transport of amino acids in the placenta. *Biochim Biophys Acta* 1985; 822(2):169–201.
30. Filshie GM, Anstey MD. The distribution of arachidonic acid in plasma and tissues of patients near term undergoing elective or emergency Caesarean section. *Br J Obstet Gynaecol* 1978; 85(2):119–23.
31. Dancis J. Why perfuse the human placenta. *Contrib Gynecol Obstet* 1985; 13:1–4.
32. Gaspari F, Marraro G, Penna GF, *et al.* Elimination kinetics of thiopentone in mothers and their newborn infants. *Eur J Clin Pharmacol* 1985; 28(3):321–5.
33. Kingston HG, Kendrick A, Sommer KM, *et al.* Binding of thiopental in neonatal serum. *Anesthesiology* 1990; 72(3):428–31.
34. Bach V, Carl P, Ravlo O, *et al.* A randomized comparison between midazolam and thiopental for elective cesarean section anesthesia: III. Placental transfer and elimination in neonates. *Anesth Analg* 1989; 68(3):238–42.
35. Bland BA, Lawes EG, Duncan PW, *et al.* Comparison of midazolam and thiopental for rapid sequence anesthetic induction for elective cesarean section. *Anesth Analg* 1987; 66(11):1165–8.
36. Gregory MA, Davidson DG. Plasma etomidate levels in mother and fetus. *Anaesthesia* 1991; 46(9):716–8.
37. Reddy BK, Pizer B, Bull PT. Neonatal serum cortisol suppression by etomidate compared with thiopentone, for elective caesarean section. *Eur J Anaesthesiol.* 1988; 5(3):171–6.
38. Dailland P, Cockshott ID, Lirzin JD, *et al.* Intravenous propofol during cesarean section: placental transfer, concentrations in breast milk, and neonatal effects. A preliminary study. *Anesthesiology* 1989; 71(6):827–34.
39. Gin T, Gregory MA, Chan K, Oh TE. Maternal and fetal levels of propofol at caesarean section. *Anaesth Intensive Care* 1990; 18(2):180–4.

40. Sanchez-Alcaraz A, Quintana MB, Laguarda M. Placental transfer and neonatal effects of propofol in caesarean section. *J Clin Pharm Ther* 1998; 23(1):19–23.
41. He YL, Tsujimoto S, Tanimoto M, *et al.* Effects of protein binding on the placental transfer of propofol in the human dually perfused cotyledon in vitro. *Br J Anaesth* 2000; 85(2):281–6.
42. Marx GF, Joshi CW, Orkin LR. Placental transmission of nitrous oxide. *Anesthesiology* 1970; 32(5):429–32.
43. Johnson RF, Herman N, Arney TL, *et al.* The placental transfer of sufentanil: effects of fetal pH, protein binding, and sufentanil concentration. *Anesth Analg* 1997; 84(6):1262–8.
44. Loftus JR, Hill H, Cohen SE. Placental transfer and neonatal effects of epidural sufentanil and fentanyl administered with bupivacaine during labor. *Anesthesiology* 1995; 83(2):300–8.
45. Volikas I, Butwick A, Wilkinson C, *et al.* Maternal and neonatal side-effects of remifentanil patient-controlled analgesia in labour. *Br J Anaesth* 2005; 95(4):504–9.
46. Kan RE, Hughes SC, Rosen MA, *et al.* Intravenous remifentanil: placental transfer, maternal and neonatal effects. *Anesthesiology* 1998; 88(6):1467–74.
47. Kopecky EA, Simone C, Knie B, *et al.* Transfer of morphine across the human placenta and its interaction with naloxone. *Life Sci* 1999; 65(22):2359–71.
48. Moya F, Kvisselgaard N. The placental transmission of succinylcholine. *Anesthesiology* 1961; 22:1–6.
49. Iwama H, Kaneko T, Tobishima S, *et al.* Time dependency of the ratio of umbilical vein/maternal artery concentrations of vecuronium in caesarean section. *Acta Anaesthesiol Scand* 1999; 43(1):9–12.
50. Johnson RF, Cahana A, Olenick M, *et al.* A comparison of the placental transfer of ropivacaine versus bupivacaine. *Anesth Analg* 1999; 89(3):703–8.
51. Kuhnert PM, Kuhnert BR, Stitts JM, *et al.* The use of a selected ion monitoring technique to study the disposition of bupivacaine in mother, fetus, and neonate following epidural anesthesia for cesarean section. *Anesthesiology* 1981; 55(6):611–17.
52. Kuhnert BR, Zuspan KJ, Kuhnert PM, *et al.* Bupivacaine disposition in mother, fetus, and neonate after spinal anesthesia for cesarean section. *Anesth Analg* 1987; 66(5):407–12.
53. Wood M, Wood AJ. Changes in plasma drug binding and alpha 1-acid glycoprotein in mother and newborn infant. *Clin Pharmacol Ther* 1981; 29(4):522–6.
54. Biehl D, Shnider SM, Levinson G, Callender K. Placental transfer of lidocaine: effects of fetal acidosis. *Anesthesiology* 1978; 48(6):409–12.

CHAPTER 4

Fetal and neonatal physiology

Thierry Girard and Thomas Erb

Fetal growth

Fetal development can be divided into different stages. During the embryonic period, which consists of the first 8 weeks, development of all major organ systems begins and crown–rump length (CRL) of the embryo is approximately 3 cm. The most accurate assessment of gestational age is by first-trimester ultrasound measurement of CRL (Tables 4.1 and 4.2).[1,2] The embryonic period is followed by the fetal period which is characterized by rapid body growth and differentiation of tissues and organ systems. Increase in weight and length is especially high during the third trimester as body stores of protein, fat, iron, and calcium are considerably enlarged.[3]

Overall, growth represents an interaction of genetic, epigenetic, and environmental factors, and endocrine and nutritional factors appear to be of critical importance. Exposure to teratogens *in utero* as well as antenatal illnesses and exposure to hazardous substances can have a negative influence on growth and development. Phases of growth occur within specific time intervals, affecting cell division and differentiation. Before and after birth, growth is mainly promoted by insulin-like growth factor 1 (IGF-1). Postnatal growth is dependent on growth and thyroid hormones.

Growth rate is highest during fetal life. Postnatally it is most pronounced directly after birth. The full-term infant adjusts growth to achieve a growth rate that will be followed for most of their childhood.

Respiratory system

The fetal lung

Developmental stages

Fetal lung development undergoes different stages, starting with the pseudoglandular period (5–16 weeks' gestation) where branching morphogenesis begins with the left and right main bronchi being formed out of the two bronchial buds. The two main bronchi then divide into secondary bronchi, which in turn continue branching into segmental and then terminal bronchi.[4] By 16 weeks, around 22 orders of branching airways are in place and major blood vessels have developed. In the canalicular period (16–26 weeks' gestation) each terminal bronchus dissects into at least two respiratory bronchioles, which consequently divide into three to six alveolar ducts. During this phase, blood supply steadily increases and a rapidly increasing number of capillaries are formed in the mesenchyme surrounding the airways. Towards the end of the canalicular period, differentiation of epithelial cells into types I and II begins. Type II epithelial cells produce surfactant, a phospholipid-rich fluid, which aids in reducing surface tension at the air–alveolar barrier.[3,5] The large majority of epithelial cells, however, thin out as type I epithelial cells. In the mature lung, these are flat cells that are part of the alveolar–capillary membrane, the blood–air barrier. By the end of the canalicular period the alveolar–capillary membrane is developed to such an extent as to enable gas exchange.

In the terminal sac or saccular period (24 weeks' gestation until birth), terminal sacs are formed as primitive alveoli. Due to their rapid maturation, fetal lungs reach a state by the 28th week of gestation where sufficient gas exchange in the primitive alveoli is possible in order for the premature infant to survive. With birth, however, lung development is not terminated, around 50 million alveoli (merely one-sixth of the alveoli found in the adult) are already developed.[6] During the alveolar period, which starts in the last few weeks of pregnancy and includes the first years after birth, the number of terminal sacs continues to grow. Millions of new primitive alveoli continually develop, which grow into respiratory bronchioles and eventually mature alveoli. The blood–air barrier continues to mature over the following years which leads to a significant gain of surface area. The large majority of primitive alveoli (around 85–90%) are formed during the first half year of life and the adult quantity of around 300 million alveoli is nearly reached at 18 months.[6] Lung growth goes on for approximately 15 more years until the chest is fully grown.

Fetal lung fluid

The fetal lung is filled with fetal lung fluid (FLF) which consists of a high chloride concentration, some protein, mucus from bronchial glands, and surfactant. It keeps the fetal lungs distended and can be thought of as a frame around which especially distal parts of the lungs can develop. Quantity and secretion rate of FLF increases with continuous growth of the fetus.[7] Volume is kept within physiological limits through distending pressure generated by liquid secretion and resistance to liquid efflux through the larynx.[8] The secreted liquid is passively moved into the trachea and oropharynx, where it is either swallowed by the fetus or released into the amniotic cavity.[3] FLF is an essential prerequisite for normal lung growth.

Changes at birth

A reduction of liquid secretion can start in the days preceding delivery and is intensified during labour[9,10] Removal of FLF occurs through a combination of mechanical drainage and liquid absorption across the lung epithelium. Only a small amount of fluid is thought to be expelled during birth.[11] Epithelial transcellular sodium channels are expressed, which drive liquid from the lumen into the interstitial space.[7] From there, pulmonary blood

Table 4.1 Crown–rump length (CRL) measured by ultrasound. Values are median, as well as 5th and 95th percentile

Gestational age (days)	CRL mean (mm)	CRL 5th/95th percentile
50	10	5/15
60	20	15/25
70	30	25/35
80	50	40/55
90	65	55/75
100	80	75/90

Reproduced with permission from Pexsters A, Daemen A, Bottomley C, Van Schoubroeck D, De Catte L, De Moor B *et al.*, New crown-rump length curve based on over 3500 pregnancies, *Ultrasound in Obstetrics and Gynaecology*, Volume 35, Issue 6, pp. 650–655, Copyright © 2010 John Wiley and Sons.

and lymph capillaries start resorbing most of the fluid. These mechanisms are activated by a raise in perinatal epinephrine, vasopressin, cortisol, and aldosterone levels characteristic for labour and delivery.[12]

Partial pressure of oxygen (PO_2) ranges from 23 to 25 mmHg (3.0–3.3 kPa) before birth and augments to about 100 mmHg postnatally. This causes an acceleration of active liquid absorption. In the term infant, all lung fluid is absorbed after 2 hours of spontaneous breathing.[7] Premature infants can have difficulties with liquid removal and infants born by elective caesarean delivery are at increased risk for postnatal respiratory problems.[13]

Surfactant

Pulmonary surfactant reduces surface tension at the physicochemical boundary between respiratory gases and respiratory epithelium in the lungs. Surfactant, which is synthesized, stored and secreted by type II alveolar epithelial cells, mainly consists of phospholipids as well as some proteins and carbohydrates.[14] Morphology of type II cells changes significantly in late gestation and surfactant production increases.[3]

Corticosteroids

Antenatal corticosteroids have been given to women at risk for preterm labour for almost 40 years. Dexamethasone and betamethasone are most commonly used and show similar results (reduction of respiratory distress syndrome and intraventricular haemorrhage). Usually two doses are administered 24 or 12 hours apart. A repeat dose of betamethasone administered to women who remain at increased risk for early birth may be beneficial.[15,16]

Glucocorticoids influence gene expression and lead to gluconeogenesis, lipolysis, and proteolysis and are immunosuppressive. In the fetal lung, protein and phospholipid synthesis are accelerated and production of surfactant is stimulated.[17] There is, however, also an influence on antioxidant enzyme production, FLF absorption, and development of the lung.[18]

Table 4.2 Table of fetal growth. Values are the 50th percentile (P10/P90)

Gestational age (weeks)	Weight (kg)	Length (cm)	Head circumference (cm)
24	0.65 (0.55/0.8)	32 (29/34.5)	22 (20.5/23.5)
28	1.15 (0.8/1.4)	38 (34.5/40.5)	26.5 (24.5/28)
32	1.85 (1.4/2.25)	43 (40/46)	30 (28/31.5)
36	2.8 (2.25/3.3)	47 (44.5/50)	33 (31/35)
40	3.6 (2.9/4.25)	51 (48.5/54)	35.5 (33.5/37.5)
44	4.3 (3.5/5.05)	54 (51.5/57.5)	37.5 (25.5/39.5)

Data from Fenton TR. A new growth chart for preterm babies: Babson and Benda's chart updated with recent data and a new format. *BMC Pediatrics*, 2003; 3:13.

Oxygen transport

Fetal oxygen transport

Fetal haemoglobin F (HbF) has a substantially higher affinity for oxygen when compared to adult haemoglobin (HbA). Fetal oxygenation occurs via the umbilical vein following placental diffusion of oxygen. The PO_2 pressure gradient directly affects mitochondrial oxygen uptake. As gestation progresses, fetal blood oxygen affinity is gradually reduced and 2,3-diphosphoglycerate (DPG) levels rise. Near-term erythropoiesis synthesizes mainly HbA. At term, HbA constitutes one-quarter of total haemoglobin.

Changes at birth

After birth, PO_2 increases significantly to values of 80 mmHg and higher and at the same time neonatal metabolism and muscle activity lead to a substantial increase in oxygen consumption. A radical change in oxygen-carrying parameters is needed. Haemoglobin oxygen affinity quickly decreases. This is partly caused by an increase of 2,3-DPG levels. P_{50} (the oxygen tension at which Hb is 50% saturated), which is at 19.4 mmHg on the first postnatal day, increases to adult values of around 27 mmHg within the first 4–6 months. HbF is continually replaced with HbA and by 12 months, HbF is reduced to 2% of total haemoglobin.[3] Low-birth-weight preterm infants have lower 2,3-DPG concentrations, lower P_{50}, and higher Hb F levels, resulting in a smaller oxygen-unloading capacity.

Control of breathing

Fetal breathing movements

The traditional belief was that breathing begins after birth, but breathing movements are already in place long before birth. Fetal breathing movements occur in episodes of rapid eye movement (REM) sleep; they are irregular and end abruptly. During fetal breathing movements, the laryngeal abductor muscles are simultaneously activated.[19] Respiratory movements stimulate lung development and condition respiratory muscles.[20] Fetal breathing movements may also serve to sustain FLF volumes and consequently help uphold the degree of lung expansion needed for normal lung growth.[21]

Spontaneous breathing

The mechanisms that initiate spontaneous breathing at birth are unknown. The widespread opinion has long been that labour and delivery cause transient fetal hypoxaemia. This was thought to stimulate peripheral chemoreceptors and consequently lead to an induction of extrauterine continuous breathing. Breathing was then thought to be continued postpartum through a series of other stimuli such as low temperatures and touch.[22] Later studies, however, have refuted this theory. Neither chemoreceptors[23] nor sensory stimuli have any influence. Breathing can already be initiated *in utero* through cord occlusion or by raising arterial PO_2.[24]

Neonatal breathing

Irregularities in breathing pattern frequently occur in neonates and especially in preterm infants.[25,26] During periodic breathing, phases of normal breathing alternate with apnoeic episodes of 5–10 seconds.[27] In term infants, periodic breathing is of no concern, as respiratory pauses are short and usually only cause a negligible decrease in heart rate. Apnoea, however, can lead to significant bradycardia especially in small preterm infants. Sleep state has a modulatory effect on quality of breathing. There are four different sleep states: quiet, REM, transitional, and indeterminate. Neonates spend around 30% of total sleep in the three phases of quiet, REM, and indeterminate sleep. With ageing, the percentage of REM sleep decreases and quiet sleep increases. During a REM sleep period, breathing can be completely irregular, leading to lower PO_2 values and hyperactive peripheral chemoreceptors.[28] Periodic breathing can be seen as a marker for apnoea, particularly in REM sleep. In healthy preterm infants, apnoea is most commonly of central origin but obstruction may contribute in a minority of cases.[29,30]

Cardiovascular system

Fetal circulation

Vascular development sets off early after gastrulation. Following differentiation and development of endothelial cell populations, two different processes are involved in blood vessel formation: vasculogenesis (*de novo* organization of blood vessels) and angiogenesis (remodelling and sprouting of pre-existing vessels.) Remodelling and maturation are mediated by molecular signals, influenced by many factors including hypoxaemia and haemodynamic forces.

Fetal circulation is unique in several aspects: on one side the fetus is connected to the placenta by two umbilical arteries and one umbilical vein. Oxygenated blood gets to the fetus via the umbilical vein and desaturated blood returns to the placenta via the umbilical arteries. On the other side, fetal circulation is characterized by three shunts, the ductus venosus, the oval foramen, and the ductus arteriosus, all serving to supply oxygen-sensitive organs (i.e. the brain and myocardium) with highly oxygenated blood (Figure 4.1).

Most of the blood from the umbilical vein bypasses the liver through the ductus venosus directly into the inferior vena cava. Only a small proportion of total blood flow goes into the liver passing the sinusoids and mixing with blood from the portal circulation. Of note, a sphincter mechanism located at the junction of the umbilical vein to the ductus venosus regulates the blood flow to the liver sinusoids. Furthermore, this mechanism is also of importance in the prevention of a sudden cardiac volume overload, as it closes if venous return following a uterine contraction is significantly increased. In the inferior vena cava, oxygen-rich blood blends with desaturated blood returning from the lower extremity and passing into the right atrium. In the heart, the majority of this blood passes through the oval foramen, an interatrial connection located in the atrial septum, to the left atrium and then left ventricle to be ejected in the ascending aorta. As the carotids and the coronary arteries are the first to diverge from the aortic arch, their areas of supply are best supplied with oxygen.

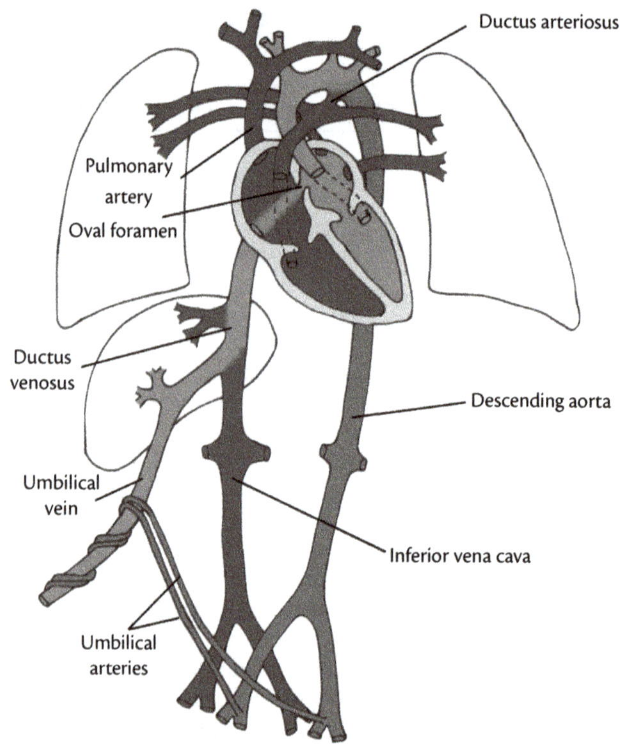

Figure 4.1 (See colour figure section). The fetal circulation before birth. Fetal circulation is characterized by three shunts: (1) ductus venosus, (2) oval foramen, and (3) ductus arteriosus. Blood flow is directed to bypass the liver in the ductus venosus. From the right atrium oxygenated blood flows through the oval foramen into the left atrium, left ventricle, and into the aorta.

The third shunt, the ductus arteriosus, is a blood vessel connecting the pulmonary artery with the aortic arch. Because pulmonary vessels in the fetus have a high resistance, most of the blood from the right ventricle bypasses the not yet functioning lungs directly to the aorta. Only a small fraction of the blood circulates through the lungs and returns via pulmonary veins to the left atrium. In the umbilical vein, the oxygen saturation of the placental blood is about 80%. This high saturation is progressively reduced as this blood progresses through the fetal circulation mixing with desaturated blood in several places, first in the liver from blood returning from the portal system, then as previously mentioned, further mixing with deoxygenated blood takes place in the inferior vena cava as well as in both atria and finally at the border where the ductus arteriosus merges with the aortic arch. Blood returning to the placenta in the umbilical arteries has a saturation of about 55–60%.

Blood pressure

Blood pressure is maintained within a physiological range by neural, hormonal, and metabolic mechanisms interacting locally and in particular on a central level.[31] A variety of peripheral sensors (arterial baroreceptors, chemoreceptors to measure PO_2, PCO_2, and pH, and mechanoreceptors to measure changes in blood volume) constantly monitor blood circulation and modulate the release of vasoactive hormones and autonomic tone to the heart and the blood vessels.[32] Reflex arcs are integrated in central nervous cardiovascular centres. These mechanisms can already be found in the fetus and subsequently in the neonate. However, the newborn's capability to maintain adequate blood pressure and blood flow to the organs can be impaired if maturation is incomplete.[3]

Arterial baroreflex

Arterial baroreceptors sense changes in vascular stretch in correlation to arterial pressure. This information is transmitted to the central nervous system, where parasympathetic and sympathetic activity is regulated.[31] Activation of the autonomic nervous system influences heart rate, contractility, peripheral vascular resistance, and effectively regulates arterial pressure oscillations.

Resets of the baroreflex to higher pressures arise at several occasions in the development (*in utero*, immediately after birth, and postnatally with increasing maturation) characterized by changes of the relationships of the arterial pressure—heart rate and of the pressure—sympathetic/parasympathetic nerve activities.[33,34]

Cardiopulmonary reflex

Cardiopulmonary mechanoreceptors located in the four cardiac chambers, the great veins, and in the lungs respond to changes in blood volume by eliciting reflexes with effects on systemic haemodynamics. However, variations of total body water and intra- and extracellular fluid composition are large during fetal development and in the newborn.[35] This also affects the sensitivity of the cardiopulmonary baroreflex which also remains immature in the neonate.[3]

Peripheral chemoreflex responses

Peripheral chemoreceptors are functional in the fetus and neonate. However, sensitivity and activity are reduced directly after delivery. This condition persists for the first postpartum days until an adaptation and resetting to higher oxygen tension levels takes place.

Sympathetic nervous system

The sympathetic nervous system is considerably activated at birth, accompanied by a significant release of catecholamines.[36,37] This contributes to a number of haemodynamic changes, in particular heart rate, peripheral vascular resistance, and redistribution of blood flow.[38] Lung inflation and increased arterial oxygen tensions appear to have a negligible effect[39] whereas the change of ambient temperature that occurs at birth has been shown to induce sympathoexcitatory responses.[40]

Humoral influences

The renin–angiotensin system is of importance during early intrauterine development, primarily influencing organogenesis.[41] With ongoing maturation, the predominant role is the adjustment of cardiovascular and renal parameters. Of note, renin plasma activity is highest during the first month of life, decreases significantly during the first year, and continues to decrease until adulthood.[42] Prematurely born children show considerably high activity levels which correlate inversely with postconceptual age. It remains obscure why renin activity is higher in young infants. Corticosteroids are essential for an infant's normal development. Endogenously produced cortisol is vital in facilitating changes in autonomic and baroreflex functions during maturation. Adrenal steroids have been shown to have a significant effect on blood pressure[43] and fetal exposure to exogenous glucocorticoids increases arterial blood pressure significantly affecting autonomic and endocrine control of cardiovascular function[44,45] which may persist after exposure. Nitric oxide (NO) is of importance in regulating fetal blood pressure and organ-specific vascular resistance. Acute blockade of endogenous NO production instantly leads to an increase of blood pressure and umbilico-placental resistance and consecutively decreases heart rate, renal blood flow velocity, and plasma renin concentration.[46]

Changes at birth

With birth, a series of alterations transform the fetal circulation into the mature pattern dividing circulation into separate pulmonary and systemic components.

Closure of ductus arteriosus

The process of closure of the ductus arteriosus starts almost directly after birth. There are two consecutive steps to the closing process. First, 'functional' closure takes place when the lumen is closed through constriction of smooth muscle in the first hours after birth.[3] This process is induced amongst other factors by an increase in arterial PO_2, a decrease in blood pressure caused by the decrease in pulmonary vascular resistance, and a decrease in prostaglandin E_2 (PGE_2) and quantity of PGE_2 receptors.[47] Over the course of the next few days, 'anatomical' closure takes place by a remodelling of the vascular walls. This includes thickening of the intima and loss of smooth muscle cells in the inner muscle media.[3] Complete obliteration takes at approximately 1–3 months, the obliterated ductus forms the ligamentum arteriosum.

Persistent ductus arteriosus

In 50% of term babies, the ductus arteriosus closes within the first 24 hours, and in almost all cases, closure has occurred within 3 days of birth. A persistent ductus arteriosus (PDA) is more commonly observed in preterm babies, especially in those with severe respiratory distress.[3] Here the down-regulation of PGE_2 receptors is reduced and local vasodilatory effects of PGE_2 persist.[3] Other factors that increase the risk of PDA are late-onset septicaemia,[48] small size for gestational age,[49] or excessive administration of fluid during first days of life.[50] Infants that are not caucasian or were given glucocorticoids before birth are less prone to be affected by PDA.[51,52]

Closure of oval foramen

With closure of the ductus arteriosus blood flow in the lungs increases heavily, consequently leading to an increased pressure in the left atrium. At the same time, the pressure in the right atrium decreases. In combination with an infant's first breath this results in the oval foramen's septum primum being pressed against the septum secundum, resulting in a functional closure. Physiologically, the oval foramen is permanently obliterated after about 1 year through fusion of the two septa. In about 20%, complete obliteration does not occur, resulting in a patent foramen ovale.

Closure of umbilical vessels and ductus venosus

Umbilical vessels are highly vasoactive and able to constrict so effectively that blood flow may become completely impaired. During normal conditions *in utero*, the umbilical vessels predominantly remain in a state of almost complete relaxation in order to guarantee an adequate supply to the fetus.[3] Within the first minute after birth, blood flow is already reduced to less than 20% of normal fetal values. Similar to the closure of the ductus arteriosus, the umbilical arteries close shortly after birth through contraction of the smooth musculature in the vessel walls. Closure is thought to be mediated by a combination of different stimuli. These include thermal and mechanical parameters and a shift in oxygen tension, which then influence vasoactive agents such as bradykinin or serotonin.[53,54] Locally produced substances such as serotonin or mechanical stretching might also be responsible for closure.[54] Permanent obliteration by fibrous proliferation occurs around 2–3 months after birth. In the neonate, proximal parts of the umbilical arteries convert to the superior vesical arteries and distal sections become the medial umbilical ligaments. Closure of the umbilical vein and the ductus venosus take place briefly after that of the umbilical arteries. The obliterated umbilical vein transforms into the ligamentum teres hepatis and the obliterated ductus venosus forms the ligamentum venosum.

Integumentary system

The skin is a complex organ with many critically important functions, some of which include maintaining fluid homeostasis, temperature regulation, and sensation. It acts as a physical barrier between the inside of the body and its environment and serves to protect an organism against possibly threatening surroundings. Besides its barrier functions it also serves as an indispensable tool in social interactions, behavioural communication, and perception.[55]

Epidermal barrier

The most outward layer, the stratum corneum, has numerous protective purposes such as ultraviolet light protection, mechanical integrity and resilience, water proofing and repellency, permeability barrier, hydration, antioxidant and xenobiote defence, and cytokine signalling.[56,57] Its unique composition is due to structural proteins and ceramides that are covalently cross-linked. Together they form a cornified envelope which is insoluble and highly complex in order to fulfil all the above-mentioned functions.[58] The stratum corneum is formed by the end of the sixth month of gestation. Epithelial surfaces are predominantly generated towards the end of gestation; their development is highly coordinated and undergoes many structural and functional changes. Antenatal exposure to hormones, for example, glucocorticoids administered to the mother, can influence these processes,[59] as can premature birth, where the stratum corneum is inadequately formed.[60] The epidermal barrier is often dysfunctional in very low-birth-weight preterm infants.

Vernix caseosa

In utero, the fetus is in a completely aqueous environment and is covered with vernix caseosa as a protective layer.[61] This complex proteolipid cellular cream has a waterproofing effect.[62] Vernix caseosa is created during the last trimester of gestation by sebaceous glands and communicates with the developing epidermis.[63]

Changes at birth

The skin's protective role is particularly apparent perinatally when a fetus undergoes the transition from the warm, wet atmosphere of the womb to the much cooler, dry, non-sterile outside world full of physical, chemical, and mechanical threats. Suddenly, the infant is exposed to high oxidative stress and ultraviolet light and must accomplish multiple mechanisms, such as thermoregulation, that were not needed before birth and were carried out by the placenta.

Temperature control

In utero, fetal temperature is approximately half a degree higher than maternal temperature with heat produced by biochemical processes only.[3] At this point, fetal thermogenesis is suppressed and excess fetal heat is eliminated either by conduction or, in much greater part (85%), by convection through blood vessels to the placenta.[64] Thermoregulatory processes develop quite early in embryogenesis. Preterm babies born as early as 25 weeks' gestation are capable of thermogenesis; however, this is not as effective as in term babies.[65]

At birth, thermogenesis is immediately activated, triggered by heat loss due to lower ambient temperatures and evaporation of amniotic fluid from the skin. Mode of delivery influences thermoregulatory processes, as lower body temperatures of around 0.3°C are seen in term infants born by caesarean delivery.[66] Mechanisms of thermogenesis can be divided into three: shivering of skeletal muscle, non-shivering thermogenesis in brown adipose tissue (BAT), and futile cycling of ions in specialized heat-producing tissues. Non-shivering thermogenesis is most significant in the neonate. Shivering can be considered as a secondary measure, a backup system for substantial hypothermia. BAT is mainly located around the kidneys, in the interscapular area of the back and on the dorsal neck. Heat is generated on the basis that energy from mitochondrial respiration is not stored as ATP but given off as heat. BAT growth and activation are regulated by a number of hormonal and nervous components.[67] Central homeothermic mechanisms are generally not well developed at birth and call for processes regulated by the autonomous nervous system such as eccrine sweating, vasodilatation, and vasoconstriction, which also need time to develop.[3] Preterm infants are even more in danger of extensive heat loss due to several reasons. They have a higher surface area to mass ratio, lower endogenous sources of heat generation such as BAT, a limited epidermal barrier, and are unable to self-regulate with flexural positioning.

Acid mantle

Human skin is physiologically covered by an acid mantle, which serves as a defence against microorganisms and helps preserve the skin's barrier function. In the newborn, skin surface pH is in a neutral range and then continually becomes more acidic over the following few weeks. Mechanisms that induce this transition are thought to include active proton pump mechanisms and endogenous factors such as lactic acid from sweat, free fatty acid generation from metabolism of triglycerides in sebum, as well as metabolic by-products of bacterial colonization.

Bacterial colonization

As the infant is no longer in the sterile environment of the uterus, skin also needs to function as a barrier against infection.

Colonization of the skin begins as soon as the infant has its first contact with the outside world.[68] The process which leads to colonization is not entirely understood. What has been shown, however, is that there is an interaction between development of the acid mantle, local microenvironmental factors, as well as microorganism growth rate. Skin care practices and products also influence colonization. In vaginally born infants, the skin is swiftly colonized with *Staphylococcus epidermidis*, the most common vaginal organism before birth and also omnipresent in the environment.[69] After a few weeks, an infant's resident bacterial flora is very similar to that of the adult and characterized as non-virulent and consistent in quantity. In very low-birth-weight preterm infants, physiological colonization may overwhelm protective capabilities; *S. epidermidis* is the most frequent cause of nosocomial sepsis.

Metabolism

Fluid homeostasis

Postnatal adaptation induces large shifts in body fluids. In early gestation, total body water (TBW) makes up around 95% of total body weight. TBW gradually decreases during development and reaches 75% at term (Figure 4.2).[35]

TBW can be divided into intra- and extracellular volume. During the early stage of gestation, growth primarily occurs through cell division and therefore extracellular volume is very large. This leads to tissues with small cells encircled by an extensive layer of extracellular fluid. Extracellular volume decreases during the course of gestation due to a reduction of hyaluronan content, which has a high water-binding capacity. Meanwhile, intracellular volume increases with physiological growth of the existing cells during the second half of gestation.[35]

The distribution of fluids is determined by the equilibrium across the capillary membrane as well as by the balance between capillary permeability and lymphatic function. The fetus and neonate have low intravascular hydrostatic and oncotic pressures,[70] high permeability of the capillary wall, and high lymphatic flow compared to the adult. When compared to adults, the interstitial space of the fetus is larger.[3]

Blood volume

Due to the volume of blood in the umbilical cord and the fetal side of the placenta, the fetus has a significantly larger blood volume when compared to the neonate. Total placentofetal blood volume at term is around 120 mL/kg, with 70 mL/kg in the fetus and 50 mL/kg being located in the placenta and umbilical cord.[71]

Changes at birth

Uterine contractions during labour and delivery lead to a shift of fluids from the plasma to interstitial compartments with a concomitant decrease in total plasma volume. The contractions lead to a direct compression of the fetus,[72] which results in an increase in blood pressure and a reduction of circulating blood volume. Vasoactive hormones such as vasopressin, norepinephrine, cortisol, and atrial natriuretic peptide are also involved and have been reported to be at increased concentrations in the umbilical cord after vaginal delivery.[3] Severe hypoxia can induce a reduction in blood volume with a translocation of blood from the placenta to the fetus.[73] The increase in blood volume causes an increased capillary pressure which in turn leads to a higher transcapillary filtration of fluid.

Placental transfusion is the most important factor to influence blood and plasma volume during the first postnatal days.[71] Obviously gravity is an important contributing factor and the

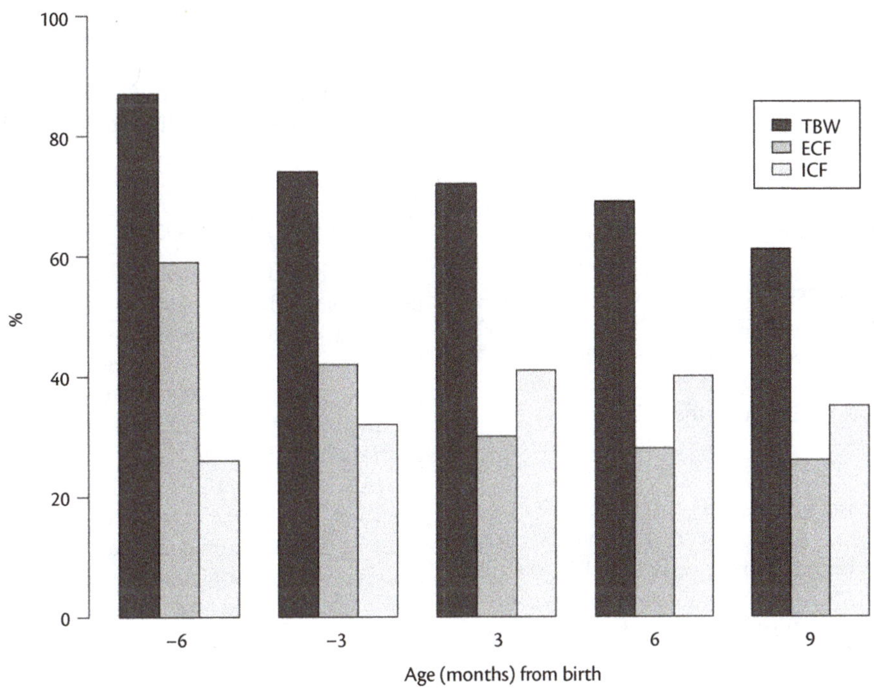

Figure 4.2 Distribution of body water for total body water (TBW), extracellular fluid (ECF), and intracellular fluid (ICF).

Data from Friis-Hansen B. Body water compartments in children: changes during growth and related changes in body composition, *Pediatrics* 1961; 28:169–81, Copyright © 1961 American Academy of Pediatrics.

position of the neonate relative to the placenta before cord clamping is of great importance for fetoplacental or placentofetal transfusions. Further contributing factors are maternal hypotension, cord compression, and caesarean delivery. Placentofetal transfusion is promoted by intrauterine asphyxia, uterine contractions, and increases in maternal uterine blood flow.[71] Timing of umbilical cord clamping critically influences neonatal blood volume. Clamping the cord directly after birth leads to a haematocrit between 0.48 and 0.51.[74] If the cord is not clamped immediately, however, and the infant is held at or below level of the placenta, there is a gradual placentofetal transfusion.[71,74] Haematocrit measured 30–120 minutes after birth is then at 0.60–0.65. Placental transfusion causes neonatal blood pressure, central venous pressure, renal blood flow and urine flow to increase and can be used therapeutically.[71] There is a reduced incidence of anaemia in early infancy in term infants and in preterm babies severity of respiratory distress syndrome, incidence of intraventricular haemorrhage, late-onset sepsis, and the need for blood transfusions is also reduced.[75–77]

In the days after birth, a weight loss of approximately 10% is normal in healthy term infants because extracellular fluid is further reduced. In low- and extremely low-birth-weight neonates weight loss is even larger.

Kidneys

Nephrogenesis undergoes different stages including a primitive kidney, the pronephros, an intermediate kidney, the mesonephros, and finally the permanent kidney, the metanephros. Renal development is completed by 34 weeks' gestation. Urine flow, renal blood flow, and glomerular filtration rate (GFR) continually increase during the second half of gestation.[78]

In utero, fetal homeostasis is mainly regulated by the placenta. During the third trimester, fetal renal function becomes more important. Function is regulated by endocrine, paracrine, and autocrine factors, and relative maturation of these determinants correlate with renal function.[3]

Changes at birth

A reduction in renal blood flow and GFR in neonates when compared to adults has to be considered especially in pharmacokinetics of renally excreted drugs.[79] Renal vascular resistance decreases immediately after birth, which leads to a continuous increase in renal blood flow. While kidneys in the fetus receive less than 5% of cardiac output, the percentage increases in the neonate to 15%. The low GFR of 5 mL/min at term increases rapidly after birth and is dependent on gestational age. It takes months for very low-birth-weight infants to achieve a normal GFR.[80]

Liver

The liver is the largest internal organ and its functions can be categorized as synthesis and secretion of serum proteins, energy metabolism, and bile secretion. During early fetal life, the liver also has a haematopoietic function which decreases towards the end of gestation. Hepatocytes mature very early and are functional as early as the second month of gestation.[81]

Changes at birth

Bilirubin is an intermediate product of haem catabolism. After hepatic conjugation it is excreted via bile and urine. Bilirubin production is higher in the neonate than in adults, and even more so in the preterm infant.[82] Conjugation and excretion, however, are less efficient due to downregulation, which leads to physiologically elevated plasma bilirubin levels during the first week of life. Jaundice is the clinical sign of hyperbilirubinaemia and visible at the skin, sclera, and mucous membranes. Unlike adults and older children, where icterus is present at bilirubin levels of 2–3 mg/dL, the concentration can increase to above 5 mg/dL in the neonate before clinical signs become visible. Jaundice can be the only indication of hepatic dysfunction, and may precede kernicterus which can lead to brain injury and must therefore be quickly identified and treated.

Glucose

In utero, fetal gluconeogenesis is virtually non-existent and the fetus is completely supplied via the placenta.[83] There is a substantial postpartum change in plasma concentration of glucoregulatory hormones. Plasma concentration of epinephrine, norepinephrine, and glucagon increase rapidly, while insulin levels decrease.[37] In the first hour after birth, plasma glucose levels reach a nadir. The subsequent rise in glucose levels reaches a plateau between 2 and 4 hours af.[84] Glucose levels partly depend on glucose intake during labour and delivery.[85] A healthy term neonate has plasma glucose levels that range between 2.2 and 4.5 mmol/L (40 and 80 mg/dL). As soon as feeding starts, glucose levels increase slightly.

Hypoglycaemia is most common during the neonatal period, particularly in the first 12–24 hours after birth. Detection and rapid treatment of hypoglycaemia are very important as failure to do so may have serious consequences. Glucose is the brain's prime energy source and lack of it can cause seizures and, if it is prolonged, permanent brain damage. There is no consensus as to what level or duration of hypoglycaemia can be determined to cause cerebral damage.[86] Hypoglycaemia is also a leading symptom of many endocrine disorders and inborn errors of metabolism, which need to be specifically diagnosed and treated.

Various clinical signs can point to hypoglycaemia including lethargy, somnolence, poor feeding, respiratory distress, apnoea, cyanotic episodes, sweating, staring spells, myoclonic jerks, and seizures.

Sensory and nervous system

Human brain development is the result of extraordinary complex processes regulated by genetic and epigenetic factors. The developmental sequence transforms a discal accumulation of undifferentiated tissue into a neuronal network capable of storing and processing a vast amount of information.

Functionally, the developing brain is considerably determined by the operational state of chemical synaptic connections between neurons. As a result of this, the biochemical features of neurotransmission may differ markedly during development. This may result in differing functional balances of multineuronal networks at different ages. At birth, the vitally important centres are functioning with limited reserve.

Pain perception

(See also Chapter 7.)

According to the International Subcommittee for the Study of Pain, pain is defined as 'an unpleasant sensory and emotional response associated with actual or potential tissue damage, or described in terms of such damage'.[87] Pain perception is dependent on nociception, which is a sensory component that is neurophysiologically determined, and emotion, which is influenced by affective state, past experience, and development.[88] Historically there was a belief that a neonate did not feel pain due to immaturity of the nervous system.[88] Therefore invasive procedures and surgery were generally undertaken without pain relief or anaesthesia. More recently, neonatal pain research has shown, however, that the neonate is fully capable of experiencing pain.[89,90] There is also evidence that a fetus may be able to respond to painful stimuli.[91] Prevention or treatment of pain leads to better outcomes and fewer undesirable long- and short-term effects.[92] Nevertheless, this discussion was revived with the latest research in anaesthesia-induced neuroapoptosis.[93]

The basic mechanisms of fetal and neonatal pain perception correlate well with adult pain perception: noxious stimuli to peripheral sensory nociceptors are transmitted to sensory areas of the cerebral cortex via the spinal cord neurons. Nonetheless, differences based on immaturity of anatomical, physiological, and chemical parameters of the nervous system exist.

By the 20th week of gestation, cutaneous nociceptors are fully formed throughout the fetus[94] and at the end of gestation the density of nociceptors is similar to that in adults. The cutaneous withdrawal reflex, development of pain pathways of the spinal cord and brainstem, and facial responses to painful stimuli can be demonstrated as early as 24 weeks' gestation.[95] Early in gestation, substance P is the primary afferent nociceptive neurotransmitter. Pain sensitivity in the neonate might be higher than in later life because of lower pain thresholds, poor discriminative abilities, and augmented tendencies to sensitization (e.g. poorly developed descending inhibitory pathways).

Markers associated with pain

Pain provokes a palette of reactions from the cardiovascular, respiratory, endocrine, metabolic, and immune system. Typically, heart rate and blood pressure increase, large fluctuations in transcutaneous oxygen tension arise, and a stress response is visible.[96] The term stress response describes hormonal and metabolic changes associated with trauma.[97,98] Pituitary, pancreatic, and adrenal hormones are released, which leads to a shift in metabolic balance.[97] There are also behavioural signs which indicate that the neonate is in pain. Responses are divided into four groups: simple motor responses, such as flexion and adduction of extremities; complex behavioural responses, such as altered sleep–wake cycles and irritability; facial expressions; and crying. There are specific expressions associated with pain, which become more distinctive as the infant ages.[99] Crying in response to pain is different from other crying behaviour and can be identified due to specific characteristics and acoustic qualities.[100]

Pain assessment

Pain assessment in infants is challenging due to the lack of direct verbal communication and absence of validated quantitative methods of measurement.[101,102] It is best to use a multidimensional approach such as the Bernese Pain Scale for Neonates.[103]

Effects of pain

Exposure to pain in the neonate may have long-term effects: the normal maturation of pain pathways is likely to be altered, and neuronal survival might be impaired by repetitive pain.[104] Cortisol levels stay elevated and changed behavioural and physiological reactivity to painful stimuli later in life have been demonstrated. This is especially the case in extremely low-birth-weight infants.[105] These are all argument supporting an adequate level of anaesthesia and analgesia in case of fetal or neonatal surgery. As previously mentioned, research in the field of anaesthesia-induced neuroapoptosis is growing.[106] Initial studies in rodents have been expanded to other species, such as primates.[107] It is far too early to draw firm conclusions about the clinical consequences of anaesthesia-induced neuronal-induced effects in the developing human being. Nevertheless, this is a topic which clearly needs further research and conclusions at this point include that unnecessary interventions must be avoided (at least in the developing brain) because we do currently not have alternatives[108] to performing anaesthesia in neonates undergoing surgical interventions.

Conclusion

In conclusion, this chapter demonstrates the complexity of fetal and neonatal physiology with a focus on the complex transition from intra- to extrauterine life. In essence, this transition involves every organ system and knowledge of the most important aspects is a prerequisite to understanding pathophysiology of this transition.

References

1. Pexsters A, Daemen A, Bottomley C, *et al.* New crown-rump length curve based on over 3500 pregnancies. *Ultrasound Obstet Gynecol* 2010; 35:650–5.
2. Fenton TR. A new growth chart for preterm babies: Babson and Benda's chart updated with recent data and a new format. *BMC Pediatr* 2003; 3:13.
3. Polin RA, Fox WW, Abman SH. *Fetal and Neonatal Physiology* (4th ed). Philadelphia: WB Saunders; 2011.
4. Kitaoka H, Burri PH, Weibel ER. Development of the human fetal airway tree: analysis of the numerical density of airway endtips. *Anat Rec* 1996; 244:207–13.
5. Frerking I, Günther A, Seeger W, *et al.* Pulmonary surfactant: functions, abnormalities and therapeutic options. *Intensive Care Med* 2001; 27:1699–717.
6. Langston C, Kida K, Reed M, *et al.* Human lung growth in late gestation and in the neonate. *Am Rev Respir Dis* 1984; 129:607–13.
7. Brown MJ, Olver RE, Ramsden CA, *et al.* Effects of adrenaline and of spontaneous labour on the secretion and absorption of lung liquid in the fetal lamb. *J Physiol* 1983; 344:137–52.
8. Harding R, Bocking AD, Sigger JN. Influence of upper respiratory tract on liquid flow to and from fetal lungs. *J Appl Physiol* 1986; 61:68–74.
9. Dickson KA, Maloney JE, Berger PJ. Decline in lung liquid volume before labor in fetal lambs. *J Appl Physiol* 1986; 61:2266–72.
10. Maloney JE. Preparation of the respiratory system for the early neonatal period. *J Dev Physiol* 1984; 6:21–30.
11. Pfister RE, Ramsden CA, Neil HL, *et al.* Volume and secretion rate of lung liquid in the final days of gestation and labour in the fetal sheep. *J Physiol* 2001; 535:889–99.
12. Bland RD. Loss of liquid from the lung lumen in labor: more than a simple "squeeze". *Am J Physiol Lung Cell Mol Physiol* 2001; 280:L602–5.
13. Levine EM, Ghai V, Barton JJ, *et al.* Mode of delivery and risk of respiratory diseases in newborns. *Obstet Gynecol* 2001; 97:439–42.
14. Possmayer F, Yu SH, Weber JM, *et al.* Pulmonary surfactant. *Can J Biochem Cell Biol* 1984; 62:1121–33.

15. Brownfoot FC. Different corticosteroids and regimens for accelerating fetal lung maturation for women at risk of preterm birth. *Cochrane Database Syst Rev* 2013; 8:CD006764.
16. Crowther CA, McKinlay CJ, Middleton P, *et al.* Repeat doses of prenatal corticosteroids for women at risk of preterm birth for improving neonatal health outcomes. *Cochrane Database Syst Rev* 2011; 6:CD003935.
17. Roberts D, Dalziel S. Antenatal corticosteroids for accelerating fetal lung maturation for women at risk of preterm birth. *Cochrane Database Syst Rev* 2006; 3:CD004454.
18. Grier DG, Halliday HL. Effects of glucocorticoids on fetal and neonatal lung development. *Treat Respir Med* 2004; 3:295–306.
19. Harding R, Bocking AD, Sigger JN. Upper airway resistances in fetal sheep: the influence of breathing activity. *J Appl Physiol* 1985; 60:160–165.
20. Dawes GSG. Breathing before birth in animals and man. An essay in developmental medicine. *N Engl J Med* 1974; 290:557–559.
21. Hooper SB, Harding R. Fetal lung liquid: a major determinant of the growth and functional development of the fetal lung. *Clin Exp Pharmacol Physiol* 1995; 22:235–47.
22. Gluckman PD, Gunn TR, Johnston BM. The effect of cooling on breathing and shivering in unanaesthetized fetal lambs in utero. *J Physiol* 1983; 343:495–506.
23. Jansen AH, Ioffe S, Russell BJ, Chernick V. Effect of carotid chemoreceptor denervation on breathing in utero and after birth. *J Appl Physiol* 1981; 51:630–633.
24. Baier RJ, Hasan SU, Cates DB, *et al.* Effects of various concentrations of O2 and umbilical cord occlusion on fetal breathing and behavior. *J Appl Physiol* 1990; 68:1597–604.
25. Kalapesi Z, Durand M, Leahy FN, *et al.* Effect of periodic or regular respiratory pattern on the ventilatory response to low inhaled CO2 in preterm infants during sleep. *Am Rev Respir Dis* 1980; 123:8–11.
26. Waggener TB, Stark AR, Cohlan BA, *et al.* Apnea duration is related to ventilatory oscillation characteristics in newborn infants. *J Appl Physiol* 1984; 57:536–44.
27. Rigatto H, Kalapesi Z, Leahy FN, *et al.* Ventilatory response to 100% and 15% O2 during wakefulness and sleep in preterm infants. *Early Hum Dev* 1982; 7:1–10.
28. Al-Matary A, Kutbi I, Qurashi M, *et al.* Increased peripheral chemoreceptor activity may be critical in destabilizing breathing in neonates. *Semin Perinatol* 2004; 28:264–72.
29. Mathew OP, Roberts JL, Thach BT. Pharyngeal airway obstruction in preterm infants during mixed and obstructive apnea. *J Pediatr* 1982; 100:964–8.
30. Miller MJ, Carlo WA, DiFiore JM, *et al.* Airway obstruction during periodic breathing in premature infants. *J Appl Physiol* 1988; 64:2496–500.
31. Persson P. Cardiopulmonary receptors and "neurogenic hypertension". *Acta Physiol Scand Suppl* 1987; 570:1–53.
32. Spyer KM. Annual review prize lecture. Central nervous mechanisms contributing to cardiovascular control. *J Physiol* 1993; 474:1–19.
33. Chapleau MW, Hajduczok G, Abboud FM. Mechanisms of resetting of arterial baroreceptors: an overview. *Am J Med Sci* 1988; 295:327–34.
34. Segar JL, Mazursky JE, Robillard JE. Changes in ovine renal sympathetic nerve activity and baroreflex function at birth. *Am J Physiol* 1994; 267:H1824–32.
35. Friis-Hansen B. Body water compartments in children: changes during growth and related changes in body composition. *Pediatrics* 1961; 28:169–81.
36. Lagercrantz H, Bistoletti P. Catecholamine release in the newborn infant at birth. *Pediatr Res* 1977; 11:889–93.
37. Padbury JF, Diakomanolis ES, Hobel CJ, *et al.* Neonatal adaptation: sympatho-adrenal response to umbilical cord cutting. *Pediatr Res* 1981; 15:1483–7.
38. Padbury JF, Martinez AM. Sympathoadrenal system activity at birth: integration of postnatal adaptation. *Semin Perinatol* 1988; 12:163–72.
39. Ogundipe OA, Kullama LK, Stein H, *et al.* Fetal endocrine and renal responses to in utero ventilation and umbilical cord occlusion. *Am J Obstet Gynecol* 1993; 169:1479–86.
40. van Bel F, Roman C, Iwamoto HS, *et al.* Sympathoadrenal, metabolic, and regional blood flow responses to cold in fetal sheep. *Pediatr Res* 1993; 34:47–50.
41. Kim S, Iwao H. Molecular and cellular mechanisms of angiotensin II-mediated cardiovascular and renal diseases. *Pharmacol Rev* 2000; 52:11–34.
42. Unno N, Wong CH, Jenkins SL, *et al.* Blood pressure and heart rate in the ovine fetus: ontogenic changes and effects of fetal adrenalectomy. *Am J Physiol* 1999; 276:H248–56.
43. Tangalakis K, Lumbers ER, Moritz KM, *et al.* Effect of cortisol on blood pressure and vascular reactivity in the ovine fetus. *Exp Physiol* 1992; 77:709–17.
44. Segar JL, Lumbers ER, Nuyt AM, *et al.* Effect of antenatal glucocorticoids on sympathetic nerve activity at birth in preterm sheep. *Am J Physiol* 1997; 274:R160–7.
45. Fletcher AJW, McGarrigle HHG, Edwards CMB, *et al.* Effects of low dose dexamethasone treatment on basal cardiovascular and endocrine function in fetal sheep during late gestation. *J Physiol* 2002; 545:649–60.
46. Yu Z-Y, Lumbers ER, Simonetta G. The cardiovascular and renal effects of acute and chronic inhibition of nitric oxide production in fetal sheep. *Exp Physiol* 2002; 87:343–51.
47. Bouayad A, Kajino H, Waleh N, *et al.* Characterization of PGE2 receptors in fetal and newborn lamb ductus arteriosus. *Am J Physiol Heart Circ Physiol* 2001; 280:H2342–9.
48. Gonzalez A, Sosenko IR, Chandar J, *et al.* Influence of infection on patent ductus arteriosus and chronic lung disease in premature infants weighing 1000 grams or less. *J Pediatr* 1996; 128:470–8.
49. Cotton RB, Lindstrom DP, Stahlman MT. Early prediction of symptomatic patent ductus arteriosus from perinatal risk factors: a discriminant analysis model. *Acta Paediatr* 1981; 70:723–7.
50. Bell EF, Acarregui MJ. Restricted versus liberal water intake for preventing morbidity and mortality in preterm infants. *Cochrane Database Syst Rev* 2001; 12:CD000503.
51. Furzan JA, Reisch J, Tyson JE, *et al.* Incidence and risk factors for symptomatic patent ductus arteriosus among inborn very-low-birth-weight infants. *Early Hum Dev* 1985; 12:39–48.
52. Clyman RI, Ballard PL, Sniderman S, *et al.* Prenatal administration of betamethasone for prevention of patient ductus arteriosus. *J Pediatr* 1980; 98:123–6.
53. McGrath JC, MacLennan SJ, Whittle MJ. Comparison of the effects of oxygen, 5-hydroxytryptamine, bradykinin and adrenaline in isolated human umbilical artery smooth muscle. *Q J Exp Physiol* 1988; 73:547–59.
54. White RP. Pharmacodynamic study of maturation and closure of human umbilical arteries. *Am J Obstet Gynecol* 1988; 160:229–37.
55. Hoath SB, Visscher M, Heaton C, *et al.* Skin science and the future of dermatology. *J Cutan Med Surg* 1998; 3:2–8.
56. Candi E, Schmidt R, Melino G. The cornified envelope: a model of cell death in the skin. *Nat Rev Mol Cell Biol* 2005; 6:328–40.
57. Kalinin A, Marekov LN, Steinert PM. Assembly of the epidermal cornified cell envelope. *J Cell Sci* 2001; 114:3069–70.
58. Hoath SB, Leahy DG. The human stratum corneum as extended, covalently cross-linked biopolymer: mathematics, molecules, and medicine. *Med Hypotheses* 2006; 66:1191–8.
59. Jain A, Rutter N, Cartlidge PH. Influence of antenatal steroids and sex on maturation of the epidermal barrier in the preterm infant. *Arch Dis Child Fetal Neonatal Ed* 2000; 83:F112–16.
60. Williams ML, Feingold KR. Barrier function of neonatal skin. *J Pediatr* 1998; 133:467–8.
61. Warner RR, Stone KJ, Boissy YL. Hydration disrupts human stratum corneum ultrastructure. *J Invest Dermatol* 2003; 120:275–84.
62. Youssef W, Wickett RR, Hoath SB. Surface free energy characterization of vernix caseosa. Potential role in waterproofing the newborn infant. *Skin Res Technol* 2001; 7:10–17.

63. Rissmann RR, Groenink HW, Weerheim AM, Hoath SB, Ponec M, Bouwstra JA. New insights into ultrastructure, lipid composition and organization of vernix caseosa. *J Invest Dermatol* 2006; 126:1823–1833.
64. Gilbert RD, Schröder H, Kawamura T, *et al.* Heat transfer pathways between fetal lamb and ewe. *J Appl Physiol* 1985; 59:634–8.
65. Watkinson M. Temperature control of premature infants in the delivery room. *Clin Perinatol* 2006; 33:43–53.
66. Christensson K, Siles C, Cabrera T, *et al.* Lower body temperatures in infants delivered by caesarean section than in vaginally delivered infants. *Acta Paediatr* 1993; 82:128–31.
67. Mostyn A, Keisler DH, Webb R, *et al.* The role of leptin in the transition from fetus to neonate. *Proc Nutr Soc* 2001; 60:187–94.
68. Sarkany I, Gaylarde CC. Bacterial colonisation of the skin of the newborn. *J Pathol* 2004; 95:115–22.
69. D'Angio CT, McGowan KL, Baumgart S, *et al.* Surface colonization with coagulase-negative staphylococci in premature neonates. *J Pediatr* 1989; 114:1029–34.
70. Takagi K, Tanaka H, Nishijima S, *et al.* Fetal blood values by percutaneous umbilical blood sampling. *Fetal Diagn Ther* 1988; 4:152–60.
71. Linderkamp O. Placental transfusion: determinants and effects. *Clin Perinatol* 1982; 9:559–92.
72. Shields LE, Brace RA. Fetal vascular pressure responses to nonlabor uterine contractions—dependence on amniotic-fluid volume in the ovine fetus. *Am J Obstet Gynecol* 1994; 171:84–9.
73. Brace RA, Cheung CY. Role of catecholamines in mediating fetal blood volume decrease during acute hypoxia. *Am J Physiol* 1987; 253:H927–32.
74. Yao AC, Moinian M, Lind J. Distribution of blood between infant and placenta after birth. *Lancet* 1969; 2:871–3.
75. Kinmond S, Aitchison TC, Holland BM, *et al.* Umbilical cord clamping and preterm infants: a randomised trial. *BMJ* 1993; 306:172–5.
76. Rabe H, Wacker A, Hülskamp G, *et al.* A randomised controlled trial of delayed cord clamping in very low birth weight preterm infants. *Eur J Pediatr* 2000; 159:775–7.
77. Mercer JS, Vohr BR, McGrath MM, *et al.* Delayed cord clamping in very preterm infants reduces the incidence of intraventricular hemorrhage and late-onset sepsis: a randomized, controlled trial. *Pediatrics* 2006; 117:1235–42.
78. Veille JC, Hanson RA, Tatum K, *et al.* Quantitative assessment of human fetal renal blood flow. *Am J Obstet Gynecol* 1993; 169:1399–402.
79. Loebstein R, Koren G. Clinical pharmacology and therapeutic drug monitoring in neonates and children. *Pediatr Rev* 1998; 19:423–8.
80. Vanpée M, Blennow M, Linné T, *et al.* Renal function in very low birth weight infants: normal maturity reached during early childhood. *J Pediatr* 1992; 121:784–8.
81. Kanamura S, Kanai K, Watanabe J. Fine structure and function of hepatocytes during development. *J Electron Microsc Tech* 1990; 14:92–105.
82. Shapiro SM. Definition of the clinical spectrum of kernicterus and bilirubin-induced neurologic dysfunction (BIND). *J Perinatol* 2004; 25:54–9.
83. Marconi AM, Cetin I, Davoli E, *et al.* An evaluation of fetal glucogenesis in intrauterine growth-retarded pregnancies. *Metabolism* 1993; 42:860–4.
84. Kalhan S, Peter-Wohl S. Hypoglycemia: what is it for the neonate? *Am J Perinatol* 1999; 17:11–8.
85. Philipson EH, Kalhan SC, Riha MM, Pimentel R. Effects of maternal glucose infusion on fetal acid-base status in human pregnancy. *Am J Obstet Gynecol* 1987; 157:866–73.
86. Williams AF. Neonatal hypoglycaemia: clinical and legal aspects. *Semin Fetal Neonat Med* 2005; 10:6.
87. International Association for the Study of Pain, *Pain Suppl* 1986; 3:S1–226.
88. Schechter NL. The undertreatment of pain in children: an overview. *Pediatr Clin North Am* 1989; 36:781–94.
89. Anand KJ, Sippell WG, Schofield NM, *et al.* Does halothane anaesthesia decrease the metabolic and endocrine stress responses of newborn infants undergoing operation? *BMJ* 1988; 296:668–72.
90. Anand KJ, Hickey PR. Halothane-morphine compared with high-dose sufentanil for anesthesia and postoperative analgesia in neonatal cardiac surgery. *N Engl J Med* 1992; 326:1–9.
91. van de Velde M, De Buck F. Fetal and maternal analgesia/anesthesia for fetal procedures. *Fetal Diagn Ther* 2012; 31:201–9.
92. American Academy of Pediatrics Committee on Fetus and Newborn, American Academy of Pediatrics Section on Surgery, Canadian Paediatric Society Fetus and Newborn Committee, *et al.* Prevention and management of pain in the neonate: an update. *Pediatrics* 2006; 118:2231–41.
93. Vutskits LL. Anesthetic-related neurotoxicity and the developing brain: shall we change practice? *Paediatr Drugs* 2012; 14:13–21.
94. Humphrey T. Some correlations between the appearance of human fetal reflexes and the development of the nervous system. *Prog Brain Res* 1964; 4:93–135.
95. Hall RW, Anand KJS. Physiology of pain and stress in the newborn. *NeoReviews* 2005; 6:e61–8.
96. Olson TL, Downey VW. Infant physiological responses to noxious stimuli of circumcision with anesthesia and analgesia. *Pediatr Nurs* 1998; 24:385–9.
97. Desborough JP. The stress response to trauma and surgery. *Br J Anaesth* 2000; 85:109–17.
98. Goldman RD, Koren G. Biologic markers of pain in the vulnerable infant. *Clin Perinatol* 2002; 29(3):415–25.
99. Grunau RV, Craig KD. Pain expression in neonates: facial action and cry. *Pain* 1987; 28:395–410.
100. Porter FLF, Miller RH, Marshall RE. Neonatal pain cries: effect of circumcision on acoustic features and perceived urgency. *Child Dev* 1986; 57:790–802.
101. Stevens B, Gibbins S. Clinical utility and clinical significance in the assessment and management of pain in vulnerable infants. *Clin Perinatol* 2002; 29:459–68.
102. Franck LS. Some pain, some gain: reflections on the past two decades of neonatal pain research and treatment. *Neonatal Netw* 2002; 21:37–41.
103. Cignacco E, Mueller R, Hamers JPH, *et al.* Pain assessment in the neonate using the Bernese Pain Scale for Neonates. *Early Hum Dev* 2004; 78:125–31.
104. Bhutta AT, Anand KJ. Vulnerability of the developing brain. Neuronal mechanisms. *Clin Perinatol* 2002; 29:357–72.
105. Grunau RE, Weinberg J, Whitfield MF. Neonatal procedural pain and preterm infant cortisol response to novelty at 8 months. *Pediatrics* 2004; 114:e77–e84.
106. Sanders RD, Hassell J, Davidson AJ, *et al.* Impact of anaesthetics and surgery on neurodevelopment: an update. *Br J Anaesth* 2013; 110 Suppl 1:i53–72.
107. Brambrink AM, Back SA, Riddle A, *et al.* Isoflurane-induced apoptosis of oligodendrocytes in the neonatal primate brain. *Ann Neurol* 2012; 72:525–35.
108. Crosby G, Davis PJ. General anesthesia in infancy is associated with learning disabilities-or not. *Anesth Analg* 2013; 117(6):1270–2.

CHAPTER 5

Maternal, fetal, and neonatal pharmacokinetics

Karel Allegaert and Kristel Van Calsteren

Introduction: clinical pharmacology in special populations

Clinical pharmacology aims to predict drug-related effects based on compound- and population-specific pharmacokinetics (PK, concentration–time), and pharmacodynamics (PD, concentration–effect). The general PK principles of disposition and elimination of drugs apply, irrespective of population-specific characteristics (Figure 5.1). Consequently, dosing should be based on the physiological characteristics of the individual patient. Pregnancy and early infancy hereby warrant focused assessment. This is because important alterations in physiology affect drug disposition up to the level of clinical relevance.[1,2] Pregnancy results in extensive alterations in PK (concentration–time profile) with a subsequent extensive interindividual variability in drug response, in part driven by the hormonal changes. In general, renal elimination capacity is increased throughout pregnancy (i.e. higher glomerular filtration rate and higher active tubular transport). Similarly, the basal metabolic activity is also increased. This commonly results in higher drug metabolism (phase I and phase II processes), although these changes are in part also iso-enzyme specific. This, although rarely, may even result in reduced enzymatic activity during pregnancy. Finally, changes in body weight or binding capacity (protein changes, pH) will likely affect the volume of distribution. Similarly, duration of pregnancy, co-morbidity (e.g. pre-eclampsia), or labour itself may further affect variability in drug disposition.

Newborns are another very specific population. When we consider the physiological changes and the subsequent between-individual variability in characteristics, we need to take into account that maturational changes are most prominent in infancy.[3–5] Consequently, drug disposition (absorption, distribution, and subsequent elimination, either through metabolic elimination or through primary renal elimination (PK) in early infancy differs substantially from children or adults. In general, neonates have an overall low clearance capacity. Between-subject variability can be explained by covariates such as size, weight, organ function, co-administration of drugs, genetic polymorphisms, growth restriction, or disease characteristics.

Maternal pharmacokinetics

Pharmacokinetic alterations due to physiological changes during pregnancy

During pregnancy, multiple changes in physiology occur, affecting the major PK processes of a drug: absorption, distribution, metabolism, and excretion (ADME) (Table 5.1).[1,2,6] This may have therapeutic and toxic consequences for both the pregnant woman and the fetus. Due to ADME changes the pregnant patient may be exposed to subtherapeutic or toxic drug levels and an unwanted amount of drug may be delivered to the fetus.

During pregnancy, an increase in progesterone level is believed to be responsible for a delayed gastrointestinal motility and increased transit time, altering the drug *absorption* and enterohepatic circulation and resulting in lower peak levels but increased exposure.

The *distribution* of drugs may be altered during pregnancy as a result of the increase in fat stores as well as extracellular fluid volume and a plasma volume expansion by 50%. As a result of this volume expansion, a decrease in the (peak) serum concentration of many drugs has been documented.[7] Furthermore, the amniotic fluid may behave as a third space for water-soluble drugs, like methotrexate, mitoxantrone, or cefazolin, with prolonged exposure and delayed elimination resulting in both maternal and potentially fetal toxicity or prolonged effects.[8] Moreover, since the protein concentration of the amniotic fluid is very low, measured drug concentrations should be considered to be free concentrations (e.g. cefazolin). As pregnancy advances, the rate of plasma volume expansion exceeds the rate of albumin production, creating physiological dilutional hypoalbuminemia (i.e. the total amount of albumin is higher, but the plasma concentration is lower when compared to the non-pregnant state). Moreover, endogenous compounds like free fatty acids, steroids, and placental hormones occupy protein-binding sites, thus decreasing the protein-binding capacity of drugs. The overall effect is a decrease in binding capacity for albumin and, therefore, an increase in unbound drug. However, as more free drug is available for either hepatic biotransformation or renal excretion, the overall effect may be an unaltered free drug concentration. In contrast to albumin, serum alpha-1-acid glycoprotein concentrations were found to remain the same as those in non-pregnancy.[7]

The increased regional blood flow, including the hepatic blood flow, will lead to higher metabolic rates, or is a reflection of this higher metabolic activity. Besides these blood flow-related changes, the increased secretion of oestrogens (e.g. oestradiol) and progesterone in normal pregnancy affects *drug metabolism* in different ways. To further illustrate this, the higher rate of hepatic metabolism of certain drugs, such as phenytoin, is possibly a result of stimulated hepatic microsomal enzyme activity (cytochrome P450 (CYP)) induced by progesterone. On the other hand, the hepatic *elimination* of other drugs, such as theophylline

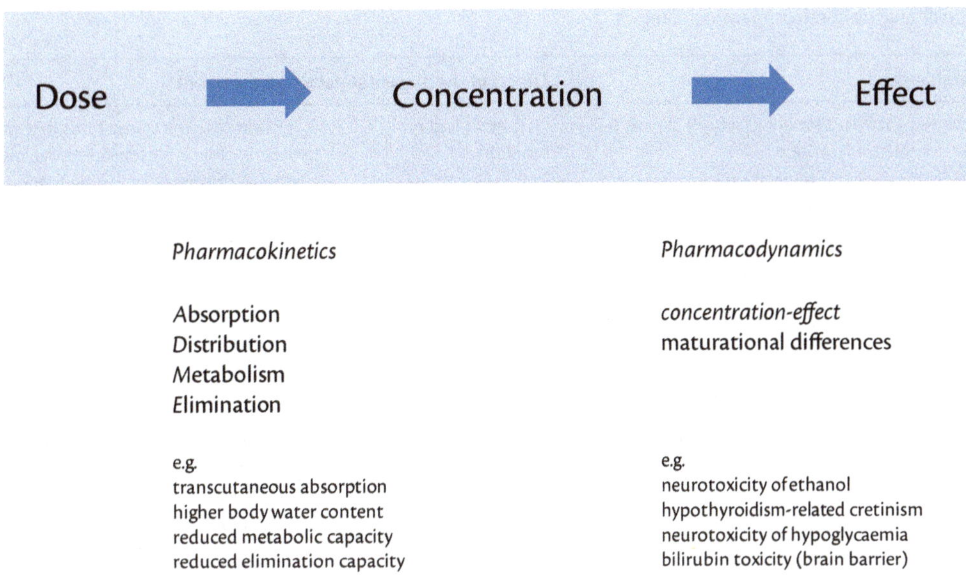

Figure 5.1 Clinical pharmacology aims to predict the concentration–time profile (pharmacokinetics) and the concentration–effect profile (pharmacodynamics).

and caffeine, is reduced secondary to competitive inhibition of microsomal oxidases by progesterone and oestradiol. Finally, oestrogens stimulate the glucuronidation (UDP glucuronosyl transferase (UGT) enzymes), but not the sulphation capacity, resulting in increased clearance of compounds (e.g. propofol, paracetamol, and lamotrigine) cleared by UGT iso-enzymes. These hepatic alterations may be detrimental for drugs that need to be metabolized to become active, like cyclophosphamide (to phosphoramide mustard and acrolein, CYP2B6) or codeine (to morphine, CYP2D6), or vice versa, for drugs that need to be metabolized to become inactive. The same holds true for paracetamol, metabolized by the liver to paracetamol glucuronide (47–62%), and paracetamol sulphate (25–36%), and about 8–10% of paracetamol is oxidized to 3-hydroxy-paracetamol and the (hepatic) toxic metabolite *N*-acetyl-P-benzoquinone-imine (NAPQI) in non-pregnant adults. The overall higher paracetamol clearance and delivery is due to both higher glucuronidation and oxidation, but not sulphation. Finally, the cholestatic effect of oestrogen may interfere with the clearance of drugs, which are secreted in the biliary system (biliary drug transporters).[1,2,6]

As renal plasma flow increases by 25–75% and glomerular filtration rate by 50%, renally cleared drugs demonstrate enhanced elimination and lower steady-state serum concentrations,[7] but the renal function can be further affected by medical conditions (e.g. preeclampsia, pre-pregnancy renal failure, and lupus nephritis).

Applications in the field of obstetric anaesthesia

Alterations in compound-specific PK and PD are in general heterogeneous, reflecting different pregnancy-related changes in each or several of the previously mentioned alterations. We aim to illustrate the pregnancy-related changes for compounds commonly administered by anaesthetists (Table 5.2). Aspects related to fetal exposure and breastfeeding will be discussed in dedicated subsections ('Transplacental Transport' and 'Applied Neonatal Pharmacology: Obstetric Anaesthesia and Breastfeeding' respectively) of this chapter.

Neuromuscular blocking agents illustrate the complexity of these changes. Plasma cholinesterase levels are decreased by 25% from early during pregnancy until the seventh day postpartum. Prolonged neuromuscular blockade with succinylcholine is uncommon, however, as the increased volume of distribution off sets the impact of decreased drug hydrolysis.[9] Vecuronium at a standard dose of 0.2 mg/kg has been shown to have a faster onset time and longer duration of action in pregnancy.[10] The onset time of rocuronium at a dose of 0.6 mg/kg is unchanged but also demonstrates a longer duration of action compared with non-pregnant patients.[11] Neuromuscular blocking agents whose elimination is organ independent also display altered PK. Cisatracurium, for example, undergoes Hoffman's elimination *in vivo*, and has a significantly more rapid onset and shorter duration of neuromuscular blockade in pregnant patients.[12] A similar exercise can be made for propofol. Due to the raised hepatic blood flow and the increased glucuronidation activity, propofol clearance is increased during pregnancy.[13] When focusing on PD, there are conflicting views regarding the half maximal effective concentration (EC_{50}) of propofol for loss of consciousness in pregnancy. Higuchi et al. reported that the EC_{50} was not different from that in non-pregnant women, indicating that there is no need to decrease the propofol concentration for loss of consciousness when inducing general anaesthesia.[14] In contrast, Mongardon et al. described that the propofol effect-site concentration is decreased during early pregnancy.[15] Combining all observations, we suggest that a higher maintenance dose will be needed to attain the same level of anaesthesia, but the extent of the increase is unclear.

Paracetamol and non-steroidal anti-inflammatory drugs (e.g. ketorolac and ibuprofen) decrease opioid consumption with the aim to reduce opioid-related side effects. Preventive analgesia using non-opioid analgesic strategies is one of the pathways to improve postoperative pain while minimizing opioid-related side effects for both mother and newborn. Since paracetamol clearance is significantly higher at delivery, it might be prudent to decrease the interval between consecutive paracetamol doses

Table 5.1 Physiological changes affecting pharmacokinetics

Maternal physiological changes		Effects of the placental–fetal compartment	
Absorption	Decreased gastrointestinal motility → slower, but more complete absorption Increased gastric pH → affects ionization (absorption) of weak acids and bases Ventilatory changes: hyperventilation and increased pulmonary blood flow → favours alveolar uptake	Placental barrier function	P-glycoprotein, multidrug resistance proteins, and breast cancer resistance protein are active transporters that work against a concentration gradient and protect the fetus against potential toxic effects of environmental toxins and other xenobiotics
Distribution	Plasma volume expansion by 50% → decrease in C_{max} Mean increase in total body water is 8 L More fat stores Amniotic fluid may behave as a third space	Acid–base equilibrium effect	Non-ionized, highly lipid-soluble molecules penetrate the placenta more quickly than less lipid-soluble ionized molecules Fetal plasma pH is slightly more acidic than the maternal → Ion trapping: weak bases in the maternal circulation will be non-ionized and easily cross the placenta, in the fetal blood they become ionized, resulting in a net movement from maternal to fetal compartment
Protein binding	Dilutional hypoalbuminemia → Increased unbound drug fraction Steroid and placental hormones occupy protein binding sites	Protein binding	Maternal plasma albumin gradually decreases during pregnancy, while fetal albumin progressively increases → Since only unbound drugs cross the placenta, protein-bound drugs reach higher total concentrations in the fetus
Metabolism	Hepatic drug metabolism alterations by increased secretion of oestrogen and progesterone (induction of microsomal enzyme activity by progesterone, or competitive inhibition of microsomal oxidases by progesterone and oestradiol) → Drug metabolism can be increased, decreased, or remain stable	Fetoplacental drug metabolism	First-pass metabolic effect by placenta Fetal liver metabolism: from 7–8 weeks postconception phase I (oxidation, dehydrogenation, reduction, and hydrolysis) and phase II (glucuronidation, methylation, and acetylation) enzymatic processes have been documented in the fetal liver; however, because of immaturity their contribution in drug elimination is marginal and most of the umbilical venous blood flow will bypass the liver via the ductus venosus to enter the fetal heart
Excretion	Increased renal blood flow and glomerular filtration rate (by 50%) Cholestatic effect of oestrogen may interfere with clearance of drugs through the biliary system	Fetoplacental elimination	Elimination of drugs from the fetus primarily occurs by diffusion back to the maternal compartment As most metabolites are more polar than their parent compounds, they are less likely to cross the placental barrier. This may result in metabolite accumulation in various fetal tissues As pregnancy progresses, higher amounts of drugs are excreted into the amniotic fluid, reflecting maturation of the fetal kidney

Data from Thomas SH, Yates LM. Prescribing without evidence – pregnancy. *Br J Clin Phamacol* 2012; 74:691–7; Pavek P, Ceckova M, Staud F. Variation of drug kinetics in pregnancy. *Curr Drug Metab* 2009; 10:520-9; and Krauer B, Krauer F, Hytten FE. Drug disposition and pharmacokinetics in the maternal-placental-fetal unit. *Pharmacol Ther* 1980; 10:301–28.

or increase the dose in the immediate postpartum to mimic the time–concentration profile aimed for in non-pregnant adults. However, increasing paracetamol dosing also results in higher oxidative metabolism during pregnancy. Consequently, we suggest that it may be more reasonable to anticipate a shorter, and less persistent analgesic effect of paracetamol in pregnant women due to the higher clearance, but not to increase the dose to avoid hepatoxicity. A similar extrapolation can be made for ketorolac. Ketorolac clearance is also significantly increased at delivery. Assuming that there is a given threshold plasma ketorolac concentration, that results in pain, the higher clearance during pregnancy will result in faster onset of pain. A decrease in the interval between consecutive administrations (at present, 8-hourly dosing) can be considered to maintain the ketorolac level above this threshold.[16–19]

Clearance of opioids will be higher at delivery. This does not necessary mean that the dose of any opioid needs to be higher, since this also includes metabolic clearance for 'prodrugs' like codeine (morphine), oxycodone (oxymorphone), or tramadol (*O*-demethyl tramadol); the phenotypic concentration–time relation will depend on simultaneous ongoing PK aspects (metabolic clearance, metabolite elimination clearance) in addition to covariates, including pharmacogenetics.[20,21] The specific risks related to maternal opioid exposure and breastfeeding are discussed in 'Transplacental Transport'.

Transplacental transport

The major function of the placenta is to transfer nutrients and oxygen from the mother to the fetus and to assist in the removal of waste products from the fetus to the mother (see also Chapter 3). In

Table 5.2 Illustrations of the impact of pregnancy on pharmacokinetics and pharmacodynamics of individual compounds commonly administered to pregnant women by anaesthetists. Issues related to placental transfer were not considered, although all compounds mentioned do cross the placental barrier

Compound	Normal dose in an adult	Pregnancy-related changes
Cefazolin	2 g, IV at induction, every 8 h prophylaxis, surgery	Higher distribution volume because of higher weight and lower albumin binding Higher clearance because of higher renal clearance and higher free concentration *Consequences*: lower peak, and shorter duration until below minimal inhibitory concentration pathogens *Suggestion*: shorter time interval for a second dose, every 6 h?
Paracetamol	2 g IV loading dose, 1 g every 8 h (postoperative) pain	Higher distribution volume because of higher weight and body composition (water-soluble) Higher clearance because of higher metabolism (glucuronidation, but also oxidation) *Consequences*: this likely results in less effective and shorter pain relief *Suggestion*: consider multimodal analgesia, higher dose may result in more toxic metabolites
Propofol	4 mg/kg or 2 mg/kg + 6 mg/kg/h	Higher clearance because of higher cardiac output/hepatic blood flow (high extraction drug) Unsure about differences in pharmacodynamics *Consequences*: recovery marginally quicker during pregnancy due to higher clearance *Suggestion*: titration to effect
Tramadol	3 mg/kg, 7 mg/kg/24 h	Higher distribution volume, higher metabolic clearance (metabolite has analgesic properties) Higher renal elimination clearance of the mother compound and the metabolite *Consequences*: higher clearance, in part compensated by higher metabolic clearance *Suggestion*: Suggested doses are 50–100 mg IV/oral, every 2 h, max. 600 mg per 24 h consider higher loading, or perhaps more appropriate higher maintenance dose

addition, it plays an important role in the synthesis of hormones, peptides, and steroids that are vital for a successful pregnancy. The placenta provides a link between the circulations of two distinct individuals but also acts as a barrier to protect the fetus from xenobiotics in the maternal blood. Similar to the blood–brain barrier, the placenta is described as an organ separating the maternal and fetal circulations. However, the term 'placental barrier' includes a false notion since the placenta is not a true barrier, but instead the placenta is the entry through which the fetus is exposed to chemicals.[22] The major and minor routes of drug disposition within the placental–fetal compartment are described in Table 5.1.

Most drugs cross the placenta by *passive diffusion*.[23] Therefore, the amount and rate of transfer is primarily determined by the concentration gradient of the drug between the maternal and fetal circulation and placental blood flow. Besides the physicochemical properties of drugs such as lipid solubility, ionization constant (pKa), molecular weight, and protein binding are critical for placental transfer. Uncharged, low-molecular-weight (<500 Da), lipid-soluble, and unbound compounds can easily cross the human placenta.[23]

While the maternal plasma albumin gradually decreases during pregnancy, fetal albumin concentration progressively increases and reaches its peak at term when it equals or even exceeds maternal albumin concentration. In contrast, fetal levels of glycoprotein alpha are much lower than maternal levels; therefore, the free fractions of basic drugs will be higher in the developing child.[7]

The maternal pH and fetal pH are significant determinants of placental transfer especially for weak acid or basic drugs with a pKa close to the plasma pH. The fetal plasma pH is usually slightly more acidic than the maternal. Consequently, weak bases will be mainly non-ionized and, therefore, able to easily penetrate the placental barrier. However, after crossing the placenta and making contact with the relatively acidic fetal blood, these molecules will become more ionized. This results in an apparent fall in fetal concentrations of the drug and leads to a concentration gradient, with subsequently a net movement from the maternal to the fetal system. This phenomenon is commonly referred to as ion trapping.[7]

Only a few drugs (e.g. ganciclovir, cephalexin, and some glucocorticoids) have been suggested to be transported across the placental barrier by *facilitated diffusion*, which requires the presence of a carrier substance within the placenta, but does not need any energy source.[22] Furthermore, *active transport* of drugs across the placental barrier has been described. It has been recognized that substrate transporting proteins are present in the fetus-derived epithelial cells that make up the exchange border between the fetal and maternal blood compartment. These include P-glycoprotein, multidrug resistance proteins, and breast cancer resistance protein. All active transporters may work against a concentration gradient but can become saturated. These protein pumps have been postulated to have evolved as a protective mechanism against the potential toxic effects of environmental toxins and other xenobiotics, and yet were shown to regulate the transfer of vinblastine, vincristine, paclitaxel, and doxorubicin.[22]

The placenta can exert a considerable first-pass *metabolic effect* on some drugs. Drugs that are not metabolized in the placenta would then enter the umbilical vein where the next fetal organ encountered is the fetal liver. However, most of the umbilical venous blood flow will bypass the liver via the ductus venosus to enter the fetal heart. Drugs that are metabolized in the fetal compartment contribute to direct fetal clearance.

Since the presence of enzymatic processes, including phase I (oxidation, dehydrogenation, reduction, and hydrolysis) and phase II reactions (glucuronidation, methylation, and acetylation by transferases), has been documented both in the placenta and the fetus, drugs can be assumed to be metabolized to some extent in the fetoplacental compartment.[22,24] CYP enzymes in particular have been well characterized in the placenta at the level of mRNA, protein, and enzyme activity. CYP1A1, -2E1, -3A4, -3A5, -3A7, and -4B1 have been detected in the term placenta. While much less is known about phase II enzymes in the placenta, some enzymes, in particular UGT iso-enzymes, have been detected and shown to have specific activity towards marker substrates, suggesting a significant role of this enzyme in placental drug detoxification. The clinical relevance is, however, poorly understood.[22]

The activity of most fetal drug-metabolizing enzyme systems that have been measured in fetal tissues is lower than the one observed in adult tissues. Neither the exact developmental time frame, nor the mechanisms by which fetal enzymes become upregulated around birth, have been delineated in primates.[23] Nevertheless, significant concentrations of drug metabolites have been found in the fetus. It should be noted that the process of biotransformation usually renders the drug more water-soluble and thus more readily excreted by the kidney. This is of concern to the fetus when the drug undergoes metabolism in the fetal compartment, because the greater water-solubility of the metabolite will decrease the ability of the compound to be cleared from the fetus across the placenta. Few studies have evaluated the potential for the accumulation of metabolites in the fetus, because most drugs lose their biological activity when they undergo metabolism. However, some drugs are activated through metabolism, like cyclophosphamide.[23]

Elimination of drugs from the fetus occurs primarily by its diffusion back to the maternal compartment. Approximately 4% of the fetal cardiac output goes to the fetal kidneys. As pregnancy progresses, higher amounts of different drugs are excreted into the amniotic fluid, reflecting maturation of the fetal kidney. It is also possible that drugs diffuse across fetal skin, umbilical cord, and the fetal surface of the placenta to reach the amniotic fluid. Because this occurs by passive diffusion, drug movement can occur in both directions, allowing drugs to be cleared form the amniotic fluid as well. Generally it is assumed that most clearance of drugs from the amniotic fluid occurs through fetal swallowing. Although drugs can be measured in meconium, most drugs swallowed by the fetus are probably reabsorbed. Thus drug excretion in fetal urine is not a true loss from the fetus. Drugs that are 'trapped', for example, in meconium, fetal hair, or bones, would be reflected in direct fetal clearance.

Concerning the blood–brain barrier, preclinical research showed the underlying morphological feature of this barrier, the tight junctions between cerebral endothelial cells and between choroid plexus epithelial cells, is present from very early in embryological development. Therefore, while the blood–cerebrospinal fluid (CSF) barrier can be considered functionally and morphologically mature, the developing barrier has different characteristics than in adults. A decrease in both CSF/plasma concentration ratios for lipid-insoluble passive markers and CSF protein concentration is seen with increasing age.[25] Saunders et al. suggested this is due to changes in transcellular transfer and volume of distribution.[26] While the exact mechanisms remain unknown, available preclinical data on actual drug transfer suggests that compared to adults a higher blood–brain transfer of drugs might be seen in foetuses.[27,28]

When focusing on compounds commonly administered by anaesthetists, there are issues related to antibiotics and analgesics and fetal exposure. Pre-incisional administration of antibiotics compared to administration of antibiotics after caesarean delivery results in a decreased risk of developing post-caesarean endometritis, but also results in fetal exposure to antibiotics (e.g. cefazolin).[29] Administration of the same compound during fetal surgery does result in sufficiently high cefazolin concentrations in the maternal and the fetal compartment, but not in the amniotic cavity.[30] Administration of systemic opioids to the mother results in concentration-dependent fetal and neonatal sedation; this is also true for the very short-acting opioids like remifentanil.

Clinical pharmacology in neonates: limited size, extensive variability

Neonatal clinical pharmacology: an introduction

When a drug is prescribed, it is with the intention of attaining an anticipated therapeutic effect (e.g. sedation, pain relief, or muscular relaxation), preferably without disproportional or unanticipated side effects (e.g. prolonged sedation, hypotension, hepatic or renal impairment, or hypoventilation). Clinical pharmacology aims to predict such (side) effects based on compound-, population-, and patient-specific PK and PD.[4] PK describes the relationship between a concentration in a given compartment (e.g. plasma, CSF, or subcutaneous fluid) and time ('what the body does to the drug'). PD describes the relationship between a concentration at a given compartment and (adverse) effects ('what the drug does to the body'). Although the general principles of clinical pharmacology also apply to neonates, their specific physiological characteristics warrant a focused approach.[5] Effective and safe pharmacotherapy in young infants should be based on integrated knowledge concerning the evolving physiological characteristics of the infant who will receive the drug, and the PK and PD characteristics of a given drug: *developmental pharmacology reflects developmental physiology.*

Consequently, clinical pharmacology in neonates is as diverse and dynamic as the neonates themselves: beyond or in addition to median estimates, covariates of variability within this population are clinically relevant.[3] Growth and development throughout paediatric human life comprise a series of simultaneously ongoing physiological events that result both in growth and maturation, commonly subdivided into subpopulations (newborn, infancy, childhood, and adolescence). Across this paediatric life span, organ size and function change as does body composition and, ultimately, cellular function and metabolic activity. This will affect population-specific PK. In addition, some tissues may be more sensitive to pharmacological effects early in life, irrespective of a given concentration or exposure whereas others will be less. This will affect population-specific PD. There is already one order of magnitude difference in weight (0.5 to 5 kg) in the neonates currently hospitalized in neonatal intensive care units. The height velocity rate (10–20 cm/year) in the last trimester of pregnancy and the first months of extrauterine life, the increase in body weight (50% increase in the first 6 weeks, and three times in the first year of life), and the energy requirements of infancy all reflect the dynamics of a rapidly evolving biological system. From a clinical pharmacology perspective, the consequence of such a rapidly evolving biology is that there is extensive within- and between-subject variability in drug disposition and effects. This maturation-related variability is further aggravated by interfering pathological processes (e.g. growth restriction, sepsis, associated cardiomyopathy, and organ failure) or treatment modalities (e.g. co-medication, extracorporeal membrane oxygenation, and surgical intervention). Maturational PK consider maturational changes in drug ADME, while maturational PD consider maturational changes in the concentration–effect profile, for example, differences in receptor expression, function, or specific tissue/organ maturational sensitivity (either more or less vulnerable). It is only after maturational PK has been considered that maturational differences in PD can be explored. The perception that the effects or side effects of a given drug are different in the newborn is often due to the fact that PK has not yet been adequately studied in this population.[3,4,5]

Absorption relates to physicochemical characteristics and patient factors that influence the translocation of a given compound from its exposure site (e.g. enteral, pulmonary, or cutaneous) to the bloodstream or another effect compartment. There is important variability in absorption characteristics in neonates. For oral bioavailability, gastric acid production, transit time, maturation of mucosal enzymes, and diet are covariates of this variability. The still absent gastric acid production in the first days of life results in faster and more extended penicillin absorption, but impairs oral absorption of some antifungal agents. Gastric emptying after breastfeeding is faster when compared to formula feeding. Rectal administration is more difficult to predict because of the shorter rectal ampulla. Percutaneous absorption is higher due to more limited keratinization of the skin together with a higher skin surface/weight ratio. This may result in population-specific side effects (e.g. iodine absorption resulting in hypothyroidism, hexachlorophene resulting in neurological deterioration, and eutectic mixture of local anaesthetics absorption resulting in methaemoglobinaemia).[4]

Distribution describes the transfer of a specific drug from one location to another (e.g. tissues, organs, and fluid spaces) within the body, and is commonly quantified by the distribution volume (Vd = total amount of drug/concentration). Body water constitutes 75–80% of body weight in the newborn while body fat is low but doubles in the first 6 months. The postnatal weight loss mainly relates to postnatal water losses.[5,31] These maturational aspects are of relevance in the distribution of either water- or fat-soluble drugs (e.g. higher distribution volume for aminoglycosides in preterm compared to term neonates). Protein-binding capacity is in general lower in neonates. Competitive binding with bilirubin on albumin may result in increased free bilirubin and subsequent kernicterus (e.g. sulphonamides and ceftriaxone). Although volume of distribution does not necessarily represent a physiological volume or space, it is commonly affected by maturational physiological changes such as body composition, regional blood flow, organ size, barriers, or plasma protein concentrations.

Metabolism and elimination clearance (i.e. excretion) together reflect the clearance capacity, that is, the volume of blood or plasma from which a drug is completely removed per unit of time. All individual iso-enzymes (e.g. cytochromes and glucuronidation enzymes) involved in drug metabolism display an iso-enzyme-specific, age-dependent phenotypic activity. Relevant alterations in drug metabolizing enzyme activity occur during development.[31] Renal elimination clearance mainly depends on glomerular filtration rate but renal tubular functions also display maturation. Glomerular filtration rate depends on age. Besides age, co-medication (e.g. indomethacin and ibuprofen) and disease characteristics (e.g. growth restriction) further contribute to the phenotypic variability.[4] Table 5.3 provides some compound-specific examples of the impact of developmental

Table 5.3 Examples of the impact of developmental pharmacokinetics (*a*bsorption, *d*istribution, *m*etabolism, *e*limination) of individual compounds commonly administered to neonates by anaesthetists

Compound	Pharmacokinetics	Relevance
Iodine disinfectant	Skin more permeable, skin surface/kg higher (*a*)	Higher absorption may suppress thyroid function
Inhalational agents	Higher alveolar ventilation/functional residual capacity ratio (*a*)	Faster wash in
Cefazolin	Lower protein-binding capacity results in higher distribution	Peak concentration is lower
	Volume (*d*), and higher free plasma fraction (*e*)	Bactericid effect relates to free concentration
	Lower glomerular filtration rate (*e*)	Lower clearance, prolonged duration of bactericid effect
Bupivacaine	Lower protein binding capacity (*d*)	Free concentration related to adverse effects
	Lower clearance (*e*)	Accumulation during continuous administration
Propofol	Lipophilic compound, lower distribution volume (*d*)	Peak concentration is higher
	Glucuronidation for metabolic clearance (*m*)	Accumulation during continuous or repeated administration
Paracetamol	Water-soluble compound, higher distribution volume (*d*)	Peak concentration is lower, less effective analgesia likely
	Glucuronidation for metabolic clearance (*m*)	Accumulation during repeated administration possible
Midazolam	Water-soluble compound, higher distribution volume (*d*)	Peak concentration is lower, effect?
	Clearance to metabolite (1-hydroxy) is low (*m*)	Metabolite is also sedative, less prolonged sedation.
	Elimination clearance of (1-hydroxy) midazolam is low (*e*)	Lower clearance results in prolonged sedation.
Codeine	Clearance to metabolite (morphine) is low (*m*)	Shorter or reduced analgesic effect
	Elimination of codeine and metabolite is low (*e*)	Accumulation of codeine or metabolite more likely, prolonged or more pronounced analgesia

PK (ADME) in neonates for drugs commonly administered by anaesthetists.

However, neonatal PK is not just miniaturized adult PK. A minor route of elimination in adults may turn out to be the most relevant elimination route in a newborn, while not all elimination processes (e.g. drug metabolism versus subsequent elimination) mature simultaneously. Consequently, the concentration–time profile of a metabolite will not only depend on the metabolite formation as well as subsequent metabolite elimination. To illustrate the clinical relevance of such an integration, we refer to published observations on tramadol (demethylation, subsequent renal elimination), morphine disposition (glucuronidation, subsequent renal elimination clearance) and midazolam (oxidation and glucuronidation, subsequent renal elimination clearance) disposition in neonates.[32–34] All metabolites have a PD (e.g. analgesia, hyperalgesia, sedation, tolerance) impact. For all these compounds, accumulation of the metabolite can be anticipated in the newborn, not because of the already very effective phenotypic drug metabolism, but because of the even more defective subsequent elimination clearance.

To further illustrate the complexity and the need for an integrated approach—including neonatal ADME aspects—we would like to summarize the available information related to the initiation, success rates, and continuation of breastfeeding with specific emphasis on the use of and the exposure to analgesia-sedatives following maternal administration. Inadequate management of maternal pain is a commonly reported risk factor for failure of breastfeeding, while maternal exposure to analgesia-sedatives is a commonly perceived risk to breastfeed without much evidence in support of this practice.

Applied neonatal pharmacology: obstetric anaesthesia and breastfeeding

Breastfeeding is the obvious reference nutrition for newborns and infants. However, initiation or continuation of breastfeeding often coexists with maternal drug use.[35] Consequently, the ultimate goal of using maternal medications during breastfeeding is dual. Firstly, one aims to provide effective and safe therapy for the maternal condition(s) for which the drug has been prescribed (e.g. post-caesarean analgesia, maternal co-morbidities, and pregnancy-related diseases). Simultaneously, one aims to assure protection of the nursing infant from any (relevant) adverse event related to the treatment of the mother. Only rarely do these goals overlap (e.g. maternal intake of galactogogues such as domperidone or metoclopramide to enhance milk production).[36] Despite the fact that lactating women are regular users of medications and that women are often advised to discontinue or stop nursing while taking a drug, there are only a limited number of drugs that have been identified as potentially harmful to the newborn.[37,38]

Using a prospective study design, Ito et al. documented in a cohort of 838 nursing infants with mothers taking medications that the incidence of adverse reactions was 11.2% (94/838).[39] All these events were classified as minor reactions, not necessitating medical attention. Antibiotics (19.3%), analgesics, including narcotics (11.2%), antihistamines (9.4%), sedatives, antidepressants, or antiepileptics (7.1%) were most commonly associated with adverse reactions. The reported adverse reactions were diarrhoea (antibiotics), drowsiness (analgesics, sedatives, antidepressants, antiepileptics), or irritability (antihistamines).[39] The incidence, the type of reactions, and the drugs associated are in line with the systematic literature review performed by Anderson et al.[37] Based on the evaluation of 100 published case reports, none were considered to be 'definite' using a standard ranking scale, while 47% were 'probable', and 53% were 'possible'. Drugs with central nervous system activity accounted for about 50% of the events.[37] These data suggest that—by taking a few simple precautions in drug selection and considering the infant's age—breastfeeding rarely needs to be discouraged or discontinued when a mother needs drug therapy.

As part of a multidisciplinary healthcare provider team, anaesthetists need to be aware of the general strategies applied to improve breastfeeding initiation and continuation rates, commonly referred to as the Baby Friendly Hospital Initiative (BFHI).[35] The ten steps to successful breastfeeding hereby provide a supportive pathway, enabling women to achieve their breastfeeding intentions as well as guidance for training of healthcare workers in breastfeeding support.[40,41] In addition, anaesthetists administer a limited number of drug classes that may warrant a focused discussion. Reading through the ten-step list (Box 5.1), some aspects are of general relevance and relate to awareness on the breastfeeding policy and the skills and knowledge needed to act and communicate in an effective and homogeneous way. Some specific issues may affect routine practices or habits of anaesthetists. This refers to the practice of *skin-to-skin* contact and the initiation of breastfeeding shortly after delivery (<0.5 hours), including after caesarean delivery.[35,42] This necessitates sufficient maternal alertness

Box 5.1 The ten steps to successful breastfeeding (Baby Friendly Hospital Initiative, BHFI)

- Have a written breastfeeding policy that is routinely communicated to all health care staff.
- Train all health care staff in skills necessary to implement this policy.
- Inform all pregnant women about the benefits and management of breastfeeding.
- Help mothers initiate breastfeeding within a half-hour of birth.
- Show mothers how to breastfeed and how to maintain lactation, even if they are separated from their infants.
- Give newborn infants no food or drink other than breast milk unless medically indicated.
- Practice rooming-in—allow mothers and infants to remain together—24 hours a day.
- Encourage breastfeeding on demand.
- Give no artificial teats or pacifiers (also called dummies or soothers) to breastfeeding infants.
- Foster the establishment of breastfeeding support groups and refer mothers to them on discharge from the hospital or clinic.

Reprinted from *Baby-Friendly Hospital Initiative (BFHI) Training Materials*, World Health Organization, UNICEF, Copyright (2009).

and short-acting, effective analgesia. The associations between maternal preferences for neuraxial techniques during labour, maternal characteristics (e.g. obesity and primiparity) or immediate skin-to-skin contact and successful breastfeeding is multifactorial, but the association between either postpartum pain or maternal sedation and breastfeeding failure has been consistently reported in the literature.[43] Consequently, obstetric anaesthesia should focus on effective, safe, reversible techniques and treatments which facilitate and do not hinder breastfeeding.

In essence, exposure of a nursing mother to any dose of drug (D_m) will result in—be it very limited—transfer of the drug into the human milk (D_i). However, concentrations reached in the human milk are usually quite low and oral bioavailability in the infant should also be considered before any relevant pharmacological exposure relative infant dose (RID) = $D_m/D_i \times$ absorption) and effect in the infant needs to be anticipated (Figure 5.2). The difference in drug level in the infant's plasma (a vs b) can be explained by the presence (a) or absence (b) of 'initial loading' related to prenatal, fetal exposure to the same compound.

Age also matters, since newborns seem to be more vulnerable to adverse effects when compared to infants and relates to the earlier discussed age-related changes in PK and PD. Finally, and often insufficiently stressed, accumulation relates to the duration of exposure and the initial concentration in the newborn. In the setting of continuation of treatment of the mother from pregnancy to postpartum, the fetus will likely already be exposed to the maternal drugs, and the newborn will already have an initial concentration of this compound at birth. The subsequent concentration will depend on the amount of exposure, the clearance capacity, and the distribution volume characteristics (e.g. postnatal weight losses).

Opioids

Over the last few decades, the rate of breastfeeding has increased steadily in the developed world. During this time, opioid use in the general population has steadily increased as well. This means that the clinical experience with these compounds is still relatively limited in time with newly emerging data on codeine, oxycodone, methadone, and tramadol in recent years.[38,44] Applying the above-mentioned ADME issues, we should be aware that absorption of opioids after oral ingestion in neonates is common while the extent of exposure through a mother's milk will depend on maternal ingestion and metabolism. Neonatal clearance relates to either metabolic or renal elimination, but will be limited.[31] Such a setting has the potential to result in unanticipated side effects.

A pivotal case report in 2006 by Koren et al. on codeine-related morphine poisoning of a 13-day-old newborn reactivated the clinical research on maternal–infant PK of opioids through breastfeeding.[45] This study reconfirmed earlier case series on the association of maternal codeine exposure, maternal side effects (drowsiness, somnolence), and neonatal side effects (poor intake, weight loss, drowsiness, somnolence). A pharmacogenetic (PG) link between maternal ultrafast metabolizer status for CYP2D6 was documented, since this results in higher and faster conversion of codeine to morphine.[45] More recently, the same group documented that a combination of maternal genetic markers (CYP2D6 and P-glycoprotein polymorphisms) predicted 87% of the infant and maternal central nervous system depression cases with a sensitivity of 80% and a specificity of 87% in a cohort of 111 breastfeeding mother–infant pairs.[46]

The incidence of central nervous system depression in neonates breastfed by mothers receiving either oxycodone, codeine, or paracetamol was retrospectively compared in 533 breastfeeding mother–infant pairs. Lam et al. clearly showed that there was a 20.1% rate of depression in infants of breastfeeding mothers taking oxycodone, as compared with 16.7% and 0.5% in mothers treated with codeine or paracetamol respectively.[47] Methadone is somewhat special, since it is commonly used in a setting of maternal opioid addiction. Methadone is excreted into human milk (2–3% of weight-adjusted maternal dose), and there are data that suggest that these infants benefit from breastfeeding (blunted opioid withdrawal syndrome).[38] Finally, using a sparse sampling study design to assess transfer of tramadol and its O-desmethyl metabolite into transitional breast milk, the combined relative infant dose of 2–3% at steady-state was low. In the absence of differences in

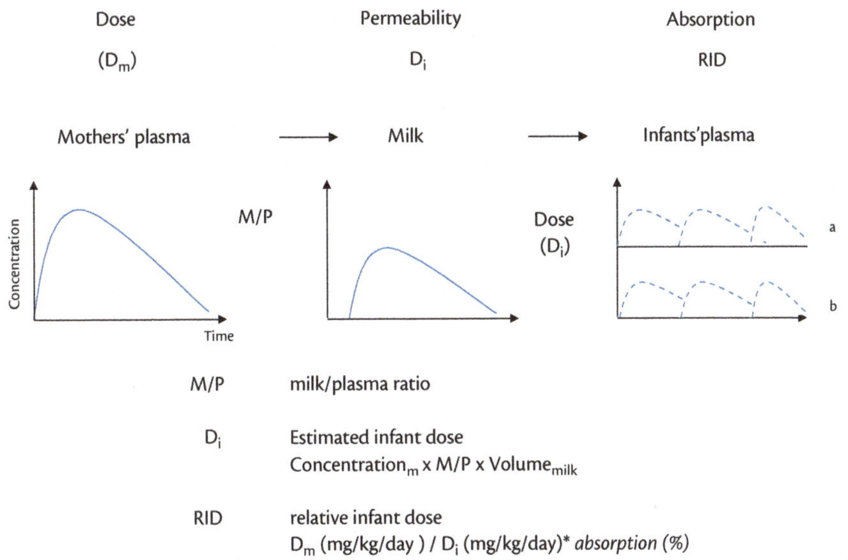

Figure 5.2 Theoretical framework to explore the extent of neonatal drug exposure through breastfeeding following maternal drug administration.

neurobehavioral scores between exposed infants and controls, the authors concluded that short-term maternal use of tramadol is compatible with breastfeeding.[48]

There are also some additional clinically useful and relevant messages in the available observations on maternal codeine and oxycodone exposure. First, there is high concordance between maternal and neonatal central nervous system depression. As a consequence, when the mother exhibits depression, the baby should be examined by a paediatrician. Second, severe depression emerged after 4 days of use, when milk output increases, exposure increases, and exposure is prolonged. Therefore, any maternal need for opioids for more than 4 days after delivery warrants focused attention while the mother's need for adequate pain control should not be neglected.[49]

Intravenous and inhalational anesthetics

Although the number of observations is limited, excretion of these compounds in human milk is not equal to infant exposure.[50] In the absence of subsequent enteral absorption, this remains without clinical symptoms. The same holds for inhalational agents in postpartum, while buccal resorption of etomidate has been observed. This only applies when these compounds are administered after delivery, since when administered during labour or delivery, placental passage and fetal accumulation may occur.

Benzodiazepines

Lorazepam, midazolam, or diazepam is commonly administered as an anxiolytic or sedation in a pre-anaesthesia setting. The mother compounds and some of the metabolites can be retrieved in human milk but concentrations remain very limited.[50,51] In 24 hours of human milk collection after a single dose in a pre-anaesthesia setting, only 0.005% of the maternal midazolam dose was retrieved. Taking the subsequent oral bioavailability (50–60%) into account, it is very reasonable to assume that the exposure will be limited when initially used after delivery. In contrast, plasma diazepam and its active metabolite (desmethyldiazepam) could be measured in neonates up to 7–10 days of postnatal age after single-dose administration to the mother during labour.[51] This relates to the much longer elimination half-life of diazepam, and when needed, short-acting benzodiazepines like midazolam are more appropriate.

Non-opioid analgesics

Human milk and plasma levels of paracetamol were monitored in three lactating women after ingestion of a 500 mg dose of paracetamol postpartum. Paracetamol concentrations remained lower in human milk (milk/plasma ratio of 0.76). Since less than 0.1% of the maternal dose would be present in 100 mL of milk, breastfeeding need not be discontinued due to maternal paracetamol exposure.[52] Similarly, ibuprofen in human milk and serum was quantified in 12 patients who had ingested one 400 mg tablet of ibuprofen every 6 hours over a 24-hour period for relief of post-caesarean delivery pain. Ibuprofen was present in the serum with a half-life of approximately 1.5 hours, but could not be quantified in human milk.[53] Based on the lower limit of quantification (1 mcg/mL), less than 1 mg of ibuprofen per day is excreted in breast milk. Similar findings have been described for ketorolac.[54] Although all these compounds may result in exposure to the newborn or infant, the extent is limited and much lower than that clinical registered dosing for analgesia or temperature reduction.[19]

Local anaesthetics

Local anaesthetics (e.g. lidocaine, bupivacaine, and ropivacaine) are commonly administered as part of regional anaesthetic techniques (e.g. regional pain block and epidural) and data are mainly available in mothers during labour or for anaesthesia during delivery.[55] Data on excretion of lidocaine and bupivacaine in human milk have been reported. Overall this exposure is limited with minor statistical significant, but clinically irrelevant differences. This is because absorption following oral ingestion is limited.

Based on the available observations, the use of systemic non-opioid analgesics, local anaesthetics as part of regional blocks, and inhalational or intravenous anaesthetics seems safe for nursing mothers. When systemic opioids are used, some clinical monitoring is warranted with specific emphasis on the duration of exposure (4 days pivotal) and the presence of any maternal sign of central nervous system depression.[49] Finally, the use of benzodiazepines should be limited with a preference for those with a shorter half-life. Under these circumstances, the most appropriate advice to a nursing mother undergoing anaesthesia is that she may reinitiate breastfeeding when she is sufficiently awake and feels strong enough to do so.

Conclusion

Maternal, fetal, and neonatal physiology affects both the PK as well as the PD of drugs administered in this population, including drugs commonly administered by anaesthetists. We illustrated the potential clinical relevance, using the available compound-specific observations. Since drug transfer through breastfeeding may be the most common, but complex pharmacological interaction between mother and infant, we focused on the available evidence on safety and risks related to analgosedatives.

References

1. Thomas SH, Yates LM. Prescribing without evidence—pregnancy. *Br J Clin Phamacol* 2012; 74:691–7.
2. Pavek P, Ceckova M, Staud F. Variation of drug kinetics in pregnancy. *Curr Drug Metab* 2009; 10:520–9.
3. Kearns GL, Abdel-Rahman SM, Alander SW, *et al.* Developmental pharmacology—drug disposition, action, and therapy in infants and children. *N Engl J Med* 2003; 349:1157–67.
4. Allegaert K, Verbesselt R, Naulaers G, *et al.* Developmental pharmacology: neonates are not just small adults. *Acta Clin Belg* 2008; 63:16–24.
5. Anderson BJ. Pharmacology in the very young: anaesthetic implications. *Eur J Anaesthesiol* 2012; 29:261–70.
6. Krauer B, Krauer F, Hytten FE. Drug disposition and pharmacokinetics in the maternal-placental-fetal unit. *Pharmacol Ther* 1980; 10:301–28.
7. Koren G (ed). *Maternal-Fetal Toxicology: A Clinician's Guide* (3rd ed). New York: Marcel Dekker, Inc; 2001.
8. Wiebe VJ, Sipila PE. Pharmacology of antineoplastic agents in pregnancy. *Crit Rev Oncol Hematol* 1994; 16:75–112.
9. Leighton BL, Cheek TG, Gross JB, *et al.* Succinylcholine pharmacodynamics in peripartum patients. *Anesthesiology* 1986; 64:202–5.
10. Baraka A, Jabbour S, Tabboush Z, *et al.* Onset of vecuronium neuromuscular block is more rapid in patients undergoing caesarean section. *Can J Anaesth* 1992; 39:135–8.
11. Pühringer FK, Sparr HJ, Mitterschiffthaler G, *et al.* Extended duration of action of rocuronium in postpartum patients. *Anesth Analg* 1997; 84:352–4.

12. Pan PH, Moore C. Comparison of cisatracurium-induced neuromuscular blockade between immediate postpartum and nonpregnant patients. *J Clin Anesth* 2001; 13:112–17.
13. Gin T, Gregory MA, Chan K, *et al.* Pharmacokinetics of propofol in women undergoing elective caesarean section. *Br J Anaesth* 1990; 64:148–53.
14. Higuchi H, Adachi Y, Arimura S, *et al.* Early pregnancy does not reduce the C(50) of propofol for loss of consciousness. *Anesth Analg* 2001; 93:1565–9.
15. Mongardon N, Servin F, Perrin M, *et al.* Predicted propofol effect-site concentration for induction and emergence of anesthesia during early pregnancy. *Anesth Analg* 2009; 109:90–5.
16. Allegaert K, van Calsteren K, Hendrickx S, *et al.* Paracetamol and ketorolac pharmacokinetics and metabolism at delivery and during postpartum. *Acta Anaesthesiol Belg* 2012; 63:121–5.
17. Kulo A, van de Velde M, van Calsteren K, *et al.* Pharmacokinetics of intravenous ketorolac following caesarean delivery. *Int J Obstet Anesth* 2012; 21:334–8.
18. Kulo A, Peeters MY, Allegaert K, *et al.* Pharmacokinetics of paracetamol and its metabolites in women at delivery and postpartum. *Br J Clin Pharmacol* 2013; 75:850–60.
19. Bloor M, Paech M. Nonsteroidal anti-inflammatory drugs during pregnancy and the initiation of lactation. *Anesth Analg* 2013; 116:1063–75.
20. Bloor M, Paech MJ, Kaye R. Tramadol in pregnancy and lactation. *Int J Obstet Anesth* 2012; 21:163–7.
21. Anderson D. A review of systemic opioids commonly used for labor pain relief. *J Midwifery Womens Health* 2011; 56:222–39.
22. Syme MR, Paxton JW, Keelan JA. Drug transfer and metabolism by the human placenta. *Clin Pharmacokinet* 2004; 43:487–514.
23. Garland M. Pharmacology of drug transfer across the placenta. *Obstet Gynecol Clin North Am* 1998; 25:21–42.
24. Polin RA, Fox WW, Abman SH (eds). *Fetal and Neonatal Physiology* (3rd ed). Philadelphia, PA: Saunders; 2004.
25. Johansson PA, Dziegielewska KM, Liddelow SA, *et al.* The blood-CSF barrier explained: when development is not immaturity. *Bioessays* 2008; 30:237–48.
26. Saunders NR, Knott GW, Dziegielewska KM. Barriers in the immature brain. *Cell Mol Neurobiol* 2000; 20:29–40.
27. Au-Yeung SC, Riggs KW, Gruber N, *et al.* The use of microdialysis for the study of drug kinetics: central nervous system pharmacokinetics of diphenhydramine in fetal, newborn, and adult sheep. *Drug Metab Dispos* 2007; 35:1285–91.
28. He K, Lago MW, Iyer RA, *et al.* Lacteal secretion, fetal and maternal tissue distribution of dasatinib in rats. *Drug Metab Dispos* 2008; 36:2564–70.
29. Heesen M, Klöhr S, Rossaint R, *et al.* Concerning the timing of antibiotic administration in women undergoing caesarean section: a systematic review and meta-analysis. *BMJ Open* 2013; 3:e002028.
30. Allegaert K, van Mieghem T, Verbesselt R, *et al.* Cefazolin pharmacokinetics in maternal plasma and amniotic fluid during pregnancy. *Am J Obstet Gynecol* 2009; 200:170.e1–7.
31. Smits A, Kulo A, de Hoon JN, *et al.* Pharmacokinetics of drugs in neonates: pattern recognition beyond compound specific observations. *Curr Pharm Des* 2012; 18:3119–46.
32. Allegaert K, Rochette A, Veyckemans F. Developmental pharmacology of tramadol during infancy: ontogeny, pharmacogenetics and elimination clearance. *Paediatr Anaesth* 2011; 21: 266–73.
33. Taylor J, Liley A, Anderson BJ. The relationship between age and morphine infusion rate in children. *Paediatr Anaesth* 2013; 23:40–4.
34. Anderson BJ, Larsson P. A maturation model for midazolam clearance. *Paediatr Anaesth* 2011; 21: 302–8.
35. Saadeh RJ. The Baby-Friendly Hospital Initiative 20 years on: facts, progress, and the way forward. *J Hum Lact* 2012; 28:272–5.
36. Forinash AB, Yancey AM, Barnes KN, *et al.* The use of galactogogues in the breastfeeding mother. *Ann Pharmacother* 2012; 46:1392–404.
37. Anderson PO, Pochop SL, Manoguerra AS. Adverse drug reactions in breastfed infants: less than imagined. *Clin Pediatr* 2003; 42:325–40.
38. Berlin CM Jr, van den Anker JN. Safety during breastfeeding: drugs, foods, environmental chemicals, and maternal infections. *Semin Fetal Neonat Med* 2013; 18:13–18.
39. Ito S, Blajchman A, Stephenson M, *et al.* Prospective follow up of adverse reactions in breast-fed infants exposed to maternal medication. *Am J Obstet Gynecol* 1993; 168:1393–9.
40. Dozier AM, Howard CR, Brownell EA, *et al.* Labor epidural anesthesia, obstetric factors and breastfeeding cessation. *Matern Child Health J* 2013; 17:689–98.
41. Gubler T, Krähenmann, Roos M, *et al.* Determinants of successful breastfeeding initiation in healthy term singletons: a Swiss university hospital observational study. *J Perinat Med* 2013; 41:331–9.
42. Hellwig JP. Encouraging breastfeeding: initiative to help hospitals become baby-friendly. *Nurs Womens Health* 2012; 16:79.
43. Woods AB, Crist B, Kowalewski S, *et al.* A cross-sectional analysis of the effect of patient-controlled epidural analgesia versus patient controlled analgesia for postcesarean pain and breastfeeding. *J Obstet Gynecol Neonatal Nurs* 2012; 41:339–46.
44. Hendrickson RG, McKeown NJ. Is maternal opioid use hazardous to breast-fed infants? *Clin Toxicol* 2012; 50:1–14.
45. Koren G, Cairns J, Chitayat D, *et al.* Pharmacogenetics of morphine poisoning in a breastfed neonate of a codeine-prescribed mother. *Lancet* 2006; 368:704.
46. Sistonen J, Madadi P, Ros CJ, *et al.* Prediction of codeine toxicity in infants and their mothers using a novel combination of maternal genetic markers. *Clin Pharmacol Ther* 2012; 91:692–9.
47. Lam J, Kelly L, Ciszkowski C, *et al.* Central nervous system depression of neonates breastfed by mothers receiving oxycodone for postpartum analgesia. *J Pediatr* 2012; 160:33–37.e2.
48. Ilett KF, Paech MJ, Page-Sharp M, *et al.* Use of a sparse sampling study design to assess transfer of tramadol and its O-desmethyl metabolite into transitional breast milk. *Br J Clin Pharmacol* 2008; 65:661–6.
49. Van den Anker JN. Is it safe to use opioids for obstetric pain while breastfeeding? *J Pediatr* 2012; 160:4–6.
50. Nitsun M, Szokol JW, Saleh HJ, *et al.* Pharmaokinetics of midazolam, propofol, and fentanyl transfer to human breast milk. *Clin Pharmacol Ther* 2006; 79:549–57.
51. Cole AP, Haley DM. Diazepam and active metabolite in breast milk and their transfert to the neonate. *Arch Dis Child* 1975; 50:741–2.
52. Bitzén PO, Gustafsson B, Jostell KG, *et al.* Excretion of paracetamol in human breast milk. *Eur J Clin Pharmacol* 1981; 20:123–5.
53. Townsend RJ, Benedetti TJ, Erickson SH, *et al.* Excretion of ibuprofen into breast milk. *Am J Obstet Gynecol* 1984; 149:184–6.
54. Wischnik A, Manth SM, Lloyd J, *et al.* The excretion of ketorolac tromethamine into breast milk after multiple oral dosing. *Eur J Clin Pharmacol* 1989; 36:521–4.
55. Ortega D, Viviand X, Lorec AM, *et al.* Excretion of lidocaine and bupivacaine in breast milk following epidural anesthesia for cesarean delivery. *Acta Anaesthesiol Scand* 1999; 43:394–7.

PART 3

Fetal and neonatal assessment and therapy

CHAPTER 6

Antenatal and intrapartum fetal evaluation

Yves Jacquemyn and Anneke Kwee

Introduction

The assessment of fetal well-being aims at reducing fetal/neonatal mortality and morbidity. The anaesthetist can be confronted with tests that evaluate fetal well-being in different ways. The results of these tests can provoke the obstetrician to decide to perform an unplanned caesarean delivery, which can result in the anaesthetist needing to provide anaesthesia for an urgent delivery. Also changes in the fetal heart rate (FHR) pattern after administration of epidural or systemic medication should be evaluated and when suspected to be abnormal the obstetrician should be informed and alerted. In this chapter, we describe different methods in use to assess fetal well-being and provide the reader with basic knowledge to aid their interpretation. We will only briefly discuss tests for fetal malformations (structural ultrasound and magnetic resonance imaging) and fetal biometry for intrauterine growth disorders. An overview of the methods discussed and their evaluation is given in Table 6.1.

Intrapartum fetal monitoring aims to identify fetuses at risk for neonatal and long-term injury due to asphyxia, triggering appropriate interventions to reduce neonatal morbidity. However, it is also important that the number of subsequent unnecessary obstetric interventions, with their associated maternal and neonatal morbidity, is limited as far as possible. The ideal method of monitoring has not yet been found, which is apparent from the fact that the number of obstetric interventions for suspected fetal distress has increased without neonatal outcomes having clearly improved.[1–3]

The terms fetal 'distress' and fetal 'compromise' are rather vague, imprecise, and non-specific. The Committee on Obstetric Practice of the American College of Obstetricians and Gynecologists has proposed using 'non-reassuring fetal status' instead.[4] For practical purposes we will consider fetal compromise as a fetus at risk of hypoxia and its consequences.[4]

Causes of fetal hypoxia are multiple but can be categorized as follows:

- Maternal: reduced maternal oxygenation such as in maternal lung disease or in case of diminished atmospheric oxygen content (e.g. living at high altitude).
- Uteroplacental: such as seen in pre-eclampsia and intrauterine fetal growth restriction due to failure of trophoblast invasion resulting in reduced maternal blood supply to the placental bed.
- Fetoplacental: impaired blood supply to the placenta such as in umbilical cord compression, maternal hypotension, or hypovolaemia.
- Fetal: intrinsic fetal diseases such as fetal anaemia and/or haemoglobinopathy.

During active labour, uteroplacental perfusion is markedly reduced since during every uterine contraction the pressure in the contracting myometrium is higher than the maternal systolic blood pressure, so blood flow to the placenta virtually ceases for the duration of a contraction. The healthy fetoplacental unit can compensate for this provided that there is a sufficient interval between contractions, which is not the case in situations of uterine hyperactivity, a frequent cause of fetal hypoxia. The accumulation of carbon dioxide will rapidly lead to respiratory acidosis (as described further) as long as aerobic metabolism is maintained. When oxygen drops further, lactate will be produced resulting in metabolic acidosis.

Cardiotocography (CTG) or electronic fetal monitoring was introduced in the 1970s without proven diagnostic accuracy, and its efficiency in improving neonatal outcome was never adequately evaluated.[5–7] A disadvantage of CTG is the high percentage of false-positive interpretations[8,9] due to high inter- and intra-observer variation.[10] In a high-risk population, during the phase of cervical dilatation the CTG shows anomalies in 10% of cases and this figure increases to 60–90% during the phase of active pushing. Without additional diagnostics, this leads to unnecessary interventions due to the large number of false-positive results and the relatively low prevalence of acidosis. With CTG anomalies, additional investigations should be performed.

Essentially, at the start of labour, women can be divided into low risk or high risk for fetal hypoxia. Examples of high-risk pregnancies are pre-existing maternal disease, complicated obstetric history, hypertensive disorders, intrauterine growth restriction (IUGR), ruptured membranes for more than 24 hours, or a post-date gestational age. During labour, women can become high risk because there is failure to progress, meconium-stained amniotic fluid, or a non-reassuring FHR. Low-risk women can be monitored by intermittent auscultation (IA), whereas high-risk women should be monitored by CTG and if non-reassuring by additional methods.

In this chapter, we provide an overview of different methods for fetal monitoring during pregnancy and labour: the screening

Table 6.1 Overview of methods for fetal monitoring in low-risk and high-risk pregnancies for developing fetal hypoxia

Method	Low risk	High risk	Comment
Antenatal			
Maternal fetal movement counting	No benefit	No data	
Biophysical profile score	No data, no indication	No benefit	
Uterine artery Doppler	Only to select high risk for development of fetal growth retardation and pre-eclampsia in later pregnancy		Does not provide information from fetus
Umbilical artery Doppler	No benefit	Reduces fetal mortality	
Middle cerebral artery Doppler	No data, no indication	No added value to umbilical artery	Can be used to diagnose and follow fetal anaemia
Ductus venosus Doppler	No data, no indication	Moderate detection of fetal compromise, no added value to umbilical artery Doppler	
Non-computerized CTG	No benefit	No benefit when used as a single test	
Computerized CTG	No data	Significant reduction in perinatal mortality	
During labour			
IA	No data when compared to no monitoring For more detail see CTG	No data	
Admission CTG	More caesarean deliveries than IA, no other differences	No data	
CTG during labour	When compared to IA: No effect on perinatal death, cerebral palsy Lowers neonatal convulsions More instrumental vaginal deliveries Non-significant rise in caesarean deliveries		No studies have been performed specifying low- or high-risk women
FBS pH	Less caesarean deliveries than CTG alone Less neonatal convulsions		No studies without CTG No studies comparing high- and low-risk pregnancies
FBS lactate	No effect on neonatal outcome No effect on instrumental deliveries		No studies without CTG No studies comparing high- and low-risk pregnancies
STAN®	Compared to CTG alone: No difference in metabolic acidosis Less operative vaginal deliveries Less need for neonatal intensive care Less use of FBS		No studies without CTG No studies comparing high- and low-risk pregnancies
Fetal pulse oximeter	No difference in caesarean deliveries No difference in metabolic acidosis		No studies without CTG No studies comparing high- and low-risk pregnancies No longer commercially available

CTG, cardiotocography; FBS, fetal blood sampling; IA, intermittent auscultation.
For details and references see text.

methods such as IA and CTG and additional methods such as fetal blood sampling (FBS) and ST-analysis of the fetal electrocardiogram (ECG). We focus on methods to detect fetal hypoxia and the pathophysiology of fetal hypoxia and refer to other chapters for a discussion on the potential causes of fetal hypoxia.

Pathophysiology of fetal compromise and relation to fetal testing

In the fetus, gas exchange occurs in the placenta, while the fetal lungs are non-functional as far as gas exchange is concerned.

The fetal circulation is different as compared to the adult, the main differences being the mixing of oxygenated and deoxygenated blood returning to the heart and differential streaming patterns allowing oxygenated blood from the placenta to reach vital organs easily. For this purpose, extracardiac shunting (ductus arteriosus and ductus venosus) and intracardiac shunting (foramen ovale) are present. Figure 6.1 represents the normal fetal circulation. Umbilical venous blood is highly oxygen-saturated blood, about half of which supplies the liver, whilst the other half enters the ductus venosus to the inferior vena cava, where it meets the less oxygen-saturated systemic venous drainage from the lower fetal body. Both streams (from the abdominal inferior cava and from the ductus venosus) do not completely mix. Oxygenated ductus venosus blood flows preferentially through the foramen ovale, left atrium, left ventricle, and ascending aorta providing oxygen to the myocardium and brain.

Both the right and left ventricles perfuse the lower body organs. The output of the right ventricle is shunted from the pulmonary artery to the aortic arch by the ductus arteriosus. The right ventricular output contains desaturated venous blood from superior and inferior vena cava and from the coronary sinus. As it passes directly through the ductus arteriosus to the descending aorta this unoxygenated venous blood is preferentially returned to the placenta for re-oxygenation.

The sympathetic innervation of the fetal myocardium is incompletely developed, even at term; beta-adrenergic receptors are present at an early age explaining the immediate fetal tachycardia seen when beta-agonists, as used for tocolysis, are administered to the mother. Vagal innervation is complete by term. As pregnancy progresses, FHR comes under increasing parasympathetic dominance, resulting in a gradual decrease in heart rate, increase in variability, and increasing responsiveness as shown by both accelerations and decelerations. The fetal heart normally appears to operate near the top of its cardiac function curve; an increase in FHR will result in only a very small increase in cardiac output, while bradycardia can result in a major decrease in cardiac output.

FHR is regulated by a variety of systems including baroreceptors, chemoreceptors, the autonomic nervous system, the adrenal medulla, hormonal influences such as renin, angiotensin, vasopressin, natriuretic peptides, prostaglandins, endothelin, and endothelium-derived nitric oxide. The magnitude and clinical relevance of the relative contribution in regulating fetal cardiac function are matters of ongoing discussion.

The baroreflex means that after an acute increase in systemic arterial pressure (as seen, for instance, when the umbilical arteries are compressed) the FHR slows. Baroreceptors are present at the carotid sinus and are active through the vagal nerve. Chemoreceptors are present in the carotid artery and in the aorta. Carotid chemoreceptor stimulation causes hypertension and tachycardia, whereas aortic chemoreceptor stimulation results in bradycardia and only a mild increase in arterial blood pressure. The carotid receptors are less sensitive than the aortic receptors which explains why bradycardia is mostly seen in cases of fetal hypoxia. The autonomic control of the FHR shows maturation with advancing gestational age. This means that interpretation of the FHR pattern should take gestational age into account. Accelerations and periods of high variability (as discussed further) are seen less frequently before 30 weeks' gestational age, their absence in preterm gestation should not be interpreted as a sign of fetal distress.[11]

The human fetus demonstrates a variety of adaptations to hypoxia, including modifying these preferential

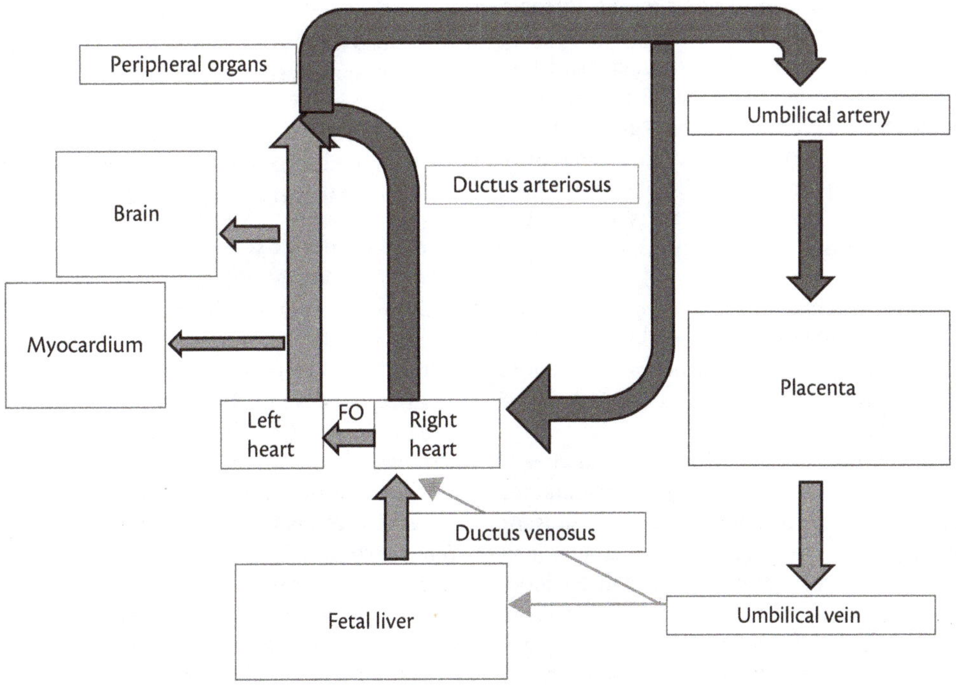

Figure 6.1 Normal fetal circulation. FO, foramen ovale.

streaming patterns. The available tests detect different aspects of these adaptations.

In the normal fetal situation, adenosine triphosphate (ATP) as an energy carrier is produced via oxidative phosphorylation mainly from glucose, although the fetus can also use fats and proteins. ATP is present in cells in small amounts, its half-life is only seconds, and ATP must be quickly regenerated to match usage by cells. Mitochondria from fetal myocardium demonstrate higher oxidative phosphorylation than from adult myocytes, reflecting increased electron transport. When the oxygen level is insufficient, anaerobic metabolism occurs, resulting in only two molecules of ATP versus 24 molecules being produced per molecule of glucose. Hypoxia also results in by-products such as lactic acid, provoking metabolic acidosis. Finally, cellular metabolism is no longer sustained, resulting in cell damage and death.

Oxygen is provided to the fetus via the maternoplacental and fetoplacental exchange. Fetal respiratory acidosis occurs when carbon dioxide cannot be washed out. This can be caused by inadequate gas exchange across the placenta, but also by a high maternal arterial PCO_2 (which blocks the diffusional transfer of CO_2 from fetus to mother), or a combination of both. As the fetal pH will be lower both during metabolic and respiratory acidosis, some other measurement of fetal acid–base balance is necessary to differentiate between the two, including fetal lactate determination or calculating fetal base excess or deficiency based on PCO_2 measurement using different algorithms.

Damage is most acute in the fetal brain, myocardium, and kidneys. When fetal hypoxia occurs, redistribution of blood is preferentially to the fetal brain ('brain sparing'), the myocardium, and adrenal glands and this is at the expense of organs such as the lungs, liver, and kidneys. Except for the fetal cerebral circulation, autoregulation (the ability to maintain constant blood flow over a wide range of perfusion pressures) is not present in the placenta-umbilico-fetal system. We will now discuss briefly the effects and clinical correlations of fetal hypoxia on the adrenals, kidney, myocardium, and brain.

In case of hypoxia, the adrenal medulla will increase circulating plasma catecholamine concentrations. Stimulation of beta-adrenoreceptors in the myocardium activates glycogenolysis and enhances myocardial work performance and is related to an increase in the fetal T-wave amplitude in the ECG, which is used in fetal ST segment monitoring. The rise in T wave is due to a shift in potassium ions (K^+) as related to lactic acid transport, affecting myocardial cell membrane potential.

Reduced renal perfusion results in oliguria. In contrast, swallowing, the mechanism for elimination of amniotic fluid, is controlled by a relatively hypoxaemia-resistant hindbrain regulatory centre. Both factors combined result in reduced amniotic fluid volume or oligohydramnios.[12]

Myocardial response to hypoxia includes T-wave rise, as already mentioned. When energy balance can no longer be maintained by anaerobic metabolism and vasodilatation, ischaemia results. As the perfusion of the myocardium is directed from the outer (epicardial) to the inner (endocardial) surface, the more distal endocardial part will suffer from ischaemia first. This causes delay in repolarization in the endocardial face as compared to the epicardial level. The change in the sequence of repolarization (the endocardial part repolarizing later than the epicardial part) is reflected as a depression of the ST segment with or without a negative T wave in the fetal ECG, which is clinically detected using ST analysis. Any other factor altering the balance of performance and repolarization through the myocardium will cause similar changes, not necessarily related to fetal hypoxia, including prematurity, infections, cardiomyopathy, and cardiac malformations.[13,14]

Fetal cerebral circulation is characterized by arterial vasodilation in case of hypoxia. Such vasodilation can be clinically measured as a reduced resistance in the middle cerebral artery (MCA) as will be discussed further. The normal human fetus develops an increasingly complicated behavioural pattern from early to late pregnancy, including gross body movements, breathing movements, fine motor movements, and even including reactions to external stimuli such as noise and vibration. Fetal movements increase FHR, FHR variation, and accelerations. In case of cerebral ischaemia, these patterns are progressively lost in the inverse sequence as they were acquired, the reaction to external stimuli disappearing first, followed by loss of fine motor movements over stopping breathing movements, and finally complete immobility without any large body movements. Presence or absence of these behavioural patterns can be evaluated using the fetal biophysical profile. A normal biophysical profile is associated with normal healthy status and absence of normality possibly equals fetal distress.

Antenatal prelabour fetal evaluation

Assessment of fetal movement by the mother

Pregnant women recognize fetal movements from the second trimester although large interindividual variation exists.

Structured fetal movement counting, such as 'count to ten' fetal kicks, has been attempted as a method to reduce variation and diminish fetal death. However, in a randomized controlled trial (RCT) including 68,000 women[15] this did not result in improved outcome as compared to informally asking for fetal movements during standard antenatal care. Fetal movement charting has not been proven to be of benefit, but only one RCT has actually been performed in low-risk women and none in high-risk women.[16]

The compromised fetus presumably reduces its activity to decrease oxygen need. Any patient reporting fetal inactivity should be further examined, including CTG and ultrasound for fetal biophysical profile, but no study has ever reported on a comparison between different methods to manage reported decreased fetal movements.[17]

Biophysical profile scoring and placental grading

Fetal behavioural state

Body movements and heart rate patterns in the human fetus reveal cyclicity that becomes more marked when reaching term. Nijhuis et al. first described four distinct behavioural states based on ultrasound and FHR recordings, which can be clearly determined at approximately 26 weeks.[18] Quiescence (state 1F) is characterized by no eye movements, no somatic movements except for the occasional startle, and a FHR pattern with little baseline variability, comparable to non-rapid eye movement (REM) sleep. When recording FHR such periods typically last for about 20 minutes, but may persist for 2 hours in normal term fetuses. State 2F is characterized by continuous eye movements, frequent bursts of somatic movements, and wide baseline variability and accelerations with movement, comparable to REM sleep. This state predominates, occurring approximately 40% of the time. State 3F shows no gross body movements, eye movements are continually present, and FHR is stable but with a wider oscillation bandwidth than for state 1F. State 3F is seldom seen and it is debated whether this is really a distinct entity. State 4F is characterized by continuous eye movements with almost continuous somatic movements and a sustained tachycardia. With advancing gestational age, state 1F increases in time without a change in 2F, but with less time spent in an unidentifiable state. In case of IUGR, as a marker of chronic hypoxaemia, fetuses show a delay in the appearance of well-delineated states, indicating subtle disturbances of the central nervous system.

Biophysical profile score

Animal studies have demonstrated that episodic fetal breathing movements (FBM) and fetal gross body movements (GBM) are inhibited by acute hypoxia.[19] This formed the basis for the development of a composite biophysical profile score (BPP) including markers of both acute (FBM, GBM, fetal tone, FHR reactivity) and chronic (amniotic fluid volume) fetal compromise.[20]

In case of IUGR and chronic fetal hypoxaemia, FBM and GBM generally decrease to minimize energy expenditure depending on the severity of the condition.[21]

The four acute markers have a different time relationship to become abnormal in case of fetal compromise. A non-reactive CTG (see 'Basic Principles' section of CTG) and absent FBM are early and sensitive, and as a consequence demonstrate a high false-positive rate; GBM and fetal tone change late. The risk for fetal metabolic acidosis and perinatal mortality increases with reductions in BPP.[22]

An overview of the scoring system as proposed by Manning et al. is given in Table 6.2.

A score of either 10 out of 10 or 8 out of 10 with normal amniotic fluid volume, or 8 out of 8 (without CTG) is indicative of fetal health and absence of distress, or better normal tissue oxygenation and absence of central acidaemia. It should be remembered that the test only represents the fetal metabolic situation at the time of the test; no good data are available to decide on the frequency at which the test should be repeated. The results are also influenced by gestational age and the normal cyclical pattern of fetal behaviour. FBM and GBM are more often absent at 26–33 weeks, resulting in falsely abnormal results.[21]

Even in the absence of metabolic acidosis, IUGR fetuses demonstrate less FBM and GFM.[23]

A score of 6/10 or less means a probability of tissue hypoxia and central acidaemia. There are no randomized trials indicating the best management in such circumstances. Clearly the BPP is more time-consuming and requires more technical skills than the CTG alone. It is accompanied by a very low false-negative rate in high-risk pregnancies (0.07%) but with a false-positive rate comparable to that of the CTG alone. In a meta-analysis of randomized trials comparing CTG alone and BPP, no difference was noted for perinatal mortality, low Apgar score, or incidence of caesarean delivery.[24] The available evidence no longer supports the use of BPP as a test for fetal well-being in high-risk pregnancies. There has been no study to evaluate BPP in low-risk pregnancies and this is not recommended.

Table 6.2 Manning biophysical profile score

Variable	Normal: score 2	Abnormal: score 0
Fetal breathing movements	1 or more episodes of ≥20 s within 30 min	Absent or no episodes of ≥20 s within 30 min
Gross body movements	2 or more discrete body/limb movements within 30 min (episodes of active continuous movement considered as a single movement)	<2 episodes of body/limb movement within 30 min
Fetal tone	1 or more episodes of active extension with return to flexion of fetal limb(s) or trunk (opining an closing of hand considered normal tone)	Slow extension with return to partial flexion, movement of limb in full extension, absent fetal movement, or partially open fetal hand
Reactive fetal heart rate	2 or more episodes of acceleration of ≥15 bpm and of >15 s associated with fetal movement within 20 min	1 or more episodes of acceleration of fetal heart rate or acceleration of <15 bpm within 20 min
Qualitative amniotic fluid volume	1 or more pockets of fluid measuring ≥2 cm in vertical axis	Either no pockets or largest pocket <2 cm in vertical axis

Adapted from *American Journal of Obstetrics and Gynecology*, Volume 151, issue 3, Manning FA, Morrisonj I, Lange IR *et al.*, Fetal assessment based on fetal biophysical profile scoring: experience in 12620 referred high risk pregnancies: I. perinatal mortality by frequency and etiology, pp. 343–50, Copyright (1985), with permission from Elsevier.

Doppler ultrasound

Basic principles

Doppler ultrasound allows non-invasive evaluation of maternal and fetal haemodynamics. Blood flow is most often quantified either by a pulsatility index or by a resistance index, reflecting the downstream vascular resistance by quantifying differences between peak systolic and end-diastolic or mean velocity.

Maternal doppler

Uterine artery

Trophoblast invasion in the uterine vessels has to occur early in the second trimester to allow increase in uterine perfusion and providing nutrient supply and gas exchange to the fetus. This invasion, destroying the muscular wall of the spiral arteries to the placenta, results in lowering the resistance to distal flow in the uterine arteries and is marked by a typical high end-diastolic velocity pattern in the uterine artery in pregnancy. Failure of trophoblast invasion of the spiral arteries results in increased resistance and decreased placental perfusion, possible fetal growth restriction, and pre-eclampsia. This results in a pathological Doppler pattern of the uterine artery with low diastolic velocity and an early diastolic notch. It has been demonstrated that screening with uterine artery Doppler is able to predict fetal growth restriction and pre-eclampsia. Uterine artery Doppler does not provide any information on the actual fetal status.

Other Doppler measurements of maternal circulation, including maternal cerebral circulation, have been studied but do not directly relate to fetal status.

Fetal doppler

Umbilical artery

Umbilical artery Doppler (Figure 6.2) is a placental function test, closely related to umbilical artery pH.[25] The resistance to flow increases in the umbilical artery as placental fetal circulation is

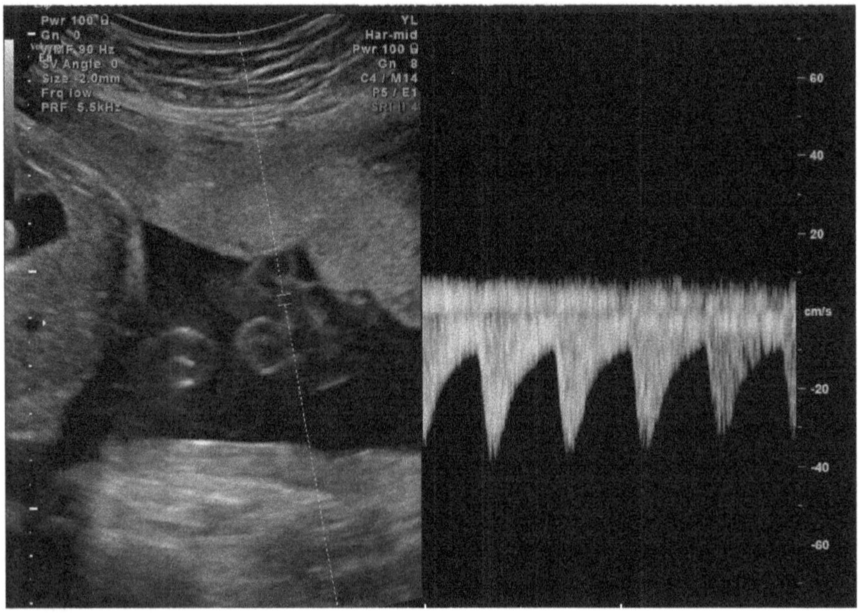

Figure 6.2 Normal umbilical artery flow pattern.

compromised (higher placental impedance) resulting in low to absent and even reversed flow in the umbilical artery during fetal diastole (Figure 6.3). Resistance to flow has been expressed in different indices such as the resistance index and the pulsatility index, a higher index indicating worse fetoplacental circulation. RCTs have demonstrated a significant association between abnormal umbilical artery Doppler and adverse perinatal outcome. Umbilical artery Doppler allows differentiation between the constitutionally small fetus and the growth-restricted fetus.

The odds ratio for perinatal mortality in growth-restricted fetuses by absent diastolic flow is 4.0, in case of reversed diastolic flow this increases to 10.6. Absence of diastolic flow has a sensitivity of 78% for detecting hypoxia and 90% for detecting fetal acidosis on fetal blood at delivery. The positive predictive value ranges from 53% to 88%, the negative predictive value from 98% to 100%.[26]

Meta-analyses have demonstrated that in high-risk (including maternal hypertension and ultrasound-proven fetal growth restriction) pregnancies, umbilical artery Doppler ultrasound significantly reduces perinatal deaths (1.2% versus 1.7%). Number needed to 'treat' to prevent 1 fetal death is 203. This is true when Doppler is combined with other tests such as CTG or BPP, when one compares Doppler alone to CTG alone no difference was noted.[27] This means that umbilical artery Doppler is by itself never an indication for immediate intervention (such as caesarean delivery); every individual case should be evaluated based on all available parameters such as fetal growth, maternal health, gestational age, and CTG. In case of fetal IUGR and absent or reversed end-diastolic umbilical artery flow hospital admission and daily CTG are advised.[28]

In low-risk unselected pregnancies, no difference in outcome is found in a meta-analysis[29] for serious neonatal morbidity, low Apgar score, caesarean delivery, operative vaginal births, induction of labour, or neonatal resuscitation and perinatal death. Neither is there any effect when using umbilical artery Doppler intrapartum as reviewed by Farrell et al.[30]

Middle cerebral artery

In the normally developing fetus, the brain is an area of low vascular impedance. In cases of hypoxia, redistribution to the fetal brain is seen, as shown by lowering of the resistance in the MCA (Figures 6.4 and 6.5). When compared to umbilical artery Doppler, adding MCA Doppler does not seem to add any clinical benefit, although it is frequently performed to demonstrate brain-sparing effects. A systematic review and meta-analysis showed low predictive accuracy for adverse perinatal outcome (positive likelihood ratio 2.77, 95% confidence interval (CI) 1.93–3.96; negative likelihood ratio 0.58, 95% CI 0.48–0.69),[31] concluding that MCA Doppler has no or very limited added value as compared to umbilical artery Doppler and CTG. Another application of MCA Doppler is in the diagnosis and management of fetal anaemia: the velocity of blood flow in the cerebral artery correlates very well with fetal haemoglobin, the lower the haemoglobin the higher the velocity. MCA velocity measurement has been the non-invasive method to diagnose fetal anaemia and determine when delivery or intrauterine transfusion is mandatory.[32]

The fetal aorta and other arteries have been studied but have no additional benefit to clinical management.

Venous fetal Doppler has also been introduced as providing information from the precordial circulation. Pulsations in the umbilical vein, caused by retrograde transmission of atrial pressure mainly in the failing heart, are related to impending fetal demise.

The flow pattern in the ductus venosus demonstrates a typical M-shaped pattern (Figure 6.6) and, in contrast to other veins, reverse flow is not present in normal fetuses. During atrial systole, reduction in forward flow always occurs, producing the characteristic negative a-wave in the ductus venosus pattern. In case of defective placentation, cardiac afterload increases and the a-wave

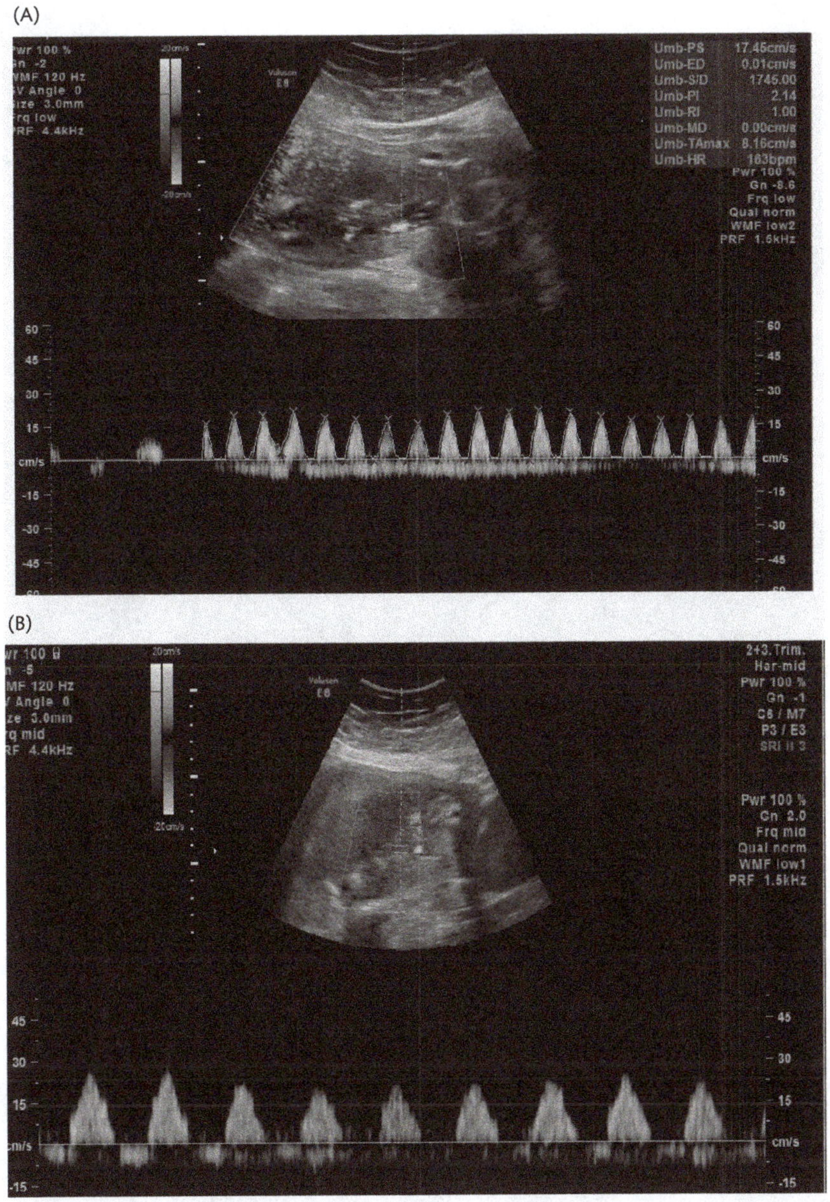

Figure 6.3 (A) Absent and (B) reversed diastolic flow in the umbilical artery.

becomes progressively steeper. When evolving to a retrograde a-wave (Figure 6.7), this signifies significant cardiac impairment. Abnormal ductus venosus Doppler showed moderate predictive accuracy for compromise of fetal/neonatal well-being overall and perinatal mortality in high-risk pregnancies with placental insufficiency.[31]

Cardiotocography

Basic principles

CTG is the continuous recording of FHR and uterine activity. In the antepartum period, with intact membranes, the FHR can be recorded from an ultrasound transducer positioned on the abdomen of the mother. Multiple attempts have been done to record the fetal ECG through electrodes placed on the maternal abdomen, even leading to small commercialized systems. But in general, the quality of the signal and the percentage of time the signal is lost (usually ~30%) are still hampering applications for daily clinical use, although recently progress in the technical aspects has been made.[33] Uterine activity is assessed from a transducer placed on the abdomen of the mother. The CTG is the reflection of the interaction of fetal neurological status to cardiovascular reflex responses.

In some machines, fetal movement detection, called actography, has been incorporated, but this technique does not improve the assessment of fetal well-being.[34]

Interpretation of the prelabour FHR pattern and management

Prelabour CTG, also called non-stress testing, has been accepted as a primary tool for pregnancies at risk. No benefit has ever been proven for routine prelabour CTG in normal low-risk pregnancies.

FHR patterns are affected by a variety of factors, as described in the paragraph on physiology, but also evolve during pregnancy with fetal maturation. Further diurnal variations are influenced by fetal behavioural states as mentioned earlier. In preterm

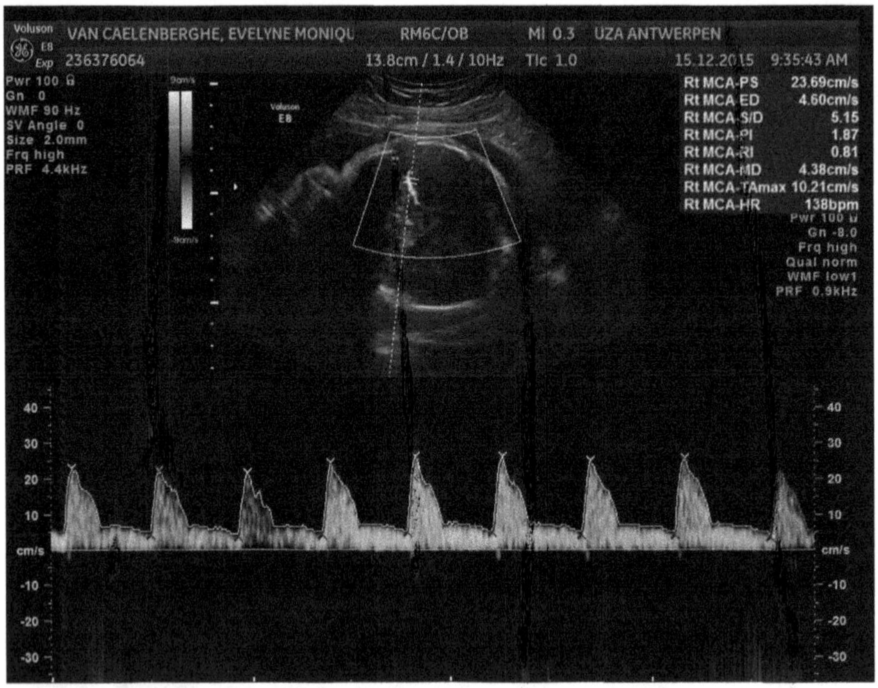

Figure 6.4 Normal middle cerebral artery flow.

pregnancies (24–32 weeks), accelerations demonstrate a lower amplitude (10 beats per minute (bpm)) and brief spontaneous decelerations, commonly called spikes, associated with movements are often recorded.[11,35]

Maternal factors also influential; medication such as narcotics, magnesium, beta-blocking agents, or corticosteroids diminish FHR variability or may lower mean heart rate. Postprandial rise in glycaemia also activates fetal heart rate variability. A non-stress test is preferably performed with the mother lying with slight left lateral tilt to avoid aortocaval compression and its resulting FHR changes.

The interpretation of an antepartum CTG includes evaluation of the timing and quality of the recording, evaluation of the basic FHR, FHR variability, accelerations, decelerations, and eventually some uterine activity.

Interpretation of a CTG trace of low technical quality should be avoided. Due to the fetal quiet sleeping state, a trace should at least be 20 minutes in duration, preferably 30 minutes.

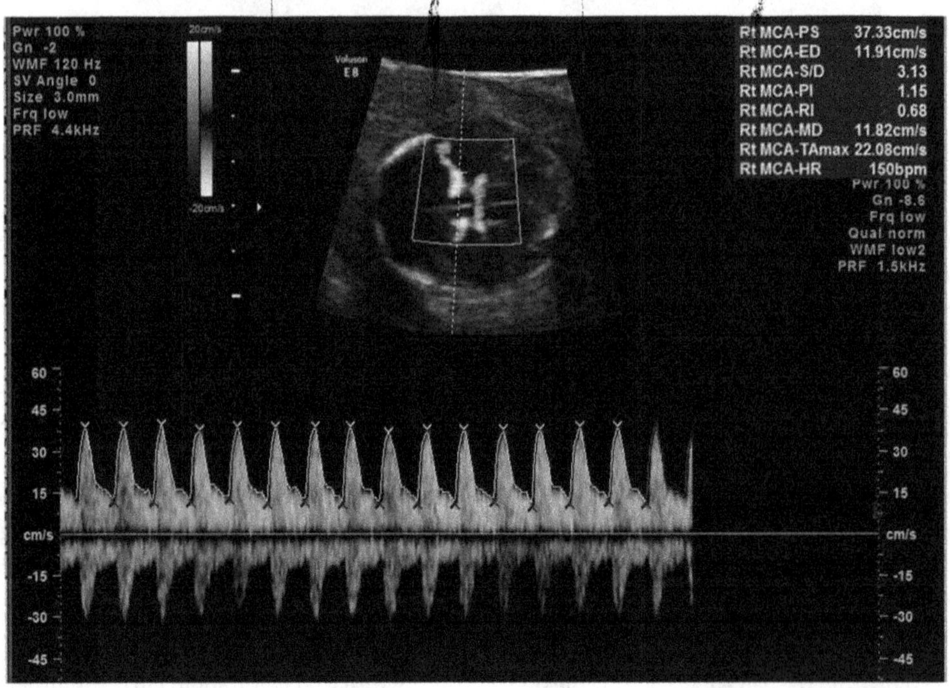

Figure 6.5 Dilated cerebral artery with decreased resistance.

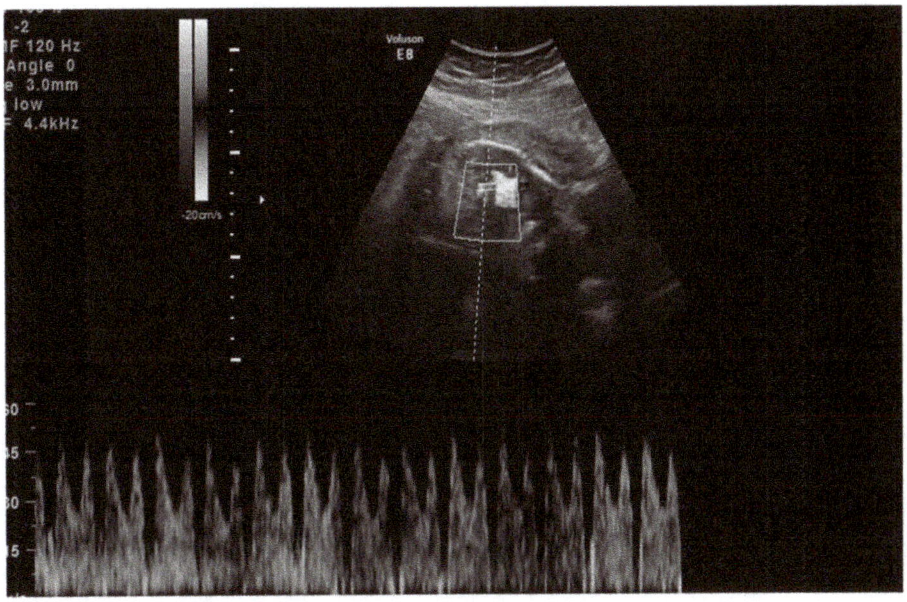

Figure 6.6 Normal M-shaped ductus venosus flow pattern.

The baseline FHR is defined as the heart rate registered for at least 10 consecutive minutes and is expressed as bpm. The basic rate diminishes during pregnancy from round 145 bpm at 24 weeks to 135 bpm at term. In a term pregnancy, normal basal FHR is between 110 and 150 bpm (Figure 6.8), tachycardia is more than 150 bpm, and bradycardia less than 110 bpm.

Tachycardia (Figure 6.9) can be transient and physiological as in fetal state 4F, but can also be associated with fetal anaemia, maternal fever, fetomaternal infection, or maternal medication such as betamimetics. A rise in maternal adrenaline due to stress or pain can also cause a period of fetal tachycardia. Maternal hyperthyroidism can also cause fetal tachycardia due to transplacental passage of thyroid hormone or thyroid stimulating antibodies. Rarely, fetal heart rhythm disorders, mainly re-entry tachycardia, cause fetal tachycardia first noticed on a CTG.

Mild bradycardia between 100 and 110 bpm is mostly benign, but if less than 100 bpm hypoxia is probable (Figure 6.10). This can be caused by diminished placental perfusion, cord compression

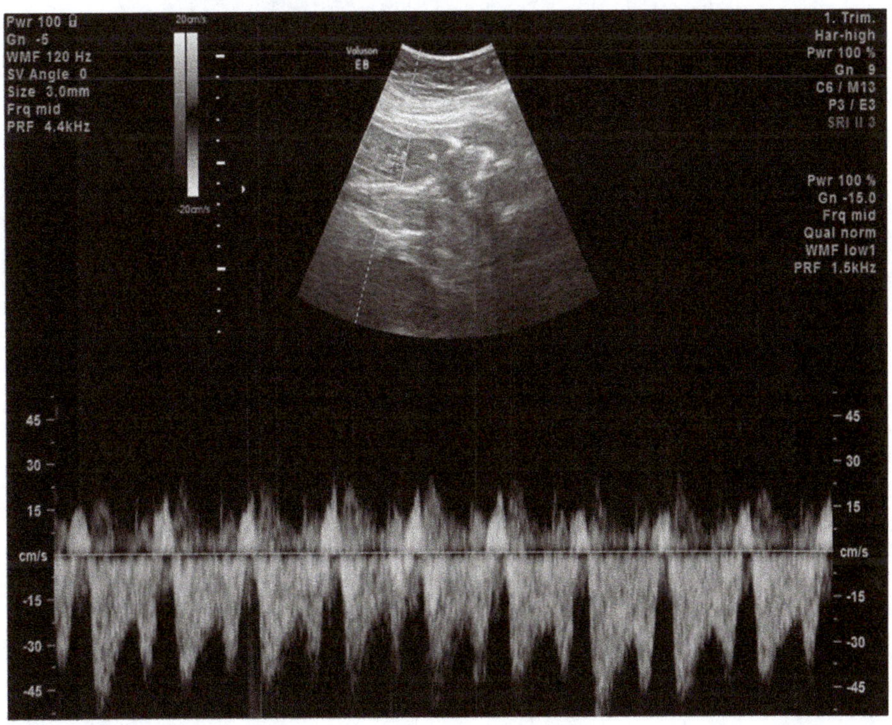

Figure 6.7 Abnormal ductus venosus flow pattern with reversed a-wave.

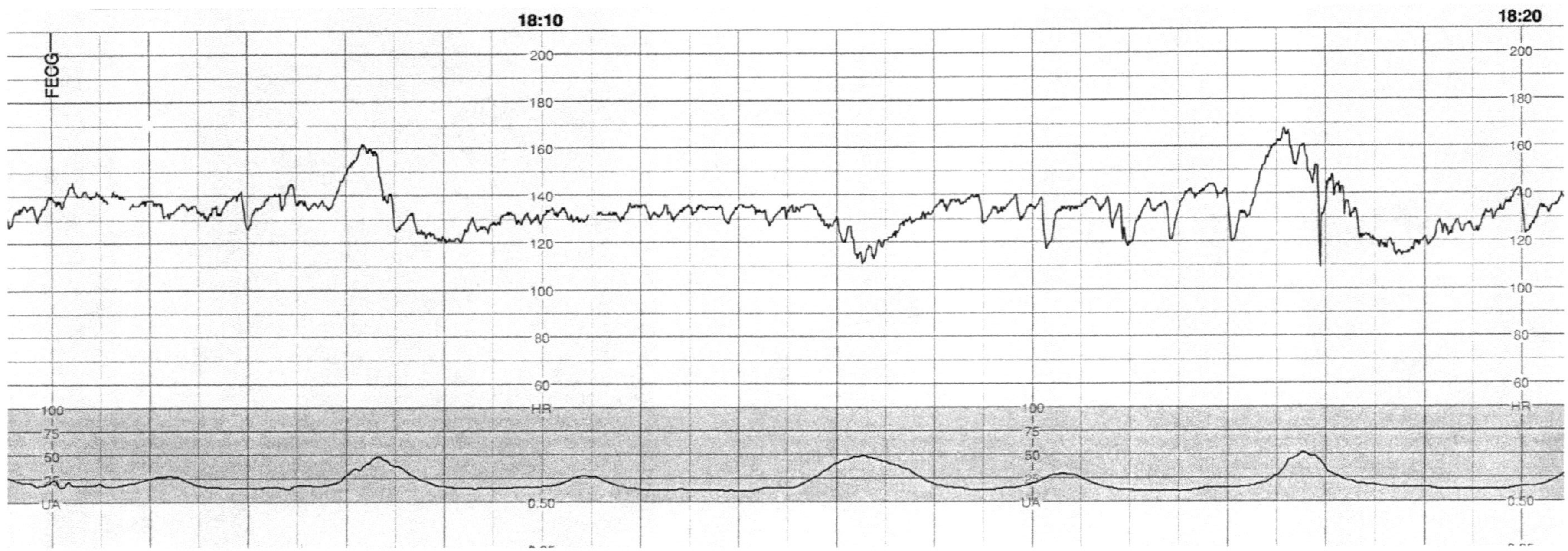

Figure 6.8 Normal cardiotocography.

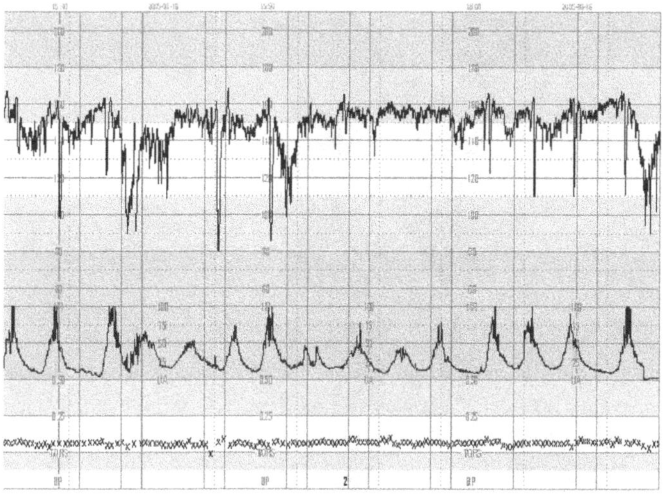

Figure 6.9 Fetal tachycardia.

(as in oligohydramnios), or maternal hypotension, the most explicit and benign demonstration of this being the aortocaval compression syndrome with the mother in dorsal decubitus. Fetal atrioventricular heart block, as can be caused by maternal systemic lupus disease, can also result in fetal bradycardia that can be further elucidated by fetal cardiac ultrasound.

FHR variability is the variation of the heart rate during 1 minute, without accelerations or decelerations. Short-term or beat-to-beat variation is the difference in interval between consecutive heart beats (expressed in milliseconds and only to be measured by computer-aided systems, see 'Computer-Aided Fetal Heart Rate Analysis'), long-term variability is presented by the bandwidth on the trace (see Figure 6.11) and is expressed in bpm. Bandwidth is normally round 6 bpm at 24 weeks and 10 bpm at 36 weeks; normal variability is considered to be between 5 and 25 bpm. Low, or minimal, variability below 5 bpm suggests fetal hypoxia but is also present in fetal sleeping behavioural states, explaining why a recording of sufficient time is necessary. Persistent low variability is the best predictor to be derived from the CTG for fetal hypoxia/metabolic acidosis. Other reasons for diminished variability include maternal medication such as hypnotics, beta-blocking agents, and fetal central nervous system disorders. Administration of betamethasone and dexamethasone to promote fetal lung maturity in the preterm fetus also results in transient (2–3 days) lowering of FHR variability.

Complete absence of variability is called a preterminal trace and is almost invariably a sign of serious fetal hypoxia or brain damage.

When bandwidth is more than 25 bpm this is called marked variability or a saltatory trace. This can represent acute fetal hypoxia due to an acute imbalance between sympathetic and parasympathetic innervations, but it can also be benign due to fetal thumb sucking or very active moving.

The sinusoidal trace is mostly a slightly tachycardic trace with an oscillating pattern demonstrating 3–5 cycles per minute for at least 20 minutes and a bandwidth of 5–15 bpm. It is seen in case of fetal anaemia but is sometimes due to medication such as meperidine and morphine. The pathophysiology behind this kind of recording is unknown, as most even severely anaemic fetuses do not develop it. In case of forceful fetal thumbsucking, a pseudosinusoidal trace can be seen.

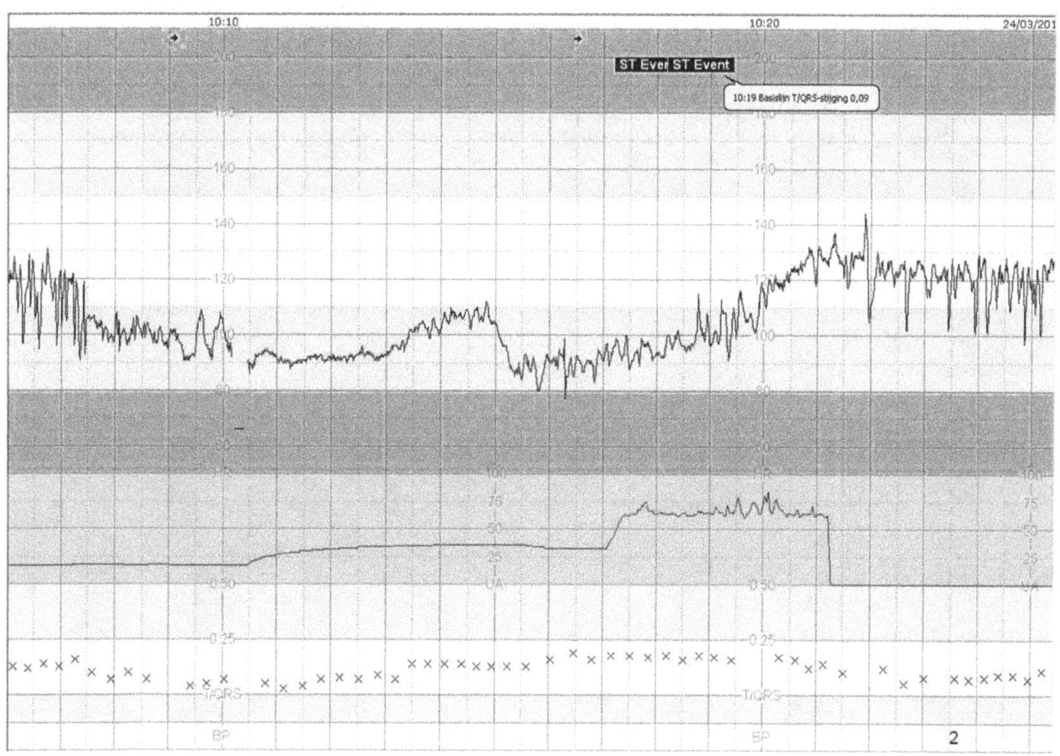

Figure 6.10 Fetal bradycardia.

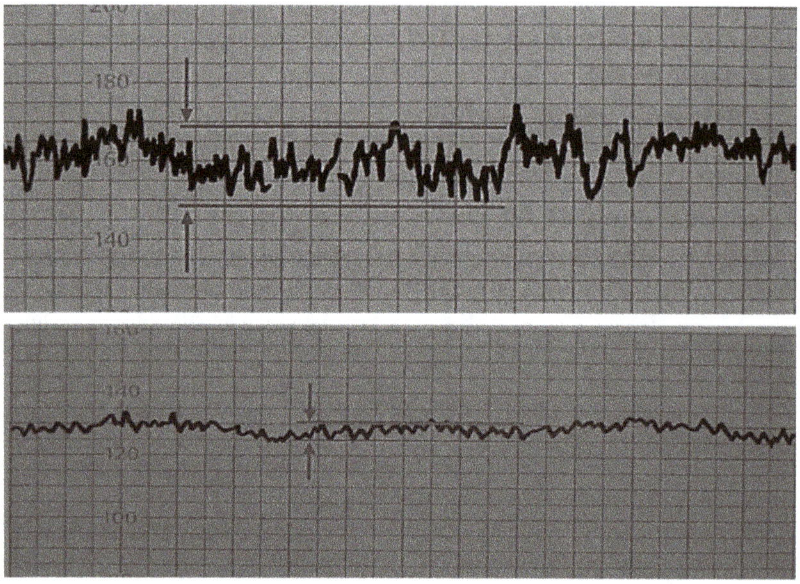

Figure 6.11 Long-term variability; variability is expressed as the bandwidth of the envelope surrounding the fetal heart rate pattern. The upper panel shows normal variability, the lower panel reduced variability.

Accelerations are defined as (from 32 weeks' gestational age) a rise in FHR for at least 15 bpm compared to the basal FHR during at least 15 seconds. These are mostly associated with fetal movements. Before 32 weeks, 10 bpm and 10 seconds are used. At least two accelerations in a 20-minute period is called a reactive stress test and almost completely excludes fetal acidosis and is related to a risk for fetal demise in the next 7 days of less than 2 per 1000. A trace without accelerations is called non-reactive.

Decelerations constitute a decrease in FHR with at least 15 bpm for at least 15 seconds. Decelerations are subdivided in uniform (early and late), variable (complicated and uncomplicated), and long decelerations.

Uniform decelerations demonstrate a rather 'rounded' pattern; if they are multiple they do have a uniform aspect. Usually the loss of heart rate is not very remarkable nor very sudden (Figure 6.6). Variable decelerations on the contrary show a steep and significant lowering. When looking at a series of variable decelerations they demonstrate changes in form, which is where the denomination 'variable' comes from. Long decelerations by definition mean less than 80 bpm for at least 2 minutes or less than 100 bpm for at least 3 minutes. When decelerations last more than 5 minutes they are called bradycardic.

Early uniform decelerations coincide with contractions (Figure 6.12); a late uniform deceleration shows the lowest point

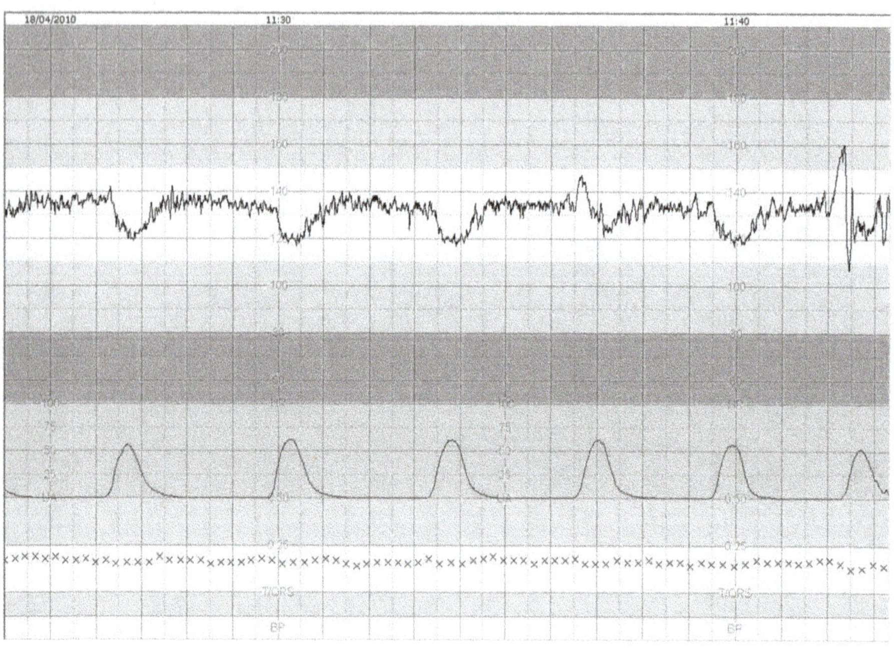

Figure 6.12 Early uniform decelerations.

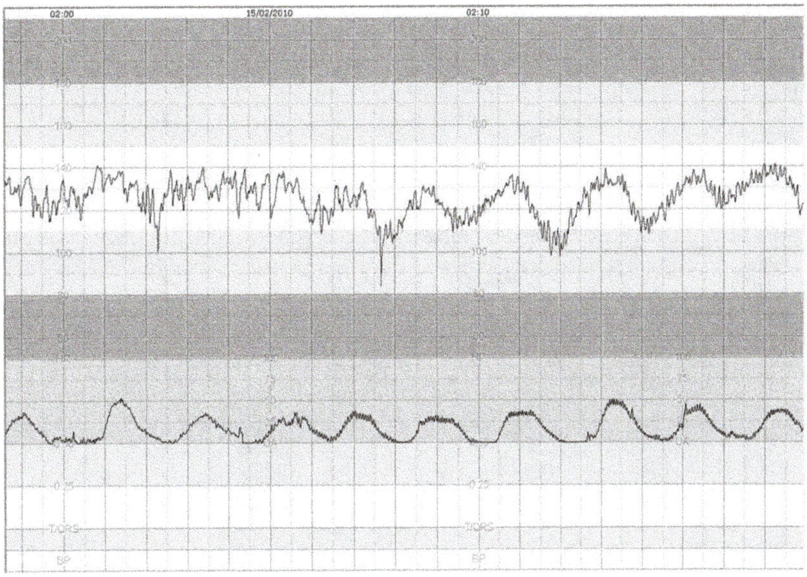

Figure 6.13 Late uniform decelerations.

after the height point (acme) of the contraction (Figure 6.13). Early uniform decelerations are not a sign of fetal hypoxia and are related to increasing pressure on the fetal skin; late uniform decelerations are due to diminished oxygen supply.

An uncomplicated variable deceleration takes less than 60 seconds (Figure 6.14) and complicated ones more than 60 seconds (Figure 6.15). Variable decelerations are mostly due to diminished blood flow to the fetus such as during a contraction or when the umbilical cord is compressed. An overview of the different deceleration types is given in Figure 6.16.

Before 30 weeks, short decelerations (<30 seconds) are frequently seen (the so-called spikes as already mentioned) and should be considered physiological.

Other influences changing the CTG pattern are discussed further later in this chapter.[36]

To aid in diagnosing fetal problems different classification systems have been developed. The system adopted by the Federation Internationale des Gynécologues et des Obstétriciens (FIGO) is most often used and is illustrated in Table 6.3.[37,38]

The system was originally developed for intrapartum monitoring but can also be used antepartum. Other systems have been and still are being proposed, but these have neither been validated nor are they used in Europe.[37]

No good data are available to guide the clinician on the interval of repeat testing.[39] Older studies have demonstrated that the rate of stillbirth after a reactive stress test within 1 week is 1.9 per 1000 compared to 26 per 1000 for a non-reactive test, increasing the rate from once to twice weekly still decreases the rate of stillbirth specifically in case of fetal growth restriction.[40,41] It should be noted that CTG is very good at ruling out fetal compromise (the negative

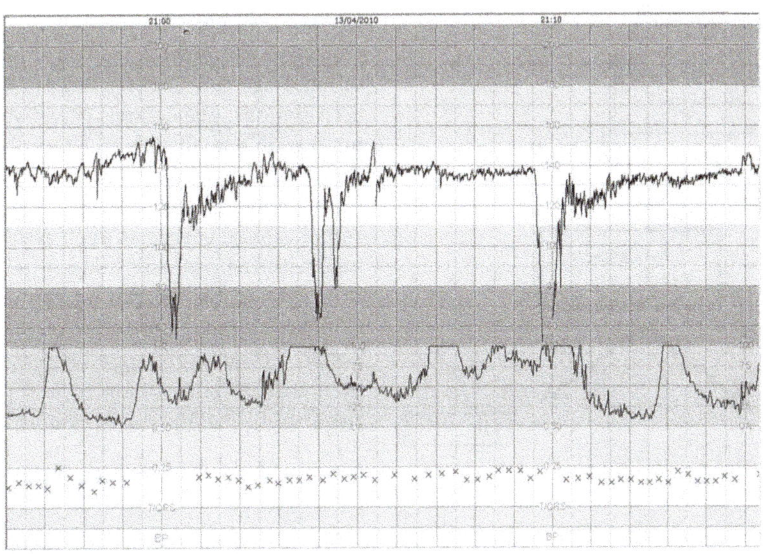

Figure 6.14 Uncomplicated variable deceleration.

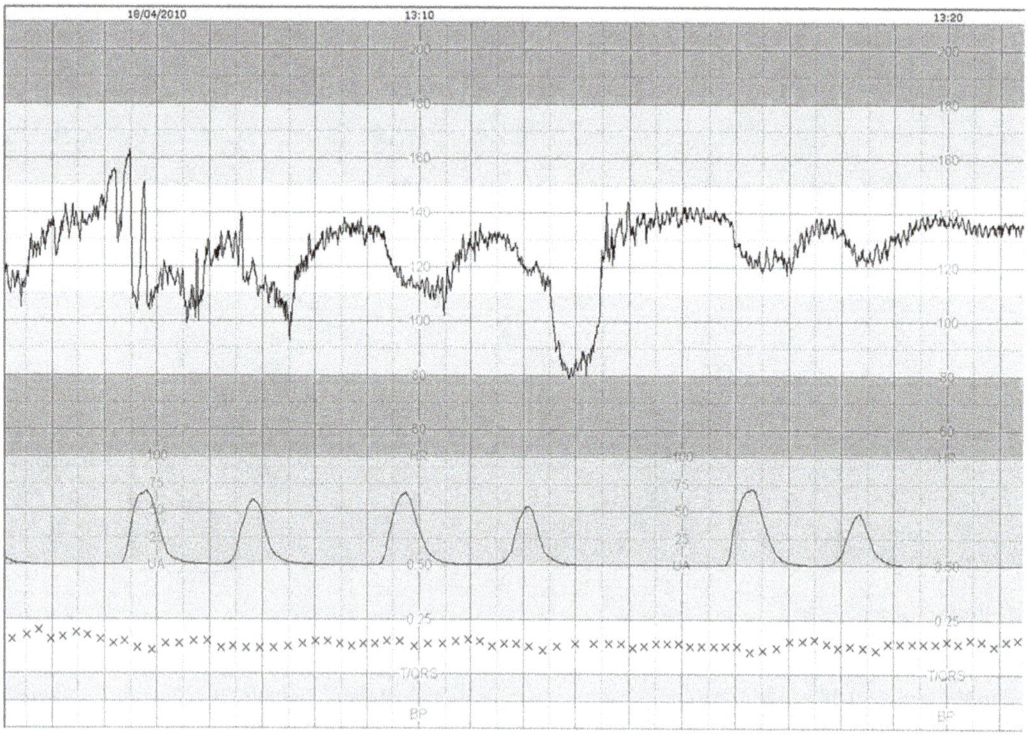

Figure 6.15 Complicated variable decelerations.

predictive value of a normal trace is higher than 90% in most studies, false negative between 0.19 and 1%) but not so good in ruling in fetal compromise (the positive predictive value is <50%, false positives ~55%). This means that most fetuses diagnosed antenatally with fetal compromise are normal. A meta-analysis of RCTs, only involving women considered at increased risk of pregnancy complications, failed to demonstrate any significant effect on perinatal mortality, low Apgar scores, admission to neonatal intensive care units, gestational age at birth, or neonatal seizures; [42,43]

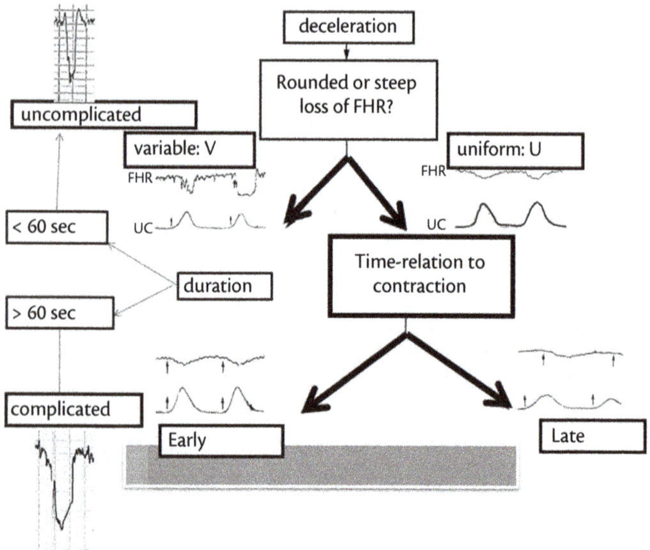

Figure 6.16 Overview of decelerations.

this means that there is no benefit of CTG used in isolation. Many factors such as fetal movements, fetal growth restriction, maternal disease, and so on guide clinical decision-making in this complex area but experience and clinical intuition also play a significant role in this imprecise situation. Studies on intuition and how to train it and on the physiology behind pattern recognition are emerging.

The contraction stress test, when uterine contractions are induced by some method to evaluate the fetal response, has little or no place in modern obstetrics. Contractions can be elicited by administration of oxytocin or by maternal nipple stimulation.

Computer-aided FHR analysis

Objective computerized FHR analysis taking into account gestational age can identify lower-amplitude FHR variability and accelerations. The systems depict variability as a continuous output variable analysing real beat-to-beat variability, also called short-term variability, but also includes accelerations, decelerations, periods of high variation, and periods of low variation using complicated algorithms. Such systems are able to correlate findings with the normal evolution related to gestational age.[45] No RCT is available comparing computerized CTG with no CTG. Comparing computerized CTG with non-computerized 'traditional' CTG interpretation demonstrated significant reduction in perinatal mortality in favour of the computerized CTG (relative risk (RR) 0.20; 95% CI 0.04–0.88).[44]

Intrapartum fetal monitoring

Introduction

In this section, an overview is presented of different techniques that are actually used in the delivery suite to monitor the fetus. CTG

Table 6.3 FIGO classification of CTG

CTG classification	Baseline of fetal heart rate	Baseline variability/accelerations	Decelerations	Contractions
Normal	110–150 bpm	5–25 bpm >2 accelerations/60 min	No decelerations Uniform, early decelerations Variable, uncomplicated decelerations with a duration <30 s and amplitude <60 bpm	5 or less contractions/10 min
Suspicious	100–110 bpm 150–170 bpm <100 bpm for ≤3 min	<5 bpm >40 min without accelerations >25 bpm (saltatory pattern/increased variability) <2 accelerations/60 min	Variable uncomplicated decelerations with duration 30–60 min and/or amplitude >60 bpm	>5 contractions/10 min
	With a combination of 2 or more suspicious/abnormal factors the CTG is classified as suspect pathological			
Pathological	>170 bpm <100 bpm for min	<5 bpm for 60 min without accelerations Sinusoidal pattern	Variable complicated decelerations with duration >60 s Uniform late decelerations Combined decelerations	
Preterminal	No variability (<2 bpm) without accelerations regardless of decelerations/heartbeat			

FIGO, International Federation of Gynecology and Obstetrics.

Reprinted from *International Journal of Gynecology & Obstetrics*, Volume 25, issue 2, Figo news, pp. 159–167, Copyright (1987), with permission from Elsevier.

is used both antenatally and during labour, but the evaluation of its effectiveness is different in both situations and adjunctive techniques can be employed during labour that are not available antenatally. In the past decade we have witnessed the rise and fall of fetal pulse oximetry; this technique will not be further discussed as it has been proven not to make any difference in terms of maternal (caesarean delivery rate) or fetal/neonatal (metabolic acidosis) outcome and is no longer commercially available.[46]

Auscultation

IA is a systematic method of listening to the fetal heart tones with an acoustic (a pinard or fetal stethoscope) device or a hand-held Doppler device. IA during labour is an accepted practice in low-risk labours in many countries. Attention is paid to rate and rhythm and eventually variability. A normal FHR is between 110 and 150 bpm at term, regular, with variation around the baseline FHR, especially an increase during fetal movements. The aim of IA is to detect late or variable decelerations and baseline bradycardia or tachycardia. The presence of any of these abnormalities is a reason to continue with CTG.

No studies have been done comparing IA with no fetal monitoring at all, and for obvious ethical reasons such studies are not expected to be realized in the future. Meta-analyses of the results of randomized clinical trials, comparing IA with CTG have failed to show any significant benefit of CTG over IA in low-risk pregnancies. Moreover, caesarean delivery rates were significantly lower in the IA arm compared with the CTG arm. This is discussed in more detail in the following 'Cardiotocography' section. It has to be mentioned that in the IA arm, IA was mostly performed every 15 minutes in the first stage and after every contraction in the second stage. The current recommendations of IA every 15 minutes in the first stage of labour is rather labour intensive for midwives and doctors and is associated with poor compliance.

Cardiotocography

In the antepartum period, only external CTG can be used. For this a Doppler device with computerized logic to interpret and count the Doppler signals is used. During labour a more direct reading from the fetal heart activity becomes possible with internal CTG, using a fetal electrode, with a spiral wire directly placed on the fetal scalp or other presenting part. The R–R interval of the extracted fetal ECG is used to calculate FHR. The recording of the contractions can also be monitored externally or internally with an intrauterine pressure catheter. There are several aspects which have to be taken into account when classifying and interpreting the CTG pattern: contractions, baseline FHR, variability, and presence of accelerations and decelerations.

Regional anaesthesia carries the potential to reduce intervillous space blood flow due to maternal hypotension as a result of sympathetic blockade. This has long been suggested as an explanation for the fetal decelerations or short periods of bradycardia noted after epidural or spinal anaesthesia. Conversely, Doppler flow measurements have actually demonstrated an increase in flow in the arcuate uterine vessels in prehydrated patients following epidural anaesthesia.

A variety of classification systems is used worldwide, an example is shown in Table 6.3 (modified FIGO classification, which is also used in the ST-analyser (STAN®) clinical guidelines). Most of them use a classification of normal CTG pattern, intermediate or suspicious CTG, abnormal or pathological CTG, and preterminal CTG pattern, based on the above-mentioned variables.

For women at low risk of intrapartum fetal hypoxia and of developing complications in labour, CTG versus IA on admission to the delivery suite demonstrated no difference in fetal/neonatal outcome, a statistically non-significant trend to more caesarean deliveries in the CTG group was noted (RR 1.20; 95% CI 1.00–1.44) and marginally more instrumental vaginal deliveries (RR 1.15; 95% CI 1.01–1.33).[40a] For women in established labour, the data from 13 randomized trials on the effectiveness of the CTG were presented in a 2013 Cochrane meta-analysis.[5] Fetal CTG monitoring, whether in combination with FBS (see later 'Fetal Blood Sampling' section) or not, was compared with IA. Continuous monitoring by means of the CTG without FBS leads to a significant increase in the number of caesarean deliveries (RR 1.63; 95% CI 1.29–2.07) and a halving of neonatal seizures (RR 0.50; 95% CI 0.31–0.80), without an effect on other neonatal outcomes including cerebral palsy and infant mortality. It has to be mentioned that IA was performed every 15 minutes during the first stage of labour and after every contraction in the second stage. Furthermore, one has to realize that these trials were mostly performed before 1980, when the caesarean delivery rate was much lower than today. Training in CTG interpretation was mostly not extensive and not uniform and classification and interpretation differs from current insights in CTG patterns. Fetal surveillance with CTG was introduced in the 1960s. Although a positive effect of CTG on neonatal outcome has never been shown, CTG is widely applied.

It is known that classification and interpretation of the CTG is difficult with large interobserver variation. For a substantial part, these problems may be solved by strict adherence to guidelines regarding classification and interpretation of the CTG, obtaining additional fetal information, and subsequent recommendations for obstetric interventions.

Fetal blood sampling

One of the techniques used to obtain additional fetal information with an abnormal CTG is FBS. FBS was introduced in the 1960s by Bretscher and Saling. Blood is obtained by means of a small incision in the skin of the fetal scalp, from which the pH, the PCO_2, and the base excess can be determined (Figure 6.17). In general, for a pH lower than 7.20 it is advised to deliver the baby within a short period of time by means of an assisted vaginal delivery

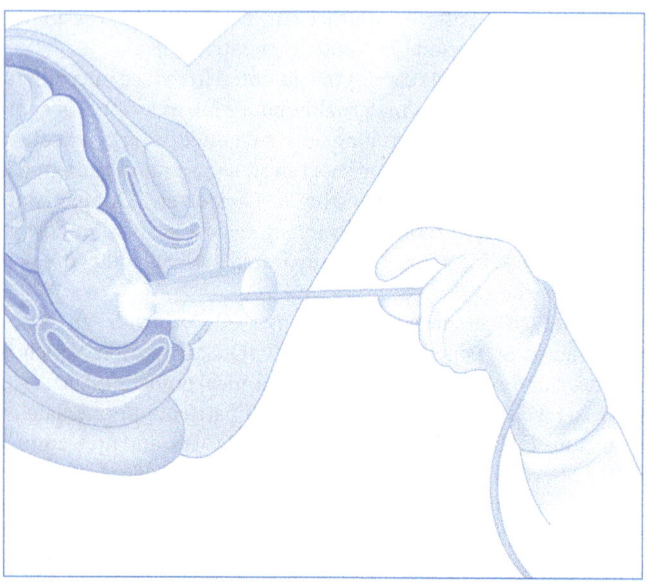

Figure 6.17 Technique of fetal blood sampling during labour.
Reproduced with permission from BRENNER MEDICAL GMBH.

or caesarean delivery. It thus offers information on the acid–base balance in the fetal blood and is regarded as the reference or 'gold standard' methodology to identify fetal distress during labour. However, FBS is inconsistently applied and not used on a large scale worldwide.[47,48] Although it is more specific than CTG alone and thus decreases the intervention rate, prevention of asphyxia is still not guaranteed.[5] Also, the technique is invasive and considered difficult, with a failure rate of at least 10%. Furthermore, the procedure has to be repeated when the CTG remains abnormal and complications have been described. FBS is never used without CTG.

Complications due to FBS occur rarely, with a reported incidence ranging from 0.4% to 6%. The most frequent is excessive fetal bleeding mostly associated with an underlying coagulopathy.[49]

In 2008, the data from 13 randomized trials on the effectiveness of the CTG with or without CTG were presented in a Cochrane meta-analysis.[5] Fetal monitoring, whether in combination with FBS or not, was compared with IA. Continuous monitoring by means of the CTG without FBS leads to a significant increase in the number of caesarean deliveries (odds ratio (OR) 1.96; 95% CI 1.24–3.09), without a positive effect on neonatal outcome. If, however, FBS was performed alongside the CTG, a less prominent increase in the number of caesarean deliveries was found (OR 1.50; 95% CI 1.10–2.06) with a 50% reduction of neonatal convulsions (OR 0.49; 95% CI 0.29–0.84).

The results on the effectiveness of monitoring by means of the CTG combined with FBS originate from six of the trials that were performed in the period 1976 to 1989. This therefore concerns results of relatively old trials in which the frequency of caesarean deliveries varies from 2.3% to 35%.

Long-term follow-up of these trials is restricted to one study, which revealed that the lower incidence of neonatal convulsions was not associated with an improved outcome over time.[7] There are no studies in which continuous CTG monitoring without FBS is compared to monitoring with FBS.

Performance of FBS has an added value compared to monitoring by CTG only and offers a solution to the large number of false-positive CTG recordings when it is compared with IA. However, in many countries it has disappeared from delivery suites. A significant reason for this is that this investigation only gives a result at a specific point in time and with a persistent anomalous CTG it must be repeated. In addition, FBS is invasive, technically difficult, and patient unfriendly. In at least 10% of attempts, performing FBS is unsuccessful and it can thus be a time-consuming procedure.[50] In addition, the training in performing FBS appears to be inadequate in many hospitals and proper logistics for determining the same are lacking.[48] The relatively large quantity of blood that is required to determine the pH is also stated as a disadvantage of FBS.

A possible alternative to the pH measurement of the FBS sample is determination of lactate concentration. For the latter, less blood is required (5 μL) than the 30–50 μL needed for the determination of the pH. A lower percentage of unsuccessful attempts for lactate determination than for pH determination has repeatedly been reported, but without this having an effect on the neonatal outcome or the number of assisted deliveries.[51] Significant differences between measurement devices have been reported and the use of intrapartum fetal scalp lactate needs more standardization and the definition of clear cut-off values before its use can be endorsed in clinical practice, until then it should only be used within a research protocol.[52,53,54]

More recently the level of lactate in amniotic fluid has been proposed to detect fetal deterioration. No prospective randomized studies have been conducted to evaluate this method.[55]

STAN® of the fetal ECG

Technique and complications

Since 2000, it has been possible via a scalp electrode not only to register the FHR but also the rest of the fetal ECG. The fetal heart and the fetal brain appear to be equally sensitive to a shortage of oxygen and thus information on myocardial function also indirectly provides information on the oxygenation of the fetal brain.

It has been shown from experimental animal research that changes in the ST segment of the ECG correlate with fetal hypoxia that occurs or worsens during labour.[14,56] The ST analyser (STAN® monitor; Neoventa Medical, Goteborg, Sweden) was developed in order to be able to combine the CTG with the analysis of the ST segment of the ECG. Changes in the shape of the ST segment are noted automatically and for a significant ST change an alarm is generated, a so-called ST event. The associated STAN® guidelines then state whether intervention is required.[57] The STAN® concept is based on the association between changes of the ST-interval of the fetal ECG and the function of the fetal myocardium during hypoxia. The changes in fetal ECG associated with fetal distress are either an increase in T-wave, quantified by the ratio T-wave to QRS-amplitude (T/QRS ratio), or a biphasic ST segment (Figure 6.18). An increase in T-wave and subsequently in T/QRS-ratio has been associated with a catecholamine surge, activation of beta-adrenoreceptors, myocardial glycogenolysis, and metabolic acidosis. A biphasic shape of the ST segment is related to two situations. First, it may occur when the fetal heart is exposed to acute hypoxic stress whereby it has had no time to respond to hypoxia or second, when the fetal heart has a reduced capacity to respond due to (chronic) stress situations and lack of or already utilized resources. Biphasic ST changes of the fetal ECG have been associated with disturbances in heart muscle function, infection, or malformations.

The STAN® concept is based on a combined interpretation of CTG and ST changes (Table 6.4). The relevance of an ST change depends on the visual assessment of the CTG that, according to FIGO criteria, is classified as 'normal', 'intermediary' (or 'suspicious'), 'abnormal' (or 'pathological'), or '(pre)terminal'.[36] If a

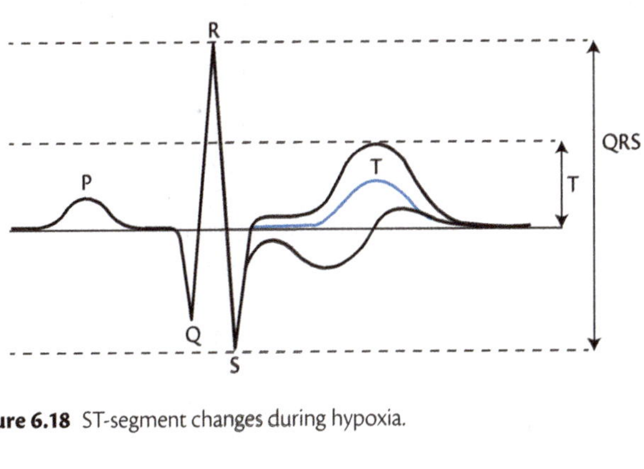

Figure 6.18 ST-segment changes during hypoxia.

CTG is normal, any ST change on the STAN® monitor can be ignored. When a CTG is (pre)terminal, immediate intervention is advised, irrespective of ST changes. In case of an intermediary or abnormal CTG, the STAN® guidelines indicate for what ST changes intervention is advised (Figure 6.19). This intervention may consist of solving a cause of fetal distress, such as hypertonia or hyperstimulation, or proceeding to delivery. The STAN® guidelines can be used from a gestational age of 36 weeks onwards.

Five RCTs, which included 15,352 patients, have been performed since 1993. Westgate et al. were the first to conduct a RCT on the effect of intrapartum fetal ECG and used absolute values of T/QRS, rather than automatically detected T/QRS changes, as described in the current STAN® clinical guidelines.[58,59,60,61,62] All five RCTs were inconclusive with four studies showing no statistically significant effect on the primary outcome, metabolic acidosis in the umbilical artery. In one study, STAN® significantly reduced the incidence of metabolic acidosis.[59]

Four meta-analyses including these five RCTs have been performed.[63–66] Compared with conventional CTG, STAN® showed no difference in metabolic acidosis (1.12% in CTG alone, 0.81% in STAN group, RR 0.80; 95% CI 0.44–1.47). STAN® significantly reduced the incidence of additional FBS, operative vaginal deliveries, and total operative deliveries with less need for neonatal intensive care. For other outcomes, no differences in effect were seen between STAN® and conventional CTG, or data were not suitable for meta-analysis. An individual patient data meta-analysis including four of the five RCTs did confirm that addition of STAN® to CTG reduces the need for instrumental vaginal delivery without changing the risk of metabolic acidosis or caesarean delivery.[67] The meta-analyses show that additional use of STAN® for intrapartum monitoring does not reduce the incidence of metabolic acidosis, but it does reduce the incidence of operative vaginal deliveries and the need for FBS. Cost-effectiveness studies are scarce but seem to provide some evidence that STAN® is a cost-effective method of intrapartum monitoring when compared with conventional CTG, when looking at both short- and long-term outcomes.[68,69] Implementation of the STAN® methodology, just like any new technology, should be performed carefully, taking into consideration that a learning curve is needed. Recent observational studies investigating the effects of long term use of STAN® have shown a decrease in incidence of metabolic acidosis$_{BDecf}$ over time.[70] Furthermore the cases of adverse neonatal outcome described in literature are mainly due to problems with the interpretation of the CTG or violation of guidelines.[71] Repeated training is crucial in the implementation of the STAN® methodology. Several studies have demonstrated that non-adherence to the clinical guidelines is the major reason for unnecessary interventions without reducing metabolic acidosis.[72–74] Nowadays, the use of the STAN® methodology is increasing and in some countries it is common practice. Fetal STAN®, scalp pH and fetal scalp stimulation are generally accepted adjunctive methods to CTG.[75]

Intrapartum maternal fever results in fetal tachycardia and an accelerated metabolism, possibly resulting in a faster development of metabolic acidosis, CTG alone can be difficult to interpret in these cases, it has been demonstrated that intrapartum fever is not associated with ST segment changes of the fetal ECG and can still

Table 6.4 The intended use of this CTG classification system is to suggest clinical conditions in which adjunctive use of ST waveform changes may aid the interpretation of specific CTG patterns

Classification of CTG	Baseline heart frequency	Variability Reactivity	Decelerations
Normal CTG	• 110–150 bpm	• Accelerations • 5–25 bpm	• Early uniform decelerations • Uncomplicated variable decelerations with a duration of <60 sec and loss of <60 beats
Intermediary CTG	• 100–110 bpm • 150–170 bpm • Short bradycardia episode (<100 bpm for ≤3 min)	• >25 bpm (saltatory pattern) • <5 bpm >40 min with absence of accelerations	• Uncomplicated variable decelerations with a duration <60 sec and loss of >60 beats
	A combination of several intermediary observations will result in an abnormal CTG		
Abnormal CTG	• 150–170 bpm and reduced variability • >170 bpm • Persistent bradycardia (<100 bpm for >3 min)	• <5 bpm for >60 min • Sinusoidal pattern	• Complicated variable decelerations with a duration of >60 sec • Repeated late uniform decelerations
Preterminal CTG	• Total lack of variability (<2 bpm) and reactivity with or without decelerations or bradycardia		

ST Analysis

These guidelines may indicate situations in which obstetric intervention[1] is required.

ST Events	Episodic T/QRS rise	Baseline T/QRS rise	Biphasic ST
Normal CTG	• Expectant management and continued observation		
Intermediary CTG	• >0.15	• >0.10	• 3 Biphasic log messages[2]
Abnormal CTG	• >0.10	• >0.05	• 2 Biphasic log messages[2]
Preterminal CTG	• Immediate delivery		

1. Intervention may include delivery or maternal-fetal resuscitation by alleviation of contributing problems such as over-stimulation or maternal hypotension and hypoxia.
2. The time span between the Biphasic messages should be related to the CTG pattern and the clinical situation.
With kind permission of Neoventa Medical

be used in these circumstances.[76] Epidural analgesia has no effect on the number or types of ST events.[77]

Fetal biometry and tests for fetal congenital anomalies relevant to the anaesthetist

Fetal growth is determined both by genetics (maternal and paternal) and by environmental factors influencing maternal nutrition and the function of the uteroplacental unit. IUGR can affect the management of the pregnant woman.

In case of pre-eclampsia, a disorder affecting all maternal organ systems based on a generalized endothelial dysfunction, IUGR is caused by a restricted perfusion of the placenta, resulting in chronic malnutrition and hypoxaemia of the fetus. The spiral arteries, perfusing the placenta, do not remodel their muscular wall in case of pre-eclampsia and remain reactive to vasoconstrictive agents. Maternal hypertension is necessary to compensate for the reduced flow through narrowed vessels. When IUGR based on uteroplacental vascular pathology has been prenatally diagnosed, care should be taken not to lower maternal blood pressure below 140 mmHg systolic and 80 mmHg diastolic as this will result in FHR decelerations due to insufficient placental perfusion.[78] In such case correcting maternal blood pressure should be aimed at first, before proceeding to an emergency delivery.

Ultrasound and, more recently, magnetic resonance imaging have facilitated the detection of a majority of placental and fetal congenital structural anomalies. In most circumstances this will not influence the management of the mother during labour and vaginal or caesarean delivery. Some exceptions should be mentioned, including a prenatally detected placenta increta, in which case one should be prepared for major haemorrhage, or if an EXIT procedure (*ex utero* intrapartum treatment) such as tracheal obstruction is planned, the immediate administration of an uterotonic agent (oxytocin, carbetocin) should be postponed in these cases.

The role of intrapartum ultrasound has been recently emerging. Traditionally the position and descent of the fetal head during labour have been determined digitally. This has been proven to be extremely inaccurate, causing up to 30% of clinically relevant missed diagnosis. Occiput posterior position, asynclytism (the oblique presentation of the fetal head to the pelvic curve), and fetal descent can be reliably diagnosed by transabdominal, transperineal, and transvaginal ultrasound during labour, clearly superior to the digital method.[79–81] It is to be expected that ultrasound will be used more frequently in the delivery suite.

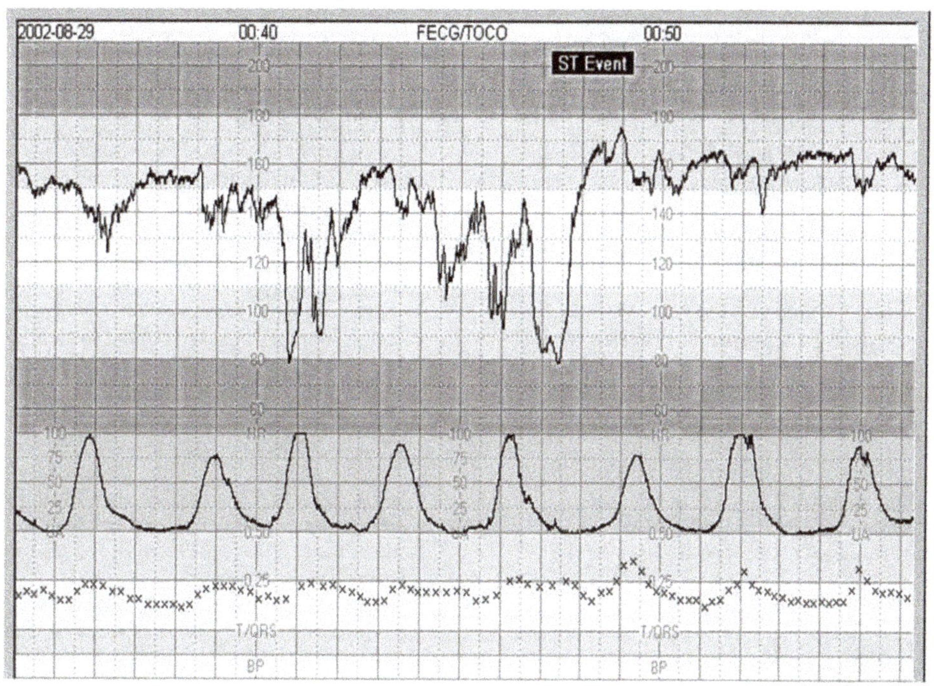

Figure 6.19 Example of STAN® recording. From top to bottom: the FHR, uterus activity and T/QRS ratio indicated as crosses. The FHR shows complicated variable decelerations resulting in classification of the CTG as abnormal. The T/QRS ratio shows a variable pattern, leading to two significant T/QRS rises indicated by the black horizontal bars stating 'ST Event'. Per ST-event exact time, type and quantification of the T/QRS rise are explained below the recording. According to the STAN® guidelines (see Appendix 1) there is an indication to intervene based on the combined presence of an abnormal CTG and significant ST-events (baseline T/QRS rise of 0.06 and 0.09).

Conclusion

In antenatal fetal monitoring, CTG and umbilical artery Doppler represent the main techniques that determine management. During labour in low-risk pregnancies, IA and CTG can be equally considered as standard; when CTG signals possible fetal hypoxia, adjunctive techniques are needed such as FBS or STAN®.

References

1. Low JA, Pickersgill H, Killen H, *et al.* The prediction and prevention of intrapartum asphyxia in term pregnancies. *Am J Obstet Gynecol* 2001; 184:724–30.
2. Parer JT, King T. Fetal heart rate monitoring: is it salvageable? *Am J Obstet Gynecol* 2000; 182:982–7.
3. Nelson KB, Dambrosia JM, Ting TY, *et al.* Uncertain value of electronic fetal monitoring in predicting cerebral palsy. *N Engl J Med* 1996; 334:613–18.
4. ACOG Committee Opinion No326. Inappropriate use of the terms fetal distress and birth asphyxia. *Obstet Gynecol* 2005; 106:1469–70.
5. Alfirevic Z, Devane D, Gyte GM. Continuous cardiotocography (CTG) as a form of electronic fetal monitoring (EFM) for fetal assessment during labour. *Cochrane Database Syst Rev* 2013; 5:CD006066.
6. Grant A, O'Brien N, Joy MT, *et al.* Cerebral palsy among children born during the Dublin randomised trial of intrapartum monitoring. *Lancet* 1989; 8674:1233–6.
7. Grant A. Monitoring of the fetus during labour. In Chalmers I, Enkin M, Keirse M (eds) *Effective Care in Pregnancy and Childbirth.* Oxford: Oxford University Press; 1991:846–82.
8. Prentice A, Lind T. Fetal heart rate monitoring during labour; too frequent intervention, too little benefit? *Lancet* 1987; 2:1375–7.
9. MacDonald D, Grant A, Sheridan-Pereira M, *et al.* The Dublin randomized controlled trial of intrapartum fetal heart rate monitoring. *Am J Obstet Gynecol* 1985; 152:524–39.
10. Nielsen PV, Stigbsy B, Nickelsen C. Intra- and interobserver variability in the assessment of intrapartum cardiotocograms. *Acta Obstet Gynecol Scand* 1987; 6:421–4.
11. Gagnon R, Campbell K, Hunse C, *et al.* Patterns of human fetal heart rate accelerations from 26 weeks to term. *Am J Obstet Gynecol* 1987; 157:743–8.
12. Manning FA. Fetal biophysical profile: a critical appraisal. *Clin Obstet Gynecol* 2002; 45:975–85.
13. Hökegard KH, Eriksson BO, Kjellmer I, *et al.* Myocardial metabolism in relation to electrocardiographic changes and cardiac function during graded hypoxia in the fetal lamb? *Acta Physiol Scand* 1981; 113(1):1–7.
14. Rosen KG, Dagbjartsson A, Henriksson BA. The relationship between circulating catecholamines and ST-waveform in the fetal lamb electrocardiogram during hypoxia. *Am J Obstet Gynecol* 1984; 149:190–5.
15. Grant A, Elbourne D, Valentin L, *et al.* Routine formal fetal movement counting and risk of antepartum late fetal death in normally formed singletons. *Lancet* 1989; 2:345–9.
16. Mangesi L, Hogmeyr GJ. Fetal movement counting for assessment of fetal well being. *Cochrane Database Syst Rev.* 2007; 1:CD004909.
17. Hofmeyr GJ, Novikova N. Management of reported decreased fetal movements for improving pregnancy outcomes. *Cochrane Database Syst Rev* 2012; 4:CD009148.
18. Nijhuis JG, Prechtl HFR, Martin CB, *et al.* Are there behavioural states in the human fetus? *Early Hum Dev* 1982; 6:177–95.
19. Natale R, Clewlow F, Dawes GS. Measurement of fetal forelimb movements in the lamb in utero *Am J Obstet Gynecol* 1981; 140:545–51.
20. Manning FA, Morrison I, Lange IR, *et al.* Fetal assessment based on fetal biophysical profile scoring: experience in 12620 referred high risk pregnancies: I. perinatal mortality by frequency and etiology. *Am J Obstet Gynecol* 1985; 151:343–50.
21. Natale R, Nasello-Paterson C, Connors G. Patterns of fetal breathing activity in the human fetus at 24 to 28 weeks. *Am J Obstet Gynecol* 1988; 72:841–6.

22. Manning FA, Snijders R, Harman CR, *et al.* Fetal biophysical profile score: VI. Correlation with antepartum umbilical venous fetal pH. *Am J Obstet Gynecol* 1993; 169:755–63.
23. Bekedam DJ, Visser GHA, de Vries JJ, *et al.* Motor behavior in the growth retarded fetus. *Early Hum Dev* 1985; 12:155–65.
24. Lalor JG, Fawole B, Alfirevic Z, *et al.* Biophysical profile for fetal assessment in high risk pregnancies. *Cochrane Database Syst Rev* 2008; 1:CD000038.
25. Alfirevic Z, Neilson JP. Doppler ultrasonography in high-risk pregnancies: systematic review with meta-analysis. *Am J Obstet Gynecol* 1995; 172:1379–87.
26. Tyrrel S, Obaid AH, Lilford RJ. Umbilical artery Doppler velocimetry as a predictor of fetal hypoxia and acidosis at birth. *Obstet Gynecol* 1989; 74(3 Pt1):332–7.
27. Alfirevic Z, Stampalija T, Gyte GM. Fetal and umbilical Doppler ultrasound in high-risk pregnancies. *Cochrane Database Syst Rev* 2010; 1:CD007529.
28. Thompson JL, Kuller JA, Rhee EH. Antenatal surveillance of fetal growth restriction. *Obstet Gynecol Survey* 2012; 67:554–65.
29. Alfirevic Z, Stampalija T, Gyte GM. Fetal umbilical Doppler ultrasound in normal pregnancy. *Cochrane Database Syst Rev* 2010; 8:CD004150.
30. Farrell T, Chien, PFW, Gordon A. Intrapartum umbilical artery Doppler velocimetry as a predictor of adverse perinatal outcome: a systematic review. *Br J Obstet Gynaecol* 1999; 106:783–92.
31. Morris RK, Say R, Robson SC, *et al.* Systematic review and meta-analysis of middle cerebral artery Doppler to predict perinatal wellbeing. *Eur J Obstet Gynecol Reprod Biol* 2012; 165:141–55.
32. Mari G, Detti L, Oz U, *et al.* Accurate prediction of fetal hemoglobin by Doppler ultrasonography. *Obstet Gynecol* 2002; 99:589–93.
33. Cohen WR, Ommani S, Hassan S, *et al.* Accuracy and reliability of fetal heart rate monitoring using maternal abdominal surface electrodes. *Acta Obstet Gynecol Scand* 2012; 91(11):1306–13.
34. Patrelli TS, D'Addetta F, Gizzo S, *et al.* Correlation between fetal movement revealed in actography and fetal-neonatal well-being: observational study on 3,805 pregnancies followed in a Northern Italy tertiary care hospital. *Clin Exp Obstet Gynecol.* 2011; 38(4):382–5.
35. Castillo RA, Devoe LD, Arthur M, *et al.* The preterm nonstress test; effects of gestational age and length of study. *Am J Obstet Gynecol* 1989; 160:172–5.
36. Giles WB, Lah FX, Trudings BJ. The effect of epidural anaesthesia for caesarean section on maternal uterine and fetal umbilical artery blood flow velocity waveform. *BJOG* 1987; 94:55–9.
37. ACOG Practice Bulletin No. 106: Intrapartum fetal heart rate monitoring: nomenclature, interpretation, and general management principles. American College of Obstetricians and Gynecologists. *Obstet Gynecol* 2009; 114(1):192–202.
38. FIGO. Guidelines for the use of fetal monitoring. *Int J Gynaecol Obstet* 1987; 25:159–67.
39. Grivell RM, Wong L, Bhatia V. Regimens of fetal surveillance for impaired fetal growth. *Cochrane Database Syst Rev* 2012; 6:CD007113.
40. Boehm FH, Salyer S, Shah DM, *et al.* Improved outcome of twice weekly nonstress testing. *Obstet Gynecol* 1986; 67:566–8.
41. Freeman RK, Anderson G, Dorchester W. A prospective multi institutional study of antepartum fetal heart rate monitoring. I. Risk of perinatal mortality and morbidity according to antepartum fetal heart rate test results. *Am J Obstet Gynecol* 1982; 143:771–7.
42. Freeman R. Intrapartum fetal monitoring: a disappointing story. *N Engl J Med* 1990; 322:364.
43. Devane D, Lalor G, Daly S, *et al.* Cardiotocography versus intermittent auscultation of fetal heart on admission to labour ward for assessment of fetal wellbeing. *Cochrane Database Syst Rev* 2012; 2:CD005122.
44. Grivell RM, Alfirevic Z, Gyte GM, *et al.* Antenatal cardiotocography for fetal assessment. *Cochrane Database Syst Rev* 2012; 1:CD007863.
45. Turan S, Turan O, Berg C, *et al.* Computerized fetal heart rate analysis, Doppler ultrasound and biophysical profile score in the prediction of acid base status of growth-restricted fetuses. *Ultrasound Obstet Gynecol* 2007; 30:750–6.
46. East CE, Chan FY, Colditz PB, *et al.* Fetal pulse oximetry for fetal assessment in labour. *Cochrane Database Syst Rev* 2007; 2:CD004075.
47. Clark SL, Paul RH. Intrapartum fetal surveillance: the role of fetal scalp bloodsampling. *Am J Obstet Gynecol* 1985; 153:717–20.
48. Westgate J, Greene K. How well is fetal blood sampling used in clinical practice? *BJOG* 1994; 101:250–1.
49. Schaap TP, Moormann KA, Becker JH, *et al.* Cerebrospinal fluid leakage, an uncommon complication of fetal blood sampling: a case report and review of the literature. *Obstet Gynecol Survey* 2011:66:42–6.
50. Tuffnell D, Haw WL, Wilkinson K. How long does a fetal scalp blood sample take? *BJOG* 2006; 113:332–4.
51. East CE, Leader LR, Sheehan P, *et al.* Intrapartum fetal scalp lactate sampling for fetal assessment in the presence of a non-reassuring fetal heart rate trace. *Cochrane Database Syst Rev* 2010; 3:CD006174.
52. Su TY, Reece M, Chua SC. Lactate using umbilical cord blood: agreement between Lactate Pro hand-held devices with blood gas analyser and evaluation of lactate stability over time. *Aust N Z J Obstet Gynaecol* 2013; 53:375–80.
53. Heinis AM, Dinnissen J, Spaanderman ME, *et al.* Comparison of two point-of-care testing (POCT) devices for fetal lactate during labor. *Clin Chem Lab Med* 2011; 50:89–93.
54. Heinis AM, Spaanderman ME, Gunnewiek JM, *et al.* Scalp blood lactate or intrapartum assessment of fetal metabolic acidosis. *Acta Obstet Gynecol Scand* 2011; 10:1107–14.
55. Wiberg-Itzel E, Pembe AB, Wray S, *et al.* Level of lactate in amniotic fluid and its relation to the use of oxytocin and adverse neonatal outcome. *Acta Obstet Gynecol Scand* 2014; 93(1):80–5.
56. Westgate JA, Bennet L, Brabyn C. ST waveform changes during repeated umbilical cord occlusions in near-term fetal sheep. *Am J Obstet Gynecol* 2001; 184:743–51.
57. Wiberg-Itzel E, Lipponer C, Norman M, *et al.* Determination of pH or lactate in fetal scalp blood in management of intrapartum fetal distress: randomised controlled multicentre trial. *BMJ* 2008; 336:1284–7.
57. Rosen KG, Luzietti R. Intrapartum fetal monitoring: its basis and current developments. *Prenat Neonat Med* 2000; 5:155–68.
58. Westgate J, Harris M, Curnow JS. Plymouth randomised trial of cardiotocogram only versus ST waveform plus cardiotocogram for intrapartum monitoring: 2400 cases. *Am J Obstet Gynecol* 1993; 169:1151–60.
59. Amer-Wåhlin I, Hellsten C, Noren H. Cardiotocography only versus cardiotocography plus ST-analysis of fetal electrocardiogram for intrapartum fetal monitoring: a Swedish randomised controlled trial. *Lancet* 2001; 358:534–8.
60. Ojala K, Vaarasmaki M, Makikallio K, *et al.* A comparison of intrapartum automated fetal electrocardiography and conventional cardiotocography—a randomised controlled study. *BJOG* 2006; 113:419–23.
61. Vayssiere C, David E, Meyer N, *et al.* A French randomized controlled trial of ST-segment analysis in a population with abnormal cardiotocograms during labor. *Am J Obstet Gynecol* 2007; 197:299–306.
62. Westerhuis ME, Visser GH, Moons KG, *et al.* Cardiotocography plus ST analysis of fetal electrocardiogram compared with cardiotocography only for intrapartum monitoring: a randomized controlled trial. *Obstet Gynecol* 2010; 115:1173–80.
63. Becker JH, Bax L, Amer-Wåhlin I, *et al.* ST analysis of the fetal electrocardiogram in intrapartum fetal monitoring: a meta-analysis. *Obstet Gynecol* 2012; 119:145–54.
64. Neilson JP. Fetal electrocardiogram (ECG) for fetal monitoring during labour. *Cochrane Database Syst Rev* 2013; 5:CD000116.
65. Salmelin A, Wiklund I, Bottinga R, *et al.* Fetal monitoring with computerised ST analysis during labor: a systematic review and meta-analysis. *Acta Obstet Gynecol Scand* 2012; 92:28–39.

66. Potti S, Berghella V. ST waveform analysis versus cardiotocography alone for intrapartum fetal monitoring: a meta-analysis of randomized trials. *Am J Perinatol* 2012; 29:657–64.
67. Schuit E, Amer-Wahlin I, Ojala K, *et al.* Effectiveness of electronic fetal monitoring with additional ST analysis in vertex singleton pregnancies at > 36 weeks of gestation: an individual participant data metaanalysis. *Am J Obstet Gynecol* 2013; 208:e1–187.
68. Vijgen SMC, Westerhuis MEMH, Opmeer BC, *et al.* Cost-effectiveness of cardiotocography plus ST-analysis of the fetal electrocardiogram compared to cardiotocography only. *Acta Obstet Gynecol Scand* 2011; 90:772–8.
69. Heintz E, Brodtkorb TH, Nelson N, *et al.* The long-term cost-effectiveness of fetal monitoring during labour: a comparison of cardiotocography complemented with ST analysis versus cardiotocography alone. *BJOG* 2008; 115:1676–87.
70. Norén H, Carlsson A. Reduced prevalence of metabolic acidosis at birth: an analysis of established STAN usage in the total population of deliveries in a Swedish district hospital. *Am J Obstet Gynecol* 2010; 202(6):546.e1–7.
71. Westerhuis MEMH, Kwee A, van Ginkel AA, *et al.* Limitations of ST-analysis in clinical practice: three cases of intrapartum metabolic acidosis. *BJOG* 2007; 114:1194–201.
72. Jacquemyn Y, Martens E, Martens G. Foetal monitoring during labour: practice versus theory in a region-wide analysis. *Clin Exp Obstet Gynecol* 2012; 39:307–9.
73. Westerhuis ME, Porath MM, Becker JH, *et al.* Identification of cases with adverse neonatal outcome monitored by cardiotocography versus ST analysis: secondary analysis of a randomized trial. *Acta Obstet Gynecol Scand* 2012; 91:830–7.
74. Massoud M, Bloc F, Gaucherand P, *et al.* How deviation from STAN guidelines contribute to operative delivery for suspected fetal distress. *Eur J Obstet Gynecol Reprod Biol* 2012; 162:45–9.
75. National Institute of Health and Care Excellence. *Intrapartum Care.* Clinical Guideline GC55. London: NICE.
76. Becker JH, van Rijswijk J, Versteijnen B, *et al.* Is intrapartum fever associated with ST-waveform changes of the fetal electrocardiogram? A retrospective cohort study. *BJOG* 2012; 119:1410–16.
77. Becker JH, Schaap TP, Westerhuis ME, *et al.* Intrapartum epidural analgesia and ST analysis of the fetal electrocardiogram. *Acta Obstet Gynecol Scand* 2011; 90:1364–70.
78. Steyn DW, Odendaal HJ. Routine or computerized cardiotocography in severe preeclampsia? A randomized controlled trial. *J Matern Fetal Invest* 1997; 7:166–71.
79. Malvasi A, Tinelli A, Barbera A, *et al.* Occiput posterior position diagnosis: vaginal examination or intrapartum sonography? A clinical review. *J Matern Fetal Neonatal Med* 2014; 27(5):520–6.
80. Tutschek B, Torkildsen EA, Eggebø TM. Comparison between ultrasound parameters and clinical examination to assess fetal head station in labor. *Ultrasound Obstet Gynecol* 2013; 41(4):425–9.
81. Ghi T, Youssef A, Maroni E, *et al.* Intrapartum transperineal ultrasound assessment of fetal head progression in active second stage of labor and mode of delivery. *Ultrasound Obstet Gynecol* 2013; 41(4):430–5.

CHAPTER 7

Fetal medicine, fetal anaesthesia, and fetal surgery

Francesca Russo, Tim Van Mieghem, and Jan Deprest

Fetal medicine

The main aim of prenatal care is to promote, protect, and maintain the health of the pregnant woman and her future child. The concept of structured prenatal surveillance to reduce maternal and perinatal mortality has been adopted in developed countries since 1920. Until recently this followed a strict schedule with monthly visits from 16 weeks, and a high number of visits in the third trimester ('pyramid of care'; Figure 7.1).[1] In the last two decades, however, several randomized trials[2–4] demonstrated that antenatal care for *low-risk* women can be effectively provided with a lower number of visits.

In contrast, the current concept of modern fetal medicine is that the risk factors for most pregnancy complications, like pre-eclampsia, gestational diabetes mellitus, fetal demise, preterm birth, fetal structural and chromosomal anomalies, fetal growth restriction, and macrosomia, are already present in the first trimester.[5–11] An early estimation of patient-specific risks is done by a combination of ultrasound, maternal biophysical parameters, maternal history, and biochemical markers. The first prenatal examination also provides an opportunity for cervical cancer screening in women who have not been screened recently, assessment of gestational age and calculation of estimated date of delivery, and education on lifestyle (tobacco smoking, food-acquired infections, physical activity, alcohol and recreational as well as medical drug use, vaccination, and food supplementation). This new strategy for pregnancy management may improve perinatal outcome by offering a more individualized care and a disease-specific approach.

At 11–13 weeks, only few women will be selected as being at high risk. In the low-risk group, the number of visits could be reduced to an additional three: one at 20–22 weeks, to evaluate fetal anatomy and growth, and reassess the individual risk for pregnancy complications; one at 37–38 weeks, to check maternal and fetal well-being and determine the timing and mode of delivery; and one at 41weeks, in case the woman has not delivered yet (Figure 7.1B).[12] High-risk patients should be referred to specialist clinics, in order to receive closer, individualized, *disease-specific* pregnancy monitoring. In the course of subsequent visits, a number of women may move between risk categories.[12]

Screening for fetal chromosomal abnormalities

In most developed countries, genetic screening tests are offered to all women in the first trimester—regardless of maternal age or other identified risk factor. In case of increased risk, a definitive diagnosis is made through further invasive testing, such as mid-trimester amniocentesis or first-trimester chorionic villus sampling (CVS) (Figure 7.2).[13,14] Usually the procedure-related risk of 0.5–1.5% for miscarriage or other pregnancy complications is taken as a guidance for the cut-off of what is considered as 'at increased risk'.[15]

Several studies demonstrated that effective screening for chromosomal abnormalities can be achieved by maternal serum free beta-human chorionic gonadotropin[16] and pregnancy-associated plasma protein-A (PAPP-A)[17] combined with ultrasound measurement of fetal nuchal translucency (NT) thickness.[18] NT is the maximum thickness of the subcutaneous translucency between the skin and the soft tissue overlying the cervical spine of the fetus. A computer algorithm integrates this information with biometry (crown–rump length[19]) and maternal characteristics, including age,[20] weight, height, the presence of type 1 diabetes, and previous history of chromosomal abnormalities.[21] The combined test has a detection rate of 93% and a false-positive rate of 5% for trisomy 21, and a slightly lower detection rate for trisomy 18, 13, or other chromosomal abnormalities.[22] For comparison, the detection rates achieved by selection of at-risk patients by maternal age alone or second-trimester maternal serum testing are 30% and 65%, respectively.[23]

Other first-trimester ultrasound markers, such as hypoplasia or absence of the nasal bone, tricuspid regurgitation, and flow in the ductus venosus and in the hepatic artery, may be added to improve the performance of the first-trimester screening, but their clinical usefulness currently remains uncertain (Figure 7.3).

Offering the first-trimester combined tests can reduce the number of women undergoing invasive diagnostic procedures,[24,25] leading to fewer losses of normal pregnancies.[26]

In the immediate future, this strategy may be revised again, when non-invasive prenatal testing via the analysis of free fetal DNA circulating in maternal blood will be routinely introduced. The technology today is ready, but cost is a limiting factor.

Screening for other fetal anomalies

Congenital malformations occur in 2–4% of all births. Despite their relatively low prevalence, fetal malformations are responsible for approximately 30% of perinatal deaths and considerable infant morbidity.[27,28] In this respect, the purpose of their prenatal diagnosis is to optimize the management of the pregnancy in terms of antenatal care, referral for planned birth at the required

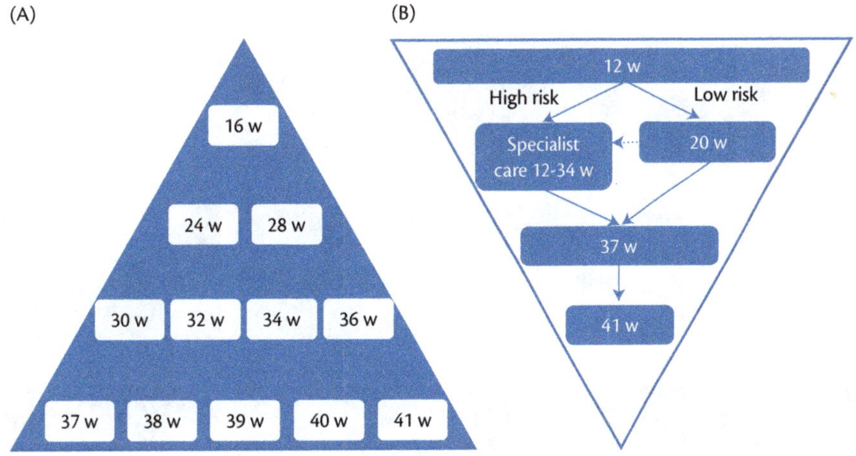

Figure 7.1 Pyramid of care. (A) Conventional follow-up scheme. (B) Inverted pyramid of care aiming at identifying the at-risk patient.
w, weeks.
Reproduced with permission from Kypros H. Nicolaides, A model for a new pyramid of prenatal care based on the 11 to 13 weeks' assessment, *Prenatal Diagnosis*, Volume 31, Issue 1, pp. 3–6, Copyright © 2011 John Wiley and Sons.

specialist level, and planning of postnatal treatment of the baby. In most European countries, parents are also given the option for termination when severe anomalies are diagnosed.

Whereas in the past these anomalies were typically diagnosed in the second trimester,[29] current resolution and skills often allow for first-trimester diagnosis. When patients opt for risk assessment, they are offered NT measurement, which will include anatomical assessment. This test has indeed been shown to pick up a whole series of gross anomalies, such as skeletal dysplasias, diaphragmatic hernia, and major cardiac defects (Table 7.1). Because a number of malformations may only develop or become visible later in pregnancy, the second-trimester '18–22-week' scan should still be offered in case of a negative first-trimester scan, in both low-risk and high-risk pregnancies.[30] When the first-trimester risk assessment is showing increased risk, yet the invasive genetic test is normal, these patients will be considered as at increased risk for structural anomalies, and will have their second-trimester anomaly scan with an expert. The risk for cardiac defects, for example, increases with fetal NT thickness and the presence of abnormal venous or cardiac Doppler in the first trimester.[31–34]

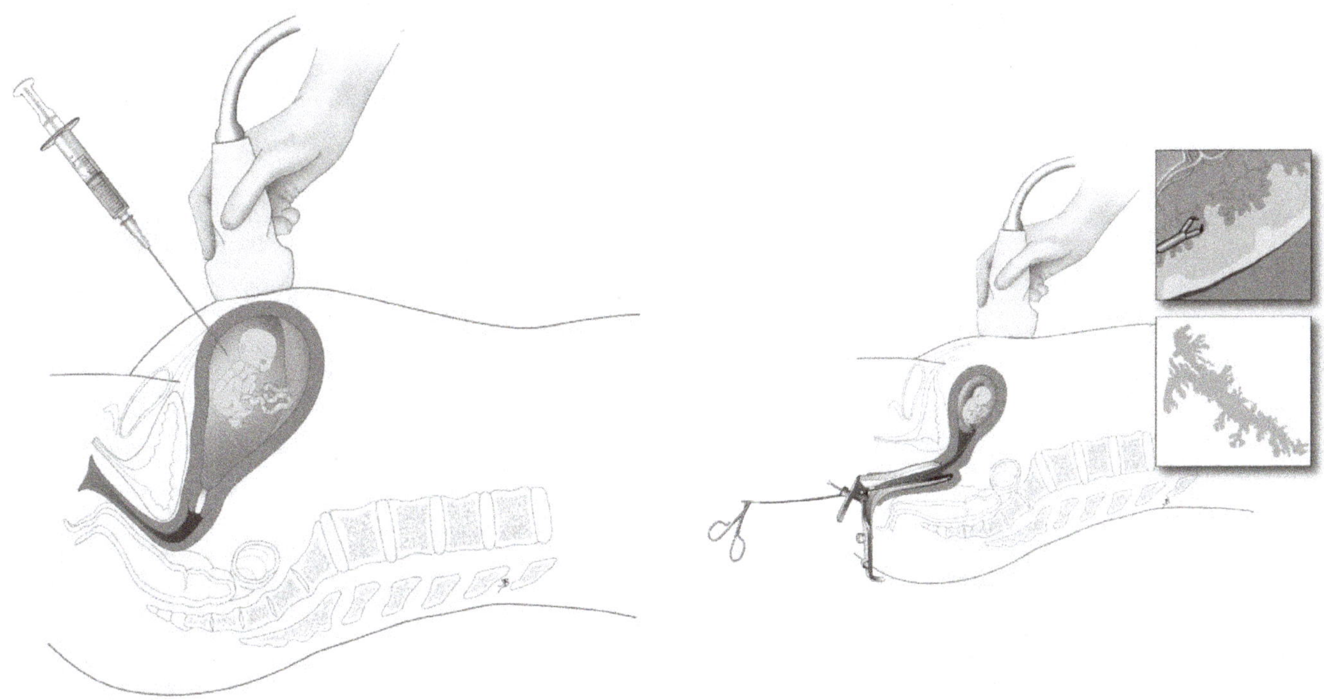

Figure 7.2 Invasive sampling for obtaining genetic fetal material, early in gestation by chorionic villus sampling (right) or from 15 weeks onwards by amniocentesis (left).
Reproduced with permission from the University Hospitals Leuven, Belgium.

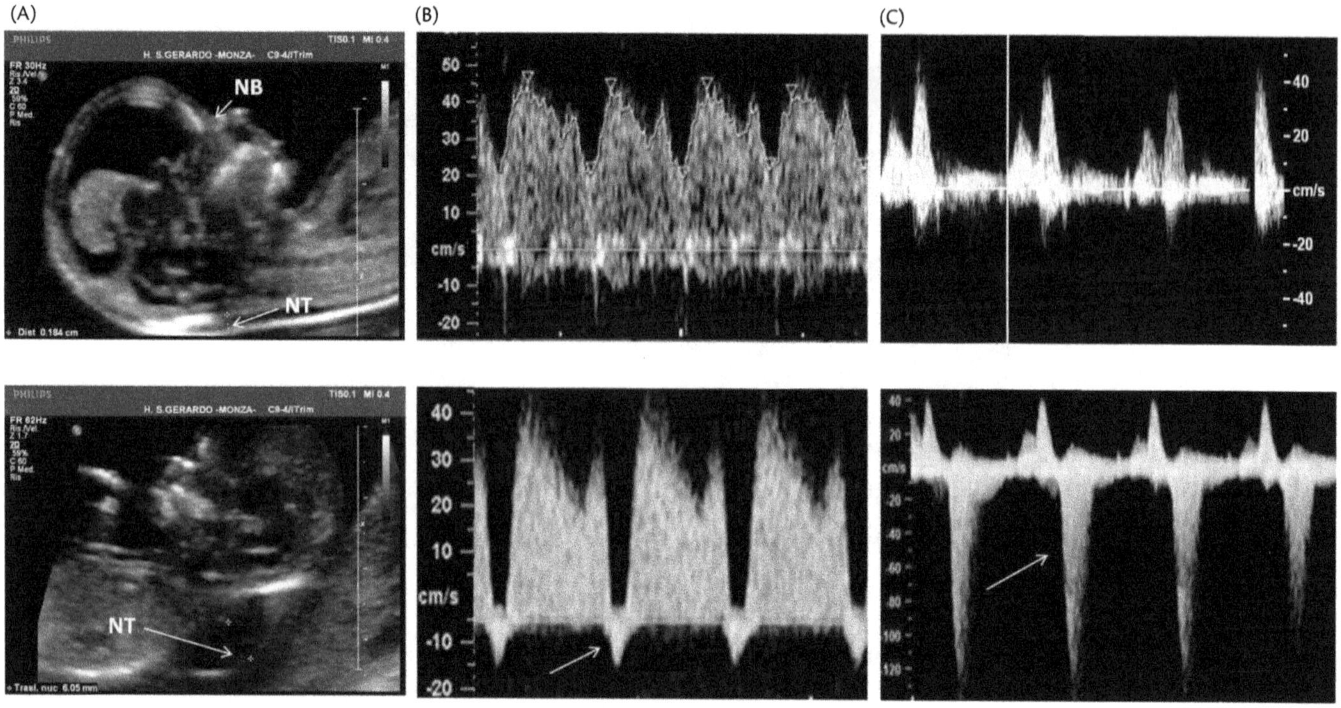

Figure 7.3 Images taken at typical first trimester screening, for identification of: (A) the nuchal translucency (NT) and the nasal bone (NB) (B) flow in the ductus venosus (C) tricuspid regurgitation. Top row: normal findings. Bottom row: abnormal findings.

Reproduced with permission from the University Hospitals San Gerardo, Monza, Italy.

Table 7.1 Summary of the most common fetal conditions amenable for therapy and outcome of interventions[a]

Pathology	Untreated leads to	Therapy	Gestational age at birth	Common complications	Outcome after therapy
Rhesus disease	High output cardiac failure and decreased tissue oxygenation	Intrauterine transfusion	36 weeks	IUFD 1.7% per procedure	Survival hydrops 74%, no hydrops 91%, CP 2.1%, developmental delay 4.8%
HLHS	Postnatal demise, univentricular circulation	Balloon valvuloplasty	88% > 36 weeks	Intrauterine resuscitation 30%, IUFD 10%	33–67% biventricular repair
Posterior urethral valves	Renal failure, pulmonary hypoplasia	Vesico-amniotic shunting	34–35 weeks	Shunt dislodgment 34%	50–90% survival, 30–40% end-stage renal failure
Pleural effusion	Cardiac failure, pulmonary hypoplasia	Thoraco-amniotic shunting	34–35 weeks	Shunt dislodgment 10–20%	Survival hydrops 55%, no hydrops 85%
CDH	Pulmonary hypoplasia	Tracheal occlusion	35 weeks	Balloon deflation 8%	50% survival
TTTS	IUFD and preterm birth	Laser ablation of anastomoses	33–34 weeks	IUFD one fetus 15%, TAPS 10%	70% double survival, 80–90% survival ≥ 1 fetus, CP 6%, mental delay 7%, motor delay 12%
Selective reduction	Neurological damage or IUFD	RFA/cord occlusion	34–35 weeks	Demise non-target fetus 15%	85% survival non-target fetus
Myelomeningocele repair	Hydrocephaly, hindbrain herniation, nerve function loss beyond lesion, cognitive and motoric impairment dependent on level of lesion	Fetal surgical closure	34 weeks	PPROM 34%, 10% uterine dehiscence	Shunt rate drops from 98% to 68%, improved Bailey score at 30 months; walking improved from 21% to 42%

CDH, congenital diaphragmatic hernia; CP, cerebral palsy; HLHS, hypoplastic left heart syndrome; IUFD, intrauterine fetal demise; PPROM, preterm premature rupture of membranes; RFA: radiofrequency ablation; TAPS, twin anaemia-polycythemia sequence; TTTS, twin-to-twin transfusion syndrome.

[a]References are provided in the text.

Adapted from *Best Practice & Research Clinical Obstetrics & Gynaecology*, Volume 26, issue 5 van Mieghem, T., *et al.*, Minimally invasive fetal therapy, pp. 711–25, Copyright (2012), with permission from Elsevier. Data from references supplied in text.

Similarly, open spina bifida is associated with caudal displacement of the brain already detectable at 11–13 weeks.[35]

Early screening for miscarriage and stillbirth

Increased risk of miscarriage and stillbirth is associated with certain maternal characteristics, including advanced maternal age, maternal weight, previous miscarriages, cigarette smoking, chronic hypertension, and African racial origin.[36–38] Analogous to aneuploidy screening, maternal characteristics are combined with biophysical measurements and biochemical testing at 11–13 weeks to allow an individualized risk estimation. However, the detection rate remains low (30%). This points to the heterogeneous aetiology of miscarriage and stillbirth. Furthermore, while early identification of the group at risk for stillbirth could lead to closer monitoring of fetal growth, well-being, and appropriate timing of delivery, no preventive interventions are known so far, so its value can be questioned.[5]

Maternal medicine

Screening for maternal diseases

Hypertensive disease occurs in 12–22% of all pregnancies and is responsible for approximately 11% of maternal deaths in developed countries. Pre-eclampsia is defined as gestational hypertension combined with proteinuria after 20 weeks' gestation.[39] It affects 5–8% of pregnancies and remains a substantial contributor to perinatal morbidity and mortality worldwide. Furthermore, it is one of the three leading causes of maternal mortality.[40] Blood pressure screening is therefore recommended at the first visit and at all subsequent visits though obviously this identifies the patient only at the onset of problems. Risk factors for pre-eclampsia should therefore be investigated during the first visit. This allows intensive maternal and fetal monitoring, leading to a timely diagnosis of pre-eclampsia, and the prompt initiation of prophylactic treatment, such as aspirin.[12] Risk calculation is based on maternal characteristics, such as age, body mass index, the presence of chronic hypertension, previous or family history of pre-eclampsia, as well as first-trimester biochemical and ultrasound parameters, which aim at measuring the degree of invasion of the placental trophoblast—which is believed to be abnormal in pre-eclampsia. Uterine artery Doppler studies can detect increased placental vascular resistance, but its sensitivity ranges from 7% to 80%.[41,42] Measurement of PAPP-A[43–45] a-disintegrin and metalloprotease 12 (ADAM12), soluble endoglin (sEng), inhibin-A, activin-A, pentraxin-3 (PTX3), P-selectin placental growth factor (PLGF), and placental protein-13 (PP13)[6,46–49] have all been associated with pre-eclampsia. Again, algorithms combining maternal characteristics, Doppler findings, and biochemical tests at 11–13 weeks can identify patients at risk for pre-eclampsia, and stratify this condition according to gestational age at onset, which correlates to the severity of the disease.[6] (See Chapter 36 for further details on pre-eclampsia.)

A similar integrated algorithm has been proposed for the first-trimester screening of gestational diabetes. Gestational diabetes is defined as a glucose intolerance occurring during pregnancy, with an incidence of about 2–3%.[50] This condition is associated with adverse perinatal outcomes (death, shoulder dystocia with or without fracture, and nerve palsy). It makes sense to diagnose diabetes, because adequate intervention, by dietary advice, blood glucose monitoring, and, if needed, metformin or insulin therapy, lowers morbidity. In low-risk patients, screening for gestational diabetes mellitus is performed at 24 to 28 weeks' gestation through an oral glucose tolerance test.[39] However, first-trimester algorithms combining maternal characteristics (body mass index, racial origin, family history, and previous macrosomic baby) and biochemical tests (serum levels of adiponectin, sex hormone-binding globulin, or visfatin) may identify about 75% of pregnancies subsequently complicated by gestational diabetes, with a false-positive rate of 20%.[51] (See chapter 47.)

Screening for preterm delivery

Infants born preterm have an increased risk of mortality and severe comorbidities, despite improved neonatal care. The risk of preterm birth has been rising in most developed countries during the past decades.[52,53] Considerable effort has been spent to investigate the pathogenesis of preterm birth and preventive measures that reduce its consequences.[54,55]

Transvaginal ultrasound of the cervix objectively measures cervical length in a standardized way, and has been shown to enable risk estimation of preterm delivery when performed at 18–22 weeks (which coincides with the anomaly scan) (Figure 7.4).[56,57] Preventive measures (e.g. by administration of progesterone) have been shown to significantly reduce the risk of delivery at less than 37 weeks.[58,59] An alternative treatment for women with a short cervix is cervical cerclage, which reduces the risk of spontaneous early preterm delivery by about 40% in women who had a previous preterm birth or second-trimester loss, but not in those without such history.[60] (See Chapter 33.)

Measuring cervical length only at 20 weeks, however, cannot prevent miscarriages due to cervical incompetence before that gestation and delays prophylactic measures. First-trimester assessment is therefore desirable. Again, it is the combination of maternal characteristics such as ethnicity, age, and socioeconomic status, previous preterm birth as well as pregnancy characteristics such as multiple pregnancy, conception after artificial reproductive technologies, and presence of urogenital tract infections which predict poor outcome.[61,62] This can be combined by measurement of endocervical length at 11–13 weeks, which has been shown to be predictive.[63] A recent study suggests that combination with PP-13, PAPP-A, and uterine artery pulsatility index are useful markers for identifying pregnancies at increased risk for early premature birth.[64]

Fetal therapy became a clinical reality after the introduction of high-resolution ultrasound. It has been boosted by the implementation of systematic pregnancy screening programmes which have led to the early detection and better understanding of the natural history of fetal anomalies. Only a limited numbers of fetal anomalies are progressive in nature, so that when left untreated, they lead to fetal and neonatal demise, or severe morbidity. Prenatal intervention aims at halting or reversing the progression of these diseases and improving the postnatal outcome. Where some fetal conditions such as open neural tube defects,[65] large solid lung masses, or sacrococcygeal teratomas[66] are still treated through maternal laparotomy and hysterotomy, we have witnessed an increased introduction of minimally invasive fetal therapeutic procedures over the last two decades. The aim of the current chapter is to present an overview of the rationale for, the technical aspects of, and outcomes of the most common minimally invasive prenatal therapeutic procedures. These are reserved for well-selected fetuses, at

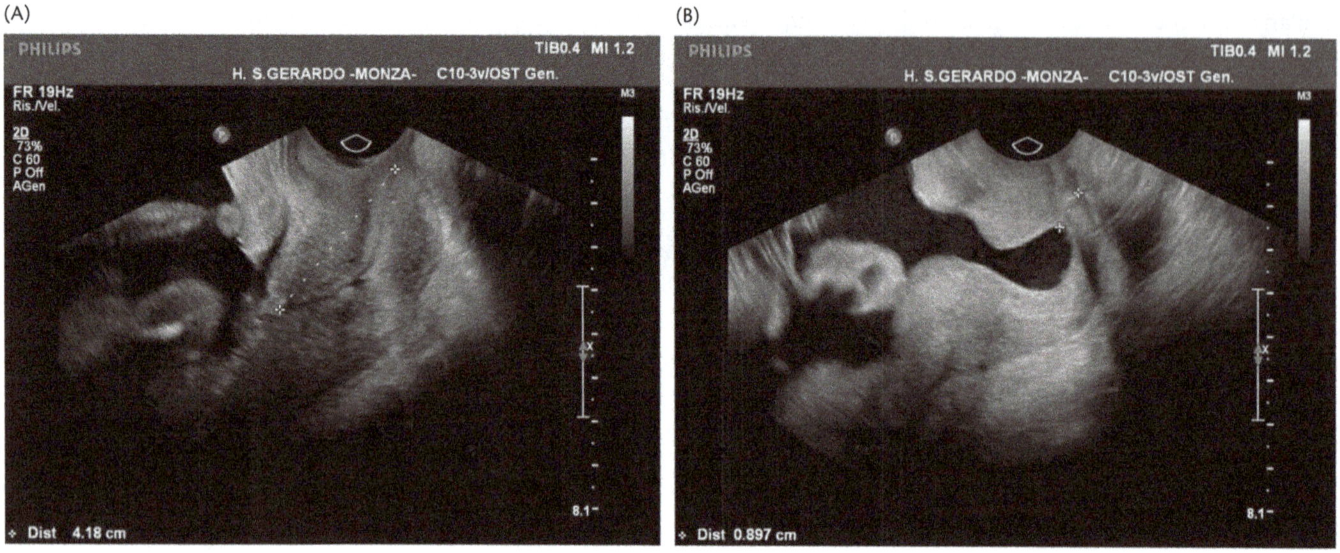

Figure 7.4 Cervical sonography for the prediction of preterm birth. (A) Normal findings. (B) Patient at high risk because of cervical incompetence.
Reproduced with permission from the University Hospitals San Gerardo, Monza, Italy.

the most severe end of the spectrum, and are only offered in a limited number of centres. Optimal patient selection, expert counselling, rigorous clinical protocols and experienced multidisciplinary teams are strict criteria for fetal therapy programmes.[67,68]

Fetal therapy

The implementation of systematic ultrasound screening leads to earlier detection of fetal anomalies. Whereas most fetal conditions are adequately treatable after birth, some disorders progress during fetal life and can lead to severe morbidity or fetal and neonatal demise. This inherently raises the question of prenatal therapy. Some fetal conditions are amenable to fetal surgical intervention, some of them by minimal access. Below we provide an overview of the rationale for, the technical aspects of, and (if available) the outcomes of the most common prenatal therapies (Table 7.1).

Intrauterine transfusion

Intrauterine transfusions are performed for severe fetal anaemia and thrombocytopenia. Technical aspects of the procedure are identical for both conditions. Fetal thrombocytopenia is very rare and for that we refer readers to the excellent recent review by Kamphuis et al.[69] This section will therefore discuss only fetal anaemia. The incidence of rhesus D (RhD) haemolytic disease has decreased dramatically since the routine administration of anti-D immunoglobulins. As a consequence, other causes of fetal anaemia, such as fetomaternal haemorrhage, twin anaemia polycythaemia sequence, parvovirus B19 infections, and haemolytic disease due to other than RhD red blood cell antigens have gained in relative importance. The severity of anaemia in a fetus at risk can be assessed by non-invasive measurement of peak systolic velocity in the middle cerebral artery. Severe anaemia, mandating antenatal intervention, is present when the peak systolic velocity is over 1.5 multiples of the median and shows an increasing trend.[70]

Intrauterine transfusions are usually performed under local anaesthesia in an outpatient setting, or when rescue delivery is anticipated under spinal or combined spinal and epidural[71] (Figure 7.5). Typically, the umbilical vein is punctured under ultrasound guidance either in its intrahepatic portion or at the placental cord root. At the start of the transfusion a blood sample is drawn for haemoglobin and haematocrit measurement and the required volume calculated to reach around 45%.[72] Pancuronium can be administered to immobilize the fetus for intrahepatic transfusions; intrahepatic vein puncture justifies the use of fetal pain relief. O rhesus-negative blood with a haematocrit of 80%, that has been screened for the most common infectious diseases, and irradiated to prevent graft-versus-host reaction, is transfused. Extremely anaemic fetuses are treated with multiple transfusions with a few days' interval. In case of persistent haemolysis, the fetal haematocrit drops around 1% per day. Therefore, repeated transfusions at 2–3-week intervals are required in rhesus disease. The last transfusion is usually given around 34 weeks of gestation to allow for a timed delivery around 36–37 weeks.

In experienced hands, intrauterine transfusions are successful in over 97% of cases.[73] The rate of severe complications is 3% per procedure in rhesus disease and the procedure-related fetal loss rate is 1.6%.[74,75] The latter increases to 10% in transfusions done before 22 weeks of gestation.[76] Overall survival after intrauterine transfusions for rhesus disease is 75% when the fetus is hydropic at the first transfusion, and over 90% in non-hydropic fetuses.[73] A large follow-up study on neurological outcomes after intrauterine transfusions for rhesus disease shows a cerebral palsy rate of 2.1% and an overall risk for developmental delay of 4.8%.[77] Neurological impairment is more likely if hydrops was present.

Fetoscopic laser coagulation of chorionic plate vessels

Twin-to-twin transfusion syndrome (TTTS) affects 9% of monochorionic twins and fetal therapy is considered when presenting between 16 and 28 weeks of gestation.[78,79] A review on the pathophysiology can be found in a recent review by Fisk et al.[80] Imbalances in vasoactive hormones and fluid shifts lead to one fetus being hypertensive and volume overloaded (the recipient fetus) and the other being volume depleted (the donor fetus). The diagnostic criteria for TTTS rely on the presence of polyuric

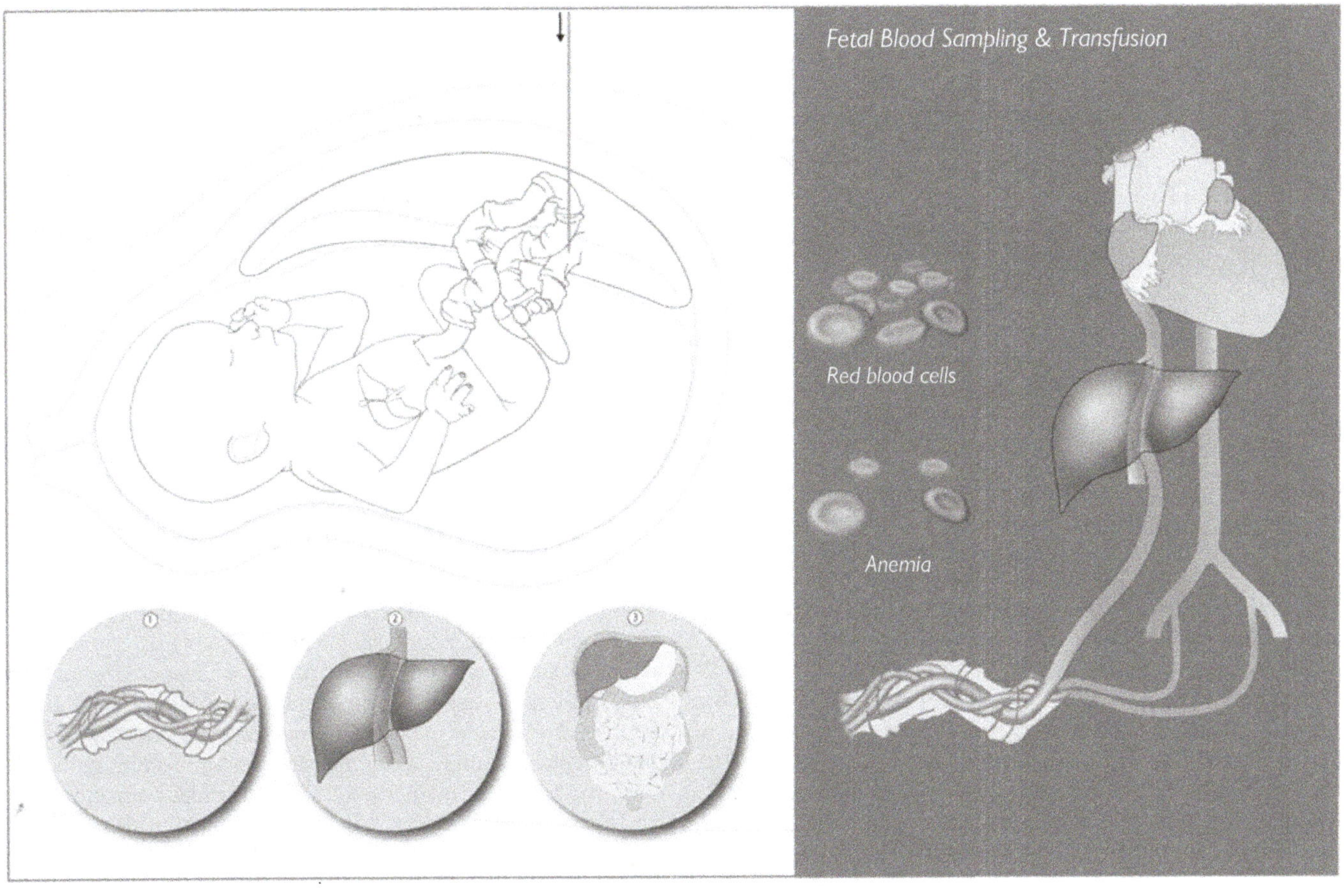

Figure 7.5 Schematic representation of an intrauterine transfusion. The fetal circulation is typically accessed at the level of the cord insertion (1), or the intra-hepatic vein (2).
Reproduced with permission from the University Hospitals Leuven, Belgium.

polyhydramnios in the recipient fetus and oliguric oligohydramnios in the donor. TTTS is further staged according to Quintero et al.[81] based on the presence (stage I) or absence (stage II) of bladder filling in the donor fetus, Doppler changes in one or both fetuses (stage III) and the presence of hydrops (stage IV), or fetal death (stage V). In a randomized controlled trial, it was shown that causative therapy, by fetoscopic laser coagulation of inter-twin anastomosis, yields better outcome than serial amniodrainages of excessive fluid.[82] Fetoscopic laser is performed under local or locoregional maternal anaesthesia (Figure 7.6). A 2–3.5 mm fetoscope with a working channel for a laser fibre[83] is introduced into the recipient's sac and all anastomosing vessels are coagulated under direct vision. The procedure is completed by amniodrainage. Recurrent TTTS and twin anaemia-polycythaemia syndrome are relatively rare complications but are amenable for therapy. Intrauterine fetal demise of one fetus, which is only partially predictable, occurs in about 15% of cases. Whereas in the earlier large series overall neonatal survival was around 55% and survival of at least one fetus around 70%,[84] these numbers increased to 70% and 80–90% respectively with increasing experience.[85,86] Mean gestational age at delivery is 33–34 weeks. In terms of long-term neurological outcome, a recent, large, multicentre follow-up study (N = 287 TTTS survivors) demonstrated that the risk for cerebral palsy in survivors is 6%.[87] Severe mental delay is observed in 7% and psychomotor impairment in 12%. This compares to the background risk of neurodevelopmental impairment (7%) and cerebral palsy (0.6%) in uncomplicated monochorionic twin pregnancies.[88] The major determinant of these adverse outcomes is prematurity[83] and the stage at the time of intervention, with poorer outcomes at an advanced stage.[89] In a very recent randomized trial, it was shown that complete separation of the placenta along the vascular equator reduces recurrence rate and improves neonatal outcome (Solomon technique—Figure 7.6B).[90]

Selective reduction in monochorionic twin gestations

In some monochorionic twin pairs, the condition of one fetus may pose a threat to the well-being of the other due to the presence of the placental anastomoses. Examples are impending demise of one fetus by selective (in one twin) intrauterine growth restriction, end-stage TTTS or after its failed therapy, and a number of discordant congenital anomalies, including twin reversed arterial perfusion (TRAP). In these circumstances, controlled fetocide of the affected fetus including obliteration of intrafetal or cord vessels can be performed to protect the healthy twin. Simultaneous arterial and venous occlusion can be achieved by cord occlusion. Bipolar cord coagulation using a 3.0 mm forceps is performed under local anaesthesia with ultrasound guidance (Figure 7.7A).[83] Thermoablation of intrafetal vessels using laser, monopolar energy, or radiofrequency needles has more recently been propagated. A straight needle or a needle equipped

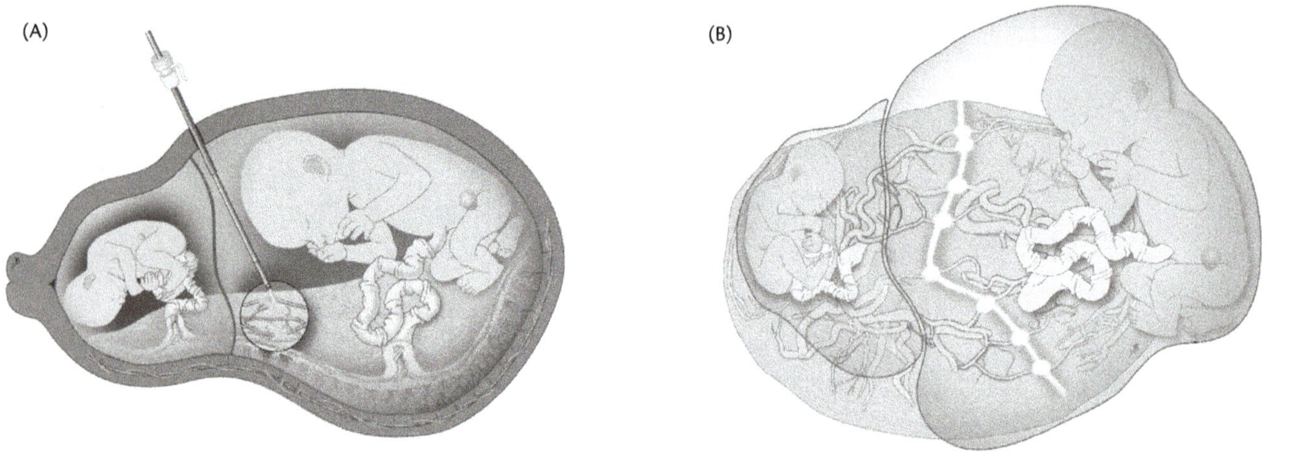

Figure 7.6 Fetoscopic laser coagulation of chorionic plate vessels for twin-to-twin transfusion syndrome, along the vascular equator (A) and completed by separation (B).
Reproduced with permission from the University Hospitals Leuven, Belgium.

with umbrella-shaped tines is inserted into the abdomen of the target fetus, close to where the cord vessels branch at the level of the umbilicus (Figure 7.7B).[91] Cord coagulation and radiofrequency ablation are equally successful in 97% of cases,[92] but survival of the non-target twin is around 80–85% because of post-procedural losses. Cases operated after 18 weeks do better than early cases.[93,94] Mean gestational age at delivery is 34–35 weeks and neurological outcome in survivors is good, with neurodevelopmental impairment in 2% of cases.[93,95]

Interventions for lower urinary tract obstruction

Fetal lower urinary tract obstruction (LUTO) occurs in about 2–3/10,000 pregnancies.[96] Many are due to isolated posterior urethral valves or urethral atresia, but associated structural or chromosomal anomalies are present in 25%.[96] Untreated, the perinatal mortality of isolated LUTO is high, primarily due to pulmonary hypoplasia secondary to the oligohydramnios, adding to the problem of severe renal failure. Survivors have a high incidence of chronic renal failure and up to 17% reach end-stage renal disease within 10 years.[97] Vesico-amniotic shunting has been proposed to improve the outcome of fetuses with severe oligohydramnios, that still have acceptable fetal renal function, based on a variety of diagnostic criteria.[98] Vesico-amniotic shunting is a percutaneous procedure using a purpose-designed cannula and trocar with echogenic tip. The instrument is advanced through the fetal abdominal wall into the bladder to deploy a catheter allowing bladder drainage into the amniotic cavity (Figure 7.8A).[83] The most frequent complication of vesico-amniotic shunting is preterm rupture of the membranes leading to a mean gestational age at delivery of 34–35 weeks.[99] Shunt dislodgment, which occurs in 34%,[99] and obstruction may mandate a repeat procedure.[100] There is evidence that vesico-amniotic shunting improves neonatal survival, especially in fetuses with poor renal function.[101] Overall survival ranges between 50% and 90% and one in three chance survivors has end-stage renal disease at a mean follow-up of 5 years.[102] Survivors may also have other respiratory and growth problems, but their self-reported quality of life falls within the normal range.

More recently intrauterine fetal cystoscopy has been proposed (Figure 7.8B).[103] The procedure, which can be done as early as 16 weeks of gestation, allows a more robust diagnosis, and in case of urethral valves, definitive treatment by laser fulguration may be attempted. A recent systematic review of four fetal cystoscopy studies[104] demonstrated that the initial diagnosis of posterior urethral valves changed in 32% (6/19) typically towards urethral

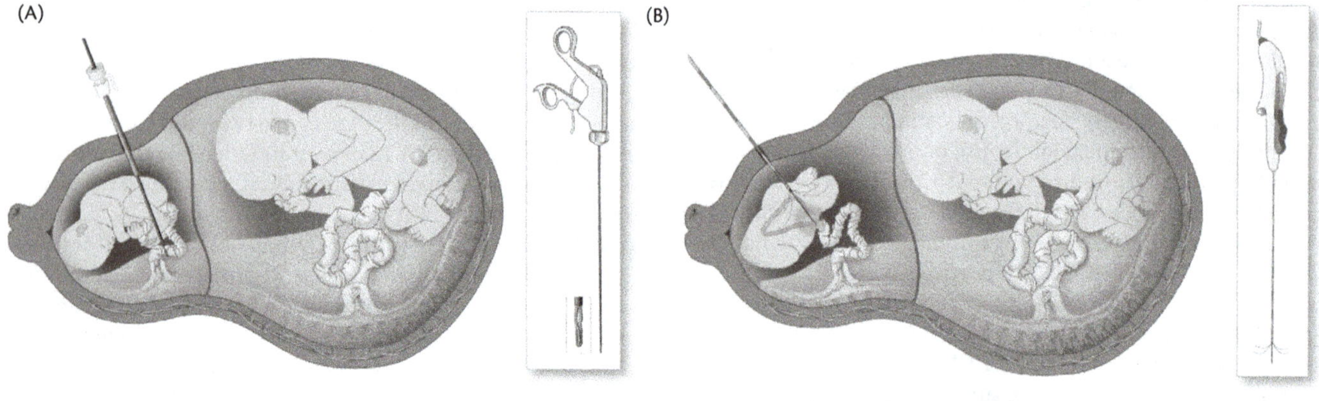

Figure 7.7 (A) Bipolar cord coagulation, using a bipolar forceps (insert). (B) Radiofrequency ablation using an RFA-device with its tines deployed.
Reproduced with permission from the University Hospitals Leuven, Belgium.

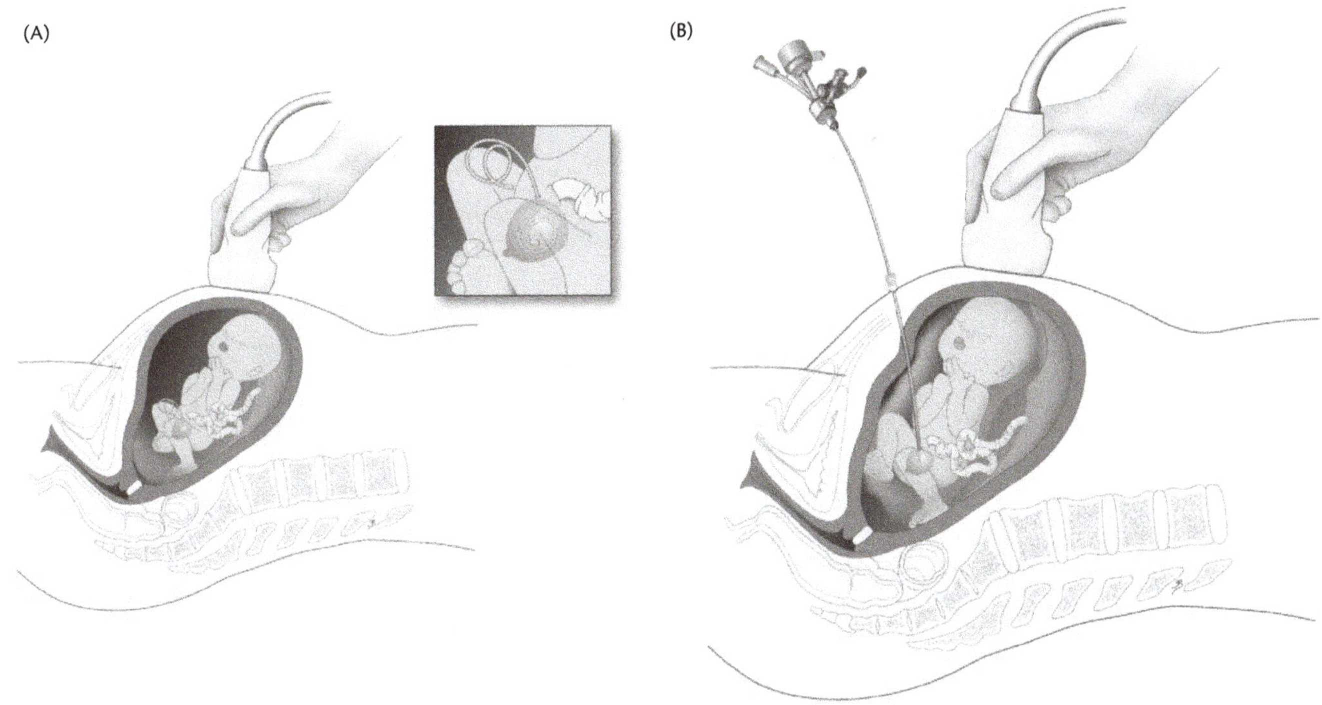

Figure 7.8 (A) Percutaneous vesico-amniotic shunting. (B) Fetal cystoscopy.
Reproduced with permission from the University Hospitals Leuven, Belgium.

atresia. In terms of postnatal survival, cystoscopic ablation of the valves was superior to expectant management yet comparable to shunting.[36]

Interventions for fetal thoracic pathology

Pleural effusions

Fetal pleural effusions can either be isolated (primary hydrothorax or chylothorax) or secondary to other conditions such as diaphragmatic hernia, bronchopulmonary sequestration, cardiac anomalies, fetal infections, and metabolic, chromosomal, or syndromal disorders. Mild to moderate primary hydrothorax, which does not lead to functional cardiac impairment, mediastinal shift, or severe lung compression, has a good outcome and hence can be managed conservatively.[105] Hydrops and association with severe pulmonary hypoplasia reduce survival rate to 25%.[105] Drainage of the effusion should theoretically alleviate intrathoracic compression and hence yield a better outcome. Such drainage can be achieved either by repeated thoracocentesis or pleuroamniotic shunting. A recent systematic review showed that outcomes of thoracocentesis and shunting were similar,[106] yet shunting is often preferred when more distant from term (Figure 7.9). The procedure is comparable to vesico-amniotic shunting. The lateral or posterior chest wall of the fetus is preferred for shunt insertion to avoid lesions to mammary gland and nipple. Shunt migration or obstruction leads to the need for repeated procedures in 10–20% of cases. Preterm premature rupture of membranes and preterm delivery are common, leading to an average gestational age at delivery of 34–35 weeks. In a recent large case series, neonatal survival was 55% in hydropic fetuses and 85% in non-hydropic fetuses.[107] Gestational age at birth and duration of shunting are both important predictors of outcome.[108]

Pulmonary parenchymal lesions

Congenital cystic adenomatoid malformation (CCAM) of the lung arises from an overgrowth of the terminal respiratory bronchioles. Bronchopulmonary sequestration (BPS) is non-functional pulmonary parenchyma that is separated from the normal lung and receives its blood supply from the systemic circulation. CCAMs are classified as microcystic, macrocystic, or mixed based on their appearance on ultrasound. Most commonly, CCAMs are small and about 50% regress in the third trimester of pregnancy.[109] Limited lesions do not compromise cardiac function or lung development and have very favourable outcomes with conservative prenatal management. Some can even be managed conservatively postnatally.[110]

More rare are the masses that grow very large and lead to pulmonary hypoplasia or hydrops, the latter being almost invariably fatal.[111] In large macrocystic CCAMs, therapeutic size reduction can be obtained by thoraco-amniotic shunting of the larger cyst. Non-hydropic fetuses with masses causing mediastinal shift that are shunted have a postnatal survival rate of 87% (gestational age at birth 37 weeks).[109] For hydropic cases, survival was only 66%. Large microcystic CCAMs are considered not to be amenable for thoraco-amniotic shunting as they are mainly solid. First, maternal administration of glucocorticoids should be attempted.[112–114] If not, surgery can be contemplated. Several minimally invasive techniques have been described but are experimental. There is more information about open fetal surgical lobectomy, which has a survival rate of 50%, yet at the cost of higher maternal morbidity.[66,115]

In view of the potential of identifying a (systemic) feeding vessel to a BPS, vascular occlusion techniques comparable to those used in twins can be used, with a greater than 90% survival rate.[109,116–121]

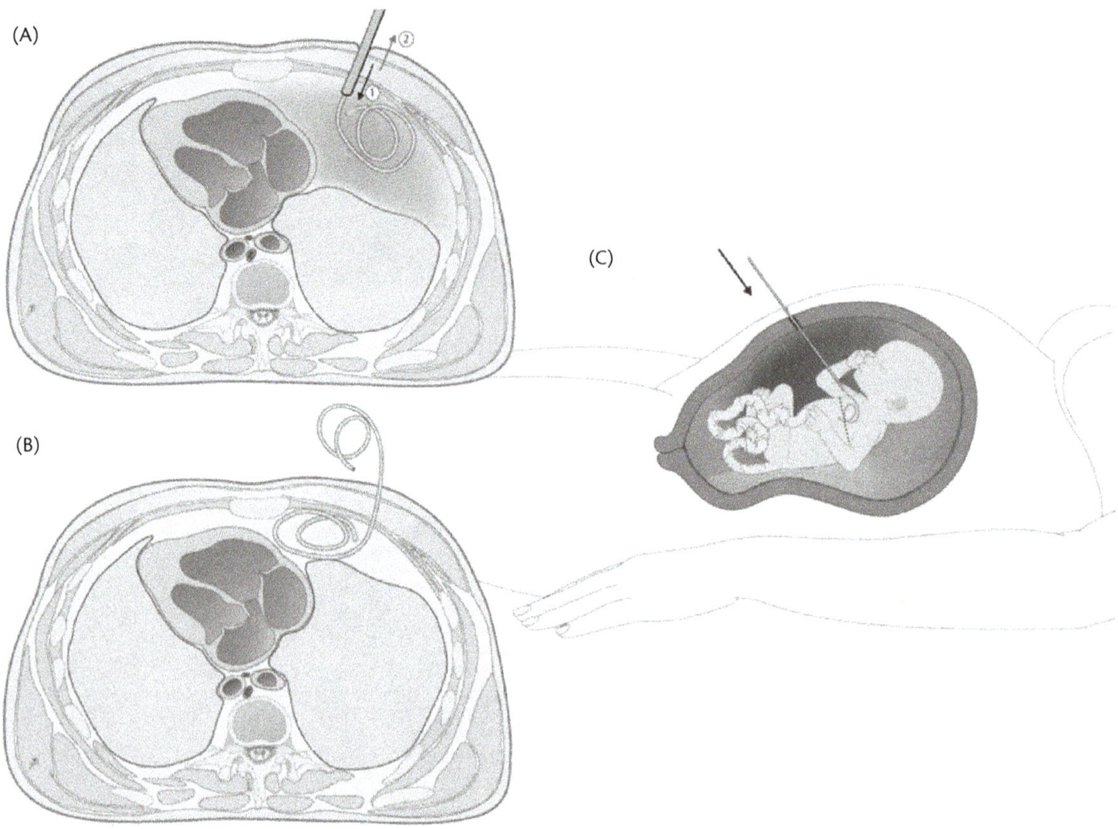

Figure 7.9 Schematic representation of a thoracic shunt being inserted (A, B) and deployed (C).
Reproduced with permission from the University Hospitals Leuven, Belgium.

Pulmonary hypoplasia due to congenital diaphragmatic hernia

Congenital diaphragmatic hernia occurs in 1/3000 pregnancies. Even when isolated (i.e. in the absence of other structural defects or chromosomal anomalies) this condition has a high neonatal mortality and morbidity due to pulmonary hypertension and hypoplasia. The prognosis of an individual fetus can be predicted prenatally based on assessment of fetal lung size and liver position.[122,123] Although the overall neonatal survival of fetuses with isolated left-sided diaphragmatic hernia approaches 70–80% in high-volume centres, fetuses with liver herniation and a contralateral lung area less than 25% of the expected area for gestational age on ultrasound have a neonatal survival of less than 25%.[124,125] Fetal lung growth can be stimulated *in utero* by tracheal occlusion (FETO). This procedure prevents the outflow of fluid produced by the lungs. As a consequence, the lungs are inflated and stretched, which is a proven strong stimulus for lung growth. Tracheal occlusion can be done fetoscopically under local anaesthesia within 10 minutes. After the fetus is anaesthetized and immobilized, a fetoscope[83] is introduced percutaneously and the fetal trachea is accessed through the mouth (as for an intubation) (Figure 7.10). A vascular occlusion balloon is delivered in the trachea, just below the vocal cords. As long as the tracheal balloon is *in situ*, the fetal airways are occluded, meaning that normal respiration cannot take place at birth. We have proposed *in utero* reversal at 34 weeks, which in animal experiments has been shown to promote lung maturation, but also allows vaginal birth and referral to a centre not familiar with FETO. Others remove the balloon at birth on placental circulation (Ex Utero Intrapartum Treatment—EXIT). The combined experience of three European centres offering FETO exceeds 200 cases.[126] The most important complications of FETO are preterm prelabour rupture of membranes and preterm delivery which occurs on average at 35 weeks. Compared to an expectantly managed historical cohort, FETO improves survival of cases with severe isolated left-sided diaphragmatic hernia from 25% to 50% and decreases neonatal morbidity.[126–128] This procedure is currently being investigated in a randomized trial (http://www.totaltrial.eu).

Fetal cardiac procedures

Despite improvements in neonatal (surgical) care and the development of dedicated follow-up programmes for infants with congenital heart disease, the outcome of fetuses with hypoplastic left heart syndrome (HLHS) remains poor. Postnatal surgery, which results in a far from optimal single-ventricle Fontan-type circulation,[129] has a considerable mortality rate leading to a total survival of less than 65%.[130] Moreover, half the long-term survivors have poor neurodevelopmental outcome[131] which may in part have an antenatal origin. Indeed, a preferential return of oxygenated blood towards the right ventricle and lower body rather than towards the left ventricle and the brain may lead to suboptimal brain oxygenation *in utero*.[132,133]

A hypoplastic heart can already be present in early pregnancy,[134] but about 5% develop in the second trimester and are progressive.[130] In these cases, which are often due to outlet valve obstruction, fetal balloon valvuloplasties may allow for intrauterine ventricular recovery and growth, and increase the chance

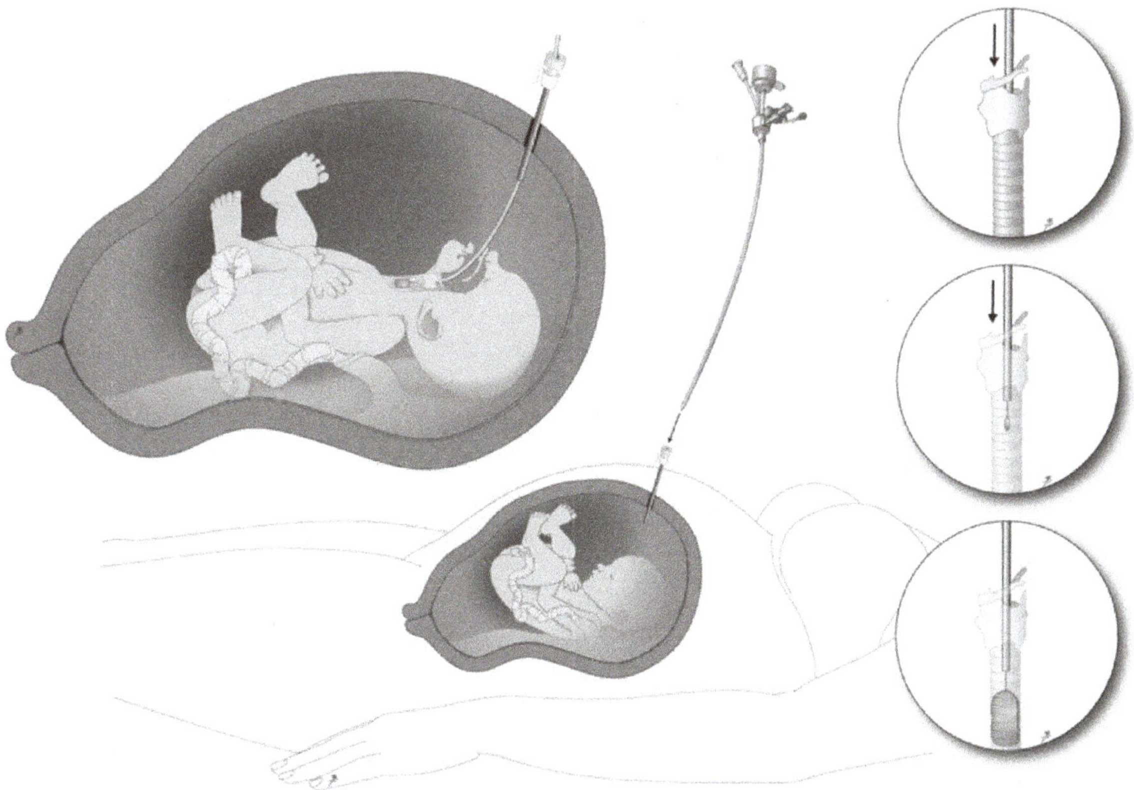

Figure 7.10 Percutaneous insertion of a balloon into the fetal trachea. Inserts show the steps for positioning a detachable balloon.
Reproduced with permission from the University Hospitals Leuven, Belgium.

of a postnatal biventricular repair. Proper patient selection and optimized techniques for needle-based access to the fetal heart have led to reasonable outcomes.[135–137] For HLHS, an 18- or 19-gauge needle is inserted into the fetal left ventricle at the level of the apex and in alignment with the left ventricular outflow tract (Figure 7.11). A guidewire and a catheter with a coronary dilatation balloon are advanced through the aortic valve, which is dilated to 120% of the valve annulus. Technical success defined as successful inflation and dilatation is achieved in 70% of cases. Perioperative complications are common. These include bradycardia necessitating fetal resuscitation (17–38%), haemopericardium (13%), ventricular thrombosis (15–20%), as well as fetal demise (8–13%).[138] Significant left ventricular growth may be observed *in utero*, yet only 33–67% of the technically successful procedures end up in a postnatal biventricular repair. Similar percutaneous cardiac balloon procedures have been proposed for HLHS with a highly restrictive foramen ovale[139] and pulmonary atresia with intact ventricular septum.[140]

Myelomeningocoele

The prevalence of neural tube defects in Europe is around 9/10,000 births making it one of the most frequent congenital anomalies affecting the central nervous system.[141] Myelomeningocele (MMC) is the most common distal closure defect and is characterized by extrusion of the meninges and the spinal cord. *In utero* exposure of the developing spinal cord and nerves causes progressive damage, whereas leakage of cerebrospinal fluid leads to hydrocephaly and downward displacement of the cerebellum and brain (Chiari malformation). This in turn affects neurocognitive prognosis and late morbidity. Over 80% of children require lifelong shunting and 50% of them will have shunt complications in the first year of life.[142] The functional impact is highly dependent on the level and extension of the lesion.[143,144]

Fetal intervention essentially aims at *isolating the defect from the toxic and traumatic intrauterine environment*. Following experimental and early clinical evaluation, the Management of Myelomeningocele Study (MOMS) demonstrated benefit of fetal rather than postnatal closure through maternal laparotomy and hysterotomy. Eligible are fetuses with lesions above S1 between 19 and 25 completed weeks of gestation.[65] This results in the *in utero* reversal of the Chiari malformation. Postnatally the need for shunting dropped by a third, and at 30 months of age, 40% of children were able to walk (control: 20%). This is in line with earlier case series that also showed that outcomes after fetal surgery are about two vertebral levels functionally better than anatomically present.

The procedure requires maternal general anaesthesia for adequate fetal anaesthesia and uterine relaxation for fetal surgery and uterine exposure. The fetus is manually positioned such that the MMC sac is in the centre of the future hysterotomy, which is made with specifically designed uterine staplers (Figure 7.12). The fetus is given an intramuscular injection of fentanyl and muscle relaxant. The actual MMC repair is not different from what is typically done after birth. The uterus is closed in two layers with prior restoration of amniotic fluid and antibiotic administration and covered with an omental patch. Prophylactic tocolytics includes magnesium sulphate (24 hours), indomethacin (48 hours), and oral nifedipine after discontinuation of magnesium sulphate until

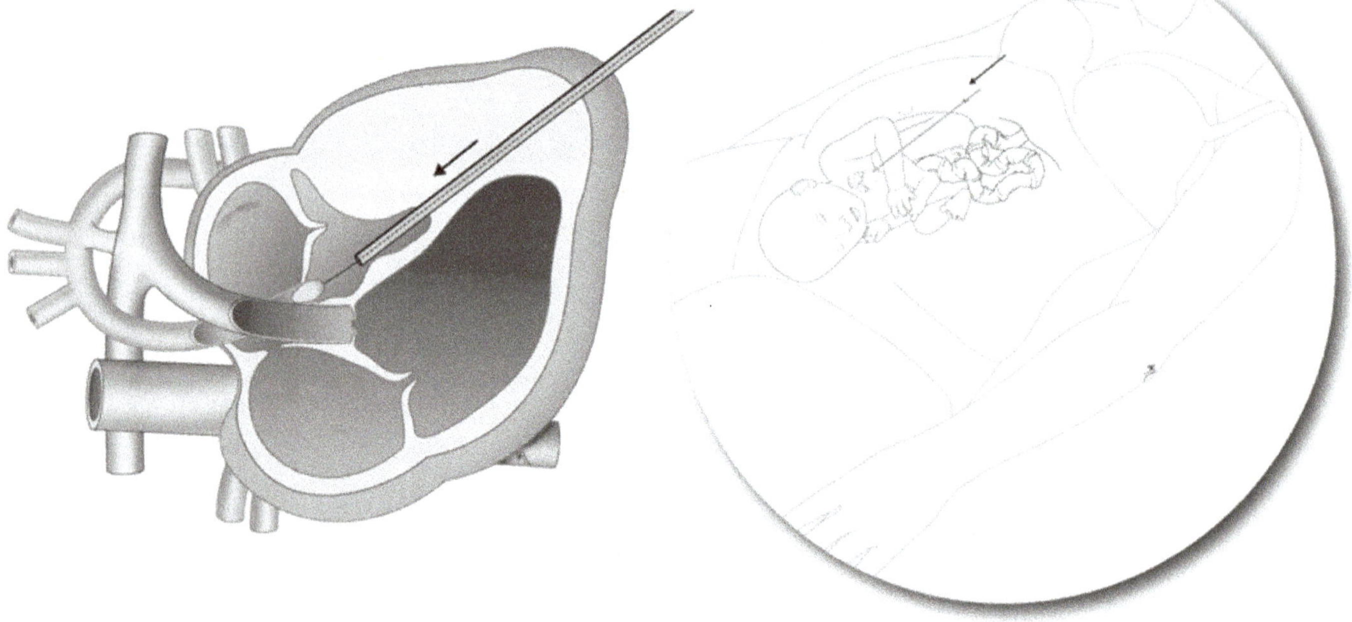

Figure 7.11 Schematic representation of a percutaneous valvuloplasty, in this case of the left ventricular outlet tract.
Reproduced with permission from the University Hospitals Leuven, Belgium.

37 weeks. Typical hospital stay is 4 days. Elective caesarean delivery by lower uterine incision is at 37 weeks.

Fetal pain

Pain is a subjective experience occurring in response to impending or actual tissue damage. The subjective experience of pain requires nociception and an emotional reaction. Nociception requires an intact sensory system, and an emotional reaction requires some form of consciousness. It is difficult to know the extent to which the fetus experiences pain. However, several indirect methods have suggested that the fetus at least *can* feel pain. Robinson and Gregory suggested the importance of providing analgesia in preterm neonates.[145] Anand et al.,[146–148] Fisk et al.,[149] and

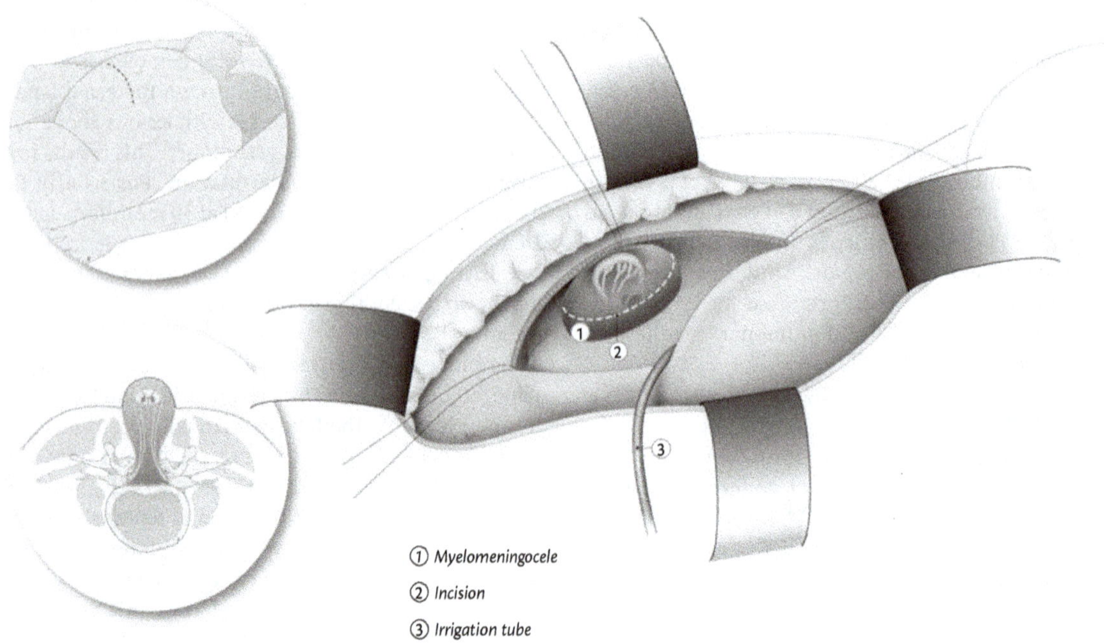

Figure 7.12 Schematic representation of a fetal myelomeningocele repair; insert: incision (top) and schematic representation of the lesion (bottom).
Reproduced with permission from the University Hospitals Leuven, Belgium.

Giannakoulopoulos et al.[150] demonstrated that premature infants and fetuses display several humoral stress responses during invasive procedures. These data indicate that the mid-gestational fetus responds to noxious stimuli by mounting a distinct stress response, as evidenced by an outpouring of catecholamines and other stress hormones as well as haemodynamic changes. And, analogous to what has been documented in neonates, prenatal stress can be expected to affect later neurodevelopment. Theoretically, *in utero* experienced pain may be 'remembered' by the fetus, which could in turn lead to altered sensory patterns or abnormal behavioural patterns in postnatal life. Consequently, management of fetal pain and associated stress response *in utero* during invasive fetal interventions is important.[149] Even if it remains unproven whether this results in improved neurodevelopment and improved long-term outcome, it is prudent to take pre-emptive action and manage potentially painful procedures accordingly.

Several treatment protocols have been proposed[151] and, in general, a policy of administration of fetal analgesics for any invasive procedures where the fetus might experience pain should be adopted, certainly from 18 to 20 weeks onward. Sufentanil (1–2 mcg/kg) or fentanyl (10 mcg/kg) can be given intramuscularly or intravenously to the fetus. Should the mother undergo general anaesthesia, the fetus should be sufficiently anaesthetized through transplacental passage.[152]

Conclusion

Advances in prenatal imaging and the introduction of screening policies enable identification of high-risk pregnancies and early diagnosis of fetal anomalies. Some of these are amenable to fetal therapy, in case treatment cannot wait until birth. Over the last two decades, fetal surgery has become a clinical reality, which was boosted by instrument development and successful clinical trials. More recently, open fetal surgery has become more widely reintroduced for *in utero* repair of neural tube defects, which remarkably is not a lethal condition. Performing prenatal surgical interventions requires adequate fetal pain relief.

References

1. Ministry of Health. *Memorandum on Antenatal Clinics: Their Conduct and Scope*. London: His Majesty's Stationery Office; 1930.
2. Villar J, Carroli G, Khan-Neelofur D, *et al.* Patterns of routine antenatal care for low-risk pregnancy. *Cochrane Database Syst Rev* 2001; 4:CD000934.
3. Carroli G, Villar J, Piaggio G, *et al.* WHO systematic review of randomised controlled trials of routine antenatal care. *Lancet* 2001; 357(9268):1565–70.
4. Dowswell T, Carroli G, Duley L, *et al.* Alternative versus standard packages of antenatal care for low-risk pregnancy. *Cochrane Database Syst Rev* 2010; 10:CD000934.
5. Akolekar R, Bower S, Flack N, *et al.* Prediction of miscarriage and stillbirth at 11–13 weeks and the contribution of chorionic villus sampling. *Prenat Diagn* 2011; 31(1):38–45.
6. Akolekar R, Syngelaki A, Sarquis R, *et al.* Prediction of early, intermediate and late pre-eclampsia from maternal factors, biophysical and biochemical markers at 11–13 weeks. *Prenat Diagn* 2011; 31(1):66–74.
7. Ashoor G, Kametas NA, Akolekar R, *et al.* Maternal thyroid function at 11–13 weeks of gestation. *Fetal Diagn Ther* 2010; 27(3):156–63.
8. Beta J, Bredaki FE, Rodriguez Calvo J, *et al.* Maternal serum alpha-fetoprotein at 11–13 weeks' gestation in spontaneous early preterm delivery. *Fetal Diagn Ther* 2011; 30(2):88–93.
9. Karagiannis G, Akolekar R, Sarquis R, *et al.* Prediction of small-for-gestation neonates from biophysical and biochemical markers at 11–13 weeks. *Fetal Diagn Ther* 2011; 29(2):148–54.
10. Nicolaides KH. Screening for fetal aneuploidies at 11 to 13 weeks. *Prenat Diagn* 2011; 31(1):7–15.
11. Syngelaki A, Chelemen T, Dagklis T, *et al.* Challenges in the diagnosis of fetal non-chromosomal abnormalities at 11–13 weeks. *Prenat Diagn* 2011; 31(1):90–102.
12. Nicolaides KH. Turning the pyramid of prenatal care. *Fetal Diagn Ther* 2011; 29(3):183–96.
13. National Collaborating Centre for Women's and Children's Health. *Antenatal Care: Routine Care for the Healthy Pregnant Woman.* London: National Collaborating Centre for Women's and Children's Health; 2008.
14. American College of Obstetricians and Gynecologists. ACOG Practice Bulletin No. 88, December 2007. Invasive prenatal testing for aneuploidy. *Obstet Gynecol* 2007; 110(6):1459–67.
15. Tabor A, Alfirevic Z. Update on procedure-related risks for prenatal diagnosis techniques. *Fetal Diagn Ther* 2010; 27(1):1–7.
16. Spencer K, Macri JN, Aitken DA, *et al.* Free beta-hCG as first-trimester marker for fetal trisomy. *Lancet* 1992; 339(8807):1480.
17. Brambati B, Macintosh MC, Teisner B, *et al.* Low maternal serum levels of pregnancy associated plasma protein A (PAPP-A) in the first trimester in association with abnormal fetal karyotype. *Br J Obstet Gynaecol* 1993; 100(4):324–6.
18. Nicolaides KH, Azar G, Byrne D, *et al.* Fetal nuchal translucency: ultrasound screening for chromosomal defects in first trimester of pregnancy. *BMJ* 1992; 304(6831):867–9.
19. Pandya PP, Snijders RJ, Johnson SP, *et al.* Screening for fetal trisomies by maternal age and fetal nuchal translucency thickness at 10 to 14 weeks of gestation. *Br J Obstet Gynaecol* 1995; 102(12):957–62.
20. Grati FR, Barlocco A, Grimi B, *et al.* Chromosome abnormalities investigated by non-invasive prenatal testing account for approximately 50% of fetal unbalances associated with relevant clinical phenotypes. *Am J Med Genet A* 2010; 152A(6):1434–42.
21. NSW Health. *Prenatal Testing/Screening for Down Syndrome & Other Chromosomal Abnormalities.* Sydney: Ministry of Health; 2007.
22. Nicolaides KH. First-trimester screening for chromosomal abnormalities. *Semin Perinatol* 2005; 29(4):190–4.
23. Nicolaides KH. First-trimester screening for Down's syndrome. *N Engl J Med* 2004; 350(6):619–21.
24. Saltvedt S, Almström H, Kublickas M, *et al.* Screening for Down syndrome based on maternal age or fetal nuchal translucency: a randomized controlled trial in 39,572 pregnancies. *Ultrasound Obstet Gynecol* 2005; 25(6):537–45.
25. Lo TK, Lai FK, Leung WC, *et al.* A new policy for prenatal screening and diagnosis of Down syndrome for pregnant women with advanced maternal age in a public hospital. *J Matern Fetal Neonatal Med* 2010; 23(8):914–19.
26. Chasen ST, McCullough LB, Chervenak FA. Is nuchal translucency screening associated with different rates of invasive testing in an older obstetric population? *Am J Obstet Gynecol* 2004; 190(3):769–74.
27. Marden PM, Smith DW, McDonald MJ. Congenital anomalies in the newborn infant, including minor variations. A study of 4,412 babies by surface examination for anomalies and buccal smear for sex chromatin. *J Pediatr* 1964; 64:357–71.
28. Todros T, Capuzzo E, Gaglioti P. Prenatal diagnosis of congenital anomalies. *Images Paediatr Cardiol* 2001; 3(2):3–18.
29. Salomon LJ, Alfirevic Z, Berghella V, *et al.* Practice guidelines for performance of the routine mid-trimester fetal ultrasound scan. *Ultrasound Obstet Gynecol* 2011; 37(1):116–26.
30. Salomon LJ, Alfirevic Z, Bilardo CM, *et al.* ISUOG practice guidelines: performance of first-trimester fetal ultrasound scan. *Ultrasound Obstet Gynecol* 2013; 41(1):102–13.
31. Hyett J, Perdu M, Sharland G, *et al.* Using fetal nuchal translucency to screen for major congenital cardiac defects at 10–14 weeks of gestation: population based cohort study. *BMJ* 1999; 318(7176):81–5.

32. Matias A, Huggon I, Areias JC, *et al.* Cardiac defects in chromosomally normal fetuses with abnormal ductus venosus blood flow at 10–14 weeks. *Ultrasound Obstet Gynecol* 1999; 14(5):307–10.
33. Martinez JM, Comas M, Borrell A, *et al.* Abnormal first-trimester ductus venosus blood flow: a marker of cardiac defects in fetuses with normal karyotype and nuchal translucency. *Ultrasound Obstet Gynecol* 2010; 35(3):267–72.
34. Pereira S, Ganapathy R, Syngelaki A, *et al.* Contribution of fetal tricuspid regurgitation in first-trimester screening for major cardiac defects. *Obstet Gynecol* 2011; 117(6):1384–91.
35. Mangione R, Dhombres F, Lelong N, *et al.* Screening for fetal spina bifida at the 11–13-week scan using three anatomical features of the posterior brain. *Ultrasound Obstet Gynecol* 2013; 42(4):416–20.
36. Smith GC, Shah I, White IR, *et al.* Maternal and biochemical predictors of antepartum stillbirth among nulliparous women in relation to gestational age of fetal death. *BJOG* 2007; 114(6):705–14.
37. Willinger M, Ko CW, Reddy UM. Racial disparities in stillbirth risk across gestation in the United States. *Am J Obstet Gynecol* 2009; 201(5):469.e1–8.
38. Spencer K, Cowans NJ, Avgidou K, *et al.* First-trimester ultrasound and biochemical markers of aneuploidy and the prediction of impending fetal death. *Ultrasound Obstet Gynecol* 2006; 28(5):637–43.
39. Akkerman D, Cleland L, Croft G, *et al. Routine Prenatal Care.* Bloomington, MN: Institute for Clinical Systems Improvement (ICSI); 2012.
40. Cantwell R, Clutton-Brock T, Cooper G, *et al.* Saving Mothers' Lives: Reviewing maternal deaths to make motherhood safer: 2006–2008. The Eighth Report of the Confidential Enquiries into Maternal Deaths in the United Kingdom. *BJOG* 2011; 118 Suppl 1:1–203.
41. Parra M, Rodrigo R, Barja P, *et al.* Screening test for preeclampsia through assessment of uteroplacental blood flow and biochemical markers of oxidative stress and endothelial dysfunction. *Am J Obstet Gynecol* 2005; 193(4):1486–91.
42. Martin AM, Bindra R, Curcio P, *et al.* Screening for pre-eclampsia and fetal growth restriction by uterine artery Doppler at 11–14 weeks of gestation. *Ultrasound Obstet Gynecol* 2001; 18(6):583–6.
43. Dugoff L, Hobbins JC, Malone FD, *et al.* First-trimester maternal serum PAPP-A and free-beta subunit human chorionic gonadotropin concentrations and nuchal translucency are associated with obstetric complications: a population-based screening study (the FASTER Trial). *Am J Obstet Gynecol* 2004;191(4):1446–51.
44. Smith GC, Stenhouse EJ, Crossley JA, *et al.* Early pregnancy levels of pregnancy-associated plasma protein a and the risk of intrauterine growth restriction, premature birth, preeclampsia, and stillbirth. *J Clin Endocrinol Metab* 2002; 87(4):1762–7.
45. Goetzinger KR, Singla A, Gerkowicz S, *et al.* Predicting the risk of pre-eclampsia between 11 and 13 weeks' gestation by combining maternal characteristics and serum analytes, PAPP-A and free beta-hCG. *Prenat Diagn* 2010; 30(12–13):1138–42.
46. Goetzinger KR, Zhong Y, Cahill AG, *et al.* Efficiency of first-trimester uterine artery Doppler, a-disintegrin and metalloprotease 12, pregnancy-associated plasma protein a, and maternal characteristics in the prediction of preeclampsia. *J Ultrasound Med* 2013; 32(9):1593–600.
47. Akolekar R, Minekawa R, Veduta A, *et al.* Maternal plasma inhibin A at 11-13 weeks of gestation in hypertensive disorders of pregnancy. *Prenat Diagn* 2009; 29(8):753–60.
48. Akolekar R, Casagrandi D, Livanos P, *et al.* Maternal plasma pentraxin 3 at 11 to 13 weeks of gestation in hypertensive disorders of pregnancy. *Prenat Diagn* 2009; 29(10):934–8.
49. Levine RJ, Lindheimer MD. First-trimester prediction of early preeclampsia: a possibility at last! *Hypertension* 2009; 53(5):747–8.
50. Stephenson MJ. Screening for gestational diabetes mellitus: a critical review. *J Fam Pract* 1993; 37(3):277–83.
51. Nanda S, Savvidou M, Syngelaki A, *et al.* Prediction of gestational diabetes mellitus by maternal factors and biomarkers at 11 to 13 weeks. *Prenat Diagn* 2011; 31(2):135–41.
52. Schaaf JM, Mol BW, Abu-Hanna A, *et al.* Trends in preterm birth: singleton and multiple pregnancies in the Netherlands, 2000–2007. *BJOG* 2011; 118(10):1196–204.
53. Ananth CV, Joseph KS, Oyelese Y, *et al.* Trends in preterm birth and perinatal mortality among singletons: United States, 1989 through 2000. *Obstet Gynecol* 2005; 105(5 Pt 1):1084–91.
54. Moons KG, Altman DG, Vergouwe Y, *et al.* Prognosis and prognostic research: application and impact of prognostic models in clinical practice. *BMJ* 2009; 338:b606.
55. Schaaf JM, Ravelli AC, Mol BW, *et al.* Development of a prognostic model for predicting spontaneous singleton preterm birth. *Eur J Obstet Gynecol Reprod Biol* 2012; 164(2):150–5.
56. Honest H, Bachmann LM, Coomarasamy A, *et al.* Accuracy of cervical transvaginal sonography in predicting preterm birth: a systematic review. *Ultrasound Obstet Gynecol* 2003; 22(3):305–22.
57. Committee opinion no. 522: incidentally detected short cervical length. *Obstet Gynecol* 2012; 119(4):879–82.
58. Meis PJ, Klebanoff M, Thom E, *et al.* Prevention of recurrent preterm delivery by 17 alpha-hydroxyprogesterone caproate. *N Engl J Med* 2003; 348(24):2379–85.
59. Mackenzie R, Walker M, Armson A, *et al.* Progesterone for the prevention of preterm birth among women at increased risk: a systematic review and meta-analysis of randomized controlled trials. *Am J Obstet Gynecol* 2006; 194(5):1234–42.
60. Berghella V, Odibo AO, To MS, *et al.* Cerclage for short cervix on ultrasonography: meta-analysis of trials using individual patient-level data. *Obstet Gynecol* 2005; 106(1):181–9.
61. Wen SW, Smith G, Yang Q, *et al.* Epidemiology of preterm birth and neonatal outcome. *Semin Fetal Neonatal Med* 2004; 9(6):429–35.
62. Goffinet, F. Primary predictors of preterm labour. *BJOG* 2005; 112 Suppl 1:38–47.
63. Greco E, Lange A, Ushakov F, *et al.* Prediction of spontaneous preterm delivery from endocervical length at 11 to 13 weeks. *Prenat Diagn* 2011; 31(1):84–9.
64. Stout MJ, Goetzinger KR, Tuuli MG, *et al.* First trimester serum analytes, maternal characteristics and ultrasound markers to predict pregnancies at risk for preterm birth. *Placenta* 2013; 34(1):14–19.
65. Adzick NS, Thom EA, Spong CY, *et al.* A randomized trial of prenatal versus postnatal repair of myelomeningocele. *N Engl J Med* 2011; 364(11):993–1004.
66. Kitano Y, Flake AW, Crombleholme TM, *et al.* Open fetal surgery for life-threatening fetal malformations. *Semin Perinatol* 1999; 23(6):448–61.
67. Harrison MR, Filly RA, Golbus MS, *et al.* Fetal treatment 1982. *N Engl J Med* 1982; 307(26):1651–2.
68. Deprest J, Toelen J, Debyser Z, *et al.* The fetal patient—ethical aspects at fetal therapy. *Facts Views Vis Obgyn* 2011; 3:7.
69. Kamphuis MM, Oepkes D. Fetal and neonatal alloimmune thrombocytopenia: prenatal interventions. *Prenat Diagn* 2011; 31(7):712–19.
70. Mari G, Deter RL, Carpenter RL, *et al.* Noninvasive diagnosis by Doppler ultrasonography of fetal anemia due to maternal red-cell alloimmunization. Collaborative Group for Doppler Assessment of the Blood Velocity in Anemic Fetuses. *N Engl J Med* 2000; 342(1):9–14.
71. Kempe A, Rösing B, Berg C, *et al.* First-trimester treatment of fetal anemia secondary to parvovirus B19 infection. *Ultrasound Obstet Gynecol* 2007; 29(2):226–8.
72. Le Ray C, Hudon L, Leduc L. Fetal transfusion of red blood cells for alloimmunization: validity of a published equation. *Fetal Diagn Ther* 2009; 25(4):379–84.
73. van Kamp IL, Klumper FJ, Meerman RH. *et al.* Treatment of fetal anemia due to red-cell alloimmunization with intrauterine transfusions in the Netherlands, 1988–1999. *Acta Obstet Gynecol Scand* 2004; 83(8):731–7.
74. van Kamp IL, Klumper FJ, Oepkes D, *et al.* Complications of intrauterine intravascular transfusion for fetal anemia due to maternal red-cell alloimmunization. *Am J Obstet Gynecol* 2005; 192(1):171–7.

75. Schumacher B, Moise KJ Jr. Fetal transfusion for red blood cell alloimmunization in pregnancy. *Obstet Gynecol* 1996; 88(1):137–50.
76. Yinon Y, Visser J, Kelly EN, *et al.* Early intrauterine transfusion in severe red blood cell alloimmunization. *Ultrasound Obstet Gynecol* 2010; 36(5):601–6.
77. Lindenburg IT, Smits-Wintjens VE, van Klink JM, *et al.* Long-term neurodevelopmental outcome after intrauterine transfusion for hemolytic disease of the fetus/newborn: the LOTUS study. *Am J Obstet Gynecol* 2012; 206(2):141.e1–8.
78. Lewi L, Jani J, Blickstein I, *et al.* The outcome of monochorionic diamniotic twin gestations in the era of invasive fetal therapy: a prospective cohort study. *Am J Obstet Gynecol* 2008; 199(5):514 e1–8.
79. Valsky DV, Eixarch E, Martinez-Crespo JM, *et al.* Fetoscopic laser surgery for twin-to-twin transfusion syndrome after 26 weeks of gestation. *Fetal Diagn Ther* 2012; 31(1):30–4.
80. Fisk NM, Duncombe GJ, Sullivan MH. The basic and clinical science of twin-twin transfusion syndrome. *Placenta* 2009; 30(5):379–90.
81. Quintero RA, Morales WJ, Allen MH, *et al.* Staging of twin-twin transfusion syndrome. *J Perinatol* 1999; 19(8 Pt 1):550–5.
82. Senat MV, Deprest J, Boulvain M, *et al.* Endoscopic laser surgery versus serial amnioreduction for severe twin-to-twin transfusion syndrome. *N Engl J Med* 2004; 351(2):136–44.
83. Klaritsch P, Albert K, Van Mieghem T, *et al.* Instrumental requirements for minimal invasive fetal surgery. *BJOG* 2009; 116(2):188–97.
84. Ville Y, Hecher K, Gagnon A, *et al.* Endoscopic laser coagulation in the management of severe twin-to-twin transfusion syndrome. *Br J Obstet Gynaecol* 1998; 105(4):446–53.
85. Chalouhi GE, Essaoui M, Stirnemann J, *et al.* Laser therapy for twin-to-twin transfusion syndrome (TTTS). *Prenat Diagn* 2011; 31(7):637–46.
86. Chmait RH, Kontopoulos EV, Korst LM, *et al.* Stage-based outcomes of 682 consecutive cases of twin-twin transfusion syndrome treated with laser surgery: the USFetus experience. *Am J Obstet Gynecol* 2011; 204(5):393.e1–6.
87. Lopriore E, Ortibus E, Acosta-Rojas R, *et al.* Risk factors for neurodevelopment impairment in twin-twin transfusion syndrome treated with fetoscopic laser surgery. *Obstet Gynecol* 2009; 113(2 Pt 1):361–6.
88. Ortibus E, Lopriore E, Deprest J, *et al.* The pregnancy and long-term neurodevelopmental outcome of monochorionic diamniotic twin gestations: a multicenter prospective cohort study from the first trimester onward. *Am J Obstet Gynecol* 2009; 200(5):494.e1–8.
89. Salomon LJ, Ortqvist L, Aegerter P, *et al.* Long-term developmental follow-up of infants who participated in a randomized clinical trial of amniocentesis vs laser photocoagulation for the treatment of twin-to-twin transfusion syndrome. *Am J Obstet Gynecol* 2010; 203(5):444 e1–7.
90. Slaghekke F, Lopriore E, Lewi L, *et al.* Fetoscopic laser coagulation of the vascular equator versus selective coagulation for twin-to-twin transfusion syndrome: an open-label randomised controlled trial. *Lancet* 2014; 383(9935):2144–51.
91. Paramasivam G, Wimalasundera R, Wiechec M, *et al.* Radiofrequency ablation for selective reduction in complex monochorionic pregnancies. *BJOG* 2010; 117(10):1294–8.
92. Roman, A, Papanna R, Johnson A, *et al.* Selective reduction in complicated monochorionic pregnancies: radiofrequency ablation vs. bipolar cord coagulation. *Ultrasound Obstet Gynecol* 2010; 36(1):37–41.
93. Lanna MM, Rustico MA, Dell'Avanzo M, *et al.* Bipolar cord coagulation for selective feticide in complicated monochorionic twin pregnancies: 118 consecutive cases at a single center. *Ultrasound Obstet Gynecol* 2012; 39(4):407–13.
94. Rossi AC, D'Addario V. Umbilical cord occlusion for selective feticide in complicated monochorionic twins: a systematic review of literature. *Am J Obstet Gynecol* 2009; 200(2):123–9.
95. van Klink JM, Koopman HM, Oepkes D, *et al.* Long-term neurodevelopmental outcome in monochorionic twins after fetal therapy. *Early Hum Dev* 2011; 87(9):601–6.
96. Anumba DO, Scott JE, Plant ND, *et al.* Diagnosis and outcome of fetal lower urinary tract obstruction in the northern region of England. *Prenat Diagn* 2005; 25(1):7–13.
97. Ylinen EM, Ala-Houhala, Wikstrom S. Prognostic factors of posterior urethral valves and the role of antenatal detection. *Pediatr Nephrol* 2004; 19(8):874–9.
98. Morris RK, Quinlan-Jones E, Kilby MD, *et al.* Systematic review of accuracy of fetal urine analysis to predict poor postnatal renal function in cases of congenital urinary tract obstruction. *Prenat Diagn* 2007; 27(10):900–11.
99. Morris RK, Malin GL, Khan KS, *et al.* Systematic review of the effectiveness of antenatal intervention for the treatment of congenital lower urinary tract obstruction. *BJOG* 2010; 117(4):382–90.
100. Irwin BH, Vane DW. Complications of intrauterine intervention for treatment of fetal obstructive uropathy. *Urology* 2000; 55(5):774.
101. Morris RK, Kilby MD. Long-term renal and neurodevelopmental outcome in infants with LUTO, with and without fetal intervention. *Early Hum Dev* 2011; 87(9):607–10.
102. Biard JM, Johnson MP, Carr MC, *et al.* Long-term outcomes in children treated by prenatal vesicoamniotic shunting for lower urinary tract obstruction. *Obstet Gynecol* 2005; 106(3):503–8.
103. Ruano R, Yoshisaki CT, Salustiano EM, *et al.* Early fetal cystoscopy for first-trimester severe megacystis. *Ultrasound Obstet Gynecol* 2011; 37(6):696–701.
104. Morris RK, Ruano R, Kilby MD. Effectiveness of fetal cystoscopy as a diagnostic and therapeutic intervention for lower urinary tract obstruction: a systematic review. *Ultrasound Obstet Gynecol* 2011; 37(6):629–37.
105. Aubard Y, Derouineau I, Aubard V, *et al.* Primary fetal hydrothorax: a literature review and proposed antenatal clinical strategy. *Fetal Diagn Ther* 1998; 13(6):325–33.
106. Deurloo KL, Devlieger R, Lopriore E, *et al.* Isolated fetal hydrothorax with hydrops: a systematic review of prenatal treatment options. *Prenat Diagn* 2007; 27(10):893–9.
107. Yinon Y, Grisaru-Granovsky S, Chaddha V, *et al.* Perinatal outcome following fetal chest shunt insertion for pleural effusion. *Ultrasound Obstet Gynecol* 2010; 36(1):58–64.
108. Bianchi S, Lista G, Castoldi F, *et al.* Congenital primary hydrothorax: effect of thoracoamniotic shunting on neonatal clinical outcome. *J Matern Fetal Neonatal Med* 2010; 23(10):1225–9.
109. Cavoretto P, Molina F, Poggi S, *et al.* Prenatal diagnosis and outcome of echogenic fetal lung lesions. *Ultrasound Obstet Gynecol* 2008; 32(6):769–83.
110. Laje P, Liechty KW. Postnatal management and outcome of prenatally diagnosed lung lesions. *Prenat Diagn* 2008; 28(7):612–8.
111. Grethel EJ, Wagner AJ, Clifton MS, *et al.* Fetal intervention for mass lesions and hydrops improves outcome: a 15-year experience. *J Pediatr Surg* 2007; 42(1):117–23.
112. Peranteau WH, Wilson RD, Liechty KW, *et al.* Effect of maternal betamethasone administration on prenatal congenital cystic adenomatoid malformation growth and fetal survival. *Fetal Diagn Ther* 2007; 22(5):365–71.
113. Morris LM, Lim FY, Livingston JC, *et al.* High-risk fetal congenital pulmonary airway malformations have a variable response to steroids. *J Pediatr Surg* 2009; 44(1):60–5.
114. Curran PF, Jelin EB, Rand L, *et al.* Prenatal steroids for microcystic congenital cystic adenomatoid malformations. *J Pediatr Surg* 2010; 45(1):145–50.
115. Crombleholme TM, Coleman B, Hedrick H, *et al.* Cystic adenomatoid malformation volume ratio predicts outcome in prenatally diagnosed cystic adenomatoid malformation of the lung. *J Pediatr Surg* 2002; 37(3):331–8.
116. Nicolini U, Cerri V, Groli C, *et al.* A new approach to prenatal treatment of extralobar pulmonary sequestration. *Prenat Diagn* 2000; 20(9):758–60.
117. Bermudez C, Pérez-Wulff J, Bufalino G, *et al.* Percutaneous ultrasound-guided sclerotherapy for complicated fetal intralobar

bronchopulmonary sequestration. *Ultrasound Obstet Gynecol* 2007; 29(5):586–9.
118. Oepkes D, Devlieger R, Lopriore E, *et al.* Successful ultrasound-guided laser treatment of fetal hydrops caused by pulmonary sequestration. *Ultrasound Obstet Gynecol* 2007; 29(4):457–9.
119. Ruano R, de A Pimenta EJ, Marques da Silva M, *et al.* Percutaneous intrauterine laser ablation of the abnormal vessel in pulmonary sequestration with hydrops at 29 weeks' gestation. *J Ultrasound Med* 2007; 26(9):1235–41.
120. Witlox RS, Lopriore E, Walther FJ, *et al.* Single-needle laser treatment with drainage of hydrothorax in fetal bronchopulmonary sequestration with hydrops. *Ultrasound Obstet Gynecol* 2009; 34(3):355–7.
121. Rammos KS, Foroulis CN, Rammos CK, *et al.* Prenatal interventional and postnatal surgical therapy of extralobar pulmonary sequestration. *Interact Cardiovasc Thorac Surg* 2010; 10(4):634–5.
122. Knox E, Lissauer D, Khan K, *et al.* Prenatal detection of pulmonary hypoplasia in fetuses with congenital diaphragmatic hernia: a systematic review and meta-analysis of diagnostic studies. *J Matern Fetal Neonatal Med* 2010; 23(7):579–88.
123. Claus F, Sandaite I, DeKoninck P, *et al.* Prenatal anatomical imaging in fetuses with congenital diaphragmatic hernia. *Fetal Diagn Ther* 2011; 29(1):88–100.
124. Jani J, Nicolaides KH, Keller RL, *et al.* Observed to expected lung area to head circumference ratio in the prediction of survival in fetuses with isolated diaphragmatic hernia. *Ultrasound Obstet Gynecol* 2007; 30(1):67–71.
125. Alfaraj MA, Shah PS, Bohn D, *et al.* Congenital diaphragmatic hernia: lung-to-head ratio and lung volume for prediction of outcome. *Am J Obstet Gynecol* 2011; 205(1):43.e1–8.
126. Jani JC, Nicolaides KH, Gratacós E, *et al.* Severe diaphragmatic hernia treated by fetal endoscopic tracheal occlusion. *Ultrasound Obstet Gynecol* 2009; 34(3):304–10.
127. Jani JC, Benachi A, Nicolaides KH, *et al.* Prenatal prediction of neonatal morbidity in survivors with congenital diaphragmatic hernia: a multicenter study. *Ultrasound Obstet Gynecol* 2009; 33(1):64–9.
128. Doné E, Gratacos E, Nicolaides KH, *et al.* Predictors of neonatal morbidity in fetuses with severe isolated congenital diaphragmatic hernia undergoing fetoscopic tracheal occlusion. *Ultrasound Obstet Gynecol* 2013; 42(1):77–83.
129. Gewillig M. The Fontan circulation. *Heart* 2005; 91(6):839–46.
130. Rychik J, Szwast A, Natarajan S, *et al.* Perinatal and early surgical outcome for the fetus with hypoplastic left heart syndrome: a 5-year single institutional experience. *Ultrasound Obstet Gynecol* 2010; 36(4):465–70.
131. Tabbutt S, Nord AS, Jarvik GP, *et al.* Neurodevelopmental outcomes after staged palliation for hypoplastic left heart syndrome. *Pediatrics* 2008; 121(3):476–83.
132. Kaltman JR, Di H, Tian Z, *et al.* Impact of congenital heart disease on cerebrovascular blood flow dynamics in the fetus. *Ultrasound Obstet Gynecol* 2005; 25(1):32–6.
133. Limperopoulos C, Tworetzky W, McElhinney DB, *et al.* Brain volume and metabolism in fetuses with congenital heart disease: evaluation with quantitative magnetic resonance imaging and spectroscopy. *Circulation* 2010; 121(1):26–33.
134. Persico N, Moratalla J, Lombardi CM, *et al.* Fetal echocardiography at 11–13 weeks by transabdominal high-frequency ultrasound. *Ultrasound Obstet Gynecol* 2011; 37(3):296–301.
135. Arzt W, Wertaschnigg D, Veit I, *et al.* Intrauterine aortic valvuloplasty in fetuses with critical aortic stenosis: experience and results of 24 procedures. *Ultrasound Obstet Gynecol* 2011; 37(6):689–95.
136. McElhinney DB, Marshall AC, Wilkins-Haug LE, *et al.* Predictors of technical success and postnatal biventricular outcome after in utero aortic valvuloplasty for aortic stenosis with evolving hypoplastic left heart syndrome. *Circulation* 2009; 120(15):1482–90.
137. Tworetzky W, Wilkins-Haug L, Jennings RW, *et al.* Balloon dilation of severe aortic stenosis in the fetus: potential for prevention of hypoplastic left heart syndrome: candidate selection, technique, and results of successful intervention. *Circulation* 2004; 110(15):2125–31.
138. Arzt W, Tulzer G. Fetal surgery for cardiac lesions. *Prenatal Diagn* 2011; 31(7):695–8.
139. Marshall AC, Levine J, Morash D, *et al.* Results of in utero atrial septoplasty in fetuses with hypoplastic left heart syndrome. *Prenatal Diagn* 2008; 28(11):1023–8.
140. Tworetzky W, McElhinney DB, Marx GR, *et al.* In utero valvuloplasty for pulmonary atresia with hypoplastic right ventricle: techniques and outcomes. *Pediatrics* 2009; 124(3):e510–8.
141. Garne E, Dolk H, Loane M, *et al.* EUROCAT website data on prenatal detection rates of congenital anomalies. *J Med Screen* 2010; 17(2):97–8.
142. Caldarelli M, Di Rocco C, La Marca F. Shunt complications in the first postoperative year in children with meningomyelocele. *Childs Nerv Syst* 1996; 12(12):748–54.
143. Mitchell LE, Adzick NS, Melchionne J, *et al.* Spina bifida. *Lancet* 2004; 364(9448):1885–95.
144. Bruner JP, Tulipan N. Tell the truth about spina bifida. *Ultrasound Obstet Gynecol* 2004; 24(6):595–6.
145. Robinson S, Gregory GA. Fentanyl-air-oxygen anesthesia for ligation of patent ductus arteriosus in preterm infants. *Anesth Analg* 1981; 60(5):331–4.
146. Anand KJ, Hickey PR. Pain and its effects in the human neonate and fetus. *N Engl J Med* 1987; 317(21):1321–9.
147. Anand KJ, Sippell WG, Aynsley-Green A. Randomised trial of fentanyl anaesthesia in preterm babies undergoing surgery: effects on the stress response. *Lancet* 1987; 1(8524):62–6.
148. Anand KJ, Barton BA, McIntosh N, *et al.* Analgesia and sedation in preterm neonates who require ventilatory support: results from the NOPAIN trial. Neonatal Outcome and Prolonged Analgesia in Neonates. *Arch Pediatr Adolesc Med* 1999; 153(4):331–8.
149. Fisk NM, Gitau R, Teixeira JM, *et al.* Effect of direct fetal opioid analgesia on fetal hormonal and hemodynamic stress response to intrauterine needling. *Anesthesiology* 2001; 95(4):828–35.
150. Giannakoulopoulos X, Sepulveda W, Kourtis P, *et al.* Fetal plasma cortisol and beta-endorphin response to intrauterine needling. *Lancet* 1994; 344(8915):77–81.
151. Myers L, Bulich LA. *Anesthesia for Fetal Intervention and Surgery.* Hamilton: BC Decker; 2005.
152. Van de Velde M, Jani J, De Buck F, *et al.* Fetal pain perception and pain management. *Semin Fetal Neonatal Med* 2006; 11(4):232–6.
153. van Mieghem T, Baud D, Devlieger R, *et al.* Minimally invasive fetal therapy. *Best Pract Res Clin Obstet Gynaecol* 2012; 26(5):711–25.

CHAPTER 8

Neonatal assessment and therapy

Ewen D. Johnston and Julie-Clare Becher

Introduction

The transition from fetal to neonatal life involves significant changes in physiology. *In utero*, life is characterized by a relatively hypoxic environment, with the lungs playing no part in gas exchange and the placenta functioning as the organ of fetal respiration. The physical effects of labour help prepare the fetus for life outside the womb, and an understanding of the processes involved in normal adaptation is essential in assessing and supporting the newborn who may not make this transition unaided.

Worldwide, neonatal mortality rates vary tenfold between developed and developing countries. The World Health Organization estimates a rate of 3/1000 live-births (high-income countries), and 32/1000 live-births (low-income countries) for this statistic.[1] Of those deaths, approximately 30% are thought to be related to birth asphyxia. It is important to appreciate that mortality alone underestimates the impact of problems at delivery on families, with around two-thirds of survivors of untreated moderate/severe hypoxic-ischaemic encephalopathy developing significant neurodisability at 18 months.[2,3]

Our training as physicians focuses on adult physiology and pathology and these concepts and considerations do not generally include the principles of newborn resuscitation and stabilization. As a consequence, even the most skilled adult (or paediatric) practitioners will naturally feel some anxiety when presented with an infant who is apnoeic and bradycardic at delivery. This need not be the case. The underlying tenets of newborn resuscitation—enabling lung aeration and optimizing temperature control—have been recognized for centuries and can be delivered with the most basic of equipment.[4] There are situations where the need for resuscitation at birth can be predicted. However, this is not always the case,[5,6] or it may not be possible to safely transfer the mother to a large unit with neonatal intensive care support before delivery. It is therefore vital that all practitioners who may be called upon to attend a delivery have the skills to provide basic newborn life support.

Delivery suite management of the newborn, once the realm of folklore and fad,[7] is now a rapidly advancing field with the International Liaison Committee on Resuscitation (ILCOR) regularly reviewing the evidence base and providing guidance on both practice and directions for future research.[8]

In this chapter, the fundamental differences between newborn infants at birth and those who have already adapted to life outside the womb will be discussed. The physiology of asphyxia will be described, and how this knowledge leads us to the development of a structured approach towards assessment and intervention when required. Delivery at preterm gestation will be covered separately, along with a number of other specific conditions requiring special consideration.

Normal physiology and transition

The fetus develops within a tightly regulated environment. Surrounded by amniotic fluid, nourished with a constant supply of glucose and oxygen through the umbilical vein, the lungs are filled with fetal lung fluid. The pulmonary vascular resistance is high, and systemic resistance low, enabling a pattern of circulation unique to this period of life where the lungs receive only 25% of the total cardiac output (at term).[9]

De-oxygenated blood returns from the fetus to the placenta through the umbilical arteries which arise from the external iliacs. (See Figure 4.1 in chapter on Fetal and Neonatal Physiology for diagram of fetal circulation) Fetal red blood cells extract oxygen from the maternal circulation at the chorionic villi, enabled by the high oxygen affinity of fetal haemoglobin. This oxygenated blood enters the umbilical vein with a saturation of approximately 85%, and travels to the ductus venosus and then the right atrium where it travels to the left side of the heart via the foramen ovale. After reaching the left side of the heart, blood follows the same course as in adult life until it returns to the umbilical arteries—the striking difference is that the healthy fetus has a PaO_2 of only 4 kPa (30 mmHg; ~60–65% saturation in the descending aorta).

Deoxygenated blood from the superior vena cava is directed from right atrium to right ventricle undergoing some mixing with the well-oxygenated flow. In the pulmonary trunk, the high pulmonary vascular resistance ensures that this blood is predominantly directed through the ductus arteriosus to join the main systemic flow.

During labour, the fetus is exposed to physical and hormonal factors which prepare them for the transition to neonatal life. Uterine contractions result in transient hypoxia as placental gas exchange is interrupted. Studies examining fetal SpO_2 during labour have demonstrated levels of 30–40% during late second stage in a group of deliveries where no additional support was required at birth.[10] These normal stresses stimulate a catecholamine response in the fetus which, coupled with the release of thyrotropin-releasing hormone in the mother, serves to stop the production of fetal lung fluid and promote its resorption prior to delivery.[11,12]

At delivery, the fetus must undergo a profound physiological change to successfully adapt to life outside the womb. Central to this are the first breaths which inflate the lungs, allowing the arteriolar bed to dilate, and deliver oxygen to the pulmonary vasculature promoting further vasodilation. The resultant drop in pulmonary vascular resistance allows blood from the right

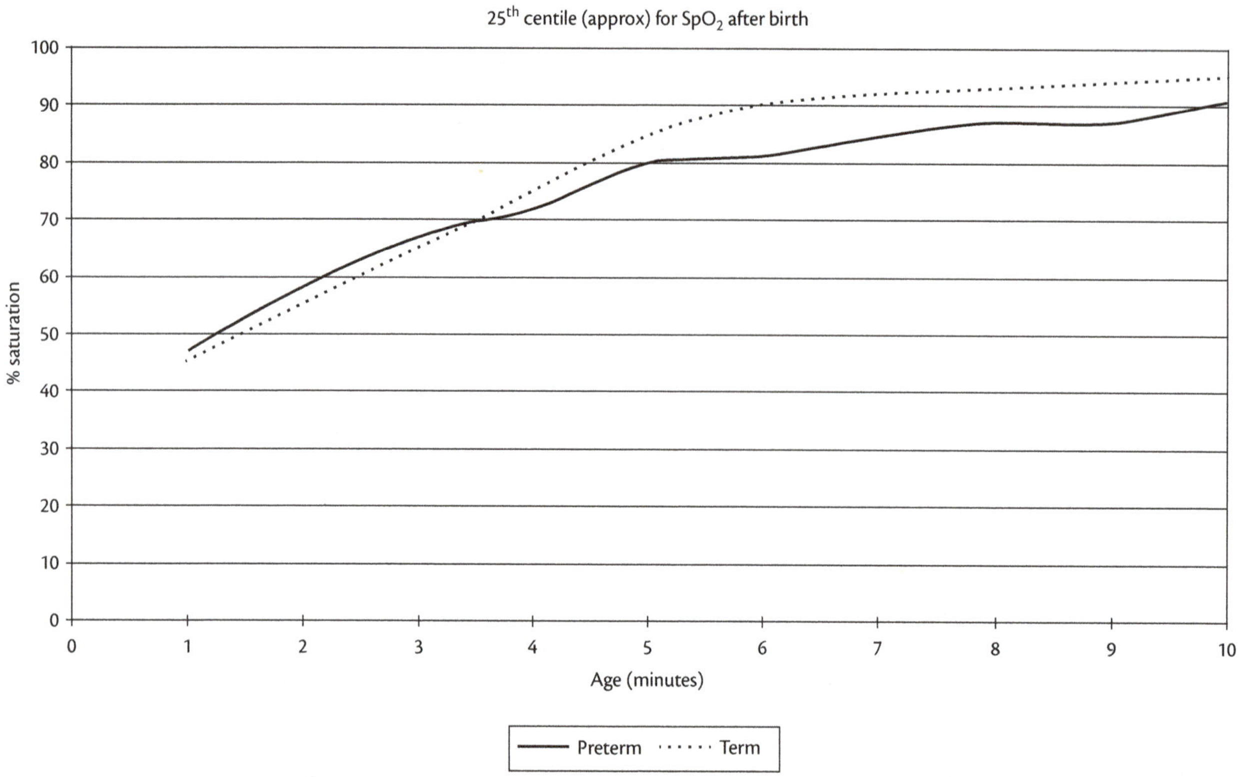

Figure 8.1 Newborn oxygen centiles.

Adapted with permission from Dawson JA, Kamlin COF, Vento M, *et al.* Defining the reference range for oxygen saturation for infants after birth. *Pediatrics* 2010;125(6):e1340–1347, Copyright © 2010 by the AAP.

ventricle to flow to the pulmonary arteries. The increased volume returning to the left atrium closes the foramen ovale, and with the low-pressure placental circuit no longer available, increased pressure in the left ventricular outflow tract now shunts oxygenated blood from left to right through the ductus arteriosus promoting constriction and closure over the coming hours to days.

From the description above it is clear that lung aeration is the key to this transition. The first breath will occur within 60 seconds in most term newborns,[13] stimulated by cold, cessation of placental circulation, and physical stimuli. Newborns must first establish and then maintain a functional residual capacity (FRC). Initial breaths are deep and long, thereafter the infant can be observed to prolong the expiratory phase after a short, deep inspiration. This 'expiratory braking', is achieved by crying and promotes an FRC when the lungs are still partially filled with fluid.[14,15]

If the heart rate has slowed, it will rapidly increase and most well infants will have a pulse of over 100 by 2 minutes.[16] Oxygen saturation will climb steadily but more slowly. It is now recognized that 'low' pre-ductal SpO_2 during this time is normal and should be tolerated without interference in an otherwise well infant. More than 25% of well term infants will take longer than 5 minutes to achieve saturations in the 90s[17] (Figure 8.1).

Almost all newborns will make this transition without any additional help—the exact numbers are unclear, but a large Swedish study from the late 1980s found that only 1.7% of infants required resuscitation.[5]

In the next section, the physiology and effects of intrauterine hypoxia will be discussed and the central role of these processes in the approach to resuscitation.

The physiology of hypoxia

The work of Dawes and Cross,[18,19] published in the 1950s and 1960s, provides the clearest description of the effects of intrauterine asphyxia.

The fetus is well adapted to tolerate the hypoxic process of delivery, and can survive periods of total asphyxia which would result in the death of an adult. This resilience is likely due to the high concentration of glycogen stored in the fetal myocardium. This reserve serves as fuel for metabolism upon which the healthy newborn relies during the first day whilst feeding is established. This glycogen can be mobilized when oxygen is not available, to sustain the fetus.[20] The process is inefficient producing only two ATP molecules for each glucose molecule entering the cycle (in comparison with aerobic respiration which produces 36 ATP per glucose) but is sufficient to maintain cardiac output and cerebral metabolism. The fetus and newborn demonstrate an enhanced ability to utilize alternate substrates for energy, particularly lactate, which may also be protective.[21]

A mammalian fetus starts breathing around 30 seconds after the placental circulation ceases (Figure 8.2). If these efforts fail to establish lung aeration and oxygenation, tachycardia and tachypnoea ensue. Blood pressure is maintained, and may rise slightly. Oxygen stores are rapidly depleted (around 2 minutes) and the fetus becomes unconscious. Breathing efforts cease after a few minutes, and the heart rate falls to about 60–80 beats per minute (bpm). This period is known as *primary apnoea*. The drop in heart rate is a chemoreflex,[9] resulting in vagal stimulation, and thereafter adrenergic vasoconstriction which redistributes the circulation

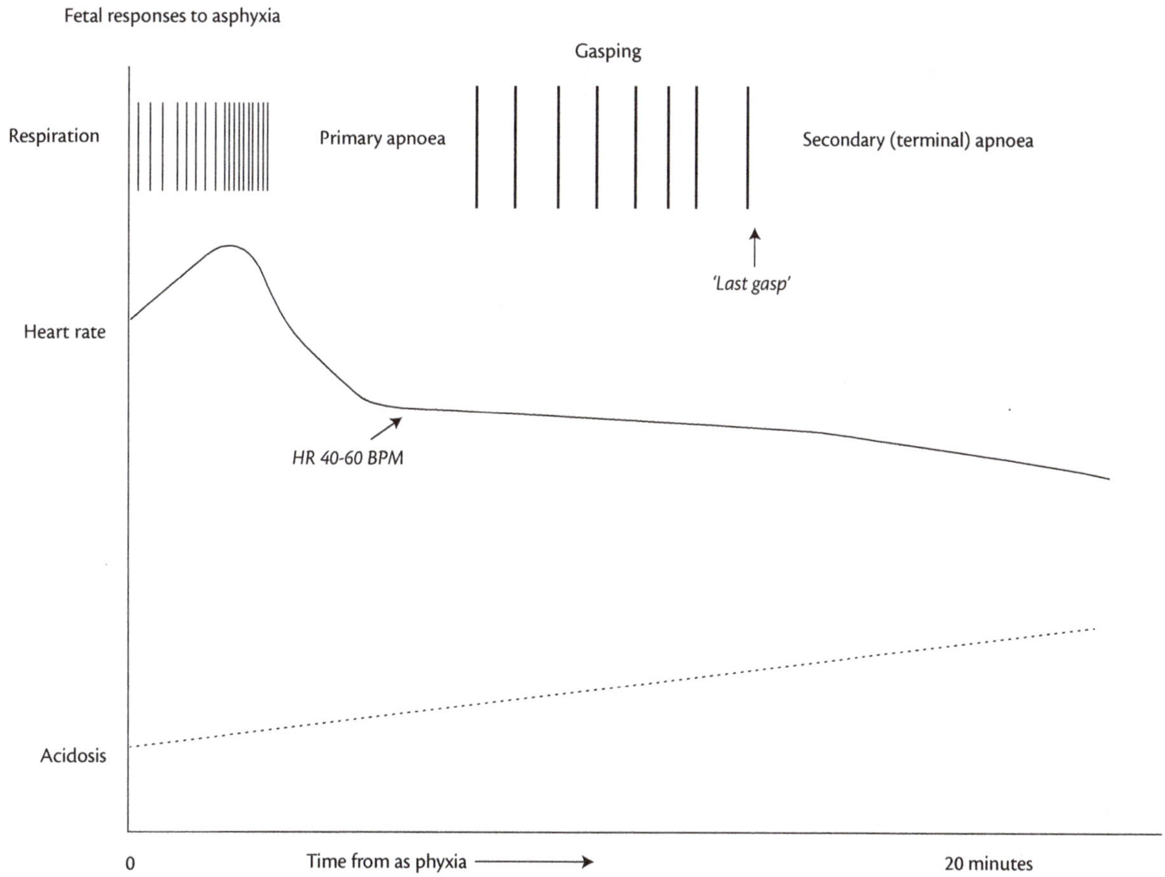

Figure 8.2 Fetal response to asphyxia.
Data from Geoffrey S. Dawes, Foetal and neonatal physiology; a comparative study of the changes at birth [by] Geoffrey S. Dawes, Chicago, US, Year Book Medical Publishers © 1968.

centrally. If oxygenation is not restored, there is a steady rise in $PaCO_2$, and lactic acid. Cyanosis is replaced by pallor as the vasoconstriction evolves, circulation to the essential organs is maintained, but in the context of increasing acidosis. *Gasping* will now ensue. Gasps are a primitive spinal reflex which are characteristic of the newborn following hypoxia. They occur when the higher cortical suppression fails, and are slow, large volume 'whole-body' breaths—it is difficult to mistake these for normal respiration.

If the asphyxia continues, gasps will become shallower, and weaker. Lactate and CO_2 accrue further and increase acidosis. Glycogen stores are exhausted and the circulation begins to fail, with a further drop in heart rate and cardiac output. Around 20 minutes after the initial insult, gasping will cease, this is *terminal apnoea*. The heart beats for around 10 minutes after this but slows steadily and is unable to sustain perfusion. Twenty to thirty minutes after complete total asphyxia, the heart stops, the fetus has a profound mixed acidosis and unless delivery with resuscitation is immediate, death is inevitable. Even if this is the case, resuscitation may not be successful, and significant brain damage may have already occurred.

There are limitations in the application of this animal model to human practice—the timing of each phase is not known with certainty, asphyxia is assumed to be constant and humans have a greater store of glycogen than rhesus monkeys. The model simulates acute, total asphyxia, which is rare, and prior to the event the experimental subjects were healthy, with no previous exposure to either partial asphyxia, or labour.

At delivery, an infant who is not breathing could be in primary or terminal apnoea, or 'between' gasps. It will be difficult to distinguish between them initially, mandating that our approach to resuscitation should be the same for all:

- The infant in *primary apnoea* will have a slow heart rate, some tone, and with gentle stimulation (e.g. drying with a warm towel), is likely to start breathing/crying and their heart rate will rapidly increase. Alternatively they will take one or two gasps which (provided the airway is clear) will inflate the lungs, followed by a rapid increase in heart rate and regular respiration.
- The infant delivered during the *gasping phase of asphyxia* will present similarly, but will be more hypotonic and pale. Gasping will be apparent, and if the airway is clear these may be sufficient to enable lung aeration and delivery of oxygen to the myocardium producing an increase in heart rate. Gasps following more prolonged asphyxia may be too weak to inflate the lungs, and a brief period of artificial ventilation may be required. However, when aeration is achieved, the heart rate will again increase rapidly (Figure 8.3). The gasps will gradually be replaced by regular respirations, over a timescale proportional to the duration of the preceding insult (the longer the asphyxia, the longer the gasping persists for after resuscitation).

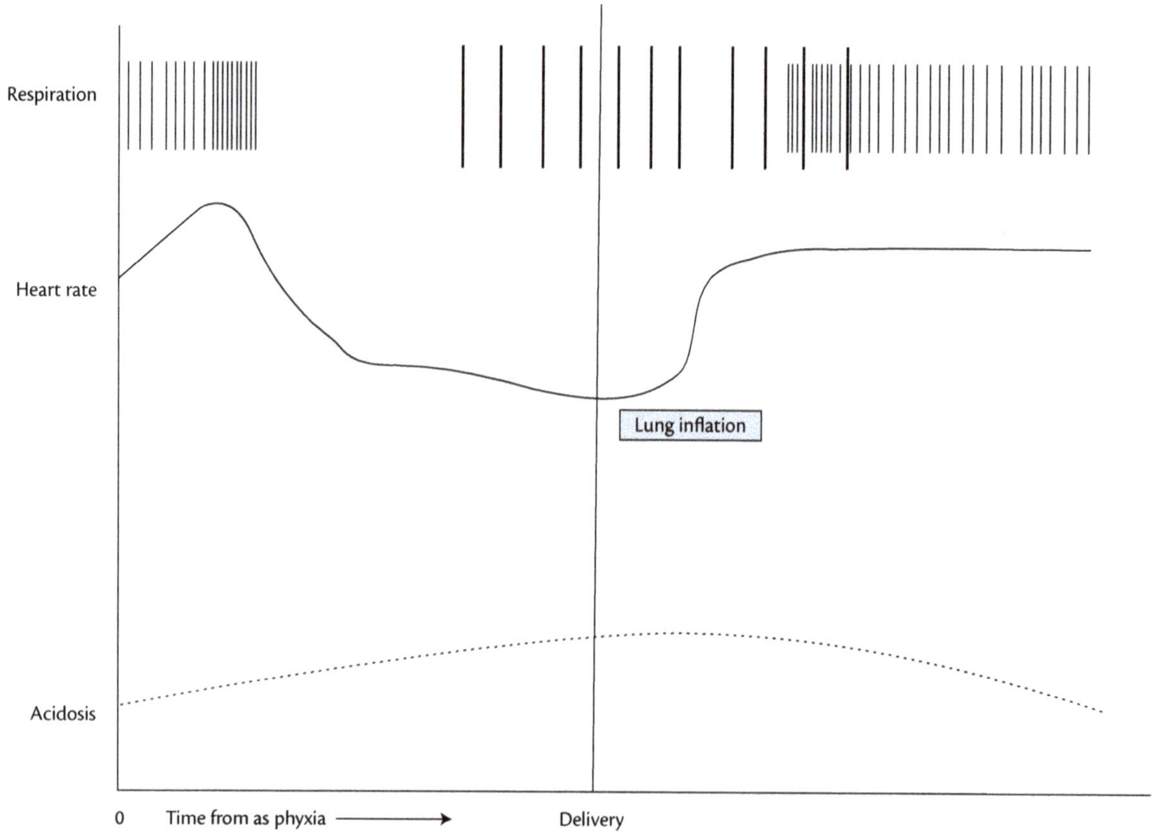

Figure 8.3 The response of an asphyxiated newborn to lung inflation.
Data from Cross KW, Resuscitation of the asphyxiated infant, *British Medical Bulletin*, Volume 22, Issue 1, pp. 73–8, Copyright © 1966 Oxford University Press.

- The infant delivered in *terminal apnoea* is pale, floppy, and bradycardic (heart rate <60 bpm). If resuscitation is not commenced, death will follow. Artificial ventilation is required to inflate the lungs, and if gasping has only just ceased, this may lead to an increase in the heart rate. Until the infant's own respiratory effort is adequate, artificial ventilation should be provided.

If the insult has continued for longer, the degree of acidosis and circulatory compromise is likely to be so great that lung aeration alone will not result in an increased heart rate—in these circumstances a brief period of cardiac compressions may be required.

Rarely it may be necessary to administer drugs (epinephrine, glucose, sodium bicarbonate) before a response in heart rate is observed. These infants will require cardiac compressions for longer before return of spontaneous circulation. These infants have experienced the greatest degree of hypoxia and acidosis, and have the highest mortality, as well as being at greatest risk of long-term neurological damage.

Equipment

Although one could provide adequate resuscitation in most cases with no more than a firm surface and a towel, in hospital, most newborn resuscitation will be undertaken on a resuscitaire (Figure 8.4), with additional equipment available. This will be situated either in the delivery suite, obstetric theatre, or a dedicated location nearby. As far as possible, equipment and layout should be standardized within each area (Table 8.1). An example of standard neonatal resuscitation equipment is shown in Figure 8.5.

Increasingly, additional monitoring (SpO_2, heart rate, temperature, exhaled CO_2) is available to support decision-making and help maintain stability, although one must recognize the potential dangers of using arbitrary, unresearched targets to guide practice.

In this section, we will discuss some considerations regarding equipment for newborn resuscitation in broad terms. However, it is best practice for clinicians to familiarize themselves with what is available within their own unit.

Resuscitaire

When stripped back to basics, the resuscitaire is simply a firm surface with a source of heat, light, and gas (Figure 8.4). Most are designed to be mobile, and are height adjustable, although they can also be fixed to the wall. Mobile models have the advantage of being able to be used for transfer between the labour suite and the neonatal unit; however, as the overhead heater will lose power when unplugged, care must be taken to ensure that the infant does not become cold. Necessary equipment on a resuscitaire is seen in Figure 8.5.

Gas supply and blender

Resuscitaires should be connected to the wall gas supply whenever possible, with cylinders kept in reserve for emergencies or transport.

Resuscitation of babies at birth should begin in air,[8,13] and if oxygen is used it should be titrated with the response monitored

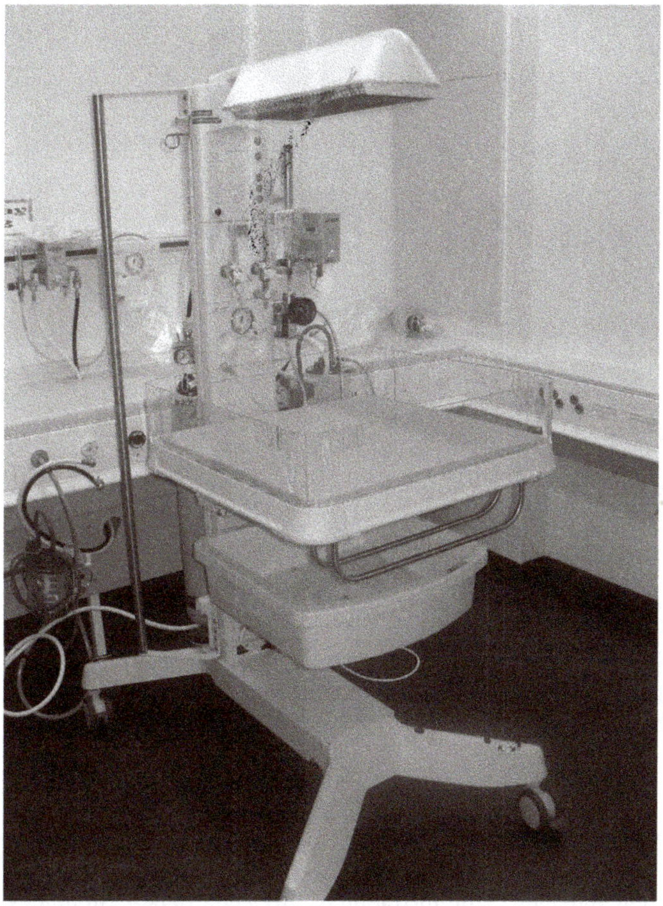

Figure 8.4 An example of a newborn resuscitaire.
Reproduced with kind permission from Laerdal Medical™.

by pulse oximetry. There is no evidence to support the targeting of oxygen saturations to any particular level or centile in any group of infants after delivery. The potential toxicity of oxygen is well recognized[22–25] and any adverse effects are likely to be greater in the two groups of newborns most likely to be given additional oxygen; those born prematurely, and those who have been asphyxiated. One should aim to avoid both hyperoxia and prolonged hypoxia.

Commonly resuscitaires in routine use do not incorporate an air/oxygen blender as standard. If a blender is not available, resuscitation with air can be provided either with a self-inflating bag, or through a T-piece connected to an appropriate air supply.

Table 8.1 Considerations and key features for a newborn resuscitation area

Considerations for a newborn resuscitation area	Key features of neonatal resuscitaire
Warm, no draughts	Built in over-head heater, light and timer/stopwatch
Good lighting	Firm, flat work surface
Means of summoning help	Access to the baby from three sides (head/left/right)
Adequate space around resuscitaire for three people	Pressure limited gas supply to T-piece ventilation circuit
Ease of access (transport incubator, emergency trolley etc.)	Air/oxygen blender (not standard, but strongly recommended)
Gas supply (air and oxygen)	Own gas supply (2 × E cylinders—1 × air/1 × O_2, or 2 × O_2)
Resuscitation algorithms easily visible (drug doses etc.)	Suction (usually gas driven—will drain cylinders quickly)

T-piece and positive end-expiratory pressure

A pressure-limited T-piece circuit with an adjustable positive end-expiratory pressure (PEEP) valve should be used to provide lung aeration and ventilation.

This system has a number of advantages over a self-inflating bag, principally:

- Can provide PEEP (or continuous positive airway pressure (CPAP))
- Operator sets peak pressure
- Easy to adjust pressure based on infant's response
- Easy to deliver timed aeration breath to set pressure.

Disadvantages:

- Gas supply needed
- Flow dependant (alterations of flow will alter previously set positive inspiratory pressure (PIP)/PEEP).

Connecting a T-piece circuit directly to a gas supply will generate dangerous pressures and must not be done. Similarly, high flow rates can overcome the safety blow-off in the resuscitaire and should be avoided. Flow rates of 8–10 L/min are acceptable.[26]

CPAP can be delivered either by mask or single- or bi-nasal prongs and is an effective way of stabilizing even the most preterm infants.[27–30]

The use of CPAP in the term infant requiring resuscitation has not been studied in humans, but there is compelling animal work suggesting a more rapid attainment of FRC after delivery with PEEP (Box 8.1).[31]

Self-inflating bags

Every resuscitation area should have a 500 mL self-inflating bag. These will allow resuscitation to continue should the gas supply fail. The bags have a pop-off valve which must be tested before every use by occluding the outflow and giving the bag a sharp squeeze. Most bags have a reservoir, but unless connected to a blended air/oxygen supply they are limited in the concentration of oxygen which can be delivered.[32] It is not possible to provide the sustained breaths required with smaller-volume bags.[33,34] There is a degree of skill required to administer a sustained aeration breath using a bag and mask, more so than using a T-piece and staff should ensure that they are familiar with both devices.

The use of larger bags in the newborn carries the risk of over-inflation (or delivery of excessive pressure); a 3 kg neonate would usually be ventilated with a tidal volume of 12–18 mL in intensive care. Vigorous squeezing of the bag can easily overcome the pop-off valve and peak pressures of greater than 60 cmH_2O can be generated relatively easily.[32,35]

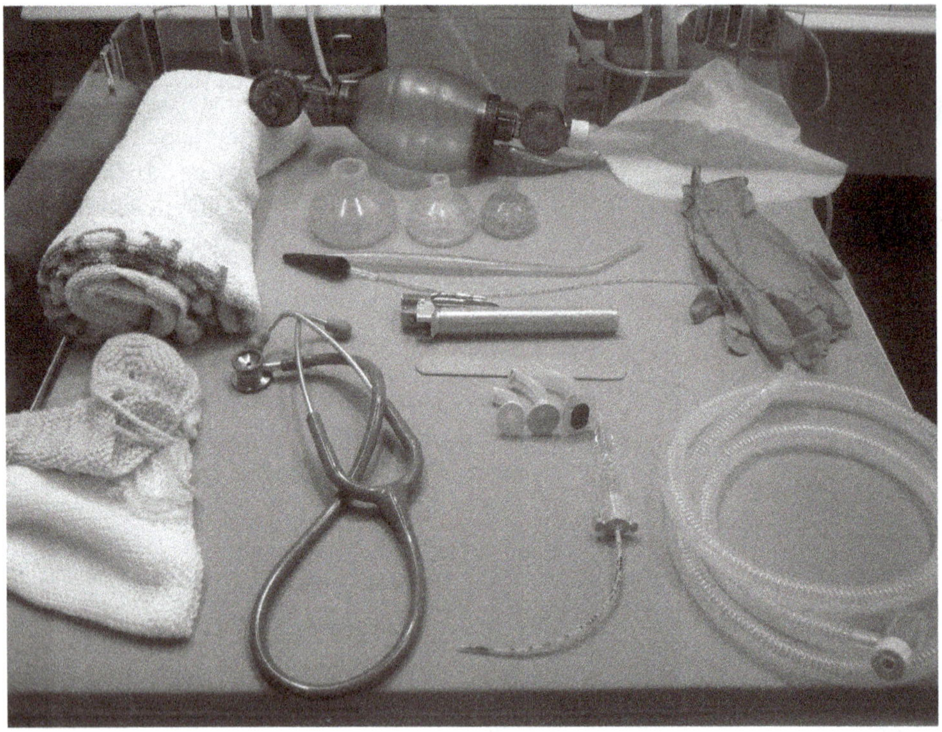

Figure 8.5 Standard neonatal resuscitation equipment.

Flow-inflating bags

These are popular in the United States,[36] and to a lesser degree in Australia and New Zealand. In experienced hands, and with a manometer attached, these are effective devices for resuscitation[35]—however, their use is not taught on the Newborn Life Support course[13] and within the United Kingdom it is unlikely that they will be available on the labour suite for neonatal use.

Masks

Most newborns do not require intubation at birth for resuscitation. The difficulties in maintaining an adequate seal with the masks available in the early days of the speciality[37] led to a perception that intubation was the preferred method of airway management for all but the most vigorous of infants.[38,39] Most facemasks for neonatal use are circular (Figure 8.6). Anatomical versions do exist, and are popular with some resuscitators. There is no evidence to support one type of modern mask over the other.[40,41] What is clear is that one must be familiar with one's own equipment. Good technique is required to minimize leak and practitioners need to use an appropriate hold, which has been shown to differ between designs (Figure 8.7 and Figure 8.8).[42]

Box 8.1 Beneficial effects of PEEP in the newborn

- Assists lung expansion
- Helps establish functional residual capacity
- Prevents collapse in end expiration
- Improves oxygenation.

Laryngoscope and blades

Intubation provides a secure airway during prolonged resuscitation and allows administration of surfactant in preterm infants. Direct visualization of the vocal cords enables suctioning of

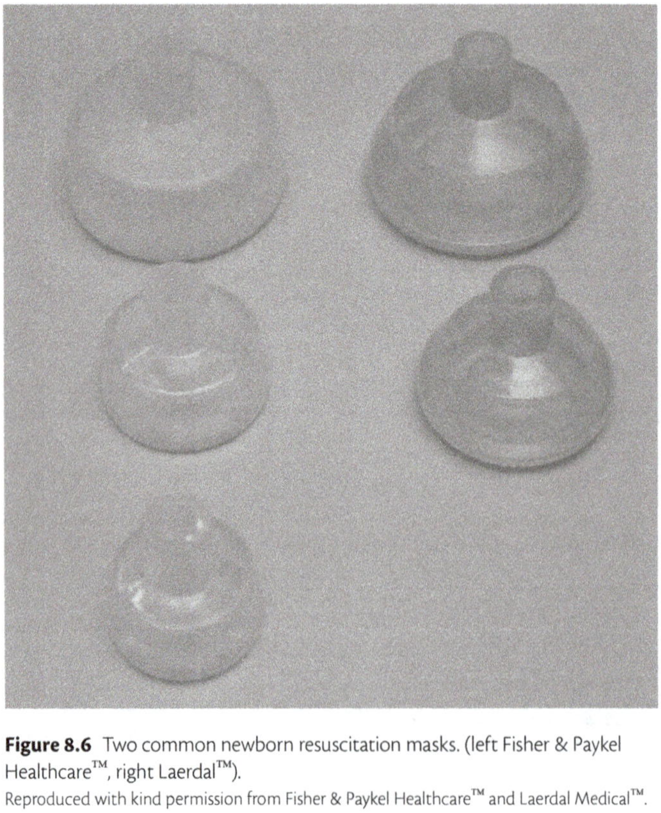

Figure 8.6 Two common newborn resuscitation masks. (left Fisher & Paykel Healthcare™, right Laerdal™).

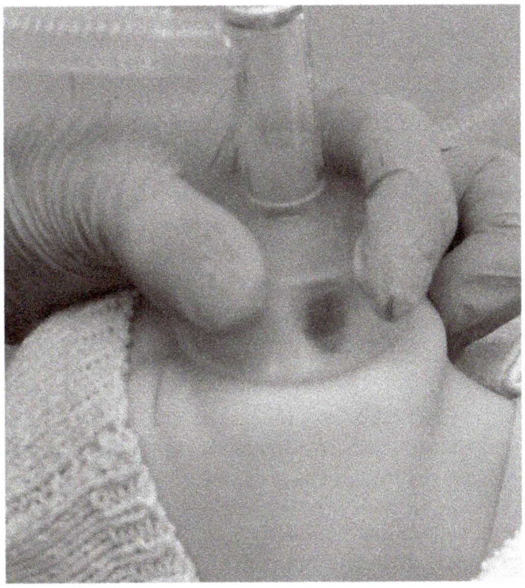

Figure 8.7 The encircling "Rim Hold" provides an optimum seal with a Fisher & Paykel Healthcare™ mask.
Reproduced with kind permission from Fisher & Paykel Healthcare™.

particulate matter (e.g. meconium), which can impede lung aeration.

Miller blades are preferred; sizes 1, 0, and 00 are used for term, preterm, and extreme preterm infants. In the smallest preterm infants (~500g), even the 00 blade may take up a large amount of space in the mouth making visualization difficult.

Endotracheal tubes

A selection of uncuffed, non-shouldered endotracheal tubes (ETTs) should be available. Routine stylet use may be associated with complications such as tracheal and pharyngeal perforation. Cold ETTs may provide sufficient rigidity should intubation prove difficult. Methods of securing tubes vary, although direct application of tape to a newborn's skin should be avoided.

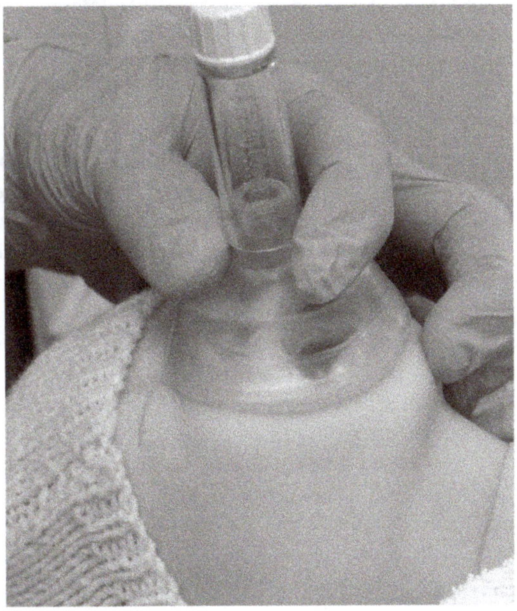

Figure 8.8 The "2-point top-hold" is recommended when a Laerdal™ mask is used.
Reproduced with kind permission from Laerdal Medical™.

Table 8.2 Suction catheters and uses for neonatal resuscitation

Device	Usage
Paediatric Yankauer	Clearing particulate matter obstructing airway
Soft French size 8–10	Removing oropharyngeal secretions/suction below cords under direct vision
Soft French size 2–3	Suctioning ETT
Meconium aspirator	Clearing particulate matter from below cords through ETT

Suction devices

A means of clearing the airway of secretions or other material is required. Most resuscitaires will incorporate their own system which is flow driven and relies on anadequate gas supply (wall or cylinder). Pressures should not exceed 200 mmHg (264 cmH_2O) but 100 mmHg should be sufficient for routine use.[43] A selection of devices should be available to enable the resuscitator to deal with different circumstances (Table 8.2).

Airway adjuncts (Guedel/laryngeal mask airway)

Oropharyngeal airways (Guedel) can be useful if the airway is difficult to maintain with other measures, and may be beneficial if there is a congenital airway abnormality (e.g. Pierre Robin sequence). A correctly sized airway will reach the angle of the jaw when the flange is positioned in the middle of the chin (Figure 8.9). Sizes 4, 5, and 6 cm are available for neonatal use, as neonates may range in size from 450 g to over 4500 g and an appropriately sized airway may not always be available. A wrongly sized or inserted Guedel will cause airway obstruction.

Insertion is best practised on a mannequin—the technique is *not* the same as in adult practice—with the airway being inserted following the curvature of the airway (rather than 'upside down' then turning, as in adults) to avoid damage to the delicate soft palate (Figure 8.10).

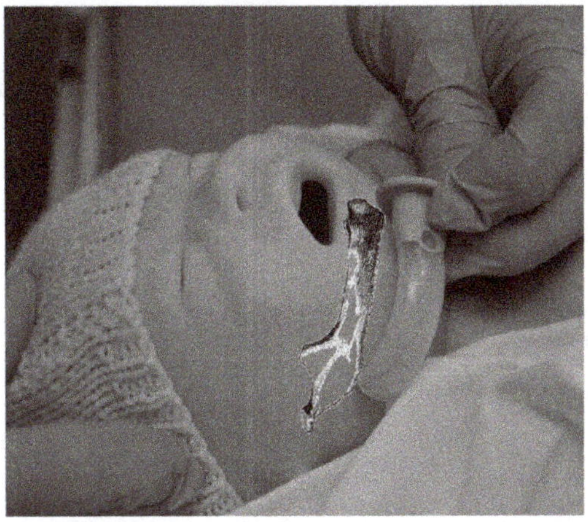

Figure 8.9 Sizing a Guedel oropharyngeal airway in relation to mandible (angle of jaw, to centre of chin).

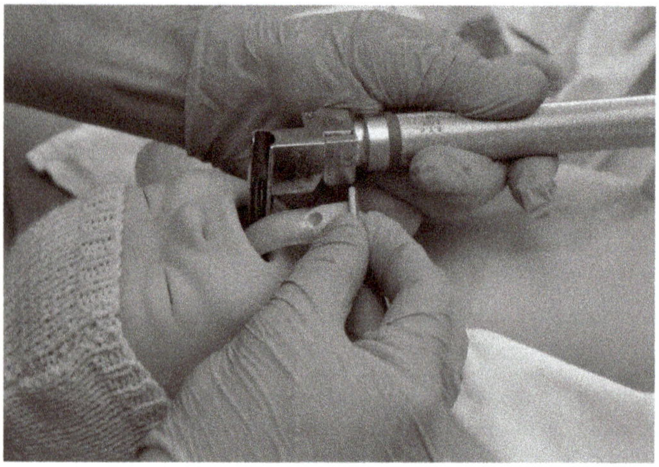

Figure 8.10 Inserting a Guedel airway in a neonate.

Laryngeal mask airways (LMAs) have been available for neonatal resuscitation since the 1990s.[44,45] Size 1 LMAs are appropriate for infants heavier than 1500 g. There is no evidence to support or reject their use over either mask ventilation or endotracheal intubation. Effective lung aeration can be provided with an LMA, however their role as a primary mode of ventilation has not been established, and is not recommended. Nevertheless the LMA may have a role in the management of an abnormal airway or when ventilation has not been possible by other means.[46]

Exhaled CO_2 detector

Disposable 'colorimetric' CO_2 detectors are now established as a means of confirming ETT position,[47–49] and are recommended by ILCOR.[8] These insert into the circuit between the ETT (or mask) and ventilation device, and cycle from purple (no CO_2 detected) to yellow (CO_2 present). There are limitations with false positive and false negatives possible (Table 8.3).[50] The detectors also prove useful in monitoring airway patency and ventilation in the non-intubated neonates receiving mask ventilation or CPAP in the delivery suite.[51,52]

Temperature monitoring

The importance of thermal control is discussed in 'Thermal Environment and Care'.

Oxygen saturation monitor

Oxygen saturation monitoring has become an established tool in the delivery suite (Box 8.2).[53] If supplemental oxygen is used,

Table 8.3 False-positive and false-negative results using a colorimetric CO_2 detector

False negative[a]	False positive
Inadequate cardiac output	Intratracheal epinephrine
Inadequate CPR	Droplet contamination by other drugs
Failure to inflate lungs	
Obstructed ETT	

[a]Detector does not change colour despite correctly sited ETT.

Box 8.2 Pulse oximeter characteristics for use in neonatal resuscitation

- Ability to obtain reading in low perfusion state/motion resistance
- Averaging time set as short as possible (≤2 seconds)
- Alarms silenced
- Pulse tone modulation
- Battery backup (can use on transfer).

one should be guided by a preductal (right wrist) SpO_2 recording rather than the subjective assessment of colour. Postductal measurements from the feet will be lower for 10–15 minutes after delivery.[54] Obtaining a recording rapidly and reliably in the delivery suite is more challenging than in other hospital environments, but speed/accuracy are improved by practice and adhering to the following sequence of events (Figure 8.11):[55]

1. Turn monitor on, silence alarms, set pulse/tone modulation to desired level.
2. Dry wrist, wrap sensor around and secure (cover from light).
3. Connect sensor to monitoring cable.

Monitoring must never take priority over the basic principles of providing warmth and inflating the lungs, but the constant feedback of heart rate and saturation provides a practical and useful adjunct to clinical assessment alone during resuscitation—although there are no trials comparing outcome after resuscitation with or without monitoring. The UK Resuscitation Council suggests administering oxygen when the saturation of an infant is below the 25th centile,[13] whereas the American Heart Association has opted for values closer to the 50th centile.[56] These centiles are derived from observations in well infants who are spontaneously breathing, and who have not required any resuscitation. There remains little data on the preterm or asphyxiated infant and none on the effect of targeting saturations to any particular centile.[17]

Future directions

The use of a respiratory function monitor (displaying flow, volume, and pressure) has been described,[57] and there are units which have established multiparameter recording of resuscitation data including video of the resuscitation,[58] which serves a training and quality improvement function, as well as enabling research.

Direct and indirect video laryngoscopy blades have been developed in neonatal sizes (0, 1) and are being used successfully in the delivery suite for training and difficult airway management.

Any advance in technology or equipment must be accompanied by research to prove its value if well-intentioned harm is to be avoided, and research in the delivery suite is subject to particular challenges.[59,60]

Team organization

The majority of newborns need no resuscitation, or lung aeration only, which can be delivered by one person. Where resuscitation is

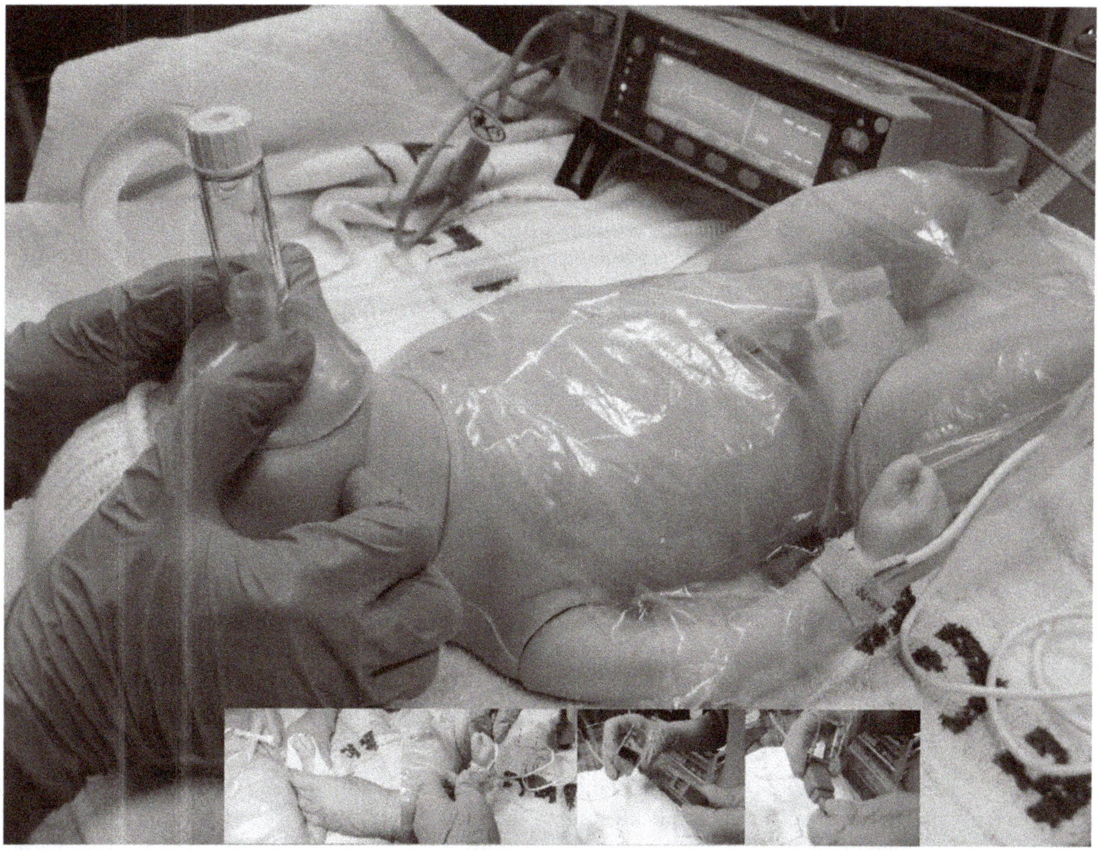

Figure 8.11 Application of a saturation monitor at delivery.

prolonged, or complex support is required (e.g. preterm, asphyxiated), additional help will be needed, and the team should be assembled in advance wherever possible.

Figure 8.12 and Figure 8.13 present one approach to team organization for newborn resuscitation, resources, and personnel. Space and experience will vary and individual units should develop their own protocols.

Anaesthetists may be called upon to support newborn resuscitation in the following scenarios:

1. No other resuscitator available
2. Need for additional help
3. Difficult airway management.

Thermal environment and care

The thermal environment of a newborn infant is key to optimal transition and stabilization. Thermal care is the first priority in the

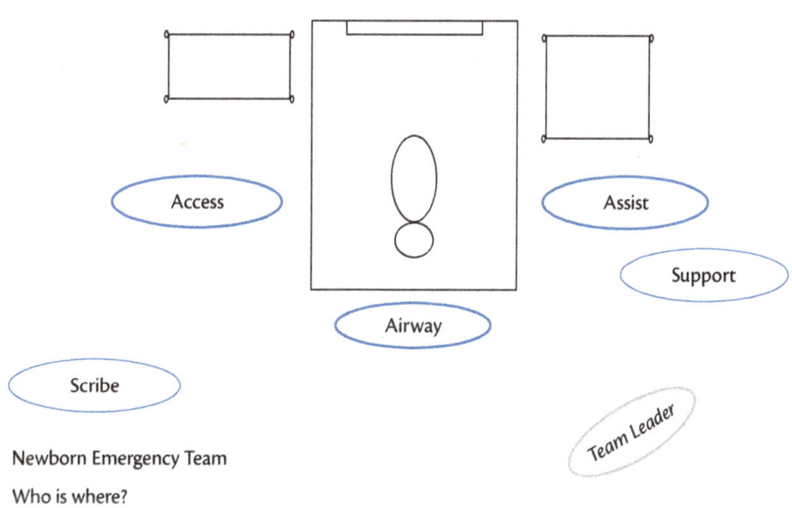

Figure 8.12 Positions of team during resuscitation.

Newborn Emergency Team

Roles and responsibilities

AIRWAY Registrar or Senior ANNP	ASSIST Nursing team leader	ACCESS SHO equivalent
1. Lead resuscitation unless dedicated "Team Leader" present 2. Start clock 3. Manage airway 4. Administer surfactant 5. Site UVC (if no other competent)	1. Provide assistance to "Airway" 2. Thermal stability (plastic bag, hat, temperature probe) 3. Apply saturation probe 4. Check and draw-up drugs/fluids 5. Chest compressions (if "Access" sitting UVC)	1. Replace metal cord clamp with plastic 2. Auscultate and tap-out HR (until monitoring in place) 3. Chest compressions (if not siting UVC) 4. Site UVC 5. Check and administer drugs/fluids

SUPPORT SHO/Midwife/NNU Nurse	Summon help if requested Fetch equipment/drugs/fluids Check drugs/fluids (if required) Chest compressions (if required)
SCRIBE SHO/Midwife/NNU Nurse	Document all events and timing
TEAM LEADER Neonatal consultant/Grid trainee/"Airway"	1. Takes leadership of resuscitation 2. Guides and supports other team members 3. Allocates tasks 4. Communicates with team 5. Communicates with parents

Figure 8.13 Roles of team during resuscitation.

approach to newborn resuscitation (Figure 8.14). Newborn infants are wet, small, and have a large surface area. They may quickly lose heat through evaporation, conduction, convection, and radiation.

Hypothermia results in exhaustion of glucose reserves leading to hypoglycaemia particularly in the preterm or growth-restricted infant who has low stores of glycogen and impaired mechanisms for glucose homeostasis. Hypothermic stress can result in hypoxia and acidosis and there is evidence from animal models that this impairs surfactant production.[61,62] Hypothermia following delivery in hospital is in most cases preventable, and where infants do become cold they are more likely to require admission to the neonatal unit which results in maternal separation, parental stress, impaired bonding and establishment of lactation, as well as increasing neonatal unit workload.[63,64]

For all infants, the resuscitation environment should be thermoneutral, that is, within a temperature range that allows the infant to maintain a normal temperature with the least amount of energy expended. A room temperature of around 25°C should be comfortable for all present at the delivery and closing doors and windows will minimize draughts and reduce convective heat loss.[65] Sufficient warm, dry towels should be available for drying and wrapping the infant as well as hats of different sizes to prevent radiant heat loss.

Infants who are well at birth should be dried and given to their mother for skin-to-skin contact. This involves placing the infant naked and prone on the mother's chest, covered with a warm blanket and hat, and is associated with improved breastfeeding and temperature homeostasis.[66] It is important to ensure that parents or staff are vigilant that the infant's mouth is able to be visualized, that breathing and colour can be easily observed, and that airway obstruction does not occur.[67]

On resuscitaires, radiant heat is provided by an overhead heater, which should be switched on in advance of birth where resuscitation is anticipated. The infant should be dried and then wrapped in a clean towel. If resuscitation is prolonged, temperature should be monitored using a probe placed between the infant's skin and the mattress. This shows good correlation with core temperature. External heat can then be titrated either manually or by servo methods to maintain normothermia.

Therapeutic hypothermia

The role of therapeutic hypothermia to 33.5°C in asphyxiated infants who develop moderate to severe hypoxic-ischaemic encephalopathy is now well established.[3]

In infants who require resuscitation for presumed intrapartum asphyxia, passive cooling may be initiated from birth. Passive cooling involves the removal of external heat sources (i.e. turning off the overhead heater) and ideally should occur in conjunction with temperature monitoring. The use of fans or gel or ice packs constitutes active cooling and should not be instituted in the delivery suite as such adjuncts can lead to rapid overcooling, which is associated with arrhythmias, cold shock, and coagulopathy.[68] Passive cooling may be continued in the neonatal unit pending a formal decision to embark on active cooling and in such cases, core temperature monitoring with a rectal probe is essential.[69,70]

Therapeutic hypothermia should only be undertaken in cooling centres which have sufficient expertise and experience to manage these critically ill infants.[71] Early liaison with neonatal transport teams[72] and the regional cooling centre may be required.

Hyperthermia should be avoided in any infant with suspected perinatal brain injury as it potentiates damage and is associated with an increased risk of adverse outcome.[73] Hyperthermia may result from external heat sources such as maximal radiant heat during a prolonged resuscitation but is also seen in maternal pyrexia secondary to infection and an association with epidural use has been reported.[74]

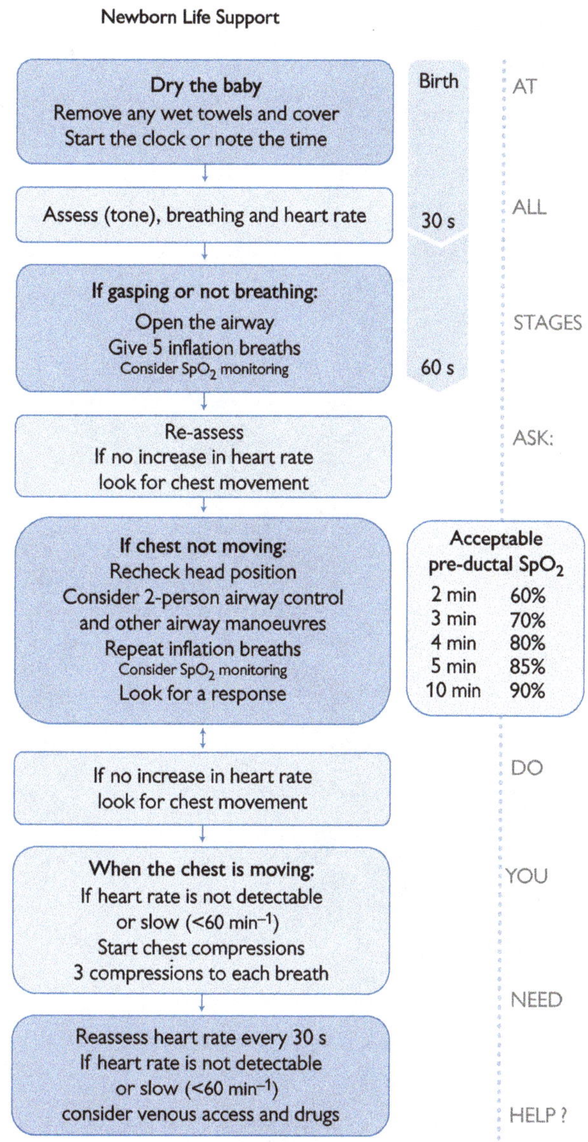

Figure 8.14 Newborn life support algorithm.
Reproduced with the kind permission of the Resuscitation Council (UK).

Preterm infants

Preterm infants (<37 completed weeks of gestation) are at increased risk from hypothermia and maintaining normothermia is challenging. They are smaller and have a larger surface area to volume ratio. The preterm skin is thin and poorly keratinized, and transepidermal water and heat loss is high. In addition to the problems described above, hypothermia on admission to the neonatal unit is associated with adverse outcomes including death and intraventricular haemorrhage.[75]

The environmental temperature should be increased to 26°C where possible. A hat is essential. In infants less than 32 weeks, use of polythene bags or film reduces the incidence of hypothermia on admission to the neonatal unit.[76] The infant is placed in a bag feet-first without drying and the bag is tucked around the neck (Figure 8.15). The infant is not covered with towels, allowing the radiant heater to warm the infant directly. Evaporative heat loss is reduced, as the humidity within the bag is high.

Auscultation of the chest and saturation monitoring can be performed through the bag without exposing the chest or limbs. The polythene bag should remain on the infant following admission until the temperature of the infant and the environment are both optimal. Chemical warming mattresses may be a useful adjunct to polythene bags.[77]

Delayed cord clamping

The practice of umbilical cord clamping within 20 seconds of delivery is widely practised as an element of active management of the third stage of labour. However, in the term infant, immediate cord clamping deprives the infant of 20–30 mg/kg of iron but delaying clamping for at least 2 minutes results

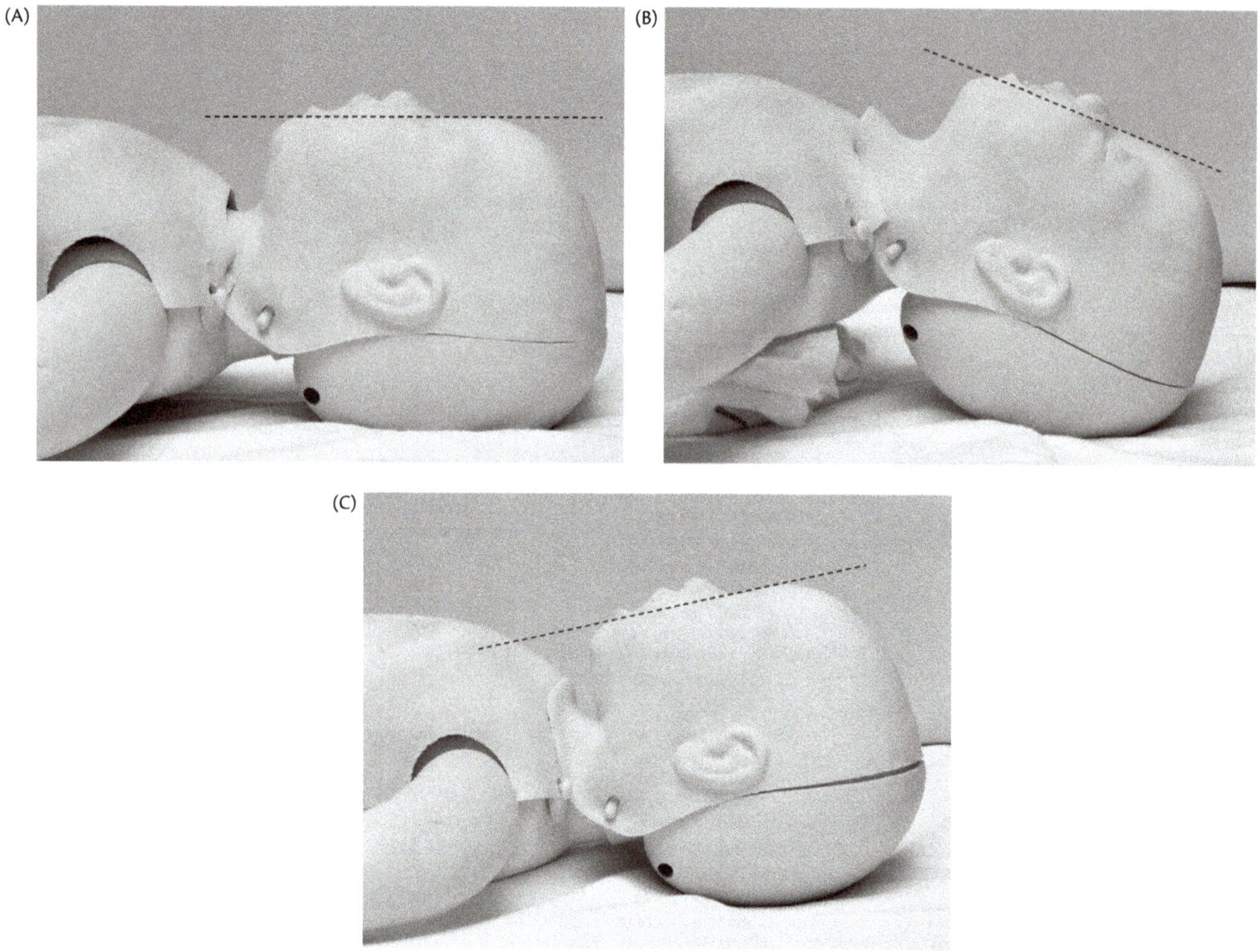

Figure 8.15 The neutral position (A) provides an open airway in the newborn. Extended (B) and flexed (C) positions will cause airway obstruction.

in increased iron stores and a reduction in iron deficiency in infancy.[78]

Preterm infants are at increased risk of risk of anaemia secondary to iatrogenic bloodletting, reduced red cell lifespan, and relatively low concentrations of erythropoietin. Blood transfusion is common in the first few weeks of life.[79] When cord clamping is delayed by 30 seconds after birth an additional 10–15 mL/kg of blood is received by the preterm infant.[80] Systematic reviews have demonstrated that a delay in cord clamping of 30–60 seconds in the preterm infant results in a reduction in the need for blood transfusion, intraventricular haemorrhage, necrotizing enterocolitis,[81,82] and results in improved cardiovascular stability in the first week of life.

There appear to be no significant adverse effects of delayed cord clamping (DCC) either to the infant (e.g. Apgar, pH, and respiratory symptoms secondary to polycythaemia), or to the mother (postpartum haemorrhage). A 2% increase in neonatal jaundice requiring phototherapy has been observed in term infants.[82]

DCC is recommended by ILCOR and the Newborn Life Support guidelines[8] for all infants not requiring resuscitation. Although professional organizations also support a delay of 30–60 seconds before clamping the cord in preterm birth,[83,84] there may be reason to be cautious in any situation where delaying resuscitation would be disadvantageous (e.g. in those infants with a heart rate of less than 60 bpm at birth or asphyxia), where placental perfusion is significantly impaired (e.g. abruption) or in monochorionic twins where placental blood supply is shared.

In all births while DCC is being undertaken, attention should be given to thermal care and airway patency.

Assessment after delivery

A structured, objective approach to newborn assessment is essential.

When presented with an infant at delivery, those who require additional support must be rapidly identified, whilst ensuring that over-zealous intervention does not compromise the infant who is spontaneously making the transition from the womb. Our knowledge of normal newborn physiology is important in this assessment.

It will not surprise readers to learn that the name most associated with neonatal resuscitation, Virginia Apgar, was an anaesthetist. Apgar's score (Table 8.4) was initially published in 1953 as a method of assessing an infant's well-being at 1 minute.[85] The '5'- and '10'-minute scores are later additions.

Table 8.4 The Apgar score

	0	1	2
Heart rate	Absent	<100 bpm	≥100 bpm
Respiratory effort	Apnoeic	Gaping/irregular	Breathing well/ crying
Colour	White/ blue	Pink centrally, blue peripheries	Pink
Reflex irritability	No response	Weak response/grimace only	Cry/withdrawal to stimuli
Muscle tone	Flaccid	Decreased tone	Good tone

The usefulness of the summed score assumes that each component is of equal importance, and is always evaluated consistently—this is an incorrect assumption. An infant in asystole at delivery has been subjected to a significant insult (Apgar score '0' for heart rate). This is in contrast to apnoea at delivery, which can occur after a relatively short period of anoxia, and may resolve spontaneously. Colour and heart rate are difficult to assess accurately,[86,87] and it is therefore unsurprising that although correlation is seen between poor outcome (death, disability, acidotic cord pH) and a low Apgar score, the predictive value is poor, with a high percentage of infants with low scores surviving with no impairment. Even when birth asphyxia leads to a clinical encephalopathy, the predictive value of the Apgar score is poor[88] until around 10 minutes.

It is now recognized that even experienced neonatologists are unable to predict outcome with any degree of accuracy based upon their assessment at delivery in the majority of circumstances.[89] The exception to this is the infant born with an obvious lethal abnormality, or those who fail to respond, and remain asystolic after 10 minutes of good quality resuscitation—in those circumstances it would be justifiable not to continue resuscitative efforts and to offer compassionate care.[8]

Apgar's achievement was in convincing those attending a delivery to focus on (and record) objective signs of well-being. Although the score consists of five components (Table 8.4), in practice it is the continued assessment of three vital signs—colour, respiratory effort, and heart rate (Table 8.5)—which provides us with the most useful information and guides our approach. Using these parameters it is possible to divide infants at delivery into three broad groups:

1. Blue, but rapidly becoming pink, with a fast heart rate, breathing well (crying) or who start breathing within 30 seconds of assessment

Table 8.5 Simplified assessment of the newborn at birth

Sign	Observation
Colour	Pink/blue/white
Respiratory effort	Regular(or crying)/gasping/absent
Heart rate	Fast/slow/very slow (or absent)

2. Blue, with a slow heart rate, and inadequate respiration or gasping
3. White, with a slow or very slow heart rate and no respiratory effort.

On the infant's arrival the clock is started and observations begin (Box 8.3). The wet towels are removed and the infant is dried while continuously assessing muscular tone and response to this stimulation. A well infant who has not cried before this time will now usually do so. Colour and respiratory effort are immediately obvious. The crying infant has an open airway, and will have a fast heart rate.

Heart rate is now assessed; auscultation over the apex is preferred as palpation can be unreliable. It will be apparent whether the rate is fast (>100 bpm), slow (60–100 bpm), or very slow (<60 bpm). It is good practice to tap this beat out so that others attending the delivery/resuscitation are immediately informed. This will have taken between 30 and 60 seconds, and you will have the information to decide whether this infant is going to require more support.

Two of the signs described above, colour and heart rate (assessed by brief auscultation or palpation), are subjective and prone to much inter-observer variability. This did not escape Apgar, who commented on colour that it was 'by far the most unsatisfactory sign and caused the most discussion among the observers'.[85] The ability of those attending a delivery to relate 'colour' to oxygen saturation is almost non-existent, with observers reporting infants to be 'pink' when saturations were generally between 60% and 80%.[86] Accurate determination of the heart rate[87] has been shown to be similarly unreliable and has no bearing on seniority or experience of the observer. Interesting though those observations are, it must be accepted that for the most part, it does not matter if an infant has a heart rate of 85 bpm which is assessed as 'fast', if they are well in all other aspects. Most newborns will not derive any benefit from improving the precision of these observations, but when resuscitation is prolonged, or in the context of a preterm infant, more accurate monitoring of heart rate and saturation (preductal pulse oximetry) can be of benefit—providing any response to the numbers displayed is tempered by an understanding that low oxygen saturations can be normal during transition.[17]

One other piece of information is often available shortly after delivery. The umbilical arterial and venous blood gas results, taken from a double-clamped section of cord will provide supportive information, particularly when there is concern about *in utero* hypoxia.

Most term babies, even those for whom neonatal support is requested, will transition without any assistance; however, a small

Box 8.3 Other observations at delivery

- Obstetric/midwifery anxiety
- Trauma/bruising
- Muscle tone
- Meconium staining (skin/cord/nails)
- Size (smaller/larger than expected)
- Obvious congenital lesions (gastroschisis, neural tube defect)
- Maturity (preterm/post-dates).

number of infants may be identified as being likely to require intervention antenatally (e.g. preterm, known anomaly), and provision must also be made to manage the infant who unexpectedly requires resuscitation at delivery. A standardized approach towards assessment enables practitioners to approach these scenarios with confidence.

Resuscitation at birth

Training in newborn resuscitation is best learned on a recognized training course, the UK Resuscitation Council's Newborn Life Support and to a lesser extent the American Heart Association's Newborn Resuscitation Program are both taught within the United Kingdom. The differences are principally around the approach to initial lung aeration and the use of oxygen. Both are valid, and reflect the relative lack of evidence of one over the other.

Preparation

When called to attend a delivery (Box 8.4), make use of the time available. Obtain as much history as possible; three key points should be elucidated:

1. Gestation
2. Presence of meconium
3. Presence of fetal distress (e.g. decelerations, bradycardia, loss of fetal heart, acidotic).

Fetal blood sample

Ensure that any windows or doors are closed to minimize heat loss. Request help if you think you may require it, and check your equipment is working and clean. Wash your hands (or use alcohol gel) and put on gloves.

- Turn on resuscitaire, turn on light, turn heater to maximum
- Towels (warm)
- Check gases (wall supply, cylinders)
- Stethoscope
- Masks—appropriate sizes
- Self-inflating bag—check pop-off
- T-piece—set pressures, 6–8 L/min flow, start in air (if possible):
  - PIP 30, PEEP 5 term
  - PIP 20, PEEP 5 preterm

Box 8.4 Situations where the need for neonatal support may be anticipated

- Preterm gestation
- Meconium staining of the liquor
- Placental abruption
- Cord prolapse
- Shoulder dystocia
- Emergency delivery for fetal distress
- Multiples (twins, triplets, etc.).

Table 8.6 Guide to ETT diameter and length of insertion by gestation and weight

Gestation	Weight in kg (50th centile)	ETT diameter (mm)	Length at lips (cm)
23–24	0.5	2.5	6
26	0.75	2.5	6.5
27	1	2.5	7
30	1.5	2.5	7.5
33	2	2.5–3.0	8
35	2.5	3.0	8.5
37	3	3.0–3.5	9
40	3.5	3.5	9.5
	4	3.5–4.0	10

- Suction working, and catheters/Yankauer suction available
- Check laryngoscope light source, and blades appropriate (Miller 1, 0, 00)
- ETT (3.5 = term, 3.0 = ~33–37 weeks, 2.5 = <33 weeks) (Table 8.6)
- Other equipment (depending on environment/situation/experience):
  - saturation monitor + probes
  - vascular access kit
  - emergency drugs/fluids/blood.

As the infant is delivered, note the time (or start timer) and dry. Assess the infant looking at *colour, breathing*, and *heart rate*. The majority of infants will not require more than warmth and provision of an open airway. If the heart rate is acceptable (>100 bpm, 'fast') there is no reason to cut the cord immediately, and 1 minute of placental transfusion (see below) should be allowed.

Resuscitation follows an ABC approach, with modifications to take the newborn physiology into account. Before effective ventilation can be delivered, the lungs must be inflated. Cardiac compressions if required may only be necessary for a short period. Preterm infants usually do not need 'resuscitation' (they have not experienced *in utero* hypoxia), but do need support to effectively transition to an *ex utero* environment which they are not well equipped to cope with.

The structured approach can be summarized as follows (see Figure 8.16):

- Thermal stability (dry and wrap)—all infants
- Lung aeration—if not breathing
- Ventilation breaths—if still not breathing after the lungs have been inflated
- Cardiac compressions—if the heart rate does not respond to lung aeration
- Drugs—if the heart rate does not respond to a short period of chest compressions.

Progression from each step is determined by ongoing assessment of the infant (colour/heart rate/breathing); an increasing heart

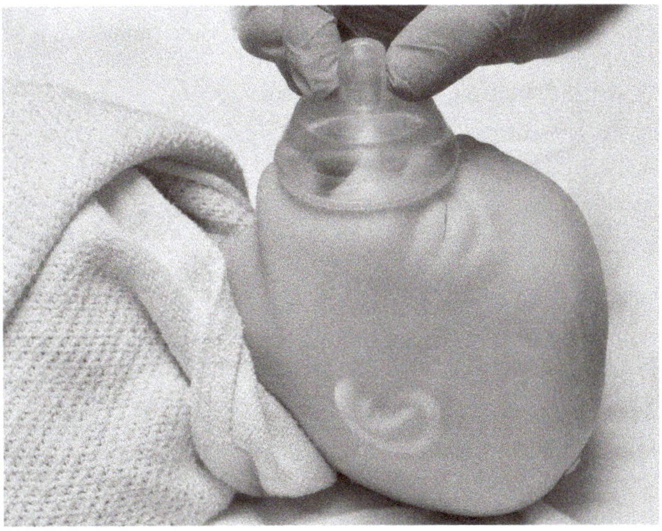

Figure 8.16 A correctly sized mask will cover the mouth and nose, without placing pressure on the eyes.

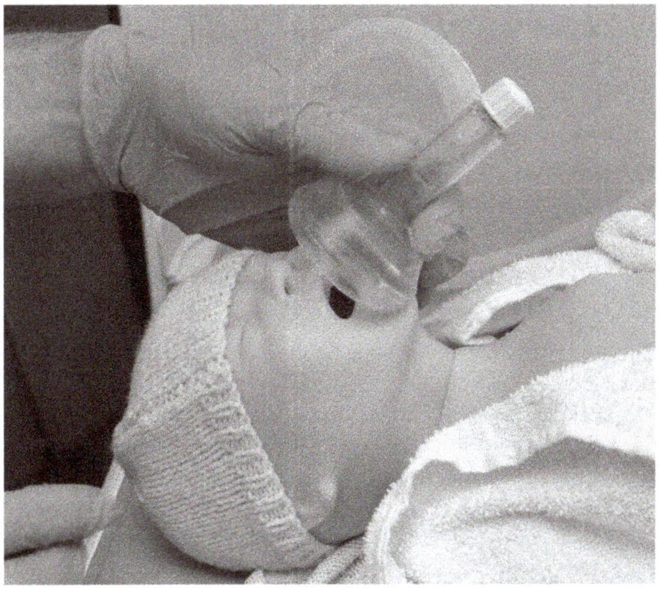

Figure 8.17 Rolling on a mask minimises leak and improves subsequent airway positioning.

rate is the first sign of improvement. Whilst all newborns will require thermal stability, very few need chest compressions and drugs.[5]

Provide warmth and a neutral airway position

On arrival at the resuscitaire, start the clock, remove any wet towels, and replace with warm dry ones. If available, put a woollen hat on the infant. Leave the chest uncovered to assess breathing whilst maintaining the airway in a neutral position (Figure 8.15). Applying 'head tilt' to a newborn will overextend the neck and cause airway obstruction. Assess the infant. If the heart rate is fast and the infant is breathing then no further intervention is required. If the heart rate is slow, or the infant does not start breathing adequately, then further support is required. Most well infants will begin breathing within 60 seconds.

Inflate the lungs

Lung aeration (also described as 'lung inflation') is the most essential manoeuvre in newborn resuscitation. No other measures will be successful if this is not achieved. Good airway positioning and minimal mask leak are key.[42,51] A hypotonic infant will obstruct their airway due to loss of pharyngeal tone, and this is overcome by maintaining a neutral position and applying a jaw thrust if required. Once an appropriately sized mask (Figure 8.16) has been chosen, it should be 'rolled' onto the face from the chin[42] using an appropriate grip (Figure 8.17). Now re-check the airway position and inflate the lungs. In Newborn Life Support practice this is done by delivering *5 breaths, each lasting 3 seconds* at a *PIP of 30* cmH_2O. This technique derives from observations that shorter breaths established a lower FRC in newborns,[90] and is supported by recent animal work.[91] Watch for chest wall rise, although this may be subtle,[92] and as the initial breaths replace lung fluid with gas then one may not observe any change with the first breaths.

Reassess the infant—if the lungs have been aerated, the heart should respond. When there is no response in heart rate the most common reason is that the lungs have not been inflated. If no chest wall movement was observed, reposition the airway and try again with jaw thrust (Figure 8.18). A persistent bradycardia with no observed chest wall movement mandates optimization of airway management (Box 8.5) and help should be summoned if not done so already.

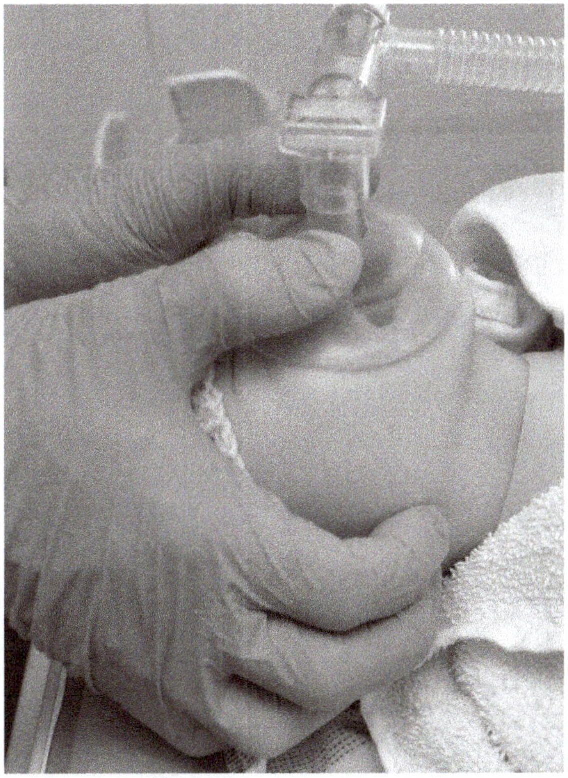

Figure 8.18 The "2 person technique" of providing mask ventilation is shown here, one person manages the airway with a jaw-thrust, the other provides ventilation. It is useful when a newborn's airway is difficult to maintain.

Box 8.5 Manoeuvres to alleviate newborn airway obstruction

- Optimize airway position (shoulder pad/towel)
- Two-person jaw thrust
- Oropharyngeal airway
- Suction under direct vision.

Meconium

The majority of infants born through meconium-stained liquor do not aspirate meconium, and routine suctioning of all infants provides no benefit, nor does suctioning on the perineum.[93] Where meconium aspiration syndrome develops after birth, meconium has already been inhaled during *in utero* gasping. Thick particulate meconium, however, may physically obstruct the trachea and prevent lung inflation causing a serious situation. If an infant with meconium staining is not immediately vigorous, inspect the oropharynx before attempting to stimulate the infant. Suction any meconium seen with a wide-bore suction catheter, then visualize the cords and suction the trachea. After suctioning, proceed to resuscitate in the usual manner, drying the infant and providing aeration breaths if required.

Suction should also be considered if no chest wall movement is seen in the absence of meconium as blood clot and vernix may also obstruct the trachea.

Ventilation breaths

Once the lungs are inflated (i.e. chest wall movement seen), in most cases the heart rate will rapidly respond and ventilation breaths are given until the infant establishes adequate respirations. In the rare event of persistent bradycardia despite good chest wall movement, ventilation breaths (Table 8.7) should be continued and cardiac compressions commenced. Ventilation breaths are delivered at a rate of 30/min (1 second in, 1 second out), lower pressures may be used now that an FRC is established (20–25 cmH_2O). Loss of ventilation due to loss of airway position or increased mask leak during resuscitation will manifest as a fall in heart rate. A colorimetric CO_2 detector can be useful during prolonged resuscitation and supplements observation of chest wall movement.[51]

Cardiac compressions

Chest compression is useless if the lungs have not been aerated.[13]

Table 8.7 Comparison of inflation and ventilation breaths

	Inflation breaths	Ventilation breaths
Indication	Establish lung aeration	Ventilation after lungs inflated
Duration	3-second inflation	1-second inflation
Pressure	PIP 30 cmH_2O	PIP 20–30 cmH_2O (chest movement)
Rate	Sets of 5 (e.g. 5 × 3 second breaths)	30/minute

Box 8.6 Considerations prior to initiation of chest compressions

- Ask 'Am I getting chest wall movement?'
- Check mask, minimize leak
- Check gases, check flow
- Consider increasing PIP and inflation time
- Check airway position
- Consider tracheal obstruction
- Confirm ETT position (if using).

If the heart rate remains undetectable or very slow (<60 bpm) and chest wall movement is seen then chest compressions should be started (Box 8.6).[8,13,56]

Cardiac compressions in the newborn may be more likely to elicit an improvement than in an adult. The infant has been subjected to an acute stress, but was in optimal physiological condition prior to this, with a physiology primed to deal with hypoxia. If oxygenated blood is delivered from the pulmonary vasculature to the coronary circulation the heart should respond and function well thereafter. The compression phase empties the chest of blood, and the relaxation phase is of paramount importance to allow refilling[94] and coronary perfusion.

Compression should be on the lower third of the sternum,[95–97] this is located by positioning one's thumbs or fingers either just below the nipple line, or a finger's breadth above the xiphisternum. Two methods are recognized (Box 8.7); the two-thumb (encircling) method and the two-finger method. The encircling method is preferred (Figure 8.19)—producing greater blood flow and pressure in experimental models when compared to two-finger compressions.[98–101] It is also less likely to cause fatigue in the resuscitator. The two-finger method is useful if one has small hands, or if access to site an umbilical venous catheter is required (Figure 8.20).

A ratio of 3:1 (compressions:breaths) should be delivered to a depth of approximately one-third of the chest's anteroposterior diameter,[102] aiming for 90 compressions and 30 breaths in 1 minute. This ratio has been demonstrated to provide more consistent compressions,[103] it allows enough time for refilling, and is supported by animal models.[104,105]

Re-assess every 30 seconds, and continue to pay close attention to airway positioning, which can become compromised during compressions. If the heart rate does not respond to a short period of compressions with adequate ventilation, the myocardium has been impaired by the degree of acidosis and exhaustion of its glycogen stores. Drugs must now be considered.

Box 8.7 Chest compressions in the newborn

- 3:1 ratio
- 30 breaths/minute (90 compressions)
- Lower third of sternum
- Two-thumb (or two-finger) technique
- Compress anteroposterior diameter by one-third
- Re-assess every 30 seconds (15 breaths).

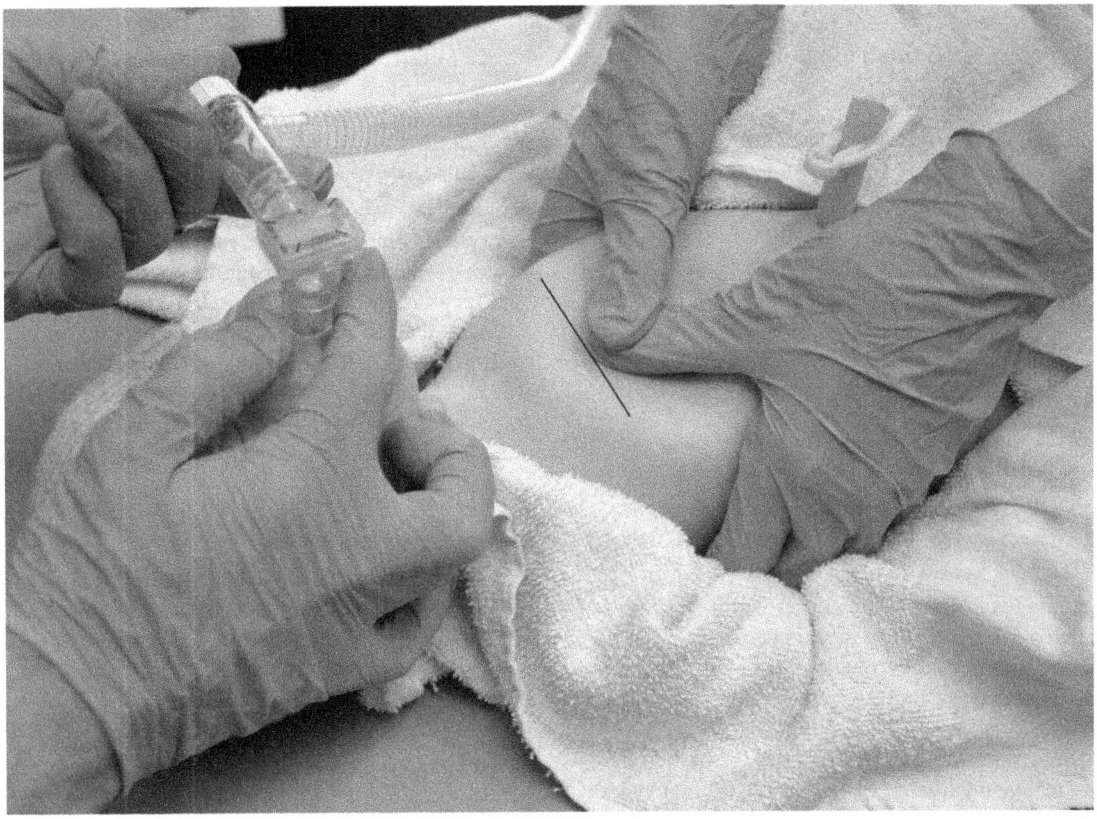

Figure 8.19 Hand position for chest compressions using the "encircling" method.

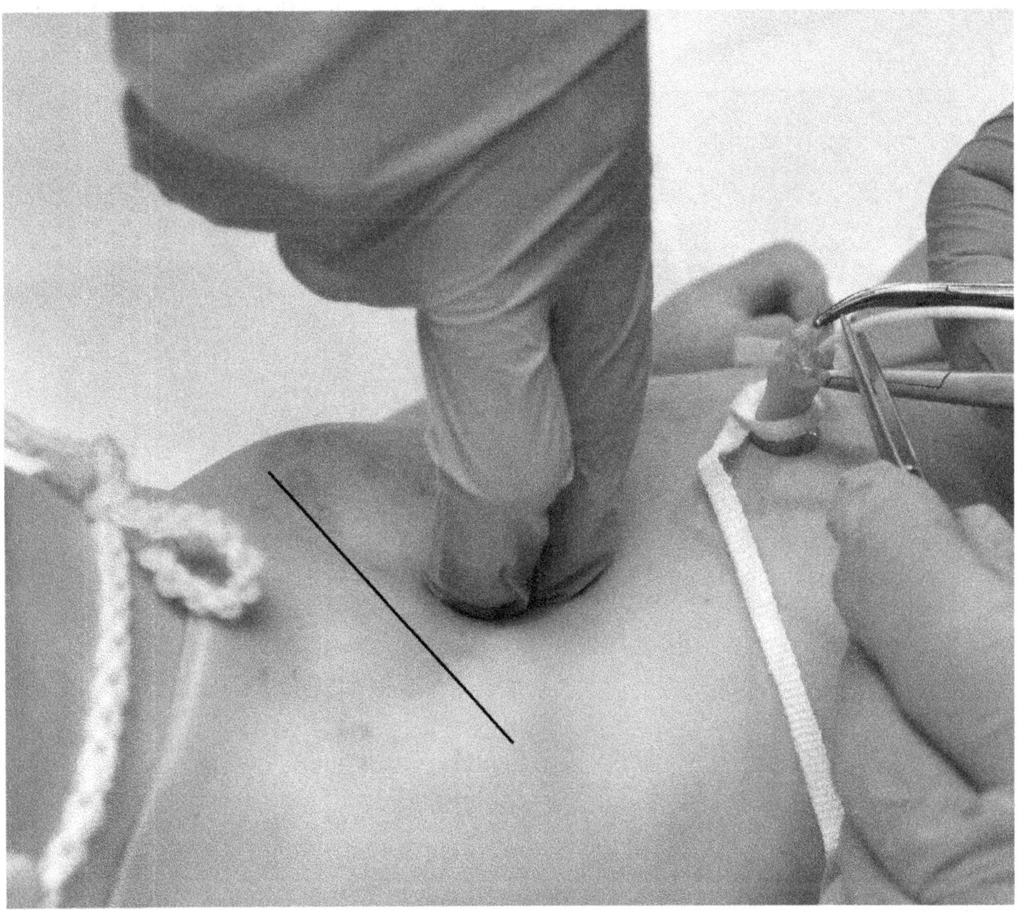

Figure 8.20 Chest compressions delivered by the "2-finger" technique are useful whilst umbilical access is being obtained.

Table 8.8 Drugs, doses and routes of administration during newborn resuscitation

Drug	Preparation	Dose	Route	Repeat?
Sodium bicarbonate	4.2% Minijet®	2–4 mL/kg	UVC	No
Epinephrine	1:10,000 (100 mcg/mL) Minijet®	0.1 mL/kg	UVC/ tracheal[a]	Yes
Glucose ('dextrose')	10% bags (10 g/100 mL)	2.5 mL/kg	UVC	No
Volume	0.9% sodium chloride, O -ve Blood	10 mL/kg	UVC	Once

[a]If the tracheal route is used a higher dose will be required (50–100 mcg/kg).

UVC, umbilical vein catheter.

Drugs

No drug can aerate the lungs, and no newborn will recover without the lungs being aerated. Failure to respond to resuscitation is almost always an airway problem, but on occasion the circulation may be so impaired that it cannot respond to lung aeration and chest compressions.

If there has been no response to 30 seconds of chest compressions, an umbilical vein catheter should be sited. Pragmatically, we would advise not to waste time trying to obtain peripheral access. The drugs used in resuscitation are shown in Table 8.8. This is an infrequent event and it is recommended that these doses are easily visible in all resuscitation areas. Measuring small doses from a Minijet® can be achieved using a three-way tap, and 1 mL syringe (Figure 8.21).

There is little evidence to support the use or sequence of any drugs during newborn resuscitation; however, epinephrine may be less effective if profound acidosis is present, and thus bicarbonate may be given concurrently. Glucose should be given too as myocardial stores will have been depleted, and volume (as saline, or blood) should be given cautiously unless there is a clear reason to suspect hypovolaemia. Although a moderate increase in filling pressure generally improves cardiac output, excess volume may overload an already compromised myocardium.

Note the time all drugs are given and follow each with a small-volume saline flush (e.g. 2 mL). Continue a cycle (30 seconds, 15 breaths) of chest compressions after each drug, and reassess response.

Stopping resuscitation

If no heart rate is detectable after 10 minutes of good quality cardiopulmonary resuscitation, the outlook is bleak and care should be reoriented.[8,106] There is little data to guide us when an infant remains persistently bradycardic, and advice should be sought from the local tertiary neonatologist.

Special considerations

Prematurity

Six to ten per cent of all births are premature—delivered before 37 completed weeks of gestation. Around 1% of infants are born at a gestation less than 28 weeks. In the developed world, the

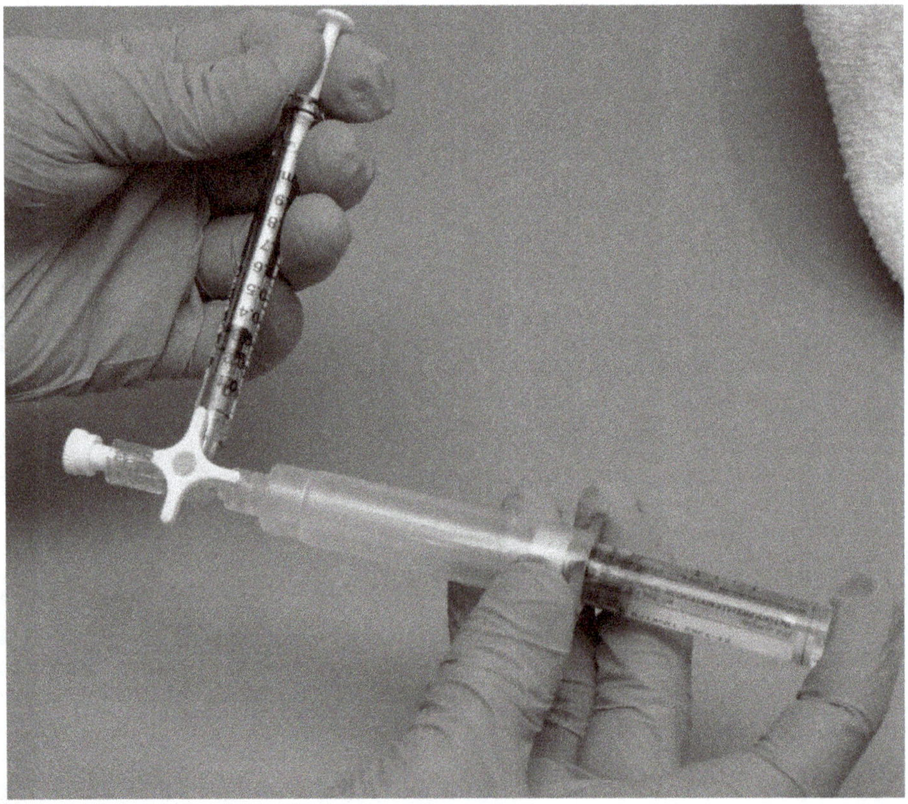

Figure 8.21 The preferred method of measuring small doses of epinephrine during resuscitation.

incidence of prematurity is rising, as is the incidence of multiple births.

Premature birth may occur following spontaneous onset of labour precipitated by maternal infection, multiple gestations, congenital anomalies in the fetus, or structural uterine abnormalities. Delivery may also be expedited in non-labouring women because of concerns about maternal health (e.g. pregnancy-induced hypertension or cardiac disease) or because of concern about fetal well-being, for example, growth restriction, maternal cholestasis, or blood group incompatibility.

Mortality

Survival is directly proportional to gestational age as are both short-term complications, such as respiratory distress syndrome, intraventricular haemorrhage, and necrotizing enterocolitis, and longer-term sequelae, such as bronchopulmonary dysplasia and neurodisability including cerebral palsy, cognitive and behavioural impairment.[107,108] Improvements in both antenatal and neonatal care in the last 20 years have resulted in improved survival such that around 90% of infants born with a birthweight less than 1500 g now survive. At extremely premature gestations, survival is less good with only 20% of infants born at 23 weeks surviving, around half suffering moderate or severe disability.[109]

Neurological morbidity

At the time of delivery and in the weeks that follow, the extreme preterm brain is undergoing a rapidly developing process of growth. The vasculature is fragile and the cellular components are vulnerable to ischaemic and inflammatory injury. Impaired cerebrovascular autoregulation means that cerebral blood flow is susceptible to swings in blood pressure including those resulting from ventilation, and changes in oxygen and carbon dioxide tension. Hallmarks of preterm brain injury therefore include periventricular haemorrhage and white matter ischaemic damage, also known as periventricular leucomalacia,[110] both of which may result in long-term cognitive and motor neurodisability.

Improving outcomes in the delivery suite

Antenatal corticosteroids

Recommendations from professional organizations state that treatment should be considered for all women at risk of preterm delivery between 24 and 36 weeks.[111,112] A course of dexamethasone or betamethasone initiated between 24 and 168 hours prior to delivery is associated with reductions in mortality (relative risk (RR) 0.69; 95% confidence interval (CI) 0.58–0.81), respiratory distress syndrome (RR 0.66; 95% CI 0.59–0.73), intraventricular haemorrhage (RR 0.48; 95% CI 0.29–0.79), pneumothorax, and necrotizing enterocolitis.[113,114]

Antenatal magnesium sulphate

Cerebral palsy develops in 15% of preterm infants with a gestational age less than 28 weeks.[108,109] Administration of antenatal magnesium sulphate shortly before preterm delivery has been shown to reduce cerebral palsy with a RR of 0.68 (95% CI 0.54–0.87[115] and is recommended by the Royal College of Obstetricians and Gynaecologists.[116] There are no associated adverse long-term fetal or maternal outcomes although some mothers may experience minor adverse symptoms associated with administration.

Delaying cord clamping

DCC reduces adverse outcomes in preterm infants (see 'Delayed cord clamping').

Table 8.9 Goals of preterm respiratory management

Aim	Rationale
Optimize early alveolar recruitment	Maximize gas exchange surface area
Avoid collapse during expiration	Prevent atelectotrauma
Avoid intubation if possible	Prevent endotrauma
Avoid excessive tidal volume	Prevent volutrauma
Avoid excess inspiratory pressure	Prevent barotrauma

Maintaining normothermia

Low temperature on admission to the neonatal unit is associated with adverse outcome in preterm infants (see 'Thermal Environment and Care').

Respiratory support of the preterm Infant

Most preterm infants regardless of gestation age require stabilization rather than resuscitation. Gentle lung recruitment rather than aggressive intervention is important in aiding transition and avoiding lung injury (Table 8.9). Following birth, infants of 32 weeks or more are generally vigorous. More immature infants may require respiratory support with or without surfactant.

Preterm infants have fragile lungs which are less compliant and therefore less able to maintain an FRC. The lung can be easily injured by over-distension and repeated re-expansion from a collapsed state. Tracheal intubation may introduce bacteria. Lung damage leads quickly to inflammation which can inhibit surfactant function and can lead ultimately to bronchopulmonary dysplasia, a chronic lung condition associated with prolonged hospital stay, reduced pulmonary function in childhood, and neurodevelopmental impairment.

Continuous positive airway pressure

CPAP reduces work of breathing by recruiting alveoli and preventing end-expiratory collapse. This aids oxygenation and prevents atelectrauma. Evidence suggests that intubation can be avoided in around 50% of infants (<750g) who can instead be managed on CPAP alone from birth with intubation for surfactant administration only if respiratory distress syndrome (RDS) develops.[37,38,126,127] Care should be taken when adopting this 'wait and watch' approach in the delivery suite that positioning of the airway is optimal and that CPAP is continuously applied, as breaks in CPAP pressure rapidly lead to alveolar de-recruitment. CPAP may be applied using a standard facemask or bi-nasal (Argyle) prongs.

Surfactant

Surfactant is a mixture of phospholipids and proteins produced by alveolar cells in increasing quantities from around 20 weeks onwards. A deficiency in surfactant results in poor lung compliance, alveolar collapse, and increased work of breathing manifest clinically as RDS. The incidence of RDS is inversely proportional to gestational age but is also more common in male infants, those of Caucasian race, and infants of diabetic mothers. Surfactant production and function is inhibited by hypothermia, infection, asphyxia, and the presence of meconium in the alveoli. Lung maturation and surfactant synthesis can be accelerated by antenatal corticosteroids.

Exogenous surfactant can be administered after birth either prophylactically or as 'rescue' treatment for RDS. Surfactant improves outcomes in infants with established RDS, resulting in a reduction in pneumothorax, mortality, and the combined outcome of mortality and bronchopulmonary dysplasia.[118]

Surfactant is normally administered to those infants most at risk of developing RDS, and may be given prophylactically in the most immature infants who require intubation in the delivery suite. More mature infants may be managed without surfactant in the delivery suite with early application of CPAP, and intervention when signs of RDS become significant in the first hours of life. Prophylactic surfactant may reduce the incidence of RDS compared to a 'rescue' therapy but results in overtreatment of infants who would not otherwise go on to develop RDS.

Oxygen

As described earlier, there is increasing evidence that a high concentration of oxygen at resuscitation is harmful to newborn infants. Preterm infants in particular have low antioxidant reserves to neutralize free radicals[119] and oxygen injury is implicated in a range of neonatal morbidities including retinopathy of prematurity, bronchopulmonary dysplasia, necrotizing enterocolitis, and brain injury. On the other hand, it has recently been shown that infants nursed at lower oxygen saturations have a higher mortality than those nursed in a higher range and this has fuelled the debate about what constitutes an appropriate saturation target range in preterm infants.[120] As with term infants, reference ranges for preterm infants have been published to guide oxygen management in the delivery suite.[17] Avoidance of both hyperoxia and hypoxia should be the goal—whilst recognizing that saturation may take 10 minutes to approach 'normal'.

The principles of stabilization of preterm infants

1. Maintenance of normothermia (see 'Thermal Environment and Care')
2. Facilitation of spontaneous respiration and supporting it with CPAP or IPPV
3. Monitoring of oxygen saturations and avoidance of hyperoxia
4. Maintenance of stability and avoidance of episodes of acute hypoxia or bradycardia.

Equipment

- Standard resuscitation equipment including appropriately sized mask, endotracheal tubes, airways, and saturation monitor
- Plastic bag or wrap
- Hats of different sizes.

Approach to resuscitation and stabilization

The approach to resuscitation/stabilization is the same as for term infants (Figure 8.14) with the following key differences:

1. Alert the neonatal unit in advance of delivery.
2. Infants under 32 weeks should be placed in a plastic bag under a radiant heater, and a hat put on them (Figure 8.22).
3. A saturation monitor and temperature probe should be applied if available.
4. Infants may have an immature respiratory drive and support of respiration is increasingly required as gestation decreases:

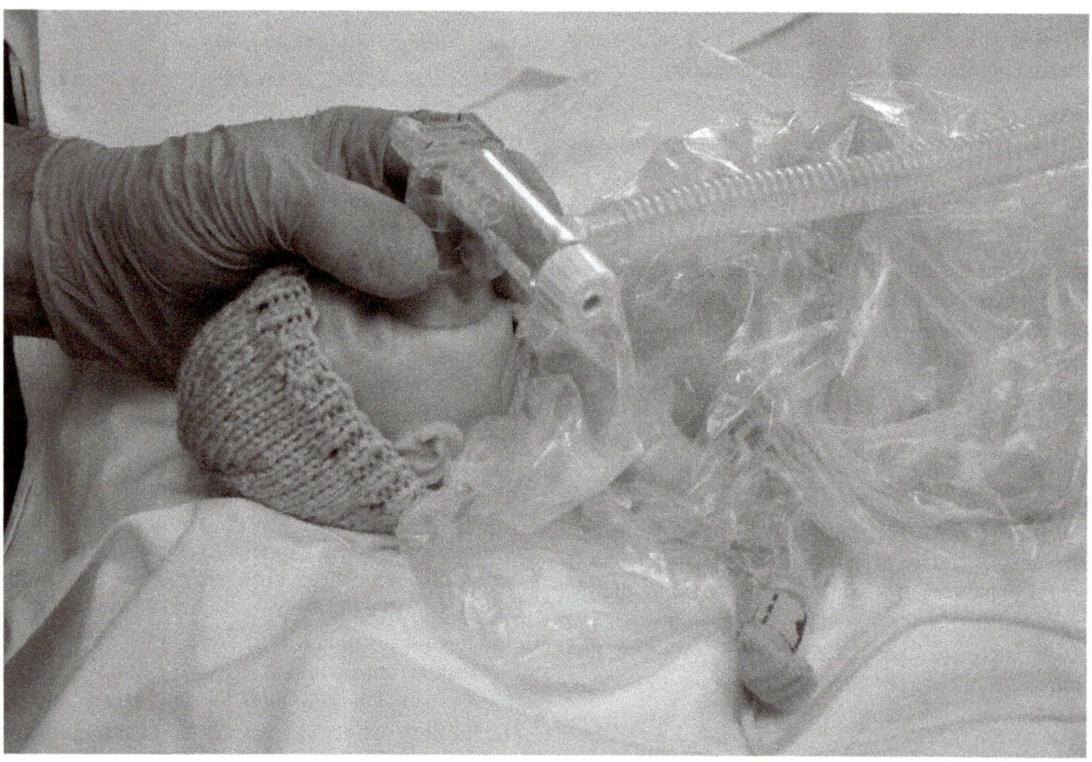

Figure 8.22 Thermal stabilisation using a clear plastic bag.

a. Preterm infants require careful positioning of their airway as they exhibit reduced tone compared to term infants with small changes in position affecting airway patency.

b. Work of breathing may be increased because of poor lung compliance secondary to surfactant deficiency, and a compliant chest wall.

5. Spontaneous breathing may be adequate to maintain a heart rate above 100 bpm and optimal saturations with minimal work of breathing, but if not, ease of respiration and alveolar recruitment is best supported by:

a. CPAP at 5 cmH_2O delivered by nasal prongs or mask through a T-piece

b. IPPV that can be delivered through a mask at starting pressures of 20/5 cmH_2O. T-piece ventilation is preferable to bag and mask ventilation as PEEP can be delivered and pressures measured and controlled:

i. Aeration and ventilation breaths should be given until spontaneous respiration is sufficient.

ii. Inspiratory pressure may need to be gradually increased if chest wall movement is not seen and there is no response in heart rate. Colorimeteric CO_2 detectors inserted into the circuit provide useful information about the patency of the airway and ability to ventilate.

iii. If manual ventilation continues to be required, intubation should be considered.

c. Intubation with an appropriate-sized ETT and IPPV delivered at initial pressures of 20/5 cmH_2O. Secure the tube carefully as accidental extubation predisposes to cardiorespiratory instability with resultant fluctuations in cerebral blood flow and this may precipitate intraventricular haemorrhage

i. Colorimetric CO_2 detectors are recommended to ensure correct tube placement.

ii. As with mask-ventilated infants, the PIP may need to be titrated to observe a response in heart rate and chest movement. Evidence of 'excellent' chest wall movement with a fast heart rate may indicate very high tidal volumes. PIP should be reduced where able to avoid lung injury.[57]

iii. Once adequate ventilation is achieved and the heart rate is stable above 100 bpm, there may be a decision to administer surfactant in the delivery suite. Surfactant is not a resuscitation drug but aids stabilization and reduces injury in the surfactant-deficient lung where positive pressure ventilation is required.[118]

Cardiac compressions

Cardiac compressions and drugs are very rarely required in the resuscitation of asphyxiated preterm infants who do not respond to ventilation and oxygenation alone. The need for these advanced resuscitation measures are associated with a high rate of mortality and neurodevelopmental impairment especially in infants with a birthweight less than 1000 g.[121] There is no evidence to support the use of chest compressions or epinephrine by any route during resuscitation in the extreme preterm infant of gestational age less than 26 weeks.[122]

Infants at the borderline of viability

Ethical concerns about the appropriateness of resuscitation of infants born at the extremes of prematurity (22–25 weeks of gestation) have led to the issue of professional guidance from the Nuffield Council of Bioethics and from the British Association of Perinatal Medicine.[122,123]

Infants born between 22 and 25 weeks of gestation have a high risk of mortality and may endure many challenging weeks of intensive care with significant morbidities both in the short term,[124] in infancy, and later in childhood when almost half of survivors born at 25 weeks or less exhibit moderate or severe impairment (Table 8.10).[109]

Current recommendations state that where infants are expected to be born at the limits of viability and if time allows, a discussion between the parents and a senior neonatologist will be had in which the risks of mortality and morbidity are discussed.

- Current evidence does not support resuscitation of infants born at 22 weeks or less of gestation, as the chances of survival are very low and the majority of survivors are likely to be seriously disabled. These infants should be offered palliative care with attention to alleviating pain and distress.
- Given the uncertainty of death and neurological sequelae in any individual infant born at 23 weeks, resuscitation should be guided by the wishes of the parents following informed and thorough discussion with a senior paediatrician. A decision not to offer resuscitation may be appropriate. Assessment of the condition of the infant at birth is not useful in predicting outcome and these decisions should be made prior to delivery where possible.[89] Active care should only be provided if parents are in clear agreement.
- Resuscitation of infants at 24 and 25 weeks is accepted neonatal practice in the United Kingdom, despite a high likelihood of some degree of disability, particularly at 24 weeks' gestation. However some parents may have views about the appropriateness of intensive care which are important to discuss.

Where an extremely premature infant of uncertain gestation delivers unexpectedly without time for parental discussion, the infant's maturity, size, and condition should be assessed by a senior paediatrician. Where only junior or non-paediatric staff are in attendance, the default position should be to proceed with resuscitation until senior advice can be sought and a more detailed discussion with parents can take place.

Table 8.10 Outcomes of delivery at extreme preterm gestation

	Gestation (completed weeks)			
	23	24	25	26
Mortality	81%	60%	44%	33%
Disability amongst survivors[a]	47%	35%	28%	20%

[a]Moderate or severe disability as classified in National Perinatal Epidemiological Unit (NPEU). *Disability and Perinatal Care.* Oxford: NPEU; 1994.

Adapted by permission from BMJ Publishing Group Limited. The *British Medical Journal*, Neurological and developmental outcome in extremely preterm children born in England in 1995 and 2006: the EPICure studies, Tamanna Moore *et al.*, volume 345, e7961, 2012.

The difficult neonatal airway

The neonatal airway is prone to obstruction even under standard physiological conditions. Predisposing factors include the following:

- Small anatomical structures including diameter of larynx (typically 4–5 mm diameter compared to 12–15 mm in adults) mean that small changes in diameter lead to significant reductions in airway calibre.
- A relatively large tongue obstructs passage of air through mouth and makes infants preferential nasal breathers.
- Large occiput favours head flexion and airway obstruction.
- Limited range of neck rotation through which the airway remains patent.
- There may be low muscular tone secondary to maternal sedation or hypoxia.
- Presence of fluid and particulate matter in the airway at birth.

Other anatomical features may make management of the airway more difficult than in older children or adults:

- High position of the larynx at C3–4 increases airway resistance and necessitates straight blade rather than curved.
- Epiglottis larger and angled over the laryngeal inlet.
- Funnel shaped airway with narrowest portion at the cricoid cartilage meaning uncuffed tubes can be successfully used to seal and protect the airway.

Structural abnormalities may further threaten airway patency and are often unexpected (Box 8.8). Large masses such as cystic hygroma or haemangiomas may be diagnosed antenatally by ultrasound scan and may be accompanied by polyhydramnios. Detailed information about the airway may be obtained by magnetic resonance imaging scan and a plan made for management at birth that may include an EXIT (*ex utero* intrapartum treatment) procedure[125] or necessitate the presence of paediatric surgical and ENT teams. Abnormalities in which cleft palate or micrognathia are prominent may also be evident antenatally (e.g. Pierre Robin sequence). Pharyngeal and laryngeal abnormalities may not be apparent until birth.

Box 8.8 Conditions which may cause airway obstruction at birth

- Beckwith–Wiedemann syndrome
- Choanal atresia
- Cleft palate
- Craniofacial dysostosis
- Cystic hygroma
- Goldenhar syndrome
- Laryngeal/tracheal webs, clefts etc.
- Mandibulofacial dysostosis
- Pierre Robin sequence
- Treacher–Collins syndrome
- Trisomy 21
- Vascular malformation.

Airway difficulties may also present following birth. Laryngomalacia classically presents in the first postnatal days with stridor and infants who have been intubated over prolonged periods of time may develop subglottic stenosis or post-extubation oedema.

Clinical signs of airway obstruction include stridor, respiratory distress with significant suprasternal tug and intercostal recession, and snorting respiration with inability to breathe through the nose. There may be an associated cleft lip or palate, a small receding chin, or an obvious neck or oral mass. On inspection of the larynx, the cords may or may not appear normal and there may be difficulty passing an ETT (laryngeal or subglottic stenosis, laryngeal or tracheal atresia), or difficulty keeping it *in situ* (laryngeal cleft). Even if the tracheal tube inserts, difficulty in ventilating may be seen with tracheal anomalies.

There is no standard protocol in the United Kingdom for the management of a difficult neonatal airway and many neonatal intensive-care units will not stock the equipment required for advanced airway techniques nor have a paediatric anaesthetist on site to offer expert support.[126]

Equipment

An easily accessible, well-maintained trolley specific to the difficult airway is central to the management of a difficult airway. Recommended contents include:

1. Oropharyngeal airways (Guedel size 000, 00, and 0)
2. Nasopharyngeal airways (size 2.0, 2.5, 3.0, 3.5)
3. Laryngeal mask airway (size 1)
4. ETTs (size 2.0, 2.5, 3.0, 3.5, 4.0)
5. Laryngoscope with straight and curved blades (size 000, 00, 0)
6. Face masks (size 00, 0/1, 2)
7. Neonatal self-inflating bag
8. Stylets
9. Sutures
10. Video laryngoscope where available (direct or indirect)
11. Algorithm and urgent referral pathway with contact list (e.g. see Figure 8.23).

Congenital diaphragmatic hernia

Congenital diaphragmatic hernia (CDH) arises from herniation of the abdominal contents into the thoracic cavity secondary to a defect in the diaphragm. The site of the defect is on the left side posteriorly in 80% (Bochdalek hernia) and more rarely may be on the right side anteriorly (Morgagni).

The prevalence of CDH in live-born (Figure 8.23) infants is between 1/2000 to 1/5000 births. With fetal anomaly screening, the majority of cases are diagnosed antenatally but some infants remain undiagnosed until birth or even into childhood. CDH may be associated with other anomalies such as aneuploidy and structural cardiac and genitourinary abnormalities. A number of different antenatal and postnatal features have been studied in an attempt to determine specific predictors of outcome although prognosis remains somewhat unpredictable. Associated abnormalities are indicative of a poor outcome.

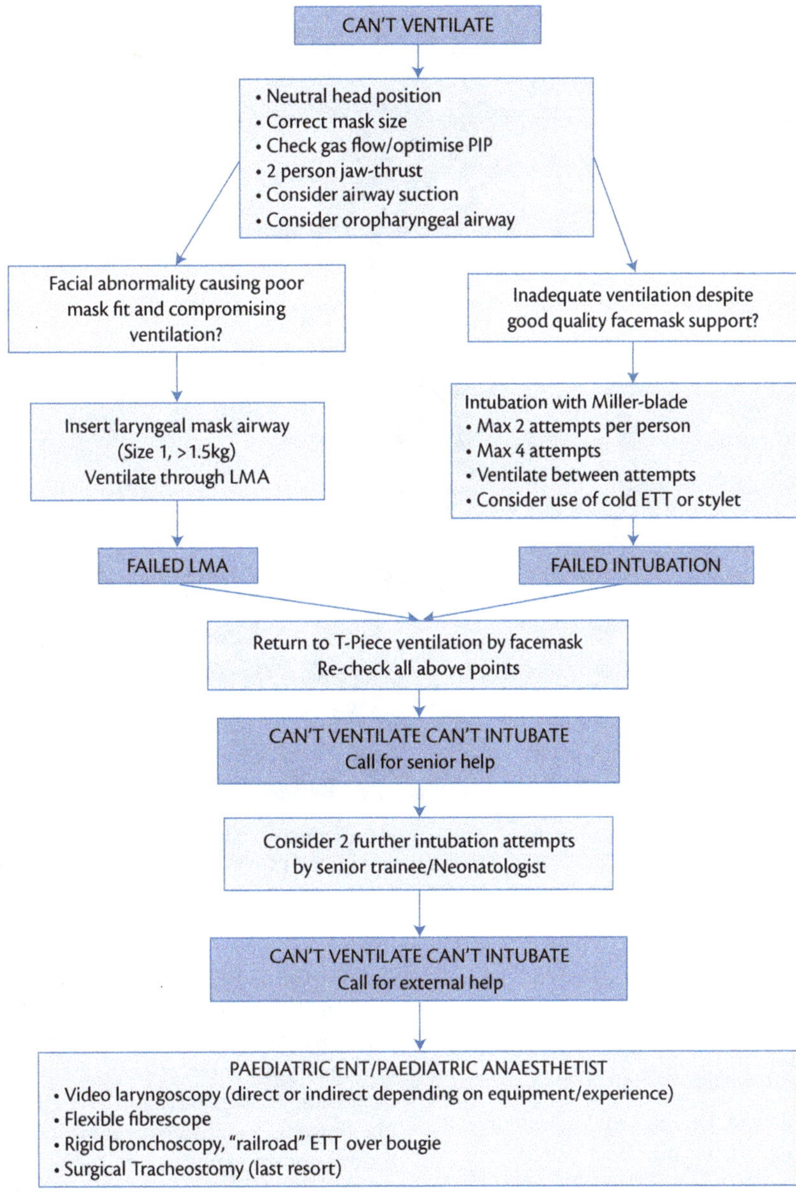

Figure 8.23 Flowchart for managing a neonatal 'Can't ventilate, can't intubate' scenar.[126]

The hernia is a space-occupying lesion which impairs lung growth and may cause mediastinal shift. There is reduction not only in lung weight and volume but also in the number of bronchial branches and alveoli. Pulmonary vessels are reduced in number and contain a high content of smooth muscle which exhibits an exaggerated response to hypoxia, acidosis, and hypercarbia and leads to pulmonary hypertension.

Internationally it has been shown that a protocol approach to management can improve some aspects of outcome with CDH.[127] Professional guidelines have recently been published in Scotland to support management decisions at birth and in the early neonatal period.[128]

The principles of resuscitation and stabilization

1. Achieve oxygenation while avoiding volutrauma/barotrauma of the existing lung tissue
2. Restore cardiac output
3. Minimize gaseous distension of the bowel

A strategy of 'gentle ventilation' with permissive hypercapnia is now standard practice, with high-frequency oscillatory ventilation (HFOV) and paralysis often required. Pulmonary hypertension is commonly treated after admission with inhaled nitric oxide. This approach, with delayed surgery may result in survival in 60–70% of cases.[129,130]

The approach to resuscitation

1. Ensure a senior paediatrician and neonatal team of appropriate skill mix are present.
2. Dry and wrap the infant.
3. Monitor SpO_2, heart rate, and temperature.

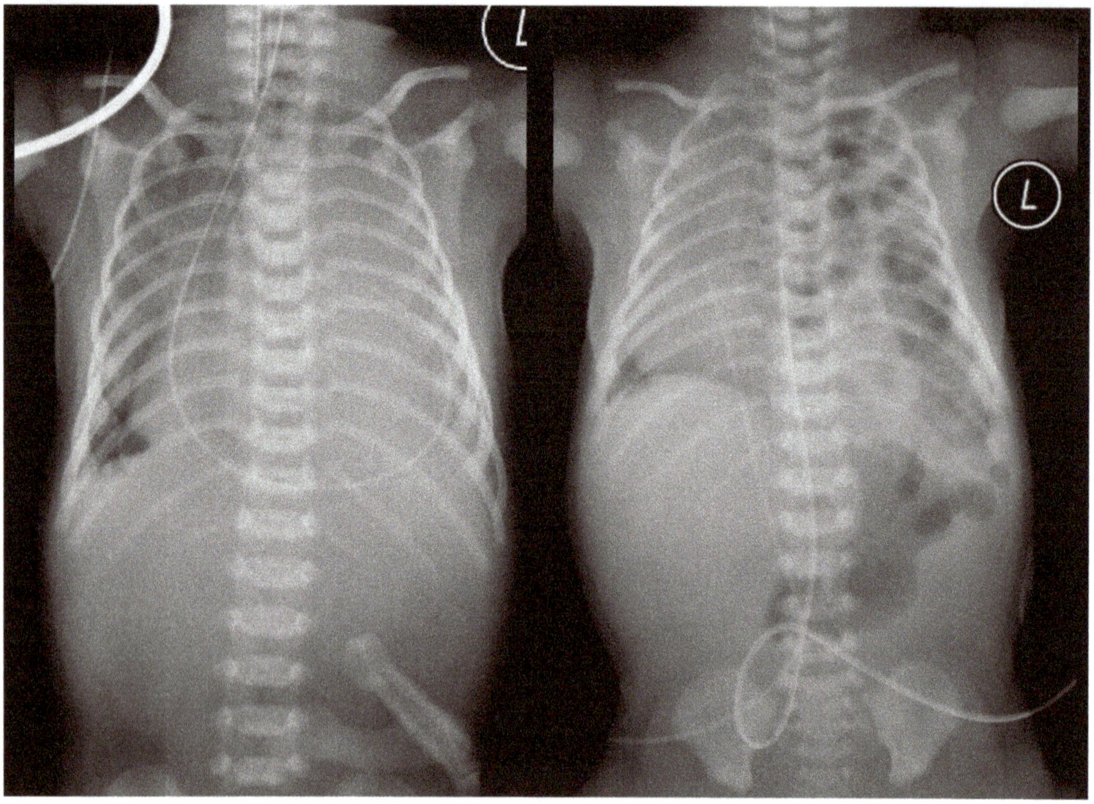

Figure 8.24 Two X-rays of infants with a congenital diaphragmatic hernia. The X-ray on the left demonstrates an infant with a left-sided diaphragmatic hernia who was intubated and paralysed from shortly after delivery. The ETT is at T1. The NGT can be seen in the intrathoracic stomach, and there is no gas in the gut. Contrast with the infant on the right, who has no gastric tube *in situ*, and a large amount of gas in the gut.

4. Intubate immediately using an appropriately sized ETT and secure.
5. Insert a large-bore (10 F) gastric tube, orally or nasally, secure, aspirate, and leave on free drainage.
6. Inflate the lungs. PIP should be limited to pressures of 25 cmH_2O or less. Higher pressures may be required initially to achieve chest wall expansion and an adequate heart rate.
7. Aim for preductal SpO_2 of 80–95%, with lower saturations acceptable if improving and the heart rate is stable.
8. Secure peripheral intravenous access and administer muscle relaxant and sedation to avoid swallowing of air and minimize respiratory asynchrony.
9. A fluid bolus of 10–20 mL/kg of intravenous 0.9% sodium chloride may be administered to improve perfusion and systemic pressure.
10. Alert the neonatal unit of delivery and transfer for admission.
11. Alert the surgical team of the birth and the condition of the infant.

Abdominal wall defects

Abdominal wall defects generally comprise two conditions: exomphalos and gastroschisis. Though such infants are usually vigorous at birth, such defects require additional care and early, if not urgent, liaison with a paediatric surgical team. As such, delivery is usually planned either in or near a surgical centre with a neonatal team in attendance at delivery.

Exomphalos results from herniation of the bowel into the umbilical cord and may range from a small cord hernia to a large defect containing bowel and liver. The prevalence is 1/5000 births. The bowel is usually covered but the exomphalos sac may sometimes rupture exposing the bowel. Exomphalos is important to distinguish from gastroschisis clinically as the former is associated with other abnormalities in around 50% of cases including structural cardiac malformations, aneuploidies and conditions such as Beckwith–Wiedemann syndrome.

The pathogenesis of gastroschisis is less clear. It is commoner in younger mothers.[131] The prevalence ranges from 1/2000 to 1/10,000 births.[132] The abdominal wall defect typically lies to the right of the umbilical cord through which small and large bowel, and gonads may prolapse.

The principles of stabilization in abdominal wall defects include:

- facilitating normal cardiorespiratory transition
- avoiding distension of the bowel with air
- avoiding ischaemic damage to the gut secondary to vascular compression at the sides of the defect
- minimizing heat and fluid loss from the gut.

The following equipment should be available in advance:

- Standard resuscitation equipment, including blankets and hat

- Plastic bag
- Equipment for venous cannulation and blood tests including blood group and save
- Wide-bore nasogastric tube (NGT) (size 10)
- Fluid bolus for use if required.

The approach to stabilization at birth:

1. Have a neonatal team in attendance with appropriate skill mix.
2. Alert the paediatric surgical team in advance of birth where possible.
3. Deliver the infant feet-first into a plastic bag secured under their arms.
4. Dry their head and arms and put a hat on them.
5. Inspect the bowel without handling it unnecessarily as this may cause vasospasm. The bowel may appear normal or thickened and covered with a fibrin peel. Poorly perfused black bowel indicates ischaemia and requires urgent discussion with the paediatric surgical team.
6. Maintain the airway in a neutral position. If resuscitation permits, it is recommended that the infant is placed in a right lateral position to avoid traction on the mesenteric vasculature or compression of the bowel beneath the body.
7. In gastroschisis, a towel over the plastic bag may protect exposed bowel from overhead radiant heating, once a satisfactory position is established. If used the towel must be periodically removed to assess gut perfusion.
8. Place a large-bore (10 F) NGT, secure and on free drainage. Regularly aspirate.
9. If the infant requires manual breaths to support respiration, mask ventilation should be avoided as this may result in gaseous bowel distension. Intubation is preferred.
10. Monitor heart rate and SpO_2.
11. Secure intravenous access in the upper limbs and replace losses as estimated by aspiration of the intestinal exudate accumulating within the bag.
    a. Assess perfusion clinically, including colour of the gut.
    b. Volume expansion may be required to optimize perfusion of the bowel and it is not unusual for infants with gastroschisis to require 20–60 mL/kg of volume in the first 6 hours of life.
12. Prophylactic systemic antibiotics may be recommended by local protocol.
13. Infants should be considered at high risk of hypoglycaemia:
    a. Increased metabolic losses
    b. Association of exomphalos with Beckwith–Wiedemann syndrome (infants may have hyperinsulinism)
14. Allow parents time to be with their baby following initial resuscitation.

Surgical repair depends on the nature and the size of the defect. For both exomphalos and gastroschisis, options include primary repair or staged silo reduction for large lesions and primary reduction of small defects. A further option in exomphalos is to promote epithelialization of the sac with a delayed ventral hernia repair.

Infants who do not respond

The commonest reason for non-response to standard resuscitative measures is inadequate airway management. Measures to optimize airway patency and ventilation are discussed in previous sections.

Cyanosis

Where infants remain blue with a good heart rate, the oxygen saturation should be checked. Many babies will only achieve saturations above 90% by 10 minutes after birth. Causes of continued low saturations include respiratory (e.g. pneumonia, pneumothorax, congenital diaphragmatic hernia) or cardiac pathology (usually mixing conditions such as atrioventricular septal defect or truncus arteriosus). Occasionally cyanosis may be due to persistence of high pulmonary artery pressure following birth, persistent pulmonary hypertension of the newborn.

Adequacy of ventilation should be assessed and optimized where necessary, oxygen should be administered to improve saturations, and the infant admitted to the neonatal unit for further assessment.

Inadequate respiratory drive

Continued poor respiratory effort following lung aeration/oxygenation may result from prolonged asphyxia, infection, prematurity, or opiate depression. Any infant who has required prolonged respiratory support in the delivery suite should be admitted to the neonatal unit for further evaluation and monitoring, and ventilatory support. Naloxone may be rarely required to reverse the effects of maternal opiates.

Prolonged asystole

The long-term outcome in surviving infants with an Apgar score of zero at 10 minutes of age is generally extremely poor and historically over 95% of such infants die or suffer severe disability.[106] The influence of therapeutic hypothermia on outcome in these infants is not clear but in one large multicentre trial, a quarter of infants who survived to receive cooling treatment in the neonatal unit were alive and well at follow-up.[133] ILCOR considers that it may be justifiable to stop resuscitation if there are no signs of life after 10 minutes of continuous and adequate resuscitation.[8] It should be appreciated that 10 minutes of age and 10 minutes of effective resuscitation are not necessarily equivalent.

Communication and record-keeping

Communication

Resuscitation

Gathering key facts about the mother and the fetus before delivery will aid the approach to resuscitation and help plan the composition of your team. Communication tools such as SBAR (Situation, Background, Assessment, and Recommendation) are increasingly used to improve timely and effective communication, a key factor in reducing risk and near miss within hospital settings (Table 8.11).[134]

Table 8.11 Example of SBAR communication

Situation Who are you? Where are you? What is happening?	'I am the senior midwife on labour ward, we have a 33-year-old woman admitted to labour ward in labour at 28 weeks' gestation'
Background Key features of the mother, pregnancy, labour or baby to date?	'The woman was discharged yesterday after presenting with ruptured membranes at 27 weeks. She received a full course of steroids, we have not had time to give magnesium'
Assessment What is the current assessment of the mother, fetus, labour, baby?	'The woman is fully dilated and starting to push. There are no fetal heart rate concerns and there is no meconium. Mum has a temperature and has had antibiotics. The resuscitaire is set up and being warmed'
Recommendation What do you want and by when?	'Please attend labour ward immediately with your senior and alert the neonatal unit'

During resuscitation, one individual, usually the most senior doctor, will take responsibility for leading the process and should ensure that both verbal instructions and responses from the team are clear and unambiguous.

Parents

It may be possible to meet with parents before the birth and explain the expected chain of events after delivery. This is a good time to discuss their expectations and concerns. Providing information in lay terminology will improve understanding and rapport.

It is increasingly common for resuscitations to take place in the delivery suite and parents may witness events which they will find frightening or which they do not understand. Information about the condition of their child should be communicated to parents as soon as possible after resuscitation. This should be done with both parents present and include the midwife looking after the mother where possible. It is critical not to offer any personal interpretation of the quality of obstetric care, instead give facts not opinions. It is good practice to check the parents' understanding of the information given. Parents may be exhausted and in a heightened state of anxiety, the mother herself may be ill, in pain, or she may have recently received analgesia or sedation—these factors may impair concentration during the discussion and comprehension of the situation.

Parents should be given the opportunity to see and touch their child even where admission to the neonatal unit is planned.

Any conversations should be documented in the infant's notes and include the information provided, questions asked, and the process of any decision-making, particularly where there has been a decision not to continue resuscitation.

If the infant dies, the role of postmortem in establishing death, and excluding other coexistent abnormalities is crucial.[135] A senior obstetrician or paediatrician should discuss postmortem and obtain consent, and in some cases where the cause of death cannot be ascertained, involvement of the relevant authorities will be necessary. Any bereaved parent should be provided with contact information and a meeting should take place with a senior paediatrician at 6 weeks.[136]

Other health professionals

All health professionals are responsible for ensuring that high-quality information is communicated in an effective way to individual parties. Verbal information should be supported by written documentation of the information shared. Where resuscitation has been difficult or unsuccessful, it is important to be aware that both junior and senior members of the team may need immediate support. It may be beneficial to recall the team at a later time for a formal debrief.

Record-keeping

All written documentation should occur as contemporaneously with events as possible in a legible form and in black ink. Entries should be signed with name and role given in block capitals (± professional registration number), and dated with the time of entry. Retrospective entries should have the time of entry recorded, as well as the time of events.

Accurate, factual accounts of the infant's condition and response should be provided along with a timeline of events, including the date and time of your summons and attendance (Box 8.9). Subjective terms such as 'Poor condition at delivery' or 'Difficult delivery' should be avoided.

Any scribing of events that has occurred during the resuscitation should be filed in the notes. As with verbal communication, avoid making assumptions about causation and ensure that if opinion is recorded that it is clearly documented as such.

Procedures

Neonatal intubation

In the delivery suite, an oral approach to intubation of the trachea is commonly practised. In infants where more long-term ventilation is anticipated, there may be conversion to a nasal tube with premedication in the neonatal unit.

Equipment

- Appropriately sized face mask
- T-piece or self-inflating bag
- Supply of air and oxygen
- Suction and large-bore catheter
- Stethoscope

Box 8.9 Key information to record after newborn resuscitation

- Condition of baby on first assessment (colour, tone, heart rate, and respirations)
- What measures of resuscitation were instituted
- When there was first good aeration of the lungs
- When the heart rate first rose above 100 bpm
- When infant made first respiratory effort
- Nature of first respiratory effort (e.g. gasp)
- Dose, route, and timing of any drugs
- Name and designation of staff present
- Cord blood gas results.

- Straight blade laryngoscope with working light and appropriately sized blade
- Range of ETT sizes (uncuffed) (Table 8.11)
- Fixation device for ETT
- Saturation monitor (if available)
- Carbon dioxide colorimeter (if available)
- Stylet introducer (optional).

Procedure

1. Prepare equipment.
2. Maintain good oxygenation and ventilation by facemask. A saturation monitor should be in place if available.
3. Place the laryngoscope in the mouth, over the tongue, guarding the gums with the thumb and forefinger of the right hand, and advance until the epiglottis is visualized. Avoid overextension of the neck as this will position the larynx very anteriorly.
4. Remove any secretions present that obscure visualization, under direct laryngoscopy. Be careful not to over-stimulate the pharyngeal wall and larynx as this may cause reflex bradycardia and spasm of the vocal cords.
5. Position oneself to ensure a view down the laryngoscope and ultimately the trachea.
6. With the laryngoscope blade in the vallecula, lift the epiglottis upward using a vertical motion of the laryngoscope blade; avoid pivoting around the end of the blade.
7. The larynx and vocal cords should be in view. Downward pressure on the cricoid may facilitate the view of the larynx.
8. With the right hand, bring the ETT in from the right angle of the mouth and not down the central groove of the laryngoscope blade where it will obscure the view.
9. If the cords are adducted, wait for them to relax, rather than forcing the tube through. Insert the tracheal tube through the cords advancing only 1–2 cm.
10. Withdraw the blade while fixing the tube against the superior alveolar ridge of the gum with the left forefinger.
11. Connect to the ventilation device and assess chest expansion. A colorimetric CO_2 detector is recommended to confirm ETT placement.
12. Auscultate for equality of air entry and heart rate. The end of the tube should be mid trachea.
13. Ensure the tube remains *in situ* while being secured.

Conclusion

In this chapter, the physiology of fetal-neonatal transition has been described, and this understanding applied to the structured approach to the newborn who does not breathe after delivery. The skills of newborn resuscitation are best learned on a recognized course, followed by a period of practice. It is hoped that this chapter has provided a useful and interesting adjunct to these courses enabling the interested reader to further explore a fascinating area of medicine.

References

1. World Health Organization. *Levels and Trends in Child Mortality 2012*. [Online] http://www.who.int/maternal_child_adolescent/documents/levels_trends_child_mortality_2012/en/
2. Azzopardi DV, Strohm B, Edwards AD, *et al.* Moderate hypothermia to treat perinatal asphyxial encephalopathy. *N Engl J Med* 2009; 361(14):1349–58.
3. Edwards AD, Brocklehurst P, Gunn AJ, *et al.* Neurological outcomes at 18 months of age after moderate hypothermia for perinatal hypoxic ischaemic encephalopathy: synthesis and meta-analysis of trial data. *BMJ* 2010; 340:c363.
4. Budin P. *Le Nourrisson* [The Nursling]. Paris: Doin; 1907.
5. Palme-Kilander C. Methods of resuscitation in low-Apgar-score newborn infants—a national survey. *Acta Paediatr* 1992; 81(10):739–44.
6. Kroll L, Twohey L, Daubeney PEF, *et al.* Risk factors at delivery and the need for skilled resuscitation. *Eur J Obstet Gynecol Reprod Biol* 1994; 55(3):175–7.
7. O'Donnell CPF, Gibson AT, Davis PG. Pinching, electrocution, ravens' beaks, and positive pressure ventilation: a brief history of neonatal resuscitation. *Arch Dis Child Fetal Neonatal Ed* 2006; 91(5):F369–F373.
8. International Liaison Committee on Resuscitation. The International Liaison Committee on Resuscitation (ILCOR) consensus on science with treatment recommendations for pediatric and neonatal patients: pediatric basic and advanced life support. *Pediatrics* 2006; 117(5):e955–e977.
9. Kiserud T, Acharya G. The fetal circulation. *Prenatal Diag* 2004; 24(13):1049–59.
10. Dildy GA, van den Berg PP, Katz M, *et al.* Intrapartum fetal pulse oximetry: fetal oxygen saturation trends during labor and relation to delivery outcome. *Am J Obstet Gynecol* 1994; 171(3):679–84.
11. Walters DV, Olver RE. The role of catecholamines in lung liquid absorption at birth. *Pediatr Res* 1978; 12(3):239–42.
12. Jain L, Eaton DC. Physiology of fetal lung fluid clearance and the effect of labor. *Semin Perinatol* 2006; 30(1):34–43.
13. Richmond S (ed). *Resuscitation at Birth: Newborn Life Support Provider Course Manual* (3rd ed). London: Resuscitation Council (UK); 2011.
14. Vyas H, Field D, Milner AD, Hopkin IE. Determinants of the first inspiratory volume and functional residual capacity at birth. *Pediatr Pulmonol* 1986; 2(4):189–93.
15. te Pas AB, Wong C, Kamlin CO, *et al.* Breathing patterns in preterm and term infants immediately after Birth. *Pediatric Res* 2009; 65(3):352–6.
16. Dawson JA, Kamlin COF, Wong C, *et al.* Changes in heart rate in the first minutes after birth. *Arch Dis Child Fetal Neonatal Ed* 2010; 95(3):F177–F181.
17. Dawson JA, Kamlin COF, Vento M, *et al.* Defining the reference range for oxygen saturation for infants after birth. *Pediatrics* 2010; 125(6):e1340–1347.
18. Dawes GS. *Foetal and Neonatal Physiology: A Comparative Study of the Changes at Birth*. Chicago, IL: Year Book Medical Publishers; 1968.
19. Cross KW. Resuscitation of the asphyxiated infant. *Br Med Bull* 1966; 22(1):73–8.
20. Shelley HJ, Neligan GA. Neonatal hypoglycaemia. *Br Med Bull* 1966; 22(1):34–9.
21. Yager JY. Hypoglycemic injury to the immature brain. *Clin Perinatol* 2002; 29(4):651–74.
22. Martin RJ, Bookatz GB, Gelfand SL, *et al.* Consequences of neonatal resuscitation with supplemental oxygen. *Semin Perinatol* 2008; 32(5):355–66.
23. Saugstad OD, Ramji S, Vento M. Resuscitation of depressed newborn infants with ambient air or pure oxygen: a meta-analysis. *Biol Neonate* 2005; 87(1):27–34.

24. Davis PG, Tan A, O'Donnell CPF, *et al.* Resuscitation of newborn infants with 100% oxygen or air: a systematic review and meta-analysis. *Lancet* 2004; 364(9442):1329–33.
25. Vento M, Asensi M, Sastre J, *et al.* Resuscitation with room air instead of 100% oxygen prevents oxidative stress in moderately asphyxiated term neonates. *Pediatrics* 2001; 107(4):642–7.
26. Hawkes CP, Oni OA, Dempsey EM, *et al.* Potential hazard of the Neopuff T-piece resuscitator in the absence of flow limitation. *Arch Dis Child Fetal Neonatal Ed* 2009; 94(6):F461–F463.
27. Ammari A, Suri M, Milisavljevic V, *et al.* Variables associated with the early failure of nasal CPAP in very low birth weight infants. *J Pediatr* 2005; 147(3):341–7.
28. Carlo WA. Gentle ventilation: the new evidence from the SUPPORT, COIN, VON, CURPAP, Colombian Network, and Neocosur Network trials. *Early Hum Dev* 2012; 88 Suppl 2:S81–S83.
29. Morley CJ, Davis PG, Doyle LW, *et al.* Nasal CPAP or intubation at birth for very preterm infants. *N Engl J Med* 2008; 358(7):700–8.
30. Support Study Group of the Eunice Kennedy Shriver NICHD Neonatal Research Network. Early CPAP versus surfactant in extremely preterm infants. *N Engl J Med* 2010; 362(21):1970–79.
31. Siew ML, Pas AB te, Wallace MJ, *et al.* Positive end-expiratory pressure enhances development of a functional residual capacity in preterm rabbits ventilated from birth. *J Appl Physiol* 2009; 106(5):1487–93.
32. Finer NN, Barrington KJ, Al-Fadley F, *et al.* Limitations of self-inflating resuscitators. *Pediatrics* 1986; 77(3):417–20.
33. Field DJ, Milner AD, Hopkin IE. Efficacy of manual resuscitation at birth. *Arch Dis Child* 1986; 61:300–2.
34. Oddie S, Wyllie J, Scally A. Use of self-inflating bags for neonatal resuscitation. *Resuscitation* 2005; 67(1):109–12.
35. Hussey SG, Ryan CA, Murphy BP. Comparison of three manual ventilation devices using an intubated mannequin. *Arch Dis Child Fetal Neonatal Ed* 2004; 89(6):F490–3.
36. Leone TA, Rich W, Finer NN. A survey of delivery room resuscitation practices in the United States. *Pediatrics* 2006; 117(2):e164–e175.
37. Milner AD, Vyas H, Hopkin IE. Efficacy of facemask resuscitation at birth. *Br Med J (Clin Res Ed)* 1984; 289(6458):1563–5.
38. Royal College of Paediatrics and Child Health, Royal College of Obstetricians and Gynaecologists (Great Britain). *Resuscitation of Babies at Birth.* London: BMJ Publishing Group; 1997.
39. Rennie JM, Roberton NRC. *Roberton's Textbook of Neonatology.* Edinburgh: Elsevier/Churchill Livingstone; 2005.
40. Wood FE, Morley CJ, Dawson JA, *et al.* Assessing the effectiveness of two round neonatal resuscitation masks: study 1. *Arch Dis Child Fetal Neonatal Ed* 2008; 93(3):F235–7.
41. O'Donnell CPF, Davis PG, Lau R, *et al.* Neonatal resuscitation 2: an evaluation of manual ventilation devices and face masks. *Arch Dis Child Fetal Neonatal Ed* 2005; 90(5):F392–6.
42. Wood FE, Morley CJ, Dawson JA, *et al.* Improved techniques reduce face mask leak during simulated neonatal resuscitation: study 2. *Arch Dis Child Fetal Neonatal Ed* 2008; 93(3):F230–4.
43. Rennie JM, Roberton NRC. *Rennie and Roberton's Textbook of Neonatology.* Edinburgh: Churchill Livingstone/Elsevier; 2012.
44. Paterson S, Byrne P, Molesky M, Seal R, Finucane B. Neonatal resuscitation using the laryngeal mask airway. *Anesthesiology* 1994; 80(6):1248–53.
45. Grein AJ, Weiner GM. Laryngeal mask airway versus bag-mask ventilation or endotracheal intubation for neonatal resuscitation. *Cochrane Database Syst Rev.* 2005; 2:CD003314.
46. Baraka A. Laryngeal mask airway for resuscitation of a newborn with Pierre-Robin syndrome. *Anesthesiology* 1995; 83(3):646–7.
47. Aziz HF, Martin JB, Moore JJ. The pediatric disposable end-tidal carbon dioxide detector role in endotracheal intubation in newborns. *J Perinatol* 1999; 19(2):110–13.
48. Kamlin CO, Colm PFO, Peter GD, *et al.* Colorimetric end-tidal carbon dioxide detectors in the delivery room: strengths and limitations. A case report. *J Pediatr* 2005; 147(4):547–8.
49. Wyllie J, Carlo WA. The role of carbon dioxide detectors for confirmation of endotracheal tube position. *Clin Perinatol* 2006; 33(1):111–19.
50. Hughes SM, Blake BL, Woods SL, *et al.* False-positive results on colorimetric carbon dioxide analysis in neonatal resuscitation: potential for serious patient harm. *J Perinatol* 2007; 27(12):800–1.
51. Finer NN, Rich W, Wang C, *et al.* Airway obstruction during mask ventilation of very low birth weight infants during neonatal resuscitation. *Pediatrics* 2009; 123(3):865–9.
52. Leone TA, Lange A, Rich W, *et al.* Disposable colorimetric carbon dioxide detector use as an indicator of a patent airway during noninvasive mask ventilation. *Pediatrics* 2006; 118(1):e202–204.
53. Dawson JA, Vento M, Finer NN, *et al.* Managing oxygen therapy during delivery room stabilization of preterm infants. *J Pediatr* 2012; 160(1):158–61.
54. Mariani GMD, Dik PBMD, Ezquer AMD, *et al.* Pre-ductal and post-ductal O2 saturation in healthy term neonates after birth. *J Pediatr* 2007; 150(4):418–21.
55. O'Donnell CPF, Kamlin COF, Davis PG, *et al.* Obtaining pulse oximetry data in neonates: a randomised crossover study of sensor application techniques. *Arch Dis Child Fetal Neonatal Ed* 2005; 90(1):F84–F85.
56. Kattwinkel J. *The Textbook of Neonatal Resuscitation* (5th ed). Elk Grove Village, IL: American Heart Association; 2006.
57. Schmolzer GM, Kamlin OF, Dawson JA, *et al.* Respiratory monitoring of neonatal resuscitation. *Arch Dis Child Fetal Neonatal Ed* 2010; 95(4):F295–303.
58. Carbine DN, Finer NN, Knodel E, *et al.* Video recording as a means of evaluating neonatal resuscitation performance. *Pediatrics* 2000; 106(4):654–8.
59. Manning DJ. Presumed consent in emergency neonatal research. *J Med Ethics* 2000; 26(4):249.
60. Johnston ED, Stenson BJ. Am I getting chest wall movement? *Arch Dis Child Fetal Neonatal Ed* 2010; 95(6):F391–F392.
61. Gluck L, Kulovich MV, Eidelman AI, *et al.* Biochemical development of surface activity in mammalian lung. IV. Pulmonary lecithin synthesis in the human fetus and newborn and etiology of the respiratory distress syndrome. *Pediatr Res* 1972; 6(2):81–99.
62. Merritt TA, Farrell PM. Diminished pulmonary lecithin synthesis in acidosis: experimental findings as related to the respiratory distress syndrome. *Pediatrics* 1976; 57(1):32–40.
63. Obeidat HM, Bond EA, Callister LC. The parental experience of having an infant in the newborn intensive care unit. *J Perinat Educ* 2009; 18(3):23–9.
64. Laptook A, Jackson GL. Cold stress and hypoglycemia in the late preterm ("near-term") infant: impact on nursery of admission. *Semin Perinatol* 2006; 30(1):24–7.
65. World Health Organization. Division of Reproductive Health. *Thermal Protection of the Newborn: A Practical Guide.* Geneva: World Health Organization; 1997.
66. Moore ER, Anderson GC, Bergman N, Dowswell T. Early skin-to-skin contact for mothers and their healthy newborn infants. *Cochrane Database Syst Rev* 2012; 5:CD003519.
67. Becher JC, Bhushan SS, Lyon AJ. Unexpected collapse in apparently healthy newborns—a prospective national study of a missing cohort of neonatal deaths and near-death events. *Arch Dis Child Fetal Neonatal Ed* 2012; 97(1):F30–4.
68. Fairchild K, Sokora D, Scott J, *et al.* Therapeutic hypothermia on neonatal transport: 4-year experience in a single NICU. *J Perinatol* 2009; 30(5):324–9.
69. Kendall GS, Kapetanakis A, Ratnavel N, *et al.* Passive cooling for initiation of therapeutic hypothermia in neonatal encephalopathy. *Arch Dis Child Fetal Neonatal Ed* 2010; 95(6):408–13.
70. Hallberg B, Olson L, Bartocci M, *et al.* Passive induction of hypothermia during transport of asphyxiated infants: a risk of excessive cooling. *Acta Paediatr* 2009; 98(6):942–6.
71. Adams E, Austin T, Becher J-C, *et al.* *Position Statement on Therapeutic Cooling for Neonatal Encephalopathy.* The British Association of Perinatal Medicine; 2010. [Online] http://www.bapm.org/publications/documents/guidelines/Position_Statement_Therapeutic_Cooling_Neonatal_Encephalopathy_July%202010.pdf

72. Johnston ED, Becher J-C, Mitchell AP, *et al.* Provision of servo-controlled cooling during neonatal transport. *Arch Dis Child Fetal Neonatal Ed* 2012; 97(5):F365–F367.
73. Perlman JM. Hyperthermia in the delivery: potential impact on neonatal mortality and morbidity. *Clin Perinatol* 2006; 33(1):55–63.
74. Greenwell EA, Wyshak G, Ringer SA, *et al.* Intrapartum temperature elevation, epidural use, and adverse outcome in term infants. *Pediatrics* 2012; 129(2):e447–54.
75. Costeloe K, Hennessy E, Gibson AT, *et al.* The EPICure study: outcomes to discharge from hospital for infants born at the threshold of viability. *Pediatrics* 2000; 106(4):659–71.
76. Cramer K, Wiebe N, Hartling L, *et al.* Heat loss prevention: a systematic review of occlusive skin wrap for premature neonates. *J Perinatol* 2005; 25(12):763–9.
77. Almeida PG, Chandley J, Davis J, *et al.* Use of the heated gel mattress and its impact on admission temperature of very low birth-weight infants. *Adv Neonatal Care* 2009; 9(1):34–9.
78. Andersson O, Hellström-Westas L, Andersson D, *et al.* Effect of delayed versus early umbilical cord clamping on neonatal outcomes and iron status at 4 months: a randomised controlled trial. *BMJ* 2011; 343:d7157.
79. Kirpalani H, Whyte RK, Andersen C, *et al.* The Premature Infants in Need of Transfusion (PINT) study: a randomized, controlled trial of a restrictive (low) versus liberal (high) transfusion threshold for extremely low birth weight infants. *J Pediatr* 2006; 149(3):301–7.
80. Aladangady N, McHugh S, Aitchison TC, *et al.* Infants' blood volume in a controlled trial of placental transfusion at preterm delivery. *Pediatrics* 2006; 117(1):93–8.
81. Rabe H, Diaz-Rossello JL, Duley L, *et al.* Effect of timing of umbilical cord clamping and other strategies to influence placental transfusion at preterm birth on maternal and infant outcomes. *Cochrane Database Syst Rev* 2012; 8:CD003248.
82. McDonald SJ, Middleton P. Effect of timing of umbilical cord clamping of term infants on maternal and neonatal outcomes. *Cochrane Database Syst Rev* 2008; 2:CD004074.
83. Committee Opinion No.543: Timing of umbilical cord clamping after birth. *Obstet Gynecol* 2012; 120(6):1522–6.
84. Royal College of Obstetricians and Gynaecologists. *RCOG Statement on BMJ Paper on the Benefits of Delayed Cord Clamping.* 2013. [Online] http://www.rcog.org.uk/what-we-do/campaigning-and-opinions/statement/rcog-statement-bmj-paper-benefits-delayed-cord-blood-c
85. Apgar V. A proposal for a new method of evaluation of the newborn infant. *Curr Res Anesth Analg* 1953; 32(4):260–7.
86. O'Donnell CPF, Kamlin CO, Davis PG, *et al.* Clinical assessment of infant colour at delivery. *Arch Dis Child Fetal Neonatal Ed* 2007; 92(6):F465–7.
87. Kamlin CO, O'Donnell CPF, Everest NJ, *et al.* Accuracy of clinical assessment of infant heart rate in the delivery room. *Resuscitation* 2006; 71(3):319–21.
88. Volpe JJ. *Neurology of the Newborn* (5th ed.) Philadelphia, PA: Saunders/Elsevier; 2008.
89. Manley BJ, Dawson JA, Kamlin CO, *et al.* Clinical assessment of extremely premature infants in the delivery room is a poor predictor of survival. *Pediatrics* 2010; 125(3):e559–64.
90. Vyas H, Milner AD, Hopkin IE, *et al.* Physiologic responses to prolonged and slow-rise inflation in the resuscitation of the asphyxiated newborn infant. *J Pediatr* 1981; 99(4):635–9.
91. te Pas AB, Siew M, Wallace MJ, *et al.* Establishing functional residual capacity at birth: the effect of sustained inflation and positive end-expiratory pressure in a preterm rabbit model. *Pediatr Res* 2009; 65(5):537–41.
92. Schmölzer GM, Dawson JA, Kamlin COF, *et al.* Airway obstruction and gas leak during mask ventilation of preterm infants in the delivery room. *Arch Dis Child Fetal Neonatal Ed* 2011; 96(4):F254–7.
93. Wiswell TE, Gannon CM, Jacob J, *et al.* Delivery room management of the apparently vigorous meconium-stained neonate: results of the multicenter, international collaborative trial. *Pediatrics* 2000; 105(1):1–7.
94. Rudikoff MT, Maughan WL, Effron M, *et al.* Mechanisms of blood flow during cardiopulmonary resuscitation. *Circulation* 1980; 61(2):345–52.
95. Finholt DA, Kettrick RG, Wagner HR, *et al.* The heart is under the lower third of the sternum: implications for external cardiac massage. *Am J Dis Child* 1986; 140(7):646–9.
96. Orlowski JP. Optimum position for external cardiac compression in infants and young children. *Ann Emerg Med* 1986; 15(6):667–73.
97. Phillips GWL, Zideman DA. Relation of infant heart to sternum: its significance in cardiopulmonary resuscitation. *Lancet* 1986; 327(8488):1024–5.
98. Dorfsman ML, Menegazzi JJ, Wadas RJ, *et al.* Two-thumb vs two-finger chest compression in an infant model of prolonged cardiopulmonary resuscitation. *Acad Emerg Med* 2000; 7(10):1077–82.
99. Houri PK, Frank LR, Menegazzi JJ, *et al.* A randomized, controlled trial of two-thumb vs two-finger chest compression in a swine infant model of cardiac arrest. *Prehospit Emerg Care* 1997; 1(2):65–7.
100. Menegazzi JJ, Auble TE, Nicklas KA, *et al.* Two-thumb versus two-finger chest compression during CPR in a swine infant model of cardiac arrest. *Ann Emerg Med* 1993; 22(2):240–3.
101. Whitelaw CC, Slywka B, Goldsmith LJ. Comparison of a two-finger versus two-thumb method for chest compressions by healthcare providers in an infant mechanical model. *Resuscitation* 2000; 43(3):213–16.
102. Meyer A, Nadkarni V, Pollock A, *et al.* Evaluation of the Neonatal Resuscitation Program's recommended chest compression depth using computerized tomography imaging. *Resuscitation* 2010; 81(5):544–8.
103. Hemway RJ, Christman C, Perlman J. The 3:1 is superior to a 15:2 ratio in a newborn manikin model in terms of quality of chest compressions and number of ventilations. *Arch Dis Child Fetal Neonatal Ed* 2013; 98(1):F42–F45.
104. Solevåg AL, Dannevig I, Wyckoff M, *et al.* Return of spontaneous circulation with a compression:ventilation ratio of 15:2 versus 3:1 in newborn pigs with cardiac arrest due to asphyxia. *Arch Dis Child Fetal Neonatal Ed* 2011; 96(6):F417–F421.
105. Berkowitz ID, Chantarojanasiri T, Koehler RC, *et al.* Blood flow during cardiopulmonary resuscitation with simultaneous compression and ventilation in infant pigs. *Pediatr Res* 1989; 26(6):558–9.
106. Harrington DJ, Redman CW, Moulden M, *et al.* The long-term outcome in surviving infants with Apgar zero at 10 minutes: a systematic review of the literature and hospital-based cohort. *Am J Obstet Gynecol* 2007; 196(5):463.e1–5.
107. Tyson JE, Parikh NA, Langer J, *et al.* Intensive care for extreme prematurity—moving beyond gestational age. *N Engl J Med.* 2008; 358(16):1672–81.
108. Doyle LW, Anderson PJ. Adult outcome of extremely preterm infants. *Pediatrics* 2010; 126(2):342–51.
109. Moore T, Hennessy EM, Myles J, *et al.* Neurological and developmental outcome in extremely preterm children born in England in 1995 and 2006: the EPICure studies. *BMJ* 2012; 345:e7961.
110. Inder TE, Volpe JJ. Mechanisms of perinatal brain injury. *Semin Neonatol* 2000; 5(1):3–16.
111. National Institutes of Health Consensus Development Conference Statement. Effect of corticosteroids for fetal maturation on perinatal outcomes. *NIH Consens Statement* 1994; 12(2):1–24.
112. Royal College of Obstetricians and Gynaecologists. *Antenatal Corticosteroids to Reduce Neonatal Morbidity.* Green-top Guideline No. 7. London: RCOG; 2014. http://www.rcog.org.uk/womens-health/clinical-guidance/antenatal-corticosteroids-prevent-respiratory-distress-syndrome-gree
113. Crowley P, Chalmers I, Keirse MJ. The effects of corticosteroid administration before preterm delivery: an overview of the evidence from controlled trials. *Br J Obstet Gynaecol* 1990; 97(1):11–25.

114. Roberts D, Dalziel S. Antenatal corticosteroids for accelerating fetal lung maturation for women at risk of preterm birth. *Cochrane Database Syst Rev* 2006; 3:CD004454.
115. Doyle LW, Crowther CA, Middleton P, *et al.* Magnesium sulphate for women at risk of preterm birth for neuroprotection of the fetus. *Cochrane Database Syst Rev* 2009; 1:CD004661.
116. Royal College of Obstetricians and Gynaecologists. *Magnesium Sulphate to Prevent Cerebral Palsy Following Preterm Birth.* Scientific Impact Paper 29. London: RCOG; 2011. http://www.rcog.org.uk/womens-health/clinical-guidance/magnesium-sulphate-prevent-cerebral-palsy-following-preterm-birth-sa
117. Dunn MS, Kaempf J, De Klerk A, *et al.* Randomized trial comparing 3 approaches to the initial respiratory management of preterm neonates. *Pediatrics* 2011; 128(5):e1069–76.
118. Seger N, Soll R. Animal derived surfactant extract for treatment of respiratory distress syndrome. *Cochrane Database Syst Rev* 2009; 2:CD007836.
119. Davis JM, Auten RL. Maturation of the antioxidant system and the effects on preterm birth. *Semin Fetal Neonatal Med* 2010; 15(4):191–5.
120. Stenson B, Brocklehurst P, Tarnow-Mordi W. Increased 36-week survival with high oxygen saturation target in extremely preterm infants. *N Engl J Med* 2011; 364(17):1680–2.
121. Wyckoff MH, Salhab WA, Heyne RJ, *et al.* Outcome of extremely low birth weight infants who received delivery room cardiopulmonary resuscitation. *J Pediatr* 2012; 160(2):239–244.e2.
122. Wilkinson AR, Ahluwalia J, Cole A, *et al.* Management of babies born extremely preterm at less than 26 weeks of gestation: a framework for clinical practice at the time of birth. *Arch Dis Child Fetal Neonatal Ed* 2008; 94(1):2–5.
123. Nuffield Council on Bioethics. *Critical Care Decisions in Fetal and Neonatal Medicine : Ethical Issues.* London: Nuffield Council on Bioethics; 2006.
124. Costeloe KL, Hennessy EM, Haider S, *et al.* Short term outcomes after extreme preterm birth in England: comparison of two birth cohorts in 1995 and 2006 (the EPICure studies). *BMJ* 2012; 345:e7976.
125. Hirose S, Farmer DL, Lee H, *et al.* The ex utero intrapartum treatment procedure: looking back at the EXIT. *J Pediatr Surg* 2004; 39(3):375–80.
126. Johansen LC, Mupanemunda RH, Danha RF. Managing the newborn infant with a difficult airway. *Infant* 2012; 8(4):116–19.
127. Reiss I, Schaible T, Van den Hout L, *et al.* Standardized postnatal management of infants with congenital diaphragmatic hernia in Europe: the CDH EURO Consortium consensus. *Neonatology* 2010; 98(4):354–64.
128. Munro FD. *Inpatient Management Standards for CDH.* Scottish Diaphragmatic Hernia Clinical Network; 2012 [Online] http://www.sdhcn.scot.nhs.uk/Documents/SDHCN%20IN-PATIENT%20GUIDELINES%2025.09.12.pdf
129. Migliazza L, Bellan C, Alberti D, *et al.* Retrospective study of 111 cases of congenital diaphragmatic hernia treated with early high-frequency oscillatory ventilation and presurgical stabilization. *J Pediatr Surg* 2007; 42(9):1526–32.
130. Boloker J, Bateman DA, Wung JT, *et al.* Congenital diaphragmatic hernia in 120 infants treated consecutively with permissive hypercapnea/spontaneous respiration/elective repair. *J Pediatr Surg* 2002; 37(3):357–66.
131. Curry JI, McKinney P, Thornton JG, *et al.* The aetiology of gastroschisis. *Br J Obstet Gynaecol* 2000; 107(11):1339–46.
132. Kilby MD. The incidence of gastroschisis. *BMJ* 2006; 332(7536):250–1.
133. Laptook AR, O'Shea TM, Shankaran S, *et al.* Adverse neurodevelopmental outcomes among extremely low birth weight infants with a normal head ultrasound: prevalence and antecedents. *Pediatrics* 2005; 115(3):673–80.
134. WHO Collaborating Centre for Patient Safety Solutions. *Communication During Patient Hand-Overs.* WHO; 2007. [Online] http://www.who.int/patientsafety/solutions/patientsafety/PS-Solution3.pdf
135. Brodlie M, Laing IA, Keeling JW, *et al.* Ten years of neonatal autopsies in tertiary referral centre: retrospective study. *BMJ* 2002; 324(7340):761–3.
136. McHaffie HE, Laing IA, Lloyd DJ. Follow up care of bereaved parents after treatment withdrawal from newborns. *Arch Dis Child Fetal Neonatal Ed* 2001; 84(2):F125–8.

PART 4

Fertility treatment, anaesthesia for non-obstetric surgery, and drugs in pregnancy and lactation

CHAPTER 9

Fertility treatment in the modern age: possibilities and anaesthesia

Diane De Neubourg and Sarah Devroe

Introduction

Assisted reproductive technology (ART) is part of medically assisted reproduction and comprises all treatments or procedures that include the *in vitro* handling of both human oocytes and sperm or of embryos for the purpose of establishing a pregnancy. This includes, but is not limited to, *in vitro* fertilization (IVF) and embryo transfer, gamete intrafallopian transfer, zygote intrafallopian transfer, tubal embryo transfer, gamete and embryo cryopreservation, oocyte and embryo donation, and gestational surrogacy.[1,2] ART does not include assisted insemination (artificial insemination) using sperm from either a woman's partner or a sperm donor or surgery.

ART is becoming increasingly important and is responsible for up to 4% of all pregnancies in Europe in 2009.[3]

In 2004, 2184 clinics from 52 countries and regions worldwide have reported their outcomes of ART to the International Committee for Monitoring Assisted Reproductive Technologies (ICMART) and are reporting on types of cycles and procedures, pregnancy, delivery and multiple birth rates, and perinatal outcomes.[4] A total of 954,743 initiated cycles resulted in an estimated 237,809 babies born. The availability of ART varied by country and ranged from 14 to 3844 treatment cycles per million inhabitants. Of all cycles, 60.6% were intracytoplasmic sperm injection (ICSI). Frozen embryo transfers (FETs) represented 31% of the initiated cycles. The overall delivery rate per fresh aspiration for IVF and ICSI was 20.2% compared with 16.6% per FET. The average number of embryos transferred was 2.35. Single (16.3%) and double embryo transfers accounted for 73.2% of cycles.

The 13th European IVF monitoring report[3] presents the results of treatments using ART initiated in Europe during 2009. From 34 countries, 1005 clinics reported 537,463 treatment cycles including IVF (135,621), ICSI (266,084), frozen embryo replacements (FERs, 104,153), egg donation (21,604), *in vitro* maturation (1334), preimplantation genetic diagnosis/screening (4389), and frozen/warmed oocyte replacements (4278). In 21 countries where all clinics reported to the ART register, a total of 399,020 ART cycles were performed in a population of 373.8 million, corresponding to 1067 cycles per million inhabitants. For IVF, the clinical pregnancy rates per aspiration and per transfer were 28.5% and 32.5%, respectively, and for ICSI the corresponding rates were 28.9% and 32.9%. In FER cycles, the pregnancy rate per thawing was 20.9%. In IVF and ICSI cycles, one, two, three, and four or more embryos were transferred in 24.2%, 57.7%, 16.9%, and 1.2%, respectively. The proportions of singleton, twin, and triplet deliveries after IVF and ICSI (combined) were 79.8%, 19.4%, and 0.8%, respectively, resulting in a total multiple delivery rate of 20.2%, compared with 21.7% in 2008, 22.3% in 2007, 20.8% in 2006, and 21.8% in 2005.

The most important complication of ART are the multiple pregnancies which have been tackled in some European countries by limiting the number of embryos for transfer, particularly in the twin-prone patient population while maintaining acceptable pregnancy rates. In Belgium, a legally enforced reduction of the number of embryos for transfer resulted in a 50% reduction of the multiple pregnancy rate from 27% to 11% since the introduction of this law in 2003 to the last assessment in 2010, without reduction of the pregnancy rate per cycle (Figure 9.1).[5]

Overview of an assisted reproductive technology procedure

An ART cycle is composed of five phases, namely controlled ovarian hyperstimulation (COH), oocyte retrieval, fertilization, embryo transfer, and luteal phase support.

Controlled ovarian hyperstimulation

Ovarian hyperstimulation has become an essential part of ART treatment. We are aiming to achieve 10–15 oocytes as this has been proven to give the highest success rates.[6] Different treatment schedules are used depending on how a premature luteinizing hormone (LH) surge is inhibited. When a gonadotropin-releasing hormone (GnRH) agonist is used, it can be done in a long down-regulation protocol or short flare-up protocol. In the long down-regulation protocol, LH and follicle-stimulating hormone (FSH) secretion are suppressed after 10–14 days after an initial flare-up. In the short flare-up protocol, gonadotropin stimulation is started during the initial flare-up of LH and FSH secretion. With GnRH antagonists, prevention of premature LH surge occurs fast and therefore no preparation in advance needs to be done. The actual stimulation of the ovaries is with gonadotrophins extracted from urine and highly purified or produced by recombinant technology. Starting doses may vary between 75 and 300 IU/day depending on age of the patient, menstrual cycle regularity, ovarian reserve testing (anti-Mullerian hormone, antral follicle count, basal FSH) and previous response to COH. The most important complication of COH is ovarian hyperstimulation syndrome (OHSS) which is a potentially very severe disease that can affect young infertile

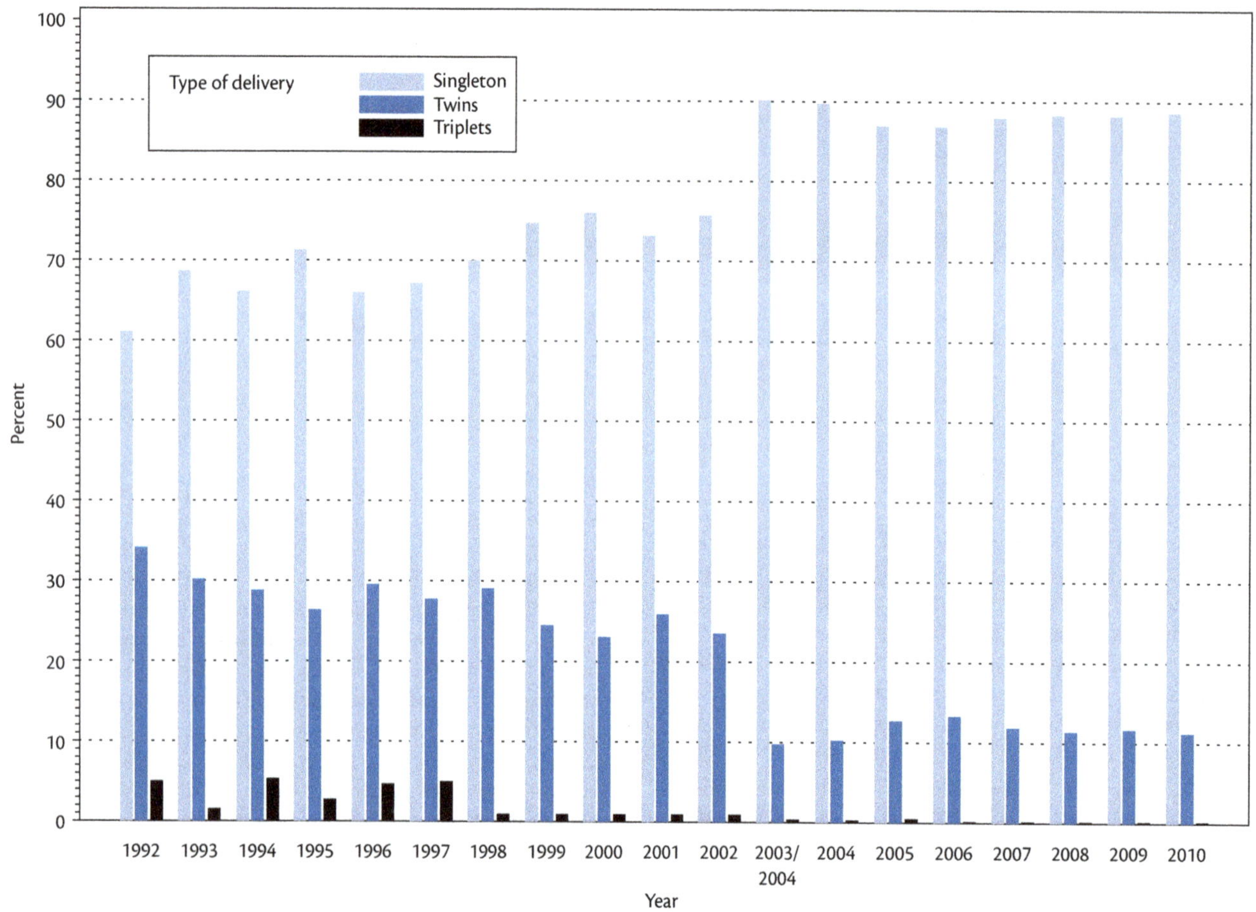

Figure 9.1 Evolution of the number of single and multiple deliveries after ART between 1992 and 2010.
http://www.Belrap.be © The College of Physicians Reproductive Medicine.

women and is characterized by enlargement of the ovaries and signs and symptoms of a fluid shift to the third space with ascites, hydrothorax, and haemoconcentration with oliguria and thromboembolic disease as a consequence.

The incidence of severe OHSS is 2% and although stimulation schedules have been adjusted and dose of gonadotrophins have been reduced, it can never be fully excluded. Therapy is usually observational and supportive. Occasionally, ascites or pleura drainage are needed for the patient's comfort and in case of severe dyspnoea.

Oocyte retrieval

Thirty-four to thirty-six hours after administration of human chorionic gonadotropin (hCG), the oocyte aspiration is planned. This interval aims at achieving maximal cytoplasmic and nuclear maturation of the oocyte to metaphase II and at being just in time before ovulation occurs. Therefore, timely initiation of the oocyte retrieval procedure is mandatory as patients may lose the whole cycle by not doing so. This will then inevitably lead to a tremendous disappointment for the couple as well as an important financial burden for the lost cycle. Nowadays, nearly all egg retrievals are performed vaginally under ultrasound guidance. A single- or double-lumen needle is introduced through a guide that is fixed on the vaginal probe of the ultrasound that is wrapped in a sterile cover. The ovaries can be reached through the lateral fornices of the vagina. Depending on the patient's characteristics, the procedure may vary from straightforward access and oocyte retrieval to a more risky intervention in some patients. This is the case in patients with obesity or prior extensive surgery in the pelvis for endometriosis or inflammatory disease of the intestine, a history of pelvic inflammatory disease, or any other event leading to an adhesive status of the ovaries. Apart from the wishes of the patient, the type of analgesia will also be dependent on the patient's history as already mentioned. Therefore, ultrasound-guided oocyte retrieval can be performed under local or locoregional anaesthesia, conscious sedation, or general anaesthesia. Gynaecological complications related to the oocyte retrieval procedure are the occurrence of bleeding and infection. In cases where a difficult procedure is anticipated or in patients with a history of important pelvic surgery or disease, antibiotics are usually given prophylactically.

Laparoscopic oocyte retrieval is rarely performed. It is used in cases where it is difficult to reach the ovaries, for example, in obese patients. However, performing a laparoscopy in this patient population is subject to an increased risk for complications as well. Therefore, in many clinics, invasive procedures such as oocyte retrieval and diagnostic and therapeutic laparoscopy will only be executed in patients with a body mass index below 35. Laparoscopic oocyte retrieval can also be part of the gamete intrafallopian transfer procedure where gametes are transferred

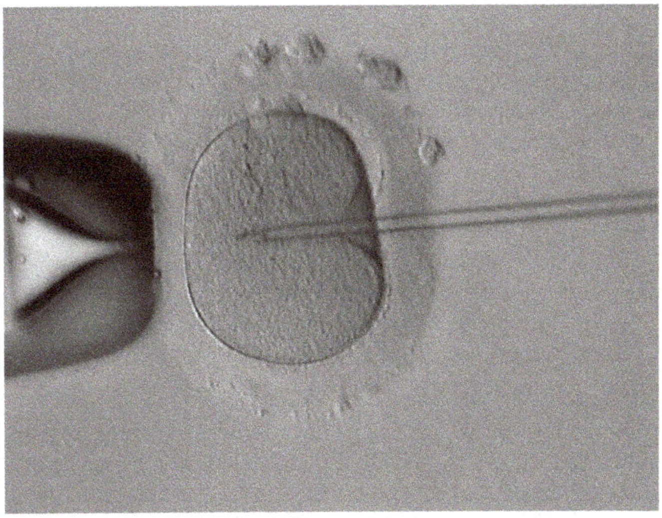

Figure 9.2 Intracytoplasmic sperm injection (ICSI) procedure: a spermatozoon is injected with a glass pipette in the cytoplasm of an oocyte under the microscope.

in the tubes via laparoscopy. However, this procedure is rarely performed in Europe nowadays as transcervical transfers are very easy and non-invasive to perform.

Fertilization

Immediately after the oocytes have been retrieved, they are placed in the incubator under ideal culture conditions. Thereafter oocytes are inseminated with approximately 20,000 spermatozoa per oocyte in the 'classical' IVF procedure or the oocytes are denudated from the cumulus cells and injected under the microscope with one sperm cell during the ICSI procedure (Figure 9.2).

Embryo culture and embryo transfer

The embryo transfer (ET) occurs at day 2, 3, 5, or 6 after oocyte aspiration yielding a cleavage stage embryo (D2, D3) or a blastocyst (D5, D6) (Figure 9.3). The timing of the transfer depends on the experience of the laboratory and the patient's characteristics. The goal is to find the best balance between selection of the embryo with the highest implantation potential and providing optimal culture conditions. The embryo transfer is usually performed transcervically after the installation of a speculum with a soft catheter loaded with one or two embryos. Quite often the embryo transfer is executed under abdominal ultrasound guidance for excellent positioning of the embryo(s). This is a minimally invasive and a nearly painless procedure and therefore no analgesia is administered. However, in a very few cases, ET is performed with analgesia for example, in patients with a history of surgery (exconization) at the cervix.

ET can be done directly in the Fallopian tube via laparoscopy. When the embryo is in the zygote stage it is named 'zygote intrafallopian transfer' (ZIFT) and when a cleavage stage embryo is transferred it is called 'embryo intrafallopian transfer' (EIFT).

Luteal phase support

The luteal phase is shortened after ART and therefore, supplementation with progesterone administered vaginally or intramuscularly or with hCG is mandatory.

The cost of an ART cycle is around €4000 in most European countries.

Anaesthetic management of the oocyte retrieval procedure

General considerations

The ideal anaesthetic method should be safe and comfortable for the patient undergoing the procedure, should not compromise the quantity or quality of the oocytes, and should have no effect on fertilization, embryo development, and pregnancy rate. It should be easy to administer and monitor, short-acting, and with few side effects.

Oocyte retrieval can be performed transvaginally or laparoscopically. Only in very few cases is a laparoscopy needed to reach the ovaries and general anaesthesia with intubation is required in these cases.

During transvaginal oocyte retrieval, the aspirating needle puncturing the vaginal fornix and the ovarian capsule, as well as the manipulation within the ovary during the procedure causes pain. It is essential to provide adequate pain relief, to immobilize the patient, and eliminate the dangers of piercing any vessel during the process of oocyte retrieval.

Since some women require high doses of sedatives and analgesics to obtain adequate pain relief while others do not, various pain-relieving methods are in use. There is currently no evidence for superiority of one procedure over another.[7,8]

Controversy exists regarding the effects of all these drugs on conception rates. In many studies, anaesthetics have been detected in follicular fluid and reported to interfere with the outcome of fertility treatment.[9] In a study published in 2012, significant differences were revealed between different anaesthetic methods for the total number of oocytes retrieved per patient, percentage

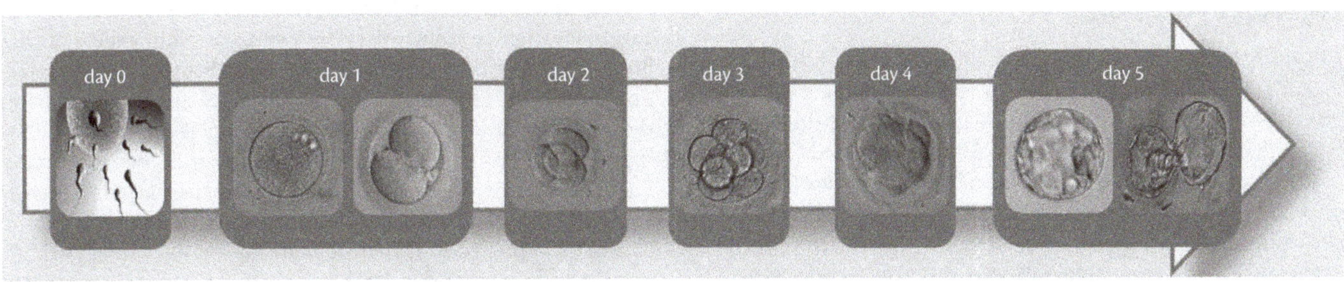

Figure 9.3 Evolution from a fertilized oocyte to a cleavage stage embryo (D2, D3) and to the blastocyst stage (D5, D6).

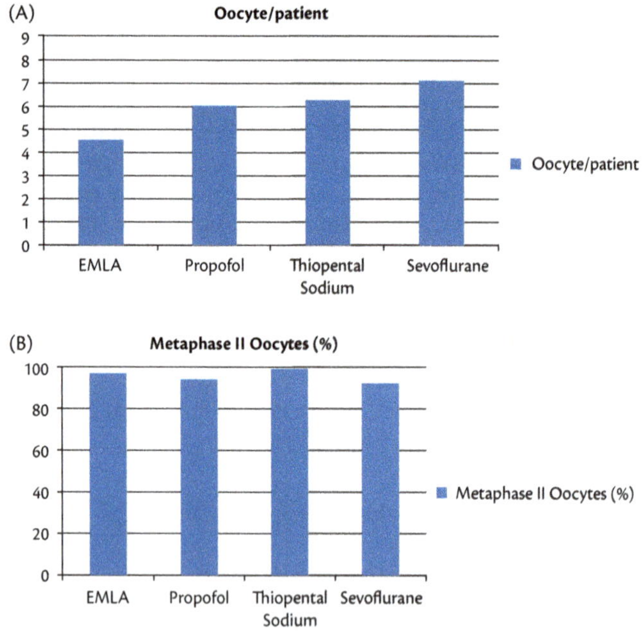

Figure 9.4 Biological parameters: number of oocytes retrieved per patient (A) and rate of metaphase II oocytes (B). In the EMLA® group they observed a lower number of retrieved oocytes when compared to the other groups. In the thiopental and sevoflurane groups, they found the highest oocytes retrieval. In the EMLA® and thiopental groups they observed more metaphase II oocytes.
Reprinted from Comparison of different anaesthetic methodologies for sedation during in vitro fertilization procedures: effects on patient physiology and oocyte competence, Alba Piroli, Roberto Marci, Franco Marinangeli, *et al*, *GYNECOLOGICAL ENDOCRINOLOGY*, volume 28, issue 10, pp. 796–9, 2012, reprinted by permission of the publisher (Taylor & Francis Ltd, http://www.tandfonline.com).

of mature oocytes in metaphase II stage, fertilization rate, and embryo development (Figure 9.4).[10]

A Cochrane analysis reviewed 21 controlled trials and concluded that there was no evidence of a significant difference in pregnancy rate or in quality of analgesia between the different methods of pain relief during oocyte pick-up. The simultaneous use of more than one method of sedation and pain relief (e.g. sedation in combination with paracervical block) resulted in better pain relief. All reviewed approaches seemed to be acceptable and were associated with a high degree of satisfaction.[8]

Different analgesia/anaesthesia techniques

Analgesia techniques that may be used for the transvaginal follicular aspiration are local anaesthesia (paracervical block or topical anaesthesia), neuraxial anaesthesia (spinal, epidural or combined), conscious sedation and general anaesthesia, or any combination of the above.

Local anaesthesia

Local paracervical anaesthesia can provide adequate pain relief for the transvaginal puncture but will not affect pain sensation when puncturing the ovaries. In a 2012 Italian study, a eutectic mixture of local anaesthetic (EMLA®) cream, a eutectic topical mixture of lidocaine and prilocaine incorporated in cream base, was administered on the vaginal fornices 1 hour before the procedure. This was compared with sedation using either propofol, sevoflurane, or thiopental. In comparison with sedation using propofol, sevoflurane, or thiopental, the authors retrieved a significantly lower number of oocytes per patient in the EMLA® cream group.[10] It was assumed that the gynaecologist performed the oocyte retrieval faster by puncturing only the largest follicles because the patients were awake during the procedure and this resulted in a high rate of mature (metaphase II) oocytes. The EMLA® cream group showed the highest fertilization rate. Anaesthesia with EMLA® cream is a possible and an acceptable alternative for anaesthesia during transvaginal oocyte retrieval in well-motivated patients.[10,11] In animal models, local anaesthetic agents seem to have an influence on the development of the early embryo. This is of minimal clinical significance because of the extreme low concentrations used in human practice.

Neuraxial anaesthesia

Neuraxial analgesia has been shown to be an effective form of pain relief during transvaginal oocyte retrieval. A spinal technique involves an injection of drugs into the cerebrospinal fluid. Epidural analgesia provides analgesia by injecting drugs into the epidural space. Both techniques have the advantage of limited absorption of the anaesthetic agent into the systemic circulation and will be associated with minimal accumulation into the follicular fluid. Of these two, spinal anaesthesia would be the advised method because a lower dose of local anaesthetic is needed, a faster onset of pain relief and recovery occurs, and there is a reduced failure rate. Hyperbaric lidocaine and bupivacaine in low dose in combination with an opioid have been successfully used in these procedures. Hyperbaric lidocaine is no longer used in current practice due to the high incidence of transient radicular irritation, but hyperbaric prilocaine could be an acceptable alternative. In addition, the risks associated with the neuraxial anaesthesia techniques must not be overlooked. Postdural puncture headache will occur in 0.5% of cases. Back pain, urinary retention, accidental intravascular injection, and anaesthesia reaching high spinal level can also occur. Apart from other more serious complications (epidural abscess or haematoma) neuraxial anaesthesia remains very time-consuming for a usually very short procedure.

Sedation and general anaesthesia

We have to differentiate moderate or conscious sedation from deep sedation or monitored anaesthesia care. Conscious sedation is a moderate sedation and defined as 'a method in which the use of drugs produce a minimally depressed level of consciousness enabling treatment to be carried out while the patient maintains an open airway continuously and responds appropriately to verbal commands' (defined by the American Society of Anesthesiologists' website in 2004, http://www.asahq.org/). This method is very popular for oocyte retrieval because it is easy to administer and safe in this mostly young, healthy and well-motivated population.

Deep sedation or monitored anaesthesia care consists of safe administration of a maximal depth of sedation in excess of that provided during conscious sedation. The ability to adjust the sedation level from full consciousness to general anaesthesia during the course of the procedure provides maximal flexibility in matching sedation levels to patients' and procedural needs. In many European countries this needs to be performed by an anaesthetist, while in some countries skilled anaesthetic personnel will take care of these procedures. There is a fine line between sedation with good pain control and general anaesthesia that requires assisted ventilation. Full monitoring of the patient with a pulse-oximeter, end-tidal CO_2, electrocardiography, and non-invasive blood pressure monitoring is necessary to ensure the patient's safety. All drugs and equipment for advanced life support should be available at the site of the procedure. The frequency of severe complications after transvaginal oocyte retrieval is very low but half of the cases with complications were anaesthesia related (bronchospasm).[12]

When selecting a desired agent for sedation, it should be considered whether it is safe for the woman and whether the substance enters the follicular fluid and has negative effects on fertilization and pregnancy rates.

Opioids

Opioids are used in moderate and deep sedation and in general anaesthesia for their analgesic effects. They should be used in a monitored way because of the dose-dependent depression of respiration. Rapid administration of opioids can also induce rigidity of the thoracic, laryngeal, or pharyngeal muscles. All equipment for respiratory support should be available, especially if a difficult airway access is expected (e.g. in obese patients). Urinary retention, pruritus, and postoperative nausea and vomiting (PONV) are also side effects of opioids.

When given during the procedure, opioids are detected in extremely low concentrations in the follicular fluid. Any potential influence on fertilization and implantation rates in these concentrations has never been substantiated.[9,13]

Remifentanil has an ultra-fast onset, organ-independent metabolism, and a very short elimination time, making it an ideal opioid for short procedures. There has been no report on negative interference with pregnancy rates or numbers and quality of retrieved oocytes using remifentanil.[14]

Alfentanil is another fast-acting opioid and is the narcotic agent most commonly used during oocyte retrieval. It has been detected in the follicular fluid but does not influence pregnancy rates even in high concentrations. It is more important to give an adequate, individualized dose of alfentanil than reducing the dose because of a potential harmful effect on the embryo.[9,15]

Benzodiazepines

Patients presenting for IVF treatment are under a high degree of stress and anxiolysis is another challenge for the anaesthetist. Benzodiazepines are used because of their sedative, anxiolytic, and amnesic effects. Additional properties of benzodiazepines include muscle relaxation and anticonvulsive effects. Midazolam is the most commonly used benzodiazepine. Although midazolam is found in the follicular fluid after a single intravenous (IV) dose, no detrimental effects have been shown.[9,15–17] Accurate respiratory monitoring is advised when these are used in combination with opioids since concurrent use may increase the incidence of apnoea and respiratory depression.

Propofol

Propofol is a short-acting anaesthetic agent for IV administration, suitable for induction and maintenance of anaesthesia and for sedation. It has a rapid onset of action and recovery and reduces PONV. An unpleasant effect for patients during intravenous administration of propofol is pain and burning at the site of injection. Propofol causes a dose-dependent decrease in systemic blood pressure and respiratory depression underlining once more the need for the presence of an anaesthetist or at least skilled anaesthetic personnel. Propofol has been reported to accumulate in the follicular fluid and these concentrations increase throughout the procedure.[18,19] At first it was suggested that propofol might have deleterious effects on reproductive outcome following IVF in animal models.[20,21] Ben-Shlomo et al. examined whether exposure to increasing concentrations of propofol had an adverse effect on fertilization and embryo development in humans. They compared oocyte quality between the first and the last oocyte retrieved in a cohort of 130 women and found no difference on fertilization rate, cleavage rate, or embryo cell number. However, they could not rule out the possibility that the short duration of their procedures and the consequent low follicular fluid concentrations contributed to this result.[22]

Ketamine

Ketamine, introduced in the 1960s, provides all components of anaesthesia necessary for oocyte retrieval: good pain-relief, loss of consciousness, and antegrade amnesia. Ketamine does not suppress the respiratory system, but it may produce unpleasant emergence reactions like vivid dreaming, 'out-of-body' experiences, and illusions within the first hours after awakening. Ketamine in combination with midazolam has been used frequently for oocyte retrieval and no differences in reproductive outcomes were observed.[23,24] To the authors' knowledge, there have been no studies measuring ketamine concentration in the follicular fluid in patients during oocyte retrieval under ketamine sedation.

Sevoflurane

In modern anaesthesia, sevoflurane is the most popular volatile anaesthetic agent. Not a lot is known about the effect of sevoflurane on the fertilization and early cleavage rate. One study conducted by Piroli et al., observed a decreased number of good quality embryos in the group of patients who received sevoflurane during oocyte retrieval[10] (Figure 9.5). The only evidence of a negative effect of sevoflurane reported in the literature is a study by Eger et al. They found that compound A, a degradation product of sevoflurane, had a genotoxic effect in Chinese hamster ovary cells.[25] A few years later, the same experiments were repeated to test sevoflurane and no genotoxicity could be found.[26] Currently sevoflurane sedation has become largely abandoned since more elegant techniques for sedation are available and the danger of inducing a general anaesthesia is substantial.

Alternative types of anaesthesia

Electroacupuncture

Recently a lot has been published in the Chinese literature about the role of electroacupuncture in the outcome of IVF procedures. There is some evidence that acupuncture treatment during ART could improve pregnancy rates in women undergoing IVF. Electroacupuncture probably has a good intraoperative supplementary analgesic effect without any extra adverse reaction and could be an adjuvant in reducing the dose of the anaesthetic drugs.[27]

Patient-controlled sedation

As the pain associated with ovum pick-up is intermittent rather than continuous, the best form of analgesia is one which allows maximal flexibility and responsiveness to the woman's needs. Patient-controlled anaesthesia could be superior to physician-administered analgesia in this context. Patient-controlled IV analgesia using opioids, propofol, or a mixture of the two has been used successfully, but satisfaction was less than conscious

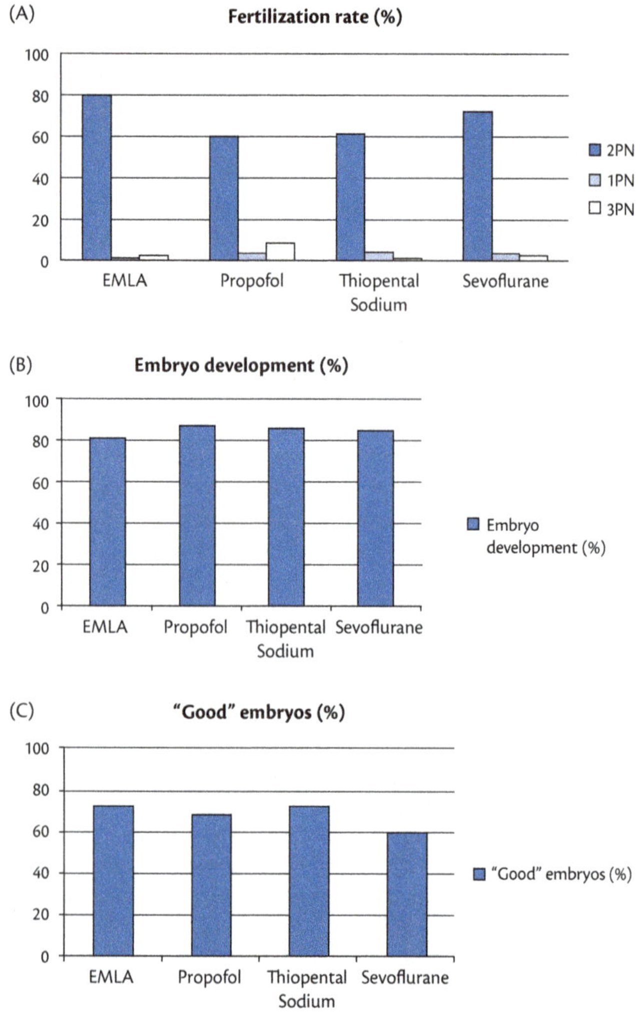

Figure 9.5 Biological parameters: fertilization rate (A), embryo development (B), and 'good embryo' rate (C). Fertilization rate was similar in EMLA® and sevoflurane groups, but significantly higher than in propofol or thiopental groups. They observed the highest rate of anomalous fertilization (defined as rate of 1PN and 3PN oocytes) in the propofol group. There was no overall difference in embryo development, but the sevoflurane group had a lower rate of 'good' embryos.

Reprinted from Comparison of different anaesthetic methodologies for sedation during in vitro fertilization procedures: effects on patient physiology and oocyte competence, Alba Piroli, Roberto Marci, Franco Marinangeli, *et al*, *GYNECOLOGICAL ENDOCRINOLOGY*, volume 28, issue 10, pp. 796–9, 2012, reprinted by permission of the publisher (Taylor & Francis Ltd, http://www.tandfonline.com).

sedation provided by a physician. A self-administered inhalational analgesic agent, such as isodesox, has potential advantages in terms of safety, ease of administration, short half-life, and minimal effects on the patient and her oocytes. Self-administered inhalation analgesia with isodesox by facemask was also associated with less effective analgesia and less patient satisfaction than physician-administered intravenous analgesia.[28,29]

Suggested anaesthetic management for transvaginal oocyte retrieval

As mentioned before, the ideal method of pain relief during oocyte retrieval should be safe and comfortable for the woman with minimal side effects, easy to administer and monitor, short acting, easily reversible, and with minimal to no effect on oocytes and embryos. Paracervical block, general anaesthesia, neuraxial anaesthesia or sedation all have advantages and disadvantages. Subsequently anaesthesia practice for IVF procedures varies in different fertility centres. In 1997, Ditkoff et al. published a US survey that demonstrated most programmes utilized anaesthesia, most commonly conscious sedation. Other types of anaesthesia used included general, neuraxial, or local anaesthesia. Anaesthesia personnel performed anaesthesia most of the time, although a significant number of IVF clinics were giving analgesia/anaesthesia without anaesthetists present. The majority of IVF personnel used a combination of meperidine and midazolam while 90% of the anaesthesiologists used midazolam and/or propofol with fentanyl. For both groups, complications were infrequent and no serious life-threatening incidents were reported.[30]

In the United Kingdom, a postal questionnaire audit was performed in 2003 by Elkington et al. which demonstrated a wide variation in personnel present during the procedure, in the drugs used, in the degree of monitoring, and the availability of emergency drugs.[31] A typical IVF procedure room in hospitals is located adjacent to the embryology laboratory and not near the general operating theatre. In the United Kingdom, more than 23% of fertility units are isolated without coverage of a resuscitation team. Remote locations should put in place regulations and protocols to maximize safety. Since the IVF population is usually young and healthy, it differs distinctly from the general population of patients requiring sedation. Serious morbidity is very rare, but women undergoing fertility procedures are increasingly older and have more frequent comorbidities (e.g. obesity, patients post chemotherapy, genetic disorders, or cystic fibrosis). It is unclear how far one should go in safety measures.[32]

The selection of the type of anaesthesia will depend on the IVF centre, and the preference of the surgeon and anaesthetist. As women vary in their experience of pain and in coping mechanisms, the optimal method should be individualized depending on the preference of both the woman and the clinician. Most centres have established protocols but the variety of methods and drugs used for this procedure raises questions about the potential advantages and disadvantages. A 2013 Cochrane review[8] aimed to assess the effectiveness and safety of different methods in terms of pain relief during and after the procedure, pregnancy outcome, patient satisfaction, and postoperative complications. It did not support one particular method or technique over another in providing effective conscious sedation and analgesia. Regardless of the nature of the drug or the dose used, opiates were effective at reducing the perception of pain. Where a second drug or intervention such as paracervical block or electroacupuncture, was associated, the simultaneous use of more than one method resulted in better pain relief than one modality alone. Patient-controlled sedation and analgesia was associated with more intraoperative pain compared with physician-administered sedation and analgesia. There was no evidence of significant difference in pregnancy rate with different methods of pain relief. High levels of satisfaction were reported in all studies. Most centres will use sedation, varying from conscious sedation to monitored anaesthesia care, provided by anaesthetists or by the fertility centre's own team (trained midwifes, nurses, or medical doctors).

A preoperative visit to the sedation team should involve a complete medical history, including patients' medication and allergies, history of PONV, motion sickness, and a clinical examination. A sedation plan should be explained to the patient and informed consent should be obtained. A good explanation of what can be expected will alleviate some of the anxiety stress associated with the procedure.

On the day of the procedure, nil per os (NPO) state and basic clinical signs should be checked. The patient is placed supine on the operating table and an IV cannula is inserted. Routine monitoring of the patient with a pulse-oximeter, end-tidal CO_2, electrocardiography, and non-invasive blood pressure monitoring is necessary to ensure the patient's safety. Oxygen is supplied by mask or nasal cannula. Sedation can be provided by intermittent titrated doses of propofol and alfentanil or fentanyl, but a continuous infusion of propofol and remifentanil is a very elegant alternative that can provide the full range of anaesthesia depth from conscious sedation, over monitored anaesthesia care to full general anaesthesia, according to the patient's need. The latter must, however, be performed by an anaesthetist. Anaesthesia managed in this way could result in higher patient acceptance than conscious sedation due to improved pain relief and less awareness during the procedure. Rarely this type of anaesthesia may require airway support. Mostly chin lift or verbal communication will be enough to encourage the patient to breathe adequately but all equipment and drugs for mask ventilation or emergency endotracheal intubation should be available. Once the desired depth of sedation is achieved, the surgeon starts the procedure. Good communication between the sedation team and the surgeon about the length of the procedure and possible additional painful stimuli will optimize the quality of sedation. At the end of the procedure, the surgeon achieves haemostasis from the vaginal wall and the patient is awakened. Paracetamol is given during the procedure and is usually enough to provide adequate analgesia in the postoperative period. Non-steroidal anti-inflammatory drugs can be added but should be avoided after the embryo transfer because changes in the prostaglandin milieu can affect embryo implantation. For antiemesis, prophylactic treatment with non-dopaminergic agents like cyclizine can be considered.

After the procedure, the patient is transferred to a recovery room and will be discharged once the discharge criteria are fulfilled. The incidence of serious postoperative complications requiring hospital admission is very low.

Conclusion

ART treatment is becoming increasingly popular to treat infertility disorders with nearly 1 million cycles reported in 2004 worldwide. Oocyte retrieval is an essential part of the *in vitro* procedure. Most oocyte retrievals are performed vaginally under ultrasound guidance. Puncturing the vaginal wall and the stimulated ovary can be painful, therefore some analgesia is usually required. The method used should be safe and comfortable for the woman with minimal side effects, easy to administer and monitor, short acting, easily reversible, and with minimal to no effect on oocytes and embryos. Topical anaesthesia, paracervical block, general anaesthesia, neuraxial anaesthesia, and sedation all have advantages and disadvantages. Most fertility clinics have chosen their method depending on patients' demands, staffing, and available facilities in the hospital or centre.

References

1. Zegers-Hochschild F, Adamson GD, de Mouzon J, *et al.* The International Committee for Monitoring Assisted Reproductive Technology (ICMART) and the World Health Organization (WHO) Revised Glossary on ART Terminology 2009. *Hum Reprod* 2009; 24:2683–87.
2. Zegers-Hochschild F, Adamson GD, de Mouzon J, *et al.* The International Committee for Monitoring Assisted Reproductive Technology (ICMART) and the World Health Organization (WHO) revised glossary of ART terminology 2009. *Fertil Steril* 2009; 92:1520–24.
3. Ferraretti AP, Goossens V, Kupka M, *et al.* Assisted reproductive technology in Europe, 2009: results generated from European registers by ESHRE. *Hum Reprod* 2013; 28(9):2318–31.
4. Sullivan EA, Zegers-Hochschild F, Mansour R, *et al.* International Committee for Monitoring Assisted Reproductive Technologies (ICMART) world report: assisted reproductive technology 2004. *Hum Reprod* 2013; 28(5):1375–90.
5. De Neubourg D, Bogaerts K, Wyns C, *et al.* The history of Belgian ART cycle registration and control: a case-study in reducing the incidence of multiple pregnancy. *Hum Reprod* 2013; 28(10):2709–19.
6. van der Gaast MH, Eijkemans MJ, van der Net JB, *et al.* Optimum number of oocytes for a successful first IVF treatment cycle. *Reprod Biomed Online* 2006; 13(4):476–80.
7. Kwan I. Conscious sedation and analgesia for oocyte retrieval during IVF procedures: a Cochrane review. *Hum Reprod* 2006; 21(7):1672–9.
8. Kwan I, Bhattacharya S, Knox F, *et al.* Pain relief for women undergoing oocyte retrieval for assisted reproduction. *Cochrane Database Syst Rev* 2013; 1:CD004829.
9. Soussis II, Boyd OO, Paraschos TT, *et al.* Follicular fluid levels of midazolam, fentanyl, and alfentanil during transvaginal oocyte retrieval. *Fertil Steril* 1995; 64(5):1003–7.
10. Piroli A, Marci R, Marinangeli F, *et al.* Comparison of different anaesthetic methodologies for sedation during in vitro fertilization procedures: effects on patient physiology and oocyte competence. *Gynecol Endocrinol* 2012; 28(10):796–9.
11. Ng E. Paracervical block with and without conscious sedation: a comparison of the pain levels during egg collection and the postoperative side effects. *Fertil Steril* 2001; 75(4):711–17.
12. Siristatidis CC, Chrelias CC, Alexiou AA, *et al.* Clinical complications after transvaginal oocyte retrieval: a retrospective analysis. *J Obstet Gynaecol* 2012; 33(1):64–6.
13. Shapira SC, Chrubasik S, Hoffmann A, *et al.* Use of alfentanil for in vitro fertilization oocyte retrieval. *J Clin Anesth* 1996; 8(4):282–5.
14. Wilhelm W, Hammadeh ME, White PF, *et al.* General anesthesia versus monitored anesthesia care with remifentanil for assisted reproductive technologies: effect on pregnancy rate. *J Clin Anesth* 2002; 14(1):1–5.
15. Gejervall AL, Lundin K, Stener-Victorin E, *et al.* Effect of alfentanil dosage during oocyte retrieval on fertilization and embryo quality. *Eur J Obstet Gynecol Reprod Biol* 2010; 150(1):66–71.
16. Chapineau J, Bazin JE, Terrisse MP, *et al.* Assay for midazolam in liquor folliculi during in vitro fertilization under anesthesia. *Clin Pharm* 1993; 12(10):770–3.
17. Swanson RJR, Leavitt MGM. Fertilization and mouse embryo development in the presence of midazolam. *Anesth Analg* 1992; 75(4):549–54.
18. Coetsier T, Dhont M, De Sutter P, *et al.* Propofol anaesthesia for ultrasound guided oocyte retrieval: accumulation of the anaesthetic agent in follicular fluid. *Hum Reprod* 1992; 7(10):1422–4.
19. Christiaens F, Janssenswillen C, Verborgh C, *et al.* Propofol concentrations in follicular fluid during general anaesthesia for transvaginal oocyte retrieval. *Hum Reprod* 1999; 14(2):345–8.
20. Alsalili M, Thornton S, Fleming S. The effect of the anaesthetic, Propofol, on in-vitro oocyte maturation, fertilization and cleavage in mice. *Hum Reprod* 1997; 12(6):1271–4.

21. Janssenswillen C, Christiaens F, Devroey P. The effect of the intravenous anesthetic propofol on fertilization and early embryo development in human in vitro fertilization (IVF) program. *Fertil Steril* 1997; 68 Suppl 1:S60.
22. Ben-Shlomo I, Moskovich R, Golan J, *et al.* The effect of propofol anaesthesia on oocyte fertilization and early embryo quality. *Hum Reprod* 2000; 15(10):2197–9.
23. Ben-Shlomo I, Moskovich R, Katz Y, *et al.* Midazolam/ketamine sedative combination compared with fentanyl/propofol/isoflurane anaesthesia for oocyte retrieval. *Hum Reprod* 1999; 14(7):1757–9.
24. Vlahos NF, Giannakikou I, Vlachos A, *et al.* Analgesia and anesthesia for assisted reproductive technologies. *Int J Gynaecol Obstet* 2009; 105(3):201–5.
25. Eger EI, Laster MJ, Winegar R, *et al.* Compound A induces sister chromatid exchanges in Chinese hamster ovary cells. *Anesthesiology* 1997; 86(4):918–22.
26. Tomioka S, Nakajo N. No genotoxic effect of propofol in Chinese hamster ovary cells: analysis by sister chromatid exchanges. *Acta Anaesthesiol Scand* 2000; 44(10):1261–5.
27. Zheng CH, Zhang MM, Huang GY, *et al.* The role of acupuncture in assisted reproductive technology. *Evid Based Complement Alternat Med* 2012; 2012:543924.
28. Bhattacharya SS, MacLennan FF, Hamilton MPM, *et al.* How effective is patient-controlled analgesia? A randomized comparison of two protocols for pain relief during oocyte recovery. *Hum Reprod* 1997; 12(7):1440–2.
29. Thompson NN, Murray SS, MacLennan FF, *et al.* A randomised controlled trial of intravenous versus inhalational analgesia during outpatient oocyte recovery. *Anaesthesia* 2000; 55(8):770–3.
30. Ditkoff ECE, Plumb JJ, Selick AA, *et al.* Anesthesia practices in the United States common to in vitro fertilization (IVF) centers. *J Assist Reprod Genet* 1997; 14(3):145–7.
31. Elkington NM, Kehoe J, Acharya U. Intravenous sedation in assisted conception units: a UK survey. *Hum Fertil (Camb)* 2003; 6(2):74–6.
32. Yasmin E, Dresner M, Balen A. Sedation and anaesthesia for transvaginal oocyte collection: an evaluation of practice in the UK. *Hum Reprod* 2004; 19(12):2942–5.

CHAPTER 10

Anaesthesia for non-obstetric surgery

Vegard Dahl and Ulrich J. Spreng

Introduction

For a pregnant woman, there is always a risk of requiring anaesthesia for non-obstetric reasons. Around 1–2% of all pregnant women will undergo non-obstetric surgery during gestation.[1] A substantial number of anaesthetic procedures and operations will be performed on women in the early stages of pregnancy who are unaware of their pregnant status at the time of intervention. Therefore pregnancy tests should be performed on all women of child-bearing age undergoing surgery. The reason for surgery may be directly related to the pregnancy, such as *in utero* operations on the fetus or cerclage; it may be indirectly related, such as, for instance, an ovarian cystectomy; or it may be coincidental, such as an appendectomy, cholecystectomy, or an injury requiring surgical intervention. In a review published in 2005 by Cohen-Kerem and colleagues including more than 12,000 non-obstetric surgical interventions in pregnancy, the reported rate of miscarriage was 5.8%, premature labour was 3.5%, and maternal deaths were as rare as 0.006%.[2]

Historically, there has been reluctance to anaesthetize pregnant patients due to a fear of jeopardizing the well-being of the fetus and mother. Although the safety of non-obstetric surgery and anaesthesia during pregnancy seems well established, there are several concerns that need to be addressed. The anaesthetist must provide safe anaesthesia for both mother and fetus. Furthermore, the anaesthesiologist must take into consideration the changes that a pregnancy induces on normal maternal physiology, and be aware of the possible hazards that anaesthesia may impose on the fetus. This includes possible teratogenic effects of drugs and diagnostic imaging, risk of preterm delivery or abortion, as well as intraoperative haemodynamic alteration of uteroplacental perfusion.

Maternal physiological changes: anaesthetic considerations

Pregnancy is associated with profound anatomical and physiological changes. Knowledge and understanding of these changes are crucial for optimal perioperative care in pregnancy.[3,4] Maternal physiological and anatomical changes requiring precautions by the anaesthetist are presented in Table 10.1.

Anaesthetic principles

Non-obstetric surgery can be carried out with either general or neuraxial anaesthesia techniques and will depend on the site of surgery, the emergency of the situation, and the choice of the anaesthetist and the pregnant patient, if possible. A multidisciplinary team approach with focus on communication and cooperation is necessary in order to minimize the risk and possible harm of the surgical and anaesthetic procedure. The multidisciplinary team should include surgeons, anaesthetists, obstetricians, and radiologists, as well as midwifes and nurses.

If possible, surgery should be performed in the second trimester because in this period the risk for preterm labour seems to be lowest. It is important to inform the patient of possible risks of anaesthesia and surgery to the fetus and pregnancy (e.g. abortion and preterm labour). The goal must, of course, be to minimize the risks of anaesthesia and surgical procedures.

The key issue during anaesthesia, no matter which technique used, is to preserve maternal haemodynamic stability. Neuraxial anaesthesia should be considered whenever possible. Accompanying maternal hypotension will reduce uteroplacental blood flow, and treatment is mandatory.[1,5] Pregnant women undergoing acute abdominal surgery will usually require general anaesthesia,[6] although some procedures like open appendectomy can be done with a regional technique.

Preoperative period

The use of tranquillizers such as midazolam and weak analgesics such as paracetamol can reduce anxiety and pain and may be beneficial in order to reduce maternal stress, which can decrease uterine blood flow. Anticholinergic medication (e.g. glycopyrrolate) will reduce oral secretions as well as prevent bradycardia during induction of anaesthesia and is recommended.[6]

Pregnancy is associated with a hormonally induced decrease in gastric motility and a cephalad displacement of the stomach. Moreover, the lower oesophagus sphincter tone is decreased in pregnant women.[7] Aspiration prophylaxis (e.g. metoclopramide, oral antacid, or H_2-receptor antagonist), especially during the third trimester, may be beneficial.[8–10] However, this is a controversial issue.[11,12] Wong et al. have shown that gastric emptying in obese, non-labouring pregnant woman is not delayed after ingestion of 300 mL of water.[13]

Intraoperative period

The risk for difficulties during intubation is higher in pregnant patients undergoing general anaesthesia compared with a general population.[4,14–16] An anaesthetist has to be prepared for a difficult airway and training in airway management is mandatory.[4,17–19]

Table 10.1 Maternal changes in anatomy and physiology and anaesthetic implications and precautions

Maternal changes	Consequences	Precautions
Venous engorgement Oedema upper airways Gain in weight Increased breast size	Intubation difficulties	Difficult airway management
Functional residual capacity ↓ Oxygen consumption ↑	Early desaturation	Preoxygenation
Hyperventilation	Respiratory alkalosis	Normoventilation[a]
Aortocaval compression (>12 weeks)	Preload ↓	Left lateral decubitus position
Systemic vascular resistance ↓	Hypotension	Fluid load Vasoconstrictor
Cardiac output ↑	Oxygen consumption ↑	FiO_2 ↑
Intra-abdominal pressure ↑	Gastric emptying delayed	Rapid sequence induction
Oesophageal sphincter tone ↓	Gastro-oesophageal reflux	Rapid sequence induction

[a]Normoventilation in pregnancy, e.g. slight hyperventilation compared with non-pregnant.

Equipment for difficult airway management should be easily accessible.[4,17]

After failed direct laryngoscopy, a device offering a view into the glottis (e.g. video laryngoscope) should be used. Moreover, the anaesthetist should be familiar with the use of an intubation laryngeal mask (e.g. LMA Fastrach™) and gum elastic bougie.[4] The management of a difficult or failed airway is discussed in Chapter 26.

Optimal positioning of the patient is important. A 15° left lateral decubitus position will help to prevent aortocaval compression (reduction in preload). Alignment of the ears with the sternal notch is advisable in order to facilitate mask ventilation, laryngoscopy, and intubation (see Figure 39.3 in Chapter 39).

Pregnancy is associated with a reduction of the functional residual capacity, which leads to a reduction in oxygen reserve. Moreover, oxygen consumption in pregnant women is increased.[3,4] Therefore, desaturation occurs faster during induction of anaesthesia.[20] Effective pre-oxygenation with a tight facemask is crucial. Several techniques can be used for optimal pre-oxygenation. The woman can either breathe with normal tidal volumes for a minimum of 3 minutes or, when time is limited, use the eight deep breaths technique.[20–22] Rapid sequence induction (RSI) is advisable and the airways should be secured with an endotracheal tube. Whether cricoid pressure should be used during RSI is controversial. On the one hand, if applied properly, it may protect against regurgitation during induction. On the other hand it may make viewing of the epiglottis and intubation more difficult. If one chooses to use a cricoid pressure or Sellick's manoeuvre during induction, it is advisable to loosen it if viewing of the epiglottis is compromised.[12,23–25]

When choosing appropriate anaesthetic drugs for pregnant women, there are three main goals:

1. Ensure maternal anaesthesia and analgesia
2. Avoid maternal hypoxia and hypocapnia
3. Avoid maternal hypotension (preserve uterine blood flow).

Induction of anaesthesia

Thiopental, propofol, etomidate, and ketamine all cause unconsciousness and can be used for induction of anaesthesia in pregnancy. Etomidate has favourable pharmacodynamic properties, causes minimal histamine release, and is suitable in haemodynamically unstable patients, especially in cardiac surgery patients.[26,27] However, etomidate supresses corticosteroid synthesis in the adrenal cortex and should be used with caution in septic patients. There is conflicting evidence whether a single dose, such as would be used for induction in the obstetric patient, is associated with increased 28-day mortality.[28,29] Clinicians should use etomidate with caution because although it may provide haemodynamic stability at induction, the long-term outcome may be worsened.[30,31] Ketamine is best suited for haemodynamically unstable patients in emergency settings and has, in addition, excellent analgesic properties.[32]

Opioids must be used to provide analgesia during intubation and surgery. The use of opioids (e.g. fentanyl, sufentanil, alfentanil, and remifentanil) may induce fetal respiratory depression. However, this is only relevant if the baby is going to be delivered during the current surgery. Moreover, opioids may decrease fetal heart rate variability during anaesthesia, and this should not be considered as a sign of impaired fetal well-being or non-reassuring fetal status.[33] This should be emphasized to the midwives and obstetricians who may assume wrongly that this is a sign of fetal distress.

The conditions for endotracheal intubation will be improved by using muscle relaxants. In RSI, succinylcholine or high-dose rocuronium should be used. Although good intubation conditions have been reported with a standard dose of rocuronium (0.6 mg/kg), 1.0–1.2 mg/kg is recommended for RSI and will give as good intubation conditions after 1 minute as a standard dose of succinylcholine.[34–36] In the rare case of a 'cannot intubate—cannot ventilation' situation[35] the muscle block induced by rocuronium can be reversed by the use of the drug sugammadex.[37] Sugammadex is especially designed to encapsulate the muscle relaxants in the steroid group. A high dose (16 mg/kg) will remove all muscle-relaxing molecules from the circulation within minutes and allows earlier re-establishment of spontaneous breathing compared with succinylcholine.[38] Due to the large molecular size of sugammadex, placental transfer is probably minimal, but data in human fetal transfer are lacking. The potential effects of sugammadex on the fetus are not known. Sugammadex as a reversal of the neuromuscular block should therefore only be used in critical situations.

Maintenance of anaesthesia

Both intravenous drugs (e.g. propofol) and volatile halogenated agents (e.g. sevoflurane, desflurane, or isoflurane) are frequently used for the maintenance of anaesthesia during pregnancy.[6,39–41] It has recently been shown that high concentrations of sevoflurane and isoflurane (minimum alveolar concentration 1.5–2.0) may induce haemodynamic instability in both the mother and the fetus[42] and that high concentrations of desflurane can reduce fetal cardiac function.[43] Nitrous oxide can be used during surgery.[37] However, it is controversial as to whether nitrous oxide should be avoided in abdominal surgery because of its ability to cause bowel distention.[44–46]

Neuraxial anaesthesia for non-obstetric surgery

Locoregional anaesthesia for non-obstetric surgical procedures during pregnancy has many advantages compared to general anaesthesia and should be preferred whenever possible. The fetus will not be exposed to drugs with possible detrimental effect and possible respiratory problems can be evaded. Neuraxial anaesthesia (spinal, epidural, or a combined spinal–epidural technique) is recommended for lower abdominal surgery and surgery in the lower extremities. When choosing neuraxial anaesthesia, posture of the patient during the procedure is important, and aortocaval compression has to be avoided (as previously discussed). The same cautions regarding fasting and preparation with antacid prophylaxis as for a general anaesthesia should be followed. It is essential to avoid hypotension in order to maintain uteroplacental blood flow. Hypotension should be treated with volume co-loading and vasoactive drugs whenever needed. Dosage of local anaesthesia needed for neuraxial anaesthesia in the second and third stages of pregnancy is reduced, and may sometimes be difficult to predict.[47] A combined spinal–epidural technique with a small dose of local anaesthesia combined with a fat-soluble opioid spinally and the possibility to top-up with local anaesthesia epidurally is probably a safe way to perform neuraxial anaesthesia in these patients. Peripheral nerve block is the method of choice for surgery in the upper extremities and surgery below knees, whenever possible.

Postoperative period

Postoperative pain should be treated adequately as pain may increase catecholamine levels with resultant placental vasoconstriction. There are many options available for treating pain after surgery, including systemic analgesia (i.e. opioid and non-opioid drugs), regional analgesic techniques (i.e. neuraxial and peripheral), local anaesthetic wound infiltration and a combination of these. It is important to assess the risks and benefits of each treatment modality. The goal is an optimized postoperative analgesic regimen for each individual patient.

Drugs used for systemic analgesia can be divided into opioid and non-opioid drugs. All opioids can induce fetal respiratory depression. However, this is only important if the surgical procedure is combined with a caesarean delivery or an immediate vaginal delivery.[6] It has been shown that the daily use of opioids in the first trimester may be associated with cardiac and neurological defects.[48] However, this has never been demonstrated for short time use of opioids in the postoperative period.

Regarding non-opioids, paracetamol (acetaminophen) is the drug of choice during pregnancy. Even in patients who have taken a paracetamol overdose the majority of pregnancies had normal outcomes.[49] Non-steroidal anti-inflammatory drugs (NSAIDs) exert their analgesic effect through inhibition of cyclooxygenase (COX) and synthesis of prostaglandins.[50] There have been several published studies reporting an increased risk for cardiac abnormalities when NSAIDs were taken during the first trimester.[51–53] Moreover, Nielsen and colleagues have recently shown that the prescription of NSAIDs may be associated with higher rates of miscarriage.[54] The use of NSAIDs during late pregnancy may lead to intrauterine constriction of the ductus arteriosus and is not recommended.[55] COX-1-mediated thromboxane facilitates platelet aggregation and haemostasis, and NSAID-derived COX inhibition may increase the risk of postoperative haemorrhage.[56] There are insufficient data regarding the use of selective COX-2 inhibitors in pregnancy.

Pregnant patients have an increased risk for thromboembolism. Therefore, it is important that these patients are mobilized as early as possible. Moreover, thrombosis prophylaxis with anticoagulants is mandatory.

Careful observation of the pregnant woman and fetus may be indicated for several days after surgery. The postoperative care unit team has to be aware of the risks of complications like preterm labour (see 'Miscarriage and Preterm Birth').

Fetal considerations for anaesthesia during pregnancy

Early period: teratogenicity of anaesthetics

In spite of fears of possible teratogenetic effects of anaesthesia no such effect has ever been demonstrated in humans in clinically relevant doses. There are, of course, no prospective comparative studies due to ethical and practical concerns. Speculation on possible harmful effects on the fetus comes either from studies on animals or from epidemiological surveys on operating theatre personnel and on outcome in women having undergone surgery during pregnancy. Studies on animals will generally include an exposure to a large dose of a drug during a long time period, and cannot be extrapolated to a short exposure with a limited concentration as in anaesthesia during surgery in humans. Nevertheless, two agents have been controversial in the last 50 years and need to be addressed:

- *Nitrous oxide* reacts with the reduced form of vitamin B_{12}, thereby inhibiting methionine synthase, which indirectly supports nucleic acid synthesis. Animal studies in the 1970s and 1980s demonstrated teratogenetic effects of nitrous oxide, which could be reversed by halothane or isoflurane but not by addition of folic acid.[57,58] Thus, from a theoretical point of view, the possible teratogenetic effect of nitrous oxide must also have a different explanation than methionine synthase inhibition. Nitrous oxide could possibly influence uterine blood flow and thus fetal oxygen supply.[59] These effects on reproduction occurred only after prolonged exposure to high concentrations of nitrous oxide and cannot be compared to real life when patients are anaesthetized for surgery in a clinical setting for relatively short periods. Large population studies from Sweden and Hungary have not found any correlation between intrauterine exposure to nitrous oxide during surgery and teratogenicity.[60,61] One may conclude that a short time exposure to nitrous oxide during pregnancy is safe. Whether exposure to nitrous oxide during a period of extensive receptogenesis later in pregnancy or in childhood results in cognitive deficits is yet to be determined (see 'Behavioural Teratogenicity'). Higher rates of spontaneous miscarriages have been observed among workers with occupational exposure to nitrous oxide such as dental assistants and operating theatre nurses.[62] When adjusted for age, smoking, and working hours, however, this association is no longer statistically significant.

- *Benzodiazepines* have been associated with a higher incidence of cleft lip and palate, pylorostenosis, and alimentary tract atresia, but the results are conflicting.[63–66] Pregnant women who use benzodiazepines long term often have multiple other confounding factors such as psychiatric disorders, social problems, multiple medication use, or epilepsy. The use of a short-acting benzodiazepine like midazolam during anaesthesia has never been associated with teratogenicity.

Behavioural teratogenicity

Lately, more focus has been set on the possible behavioural teratogenic effect of anaesthetics, defined as the possibility of permanent changes in behaviour without significant structural changes. The pathophysiology seems to include an increase in neuronal death, decreased neural stem cell migration, and a possible altered cytoskeletal structure of glia cells when exposed to anaesthetics in periods with high synaptogenesis. The human brain is developing throughout gestation and for many years after birth. During this period of extensive receptogenesis, an exposure to drugs interacting with GABA (gamma-aminobutyric acid) and NMDA (*N*-methyl D aspartate) receptors has, in animal models, been shown to enhance apoptosis or programmed cell death with persistent learning deficits.[67,68] The anaesthetic drugs that interfere with either the GABA or the NMDA receptors include most widely used anaesthetic drugs like nitrous oxide, midazolam, ketamine, and volatile agents. As an example, isoflurane has been shown to decrease proliferation and inhibit neuron growth in a dose-dependent matter in a cell culture model.[69] These data, although disturbing, must be analysed with caution. It is important to know that the period of extensive receptogenesis is weeks in rats, compared to many years in humans. The average rat brain has 70–200 million neurons, compared to 86,000 billion in the developed human brain. Therefore, these experimental models in rodents cannot be compared to human exposure to anaesthetic drugs. The doses used in the animal models would represent continuous exposure for several weeks without any surgical stimulation in humans, and thus cannot be extrapolated to a short exposure during pregnancy. Some epidemiological studies on humans may, however, support the hypothesis that extensive exposure to anaesthesia has a negative influence on human brain development. A population-based, retrospective cohort study from Minnesota, United States, compared 593 children, who had received general anaesthesia before the age of 4 years to 4764 children without anaesthesia exposure. Results have shown that multiple exposures to anaesthesia revealed an increased risk of learning disabilities.[70] It is impossible to say whether anaesthesia by itself may be harmful or the need for anaesthesia is a marker for other causes. This has been heavily debated during the last decade. One must also take into consideration that painful procedures and stress in itself may influence neurodevelopment in a negative way. Data on exposure to anaesthetic drugs during pregnancy and behavioural teratogenicity in humans are sparse. One other population-based study also from Minnesota found no differences in learning abilities between children who had been exposed to general anaesthesia during a caesarean delivery compared to those who had been delivered vaginally.[71]

One may hope that our future knowledge regarding the influence of anaesthetics on human brain development will enable us to take measures in order to minimize the possible harmful effects. In the meantime, it is advisable to have in mind that general anaesthesia is potentially harmful to the developing fetal brain. Therefore, general anaesthesia should be used with care and prolonged periods of exposure to anaesthetic drugs should be minimized if possible. This is in addition to the risks of general anaesthesia for the pregnant mother herself.

When informing the pregnant woman about possible harmful effects of anaesthesia to the fetus one should emphasize that the risks for damage are very small. There is no evidence for teratogenicity with a single anaesthetic exposure during the first trimester of pregnancy, and no risks for adverse effects during third-trimester exposure. Possible negative effects on learning and behaviour are based on animal data and of little relevance.

Perioperative fetal monitoring

Interdisciplinary cooperation between anaesthetist, obstetrician, and midwife is important regarding fetal monitoring. The well-being of the fetus should be verified by an obstetric consultation before induction of anaesthesia. Fetal heart rate and uterine activity should be monitored and documented before induction and, if possible, throughout the whole surgical procedure until emergence from anaesthesia. It is important to know that loss of beat-to-beat variability is normal during anaesthesia. However, fetal bradycardia is a serious sign, which must initiate immediate reactions. It is advisable to continue fetal monitoring into the postoperative period in order to document the well-being of the fetus and reassure the mother.

Miscarriage and preterm birth

Non-obstetric surgery during pregnancy will increase the risk of abortion and preterm delivery. It is still unclear whether the disease itself, the surgery, or the anaesthesia is responsible for the increased risk. In a large systematic review published in 2005 encompassing more than 12,000 pregnant women, Cohen-Kerem and colleagues found the overall percentage of reported miscarriages to be 5.8% of pregnant women undergoing a surgical intervention.[2] The risk was especially high during the first trimester (10.5%). The rate of delivery induced by surgical intervention was 3.5%. A subanalysis indicated that the type of surgery was an important factor. Appendectomy seemed to be associated with the highest risk of miscarriages and preterm labour. The gravity of the disease, as well as early diagnosis and management, will influence on the frequency. There are no major differences between open and laparoscopic surgery related to miscarriage and preterm delivery.[2] From a theoretical point of view one would think that the use of volatile agents, which are known to be uterorelaxant, would be advantageous. This has, however, never been proven. No evidence supports one anaesthetic drug as superior to another in the prevention of preterm labour or miscarriage, and neither is there evidence that one tocolytic drug is better than another. In order to minimize the risk of preterm labour and miscarriage, it is important for the anaesthetist to balance anaesthesia as careful as possible. Measures should be taken in order to maintain uteroplacental blood flow by ensuring a haemodynamically stable woman.

The pregnant patient should be kept normoventilated (for pregnancy) and normovolaemic. Surgery should be done gently with as little manipulation of the uterus as possible. The risk of preterm labour or miscarriage necessitates careful observation of the pregnant woman, also in a prolonged postoperative period. Treatment with a tocolytic agent in this period may be necessary, and the new oxytocin antagonist atosiban is recommended.[72] Tocolysis by prostaglandin inhibition, using an NSAID such as indomethacin, although controversial, is an option during the first trimester.

Diagnostic imaging in pregnancy

Pregnant women with a condition that requires anaesthesia and surgery are often in need of diagnostic imaging in order to establish a diagnosis.[73] Exposure to radiation has been a source of much speculation and anxiety among patients and healthcare professionals. As an example, the pregnancy website of the American Health Physics Society (http://www.HPS.org) received 1.3 million visits in 2007, most of them concerning risks of environmental xenobiotic exposure during pregnancy.[74] Potential risks include teratogenicity, intrauterine death, genetic damage, and risk of malignancy later in life. Indeed, older studies seemed to confirm that exposure to radiation *in utero* augments the risk of post-exposure malignancies in childhood such as leukaemia and intracerebral tumours.[75,76] However, modern, better-designed studies have failed to replicate these associations, both to X-ray in general and to abdominal and pelvic X-rays.[77]

Radiation can be divided into either ionizing or non-ionizing radiation. Ultrasound imaging and magnetic resonance imaging (MRI) are examples of the latter, while diagnostic X-ray is an example of ionizing radiation. When describing ionizing radiation exposure from medical diagnostic equipment, the amount is described in the SI unit gray (Gy) or milligray (mGy). The use of absorbed dose of radiation (rad) is also common. The possible detrimental effect on the fetus will depend on the radiation dose and the gestational age.[78] Studies on animals seem to indicate that doses of 100–200 mGy (10–20 rad) can be lethal during the first weeks of gestation (3–4 weeks' gestational age). The lethal doses increase rapidly and are similar to the mother at birth (20,000 mGy or 2000 rad). High doses of exposure are also necessary in order to induce malformations, neurobehavioral abnormalities, or cancer.[79]

Table 10.2 Estimated radiation to the fetus according to imaging procedure

Imaging procedure	Estimated fetal absorption	
	mGy	Rad
X-ray of the chest	<0.01	0.001
CT scan of the chest	0.06–0.96	0.006–0.096
X-ray of the abdomen	1–4.2	0.1–0.42
X-ray lumbar spine	8–49	0.8–4.9
CT-scan of the abdomen	8–49	0.8–4.9
X-ray of the pelvis	1.1–4	0.11–0.4
MRI	Non-ionizing radiation	Non-ionizing radiation
Ultrasound	Non-ionizing radiation	Non-ionizing radiation

Adapted from the *American Journal of Obstetrics and Gynecology*, volume 206, issue 6, Groen RS *et al.*, Fear of the unknown: ionizing radiation exposure during pregnancy, pp. 456–62. Copyright (2012) with permission from Elsevier.

The doses that a fetus is exposed to during diagnostic imaging vary from less than 0.01 mGy for a chest X-ray to 10–50 mGy for an abdominal computed tomography (CT) scan (Table 10.2). Although reassuring, there are controversies regarding the safety limit of radiation exposure. The International Commission on Radiological Protection has estimated that a intrauterine exposure of less than 100 mGy is safe, while the American College of Obstetricians and Gynaecologists has set the limit, particularly regarding the risk of congenital malformations, to 50 mGy.[80] Taking these safety limits into consideration, one should be cautious with repeated CT scans and/or fluoroscopically guided procedures during pregnancy. With the exception of the above-mentioned procedures, women should be reassured that the hazards of diagnostic imaging during pregnancy are far outweighed by the benefit of an accurate diagnosis,[73,81] for example, in thromboembolic disease (see Chapter 37).

Diagnostic ultrasound has, during the last five decades, become an essential tool in obstetrics. The original analogue imaging devices have developed to digital two-dimensional (2D) imagers, and subsequently into 3D (4D with motion). Safety limits for thermal and mechanical exposures have been gradually relaxed during the last decades. Considering the huge amount of ultrasound imaging that has been performed without ever demonstrating any harm to the mother or fetus, it seems safe to assume that ultrasound can be used in any medical examination of the pregnant woman.[82] Ultrasound is a very useful tool in diagnosis of the acute abdomen in pregnancy,[83] and is now considered the modality of choice for a suspected appendicitis in pregnancy.[84]

As radiologists gain more knowledge, the use of MRI in diagnosing abdominal pathology in pregnancy is growing. MRI without intravenous contrast is safe for mother and child, and provides excellent anatomical resolution.[85–87] If contrast enhancing is indicated, gadolinium-containing contrast media are contraindicated and should only be used if absolutely essential. Iodine-containing contrast media may lead to a transient hypothyroidism in the newborn.[88]

In summary, there is no evidence of any major risk to the developing fetus from a single exposure to any diagnostic imaging modality.

Laparoscopic surgery during pregnancy

Pregnancy used to be considered as an absolute contraindication to laparoscopic procedures. This has been challenged during the last decades, and laparoscopy is now considered as a safe alternative to open surgery in pregnant women. The possible benefits include better intraoperative visualization, less surgical trauma, less uterine manipulation, and faster recovery.[89,90] Laparoscopic procedures are safest when performed in the second trimester, when the uterus is smaller and less susceptible to trauma from the instruments.[90]

The access to the abdomen should be performed with an open technique as suggested by the Society of American Gastrointestinal Endoscopic Surgeons (SAGES),[91] thus avoiding direct injury to the gravid uterus. The use of CO_2 to achieve pneumoperitoneum will lead to possible ventilation problems, and is a potential risk for acidosis in the fetus. The pressure should therefore be as low as possible (10–12 mmHg).[91] Great care should be taken in order to minimize manipulation of the uterus. Intraoperative and postoperative preventive measures should be followed in order to avoid thromboembolic complications.[90]

Electroconvulsive therapy during pregnancy

Serious mental disorders requiring treatment may occur during pregnancy. Postpartum depression is a common disorder, and studies indicate that in women who experienced postpartum depression, more than 50% were also depressed during the pregnancy itself.[92] Treatment of serious mental illness during pregnancy represents a special challenge since the well-being of at least two individuals has to be taken into consideration. Pharmacological treatment of the mother may pose a threat to the fetus, especially during the first trimester. In this context, electroconvulsive therapy (ECT) seems to have a role in the treatment of serious conditions of perinatal depression. ECT does not generate electric current directly through the uterus. Possible harm to the fetus may occur due to hypertension and/or hypoxia during seizure. There are no randomized controlled studies comparing ECT with other treatment modalities for mental disorders in pregnancy. In a review article published in 2007 encompassing 339 pregnant women who underwent ECT series, remission or partial remission was reported in 78% of the cases. There were 25 fetal and neonatal complications, but only 11 of these were possibly related to the ECT treatment and only one was believed to be the direct result of the ECT.[93] Anaesthesia during ECT is normally induced by propofol or thiopentone. Motor activity is limited by the use of low-dose succinylcholine (0.5–1 mg/kg), thus preventing the patient harming herself or the fetus by vigorous muscle contractions. None of above-mentioned drugs are considered harmful to the neonate as long as they are administered before delivery. Theoretically, the risk of pulmonary aspiration during the procedure is higher in pregnant patients than in a non-pregnant population. However, in the review there were no reports of pulmonary aspiration among the 339 cases. This review, however, does not state whether the patients had cricoid pressure applied or indeed were intubated. In conclusion, ECT for serious mental disorders during pregnancy is often the preferred method of treatment. It does not seem to have any harmful effect on the fetus.

Electric cardioversion during pregnancy

Arrhythmias during pregnancy are not uncommon.[94] Often, arrhythmias are diagnosed for the first time in pregnancy. Although some cases are due to underlying cardiac diseases, most cases are benign and do not need medical intervention. However, sustained arrhythmias with symptoms may require treatment. The treatment of arrhythmias in the pregnant population is similar to the treatment in non-pregnant people, and when medical treatment fails or the situation becomes life-threatening, electric cardioversion should be considered.[95] It is recommended to use a smaller dose of energy, 50–100 joules at least as the first application of current.[96] A review of the literature seems to indicate that the success rate of cardioversion is greater (>90%) in pregnancy compared to a non-pregnant population (success rate of 40–90%).[95] Very little current reaches the uterus, and the small size of the fetal heart implies a high fibrillation threshold.[97,98]

As for the non-pregnant population requiring cardioversion, anaesthesia is induced with small to medium doses of propofol or thiopentone. Due to the physiological changes during pregnancy, preoxygenation should be performed.[20] Endotracheal intubation is recommended after the first trimester.

Cardiac surgery during pregnancy

Cardiac disorders may complicate pregnancy. However, the prevalence of clinically significant cardiac disease in pregnancy is low (<1%).[99] Women with pre-existing cardiac disease can develop acute heart failure during pregnancy.[100] Medical therapy is the first-line treatment. However, rarely, cardiac surgery is necessary. A multidisciplinary approach including the obstetrician, the cardiologist, cardiac surgeon, and anaesthetist, with close communication is necessary. Cardiac valve disease is the most frequent pathology and mitral valve disease is most prevalent.[101] Pregnancy is associated with profound physiological changes (as earlier described; Table 10.1). Both cardiac output and maternal blood volume are significantly increased. It is essential to maintain adequate preload and systemic vascular resistance. Aortocaval compression must be avoided. Moreover, hypoxaemia and myocardial depression during general anaesthesia should be avoided.

Cardiac surgery requiring cardiopulmonary bypass increases both maternal and fetal mortality.[100] The use of hypothermia decreases oxygen exchange through the placenta and may result in fetal bradycardia. It is important to maintain adequate uteroplacental flow and the pump flow should be increased by up to 50% during cardiopulmonary bypass. Moreover, the mean arterial pressure should be above 60 mmHg.

The use of perioperative fetal monitoring is advisable during cardiac surgery.

Neurosurgery during pregnancy

Cerebrovascular disease such as haemorrhage, arterial infarction, and venous thrombosis can occur during pregnancy. It is unclear if the incidence of intracerebral haemorrhage is increased in pregnancy. Bateman and colleagues found a frequency of 7.1/100,000 person-years in pregnant woman compared to 5/100,000 person-years in non-pregnant woman.[102] In contrast to this, Kim and colleagues recently have shown that the risk of rupture of cerebral aneurysms is not increased during pregnancy.[103] Intracerebral haemorrhage is the cause for about 7% of all pregnancy-related mortality.[102]

Anaesthetic management in patients undergoing neurosurgical procedures should be similar to that described for other obstetric patients. Maintenance of uteroplacental flow is essential. Pregnant women with untreated aneurysms should be managed in such a way that haemodynamic stability is maintained. Hypertension should be avoided. Many have their surgery/interventional radiology postponed till after delivery.

Anaesthetic management of the traumatized pregnant woman

Trauma is one of the most common causes of non-obstetric maternal morbidity and mortality during pregnancy. In some reports, as many as 40–50% of maternal deaths are related to trauma and it represents one of the leading causes of death due to non-obstetric reasons in pregnant women.[104] The incidence of major trauma varies in the literature between 2% and 7% of all pregnancies,[105,106] and is highest in the last trimester. Motor vehicle accidents, domestic violence, and/or intimate partner violence are the leading causes. Injuries from falls are also common. As in the non-pregnant population, socioeconomic status, level of education, and the use of toxic substances are strongly correlated to incidents of domestic violence.

When exposed to trauma, the risk for the fetus may result from direct force or by the changes imposed on the mother. In motor vehicle accidents, incorrect use of a safety belt may expose the fetus to coup/contre-coup forces leading to high intrauterine pressure and the risk of uterine rupture, bleeding, and abruption. Complications for the fetus encompass spontaneous abortion, placental abruption, premature birth, uterine rupture, fetal-maternal haemorrhage, and stillbirth. The risk of intrauterine death is correlated to the severity of the trauma. High maternal injury severity score, severe haemorrhage and hypovolaemia, an established abruption placenta, and maternal disseminated intravascular coagulation are all strong predictors of intrauterine death.[107–109]

Trauma management should primarily focus on stabilizing the mother, as the fetus is highly dependent on the mother's haemodynamic stability. The trauma team should initially follow a standard, well-established algorithm like the advanced trauma life support (ATLS).[110] When following the ABCDE of advanced life support, one should remember the many physiological changes that a pregnancy induces. Left lateral tilt should be established in order to avoid aortocaval compression if the woman is more than 20 weeks pregnant. If a chest tube is indicated it should be placed one or two intercostal areas higher than normal in order to avoid intra-abdominal placement, and guidance by ultrasound is advisable. As for all anaesthesia inductions in the pregnant woman, one should be prepared for a difficult intubation. An obstetrician should be part of the initial trauma team, and if the fetus is viable (>24 weeks), a neonatologist should also be present whenever possible. Fetal monitoring must be established as quickly as possible after the initial stabilization of the mother. An early ultrasound is indicated in order to establish the state of the fetus. If the pregnancy by itself makes resuscitation and stabilization of the woman difficult, especially during emergency intra-abdominal procedures, a termination of the pregnancy or an emergency caesarean delivery must be considered. If the mother is dead one must consider perimortem caesarean delivery as early as possible during resuscitation, preferably within 4 minutes.[111] A possible algorithm for guiding care of the pregnant trauma victim, including the letter F for Fetus, is shown in Table 10.3.

Conclusion

Surgery for non-obstetric reasons will be performed in 1–2% of all pregnant women. A careful evaluation of these patients and a good multidisciplinary preparation will reduce the risks for preterm labour, miscarriage, or abortions. Preventive measures should encompass a thorough evaluation of the airways, aspiration prophylaxis, and aortocaval displacement in order to prevent hypotension. The anaesthetic management should focus on maintenance of maternal haemodynamic stability and normoventilation. Locoregional anaesthetic techniques should be preferred whenever possible.

Table 10.3 Algorithm for guiding care of the pregnant trauma victim

Advanced trauma life support		**Management**
A	Airway	Secure airway Protect cervical spine Prepare for a difficult airway
B	Breathing	Check respiration Avoid maternal hypoxia Avoid maternal hypocapnia
C	Circulation	Identify and control bleeding Maintain adequate blood pressure (systolic blood pressure > 100 mmHg) Left lateral tilt (on backboard) Consider emergency caesarean delivery to save the mother
D	Disability	Examine neurology Glasgow Coma Scale score
E	Exposure	Undress patient Prevent hypothermia
F	Fetus	Establish fetal monitoring as quickly as possible Perform early ultrasound Carry out emergency caesarean delivery if necessary

References

1. Goodman S. Anesthesia for nonobstetric surgery in the pregnant patient. *Semin Perinatol* 2002; 26(2):136–45.
2. Cohen-Kerem R, Railton C, Oren D, *et al.* Pregnancy outcome following non-obstetric surgical intervention. *Am J Surg* 2005; 190(3):467–73.
3. Palmer CM, D'Angelo R, Paech MJ. *Handbook of Obstetric Anesthesia.* Oxford: BIOS; 2002.
4. Biro P. Difficult intubation in pregnancy. *Curr Opin Anaesthesiol* 2011; 24(3):249–54.
5. Kunitz O, Rossaint R. [Anesthesia during pregnancy]. *Chirurg* 2005; 76(8):737–43.
6. Kuczkowski KM. The safety of anaesthetics in pregnant women. *Expert Opin Drug Saf* 2006; 5(2):251–64.
7. Van Thiel DH, Gavaler JS, Joshi SN, *et al.* Heartburn of pregnancy. *Gastroenterology* 1977; 72(4 Pt 1):666–8.
8. Everson GT. Gastrointestinal motility in pregnancy. *Gastroenterol Clin North Am* 1992; 21(4):751–76.
9. Hong JY, Park JW, Oh JI. Comparison of preoperative gastric contents and serum gastrin concentrations in pregnant and nonpregnant women. *J Clin Anesth* 2005; 17(6):451–5.
10. Practice guidelines for obstetric anesthesia: an updated report by the American Society of Anesthesiologists Task Force on Obstetric Anesthesia. *Anesthesiology* 2007; 106(4):843–63.
11. Levy DM, Williams OA, Magides AD, *et al.* Gastric emptying is delayed at 8-12 weeks' gestation. *Br J Anaesth* 1994; 73(2):237–8.
12. de Souza DG, Doar LH, Mehta SH, *et al.* Aspiration prophylaxis and rapid sequence induction for elective cesarean delivery: time to reassess old dogma? *Anesth Analg* 2010; 110(5):1503–5.

13. Wong CA, McCarthy RJ, Fitzgerald PC, *et al.* Gastric emptying of water in obese pregnant women at term. *Anesth Analg* 2007; 105(3):751–5.
14. McDonnell NJ, Paech MJ, Clavisi OM, *et al.* Difficult and failed intubation in obstetric anaesthesia: an observational study of airway management and complications associated with general anaesthesia for caesarean section. *Int J Obstet Anesth* 2008; 17(4):292–7.
15. Djabatey EA, Barclay PM. Difficult and failed intubation in 3430 obstetric general anaesthetics. *Anaesthesia* 2009; 64(11):1168–71.
16. Gerlach K, Dorges V, Uhlig T. [Difficult airway management]. *Anasthesiol Intensivmed Notfallmed Schmerzther* 2006; 41(2):93–118.
17. Mhyre JM, Healy D. The unanticipated difficult intubation in obstetrics. *Anesth Analg* 2011; 112(3):648–52.
18. Munnur U, de Boisblanc B, Suresh MS. Airway problems in pregnancy. *Crit Care Med* 2005; 33(10 Suppl):S259–68.
19. Munnur U, Suresh MS. Airway problems in pregnancy. *Crit Care Clin* 2004; 20(4):617–42.
20. McClelland SH, Bogod DG, Hardman JG. Pre-oxygenation and apnoea in pregnancy: changes during labour and with obstetric morbidity in a computational simulation. *Anaesthesia* 2009; 64(4):371–7.
21. Chiron B, Laffon M, Ferrandiere M, *et al.* Standard preoxygenation technique versus two rapid techniques in pregnant patients. *Int J Obstet Anesth* 2004; 13(1):11–14.
22. Tanoubi I, Drolet P, Donati F. Optimizing preoxygenation in adults. *Can J Anaesth* 2009; 56(6):449–66.
23. Lerman J. On cricoid pressure: "may the force be with you". *Anesth Analg* 2009; 109(5):1363–6.
24. Ovassapian A, Salem MR. Sellick's maneuver: to do or not do. *Anesth Analg* 2009; 109(5):1360–2.
25. Fenton PM, Reynolds F. Life-saving or ineffective? An observational study of the use of cricoid pressure and maternal outcome in an African setting. *Int J Obstet Anesth* 2009; 18(2):106–10.
26. Bergen JM, Smith DC. A review of etomidate for rapid sequence intubation in the emergency department. *J Emerg Med* 1997; 15(2):221–30.
27. Wagner CE, Bick JS, Johnson D, *et al.* Etomidate use and postoperative outcomes among cardiac surgery patients. *Anesthesiology* 2014; 120(3):579–89.
28. Chan CM, Mitchell AL, Shorr AF. Etomidate is associated with mortality and adrenal insufficiency in sepsis: a meta-analysis. *Crit Care Med* 2012; 40(11):2945–53.
29. McPhee LC, Badawi O, Fraser GL, *et al.* Single-dose etomidate is not associated with increased mortality in ICU patients with sepsis: analysis of a large electronic ICU database. *Crit Care Med* 2013; 41(3):774–83.
30. Legrand M, Plaud B. Etomidate and general anesthesia: the butterfly effect? *Anesth Analg* 2013; 117(6):1267–9.
31. Komatsu R, You J, Mascha EJ, *et al.* Anesthetic induction with etomidate, rather than propofol, is associated with increased 30-day mortality and cardiovascular morbidity after noncardiac surgery. *Anesth Analg* 2013; 117(6):1329–37.
32. Sih K, Campbell SG, Tallon JM, *et al.* Ketamine in adult emergency medicine: controversies and recent advances. *Ann Pharmacother* 2011; 45(12):1525–34.
33. Fedorkow DM, Stewart TJ, Parboosingh J. Fetal heart rate changes associated with general anesthesia. *Am J Perinatol* 1989; 6(3):287–8.
34. McGuigan PJ, Shields MO, McCourt KC. Role of rocuronium and sugammadex in rapid sequence induction in pregnancy. *Br J Anaesth* 2011; 106(3):418–19.
35. Williamson RM, Mallaiah S, Barclay P. Rocuronium and sugammadex for rapid sequence induction of obstetric general anaesthesia. *Acta Anaesthesiol Scand* 2011; 55(6):694–9.
36. Perry JJ, Lee JS, Sillberg VA, *et al.* Rocuronium versus succinylcholine for rapid sequence induction intubation. *Cochrane Database Syst Rev* 2008; 2:CD002788.
37. Sharp LM, Levy DM. Rapid sequence induction in obstetrics revisited. *Curr Opin Anaesthesiol* 2009; 22(3):357–61.
38. Sorensen MK, Bretlau C, Gatke MR, *et al.* Rapid sequence induction and intubation with rocuronium-sugammadex compared with succinylcholine: a randomized trial. *Br J Anaesth* 2012; 108(4):682–9.
39. Abboud TK, Zhu J, Richardson M, *et al.* Desflurane: a new volatile anesthetic for cesarean section. Maternal and neonatal effects. *Acta Anaesthesiol Scand* 1995; 39(6):723–6.
40. Chin KJ, Yeo SW. Bispectral index values at sevoflurane concentrations of 1% and 1.5% in lower segment cesarean delivery. *Anesth Analg* 2004; 98(4):1140–4.
41. Dwyer R, Fee JP, Moore J. Uptake of halothane and isoflurane by mother and baby during caesarean section. *Br J Anaesth* 1995; 74(4):379–83.
42. Okutomi T, Whittington RA, Stein DJ, *et al.* Comparison of the effects of sevoflurane and isoflurane anesthesia on the maternal-fetal unit in sheep. *J Anesth* 2009; 23(3):392–8.
43. Boat A, Mahmoud M, Michelfelder EC, *et al.* Supplementing desflurane with intravenous anesthesia reduces fetal cardiac dysfunction during open fetal surgery. *Paediatr Anaesth* 2010; 20(8):748–56.
44. Cunningham AJ. Laparoscopic surgery—anesthetic implications. *Surg Endosc* 1994; 8(11):1272–84.
45. El-Galley R, Hammontree L, Urban D, *et al.* Anesthesia for laparoscopic donor nephrectomy: is nitrous oxide contraindicated? *J Urol* 2007; 178(1):225–7.
46. Brodsky JB, Lemmens HJ, Collins JS, *et al.* Nitrous oxide and laparoscopic bariatric surgery. *Obes Surg* 2005; 15(4):494–6.
47. Kestin IG. Spinal anaesthesia in obstetrics. *Br J Anaesth* 1991; 66(5):596–607.
48. Brennan MC, Rayburn WF. Counseling about risks of congenital anomalies from prescription opioids. *Birth Defects Res A Clin Mol Teratol* 2012; 94(8):620–5.
49. McElhatton PR, Sullivan FM, Volans GN. Paracetamol overdose in pregnancy analysis of the outcomes of 300 cases referred to the Teratology Information Service. *Reprod Toxicol* 1997; 11(1):85–94.
50. Miller RD. *Miller's Anesthesia* (7th ed.). Philadelphia, PA: Churchill Livingstone/Elsevier; 2010.
51. Adams K, Bombardier C, van der Heijde DM. Safety of pain therapy during pregnancy and lactation in patients with inflammatory arthritis: a systematic literature review. *J Rheumatol Suppl* 2012; 90:59–61.
52. Ericson A, Kallen BA. Nonsteroidal anti-inflammatory drugs in early pregnancy. *Reprod Toxicol* 2001; 15(4):371–5.
53. Ofori B, Oraichi D, Blais L, *et al.* Risk of congenital anomalies in pregnant users of non-steroidal anti-inflammatory drugs: a nested case-control study. *Birth Defects Res B Dev Reprod Toxic*ol 2006; 77(4):268–79.
54. Nielsen GL, Sorensen HT, Larsen H, *et al.* Risk of adverse birth outcome and miscarriage in pregnant users of non-steroidal anti-inflammatory drugs: population based observational study and case-control study. *BMJ* 2001; 322(7281):266–70.
55. Moise KJ Jr. Effect of advancing gestational age on the frequency of fetal ductal constriction in association with maternal indomethacin use. *Am J Obstet Gynecol* 1993; 168(5):1350–3.
56. Schafer AI. Effects of nonsteroidal antiinflammatory drugs on platelet function and systemic hemostasis. *J Clin Pharmacol* 1995; 35(3):209–19.
57. Brodsky JB, Cohen EN. Adverse effects of nitrous oxide. *Med Toxicol* 1986; 1(5):362–74.
58. Fujinaga M, Baden JM, Yhap EO, *et al.* Reproductive and teratogenic effects of nitrous oxide, isoflurane, and their combination in Sprague-Dawley rats. *Anesthesiology* 1987; 67(6):960–4.
59. Polvi HJ, Pirhonen JP, Erkkola RU. Nitrous oxide inhalation: effects on maternal and fetal circulations at term. *Obstet Gynecol* 1996; 87(6):1045–8.
60. Czeizel AE, Pataki T, Rockenbauer M. Reproductive outcome after exposure to surgery under anesthesia during pregnancy. *Arch Gynecol Obstet* 1998; 261(4):193–9.
61. Mazze RI, Kallen B. Reproductive outcome after anesthesia and operation during pregnancy: a registry study of 5405 cases. *Am J Obstet Gynecol* 1989; 161(5):1178–85.
62. Olfert SM. Reproductive outcomes among dental personnel: a review of selected exposures. *J Can Dent Assoc* 2006; 72(9):821–5.

63. Bonnot O, Vollset SE, Godet PF, *et al.* [In utero exposure to benzodiazepine. Is there a risk for anal atresia with lorazepam?]. *Encephale* 2003; 29(6):553–9.
64. Enato E, Moretti M, Koren G. The fetal safety of benzodiazepines: an updated meta-analysis. *J Obstet Gynaecol Can* 2011; 33(1):46–8.
65. McElhatton PR. The effects of benzodiazepine use during pregnancy and lactation. *Reprod Toxicol* 1994; 8(6):461–75.
66. Wikner BN, Stiller CO, Bergman U, *et al.* Use of benzodiazepines and benzodiazepine receptor agonists during pregnancy: neonatal outcome and congenital malformations. *Pharmacoepidemiol Drug Saf* 2007; 16(11):1203–10.
67. Jevtovic-Todorovic V, Hartman RE, Izumi Y, *et al.* Early exposure to common anesthetic agents causes widespread neurodegeneration in the developing rat brain and persistent learning deficits. *J Neurosci* 2003; 23(3):876–82.
68. Ikonomidou C, Bosch F, Miksa M, *et al.* Blockade of NMDA receptors and apoptotic neurodegeneration in the developing brain. *Science* 1999; 283(5398):70–4.
69. Sall JW, Stratmann G, Leong J, *et al.* Isoflurane inhibits growth but does not cause cell death in hippocampal neural precursor cells grown in culture. *Anesthesiology* 2009; 110(4):826–33.
70. Wilder RT, Flick RP, Sprung J, *et al.* Early exposure to anesthesia and learning disabilities in a population-based birth cohort. *Anesthesiology* 2009; 110(4):796–804.
71. Sprung J, Flick RP, Wilder RT, *et al.* Anesthesia for cesarean delivery and learning disabilities in a population-based birth cohort. *Anesthesiology* 2009; 111(2):302–10.
72. Usta IM, Khalil A, Nassar AH. Oxytocin antagonists for the management of preterm birth: a review. *Am J Perinatol* 2011; 28(6):449–60.
73. Patel SJ, Reede DL, Katz DS, *et al.* Imaging the pregnant patient for nonobstetric conditions: algorithms and radiation dose considerations. *Radiographics* 2007; 27(6):1705–22.
74. Brent RL. Saving lives and changing family histories: appropriate counseling of pregnant women and men and women of reproductive age, concerning the risk of diagnostic radiation exposures during and before pregnancy. *Am J Obstet Gynecol* 2009; 200(1):4–24.
75. Bross ID, Natarajan N. Risk of leukemia in susceptible children exposed to preconception, in utero and postnatal radiation. *Prev Med* 1974; 3(3):361–9.
76. Stewart A, Webb J, Hewitt D. A survey of childhood malignancies. *Br Med J (Clin Res Ed)* 1958; 1(5086):1495–508.
77. Smits AK, Paladine HL, Judkins DZ, *et al.* Clinical inquiries. What are the risks to the fetus associated with diagnostic radiation exposure during pregnancy? *J Fam Pract* 2006; 55(5):441–2, 444.
78. Tremblay E, Therasse E, Thomassin-Naggara I, *et al.* Quality initiatives: guidelines for use of medical imaging during pregnancy and lactation. *Radiographics* 2012; 32(3):897–911.
79. Groen RS, Bae JY, Lim KJ. Fear of the unknown: ionizing radiation exposure during pregnancy. *Am J Obstet Gynecol* 2012; 206(6):456–62.
80. ACOG Committee Opinion. Number 299, September 2004 (replaces No. 158, September 1995). Guidelines for diagnostic imaging during pregnancy. *Obstet Gynecol* 2004; 104(3):647–51.
81. McCollough CH, Schueler BA, Atwell TD, *et al.* Radiation exposure and pregnancy: when should we be concerned? *Radiographics* 2007; 27(4):909–17.
82. Miller DL. Safety assurance in obstetrical ultrasound. *Semin Ultrasound CT MR* 2008; 29(2):156–64.
83. Katz DS, Klein MA, Ganson G, *et al.* Imaging of abdominal pain in pregnancy. *Radiol Clin North Am* 2012; 50(1):149–71.
84. Parks NA, Schroeppel TJ. Update on imaging for acute appendicitis. *Surg Clin North Am* 2011; 91(1):141–54.
85. Chen MM, Coakley FV, Kaimal A, *et al.* Guidelines for computed tomography and magnetic resonance imaging use during pregnancy and lactation. *Obstet Gynecol* 2008; 112(2 Pt 1):333–40.
86. Hibbeln JF, Shors SM, Byrd SE. MRI: is there a role in obstetrics? *Clin Obstet Gynecol* 2012; 55(1):352–66.
87. Brown MA, Birchard KR, Semelka RC. Magnetic resonance evaluation of pregnant patients with acute abdominal pain. *Semin Ultrasound CT MR* 2005; 26(4):206–11.
88. Ahmet A, Lawson ML, Babyn P, *et al.* Hypothyroidism in neonates post-iodinated contrast media: a systematic review. *Acta Paediatr* 2009; 98(10):1568–74.
89. Chung JC, Cho GS, Shin EJ, *et al.* Clinical outcomes compared between laparoscopic and open appendectomy in pregnant women. *Can J Surg* 2013; 56(5):341–6.
90. Kirshtein B, Perry ZH, Avinoach E, *et al.* Safety of laparoscopic appendectomy during pregnancy. *World J Surg* 2009; 33(3):475–80.
91. Yumi H. Guidelines for diagnosis, treatment, and use of laparoscopy for surgical problems during pregnancy: this statement was reviewed and approved by the Board of Governors of the Society of American Gastrointestinal and Endoscopic Surgeons (SAGES), September 2007. It was prepared by the SAGES Guidelines Committee. *Surg Endosc* 2008; 22(4):849–61.
92. Dietz PM, Williams SB, Callaghan WM, *et al.* Clinically identified maternal depression before, during, and after pregnancies ending in live births. *Am J Psychiatry* 2007; 164(10):1515–20.
93. Anderson EL, Reti IM. ECT in pregnancy: a review of the literature from 1941 to 2007. *Psychosom Med* 2009; 71(2):235–42.
94. Robins K, Lyons G. Supraventricular tachycardia in pregnancy. *Br J Anaesth* 2004; 92(1):140–3.
95. Tromp CH, Nanne AC, Pernet PJ, *et al.* Electrical cardioversion during pregnancy: safe or not? *Neth Heart J* 2011; 19(3):134–6.
96. Trappe HJ. [Arrhythmias during pregnancy]. *Dtsch Med Wochenschr* 2008; 133(36):1799–804.
97. Page RL. Treatment of arrhythmias during pregnancy. *Am Heart J* 1995; 130(4):871–6.
98. Wang YC, Chen CH, Su HY, *et al.* The impact of maternal cardioversion on fetal haemodynamics. *Eur J Obstet Gynecol Reprod Biol* 2006; 126(2):268–9.
99. Hameed AB, Sklansky MS. Pregnancy: maternal and fetal heart disease. *Curr Probl Cardiol* 2007; 32(8):419–94.
100. Pomini F, Mercogliano D, Cavalletti C, *et al.* Cardiopulmonary bypass in pregnancy. *Ann Thorac Surg* 1996; 61(1):259–68.
101. Arnoni RT, Arnoni AS, Bonini RC, *et al.* Risk factors associated with cardiac surgery during pregnancy. *Ann Thorac Surg* 2003; 76(5):1605–8.
102. Bateman BT, Schumacher HC, Bushnell CD, *et al.* Intracerebral hemorrhage in pregnancy: frequency, risk factors, and outcome. *Neurology* 2006; 67(3):424–9.
103. Kim YW, Neal D, Hoh BL. Cerebral aneurysms in pregnancy and delivery: pregnancy and delivery do not increase the risk of aneurysm rupture. *Neurosurgery* 2013; 72(2):143–50.
104. Romero VC, Pearlman M. Maternal mortality due to trauma. *Semin Perinatol* 2012; 36(1):60–7.
105. Einav S, Sela HY, Weiniger CF. Management and outcomes of trauma during pregnancy. *Anesthesiol Clin* 2013; 31(1):141–56.
106. Mendez-Figueroa H, Dahlke JD, Vrees RA, *et al.* Trauma in pregnancy: an updated systematic review. *Am J Obstet Gynecol* 2013; 209(1):1–10.
107. Melamed N, Aviram A, Silver M, *et al.* Pregnancy course and outcome following blunt trauma. *J Matern Fetal Neonatal Med* 2012; 25(9):1612–17.
108. Trivedi N, Ylagan M, Moore TR, *et al.* Predicting adverse outcomes following trauma in pregnancy. *J Reprod Med* 2012; 57(1–2):3–8.
109. Schiff MA, Holt VL. The injury severity score in pregnant trauma patients: predicting placental abruption and fetal death. *J Trauma* 2002; 53(5):946–9.
110. van Olden GD, Meeuwis JD, Bolhuis HW, *et al.* Clinical impact of advanced trauma life support. *Am J Emerg Med* 2004; 22(7):522–5.
111. Warraich Q, Esen U. Perimortem caesarean section. *J Obstet Gynaecol* 2009; 29(8):690–3.

CHAPTER 11

Drugs in pregnancy and lactation

Oliver Kraemer and Timothée Fraisse

Drugs during pregnancy

Whereas during normal, uncomplicated pregnancy few drugs are usually required, a wide range of drugs might be necessary during high-risk or complicated pregnancies. This can lead to complex or controversial decisions.[1,2] Besides herbal and over-the-counter drugs, it is estimated that more than half of pregnancies in developed countries are exposed to one or more prescribed drugs, with 7–10% of exposed pregnancies being exposed to drugs labelled D or X, based on the US Food and Drug Administration (FDA) classification (Figure 11.1).[3] However, drug safety classification gives a very crude estimation of risks and should only be used as a general guideline when planning treatment.[4] This chapter will provide the basis for understanding the principles of reproductive and developmental toxicology and elaborate on strategies for use of some of the most common drugs in obstetric anaesthesia. It should neither be considered as an exhaustive description of the potential side effects nor as a prescription guide for specific situations.

Scientific knowledge evolves continuously with the emergence of new drugs and reports of newly observed side effects based on pharmacovigilance follow-up. One should always refer to up-to-date international references when administering drugs to pregnant women, especially with newly marketed compounds. Literature references typically include Schaefer et al.'s *Drugs During Pregnancy and Lactation*[5] and Briggs and Freeman's *Drugs in Pregnancy and Lactation*[2], also available as an iPhone app. Web-based public sources include the Organization of Teratology Information Specialists (http://www.otispregnancy.org/), the Drugs and Lactation Database (LactMed; http://toxnet.nlm.nih.gov/newtoxnet/lactmed.htm), the Toxnet Toxicology data network (http://toxnet.nlm.nih.gov), and the European Network of Teratology Information Services (ENTIS; http://www.entisorg.org) which provide useful guidelines for most common prescription drugs, herbals, and other chemicals (e.g. drugs of abuse).

Additionally, specialized units in most university hospitals and poison control centres will provide useful recommendations in cases of atypical situations.

Basic principles of reproductive and developmental toxicology

A drug's ability to induce developmental or fetotoxic disorders depends upon four fundamental variables:

- Developmental stage of the embryo/fetus
- Genetic susceptibility (as for codeine metabolism)
- Dose
- Mechanism of action.

The complex interaction of all four variables leads to a great variability in the observed effects of a given drug. Hence it is difficult to extrapolate the data obtained in toxicological animals experiments to humans. Moreover, because of the ethical limitations to conduct clinical trials in the pregnant population, most relevant evidence is obtained following clinical monitoring of drugs inadvertently administered to women at various pregnancy stages. In order to assess the potential reproductive and developmental toxicity of a drug in humans, all available data sets should be taken into account prior to a decision (animal reprotoxicological studies as well as epidemiological data).[6] Epidemiological observations such as case registries are essentially limited in number and subject to various biases. Cohort studies and case–control cohort studies have been commonly used since the 1980s to establish statistical associations between drug exposure and various pregnancy outcomes.[7–11]

Pharmacokinetic changes during pregnancy

During pregnancy, several ADME parameters are modified that can lead to different risks for the embryo/fetus (i.e. absorption, distribution, metabolism, and excretion). The final concentration of a given drug in the embryo is therefore affected by four main consecutive factors: drug distribution in the mother, maternal drug metabolism and passage through the placental barrier (Chapter 3 has more detailed information on drug passage through the placenta), drug distribution in the embryo/fetus, and reabsorption from the amniotic fluid. Dosages must therefore be carefully adapted (often increased) during pregnancy in order to meet the therapeutic range required for the mother. However, when increasing dosages of drugs easily crossing the placental barrier, the prescribing physician should be particularly cautious regarding potential embryo- or fetotoxicity and always favour drugs that are known to be the safest:

- Drug distribution in the mother is affected by physiological changes which can be summarized by an increase in resorption (decrease in peristalsis of the intestines and increase in skin and lung blood flow), an increase in volume of distribution (plasma, total body water increases up to 8 L at the end of pregnancy, and fat deposition), a decrease in plasma proteins concentration to which drugs are non-covalently linked (especially albumin that decreases up to 10 g/L), changes in metabolism (the different liver metabolic pathways are activated when increasing the female hormone production), and an enhanced excretion through glomerular filtration (almost double the renal plasma flow).[12]

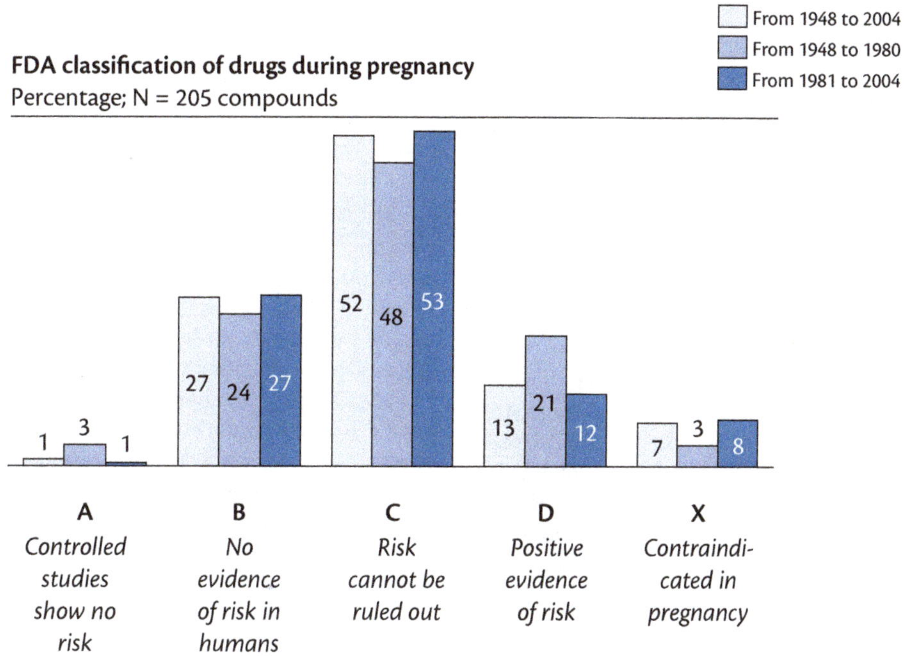

Figure 11.1 The sole FDA classification of drugs does not provide sufficient information to support informed prescription in most cases.
Data from the U.S. Food and Drug Administration.

- The passage to the placenta has been extensively studied at the time of delivery. The maternal/placental blood–blood barrier allows selective diffusion of drugs. One should consider that most molecules will achieve equilibrium on both sides of the placenta over time and that transfer of most drugs to the fetus is certain. Small (molecular weight < 600–800 Da), lipophilic, non-ionized molecules tend to cross the placenta more easily than others. Larger molecules with molecular weight around 5000 Da (such as insulin), hydrophilic, ionized, or linked to plasma proteins will cross the barrier to a lesser extent. Therefore, most anaesthetics will easily cross the placental barrier due to their high hydrophobic/lipophilic profile. Some other drugs cross through specific transport mechanisms (e.g. immunoglobulins). Little is known regarding *in vivo* drug transport through the yolk sac and the placenta at earlier stages of pregnancy. Most early-stage studies have been performed with *in vitro* models allowing a better understanding of single-dose transfer but not capturing the complexity of multiple-dose administration, and potential accumulation (depending on biodistribution and pharmacokinetics of the drugs in mother).[5,13]
- Accumulation of the parent drug or its metabolites is likely to occur in the fetal compartment (embryo/fetus and the amniotic fluid) because of the limited fetal metabolism.[14] While this is in most cases detrimental to the fetus, it is considered beneficial in the prevention of mother-to-child infections transfer (e.g. with certain antiretrovirals or antibiotics).

Anaesthetic drugs: local anaesthetics, hypnotics, and muscle relaxants

Major stages of fetal brain development occur during the last trimester of intrauterine life, with the human brain being not fully developed at birth and continuing to grow over the first few years of postnatal life.[15] There is a current debate on whether general anaesthesia can cause cognitive and mild neurocognitive effects due to neuronal apoptosis in newborns during their neonatal period.[16] Few epidemiological studies have specifically focused on individual anaesthetic drugs. However, several studies did not exert negative outcomes after a range of surgical procedures, which used a variety of anaesthetic agents.[8,10,17,18] The potential impact of surgery on neurodevelopment is not the purpose of this chapter.[19]

None of the commonly used anaesthetics induce an increase in congenital malformations. However, particular attention should be paid to avoid otherwise common anaesthesia-related side effects occurring in the mother that might be detrimental to the fetus (e.g. hypoventilation and malignant hyperthermia):

- Widely used local anaesthetics (ropivacaine, bupivacaine, levobupivacaine, lidocaine, and chloroprocaine) are generally considered safe during pregnancy and labour. Both ropivacaine and bupivacaine are highly bound to plasma proteins (94–95%) which leads to low placental transfer (equilibrium in the fetus occurs at roughly one-third of the mother's blood concentration). Both drugs exert extended half-lives in neonates.
- Bupivacaine's half-life in adults and neonates is 2.7 and 8.1 hours, respectively. Ropivacaine's milk transfer is very low and probably lower than that of bupivacaine and lidocaine.[20] Lidocaine has been widely studied in humans and rats at various pregnancy stages and does not demonstrate higher teratogenic risks in humans.[21,22] However, because of its lower protein binding (60–80%), lidocaine (FDA Pregnancy Category B) easily transfers through the placenta and achieves high concentration equilibrium in the fetus. Several side effects have been observed, all occurring at a very low frequency (e.g. transient neurobehavioral or cardiopulmonary impairments in the neonates). However, the total amount needed should be as little as possible when procedures (e.g. dental) are required in pregnant women, and should be postponed if not required.

- Most intravenous hypnotics may be used during pregnancy and labour, with particular caution for specific molecules:
  - Propofol (molecular weight 179 Da) can be administered during the entire pregnancy (from oocyte retrieval in the fertility laboratory to labour and delivery). It is highly bound to plasma protein (95–99%) but highly lipophilic/hydrophobic (3.842) and therefore reaches fairly high levels in the fetus at all stages of pregnancy (~70% of the mother's blood concentration). When used during the period of delivery, and because of its respiratory depressant effects, specific care should be given to monitoring of the neonate.[23–25]
  - Thiopental is considered safe for use at all stages of pregnancy. There is, however, less epidemiological data available regarding its use at early pregnancy stages. Thiopental achieves a fast equilibrium (1:1) between maternal and fetal blood as it binds to a lesser extend with plasma proteins (80%). Similarly to propofol, specific attention should be paid to monitoring the neonate when administered around the time of delivery.[22]
  - Etomidate is generally considered safe during pregnancy despite the fact that there is only limited epidemiological data available. When administered at the time of delivery, main adverse effects are a transient decrease in newborn cortisol levels (with no clinical impact) and possible respiratory distress.[26]
  - Ketamine should, when possible, be avoided during pregnancy (limited epidemiological data) and labour, as several adverse effects can occur, such as increased uterine tone and neonatal behavioural impairment. Additionally, ketamine should be clearly contraindicated in the following occurrences: maternal hypertension and/or (pre-)eclampsia, uterine hypertonicity, and intermediate to pathological fetal cardiotocography patterns.
- Halogenated agents are commonly used during pregnancy and delivery. These agents may be considered safe at any time during pregnancy. However, a careful monitoring of the newborn should be done when used at the time of delivery (possible respiratory and circulatory depression). These agents are considered non-teratogenic.[5,27,28] Sevoflurane, desflurane, and halothane have a uterine relaxant effect through activation of ATP-dependent potassium channels, and their ability to reduce uterine tone is well known to obstetricians.[29,30] This may result in a higher risk of blood loss at caesarean delivery. The use of isoflurane may cause an increase in bilirubin levels in the newborn.[31] Limited human data are available on the use of desflurane and sevoflurane during pregnancy, which are nonetheless routinely used at various stages of pregnancy. Sporadic cases of malignant hyperthermia and fetal bradycardia have been reported with the use of desflurane and sevoflurane respectively.[32,33]
- Nitrous oxide is generally a well-tolerated anaesthetic, with a mild effect on the circulatory system or the uterine tone. When used during pregnancy,[22,34] no increase in the incidence of malformations was demonstrated. Nevertheless several anaesthetists do not use it in pregnant patients, as it interacts with vitamin B_{12} resulting in a selective inhibition of methionine synthase, a key enzyme in methionine and folate metabolism. When used at the time of delivery, the newborn should be monitored for possible respiratory distress.
- Most common muscle relaxants (e.g. atracurium, rocuronium, suxamethonium, and vecuronium) may be safely used at various stages of pregnancy, including during delivery. Only limited amounts of these drugs cross the placental barrier, because of their short half-lives and low hydrophobic and high ionization profiles. Concentration in the umbilical cord accounts for 10–20% of maternal plasma concentration.[35–38]

Contrary to what has long been thought, several studies did not demonstrate an association between occupational exposure to volatile anaesthetics and abortion or malformative rates,[39,40] despite workplace concentrations that often exceed legal requirements. On the other hand, occupational exposure to nitrous oxide has been retrospectively associated with increased abortion rates and decreased fertility, both of which may be mitigated by the use of scavenging devices.[41,42] These results may have been biased by several confounding factors and should therefore be considered with all due caution.

Analgesics and anti-inflammatory drugs

- Paracetamol (acetaminophen) is considered safe at all stages of pregnancy. It is the first-line analgesic and antipyretic treatment in pregnant women.[43–45] Because of its low protein binding (~25%) and small molecular weight (151 Da), paracetamol easily crosses the placental barrier and achieves high concentrations in the fetal compartment. Maternal intake of paracetamol for more than 4 weeks during pregnancy, especially during the first and second trimesters, may moderately increase the occurrence of cryptorchidism.[46]
- Codeine may be used during pregnancy when therapeutic doses of paracetamol do not achieve sufficient pain relief, and also as a third-line treatment (after non-steroidal anti-inflammatory drugs (NSAIDs)). Animal studies have not shown any hazards, but there is inadequate evidence of safety during pregnancy. A few unconfirmed retrospective studies indicated a possible teratogenic effect. These were not confirmed by more recent cohort studies.[47] Administration at the time of delivery may trigger respiratory depression and suckling difficulties in the newborn. Additionally, withdrawal symptoms may appear after chronic *in utero* exposure (e.g. abuse). Recent studies outlined a possible link between codeine intake during pregnancy, caesarean delivery, and postpartum haemorrhage.[47] According to a 2013 update from the UK Medicines & Healthcare products Regulatory Agency (MHRA) (https://www.gov.uk/drug-safety-update), the use of codeine during pregnancy and lactation should be balanced between risks and benefits, and is considered acceptable if there is no safer alternative. Similarly, the MHRA has said that codeine is contraindicated in children under the age of 12 because of an increased risk of serious and life-threatening adverse reactions, including loss of consciousness and respiratory arrest.
- Fentanyl, sufentanil, and alfentanil are commonly used during all pregnancy stages, either through intravenous, spinal, or epidural administration.[5,48] They easily cross the trophoblast membrane and the placenta.[49,50] There is only limited epidemiological data available in humans, especially regarding pregnancy outcome after administration during the first trimester.
- Chronic morphine use should, when possible, be avoided during pregnancy. Developmental studies in mice and hamsters

demonstrated an increased teratogenicity,[48] with increased neurological, soft tissue, and skeletal abnormalities, when used at a maternal toxic dose. Available epidemiological data in humans does not confirm an increase in malformations or in behavioural anomalies in newborns exposed during pregnancy. As for codeine and other opioids, specific attention should be paid when administered chronically *in utero* and at the time of delivery (respiratory depression and psychophysiological effects can occur in neonates, and naloxone and resuscitative equipment should be available).

- Pethidine should not be used as an analgesic during pregnancy because of fetal:maternal concentration ratios greater than 1. It is, however, widely used during labour for pain relief (with no negative effects on labour duration nor on postpartum bleeding). Poorly metabolized by the newborn, it may trigger respiratory depression and breastfeeding difficulties and neonates should be appropriately monitored when pethidine is administered 1–4 hours before delivery, especially after administration of repeated doses (accumulation in the maternal and fetal compartments) or in premature births (for which it should be contraindicated).
- Tramadol use should, when possible, be avoided during conception and early pregnancy. There is no proper evaluation or clear evidence of fetal or neonatal harm, despite sporadic fetal losses being reported. At the time of parturition, and following chronic maternal use, there is a risk of neonatal withdrawal syndrome, with the molecule easily crossing the placental barrier and achieving equilibrium in the fetal compartment.
- Naloxone may be administered at all stages of pregnancy. Animal data does not suggest any teratogenic effect. Human data are sporadic but reassuring.
- Ibuprofen and other commonly used NSAIDs (i.e. diclofenac) may be used for anti-inflammatory or analgesic indications before 24 weeks' gestation.[46,51] After 24 weeks, all NSAIDs are contraindicated whatever the route of administration because of pulmonary and renal vasoconstriction in the fetus that can lead to oligoamnios or fetal death following the closure of the ductus arteriosus. In a recent Norwegian cohort study, use of ibuprofen or diclofenac in the second trimester was significantly associated with low birthweight, and ibuprofen use in the second and third trimesters was significantly associated with asthma in 18-month-old children.[51] This large cohort study assessed infant survival, congenital malformations, structural heart defects, neonatal complications, haemorrhage during pregnancy and postpartum, as well as asthma at the age of 18 months. It did not find any effect on rates of infant survival, congenital malformation, or structural heart defects. There was, however, a significant association between diclofenac and ibuprofen use late in pregnancy, and maternal bleeding and asthma in the child, respectively.
- Aspirin is not considered as the analgesic or antipyretic of choice but may still be used at various stages of pregnancy.[52,53] Large retrospective and prospective studies in humans did not demonstrate an increase in malformation rates, despite evidence of birth defects in the animal models. Aspirin may be used at therapeutic doses during pregnancy with the following restrictions:
  - Doses greater than 500 mg/day are contraindicated after 24 weeks gestation. Special caution should be paid during the last weeks of the pregnancy, since even low-dose administration will decrease platelet adhesiveness and may trigger newborn intracranial bleeding and increased postpartum bleeding.
- Selective cyclooxygenase (COX)-2 inhibitors should be avoided during pregnancy because of the lack of human data to support their use. Use of diclofenac systemic formulations during pregnancy has recently raised concerns in the United Kingdom, despite a reassuring prospective observational cohort study.[54] As for other NSAIDs, administration should be contraindicated after 24 weeks' gestation.

Anti-infective agents during pregnancy: antibiotics, antimycotics, and antivirals

- Penicillins and other beta-lactam antibiotics are classified as bactericidal. As penicillin interacts with bacterial wall synthesis (this mechanism does not exist in humans) it is the first-line antibiotic treatment for many common infectious problems in pregnancy. There exists sufficient clinical proof that there is neither embryo- nor fetotoxicity even though penicillin has rapid transplacental passage.[55,56] This is also true for combination therapy with clavulanic acid and also beta-lactamase inhibitors, which are considered safe for use during pregnancy.
- Cephalosporins such as penicillin are commonly used during pregnancy. They have a higher clearance during pregnancy and a dosage adaption is needed. Almost a complete transplacental passage occurs for all generations of cephalosporins.[57] However, as second- and third-generation are associated with cases of immunohaemolysis,[58] most clinicians prefer the older cephalexin and cefuroxime. There is no evidence for teratogenicity in the first trimester.[59,60]
- Erythromycin and other macrolide antibiotics are bacteriostatic, and are commonly used in case of known allergy to penicillin. They interact with bacterial protein synthesis. There are reports of maternal hepatotoxicity in the second half of pregnancy for erythromycin estolate or troleandomycin and therefore these two macrolides are to be avoided during the second and third trimester. The placental passage is low (5–20%) during the third trimester for erythromycin, and it is therefore not recommended in the treatment of fetal or amniotic infections. No macrolides have demonstrated teratogenicity,[61,62] and clindamycin and lincomycin do not cause embryo- or fetotoxicity.[63–66] Spiramycin is the treatment of choice for toxoplasmosis in the first trimester. Clindamycin and lincomycin are used second line, because they are less effective in bacterial vaginal infection and should be used only after penicillins, cephalosporins, or other macrolides failures. They do present with high maternal resorption and there is a 50% passage across the placental barrier.
- Tetracyclines are only used in a second intention, as broad-spectrum antibiotics, and can be used, for example, for treating urinary tract infections in the first trimester. They are contraindicated after the 16th week of gestation because of their accretion to teeth and bones that is clearly demonstrated in animals. In the 1950s they were often used, and are associated with

yellow discoloured teeth. They are bacteriostatic, affect protein synthesis, and no teratogenicity has been reported.[2]

- Sulphonamides, trimethoprim, and co-trimoxazole (single or combination use) are also used as a second choice during pregnancy for urinary tract infections. There is no evidence for teratogenicity. Sulphonamides are bacteriostatic and 50–90% accumulates in the fetal compartment. They do suppress bilirubin from their plasma protein binding. Trimethoprim is a folic acid antagonist, and its use can be considered, when combined with folic acid substitution, in specific situations such as *Pneumocystis jirovecii* pneumonia (AIDS setting) during the first trimester.
- Gyrase antagonists (4-quinolones) interact with a bacterial-specific topoisomerase enzyme and therefore have theoretically no interaction in humans. They are used when first-line therapy for enteral bacteria such as pseudomonas fails or when resistance to better agents is identified (e.g. ciprofloxacin and norfloxacin). However, routine use of these agents is not recommended despite reassuring reports. In cases of occasional use in the first trimester, a high-definition ultrasound is recommended to evaluate malformative risk in the embryo/fetus.
- Nitrofurantoin, fosfomycin, and methenamine, used for urinary tract infections, are not recommended except in very specific situations.
- Nitroimidazole antibiotics are indicated in trichomonas or anaerobe infections. Metronidazole reaches higher concentrations in the fetal compartment than in the maternal compartment. As it presents mutagenic and carcinogenic potential, following toxicological *in vitro* and *in vivo* evaluation, a cautious approach is advised when used during pregnancy. Its vaginal use is not indicated.
- Aminoglycosides have bactericidal interaction on (Gram-negative) bacterial protein synthesis. Concentration in the fetal compartment does reach up to 20–40% of maternal concentrations after parenteral administration. No teratogenicity has been reported, but because of ototoxicity, their indications are limited to life-threatening infections or after first-line treatment failure. Maternal plasma concentrations should be regularly monitored.
- Chloramphenicol presents a bacteriostatic action, and is clearly contraindicated in pregnancy because of its known risks of potentially lethal agranulocytosis or Grey syndrome.
- Polypeptides antibiotics are used against Gram-positive bacteria as multiresistant staphylococci, but remain limited to life-threatening infections.
- Tuberculostatics such as isoniazid, rifampicin, and ethambutol are first-line treatment against mycobacteria and are not considered teratogenic. Vitamin B_6 must be administered to the mother treated with isoniazid. Vitamin K must be administered to the newborn of mothers treated by rifampicin. Pyrazinamide and dapsone are second-choice treatments.
- Local antimycotics:
    - Nystatin is the first-choice agent for non-systemic, local treatment during pregnancy, with limited feto- or embryotoxicity reported.[67,68] There might be a possible, yet unconfirmed, association between hypospadias and nystatin.
    - Clotrimazole is a good choice in local antimycotic treatment in pregnancy, as there is limited systemic absorption, and with limited feto- or embryotoxic effects reported.[68] Other imidazole derivatives are considered second-choice alternatives in the second and third trimesters.
    - There is only limited human data available regarding the use of other local antimycotics during pregnancy (amorolfine, ciclopirox, naftifine, terbinafine, tolciclate, and tolnaftate), that are hence not recommended as first-line therapies.
- Systemic antimycotics:
    - Conazole antimycotics: in animal models these drugs are described to pass the fetoplacental barrier, but they have shown a limited teratogenic potential in humans (http://www.entisorg.org). Their use can be allowed during the first trimester when systemic treatment cannot be avoided. Regular ultrasound for organogenesis confirmation should be performed by a trained physician.
    - Amphotericin B is only considered for local use. The parenteral route is only used in cases of threatening, generalized mycosis. Regular ultrasound to check organogenesis should be performed by a trained physician.
- Antivirals—antiretroviral drugs/HIV drugs during pregnancy and during labour/postpartum:
    - Aciclovir: there is no data on embryo- or fetotoxicity. Local application is possible.
    - Famciclovir, ganciclovir, valaciclovir, and the prodrugs of these virostatics are inadequately investigated to allow unequivocal statements for use in pregnancy.
    - A more detailed account of antivirals is presented in Chapter 50.

Other drugs of interest during anaesthesia

- Epinephrine may be used during pregnancy either via epidural administration associated with a local anaesthetic or through intravenous administration. Epidemiological data does not suggest an increased teratogenic risk. However, epinephrine can have significant effects on uteroplacental perfusion. Nevertheless, its administration should not be delayed if life-saving, as in the setting of resuscitation.
- Ephedrine, phenylephrine, pseudoephedrine, and similar drugs should be avoided during pregnancy whatever their administration route, as they induce fetal vascular system abnormalities.[69] Appropriate ultrasound monitoring is suggested after accidental use during the first trimester. Low-dose nasal administration may be considered provided that the treatment is only for a short duration. Using these drugs in a perioperative setting or at the time of delivery to maintain blood pressure is of course acceptable and often required.
- Atropine may be used during pregnancy at the therapeutic recommended doses. Epidemiological data is rare but reassuring regarding embryotoxicity potential. Atropine easily crosses the placenta and reaches concentrations in the fetus that are similar to the mother. Its use should be limited to clear therapeutic indications.

- Glycopyrrolate, on the other hand, does not cross the placenta and is the drug of choice for maternal bradycardia.

Drugs during lactation

Multiple studies demonstrate that breastfeeding is beneficial for both the mother (reduced blood loss, reduced incidence of postpartum depression, etc.) and the breastfed infant (respiratory, gastrointestinal, meningeal and urinary infection protection, better developmental scores, auditory and visual acuity, etc.). The World Health Organization and the Innocenti Declaration therefore both promote breastfeeding over bottle-feeding.[70] However, medical interventions requiring appropriate sedation and/or analgesia are fairly frequent during the perinatal and immediate postpartum periods and, to a lesser extent, during the late postpartum. It thus becomes the responsibility of the anaesthetist, together with the obstetrician and/or paediatrician, to assess and balance the risks associated with each drug for both the mother and infant. Pharmacological risks to the lactating mother (e.g. linked to pharmacokinetic changes) are quite rare, especially when compared to the risks stemming from not treating or undertreating. Risks to the breastfed infant are most commonly linked to the amount of drug received (i.e. volume ingested multiplied by milk concentration) and drug disposition in the infant (which depends upon the absorption and clearance rates of the specific drug). For some drugs, it may however be totally or partially unrelated to the drug amount. Therefore, any clinical decision should be scientifically supported and appropriately documented in the patient's medical record in order to mitigate legal risk and ensure optimal care is provided.

This section aims at providing the clinician with a better understanding of the underlying mechanisms of blood–milk transportation of drugs as well as a description of the current consensus for most commonly encountered anaesthetics and analgesics. It will not discuss the rational of breastfeeding versus traditional formulas outside the context of the postpartum surgery nor will it be exhaustive in the description of the therapeutic classes. The reader will find mention of Internet and printed references at the beginning of this chapter that may come useful in atypical situations.

Functional anatomy of the breast during pregnancy and lactation

The mammary gland consists of 10–15 ducts extending from the nipple together with alveolar complexes at the termination of every duct. The areola has multiple physiological roles. It contains sebaceous and sweat glands, serves as the termination point for the fourth intercostal nerve, and regulates oxytocin secretion from the posterior pituitary gland as well as prolactin secretion from the anterior pituitary gland. During pregnancy, alveolar complexes increase in number and intricacy while milk secretion is kept low by sex steroids (primarily by progesterone). At parturition, a series of changes called 'lactogenesis' transforms the cells into the fully secretory state. These include closing of apical tight junctions, increasing blood flow, and so on.

Five different ways for molecules to cross the milk–blood barrier

As for most blood barriers, there are five mechanisms involved in the transfer of drugs from blood to milk: exocytosis (apical secretion through vesicles), lipidic transport (apical secretion in lipidic vesicles), apical transport (passive diffusion through the cell), transcytosis (active transport mechanisms), and paracellular pathway (diffusion of large molecules through intercellular spaces). While the paracellular pathway is clearly the dominant pathway during pregnancy, a few days after parturition the apical tight junctions close, therefore limiting the drug transfer to apical transport and, to a lesser extent, transcytosis. The paracellular pathway is again involved during involution, at the end of the lactation period, or in the event of mastitis.

Main physicochemical properties influencing drug transfer during lactation

During lactation, most blood–milk transfer occurs through apical transport, which is a passive diffusion of the drugs through the mammary cells. The extent to which a drug will be transported through the cell is driven by the molecule's physicochemical properties, namely:

- Molecular weight: molecules under 300 Da are likely to cross easily (e.g. ethanol and amphetamines) whereas large molecules simply cannot (e.g. heparin and insulin).
- Lipid solubility: highly lipophilic drugs are likely to achieve a quick equilibrium between blood and milk concentrations. This implies that most anaesthetics and central nervous system (CNS) drugs are likely to easily cross the milk–blood barrier.
- pH ionization: the milk's pH is slightly lower than blood's (pH = 7.2 vs 7.4). Weak bases are likely to be sequestered in the milk (barbiturates, antihistamines, and erythromycin) whereas weak acids are less likely to cross (penicillins).
- Plasma protein binding: highly bound molecules are less likely to cross and therefore milk/plasma (M/P) ratio is likely to decrease sharply as plasmatic protein binding increases. For example: sulphanilamide (protein binding = 8%, M/P ratio = 1), sulfathiazole (protein binding = 50%, M/P ratio = 0.36), and warfarin (protein binding > 90%, M/P ratio = 0.03).

Physiological co-factors influencing the milk/plasma ratio

Besides the drug's intrinsic ability to cross the milk–blood barrier, several physiological co-factors influence the M/P ratio for any given drug:

- The drug's dose and bioavailability: the level to which any given drug will be found in the mother's blood will influence the milk equilibrium level. Drugs such as aminoglycosides, vancomycin, or cephalosporin are poorly absorbed and therefore less likely to be found in the milk. Additionally, fed or fasted mothers will absorb a given drug at different rates, resulting in different M/P ratios.
- The drug's maternal clearance: the mother's kidney and liver metabolism will influence the rate at which a drug will be cleared from the blood. An altered clearance will trigger a prolonged plasma half-life and hence a potentially higher milk concentration.
- Timing of medication: this is clearly the most complex influencing factor, given the variability in milk composition and production during the postpartum period as well as during the

circadian cycle. However, in most cases, the preferred timing for drug administration is just after breastfeeding.

- Drug administration immediately postpartum: the breastfed infant will only ingest small volumes of milk during the immediate postpartum (which does not imply small concentrations or small quantities of drugs because of the predominance of the paracellular pathway at this stage of the lactation).

Milk secretion increases sharply in the first postpartum days (from 50 mL on day 1 to >600 mL on day 5) and quickly reaches a plateau (usually limited to a maximum of about 1.5 mL of milk per gram of tissue per day). Meanwhile, milk composition varies drastically with lactose concentration increasing sharply and sodium and chloride concentration dropping rapidly.

Local anaesthetics, hypnotics, and muscle relaxants

Local anaesthetics are widely used and generally considered safe during all stages of breastfeeding, including when added to epinephrine. Lidocaine and bupivacaine have been extensively tested in lactating mothers, including at high intravenous dosages, for example, for cardiac arrhythmia. Despite a rather quick milk:blood equilibrium, relatively small amounts of the drugs are ingested by the suckling infant. Ropivacaine's milk transfer is very low and probably lower than that of bupivacaine and lidocaine.[20,71] Articaine has an even shorter half-life associated with a higher plasmatic binding probably resulting in an even lower milk concentration. Considering the poor absorption patterns of these drugs and their metabolites it is not surprising that clinical observation does not report any serious adverse events.[72–74] The addition of epinephrine to any of the previous drugs should not be considered problematic as it will in any case limit the passage of the drugs from the mother's blood to the milk. Prilocaine is the only local anaesthetic that should be avoided because it may create more methaemoglobin, however its accidental use should not be an indication to breastfeeding interruption.

It is now widely accepted that mothers may breastfeed their infant as soon as they recover from general anaesthesia. Methohexital, thiopental, and halothane are the drugs of choice according to the American Association of Pediatrics (AAP). Because of their physiochemical properties and despite the absence of studies, sevoflurane and isoflurane are believed to be excreted into the milk. However, since there has been no report of adverse effects to the breastfed infant their use might be considered compatible with breastfeeding. Methohexital passes into the milk in negligible amounts, resulting in extremely low infant exposure.[75] Thiopental has a rather long half-life of approximately 10 hours but a M/P ratio of about 0.5 which leads to negligible amounts ingested by the breastfed infant. No toxic effect is expected despite its prolonged half-life in the infant after single-dose administration.[76] Halothane and other volatile agents easily cross the milk–blood barrier but no adverse clinical outcomes have been yet reported after anaesthesia of a lactating mother or after prolonged occupational exposure.[77,78]

Propofol may be safely used for general anaesthesia induction. It has a short half-life and an extremely high plasma binding (95–99%). Despite its small molecular weight, high pKa, and hydrophobicity, the amount ingested by the infant is considered negligible.[25,79]

Most commonly used muscle relaxants (e.g. atracurium, pancuronium, rocuronium, suxamethonium, and vecuronium) may be safely prescribed at various stage of lactation. Only limited amounts of these drugs cross the milk–blood barrier, because of their low hydrophobic and high ionization structures. Moreover, all these drugs demonstrate an extremely limited intestinal absorption profile.

Analgesics and anti-inflammatory drugs

Paracetamol is the analgesic and antipyretic drug of choice during lactation. It is excreted at a very low rate into the milk, with a peak level occurring 1–2 hours after a single oral dose. A suckling infant will receive 1–2% of the weight-adjusted maternal dose. There has been only one adverse event reported so far (a maculopapular rash which resolved within 24 hours after discontinuation of the treatment and resumed when the treatment was reintroduced).[80–82]

Codeine may only be used as a third-line treatment and for a short duration (up to four times at 60 mg). Specific attention should be taken with children with a risk for apnoea. Breastfeeding should be stopped if the mother or the child demonstrates symptoms of opioid toxicity (sedation, constipation, poor milk intake, or poor body weight gain). There is a clear dose–effect correlation between maternal treatment and CNS depression in the infant. Moreover, it should be contraindicated in known or suspected ultrarapid metabolizers (cytochrome P450 2D6 ultrarapid metabolizers) (high sedation and constipation) as a case report from 2006 shows.[83–85] In 2013, the MHRA issued a recommendation to avoid codeine during lactation and to reserve its use to third-line indications, after use of paracetamol and NSAIDs (https://www.gov.uk/drug-safety-update).

Fentanyl and associated drugs (sufentanil, alfentanil, etc.) are considered safe for use during lactation. Fentanyl easily crosses the milk–blood barrier with a peak concentration occurring 0.75 hours after a single administration and a milk/blood ratio greater than 1. Because of the rapidly decreasing colostrum concentration and its low oral bioavailability, fentanyl is considered compatible with breastfeeding.[86]

Use of morphine should be limited to single administration or short duration treatments, with specific CNS monitoring of the infant. Morphine easily crosses the blood–milk barrier due to its low molecular weight and intermediate plasma binding (30–40%). There is no available clinical data regarding the neurobehavioral and developmental effects over the long term. It is nonetheless considered compatible with breastfeeding by the AAP.[87–89]

Pethidine is widely used at the time of parturition. It triggers higher saliva levels in infants up to 48 hours after birth with no significant adverse effects reported. It is considered compatible with lactation by the AAP. As for all opioid drugs, and because of the very long half-lives of pethidine and its metabolite in neonates (13 and 63 hours, respectively), particular attention should be paid to CNS monitoring when administered 1–4 hours before delivery, especially after repeated doses (accumulation in maternal and fetal compartments). It is contraindicated in preterm infants.[75,89–91]

Tramadol may be used during breastfeeding for short-duration periods and in case of mild to severe pain after delivery, especially in case of poor opioids tolerance. Both tramadol and its active metabolite are excreted into breast milk to a limited extent. There has been no evidence of fetal or neonatal negative outcomes when used during labour (however, the analgesic effect of tramadol is limited during labour).

Naloxone is supposed to be compatible with lactation, despite the fact that there is no human data available. In the absence of consensus, and because of its rather short adult half-life (30–81 minutes), one may consider to avoid breastfeeding for 12–24 hours after single-dose administration.

Ibuprofen and other commonly used NSAIDs (e.g. diclofenac) do not cross easily the milk–blood barrier (M/P ratio < 1). These drugs have very short half-lives, are highly bound to plasma proteins (99%) and are polarized (acidic profiles). Ibuprofen is the NSAID of choice as it is very poorly excreted into milk and widely used with no significant adverse events reported.[92,93] Other common NSAIDs may also be used occasionally but should not be considered as safe as ibuprofen or flurbiprofen. Diclofenac and its numerous metabolites have not been studied in humans. One may want to consider indomethacin as a valid alternative to diclofenac despite one reported seizure case possibly attributed to the drug. Indomethacin is considered compatible with breastfeeding by the AAP and should be preferred over diclofenac[94] despite reported cases of convulsions in newborns associated with its use.[95,96] Accidental exposure to the other NSAIDs does not require weaning but the medication should be adapted.

Acetyl salicylic acid is very poorly excreted into milk but is trapped in this compartment (M/P ratio ~0.05 at plasmatic peak level 3 hours after administration reaches ~0.3 after 12 hours). There has been one reported case of metabolic acidosis in a breastfed infant. The AAP does not ban aspirin but calls for particular caution.[97,98]

Ketorolac has been studied after oral administration in breastfeeding mothers 2–6 days after parturition. It reached extremely small concentrations in milk. It is approved by the AAP.[99]

There are not sufficient data available with selective COX2 inhibitors to support their use during lactation. Because celecoxib and rofecoxib are poorly excreted into milk and are unlikely to pose a significant risk, an accidental single-dose administration does not require any limitation of breastfeeding. It is believed that celecoxib is eliminated from the breast milk 24 hours after a single-dose administration. On the other hand, rofecoxib has a rather long adult serum half-life (~17 hours) and may trigger accumulation in both serum and milk compartments.[100–103]

Anti-infective agents during lactation: antibiotics, antimycotics, and antivirals

Most antibiotics pass in minimal concentration (< 1% of newborn body weight adjusted dosage during therapeutic use) into the suckling infant. Theoretically side effects to the infant are changes in defaecation, formation of antibiotic resistances, and sensibility. None of them is considered clinically relevant.

- Penicillins and cephalosporins are all considered as first choice in lactation, especially second-generation cephalosporins. Combinations with or single use of clavulanic acid can be used when necessary.
- Erythromycin and roxithromycin are again first choice in lactation. Other macrolide antibiotics remain second choice. It should be used with caution if there is hyperbilirubinaemia of the newborn.
- Tetracyclines remain second-line treatment.
- Sulphonamides and nitrofurantoin cross the milk–blood barrier. Special attention should be paid in case nitrofurantoin use when the infant has a G6PD deficiency, as cases of haemolytic anaemia were reported.
- Dapsone has been associated with one reported case of haemolytic anaemia in a breastfed infant.[104]
- Clindamycin and vancomycin are excreted into the milk but poorly absorbed in the infant bowel. Clindamycin is approved by the AAP. Vancomycin is considered safe but was not reviewed by the AAP. The main side effect for both drugs is a modification of the bowel flora. There was one reported case of haemorrhagic enteritis with clindamycin.
- Chloramphenicol seems to have a bone marrow depressant effect and is therefore not recommended in breastfeeding mothers.[105]
- Metronidazole is considered compatible with breastfeeding.
- Aminoglycosides (e.g. gentamicin) are absorbed by the infant gut and can accumulate.
- Antimycotics in lactation: in general, local therapy is not considered harmful during lactation. Systemic therapy should only be considered if there is a clear clinical indication. In breast skin/nipple mycosis, the germ reservoir is the oral cavity of the suckling infant. Therefore treatment of mother and child is necessary. Nystatin and clotrimazole or miconazole are first choice for local treatment, but depending on the indication other antimycotics might be used temporarily or on small localizations.

Other drugs of interest during anaesthesia

Epinephrine may be used during lactation when associated with local anaesthetics. There are no human data available regarding its use following intravenous administration in emergency situations but there is a suspected toxicity for the infant. Under these emergency circumstances, one should temporarily avoid breastfeeding.

There are very scarce data regarding human exposure to ephedrine during lactation with only one case report presenting an irritability and disturbed sleeping pattern in a 3-month-old suckling infant.

Atropine is approved for use during lactation by the AAP. Its passage through the milk–blood barrier has not been extensively studied but no clinical adverse effects have been reported so far.

Conclusion

With drug safety classification only providing a very crude estimation of maternal, fetal, and neonatal risks, physicians, and especially anaesthetists, often face complex or controversial decisions during pregnancy and lactation.

There are a few basic rules applicable to most cases in order to limit risks to the fetus or the suckling infant:

- Limit prescription to what is truly necessary.
- Do not prescribe lower/higher doses than necessary.
- Avoid newly released medications or medications known to be at risk (e.g. cytotoxic agents, radioactive compounds, CNS active drugs, active metabolites of the parent drug, drugs that have long paediatric half-lives such as barbiturates and benzodiazepines, and all drugs of abuse).
- Choose drugs that are poorly excreted into the fetal compartment or into the milk.

- Additionally, during lactation one should:
  - avoid drugs that are poorly eliminated by the infant, especially for premature or sick infants
  - adapt formulation and route of administration so that the plasma concentration is low at the time of breastfeeding and preferably breastfeed just before drug administration
  - advise the paediatrician and nurses in charge of the suckling infant when particular surveillance is needed.

In any case, as scientific knowledge evolves continuously with the emergence of new drugs and reports of newly observed side effects, one should always refer to up-to-date best standard of care and review references, which should be clearly documented in the patient's medical record, especially with respect to newly marketed compounds. Specialized units in most university hospitals and poison control centres will always provide useful recommendations in cases of atypical situations.

References

1. Chamberlain, G. ABC of antenatal care. Organisation of antenatal care. *BMJ* 1991; 302(6777):647–50.
2. Briggs GG, Freeman RK. *Drugs in Pregnancy and Lactation: A Reference Guide to Fetal and Neonatal Risk* (10th ed). Philadelphia, PA: Lippincott, Williams & Wilkins; 2014.
3. Daw JR, Mintzes B, Law MR, *et al.* Prescription drug use in pregnancy: a retrospective, population-based study in British Columbia, Canada (2001–2006). *Clin Ther* 2012; 34(1):239–49.e2.
4. Malm H, Martikainen J, Klaukka T, *et al.* Prescription of hazardous drugs during pregnancy. *Drug Saf* 2004; 27(12):899–908.
5. Schaefer C, Peters PWJ, Miller RK. *Drugs During Pregnancy and Lactation: Treatment Options and Risk Assessment* (3rd ed.) Amsterdam: Elsevier Academic Press; 2014.
6. Shepard TH. "Proof" of human teratogenicity. *Teratology* 1994; 50(2):97–8.
7. Kallen B. Case control study of hypospadias, based on registry information. *Teratology* 1988; 38(1):45–50.
8. Mazze RI, Kallen B. Reproductive outcome after anesthesia and operation during pregnancy: a registry study of 5405 cases. *Am J Obstet Gynecol* 1989; 161(5):1178–85.
9. Andrews EB, Tilson HH, Hurn BA, *et al.* Acyclovir in Pregnancy Registry. An observational epidemiologic approach. *Am J Med* 1988; 85(2A):123–8.
10. Mazze RI, Kallen B. Appendectomy during pregnancy: a Swedish registry study of 778 cases. *Obstet Gynecol* 1991; 77(6):835–40.
11. Albano JD, Tilson H. No evidence for increased risk of cleft lip or cleft palate among infants exposed to antiretroviral drugs during pregnancy in the antiretroviral pregnancy registry. *Cleft Palate Craniofac J* 2013; 50(3):376–7.
12. Loebstein R, Lalkin A, Koren G. Pharmacokinetic changes during pregnancy and their clinical relevance. *Clin Pharmacokinet* 1997; 33(5):328–43.
13. Miller RK, Genbacev O, Turner MA, *et al.* Human placental explants in culture: approaches and assessments. *Placenta* 2005; 26(6):439–48.
14. Juchau MR. Bioactivation in chemical teratogenesis. *Annu Rev Pharmacol Toxicol* 1989; 29:165–87.
15. Dobbing J, Sands J. Comparative aspects of the brain growth spurt. *Early Hum Dev* 1979; 3(1):79–83.
16. Reddy SV. Effect of general anesthetics on the developing brain. *J Anaesthesiol Clin Pharmacol* 2012; 28(1):6–10.
17. Rice SA, Fish KJ. *Anesthetic Toxicity.* New York: Raven Press; 1994.
18. Bonnin M, Mercier FJ, Sitbon O, *et al.* Severe pulmonary hypertension during pregnancy: mode of delivery and anesthetic management of 15 consecutive cases. *Anesthesiology* 2005; 102(6):1133–7.
19. Sanders RD, Hassell J, Davidson AJ, *et al.* Impact of anaesthetics and surgery on neurodevelopment: an update. *Br J Anaesth* 2013; 110 Suppl 1:i53–72.
20. Matsota PK, Markantonis SL, Fousteri MZ, *et al.* Excretion of ropivacaine in breast milk during patient-controlled epidural analgesia after cesarean delivery. *Reg Anesth Pain Med* 2009; 34(2):126–9.
21. Fragneto RY, Bader AM, Rosinia F, *et al.* Measurements of protein binding of lidocaine throughout pregnancy. *Anesth Analg* 1994; 79(2):295–7.
22. Heinonen OP, Slone D, Shapiro S. *Birth Defects and Drugs in Pregnancy.* Littleton, MA: Publishing Sciences Group; 1977.
23. Gin T, O'Meara ME, Kan AF, *et al.* Plasma catecholamines and neonatal condition after induction of anaesthesia with propofol or thiopentone at caesarean section. *Br J Anaesth* 1993; 70(3):311–16.
24. D'Alessio JG, Ramanathan J. Effects of maternal anesthesia in the neonate. *Semin Perinatol* 1998; 22(5):350–62.
25. Dailland P, Cockshott ID, Lirzin JD, *et al.* Intravenous propofol during cesarean section: placental transfer, concentrations in breast milk, and neonatal effects. A preliminary study. *Anesthesiology* 1989; 71(6):827–34.
26. Reddy BK, Pizer B, Bull PT. Neonatal serum cortisol suppression by etomidate compared with thiopentone, for elective caesarean section. *Eur J Anaesthesiol* 1988; 5(3):171–6.
27. Cohen-Kerem R, Railton C, Oren D, *et al.* Pregnancy outcome following non-obstetric surgical intervention. *Am J Surg* 2005; 190(3):467–73.
28. Kuczkowski KM. The safety of anaesthetics in pregnant women. *Expert Opin Drug Saf* 2006; 5(2):251–64.
29. Hood DD, Holubec DM. Elective repeat cesarean section. Effect of anesthesia type on blood loss. *J Reprod Med* 1990; 35(4):368–72.
30. Yoo KY, Lee JC, Yoon MH, *et al.* The effects of volatile anesthetics on spontaneous contractility of isolated human pregnant uterine muscle: a comparison among sevoflurane, desflurane, isoflurane, and halothane. *Anesth Analg* 2006; 103(2):443–7.
31. De Amici D, Delmonte P, Martinotti L, *et al.* Can anesthesiologic strategies for caesarean section influence newborn jaundice? A retrospective and prospective study. *Biol Neonate* 2001; 79(2):97–102.
32. Ong BY, Baron K, Stearns EL, *et al.* Severe fetal bradycardia in a pregnant surgical patient despite normal oxygenation and blood pressure. *Can J Anaesth* 2003; 50(9):922–5.
33. Allen GC, Brubaker CL. Human malignant hyperthermia associated with desflurane anesthesia. *Anesth Analg* 1998; 86(6):1328–31.
34. Crawford JS, Lewis M. Nitrous oxide in early human pregnancy. *Anaesthesia* 1986; 41(9):900–5.
35. Abouleish E, Wingard LB Jr, de la Vega S, *et al.* Pancuronium in caesarean section and its placental transfer. *Br J Anaesth* 1980; 52(5):531–6.
36. Dailey PA, Fisher DM, Shnider SM, *et al.* Pharmacokinetics, placental transfer, and neonatal effects of vecuronium and pancuronium administered during cesarean section. *Anesthesiology* 1984; 60(6):569–74.
37. Demetriou M, Depoix JP, Diakite B, *et al.* Placental transfer of Org NC 45 in women undergoing Caesarean section. *Br J Anaesth* 1982; 54(6):643–5.
38. Kaneko T, Iwama H, Tobishima S, *et al.* [Placental transfer of vecuronium administered with priming principle regimen in patients undergoing cesarean section]. *Masui* 1997; 46(6):750–4.
39. Terrana T, Radice L, Cirla AM, *et al.* [Occupational exposure to volatile anesthetics and reproductive effects: a bibliographic review of epidemiological studies]. *G Ital Med Lav* 1992; 14(1–6):43–7.
40. Tannenbaum TN, Goldberg RJ. Exposure to anesthetic gases and reproductive outcome. A review of the epidemiologic literature. *J Occup Med* 1985; 27(9):659–68.
41. Rowland AS, Baird DD, Shore DL, *et al.* Nitrous oxide and spontaneous abortion in female dental assistants. *Am J Epidemiol* 1995; 141(6):531–8.

42. Rowland AS, Baird DD, Weinberg CR, *et al.* Reduced fertility among women employed as dental assistants exposed to high levels of nitrous oxide. *N Engl J Med* 1992; 327(14):993–7.
43. Feldkamp ML, Meyer RE, Krikov S, *et al.* Acetaminophen use in pregnancy and risk of birth defects: findings from the National Birth Defects Prevention Study. *Obstet Gynecol* 2010; 115(1):109–15.
44. Scialli AR, Ang R, Breitmeyer J, *et al.* A review of the literature on the effects of acetaminophen on pregnancy outcome. *Reprod Toxicol* 2010; 30(4):495–507.
45. Rebordosa C, Kogevinas M, Bech BH, *et al.* Use of acetaminophen during pregnancy and risk of adverse pregnancy outcomes. *Int J Epidemiol* 2009; 38(3):706–14.
46. Jensen MS, Rebordosa C, Thulstrup AM, *et al.* Maternal use of acetaminophen, ibuprofen, and acetylsalicylic acid during pregnancy and risk of cryptorchidism. *Epidemiology* 2010; 21(6):779–85.
47. Nezvalova-Henriksen K, Spigset O, Nordeng H. Effects of codeine on pregnancy outcome: results from a large population-based cohort study. *Eur J Clin Pharmacol* 2011; 67(12):1253–61.
48. Ciociola AA, Gautieri RF. Evaluation of the teratogenicity of morphine sulfate administered via a miniature implantable pump. *J Pharm Sci* 1983; 72(7):742–5.
49. Cooper J, Jauniaux E, Gulbis B, *et al.* Placental transfer of temazepam and fentanyl in early human pregnancy. *Reprod Biomed Online* 2001; 2(3):165–71.
50. Shannon C, Jauniaux E, Gulbis B, *et al.* Placental transfer of fentanyl in early human pregnancy. *Hum Reprod* 1998; 13(8):2317–20.
51. Nezvalova-Henriksen K, Spigset O, Nordeng H. Effects of ibuprofen, diclofenac, naproxen, and piroxicam on the course of pregnancy and pregnancy outcome: a prospective cohort study. *BJOG* 2013; 120(8):948–59.
52. Low dose aspirin in pregnancy and early childhood development: follow up of the collaborative low dose aspirin study in pregnancy. CLASP collaborative group. *Br J Obstet Gynaecol* 1995; 102(11):861–8.
53. CLASP: a randomised trial of low-dose aspirin for the prevention and treatment of pre-eclampsia among 9364 pregnant women. CLASP (Collaborative Low-dose Aspirin Study in Pregnancy) Collaborative Group. *Lancet* 1994; 343(8898):619–29.
54. Cassina M, De Santis M, Cesari E, *et al.* First trimester diclofenac exposure and pregnancy outcome. *Reprod Toxicol* 2010; 30(3):401–4.
55. Berkovitch M, Diav-Citrin O, Greenberg R, *et al.* First-trimester exposure to amoxycillin/clavulanic acid: a prospective, controlled study. *Br J Clin Pharmacol* 2004; 58(3):298–302.
56. Jepsen P, Skriver MV, Floyd A, *et al.* A population-based study of maternal use of amoxicillin and pregnancy outcome in Denmark. *Br J Clin Pharmacol* 2003; 55(2):216–21.
57. Stewart KS, Shafi M, Andrews J, *et al.* Distribution of parenteral ampicillin and cephalosporins in late pregnancy. *J Obstet Gynaecol Br Commonw* 1973; 80(10):902–8.
58. Garratty G, Leger RM, Arndt PA. Severe immune hemolytic anemia associated with prophylactic use of cefotetan in obstetric and gynecologic procedures. *Am J Obstet Gynecol* 1999; 181(1):103–4.
59. Berkovitch M, Segal-Socher I, Greenberg R, *et al.* First trimester exposure to cefuroxime: a prospective cohort study. *Br J Clin Pharmacol* 2000; 50(2):161–5.
60. Czeizel AE, Rockenbauer M, Sørensen HT, *et al.* Use of cephalosporins during pregnancy and in the presence of congenital abnormalities: a population-based, case-control study. *Am J Obstet Gynecol* 2001; 184(6):1289–96.
61. Cooper WO, Ray WA, Griffin MR. Prenatal prescription of macrolide antibiotics and infantile hypertrophic pyloric stenosis. *Obstet Gynecol* 2002; 100(1):101–6.
62. Louik C, Werler MM, Mitchell AA. Erythromycin use during pregnancy in relation to pyloric stenosis. *Am J Obstet Gynecol* 2002; 186(2):288–90.
63. Czeizel AE, Rockenbauer M, Olsen J, *et al.* A teratological study of aminoglycoside antibiotic treatment during pregnancy. *Scand J Infect Dis* 2000; 32(3):309–13.
64. Czeizel AE, Rockenbauer M, Sørensen HT, *et al.* A teratological study of lincosamides. *Scand J Infect Dis* 2000; 32(5):579–80.
65. Mickal A, Panzer JD. The safety of lincomycin in pregnancy. *Am J Obstet Gynecol* 1975; 121(8):1071–4.
66. Weinstein AJ, Gibbs RS, Gallagher M. Placental transfer of clindamycin and gentamicin in term pregnancy. *Am J Obstet Gynecol* 1976; 124(7):688–91.
67. Czeizel AE, Kazy Z, Puho E. A population-based case-control teratological study of oral nystatin treatment during pregnancy. *Scand J Infect Dis* 2003; 35(11–12):830–5.
68. King CT, Rogers PD, Cleary JD, *et al.* Antifungal therapy during pregnancy. *Clin Infect Dis* 1998; 27(5):1151–60.
69. Werler MM. Teratogen update: pseudoephedrine. *Birth Defects Res A Clin Mol Teratol* 2006; 76(6):445–52.
70. Nutrition. The Innocenti Declaration: progress and achievements. Part I. *Wkly Epidemiol Rec* 1998; 73(5):25–30.
71. Bailey DN, Briggs JR. The binding of acetaminophen, lidocaine, and valproic acid to human milk. *Am J Clin Pathol* 2004; 121(5):754–7.
72. Zeisler JA, Gaarder TD, De Mesquita SA. Lidocaine excretion in breast milk. *Drug Intell Clin Pharm* 1986; 20(9):691–3.
73. Ortega D, Viviand X, Lorec AM, *et al.* Excretion of lidocaine and bupivacaine in breast milk following epidural anesthesia for cesarean delivery. *Acta Anaesthesiol Scand* 1999; 43(4):394–7.
74. Giuliani M, Grossi GB, Pileri M, *et al.* Could local anesthesia while breast-feeding be harmful to infants? *J Pediatr Gastroenterol Nutr* 2001; 32(2):142–4.
75. Borgatta L, Jenny RW, Gruss L, *et al.* Clinical significance of methohexital, meperidine, and diazepam in breast milk. *J Clin Pharmacol* 1997; 37(3):186–92.
76. Andersen LW, Qvist T, Hertz J, *et al.* Concentrations of thiopentone in mature breast milk and colostrum following an induction dose. *Acta Anaesthesiol Scand* 1987; 31(1):30–2.
77. Lee JJ, Rubin AP. Breast feeding and anaesthesia. *Anaesthesia* 1993; 48(7):616–25.
78. Cote CJ, Kenepp NB, Reed SB, *et al.* Trace concentrations of halothane in human breast milk. *Br J Anaesth* 1976; 48(6):541–3.
79. Nitsun M, Szokol JW, Saleh HJ, *et al.* Pharmacokinetics of midazolam, propofol, and fentanyl transfer to human breast milk. *Clin Pharmacol Ther* 2006; 79(6):549–57.
80. Bitzen PO, Gustafsson B, Jostell KG, *et al.* Excretion of paracetamol in human breast milk. *Eur J Clin Pharmacol* 1981; 20(2):123–5.
81. Berlin CM Jr, Yaffe SJ, Ragni M. Disposition of acetaminophen in milk, saliva, and plasma of lactating women. *Pediatr Pharmacol (New York)* 1980; 1(2):135–41.
82. Findlay JW, DeAngelis RL, Kearney MF, *et al.* Analgesic drugs in breast milk and plasma. *Clin Pharmacol Ther* 1981; 29(5):625–33.
83. Meny RG, Naumburg EG, Alger LS, *et al.* Codeine and the breastfed neonate. *J Hum Lact* 1993; 9(4):237–40.
84. Koren G, Cairns J, Chitayat D, *et al.* Pharmacogenetics of morphine poisoning in a breastfed neonate of a codeine-prescribed mother. *Lancet* 2006; 368(9536):704.
85. Madadi P, Moretti M, Djokanovic N, *et al.* Guidelines for maternal codeine use during breastfeeding. *Can Fam Physician* 2009; 55(11):1077–8.
86. Steer PL, Biddle CJ, Marley WS, *et al.* Concentration of fentanyl in colostrum after an analgesic dose. *Can J Anaesth* 1992; 39(3):231–5.
87. Oberlander TF, Robeson P, Ward V, *et al.* Prenatal and breast milk morphine exposure following maternal intrathecal morphine treatment. *J Hum Lact* 2000; 16(2):137–42.
88. Robieux I, Koren G, Vandenbergh H, *et al.* Morphine excretion in breast milk and resultant exposure of a nursing infant. *J Toxicol Clin Toxicol* 1990; 28(3):365–70.
89. Wittels B, Scott DT, Sinatra RS. Exogenous opioids in human breast milk and acute neonatal neurobehavior: a preliminary study. *Anesthesiology* 1990; 73(5):864–9.
90. Bar-Oz B, Bulkowstein M, Benyamini L, *et al.* Use of antibiotic and analgesic drugs during lactation. *Drug Saf* 2003; 26(13):925–35.

91. Peiker G, Müller B, Ihn W, *et al.* [Excretion of pethidine in mother's milk (author's transl)]. *Zentralbl Gynakol* 1980; 102(10):537–41.
92. Townsend RJ, Benedetti TJ, Erickson SH, *et al.* Excretion of ibuprofen into breast milk. *Am J Obstet Gynecol* 1984; 149(2):184–6.
93. Ito S, Blajchman A, Stephenson M, *et al.* Prospective follow-up of adverse reactions in breast-fed infants exposed to maternal medication. *Am J Obstet Gynecol* 1993; 168(5):1393–9.
94. Lebedevs TH, Wojnar-Horton RE, Yapp P, *et al.* Excretion of indomethacin in breast milk. *Br J Clin Pharmacol* 1991; 32(6):751–4.
95. Eeg-Olofsson O, Malmros I, Elwin CE, *et al.* Convulsions in a breast-fed infant after maternal indomethacin. *Lancet* 1978; 2(8082):215.
96. Fairhead FW. Convulsions in a breast-fed infant after maternal indomethacin. *Lancet* 1978; 2(8089):576.
97. Clark JH, Wilson WG. A 16-day-old breast-fed infant with metabolic acidosis caused by salicylate. *Clin Pediatr (Phila)* 1981; 20(1):53–4.
98. Erickson SH, Oppenheim GL. Aspirin in breast milk. *J Fam Pract* 1979; 8(1):189–90.
99. Wischnik A, Manth SM, Lloyd J, *et al.* The excretion of ketorolac tromethamine into breast milk after multiple oral dosing. *Eur J Clin Pharmacol* 1989; 36(5):521–4.
100. Gardiner SJ, Begg EJ, Zhang M, *et al.* Transfer of rofecoxib into human milk. *Eur J Clin Pharmacol* 2005; 61(5–6):405–8.
101. Gardiner SJ, Doogue MP, Zhang M, *et al.* Quantification of infant exposure to celecoxib through breast milk. *Br J Clin Pharmacol* 2006; 61(1):101–4.
102. Zhang M, Moore GA, Gardiner SJ, *et al.* Determination of celecoxib in human plasma and breast milk by high-performance liquid chromatographic assay. *J Chromatogr B Analyt Technol Biomed Life Sci* 2006; 830(2):245–8.
103. Knoppert DC, Stempak D, Baruchel S, *et al.* Celecoxib in human milk: a case report. *Pharmacotherapy* 2003; 23(1):97–100.
104. Sanders SW, Zone JJ, Foltz RL, *et al.* Hemolytic anemia induced by dapsone transmitted through breast milk. *Ann Intern Med* 1982; 96(4):465–6.
105. Plomp TA, Thiery M, Maes RA. The passage of thiamphenicol and chloramphenicol into human milk after single and repeated oral administration. *Vet Hum Toxicol* 1983; 25(3):167–72.

PART 5

Obstetric management of labour and labour analgesia

CHAPTER 12

Obstetric management of labour, delivery, and vaginal birth after caesarean delivery

Roland Devlieger and Maria-Elisabeth Smet

Introduction

Due to Eve's disobedience in the Garden of Eden, God condemned not only her, but all women, to painful labour for many generations. In view of this religious conviction and partly due to the fallacy that it supports bonding between mother and child, one can understand the acceptance with which many women over the centuries gave birth without pain relief. Fortunately, nowadays divine condemnation is considered outdated by most and analgesia in labour is accepted practice in many cultures.

The first anaesthetic used in labour was nitrous oxide. This 'laughing gas' was discovered in 1799 by Sir Humphrey Davy. In 1847, Sir James Young Simpson discovered the anaesthetic possibilities of chloroform. This was given to numb Queen Victoria during the deliveries of her two youngest children. Hence the name, anaesthetic 'à la reine'.

More recently, the paracervical block was introduced. Today, this technique has been largely abandoned even though it is a relatively simple way to relieve pain during the first stage of labour. It is limited in its use mostly because of its short duration of action and the fact that fetal bradycardia has been described after inadvertent intravascular injection, in some cases with fatal outcome. The history of obstetric anaesthesia is detailed in Chapter 1.

With the improvements in efficacy and safety of neuraxial techniques for pain relief during labour, the demands on the obstetric anaesthetist increase. Moreover, the role of the anaesthetist extends beyond pain relief. As labour and delivery can be complicated by many life-threatening emergencies (fetal distress, amniotic fluid embolism, postpartum haemorrhage (PPH), etc.) obstetricians often rely on their anaesthetic colleagues who have become important players in the multidisciplinary obstetric management team. Therefore, an optimal bilateral understanding between obstetrician and anaesthetist is of utmost importance for the well-being of women in labour, and some insight into normal and abnormal labour and delivery is helpful for anaesthetists.

Normal labour and delivery

Labour is the process where uterine contractions lead to effacement and progressive dilation of the cervix. The cervix dilates until it is fully confluent with the vagina (Figure 12.1). The fetus can then descend through the birth canal. Delivery of the baby is followed by delivery of the placenta.

Labour in humans is typically divided into three phases or stages:[1] during the *first stage* the cervix progressively dilates as a result of regular uterine contractions to full dilatation (referred to as 10 cm). The cervix starts off as closed, firm, posterior, and approximately 3 cm long. This first stage begins with a *latent phase*, which is very variable in duration. It represents the early stage of labour that is characterized by irregular, infrequent, and mild contractions and little or no dilation of the cervix or descent of the fetus. In this phase, the cervix becomes softer, shorter, and more anteriorly situated into the vagina while the fetal head descends. This phase can last for days, may or may not be associated with painful contractions, and ends when the cervix is fully effaced and around 3 cm dilated. There is strong evidence that the first stage of labour is 1 hour shorter when women are stimulated to assume upright positions (standing, sitting, kneeling, walking, etc.) in comparison with a recumbent position.[2] Once the contractions are regular and powerful, resulting in cervical effacement, dilatation of 3 cm and more, the so-called active first phase of labour has been reached. The *active phase* of labour is more predictable in timing and is associated with increasingly powerful contractions. During this active phase, the cervix dilates at a rate of about 1 cm per hour but faster progression is common, especially in multiparous women. The *second stage* of labour is from when the cervix is fully dilated until the baby is born. The *third stage* of labour ends with the delivery of the placenta.

Traditionally labour has three components (the three 'Ps'); the passage (pelvis), the passenger (baby) and the powers (uterine contractions and maternal effort). Each of these can contribute to the labour and delivery, to deviate from the physiological situation, thereby causing a prolonged or obstructed labour (see later sections).

Cervical dilatation and other cardinal maternal and fetal parameters are recorded during labour using a composite graphical representation over time on a sheet of paper: the partogram (Figure 12.2). Relevant measurements might include statistics such as cervical dilatation, fetal heart rate (FHR), duration of labour, and vital signs. It is intended to provide an accurate record

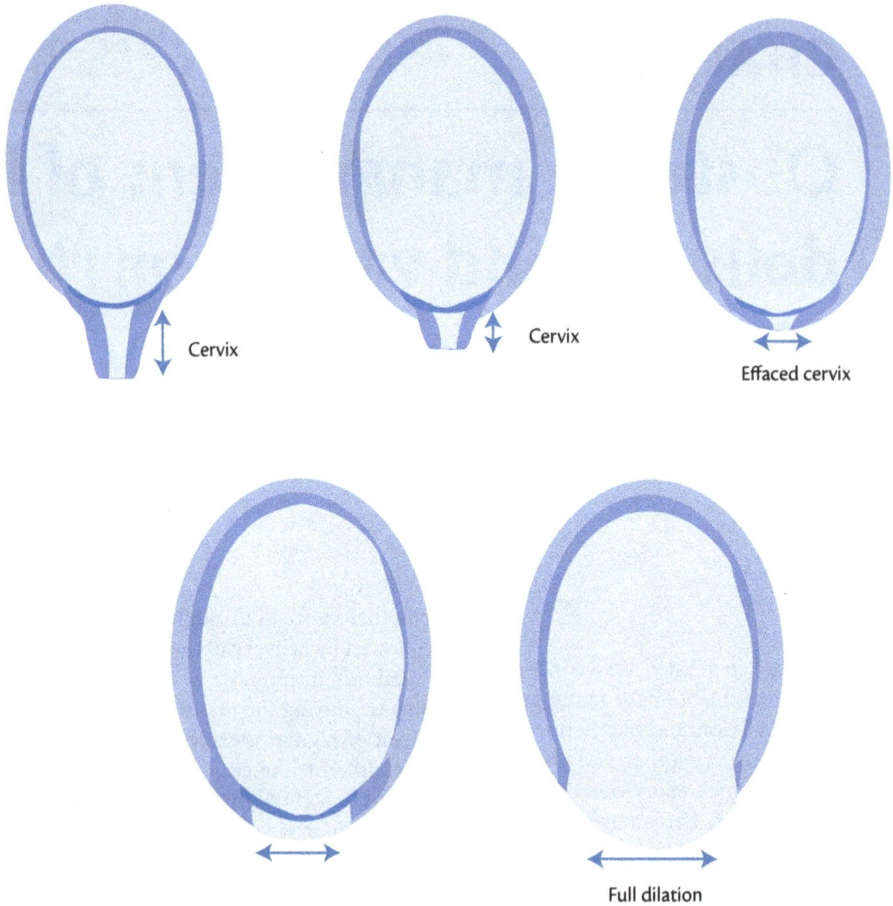

Figure 12.1 Cervical changes during labour.

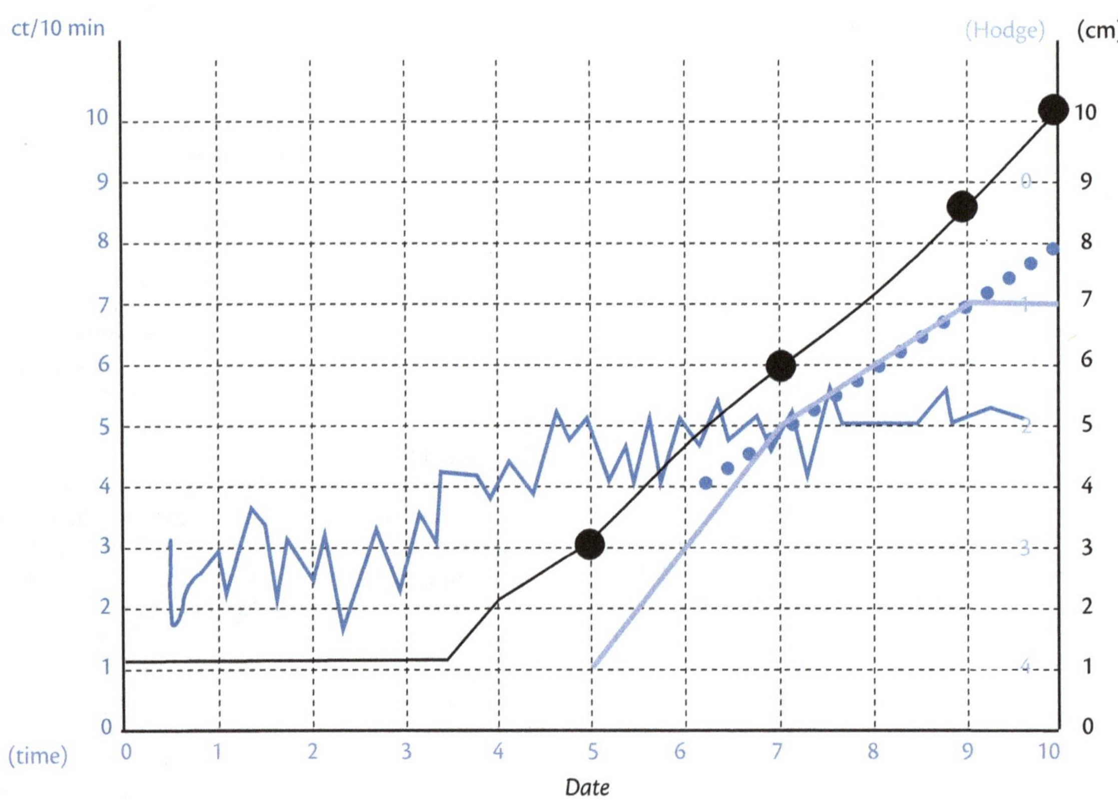

Figure 12.2 Intrapartum information.

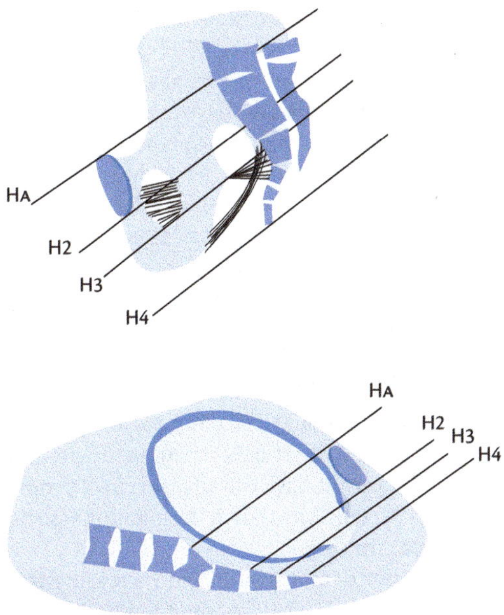

Figure 12.3 Hodge planes.

of the progress in labour, so that any delay or deviation from normal may be detected quickly and treated accordingly. The use of a partogram in established labour is recommended by the *Intrapartum Care* guideline from the UK National Institute for Health and Care Excellence (NICE).[3]

Nowadays, intrapartum information including maternal parameters and partogram is available electronically in most units (Figure 12.2). During labour, the attendant midwifery or medical staff will evaluate the patient at regular intervals. This will include a vaginal examination during established labour to assess:

- cervical dilatation, softening, effacement, and position (modified Bishop's score)
- presenting fetal part (cephalic, breech, other)
- engagement and descent of the presenting parts in Hodge planes I, II, III, and IV (Figure 12.3)
- position (occiput anterior, occiput posterior, occiput transverse) and flexion (occiput, vertex, brow, face) of the fetal head in the pelvis.

In case of inconclusive vaginal examination, ultrasound is increasingly being utilized to evaluate the position of the fetus. Besides regular vaginal examination, the assessment of progress in labour depends on the assessment of effective contractions. The nature and timing of contractions can be evaluated clinically by abdominal palpation or can be recorded using a tocograph, usually in combination with FHR monitoring: cardiotocography (CTG) (Figure 12.4).

External tocodynamometry or tocography does not, however, provide detailed information on the strength of the contractions. In contrast, internal tocodynamometry using invasive intrauterine pressure sensors is able to detect normal and abnormal intrauterine pressure levels. Monitoring of the frequency of contractions is important especially when intravenous (IV) oxytocin is used as excessive uterine activity (hyperstimulation or tachysystole) can cause fetal distress. As the insertion of an intrauterine catheter has higher costs and also potential risks for mother and child and no benefit was shown in a recent Cochrane review, the use of internal uterine pressure sensors is not advised in routine practice.[4]

The *second stage* of labour starts at full dilation of the cervix, includes the descent of the fetus in the birth canal, and ends with the birth of the newborn. Active pushing is best started when the parturient feels the urge to push due to the pressure of the descending fetal head on the cervix and on the rectum (Ferguson reflex). It is therefore advised to wait for approximately 1 hour, after full dilatation of the cervix is achieved, in order to allow for the spontaneous descent of the fetal head. The latter is especially advised in nulliparous women.[1] In a patient with neuraxial anaesthesia in labour and a term, singleton fetus, the second stage can be prolonged by approximately 1 hour. Delayed pushing (waiting 1–3 hours or until urge to push) is associated with higher incidence of spontaneous vaginal delivery in these patients compared to pushing immediately upon entering the second stage.[5]

Women should be encouraged to give birth in the position they find most comfortable. Care should be taken when positioning a patient in supine or lithotomy positions to avoid maternal hypotension and decreased uterine perfusion compression of the great vessels by the gravid uterus ('aortocaval compression syndrome'). This is best achieved by slightly tilting the parturient towards the left lateral position.

As the fetus descends through the pelvis, initially with the sagittal suture in the transverse direction, it will perform an internal

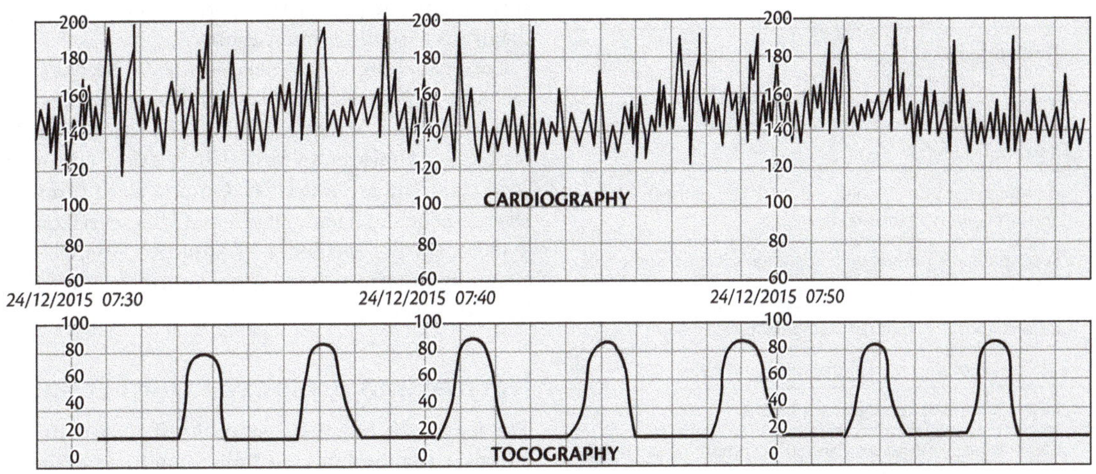

Figure 12.4 Cardiotocography.

rotation at the level of Hodge III, thereby turning the occiput to an anterior position. The reason for this rotation lies in the anatomy of the human female pelvis offering the largest transverse diameter at the pelvic inlet, and the anteroposterior, vertical diameter at the outlet. As a result, after the delivery of the head, the head will reposition with an external rotational movement to enable the shoulders to pass through the pelvic outlet.[1] There are no clear data on whether an episiotomy influences the fetal outcome.

After the fetal head descends, flexes, and rotates to the occiput anterior position, the labia minora will distend, and crowning will occur. At this time, an opening of approximately 3–4 cm will be seen at the introitus. Should episiotomy be deemed necessary, it should be performed at this stage. The use of episiotomy, however, remains controversial, as it does not appear to protect against sphincter damage in a systematic review by Hartmann et al.[6] The routine use of episiotomy should therefore be avoided.

When the head is delivered, the birth attendant examines the neck of the newborn for the presence of a nuchal cord. If tightly entwined, the cord is cut by the obstetrician at that point. Subsequently, the head is gently pulled towards the sacrum, allowing the anterior shoulder to be born. When moved upwards in the direction of the pubic symphysis, the posterior shoulder follows. In the so-called hands-on method, the perineum is supported by the hand of the birth attendant both during the passage of the head through the perineum, as well as during delivery of the posterior shoulder. Although this method was developed to prevent severe (third- and fourth-degree) perineal tears (Table 12.1), this was not confirmed in comparative studies.[7] In contrast, the use of warm compresses on the perineum is associated with a decreased occurrence of perineal trauma and should be offered to labouring women.[8]

The *third stage* of labour comprises the delivery of the placenta. Although this happens spontaneously in most cases, an active management of the third stage of labour is advisable. This includes:[9]

- prophylactic oxytocin (5–10 units intramuscular (IM) or slowly IV) at delivery of the anterior shoulder
- uterine massage
- controlled cord traction.

Table 12.1 Degree of perineal tears

Degree of laceration	Description
First degree	Superficial laceration limited to the perineal skin or vaginal mucosa
Second degree	First-degree rupture with laceration of the perineal muscles and fascia, with intact anal sphincter
Third degree	Second-degree rupture with laceration comprising the anal sphincter
3a	Laceration of the external anal sphincter < 50%
3b	Laceration of the external anal sphincter > 50%
3c	Laceration of the internal anal sphincter
Fourth degree	Third-degree rupture with laceration comprising the rectal mucosa

Active management of the third stage was shown to shorten the third stage, to reduce blood loss and PPH (>1000 mL), and therefore to reduce the incidence of maternal anaemia (haemoglobin <9 g/dL).[9] Randomized trials also have examined the use of oxytocin alone, ergometrine alone, misoprostol alone, and combinations of oxytocin and ergometrine (syntometrine) in active management protocols compared with physiological management where a spontaneous delivery of the placenta is awaited. Trials have also compared the various uterotonics in active management protocols and this has been the subject of a meta-analysis in an extensive recent Cochrane review.[9]

These findings suggest that syntometrine may have a slight advantage in reducing PPH by 500 mL or more (relative risk (RR) 0.74; 95% confidence interval (CI) 0.65–0.85) and possibly by 1000 mL or more (RR 0.79; 95% CI 0.59–1.06), oxytocin alone is also very effective and does not have the adverse effect profile (nausea, vomiting, and hypertension) that is frequently associated with preparations containing ergot.

This review further demonstrates that increasing the IM dose of oxytocin from 5 IU to 10 IU raises the effectiveness of oxytocin. However, no more than 5 IU of oxytocin as a single IV bolus should be given, although it may be repeated after an interval. All IV oxytocin boluses should be administered slowly over several minutes to avoid cardiovascular side effects.

Trials using oxytocin alone showed reduced rates of manual removal of the placenta, whereas those using ergot preparations demonstrated increased rates.

More recently, trials have been performed using a synthetic oxytocin analogue, carbetocin (Pabal®), which has a prolonged action. A review on the subject showed a decreased need for additional uterotonic drugs after a bolus of carbetocin.[10] However, a Cochrane review concluded that carbetocin should not be used as a first-line agent compared to other proven uterotonic agents, in view of the reduced availability and increased costs associated with carbetocin.[11]

Misoprostol is a low-cost, heat-stable uterotonic drug in pill form and therefore potentially an excellent agent for prophylaxis in the third stage of labour. Unfortunately, randomized trials have shown it to be inferior to injectable uterotonics.[12] Adverse effects, such as shivering and fever, are common and in regimens using higher doses, nausea, vomiting, and diarrhoea occur more frequently. The presence of prostaglandin-induced pyrexia and shivering in the postpartum period may lead to confusion in the diagnosis of septic complications.[13]

Cord clamping is best delayed (30–90 seconds, maximum 120 seconds) in preterm neonates as it is associated with fewer neonatal transfusions, less hypotension, and less intraventricular haemorrhages.[14] However, in term deliveries the advantages of delayed cord clamping are less clear. On one hand it results in a higher level of neonatal haemoglobin and iron levels, on the other hand it increases the incidence of jaundice. Therefore, delayed cord clamping in term infants, is not routinely advised and should be individualized.[15]

Normal and prolonged third stage

The length of the third stage itself is usually 5–15 minutes. However, the absolute time limit for delivery of the placenta, without significant bleeding, remains unclear. Placental retention or prolonged third stage is defined as a placenta that is not delivered 30 minutes after the birth of the baby.[1] The main complications associated with this condition are uterine atony, maternal PPH, and subsequent hypotension. PPH may cause anaemia and should be corrected with oral or IV iron or by transfusion if appropriate (see Chapter 35 and Chapter 48). The duration of hospitalization may be prolonged if the patient is anaemic, and the establishment of effective breastfeeding may be hampered.[16]

The pregnancy-related (direct) maternal mortality rate in the United States is approximately 7–10 women per 100,000 live births and it is estimated that 8% of these deaths are caused by PPH.[17] In the developing world, several countries have maternal mortality rates in excess of 1000 women per 100,000 live births, and World Health Organization statistics suggest that 25% of maternal deaths are due to PPH. Therefore, an active management of the third stage is advised as discussed previously. Emptying the bladder and actively rubbing the uterus are an integral part of active management. If despite these measures the placenta is not delivered after 1 hour, additional uterotonic drugs (prostaglandins)[18] and operative manual removal of placenta and exploration of the uterine cavity needs to be considered. The clinical management in case of retained placenta is summarized in Box 12.1.

As mentioned earlier in this section, the most common definition for placental retention is non-delivery of the placenta for more than 30 minutes. This is an arbitrary definition, and management is greatly influenced by the clinical assessment of whether significant bleeding is occurring. This bleeding may be visible or may manifest only by the increasing size of the uterus, filled with blood and clots. In the absence of any evidence of placental detachment,

Box 12.1 Management summary for retained placenta

1. Empty bladder and massage uterus
2. Consider umbilical vein injection of oxytocin (10 IU in 1–2 mL saline) in stable women
3. Consider alternative uterotonics (sulprostone, Hemabate®, misoprostol)
4. Insert IV line (2 large-bore cannula if bleeding actively) and take blood samples for haemoglobin, clotting and cross match)
5. Provide adequate anaesthesia in theatre
6. Attempt manual removal
7. Check the uterine cavity using ultrasound to ascertain that all placenta and fetal membranes have been removed
8. Palpate and massage uterus until firm, continue uterotonic drugs
9. Proceed to curettage, preferably under direct ultrasound visualization if incomplete manual removal
10. Consider diagnosis of placenta accreta
11. Administer antibiotics
12. Quantify fetomaternal transfusion in Rhesus D-negative patients before anti-D administration
13. Monitor patient for increased risk of PPH.

one should also consider the diagnosis of complete placenta accreta or a variant. This condition may present with bleeding if only a portion of the placenta is abnormally implanted.

Ensuring that the bladder is empty speeds up the delivery of the placenta and at least aids in the assessment and control of the uterus. Ideally, women should have an empty bladder at the start of the active second stage of labour. This usually occurs naturally because of pressure from the presenting part and maternal expulsive effort. Encouraging the woman to attempt to void late in the second stage or following delivery is not unreasonable, although this may be difficult. Alternatively, a single sterile catheterization can be performed. Emptying the bladder is mandatory before any attempt at assisted vaginal delivery.

A number of trials have evaluated the role of injection drugs and/or fluids into the umbilical cord in the management of retained placenta. This procedure takes time and should only be attempted in women not experiencing significant bleeding. Tested injection fluids into the umbilical cord vein include isotonic sodium chloride solution (normal saline), oxytocin and saline, prostaglandin and saline, misoprostol and saline, and dextran-70. The studies comparing injection of oxytocin (commonly, 10 IU) and saline (commonly, 20 mL) with expectant management (odds ratio (OR) 0.7; 95% CI 0.48–1.02) or saline injection alone (OR 0.59; 95% CI 0.43–0.82 and number needed to treat 8; 95% CI 5–20) suggest that this practice indeed reduces the need for manual removal of the placenta. However, misoprostol (oral or rectal) could be at least as effective in this setting and the effect of injecting oxytocin in the umbilical vein showed little or no effect in the high-quality trials.[19,20] This intervention seems therefore only reasonable in stable women with minimal bleeding while preparations for a manual removal are being made.

Manual removal of the placenta (Figure 12.5) is warranted if the above manoeuvers have failed to deliver the placenta or if significant bleeding occurs. The retained or partially detached placenta interferes with uterine contraction and retraction and leads to bleeding. The risk of significant PPH increases the longer the placenta remains *in situ* and is increased sixfold if the placenta remains undelivered after 30 minutes.

To safely perform a manual placental removal, it is mandatory to perform this in an operation theatre. The choice of type of anaesthesia (neuraxial or general) that is required should depend upon the clinical urgency of the situation and the presence of

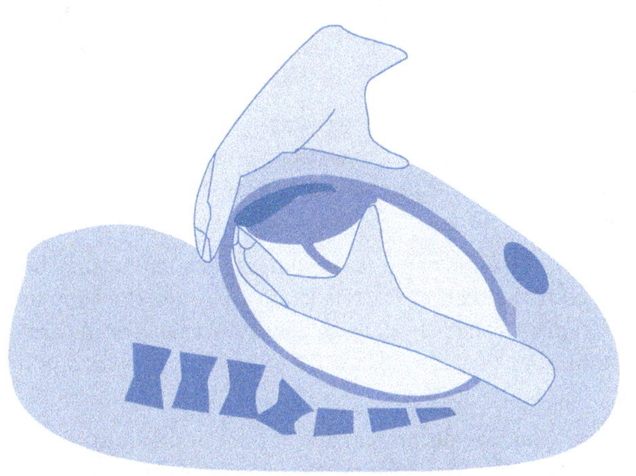

Figure 12.5 Manuel removal of the placenta (manoeuvre of Credé).

contraindications to neuraxial anaesthesia such as hypovolaemia or coagulation abnormalities. If spinal anaesthesia is chosen, inexperienced anaesthetists often block too low, thinking that only uterine anaesthesia is required. The block should be high enough for the patient to tolerate the hand in the fundus (e.g. 2.4 mL 0.5% bupivacaine). The cessation of an oxytocin infusion or the administration of uterine relaxants to promote uterine exploration and manual removal is of questionable value and may lead to increased bleeding. Ultrasonography is useful in many cases in order to evaluate the uterine cavity, to instrument the uterus without the risk of perforation, and to assess the completeness of the removal after the procedure.

When possible, an elbow-length glove is worn and attention is paid to asepsis. Antibiotic prophylaxis (cefazolin 2 g IV) is best administered in the absence of contraindications. The perineum and vagina must be prepared and disinfected. The vaginal hand may be immersed in povidone-iodine solution (Proviodine®) or in a chlorhexidine crème (Hibitane®) to facilitate entry. The hand is passed into the vagina through the cervix and into the lower segment following the umbilical cord. Care is taken to minimize the profile of the hand as it enters, keeping the thumb and fingers together in the shape of a cone to avoid damage to the soft tissues, especially the cervix.

The non-vaginal hand is used to hold the uterus at its fundal part. If the placenta is encountered in the lower segment, it is removed. If the placenta is not encountered, the placental edge is sought. Once found, the fingers gently expand the space between the placenta and uterus and shear off the placenta. The placenta is pushed to the palmar aspect of the hand and wrist; and when it is entirely separated, the hand is withdrawn. Ensure that an oxytocin infusion (e.g. 40 IU/1 L Ringers' lactate at 125 mL/unit) is running rapidly as the hand is withdrawn in order to encourage strong uterine contraction and subsequently perform uterine massage. Care must be taken to remove all the fetal membranes. Once uterine contraction is established, the placenta and membranes are examined by the operator to determine whether further exploration or curettage is necessary.

Obstructed labour and delivery

Obstructed labour is a first- or second-stage phenomenon in women whose labour is prolonged. A prolonged first stage exists when no progression in dilatation and descent occurs during 2–4 hours.[1] The reason why labour becomes prolonged or obstructed may be due to one of the 'Ps' referred to earlier—passenger, passage, and powers—and is summarized in Table 12.2:

- *Passenger*: the fetus is the 'passenger' travelling down the birth canal. Prolonged labour may occur if the fetal head is too large to pass through the mother's pelvis, or the fetal presentation is abnormal.
- *Passage*: the birth canal is the 'passage', so labour may be prolonged if the mother's pelvis is too small for the baby to pass through or if the pelvis has an abnormal shape, or in case there is a tumour (e.g. fibroids) or other physical obstruction in the pelvis.
- *Powers*: inadequate 'power', due to poor or uncoordinated uterine contractions, is a major cause of prolonged labour. Either the uterine contractions are not strong enough to efface and dilate the cervix in the first stage of labour, or the muscular effort of the uterus is insufficient to push the baby down the birth canal during the second stage. Another important component of the 'power' is the active maternal 'pushing' effort during the active second stage. This can be reduced due to maternal exhaustion or interfering muscular, respiratory, or cardiovascular conditions.

Table 12.2 Causes of prolonged or obstructed labour

Passenger	Passage	Powers
Large head (cephalopelvic disproportion): ◆ Macrosomia ◆ Macrocephaly ◆ Hydrocephaly	Bony pelvis abnormalities: ◆ Malnutrition ◆ Deformation (trauma, poliomyelitis, etc.)	Inadequate contractions: ◆ Regional anaesthesia ◆ Induced labour (less effective contractions)
Malpresentation, malpositioning, multiple pregnancies: ◆ Brow, face, shoulder ◆ Persistent malposition ◆ Locked twins ◆ Conjoined twins	Soft tissue abnormalities: ◆ Tumour (fibroids) ◆ Infections ◆ Scars (genital mutilation)	Insufficient/ineffective maternal effort: ◆ Maternal exhaustion, ◆ Maternal respiratory, neuromuscular or cardiovascular condition

A cardinal clinical sign for the diagnosis of obstructed labour is when the widest diameter of the fetal skull remains *stationary* above the pelvic brim because it is unable to descend. This can be clinically detected by careful palpation of the mother's abdomen as the uterus relaxes and softens between contractions, but an internal examination is usually required to confirm the diagnosis and determine the cause of the arrest.

Uterine contractions are considered adequate when they occur every couple of minutes and last for at least 30 seconds. Insufficiently frequent or strong uterine contractions are more often seen in a patient with neuraxial analgesia containing opioids.[21] The contractions can then be optimized either by artificially rupturing the fetal membranes (AROM; see 'Induction of Labour') (Figure 12.6) if the membranes are still intact, or by exogenous administration of oxytocin according to local institutional protocols.

Oxytocin (derived from the Greek word *oxys tocos*, meaning 'fast birth') is a mammalian neuropituitary hormone that acts primarily as a neuromodulator in the brain but also plays roles in sexual reproduction, in particular during and after childbirth. It is released in large amounts after distention of the cervix and uterus during labour, facilitating birth, maternal bonding, and, after stimulation of the nipples, breastfeeding. Oxytocin effects are regulated by complex positive feedback mechanisms (Figure 12.7).[22]

Cephalo-pelvic disproportion (CPD) is present when there is a disproportion between the head of the fetus and the birth canal. CPD means it is difficult or impossible for the fetus to pass safely through the mother's pelvis due either to a maternal pelvis that is too narrow for that fetal head, or due to a fetal head that is relatively too large for the mother's pelvis. Small (or contracted) pelvises are more frequent in developing countries, on one the hand due to malnutrition in childhood persisting into adult life, and on the other hand due to underage sex and marriage. CPD causes

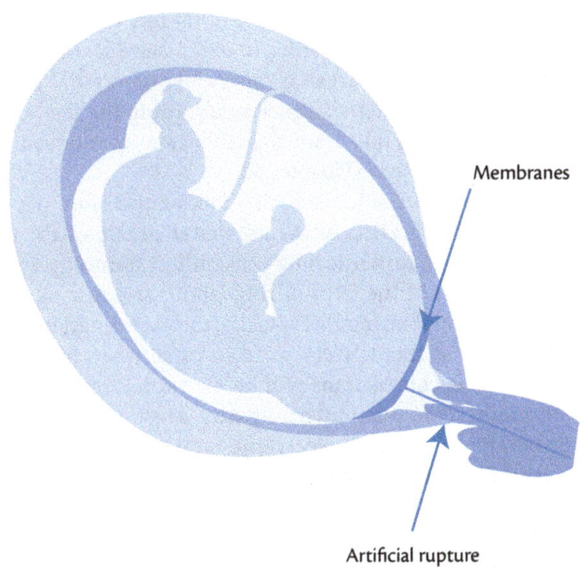

Figure 12.6 Artificial rupture of membranes (AROM).
Courtesy of S. De Bisschop.

a prolonged first and second stage, which yields an increased risk for fetal and maternal complications. A longer second stage is accompanied by increased occurrence of fetal asphyxia, PPH, perineal laceration, infection of mother and fetus, and is a good predictor for shoulder dystocia (see 'Shoulder Dystocia').

Therefore, if despite adequate stimulation no progression in the partogram is obtained and labour is obstructed during the first stage, the safest management plan is to perform a caesarean delivery (CD). In case of arrest of labour during the second stage, the physician needs to evaluate the possibility of performing an operative or instrumental vaginal delivery as an alternative for CD.

Induction of labour

Overall, induction of labour should be restricted to medical conditions in which the prolongation of pregnancy yields significant risks for mother or fetus (e.g. post-term pregnancies pursuing 10 days beyond the due date). If induction of labour is performed solely for non-obstetric reasons (e.g. for the convenience of the patient or the caregiver) it will result in increased rates of failures, complications, and morbidity.

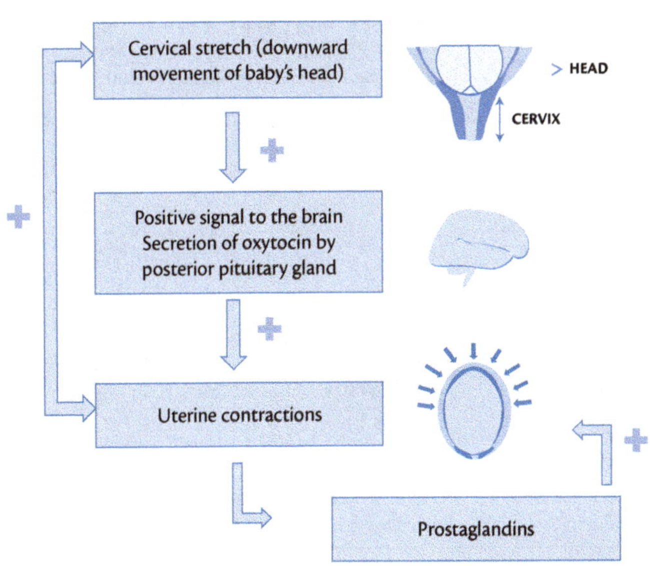

Figure 12.7 Positive feedback mechanism oxytocin.

If the cervix is unfavourable, labour can be induced by exogenous administration of prostaglandin E_2 (PGE_2), the synthetic form of the natural hormone involved in the normal initiation of labour.

If, however, the cervix is already partially dilated (2–3 cm) and effaced, labour can be induced by membrane sweeping or amniotomy (Figure 12.6) alone. In many cases, contractions will follow AROM.

If contractions are poor or the cervix fails to dilate, IV oxytocin can augment the induced contractions. This is best preceded by AROM as the uterus responds poorly to exogenous oxytocin in the presence of intact membranes.[23]

There is currently insufficient evidence to assess how to best use oxytocin for augmentation of labour. Based mostly on physiological studies, an oxytocin dilution of 10 mU/mL, initial dose of 2 mU/min (12 mL/h) with incremental increase of 2 mU/min (12 mL every 30–45 minutes until adequate labour) and maximum dose of 16 mU/min have been proposed.[24]

There is significant debate about the ideal setting and timing of induction of labour. Limited information is available on the safety of outpatient management of induction of labour, and larger controlled studies are needed to establish an effective and safe dose and vehicle for PGE_2 before use on an outpatient basis can be recommended.

Membrane sweeping

Membrane sweeping or 'stripping' is commonly practised to induce labour. According to the American College of Obstetricians and Gynecologists (ACOG), stripping membranes increases the likelihood of spontaneous labour within 48 hours and reduces the incidence of induction with other methods.[25] NICE notes that membrane sweeping should be regarded as an adjunct to induction of labour rather than an actual method of induction.[26] It recommends membrane sweeping be offered to all women prior to formal induction of labour, to nulliparous women at 40 weeks of gestational age, and to all women at 41 weeks of gestational age.

Amniotomy

Amniotomy (Figure 12.6) alone for labour induction is not recommended in most leading guidelines on the subject. According to ACOG, amniotomy used alone for inducing labour can be associated with unpredictable and sometimes long intervals before the onset of contractions.[25] There is therefore insufficient evidence on the efficacy and safety of amniotomy alone for labour induction. Amniotomy combined with early oxytocin infusion compared with amniotomy alone reduces the induction-to-delivery interval significantly. Amniotomy should be postponed if the baby's head is high and the physician/midwife should palpate for the umbilical cord and vasa previa and avoid dislodging the fetal head when performing amniotomy. If amniotomy has to be performed with a high fetal head, this is best done in theatre where there are all the facilities for immediate delivery if cord prolapse occurs.

Induction in women with ruptured membranes

For women with premature rupture of membranes (PROM) at term, labour is usually induced at the time of presentation, or within 48 hours of presentation, to reduce the risk of chorio-amnionitis. Oxytocin is the method of choice, especially if the Bishop score is favourable. Vaginal PGE_2 is globally regarded as an appropriate, safe, and effective induction method for women with PROM. In a randomized study of labour induction in women with PROM at term, a single dose of intravaginal misoprostol was necessary for successful labour induction in 86% of the patients.[27] The same precautions should be exercised when prostaglandins are used for induction of labour with ruptured membranes as for intact membranes.

For women with preterm pre-labour rupture of membranes (PPROM), induction should not be carried out before 34 weeks unless there are additional obstetric indications (like infection or fetal compromise). After 34 weeks, the maternity team and mother should discuss risks to both woman and baby, as well as local availability of neonatal intensive care facilities, before a decision is made about whether to induce labour, using vaginal PGE_2.[25] (See also Chapter 33.)

Mechanical methods

Although they are debated in some countries like the United Kingdom,[26] mechanical dilation methods are effective in ripening the cervix and include hygroscopic dilators, osmotic dilators (*Laminaria japonicum*), Foley catheters, and double-balloon devices. In women undergoing induction with an unfavourable cervix, mechanical methods are associated with a decreased CD rate when compared with oxytocin alone. Multiple studies have demonstrated the efficacy of mechanical cervical dilators but there is insufficient evidence to assess how effective (vaginal delivery within 24 hours) mechanical methods are compared with prostaglandins. Potential advantages of a mechanical method like the Foley bladder catheter include low cost compared with prostaglandins, stability at room temperature, and reduced risk of uterine hyperstimulation with or without FHR changes.[25]

Prostaglandins

Recommendations for pharmacological induction of labour with prostaglandins also differ. Both prostaglandin analogues (misoprostol and dinoprostone) are regarded as effective for cervical ripening and induction of labour according to ACOG. ACOG states that there is extensive clinical experience with misoprostol and a large body of published reports supporting its safety and efficacy when used appropriately.[25] The US Food and Drug Administration in 2002 approved a new label on the use of misoprostol during pregnancy for cervical ripening and for the induction of labour. In contrast, the UK NICE, states that vaginal PGE_2 (dinoprostone) is the preferred method of induction of labour and that misoprostol should only be offered as a method of induction of labour to women who have intrauterine fetal death or in the context of a clinical trial. While, extensively used in clinical practice, Misoprostol is not officially licensed for use in pregnancy in the United Kingdom, because of marketing reasons.[26]

Intrapartum fetal monitoring

Monitoring of fetuses in labour aims to identify hypoxia before it is sufficient to lead to damaging acidosis and long-term neurological adverse outcome for the baby.[1] The limitations of the different tests available mean that, in order to avoid significant hypoxia, interventions such as caesarean or instrumental vaginal delivery are undertaken when there is concern regarding the fetal condition. Fetal monitoring thus leads to higher rates of interventions. (For greater detail, refer to Chapter 6.)

The assessment of the fetus during labour therefore depends on a careful consideration of the antenatal course of the pregnancy, the liquor or amniotic fluid (meconium staining), and the heart rate changes of the fetus during labour (reassuring versus non-reassuring or abnormal). Typically, once a woman in labour presents herself at the delivery ward in established labour, the FHR and uterine contractions will be monitored by CTG for at least 30 minutes, and then intermittently. Most accepted lists of indications for *continuous* electronic fetal monitoring during labour include neuraxial analgesia and are listed in Table 12.3.[27]

A normal FHR at term should be between 110 and 150 beats per minute (bpm). A reassuring FHR (Figure 12.4) trace shows normal variability and the presence of accelerations. Variability (Figure 12.8) is defined as a short term ('beat-to-beat') change in FHR and should normally be between 5 and 25 bpm.[28] An acceleration (Figure 12.8) is defined as an increase of the FHR from baseline with 15 bpm lasting for at least 15 seconds. A deceleration is defined as a decrease of the FHR with 15 bpm during at least 15 seconds. A baseline greater than 160 bpm during 10 minutes is defined as tachycardia (Figure 12.9). A baseline beneath 110 bpm during at least 5 minutes or a decline in FHR of 40 bpm, is defined as a bradycardia (Figure 12.10). Decreased variability and so-called late decelerations (Figure 12.11), with a nadir after the contraction has passed, have the strongest relationship with fetal acidosis and

Table 12.3 Indications for continuous electronic fetal monitoring during labour

Risk factor	Example
High-risk pregnancy identified before labour	Intrauterine growth restriction, preterm labour, post-term pregnancy (>42 weeks), poly/oligohydramnios, multiple gestation, suspicion of (partial) abruption (more than average vaginal blood loss, sonographical presumption, non-reassuring intermittent auscultation)
Induced or augmented labour	
Obstructed labour	
Abnormal fetal presentation	Breech
Neuraxial analgesia	Epidural, combined spinal–epidural analgesia
Significant maternal condition	Renal disease, diabetes, cardiovascular disease, pre-eclampsia, HELLP syndrome
Previous caesarean delivery	
Threatened fetal condition	Non-reassuring intermittent auscultation, meconial amniotic fluid, increasing blood loss

Adapted with permission from G Justus Hofmeyr, A Metin Gülmezoglu, Cynthia Pileggi, Vaginal misoprostol for cervical ripening and induction of labour, *Cochrane Database of Systematic Reviews*, Copyright © 2010 John Wiley and Sons.

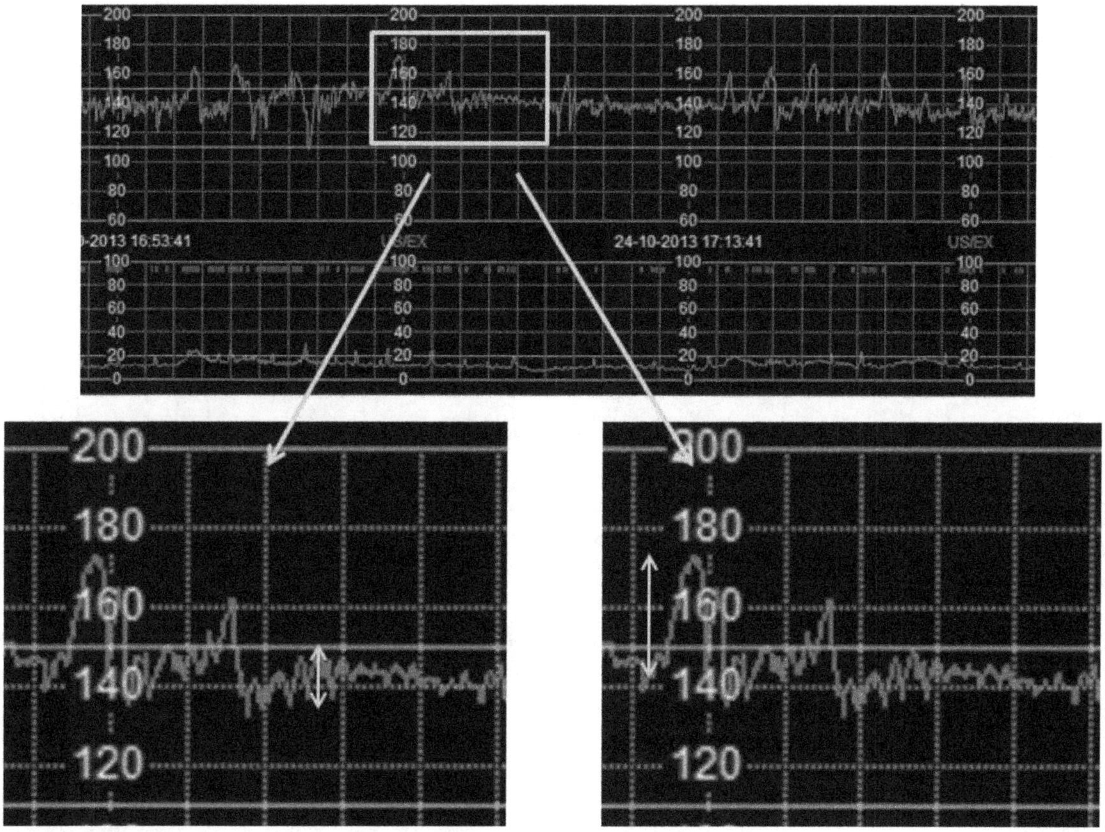

Figure 12.8 (Lower left) Beat-to-beat variability (5–25 bpm) and (lower right) acceleration.

hypoxia.[28] In case there is no variability or reactivity left, the CTG has become pre-terminal and immediate delivery is mandatory (Figure 12.12).

In case of non-reassuring CTG, fetal scalp sampling for determination of the fetal acid–base state, or more recently fetal electrocardiography with ST analysis (STAN®) can help to identify compromised fetuses at risk for perinatal asphyxia. A normal ST waveform demonstrates a sufficient fetal oxygen supply. During hypoxia the T-wave amplitude of the ECG increases and the STAN® monitor displays an automatic 'ST Event' alert (Figure 12.13).

The STAN® method is a combination of standard CTG parameters and ST analysis. If there is a significant change in the ST interval and a 'ST event' alert is displayed, actions are recommended according to clinical guidelines. A recent Swedish meta-analysis comparing CTG plus ST analysis with CTG alone concluded that there is currently no evidence that STAN® reduces the incidence

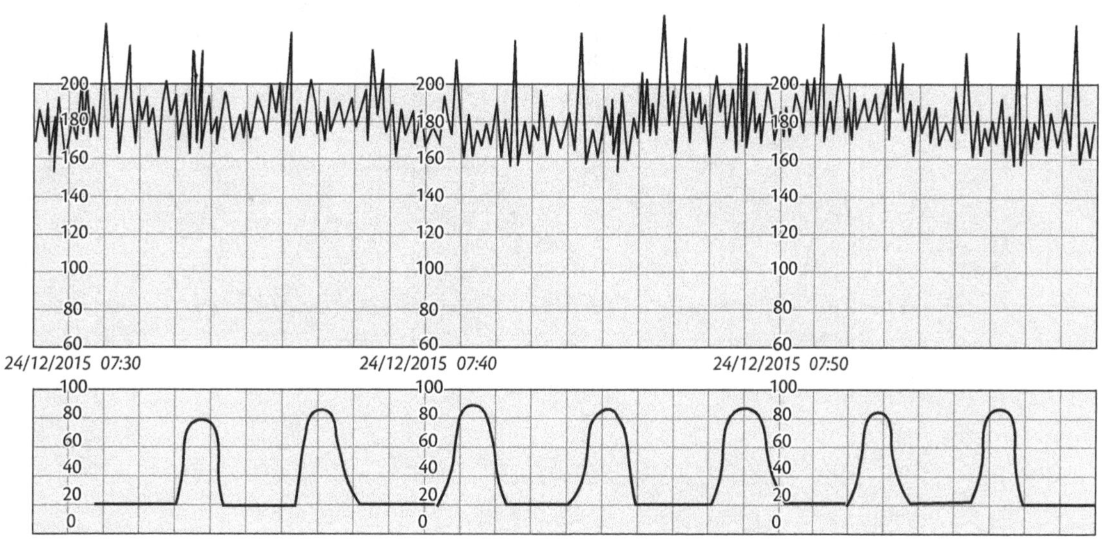

Figure 12.9 Fetal tachycardia.

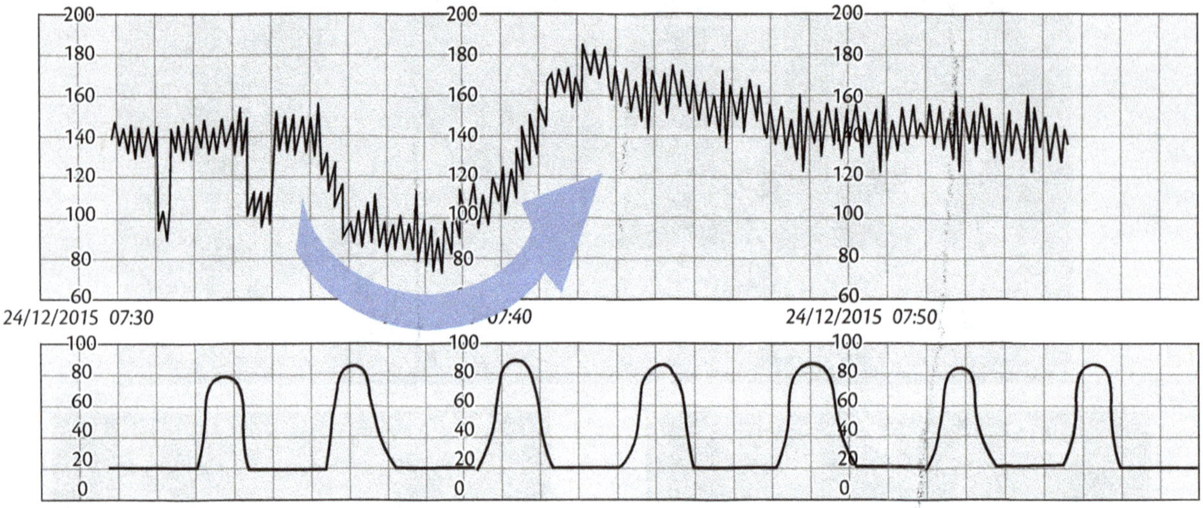

Figure 12.10 Fetal bradycardia.

of metabolic acidosis (RR 0.96; 95% CI 0.49–1.88). Caesarean and instrumental vaginal deliveries due to fetal distress or other indications were also comparable in both groups but STAN® reduced the number of instances which require scalp blood sampling.[29]

Shoulder dystocia

Shoulder dystocia is a specific case of dystocia. It occurs when after delivery of the head, the anterior shoulder cannot pass or requires significant manipulation to pass below the pubic symphysis (Figure 12.14), prolonging the head-to-shoulder interval. It occurs in approximately 1% (range 0.6–1.4%) of deliveries.[1] Clinically, shoulder dystocia is recognized by non-emergence of the anterior shoulder during a routine delivery and is sometimes preceded by the so-called turtle sign (the 'bobbing' or appearance and immediate retraction of the fetal head during maternal effort and expulsion).

In shoulder dystocia, it is the chin that presses against the walls of the perineum of the parturient due to the shoulder being impacted behind the pubic symphysis, causing the so-called turtle sign (Figure 12.14).

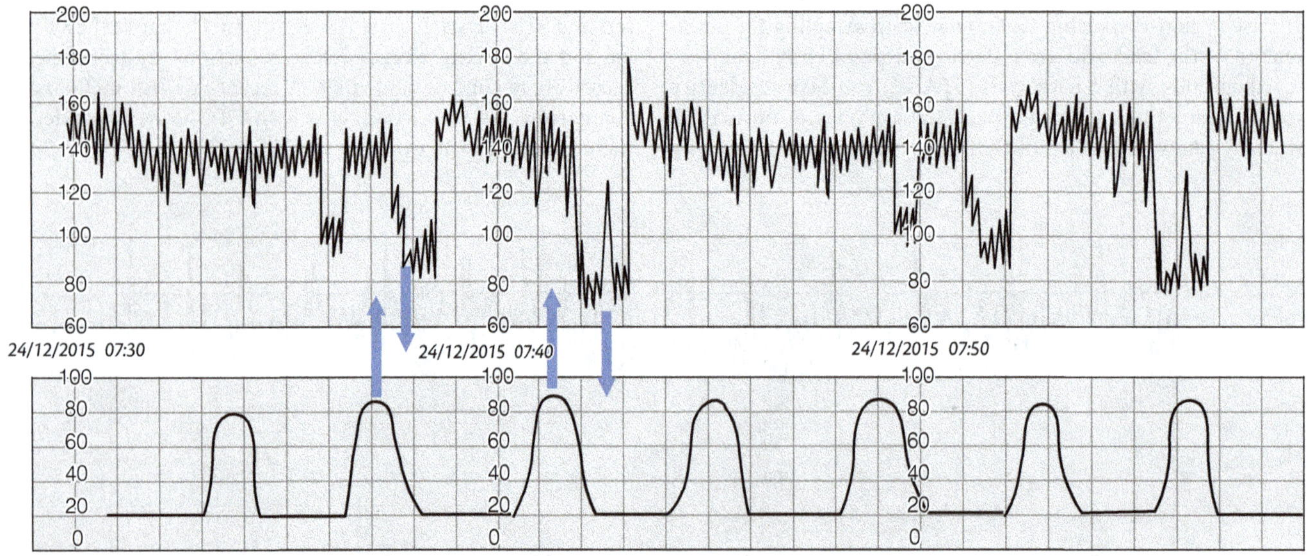

Figure 12.11 Late deceleration.

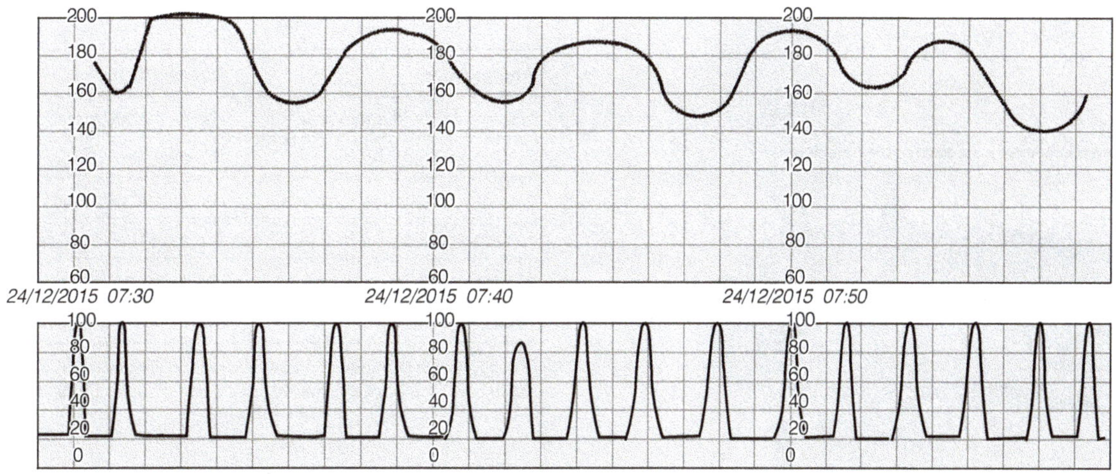

Figure 12.12 Preterminal cardiotocography.

Shoulder dystocia is an obstetric emergency, and fetal demise can occur if the infant is not delivered within minutes. Indeed, once the head is born, the umbilical cord is being compressed within the birth canal with almost complete cessation of blood flow. As a result, the cord blood pH declines by approximately 0.04 units/min. On the one hand this means the obstetrician has time to resolve the dystocia, on the other hand it means that if the interval is prolonged, severe damage to the fetus can occur as a result of decreased umbilical blood flow. Additional morbidity can be the result of inadvertent excessive pulling on the fetal head, or result from the manipulation and manoeuvers required to deliver the shoulder and complete the delivery (Box 12.2).

The major concern of shoulder dystocia is damage to the upper brachial plexus supplying the sensory and motor components of the shoulder, arm, and hands. The ventral roots (motor pathway) are most prone to injury, as they are in the plane of greatest tension (anterior, sensory nerves are somewhat protected due to the usual inward movement of the shoulder).

The major risk factors for shoulder dystocia are summarized in Table 12.4.[30] Shoulder dystocia often (50%) occurs in the absence of any risk factor. Therefore, it is advised that all personnel assisting childbirth should be trained in managing cases of shoulder dystocia and that at least one clinician experienced in the management of shoulder dystocia is available at every delivery.

The most studied risk factors for shoulder dystocia are maternal diabetes and fetal macrosomia. If the birth weight of the infant was between 4250 and 4500 g, the frequency of shoulder dystocia

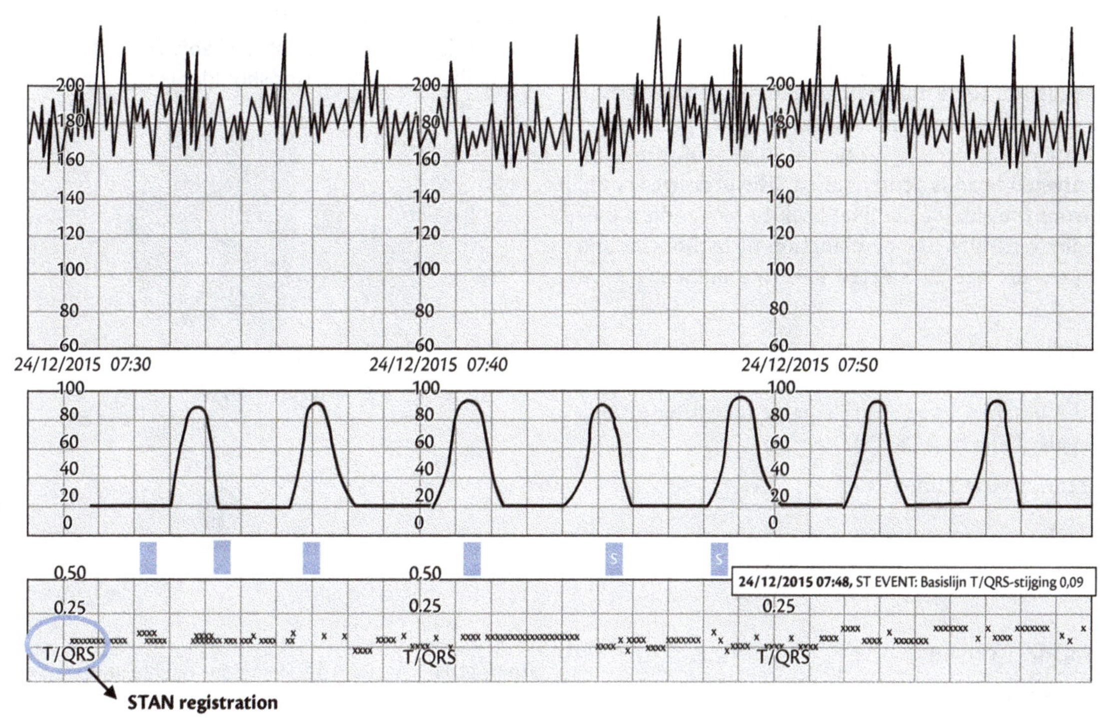

Figure 12.13 ST event.

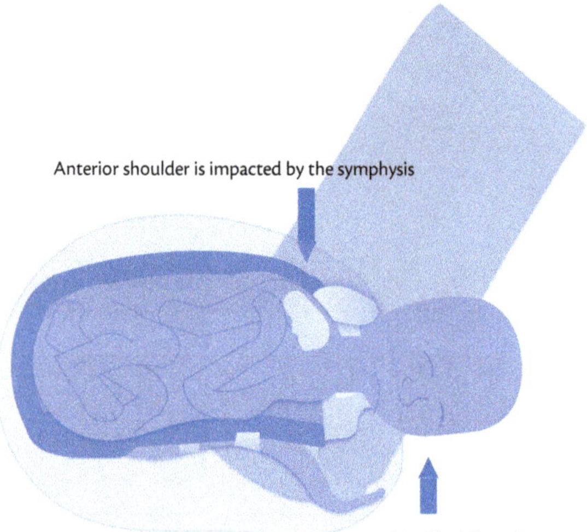

Figure 12.14 Turtle sign.

was 9.1% if the mother was not diabetic and 16.7% in diabetic mothers in a large Californian cohort.[31]

Many manoeuvers have been developed and modified to facilitate the delivery of the anterior shoulder in cases of shoulder dystocia including:

- *Episiotomy*: although the problem of shoulder dystocia is related to the bony pelvis and not the soft tissues, the space created with an episiotomy (Figure 12.15) may facilitate further internal manoeuvers. An episiotomy can be difficult to perform in these cases due to the impaction of the fetal head tightly to the perineum. In these cases, a scalpel may be helpful.
- *McRoberts' manoeuver*: this manoeuver involves hyperflexion and exorotation of the maternal legs, placing the mother's legs tightly to her abdomen with flexed knees (Figure 12.16). This manoeuver widens the pelvis, and flattens the spine in the lower back (lumbar spine level).[32]
- *Suprapubic pressure* (or Rubin I manoeuvre): if McRoberts' manoeuver does not succeed, an assistant applies pressure on the lower abdomen (Figure 12.17, external suprapubic pressure) while the delivered head is gently pulled. The pressure should be applied from the side of the fetal back to move the shoulder of the baby ventrally. The combination of McRoberts and suprapubic pressure are considered first-line manoeuvers in the management of shoulder dystocia and these will resolve the shoulder dystocia in more than 50% of cases.[34,35]

If not successful, it is advised to proceed to second-line manoeuvres:

- *Rubin II manoeuvre*: in this manoeuvre (Figure 12.18) the operator will enter vaginally from the back of the delivered head and posterior pressure is applied on the anterior shoulder, which brings the fetus in an oblique position with the head somewhat towards the vagina.
- *Woods' screw manoeuver*: in this manoeuvre the operator enters and applies pressure to the dorsal part of the posterior shoulder, which leads to turning the anterior shoulder to the posterior and vice versa (somewhat the opposite of Rubin II manoeuvre).
- *Removal of the posterior arm* (Jacquemier's or Barnum's manoeuvre): this manoeuvre implies delivery of the posterior shoulder first (Figure 12.19). This is realized by entering the operator's hand and ventrally from the baby, identifying the forearm and hand in the birth canal and gently pulling the posterior arm ventrally over the face of the baby. Once the posterior shoulder is delivered, the anterior shoulder is usually disimpacted easily.

Box 12.2 Complications associated with shoulder dystocia

- Injury of the brachial plexus: Erb's palsy (affecting C5/6), Klumpke's palsy (affecting C8/T1).
- Fracture of the clavicle/humerus
- Cerebral palsy
- Fetal hypoxia
- Fetal demise
- Maternal vaginal lacerations
- Postpartum haemorrhage.

Table 12.4 Risk factors for shoulder dystocia

Antepartum	Intrapartum
History of shoulder dystocia	Labour induction/augmentation
Prior macrosomic baby	Dysfunctional labour
Excessive weight gain	Prolonged first stage
Maternal obesity	Prolonged second stage
Maternal diabetes	Neuraxial analgesia
Fetal macrosomia	Operative vaginal delivery

Reproduced with permission from ACOG Practice Bulletin No. 40: Shoulder Dystocia, *Obstetrics & Gynecology*, Volume 100, Issue 5, pp. 1045–50, Copyright © 2002 Wolters Kluwer Health, Inc.

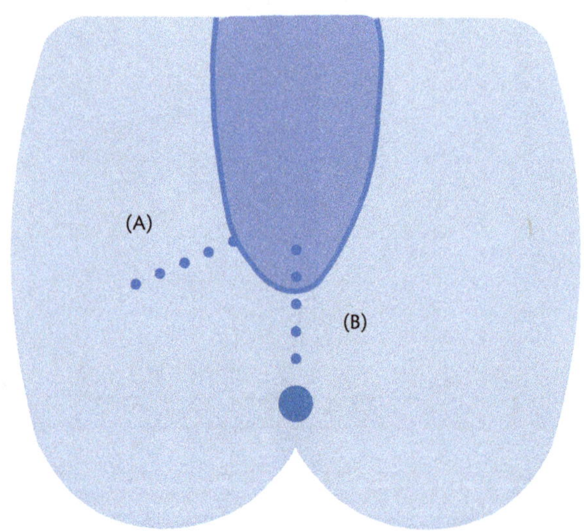

Figure 12.15 Episiotomy. The dotted line indicates the possible routes of an episiotomy. (A) Mediolateral episiotomy (preferable). (B) Median episiotomy.

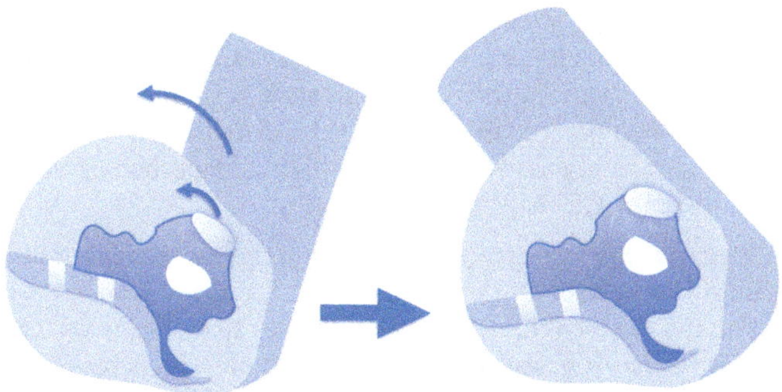

Figure 12.16 McRoberts manoeuver.
Reproduced From Jacquemyn Y. *Procedureboek Verloskunde. Praktische richtlijnen bij verloskundige problemen*. Leuven: Acco; 2007.

- *Positioning on 'all fours'* (Gaskin's manoeuvre): this manoeuver is named after a midwife, Ina May Gaskin. It involves moving the mother to an all-fours position with the back arched, widening the pelvic outlet. The realization of this measure requires sufficient mobility of the patient and is not always feasible in most patients with neuraxial analgesia.

If the baby is still not delivered despite attempting the second-line manoeuvres described above and after considering repeating the prior steps, more aggressive third-line manoeuvers can be attempted:

- *Zavanelli's manoeuver*: this involves internal cephalic replacement followed by CD. It is realized by flexing the fetal delivered head and correcting the external rotation. Uterine relaxation is usually required.[36]

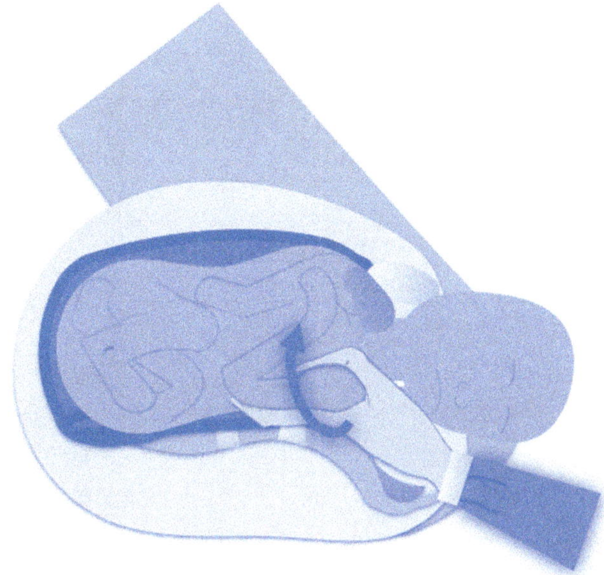

Figure 12.18 Rubin II manoeuver.
Reproduced From Jacquemyn Y. *Procedureboek Verloskunde. Praktische richtlijnen bij verloskundige problemen*. Leuven: Acco; 2007.

- *Intentional fetal clavicular fracture*: this manoeuver involves applying pressure on the fetal anterior clavicle in order to fracture it. This reduces the diameter of the shoulder girdle, required for passage through the birth canal.[37]
- *Maternal symphysiotomy*: this manoeuvre involves surgical or traumatic separation of the pubis symphysis which makes the opening of the birth canal laxer by breaking the connective tissue between the two pubic bones and facilitates the disimpaction of the fetal shoulders.

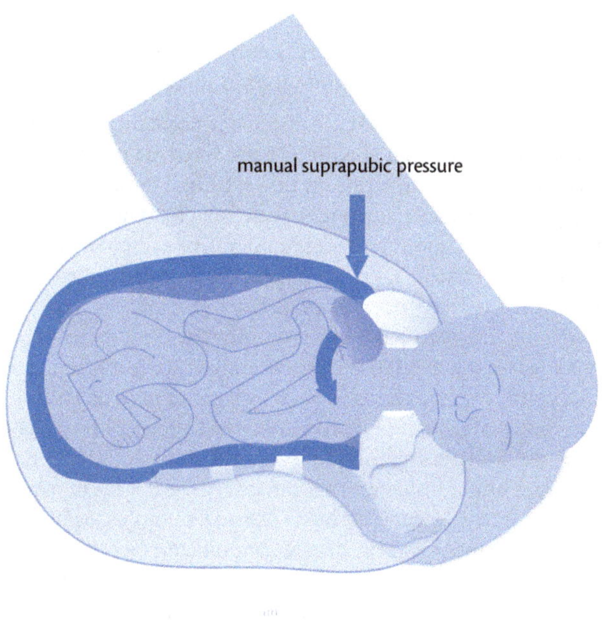

Figure 12.17 Suprapubic pressure.
Reproduced From Jacquemyn Y. *Procedureboek Verloskunde. Praktische richtlijnen bij verloskundige problemen*. Leuven: Acco; 2007.

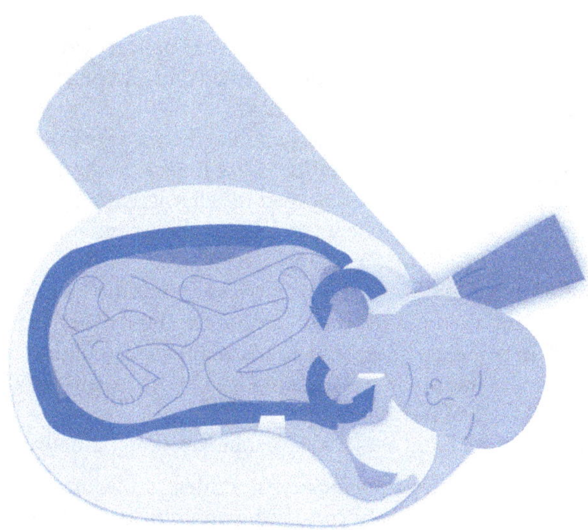

Figure 12.19 Jacquemier's manoeuver.
Reproduced From Jacquemyn Y. *Procedureboek Verloskunde. Praktische richtlijnen bij verloskundige problemen*. Leuven: Acco; 2007.

Table 12.5 Mnemonics

HELPERR
Call for **H**elp
Evaluate for **E**pisiotomy
Legs
Suprapubic **P**ressure
Enter manoeuvres (internal rotation)
Remove the **P**osterior arm
Roll the patient

HELPERR © ALSO (Advanced Life Support in Obstetrics).

- *Abdominal rescue*, described by O'Shaughnessy:[38] this technique involves performing a hysterotomy to facilitate vaginal delivery of the impacted shoulder.

Different mnemonics (Table 12.5) have been developed to facilitate a systematic approach for training and management of shoulder dystocia. The advantage of proceeding in the order of a logical sequence of action like HELPERR (Advanced Life Support in Obstetrics®) is that it goes from least to most invasive, thereby reducing harm to the mother in the event that the infant delivers with one of the earlier manoeuvers. In case these manoeuvers are unsuccessful, a skilled obstetrician may attempt some of the additional third-line procedures listed above. Intentional clavicular fracture is a final attempt at non-operative vaginal delivery prior to Zavanelli's manoeuver or symphysiotomy, both of which are considered extraordinary treatment measures. Finally, detailed and systematic notification of the order and duration of manipulations reduces the risk for litigation, which is high in obstetric trauma. Specific checklist and forms are available in some units to facilitate this.

Operative vaginal delivery

Operative vaginal delivery or instrumental delivery refers to a vaginal delivery in which the operator uses a forceps or a vacuum device to assist the delivery of the baby.

Decisions regarding use of instrumental delivery are based primarily upon the maternal/fetal/neonatal impact of these procedures and are always weighed against the alternative options such as CD, expectant management (prolonging the second stage), and augmentation of contractions using oxytocin.[1]

In the United States, forceps deliveries account for 1% of vaginal births and vacuum deliveries account for about 4% of vaginal births.[39] In some countries, like the Scandinavian countries, the use of forceps has been largely abandoned at the expense of vacuum (ventouse) delivery.

There are three main *indications* for operative vaginal delivery:[39]

- *Prolonged second stage of labour*: in nulliparous women, this is usually defined as lack of continuing progress for 3 hours with neuraxial analgesia or 2 hours without analgesia. In multiparous women, it refers to lack of continuing progress for 2 hours with neuraxial analgesia or 1 hour without analgesia.
- *Non-reassuring fetal condition*: suspicion of immediate or potential fetal compromise (e.g. non-reassuring FHR pattern, abruption) is an indication for operative vaginal delivery. The condition to proceed to operative vaginal delivery is that expeditious vaginal delivery can be readily accomplished. If this is not the case, CD may be the safer option.
- *Maternal indications to shorten the active phase*: forceps or vacuum can be used to shorten the second stage of labour if the Valsalva manoeuvre is contraindicated because of maternal cardiovascular or neurological disease, or if pushing is ineffective because of exhaustion or a history of maternal neurological or muscular disease.

To safely perform an instrumental delivery, the operator should be experienced in operative vaginal delivery and the following *prerequisites* should be present:[39]

- The fetal position is cephalic, with the vertex presenting (exception: forceps delivery to assist in the delivery of an after-coming head in vaginal breech delivery (see 'Breech Delivery').
- The cervix is fully dilated.
- The fetal membranes are ruptured.
- The head is engaged in the maternal pelvis, meaning that the largest diameter of the fetal head is below the level of the ischial spine (below Hodge II). With abdominal examination, no more than one-fifth of the fetal head should be palpable abdominally if the vertex is engaged.
- The fetal size has been estimated at less than 4500 g and clinical pelvimetry shows adequate mid and outlet pelvic dimensions.
- Maternal analgesia is satisfactory.
- Maternal bladder is empty.
- The patient consents to the procedure.
- The option of performing an immediate CD should be available if complications arise.
- The operator is experienced and ready to stop the procedure if a reasonable number of attempts are not successful.

If the fetal presentation or position is uncertain, intrapartum ultrasound examination should be performed, as it is more accurate than digital examination in this setting. Studies have shown that digital examination incorrectly defined fetal head position in over 25% of cases about to undergo operative vaginal delivery.[40]

Factors associated with an increased risk of failed operative delivery include occiput posterior position (Figure 12.20), one-fifth of the head palpable abdominally, the presenting part only as far as the ischial spines, excessive moulding of the fetal head, protracted labour, maternal obesity, and macrosomia.

The choice of instrument is determined by level of training and experience, availability, and the specific clinical situation. Further factors that might influence this choice are the degree of maternal analgesia and knowledge of the risks and benefits associated with each instrument. Vacuum devices should not be used to assist delivery prior to 34 weeks of gestation because of the risk of fetal intraventricular haemorrhage. Prior fetal scalp blood sampling or multiple attempts at fetal scalp electrode placement are also relative contraindications to vacuum extraction since these procedures may increase the risk of cephalohaematoma or external

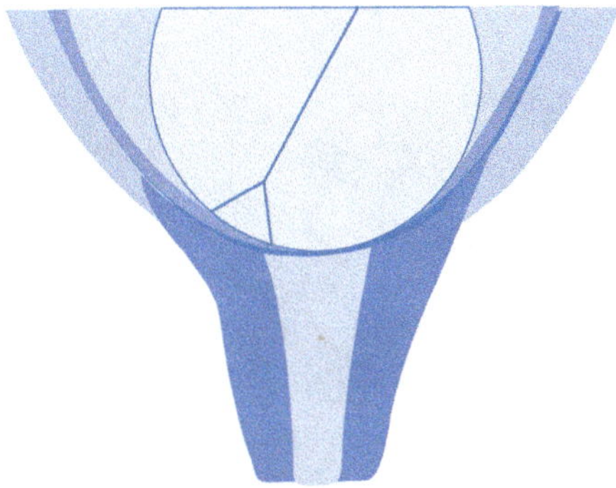

Figure 12.20 Occiput posterior position.

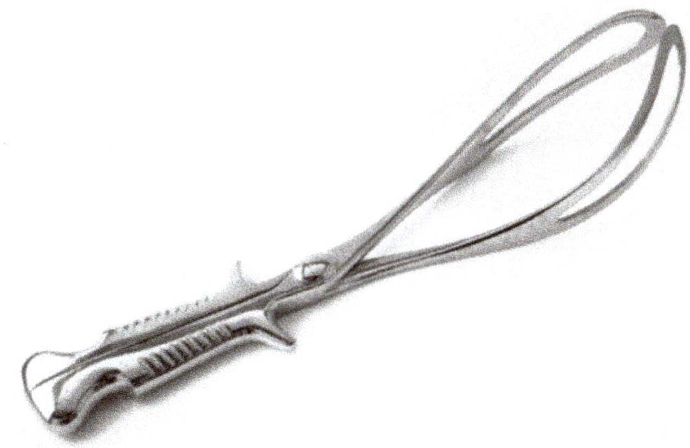

Figure 12.21 Forceps.
Courtesy of Fransesca Ferrando.

bleeding from the scalp wound. Overall, vacuum delivery is probably safer than forceps for the mother, while forceps delivery is probably safer than vacuum for the fetus. Vacuum devices are easier to apply, place less force on the fetal head, require less maternal analgesia, result in less maternal soft tissue trauma, and do not affect the diameter of the fetal head compared to forceps. By comparison, the advantages of forceps are that they are unlikely to detach from the head, can be used on premature fetuses, result in less cephalohaematoma and retinal haemorrhage, and do not aggravate bleeding from scalp lacerations (Table 12.6).[39]

There are many different designs for forceps, but all consist of two separate blades that each have the same four components: blade, shank, lock, and handle (Figure 12.21).

There is insufficient evidence to compare different types of forceps.[40] Specific types exist for rotational applications (e.g. Kielland) and forceps application in case of an after-coming head during a vaginal breech delivery (e.g. Piper).

Vacuum devices include soft (silicone, plastic, rubber) and rigid (metal, plastic) cups (Figure 12.22). Smaller disposable hand-pumped devices are also becoming widely available (e.g. Kiwi® omnicup; Figure 12.23).

A meta-analysis of eight trials involving 1076 women compared soft (silicone, plastic, rubber) vacuum extractor cups to rigid (metal, plastic) showed that soft cups were more likely to fail in achieving vaginal delivery (OR 1.63; 95% CI 1.17–2.28).[41] However, there were fewer scalp injuries and cephalohaematomas with the soft cup and no differences between groups with regard to maternal injury.

Trials comparing conventional vacuum devices to the Kiwi Omnicup® showed a statistically significant higher failure rate with the Kiwi Omnicup® compared to conventional vacuum (30.1 versus 19.2% (RR 1.58; 95% CI 1.10–2.24)).[42] It was also associated with a greater number of cup detachments (mean 0.68 compared with 0.28, with 44% compared with 18% having at least one detachment; P < 0.0001). There was no difference in the incidence of severe maternal trauma, and there were no cases of serious neonatal injury. Therefore, most obstetricians will only use the elegant but expensive Kiwi Omnicup® device for the 'easier' procedures.

There is paucity of data to assess the benefits and risks of episiotomy in operative vaginal delivery. A large observational study demonstrated that mediolateral episiotomy (Figure 12.15) significantly protected against anal sphincter damage in both vacuum and forceps delivery.[42] Long-term maternal sequelae from operative delivery are primarily related to potential disturbances in urinary and anal function, such as urinary incontinence, faecal

Table 12.6 Advantages of forceps and vacuum delivery

Favours vacuum	Favours forceps
Less third and fourth degree tears (7.5% vs 14%)	Can be used before 34 weeks
Less vaginal wall lacerations (8% vs 26%)	Less cephalohaematoma (5% vs 9%)
Less severe postoperative pain (9 vs 15%)	Less retinal bleeding 5% vs 8%)
Easier to apply, less training required, less anaesthesia required	Less likely to fail (9% vs 14%)
Less facial injury (0.2% vs 1.7%)	Less maternal concern about the babies appearance (see above, cephalohaematoma)

Reproduced with permission from Goldberg J and Glazer AB, Operative vaginal delivery, pp. 116–119, In Berghella V (ed) *Obstetric evidence based guidelines*, Informa Healthcare, UK, Copyright © 2012.

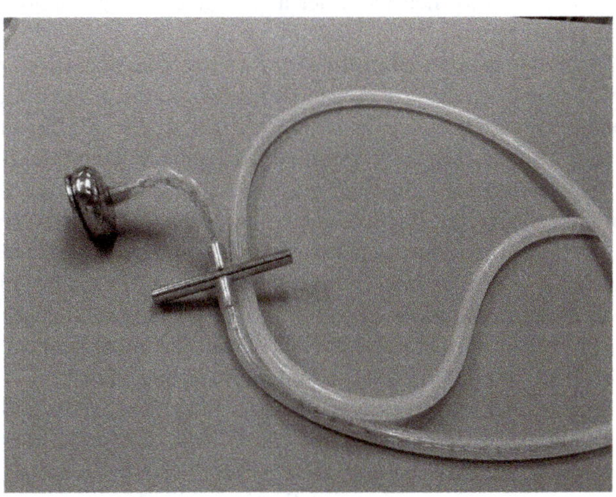

Figure 12.22 Ventouse.

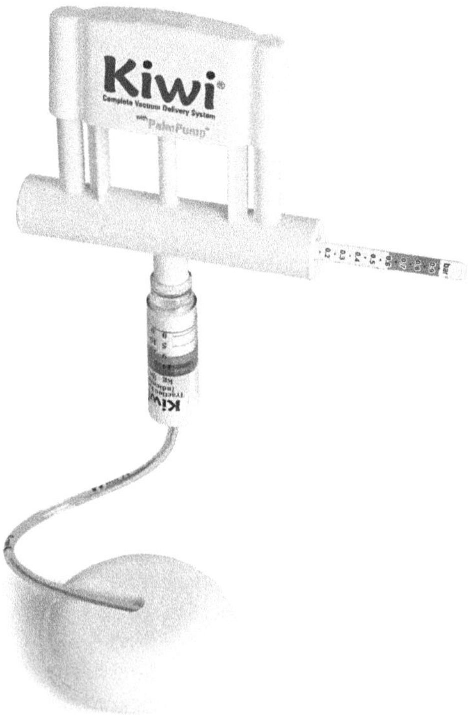

Figure 12.23 Kiwi Omnicup® device.
Courtesy of Clinical Innovations LLC.

incontinence, pelvic organ prolapse, and, occasionally, fistula formation.

If performed, vacuum application should begin with low suction and be slowly increased to 0.7–0.8 kg/cm^2. Traction should only be in the direct line of the vaginal canal and the cup should be positioned correctly to the fetal occiput, at the so-called flexion point. Ideally, vacuum application should not last longer than 5 minutes as the risk for cephalohaematomas increases with increasing duration of application of the vacuum.[42]

After delivery, the neonatal care provider should be informed that the birth was attempted or assisted by vacuum or forceps. Since a serious complication, such as a subgaleal haematoma, can occur within hours of delivery, it is important that the infant care providers be informed by either a reliable charting method or direct notification.

The short-term complications to the fetus from operative vaginal delivery are usually caused by head compression and traction on the fetal intracranial structures, face, and scalp. The most serious complication is intracranial haemorrhage. Virtually all of these complications can also occur in the course of a spontaneous vaginal delivery, but the incidence is lower than with instrumental delivery. The reported incidence of each complication varies widely and depends on a number of factors, such as the equipment used (metal, plastic, vacuum, forceps), fetal station, and the experience of the operator. Developmental outcome appears to be equivalent for both forceps- and vacuum-assisted births.[42]

Recently, next to forceps and vacuum, a new alternative instrument, the Odón device (Figure 12.24), was developed. It is a low-cost device that may be safer and easier to apply than forceps/vacuum extractor for assisted deliveries in developing countries but needs extensive clinical evaluation first.[43]

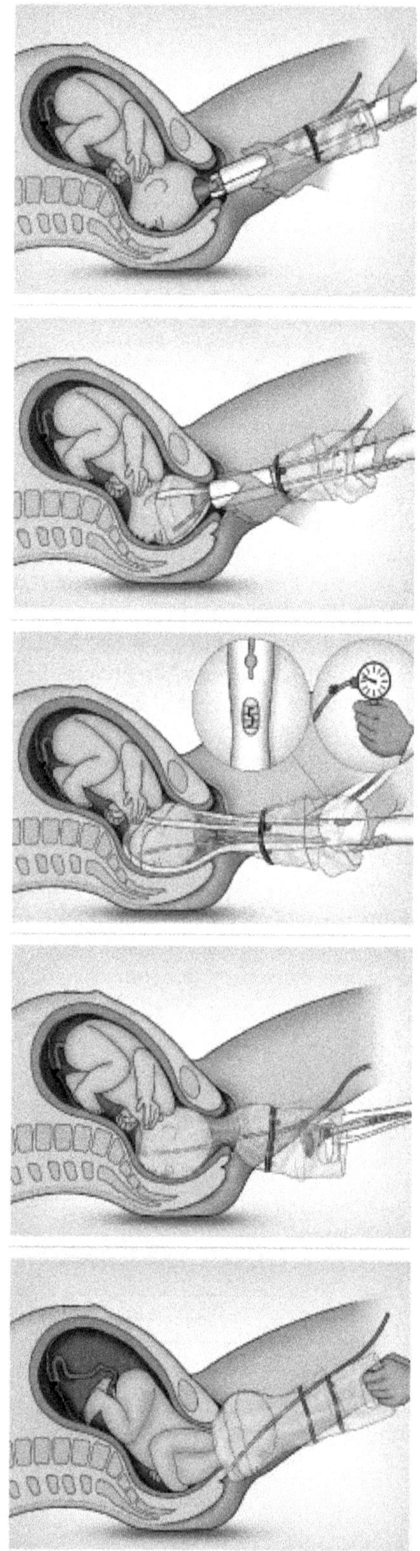

Figure 12.24 Odón device.
Adapted from World Health Organization Odon Device Research Group. Feasibility and safety study of a new device (Odón device) for assisted vaginal deliveries: study protocol. *Reproductive Health*, volume 10, issue 33. 2013.

Breech delivery

Breech presentation complicates 3–4% of all pregnancies at term (>37 weeks). The problem with vaginal breech delivery is that the head, usually the biggest part of the fetus, has to pass through the pelvis after the body has delivered. The term breech trial[44] has resulted in a change in practice in most countries, and it is now largely recommended that a breech baby is delivered by CD. It is also advised that women presenting with a fetus in breech at 36–37 weeks of gestation should be offered the opportunity to have their baby turned to cephalic near term (external cephalic version).[45] The management summary of breech presentation at term is presented in Box 12.3.

Despite this, vaginal breech deliveries will continue to occur, even in institutions with a policy of routine CDs for breech presentation, because of situations such as precipitous delivery, out-of-hospital delivery, severe fetal anomaly or fetal death, and mother's preference for vaginal birth. Therefore, it is essential for clinicians to maintain the skills of breech delivery. (For greater detail see Chapter 33.)

Delivery in twins

Twin pregnancies, either monochorionic or dichorionic, are at increased risk of intrapartum complications compared to singletons.[47] The most frequent problems encountered are FHR abnormalities and complications related to dystocia and malpresentation. The delivery of twins therefore requires properly trained staff and a multidisciplinary approach. Globally, the feeling is that twins should be delivered by CD if the presenting twin (twin I) does not have a cephalic presentation.[48] If twin I is cephalic, in the small majority of cases twin II will also be cephalic but the head will be obliquely placed. In other cases, twin II will be breech or transverse. Generally, twin II is the smaller of the twins. Chorionicity is another important determinant of the perinatal risks in twins and should also be taken into account in the decision process of how and when to deliver twins.[49] (See Chapter 33 for more details of the management of twins.)

Box 12.3 Management of breech presentation at term

- Offer and encourage external cephalic version (ECV) at term.
- There is no simple algorithm for predicting ECV success.
- Tocolysis with a betamimetic drug appears to increase ECV rates.
- If vaginal delivery of breech presentation is chosen, ensure involvement of adequate staff.
- Assisted breech delivery or Bracht manoeuvre may be equally effective.
- Ensure that drill for nuchal arm and entrapped head is in place.
- Maintain competencies through practice at caesarean delivery for breech and through regular manikin training.
- Audit uptake and success rates of ECV.

Adapted with permission from Kate Grady, Charlotte Howell and Charles Cox, *Managing Obstetric Emergencies and Trauma: The MOET Course Manual*, Second Edition, Cambridge University Press, Cambridge, UK, Copyright © 2007.

Caesarean delivery

A CD is a surgical operative procedure in which one or more incisions are made through the mother's abdomen (laparotomy) and uterus (hysterotomy) to deliver one or more babies, or to remove a dead fetus. The first modern CD was performed by German gynaecologist Ferdinand Adolf Kehrer in 1881.

Technique

A number of different techniques for CD have been described and compared to each other.

While most CDs are performed under neuraxial blockade, patients should be given a prophylactic histamine 2 receptor antagonist like ranitidine. In some units, oral sodium citrate is given as well. Prior to skin incision, antibiotic prophylaxis should routinely be administered in order to reduce the incidence of endometritis and wound infection (e.g. cefazolin 2 g IV).[50]

The skin incision can be transverse or vertical. In general, a transverse (e.g. Pfannenstiel or Joel–Cohen) incision of approximately 15 cm is preferred for CD. This type of incision results in less postoperative pain, greater wound strength, and better cosmetic results than a vertical incision. On the other hand, vertical incisions sometimes allow faster abdominal entry cause less bleeding and nerve injury, and can be more easily extended if more space is required for access in specific cases (fibroids, abnormal placentation, etc.).

Incision and dissection is performed using the scalpel for sharp dissection or electrocautery device in accordance with the surgeon's preference. The dissection of the subcutaneous tissue layer can be performed blunt (with fingers) of sharp (with knife, dissection scissors of electrocautery). Blunt dissection (Misgav–Ladach technique) is probably the method of choice as it has been associated with shorter operative times and decreased risk of vessel injury.[51]

For the opening of the fascial layer, a small transverse incision is usually made medially with and then extended laterally using blunt digital dissection or surgically using scissors. The rectus muscles are preserved and separated bluntly. Most authors favour using the fingers to bluntly open the peritoneum to minimize the risk of inadvertent injury to bowel, bladder, or other organs that may be adherent to the underlying surface. The abdominal incision should be adequate to allow atraumatic delivery of the fetus. The surgeon and the assistant can manually stretch apart the opening at the angles of the incisions if necessary. Also, sharp additional dissection may be necessary at this point. A routine bladder flap is not required, but some obstetricians choose to perform a bladder flap when a difficult delivery is anticipated (e.g. deeply engaged or large head). In these cases, creation of the bladder flap may help to keep the bladder dome out of the surgical field. In some patients, such as those who are not in labour, it may not be possible to make an incision in the lower uterine segment without first creating a bladder flap. Prior to opening the uterus (hysterotomy), the surgeon should determine the location of the placenta and the fetal lie. A correct estimation of the position can usually be obtained by palpating the uterus. If not, ultrasound (sterile probe) can be

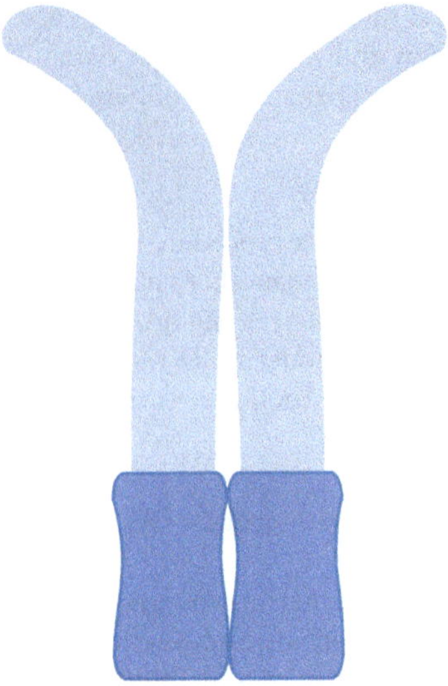

Figure 12.25 Uterus didelphys.

useful if it is important to avoid lacerating the placenta. The size of the hysterotomy should be large enough to allow atraumatic delivery of the fetus. A transverse lower uterine incision (i.e. Monroe–Kerr or Kerr incision) is generally performed but the type of incision (vertical or horizontal) may vary depending on the position and size of the fetus(es), the location of the placenta, presence of uterine anomalies (didelphys (Figure 12.25), myomata (Figure 12.26)), and the development of the lower uterine segment.

Compared with vertical incisions, transverse incisions result in less blood loss, less need for bladder dissection, easier approximation, and a lower risk of rupture in subsequent pregnancies.[52] If extension of the transverse incision is required, a 'J' or inverted 'T' extension is used as lateral extension is not possible without the risk of laceration of large blood vessels.

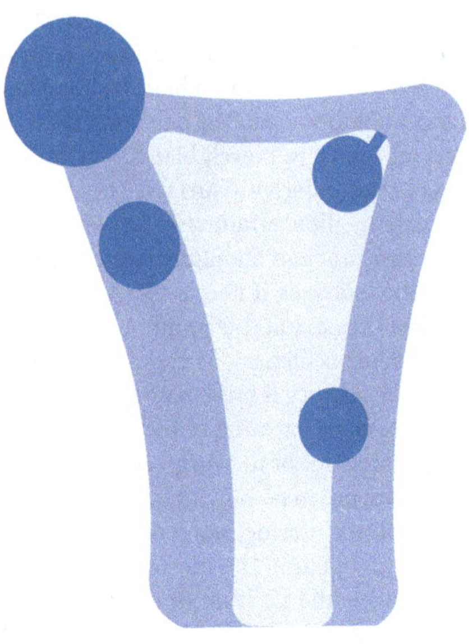

Figure 12.26 Example of a uterus myomatosus.

A 'classical' incision is a vertical incision that extends into the upper uterine segment/fundus. This type of incision is only rarely performed at or near term because it is associated with more maternal morbidity. In subsequent pregnancies, it is also associated with a higher risk of uterine dehiscence or rupture (4–9%) compared with low vertical (1–7%) and low transverse (0.2–1.5%).

The uterus is opened with a scalpel and care should be taken at that point not to injure the baby or the umbilical cord. Various techniques have been described to perform this safely. The uterine muscle is elevated and carefully thinned, separating the uterine tissue from the fetal membranes or skin. If possible, the fetal membranes are left intact until complete extension of the incision. Once the uterine cavity is entered, the hysterotomy incision can be extended using scissors or blunt expansion with the surgeon's fingers. The latter technique is faster, has less risk of inadvertent trauma to the fetus, and may reduce blood loss and extension of the incision. The use of absorbable staples is not advocated and should be restricted to specific situations (e.g. open fetal surgery and *ex utero* intrapartum treatment (EXIT) procedure).

As a result of impaired uteroplacental blood flow after incision of the uterus, the time lag between the uterine incision and the delivery of the baby influences the blood gases and Apgar scores of the baby and should be kept as short as possible. At the same time, the extraction should be atraumatic for both the mother and baby. Extraction of the baby at CD is usually uncomplicated, but may be made more difficult in cases of oligo- or anhydramnion, extreme prematurity, a deeply impacted or floating fetal head, or an abnormal lie (breech, transverse). For each of these situations, specific techniques have been described, that go beyond the scope of this chapter.

However, in certain circumstances to aid delivery, the obstetrician may request that the anaesthetist relax the uterus. This can be achieved by increasing the volatile agent if a general anaesthetic has been administered. Alternatively, sublingual glyceryl trinitrate two puffs or subcutaneous terbutaline 250 mcg can be given if the patient is awake.

Once the baby is born, the cord is clamped and the baby is handed to a paediatrician or appropriately trained clinician for initial evaluation and stabilization depending on the (expected) condition of the neonate. Especially in premature babies, delayed clamping of the cord could be beneficial.[53]

Once the baby is delivered, IV oxytocin is administered by the anaesthetist to promote uterine contraction. Different regimens have been proposed (Table 12.7), but in order to avoid maternal cardiovascular complications, a slow continuous rather than fast bolus is advocated (5 IU slow IV over 10 minutes).

Manual extraction of the placenta results in more maternal morbidity (bleeding, endometritis, and low haemoglobin) and should be avoided when possible. Instead, gentle cord traction together with massage of the uterus and the use of oxytocin to enhance the contractile expulsion should be used to deliver the placenta. The surgeon then inspects the placenta for abnormalities and completeness. Subsequently, the uterine cavity is explored to ensure that the entire placenta has been removed and no parts of placenta or membranes are left.

Recently, carbetocin (Pabal®) has become available. Its use after CD has been associated with lower need for additional uterotonics

Table 12.7 Proposed oxytocin regimens after caesarean delivery

Bolus	Infusion	Combination
5 IU slow IV/10 min	Initial dose: 80 IU in 500 mL Ringer's lactate over 30 min Subsequent dose: 20 IU in 1L Ringer's lactate at 125 mL/h	Oxytocin + ergometrine (0.5 mg) No significant reduction in blood loss Oxytocin + misoprostol (200–800 mcg rectal or sublingual). Reduces the need for additional uterotonics Oxytocin + tranexamic acid (10 mg/kg) given before caesarean delivery. Reduces the need for additional uterotonics and the amount of blood loss

but the higher costs and restricted availability have so far limited the use of this drug.[54]

Closure of the uterus can be performed with or without exteriorizing the uterus based on individual clinical circumstances and personal preference. However, communication between the obstetrician and anaesthetist is important before this manoeuvre is carried out as the peritoneal stretching during exteriorization can cause considerable discomfort if the CD is under epidural and the patient should be warned. Spinal anaesthesia is usually of sufficient density that the patient will not experience painful sensation.

For closure of the uterine incision, a single- or double-layer continuous closure can be opted for. The suture material used is often an absorbable synthetic monofilament (e.g. Monocryl®) or braided (e.g. Vicryl®) suture with sharp or blunt tip needles. The latter type of needle results in less glove perforation incidents, but reduced operative performance. Full thickness suturing, involving the endometrial layer results in less wedge-type healing defects 6 weeks postpartum and may be beneficial. There is significant debate on whether a single- or a double-layer closure of the uterine incision should be performed, and the literature contains conflicting evidence. Single-layer closure results in decreased operation time, but may be associated with increased risk for uterine dehiscence or rupture during a subsequent pregnancy. In a recent systematic review, a locked single-layer closure was associated with a significantly increased risk for uterine rupture compared to a double-layer closure (OR 4.96; 95% CI 2.58–9.52), but the authors of the review suggest that further study in a well-designed randomized trial is necessary on the risks of single-layer uterine closure, given the limitations of the studies in this meta-analysis.[55] There is good evidence for the benefit of non-closure of the visceral and parietal peritoneum (decreased operating time) without clear indications for increased risk for adhesion formation or any other associated complication.[56]

The technique of fascial closure is critical as this provides the majority of wound tensile strength during healing. Care should be taken to avoid too much tension as strangulation of the wound edges could result in more postoperative pain and reduced wound healing quality. For transverse fascial incisions, a continuous closure with slowly absorbable braided suture (e.g. #0 or #1 polyglactin 910) is a common approach among general surgeons and obstetricians also commonly use this technique.[57] The subcutaneous adipose layer is closed with interrupted delayed-absorbable sutures if the layer is 2 cm or more in thickness to avoid the formation of a wound seroma.[58]

Reapproximation of the skin edges may be performed with staples or subcuticular suture; available data from randomized trials do not allow a strong recommendation for one method over the other both in terms of cosmetic result as well as postoperative complications.[59]

Indications for caesarean delivery

While most CDS were performed traditionally for situations in which a vaginal delivery would jeopardize the health of the baby, the mother, or both, today, an increasing number of women are requesting a CD without medical indication. This 'caesarean on request' procedure is at the centre of a heated debate amongst health professionals and patients. As a result, CD rates have risen all over the world, both in developed as well as in developing countries. In China, a record level of 46% was recorded and many Asian, European, and Latin American countries report levels of 25% and above. In the United States, the rate has also increased significantly, from 21% in 1996 to 33% of all births in 2011. Also, in the United States the rate varied widely between hospitals in 2009 (range 6.9–69.9% of births). In Europe, there are significant differences between countries with the highest figures found in southern European countries: in Italy the CD rate is 40%, in Belgium, it is just below 20%, while in the Nordic countries it is around 15%. Strict guidelines for non-medically indicated CD before 39 weeks have been established[60] (NICE guidelines, ACOG guidelines, Roshan guidelines), as these procedures increase the risk for neonatal morbidity, especially respiratory adaptive problems.

Table 12.8 Factors affecting the probability of a successful VBAC

Decreased probability	Increased probability
Hispanic ethnicity, African American race	History of prior vaginal delivery
Increased maternal age	History of prior VBAC
Single marital status	Non-recurring indication for prior caesarean (malpresentation, non-reassuring fetal heart pattern, etc.)
<12 years of education	Greater cervical dilation/effacement at admission or rupture of membranes
Obesity (BMI ≥ 30 kg/m^2)	Spontaneous labour
Maternal disease (e.g. hypertension, diabetes)	
Delivery at a rural or private hospital	
Gestational age > 40 weeks	
Labour induction or augmentation	
Estimated fetal weight > 4000 g	

Data from Eden KB, McDonagh M, Denman MA, *et al.* New insights on vaginal birth after cesarean: can it be predicted? *Obstet Gynecol* 2010:116:967–981.

Table 12.9 Risk factors for uterine rupture in the context of VBAC

Risk factor	Incidence of uterine rupture	References
Labour induction (prostaglandins)	2.4%	Scott et al.[67]
Labour induction (oxytocin)	1.1%	Landon et al.[66]
Labour augmentation (oxytocin)	0.9%	Landon et al.[66]
Interval between deliveries < 18 months	2.25%	Ship et al.[68]
Maternal age > 30 years	–	
Fetal macrosomia	Relative risk 2.3 3.6% after 1 caesarean delivery with no prior vaginal delivery	Elkousy et al. 2003[69]
Single layer closure versus double layer closure	≥ 2-fold increase	Bujold et al.[70]
Fever at time of caesarean delivery	Increase Odds ratio 3.5%; 95% confidence interval 1.2–11.3	Ship et al.[71]
Prior uterine rupture (lower segment)	6%	Ritchie et al.[72]
Prior uterine rupture (upper segment)	32%	Ritchie et al.[72]
Induction > 40 weeks	3.2%	Bangdiwala et al.[62]

Data from various sources (see references).

Vaginal birth after caesarean delivery

A woman with a previous CD has two options for mode of delivery in the subsequent pregnancy: a planned CD or a trial of labour after caesarean in order to try to achieve a vaginal birth after caesarean (VBAC). A trial of labour appears to be a reasonable option for most women with a single prior low transverse CD with no other contraindications to vaginal delivery. Contraindications for trial of labour after caesarean include:[61]

- prior uterine rupture
- classical (vertical) uterine scar or complete (from endometrium to serosa) uterine scar from other surgery (myomectomy, interstitial pregnancy, etc.)
- Medical or obstetrical complication precluding vaginal birth
- inability to perform emergency CD
- multiple uterine scars.

VBAC success rates vary in the general population from 60% to 80%.[60] Obese (body mass index (BMI) > 30) women, women with more than one CD in history and women with macrosomic fetuses (>4000 g) have lower success rates.[62] Much research has been dedicated to the development of tools to predict the success rate for VBAC in an individual patient. Most screening tools are not sensitive enough to be clinically useful. One available for clinical use can be accessed freely at www.bsc.gwu.edu/mfmu/vagbirth.html and is based on a large multicentric cohort.[63] Factors affecting the probability of VBAC are listed in Table 12.8.[64]

Complications and safety of VBAC are especially related to the risk of uterine rupture. The overall risk of uterine rupture during trial of labour after CD at term is 0.7% after one previous low transverse CD versus 0.026% with a planned repeat CD.[65] This means that overall there are about five to six additional ruptures per 1000 women undergoing trial of labour after caesarean. The lowest risk is present when labour occurs spontaneously (0.4%). Induction of labour without prior history of vaginal birth, especially when using prostaglandins for cervical ripening, strongly increases the risk for uterine rupture.[66] Other factors associated with an increased risk for uterine rupture are listed in Table 12.9.[62,66–72]

Fetal loss occurs in about 6% of women with uterine rupture at term which translates to an overall risk of intrapartum fetal death rate of about 20/100.000 in women attempting VBAC.[62]

Conclusion

While the physical process of labour and subsequent delivery has largely remained unchanged over the last centuries, the circumstances and medical monitoring have evolved towards a safe environment for both mother and child.

The role of the anaesthesiologist in the birth process has become crucial not only in providing pain relief when requested or medically indicated, but also in contributing to the multidisciplinary team approach to rare, but potentially fatal obstetrical emergencies.

We hope this chapter helped to familiarize readers with the normal and dysfunctional birth and to enthuse anaesthetists, obstetricians, midwives, and other caregivers to further improve collaboration and qualitative care for the sake of mothers and children.

References

1. Cunningham FG, Levano KJ, Bloom S, *et al.* (eds). *Williams Obstetrics* (23rd ed). New York: McGraw-Hill Medical; 2009.
2. Lawrence A, Lewis L, Hofmeyr GJ, *et al.* Maternal positions and mobility during first stage labour. *Cochrane Database Syst Rev* 2013; 10:CD003934.
3. National Institute of Health and Care Excellence. *Intrapartum Care: Care of Healthy Women and Their Babies During Childbirth.* Clinical Guideline 190. London: NICE; 2014.
4. Bakker JJ, Janssen PF, van Halem K, *et al.* Internal versus external tocodynamometry during induced or augmented labour. *Cochrane Database Syst Rev* 2013; 8:CD006947.
5. Roberts CL, Torvaldsen S, Cameron CA, *et al.* Delayed versus early pushing in women with epidural analgesia: a systematic review and meta-analysis. *BJOG* 2004; 111(12):1333–40.
6. Hartmann K, Viswanathan M, Palmieri R, *et al.* Outcomes of routine episiotomy: a systematic review. *JAMA* 2005; 293(17):2141–8.
7. Mayerhofer K, Bodner-Adler B, Bodner K, *et al.* Traditional care of the perineum during birth. A prospective, randomized, multicenter study of 1,076 women. *J Reprod Med* 2002; 47(6):477–82.
8. Aasheim V, Nilsen AB, Lukasse M, *et al.* Perineal techniques during the second stage of labour for reducing perineal trauma. *Cochrane Database Syst Rev* 2011; 12:CD006672.
9. Begley CM, Gyte GM, Devane D, *et al.* Active versus expectant management for women in the third stage of labour. *Cochrane Database Syst Rev* 2011; 11:CD007412.
10. Boucher M, Nimrod CA, Tawagi GF, *et al.* Comparison of carbetocin and oxytocin for the prevention of postpartum hemorrhage following vaginal delivery: a double-blind randomized trial. *J Obstet Gynaecol Can* 2004; 26(5):481–8.

11. Su LL, Chong YS, Samuel M. Carbetocin for preventing postpartum haemorrhage. *Cochrane Database Syst Rev* 2012; 4:CD005457.
12. Tunçalpö, Hofmeyr GJ, Gülmezoglu AM. Prostaglandin for preventing postpartum haemorrhage. *Cochrane Database Syst Rev* 2012; 8:CD000494.
13. Elati A, Weeks A. Risk of fever after misoprostol for the prevention of postpartum hemorrhage: a meta-analysis. *Obstet Gynecol* 2012; 120(5):1140–8.
14. Rabe H, Diaz-Rossello JL, Duley L, *et al.* Effect of timing of umbilical cord clamping and other strategies to influence placental transfusion at preterm birth on maternal and infant outcomes. *Cochrane Database Syst Rev* 2012; 8:CD003248.
15. Committee on Obstetric Practice, American College of Obstetricians and Gynecologists. Committee Opinion No. 543: Timing of umbilical cord clamping after birth. *Obstet Gynecol* 2012; 120:1522–6.
16. Henly SJ, Anderson CM, Avery MD, *et al.* Anemia and insufficient milk in first-time mothers. *Birth* 1995; 22(2):86–92.
17. Confidential Enquiries into Maternal and Child Health. Saving Mothers' Lives Reviewing maternal deaths to make motherhood safer: 2006–2008. *BJOG* 2011; 118 Suppl 1:1–203.
18. van Beekhuizen HJ, de Groot AN, De Boo T, *et al.* Sulprostone reduces the need for the manual removal of the placenta in patients with retained placenta: a randomized controlled trial. *Am J Obstet Gynecol* 2006; 194(2):446–50.
19. Güngördük K, Asicioglu O, Besimoglu B, *et al.* Using intraumbilical vein injection of oxytocin in routine practice with active management of the third stage of labor: a randomized controlled trial. *Obstet Gynecol* 2010; 116(3):619–24.
20. Mori R, Nardin JM, Yamamoto N, *et al.* Umbilical vein injection for the routine management of third stage of labour (review). *Cochrane Database Syst Rev* 2012; 3:CD006176
21. Poole JH. Neuraxial analgesia for labor and birth: implications for mother and fetus. *J Perinat Neonatal Nurs* 2003; 17(4):252–67.
22. Lee HJ, Macbeth AH, Pagani JH, *et al.* Oxytocin: the great facilitator of life. *Prog Neurobiol* 2009; 88(2):127–51.
23. Gagnon-Gervais K, Bujold E, Iglesias MH, *et al.* Early versus late amniotomy for labour induction: a randomized controlled trial. *J Matern Fetal Neonatal Med* 2012; 25(11):2326–9.
24. Hayes EJ, Weinstein L. Improving patient safety and uniformity of care by a standardized regimen for the use of oxytocin. *Am J Obstet Gynecol* 2008; 198(6):622.e1–7.
25. American College of Obstetricians and Gynecologists. ACOG Practice Bulletin No. 107: Induction of labor. *Obstet Gynecol* 2009; 114(2 Pt 1):386–97.
26. National Collaborating Centre for Women's and Children's Health/ National Institute for Health and Clinical Excellence (NCCWCH/ NICE). *Induction of Labour.* London: NICE.
27. Hofmeyr GJ, Gülmezoglu AM, Pileggi C. Vaginal misoprostol for cervical ripening and induction of labour. *Cochrane Database Syst Rev* 2010; 10:CD000941.
28. Royal College of Obstetricians and Gynaecologists. *Fetal Monitoring in Labour.* London: Royal College of Obstetricians and Gynaecologists; 2001.
29. Salmelin A, Wiklund I, Bottinga R, *et al.* Fetal monitoring with computerized ST analysis during labor: a systematic review and meta-analysis. *Acta Obstet Gynecol Scand* 2013; 92(1):28–39.
30. American College of Obstetricians and Gynecologists. ACOG practice bulletin clinical management guidelines for obstetrician-gynecologists. Number 40, November 2002. *Obstet Gynecol* 2002; 100(5 Pt 1):1045–50.
31. Nesbitt TS, Gilbert WM, Herrchen B. Shoulder dystocia and associated risk factors with macrosomic infants born in California. *Am J Obstet Gynecol* 1998; 179(2):476–80.
32. Gherman RB, Tramont J, Muffley P, Goodwin TM. Analysis of McRoberts' maneuver by x-ray pelvimetry. *Obstet Gynecol* 2000; 95(1):43–7.
33. Jacquemyn Y. *Procedureboek Verloskunde. Praktische richtlijnen bij verloskundige problemen.* Leuven: Acco; 2007.
34. McFarland MB, Langer O, Piper JM, *et al.* Perinatal outcome and the type and number of maneuvers in shoulder dystocia. *Int J Gynecol Obstet* 1996; 55:219–24.
35. Blackwell SC. Shoulder dystocia. In Berghella V (ed) *Obstetric Evidence Based Guidelines.* London: Informa Healthcare; 2012:216–23.
36. Sandberg EC. The Zavanelli maneuver: 12 years of recorded experience. *Obstet Gynecol* 1999; 93:312–17.
37. Del Portal DA, Horn AE, Vilke GM, *et al.* Emergency department management of shoulder dystocia. *J Emerg Med* 2014; 46(3):378–82.
38. O'Shaughnessy MJ. Hysterotomy facilitation of the vaginal delivery of the posterior arm in a case of severe shoulder dystocia. *Obstet Gynecol* 1998; 92(4 Pt 2):693–5.
39. American College of Obstetricians and Gynecologists. ACOG Practice bulletin operative vaginal delivery. ACOG Practice Bulletin No. 17: Operative vaginal delivery *Obstet Gynecol* 2000; 95(6):998–1005.
40. Molina FS, Nicolaides KH. Ultrasound in labor and delivery. *Fetal Diagn Ther* 2010; 27(2):61–7.
41. Goldberg J, Glazer AB. Operative vaginal delivery. In Berghella V (ed) *Obstetric Evidence Based Guidelines.* London: Informa Healthcare; 2012:116–19.
42. Groom KM, Jones BA, Miller N, *et al.* A prospective randomised controlled trial of the Kiwi Omnicup versus conventional ventouse cups for vacuum-assisted vaginal delivery. *BJOG* 2006; 113(2):183–9.
43. World Health Organization Odon Device Research Group. Feasibility and safety study of a new device (Odón device) for assisted vaginal deliveries: study protocol. *Reprod Health* 2013; 10:33.
44. Hannah ME, Hannah WJ, Hewson SA, *et al.* Planned caesarean section versus planned vaginal birth for breech presentation at term: a randomized multicenter trial. Term Breech Trial Collaborative Group. *Lancet* 2000; 356(9239):1375–83.
45. Hofmeyr GJ, Kulier R. External cephalic version for breech presentation at term. *Cochrane Database Syst Rev* 2012; 10:CD000083.
46. Grady K, Howell C, Cox C. *Managing Obstetric Emergencies and Trauma: The MOET Course Manuel* (2nd ed). London: Royal College of Obstetricians and Gynaecologists; 2007
47. Chauhan SP, Scardo JA, Hayes E, *et al.* Twins: prevalence, problems, and preterm births. *Am J Obstet Gynecol* 2010; 203(4):305–15.
48. Rossi AC, Mullin PM, Chmait RH. Neonatal outcomes of twins according to birth order, presentation and mode of delivery: a systematic review and meta-analysis. *BJOG* 2011; 118(5):523–32.
49. Lewi L, Gucciardo L, Van Mieghem T, *et al.* Monochorionic diamniotic twin pregnancies: natural history and risk stratification. *Fetal Diagn Ther* 2010; 27(3):121–33.
50. Smaill FM, Gyte GM. Antibiotic prophylaxis versus no prophylaxis for preventing infection after cesarean section. *Cochrane Database Syst Rev* 2010; 1:CD007482.
51. Holmgren G, Sjöholm L, Stark M. The Misgav Ladach method for cesarean section: method description. *Acta Obstet Gynecol Scand* 1999; 78(7):615–21.
52. Dahlke JD, Mendez-Figueroa H, Rouse DJ, *et al.* Evidence-based surgery for cesarean delivery: an updated systematic review. *Am J Obstet Gynecol* 2013; 209(4):294–306.
53. Menget A, Mougey C, Thiriez G, *et al.* Advantage of delayed umbilical cord clamping in newborn infant. *Arch Pediatr* 2013; 20(9):1022–7.
54. Holleboom CA, van Eyck J, Koenen SV, *et al.* Carbetocin in comparison with oxytocin in several dosing regimens for the prevention of uterine atony after elective caesarean section in the Netherlands. *Arch Gynecol Obstet* 2013; 287(6):1111–17.
55. Roberge S, Chaillet N, Boutin A, *et al.* Single- versus double-layer closure of the hysterotomy incision during cesarean delivery and risk of uterine rupture. *Int J Gynaecol Obstet* 2011; 115(1):5–10.
56. Bamigboye AA, Hofmeyr GJ. Closure versus non-closure of the peritoneum at caesarean section. *Cochrane Database Syst Rev* 2003; 4:CD000163.
57. Rahbari NN, Knebel P, Diener MK, *et al.* Current practive of abdominal wall closure in elective surgery—is there any consensus? *BMC Surg* 2009; 9:8

58. Chelmow D, Rodriguez EJ, Sabatini MM. Suture closure of subcutaneous fat and wound disruption after cesarean delivery: a meta-analysis. *Obstet Gynecol* 2004; 103(5 Pt 1):974–80.
59. Mackeen AD, Berghella V, Larsen ML. Techniques and materials for skin closure in caesarean section. *Cochrane Database Syst Rev* 2012; 9:CD003577.
60. American College of Obstetricians and Gynecologists. ACOG Committee Opinion No. 559: Cesarean delivery on maternal request. *Obstet Gynecol* 2013; 121(4):904–7.
61. Signore C. VBAC: What does the evidence show? *Clin Obstet Gynaecol* 2012; 55(4):961–8.
62. Bangdiwala SI, Brown SS, Cunningham FG. NIH consensus development conference draft statement on vaginal birth after cesarean: new insights. *NIH Consensus Statement Sci Statements* 2010; 27(3):1–42.
63. Grobman WA, Lai Y, Landon MB, *et al.* Development of a nomogram for prediction of vaginal birth after cesarean delivery. *Obstet Gynecol* 2007; 109(4):806–12.
64. Eden KB, McDonagh M, Denman MA, *et al.* New insights on vaginal birth after cesarean: can it be predicted? *Obstet Gynecol* 2010; 116:967–81.
65. Guise JM, Denman MA, Emeis C, *et al.* Vaginal birth after cesarean: new insights on maternal and neonatal outcomes. *Obstet Gynecol* 2010; 115:1267–78.
66. Landon MB, Hauth JC, Leveno KJ, *et al.* Maternal and perinatal outcomes associated with a trial of labor after prior cesarean delivery. *N Engl J Med* 2004; 351(25):2581–9.
67. Scott J. Intrapartum management of trial of labour after caesarean delivery: evidence and experience. *BJOG* 2014; 121(2):157–62.
68. Ship TD, Zelop CM, Repke JT, *et al.* Interdelivery interval and risk of symptomatic uterine rupture. *Obstet Gynecol* 2001; 97(2):175–7.
69. Elkousy MA, Sammel M, Stevens E, *et al.* The effect of birth weight on vaginal birth after cesarean delivery success rates. *Am J Obstet Gynecol* 2003; 188(3):824–30.
70. Bujold E, Goyet M, Marcoux S, *et al.* The role of uterine closure in the risk of uterine rupture. *Obstet Gynecol* 2010; E116(1):43–50.
71. Ship TD, Zelop C, Cohen A, *et al.* Post-cesarean delivery fever and uterine rupture in a subsequent trial of labour. *Obstet Gynecol* 2003; 101(1):136–9.
72. Ritchie EH. Pregnancy after rupture of the pregnant uterus. A report of 36 pregnancies and a study of cases reported since 1932. *J Obstet Gynaecol Br Commonw* 1971; 78:642–8.

CHAPTER 13

Non-pharmacological methods of pain relief and systemic analgesia in labour

Grace McClune and David Hill

Introduction

Pain in labour is a nearly universal experience for childbearing women; for many it is the most severe pain they will feel during their lifetime.[1] The management of labour pain, however severe, is one of the major goals of intrapartum care. The experience of labour pain is complex and individual. Women's desires for and expectations of pain relief during labour and delivery differ widely. Fortunately there are many options, both pharmacological and non-pharmacological, for the modification and relief of this pain. Epidural analgesia remains the most effective method of pain control and is a popular choice for many women, but it is not a universal solution.[2] Many women wish to avoid the risks of this invasive procedure and opt for other pharmacological solutions to reduce pain. Others prefer to completely avoid the pharmacological approach if possible, instead opting for complementary approaches to the reduction of pain and suffering. Their choice may be influenced by many factors including availability, possible side effects on themselves, their baby, or both, and the potential influence their chosen mode of pain relief may have on the birth process itself.[3]

A 2008 systematic review of women's expectations and experiences of pain relief in labour demonstrated that women were inadequately prepared for the reality of labour pain. They were therefore unable to make informed choices about pain relief. Women need to be informed antenatally about the options for pain relief in labour and the risks and benefits of the choices available.[4]

As part of the delivery suite team, anaesthetists should appreciate the need for labour analgesia and the merits and drawbacks of the varying options. This chapter will discuss the physiology behind labour pain, the history of analgesia in labour, the current non-pharmacological methods of pain relief available, and the use of systemic analgesia in labour.

Pain in labour

The International Association for the Study of Pain describes pain as 'an unpleasant sensory and emotional experience associated with actual or potential tissue damage, or described in terms of such damage'.[5] The ability of the body to detect potentially tissue-damaging stimuli is an important protective mechanism that involves multiple interacting peripheral and central mechanisms. However, unlike other acute and chronic pain experiences, labour pain is not in most cases associated with pathology, but with the birth of a baby, one of the most basic and fundamental of life's experiences.[6]

Historically, pain was considered by the medical profession to be an inevitable response to tissue damage. No consideration was given to the roles of emotion, past experience, anxiety, or expectation. It would be a mistake to view pain simply as a sensory message of peripheral tissue trauma, coded in peripheral nerves, transmitted in central neural pathways, and decoded in the brain. If this were the only view taken then the management of pain in labour would concentrate on eradication of pain sensation through pharmacological means as the only relevant technique. Methods of decreasing the affective component of pain or of decreasing but not eliminating the sensory component may be dismissed as ineffective if a purely neurophysiological model is adopted.[7]

The gate control theory of pain, first proposed in 1965, suggested that the transmission of pain signals from peripheral nerves through the spinal cord is regulated by other peripheral nerves and by interneurons in the spinal cord and central supraspinal centres. Local processes within the spinal cord either 'open the gate', and allow for transmission to higher centres, or 'close the gate', preventing transmission of the signal. This emphasis on central neural mechanisms forced the medical and biological science worlds to accept the brain and spinal cord as active systems that filter, select, and modulate inputs. This hypothesis has been revised and expanded since its inception; the current theory describes pain as a neuromatrix that integrates multiple sensory and cognitive inputs to produce an output that is recognizable as the sensation of pain. This neuromatrix includes somatosensory, thalamocortical, and neurohumoral components that interact with the emotional and cognitive components of the limbic system and higher cortical centres (Figure 13.1).[8–10]

Peripheral pain pathways in labour

The detection of noxious stimuli requires activation of peripheral nociceptors and signal transduction into action potentials for conduction to the central nervous system. Nociceptive afferents are widely distributed throughout the body and comprise

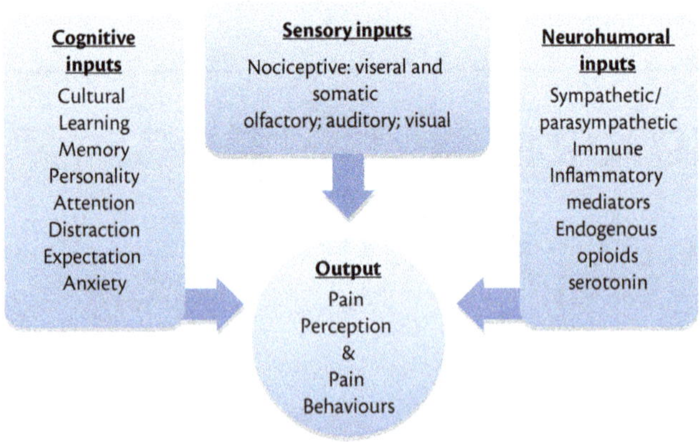

Figure 13.1 Schematic representation of pain neuromatrix.

Data from Melzack R. From the gate to the neuromatrix, *Pain*, 1999; 6:S121–S126, Copyright © 1999 Elsevier.

both medium-diameter, lightly myelinated A-delta fibres and small-diameter, slow-conducting, unmyelinated C fibres. Polymodal C-fibre nociceptors, which respond to a broad range of physical and chemical stimuli, are responsible for the majority of labour pain.[11]

Pain originates from different sites as the process of labour progresses (Table 13.1). This process can be divided into three stages: the first stage from the onset of cervical change until 10 cm or full dilatation; the second stage from full cervical dilatation until delivery of the baby; and the third stage from delivery of the baby to expulsion of the placenta and membranes. Pain in the first and second stages is considered below.

Table 13.1 Peripheral pathways and mechanisms of labour pain

Site of stimulus	Mechanism of stimulus	Peripheral pathway	Site of pain sensation
Uterus	Pressure, distension, and ischaemia leading to release of inflammatory mediators	Visceral afferent fibres accompanying sympathetic nerves to dorsal rami of T10–L1	Abdomen (upper, mid, and lower) Groin Lower back
Cervix	Pressure, dilatation, tearing of tissues, and release of inflammatory mediators	Visceral afferent fibres accompanying sympathetic fibres to dorsal rami of T10–L1	Groin Lower back
Lumbosacral region	Pressure (fetal malposition)	Lumbosacral plexus L5–S1	Lower back Thigh
Bladder	Pressure	Visceral afferent fibres accompanying sympathetic fibres to dorsal rami of T10–L1	Suprapubic
Vagina	Distension and tearing of tissues	Somatic afferent fibres accompanying parasympathetic nerves to dorsal rami of S2–4	Vagina
Perineum	Pressure and tearing of tissues	Pudendal nerve (S2–4)	Perineum

First stage of labour

Pain in labour begins with diffuse, poorly localized, cramping visceral sensations. The pressure generated during contractions of the uterus and in stretching of the cervix stimulates high-threshold mechanoreceptors.[12] At the same time, uterine chemoreceptors are activated by the release of bradykinin, histamine, serotonin, acetylcholine, and potassium ions from uterine myocytes due to ischaemia of the tissues during contractions, and to aid cervical ripening and dilatation.[13] Following stimulation of these mechano- and chemoreceptors, the pain signal is transmitted through A-delta and C primary afferent nerve fibres from the uterus to the spinal cord. These fibres accompany sympathetic nerves through the inferior and superior hypogastric plexus, and the lumbar and lower thoracic sympathetic chains; they end in communication with the dorsal rami of T10–L1 (Figure 13.2).[14]

Similar to other types of visceral pain, labour pain may be referred to the abdominal wall, lumbosacral region, iliac crests, gluteal areas, and thighs.[12] Many women experience contraction-related low back pain, for some this becomes continuous between contractions. Some women experience very widespread and diffuse pain sensations, whereas others may feel very localized pain in specific, well-defined areas.[6]

Second stage of labour

Towards the end of the first stage of labour and during the second stage of labour, distension and traction on the pelvic structures, the pelvic floor, and the perineum results in predominately somatic pain. These stimuli are carried via mostly A-delta fibres passing in the parasympathetic bundle of the pudendal nerve to the dorsal rami of S2–4 and result in sharp well-localized pain.[15] In addition, the parturient experiences rectal pressure and an urge to 'bear down' as the presenting part of the fetus descends into the pelvic outlet (Figure 13.2).[16]

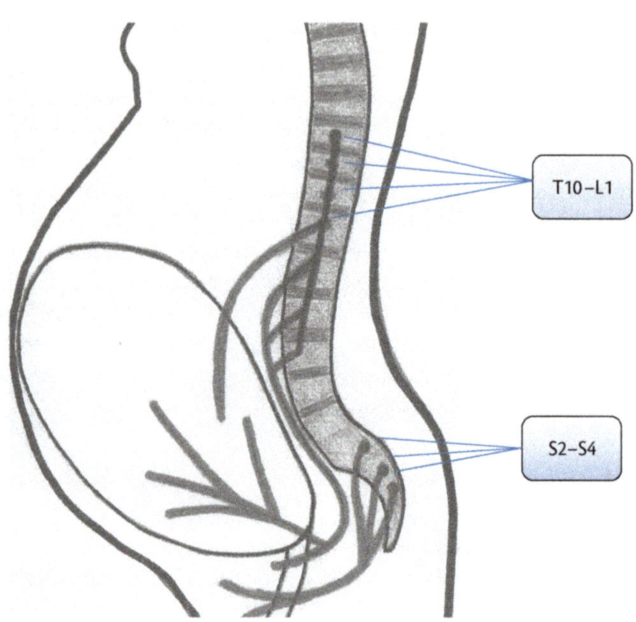

Figure 13.2 Peripheral pain pathways in labour.

Sensitization

The increasing intensity of pain commonly observed in labour may be partially attributable to a lowered activation threshold in the mechanoreceptors, and to chemoreceptor stimulation produced by the repeated uterine contractions. This process of sensitization of peripheral nociceptors occurs by way of the inflammatory products released from uterine myocytes during labour and in the process of cervical dilatation. These substances (prostaglandins, cytokines, and growth factors) result in a change in dorsal root ganglion cell numbers, peptide expression and release, receptor, and ion channel expression. For example, inflammatory mediators alter the expression of sodium channels subtypes resulting in more rapid, repetitive firing capabilities and spontaneous afferent activity.[8]

Central pain pathways in labour

Labour pain transmission includes both the ascending and descending pathways of the central nervous system (Figure 13.3).

Ascending pathways

Primary afferent terminals in the spinal cord contain excitatory amino acids, peptides, and neurotrophic factors, which act as neurotransmitters and are released by different intensity stimuli.[17] Most of the primary afferent neurons synapse initially in the substantia gelatinosa (the superficial laminae I and II) of the dorsal horn in the spinal cord. Locally projecting interneurons then synapse with the deeper wide dynamic range neurons of lamina V. Secondary neurons whose cell bodies lie in the dorsal grey matter of the spinal cord transmit the stimuli via the spinothalamic tract to the thalamus. There another synapse occurs before transmission reaches the brainstem and cerebellum, where spatial and temporal analysis occurs, and the hypothalamic and limbic systems, where emotional and autonomic responses originate.[18]

Descending pathways

At the level of the dorsal horn, motor and sympathetic reflex activity is stimulated. Modulation of nociceptive impulse transmission may occur through several complex inhibitory systems activated at many levels of the central nervous system. Inhibitory modulation within the dorsal horn and can be mediated by non-nociceptive peripheral inputs, local inhibitory interneurons, descending bulbospinal tracts, and higher-order brain functions.[6,11]

Psychological and environmental factors

Psychological factors that influence the experience of pain include attention, memory, or learning, thought processing, beliefs, mood, behavioural responses, and interactions with the environment. In comparison to the non-pregnant state there are a number of factors that can influence the perception of pain in pregnancy. Fear may be intense, particularly in nulliparous women, or in those with a previous bad experience. Generalized anxiety related to the pregnancy, its outcome, or its implications for the woman may enhance her perception of pain. Poor knowledge and/or misinformation may exacerbate this situation. Certain cultures are more emotive and expressive than other, more stoic ones, leading possibly to differences in pain behaviours rather than in the extent of pain felt.[19] Fatigue and general debility, common in late pregnancy, may also contribute to the experience of labour pain. Positive attitudes to pregnancy on the other hand, may increase tolerance to pain, with labour pain being seen as a positive force rather than a destructive one. For example, younger women have a physiological advantage in their tolerance to pain, but older or multiparous women may be more relaxed and less fearful, leading them to tolerate pain better.[11]

In summary, pain is a highly abstract and subjective experience, not simply the transmission of stimuli from nociceptors. Noxious or nociceptive stimuli are centrally received and interpreted through the interaction of a wide variety of emotional,

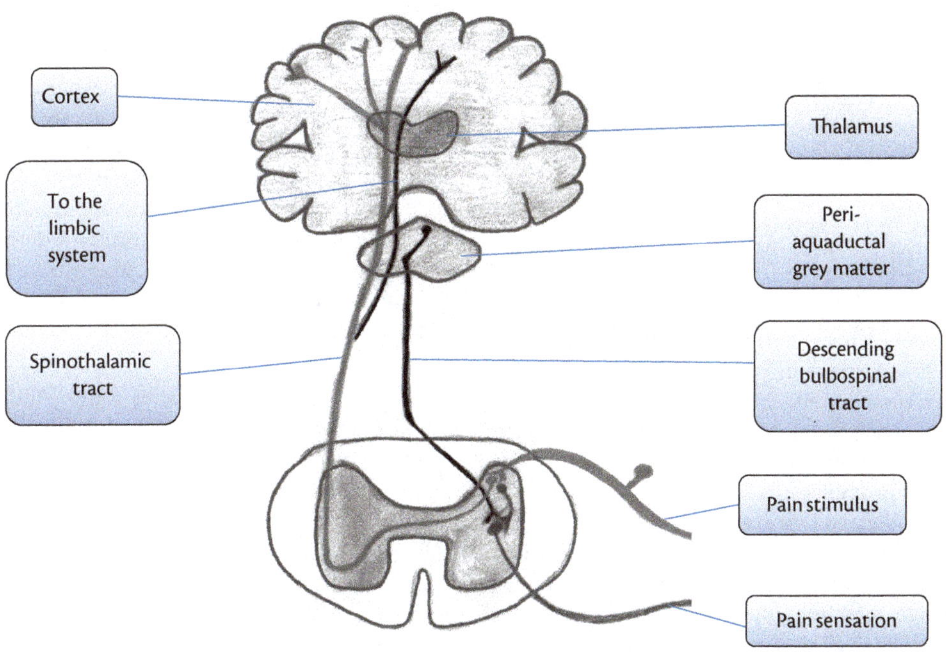

Figure 13.3 Central pain pathways in labour.

motivational, social, cultural, and cognitive variables unique to the individual. It is this intensely personal interpretation of noxious sensory stimuli transmitted during labour that determines a woman's private experience of pain.[6,12]

Adverse consequences of labour pain

Pain is undesirable due to its unpleasant physical sensations and emotional effects but also because of a variety of potential adverse physiological and psychological consequences.

Hyperventilation

Hyperventilation in labour is common and can lead to hypocapnia and respiratory alkalosis. Profound hypocapnia may inhibit ventilatory drive between contractions leading to hypoxia, dizziness, and loss of consciousness. Maternal alkalosis decreases placental blood flow due to uteroplacental vasoconstriction and impairs the transfer of oxygen to the fetal circulation due to an increased affinity for oxygen by maternal haemoglobin and therefore decreased off-loading to the fetus (a shift in the oxygen dissociation curve to the left).[16,20]

Hypertension

Increases in cardiac output and blood pressure via sympathetic activity and increased venous return associated with uterine contractions may cause hypertension, which can be problematic in cardiac disease and pre-eclampsia.[11]

Catecholamine release

The neuroendocrine responses to pain and stress (increased maternal catecholamine secretion) can cause vasoconstriction and reduced placental perfusion; reduced fetal oxygenation; fetal acidosis; and fetal bradycardia.[16]

Delayed gastric emptying

The effect of labour on gastric emptying and acidity is unclear; delayed emptying and increased acid secretion have been suggested.[11]

Psychological

Severe labour pain has been implicated in contributing to long-term emotional stress, with potential adverse consequences on maternal mental health and family relationships. Women who experience unrelieved pain during labour may be more likely to develop postpartum depression and it is a recognized risk factor for post-traumatic stress disorder.[21,22]

Non-pharmacological methods of pain relief in labour

There are a wide variety of non-pharmacological approaches to the relief of pain in labour, many of which are taught to women and their birthing partners at antenatal classes. Some methods reduce pain while others help women cope better with their pain by enhancing the psycho-emotional and spiritual components of care. Any technique that promotes mental and physical relaxation will decrease anxiety and catecholamine levels, and should promote increased uterine perfusion, more efficient and less painful uterine contractions, and less fetal distress. Some techniques are simple and can be performed by midwives or birthing partners with little training, others such as acupuncture require specialized accreditation and therefore have larger cost implications.

Table 13.2 Non-pharmacological methods of pain relief in labour

Reduction of painful stimuli	Activation peripheral sensory receptors	Enhancement of descending inhibitory neural pathways
Movement and positioning	Temperature modulation	Childbirth education
Counter-pressure	Hydrotherapy	Attention focusing and distraction
	Massage and reflexology	Relaxation, music, and audioanalgesia
	Acupuncture and acupressure	Hypnosis
	TENS	Biofeedback
	Sterile water injections	
	Aromatherapy	

Non-pharmacological forms of pain relief can be classified as techniques that reduce painful stimuli, techniques that activate peripheral sensory receptors, and techniques that enhance descending inhibitory neural pathways (Table 13.2).[23] In most cases, there are few randomized control trials supporting the use of these techniques but maternal satisfaction is often high with almost half of women reporting the use of complementary therapies in labour.[24]

The reduction of painful stimuli

Completely avoiding the painful stimuli that arise from uterine contractions or from pressure on maternal tissues by the fetus is not feasible without pharmacological intervention but techniques to reduce the extent of this stimulation do exist. This is the purpose of practices such as variations in maternal positioning, movement, and counter-pressure.

Maternal movement and positioning

Labouring women find that they experience less pain in some positions than in others and consequently walk, move, and change positions spontaneously to make themselves more comfortable.[25] Pelvic dimensions vary with differences in maternal position and these changes may help to reduce labour pain. For example, pressure of the fetal head on the sacroiliac joint may be relieved if the parturient moves from a lying down position to being on her hands and knees. Changes in position may also help to accelerate labour by increasing pelvic diameter and facilitating the rotation and engagement of the fetal head.[26] The 'birth ball' is a large inflated exercise ball that has been adopted by many maternity units to aid movement of women in labour and help relaxation. The ball expands the number of positions women can use and offers support for movement, for example, bouncing during contractions.

Efficacy

Most trials of movement and positioning during the first stage of labour have compared various upright positions with horizontal positions for their effects on pain and labour progress. Women consistently find sitting or standing positions more comfortable than being supine, though they do favour lying on one side with advanced labour.[27] Studies have also shown reduced pain scores in labour and at delivery in women who use birthing balls.[28,28] Despite anecdotal evidence, there is no trial confirmation that walking produces shorter labours.[30] A 2012 systematic review evaluated the routine use of the supine position during the second stage of labour to other positions and found that women experienced more severe pain in the supine position and had a preference for other birthing positions.[31]

Limitations

Many labouring women are restricted to bed due to the need for fetal heart rate monitoring or intravenous (IV) fluid and drug administration. In addition, midwives often need to suggest specific positions to accelerate labour or correct fetal or maternal problems (e.g. fetal heart rate decelerations or maternal hypotension). A survey in 2005 found that more than 75% of women did not walk around while in labour. Aside from those who were receiving pharmacological analgesia restricting them to bed, the most common reason women gave for not walking was: being 'connected to things' (e.g. fetal heart rate monitor), or being 'told not to walk around'. However, 60% of the women did report changing positions while in bed to relieve pain during labour.[32]

Implications for practice

Evidence suggests that in the first stage of labour the use of upright positions, interspersed with other positions, is associated with less painful labour; one popular option for achieving this is the use of birthing balls. Where possible, delivery in a position other than supine produces less discomfort.

Counter-pressure

Counter-pressure consists of a steady strong pressure applied to the lower back or each side of the hips during contractions. This appears to alleviate back pain in some women particularly when pain is related to an occiput posterior position. There are currently no trials evaluating the effectiveness of this technique.

Activation of peripheral sensory receptors

The transmission of pain from the uterus, cervix, and pelvic joints is potentially inhibited by the stimulation of large, afferent sensory nerve fibres, which carry impulses towards the central nervous system, and by the release of endorphins and encephalins, which mediate the experience of pain. There are a number of complementary therapies that utilize this process.

Temperature modulation

Hot packs to the abdomen, back, or perineum or a warm blanket over the entire body in the second stage of labour have the potential to relieve the burning sensation of pain. Hot baths or showers produce a number of beneficial effects including relaxation and increased well-being. A reduction in pain perception occurs as a result of the stimulation of tactile and thermal receptors by warm water.[23] For some women, the use of extreme cold may be similarly useful in decreasing pain perception.

Implications for practice

The effects of temperature modulation have not been evaluated in controlled trials but observational evidence suggests that these techniques are effective. Provided care is taken not to cause burns to the skin, this practice is simple, inexpensive, and safe.[33]

Hydrotherapy

Women labour in warm water for mental and physical relaxation and pain relief. Immersion takes place in a pool, tub, or bath, which is larger than a normal domestic bath, and may be use for one or more stages of labour, and for any duration.

Maternal effects

There are many proposed advantage to hydrotherapy in labour. The buoyancy of water enables women to move more easily. The warmth of the water may induce muscle relaxation and reduce anxiety, decreasing release of catecholamines and stimulating the release of endorphins. Water immersion is associated with improved uterine perfusion, less painful contractions, and potentially a shorter labour with fewer interventions.[34–36] Hydrotherapy also has marked physiological effects on the cardiovascular system; shoulder-deep warm water immersion reduces blood pressure due to vasodilatation of the peripheral vessels and redistribution of blood flow.[37] Immersion during labour also increases maternal satisfaction and sense of control. Subsequently, if the mother is not fearful, oxytocin release is optimized, stimulating effective contractions. In addition, the ease of mobility that water immersion offers may optimize fetal position.[38]

A number of potential maternal adverse effects of water immersion during labour have, however, also been proposed. There is the possibility that it may promote unrealistic expectations about labour, restrict choice of analgesia, reduce contraction effectiveness, and increase perineal trauma, an increased risk to the mother of infection caused by water entering the uterus. Potentiation of bleeding after delivery of the placenta and an increase in the incidence of manual removal of the placenta is also a concern. Injuries to women may occur when attempting to get out of the bath quickly and emergency interventions may be delayed if it is difficult to get the mother out of the bath or if the water does not flow out quickly.[39–41]

Efficacy

A 2009 systematic review stated that most of the evidence on the use of water immersion is based on observational studies with few randomized controlled trials. These have nevertheless shown immersion in water to significantly reduce maternal pain, the use of epidural/spinal analgesia, and blood pressure as well as demonstrating a decreased incidence in operative delivery and perineal trauma.[42] Factors such as depth of water, size of the pool, and whether the water is still or aerated/whirlpool water have not been compared, as pool design and practice have tended to be based on local availability and customs. Although the use of additives to the water, such as essential oils, appears to be gaining popularity, to date no trial has generated reliable evidence to support or refute the use of any additive.

Neonatal effects

The fetus potentially benefits from hydrotherapy by way of a relaxed mother, as this maximizes placental oxygen perfusion.[43] Concerns have been raised, however, in regard to neonatal respiratory difficulties, thermoregulation during labour, and infection. The diving reflex (apnoea on expiration with a closed larynx) prevents a healthy baby born in water from drowning. This reflex is stimulated via facial skin receptors triggered as the skin makes contact with the water. Fetal breathing is also inhibited by way of sensors in the oral pharynx, including free nerve endings/taste buds, which prevents aspiration. Conversely, a compromised neonate born underwater has the potential to gasp before the nose and mouth are above the surface, inhaling bath water into the lungs. Inhalation of even a small quantity of fresh water can be absorbed quickly into the circulation causing appreciable haemodilution and fluid overload.[44] There have been two reports of neonatal death following water-birth attended by a midwife.[42] However, a direct causal link cannot be assumed on the limited evidence available in these cases.

The water temperature of a pool should not exceed the maternal body temperature, as immersing a woman in water above her natural core temperature will result in fetal hyperthermia. High temperatures have been identified as a safety issue by several authors as being associated with fetal mortality and morbidity, based on individual case studies and/or theory.[44–46] It has been suggested that neonatal infection may occur due to cross-contamination from the water and pool, and from the mother. However, a 2009 systematic review concluded there was not a significantly increased risk of infection for the fetus/neonate.[42]

Implications for practice

Overall, the evidence indicates that hydrotherapy decreases maternal pain levels and reduces the uptake of pharmacological analgesia. There is little evidence to support the concerns over adverse neonatal effects. The UK Department of Health currently recommends that a pool facility should be an option available to women in all UK maternity units, and is promoting water immersion during labour and water-birth as a means of empowering women and is consistent with the current agenda of normalizing birth.[47,48] Hydrotherapy during the first stage of labour can be supported for women at low risk of complications. There is no clear evidence to support or discourage a woman's decision to give birth in water.

Massage and reflexology

Massage involves manipulation of the body's soft tissues. It is an ancient technique that has been widely employed during labour, to help relax tense muscles and to soothe and calm the individual. However, relatively little study has been undertaken examining its effects in the intrapartum period. Different massage techniques may suit different women: a woman who is experiencing backache during labour may find massage over the lumbosacral area soothing; others find light abdominal massage comforting. Women may vary in their response to massage. Some prefer to be massaged during contractions, which helps to 'spread the pain' while some prefer to be massaged after each contraction to relax and soothe tired muscles. Massage may help to relieve pain by relieving muscle spasm, distracting from pain, providing a sense of relaxation and reducing anxiety, decreasing pain intensity by inhibiting sensory transmission in the pain pathways, or by improving blood flow and oxygenation of tissues.[49]

Pressure applied to the feet has been shown to result in an anaesthetizing effect on other parts of the body. Reflexologists propose that these effects are due to reflex points on the feet corresponding to organs and structures of the body and that pain may be reduced by gentle manipulation or pressing certain parts of the foot.[50] It is claimed that by applying pressure to 'reflex zones', energy blocks or disturbances such as calcium, lactate, or uric acid crystals are reabsorbed and later eliminated. This process is more commonly known as detoxification. Reflexology may also reduce stress and tension.[51]

Implications for practice

There are few trials evaluating the benefits of massage therapy in labour, those that do exist suggest that massage is a useful therapy in alleviating pain for some women in labour without the risk of adverse effects.[52,53] There is only anecdotal evidence supporting the use of reflexology.[54] Professional training programmes for massage and reflexology therapists vary from country to country and may be undertaken as part of a broader health professional training or as a profession in their own right.[55]

Acupuncture and acupressure

Acupuncture involves the insertion of fine needles into different, specific parts of the body. Other related techniques include acupressure—applying pressure on the acupuncture point. It uses fingers or small beads instead of needles at the same points on the skin. These techniques are ancient healing arts, which are regarded as conventional medicine in the Far East. The aim is that by stimulating acupuncture points located on the hands, feet, and ears, labour pain is reduced. Several ideas have been presented to explain how acupuncture works. Traditionally acupuncturists believed that health was dependent on the correct flow of energy through the meridians (invisible tracts running through the body). The strength and clarity of these meridians govern the vital health of all the vital organs in the body. If the person is ill, then the energy flow is blocked or unbalanced. The aim is to stimulate the appropriate meridians by using needles, heat, electricity, and pressure at certain points. When these blocks are removed, energy can flow and the body can heal itself.

Since most acupuncture points are either connected to, or located near, neural structures, this suggests that acupuncture stimulates the nervous system, supporting the gate control theory of pain modulation.[56,57]

Efficacy

For labour pain, the ideal placement of needles depends on the degree and location of pain, the stage of labour and a variety of other factors such as anxiety and fatigue.[56] The evidence for the use of acupuncture in labour is conflicting. Studies into its use have given conflicting results, with some concluding that it is ineffective, while others that it is a valuable analgesic technique. One reason for this may be the lack of standardization of acupuncture points and methods used.[58,59] Recent systematic reviews (2010, 2011, and 2012) of studies into complementary therapies for labour all concluded that acupuncture might play a role in increasing patient satisfaction with pain relief and in reducing the use of other analgesia; but it is unlikely to help reduce pain intensity. When asked, women receiving acupressure state that they experience less pain when compared with controls, but their use of pharmacological analgesia or satisfaction with this analgesia does not seem to be influenced. Acupuncture or acupressure may have different effects at different time-points and these effects may only be transient; increased maternal satisfaction with other methods of analgesia may be the real benefit.[54,60,61]

Implications for practice

The systematic reviews conclude that there is insufficient evidence on acupuncture to make firm clinical recommendations. This view is supported by the UK's National Institute for Health and Care Excellence clinical guideline on intrapartum care, which state that 'acupuncture, acupressure should not be provided (as routine care), but women who wish to use these techniques should not be prevented from doing so'.[62]

Transcutaneous electrical nerve stimulation

A transcutaneous electrical nerve stimulator (TENS) is a device that emits low-voltage pulsatile electrical impulses, which vary in frequency and intensity. In labour, the electrodes from the TENS machine are attached to the lower back, placed about 2 cm over the T10–L1 dermatomes either side of the spinous processes to provide analgesia for the first stage of labour. A second set of electrodes is placed over the S2–4 dermatomes for second-stage pain relief. Low-intensity, high-frequency (100–200 Hz) TENS stimulates the A fibres at these dermatomes blocking pain transmission to the brain. Lower frequency stimulation at 40–60 Hz, causes the release of endorphins, which bind to opiate receptors, increasing pain tolerance.[63,64] Women can alter the amount of current supplied to the electrodes providing some degree of control throughout their labour. TENS can also be applied to acupuncture points or directly to the head by trained staff.

TENS has minimal side effects and may be appropriate for women who have contraindications to other methods of pain relief or where other methods are not available. By reducing anxiety, increasing a sense of control, and by providing distraction, TENS increases a woman's sense of well-being and thereby also reduces pain in labour. TENS may also reduce the length of labour by suppressing the release of catecholamines, which can inhibit the contraction of the uterus and thereby, delay progress. It is contraindicated in patients with a cardiac pacemaker and is not advisable for use in patients with epilepsy and should be discontinued should any skin irritation occur on the electrode sites.[56,65]

Efficacy

A 1997 systematic review of the evidence for TENS in labour found little evidence for the use of TENS.[66] One study, however, found that women reported moderate to good pain relief from TENS when surveyed post delivery, but that pain scores while in labour did not differ when compared to sham TENS. A significantly bigger proportion of women in the TENS treatment group claimed that they would chose to use TENS in future labours compared with those in the sham TENS control group. When considering the use of additional analgesia as a secondary measure of effectiveness there was a small but demonstrable benefit to TENS in a number of studies.[66,67]

Implications for practice

The evidence from randomized trials for analgesic benefits from TENS during labour is not compelling but does hint towards an analgesic-sparing effect and a positive response from women with many choosing to use it again for future births. Experienced practitioners state that TENS may be more effective if initiated in early labour, to allow for the build-up of endorphin production before the pain becomes severe.[67]

Sterile water injections

The incidence of low back pain in labour is estimated to be anything up to 75%. Sterile water administered intradermally can be used to reduce this pain. Intracutaneous injections of sterile water are used at four sites in the lower back, approximately corresponding to the borders of the sacrum. A small bleb is produced by injection of approximately 0.1 mL of water between the dermal layers of the skin. Two are placed 3–4 cm either side of the lumbar-sacral spine, with the other two sites 2–3 cm below and 1–2 cm medial to the original injection points. Injections may also be given subcutaneously. The exact location of injections does not appear to be critical to their success.[68] The injections themselves are associated with acute somatic pain so they are usually given at the height of a contraction, either sequentially or simultaneously. The injection site pain lasts around 30 seconds and as it begins to subside, so does the referred pain from the viscera, with the analgesic effect lasting for 2–3 hours.[69]

The mechanism of action of this therapy is not well understood. The injection of intradermal sterile water produces irritation in the skin; these changes may trigger the A-delta cutaneous afferent pain fibres leading to endorphin release similar to that seen with acupuncture. Alternatively, hyperstimulation of somatic nerves may overwhelm the visceral component; referred stimulation to relieve referred pain. Another explanation is that it may exert its effect through physiological distraction.[70] Similar injections of normal saline are not associated with such intense pain but do not then produce the subsequent analgesia effects.

Efficacy

Several randomized control trials comparing the effects of intradermal water blocks to placebo or to an alternative non-pharmacological method for the treatment of low back pain in labour have reported that water blocks decrease low back pain in labour.[71–76] However, the authors of a 2012 systematic review of all studies to date felt that the comparatively low total number of participants severely limited the applicability of the evidence to clinical practice.[70]

Implications for practice

Despite this rapidly becoming a popular form of analgesia, there is no robust evidence that it is effective for either intractable back pain in labour or the pain associated with uterine contractions.

Aromatherapy

Aromatherapy is the use of essential oils, highly concentrated aromatic substances extracted from plants by a process of distillation or cold compression. The mechanism of action for aromatherapy is unclear: the oils are thought to increase the secretion of the body's own sedative, stimulant, and relaxing neurotransmitters (paracrine and endocrine) by activation of the limbic system. They may be massaged into the skin, or inhaled by using a steam infusion or burner.[65]

Efficacy

Studies (in areas outside of obstetrics) investigating psychological and physiological effects of essential oils showed no change on physiological parameters such as blood pressure or heart rate but did indicate psychological improvement in mood and anxiety.[77] One large study looking at the use of aromatherapy in labour reported that half of the women found it 'helpful' in reducing fear anxiety and pain.[78] A 2011 systematic review reported no difference in pain intensity or the use of pharmacological agents when using aromatherapy.[79]

Implications for practice

As aromatherapy is increasing in popularity among midwives and nurses, it is important to note that it may have undesirable side effects such as nausea and headache. Some experts have stated that 'essential oils are as potent as pharmacological drugs and are equally open to misuse or abuse, whether intended or not … and until more clinical research trials have been undertaken, it would be prudent for midwives to work cautiously with essential oils, using the lowest possible dose and on the least number of occasions'.[80]

Enhancement of descending inhibitory pathways

Techniques such as antenatal education, relaxation, music, and hypnotherapy aim to engage the brain's inhibitory response to pain, either consciously or subconsciously, potentially reducing the severity of the sensations and helping the parturient to cope with the pain.

Childbirth education

Antenatal education consisting of individual or group classes is partly designed to inform pregnant women and their partners about the labour and birth process. Amongst other things this education covers analgesia options and 'self-help' measures. The content of these classes and other research done by expectant mothers can help them to identify and understand their own coping styles and preferences and develop their own coping strategies for labour. This influences expectations of labour pain and can therefore be beneficial in helping them to cope with the experience.[56] In one trial, women who received education in the antenatal period were less likely to request epidural analgesia in labour but not less likely to request some form of systemic analgesia.[81]

Attention focusing and distraction

Many methods of coping with pain involve the conscious participation of the individual in activities that are designed to take their mind off the pain. Attention focusing activates include verbal coaching, visualization, concentration on visual, auditory, or tactile stimuli, and patterned breathing. Most antenatal classes advocate patterned breathing as a means of distraction and of increasing the sense of control women feel in labour.[56] There are no studies that evaluate these techniques as independent variables but surveys would suggest that the majority of women do find them helpful.[82]

Relaxation, music, and audioanalgesia

Relaxation techniques are based on the practice of developing conscious awareness of muscular tension, releasing that tension, and then maintaining relaxation. Yoga, meditation, and music techniques may all have a calming effect and provide a distraction from pain and tension. Audioanalgesia is the use of music, white noise, or environmental sounds to decrease pain perception. Although there is no strong evidence that it significantly reduces pain intensity and analgesic requirements in labour, there are no adverse effects and it is a popular option for labouring women.[56,83]

Hypnosis

Hypnosis has been described as a state of narrow focused attention, reduced awareness of external stimuli, and an increased response to suggestions—positive statements used in order to achieve specific therapeutic goals.[84] These suggestions may be verbal or non-verbal and result in apparent spontaneous changes in perception, mood, or behaviour. These therapeutic communications are directed to the person's subconscious and the responses are independent of any conscious effort or reasoning. Women can learn self-hypnosis, which can be used in labour to reduce pain from contractions. Common hypnotic pain relief techniques are 'glove anaesthesia', in which the woman imagines that they have a numb hand that can be used to relieve pain in other areas, or 'time distortion', which allows the women to imagine the contractions becoming shorter and further apart.[85] Recent advances in neuroimaging have led to increased understanding of the neurophysiological changes occurring during hypnosis.[86]

Efficacy

A 2011 systematic review of trials using hypnosis found that the use of hypnosis was associated with a strong trend in the reduction of requests for pharmacological intervention. In comparison to education and counselling alone, several studies have shown hypnosis to be superior in reducing pain.[56,85,87]

Implications for practice

There is little or no risk to the use of self-hypnosis in labour in women without a history of psychosis but it requires antenatal training by a trained hypnotherapist.

Biofeedback

Biological feedback is a term that describes a therapeutic technique where individuals are trained to improve their health and well-being through signals coming from their own bodies, for example, temperature, heart rate, and muscular tension. The aim is that with the aid of electrical instruments to measure response, conscious changes in thoughts and emotions help the individual to gain control over physiological responses. Electromyography, measuring muscle tension, appears to have some positive effects in early labour but shows no benefit as labour progresses.[56]

Birthing partners and doula

Many women like to have a birthing partner with them during labour and delivery. They provide both physical support, for example, massaging shoulders, help with positioning, support with breathing techniques; and emotional support, for example, reassurance, comfort, listening, and support with decision-making. Many different people can provide this help including fathers, other relations, and friends. Historically, women have been attended and supported by other women during labour. Some women therefore chose to employ the services of a doula, a professional who is trained in childbirth and provides continuous support to a mother before, during, and just after birth. Doula comes from a Greek word that means 'a woman who serves' or 'handmaiden'.[88,89]

Efficacy

A 2012 Cochrane review on the use of continuous support in childbirth evaluated evidence from 22 randomized controlled trials from 16 countries. Overall, women allocated to continuous support were more likely to have a spontaneous vaginal birth and less likely to have intrapartum analgesia or to report dissatisfaction. In addition, their labour was on average 40 minutes shorter and they were less likely to have a caesarean delivery or instrumental vaginal birth, neuraxial analgesia, or a baby with a low 5-minute Apgar score. The subgroup analyses suggested that continuous support was most effective when provided by someone neither part of the hospital staff nor the woman's social network, and in settings in which epidural analgesia was not routinely available. The review concluded that continuous support from a person who is present solely to provide support, is not a member of the woman's social network, is experienced in providing labour support, and has at least a modest amount of training, appears to be most beneficial.[90]

Non-pharmacological approaches to labour pain: summary of key points

- May reduce the intensity of pain sensation but are unlikely to entirely relieve pain. There is limited evidence for their efficacy.
- May help women maintain a sense of control in labour and subsequently cope better with labour pain.
- Have few serious side effects.
- May be combined or used alongside systemic analgesia to increase effectiveness.

Systemic analgesia for labour

Systemic medications are the most common form of analgesia in labour. These medications are diverse in their mechanisms of action (Figure 13.4). Consequently they display varying efficacy and side effect profiles both for mother and baby.

Inhalational agents

Inhalation labour analgesia involves the intermittent use of subanaesthetic concentrations of nitrous oxide or other volatile agents. Pain can be relieved while maintaining maternal consciousness and avoiding regurgitation or aspiration of stomach contents. Inhalational agents readily cross the placenta and the concentration in fetal blood soon approaches that of the mother but, since these agents are excreted almost entirely through the lungs, they are readily excreted from the newborn. The efficacy of inhalational analgesia depends on the analgesic strength of the agent and on how quickly it reaches analgesic concentration after the start of inspiration. A rapid offset with complete elimination between contractions would prevent accumulation completely. Nitrous oxide is the best match in current use.

Nitrous oxide

Intermittent inhaled nitrous oxide was first introduced to provide labour analgesia in the late nineteenth century and became routine in the 1930s. The precise mechanism of action for nitrous oxide analgesia remains uncertain but it appears to modulate pain stimuli by way of descending spinal cord nerve pathways.[91] Nitrous oxide has a low blood–gas partition coefficient (0.47) and so equilibrates rapidly with arterial concentration, thus the peak analgesic effect of nitrous oxide is at approximately 50 seconds. As the peak effect of uterine contractions is typically at 30 seconds the analgesic effects of nitrous oxide may be out of phase with the pain of contractions. Nitrous oxide can be used alone or to supplement other methods of analgesia.

Worldwide the use of nitrous oxide is very variable. It is widely available in Europe, and in the United Kingdom 60% of parturients choose to use it. This largely results from the ease with which midwives in the United Kingdom can prescribe Entonox® (a 50:50 blend with oxygen, in a pre-mixed cylinder) without involving a physician. Similarly, uptake in Australia and Canada is about 50%. However, nitrous oxide is not routinely available in many European countries (it is only available in one centre in Belgium, for example) or in the United States where only 1% of parturients uses this method of analgesia.[92–95] A reducing valve fitted to the nitrous oxide/oxygen cylinder or to a blender that mixes the two gases from separate cylinders connects to a breathing circuit that has a demand valve connected to a facemask or mouthpiece. This demand valve opens only when the parturient applies negative pressure by inspiring through the mouthpiece or a well-sealed mask covering her nose and mouth.

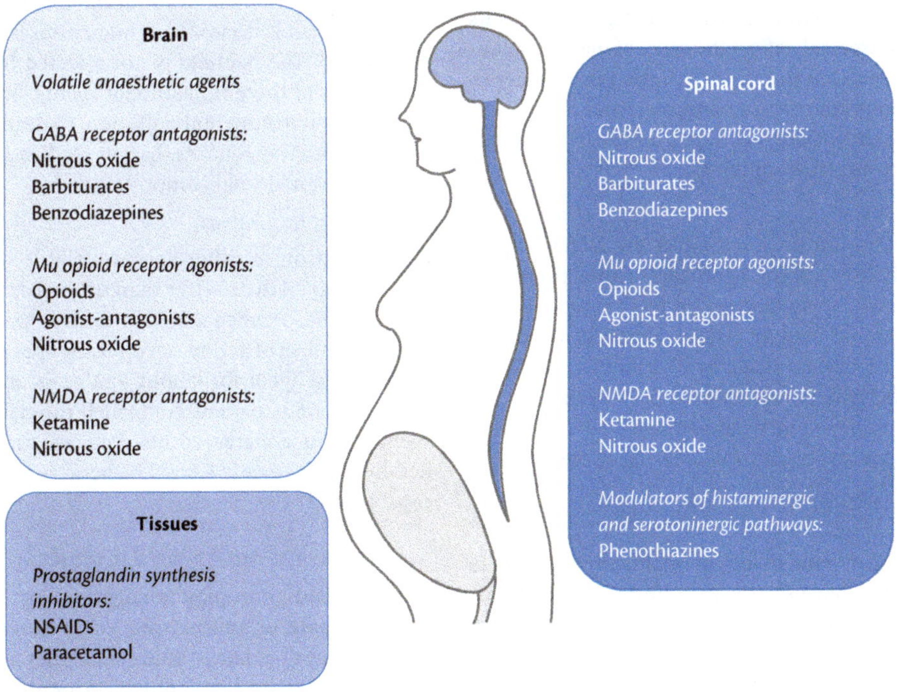

Figure 13.4 Sites of action of systemic analgesia.

Efficacy

Most efficacy studies of nitrous oxide have compared either its use to placebo (inhaled air), the analgesic benefit of increasing the inhaled concentration, or the effects of adding other volatile agents to the inhaled mixture. A 2002 systematic review of randomized controlled trials looking at the efficacy of inhaled nitrous oxide as labour analgesia concluded that current published work does not provide clear quantitative objective evidence of its efficacy.[91] A consistent finding in studies and surveys of nitrous oxide has been that 30–40% of mothers find its use of no benefit. Studies report conflicting results with regard to any improvement in pain scores of parturients but even those with negative results about analgesia report that many subjects wished to continue to use nitrous oxide after the study period. The majority of women who do report significant benefit state that they would choose nitrous oxide as a form of pain relief for subsequent labours.[91,92,96,97] This suggests that although it may not produce measurable analgesia for labour pain, nitrous oxide does have some benefits, though this may be in part a placebo effect.

Studies of non-pharmacological methods of pain relief suggest that the analgesia from TENS or sterile water injections may be similar to that associated with nitrous oxide use with comparable levels of patient satisfaction. One study found that 90% of women reported similar levels of partial relief from either TENS or nitrous oxide.[98–100] Reductions in pain with inhaled nitrous oxide use seem similar to that of systemic opioids, but inferior to those achieved with epidural analgesia.[101–103] One study directly compared the efficacy of self-administered nitrous oxide to intermittent patient-controlled administration of IV remifentanil. It found the analgesic benefit of nitrous oxide to be inferior to remifentanil.[104]

Maternal side effects

Inhaled nitrous oxide analgesia for labour displays good safety outcomes for both mother and baby. Some women experience significant nausea with the use of nitrous oxide; however, in trials its use does not seem to appreciably affect the rates of maternal nausea or vomiting. It may increase the rate of maternal oxygen desaturation in between labour contractions and maternal drowsiness increases in a dose-dependent fashion. Long-term use of nitrous oxide may result in bone marrow suppression.[91,103,105,106]

Fetal and neonatal effects

Nitrous oxide administration does not adversely affect uterine activity. Studies have failed to show significant neonatal respiratory depression, reduced Apgar scores, or fetal acidosis.[107,108] However, the full effects on human fetuses exposed to nitrous oxide or other anaesthetic agents *in utero* are unknown. Recently neurotoxic effects of anaesthetic agents have been demonstrated in the developing brains of rodents and primates. Nitrous oxide administration may have more risk for creating these changes than other agents.[109–111]

Effects on staff

The long-term effects of nitrous oxide on healthcare workers is unclear; however, studies have shown that midwives are regularly exposed to levels of nitrous oxide higher than permitted by the Control of Substances Hazardous to Health (COSHH) regulations and may be at an increased risk of adverse reproductive outcomes. COSHH exposure limits mirror the Indicative Occupational Exposure Limit Values set out by the European Commission.[112–114]

Implications for practice

Despite a lack of clear evidence supporting the efficacy of nitrous oxide in providing adequate analgesia in labour, it remains in widespread use and a popular choice for many women.

Volatile anaesthetic agents

Although most inhalation anaesthetic agents have been studied for labour analgesia, they have not been adopted in recent years for widespread use. An anaesthetist must be present for their use, which undoubtedly reduces application. Halogenated hydrocarbons are slightly more effective than nitrous oxide for the reduction of pain and are less likely to precipitate nausea. The mechanism of action for these agents (e.g. trichloroethylene, methoxyflurane, cyclopropane, enflurane, isoflurane, and desflurane) is not well understood. Evidence suggests that they act by binding to proteins and selectively targeting synaptic ion channels, resulting in central nervous system depression.

Ether was the first volatile to be used as an anaesthetic but is unsuitable for labour analgesia as it is a potent emetic with an unpleasant pungent odour, is irritating to the respiratory tract, and is explosive. Chloroform has a pleasant odour, is non-irritant, more potent and faster acting than ether, but has undesirable, dose-related side effects, such as arrhythmias and hepatic damage. Methoxyflurane and trichloroethylene were used for analgesia in labour in the past but have been withdrawn for other, non-obstetric, reasons.[115]

Isoflurane (0.25%), when added to Entonox® produces superior analgesia than Entonox® alone but does not produce more maternal satisfaction. This concentration will not change uterine contractility or responsiveness to oxytocin. Desflurane, while having the advantage of rapid onset and offset of action, produces similar analgesic results as Entonox®, causes amnesia in a significant proportion of women. Sevoflurane 0.8% (Sevox) produces better analgesia than Entonox® but higher doses only increase maternal sedation.[116] The neonate is not affected by these analgesic concentrations of these inhalational agents. There is, however, a concern over environmental pollution, maternal amnesia, and loss of protective airway reflexes. Larger studies are needed to assess the incidence of maternal compromise.[117]

Implications for practice

In comparison to other agents, volatile inhaled agents provide analgesia equal to or better than nitrous oxide either when administered alone, or when added to nitrous oxide. Because of its short onset and offset of action, sevoflurane appears to be the best-suited inhalational agent for labour analgesia and could potentially be administered as patient-controlled inhalation analgesia. Volatile agents produce increased maternal sedation and their use is limited by requirements for anaesthetic supervision and scavenging capabilities.[91]

Sedatives and non-opioid analgesia

Sedatives and non-opioid analgesics may be effective for mild to moderate pain or alternatively can be used in combination with opioid drugs to enhance pain relief. They act in a variety of different ways and many have antipyretic or anti-inflammatory actions, as well as sedative or analgesic properties.

Paracetamol

Paracetamol is a widely used and effective antipyretic and analgesic medication with well-established tolerability. It has a favourable safety profile when compared with other analgesics, opioids, and non-steroidal anti-inflammatory drugs and when used in pregnancy has been reported not to be associated with an increased risk of congenital anomalies.[118–120]

Dosage

Paracetamol 1 g (if >50 kg) orally or IV, 4–6-hourly with a maximum of 4 g in 24 hours.

Efficacy

Oral administration of paracetamol in labour does not appear to confer significant analgesic benefit; however, the investigation of IV paracetamol in labour is relatively recent. One study found the effectiveness of IV paracetamol to be comparable to that of IV pethidine with duration of action of up to 2 hours. Paracetamol had fewer maternal adverse effects than pethidine. A further study is currently ongoing aiming to assess the efficacy of IV infusion of paracetamol in comparison with placebo.[121,122]

Implications for practice

Paracetamol appears to be safe to use, however, its place in providing analgesia in labour is not yet established.

Non-steroidal anti-inflammatory drugs

The primary mechanism of action of non-steroidal anti-inflammatory drugs (NSAIDs) is inhibition of prostaglandin formation. Blockade of the pro-inflammatory mediators by NSAIDs will reduce the inflammatory response and subsequent pain. Classically, their effect is anti-inflammatory, analgesic, and antipyretic.

Efficacy

A 2012 systematic review of non-opioid drugs for pain management in labour reported on several trials comparing NSAIDs with other forms of labour analgesia. One trial comparing ketorolac (NSAID) to pethidine found that for all measures of efficacy, the patients in the ketorolac group consistently reported higher pain severity compared to pethidine. In another study, women in the NSAID group were less likely to express satisfaction with pain relief when compared with the opioid group.[123]

Maternal and neonatal effects

As inhibitors of cyclooxygenase, NSAIDs given during pregnancy have the potential to cause adverse maternal and fetal effects. Maternal effects include prolongation of labour, whereas constriction of the ductus arteriosus, renal dysfunction, and haemostatic abnormalities can occur in the fetus and neonate.[124]

Implications for practice

NSAIDs may have a subsidiary role in the management of labour pain but they do not appear to be effective as sole agents.

Ketamine

Ketamine is a phencyclidine derivative which when administered in small doses produces a dissociative state of analgesia. Some clinicians have promoted it as a suitable analgesic for labour, but although it has a rapid onset of action (~30 seconds) its effects are of short duration, up to 5 minutes, meaning frequent repeated administration is necessary.

Dosage

Ketamine 10–20 mg IV or intramuscularly (IM) repeated at intervals of 2–5 minutes. Maximum dose in 30 minutes should not exceed 1 mg/kg.

Maternal side effects

At higher doses (i.e. >1 mg/kg) ketamine can be used to induce general anaesthesia; it is therefore important that verbal contact must be maintained with the parturient at all times as excessive sedation may lead to airway compromise. At low doses, however, ketamine may still be the cause of maternal hallucinations and frequently causes amnesia.[125] It should be avoided in pre-eclampsia as it may exacerbate hypertension by stimulation of the sympathetic nervous system. Ketamine produces a dose-dependent increase in uterine tone, which at these doses is not clinically significant.[126]

Fetal and neonatal effects

High doses of ketamine have been associated with abnormal neonatal muscle tone but low doses do not result in neonatal depression.[127]

Implications for practice

The short duration of action of ketamine makes it unsuitable for analgesia during the first stage of labour but it may have a role immediately prior to delivery.

Barbiturates

Barbiturates such as phenobarbital have a primarily sedative effect on the central nervous system. They may be used in the early phase of labour to decrease anxiety but lack analgesic properties and may heighten the perception of pain when given in the absence of opioid analgesia. Their use in labour is minimal as barbiturates are lipid soluble so readily cross the placenta; most have long elimination half-lives leading to prolonged neonatal depressive effects if given in repeated doses or close to the time of delivery.[128]

Phenothiazines

Phenothiazines, such as chlorpromazine, prochlorperazine, or promethazine, are a group of drugs used primarily as antipsychotic and sedative drugs. They also have antimuscarinic, antiemetic, antihistamine, antidopaminergic, and alpha-adrenoceptor antagonist properties. They are used in combination with opioids in some obstetric patients to provide sedation and decrease nausea. They rapidly cross the placenta and may result in decreased fetal heart rate variability but do not seem to cause neonatal respiratory depression.[126]

Benzodiazepines

Benzodiazepines may decrease opioid requirements during labour but at a cost of significant maternal sedation and neonatal respiratory depression, reduced tone, and impaired temperature control. They are not recommended for use as a sedative in labour.[128]

Systemic opioids

Obstetric anaesthesia has an uneasy relationship with systemic opioids. While they are the most widely used systemic analgesia in labour, the variable efficacy of these drugs combined with a broad range of maternal side effects and concerns over neonatal depression have limited their use.[101,129] Until recently there has been little evidence to suggest that one agent or mode of administration is intrinsically superior to the others; consequently the choice of opioid analgesic in labour is dictated largely by institutional tradition and/or personal preference.

Opioid drugs act by binding to opioid receptors, which are found principally in the central and peripheral nervous system and the gastrointestinal tract. Maternal side effects of opioids include nausea, vomiting, delayed gastric emptying, sedation, disorientation, pruritus, and respiratory depression. There is variable susceptibility amongst parturients towards these adverse effects, which are predominantly dose dependent rather than drug dependent.[130]

Opioids may affect the fetus directly by placental transfer or indirectly though effects on the mother, for example, by altered minute ventilation or uterine tone. As a group, opioid medications by virtue of their low molecular weight and high lipid solubility readily cross the placenta by diffusion.[131] The amount of free drug delivered to the placenta depends on placental blood low and maternal protein binding, and the amount of drug available to the fetus depends on the degree of placental uptake, fetal metabolism, and clearance (Figure 13.5).[132] The speed and amount of placental transfer and consequent umbilical vein to maternal artery concentration ratios vary with different drugs and modes of administration. Opioids are primarily associated with neonatal respiratory depression and decreased beat-to-beat fetal heart rate variability. However, subtle neurobehavioural changes may also be observed in the early neonatal period, for example, decreased alertness and a delay in effective feeding due to the inhibition of sucking reflexes. The long-term significance of these neurobehavioural changes remains unclear.[133] Maternal administration of an opioid antagonist during labour or immediately prior to delivery has not been shown to have any substantial neonatal benefit and only serves to reduce maternal analgesic benefit. Naloxone is best administered directly to the neonate if required (Figure 13.5).[134]

A link between opioids and an alteration in immune function is often referred to in the literature and extensive research has been directed at investigating the immunomodulatory effects of opioids. There appear to be differences amongst opioids in immunomodulatory effects with several proposed mechanisms and sites of action including: the mu opioid receptors, a direct action on the immunocyte, modulation of the hypothalamic–pituitary–adrenal axis and modulation of sympathetic activity.[135] The clinical significance of these effects, however, has not yet been fully established but it would be sensible to consider the potential for immunomodulation particularly in those already immunosuppressed.[136]

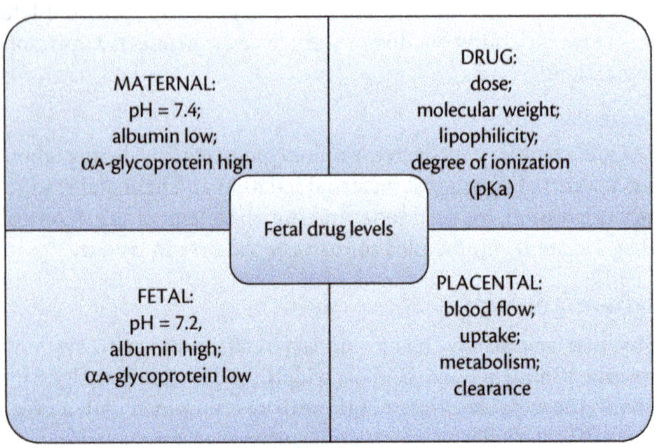

Figure 13.5 Factors affecting fetal opioid levels after systemic administration.
Data from Ala-Kokko T, Vähäkangas K, Pelkonen O. Placental function and principles of drug transfer. *Acta Anaesthesiologica Scandinavica* 1993; 37 (s100):47–49, Copyright © 1993 John Wiley and Sons.

Modes of administration

Intermittent bolus

Opioid analgesia may be administered by any number of different routes: transdermal, buccal, oral, subcutaneous, IM, IV, epidural, or intrathecal. For the purposes of labour analgesia the IM, IV, and neuraxial routes are most common. Intermittent IM injections have the advantage of being midwife delivered and thus readily available but may be painful. There is variable drug absorption depending on the site of injection and an inevitable delay between time of injection and onset of action. The quality and duration of IM analgesia is inconsistent. By contrast, opioids given via IV injection have the advantage of quicker onset, the ability to titrate to effect, and more predictable quality and duration of analgesia (Table 13.3). In many institutions, however, IV administration of opioids requires the presence of a physician, so limiting ready availability.

Patient-controlled analgesia

The use of intermittent bolus or continuous IV infusion of opioids for postoperative pain has largely given way to patient-controlled (IV) analgesia (PCA). Good analgesia has been shown to be achievable with lower drug doses, thus reducing side effects and improving patient satisfaction. Patient satisfaction in childbirth is important and though the use of PCA does not lead to the complete absence of pain the benefit of a perceived sense of control during

Table 13.3 Examples of intermittent IV/IM bolus opioid analgesia for labour

Drug	Dose (IV/IM)	Onset (IV/IM)	Duration of action	Frequency of administration
Pethidine[142]	25–50 mg IV 50–100 mg IM	5–10 min IV 40–45 min IM	2–3 h	2–4-hourly
Codeine[171]	30–60 mg IM	10–30 min IM	3–4 h	4–6-hourly
Tramadol[171]	50–100 mg IV/IM	<60 min	3–4 h	4–6-hourly
Morphine[142]	2–5 mg IV 5–10 mg IM	2–3 min IV 20–40 min IM	3–4 h	4–6-hourly
Diamorphine[142]	1–2.5 mg IV 2.5–5 mg IM	2–3 min IV 5–10 min IM	3–4 h	4–6-hourly
Nalbuphine[142]	10–20 mg IV/IM	2–3 min IV 15 min IM	3–6 h	3–4-hourly
Butorphanol[171]	1–2 mg IV/IM	5–10 min IV 10–30 min IM	3–4 h	6–8-hourly
Pentazocine[171]	30–60 mg IV/IM	2–3 min IV 15–20 min IM	2–3 h	3–4-hourly
Fentanyl[189]	25–50 mcg IV 50–100 mcg IM	2–3 min IV 10 min IM	30–60 min	>60 min

Data from various sources (see references).

labour has been demonstrated in a number of studies.[137–139] This advantage, along with a growing need to find an effective alternative to neuraxial analgesia for those who do not want, cannot have, or simply do not need an epidural, has led to the increasing use of PCA systems for analgesia in labour. Frequent smaller doses of opioid result in more uniform analgesia and, through a more steady plasma drug concentration, may result in reduced placental transfer when compared to intermittent bolus IV administration. Various opioids have been suggested for PCA use in labour (Table 13.4); however, due to the changing nature, frequency, and intensity of labour pain, rapid-onset and short-acting agents such as remifentanil are most suitable. An ideal IV opioid should have an onset and offset that can match the time course of uterine contractions, so that the parturient experiences worthwhile analgesia. Uterine contractility and fetal heart rate variability should be preserved and there should be minimal respiratory depressive maternal and neonatal side effects so that administration can be continued up to and during delivery. Gastric emptying should not be delayed in case general anaesthesia is required.[140]

Pethidine

Pethidine (meperidine) is a synthetic opioid. It is a weakly basic phenylpiperidine derivative related to fentanyl and sufentanil. It is legally available for independent use by midwives in the United Kingdom, and worldwide is the most extensively used and investigated opioid analgesic in labour. A recent survey of units in the United Kingdom reported that 95% are using IM pethidine.[141] It is approximately 28 times more lipid-soluble than morphine and 90% metabolized by the liver to the active metabolite norpethidine.

Dosage

Pethidine is ten times less potent than morphine. The usual dose in labour is 50–100 mg or 1 mg/kg (maximum 200 mg) IM every 2–4 hours with half the dose being administered if the IV route is preferred. IV administration gives more predictable blood concentrations and a faster onset of analgesia when compared with the IM route (5 vs 45 minutes).[142]

Table 13.4 Examples of intravenous patient-controlled analgesia regimens for labour

Drug	Patient-controlled dose	Lockout time
Pethidine (bolus only)[155]	15 mg	10 min
Pethidine (loading dose with bolus)[155]	49.5 mg loading dose plus 5 mg bolus	10 min
Morphine[169]	1 mg	5 min
Diamorphine[169]	0.5 mg	5 min
Nalbuphine[187]	1 mg	6–10 min
Fentanyl[193]	50 mcg loading dose plus 20 mcg bolus	5 min
Remifentanil (bolus dose by weight)[210]	0.25–0.5 mcg/kg	2–3 min
Remifentanil (fixed bolus dose)[210]	40 mcg	2 min
Remifentanil (infusion with bolus)[219]	0.025–0.1 mcg/kg/min infusion plus 0.25 mcg/kg bolus	5 min

Data from various sources (see references).

Efficacy

Studies on pethidine have consistently cast doubts on its effectiveness as a labour analgesic and there are concerns about its maternal, fetal, and neonatal side effect profile.[143,144] Maternal satisfaction with pethidine is historically poor with a UK National Birthday Trust survey in 1990 reporting only 16% of women rating it as helpful with 25% rating it as unhelpful. A 2002 randomized controlled trial comparing IV pethidine with placebo found that pethidine provided effective pain relief in only 23.8% of patients. Midwives rate the efficacy of pethidine better than the women receiving it though this may be attributable to misinterpretation of sedation for analgesia.[101,116,145]

Maternal side effects

Pethidine decreases gastric emptying in 70% of women by at least 5 hours and increases gastric volumes in labour. It causes dose-dependent respiratory depression with desaturation having been shown to occur between contractions, particularly when used in combination with Entonox®. Neurological effects include confusion, loss of control, and sedation. Norpethidine, the active metabolite, has proconvulsant properties making pethidine potentially unsuitable for use in parturients at increased risk of seizure activity such as those with pre-eclampsia. Although research into the effects of pethidine on the duration of labour is limited there is a strong suggestion in the literature that the use of this drug is associated with a lengthening of labour and that this association is dose related.[146]

Fetal and neonatal effects

Both pethidine and norpethidine readily cross the placenta and equilibrium between the maternal and fetal compartments can be achieved in 6 minutes with an umbilical vein/maternal artery ratio of 0.61.[147] The dosage and timing of maternal administration of pethidine are the most important determinants of effects on the fetus and neonate. The highest fetal plasma concentration of pethidine occurs 2–3 hours after maternal IM administration. Pethidine has been shown to significantly affect fetal heart rate variability during labour with reduced variability being seen approximately 25 minutes after IV administration and 40 minutes after IM administration. Variability of the fetal heart rate typically recovers within 60 minutes.[148,149]

The fetal circulation is more acidic than the maternal, so pethidine is more ionized in this environment leading to accumulation. This phenomenon of ion trapping along with a greater free drug concentration caused by lower plasma protein concentrations and an immature respiratory centre make respiratory depression more likely in the neonate than in the mother.[150] The neonatal effects of pethidine are compounded by the metabolism in the neonate of pethidine to norpethidine. The half-lives of pethidine and norpethidine are 4 and 20 hours, respectively, in the parturient but two to seven times longer in the neonate.[147] The babies of women who have received pethidine in labour have been shown to be sleepier, less attentive, and less able to establish breastfeeding, despite normal Apgar scores at birth.[148,151] These neonatal effects are minimal if pethidine is given within 1 hour of delivery. Concerns over long-term risk of substance abuse in adult offspring after intrapartum pethidine were proven to be unfounded in a 2012 Dutch 20-year follow-up cohort study.[152]

Implications for practice

Pethidine has questionable efficacy and significant side effects. However, with easy of availability, familiarity, and low cost it has continued to be the opioid of choice in many institutions and the standard that other analgesic options are measured against. With the emergence of viable alternatives, however, it may be time to consider abandoning the use of pethidine in the developed world.

Patient-controlled analgesia

Pethidine has been used successfully for PCA in the postoperative setting; however, its use in labour has yielded unimpressive results with higher total doses of pethidine being administered compared to midwife-administered intermittent boluses and no significant change in the maternal or neonatal side effect profiles seen.[153]

Various different dosing regimens have been used, for example:

- Pethidine 49.5 mg loading dose and 5 mg boluses with a lockout of 10-minute and a maximum overall dose limit of 200 mg.
- Pethidine 15 mg bolus dose with 10-minute lockout.

Recent comparisons of pethidine PCA, with remifentanil and fentanyl in labour have favoured these shorter-acting agents for both analgesic effect and side effect profile.[154–156]

Codeine

Codeine is a naturally occurring opioid with reduced potency and efficacy when compared to morphine. It can be administered orally or IM as a sole agent in doses of up to 60 mg 4–6-hourly. It is also available in combination with paracetamol. It is not commonly the opioid of choice in active labour due to an inability to achieve adequate analgesia yet still being associated with a risk of neonatal respiratory depression. If used long term during pregnancy, neonatal withdrawal symptoms may occur.[157] The use of codeine in children under 12 years of age and in breastfeeding mothers have recently been discouraged by the European Medicines Agency and Medicines and Healthcare products Regulatory Agency because of concerns over respiratory depression in individuals who have ultra-rapid metabolizer form of the enzyme CYP2D6.[158] Although no new recommendations have as yet been made regarding its use in pregnancy, it would be sensible to consider this potential effect if prescribing codeine to a labouring woman or breastfeeding mother.

Tramadol

Tramadol is a synthetic opioid that acts as a mu-receptor agonist while also inhibiting serotonin and noradrenaline reuptake.

Dosage

It has been used successfully in labour at doses of 50–100 mg, 4-hourly, and can be administered orally, IM, or IV.

Efficacy

Studies comparing bolus tramadol with bolus pethidine for labour analgesia and have concluded that tramadol offers an analgesic effect similar to pethidine.[159,160]

Maternal side effects

Studies of the general adult population would suggest that tramadol does not exhibit the same level of respiratory depression or delay of gastric emptying as morphine or pethidine.[161,162] However, other mu-receptor associated side effects such as dizziness, nausea and constipation do occur; tramadol is also a proconvulsant.

Fetal and neonatal effects

In comparison to pethidine, tramadol has less potential for respiratory depressive effect on the neonate.[159,160]

Patient-controlled analgesia

Like pethidine, tramadol PCA systems have been successfully used in non-obstetric situations. However, there is a paucity of published information regarding its use in labour with at present just one study comparing tramadol PCA use with combined spinal–epidural (CSE) analgesia. This study reported significantly better pain scores in the CSE group and significantly worse neonatal Apgar scores in the tramadol group. Therefore, despite the ability of tramadol PCA to provide moderate analgesic effect while causing less maternal respiratory depression, its adverse effect on Apgar scores and proconvulsant properties make tramadol an unsuitable agent for labour analgesia in PCA form.[163,164]

Implications for practice

Tramadol does not appear to have significant benefits over pethidine and therefore has not become commonly used in practice.

Morphine and diamorphine

Morphine is a mu-receptor agonist acting primarily in the central nervous system. It is metabolized by the liver to an inactive metabolite, morphine-3-glucuronide and the active metabolite morphine-6-glucuronide and is rapidly cleared by the kidneys from the maternal circulation. Diamorphine is semi-synthetic opioid, the diacetylated analogue of morphine. It is a pro-drug and is converted the active components of acetylmorphine and morphine by esterases in liver, plasma, and central nervous system. It is 1.5–2 times more potent than morphine and has a more rapid onset of action.

Dosage

Morphine is ten times more potent than pethidine; the dose for maternal analgesia is 2–5 mg IV or 5–10 mg IM. When given IV it has an onset time of 2–3 minutes with a peak effect at 10–20 minutes, the onset of effect after IM injection is slower at 20–40 minutes with a peak effect at 1–2 hours.[154] Diamorphine is administered IM at a dose of 2.5–5 mg, half that of morphine.

Efficacy

A small randomized controlled study comparing the efficacy of morphine and pethidine in labour showed little difference between the two drugs. It found that neither agent reduced pain scores but both increased sedation with increasing dosage. It has therefore been argued that both pethidine and morphine merely provide sedation rather than analgesia in labour with the authors of one review going as far as to say that it seems 'unethical and medically incorrect to meet parturients' requests for pain relief by giving them sedation'.[101,150]

Diamorphine is used in over a third of institutions in the United Kingdom and is the most commonly used opioid for analgesia in labour in Scotland.[165] The 1990 UK National Birthday Trust survey found that both midwives and parturients rated it as more effective than pethidine.[116] A small trial comparing IM pethidine with diamorphine, showed diamorphine to have some benefits over pethidine when used for labour analgesia but the trial did not study the potential adverse effects of either opioid.[166]

Maternal side effects

The maternal side effects of morphine are dose related and similar to pethidine but its metabolites do not have proconvulsant effects.

Diamorphine has been reported to provide effective analgesia associated with euphoria and less maternal vomiting than traditionally associated with pethidine use.[166]

Fetal and neonatal effects

Morphine is primarily bound to albumin and although it readily crosses the placenta with an umbilical vein/maternal artery ratio of 0.96 at 5 minutes, rapid maternal elimination reduced the overall fetal drug load.[167,168] The effect of drug transfer to the fetus depends on dose and gestational age with morphine metabolism being reduced in the immature fetal liver. As with pethidine, maternal administration of morphine may result in neonatal respiratory depression and decreased fetal heart rate variability. A 2010 Cochrane review found that diamorphine produces less neonatal respiratory depression than pethidine.[144]

Patient-controlled analgesia

The use of morphine and diamorphine in PCA for labour has not been shown to offer any significant advantages over IM administration.[169]

Implications for practice

Morphine does not display any real advantages over pethidine and therefore is not in common use. Diamorphine is widely used in some areas and a large randomized controlled trial to comparing IM diamorphine and pethidine in terms of their analgesic efficacy in labour and their side effects in mother, fetus, and neonate is current ongoing (2012). If this trial yields positive results, it may lead to more widespread use of diamorphine in clinical practice.[170]

Nalbuphine, butorphanol, and pentazocine

Nalbuphine, butorphanol, and pentazocine are synthetic opioid agonist/antagonists. They are partial agonists at kappa and sigmoid opioid receptors but display antagonistic or partial agonist properties at mu opioid receptors. The hope that they would provide good analgesia without the same degree of adverse effects when compared to pure mu agonists initially prompted studies into their potential as labour analgesics.

Dosage and efficacy

When compared to morphine 10 mg, nalbuphine is less potent with a dose of 10–20 mg being required every 4–6 hours. The onset of analgesia is 2–3 minutes with IV administration and within 15 minutes of IM injection. Nalbuphine has a plasma half-life of 5 hours, and in clinical studies the duration of analgesic activity has been reported to range from 3 to 6 hours.[142] Butorphanol is five times more potent than morphine with a typical dose of 1–2 mg given either IV or IM. It has a longer duration of action, of up to 10 hours due to receptor binding.[171] Pentazocine is less potent with a dose of 30–60 mg being required to achieve analgesic effects similar to that to morphine 10 mg. Peak analgesia occurs at 10 minutes after IV administration and within 60 minutes of IM injection.[172] The analgesic effects of nalbuphine and butorphanol are similar to pethidine in IM administration with pentazocine appearing to have inferior labour analgesic properties.[173–176]

Maternal side effects

Despite being mixed mu agonist/antagonists these opioids still exhibit many of the mu-associated side effects. When compared to morphine these opioids result in similar maternal respiratory depression at equivalent analgesic doses but a ceiling effect is noted with increased dose and repeated administration. In comparison to pethidine, they produce less nausea and vomiting but more sedation and dizziness. One study comparing their use for labour analgesia determined that they caused significant maternal respiratory acidosis. These acidotic changes were most marked with pentazocine, moderate with nalbuphine, and minimal with butorphanol.[173,177,178] Pentazocine has limited popularity in obstetrics due to unpleasant psychomimetic effects.[179] A 2011 pilot study suggested that nalbuphine reduced duration of the labour regardless of oxytocin infusion and was without significant risks.[180]

Fetal and neonatal effects

Placental transfer of nalbuphine occurs rapidly. Measurements of umbilical cord blood of nalbuphine levels demonstrate that newborn concentrations vary substantially, ranging from one-third to six times the simultaneous maternal concentration.[173] When comparing nalbuphine with pethidine, studies give some conflicting results regarding adverse effects on the fetus. Some cite nalbuphine as being associated with a decrease in Apgar scores, fetal acidosis, increase in incidences of fetal bradycardia and neonatal hypoxia requiring supplemental oxygen therapy, and even mechanical ventilation, while others do not demonstrate a significant difference in these factors.[181–184] One advantage of nalbuphine over pethidine is the absence of active metabolites, thus, the adverse effects on the neonate are much shorter in duration with nalbuphine than seen with pethidine. Butorphanol also undergoes rapid placental transfer but has a less pronounced acidotic effect on fetal blood gases when compared to nalbuphine and pentazocine. When compared to pethidine, no significant differences in fetal heart rate variability, Apgar scores or neurobehavioural effects have been shown.[174,175,178,185] Pentazocine has similar neonatal depressive effects as pethidine after a single-dose administration, but repeated doses do not have a similar cumulative effect.[186]

Patient-controlled analgesia

In contrast to IV or IM bolus administration, a study comparing nalbuphine PCA, at a dose of 1 mg bolus with 6–10-minute lockout, against IV bolus nalbuphine found that while both methods produced effective pain relief, more satisfactory analgesia was obtained with PCA delivery.[187] When nalbuphine PCA is compared to pethidine PCA, nalbuphine provides more effective maternal analgesia without adverse fetal/neonatal effects.[183] There do not appear to be any studies considering butorphanol or pentazocine PCA for labour analgesia.

Implications for practice

The use of synthetic opioid agonist/antagonists in labour is limited, despite the analgesic effects of nalbuphine and butorphanol being similar to pethidine in IM administration.[173–176] Overall, their side effect profiles do not confer a benefit when compared with pethidine.

Fentanyl

Fentanyl is a phenylpiperidine derivative and is highly protein bound to albumin. It is about 50 times more lipid-soluble than morphine with potency 75–100 times that of morphine and 800 times that of pethidine. Its advantages include rapid onset with a peak effect after 3–4 minutes and lack of active metabolites but its terminal half-life of about 8 hours is longer than that of morphine or pethidine.[116]

Dosage and efficacy

Studies into the use of intermittent bolus fentanyl in labour have typically given parturients 25–50 mcg IV as frequently as every hour with cumulative doses reaching 600 mcg. Parturients experienced worthwhile but transient analgesia, with peak effect at 3–4 minutes and effects lasting up to 45 minutes.[188–190] In one study the effects of fentanyl were rated equivalent to those of pethidine.[191]

Maternal side effects

Maternal nausea, vomiting, and prolonged sedation occur less frequently with fentanyl when compared to pethidine.[191]

Fetal and neonatal effects

Fentanyl crosses the placenta rapidly, with peak fetal concentrations at 5 minutes and an umbilical vein/maternal artery ratio of 0.31.[192] It produces a reduction in baseline fetal heart rate and in beat-to-beat variation lasting for up to 30 minutes and has a temporary respiratory depressant effect on the fetus, particularly with regard to breathing movements, which are abolished at 10 minutes after administration, but return to baseline by 20 minutes.[188,189] However, neonatal assessment of Apgar scores and incidence of respiratory depression show no difference between infants exposed to fentanyl and those with no opioid exposure. Neonates who have been exposed to fentanyl are less likely to require naloxone administration than those exposed to pethidine.[189,191]

Implications for practice

Intermittent bolus fentanyl is not widely used in labour due primarily to its short duration of action.

Patient-controlled analgesia

Fentanyl PCA first was reported in a case report in 1992 for a parturient with thrombocytopenia in which neuraxial blockade was contraindicated. Using a regimen of a fentanyl PCA bolus of 25 mcg with a 10-minute lockout and a background IV infusion of fentanyl at 25 mcg per hour effective analgesia was achieved over almost 12 hours of labour reporting Apgar scores of 9 at 1 and 5 minutes and no adverse effects on the neonate.[192]

Dosage

A dose-finding study for the use of fentanyl PCA as an analgesic option for induced second-trimester termination of pregnancy (TOP) determined that a fentanyl 50 mcg demand bolus with a 6-minute lockout provided satisfactory analgesia for second-trimester labour. This obviously did not assess effects of fentanyl PCA on the fetus and could not be applied directly to normal live birth labour analgesia.[193] A suggested regimen for fentanyl PCA for normal live births consists of a 50 mcg loading dose, 20 mcg bolus, and a lockout period of 5 minutes, although no formal trials for a dose-finding study for fentanyl have been undertaken and published.

Efficacy

An initial study into the use of fentanyl PCA assessed its usefulness for labour analgesia and safety for the newborn when compared with epidural analgesia. In one study, epidural analgesia was found to be significantly more effective with a 30% conversion rate from the PCA fentanyl group to the epidural group due to unsatisfactory pain relief. However, the overall satisfaction between the two groups did not differ.[194] A study comparing fentanyl PCA, with a 10 mch/h continuous infusion and a 10 mcg bolus with 12-minute lockout, with intermittent fentanyl boluses of 50–100 mcg/h, found analgesia, sedation levels, and neonatal to be equivalent for the two groups.[195] In a recent study, despite parturients receiving fentanyl PCA showing significantly longer labour and more need of oxytocin augmentation, compared to controls women expressed their satisfaction with fentanyl PCA use.[196]

Maternal, fetal, and neonatal effects

Fentanyl PCA did not produce any serious maternal side effects and no significant differences in cardiotocography (CTG) abnormalities, Apgar scores, or fetal pH were reported in a 1997 study. However, during 12-hour postpartum monitoring of the neonates a significant number recorded lower SpO_2 levels after fentanyl PCA compared to epidural analgesia.[194] Two further retrospective studies have shown conflicting neonatal outcomes; one found there to be a 44% increase in 'moderately depressed' neonates with neurobehavioral effects lasting up to 7 days post delivery. The total maternal dose of fentanyl in this study was significantly higher for neonates who required naloxone administration. The second study reported no neonatal complications of fentanyl PCA use despite comparable fentanyl doses. The authors of the second study theorized that the major factor behind this difference was the last dose to delivery interval, which was increased from approximately 30 minutes in the first study to 82 minutes in the second.[197,198]

Implications for practice

Fentanyl PCA has a role in clinical practice but it needs to be appreciated that the neonatal effects of fentanyl may persist for a significant period after delivery. If used, the fetus and neonate must be appropriately monitored and naloxone and oxygen should be available if neonatal distress occurs.

Alfentanil and sufentanil

Alfentanil and sufentanil, like fentanyl, are phenylpiperidine derivatives. Alfentanil is highly bound to α_1-glycoprotein and is less lipophilic than fentanyl. Due to its low volume of distribution it has a rapid onset of action, approximately 1 minute, and a shorter duration of action than fentanyl.[199] Theoretically, it therefore should be ideal for labour pain where there is a short period of intense pain easing off over several minutes. However, alfentanil performs disappointingly when tested clinically. Comparison of equipotent doses of alfentanil PCA and fentanyl PCA for labour analgesia found that fentanyl provided more effective analgesia in the first stage of labour than alfentanil PCA with no significant differences in side effects to the parturient or to the fetus/neonate.[200]

Sufentanil is more potent and lipophilic than fentanyl with a shorter duration of action. It has been studied extensively for epidural and intrathecal administration for labour analgesia but its potency limits systemic use in labour. One study comparing its effect for labour analgesia when delivered via intrathecal, epidural, and IV routes concluded that epidural and IV sufentanil did not provide evidence of satisfactory labour analgesia.[201]

Implications for practice

Alfentanil and sufentanil offer less of an analgesic effect than pethidine with no benefit in maternal or neonatal safety profile and in fact alfentanil results in lower neonatal neurobehavioral scores than those parturients who received pethidine.[202] They are therefore not a viable alternative in clinical practice.

Remifentanil

Remifentanil is an ultra-short-acting synthetic phenylpiperidine and a pure mu agonist. It is a derivative of fentanyl with similar potency, but a more rapid onset and offset of action. It exhibits onset of effect at around 1 minute, rapid metabolism by tissue and plasma esterase to inactive metabolites, and has a context-sensitive half-life of 3 minutes. Consequently, there is no accumulation, even after prolonged administration, giving this agent an advantage over other opioids for labour PCA. These properties predict that IV remifentanil could be suitable for the cyclical pain of uterine contractions. Because of this its introduction in the early 1990s heralded a growing interest among obstetric anaesthetists.[203]

Suitability for labour analgesia

At the outset, computerized simulations of the effect site concentrations of remifentanil predicted that the half time for blood effect site equilibration was 1.3–1.6 minutes.[204] A study recording effects on ventilation in volunteers following a 0.5 mcg/kg bolus over 5 seconds reported onset of effect at 30 seconds and peak effect at 2.5 minutes.[205] This suggested that it would be difficult, if not impossible, to coincide peak effect with each uterine contraction with the peak effect being more likely to coincide with the second or subsequent contraction. This may explain why the first published attempt to use remifentanil for labour analgesia fell short of expectations.[206] However, in this study a third party administered the bolus doses of remifentanil, which inevitably lead to a delay in dosing. Though the investigators concluded that remifentanil was ineffective, it is likely that the peak effect occurred in the period between contractions.

Subsequent case reports[207–209] and studies[155,210–214] employing PCA IV devices were more successful. With tutoring, the parturients were able to learn to anticipate the next contraction and to make an early effective demand.[215,216]

Dosage

The efficacy of remifentanil depends on both the dose and the manner in which it is administered. Two feasibility/dose-finding studies have been carried out regarding remifentanil PCA use. In the feasibility study, a bolus dose range of 0.25 to 0.5 mcg/kg produced a median reduction in pain score of 30 mm compared with baseline.[210] The dose-finding study reported a median reduction in pain scores of 42 mm with a median dose of 0.4 mcg/kg.[211] There is, however, no consensus on the optimal dosing regimen for remifentanil with each subsequent study using its own dosing schedule with bolus doses ranging from 0.2 to 0.93 mcg/kg (Table 13.5). The most popular dose by weight used in clinical practice is 0.5 mcg/kg, or for a fixed dose regimen of 40 mcg. Some investigators have commented on the wide individual variation of bolus dose required to achieve effective analgesia. This would suggest a fixed-dose regimen could under-dose and lead to failure of analgesia or could overdose and lead to maternal oxygen desaturation.

Variable dosing regimens may improve matters, particularly during the second stage when reported pain scores are high. However, this would require physician attendance to ensure appropriate monitoring. Two recent randomized crossover studies compared a set bolus dose and infusion rate regimen with a variable dose and infusion rate as it is not only the dose but also the bolus infusion rate and delivery time that are important for efficient pain relief for the developing contraction. They both found that the variable dose and infusion rate regimen was better titrated to individuals' remifentanil requirement, as shown by a lower rate of analgesic requests within the lockout period on the PCA pump.[217,218] The introduction of a background infusion has also been studied. In the feasibility study, which recommended a PCA bolus dose of 0.25–0.5 mcg/kg, the introduction of a background infusion of remifentanil did not improve analgesia, but caused excessive maternal sedation and oxygen desaturation.[210] In contrast, a Canadian study has recommended a PCA bolus of 0.25 mcg/kg with a background infusion of 0.025 to 0.1 mcg/kg/min.[219]

Reported lockout times have also varied, some described lockout times of 2 minutes while others describe a bolus dose delivered over 1 minute with a 1-minute lockout time. With an average uterine contraction time of 70 seconds, it would seem prudent to allow a dose every 2 minutes[220] but a recent editorial recommended a minimum 3-minute lockout time to prevent the administration of additional doses before the peak analgesic effects of a bolus has occurred.[221]

Efficacy

Initial case reports involving women who could not have an epidural for one reason or another reported ineffective analgesia and doubts were raised concerning the effectiveness of IV remifentanil for labour pain.[222] In addition to the dose-finding studies there are three published observational studies regarding the efficacy remifentanil PCA in labour. The dosing regimen in these studies varied, with investigation of a fixed dose of 0.5 mcg/kg; a fixed background infusion dose and an escalating PCA bolus dose; a fixed bolus dose and an escalating background infusion dose and an escalating bolus dose. All of the observational studies reported analgesia with remifentanil with a reduction in significant pain scores from baseline (Table 13.5).[213,219,223]

A number of studies have evaluated remifentanil PCA to IM or IV pethidine, pethidine PCA and fentanyl PCA.[154,155,212,224–225] A recent meta-analysis evaluating randomized controlled trials investigating efficacy and safety of remifentanil administered via a PCA compared with any other analgesic technique for labour pain concluded that remifentanil PCA provided superior analgesia and higher patient satisfaction compared with pethidine with a comparable degree of adverse events.[226] In the most relevant studies where both drugs were administered by PCA, similar mean pain scores were reported with both drugs.

The analgesia provided by IV remifentanil PCA is not complete. In comparison to epidural anaesthesia, randomized control trials have confirmed that epidural analgesia provides superior pain relief, but remifentanil does achieve a reduction in pain scores particularly during the first stage of labour. Despite incomplete analgesia a common theme among all the studies was high maternal satisfaction with remifentanil.[227–231] Further studies are ongoing.[232]

Opioid analgesia in labour, originally introduced as an alternative to inhalational analgesia, does not provide complete analgesia. As a result, Entonox® and opioid analgesia together has become popular when neuraxial analgesia is not used. If remifentanil could provide worthwhile analgesia without the need for Entonox®, this would be a considerable advantage. There is evidence that remifentanil can provide superior analgesia to Entonox® alone.[104] However, it appears that, if given the choice, women would opt to use Entonox® concomitantly despite using remifentanil.[155]

Table 13.5 Remifentanil studies for labour analgesia

Study	Remifentanil PCA dose	Background remifentanil infusion	Lockout interval (min)	Comparison group	Nitrous oxide used	Median or reduction in pain scores with remifentanil	Conversion to neuraxial analgesia
Volmanen et al.[104]	0.4 mcg/kg	None	1	Nitrous Oxide	No	Reduction of 15 mm	Not reported
Douma et al.[154]	40 mcg	No	2	PCA pethidine PCA fentanyl	No	Reduction of 32 mm	Not reported
Blair et al.[155]	40 mcg	None	2	PCA pethidine	Yes	Median 64 mm	2 of 20
Blair et al.[210]	0.25–0.5 mcg/kg	0.025–0.05 mcg/kg/min	2	None	No	Reduction of 30 mm	4 of 21
Volmanen et al.[211]	0.2–0.8 mcg/kg	None	1	None	No	Reduction of 42 mm	Not reported
Thurlow et al.[212]	0.2 mcg/kg	None	3	IM pethidine	Yes	Median 48 mm	7 of 18
Volikas et al.[213]	0.5 mcg/kg	None	2	None	No	Reduction of 23 mm	7 of 50
Evron et al.[214]	0.27–0.93 mcg/kg	None	3	Pethidine infusion	No	Median 35 mm	4 of 43
Buehner et al.[217]	0.5–1 mcg/kg	None	1–2	None	No	94% rated analgesia as good—excellent	9 of 153
Jost et al.[218]	20–55 mcg	50 mcg/hour	1	None	No	Reduction of 25 mm	Not reported
Balki et al.[219]	0.25–1 mcg/kg	0.025 mcg/kg/min (fixed)	2	0.25 mcg/kg + 0.025–0.1 mcg/kg/min (variable)	No	Reduction of 56 mm versus 41 mm in 2 groups	1 of 20
Tveit et al.[223]	0.15–1.05 mcg/kg	None	2	None	No	Reduction of 47 mm	3 of 41
Ng et al.[224]	25–30 mcg	None	4	IM pethidine	No	Reduction of 19 mm	Not reported
Volikas et al.[225]	0.5 mcg/kg	None	2	PCA pethidine	Yes	Reduction of 25 mm	1 of 9
Stourac et al.[227]	20 mcg	None	2	Epidural	No	Reduction of 59 mm	None
Douma et al.[228]	40 mcg	None	2	Epidural	No	Reduction of 38 mm	None
Volmanen et al.[229]	0.3–0.7 mcg/kg	None	1	Epidural	No	Reduction of 25 mm	Not reported
Marwah et al.[230]	0.25 mcg/kg	None	2	PCA fentanyl	No	Reduction of 45 mm	3 of 47
Stocki et al.[231]	20–60 mcg/kg	None	2	Epidural	No	Reduction of 45 mm	Not reported

Data from various sources (see references).

Maternal effects, safety, supervision, and monitoring

Like with other opioid analgesics the major concern is the potential for maternal sedation, respiratory depression, and oxygen desaturation. Virtually all studies report episodes of maternal oxygen desaturation yet comment that they were transient and easily corrected with nasal oxygen or reduction in dose.[233] The comparative studies found that remifentanil PCA caused incidences of maternal oxygen desaturation similar to that for pethidine PCA and slightly higher than that of fentanyl PCA. An appraisal of the literature suggests that 32% of patients in the published studies had some degree of ventilatory depression.[234] Although these findings are comparable to a study that included women with no analgesia where episodes of oxygen desaturation in labour occurred in 46% of women for between 30 seconds to 6 minutes per hour in the second stage of labour, both the timing and the mechanisms are clearly different.[218] A 2013 study comparing the efficacy and respiratory effects of remifentanil PCA with epidural analgesia showed evidence of apnoeic episodes in women without concurrent desaturation. This led the authors to suggest the use of capnography to identify respiratory depression in addition to saturation monitoring.[231] Sedation is also widely reported during remifentanil administration with one study in particular reporting an excessively sedated woman who subsequently desaturated[223] (Table 13.6). Nausea and vomiting is variously reported though as it is endemic in childbirth it is difficult to distinguish a true opioid effect. The highest incidence reported was 48%.[211]

Table 13.6 Maternal and neonatal effects of remifentanil

Study	Remifentanil bolus PCA dose	Maternal desaturation	Maternal sedation	Apgar scores at 1 and 5 minutes
Volmanen et al.[104]	0.4 mcg/kg	None SaO_2 < 93% All given supplemental O_2	Increased sedation scores versus N_2O	9, 9
Douma et al.[154]	40 mcg	37 of 50 (SaO_2 < 95%) 6 of 50 supplemental O_2	Mild to moderate sedation	9, 10
Blair et al.[155]	40 mcg	Similar to pethidine	Similar to pethidine	8, 9
Blair et al.[210]	0.25–0.5 mcg/kg	4 of 21 (SaO_2 < 90%)	2 of 21	8, 9
Volmanen et al.[211]	0.2–0.8 mcg/kg	10 of 17 (SaO_2 < 94%)	Mild sedation	8, 10
Thurlow et al.[212]	0.2 mcg/kg	7 of 18 (SaO_2 < 94%)	Not reported	Not reported
Volikas et al.[213]	0.5 mcg/kg	None SaO_2 < 93%	Mild sedation	9, 9
Evron et al.[214]	0.27–0.93 mcg/kg	None SaO_2 < 94%	None reported	None < 7
Buehner et al.[217]	0.5–1 mcg/kg	16% (SaO_2 < 90%)	Mild to moderate sedation	9, 10
Jost et al.[218]	20–55 mcg	None SaO_2 < 93%	Moderate sedation	Not reported
Balki et al.[219]	0.25–1 mcg/kg	6 of 10	Mild sedation in all	>7
Tveit et al.[223]	0.15–1.05 mcg/kg	None SaO_2 < 91% 11 of 19 supplemental O_2	9 of 19 sedation score > 2	9, 9
Ng et al.[224]	25–30 mcg	None reported	None reported	8, 9
Volikas et al.[225]	0.5 mcg/kg	Not reported	Not reported	9, 10
Stourac et al.[227]	20 mcg	Not reported	Mild sedation	9, 9
Douma et al.[228]	40 mcg	None SaO_2 < 92%	Minimal sedation	8, 9
Volmanen et al.[229]	0.3–0.7 mcg/kg	13 of 24 (SaO_2 < 94%)	13 of 24	9, 9
Marwah et al.[230]	0.25 mcg/kg	6 of 47 (SaO_2 < 90%) 15 of 47 supplemental O_2	4 of 47	9, 9
Stocki et al.[231]	20–60 mcg/kg	13 of 19 (SaO_2 < 94%) All given supplemental O_2 Evidence of apnoea without desaturation	6 of 19 sedation at 1 hour	9, 10

Data from various sources (see references).

As the use of remifentanil for labour analgesia has become more widespread there have been increasing questions asked about its safety profile with some calling for its use to be discontinued.[235–236] The incidence of maternal desaturation shown in the various studies highlights the need for appropriate monitoring, supervision, and training for the caregiver to manage potential adverse events. A recent survey of all UK delivery suites showed that 11% of respondents reported critical incidents related to the use of remifentanil, mostly respiratory depression.[237] Remifentanil is a potent agent and there is the potential for significant harm. To date there have been four case reports describing respiratory arrests with remifentanil PCA.[238–241] While each has their own set of circumstances and potentially confounding factors, their existence cannot and should not be ignored.

In contrast, with appropriate monitoring there is a reasonable volume of study and audit data to support the safe use of remifentanil PCA in labour,[242–243] but high standards must be maintained. There is potentially a temptation to view remifentanil as a cheap and therefore attractive option for labouring women but the appropriate resources and staffing must be available to ensure safety. As one 2013 article put it 'Remifentanil should be viewed as a complimentary method to the more potent neuraxial techniques and not as a "poor man's epidural"'.[244] The view expressed in a 2013 editorial that if appropriate monitoring and supervision of patients cannot be guaranteed at all times then units should not offer remifentanil as an option for labouring women, is a good one.[221] Units choosing to use remifentanil should have stringent guidelines in place to ensure appropriate safeguards for women and regular audit processes to ensure compliance. Women receiving remifentanil PCA must have continuous one-to-one nursing or midwifery care from appropriately trained staff, routine oxygen saturation monitoring, and oxygen supplementation if needed to treat maternal desaturation.[233]

Fetal and neonatal effects

Fundamental to the use of remifentanil in obstetrics were data published in 1998 and 2001. The first study reported placental transfer of an IV remifentanil infusion during caesarean delivery under epidural anaesthesia. Remifentanil readily crossed the placenta with an umbilical vein/maternal artery ratio of 0.82 and, if administered close to the delivery of the neonate, the umbilical artery/vein ratio was 0.29, suggesting rapid metabolism and redistribution in the neonate.[245] The second study reported the pharmacokinetics of remifentanil when used for postoperative pain relief in neonates. The pharmacokinetics was found to be similar to those for older children and adults.[243]

Studies have to date reported reassuring neonatal outcomes. No studies have identified an excess of non-reassuring CTG traces with remifentanil. No association has been found between commencement of PCA and deterioration in the CTG requiring intervention or fetal blood gas sampling. Apgar scores and cord blood gases, where reported, did not show any unexpected deviations from normal practice (Table 13.6). The comparative study of PCA remifentanil with PCA pethidine found fewer non-reassuring CTGs and better neurobehavioral scores in the remifentanil group, and in comparison to fentanyl PCA less neonatal resuscitation was required.[212,214,246] These results seem to confirm remifentanil's rapid metabolism and redistribution in the neonate following placental transfer.

Off-label use

Remifentanil is not licensed for use in obstetric patients. However, the administration of drugs outside their product licence is common in obstetric anaesthesia.[247] Opioids by the spinal and epidural route, as well as all self-prepared mixtures of drugs, are not licensed. Propofol and doses above 250 mg of thiopentone are not licensed either. However, most obstetric anaesthetists are content to use drugs outside the product licence with almost all of the 169 members of the Obstetric Anaesthetists' Association surveyed in 1997 admitting to using drugs outside the product licence in obstetric anaesthesia.[91] It is unlikely that the manufacturers of remifentanil will invest in the cost of obtaining a licence for obstetric use. The onus remains on each clinician to assess the risk:benefit ratio.

Practical experience and implications for practice

In the authors' institution, IV remifentanil PCA is offered for routine use as a labour analgesic. The dosing regimen is a fixed bolus of 40 mcg delivered over 20 seconds with a 2-minute lockout. Supervision is by trained midwives who give one-to-one care with a protocol that includes continuous oxygen saturation monitoring, the constant presence of a midwife, regular documentation of pain scores, respiratory rate, and sedation level, and use of a dedicated cannula with an anti-syphon valve. As with all areas where strong parenteral opioids are administered, full resuscitation equipment is immediately available, with supplemental oxygen and 'bag-valve-mask' apparatus in the room. Other aspects of antepartum care are normal, with intermittent monitoring of CTG unless otherwise indicated. Our continuous audit process has also demonstrated high levels of satisfaction with remifentanil PCA, with many women returning to the unit and choosing the same method of analgesia for subsequent labours. Remifentanil PCA is now the analgesic choice in almost 30% of our deliveries, and since its introduction, the epidural rate in our unit has dropped by one-third.[248] The safety aspects of our institution's guidelines for the administration of remifentanil for labour analgesia are summarized in Table 13.7.

Currently evidence would suggest that remifentanil is more suited than any other systemic opioid to obstetric anaesthesia. It is currently available in over a third of units in the United Kingdom.[238] Time will tell whether its use will become routine elsewhere. Particular care must be taken when other opioids have previously been administered in labour. Continued appraisal and study of administration techniques is needed, particularly in relation to safety, and adverse event reporting should be encouraged. Remifentanil is a potent opioid and its side effect profile demands guidelines and strict adherence to them to ensure maternal and neonatal safety. The risks and benefits of its use should therefore be jointly considered.

Table 13.7 Guidelines for the safe administration of remifentanil patient-controlled intravenous analgesia

	Criteria
Prescription and training	◆ Prescribed by an anaesthetist ◆ Only nurses/midwives who have undergone a period of supervised practice and have been deemed competent may administer this infusion
Eligibility	◆ 36 weeks' gestation ◆ In established labour ◆ Informed consent
Contraindications	◆ Other opioid use in preceding 4 hours ◆ Allergy to opioids ◆ Multiple pregnancy ◆ Pre-eclampsia
Supervision and monitoring	◆ Continuous one-to-one nursing/midwifery supervision ◆ Continuous SaO_2 pulse-oximetry established prior to first administration ◆ 30-minute observations: respiratory rate, sedation score, pain score
Equipment	◆ Dedicated IV cannula ◆ Dedicated PCA administration pump ◆ Unidirectional anti-syphon valve on administration set
Indications for contacting anaesthetist	◆ Excessive sedation score (not rousable to voice) ◆ Respiratory rate < 8 breaths per minute ◆ SaO_2 < 90% despite oxygen via nasal specs

Data from D. Hill & E. Madden, Guideline: Remifentanil controlled analgesia for labour, Ulster Community & Hospitals Trust, Women & Child Health Directorate. 2005.

Systemic analgesia for labour: summary of key points

- Systemic analgesic drugs have variable efficacy and side effect profiles. None produce complete analgesia.
- Inhaled nitrous oxide provides modest analgesic effects for some parturients and may be used either alone or in combination with other forms of analgesia.
- Simple non-opioid analgesics have a place in obstetric analgesia but are likely to be ineffective if used in isolation.
- Sedative drugs have limited application in early labour but are inappropriate as a substitute for analgesia; ketamine may have a role at the time of delivery but is unsuitable for use throughout the course of labour.
- All opioid analgesics readily cross the placenta and therefore all have the potential to cause fetal effects such as reduced heart

rate variability, neonatal respiratory depression, sedation, and neurobehavioural effects.

- Intermittent bolus delivery of opioids such as pethidine has traditionally been the mostly commonly used mode of administration of systemic opioids in labour.
- PCA with short-acting agents such as remifentanil is becoming increasingly popular and offers the parturient more effective analgesia with a greater sense of control in labour.
- PCA in the setting of on-to-one midwifery care is becoming a safe and viable alternative to neuraxial analgesia in for women provided that appropriate monitoring and resources are available and used to safeguard against the risk of respiratory depression.

References

1. Melzach R. The myth of painless childbirth. *Pain* 1984; 19:321–7.
2. Anim-Somuah M, Smyth R, Howell C. Epidural versus non-epidural or no analgesia in labour. *Cochrane Database Syst Rev* 2005; 4:CD000331.
3. Raynes-Greenow CH, Nassar N, Torvaldsen S, *et al.* Assisting informed decision making for labour analgesia: a randomised controlled trial of a decision aid for labour analgesia versus a pamphlet. *BMC Pregnancy Childbirth* 2010; 10:15–27.
4. Lally JE, Murtagh MJ, Macphail S, *et al.* More in hope than expectation: a systematic review of women's expectations and experience of pain relief in labour. *BMC Med* 2008; 6:7.
5. Merskey H, Bogduk N. *Classification of Chronic Pain: IASP Task Force on Taxonomy.* Seattle, WA: IASP Press; 1994.
6. Lowe NK. The nature of labour pain. *Am J Obstet Gynecol* 2002; 1865:S16–S24.
7. Chapman CR, Nakamura Y. A passion of the soul: an introduction to pain for consciousness researchers. *Conscious Cogn* 1999; 8:391–422.
8. Eisenach JC. The pain of childbirth and its effect in the mother and foetus. In Chestnut D (ed). *Obstetric Anesthesia: Principles and Practice* (3rd ed). Philadelphia, PA: Elsevier Mosby, 2004:288–301.
9. Melzack R, Wall PD. Pain mechanisms: a new theory. *Science* 1965; 150:971–5.
10. Melzack R. From the gate to the neuromatrix. *Pain* 1999; 6:S121–S126.
11. Macintyre PE, Schug SA, Scott DA, *et al. Acute Pain Management: Scientific Evidence* (3rd ed). Melbourne: Australian and New Zealand College of Anaesthetists and Faculty of Pain Medicine; 2010.
12. Bonica JJ. Definitions and taxonomy of pain. In Bonica JJ (ed) *The Management of Pain* (2nd ed). Philadelphia, PA: Lea & Febiger, 1990:18–27.
13. Crawford JS. *Principles and Practice of Obstetric Analgesia and Anaesthesia* (5th ed). Oxford: Blackwell Publishing; 1985.
14. Brownridge P. The nature and consequences of childbirth pain. *Eur J Obstet Gynecol Reprod Biol* 1995; 59:S9–S15.
15. McDonald JS. Pain of childbirth. In Loeser JD (ed) *Bonica's Management of Pain* (3rd ed). Philadelphia, PA: Lippincott Williams and Wilkins, 2001:1388–414.
16. Grant GJ. Pharmacologic management of pain during labour and delivery. *UptoDate®* 2013. [Online] http://www.uptodate.com/contents/pharmacologic-management-of-pain-during-labor-and-delivery
17. Sandkuhler J. Models and mechanisms of hyperalgesia and allodynia. *Physiol Rev* 2009; 89(2):707–58.
18. Terman GW, Bonica JJ. Spinal mechanisms and their modulation. In Loeser JD (ed) *Bonica's Management of Pain* (3rd ed). Philadelphia, PA: Lippincott Williams and Wilkins, 2001:73–152.
19. Green CR, Anderson KO, Baker TA, *et al.* The unequal burden of pain: confronting racial and ethnic disparities in pain. *Pain Med* 2003; 4(3):277–94.
20. Burden RJ, Janke EL, Brighouse D. Hyperventilation-induced unconsciousness during labour. *Br J Anaesth* 1994; 73(6):838–9.
21. Hiltunen P, Raudaskoski T, Ebeling H, *et al.* Does pain relief during labour decrease the risk of postnatal depression? *Acta Obstet Gynecol* 2004; 83(3):257–61.
22. Soet JE, Brack GA, Dilorio C. Prevalence and predictors of women's experience of psychological trauma during childbirth. *Birth,* 2003; 30(1):36–46.
23. Enkin M, Keirse MJN, Neilson J, *et al. A Guide to Effective Care in Pregnancy and Childbirth* (3rd ed). Oxford: Oxford University Press; 2000.
24. Porter J. Analgesia in labour: alternative techniques. *Anaesth Intensive Care Med* 2004; 5:235.
25. Carlson, JM, Diehl, JA, Sachtleben-Murray, M, *et al.* Maternal position during parturition in normal labor. *Obstet Gynecol* 1986; 684:443–7.
26. Michel, SC, Rake, A, Treiber, K, *et al.* MR obstetric pelvimetry: effect of birthing position on pelvic bony dimensions. *AJR Am J Roentgenol* 2002; 179(4):1063–7.
27. Simkin, P, O'Hara, M. Non-pharmacologic relief of pain during labor: Systematic reviews of five methods. *Am J Obstet Gynecol* 2002; 186(5):S131–59.
28. Gau ML, Chang CY, Tian SH, *et al.* Effects of birth ball exercises on pain and self-efficacy during childbirth: a randomised controlled trial in Taiwan. *Midwifery* 2011; 27(6):e293–300.
29. Taavoni S, Abdolahian S, Haghani H, *et al.* Effect of birth ball usage on pain in the active phase of labour in the upright delivery positions—a randomised controlled trial. *J Midwifery Womens Health* 2001; 56(2):137–40.
30. Bloom SL, McIntire DD, Kelley MA, *et al.* Lack of effect of walking on labour and delivery. *N Engl J Med* 1998; 339(2):76–9.
31. Gupta, J, Hofmeyr, G, Shehmar M. Position in the second stage of labour for women without epidural anaesthesia. *Cochrane Database Syst Rev* 2012; 5:CD002006.
32. DeClercq, ER, Sakala, C, Corry, MP, *et al.* Listening to Mothers II: Report of the Second National Survey of Women's Childbearing Experiences. *J Perinat Educ* 2007; 16(4):15–17.
33. Simpkin P. Reducing pain and enhancing progress in labour: a guide to non-pharmacological methods for maternity caregivers. *Birth,* 1995; 22(3):161–71.
34. Church LK. Water birth: one birthing center's observations. *J Nurse Midwifery* 1989; 34(4):165–70.
35. Ginesi L, Niescierowicz R. Neuroendocrinology and birth 1: stress. *Br J Midwifery* 1998; 6(10):659–63.
36. Geissbuehler V, Eberhard J. Waterbirths: a comparative study. A prospective study on more than 2,000 waterbirths. *Fetal Diagn Ther* 2000; 15(5):291–300.
37. Cefalo RC, Andre U, Hellgers E. The effects of maternal hyperthermia on maternal and fetal cardiovascular and respiratory function. *Am J Obstet Gynecol* 1978; 131(6):687–94.
38. Richmond H. Women's experiences of waterbirth. *Pract Midwife* 2003; 6(3):26–31.
39. McCandlish R, Renfrew M. Immersion in water during labor and birth: the need for evaluation. *Birth* 1993; 20(2):79–85.
40. Hawkins S. Water versus conventional birth: infections rates compared. *Nurs Times* 1995; 91(15):38–40.
41. Zimmerman R, Huch A, Huch R. Water birth—is it safe? *J Perinat Med* 1993; 21:5–11.
42. Cluett ER, Burns E. Immersion in water in labour and birth. *Cochrane Database Syst Rev* 2009; 2:CD000111.
43. Ohlsson G, Buchhave P, Leandersson U, *et al.* Warm tub bathing during labor: maternal and neonatal effects. *Acta Obstet Gynecol Scand* 2001; 80(4):311–14.

44. Johnson P. Birth under water—to breathe or not to breathe. *Br J Obstet Gynecol* 1996; 103(3):202–8.
45. Rosevear SK, Fox R, Marlow N, *et al.* Birthing pools and the fetus. *Lancet* 1993; 342:1048–9.
46. Deans AC, Steer PH. Temperature of pool is important. *BMJ* 1995; 311:390–1.
47. Department of Health. *National Service Framework for Children, Young People and Maternity Service.* London: Department of Health; 2004. http://www.dh.gov.uk/prod_consum_dh/groups/dh_digitalassets/@dh/@en/documents/digitalasset/dh_4090552.pdf
48. Schmid V, Downe S. Midwifery skills for normalising unusual labours. In Walsh D, Downe S (eds) *Essential Midwifery Practice: Intrapartum Care.* Chichester: Blackwell Publishing; 2010:159–90.
49. Vickers A, Zollman C. ABC of complementary therapies: massage therapies. *BMJ* 1999; 319:1254–7.
50. Ernst E, Koeder K. An overview of reflexology. *Eur J Gen Pract* 1997; 3:52–7.
51. Botting D. Review of literature on the effectiveness of reflexology. *Complement Ther Nurs Midwifery* 1997; 3:123–30.
52. Chang MY, Wang SY, Chen CH. Effects of massage on pain and anxiety during labour: a randomized controlled trial in Taiwan. *J Adv Nurs* 2002; 38:68–73.
53. Kimber l, McNabb, M, McCourt C, *et al.* Massage or music for pain relief in labour: a pilot randomised placebo controlled trial. *Eur J Pain* 2008; 12(8):961–9.
54. Smith CA, Levett KM, Collins CT, *et al.* Massage, reflexology and other manual methods for pain management in labour. *Cochrane Database Syst Rev* 2012; 2:CD009290.
55. Rich GJ. *Massage Therapy: The Evidence for Practice.* Philadelphia, PA: Elsevier; 2002.
56. Simkin P, Klein MC. Non-pharmacological approaches to management of labour pain. *UptoDate®* 2012. [Online] http://www.uptodate.com/contents/nonpharmacological-approaches-to-management-of-labor-pain
57. Ahn AC. Acupuncture. *UptoDate®* 2012. [Online] http://www.uptodate.com/contents/acupuncture
58. Umeh BUO. Sacral acupuncture for pain relief in labour: Initial clinical experience in Nigerian women. *Acupunct Electrother Res* 1986; 11:147–51.
59. Wallis L, Shnider SM, Palahniuk RJ, *et al.* An evaluation of acupuncture analgesia in obstetrics. *Anaesthesiology* 1974; 416:596–601.
60. Cho SH, Lee H, Ernst E. Acupuncture for pain relief in labour: a systematic review and meta-analysis. *Br J Obstet Gynecol* 2010; 117(8):907–20.
61. Lee H, Cho SH, Ernst E. Meta-analysis of randomised controlled trials (RCTs) involving acupuncture for labour pain shows acupuncture to be more effective than comparison treatments in analgesic consumption but the overall evidence is still limited, calling for further investigations. *Br J Obstet Gynecol* 2011; 118(2):101–2.
62. National Institute for Health and Clinical Excellence. *Intrapartum Care: Care of Healthy Women and Their Babies during Childbirth.* Clinical Guideline 55. London: National Institute for Health and Clinical Excellence; 2007.
63. Janco M, Trontelj J. TENS: a microneurographic and perceptual study. *Pain* 1980; 9:219–30.
64. Salar G, Job I, Mingrino S, Bosio A, *et al.* Effects of transcutaneous electrotherapy on CSF beta-endorphin content in patients without pain problems. *Pain,* 1981; 10:169–72.
65. Habanananda T. Non-pharmacological pain relief in labour. *J Med Assoc Thai* 2004; 87(3):S194–202.
66. Carroll D, Tramèr M, McQuay H, *et al.* Transcutaneous electrical nerve stimulation in labour pain: a systematic review. *Br J Obstet Gynecol* 1997; 104:169–75.
67. Thomas IL, Tyle V, Webster J, *et al.* An evaluation of transcutaneous electrical nerve stimulation for pain relief in labour. *Aust N Z J Obstet Gynaecol* 1988; 28:182–9.
68. Reynolds JL. Practice tips. Intracutaneous sterile water injections for low back pain during labour. *Can Fam Physician* 1998; 44:2391–2.
69. Huntley AL, Coon JT, Ernst E. Complementary and alternative medicine for labor pain: a systematic review. *Am J Obstet Gynecol* 2004; 191(1):36–44.
70. Derry S, Straube S, Moore RA, *et al.* Intracutaneous or subcutaneous sterile water injection compared with blinded controls for pain management in labour. *Cochrane Database Syst Rev* 2012; 1:CD009107.
71. Mårtensson L, Wallin G. Sterile water injections as treatment for low-back pain during labour: a review. *Aust N Z J Obstet Gynaecol* 2008; 48(4):369–74.
72. Bahasadri S, Ahmadi-Abhari S, Dehghani-Nik M, *et al.* Subcutaneous sterile water injection for labour pain: a randomised controlled trial. *Aust N Z J Obstet Gynaecol* 2006; 46(2):102–6.
73. Ader L, Hansson B, Wallin G. Parturition pain treated by intracutaneous injections of sterile water. *Pain* 1990; 41:133–8.
74. Wiruchpongsanon P. Relief of low back labor pain by using intracutaneous injections of sterile water: a randomized clinical trial. *J Med Assoc Thai* 2006; 89(5):571–6.
75. Trolle B, Moller M, Kronborg H, *et al.* The effect of sterile water blocks on low back labor pain. *Am J Obstet Gynecol* 1991; 164:1277–81.
76. Labrecque M, Nouwen A, Bergeron M, *et al.* A randomized controlled trial of non-pharmacologic approaches for relief of low back pain during labor. *J Fam Pract* 1999; 48(4):259–63.
77. Stevensen CJ. The psychophysiological effects of aromatherapy massage following cardiac surgery. *Complement Ther Med* 1995; 2:27–35.
78. Burns EE, Blamey C, Ersser SJ, *et al.* An investigation into the use of aromatherapy in intrapartum midwifery practice. *J Altern Complement Med* 2000; 6(2):141–7.
79. Smith CA, Collins CT, Crowther CA. Aromatherapy for pain management in labour. *Cochrane Database Syst Rev* 2011; 7:CD009215.
80. Tiran D. Massage and aromatherapy. In Tian D, Mack S (eds) *Complementary Therapies for Pregnancy and Childbirth* (2nd ed). New York: Balliere Tindal; 2000:129–68.
81. Maimburg RD, Vaeth M, Durr J, *et al.* Randomised trial of structured antenatal training sessions to improve the birth process. *Br J Obstet Gynaecol* 2010; 117(8):921–8.
82. Smith CA, Levett KM, Collin CT, *et al.* Relaxation techniques for pain management in labour. *Cochrane Database Syst Rev* 2011; 12:CD009514.
83. Phumdoung S, Good M. Music reduces sensation and distress of labour pain. *Pain Manag Nurs* 2003; 4(2):54–61.
84. Mantle F. The role of hypnosis in pregnancy and childbirth. In Tian D, Mack S (eds) *Complementary Therapies for Pregnancy and Childbirth* (2nd ed). New York: Balliere Tindal; 2000:215–24.
85. Madden K, Middleton P, Cyna AM, *et al.* Hypnosis for pain management during labour and childbirth. *Cochrane Database Syst Rev* 2011; 11:CD009356.
86. Oakley DA. Hypnosis, trance and suggestion: evidence from neuroimaging. In Nash MR, Barnier AJ (eds) *The Oxford Handbook of Hypnosis: Theory, Research and Practice.* Oxford: Oxford University Press; 2008:365–92.
87. Landolt AS, Milling LS. The efficacy of hypnosis as an intervention for labour and delivery pain: a comprehensive methodological review. *Clin Psychol Rev* 2011; 31(6):1022–31.
88. Doula UK. [Website] www.doula.org.uk
89. Evidence Based Birth. [Website] www.evidencebasedbirth.com
90. Hodnett ED, Gates S, Hofmeyr GJ, *et al.* Continuous support for women during childbirth. *Cochrane Database Syst Rev* 2012; 10:CD003766.
91. Rosen MA. Nitrous oxide for relief of labor pain: a systematic review. *Am J Obstet Gynecol* 2002; 186:S110–26.
92. Clyburn P. The use of Entonox for labour pain should be abandoned. Opposer. *Int J Obstet Anesth* 2001; 10:25–39.

93. Australian Institute of Health and Welfare. *Australian Mother and Babies 2007: Perinatal Status Report.* [Online] http://www.preru.unsw.edu.au/PRERUWeb.nsf/page/ps23
94. Rooks JP. Nitrous oxide for pain in labor-why not in the United States? *Birth* 2007; 34(1):3–5.
95. Gibbs CP, Krischer J, Peckham BM, *et al.* Obstetric anesthesia: a national survey. *Anesthesiology* 1986; 65(3):298–306.
96. Wong CA. Epidural and spinal analgesia/anesthesia for labor and vaginal delivery. In Chestnut DH, Polley LS, Tsen LC, *et al.* (eds) *Chestnut's Obstetric Anesthesia: Principles and Practice.* Philadelphia, PA: Mosby Elsevier; 2009:429–92.
97. Westling F, Milsom I, Zetterstrom H, *et al.* Effects of nitrous oxide oxygen inhalation on the maternal circulation during vaginal delivery. *Acta Anaesthesiol Scand* 1992; 36(2):175–81.
98. Minnich ME. Childbirth preparation and non-pharmacologic analgesia. In Chestnut DH, Polley LS, Tsen LC, *et al.* (ed). *Chestnut's Obstetric Anesthesia: Principles and Practice.* Philadelphia, PA: Mosby Elsevier; 2009:405–14.
99. Ranta P, Jouppila P, Spalding M, *et al.* Parturients' assessment of water blocks, pethidine, nitrous oxide, para-cervical and epidural blocks in labour. *Int J Obstet Anesth* 1994; 3(4):193–8.
100. Harrison RF, Shore M, Woods T, *et al.* A comparative study of transcutaneous electrical nerve stimulation (TENS) entonox, pethidine + promazine, and lumbar epidural for pain relief in labor. *Acta Obstet Gynecol Scand* 1987; 66(1):9–14.
101. Olofsson C, Ekblom A, Ekman-Ordeberg G, *et al.* Lack of analgesic effect of systemically administered morphine or pethidine on labour pain. *Br J Obstet Gynecol* 1996; 103:968–72.
102. Carstoniu J, Levytam S, Norman P, *et al.* Nitrous oxide in early labor: safety and analgesic efficacy assessed by a double-blind, placebo-controlled study. *Anesthesiology* 1994; 80:30–5.
103. Yentis SM. The use of Entonox for labour pain should be abandoned. Proposer. *Int J Obstet Anesth* 2001; 10(1):25–9.
104. Volmanen P, Akural E, Raudaskoski T, *et al.* Comparison of remifentanil and nitrous oxide in labour analgesia. *Acta Anaesthesiol Scand* 2005; 49(4):453–8.
105. Lucas DN, Siemaszko O, Yentis SM. Maternal hypoxemia associated with the use of Entonox in labour. *Int J Obstet Anesth* 2000; 9(4):270–2.
106. McAneny T, Doughty AG. Self-administration of nitrous oxide/oxygen in obstetrics. *Anaesthesia* 1963; 18:488–97.
107. Stefani S, Hughes S, Shnider S, *et al.* Neonatal neurobehavioral effects of inhalation analgesia for vaginal delivery. *Anesthesiology* 1982; 56(5):351–5.
108. Griffin RP, Reynolds F. Maternal hypoxemia during labour and delivery: the influence of analgesia and effect on neonatal outcome. *Anaesthesia* 1995; 50(2):151–6.
109. Creely CE, Olney JW. The young: neuroapoptosis induced by anesthetics and what to do about it. *Anesth Analg* 2010; 110(2):442–8.
110. Bambrink AM, Evers AS, Avidan MS, *et al.* Isoflurane-induced neurapoptosis in the neonatal rhesus macaque brain. *Anesthesiology,* 2010; 112(4):834–41.
111. Sanders RD, Weimann J, Maze M. Biologic effects of nitrous oxide. *Anesthesiology,* 2008; 109(4):707–22.
112. Mills GG, Singh D, Longan M, *et al.* Nitrous oxide exposure on the labour ward. *Int J Obstet Anesth* 1996; 5(3):160–4.
113. Rowland AS, Baird DD, Weinberg CR, *et al.* Reduced fertility among women employed as dental assistants exposed to high levels of nitrous oxide. *N Engl J Med* 1992; 327(14):993–7.
114. Health and Safety Executive. *EH 40/2005. Workplace Exposure Limits.* [Online] www.hseni.gov.uk/eh40_2005.pdf
115. Rudra A. Pain relief in labour—review article. *Update Anaesth* 2004; 18:3.
116. Wee, M. Analgesia in labour: inhalational and parenteral. *Anaesth Intensive Care Med* 2004; 5(7):233–4.
117. Yeo ST, Holdcroft A, Yentis SM, *et al.* Analgesia with sevoflurane in labour. II. Sevoflurane compared with entonox for labour analgesia. *Br J Anaesth* 2007; 98:110–15.
118. Malaise O, Bruyere O, Jean-Yves R. Intravenous paracetamol: a review of efficacy and safety in therapeutic use. *Future Neurol* 2007; 2(6):673–88.
119. Graham GG, Scott KF, Day RO. Tolerability of paracetamol. *Drug Safety* 2005; 28(3):227–40.
120. Hyllested M, Jones S, Pedersen JL, *et al.* Comparative effect of paracetamol, NSAIDs or their combination in postoperative pain management: a qualitative review. *Br J Anaesth* 2002; 88(2):199–214.
121. Elbohoty AEH, Abd-Elrazek H, Abd-El-Gawad M, *et al.* Intravenous infusion of paracetamol versus intravenous pethidine as an intrapartum analgesic in the first stage of labor. *Int J Gynecol Obstet* 2012; 118(1):7–10.
122. Elbohoty AEH. Intravenous infusion of paracetamol for intrapartum analgesia of labor. *ClinicalTrials.gov,* Identifier: NCT01428375. [Online] http://clinicaltrials.gov/ct2/show/NCT01428375
123. Othman M, Jones L, Neilson JP. Non-opioid drugs for pain management in labour. *Cochrane Database Syst Rev* 2012; 11CD009223.
124. Ostensen ME. Safety of non-steroidal anti-inflammatory drugs during pregnancy and lactation. *Inflammopharmacology* 1996; 4:31–41.
125. Ganla KN, Deshmukh S, Bhide A, *et al.* Analgesia in labor by intermittent intravenous bolus. *J Obstet Gynecol* 2000; 4:60–2.
126. Wakefield ML. Systemic analgesia: parenteral and inhalational agents. In Chestnut D (ed) *Obstetric Anesthesia: Principles and Practice* (3rd ed). Philadelphia, PA: Mosby Elsevier; 2004:311–23.
127. Stevenson C. Ketamine—a review. *Update Anaesth* 2005; 20:25–9.
128. Hawkins JL. Obstetric analgesia and anesthesia. In Gibbs RS, Karlan BY, Kaney AF, *et al.* (eds) *Danforth's Obstetrics and Gynecology* (10th ed). Philadelphia, PA: Lippincott, Williams, and Wilkins; 2008:43–59.
129. Elbourne D, Wiseman RA. Types of intra-muscular opioids for maternal pain relief in labour. *Cochrane Database Syst Rev* 1998; 4:CD001237.
130. Benyamin R, Trescot AM, Datta A, *et al.* Opioid complications and side effects. *Pain Physician* 2008; 11:S105–S120.
131. Bailey PL, Egan TD, Stanley TH. Intravenous opioid anesthetics. In Miller RD (ed) *Anesthesia* (5th ed, Volume 1). Philadelphia, PA: Churchill Livingstone 2000:273–376.
132. Ala-Kokko T, Vähäkangas K, Pelkonen O. Placental function and principles of drug transfer. *Acta Anaesthesiol Scand* 1993; 37:47–9.
133. Littleford J. Effects on the fetus and newborn of maternal analgesia and anesthesia: a review. *Can J Anaesth* 2004; 51(6):586–609.
134. Maguie W, Fowlie PW. Naloxone for narcotic exposed newborn infants. *Cochrane Database Syst Rev* 2002; 4:CD003483.
135. Al-Hashimi M, Scott SWM, Thompson JP, *et al.* Opioids and immune modulation: more questions than answers. *Br J Anaesth* 2013; 111(1):80–8.
136. Budd K. Pain management: is opioid immunosuppression a clinical problem? *Biomed Pharmacother* 2006; 60(7):310–17.
137. Brewin C, Bradley C. Perceived control and the experience of childbirth. *Br J Clin Psychol* 1982; 21:263–9.
138. Green J. Expectations and experiences of pain in labour—findings from a large prospective study. *Birth* 1993; 20:65–72.
139. McCrea HB, Wright M. Satisfaction in childbirth and perceptions of personal control in pain relief during labour. *J Adv Nurs* 1999; 29(4):877–84.
140. Hill D. The use of remifentanil in obstetrics. *Anesthesiol Clin* 2008; 26:169–82.
141. Saravanakumar K, Garstang J S, Hasan K. Intravenous patient-controlled analgesia for labour: a survey of UK practice. *Int J Obstet Anesth* 2007; 16(3):221–5.
142. Yentis SM, Hirsch NP, Smith GP. *Anaesthesia and Intensive Care A-Z: An Encyclopedia of Principles and Practice* (3rd ed). London: Elsevier; 2004.
143. Bricker L, Lavender T. Parenteral opioids for labor pain relief: a systematic review. *Am J Obstet Gynecol* 2002; 186(5):S94–S109.
144. Ullman R, Smith LA, Burns E, *et al.* Parenteral opioid for maternal pain relief in labour. *Cochrane Database Syst Rev* 2010; 9:CD007396.

145. Soontrapa S, Somboonporn W, Komwilaisak R, *et al.* Effectiveness of intravenous meperidine for pain relief in the first stage of labour. *J Med Assoc Thai* 2002; 85:1169–75.
146. Thomson AM, Hillier VF. A re-evaluation of the effect of pethidine on the length of labour. *J Adv Nurs* 1994; 19(3):448–56.
147. Morselli PL, Rovei V. Placental transfer of pethidine and norpethidine and their pharmacokinetics in the newborn. *Eur J Clin Pharmacol* 1980; 18(1):24–30.
148. Jones L, Othman JL, Dowswell T, *et al.* Pain management for women in labour: an overview of systematic reviews. *Cochrane Database Syst Rev* 2012; 3:CD009234.
149. Kariniemi V, ÄMmälä P. Effects of intramuscular pethidine on fetal heart rate variability during labour. *Br J Obstet Gynecol* 1981; 88(7):718–20.
150. Fortescue C, Wee M. Analgesia in labour: non-regional techniques. *CEACCP* 2005; 5(1):9–13.
151. Nissen E, Widstrom AM, Lilja G, *et al.* Effects of routinely given pethidine during labour on infants' developing breastfeeding behaviours. Effects of dose-delivery time interval and various concentrations of pethidine/norpethidine in cord plasma. *Acta Paediatri* 1997; 86(2):201–8.
152. Pereira RR, Kanhai H, Rosendaal F, *et al.* Parenteral pethidine for labour pain relief and substance use disorder: 20-year follow-up cohort study in offspring. *BMJ Open,* 2012; 2(3):1–4.
153. Rayburn W, Leuschen MP, Earl R, *et al.* Intravenous meperidine during labour: a randomised comparison between nursing and patient controlled administration. *Obstet Gynecol* 1989; 74(5):702–6.
154. Douma MR, Verwey RA, Kam-Endtz CE, *et al.* Obstetric analgesia: a comparison of patient-controlled meperidine, remifentanil, and fentanyl in labour. *Br J Anaesth* 2010; 104(2):209–15.
155. Blair JM, Dobson GT, Hill DA, *et al.* Patient controlled analgesia for labour: a comparison of remifentanil with pethidine. *Anaesthesia* 2005; 60(1):22–7.
156. Leong WL, Sng BL, Sia AT. A comparison between remifentanil and meperidine for labor analgesia. *Anesth Analg* 2011; 113(4):818–25.
157. Khan K, Chang J. Neonatal abstinence syndrome due to codeine. *Arch Dis Child Fetal Neonat Ed* 1997; 76(1):F59–F60.
158. Medicines and Healthcare products Regulatory Agency. *Codeine: Restricted Use as Analgesic in Children and Adolescents after European Safety Review.* [Online] www.mhra.gov.uk/safetyinformation/drugsafetyupdate/CON287006
159. Husslein P, Kubista E, Egarter C. Obstetrical analgesia with tramadol—results of a prospective randomized comparative study with pethidine. *Z Geburtshilfe Perinatol* 1987; 191(6):234–7.
160. Viegas OAC, Khaw B, Ratnam SS. Tramadol in labor pain in primiparous patients. A prospective comparative clinical trial. *Eur J Obstet Gynecol Reprod Biol* 1993; 49(3):131–5.
161. Houmes R-JM, Voets MA, Verkaaik A, *et al.* Efficacy and safety of tramadol versus morphine for moderate and severe postoperative pain with special regard to respiratory depression. *Anesth Analg* 1992; 74(4):510–14.
162. Crighton IM, Martin PH, Hobbs GJ, *et al.* A comparison of the effects of intravenous tramadol, codeine, and morphine on gastric emptying in human volunteers. *Anesth Analg* 1998; 87(2):445–9.
163. Vickers MD, O'Flaherty D, Szekely SM, *et al.* Tramadol: pain relief by an opioid without depression of respiration. *Anaesthesia* 1992; 47(4):291–6.
164. Long J, Yue Y. Patient controlled intravenous analgesia with tramadol for labor pain relief. *Chin Med J* 2003; 116(11):1752–5.
165. Tuckey JP, Prout RE, Wee MYK. Prescribing intramuscular opioids for labour analgesia in consultant-led maternity units: a survey of UK practice. *Int J Obstet Anesth* 2008; 17(1):3–8.
166. Fairlie FM, Marshall L, Walker JJ, *et al.* Intramuscular opioids for maternal pain relief in labour: a randomised controlled trial comparing pethidine with diamorphine. *Br J Obstet Gynecol* 1999; 106(11):1181–7.
167. Gerdin A, Salmonson T, Lindberg B, *et al.* Maternal kinetics of morphine during labour. *J Perinat Med* 1990; 18(6):479–87.
168. Gerdin E, Rane A, Lindberg B. Transplacental transfer of morphine in man. *J Perinat Med* 1990; 18(4):305–12.
169. McInnes RJ, Hillan E, Clark D, *et al.* Diamorphine for pain relief in labour: a randomised controlled trial comparing intramuscular injection and patient controlled analgesia. *Br J Obstet Gynaecol* 2004; 111(10):1081–9.
170. Wee M, Tuckey, JP, Thomas P, *et al.* The IDvIP Trial: a two-centre randomized double-blind controlled trial comparing intramuscular diamorphine and intramuscular pethidine for labour analgesia. *BMC Pregnancy Childbirth* 2011; 11:51.
171. Peck TE, Will SA, Williams M. *Pharmacology for Anaesthesia and Intensive Care* (2nd ed). Cambridge: Cambridge University Press; 2004.
172. Jaffe JH, Martin WR. Opioids with mixed actions: partial agonists. In Gilman AG, Rall TW, Nies AS, *et al.* (ed) *The Pharmacological Basis of Therapeutics* (8th ed). New York: Pergamon Press; 1990:512–14.
173. Wilson SJ, Errick JK, Balkon J. Pharmacokinetics of nalbuphine during parturition. *Am J Obstet Gynaecol* 1986; 155(2):340–4.
174. Maduska AL, Hajghassemali M. A double blind comparison of butorphanol and meperidine in labour: maternal pain relief and effects on the newborn. *Can Anaesth Soc J* 1978; 25(5):398–404.
175. Hodgkinson R, Huff RW, Hayashi RH, *et al.* Double-blind comparison of maternal analgesia and neonatal behavior following intravenous butorphanol and meperidine. *J Int Med Res* 1979; 7(3):224–30.
176. Dan U, Rabinovici Y, Barkai G, *et al.* Intravenous pethidine and nalbuphine during labor: a prospective double-blind comparative study. *Gynecol Obstet Invest* 1991; 32(1):39–43.
177. Wahab SA, Askalani AH, Amar RA, *et al.* Effect of some recent analgesics on labor pain and maternal and fetal blood gases and pH. *Int J Gynecol Obstet* 1988; 26(1):75–80
178. Kallos T, Caruso FS. Respiratory effects of butorphanol and pethidine. *Anaesthesia* 1979; 34(7):633–7.
179. Taylor M, Galloway DB, Petrie JC, *et al.* Psychomimetic effects of pentazocine and dihydrocodeine tartrate. *Br Med J* 1978; 2:1198.
180. Kim, TH, Kim JM, Lee HH, *et al.* Effect of nalbuphine hydrochloride on the active phase during first stage labour: a pilot study. *J Obstet Gynaecol* 2011; 31(8):724–7.
181. Guillonneau M, Jacqz-Aigrain E, de Crepy A, *et al.* Perinatal adverse effects of nalbuphine given during parturition. *Lancet* 1990; 335:1588.
182. Nicolle E, Devillier P, Delanoy B, *et al.* Therapeutic monitoring of nalbuphine: Transplacental transfer and estimated pharmacokinetics in the neonate. *Eur J Clin Pharmacol* 1996; 49(6):485–9.
183. Frank M, McAteer EJ, Cattermole R, *et al.* Nalbuphine for obstetric analgesia. A comparison of nalbuphine with pethidine for pain relief in labour when administered by patient-controlled analgesia (PCA). *Anaesthesia* 1987; 42(7):697–703.
184. Quilligan EJ, Keegan KA, Donahue MJ. Double blind comparison of intravenously injected butorphanol and meperidine in parturients. *Int J Obstet Gynecol* 1980; 18(5):363–7.
185. Giannina G, Guzman ER, Lai Y-L, *et al.* Comparison of the effects of meperidine and nalbuphine on intrapartum fetal heart rate tracings. *Obstet Gynecol* 1995; 86(3):441–5.
186. Refstad SO, Lindbaek E. Ventilatory depression of the newborn of women receiving pethidine or pentazocine. *Br J Anaesth* 1980; 52(3):265–71.
187. Podlas J, Breland BB. Patient-controlled analgesia with nalbuphine during labor. *Obstet Gynecol* 1987; 70(2):202–4.
188. Smith CV, Rayburn WF, Allen KV, *et al.* Influence of intravenous fentanyl on fetal biophysical parameters during labour. *J Matern Fetal Med*1996; 5(2):89–92.
189. Rayburn WF, Rathke A, Leuschen P, *et al.* Fentanyl citrate analgesia during labour. *Am J Obstet Gynaecol* 1989; 161(1):202–6.
190. Shafer SL, Varvel JR. Pharmacokinetic, pharmacodynamics and rational opioid selection. *Anaesthesiology* 1991; 74(1):53–63.

191. Rayburn WF, Smith CV, Parriott JE, *et al.* Randomised comparison on meperidine and fentanyl during labour. *Obstet Gynaecol* 1989; 74(4):604–6.
192. Rosaeg OP, Kitts JB, Koren G, *et al.* Maternal and fetal effects of intravenous patient-controlled fentanyl analgesia during labour in a thrombocytopenic parturient. *Can J Anaesth* 1992; 39(3):277–81.
193. Castro C, Tharmaratnam U, Brockhurst N, *et al.* Patient controlled analgesia with fentanyl provides effective analgesia for second trimester labour: a randomized controlled study. *Can J Anaesth* 2003; 50(10):1039–46.
194. Nikkola EM, Ekblad UU, Kero PO, *et al.* Intravenous fentanyl PCA during labour. *Can J Anaesth* 1997; 44(12):1248–55.
195. Rayburn WF, Smith CV, Leuschen MP, *et al.* Comparison of patient controlled and nurse administered analgesia using intravenous fentanyl during labour. *Anaesthesiol Rev* 1991; 18(1):31–6.
196. Miyakoshi K, Tanaka M, Morisaki H, *et al.* Perinatal outcomes: Intravenous patient controlled fentanyl versus no analgesia in labour. *J Obstet Gynaecol Res* 2013; 39(4):783–9.
197. Morley-Forster PK, Weberpals J. Neonatal effects of patient controlled analgesia using fentanyl in labour. *Int J Obstet Anesth* 1998; 7(2):103–7.
198. Hosokawa Y, Morisaki H, Nakatsuka I, *et al.* Retrospective evaluation of intravenous fentanyl patient controlled analgesia during labour. *J Anaesth* 2012; 26(2):219–24.
199. Shafer SL, Varvel JR. Pharmacokinetics, pharmacodynamics, and rational opioid selection. *Anesthesiology* 1991; 74(1):53–63.
200. Morley-Forster PK, Reid DW, Vandeberghe H. A comparison of patient controlled analgesia fentanyl and alfentanil for labour analgesia. *Can J Anaesth* 2000; 47(2):113–19.
201. Camann WR, Denney RA, Holby ED, *et al.* A comparison of intrathecal, epidural and intravenous sufentanil for labour analgesia. *Anesthesiology* 1992; 77(5):884–7.
202. Shannon KT, Ramanathan S. Systemic medication for labour analgesia. *Obstet Pain Manage* 1995; 2:1–6.
203. Egan TD. Pharmacokinetics and pharmacodynamics of remifentanil: an update in the year 2000. *Curr Opin Anaesthesiol* 2000; 13(4):449–55.
204. Egan TD, Minto CF, Hermann DJ, *et al.* Remifentanil versus alfentanil: comparative pharmacokinetics and pharmacodynamics in healthy adult male volunteers. *Anesthesiology* 1996; 84(4):821–33.
205. Babenco HD, Conard PF, Gross JB. The pharmacodynamics effect of a remifentanil bolus on ventilatory control. *Anesthesiology* 2000; 92(2):393–8.
206. Olufolabi AJ, Booth JV, Wakeling HG, *et al.* A preliminary investigation of remifentanil as a labor analgesic. *Anesth Analg* 2000; 91(3):606–8.
207. Thurlow JA, Waterhouse P. Patient-controlled analgesia in labour using remifentanil in two parturients with platelet abnormalities. *Br J Anaesth* 2000; 84(3):411–13.
208. Jones R, Pegrum A, Stacey RG. Patient-controlled analgesia using remifentanil in the parturient with thrombocytopenia. *Anaesthesia* 1999; 54(5):461–5.
209. Owen MD, Poss MJ, Dean LS, *et al.* Prolonged intravenous remifentanil infusion for labor analgesia. *Anesth Analg* 2002; 94(4):918–19.
210. Blair JM, Hill DA, Fee JP. Patient controlled analgesia for labour using remifentanil: a feasibility study. *Br J Anaesth* 2001; 87(3):415–20.
211. Volmanen P, Akural EI, Raudaskoski T, *et al.* Remifentanil in obstetric analgesia: a dose- finding study. *Anesth Analg* 2002; 94(4):913–17.
212. Thurlow JA, Laxton CH, Dick A, *et al.* Remifentanil by patient controlled analgesia compared with intramuscular meperidine for pain relief in labour. *Br J Anaesth* 2002; 88(3):374–8.
213. Volikas I, Butwick A, Wilkinson C, *et al.* Maternal and neonatal side effects of remifentanil patient-controlled analgesia in labour. *Br J Anaesth* 2005; 95(4):504–9.
214. Evron S, Glezerman M, Sadan O, *et al.* Remifentanil: a novel systemic analgesic for labor pain. *Anesth Analg* 2005; 100(1):233–8.
215. Volmanen P, Alahuhta S. Will remifentanil be a labour analgesic? *Int J Obstet Anesth* 2004; 13(1):1–4.
216. Dhileepan S, Stacey RG. A preliminary investigation of remifentanil as a labor analgesic. *Anesth Analg* 2001; 92(5):1358–9.
217. Buehner U, Broadbent JR, Chesterfield B. Remifentanil patient controlled analgesia for labour: a complete audit cycle. *Anaesth Intensive Care* 2011; 39(4):666–70.
218. Jost A, Ban B, Kamenik M. Modified patient-controlled remifentanil bolus delivery regimen for labour pain. *Anaesthesia* 2013; 68(3): 245–52.
219. Balki M, Kasodekar S, Dhumne S, *et al.* Remifentanil patient-controlled analgesia for labour: optimizing drug delivery regimens. *Can J Anaesth* 2007; 54(8):626–33.
220. Caldero-Barcia, Poseiro JJ. Physiology of the uterine contraction. *Clin Obstet Gynecol* 1960; 3:386–408.
221. Machatuta NA, Kinsella SM. Remifentanil for labour analgesia: time to draw breath? *Anaesthesia* 2013; 68(3):231–5.
222. Lacassie HJ, Olufolabi AJ. Remifentanil for labor pain: Is the drug or the method the problem? *Anesth Analg* 2005; 101(4):1242–3.
223. Tveit TO, Halvorsen A, Seiler S, *et al.* Efficacy and side effects of intravenous remifentanil patient controlled analgesia used in a stepwise approach for labour: an observational study. *Int J Obstet Anesth* 2013; 22(1):19–25.
224. Ng TK, Cheng BC, Chan WS, *et al.* A double blind randomised comparison of intravenous patient controlled remifentanil with intramuscular pethidine for labour analgesia. *Anaesthesia* 2011; 66(9):796–801.
225. Volikas I, Male D. A comparison of pethidine and remifentanil patient controlled analgesia in labour. *Int J Obstet Anesth* 2001; 10(2):86–90.
226. Schnabel A, Hahn N, Broscheit J, *et al.* Remifentanil for labour analgesia: a meta-analysis of randomised controlled trials. *Eur J Anaesthesiol* 2012; 29(4):177–85.
227. Stourac P, Suchomelova H, Stodulkova M, *et al.* Comparison of parturient—controlled remifentanil with epidural bupivacaine and sufentanil for labour analgesia: randomised controlled trial. *Biomed Pap Med Fac Univ Palacky Olomouc Czech Repub* 2014; 158(2):227–32.
228. Douma MR, Middledorp JM, Verwey RA, *et al.* A randomised comparison of intravenous remifentanil patient—controlled analgesia with epidural ropivicaine/sufentanil during labour. *Int J Obstet Anaesth* 2011; 20(2):118–23.
229. Volmanen P, Sarvela J, Akural EL, *et al.* Intravenous remifentanil vs epidural levobupivicaine with fentanyl for pain relief in early labour: a randomised, controlled, double-blinded study. *Acta Anaesthesiol Scand* 2008; 52(2):249–55.
230. Marwah R, Hassan S, Carvalho JC, *et al.* Remifentanil versus fentanyl for intravenous patient-controlled labour analgesia: an observational study. *Can J Anaesth* 2012; 59(3):246–54.
231. Stocki D, Matot I, Einav S, *et al.* A randomized controlled trial of the efficacy and respiratory effects of patient-controlled intravenous remifentanil analgesia and patient-controlled epidural analgesia in laboring women. *Anaesth Analg* 2013; 118(3):589–97.
232. Freeman LM, Bloemenkamp KW, Franssen MT, *et al.* Remifentanil patient controlled analgesia versus epidural analgesia in labour. A multicentre randomized controlled trial. *BMC Pregnancy Childbirth* 2012; 12:63.
233. Hinova A, Fernando R. Systemic remifentanil for labour analgesia. *Anesth Analg* 2009; 109:1925–9.
234. Van de Velde M. Remifentanil patient- controlled analgesia should be routinely available for use in labour. *Int J Obstet Anesth* 2008; 17: 339–42.
235. Sneyd R. Remifentanil on the labour ward, *Anaesthesia* 2012; 67(9):1045–6.

236. Kan RE, Hughes SC, Rosen MA, *et al.* Intravenous remifentanil: placental transfer, maternal and neonatal effects. *Anesthesiology,* 1998; 88(6):1467–74.
237. Howie KM, Millar S. Usage of remifentanil patient controlled analgesia in labour in the UK. *Int J Obstet Anesth* 2011; 20:S36.
238. Bonner JC, McClymont W. Respiratory arrest in an obstetric patient using remifentanil patient-controlled analgesia. *Anaesthesia* 2012; 67(5):538–40.
239. Pruefer C, Bewlay A. Respiratory arrest with remifentanil patient-controlled analgesia—another case. *Anaesthesia* 2012; 67(9):1044–5.
240. Marr R, Hyams J, Bythell V. Cardiac arrest in an obstetric patient using remifentanil patient-controlled analgesia. *Anaesthesia* 2013; 68(3):283–7.
241. Kinney MA, Rose CH, Traynor KD, *et al.* Emergency bedside cesarean delivery: lessons learned in teamwork and patient safety. *BMC Res Notes* 2012; 5:412.
242. McMackin P, Hodgkinson P, Foley P, *et al.* Remifentanil PCA for labour: completing the audit cycle. Abstracts of free papers presented at the annual congress of the AAGBI, Edinburgh. *Anaesthesia* 2011; 66:S1.
243. Laird R, Hughes D, Hill D. Audit of remifentanil patient-controlled analgesia for labour. Abstracts of free papers presented at the annual meeting of the Obstetric Anaesthetists Association, Sheffield. *Int J Obstet Anesth* 2007; 16:S43.
244. Kranke P, Girard T, Lavand'homme P, *et al.* Must we press on until a young mother dies? Remifentanil patient-controlled analgesia in labour may not be suited as a "poor man's epidural". *BMC Pregnancy Childbirth* 2013; 13:139.
245. Ross AK, Davis PJ, Dear GL, *et al.* Pharmacokinetics of remifentanil in anesthetized pediatric patients undergoing elective surgery or diagnostic procedures. *Anesth Analg* 2001; 93(6):1393–401.
246. Griffin RP, Reynolds F. Maternal hypoxemia during labour and delivery: the influence of analgesia and effect on neonatal outcome. *Anaesthesia* 1995; 50(2):151–6.
247. Howell PR, Madej TH. Administration of drugs outside of product license: awareness and current practice. *Int J Obstet Anesth* 1999; 8(1):30–6.
248. Hughes D, Hodgkinson P. Remifentanil PCA for labour analgesia. *Anaesthesia* 2013; 68(3):298.

CHAPTER 14

Initiation of neuraxial labour analgesia

Eva Roofthooft, Sarah Devroe, and Marc Van de Velde

Introduction

Labour, although a natural process, can be very painful and lengthy. Many parturients will request some form of analgesia. Labour analgesia can be non-pharmacological (see Chapter 13) or pharmacological. Pharmacological options include inhalational analgesia with nitrous oxide and/or volatile anaesthetics (Chapter 13), parenteral opioids (pethidine, fentanyl, alfentanil, sufentanil, morphine, diamorphine, or remifentanil—see Chapter 13) or central neuraxial techniques (epidural, spinal or combined spinal–epidural (CSE)—see Chapters 14–19). Neuraxial labour analgesia has been extensively researched and debated in the recent decades. Arguably, neuraxial analgesia is the most effective strategy to manage labour pain in contemporary clinical obstetric practice.[1–3] It is the only method that can block both the impulses from the first stage of labour entering the spinal cord at T10–L1 and the impulses of the second stage of labour entering the spinal cord via sacral roots S2–S4 (see Chapter 13). Effective analgesia has significant maternal and fetal/neonatal advantages in terms of reducing the negative effects of stress. However, neuraxial analgesia is also associated with side effects which impact on mother, fetus, neonate, and the process of labour.[2–4]

When anaesthetists plan for a central neuraxial analgesic strategy, several vital choices have to be made (Figure 14.1):

- How should analgesia be initiated?
- How should analgesia be maintained (see Chapter 15)?
- What is the dose and concentration of the local anaesthetic that is used (see Chapter 16)?
- Which local anaesthetic agent (see Chapter 16) and which adjuvant drugs (see Chapter 17) should be used for initiation and maintenance of analgesia?

In this chapter we will discuss the various options of labour analgesia initiation.

Most commonly neuraxial analgesia is initiated using a conventional epidural approach in which an epidural catheter is threaded into the epidural space and used for initiation and maintenance. In the last 25 years, CSE analgesia has gained widespread acceptance and popularity. With a spinal injection, analgesia is rapidly achieved and the epidural catheter is used only for maintenance. Initiating analgesia using a single-shot spinal injection is less common and is usually reserved for very specific indications (such as full cervical dilatation). Also, continuous spinal analgesia using intrathecally inserted catheters has been used for labour analgesia, but is only recommended in very specific high-risk patients or following an accidental dural puncture.

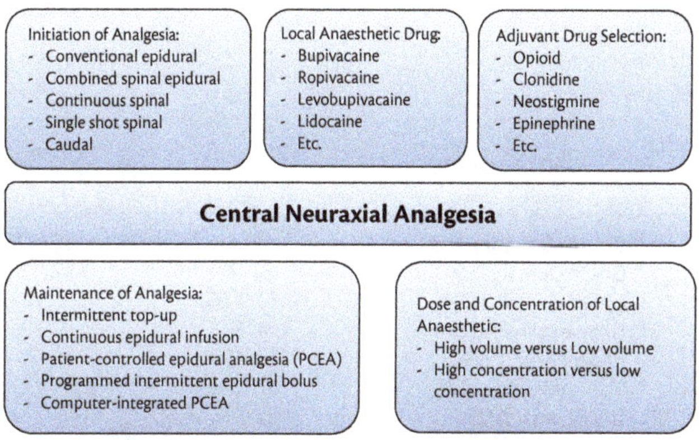

Figure 14.1 When central neuraxial analgesia is performed to alleviate labour pain, anaesthetists need to make several decisions and have several choices: how is analgesia initiated? Which local anaesthetic and adjuvant drug is used? How is analgesia maintained? Which dose and concentration of local anaesthetic is used?

Preparation for initiation of neuraxial analgesia

Indications and contraindications

Whenever women in labour experience pain, analgesia should be offered. Neuraxial blockade is one of the options available and modern clinical guidelines clearly state that no women in labour, when requesting neuraxial analgesia, should be denied receiving it. In 2007, the National Institute of Clinical Excellence (now the National Institute of Health and Care Excellence (NICE)) first published its guideline on *Intrapartum Care: Care of Healthy Women and their Babies during Childbirth* and stated 'Women in labour who desire regional analgesia should not be denied it, including women in severe pain in the latent first stage of labour'.[5] The American College of Obstetricians and Gynecologists (ACOG) in 2006 and the American Society of Anesthesiologists in 2007 stated that in the absence of contraindications, a maternal request for analgesia is a sufficient enough reason to receive it and that neuraxial analgesia is an appropriate method of labour pain relief.[6,7] It used to be thought that initiating labour analgesia early

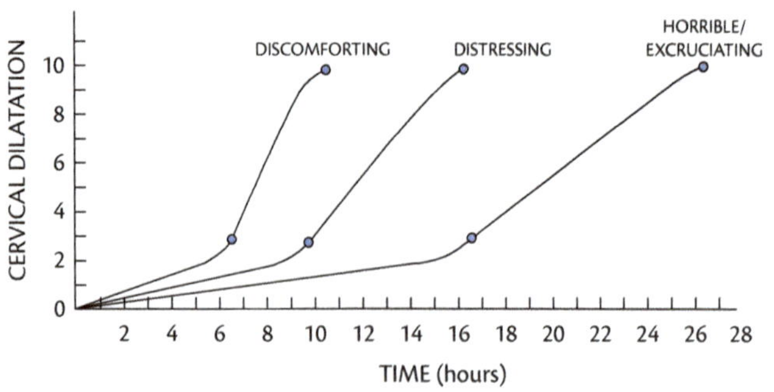

Figure 14.2 Relationship between pain intensity in latent, early labour and speed of cervical dilatation. Severe pain in early labour also resulted in more instrumental deliveries and hence is an indicator of dystocia.

would have a detrimental effect on the course of labour. However, severe pain early in labour is an independent indicator of dystocia or difficult, prolonged labour, often resulting in an instrumental delivery (Figure 14.2).[8] It has also been clearly demonstrated that neuraxial labour analgesia initiated during early labour, does not impact on labour outcome (Figure 14.3).[9,10]

Although many contraindications exist for neuraxial anaesthesia, several contraindications are relative and an individualized risk/benefit analysis, especially in obstetric patients, should be considered. Absolute and relative contraindications are listed in Box 14.1. However, in most instances experienced obstetric anaesthetists will, based on an individualized risk assessment, initiate neuraxial analgesia.

Preoperative assessment

Ideally every parturient undergoing peripartum neuraxial analgesia should be screened preoperatively for informed consent

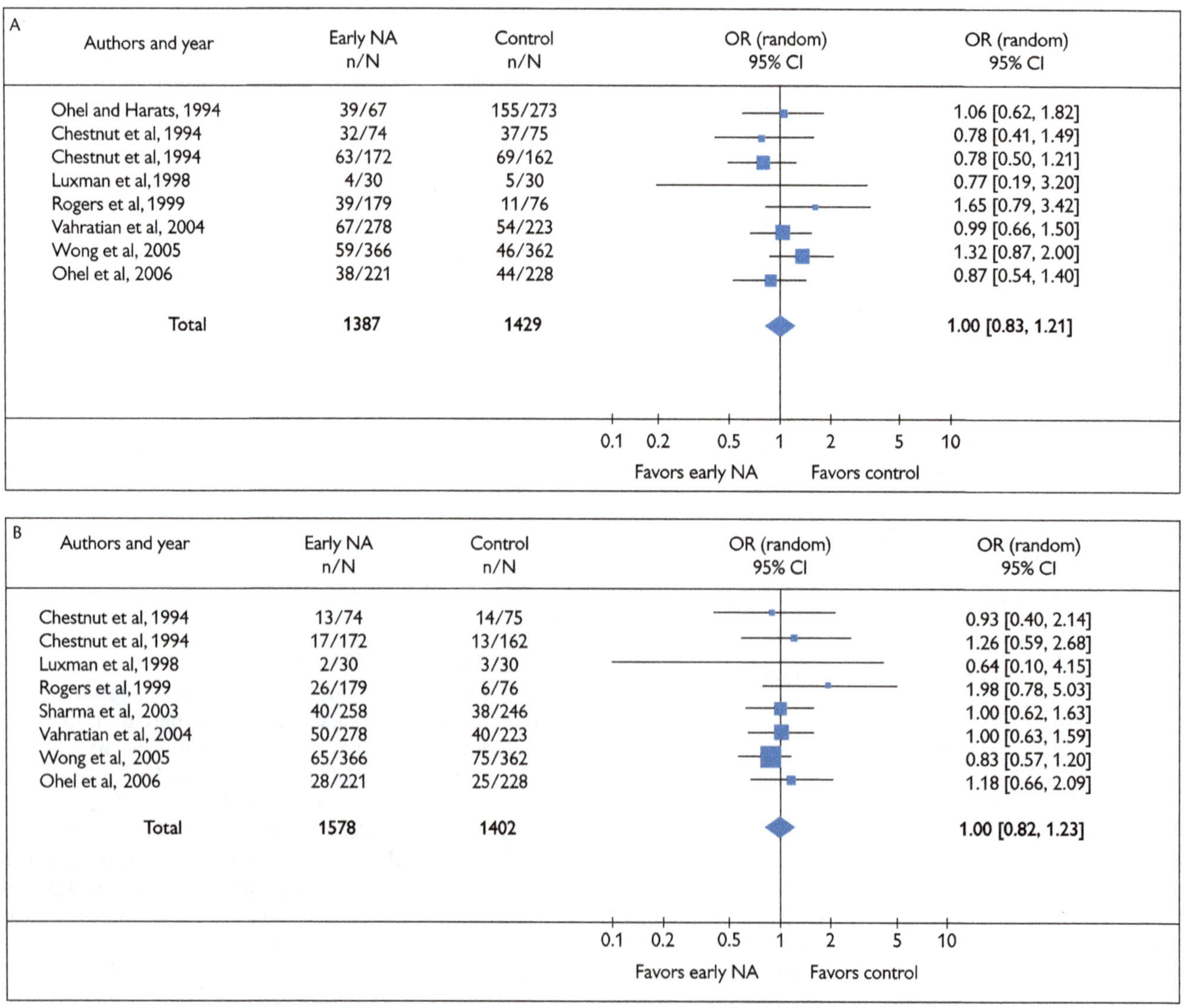

Figure 14.3 Rates of instrumental vaginal delivery (A) and caesarean delivery (B) for each of the studies with odds ratios (ORs) and 95% confidence intervals (CI). The diamond represents the point estimate of the pooled OR, and the length of the diamond is proportional to the CI. Neuraxial analgesia on patient request did not increase the chance of an instrumental vaginal delivery or caesarean delivery. Please refer to original paper for references.

n = number of events in treatment or control group; N = total number of patients in treatment or control group; NA = neuraxial analgesia.

Box 14.1 Absolute and relative contraindications to neuraxial anaesthesia/analgesia in the parturient

Of note: experienced anaesthesiologists will often insert, based on an individualized risk/benefit assessment, neuraxial anaesthesia in patients with relative contraindications.

Absolute contraindications

- Overt coagulopathy
- Infection at puncture site
- Acutely raised intracranial pressure
- Uncorrected, severe hypovolaemia
- Patient refusal
- Patient inability to cooperate.

Relative contraindications

- Mild or single-factor coagulopathy
- Chronic raised intracranial pressure
- Corrected hypovolaemia
- Systemic infection
- Stenotic valvular lesions
- Pulmonary hypertension (Eisenmenger type)
- Pre-existing neurological disease.

and to identify risks. In some countries, every parturient is seen antenatally prior to delivery. However, in everyday routine clinical practice in many regions, parturients are first seen by the anaesthetist on the day of labour. A focused history and short clinical examination should be made as well as a review of the patient's obstetric history.[11–13] According to the American Society of Anesthesiologists guidelines, the short clinical examination should include a baseline blood pressure measurement and airway, heart, lung, and back examinations. In healthy parturients, no laboratory investigations are required (also a routine platelet count is not necessary), but these may become necessary in selected patients.[11,12,14] All guidelines agree that close communication between obstetricians, midwives, and anaesthetists must be maintained, focusing on adequate handovers and early labour ward rounds to identify parturients at high risk for complications or operative delivery. Pre-anaesthetic assessment of fetal well-being by recording the fetal heart rate by a qualified individual is recommended.

Informed consent

To inform parturients about neuraxial analgesia risks and benefits, structured information should be available in every unit that offers neuraxial analgesia (patient information sessions or antenatal classes, printed leaflets, possibility for an individualized pre-delivery consult, etc.). However, as already mentioned, patients will often not have received information about analgesia before entering the labour process. Information of risks should be given as well as advantages.[15] Several authors have questioned the women's capacity, especially when being distressed and in pain, to fully understand the information provided and to give consent.[16,17] However, anaesthetists act in the best interest of the patient and this should be made clear to the patient and her partner. For further information we refer to Chapter 29.

Intravenous lines and fluids

All parturients undergoing neuraxial analgesia should have an intravenous (IV) line established. Most guidelines do not recommend a fixed amount of fluid, especially in circumstances when low-dose CSE or epidural analgesia is used.[5,7,12] However, many practitioners will prehydrate the patient with 500–1000 mL crystalloid solution. A bolus of glucose-containing fluids is best avoided.

Necessary equipment and safety precautions

Equipment to resuscitate a patient and airway equipment should be readily available. Drugs to induce general anaesthesia (propofol, thiopental, ketamine, midazolam), opioid reversal (naloxone), cardiovascular support (ephedrine, phenylephrine, atropine, epinephrine, calcium) and treatment of local anaesthetic systemic toxicity (LAST; Intralipid® 20%) should be available in the labour and delivery area.[18,19] Cardiotocographic monitors should be available to monitor uterine activity and fetal heart rate immediately after initiation of analgesia. During initiation, fetal heart rate monitoring is not absolutely mandatory provided the pregnant patient is healthy and the fetal status was reassuring prior to initiation. However in some countries or regions, local guidelines may request cardiotocographic monitoring during neuraxial analgesia initiation. Non-invasive maternal blood pressure and heart rate monitoring should be instituted during neuraxial analgesia initiation.

Patient positioning

Patient and anaesthetist preference should guide the best position to perform the neuraxial procedure. Both the lateral decubitus and the sitting position are widespread. However, both positions have advantages and disadvantages (Box 14.2). Immediately following the procedure the patient can be placed in the left lateral

Box 14.2 Advantages of the lateral decubitus or sitting position to perform neuraxial analgesia in labour

Advantages of lateral position

- Less hypotension
- Increased parturient comfort
- Better continuous fetal heart rate monitoring
- Less venous cannulation by the epidural catheter.

Advantages of sitting position

- Better and more reliable identification of Tuffier's line.
- Better anatomical landmark identification in 'difficult back' patients (obesity, back surgery, scoliosis)
- Improved respiratory mechanics
- Better and more reliable identification of Tuffier's line.

position or wedged supine position. Careful attention is required to avoid aortocaval compression, essential to maintain cardiac output and uteroplacental perfusion.[20] The wedged supine position is often preferred with conventional epidural analgesia to enhance bilateral local anaesthetic spread. With CSE, spread of the intrathecal dose is excellent and bilateral irrespective of the position employed, therefore maintaining the left lateral position might be preferred.

Aseptic technique

Before initiating neuraxial analgesia and placing spinals or epidurals, careful disinfection of the skin is required using either povidone-iodine or chlorhexidine 0.5% in alcohol. Checketts et al. showed that chlorhexidine is more effective then povidone-iodine.[21] However, it must be remembered that these substances are potentially neurotoxic and recently catastrophic cases of inadvertent administration of disinfectant into the epidural and spinal space have been reported, resulting in progressive quadriplegia.[22,23] Therefore, care must be taken not to contaminate needles with disinfectant so as not to introduce the disinfectant into the epidural or subarachnoid space. Hence the neuraxial analgesia procedure should only be started when the disinfectant has dried onto the skin, thus minimizing the risk of inadvertent transfer of disinfectant into the epidural or spinal space.

Different options of neuraxial analgesia initiation

Several options to initiate analgesia exist with conventional epidural analgesia being the most popular and most widely employed technique (Boxes 14.3 and 14.4). Since the early 1990s, the CSE technique for labour analgesia has gained worldwide acceptance and is an established method of labour pain relief.[24,25] In certain institutions and countries, it is even as popular as an epidural.[26] Rarely used methods to initiate labour analgesia are the caudal, continuous spinal, and single-shot spinal technique. We refer to other textbooks for extensive information regarding the technical aspects of the different neuraxial techniques.

Box 14.3 Possible procedure to initiate epidural analgesia

1. Site IV line and administer crystalloid IV fluid load (500 mL).
2. Position patient sitting or full left lateral.
3. Have assistant disinfect the skin (with chlorhexidine solution). No disinfectant should be on the epidural tray. Only initiate neuraxial anesthesia when skin is dry.
4. Prepare epidural set and prepare necessary drugs in a sterile fashion.
5. Site epidural catheter.
6. Administer test dose (note: this is questioned by many practitioners).
7. Fixate epidural catheter.
8. Position parturient supine with left lateral tilt.
9. Administer low-concentration local anaesthetic solution with adjuvant (usually opioid) in a volume of 10–20 mL in incremental doses.
10. Have maternal vital signs and fetal heart rate monitored for at least 30–45 minutes.
11. Assess efficacy of epidural analgesia and initiate appropriate measures if pain relief is not achieved after 30 minutes.
12. Start maintenance analgesia (see Chapter 15).

Box 14.4 The ideal drug or drug combination for labour analgesia

- Rapid onset of analgesia
- Large sensory–motor separation thus avoiding motor block
- Long-acting drug
- Low risk of local anaesthetic systemic toxicity (LAST)
- No effect on uterine activity
- No effect on uteroplacental perfusion
- Limited transplacental passage
- No direct effects on the fetus.

To perform safe neuraxial analgesia or anaesthesia, a thorough understanding of the anatomy of the vertebral column, the spinal canal, and epidural space is required. Seven cervical, 12 thoracic, 5 lumbar, 5 fused sacral, and 3–5 (most commonly 4) fused coccygeal vertebrae comprise the vertebral column. The spinal cord comes down from the brainstem and terminates as the conus medullaris at the lower border of the L1 vertebral body (and even lower in at least 5% of individuals).[27] The lower lumbar and sacral nerve roots run down to the coccyx as the cauda equina. Three membranes surround the spinal cord within the vertebral column: the pia mater, the arachnoid mater, and the dura mater. In between the pia mater and the arachnoid mater lies the subarachnoid space containing cerebrospinal fluid (CSF) which runs down to the level of S2. Spinal anaesthesia is performed by injecting anaesthetics in this space. Between the arachnoid mater and the dura mater, lies a potential space called the subdural space, which can be created by traumatic punctures and this may explain patchy or failed epidural blocks with higher than expected cephalad spread.[28,29] The epidural space surrounds the dura mater circumferentially and extends from the foramen magnum, where the dura mater and periosteum fuse, to the sacrococcygeal ligament. The space contains adipose tissue, blood vessels, nerve roots, and loose connective tissue in a non-uniform distribution. The ligamentum flavum is the posterior boundary of the epidural space. Epidural anaesthesia/analgesia is performed by inserting a catheter and/or injecting drugs into the epidural space.

Initiation using conventional epidural analgesia

Epidural anaesthesia technique

To identify the epidural space, special equipment is required, including an epidural needle, an epidural catheter, and a loss of resistance (LOR) syringe. The epidural needle is usually a 16 G to 18 G needle with an end opening and Huber tip (Tuohy needle). The epidural catheter is made out of plastic and depending on the type and manufacturer has varying degrees of stiffness. Another difference between various epidural catheters is that they can be single-orifice catheters or multi-orifice catheters. Advantages of multi-orifice catheters include better spread of local anaesthetic and the ability to aspirate blood or CSF to identify inappropriate location of the catheter. The epidural space is usually identified using the LOR technique. The medium used for LOR is either saline or air. Several investigators have suggested that the LOR to air technique should no longer be used because of a higher incidence of accidental dural puncture,[30,31] more postdural puncture headache (PDPH),[32] more pneumocephalus, more risk for patchy analgesia,[31] and more paraesthesias. However, in experienced hands, LOR to air is a safe technique.[33]

The epidural needle is advanced into the interspinous ligament and gradually advanced by the operator's non-dominant hand while the thumb of the operator's dominant hand applies constant or intermittent pressure to the LOR syringe. Upon entering the epidural space, the content of the LOR syringe flows easily into the epidural space. Then a catheter is advanced into the epidural space, and the needle pulled back, after which the catheter is pulled back until the catheter remains 3–5 cm in the epidural space. In many institutions, micropore filters are used in between the epidural catheter and the infusion fluid to protect against infection. However, there is no evidence that they actually do have a protective effect.[34] It must be emphasized that filters may hamper the aspiration of CSF or blood, hence aspiration, using a 2 mL syringe needs to be performed without a filter. Following fixation of the epidural catheter, the patient is positioned supine with left lateral tilt.

Test dose

Following insertion of an epidural catheter, the catheter can accidentally have been placed intrathecally or intravascularly. Intravascular cannulation of the epidural catheter occurs in up to 9% of obstetric patients.[35,36] Especially when high doses of local anaesthetic are administered, the risk of LAST or high/total spinal anaesthesia is significant and potentially life-threatening. Therefore, identification of catheter misplacement is crucial. For this purpose a so-called test dose is administered (Box 14.5). Ideally a test dose should have a high specificity (low false-positive rate) and high sensitivity (low false-negative rate). Unfortunately no test dose is 100% full proof. A negative response to a test dose decreases the chance of catheter malpositioning, but does not exclude it. Also throughout the course of labour, epidural catheter migration has been described.[37,38] Hence a catheter tested following placement, should always be re-tested when high doses of local anaesthetic are administered as a bolus (e.g. when topping up a labour epidural for caesarean delivery).

When dilute epidural analgesic solutions are used, several obstetric anaesthetists question the need to use a formal test dose. They argue that the risk of LAST or high spinal block is virtually non-existent when low-concentration epidural solutions are given and incremental dosing is used when top-ups are given. The first dose then serves as a test dose. Moreover, an epinephrine-containing test dose may increase the risk of motor block in the parturient[39] and detrimentally affects uteroplacental perfusion,[40] while lidocaine 40–60 mg intrathecally will produce some degree of motor block which is undesirable in labour.[41] Furthermore, during CSE analgesia, because of the immediate effect of the spinal component, a test dose to assess intrathecal placement of the epidural catheter is not useful. Finally, in labouring patients, test doses that rely on a tachycardic response to evaluate intravascular catheter placement are found to be difficult to interpret, because of significant maternal heart rate variability during labour. Additionally, when multi-orifice catheters are used, careful aspiration of the catheter (without a micropore filter) will in many instances allow identification of misplacement since CSF or blood will be aspirated. Therefore, many practitioners will not give a formal test dose when low-concentration epidural solutions are used for labour pain relief.[42] They will aspirate the catheter and give the first therapeutic dose fractionated and consider this the test dose.

However, when large doses are given, a test dose is necessary. Table 14.1 gives an overview of the various testing modalities of an epidural catheter and the expected response when the catheter is intravascular or intrathecal.

Box 14.5 Disadvantages of a formal test dose to evaluate intravascular or intrathecal placement of the epidural catheter

- Low specificity: large heart rate variability in labour resulting in a false-positive test dose
- Effects of epinephrine on uteroplacental perfusion
- Effects of lidocaine and epinephrine on motor function
- Difficulty testing the catheter when placed as part of a CSE.

Choice of local anaesthetic: drug, concentration, and dose

We refer to more detailed information in Chapter 16. Although theoretically all local anaesthetics can be used for epidural labour analgesia, in clinical practice the choice is limited to one of four local anaesthetics: lidocaine, bupivacaine, levobupivacaine, and ropivacaine. In contemporary obstetric anaesthesia practice, lidocaine is rarely used for neuraxial labour pain relief because of its short duration and concerns about neonatal neurobehavioral scores.[43–47]

Bupivacaine is probably the most popular local anaesthetic worldwide for neuraxial labour analgesia. The advantages of high-volume, low-concentration solutions to initiate epidural analgesia have been clearly demonstrated. Less motor block and better labour outcome of lower epidural local anaesthetic concentrations were well demonstrated by the Comparative Obstetric Mobile Epidural Trial (COMET) trial.[48] Christiaens et al. and Lyons et al. in two methodologically different studies elegantly showed that high-volume analgesia results in better quality analgesia with less local anaesthetic consumption probably due to better epidural sacral spread.[49,50]

It has been shown, using the up-and-down sequential allocation methodology, that ropivacaine and levobupivacaine are less potent then bupivacaine at the effective dose in 50% of subjects (ED_{50}).[51–53] However, more recent work by Ngan Kee et al. showed that at the ED_{95} this difference was much smaller and not statistically significant[54] (Figure 14.4). Theoretically ropivacaine

Table 14.1 Epidural catheter testing modalities

Testing modality	Result when IV catheter	Result when IT catheter
Lidocaine 1.5% with epinephrine 5 mcg/mL (1:200,000) 3–4 mL	An increase in heart rate of 20 bpm within 60 seconds	Motor blockade (reduced hip flexion) within 5 minutes
Bupivacaine 0.25% with epinephrine 5 mcg/mL (1:200,000) 3–4 mL	Increase in heart rate of 20 bpm within 60 seconds	Motor blockade (reduced hip flexion) within 5 minutes
Lidocaine 100 mg	Tinnitus, circumoral paraesthesia	Motor blockade (reduced hip flexion) within 5 minutes
Ropivacaine 25 mg	Tinnitus, circumoral paraesthesia	Motor blockade (reduced hip flexion) within 5 minutes
Fentanyl 100 mcg	Dizziness, sleepy feeling	No effect
Air 1 mL	Doppler heart sound changes	
Lidocaine 40–60 mg	No effect	Motor blockade (reduced hip flexion) within 5 minutes
Bupivacaine 7.5 mg	No effect	Motor blockade (reduced hip flexion) within 5 minutes
Aspiration of catheter	Blood	Cerebrospinal fluid

Note that an epidural catheter can migrate and re-testing is required whenever a large bolus dose is administered.

bpm, beats per minute; IT, intrathecal, IV, intravascular.

and levobupivacaine produce less systemic toxicity and have the potential for reduced motor block, which is especially important in labouring patients.

All local anaesthetics can produce systemic toxicity by direct and indirect mechanisms that derive from their mode of action, that is, inhibition of voltage-gated ion channels.[55–57] Furthermore, local anaesthetics also interfere with mitochondrial respiration by impeding oxidative phosphorylation, thus depleting the cell's energy reserve. Ropivacaine and levobupivacaine both have lower systemic toxicity then bupivacaine.[55–57] Evidence from *in vitro* studies, *ex vivo* whole-organ studies, animal studies, studies in volunteers, and case reports shows that ropivacaine is the least toxic, levobupivacaine has intermediate toxicity, and bupivacaine is the most toxic.[58] Reduced systemic toxicity has also been demonstrated in pregnant animals.[59]

Halpern and Walsh performed a meta-analysis of 23 randomized trials that compared ropivacaine and bupivacaine during labour analgesia.[60] Onset, duration, and quality of analgesia were similar between the two local anaesthetics. No differences in mode of delivery or other outcome parameters were identified, except for a more frequent incidence of motor block with bupivacaine. Several individual studies using low concentrations of local anaesthetic (≤0.125%) did demonstrate differences in motor block with ropivacaine producing less motor block then bupivacaine.[61–69] This difference in motor block especially becomes apparent when

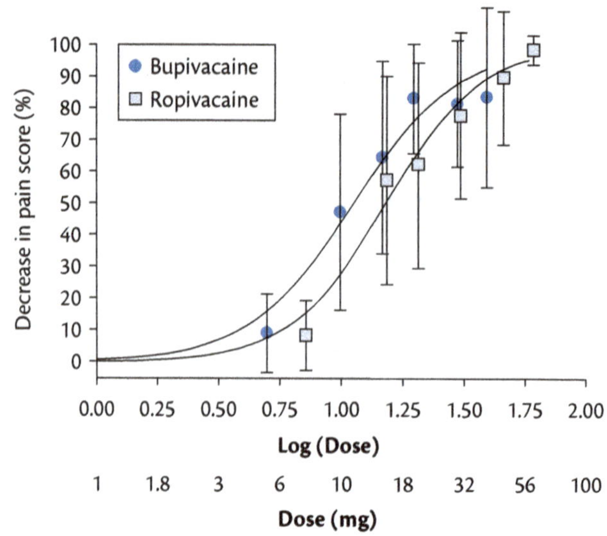

Figure 14.4 Dose–response curves for effective analgesia in labour comparing bupivacaine and ropivacaine. At the ED_{95} both drugs had similar potency.
Data from Scanlon JW, Brown WU Jr, Weiss JB, Alper MH. Neurobehavioral responses of newborn infants after maternal epidural anesthesia. *Anesthesiology*, 1974, volume 40, issue 2, pp. 121–128.

analgesia is required for more than 4–5 hours as Gautier et al. and Halpern et al. clearly demonstrated (Figure 14.5).[63,69] In the study by Gautier et al.,[63] this difference persisted even if lower concentrations of epidural bupivacaine were used to provide analgesia. Table 14.2 gives an overview of motor block reported in several studies that compared low and similar concentrations of ropivacaine and bupivacaine during labour analgesia. However, for completeness, most studies were not powered to evaluate motor block effects.

This has been confirmed using the minimum local anaesthetic concentration (MLAC) methodology. Lacassie et al. determined the motor block MLAC concentration of ropivacaine,

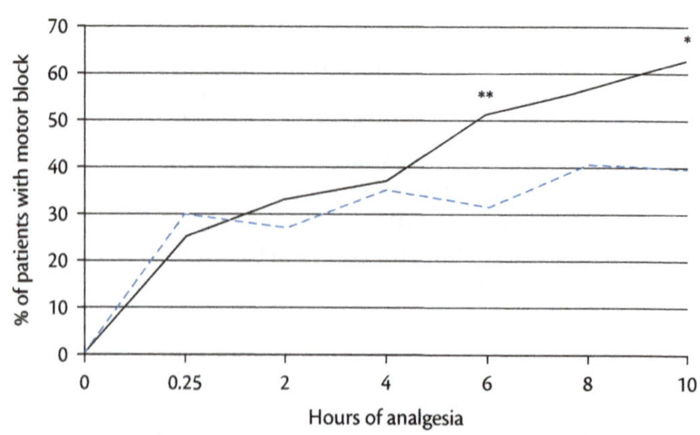

Figure 14.5 Percentage of patients over time with any motor block in a multicentre trial comparing ropivacaine 0.1% and bupivacaine 0.1% both combined with fentanyl 5 mcg/mL for labour analgesia. Especially with prolonged labour, ropivacaine is less potent in terms of motor blocking properties.
Dotted line is ropivacaine; solid line is bupivacaine.
Reproduced with permission from Halpern SH, Breen TW, Campbell DC, Muir HA, Kronberg J, Nunn R, Fick GH., A multicenter, randomized, controlled trial comparing bupivacaine with ropivacaine for labor analgesia, *Anesthesiology*, Volume 98, pp. 1431–1435, Copyright © 2003 Wolters Kluwer Health.

Table 14.2 Number of parturients developing any degree of motor block throughout labour with epidural analgesia using similar and low concentration (0.125% or less) local anaesthetic solutions with or without opioid

Study	Bupivacaine (n)	Ropivacaine (n)	Number of patients in total in the study
Campbell et al.[61]	5	0[a]	40
Meister et al.[62]	18	8[a]	50
Gautier et al.[63]	15	3[a]	90
Lee et al.[64]	21	10	346
Owen et al.[65]	12	8	50
Gogarten et al.[66]	11	4	109
Chua et al.[67]	5	3	32
Fischer et al.[68]	19	10	189
Halpern et al.[69]	47	29[a]	186
Total	**153**	**75**	**1092**

Data from various sources (see references).

levobupivacaine, and bupivacaine using a model of up-and-down sequential allocation.[70,71] The authors noted that at equianalgesic doses, if motor block with racemic bupivacaine was 1.0, motor block with ropivacaine was 0.66 and with levobupivacaine was 0.87.

Choice of adjuvant drug in epidural solutions

Opioids

Opioids used for labour pain relief act through mechanisms in the dorsal horn. Activation of μ, δ, and κ-receptors induces presynaptic inhibition of neurotransmitter release and produces postsynaptic neuronal membrane hyperpolarization. Pure epidural opioid analgesia is feasible in the early stages of labour. Capogna et al. determined the ED_{50} of epidural fentanyl and sufentanil using the MLAC methodology.[72] To produce analgesia in 50% of patients a dose of 124 mcg fentanyl and 21 mcg sufentanil was required, establishing a potency ratio of 5.9 between sufentanil and fentanyl. However, usually opioids are combined with local anaesthetics. It has been repeatedly shown that opioids have a synergistic effect with various local anaesthetic agents. Opioids reduce the ED_{50} of different local anaesthetics.[73] Buyse et al. showed that sufentanil reduced local anaesthetic consumption fourfold.[74] In clinical practice, the addition of opioids reduces the onset of analgesia, prolongs the duration of initial epidural analgesia, reduces local anaesthetic consumption, and decreases the incidence of patients with insufficient analgesia.[75] The incidence of troublesome motor block is reduced and the rate of spontaneous vaginal delivery is increased.[75] Unfortunately, more patients experience pruritus.[75]

Clonidine

Clonidine, an α_2-receptor agonist, acts through α_2-receptors located in the dorsal horn to produce labour analgesia. Presynaptic stimulation of α_2-receptors inhibits neurotransmitter release and postsynaptic stimulation prevents neuronal transmission through hyperpolarization. Animal safety studies established that clonidine was not neurotoxic and did not affect spinal cord blood flow.[76,77] Several clinical trials have studied various doses (30–150 mcg) of epidural clonidine during labour.[78–81] Doses above 100 mcg induce maternal hypotension, bradycardia, and sedation and in some trials also new-onset fetal heart rate changes.[79] Based on work by Landau et al. the optimal epidural dose of clonidine is probably 75 mcg.[81] Prolonged analgesia, reduced local anaesthetic consumption, and less epidural top-ups for breakthrough pain without an increase in side effects were noted. However, Nakamura et al. reported worse neonatal adaptive capacity scores when clonidine 75 mcg was added to an epidural ropivacaine mixture.[82]

Epinephrine

Epinephrine also acts through α_2-receptors. However, vascular effects, especially with epidural administration, might also be involved. Epidurally administered epinephrine significantly reduces the MLAC concentration of bupivacaine in labouring patients and improves the quality of analgesia.[83] Unfortunately, epinephrine also induces an increased incidence of maternal motor deficit.[84,85] Epidural epinephrine might also prolong labour duration by β-agonist effects, especially when higher doses are infused in the epidural space.[86–88] Furthermore, adding epinephrine to pharmacist pre-prepared solutions complicates storage and significantly increases the price of handling and preparation. Thus, this author has abandoned the addition of epinephrine from the local anaesthetic solution used for spinal and epidural administration when used for labour analgesia.

Neostigmine

Acetylcholine is an important neurotransmitter in the dorsal horn of the spinal cord for the descending inhibitory pathways. Neostigmine, a cholinesterase inhibitor, increases the concentration of acetylcholine in the synapses and this produces analgesia by stimulating acetylcholine-mediated mechanisms. Naguib and Yaksh demonstrated that the analgesic effects of neostigmine and clonidine are synergistic.[89] Following reassuring safety studies, in which no neurotoxic effects and no detrimental effects on spinal cord perfusion were identified, neostigmine has been evaluated for labour pain relief.[90,91] Although not a potent analgesic as a single drug, it does have analgesic effects when combined with other drugs such as opioids, clonidine, and local anaesthetics.[92–94]

Van de Velde et al. evaluated the combination of clonidine 75 mcg with neostigmine 500 mcg given epidurally following the spinal component of a CSE.[95] They noted a local anaesthetic-sparing effect, increased duration of initial spinal analgesia, and fewer problems with breakthrough pain. Ross et al. noted that adding neostigmine to the patient-controlled epidural analgesia (PCEA) mixture reduced bupivacaine consumption during labour.[96] Eisenach, along with Paech and Pan, concluded that neostigmine is a promising adjuvant drug to assist in managing labour pain but that further research is required.[97,98]

Initiation using combined spinal–epidural analgesia

Technique

The CSE technique combines the advantages of a conventional epidural technique with the advantages of single-shot spinal (SSS) technique. Most practitioners use the single interspace needle-through-needle CSE technique. Following identification of the epidural space, a longer spinal needle is advanced through the epidural needle into the subarachnoid space. An initial dose of drug is administered. The spinal needle is removed and an epidural catheter advanced as in a conventional epidural technique. Alternatively, but currently rarely used, is the double-space CSE technique in which a SSS is performed followed by an epidural at a different interspace. The double-space technique has advantages (time to redo the epidural if required and easier testing of the epidural catheter) and disadvantages (two punctures; higher chance of damaging the conus if a lower interspace cannot be used for the spinal).

Testing the epidural catheter following CSE

Since epidural catheters can inadvertently be misplaced in either the CSF or in an epidural vein, anaesthetists have been using test doses to verify the correct position of the catheter. Unfortunately, test doses are neither sensitive nor specific[99,100] (Table 14.1). Furthermore epinephrine-containing test doses can induce motor impairment and thus reduce ambulation during labour. Some authors also suggested that an epinephrine-containing test dose has potential adverse effects on uteroplacental perfusion. As a result, several authors have abandoned routine testing of the epidural catheter and look for signs of IV or intrathecal injection with each bolus given through the catheter.[101]

With CSE, analgesia occurs rapidly and testing the functionality of the epidural catheter is not possible until the initial spinal dose wears off. Many anaesthetists consider the fact that the reliability of the epidural catheter is uncertain during this period as a major disadvantage. Their concern is related to the possibility that the catheter may be dysfunctional when an emergency caesarean section is required. Especially in high-risk pregnancies this is considered a major drawback. However, it is important to note that even with a well-tested epidural catheter, it can never be absolutely sure that several hours later the catheter remains correctly positioned.[37,38] Even with conventional epidural catheters, fractionated dosing or a *de novo* test dose are required the moment the catheter is used for the injection of high doses of local anaesthetics.

A second concern involves the fact that some anaesthetists do not want to initiate epidural analgesia immediately after the spinal dose. Only once the spinal dose has worn off, the epidural catheter is formally tested and used throughout labour. As a result most patients will experience breakthrough pain until the epidural dose is effective. However, several authors initiate an epidural infusion immediately following the initial spinal dose.[102] With low-volume, low-dose techniques, the risk of total spinal anaesthesia or toxic side effects is minimal. However, if continuous epidural infusion or patient-controlled epidural analgesia does not produce adequate analgesia, one must consider an intravascular position of the catheter and resite the catheter.

Choice of intrathecal drug combinations

Plain intrathecal opioids are successful in producing labour analgesia. Palmer et al. established that fentanyl 25 mcg, used alone, was the optimal intrathecal dose.[103] Increasing the dose above 25 mcg did not improve the duration or quality of analgesia, but increased the incidence of side effects. For sufentanil, an ED_{95} of 8.9 mcg was established.[104] However, certainly in Europe, most anaesthetists prefer the intrathecal combination of local anaesthetics and opioids, often pre-mixed solutions, prepared by the hospital pharmacy.[105] Adding opioids to the spinal mixture, reduces the ED_{50} of the local anaesthetic agent and prolongs in a dose-dependent manner the duration of initial spinal analgesia.[106] Respiratory depression following intrathecal opioids has been described. This occurred usually in short-stature patients receiving high doses of opioids following initial parenteral opioid analgesia. Respiratory depression occurred within 30 minutes from injection. Vigilance following the intrathecal injection of opioids is therefore required. During labour analgesia, intrathecal opioids have been associated with new-onset fetal heart rate changes.[107,108] Usually these changes were related to uterine hyperactivity and not maternal hypotension. Several authors postulated that an imbalance between maternal catecholamines following rapid spinal analgesia produces uterine hypertonicity. It remains unclear why this only occurs following high-dose intrathecal opioids and not following the combination of lower doses of opioids and local anaesthetics.[109]

Chiari et al. studied the use of pure spinal clonidine labour analgesia.[110] This is not feasible since doses producing adequate analgesia also induce unacceptable hypotension. Adding lower doses of clonidine (15–45 mcg) to spinal analgesics does improve the duration and quality of initial spinal analgesia, but hypotension remains problematic.[111,112]

Nelson et al. investigated the analgesic potential and side effect profile of 5, 10, or 20 mcg intrathecal neostigmine alone.[113] Ten mcg was considered the optimal dose to be added to intrathecal sufentanil. The ED_{50} of spinal sufentanil with and without neostigmine was determined. Neostigmine successfully reduced the ED_{50} of spinal sufentanil. In a further step, they compared twice the ED_{50} of spinal sufentanil with neostigmine to twice the ED_{50} of plain spinal sufentanil. A synergistic effect on duration of analgesia of neostigmine was observed. D'Angelo et al., however, reported no increase in analgesic duration with neostigmine as part of a multidrug combination (local anaesthetic, opioid, clonidine, and neostigmine).[114] Furthermore, several authors reported a very high incidence of severe nausea and vomiting.[115]

Currently bupivacaine is mostly used for intrathecal labour analgesia, usually in combination with opioids. Also levobupivacaine and ropivacaine have been used successfully during labour analgesia. Lim et al. compared 2.5 mg bupivacaine with 2.5 mg ropivacaine and 2.5 mg levobupivacaine.[116] Bupivacaine produced the longest duration of analgesia but with the highest incidence of motor block. These results were not confirmed by Sah et al. who found no difference between levobupivacaine and bupivacaine.[117] Camorcia and co-workers described the minimum local analgesic doses of all three local anaesthetics and suggested a potency hierarchy of spinal bupivacaine > levobupivacaine > ropivacaine.[118] Whitty et al. described the ED_{95} of spinal bupivacaine combined with fentanyl.[119] Van de Velde et al. were the first to construct the full dose–response relationship of spinal ropivacaine, levobupivacaine, and bupivacaine combined with opioids for labour analgesia.[120] They noted that bupivacaine was significantly more potent than both the other local anaesthetics, but that ropivacaine and levobupivacaine were of similar analgesic potency (Figure 14.6).[120]

Initiation using single-shot spinal, continuous spinal, or caudal analgesia

Single-shot spinal

SSS anaesthesia is a simple and highly effective technique using a spinal needle which can be cutting (e.g. Quincke) or non-cutting

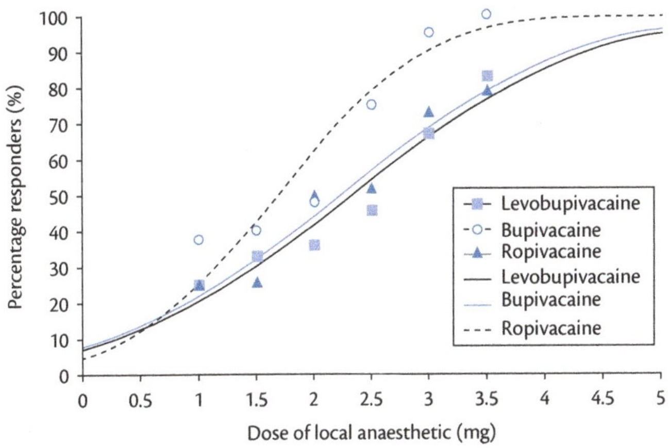

Figure 14.6 Full dose–response curves for bupivacaine, ropivacaine, and levobupivacaine combined with sufentanil throughout all stages of labour. Bupivacaine is significantly more potent then both other agents.

(e.g. Whitacre/pencil-point). Cutting needles produce a high incidence of PDPH especially in obstetric patients and are currently rarely used in obstetric anaesthesia. Spinal needles also vary in size between 24 and 29 G needles. SSS is rarely used for labour analgesia and usually only in situations where brief analgesia is required shortly before anticipated delivery or when patients have difficulty in remaining immobile during neuraxial insertion.

Continuous spinal

In rare situations, continuous spinal anaesthesia can be used. A spinal needle punctures the dura and a catheter is threaded into the subarachnoid space. This can be done using the Tuohy epidural needle and the epidural catheter following accidental dural puncture or by using specifically designed spinal catheter sets. However, especially in obstetric patients, a very high incidence of PDPH occurs following continuous spinal analgesia.[121] Additional risks include technical difficulties inserting the catheters, unreliability of the catheters, and injecting an accidental epidural dose intrathecally. Therefore this technique is reserved for high-risk patients in which pure opioid analgesia is useful.[122]

Choosing between combined spinal–epidural and conventional epidural analgesia

Obstetric anaesthetists are divided when questioned on the place of CSE in labour analgesia. In a 2012 Cochrane review, it was concluded that CSE offers little benefit as compared to conventional epidural analgesia.[123] However, it was acknowledged that CSE produces faster analgesia. Side effects on mother, infant, and labour were similar between techniques, apart from a slight increase in the incidence of pruritus with CSE. However, because of this ongoing discussion, we feel that a more detailed overview of the available literature is required. Also perhaps this more detailed discussion might aid clinicians in choosing one over the other technique for individual patients and situations.

Onset Time of Analgesia

Arguably the most obvious advantage of the CSE technique is the rapid onset of effective analgesia.[123] Consistently, effective labour analgesia is accomplished within 4–8 minutes following the intrathecal injection of drugs.[123–139] Following conventional epidural analgesia, initial analgesia is usually achieved within 10 to 25 minutes[133,134] (Figure 14.7).

It is important to note, however, that although the onset time of epidural analgesia might be reasonable, a wide interpatient variability exists depending on parity, stage of labour and other relevant obstetric and non-obstetric factors. Especially during late or active labour, analgesia following an epidural is often delayed and always requires local anaesthetics. With CSE, onset time is short in all patients irrespective of the stage of labour and can be achieved using pure opioid analgesia. Importantly, in many studies, epidural mixtures used relatively high concentrations of local anaesthetic (>0.2%).

Quality of pain relief: visual analogue scale scores, satisfaction, and anaesthetist intervention rate

Several trials demonstrated lower visual analogue scale (VAS) scores for labour pain during the first hours after initiation with CSE,[140–143] whilst other comparative trials could not demonstrate a difference in VAS scores.[144,145] No trials report higher VAS scores with CSE. A recent trial by Gambling et al. demonstrated better first-stage analgesia with CSE, despite fewer epidural top-ups.[146]

Less unilateral analgesia with CSE was reported as compared to conventional epidural analgesia.[138] Interestingly, Hess et al. found that patients treated with conventional epidural analgesia experienced more recurrent breakthrough pain as compared to CSE-treated women.[147] Goodman et al., however, failed to corroborate these findings.[142]

The presence of a dural puncture may facilitate the passage of epidurally administered drugs during maintenance of analgesia to the CSF; at least in animals, such an effect has been reported.[148] In patients, Leighton et al. also reported that epidural bupivacaine blocked more dermatomes when administered following an initial dural puncture as compared to epidural bupivacaine administered without prior dural puncture.[149] Cappiello et al. perforated the dura with a 25 G Whitacre needle without administration of spinal drugs.[150] The control group had no dural puncture. In both groups, analgesia was initiated with an epidural local anaesthetic/opioid mixture. Patients treated with a dural puncture had better sacral spread, shorter onset of analgesia, and better quality pain relief. In a similar study using a 27 G Whitacre needle, no difference between patients treated with or without a dural puncture could be identified.[151]

Local anaesthetic consumption

Local anaesthetic requirements are significantly reduced with CSE as compared to low-dose epidural techniques.[133,137,138,141,143] Discussion is ongoing as to whether this is the result of the omission of the initial epidural bolus or that also during labour a dose-sparing effect persists (as a result of the dural hole).

However, a recent trial by Patel et al., using the MLAC methodology, determined that with CSE local anaesthetic requirements might be increased for the second epidural injection as compared to conventional epidural analgesia.[152] However, it must be noted

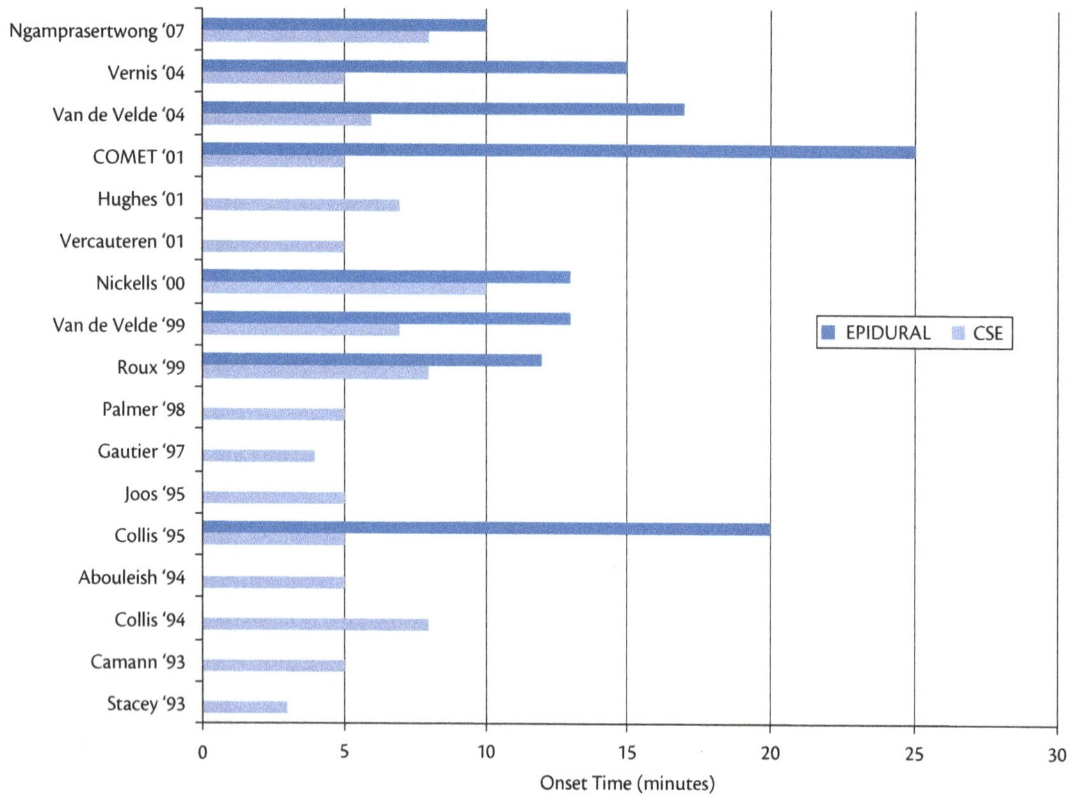

Figure 14.7 Onset time of analgesia in different studies in patients treated either with combined spinal epidural analgesia (CSE, light blue bars) or conventional epidural analgesia (dark blue bars).
Data from various studies (see references).

that the effect was marginal and that the methodology of the study does not reflect clinical practice in which the epidural maintenance strategy is started immediately following the initial dose and not when the patient has pain once again.

Duration of initial analgesia

Spinal analgesia typically lasts for 90–150 minutes, but a wide variety exists depending on administered spinal drugs and pain-modulating factors such as parity, stage of labour, type of labour, frequency, and strength of contractions. The initial duration of the spinal dose is similar to an initial epidural bolus.[153–163] In ideal circumstances using multidrug combinations, spinal analgesia can last more than 4 hours.[156,160] Many authors continue the search for long-lasting spinal analgesia, hoping that SSS analgesia will ultimately be achieved. Despite extensive research, disappointingly, no more (and often less) than 50% of patients deliver during initial spinal analgesia.

Epidural catheter reliability

Following the initial spinal injection, due to bilateral analgesia and sensory changes, testing of the epidural catheter can be difficult and one is unsure if the epidural is in the correct space. Furthermore, the reliability of the catheter to achieve bilateral analgesia once the spinal dose has worn off has not been proven until used. However, various investigators noted that the reliability of epidural catheters following CSE was similar or increased as compared to stand-alone epidural catheters.[138,150,164–170] There was less need for epidural catheter replacement and there was less unilateral analgesia requiring catheter manipulation. Unfortunately many of these studies are retrospective or have catheter reliability as a secondary outcome factor.

When using a CSE technique, a perfect midline approach is required to identify the subarachnoid space and consequently more epidural catheters are positioned reliably into the epidural space. Interestingly, Thomas et al. noted that when no CSF was obtained following attempted CSE, subsequently much more epidural catheters required replacement as compared to those catheters placed when CSF was noted.[151]

Failed spinal component

Failure to identify the spinal space and produce good spinal analgesia is reported in 0–18% of patients.[151] As with every technique, failure may occur, but in these instances the epidural catheter can still be used to provide analgesia. Failure of the spinal component indicates that the epidural needle is not perfectly situated on the midline and is a risk factor for subsequent epidural catheter failure.[151]

Side effects of neuraxial analgesia initiation

Pruritus

This is the most common side effect of neuraxial opioids, occurring in almost all patients. In the most recent Cochrane review, pruritus was more frequent following CSE and was reported to be the only complication occurring more frequently with CSE.[123] It usually develops shortly after analgesia. It is mild and hardly ever requires antipruritic therapy.

Nausea

Nausea and vomiting are very rare complications during CSE and conventional epidural analgesia. No differences in the incidence of nausea have between reported when comparing the two techniques, except in the retrospective trial by Miro et al. who reported more nausea and vomiting in patients treated with epidural analgesia.[166] We must remember that nausea is a part of the birth process especially during induced labour.

Hypotension

As with any neuraxial technique, hypotension can occur following labour analgesia. Both CSE and conventional epidural analgesia have been associated with usually mild hypotension, which is easily treated.[133] Hypotension following the spinal injection is transient and occurs within the first 30 minutes following initiation of analgesia. In clinical, routine practice it is important to avoid the supine position. Although opioids do not produce sympatholysis, hypotension is observed with pure intrathecal opioid analgesia.[171] When local anaesthetics are combined, hypotension seems to be more pronounced, but clinically is usually easily treated. Intrathecal clonidine, however, is often associated with severe hypotension and this author cannot recommend its routine use based on his personal experience with this drug. Hypotension can be severe and is often protracted requiring prolonged supportive vasopressor therapy.[172]

Respiratory depression

Several case reports have demonstrated that lipid-soluble opioids may induce respiratory depression.[173] In some, but not all, cases respiratory arrest occurred in relatively short-stature women who had received parenteral or epidural opioids prior to the spinal injection. Fortunately, respiratory depression occurred typically within the first 30 minutes and was easily treated and reversed using naloxone. In one patient, chest compressions and resuscitation were required.[173] Ferrouz et al. performed a retrospective chart analysis and reported one respiratory arrest in over 5000 CSEs performed with 10 mcg spinal sufentanil.[174] As this complication is rare, most authors advocate vigilance and advise using lower doses of intrathecal opioids than those initially used on empirical grounds.

Other complications related to excessive rostral spread of opioids and local anaesthetics have been described and include aphonia, aphagia, dysphagia, altered levels of consciousness, high sensory block, and transient swallowing difficulties. Sudden hypoglycaemia has also been described.[175]

Motor block

For many years, strategies to reduce the incidence and severity of motor block, associated with epidural analgesia, have been designed. Lower concentrations of local anaesthetics, the addition of opioids and other adjuvant drugs, the introduction of patient-controlled epidural analgesia, and the use of newer local anaesthetics have been instrumental in reducing problematic motor block. Low-dose epidurals are successfully used to allow labouring women to maintain mobility whilst being completely pain free.[137] With CSE it is easier to provide effective analgesia with no or very minute doses of local anaesthetics. As already described, CSE decreases both the total local anaesthetic consumption[133,137] and the occurrence of motor block compared to standard epidural techniques.[133,137]

Some have questioned the safety of walking during labour and neuraxial analgesia.[176] However, several authors demonstrated that with CSE and epidurals motor function and balance remained intact, similar to pregnant patients without neuraxial analgesia.[177]

Although reduced motor block and ambulation during neuraxial analgesia are certainly feasible, controversy concerning the benefits of ambulation remains. Several trials demonstrated that ambulation during labour does not affect the outcome of labour,[178] whilst others did note a beneficial effect of ambulation. In patients without epidural analgesia, ambulation halved the operative delivery rate.[179] Ambulation also reduced the length of the second stage of labour.[180] In the COMET trial, mobile techniques for labour analgesia were associated with an improved labour outcome.[137,164]

Fetal heart rate changes

Abnormal fetal heart rate recordings and fetal bradycardia are worrying side effects that may follow any type of effective labour analgesia. Wong et al. reported more abnormal cardiotocographic readings following CSE as compared to systemic analgesia.[9] Some authors reported that this complication could be more common following intrathecal opioids than following conventional epidural analgesia.[107,108] Clarke et al. were the first to describe in detail the association between intrathecal opioids, uterine hyperactivity, and fetal bradycardia in the absence of maternal hypotension.[107]

Mardirossof et al. performed a meta-analysis of several prospective trials comparing intrathecal opioid analgesia with non-intrathecal opioid analgesia with respect to fetal bradycardia (Figure 14.8).[181] It was concluded that intrathecal opioids were associated with significantly more fetal heart rate abnormalities. Vercauteren et al. suggested that the incidence of fetal bradycardia depended on the dose of the intrathecal opioid.[182] Van de Velde et al. performed a prospective, randomized trial specifically designed to evaluate the effects of intrathecal opioids on the incidence of non-reassuring fetal heart rate changes.[109] These authors concluded that high doses of intrathecal opioids increased the incidence of fetal heart rate abnormalities despite a reduced incidence of hypotension. The presumed mechanism of opioid-induced non-reassuring fetal heart rate tracings is uterine hyperactivity caused by rapid analgesia and, as a result, a rapid decrease in maternal circulating catecholamines.

Recently, Patel et al. compared CSE and conventional epidural analgesia and found that both techniques influenced the fetal heart rate, but that there was no difference between the two techniques with respect to inducing non-reassuring fetal heart rate changes.[183]

Postdural puncture headache

Since CSE includes a dural puncture, there is a theoretical risk of PDPH. This is a devastating complication in an otherwise healthy mother, keen on taking care for her newborn child. However the use of small-gauge atraumatic spinal needles (26–29 G) has dramatically decreased the problem. From the available literature it seems that PDPH due to neuraxial analgesia occurs in no more than 1% of patients. Furthermore, the incidence is not increased as compared to conventional epidural analgesia.[132,184] Norris et al. reported that unintended dural puncture with the

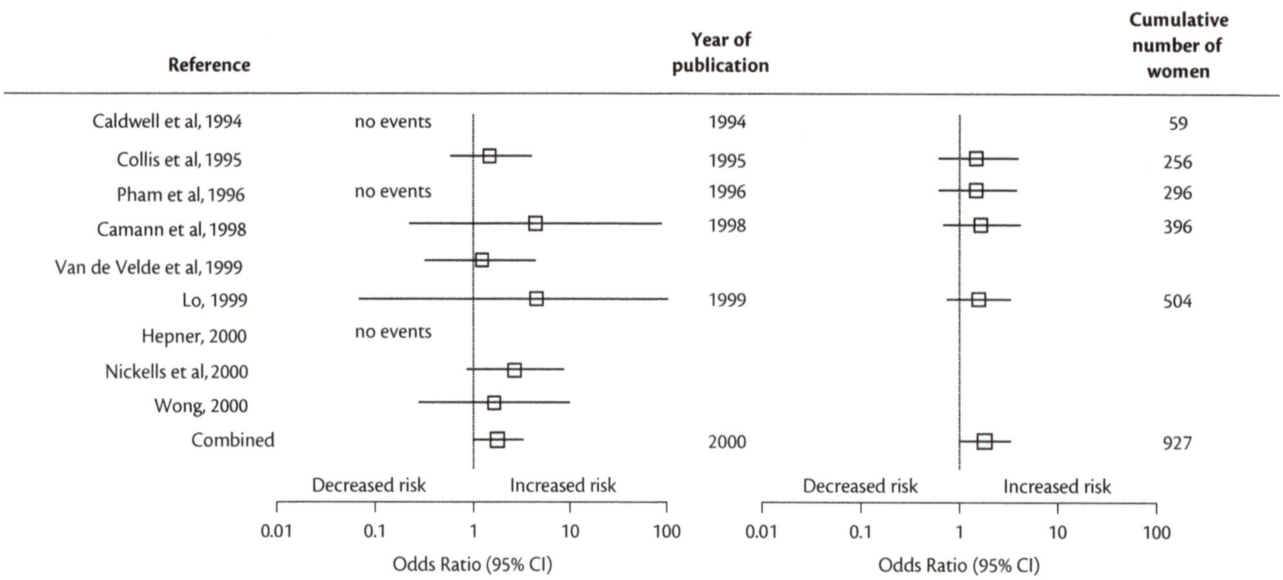

Figure 14.8 Meta-analysis of randomized, double-blind trials evaluating the effect of intrathecal opioids on fetal heart rate changes as compared to analgesia without intrathecal opioids. Please refer to original paper for references.

Reproduced with permission from Chahé Mardirosoff, Lionel Dumont, Michel Boulvain, Martin R. Tramèr, Fetal bradycardia due to intrathecal opioids for labour analgesia: a systematic review, *BJOG: An International Journal of Obstetrics and Gynaecology*, Volume 109, Issue 3, pp. 274–281, Copyright © 2003 John Wiley and Sons.

[a]$P < 0.05$ versus bupivacaine.

epidural needle occurs much more frequently when using conventional epidural analgesia as compared to CSE.[184] Rarely the spinal needle itself is responsible for PDPH. Usually a dural tap with either the Tuohy needle or the epidural catheter causes postural headache. It is also worthwhile to mention several reports advising the insertion of the epidural catheter in the subarachnoid space following an accidental dural tap. The incidence of PDPH and blood patching seems reduced when the epidural catheter is threaded intrathecally, although the evidence is conflicting.[185–187]

Neurological deficit

With any central neuraxial technique permanent neurological deficit is a rare but devastating possibility. If a CSE is inserted at a level higher then L3–4 interspace, direct trauma to the conus medullaris is possible by the spinal needle. Reynolds published a series of seven obstetric patients who had damage to the conus following a CSE performed at a much higher interspace.[188] Anaesthetists are notoriously poor in identifying the correct interspace using landmarks and usually miss the correct interspace by one or more segments cranially.[189] Hence caution when determining the correct interspace is absolutely mandatory.

In 2009, the 3rd National Audit Project of the Royal College of Anaesthetists was published.[190] The report gathered data from hospitals in the United Kingdom over a 2-week period and extrapolated it for 1 year. It looked at major complications following central neuraxial blocks in the United Kingdom, both in obstetric and non-obstetric patients. The report indicated that CSE might carry a higher risk of permanent injury as compared to epidural anaesthesia as it was used in less than 6% of cases but resulted in 13–14% of major complications.

Meningitis

Several case reports have been published in which meningitis developed after CSE.[191–194] In at least some of these cases an inappropriate aseptic technique was possibly involved. However breaching of the dura carries a theoretically higher risk of infection than when the dura is not perforated. Infectious complications have also been described with epidural techniques. Therefore it must be emphasized that with both CSEs and epidurals a scrupulous aseptic technique is mandatory.

Conclusion

Epidural analgesia is the most popular method to initiate neuraxial analgesia for labour. However, CSE analgesia is also a very popular technique for labour pain relief and in some parts of Europe (e.g. Belgium) is as common as standard epidurals for initiation of labour analgesia. Epidural analgesia is reliable, relatively simple, and with modern approaches (e.g. drugs, adjuvants, and maintenance strategies) has limited effects on the labour process. However, its onset is relatively slow and a high percentage of epidural catheter failures have been described. A recent Cochrane review suggests that CSE produces much faster analgesia then conventional epidural analgesia. Although various authors limit the use of the technique to specific indications, a wide variety of indications have been described by different authors (Box 14.6). CSE analgesia provides rapid, highly effective analgesia with minimal motor block and low local anaesthetic consumption. Maternal satisfaction is improved. A possible important advantage of the CSE technique is enhanced epidural catheter reliability, but this needs further study and confirmation. PDPH and infections do not occur more frequently than with conventional

Box 14.6 Indications reported in the literature for the CSE technique to initiate labour analgesia

- Advanced labour with greater than 6 cm cervical dilation
- Rapidly advancing labour such that the mother is severely distressed
- Pushing against a cervix that is not fully dilated
- Repeated epidural failures or attempts
- Ruptured membranes
- Distressed mothers
- Full cervical dilation
- Early labour to produce analgesia without local anaesthetics to minimize motor block or to minimize haemodynamic side effects
- High-risk pregnancies (cardiac, preeclampsia, twins, etc.)
- Obese parturients.

Data from Simmons SW, Taghizadeh N, Dennis AT, Hughes D, Cyna AM. Combined spinal-epidural versus epidural analgesia in labour. *Cochrane Database Syst Rev*, 2012.

epidural analgesia. However, non-reassuring fetal heart rate tracings occur significantly more frequently following high doses of intrathecal opioids in CSE and occasionally, respiratory depression, also following high doses of opioids intrathecally, can occur.

References

1. Schrock SD, Harraway-Smith C. Labor analgesia. *Am Fam Physician* 2012; 85:447–54.
2. Jones L, Othman M, Dowsell T, *et al.* Pain management for women in labour: an overview of systematic reviews. *Cochrane Database Syst Rev* 2012; 3:CD009234.
3. Anim-Somuah M, Smyth RM, Jones L. Epidural versus non-epidural or no analgesia in labour. *Cochrane Database Syst Rev* 2011; 12:CD000331.
4. Simkin P. Moving beyond the debate: a holistic approach to understanding and treating effects of neuraxial analgesia. *Birth* 2012; 39:327–32.
5. National Institute of Clinical Excellence. *Intrapartum Care: Care of Healthy Women and their Babies During Childbirth.* Clinical Guideline 55. London: NICE; 2007.
6. American College of Obstetricians and Gynecologists Committee on Obstetric Practice. ACOG Committee Opinion no. 339. Analgesia and cesarean delivery rates. *Obstet Gynecol* 2006; 107:1487–9.
7. American Society of Anesthesiologists. *Statement on Pain Relief During Labor,* 1999 (and last amended 2010). [Online] http://www.asahq.org
8. Wuitchik M, Bakal D, Lipshitz J. The clinical significance of pain and cognitive activity in latent labor. *Obstet Gynecol* 1989; 73:35–42.
9. Wong CA, Scavone BM, Peaceman AM, *et al.* The risk of Cesarean delivery with neuraxial analgesia given early versus late in labor. *N Engl J Med* 2005; 352:655–65.
10. Marucci M, Cinnella G, Perchiazzi G, *et al.* Patient-requested neuraxial analgesia for labor: impact on rates of cesarean and instrumental vaginal delivery. *Anesthesiology* 2007; 106:1035–45.
11. ASA Task Force on Obstetric Anesthesia. Practice guidelines for obstetric anesthesia. *Anesthesiology* 2007; 106:843–63.
12. Working Party on Obstetric Anesthesia of the Belgian Association of Regional Anesthesia (BARA). Belgian Guidelines and Recommendations for Safe Practice in Obstetric Anesthesia. *Acta Anaesthesiol Belg* 2003; 54:119–25.
13. Association of Anaesthetists of Great Britain & Ireland Obstetric Anaesthetists' Association. *OAA/AAGBI Guidelines for Obstetric Anaesthetic Services 2005.* London: Association of Anaesthetists of Great Britain & Ireland Obstetric Anaesthetists' Association; 2005.
14. Wallenborn J, German Society for Anesthesiology and Intensive Care Medicine; Professional Association of German Anesthetists, *et al.* [Execution of analgesia and anesthesia procedures in obstetrics : Second revised recommendations of the German Society for Anesthesiology and Intensive Care Medicine and the Professional Association of German Anesthetists in cooperation with the German Society for Gynecology and Obstetrics]. *Anaesthesist* 2010; 59:250–4.
15. Bethune L, Harper N, Lucas DN, *et al.* Complications of obstetric regional analgesia: how much information is enough? *Int J Obstet Anesth* 2004; 13:30–4.
16. Jackson GN, Sensky T, Reide P, *et al.* The capacity of consent to epidural analgesi in labour. *Int J Obstet Anesth* 2011; 20:269–70.
17. Broaddus BM, Chandrasekhar S. Informed consent in obstetric anesthesia. *Anesth Analg* 2011; 112:912–15.
18. The Association of Anaesthetists of Great Britain & Ireland. *AAGBI Safety Guideline. Management of Severe Local Anaesthetic Toxicity.* 2010. [Online] http://www.aagbi.org/sites/default/files/la_toxicity_2010_0.pdf
19. Neal J, Bernards CM, Butterworth JF, *et al.* ASRA practice advisory on local anesthetic systemic toxicity. *Reg Anesth Pain Med* 2010; 35:152–61.
20. Armstrong S, Fernando R, Columb M, *et al.* Cardiac index in term pregnant women in the sitting, lateral, and supine positions: an observational, crossover study. *Anesth Analg* 2011; 113:318–22.
21. Checketts MR. Wash and go—but with what? Skin antiseptic solutions for central neuraxial block. *Anaesthesia* 2012; 67:819–22.
22. Bogod D. The sting in the tail: antiseptics and the neuraxis revisited. *Anaesthesia* 2012; 67:1305–9.
23. Killeen T, Kamat A, Walsh D, *et al.* Severe adhesive arachnoiditis resulting in progressive paraplegia following obstetric spinal anaesthesia: a case report and review. *Anaesthesia* 2012; 67:1386–94.
24. Collis RE, Baxandall ML, Srikantharajah ID, *et al.* Combined spinal epidural analgesia: technique, management and outcome of 300 mothers. *Int J Obstet Anesth* 1994; 3:75–81.
25. Camann WR, Mintzer BH, Denney RA, *et al.* Intrathecal sufentanil for labor analgesia. *Anesthesiology* 1993; 78:870–4.
26. Van Houwe P, Heytens L, Vercruysse P. A survey of obstetric anaesthesia practice in Flanders. *Acta Anaesthesiol Belg* 2006; 57:29–37.
27. Reynolds F. Damage to the conus medullaris following spinal anaesthesia. *Anaesthesia* 2001; 56:238–47.
28. Collier CB. Accidental subdural injection during attempted lumbar epidural block may present as a failed or inadequate block: radiographic evidence. *Reg Anesth Pain Med* 2004; 29:45–51.
29. Reina MA, Collier CB, Prats-Galino A, *et al.* Unintentional subdural placement of epidural catheters during attempted epidural anesthesia: an anatomic study of spinal subdural compartment. *Reg Anesth Pain Med* 2011; 36:537–41.
30. Paech M, Banks S, Gurrin L. An audit of accidental dural puncture during epidural insertion of a Tuohy needle in obstetric patients. *Int J Obstet Anesth* 2001; 10:162–7.
31. Evron S, Sessler D, Sadan O, *et al.* Identification of the epidural space: loss of resistance with air, lidocaine or the combination of air and lidocaine. *Anesth Analg* 2004; 99:245–50.
32. Schier R, Guerra D, Aguilar J, *et al.* Epidural space identification: a meta-analysis of complications after air versus liquid as the medium for loss of resistance. *Anesth Analg* 2009; 109:2012–21.
33. Hinova A, Fernando R. Air vs. normal saline for the loss of resistance technique during epidural insertion. In McConachie I (ed) *Controversies in Obstetric Anesthesia.* Cambridge University Press; 2013:122–30.

34. Tyagi A, Kumar R, Bhattacharya A, *et al.* Filters in anaesthesia and intensive care. *Anaesth Intensive Care* 2003; 31:418–33.
35. Mulroy MF, Norris MC, Liu SS. Safety steps for epidural injection of local anesthetics: review of the literature and recommendations. *Anesth Analg* 1997; 85:1346–56.
36. Camorcia M. Testing the epidural catheter. *Curr Opinion Anaesthesiol* 2009; 22:336–40.
37. Richardson MG, Wissler RN. Unexpected high spinal block in obstetrics. *Br J Anaesth* 1996; 77:806–7.
38. Fivez T, Deblonde S, Van de Velde M. Late intravascular migration of a previously well functioning labour epidural catheter. *Eur J Anaesthesiol* 2010; 27:634–6.
39. Cohen SE, Yeh JY, Riley ET, *et al.* Walking with labor epidural analgesia: the impact of bupivacaine concentration and a lidocaine-epinephrine test-dose. *Anesthesiology* 2000; 92:387–92.
40. Marcus MA, Vertommen JD, Van Aken H, *et al.* Hemodynamic effects of intravenous isoproterenol versus epinephrine in the chronic maternal-fetal sheep preparation. *Anesth Analg* 1996; 82:1023–6.
41. Calimaran AI, Strauss-Hoder TP, Wang WY, *et al.* The effect of epidural test dose on motor function after a combined spinal epidural technique for labor analgesia. *Anesthesiology* 2003; 96:1167–72.
42. Van Zundert A, Vaes L, Soetens M, *et al.* Every dose given in epidural analgesia for vaginal delivery can be a test dose. *Anesthesiology* 1987; 67:436–40.
43. Milaszkiewicz R, Payne N, Loughnan B, *et al.* Continuous extradural infusion of lignocaine 0.75% vs bupivacaine 0.125% in primiparae: quality of analgesia and influence on labour. *Anaesthesia* 1992; 47:1042–6.
44. Kennedy RL, Bell JU, Miller RP, *et al.* Uptake and distribution of lidocaine in fetal lambs. *Anesthesiology* 1990; 72:483–9.
45. Reynolds F, Taylor G. Maternal and neonatal blood concentrations of bupivacaine: a comparison of lignocaine during continuous extradural analgesia. *Anaesthesia* 1970; 25:14–23.
46. Scanlon JW, Brown WU Jr, Weiss JB, *et al.* Neurobehavioral responses of newborn infants after maternal epidural anesthesia. *Anesthesiology* 1974; 40:121–8.
47. Abboud TK, Afrasiabi A, Sarkis F, *et al.* Continuous infusion epidural analgesia in parturients receiving bupivacaine, chloroprocaine, or lidocaine: maternal, fetal, and neonatal effects. *Anesth Analg* 1984; 63:421–8.
48. Comparative Obstetric Mobile Epidural Trial (COMET) Study Group UK. Effect of low dose mobile versus traditional epidural techniques on mode of delivery: a randomised controlled trial. *Lancet* 2001; 358:19–23.
49. Christiaens F, Verborgh C, Dierick A, *et al.* Effects of diluent volume of a single dose of epidural bupivacaine in parturients during the first stage of labor. *Reg Anesth Pain Med* 1998; 23:134–41.
50. Lyons GR, Kocarev MG, Wilson RC, *et al.* A comparison of minimum local anesthetic volumes and doses of epidural bupivacaine (0.125% w/v and 0.25% w/v). *Anesth Analg* 2007; 104:412–15.
51. Capogna G, Celleno D, Fusco P, *et al.* Relative potencies of bupivacaine and ropivacaine for analgesia in labour. *Br J Anaesth* 1999; 82:371–3.
52. Polley LS, Columb MO, Naughton NN, *et al.* Relative analgesic potencies of ropivacaine and bupivacaine for epidural analgesia in labour. *Anesthesiology* 1999; 90:944–50.
53. Polley LS, Columb MO, Naughton NN, *et al.* Relative analgesic potencies of levobupivacaine and ropivacaine for epidural analgesia in labor. *Anesthesiology* 2003; 99(6):1354–8.
54. Ngan Kee WD, Ng FF, Khaw KS, *et al.* Determination and comparison of graded dose-response curves for epidural bupivacaine and ropivacaine for analgesia in laboring nulliparous women. *Anesthesiology* 2010; 113:445–53.
55. Groban L, Dolinski SY. Differences in cardiac toxicity among ropivacaine, levobupivacaine, bupivacaine, and lidocaine. *Techn Reg Anesth Pain Manag* 2001; 5:48–55.
56. Stienstra R. Ropivacaine for obstetric use. *Techn Reg Anesth Pain Manag* 2001; 5:60–3.
57. Mather LE, Chang DHT. Cardiotoxicity with modern local anaesthetics. Is there a safer choice? *Drugs* 2001; 61:333–42.
58. Groban L, Dolinski SY. Differences in cardiac toxicity among ropivacaine, levobupivacaine, bupivacaine, and lidocaine. *Techn Reg Anesth Pain Manag* 2001; 5:48–55.
59. Santos AC, Arthur GR, Wlody D, *et al.* Comparative systemic toxicity of ropivacaine and bupivacaine in nonpregnant and pregnant ewes. *Anesthesiology* 1995; 82:734–40.
60. Halpern SH, Walsh V. Epidural ropivacaine versus bupivacaine for labor: a meta-analysis. *Anesth Analg* 2003; 96:1473–9.
61. Campbell DC, Zwack RM, Crone LA, *et al.* Ambulatory labor epidural analgesia: bupivacaine versus ropivacaine. *Anesth Analg* 2000; 90:1384–9.
62. Meister GC, D'Angelo R, Owen M, *et al.* comparison of epidural analgesia with 0.125% ropivacaine with fentanyl versus 0.125% bupivacaine with fentanyl during labor. *Anesth Analg* 2000; 90:632–7.
63. Gautier P, De Kock M, Van Steenberge A, *et al.* A double blind comparison of 0.125% ropivacaine with sufentanil and 0.125% bupivacaine with sufentanil for epidural labor analgesia. *Anesthesiology* 1999; 90:772–8.
64. Lee BB, Ngan Kee WD, Ng FF, *et al.* Epidural infusions of ropivacaine and bupivacaine for labor analgesia: a randomized, double blind study of obstetric outcome. *Anesth Analg* 2004; 98:1145–52.
65. Owen MD, Thomas JA, Smith T, *et al.* Ropivacaine 0.075% and bupivacaine 0.075% with fentanyl 2 μg/ml are equivalent for labor epidural analgesia. *Anesth Analg* 2002; 94:179–83.
66. Gogarten W, Van de Velde M, Soetens F, *et al.* A multicentre trial comparing different concentrations of ropivacaine plus sufentanil with bupivacaine plus sufentanil for patient controlled epidural analgesia in labour. *Eur J Anaesthesiol* 2004; 21:38–45.
67. Chua NP, Sia AT, Ocampo CE. Parturient controlled epidural analgesia during labour: bupivacaine vs ropivacaine. *Anaesthesia* 2001; 56:1169–73.
68. Fischer C, Blanie P, Jaouen E, *et al.* Ropivacaine 0.1% plus sufentanil 0.5 μg/ml versus bupivacaine 0.1% plus sufentanil 0.5 μg/ml using patient controlled epidural analgesia for labor. *Anesthesiology* 2000; 92:1588–93.
69. Halpern SH, Breen TW, Campbell DC, *et al.* A multicenter, randomized, controlled trial comparing bupivacaine with ropivacaine for labor analgesia. *Anesthesiology* 2003; 98:1431–5.
70. Lacassie HJ, Columb MO, Lacassie HP, *et al.* The relative motor blocking potencies of epidural bupivacaine and ropivacaine in labor. *Anesth Analg* 2002; 95:204–8.
71. Lacassie HJ, Columb MO. The relative motor blocking protencies of bupivacaine and levobupivacaine. *Anesth Analg* 2003; 97:1509–13.
72. Capogna G, Camorcia M, Columb MO. Minimum analgesic dose of fentanyl and sufentanil for epidural analgesia in the first stage of labor. *Anesth Analg* 2003; 96:1178–82.
73. Polley LS, Columb MO, Wagner DS, *et al.* Dose-dependent reduction of the minimum local analgesic concentration of bupivacaine by sufentanil for epidural analgesia in labor. *Anesthesiology* 1998; 8:626–32.
74. Buyse I, Stockman W, Columb M, *et al.* Effect of sufentanil on minimum local analgesic concentrations of epidural bupivacaine, ropivacaine and levobupivacaine in nullipara in early labour. *Int J Obstet Anesth* 2007; 16:22–8.
75. Vertommen JD, Vandermeulen E, Van Aken H, *et al.* The effects of the addition of sufentanil to 0.125% bupivacaine on the quality of analgesia during labor and on the incidence of instrumental deliveries. *Anesthesiology* 1991; 74:809–14.
76. Gordh T, Post C, Olsson Y. Evaluation of the toxicity of subarachnoid clonidine, guanfacine, and a substance P-antagonist on rat spinal cord and nerve roots. *Anesth Analg* 1986; 65:1303–11.

77. Eisenach JC, Grice SC. Epidural clonidine does not decrease blood pressure or spinal cord blood flow in awake sheep. *Anesthesiology* 1988; 68:335–40.
78. Aveline C, El Metaoua S, Masmoudi A, *et al.* The effect of clonidine on the minimum local analgesic concentration of epidural ropivacaine during labor. *Anesth Analg* 2002; 95:735–40.
79. Chassard D, Mathon L, Dailler F, *et al.* Extradural clonidine combined with sufentanil and 0.0625% bupivacaine for analgesia in labour. *Br J Anaesth* 1996; 77:458–62.
80. Brichant JF, Bonhomme V, Mikulski M, *et al.* Admixture of clonidine to epidural bupivacaine for analgesia during labor: effect of varying clonidine doses. *Anesthesiology* 1994; 81:A1136.
81. Landau R, Schiffer E, Morales M, *et al.* The dose sparing effect of clonidine added to ropivacaine for labor epidural analgesia. *Anesth Analg* 2002; 95:728–34.
82. Nakamura G, Ganem EM, Pinheiro Modolo NS, *et al.* Labor analgesia with ropivacaine added to clonidine: a randomized clinical trial. *Sao Paulo Med J* 2008; 126:102–6.
83. Polley LS, Columb MO, Naughton NN, *et al.* Effect of epidural epinephrine on the minimum local analgesic concentration of epidural bupivacaine in labor. *Anesthesiology* 2002; 96:1123–8.
84. Gautier PE, Debry F, Fanard L, *et al.* Ambulatory combined spinal epidural analgesia for labor. Influence of epinephrine on bupivacaine-sufentanil combination. *Reg Anesth* 1997; 22:143–9.
85. Cohen SE, Yeh JY, Riley ET, *et al.* Walking with labor epidural analgesia. The impact of bupivacaine concentration and a lidocaine-epinephrine test dose. *Anesthesiology* 2000; 92:387–92.
86. Okutomi T, Mochizuki J, Amano K, *et al.* Effect of epidural epinephrine infusion with bupivacaine on labor pain and mother-fetus outcome in humans. *Reg Anesth Pain Med* 2000; 25:228–34.
87. Okutomi T, Amano K, Morishima HO. Effect of standard diluted epinephrine infusion on epidural anesthesia in labor. *Reg Anesth Pain Med* 2000; 25:529–34.
88. Dounas M, O'Kelly BO, Jamali S, *et al.* Maternal and fetal effects of adrenaline with bupivacaine for epidural analgesia during labour. *Eur J Anaesth* 1996; 13:594–8.
89. Naguib M, Yaksh TL. Antinociceptive effects of spinal cholinesterase inhibition and isobolographic analysis of the interaction with μ and α2 receptor systems. *Anesthesiology* 1994; 80:1338–48.
90. Yaksh TL, Grafe MR, Malkmus S, *et al.* Studies on the safety of chronically administered intrathecal neostigmine methylsulfate in rats and dogs. *Anesthesiology* 1995; 82:412–27.
91. Hood DD, Eisenach JC, Tong C, *et al.* Cardiorespiratory and spinal cord blood flow effects of intrathecal neostigmine methylsulfate, clonidine and their combination in sheep. *Anesthesiology* 1995; 82:428–35.
92. Roelants F, Rizzo M, Lavand'homme P. The effect of epidural neostigmine combined with ropivacaine and sufentanil on neuraxial analgesia during labor. *Anesth Analg* 2003; 96:1191–6.
93. Roelants F, Lavand'Homme PM. Epidural neostigmine combined with sufentanil provides balanced and selective analgesia in early labor. *Anesthesiology* 2004; 101:439–44.
94. Roelants F, Lavand'Homme PM, Mercier-Fuzier V. Epidural administration of neostigmine and clonidine to induce labor analgesia. *Anesthesiology* 2005; 102:1205–10.
95. Van de Velde M, Berends N, Kumar A, *et al.* Effects of epidural clonidine and neostigmine following intrathecal labour analgesia: a randomised, double-blind, placebo controlled trial. *Int J Obstet Anesth* 2009; 18:207–14.
96. Ross VH, Pan PH, Owen MD, *et al.* Neostigmine decreases bupivacaine use by patient-controlled epidural analgesia during labor: a randomized controlled study. *Anesth Analg* 2009; 109:524–31.
97. JC Eisenach. Epidural neostigmine: will it replace lipid soluble opioids for postoperative and labor analgesia? *Anesth Analg* 2009; 109:293–5.
98. Paech M, Pan P. New recipes for neuraxial labor analgesia: simple fare or gourmet combos? *Int J Obstet Anesth* 2009; 18:201–3.
99. Colonna-Romano P, Lingaraju N, Godfrey SD. Epidural test dose and intravascular injection in obstetrics: sensitivity, specificity, and lowest effective dose. *Anesth Analg* 1992; 75:372–6.
100. Norris MC, Ferrenbach D, Dalman H, *et al.* Does epinephrine improve the diagnostic accuracy of aspiration during labor epidural analgesia? *Anesth Analg* 1999; 88:1073–6.
101. Birnbach DJ, Chestnut DH. The epidural test dose in obstetric patients: has it outlived its usefulness? *Anesth Analg* 1999; 88:971–2.
102. Gaiser RR, Lewin SB, Cheek TG, *et al.* Effects of immediately initiating an epidural infusion in the combined spinal epidural technique in nulliparous parturients. *Reg Anesth Pain Med* 2000; 25:223–7.
103. Palmer CM, Cork RC, Hays R, *et al.* The dose response relation of intrathecal fentanyl for labor analgesia. *Anesthesiology* 1998; 88:355–61.
104. Herman NL, Calicott R, Van Decar TK, *et al.* Determination of the dose response relationship for intrathecal sufentanil in labouring patients. *Anesth Analg* 1997; 84:1256–61.
105. Vercauteren M, Bettens K, Van Springel G, *et al.* Intrathecal labour analgesia: do we need another combination than used epidurally? *Int J Obstet Anesth* 1997; 6:242–6
106. Stocks GM, Hallworth SP, Fernando R, *et al.* Minimum local analgesic dose of intrathecal bupivacaine in labor and the effect of intrathecal fentanyl. *Anesthesiology* 2001; 94:593–8.
107. Clarke VT, Smiley RM, Finster M. Uterine hyperactivity after intrathecal injection of fentanyl for analgesia during labor: a cause of fetal bradycardia? *Anesthesiology* 1994; 81:1083.
108. Van de Velde M, Vercauteren M, Vandermeersch E. Fetal heart rate abnormalities after regional analgesia for labor pain: the effect of intrathecal opioids. *Reg Anesth Pain Med* 2001; 26:257–62.
109. Van de Velde M, Teunkens A, Hanssens M, *et al.* Intrathecal sufentanil and fetal heart rate abnormalities: a double blind, double placebo controlled trial comparing two forms of combined spinal epidural analgesia with epidural analgesia in labor. *Anesth Analg* 2004; 98:1153–9.
110. Chiari A, Lorber C, Eisenach JC, *et al.* Analgesic and hemodynamic effects of intrathecal clonidine as the sole analgesic agent during first stage labor. *Anesthesiology* 1999; 91:388–96.
111. Mercier FJ, Dounas M, Bouaziz H, *et al.* The effect of adding a minidose of clonidine to intrathecal sufentanil for labor analgesia. *Anesthesiology* 1998; 89:594–601.
112. Paech MJ, Banks SL, Gurrin LC, *et al.* A randomized, double blind trial of subarachnoid bupivacaine and fentanyl, with or without clonidine, for combined spinal/epidural analgesia during labor. *Anesth Analg* 2002; 95:1396–401.
113. Nelson KE, D'Angelo R, Foss ML, *et al.* Intrathecal neostigmine and sufentanil for early labor analgesia. *Anesthesiology* 1999; 91:1293–8.
114. D'Angelo R, Dean LS, Meister GC, *et al.* Neostigmine combined with bupivacaine, clonidine and sufentanil for spinal labor analgesia. *Anesth Analg* 2001; 93:1560–4.
115. Owen MD, Ozsarac O, Sahin S, *et al.* Low dose clonidine and neostigmine prolong the duration of intrathecal bupivacaine-fentanyl for labor analgesia. *Anesthesiology* 2000; 92:361–6.
116. Lim Y, Ocampo CE, Sia AT. A comparison of duration of analgesia of intrathecal 2.5 mg of bupivacaine, ropivacaine, and levobupivacaine in combined spinal epidural analgesia for patients in labor. *Anesth Analg* 2004; 98:235–9.
117. Sah N, Vallejo MC, Ramanathan S, *et al.* Bupivacaine versus L-bupivacaine for labor analgesia via combined spinal-epidural: a randomized, double-blinded study. *J Clin Anesth* 2005; 17:91–5.
118. Camorcia M, Capogna G, Columb MO. Minimum local analgesic doses of ropivacaine, levobupivacaine, and bupivacaine for intrathecal labor analgesia. *Anesthesiology* 2005; 102:646–50.

119. Whitty R, Goldszmidt E, Parkes RK, *et al.* Determination of the ED95 for intrathecal plain bupivacaine combined with fentanyl in active labor. *Int J Obstet Anesth* 2007; 16:341–5.
120. Van de Velde M, Dreelinck R, Dubois J, *et al.* Determination of the full dose-response relation of intrathecal bupivacaine, levobupivacaine, and ropivacaine, combined with sufentanil, for labor analgesia. *Anesthesiology* 2007; 106:149–56.
121. Arkoosh VA, Palmer CM, Yun EM, *et al.* A randomized, double-masked, multicenter comparison of the safety of continuous intrathecal labor analgesia using a 28-gauge catheter versus continuous epidural labor analgesia. *Anesthesiology* 2008; 108:286–98.
122. Van de Velde M, Budts W, Vandermeersch E, *et al.* Continuous spinal analgesia for labor pain in a parturient with aortic stenosis. *Int J Obstet Anesth* 2003; 12:51–4.
123. Simmons SW, Taghizadeh N, Dennis AT, *et al.* Combined spinal-epidural versus epidural analgesia in labour. *Cochrane Database Syst Rev* 2012; 10:CD003401.
124. Stacey RGW, Watt S, Kadim MY, *et al.* Single space combined spinal extradural technique for analgesia in labour. *Br J Anaesth* 1993; 71:499–502.
125. Camann WR, Mintzer BH, Denney RA, *et al.* Intrathecal sufentanil for labor analgesia. *Anesthesiology* 1993; 78:870–4.
126. Collis RE, Baxandall ML, Srikantharajah ID, *et al.* Combined spinal epidural analgesia: technique, management and outcome of 300 mothers. *Int J Obstet Anesth* 1994; 3:75–81.
127. Collis RE, Davies DWL, Aveling W. Randomised comparison of combined spinal epidural and standard epidural analgesia in labour. *Lancet* 1995; 345:1413–16.
128. Abouleish A, Abouleis E, Camann W. Combined spinal epidural analgesia in advanced labour. *Can J Anaesth* 1994; 41:575–8.
129. Joos S, Servais R, Van Steenberge A. Sequential spinal epidural analgesia for pain relief in labour. *Int J Obstet Anesth* 1995; 4:155–7.
130. Gautier PE, Debry F, Fanard L, *et al.* Ambulatory combined spinal epidural analgesia for labor. Influence of epinephrine on bupivacaine-sufentanil combination. *Reg Anesth* 1997; 22:143–9.
131. Palmer CM, Cork RC, Hays R, *et al.* The dose response relation of intrathecal fentanyl for labor analgesia. *Anesthesiology* 1998; 88:355–61.
132. Van de Velde M, Mignolet K, Vandermeersch E, *et al.* Prospective, randomized comparison of epidural and combined spinal epidural analgesia during labor. *Acta Anaesth Belg* 1999; 50:129–36.
133. Van de Velde M, Teunkens A, Hanssens M, *et al.* Intrathecal sufentanil and fetal heart rate abnormalities: a double blind, double placebo controlled trial comparing two forms of combined spinal epidural analgesia with epidural analgesia in labor. *Anesth Analg* 2004; 98:1153–9.
134. Nickells JS, Vaughan DJA, Lillywhite NK, *et al.* Speed of onset of regional analgesia in labour: a comparison of the epidural and spinal routes. *Anaesthesia* 2000; 55:17–20.
135. Vercauteren M, Jacobs J, Jacquemyn Y, *et al.* Intrathecal labor analgesia with bupivacaine and sufentanil: the effect of adding 2.25 µg epinephrine. *Reg Anesth Pain Med* 2001; 26:473–7.
136. Hughes D, Hill D, Fee JPH. Intrathecal ropivacaine or bupivacaine with fentanyl for labour. *Br J Anaesth* 2001; 87:733–7.
137. COMET study group UK. Effect of low dose mobile versus traditional epidural techniques on mode of delivery: a randomised controlled trial. *Lancet* 2001; 358:19–23.
138. Vernis L, Duale C, Storme B, *et al.* Perispinal analgesia followed by patient-controlled infusion with bupivacaine and sufentanil: combined spinal epidural vs epidural analgesia alone. *Eur J Anaesthesiol* 2004; 21:186–92.
139. Roux M, Wattrisse G, Tai RB, Dufossez F, *et al.* Obstetric analgesia: peridural analgesia versus combined spinal and epidural analgesia. *Ann Fr Anesth Reanim* 1999; 18:487–98.
140. Ngamprasertwong P, Kumwilaisakmd K, Indrambarya T, *et al.* Combined spinal-epidural analgesia and epidural analgesia in labor: effect of intrathecal fentanyl vs epidural bupivacaine as a bolus. *J Med Assoc Thai* 2007; 90:1368–74.
141. Collis RE, Davies DWL, Aveling W. Randomised comparison of combined spinal epidural and standard epidural analgesia in labour. *Lancet* 1995; 345:1413–16.
142. Goodman SR, Smiley RM, Negron MA, *et al.* A randomized trial of breakthrough pain during combined spinal-epidural versus epidural labor analgesia in parous women. *Anesth Analg* 2009; 108:246–51.
143. Kayacan N, Ertugrul F, Cete N, *et al.* Comparison of epidural and combined spinal epidural analgesia in the management of labour without pain. *J Int Med Res* 2006; 34:596–602.
144. Hepner DL, Gaiser RR, Cheek TG, *et al.* Comparison of combined spinal epidural and low dose epidural for labour analgesia. *Can J Anaesth* 2000; 47:232–6.
145. Price C, Lafreniere L, Brosnan C, *et al.* Regional analgesia in early labour: combined spinal epidural versus epidural. *Anaesthesia* 1998; 53:951–5.
146. Gambling D, Berkowitz J, Farrell TR, *et al.* A randomized comparison of epidural analgesia and combined spinal-epidural analgesia in a private setting: pain scores during first and second stages of labor and at delivery. *Anesth Analg* 2013; 116:636–43.
147. Hess PE, Pratt SD, Lucas TP, *et al.* Predictors of breakthrough pain during labor epidural analgesia. *Anesth Analg* 2001; 93:414–18.
148. Swenson JD, Wisniewski M, McJames S, *et al.* The effect of prior dural puncture on cisternal cerebrospinal fluid morphine concentration in sheep after administration of lumbar epidural morphine. *Anesth Analg* 1996; 83:523–5.
149. Leighton BL, Arkoosh VA, Huffnagle S, *et al.* The dermatomal spread of epidural bupivacaine with and without prior intrathecal sufentanil. *Anesth Analg* 1996; 83:526–9.
150. Cappiello E, O'Rourke N, Segal S, *et al.* A randomized trial of dural puncture epidural technique compared with the standard epidural technique for labor analgesia. *Anesth Analg* 2008; 107:1646–51.
151. Thomas JA, Pan PH, Harris LC, *et al.* Dural puncture with a 27-Gauge Whitacre needle as part of a combined spinal-epidural technique does not improve labor epidural catheter function. *Anesthesiology* 2005; 103:1046–51.
152. Patel NP, Armstrong SL, Fernando R, *et al.* Combined spinal epidural vs epidural labour analgesia: does initial intrathecal analgesia reduce the subsequent minimum local analgesic concentration of epidural bupivacaine? *Anaesthesia* 2012; 67:584–93.
153. Viscomi CM, Rathmell JP, Pace NL. Duration of intrathecal labor analgesia: early versus advance labour. *Anesth Analg* 1997; 84:1108–12.
154. Amor MB, Draief A, Ouezini R, *et al.* Thirty µg intrathecal clonidine prolongs labour analgesia, but increases the incidence of hypotension and abnormal foetal heart rate patterns. *Ann Fr Anesth Reanim* 2007; 26:916–20.
155. Chiari A, Lorber C, Eisenach JC, *et al.* Analgesic and hemodynamic effects of intrathecal clonidine as the sole analgesic agent during first stage labor. *Anesthesiology* 1999; 91:388–96.
156. D'Angelo R, Evans E, Dean LA, *et al.* Spinal clonidine prolongs labour analgesia from spinal sufentanyl and bupivacaine. *Anesth Analg* 1999; 88:573–6.
157. Eisenach JC. Additives for epidural analgesia for labor: why bother? *Reg Anesth Pain Med* 1998; 23:531–2.
158. Hughes D, Hill D, Fee JPH. Intrathecal ropivacaine or bupivacaine with fentanyl for labour. *Br J Anaesth* 2001; 87:733–7.
159. Mercier FJ, Dounas M, Bouaziz H, *et al.* The effect of adding a minidose of clonidine to intrathecal sufentanyl for labour analgesia. *Anesthesiology* 1998; 89:594–601.
160. Owen MD, Ozsarac O, Sahin S, *et al.* Low dose clonidine and neostigmine prolong the duration of intrathecal bupivacaine-fentanyl for labor analgesia. *Anesthesiology* 2000; 92:361–6.
161. Paech MJ, Banks SL, Gurrin LC, *et al.* A randomised, double blinded trial of subarachnoid bupivacaine and fentanyl, with or

without clonidine, for combined spinal/epidural analgesia during labour. *Anesth Analg* 2002; 95:1396–401.
162. Sia ATH. Optimal dose of intrathecal clonidine added to sufentanil plus bupivacaine for labour analgesia. *Can J Anaesth* 2000; 47:875–80.
163. Viscomi CM, Rathmell JP, Pace NL. Duration of intrathecal labor analgesia: early versus advance labour. *Anesth Analg* 1997; 84:1108–12.
164. COMET study group. Randomized controlled trial comparing traditional with two mobile epidural techniques. *Anesthesiology* 2002; 97:1567–75.
165. Lee S, Lew E, Lim Y, *et al.* Failure of augmentation of labor epidural analgesia for intrapartum cesarean delivery: a retrospective review. *Anesth Analg* 2009; 108:252–4.
166. Miro M, Guasch E, Gilsanz F. Comparison of epidural analgesia with combined spinal epidural analgesia for labor: a retrospective study of 6497 cases. *Int J Obstet Anesth* 2008; 17:15–19.
167. Norris MC. Are combined spinal epidural catheters reliable? *Int J Obstet Anesth* 2000; 9:3–6.
168. Norris MC, Fogel ST, Conway-Long C. Combined spinal epidural versus epidural analgesia. *Anesthesiology* 2001; 95:913–20.
169. Thomas JA, Pan PH, Harris LC, *et al.* Dural puncture with a 27-Gauge Whitacre needle as part of a combined spinal-epidural technique does not improve labor epidural catheter function. *Anesthesiology* 2005; 103:1046–51.
170. Van de Velde M, Teunkens A, Hanssens M, *et al.* Post dural puncture headache following combined spinal epidural or epidural anaesthesia in obstetric patients. *Anaesth Intensive Care* 2001; 29:595–9.
171. Riley ET, Ratner EF, Cohen SE. Intrathecal sufentanil for labor analgesia: do sensory changes predict better analgesia and greater hypotension? *Anesth Analg* 1997; 84:346–51.
172. Missant C, Teunkens A, Vandermeersch E, *et al.* Intrathecal conidine prolongs labour analgesia but worsens fetal outcome: a pilot study. *Can J Anaesth* 2004; 51:696–701.
173. Pan PH, Moore CH, Ross VH. Severe maternal bradycardia and asystole after combined spinal epidural labor analgesia in a morbidly obese parturient. *J Clin Anesth* 2004; 16:461–4.
174. Ferouz K, Norris MC, Leighton BL. Risk of respiratory arrest after intrathecal sufentanil. *Anesth Analg* 1997; 85:1088–90.
175. Crites J, Ramanathan J. Acute hypoglycemia following combined spinal epidural anesthesia (CSE) in a parturient with diabetes mellitus. *Anesthesiology* 2000; 93:591.
176. Buggy D, Hughes N, Gardiner J. Posterior column sensory impairment during ambulatory extradural analgesia in labour *Br J Anaesth* 1994; 73:540–2.
177. Davies J, Fernando R, McLeod A, *et al.* Postural stability following ambulatory regional analgesia for labor. *Anesthesiology* 2002; 97:1576–81.
178. Nageotte MP, Larson D, Rumney PJ, *et al.* Epidural analgesia compared with combined spinal epidural analgesia during labor in nulliparous women. *N Engl J Med* 1997; 337:1715–19.
179. Albers LL, Anderson D, Cragin L, *et al.* The relationship of ambulation in labor to operative delivery. *J Nurse Midwifery* 1997; 42:4–8.
180. Golara M, Plaat F, Shennan AH. Upright versus recumbent position in the second stage of labour in women with combined spinal epidural analgesia. *Int J Obstet Anesth* 2002; 11:19–22.
181. Mardirossof C, Dumont L, Boulvain M, *et al.* Fetal bradycardia due to intrathecal opioids for labour analgesia: a systematic review. *BJOG* 2002; 109:274–81.
182. Vercauteren M, Bettens K, Van Springel G, *et al.* Intrathecal labor analgesia: can we use the same mixture as is used epidurally? *Int J Obstet Anesth* 1997; 6:242–6.
183. Patel NP, El-Wahab N, Fernando R, *et al.* Fetal effects of combined spinal epidural versus epidural labour analgesia: a prospective, randomised and double-blind study. *Anaesthesia* 2014: 69:458–67
184. Norris MC, Grieco WM, Borkowski M, *et al.* Complications of labor analgesia: epidural versus combined spinal epidural techniques. *Anesth Analg* 1994; 79:529–37.
185. Heesen M, Klohr S, Roissant R, *et al.* Insertion of an intrathecal catheter following accidental dural puncture: a meta-analysis. *Int J Obstet Anesth* 2013; 22:26–30.
186. Apfel CC, Saxena A, Cakmakkaya OS, *et al.* Prevention of postdural puncture headache after accidental dural puncture: a quantitative systematic review. *Br J Anaesth* 2010; 105:255–63.
187. Bradbury CL, Singh SI, Badder SR, *et al.* Prevention of post-dural puncture headache in parturients: a systematic review and meta-analysis. *Acta Anaesthesiol Scand* 2012; 57:417–30.
188. Reynolds F. Damage to the conus medullaris following spinal anaesthesia. *Anaesthesia* 2001; 56:238–47.
189. Broadbent CR, Maxwell WB, Ferrie R, *et al.* Ability of anaesthetists to identify a marked interspace. *Anaesthesia* 2000; 55:1122–6.
190. Royal College of Anaesthetists. *3rd National Audit Project (NAP3): National Audit of Major Complications of Central Neuraxial Block in the United Kingdom*. London: Royal College of Anaesthetists; 2009. http://www.rcoa.ac.uk/node/4207
191. Cascio M, Heath G. Meningitis following a combined spinal-epidural technique in a labouring term parturient. *Can J Anaesth* 1996; 43:399–402.
192. Stallard N, Barry P. Another complication of the combined extradural-subarachnoid technique. *Br J Anaesth* 1995; 75:370–1.
193. Harding SA, Collis RE, Morgan BM. Meningitis after combined spinal-extradural anaesthesia in obstetrics. *Br J Anaesth* 1994; 73:545–7.
194. Pinder AJ, Dresner M. Meningococcal meningitis after a CSE. *Int J Obstet Anesth* 2002; 12:183–7.

CHAPTER 15

Maintenance of neuraxial labour analgesia

Alex Tiong Heng Sia, Ban Leong Sng, and Serene Leo

Introduction

Labour pain is one of the most painful experiences a woman can undergo;[1] physical and psychological factors have been shown to influence the extent and severity of pain suffering.[2] Although neuraxial analgesia is relatively invasive, with years of medical research and improved safety, epidural analgesia is now considered the gold standard of labour pain relief. It is the only method that provides excellent analgesia without significant maternal and fetal sedation. Understanding the dynamic and multifaceted nature of labour pain is essential to providing the optimal regimen in the maintenance of analgesia.

Apart from providing the desired degree of pain relief, the other objectives of maintaining an effective neuraxial block would give the mother the ability to titrate the most satisfactory level of pain relief and minimal side effects such as motor blockade. With the introduction of patient-controlled epidural analgesia (PCEA) by Gambling et al. in 1988, parturient 'self-titration' of epidural analgesia was made possible.[3] In spite of that, some women may still require rescue epidural supplementation from 'breakthrough' pain due to a multitude of factors, including misplaced epidural catheters producing inadequate blockade as well as dysfunctional labour and cephalopelvic disproportion that may predispose women to increased pain during labour. The effectiveness of the maintenance of neuraxial blocks is dependent on a variety of factors. The effective and correct placement of the epidural catheter in the epidural space, the use of an appropriate epidural maintenance analgesic drug solution, and the utilization of newer drug delivery systems and technology will contribute to the effectiveness and the ability to individualize therapy.

The initiation of neuraxial block

An effective induction of labour analgesia is critical to allow a successful continued maintenance of epidural analgesia (see also Chapter 14). There has been an ongoing debate regarding the advantages and disadvantages of epidural labour analgesia versus the newer combined spinal–epidural (CSE) technique. Indeed, the induction of labour analgesia using the CSE technique has gained much popularity in recent years. The advantages of a CSE include a rapid onset of uniform analgesia and minimal motor blockade with the judicious use of small analgesic doses of local anaesthetic and opioid. Consequently, CSE is able to achieve a reliable block of sacral nerve roots with minimal maternal and umbilical cord blood concentrations of analgesics.[4–6] The CSE technique employing the 'needle-through-needle' technique has also been thought to improve the chances of the placement of a properly functioning epidural catheter by prior verification of the subarachnoid space with the spinal needle.[6–8] In addition, the dural puncture created during the CSE technique is thought to allow some subarachnoid transfer of epidurally administered drugs and thus improve the quality of epidural analgesia.[9]

There is also evidence to suggest that blocks initiated by CSE could potentially reduce the risk of breakthrough pain during the subsequent maintenance of epidural analgesia.[10] In a randomized controlled trial of 100 women, Goodman et al.[10] compared initiation of neuraxial analgesia with epidural analgesia (3 mL of epidural bupivacaine 2.5 mg/mL, followed by 10 mL of bupivacaine 1.25 mg/mL with 50 mcg fentanyl) to CSE (intrathecal bupivacaine 2.5 mg with 25 mcg fentanyl). Both groups received epidural infusions of bupivacaine 0.625 mg/mL with 2 mcg/mL fentanyl at 12 mL/h. The visual analogue scale scores for pain were lower in the CSE group at 10 minutes and 30 minutes after initiation of neuraxial analgesia, although subsequent analgesia was comparable.

The potential benefits of CSE are also supported by a retrospective observational study of 6497 parturients; the authors concluded that though comparable in terms of safety, the quality of analgesia was better in patients who received CSE when compared to conventional epidural analgesia.[11] While the current literature supports a faster onset time to effective analgesia when the CSE technique is used for initiation of labour analgesia as compared with epidural analgesia, it is still equivocal with regard to the impact of CSE on overall maternal satisfaction with analgesia.[12,13]

The latest Cochrane systematic review by Simmons et al. has shown that CSE confers no advantage over epidural analgesia in terms of maternal satisfaction scores or the percentage of patients requiring physician-administered top-up doses[14] for breakthrough pain. Moreover, there were no differences in the incidence of maternal side effects such as motor block, hypotension, post-dural puncture headache, or adverse effects on the neonate.[10,12]

CSE may be associated with a greater incidence of pruritus compared to epidural analgesia owing to the administration of intrathecal opioids.[5,11,12] There were earlier concerns of the effects of the spinal component of CSE on fetal heart rate abnormalities. Van de Velde et al. showed that the use of intrathecal opioids could be related to a higher incidence of non-reassuring fetal heart rate patterns, particularly in those who had received an analgesic mixture that contained a relatively higher dose of intrathecal opioids, that is, sufentanil 7.5 mcg versus 1.5 mcg.[15] This could be attributed to the rapid onset of pain relief associated with a higher dose of intrathecal opioids leading to a more sudden decrease in plasma epinephrine and beta-endorphins; this imbalance causes an unopposed action of oxytocin and norepinephrine, with the resultant uterine hypertonus and reduced blood flow, respectively. A smaller dose of intrathecal opioid may reduce the risk of uterine hypertonus. A meta-analysis by Mardirosoff et al. concluded that only 28 women need to receive intrathecal opiates for one fetal bradycardia to occur.[16]

However, Skupski et al.[17] found that there were no differences between epidural and CSE analgesia with similar outcomes in the rate of caesarean delivery and presence of prolonged decelerations in a randomized non-blinded trial. More recently, Patel et al. conducted a double-blinded randomized controlled trial comparing CSE with epidural analgesia.[18] CSE analgesia during the first stage of labour did not increase fetal heart rate abnormalities or have an adverse effect on neonatal or obstetric outcomes when compared to epidural analgesia. However, these authors admitted that only two of the studies in the Mardirosoff meta-analysis were directly comparable with their study, which could explain the different conclusions.

The role of drugs used for epidural analgesic solutions

When the effect of the induction dose of neuraxial blocks wears off, the maintenance of labour epidural analgesia largely depends on the mode of administration of drugs through the indwelling epidural catheter. Over the past decade, labour epidural research has been focused on maintaining effective pain relief throughout labour while minimizing the undesirable effects of maternal motor blockade to preserve maternal comfort and retaining the option of ambulation. Reducing motor blockade also retains perineal muscle power to perform expulsive efforts at the time of delivery.

The choice of drugs for labour epidural analgesia should be safe for mother and fetus, and ideally not affect the progression of labour.[19] Historically, undiluted plain bupivacaine (0.5%) was used for the maintenance of epidural analgesia and resulted in dense motor blockade. The addition of a short-acting opioid (e.g. fentanyl) to the local anaesthetic solution permitted a significant reduction in the effective concentration of bupivacaine, so alleviating the problem of dense motor blockade. Chestnut and colleagues[20] reported effective analgesia with concentrations as low as 0.0625% bupivacaine when combined in a solution with 2 mg/mL fentanyl. In the Comparative Obstetric Mobile Epidural Trial (COMET)[19] conducted in the United Kingdom, traditional epidural labour analgesia (using 0.25% bupivacaine) was compared with low-dose CSE and a low-dose epidural infusion (using 0.1% bupivacaine and 2 mg/mL fentanyl). The investigators randomly assigned 1054 nulliparous women requesting epidural pain relief to traditional epidural (n = 353), low-dose CSE (n = 351), or low-dose infusion epidural (n = 350). The authors found that the use of a low-dose maintenance infusion after the induction of labour analgesia with either CSE or plain epidural led to higher rates of spontaneous vaginal delivery. The spontaneous vaginal delivery rate was 35.1% in the traditional epidural group, 42.7% in the low-dose CSE group (odds ratio (OR) 1.38; 95% confidence interval (CI) 1.01–1.89; P = 0.04) and 42.9% in the low-dose epidural group (OR 1.39; 95% CI 1.01–1.90; P = 0.04). These differences were accounted for by a reduced incidence of instrumental vaginal delivery in the low-dose groups, most likely due to better preservation of motor function during labour and delivery. Analgesic efficacy was similar in all three groups and there was no difference in the rates of caesarean delivery. In current obstetric anaesthetic practice, continued routine use of traditional epidurals using concentrated solutions of local anaesthetics cannot be justified, and the use of low-dose epidurals for labour analgesia maintenance has since gained popularity.

A combination of a low-dose local anaesthetic with a lipid-soluble opioid is commonly administered as the spinal component of the CSE technique. A recent review has found that the dose of 2.5 mg intrathecally of bupivacaine, ropivacaine, and levobupivacaine used for CSE labour analgesia, with or without lipophilic opioids, should provide adequate analgesia[5] (Table 15.1). Bupivacaine, in concentrations from 0.0625% to 0.125%, is a very commonly used local anaesthetic for epidural analgesia. It is often used in combination with fentanyl (1.5–3.0 mcg/mL) and sufentanil (0.2–0.33 mcg/mL) for the maintenance of epidural and CSE analgesia. Levobupivacaine is the S enantiomer of bupivacaine with comparable potency. However, levobupivacaine may have the advantage of being potentially less cardiotoxic, even though this may not be clinically relevant since low concentrations are typically used in modern labour epidurals.

Ropivacaine is another popular local anaesthetic that confers a lower potential for cardiotoxicity and less motor blockade when compared to bupivacaine. Although early studies on ropivacaine have suggested that its potency is 60% of bupivacaine, recent evidence concluded that ropivacaine is equipotent with bupivacaine to produce sensory blockade at clinically relevant doses.[21] The maintenance epidural concentration with ropivacaine is recommended to be 0.08% and 0.2%.[22] Ropivacaine has limited transfer across the placenta, reducing fetal exposure similar to bupivacaine, possibly due to its high protein binding limiting uteroplacental transfer.[23] There could be an increased incidence of motor blockade in parturients receiving bupivacaine compared to ropivacaine, although this difference may not be clinically significant during a relatively short labour.[24–28] However, in prolonged labour, bupivacaine may result in a significantly higher incidence of motor blockade.[29]

Typically, the combination of local anaesthetic with lipid-soluble opioids such as fentanyl or sufentanil allows the use of lower doses of both agents and minimizes the adverse effects such as motor blockade and other risks due to systemic absorption. The use of opioids in combination with local anaesthetics is common practice and confers a synergistic effect.[30] Both fentanyl and sufentanil are suitable when used with epidural local anaesthetics for neuraxial analgesia.[31] The doses of epidural fentanyl (commonly about 2 mcg/mL) and epidural sufentanil (commonly up to 1 mcg/mL) used in labour analgesia are safe and effective for both mother and neonate.[32,33] For instance, a continuous epidural infusion (CEI) with 0.125% bupivacaine with 2 mcg/mL fentanyl at a rate of 10 mL/h showed a constant maternal and neonatal drug concentration with no fetal accumulation; the umbilical gas values and neurobehavioural scores were within normal limits with no significant neonatal adverse effects.[32]

Epidural clonidine (an alpha-2-receptor agonist that modulates pain perception at the spinal level) has shown some promise in

Table 15.1 Trials determining the ED_{95} for spinal local anaesthetics administered as part of combined spinal epidural regimen for labour analgesia

Reference	N	Groups; drugs	ED_{95} (mg)	Definition of efficacy	Comments
Sia et al. **[A]**	100	N=50; "L" N=50; "R"	1.61 (CI95:1.37–2.14) 2.12 (CI95:1.81–2.81)	VAPS ≤ 10 at 10 min. PI	No block failure in patient who received 2.5 mg or more of both LA
Whitty et al. **[B]**	40	N=40; "B"+"F" 15 µg	1.66 (CI95:1.50–482.5)	VAPS ≤ 10 at 10 min. PI	100 % success with 1.75 mg No motor block
Van de Velde et al. **[C]**	433	N=145; "B"+"S" 1.5 µg N=142; "R"+"S" 1.5 µg N=146; "L"+"S" 1.5 µg	3.3 (CI95:2.9–4.1) 4.8 (CI95:4.0–6.7) 5.0 (CI95:4.1–7.0)	VAPS < 25 at 15 min. PI and for 45 min. PI	The ED_{95} was extrapolated from probit regression after the patients were randomly allocated to receive one of 6 doses (1, 1.5, 2, 2.5, 3 or 3.5 mg) of the respective LA Analgesic potency ratio at ED_{95}: * "L":"R" = 1.0 (CI95:0.7–1.4) "B":"R" = 0.71 (CI95: NA) "B":"L" = 0.67 (CI95: NA) Duration of analgesia determined by the dose used, not the drug. Onset of analgesia faster with "B" than with "R" and "L"
Parpaglioni et al. **[D]**	70	N=35; "L", spontaneous labour N=35; "L", induced labour	1.56 (CI95:±0.25) 2.27 (CI95=±0.33)	VAPS ≤ 10 at 20 min. PI	Data expressed as ED_{95} in 10 mL: for spontaneous labour, MLAC was 0.0156% and for induced labour, MLAC was 0.0227% ED_{95} extrapolated from MLAC ? Statistical methodology not clear

"B" = bupivacaine: "L" = Levobupivacaine: "R" = Ropivacaine: "F" = Fentanyl: "S" = Sufentanil; ED_{95} = Effective dose in 95% of the population; VAPS = Visual analogue pain score; CI95 = 95% confidence interval; LA = Local anaesthetic; PI = Post-spinal injection; NA= Not available.

*The analgesic potency ratio is determined by dividing the MLAD of one LA by the other. The smaller the ratio, the greater the analgesic potency of the first LA compared to the second. A ratio of 1 indicates equal potencies.

Reproduced with permission from Loubert C, Hinova A, Fernando R., Update on modern neuraxial analgesia in labour: a review of the literature of the last 5 years, *Anaesthesia*, Volume 66, Issue 3, pp. 191–212, Copyright © 2011 John Wiley and Sons. Data from Sia AT, Goy RW, Lim Y, Ocampo CE. A comparison of median effective doses of intrathecal levobupivacaine and ropivacaine for labor analgesia. *Anesthesiology* 2005 Mar;102(3):651–6; Whitty R, Goldszmidt E, Parkes RK, Carvalho JC. Determination of the ED95 for intrathecal plain bupivacaine combined with fentanyl in active labor. *Int J Obstet Anesth* 2007 Oct;16(4):341–5; Van de Velde M, Dreelinck R, Dubois J, Kumar A, Deprest J, Lewi L, Vandermeersch E. Determination of the full dose-response relation of intrathecal bupivacaine, levobupivacaine, and ropivacaine, combined with sufentanil, for labor analgesia. *Anesthesiology* 2007 Jan;106(1):149–56; Parpaglioni R, Frigo MG, Sebastiani M, Lemma A, Barbati G, Celleno D. High volume of subarachnoid levobupivacaine decreases drug requirement in first stage labor analgesia. *Minerva Anestesiol* 2004 Dec;70(12):809–21.

recent research as an adjuvant for labour epidural analgesia; the addition of clonidine to a bupivacaine–adrenaline–sufentanil mixture improved the quality and duration of analgesia as compared with solutions not containing clonidine.[34] Epidural clonidine 2 mcg/mL when added to levobupivacaine 0.0625% with sufentanil 0.25 mcg/mL using PCEA has been shown to improve labour analgesia, reduce manual supplementation for rescue analgesia, and reduce pruritus.[35] However, there was no improvement in maternal satisfaction using this regimen. Furthermore, blood pressure was found to be lower in the clonidine group but without adverse clinical consequences. Epidural clonidine (75 mcg) when given with neostigmine 500 mcg after intrathecal ropivacaine and sufentanil via a CSE technique resulted in significantly prolonged initial analgesia 114 (105–163) minutes compared to placebo 95 (70–120) minutes.[36] There was also a reduced hourly ropivacaine consumption. Therefore, epidural clonidine may have distinct advantages to improve the quality of labour neuraxial analgesia, although its routine use is generally not recommended due to the potential risk of hypotension and sedation.

Spinal clonidine has been investigated also for its efficacy and safety during initiation of neuraxial analgesia.[37] Spinal clonidine 50 mcg has been shown to prolong analgesia when added to sufentanil 7.5 mcg and bupivacaine 2.5 mg early in the first stage of labour. This was achieved with similar pain scores and side effects, including motor block, sedation, and hypotension. However, there is more evidence to suggest that spinal clonidine may not be recommended for routine use.[38] There is an increased risk of hypotension and abnormal fetal heart tracing patterns with the use of low-dose spinal clonidine.[38] Other studies have suggested that spinal clonidine may not increase the duration or quality of analgesia when used for initiation of labour neuraxial analgesia.[39]

Similarly, a continuous epidural administration of neostigmine has been shown to result in a bupivacaine-sparing effect.[40] The addition of epidural neostigmine 4 mcg/mL reduces the hourly consumption of bupivacaine by 19–25% with PCEA during labour. There was no increased risk of nausea, uterine hypertonus, or fetal heart rate abnormalities. However, mild sedation was present. Despite studies reporting the advantages of using epidural clonidine and neostigmine for epidural labour analgesia, safety concerns have been raised on their use for neuraxial labour analgesia.[41,42]

The role of epidural drug delivery systems: patient-controlled epidural analgesia

The earliest method of maintaining labour epidural analgesia was via manually administered epidural boluses, a practice that is certainly labour intensive and cumbersome.[43] With the advent of automated infusion pumps, it became possible to administer a continuous infusion of an analgesic solution via an indwelling epidural catheter. Recently, due to increasing awareness of the benefits of providing parturients greater autonomy over their own labour analgesic regimens, more interactive and flexible analgesic modalities have been developed.

PCEA is a mode of epidural drug delivery that allows the parturient to administer intermittent boluses of epidural solution herself. This provides flexibility to accommodate her escalating analgesic requirements as labour progresses or as labour augmentation regimens are started. PCEA programme settings such as demand bolus, lockout interval, background infusion rate, and hourly maximum dose limits are usually decided upon by the attending anaesthetist.

The earliest study comparing PCEA with CEI was published in 1988 by Gambling et al.[3] Since then, there have been numerous studies confirming the various advantages of PCEA over CEI as a mode of labour epidural drug delivery. The use of PCEA has been shown to reduce the total volume of local anaesthetic solution used without compromising quality of analgesia, resulting in a lower incidence of side effects and greater maternal satisfaction with labour analgesia.[43]

An earlier meta-analysis by Van der Vyver et al.[44] reviewed nine studies involving a total of 640 parturients, which compared demand-only PCEA (without background infusion) with CEI. The authors found that parturients in the PCEA group required lower total doses of local anaesthetic solution, had less lower limb motor blockade, and were less likely to require epidural rescue medication than parturients in the CEI group. D'Angelo[45] conducted another review of 19 PCEA studies, which demonstrated that PCEA had several advantages over CEI and intermittent epidural boluses. These include reduced consumption of local anaesthetics, reduced motor blockade, reduced pain scores, reduced clinician and midwife workload, and increased maternal satisfaction.

Although PCEA for labour analgesia has gained widespread acceptance, research to optimize the PCEA programme settings are still ongoing. The need for a basal infusion, in particular, had been a topic of much debate. Some studies found that a background infusion helped to reduce the incidence of breakthrough pain requiring clinician supplementation and reduce pain scores without any increase in local anaesthetic consumption.[46–48] On the other hand, other studies found that a background infusion led to an increase in local anaesthetic consumption without any improvement in analgesic efficacy.[49–51]

Common PCEA parameters include a background infusion of 5–8 mL/h, a bolus dose of 5–10 mL, and a lock-out interval of between 10 to 20 minutes.[22] A review by Halpern et al. also suggested that administration of approximately one-third of the hourly dose via a continuous infusion may minimize the risk of breakthrough pain, whilst optimizing dose titration for the parturient.[52] Furthermore, a meta-analysis reported in the American Society of Anesthesiologists practice guidelines for obstetric anaesthesia suggested that a background infusion as part of a PCEA regimen does provide better analgesia (OR 3.33; 95% CI 1.87–5.92).[13] Although many of studies report a decrease in consumption of local anaesthetic without the basal infusion, there are no reports of toxicity or excessive motor block associated with the use of a basal infusion.

This conclusion was shared by Loubert et al. who in a review, reported that most studies seem to recommend a moderate basal infusion (around 4–6 mL/h) for benefits of reduced pain scores and reduced incidence of breakthrough pain without increasing the risk of side effects or overall local anaesthetic consumption.[5] However, increasing background infusion rates may lead to greater local anaesthetic consumption. To find a balance between fewer physician interventions and reducing local anaesthetic use, Smiley and Stephenson have suggested a strategy that consists of administering about a third of the expected local anaesthetic hourly demand as a background infusion.[53]

Unfortunately, the ideal bolus dose and lockout interval for PCEA remain unknown. Stratmann et al. compared a 5- versus 15-minute lock-out interval and concluded that the shorter lock-out interval resulted in a better bolus-delivered-to-bolus-attempted ratio, which is thought to be an index of PCEA efficiency. However, there was no demonstrable improvement in any other outcomes such as pain scores, physician intervention, or maternal satisfaction.[54] Halpern and Carvalho compared six studies with various PCEA settings to determine the ideal bolus volume and lock-out interval.[52] They suggested that larger boluses (with a corresponding longer lock-out interval) may improve spread of the local anaesthetic solution in the epidural space with a potential for better analgesia. However, there were no significant improvements in outcomes such as analgesic efficacy, maternal satisfaction, or physician top-up requirements. They concluded that there was no ideal bolus dose or lock-out interval setting for labour PCEA. Loubert and colleagues shared a similar opinion, concluding that there is no strong evidence to favour one regimen over another.[5]

The role of automated mandatory boluses

After PCEA gained popularity and became established, interest was shown in administering epidural solutions as automated mandatory boluses or programmed intermittent boluses instead of a slow continuous infusion. In a laboratory experiment, Kaynar et al. found that a bolus injection, administered at greater injection pressures, allowed drug exit from all holes of a multi-orifice catheter, whereas a slow continuous infusion, given at lower injection pressures, caused the drug to exit almost exclusively from the most proximal hole.[55] Based on his study in human cadavers, Hogan also suggested that the use of intermittent boluses could produce a more uniform epidural block due to an increased injectate pressure compared to a continuous infusion.[56]

The above experimental evidence has been explored in a clinical setting in several trials. Fettes et al. recruited 40 primigravidae who after initiation of epidural analgesia were randomized to receive either an infusion of 0.2% ropivacaine with fentanyl 2 mg/mL at 10 mL/h, or hourly boluses of 10 mL of the same solution.[57] Their results showed that regular intermittent epidural injections were associated with a reduced need for epidural rescue medication, less epidural drug use, and a longer time to first rescue bolus, while providing equivalent pain relief, than continuous infusion of the same solution of ropivacaine and fentanyl. Chua and Sia randomized 42 nulliparous parturients who initially received CSE analgesia, to receive either automated intermittent boluses of 0.1% ropivacaine with fentanyl 2 mcg/mL at 5 mL every hour, or a continuous infusion of the same solution at 5 mL/h.[58] Their results showed that parturients in the intermittent bolus group had a longer duration of analgesia after CSE, reported lower pain scores, and achieved a higher sensory block than those in the continuous infusion group.

Lim et al. went on to investigate the effect of administering automated mandatory boluses in a smaller volume.[59] The authors randomized 50 parturients after induction of analgesia with a CSE technique to receive either automated intermittent boluses of 2.5 mL every 15 minutes or a continuous infusion of 10 mL/h. In both groups, the epidural solution consisted of 0.1% ropivacaine with fentanyl 2 mcg/mL. The results showed that there were no significant differences between the two groups in terms of breakthrough pain and that the low-volume bolus did not appear to improve analgesic efficacy compared to a continuous epidural infusion.

Attempts were soon made to incorporate background automated mandatory boluses into a PCEA programme. Wong et al. investigated 158 multiparous women scheduled for induction of labour at cervical dilation between 2 and 5 cm to receive CSE analgesia. The two groups received either boluses of 6 mL every 30 minutes in conjunction with PCEA or continuous basal infusion of 12 mL/h with PCEA, using a dual pump system.[60] The epidural solution used for the basal infusion was bupivacaine 0.0625% and fentanyl 2 mcg/mL. The bolus group had less bupivacaine consumption, similar analgesic efficacy, and higher patient satisfaction scores compared to those in the infusion group.

Sia et al. devised a computer program that allowed a single infusion pump to function as a PCEA pump with the ability to deliver either background intermittent boluses or a basal infusion in addition to patient-demand boluses.[61,62] This was achieved by uploading pre-programmed PCEA algorithms into a personal digital assistant that was connected to a normal infusion pump. Their initial study was done on 42 parturients whom after successful induction of CSE analgesia, were randomized to receive either a PCEA with a continuous basal infusion of 5 mL/h or PCEA with automated boluses of 5 mL every 60 minute.[61] They found that the automated bolus group had a reduced overall consumption of ropivacaine, longer duration of analgesia before the first PCEA self-bolus, as well as a smaller proportion of patients who self-administered PCEA boluses compared to the infusion group. There was, however, no difference in the need for clinician interventions between both groups. A follow-up study using a modified version of the original algorithm demonstrated very similar results to the first study, suggesting that further refinement of the automated bolus PCEA regimen was needed in order to reduce the incidence of breakthrough pain requiring clinician intervention.[62]

Capogna et al. performed a double-blind randomized controlled trial in which 145 women in labour, after initiation of epidural analgesia, were randomly assigned to receive 10 mL boluses of levobupivacaine 0.0625% with sufentanil 0.5 mcg/mL every hour or a continuous epidural infusion of 10 mL/h.[63] A second pump functioning as a PCEA pump containing levobupivacaine 0.125% was used to treat breakthrough pain. The outcome of interest was the degree of maternal motor blockade as assessed in both lower extremities using the modified Bromage score. The authors found that motor block was reported in 37% of patients in the infusion group and in 2.7% in the intermittent bolus group ($P < 0.001$; OR 21.2; 95% CI 4.9–129.3). Also, motor block occurred earlier and was more frequent at full cervical dilation in the infusion group. The incidence of instrumental delivery was 20% for the infusion group and 7% for the bolus group ($P < 0.03$). Total levobupivacaine consumption, number of patients requiring additional PCEA boluses, and mean number of PCEA boluses per patient were lower in the bolus group. There were no observed differences in pain scores. The authors concluded that maintenance of epidural analgesia with intermittent boluses compared with a continuous infusion resulted in a lower incidence of maternal motor block and instrumental vaginal delivery.

Attempts have also been made to study the effects of manipulating the programmed intermittent bolus time interval and injection volume on total drug use for labour analgesia. Wong et al. randomized 190 nulliparous patients in labour to a PCEA regimen along with either one of the three bolus dose regimens for maintenance of labour analgesia: 2.5 mL every 15 minutes, 5 mL every 30 minutes, or 10 mL every 60 minutes.[64] They found that the total bupivacaine consumption decreased significantly when the bolus time interval and bolus volumes were increased. However, there was no difference in pain scores, PCEA demands or administrations, incidence of breakthrough pain requiring physician top-ups, time to first PCEA self-bolus, and patient satisfaction in all three groups.

The studies discussed in the previous paragraphs have investigated fixed doses of automated boluses in combination with a PCEA program for labour analgesia. However, it is known that labour pain intensifies with progressive cervical dilatation and hence the parturient's analgesic needs may escalate as her labour progresses or as augmentation regimens are started. Hence, a variable frequency of background automated boluses that is responsive to the patient's needs may provide more efficacious analgesia[65] (Figure 15.1). Novel software enables a PCEA pump to determine the patient's analgesic usage over the past hour and deliver 5 mL machine boluses once, twice, three, or four times per hour depending on the patient's most recent analgesic usage (hence the term variable frequency). The trial included 102 nulliparous women in labour who were randomized to receive either a PCEA with variable frequency automated mandatory boluses or a PCEA with a basal infusion of 5 mL/h following initiation of labour analgesia with a CSE technique. The epidural solution was ropivacaine 0.1% with fentanyl 2 mcg/mL. Patients in the automated bolus group were found to have a significantly lower incidence of breakthrough pain requiring clinician intervention (5.9% vs 23.5%; $P = 0.023$) as well as higher maternal satisfaction scores. There were no differences in mean hourly consumption of ropivacaine, mean hourly pain scores or sensory levels, maternal side effects, mode of delivery, or neonatal outcomes.

George, et al. performed a systematic review and meta-analysis comparing the automated mandatory bolus technique with the use of basal infusion during maintenance of epidural analgesia for labour pain.[66] The review did not find any statistical difference in the rate of caesarean delivery (OR 0.87; 95% CI 0.56–1.35), duration of labour (mean difference (MD), −17 minutes; 95% CI −42 to 7), or the need for anaesthetic intervention (OR 0.56; 95% CI 0.29–1.06). However, the bolus group did result in a small but statistically significant reduction in local anaesthetic usage (MD −1.2 mg bupivacaine equivalent per hour; 95% CI −2.2 to −0.3). Maternal satisfaction score (100 mm visual analogue scale) was higher with the bolus technique (MD 7.0 mm; 95% CI 6.2–7.8).

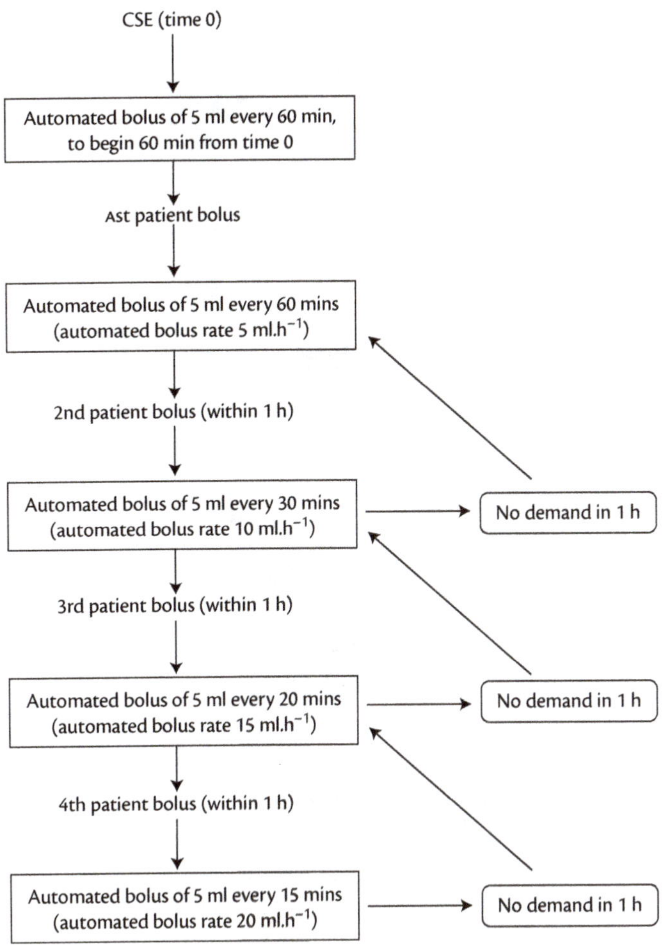

Figure 15.1 Flowchart of variable frequency automated mandatory bolus regimen.

Computer integrated patient-controlled epidural analgesia

Despite having patient feedback on analgesic demands on the PCEA, the conventional PCEA still lacks the flexibility to vary its basal infusion rate. The role of a basal infusion is likely to become increasingly important as pain intensifies with labour progresses or when labour oxytocin augmentation is instituted.

The novel clinical algorithm using smart pump technology was devised in 2005. This converts an ordinary continuous infusion pump into a computer-integrated PCEA (CIPCEA) that is more responsive to the parturient's needs. The CIPCEA hardware utilizes a laptop computer with a programmed algorithm to run a standard epidural infusion pump for research (Figure 15.2). This interactive program records the history of the patient's analgesic requirements over the past hour and increases the magnitude of its basal infusion proportionally to the number of demand boluses made. The CIPCEA algorithm adjusts the background infusion to 5, 10, or 15 mL/h if the patient required one, two, or three demand boluses respectively in the last hour and decreases the background

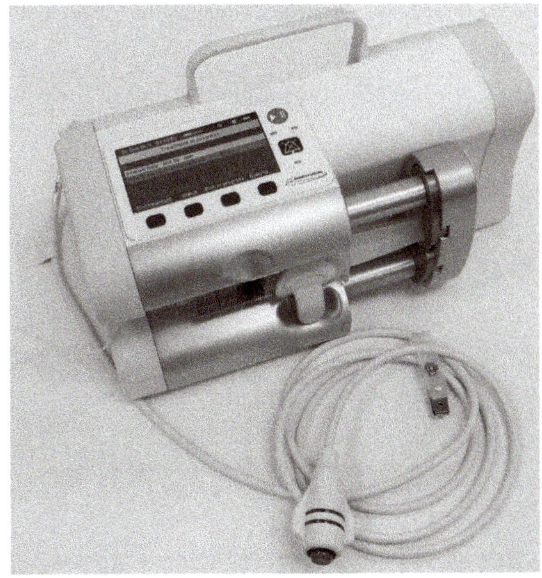

Figure 15.2 Computer integrated patient-controlled epidural analgesia pump.

infusion by decrements of 5 mL/h if there were no bolus demands in the preceding hour[67] (Figure 15.3). The algorithm is designed to respond to the patient's analgesic requirement to improve analgesic efficacy whilst minimizing increases in local anaesthetic use-associated background infusions.[68]

The feasibility of the CIPCEA was assessed in a pilot study by Sia et al. involving 40 parturients in early labour who were randomized to receive either CEI of ropivacaine 0.1% with 2 mcg/mL with a continuous infusion of 10 mL/h or the CIPCEA regimen following successful induction with CSE analgesia.[69] The CIPCEA regimen was associated with a significant reduction in the incidence of breakthrough pain without increasing local anaesthetic consumption or incidence of side effects.

In a follow-up study, Lim et al. compared the CIPCEA pump with a conventional demand-only PCEA pump, looking specifically at epidural drug consumption.[67] There was no difference in the time-weighted consumption of local anaesthetic between the two groups. The incidence of breakthrough pain requiring unscheduled anaesthetist supplementation was 35% in the conventional PCEA group and 15% in the CIPCEA group, although this difference did not reach statistical significance. The CIPCEA group had significantly higher maternal satisfaction scores.

Sng et al. investigated the administration of CIPCEA versus PCEA with a moderate fixed 5 mL/h basal infusion.[68] The results showed a higher maternal satisfaction with the CIPCEA regimen. Local anaesthetic consumption, visual analogue pain scale scores, and incidence of breakthrough pain were similar in the two groups. The CIPCEA group had a higher basal infusion rate during the second stage of labour, compared with PCEA with moderate fixed basal infusion. This may support earlier findings by Capogna et al. who showed an increased epidural local anaesthetic requirement as labour progresses.[70]

From the studies, the CIPCEA program appears to reduce the incidence of breakthrough pain during maintenance of labour epidural analgesia and increases the maternal satisfaction. There was no increased local anaesthetic consumption or side effects.

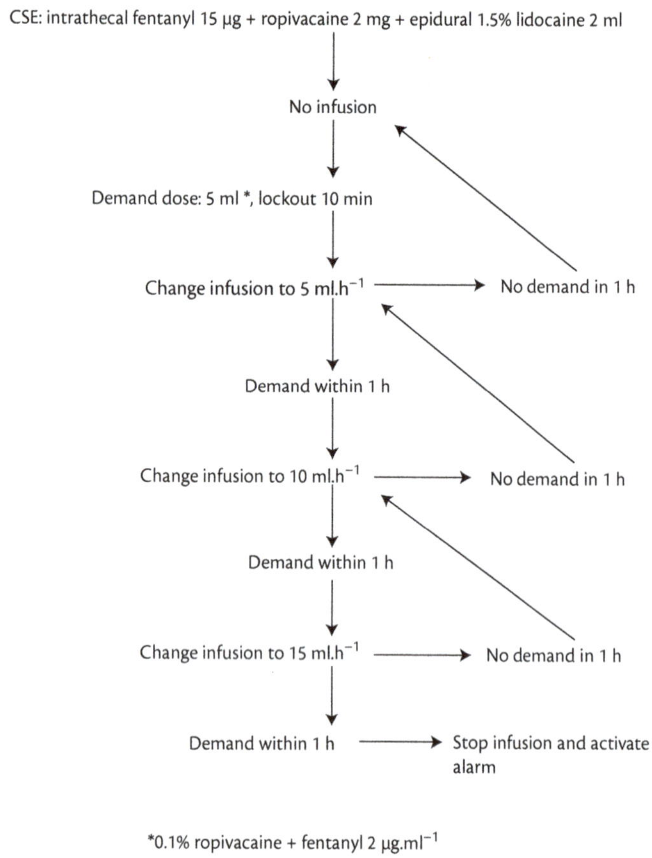

Figure 15.3 Flowchart of computer integrated patient-controlled epidural analgesia regimen.

Reproduced with permission from Y. Lim, A. T. Sia, C. E. Ocampo, Comparison of computer integrated patient controlled epidural analgesia vs. conventional patient controlled epidural analgesia for pain relief in labour, *Anaesthesia*, Volume 61, Issue 4, pp. 339–344, Copyright © 2006 John Wiley and Sons.

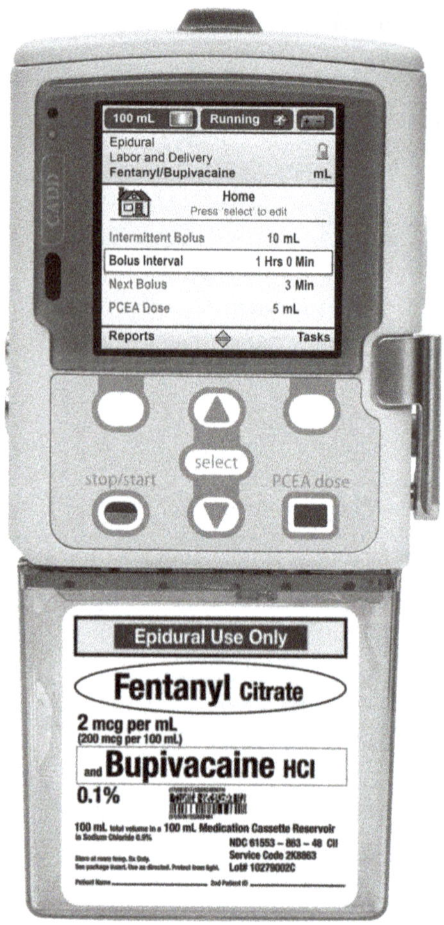

Figure 15.4 A modern smart epidural pump capable of delivering boluses in a patient-controlled epidural analgesia/programmed intermittent epidural bolus mode.

Reproduced with permission from Smiths Medical.

Pump technology has progressed and improved to enable novel algorithms to deliver smart interactive systems such as the CIPCEA and variable frequency automated mandatory bolus regimens. Commercially available systems delivering programmed intermittent epidural boluses incorporating programmed boluses and patient boluses are also available (Figure 15.4).

Conclusion

Labour pain is an extremely subjective and constantly evolving experience. It would be simplistic to apply one epidural regimen to suit all parturients. Instead, individualization of therapy is imperative in providing effective labour analgesia. There have been recent advances in clinical research and medical technology which could aid clinicians in administering the seamless labour epidural analgesia that will hopefully enable every parturient to have a relatively pain-free birthing experience.

Conflict of interest

Professor Alex Sia has filed for a patent for the variable frequency automated mandatory bolus regimen.

References

1. Melzack R. The myth of painless childbirth (the John J. Bonica lecture). *Pain* 1984; 19(4):321–37.
2. Melzack R, Kinch R, Dobkin P, *et al.* Severity of labour pain: influence of physical as well as psychologic variables. *Can Med Assoc J* 1984; 130(5):579–84.
3. Gambling DR, Yu P, Cole C, *et al.* A comparative study of patient controlled epidural analgesia (PCEA) and continuous infusion epidural analgesia (CIEA) during labour. *Can J Anaesth* 1988; 35(3 (Pt 1)):249–54.
4. Leo S, Sia AT. Maintaining labour epidural analgesia: what is the best option? *Curr Opin Anaesthesiol* 2008; 21(3):263–9.
5. Loubert C, Hinova A, Fernando R. Update on modern neuraxial analgesia in labour: a review of the literature of the last 5 years. *Anaesthesia* 2011; 66(3):191–212.
6. Albright GA, Forster RM. The safety and efficacy of combined spinal and epidural analgesia/anesthesia (6,002 blocks) in a community hospital. *Reg Anesth Pain Med* 1999; 24(2):117–25.
7. Norris MC, Fogel ST, Conway-Long C. Combined spinal-epidural versus epidural labor analgesia. *Anesthesiology* 2001; 95(4):913–20.
8. Van de Velde M. Combined spinal-epidural analgesia in labor. *Anesthesiology* 2000; 92(3):869–70.
9. Beaubien G, Drolet P, Girard M, *et al.* Patient-controlled epidural analgesia with fentanyl-bupivacaine: influence of prior dural puncture. *Reg Anesth Pain Med* 2000; 25(3):254–8.

10. Goodman SR, Smiley RM, Negron MA, *et al.* A randomized trial of breakthrough pain during combined spinal-epidural versus epidural labor analgesia in parous women. *Anesth Analg* 2009; 108(1):246–51.
11. Miro M, Guasch E, Gilsanz F. Comparison of epidural analgesia with combined spinal-epidural analgesia for labor: a retrospective study of 6497 cases. *Int J Obstet Anesth* 2008; 17(1):15–19.
12. Simmons SW, Cyna AM, Dennis AT, *et al.* Combined spinal-epidural versus epidural analgesia in labour. *Cochrane Database Syst Rev* 2007; 3:CD003401.
13. Practice guidelines for obstetric anesthesia: an updated report by the American Society of Anesthesiologists Task Force on Obstetric Anesthesia. *Anesthesiology* 2007; 106(4):843–63.
14. Simmons SW, Taghizadeh N, Dennis AT, *et al.* Combined spinal-epidural versus epidural analgesia in labour. *Cochrane Database Syst Rev* 2012; 10:CD003401.
15. Van de Velde M, Teunkens A, Hanssens M, *et al.* Intrathecal sufentanil and fetal heart rate abnormalities: a double-blind, double placebo-controlled trial comparing two forms of combined spinal epidural analgesia with epidural analgesia in labor. *Anesth Analg* 2004; 98(4):1153–9.
16. Mardirosoff C, Dumont L, Boulvain M, *et al.* Fetal bradycardia due to intrathecal opioids for labour analgesia: a systematic review. *BJOG* 2002; 109(3):274–81.
17. Skupski DW, Abramovitz S, Samuels J, *et al.* Adverse effects of combined spinal-epidural versus traditional epidural analgesia during labor. *Int J Gynaecol Obstet* 2009; 106(3):242–5.
18. Patel NP, El-Wahab N, Fernando R, *et al.* Fetal effects of combined spinal-epidural versus epidural labour analgesia: a prospective, randomised double-blind study. *Anaesthesia* 2014; 69(5):458–67.
19. Effect of low-dose mobile versus traditional epidural techniques on mode of delivery: a randomised controlled trial. *Lancet* 2001; 358(9275):19–23.
20. Chestnut DH, Owen CL, Bates JN, *et al.* Continuous infusion epidural analgesia during labor: a randomized, double-blind comparison of 0.0625% bupivacaine/0.0002% fentanyl versus 0.125% bupivacaine. *Anesthesiology* 1988; 68(5):754–9.
21. Polley LS, Columb MO, Naughton NN, *et al.* Relative analgesic potencies of ropivacaine and bupivacaine for epidural analgesia in labor: implications for therapeutic indexes. *Anesthesiology* 1999; 90(4):944–50.
22. Wong CA. Advances in labor analgesia. *Int J Womens Health* 2010; 1:139–54.
23. Johnson RF, Cahana A, Olenick M, *et al.* A comparison of the placental transfer of ropivacaine versus bupivacaine. *Anesth Analg* 1999; 89(3):703–8.
24. Campbell DC, Zwack RM, Crone LA, *et al.* Ambulatory labor epidural analgesia: bupivacaine versus ropivacaine. *Anesth Analg* 2000; 90(6):1384–9.
25. Evron S, Glezerman M, Sadan O, *et al.* Patient-controlled epidural analgesia for labor pain: effect on labor, delivery and neonatal outcome of 0.125% bupivacaine vs 0.2% ropivacaine. *Int J Obstet Anesth* 2004; 13(1):5–10.
26. Fischer C, Blanie P, Jaouen E, *et al.* Ropivacaine, 0.1%, plus sufentanil, 0.5 microg/ml, versus bupivacaine, 0.1%, plus sufentanil, 0.5 microg/ml, using patient-controlled epidural analgesia for labor: a double-blind comparison. *Anesthesiology* 2000; 92(6):1588–93.
27. Halpern SH, Breen TW, Campbell DC, *et al.* A multicenter, randomized, controlled trial comparing bupivacaine with ropivacaine for labor analgesia. *Anesthesiology* 2003; 98(6):1431–5.
28. Meister GC, D'Angelo R, Owen M, *et al.* A comparison of epidural analgesia with 0.125% ropivacaine with fentanyl versus 0.125% bupivacaine with fentanyl during labor. *Anesth Analg* 2000; 90(3):632–7.
29. Gautier P, De Kock M, Van Steenberge A, *et al.* A double-blind comparison of 0.125% ropivacaine with sufentanil and 0.125% bupivacaine with sufentanil for epidural labor analgesia. *Anesthesiology* 1999; 90(3):772–8.
30. Pert CB, Kuhar MJ, Snyder SH. Opiate receptor: autoradiographic localization in rat brain. *Proc Natl Acad Sci U S A* 1976; 73(10):3729–33.
31. Cheng CJ, Sia AT, Lim EH, *et al.* Either sufentanil or fentanyl, in addition to intrathecal bupivacaine, provide satisfactory early labour analgesia. *Can J Anaesth* 2001; 48(6):570–4.
32. Bader AM, Fragneto R, Terui K, *et al.* Maternal and neonatal fentanyl and bupivacaine concentrations after epidural infusion during labor. *Anesth Analg* 1995; 81(4):829–32.
33. Porter JS, Bonello E, Reynolds F. The effect of epidural opioids on maternal oxygenation during labour and delivery. *Anaesthesia* 1996; 51(10):899–903.
34. Claes B, Soetens M, Van Zundert A, *et al.* Clonidine added to bupivacaine-epinephrine-sufentanil improves epidural analgesia during childbirth. *Reg Anesth Pain Med* 1998; 23(6):540–7.
35. Wallet F, Clement HJ, Bouret C, *et al.* Effects of a continuous low-dose clonidine epidural regimen on pain, satisfaction and adverse events during labour: a randomized, double-blind, placebo-controlled trial. *Eur J Anaesthesiol* 2010; 27(5):441–7.
36. Van de Velde M, Berends N, Kumar A, *et al.* Effects of epidural clonidine and neostigmine following intrathecal labour analgesia: a randomised, double-blind, placebo-controlled trial. *Int J Obstet Anesth* 2009; 18(3):207–14.
37. D'Angelo R, Evans E, Dean LA, *et al.* Spinal clonidine prolongs labor analgesia from spinal sufentanil and bupivacaine. *Anesth Analg* 1999; 88(3):573–6.
38. Belhadj Amor M, Draief A, *et al.* [30 microg intrathecal clonidine prolongs labour analgesia, but increases the incidence of hypotension and abnormal foetal heart rate patterns]. *Ann Fr Anesth Reanim* 2007; 26(11):916–20.
39. Cardoso MM, Papa FV, Vieira RF, *et al.* [The effect of adding subarachnoid clonidine to hyperbaric bupivacaine and sufentanil during labor analgesia.]. *Rev Bras Anestesiol* 2006; 56(2):119–25.
40. Ross VH, Pan PH, Owen MD, *et al.* Neostigmine decreases bupivacaine use by patient-controlled epidural analgesia during labor: a randomized controlled study. *Anesth Analg* 2009; 109(2):524–31.
41. Eisenach JC. Epidural neostigmine: will it replace lipid soluble opioids for postoperative and labor analgesia? *Anesth Analg* 2009; 109(2):293–5.
42. Paech M, Pan P. New recipes for neuraxial labor analgesia: simple fare or gourmet combos? *Int J Obstet Anesth* 2009; 18(3):201–3.
43. Haydon ML, Larson D, Reed E, *et al.* Obstetric outcomes and maternal satisfaction in nulliparous women using patient-controlled epidural analgesia. *Am J Obstet Gynecol* 2011; 205(3):271 e1–6.
44. van der Vyver M, Halpern S, Joseph G. Patient-controlled epidural analgesia versus continuous infusion for labour analgesia: a meta-analysis. *Br J Anaesth* 2002; 89(3):459–65.
45. D'Angelo R. New techniques for labor analgesia: PCEA and CSE. *Clin Obstet Gynecol* 2003; 46(3):623–32.
46. Ferrante FM, Rosinia FA, Gordon C, *et al.* The role of continuous background infusions in patient-controlled epidural analgesia for labor and delivery. *Anesth Analg* 1994; 79(1):80–4.
47. Missant C, Teunkenst A, Vandermeersch E, *et al.* Patient-controlled epidural analgesia following combined spinal-epidural analgesia in labour: the effects of adding a continuous epidural infusion. *Anaesth Intensive Care* 2005; 33(4):452–6.
48. Bremerich DH, Waibel HJ, Mierdl S, *et al.* Comparison of continuous background infusion plus demand dose and demand-only parturient-controlled epidural analgesia (PCEA) using ropivacaine combined with sufentanil for labor and delivery. *Int J Obstet Anesth* 2005; 14(2):114–20.
49. Petry J, Vercauteren M, Van Mol I, *et al.* Epidural PCA with bupivacaine 0.125%, sufentanil 0.75 microgram and epinephrine 1/800.000 for labor analgesia: is a background infusion beneficial? *Acta Anaesthesiol Belg* 2000; 51(3):163–6.
50. Boselli E, Debon R, Cimino Y, *et al.* Background infusion is not beneficial during labor patient-controlled analgesia with 0.1% ropivacaine plus 0.5 microg/ml sufentanil. *Anesthesiology* 2004; 100(4):968–72.
51. Vallejo MC, Ramesh V, Phelps AL, *et al.* Epidural labor analgesia: continuous infusion versus patient-controlled epidural analgesia

with background infusion versus without a background infusion. *J Pain* 2007; 8(12):970–5.
52. Halpern SH, Carvalho B. Patient-controlled epidural analgesia for labor. *Anesth Analg* 2009; 108(3):921–8.
53. Smiley RM, Stephenson L. Patient-controlled epidural analgesia for labor. *Int Anesthesiol Clin* 2007; 45(1):83–98.
54. Stratmann G, Gambling DR, Moeller-Bertram T, *et al.* A randomized comparison of a five-minute versus fifteen-minute lockout interval for PCEA during labor. *Int J Obstet Anesth* 2005; 14(3):200–7.
55. Kaynar AM, Shankar KB. Epidural infusion: continuous or bolus? *Anesth Analg* 1999; 89(2):534.
56. Hogan Q. Distribution of solution in the epidural space: examination by cryomicrotome section. *Reg Anesth Pain Med* 2002; 27(2):150–6.
57. Fettes PD, Moore CS, Whiteside JB, *et al.* Intermittent vs continuous administration of epidural ropivacaine with fentanyl for analgesia during labour. *Br J Anaesth* 2006; 97(3):359–64.
58. Chua SM, Sia AT. Automated intermittent epidural boluses improve analgesia induced by intrathecal fentanyl during labour. *Can J Anaesth* 2004; 51(6):581–5.
59. Lim Y, Sia AT, Ocampo C. Automated regular boluses for epidural analgesia: a comparison with continuous infusion. *Int J Obstet Anesth* 2005; 14(4):305–9.
60. Wong CA, Ratliff JT, Sullivan JT, *et al.* A randomized comparison of programmed intermittent epidural bolus with continuous epidural infusion for labor analgesia. *Anesth Analg* 2006; 102(3):904–9.
61. Sia AT, Lim Y, Ocampo C. A comparison of a basal infusion with automated mandatory boluses in parturient-controlled epidural analgesia during labor. *Anesth Analg* 2007; 104(3):673–8.
62. Leo S, Ocampo CE, Lim Y, *et al.* A randomized comparison of automated intermittent mandatory boluses with a basal infusion in combination with patient-controlled epidural analgesia for labor and delivery. *Int J Obstet Anesth* 2010; 19(4):357–64.
63. Capogna G, Camorcia M, Stirparo S, *et al.* Programmed intermittent epidural bolus versus continuous epidural infusion for labor analgesia: the effects on maternal motor function and labor outcome. A randomized double-blind study in nulliparous women. *Anesth Analg* 2011; 113(4):826–31.
64. Wong CA, McCarthy RJ, Hewlett B. The effect of manipulation of the programmed intermittent bolus time interval and injection volume on total drug use for labor epidural analgesia: a randomized controlled trial. *Anesth Analg* 2011; 112(4):904–11.
65. Sia AT, Leo S, Ocampo CE. A randomised comparison of variable-frequency automated mandatory boluses with a basal infusion for patient-controlled epidural analgesia during labour and delivery. *Anaesthesia* 2013; 68(3):267–75.
66. George RB, Allen TK, Habib AS. Intermittent epidural bolus compared with continuous epidural infusions for labor analgesia: a systematic review and meta-analysis. *Anesth Analg* 2013; 116(1):133–44.
67. Lim Y, Sia AT, Ocampo CE. Comparison of computer integrated patient controlled epidural analgesia vs. conventional patient controlled epidural analgesia for pain relief in labour. *Anaesthesia* 2006; 61(4):339–44.
68. Sng BL, Sia AT, Lim Y, *et al.* Comparison of computer-integrated patient-controlled epidural analgesia and patient-controlled epidural analgesia with a basal infusion for labour and delivery. *Anaesth Intensive Care* 2009; 37(1):46–53.
69. Sia AT, Lim Y, Ocampo CE. Computer-integrated patient-controlled epidural analgesia: a preliminary study on a novel approach of providing pain relief in labour. *Singapore Med J* 2006; 47(11):951–6.
70. Capogna G, Celleno D, Lyons G, *et al.* Minimum local analgesic concentration of extradural bupivacaine increases with progression of labour. *Br J Anaesth* 1998; 80(1):11–13.

CHAPTER 16

Labour analgesia: choice of local anaesthetics

Giorgio Capogna

Introduction

Local anaesthetics were the mainstay of epidural labour analgesia in the past. The ideal local anaesthetic agent would provide a rapid onset of effective analgesia, with minimal motor block, risk of maternal toxicity, placental transfer, and effects on labour and the fetus, as well as a long duration of action. Traditionally, for many years racemic bupivacaine (hereafter referred to as 'bupivacaine') has been, and is still, the most widely used local anaesthetic for labour analgesia. Bupivacaine provides effective epidural analgesia but produces dose-dependent motor block and has a poor safety profile, causing life-threatening cardiovascular and neurological sequelae if given in overdose. In order to overcome these two problems, opioids were introduced to be added to local anaesthetics because they interact synergistically to provide analgesia. An opioid combination allows for a decreased concentration of local anaesthetic, and so reduces motor block.[1] Nowadays with the widespread use of ultralow-dose epidural infusions of bupivacaine and opioid and in some units, with the use of the combined spinal–epidural (CSE) technique, it is very unlikely that systemic toxicity will be a problem during labour epidural analgesia.[2] Concerns about bupivacaine cardiac toxicity and the intensity of its motor block have also led to the investigation of other agents. The two new local anaesthetics, levobupivacaine and ropivacaine, have been compared to bupivacaine and have been proposed as alternatives, to provide satisfactory labour analgesia with a possible reduced incidence of motor blockade and decreased cardiotoxicity.

Unfortunately the research into local anaesthetic dosing requirements and the effects of other analgesics such as opioids initially took the form of 'recipe' designs or methodology containing comparisons of fixed combinations of drugs.[3–5] These early studies assumed that the new local anaesthetics (ropivacaine and levobupivacaine) were equipotent with bupivacaine. In addition, all too frequently, comparative studies using protocols with combinations of drugs have been carried out without fully understanding the relative potencies or the dose–response curves of the drugs under examination. In these studies,[3–5] any differences in potency may have been imperceptible owing to the use of local anaesthetics at relatively high concentrations, above the 95th centile for efficacy, and therefore clinically effective in almost all cases.

It is now clear that although bupivacaine and levobupivacaine may be equipotent,[10] this may not be the case with ropivacaine.[7,8] It has therefore been argued that the modest motor-sparing properties and even the reduced systemic toxicity of ropivacaine shown in some initial studies may merely reflect the potency difference (i.e. ropivacaine is a less potent drug), and should be re-evaluated.

The dose-varying methodologies would obviously be more informative than the fixed-dose alternative allowing for the calculation of any type of effect. The introduction of the minimum local analgesic concentration (MLAC) model[9–10] designed for a clinical setting, for example, epidural analgesia in the first stage of labour, has allowed the evaluation of the concentration–response relationship of local anaesthetic drugs.

The analgesic level

Local anaesthetics have been shown to be active in the dorsal horn of the cord, but the main action is actually the conduction blockade of the nerve root. A band of analgesia with definable upper and lower limits can be achieved through epidural administration. Experimenting with different doses of lidocaine, the pioneers of epidural anaesthesia, Bromage and Covino,[11] discovered that, in terms of dermatomes, the size of the dermatomal area was proportional to the mass of local anaesthetic administered. However, this original idea of dermatomal spread being only dependent on the dose was later re-evaluated. Columb et al.[12] gave a fixed dose of chloroprocaine in different dilutions to parturients and found that the analgesia no longer proved effective when the concentration was below 0.5%. This indicates that a desired analgesic effect can be obtained by considering not only the local anaesthetic dose but also the concentration to be given.

Differential block

The impulse conduction block by local anaesthetics is a complex and dynamic process. In non-myelinated axons, the nerve impulse is propagated slowly by the progressive spread of the depolarization front along the membrane. In myelinated axons, the insulating properties of myelin allow the impulse to travel rapidly by jumping from (Ranvier) node to node (saltatory conduction). The block of at least three nodes of Ranvier is necessary to obtain an almost complete conduction block.

Ideally if all the axons in a nerve bundle (such as spinal roots) are exposed to a concentration of local anaesthetic greater than the minimum blocking concentration (the lowest concentration of local anaesthetic that blocks impulse conduction within a specified time) and to a sufficient volume to affect three or more successive nodes of Ranvier, the nerve is completely blocked. The innervated parts are anaesthetized and the muscles are paralysed.[13] In non-myelinated axons, the impulse is propagated slowly by progressive spread of the depolarization front along the membrane.

Effects of the local anaesthetic depends on where and what kind of nerve fibres are involved. Differential block occurs when an impulse in one nerve fibre is completely blocked while in another fibre it continues wholly or in part resulting, for example, in the occurrence of analgesia without motor block. This differential block may be due to differences in nerve properties or to a non-uniform local anaesthetic distribution, where a fibre totally immersed by local anaesthetic may be blocked while a similar fibre lying deeper may remain unblocked. Differential block may also be achieved by lowering the concentration of the local anaesthetic solution in order to mainly block the small fibres (pain sensation) rather than the larger ones (motor function). In fact, sensory inputs related to pain are carried by two separate conduction systems: one relaying signals rapidly via myelinated, small A-delta fibres and the other conveyed via slowly conducting, non-myelinated, very small C-fibres. Motor function is supported by the myelinated, large, and fast A fibres, in particular by A-alpha and A-beta fibres.

Ideally the best solution in labour would be to block all the nociceptive afferent transmission while at the same time sparing all non-nociceptive fibres. This may be accomplished, in clinical practice, by using very dilute local anaesthetic solutions with or without the addition of opioids

The visceral pain experienced in the first stage of labour might be C-fibre mediated, while the A fibres may play a larger role in the somatic pain of the second stage. Capogna et al.[5] demonstrated that more local anaesthetic is needed as labour progresses. This may be the result of increasing A-fibre recruitment as the fetal head descends. This is confirmed by the observation that intrathecal or epidural opioids, which typically affect the C fibres, work well in the first stage, where the pain is mostly mediated by C fibres, but not in the second stage of labour where the A fibres are much more involved.[15]

Addition of opioids

Opioids are usually added to the analgesic mixture to allow for the use of a very diluted concentration of local anaesthetic, so reducing the occurrence of motor block.

Adding an opioid to bupivacaine when bupivacaine is used at a concentration equal to or higher than 0.125% is of no benefit since this concentration corresponds approximately to the EC_{95} of bupivacaine, that is, the concentration at which 95% of mothers are pain free.[16] Conversely when using a bupivacaine concentration lower than 0.125%, an opioid must be added to provide satisfactory and reliable analgesia.[16] The addition of epidural opioids to epidural local anaesthetic solution also reduces the amount of local anaesthetic needed to produce analgesia and so, in turn, reduces motor block and the likelihood of operative delivery.[17]

Role of volume

One of the least researched areas of epidural dosing is the need for epidural drugs to be administered in liquid form in order to effect an adequate spread to the nerve roots. Often the dose creates more problems than volume. Anaesthetists, for example, may give 10 mL of 0.25% bupivacaine more readily to treat a suboptimal labour analgesic block instead of giving a larger volume of a more dilute solution. However, bupivacaine 0.125% when compared with 0.25% produced equivalent analgesia at an increased volume but with a reduced total drug dose.[18] Certainly reducing the dose of local anaesthetic with no loss of analgesic efficacy can only be beneficial. It must be remembered that any dose reduction, without loss of efficacy, reduces the risk of toxicity, improves safety, and may also reduce the likelihood of motor block. With the use of a dilute local anaesthetic solution the mother can ambulate and this is also commonly perceived as leading to a reduced risk of perineal motor block, so favouring a spontaneous vaginal delivery.

The dose/concentration–response curve

To identify the best analgesic solution for labour analgesia, several comparative studies have been performed, but unfortunately many of them were clinically of little value because of the inability to identify equivalent analgesia between differing combinations of local anaesthetic and opioid or other analgesic adjuvants.

In effect, in the past, there has been a scarcity of pharmacodynamic information about the analgesic dose–response relationship of epidural local anaesthetics in labour. This has led to a clinical model being developed which determines the MLAC based on an up–down sequential allocation method.[9]

The up-down method was originally developed for explosives research in the 1940s and has subsequently been applied to many fields of research including engineering, psychology, poisons, and volatile anaesthetics (minimum alveolar concentration (MAC)). This methodology has been extensively described by Dixon and Massey.[10]

This model has been applied to local anaesthetic drugs, similarly to that which was in routine use for inhalation anaesthetics, the MAC. Before this, much of the clinical research into local anaesthetic drugs involved comparisons of fixed doses or combinations with other adjuvants. Most of these studies used supramaximal doses with the resulting conclusions of similar efficacy being difficult to interpret correctly.[3–5]

The MLAC model uses 'up-and-down' sequential allocation to identify the median effective concentration (EC_{50}) or dose (ED_{50}) of local anaesthetic in a given clinical scenario. This is an experimental design in which the dose received by a subject is determined by the response of the previous subject. For the model to apply, the response being measured must be 'all-or-none' in nature, for example, yes or no, effective or ineffective. If a subject's response to a given dose level is above threshold (an effective outcome), there is a step-by-step reduction in the dose given to the subsequent subject. A below-threshold response (an ineffective outcome) leads to an increase by the same amount. Using this approach, testing is eventually centred on the median threshold (EC_{50} or ED_{50}) for the response, above which 50% of subjects will respond and below which 50% will not (Figure 16.1).

The ED_{50} is the point at which the pharmacological strength/potency is defined, so it is here that the dose–response relationship is established with the greatest accuracy Comparisons between different ED_{50s} should therefore permit:

- the comparison between the potency ratio of two different local anaesthetics
- the local anaesthetic-sparing effect of other adjuvant drugs
- the calculation of the effects on requirements due to non-pharmacological or obstetric factors.

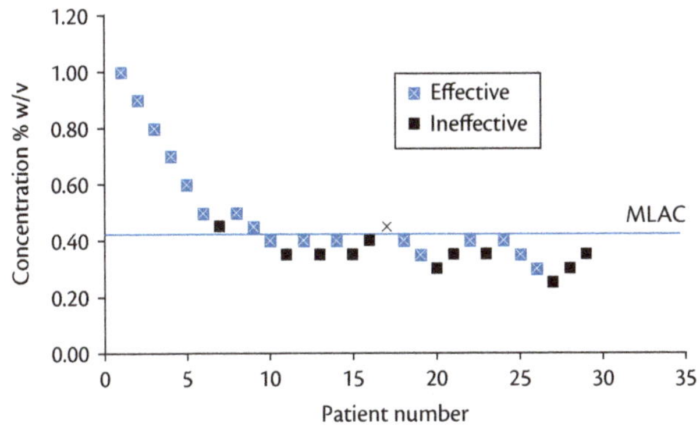

Figure 16.1 The up–down sequential allocation study design.

The concept was initially created to study epidural drugs but can now also be used in a similar way for intrathecal local anaesthetics.

Box 16.1 lists the main findings using the MLAC method.

EC_{50} and the relative potency of epidural bupivacaine, ropivacaine, and levobupivacaine

There has been an interesting controversy around the studies which address the epidural analgesic potency issue of bupivacaine, ropivacaine, and levobupivacaine. The potency ratio between bupivacaine and ropivacaine for analgesia given in the first stage of labour was found to be 0.60 in two MLAC studies carried out in 1999 in both Italy and the United States.[7,8] The studies therefore showed that ropivacaine was approximately 40% less potent than bupivacaine.

Another study compared the effectiveness of the pain relief in the first stage of labour, by examining the epidural analgesia potency of both levobupivacaine and bupivacaine and found the potency ratio to be 0.98.[19]

Taking into consideration the two MLAC studies which compared the potency ratio between the three local anaesthetics, the results showed that bupivacaine is considerably more potent than ropivacaine and slightly more potent than levobupivacaine so permitting the conclusion that levobupivacaine is more potent than ropivacaine (Table 16.1).[6,20]

This potency hierarchy, confirmed by additional clinical studies,[21–25] is no more evident where the three local anaesthetics are compared at equipotent concentration.[23,24]

Box 16.1 The main findings obtained by using the MLAC method

- EC_{50} and relative potency of **epidural** bupivacaine, ropivacaine, and levobupivacaine
- Differential blockade
- ED_{50} and relative potency of **spinal** bupivacaine, ropivacaine, and levobupivacaine
- ED_{50} of opioids and sparing effect on local anaesthetic requirement
- MLAC and obstetric variables:
  - Progression of labour
  - Dystocia
  - Induced labour.

Table 16.1 Relative potencies for analgesia and for motor block of epidural bupivacaine, levobupivacaine and ropivacaine

	Relative potencies (95% CI)	Reference
Analgesia		
Bupivacaine: ropivacaine	0.60 (0.47–0.75)	7,8
Bupivacaine: levobupivacaine	0.98 (0.67–1.41)	19
Motor block		
Bupivacaine: ropivacaine	0.66 (0.52–0.82)	26
Bupivacaine: levobupivacaine	0.87 (0.77–0.98)	27

CI, confidence interval.

Data from various sources (see references).

Differential blockade

It is widely understood that the differential blockade of sensory and motor fibres can be brought about by the three local anaesthetics, bupivacaine, ropivacaine and levobupivacaine, all members of the chemical family of the pipecoloxylidines.

As previously indicated, early traditional studies[3–5] showed that racemic bupivacaine demonstrated a worse clinical profile than ropivacaine or levobupivacaine as it seemed to produce more motor block. Lacassie et al.[26,27] set out in two studies to specifically assess the epidural motor blocking potency of the three local anaesthetics and their relative potency ratio for motor block using a modification of the MLAC design.

When investigating relative potencies, one intuitively assumes that motor block will be less affected by obstetric variables such as the progression of labour, which can in turn affect analgesia, which is the end point of the potency ratio studies.

The motor block potency ratios shown in Table 16.1[26,27] are very similar to the analgesic potency ratios in the previous MLAC studies.[6–8,19,20] Once again it is because ropivacaine is less potent in that it causes less motor block of the lower limbs compared to bupivacaine and levobupivacaine. It can therefore be concluded that when traditional comparative studies reported less motor block for ropivacaine and levobupivacaine it could only have been due to differences in analgesic potency and not to some intrinsic drug property (pharmacological effects).

ED_{50} and relative potency of spinal bupivacaine, ropivacaine, and levobupivacaine

The pharmacodynamics of intrathecal local anaesthetics and their relative potency ratio have also been investigated by a modified up–down technique. Since the pharmacodynamics for intrathecal drugs depend on dose rather than on the concentration, the most suitable term to use is the minimum local analgesic dose (MLAD) rather than concentration (MLAC).

The intrathecal MLAD studies observed a potency hierarchy between the three local anaesthetics, which has been confirmed for both analgesia and motor block[28,29] as shown in Table 16.2.

The intrathecal MLAD studies show that the hierarchy between intrathecal bupivacaine levobupivacaine and ropivacaine in terms of the potency ratio values for analgesia and those for motor block are approximately the same as those found for epidural use.

Epidural and spinal sensory motor separation

Bupivacaine, levobupivacaine, and ropivacaine have a wide sensory–motor separation when given epidurally, and this means

Table 16.2 Relative potencies for analgesia and for motor block of spinal bupivacaine, levobupivacaine and ropivacaine

	Relative potencies (95% CI)	Reference
Analgesia		
Bupivacaine: ropivacaine	0.59 (0.42–0.82)	28
Bupivacaine: levobupivacaine	0.71 (0.51–0.98)	28
Levobupivacaine: ropivacaine	0.83 (0.64–1.09)	28
Motor block		
Bupivacaine: ropivacaine	0.65 (0.56–0.76)	29
Bupivacaine: levobupivacaine	0.81 (0.69–0.94)	29
Levobupivacaine: ropivacaine	0.80 (0.70–0.92)	29

CI, confidence interval.

Data from various sources (see references).

that there will rarely be motor block when these local anaesthetics are administered for labour epidural analgesia at ultralow concentrations. However the sensory-motor separation advantages observed with epidural administration are considerably less with the intrathecal administration.

The opioid-sparing effect on local anaesthetic requirement and the ED_{50} of opioids

Previous traditional studies were not able to show differences in analgesic efficacy between a full analgesic supramaximal dose of local anaesthetic and the addition of a single opioid.[30,31] Furthermore these studies used local anaesthetics at high concentrations, such as bupivacaine 0.25% or 0.125%, which appear at the top of the dose–response curve and need no additional drugs to provide effective analgesia. After examining a number of different adjuvants the results show that only opioids have significant local anaesthetic-sparing effects that can be used in routine clinical practice.

This sparing effect was seen using both fentanyl and sufentanil, in fact up to a 90% reduction in the EC_{50} with both epidural and intrathecal local anaesthetics.[32–38] A reduction in EC_{50} for fentanyl and sufentanil also indicated a clear dose-dependent sparing effect (Figure 16.2).[16,38]

The potency ratio between two single opioids without adding any local anaesthetic can also be determined by using the MLAC method and Capogna et al.[39] observed that the potency ratio between epidural sufentanil and fentanyl for labour analgesia is 5.9.

MLAC and obstetric variables

Because the standardization of labour pain is difficult, being a subjective and dynamic process, it is not surprising to find differences in MLAC estimates and relative potencies.[14,40] This is also true in most areas of research, including human toxicity studies.

Parity and cervical dilation at the moment of epidural insertion plus other obstetric variables should be considered. The comparison of drugs should be undertaken using parturients at similar points of their labour as the analgesic effectiveness of a drug is often related to the progress in labour when it is administered. A reasonable approach would therefore be to standardize the progression of labour using only parturients with a comparable dilation and fetal head descent and excluding those with scores less than 30 (0–100 mm) on a visual analogue pain scale.

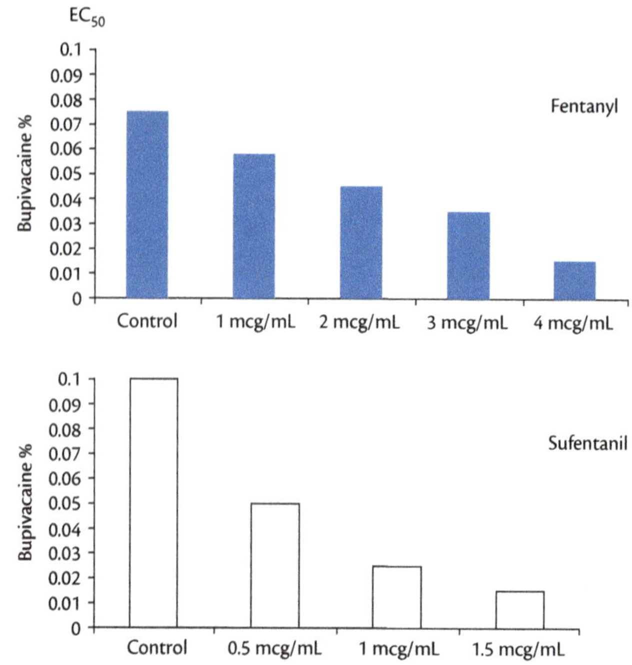

Figure 16.2 Dose-dependent sparing effect of opioids on EC_{50} of bupivacaine.
Data from G Lyons, MO Columb, L Hawthorne *et al.* Epidural pain relief in labour: bupivacaine sparing by epidural fentanyl is dose dependent, *British Journal of Anaesthesia*, volume 78, pp. 493–497, Copyright © 1997 Oxford University Press. Data from Polley LS, Columb MO, Wagner DS, Naughton NN. Dose-dependent reduction of minimum local analgesic concentration of bupivacaine by sufentanil for epidural analgesia in labor. *Anesthesiology*, volume 89, pp. 626–632, Copyright © 1998 Wolters Kluwer.

Several obstetric variables may have an effect on the level of labour pain and the subsequent local anaesthetic requirement. The MLAC method has also been used to investigate these variables, which can include the occurrence of dystocia, the progression of labour, and its induction.

One MLAC study examined the effect of a cervical dilation (less or greater than 5 cm) on the EC_{50} of epidural bupivacaine.[14] The results indicated that three times more bupivacaine is needed as the cervix dilates and labour progresses (Figure 16.3).[14]

The need for local anaesthetic has been shown to be significantly higher in dystocic labours. When comparing women who eventually delivered by caesarean as a result of dystocia with those who delivered spontaneously, an interesting MLAC study[40] showed that the EC_{50} of bupivacaine was higher in parturients with dystocia where the labour was more painful (Figure 16.4). A possible inference from these results may be that the local anaesthetic consumption could be a possible indicator for dystocia.

Capogna et al.[41] have also shown that there is a significantly higher analgesic requirement in induced parturients when compared to women who deliver spontaneously. Induced labour was therefore found to be more painful, with patients needing a higher ED50 of epidural sufentanil.

MLAC and other issues

Second epidural dose

Utilizing the MLAC method it has been possible to determine if subsequent epidural requirements are reduced by using an initial epidural bolus for establishing labour analgesia compared to an initial spinal bolus using a CSE technique. Patel et al.[42] compared the MLAC of epidural bupivacaine given after first administering

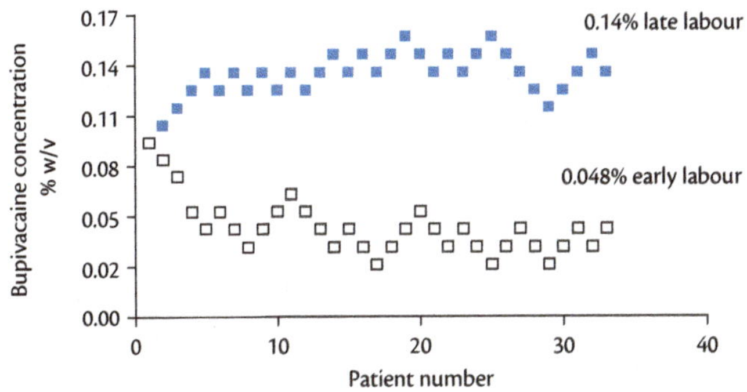

Figure 16.3 MLAC of epidural bupivacaine and progression of labour.
Data from Capogna G, Celleno D, Lyons G, *et al.* Minimum local analgesic concentration of extradural bupivacaine increases with progression of labour. *British Journal of Anaesthesia*, volume 80, pp. 11–13, Copyright © 1998 Oxford University Press.

an intrathecal (bupivacaine 2.5 mg and fentanyl 5 mcg) or epidural (bupivacaine 20 mg and fentanyl 40 mcg) injection. The MLAC method was used to assess the bupivacaine requirements for the second (epidural) injection. The results showed that when compared with epidural analgesia, the requirements increased after intrathecal analgesia by a factor of 1.45. This was surprising and although interesting statistically, these results will probably not be clinically important as the doses used in routine clinical practice are on the upper flat portion of the dose–response curve so the above-noted effect will probably not be realized. It does, however, indicate that any differences seen by clinicians between CSE and epidural analgesia are not the result of a reduction in drug requirement in the maintenance period of epidural analgesia.

Dose, volume, and concentration in the intrathecal space

Traditionally dose has always been thought to be the most important factor affecting the characteristics of the intrathecal block.[43] One study conducted by Camorcia et al.[44] has, however, shown that the characteristics of the block may also be affected by the concentration of local anaesthetic when administered in the intrathecal space. This study demonstrated that the ED_{50} of intrathecal 0.1% ropivacaine caused 50% less motor block when compared to the 1% solution suggesting that considerably less motor block is caused by a more diluted local anaesthetic solution in the subarachnoid space. This might be very useful information when using the CSE technique to reduce motor block.

Effect of gender on local anaesthetic requirement

Studies show that females show a higher sensitivity to noxious stimuli than males, and that there are also different responses to non-opioid drugs between the sexes.[45] Anaesthetic requirements, particularly for morphine, may also importantly depend on gender.[46] It has been found that female patients also need more propofol for general anaesthesia than men.[46]

Camorcia et al. investigated how the intrathecal bupivacaine requirement changes with gender and pregnancy.[47] The study results showed that the ED_{50} needed to achieve motor block in term pregnancy was considerably reduced and it was also greater (30%) in males than in females (Figure 16.5).[47] Another study[48] confirmed these findings, their results indicating that the ropivacaine MLAC for caudal anaesthesia in male patients was 31% less than in female patients. Physical differences of weight and height must of course have an effect on the MLAC of local anaesthetics and further studies should investigate the different responses of men and women to local anaesthetics given for both neuraxial and peripheral nerve blocks.

Pharmacogenetics

The focal point of many genetic studies has been the mu-opioid receptor (μOR), encoded by the gene *OPRM1* because a large number of endogenous opioid peptides, among which are beta-endorphin and encephalin, have this receptor as their main point of action. It is also the principal target for opioid analgesics.[49]

Landau et al.[50] used two distinct methodologies in two different groups to calculate the ED_{50} and showed that labouring women carrying the 304G allele of *OPRM1* responded much more sensitively to the analgesia provided by intrathecal fentanyl. In this study, women were genotyped in late pregnancy, and this allowed the researchers to enrol patients in two separate groups according to their genotype at the time of the labour analgesia request. They reported that 304A homozygous women needed much more fentanyl to achieve labour analgesia and this result was similar to that obtained in another study[51] where there was a pharmacogenetic effect of μOR on ED_{50} of epidural sufentanil.

The analgesic response to neuraxial opioids can be considerably influenced not only by the complexity of different labour and obstetric considerations but also by the labour pain itself and the

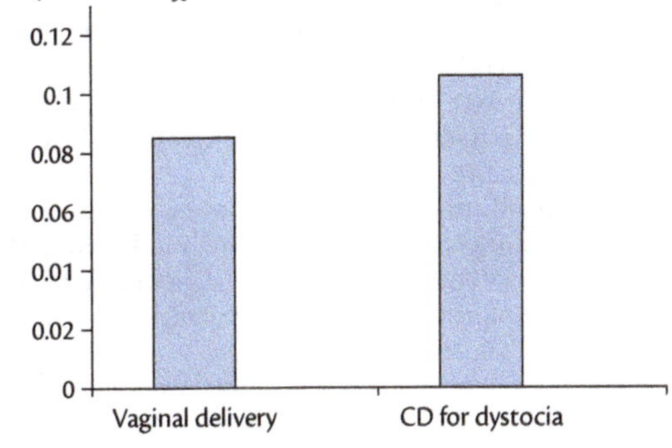

Figure 16.4 EC_{50} of bupivacaine in women who deliver by caesarean delivery (CD) for dystocia.
Data from Panni MK, Segal S. Local anesthetic requirements are greater in dystocia than in normal labor. *Anesthesiology*, volume 98, pp. 957–963 Copyright © 2003 Wolters Kluwer.

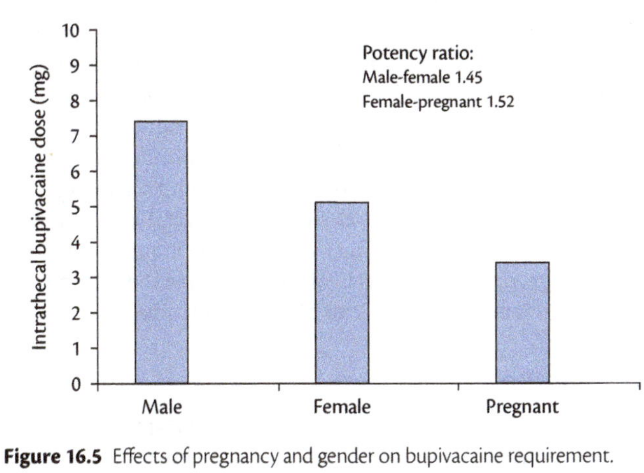

Figure 16.5 Effects of pregnancy and gender on bupivacaine requirement.
Data from Camorcia M, Capogna G, Columb MO. Effect of sex and pregnancy on the potency of intrathecal bupivacaine: determination of ED_{50} for motor block with the up-down sequential allocation method. *European Journal of Anaesthesiology*, volume 28, pp. 240–4, Copyright © 2011 Wolters Kluwer.

diversity found in labour management. It is therefore difficult to judge what part this polymorphism or any genetic variant plays in the clinical efficacy of opioids.

Caucasian parturients show a high incidence of genetic polymorphism for opioid receptors[52] but whether this is clinically important or if it influences the dose of opioid administered epidurally or intrathecally to the subset of women carrying the genetic variant must still be proven.

Caesarean delivery

The dose of the intrathecal local anaesthetic for caesarean delivery has been calculated using a MLAC design.[53–56] These studies consider a dose to be effective when it gives satisfactory sensory dermatomal anaesthesia to a definite dermatomal level with no additional need for other analgesic medications during surgery, which must continue unimpeded for a definite length of time after the intrathecal injection.

It should, however, be said that using the MLAC design in these kinds of studies in a surgical setting, may create ethical problems if patients are exposed to intraoperative pain during their caesarean delivery but these can be overcome by using a CSE technique where the epidural can be used if the intrathecal component is insufficient.

Criticism of minimum local analgesic concentration studies

MLAC studies have shown that there are potency differences among local anaesthetics, but the real significance of these differences as demonstrated by the up–down studies is unclear. Until this uncertainty is answered, prospective randomized (dose–response) clinical studies should not be replaced by data arising from up–down studies.

One of the major criticisms of MLAC studies is that the function of MLAC, EC_{50}, and ED_{50} is to simply describe pharmacologically the measurement of the median of a dose–response distribution.[57–59] As such, they are in essence mathematically comparable to the means or medians used in almost every other study design. An example of this are local anaesthetic toxicity studies which are really ED_{50} estimates as they compare the mean or median tolerated doses, although they are never specifically described as such. However, even if the EC_{50} or ED_{50} are very useful and precise to estimate the potency ratios and therefore to evaluate differences in potency between two drugs, they may not be so precise in estimating the ED_{95} or EC_{95} which is approximately the therapeutic dose.

New study designs are needed and their results validated by further trials.[60,61,62] Until this time care should be taken when taking information from up–down studies and applying it to clinical situations. These studies should, however, be used to help determine clinical practice. Their information should be the first step in designing good clinical trials that examine the relationship between drugs and anaesthetic or obstetric outcomes.

Conclusion

Local anaesthetics vary in their potency and motor–sensory separation and knowledge of these are important for clinicians to achieve the type of analgesia and anaesthesia they require. The MLAC model has enabled clinical comparisons of local anaesthetics at equipotent concentrations. It has quantified what contribution opioids make to the overall effectiveness of the analgesic mixture and provided a means of optimizing combinations of local anaesthetic–opioid solutions. MLAC has also demonstrated the effect of inter-individual and obstetric variables on local anaesthetic potency and provided a pharmacological-based rationale for analgesia solutions used for labour analgesia. Importantly, MLAC studies confirm that the intensity and nature of labour pain is always changing, as labour progresses, and therefore the analgesic approach should be equally dynamic. Although various controversial issues still exist with the MLAC methodology, it has firmly become established in determining local anaesthetic dosing in clinical practice.

References

1. Ostheimer GW, Leavitt KA. Epidural anesthesia. In Van Zundert A, Ostheimer GW (eds) *Pain Relief & Anesthesia in Obstetrics*. New York: Churchill Livingstone; 1996:285–305.
2. McGrady E. Epidural analgesia in labour. *Contin Educ Anaesth Crit Care Pain* 2004; 4: 114–17.
3. Burke D, Henderson DJ, Simpson AM, *et al.* Comparison of 0.25% S(-)-bupivacaine with 0.25% RS-bupivacaine for epidural analgesia in labour. *Br J Anaesth* 1999; 83:750–5.
4. Gaiser RR, Venkateswaren P, Cheek TG, *et al.* Comparison of 0.25% ropivacaine and bupivacaine for epidural analgesia for labor and vaginal delivery. *J Clin Anesth* 1997; 7:564–8.
5. Writer D, Stienstra R, Eddleson JM, *et al.* Neonatal outcome and mode of delivery after epidural analgesia for labor with ropivacaine and bupivacaine: a double-blind comparison. *Anesth Analg* 1995; 80:285–9.
6. Benhamou D, Ghosh C, Mercier FJ. A randomized sequential allocation study to determine the minimum effective analgesic concentration of levobupivacaine and ropivacaine in patients receiving epidural analgesia for labor. *Anesthesiology* 2003; 99:1383–6.
7. Capogna G, Celleno D, Fusco P, *et al.* Relative potencies of bupivacaine and ropivacaine in labour. *Br J Anaesth* 1999; 82:371–3.
8. Polley LS, Columb MO, Naughton NN, *et al.* Relative analgesic potencies of ropivacaine and bupivacaine for epidural analgesia in labour: implications for therapeutic indexes. *Anesthesiology* 1999; 90: 944–50.
9. Columb MO, Lyons G. Determination of the minimum local analgesic concentrations of epidural bupivacaine and lidocaine in labor. *Anesth Analg* 1995; 81:833–7.
10. Dixon WJ, Massey FJ. The up-and-down method. In *Introduction to Statistical Analysis* (4th ed). New York: McGraw-Hill; 1983:428–39.
11. Cousins MJ, Bromage PR. Epidural neural blockade. In Cousins MJ, Bridenbaugh PO (eds) *Neural Blockade in Clinical Anaesthesia and Pain Management*. Philadelphia, PA: Lippincott; 1988:253–60.
12. Columb MO, Lyons G, Naughton NN, *et al.* Determination of the minimum local analgesic concentration of epidural chloroprocaine in labor. *Int J Obstet Anesth* 1997; 6:39–42.
13. Fink BR. Towards the mathematization of spinal anesthesia. *Reg Anesth* 1992; 17:263–73.
14. Capogna G, Celleno D, Lyons G, *et al.* Minimum local analgesic concentration of extradural bupivacaine increases with progression of labour. *Br J Anaesth* 1998; 80:11–13.
15. Mather LE. Opioid analgesic drugs. In Nimmo WS, Rowbotham DJ, Smith G (eds) *Anaesthesia* (2nd ed). Oxford: Blackwell; 1994:132–65.
16. Lyons G, Columb MO, Hawthorne L, *et al.* Epidural pain relief in labour: bupivacaine sparing by epidural fentanyl is dose dependent. *Br J Anaesth* 1997; 78:493–7.
17. Amer-Wahlin I, Christoffersson M, Dahlgren N, *et al.* Epidural analgesia with sufentanil during labor and operative delivery. *Acta Obstet Gynecol Scand* 2000; 79:538–42.
18. Lyons G, Kocarev MC, Wilson RC, *et al.* Comparison of minimum local analgesic volumes of epidural bupivacaine (0.125% w/v and 0.25% w/v) for analgesia in labor. *Anesth Analg* 2007; 104:12–15.

19. Lyons G, Columb MO, Wilson RC, *et al.* Epidural pain relief in labour: potencies of levobupivacaine and racemic bupivacaine. *Br J Anaesth* 1998; 81:899–901.
20. Polley LS, Columb MO, Naughton NN, *et al.* Relative analgesic potency of levobupivacaine and ropivacaine for epidural analgesia in labor. *Anesthesiology* 2003; 99:1354–8.
21. Gautier PE, de Kock M, van Steenberge A, *et al.* Intrathecal ropivacaine for ambulatory surgery. *Anesthesiology* 1999; 91:1239–45.
22. Bolukbasi D, Sener EB, Sarihasan B, *et al.* Comparison of maternal and neonatal outcomes with epidural bupivacaine plus fentanyl and ropivacaine plus fentanyl for labor analgesia. *Int J Obstet Anesth* 2005; 14:288–93.
23. Fernandez-Guisasola J, Serrano ML, Cobo B, *et al.* A comparison of 0.0625% bupivacaine with fentanyl and 0.1% ropivacaine with fentanyl for continuous epidural labor analgesia. *Anesth Analg* 2001; 92:1261–5.
24. Camorcia M, Capogna G. Epidural levobupivacaine, ropivacaine and bupivacaine in combination with sufentanil in early labor. *Eur J Anaesth* 2003; 20:1–4.
25. Sah N, Vallejo M, Phelps A, *et al.* Efficacy of ropivacaine, bupivacaine, and levobupivacaine for labor epidural analgesia. *J Clin Anesth* 2007; 19:214–17.
26. Lacassie HJ, Columb MO, Lacassie HP, *et al.* The relative motor blocking potencies of epidural bupivacaine and ropivacaine in labor. *Anesth Analg* 2002; 95:204–8.
27. Lacassie HJ, Columb MO. The relative motor blocking potencies of bupivacaine and levobupivacaine in labor. *Anesth Analg* 2003; 97:1509–13.
28. Camorcia M, Capogna G, Columb MO. Minimum local analgesic doses of ropivacaine, levobupivacaine and bupivacaine for intrathecal labor analgesia. *Anesthesiology* 2005; 102:646–50.
29. Camorcia M, Capogna G, Berritta C, *et al.* The relative potency for motor block after intrathecal bupivacaine, ropivacaine and levobupivacaine. *Anesth Analg* 2007; 104:904–7.
30. Celleno D, Capogna G. Epidural fentanyl plus bupivacaine 0,125% per cent for labour: analgesic effects. *Can J Anaesth* 1988; 35:375–8.
31. Scrutton MJL, Porter JS, O'Sullivan G. Comparison of three different loading doses to establish epidural analgesia in labour. *Int J Obstet Anesth* 1998; 7:165–9.
32. Polley LS, Columb MO, Lyons G, *et al.* The effect of epidural fentanyl on the minimum local analgesic concentration of epidural chloroprocaine in labor. *Anesth Analg* 1996; 83:987–90.
33. Lyons G, Columb MO, Hawthorne L, *et al.* Extradural pain relief in labour. Bupivacaine sparing by extradural fentanyl is dose dependent. *Br J Anaesth* 1997; 78:493–7.
34. Palm S, Gertzen W, Ledowski T, *et al.* Minimum local analgesic dose of plain ropivacaine vs. ropivacaine combined with sufentanil during epidural analgesia for labour. *Anaesthesia* 2001; 56:526–9.
35. Stocks GM, Hallworth SP, Fernando R, *et al.* The minimum local analgesic dose of intrathecal bupivacaine in labor and the effect of intrathecal fentanyl. *Anesthesiology* 2001; 94:987–90.
36. Robinson AP, Lyons G, Wilson RC. Levobupivacaine for epidural analgesia in labor: the sparing effect of extradural fentanyl. *Anesth Analg* 2001; 92:410–14.
37. Buyse I, Stockman W, Columb MO, *et al.* Effect of sufentanil on minimum local analgesic concentrations of epidural bupivacaine, ropivacaine and levobupivacaine in nullipara in early labour. *Int J Obstet Anesth* 2007; 16:22–8.
38. Polley LS, Columb MO, Wagner DS, *et al.* Dose-dependent reduction of minimum local analgesic concentration of bupivacaine by sufentanil for epidural analgesia in labor. *Anesthesiology* 1998; 89:626–32.
39. Capogna G, Camorcia M, Columb MO. Minimum local analgesic doses of fentanyl and sufentanil for epidural analgesia in the first stage of labor. *Anesth Analg* 2003; 96:1178–82.
40. Panni MK, Segal S. Local anesthetic requirements are greater in dystocia than in normal labor. *Anesthesiology* 2003; 98:957–63.
41. Capogna G, Parpaglioni R, Lyons G, *et al.* Minimum local analgesic dose of epidural sufentanil for first stage labor analgesia: a comparison between spontaneous and prostaglandin induced labor in nulliparous women. *Anesthesiology* 2001; 94:740–4.
42. Patel NP, Armstrong SL, Fernando R, *et al.* Combined spinal epidural vs. epidural labour analgesia: does initial intrathecal analgesia reduce the subsequent minimum local analgesic concentration of epidural bupivacaine? *Anaesthesia* 2012; 67:584–93.
43. Van Zundert AA, Grouls RJ, Korsten HH, Lambert DH. Spinal anesthesia: volume or concentration-what matters? *Reg Anesth* 1996; 21:112–18.
44. Camorcia M, Capogna G, Columb MO. The relative motor blocking potencies of intrathecal ropivacaine: effects of concentration. *Anesth Analg* 2004; 98:1779–82.
45. Sun LS. Gender differences in pain sensitivity and responses to analgesia. *J Gend Specif Med* 1998; 1:28–30.
46. Pleym H, Spigset O, Kharasch ED, *et al.* Gender differences in drug effects: implications for anesthesiologists. *Acta Anaesthesiol Scand* 2003; 47:241–59.
47. Camorcia M, Capogna G, Columb MO. Effect of sex and pregnancy on the potency of intrathecal bupivacaine: determination of ED50 for motor block with the up-down sequential allocation method. *Eur J Anaesthesiol* 2011; 28:240–4.
48. Li Y, Zhou Y, Chen H, *et al.* The effect of sex on the minimum local analgesic concentration of ropivacaine for caudal anesthesia in anorectal surgery. *Anesth Analg* 2010; 1:1490–3.
49. Flores CM, Mogil JS. The pharmacogenetics of analgesia: toward a genetically-based approach to pain management. *Pharmacogenomics* 2001; 2:177–94.
50. Landau R, Kern C, Columb MO, *et al.* Genetic variability of the μ-opioid receptor influences intrathecal fentanyl analgesia requirements in laboring women. *Pain* 2008; 30; 139:5–14.
51. Camorcia M, Capogna G, Stirparo S, *et al.* Effect of μ-opioid receptor A118G polymorphism on the ED50 of epidural sufentanil for labor analgesia. *Int J Obstet Anesth* 2012; 21:40–4.
52. Landau R, Cahana A, Smiley R, *et al.* Genetic variability of mu-opioid receptor in an obstetric population. *Anesthesiology* 2004; 100:1030–3.
53. Parpaglioni R, Baldassini B, Barbati G, *et al.* Adding sufentanil to levobupivacaine or ropivacaine intrathecal anaesthesia affects the minimum local anaesthetic dose required. *Acta Anaesthesiol Scand* 2009; 53:1214–20.
54. Parpaglioni R, Frigo MG, Lemma A, *et al.* Minimum local anaesthetic dose (MLAD) of intrathecal levobupivacaine and ropivacaine for caesarean section. *Anaesthesia* 2006; 61:110–15.
55. Geng ZY, Wang DX, Wu XM. Minimum effective local anesthetic dose of intrathecal hyperbaric ropivacaine and bupivacaine for cesarean section. *Chin Med J (Engl)* 2011; 124:509–13.
56. Bouvet L, Da-Col X, Chassard D, *et al.* ED50 and ED95 of intrathecal levobupivacaine with opioids for Caesarean delivery. *Br J Anaesth* 2011; 106:215–20.
57. Columb MO. Pro-Con debate: MLAC studies: more ups than down? In *Society for Obstetric Anesthesia and Perinatology Syllabus*. Milwaukee, WI: SOAP; 2004:23–31.
58. D'Angelo R, James RL. Is ropivacaine less potent than bupivacaine? *Anesthesiology* 1999; 90:941–3.
59. D'Angelo R, Shafer S, Clyne B, *et al.* Efficiency and accuracy of up-down vs random allocation to determine analgesic potency and dose response. *Anesthesiology SOAP Abstract Suppl* 2005; 102:A-24.
60. Ingelmo P, Frawley G, Astuto M, *et al.* Relative analgesic potencies of levobupivacaine and ropivacaine for caudal anaesthesia in children. *Anesth Analg* 2009; 108:805–13.
61. Ngan Kee W, Ng FF, Khaw KS, *et al.* Determination and comparison of graded dose-response curves for epidural bupivacaine and ropivacaine for analgesia in laboring nulliparous women. *Anesthesiology* 2010; 113:445–53.
62. Ngan Kee WD, Lee A. Multi-dimensional response-probability-dose curves for bupivacaine and ropivacaine epidural labour analgesia. *Anaesthesia* 2013; 68:368–76.

CHAPTER 17

Adjuvant drugs in neuraxial anaesthesia

Catherine Cromey and Susan Catling

Introduction

An adjuvant is defined as a substance that enhances the activity of another substance.[1] In obstetrics, neuraxial (spinal and epidural) local anaesthetics provide effective analgesia and anaesthesia when used alone as single agents, but can cause dose-related undesirable side effects such as maternal hypotension[2,3] and motor blockade, with its associated higher risk of instrumental delivery.[4] An alternative to single-agent therapy is the use of adjuvants from different pharmacological classes.

When two or more drugs are administered together their effects may be:

- additive (the sum of the effects produced by each agent alone)
- subadditive (i.e. less than the sum of effects from each agent alone)
- supra-additive (i.e. synergistic; greater than the sum of the effects of each agent alone).[5]

By combining drugs with additive or synergistic effects, maximal efficacy can be obtained whilst simultaneously limiting the dose of each individual drug to minimize side effects.

Neuraxial adjuvants in the context of local anaesthetics reduce the amount of drug required, so lessening side effects (e.g. motor block and hypotension), or provide better analgesia by increasing the efficacy of the technique

Neuraxial adjuvants can be classified as opioid and non-opioid drugs:

- Opioid:
  - morphine
  - fentanyl
  - sufentanil
  - alfentanil
  - pethidine
  - diamorphine

  Many of the opioid neuraxial adjuvants have a long established role in anaesthetic obstetric practice with well-defined safety profiles
- Non-opioid—this is a diverse group of substances including:
  - simple chemicals (e.g. bicarbonate, magnesium)
  - alpha-adrenergic agonists (e.g. clonidine, epinephrine, droperidol)
  - cholinesterase inhibitor (e.g. neostigmine)
  - gamma-aminobutyric acid (GABA) receptor agonists (e.g. midazolam)
  - *N*-methyl-D-aspartate (NMDA) receptor antagonists (e.g. ketamine)
  - steroids (e.g. dexamethasone)

  Many of these non-opioid agents remain largely theoretical or experimental, or have an unacceptable or undefined safety profile.

Most neuraxial adjuvants are not licensed and each agent has side effects. Preservative-free agents must be used to minimize the risks of neurotoxicity. This chapter will discuss the mechanism of action, efficacy, safety, and practical uses of each adjuvant.

Adjuvants: mechanisms of action and routes of administration

Several mechanisms to explain antinociceptive interactions between drugs in the spinal cord[6–8] have been suggested:

- Pharmacokinetic mechanisms—addition of the adjuvant drug can change the physical properties of the injectate[9,10] by affecting:
  - density—for example, changed by hypertonic dextrose, which is used therapeutically to make 'heavy' bupivacaine. It has also been demonstrated that the addition of fentanyl reduces the density of plain 0.5% bupivacaine *in vitro* sufficiently to alter its movement in simulated cerebrospinal fluid (CSF)[9]
  - ionization—for example, changed by addition of bicarbonate to alter pH
  - vascular absorption—epidurally administered drugs must first diffuse through the dura to gain access to the intrathecal space and hence their site of action in the spinal cord, and this is affected by local vasoconstriction, for example, by addition of epinephrine to the injectate.

  These pharmacokinetic effects of the adjuvant will change the concentrations of injected local anaesthetic at the spinal effector sites, thus increasing or prolonging antinociception.[9] The effective dose, speed of onset, duration of action, and side effect profile of the local anaesthetic can be changed to produce a more intense, reliable sensory block to permit instrumental delivery or surgery with smaller doses of local anaesthetic.[11] These mechanisms are discussed in detail for each individual agent later in this chapter.

- Pharmacodynamic mechanisms—a pool of second-messenger molecules are coupled to a single class of ion channels.[5] Different opioid (and α_2-adrenoceptor) receptor subtypes activate these second-messenger molecules leading to the same outcome via different activity causing multiplication of effect. These exist together on individual neurons and share second-messenger mechanisms.[12,13] For example, clonidine appears to act synergistically with opioids at the delta (δ)-opioid receptor[5] but not mu (μ)- or kappa (κ)-opioid receptors. There is also synergism between μ-opioid and δ-opioid receptor agonists, due to allosteric change in the receptor binding site, which leads to greater binding affinity of the next agonist.[5]
- There may be interaction from different drugs inhibiting spinal nociceptive processing at different sites leading to a multiplied effect. For example, presynaptic (inhibition of transmitter release) and postsynaptic (hyperpolarization of rostral transmission neurons) sites of action have been identified for opioids and α_2-adrenoceptor agonists in the spinal cord.[14]

Clinical uses of various adjuvants

So far, non-opioid intrathecal adjuncts have shown limited clinical application and are not in general use in most delivery suites, whereas opioids increase duration and quality of spinal block without delaying recovery and have become 'standard practice' in most maternity units. In 2010, Wahlen and colleagues investigated 'standard practice' in Germany and Austria using an online survey of 39 university hospitals (Table 17.1).[15,17,18]

This is in contrast to practice in the United Kingdom, where sufentanil is unlicensed and therefore not used. In 2011, Jagannatha showed in an electronic survey that fentanyl (78.8%) and diamorphine (79.1%) were the more commonly used adjuvants for neuraxial block in the United Kingdom, with morphine used in 14.9%.[16] The commonly used doses of fentanyl, diamorphine, and morphine were 15–25 mcg, 200–300 mcg, and 100–200 mcg respectively. Most of the patients with spinal opioids including morphine were sent straight back to the ward postoperatively, but the lack of a high dependency unit prevented the use of opioids in epidurals in 46%. Interestingly, this survey showed that more than 70% of anaesthetists were unsure about the licence for the use of neuraxial opioids.

Table 17.1 Neuraxial opioid adjuvant use in Germany/Austria 2010[15–18]

Drug	Spinal for CD	Epidural for CD	Epidural for labour
Sufentanil	63	51	84.3
Fentanyl	12	3	3.1
Morphine	3	0	0
No adjuvant	22	46	12.5

Data refers to the % of each opioid used as a total of all opioid adjuvants used.
Data from various sources (see references).

This differing pattern of opioid use in Germany and the United Kingdom has remained constant over the last decade. In Germany in 1996, Stamer and colleagues showed that 62% of units added an intrathecal opioid adjuvant for caesarean delivery (CD), of these, 56.5% were sufentanil, 5% fentanyl and 1.3% morphine, and these figures have hardly changed.[17] The pattern of neuraxial opioid use seems to vary significantly between and within European countries. Rawal and Allvin conducted an electronic survey of 105 European hospitals and found that in 1 year, 55,117 patients (7% of all surgical patients) received neuraxial opioid analgesia.[18] The most common spinal opioid was morphine, followed by fentanyl but 12 different opioids and 8 non-opioids were mentioned. Epidural opioid administration was far more common than intrathecal (89% vs 11%). By contrast, two surveys in 1996 in the United Kingdom showed that fentanyl was the lipophilic opioid most often used for labour epidurals, with alfentanil and diamorphine used infrequently.[19,20] In the nearly 20 years since this survey, the use of alfentanil and diamorphine in labour epidurals has declined even further and they can be regarded as obsolete in this context.

Opioid adjuvants

Opioid receptors

Opioid receptors span the membrane seven times and are linked to inhibitory G-proteins.[21] Specific opioid receptors are classically grouped according to their agonists—mu (μ), kappa (κ), and delta (δ)—and the non-classical (nociception, opioid receptor-like 1) receptor. New terminology has renamed them according to their receptor type as MOPr (μ), DOPr (δ), KOPr (κ), and NOPr (ORL_1). When an opioid agonist stimulates the receptor, voltage sensitive calcium channels are closed and potassium flows out of the cell causing hyperpolarization and reduced cAMP. This leads to inhibition of neurotransmitter release.

μ-receptors are found throughout the central nervous system (CNS) and are responsible for most of the analgesic effects of opioids. In the spinal cord, they are located presynaptically on primary afferent neurons within the dorsal horn.[22] Apart from analgesia, μ-receptor stimulation produces respiratory depression (by reducing chemoreceptor sensitivity to carbon dioxide), constipation (by reducing secretions and peristalsis), and cardiovascular depression.

KOP or κ-receptor stimulation produces analgesia at the spinal level but may cause sedation, dysphoria, and hallucinations. κ-receptor agonists have the advantage that they do not cause respiratory depression but their action as antagonists at μ-receptors limits their usefulness.

The δ-receptor is spread widely throughout the CNS, and when stimulated causes inhibition of neurotransmitter release. It may be involved in regulating mood and movement but its stimulation may be proconvulsant.[23]

Opioid receptor mechanisms in the spinal cord

Opioids injected intrathecally access opioid receptors in three different areas:

1. The major site is direct interaction with presynaptic primary afferent nerve terminals in the substantia gelatinosa of the dorsal horn of the spinal cord inhibiting neurotransmitter release.[14] This reduces signalling between primary and

secondary afferent neurons, thereby inhibiting transmission of nociceptive impulses through the dorsal horn and suppressing nociceptive spinal reflexes. There is also postsynaptic binding to receptors on the secondary afferent neurons, causing hyperpolarization and decreasing excitability. Opioids vary in their receptor specificity and in their efficacy at the different types of receptor,[24] so that some opioids can be agonists or partial agonists on one type of receptor, and antagonists or partial agonists at another. Intrathecal opioids preferentially modulate transmission in C- and A-fibres, with little effect on dorsal root axons, and different opioid agonists can act synergistically when co-administered.[25] Opioids (with the exception of pethidine (meperidine)) have no effect on nerve conduction.

2. CSF flow causes cephalad movement of intrathecally injected opioids, which then act supraspinally on descending inhibitory pathways. Endogenous opioid peptides may be released both at supraspinal and spinal sites, and at the spinal level analgesia also results from the release of serotonin (5-HT) from descending inhibitory fibres.[22]
3. A minimal amount will diffuse into the epidural space and be absorbed systemically through the epidural venous plexus, causing centrally mediated analgesia. Epidural administration of sufentanil, fentanyl, and morphine produces plasma levels equivalent to intramuscular injection of similar doses.[14]

Neuraxial opioids: clinical uses

Numerous trials have shown that the addition of opioids to local anaesthetic solutions significantly improves pain relief, permits smaller doses of local anaesthetic with subsequent reduced motor block and hypotension, reduces postoperative analgesic requirements, and reduces the frequency of patchy block.[26,27] Individual opioids vary in their potency, lipophilicity, and side effect profile—these are discussed later, but some general principles apply. The dose of epidural opioid is usually about five to ten times that needed for intrathecal use.[14] See Table 17.2.[28–43]

Table 17.2 Equivalent spinal and epidural doses of commonly used neuraxial opioids[28–43]

Drug	Clinical intrathecal dose range	Clinical epidural dose range
Fentanyl	*10–25 mcg*	*50–100 mcg (1 mcg/kg)*
	Labour (sole agent) ED_{95} 17.4 mcg (95% CI 13.8–27.1 mcg)[28]	33–92 mcg[36] (*'optimal' 50–100 mcg)*
	Labour (with bupivacaine) 10–15 mcg[29]	Labour (sole agent): ED_{50} 124 mcg[37]
	CD (with bupivacaine) 10–25 mcg[30]	Labour (with bupivacaine): ED_{95} 50 mcg[38]
		C.D ED_{95} 92 mcg[36]
Sufentanil	*2.5–20 mcg*	*25–60 mcg*
	Labour ED_{95} 8–10 mcg[28,31]	Labour: ED_{50} (alone) 21 mcg[37]
	Labour (with bupivacaine) 'optimal' 1.5–2 mcg[32]	Labour: ED_{95} (with bupivacaine) 8 mcg[28]
	CD (with bupivacaine) 2.5–20 mcg 'Optimal' 5 mcg[33]	CD: (with bupivacaine) 10–20 mcg[39,36]
Morphine	*50–500 mcg*[34]	*3.75–5.0 mg*
	(CD with bupivacaine)	*'Optimal' 3.75 mg* (postop CD)[40]
Diamorphine	*0.3–0.4 mg*[35]	*2.0–5.0 mg*[41]
	(CD with bupivacaine)	(CD with bupivacaine)
		Labour (with bupivacaine) 250–500 mg/h[42,43]

CD, caesarean delivery; ED_{50}, effective dose required for desired effect in 50% of people receiving the drug; ED_{95}, effective dose required for desired effect in 95% of people receiving the drug.

Data from various sources (see references).

Side effects/disadvantages of opioid adjuvants

The addition of opioid adjuvants to neuraxial solutions has several disadvantages. Extra time will be required to draw up, mix, and administer controlled drugs and their use must be properly documented. The use of multiple drugs increases the chance of drug errors and cautious rechecking of drug ampoules must occur.

The other disadvantage of using opioids as neuraxial adjuvants are the side effects that their addition brings. All complications of opioids, such as nausea, vomiting, pruritus, and respiratory depression, are dose dependent[44] and each is discussed in detail in the following sections. High opioid doses may also lead to decreased fetal heart rate (FHR) variability.[45]

Pruritus

This is seen in up to 70% of patients receiving neuraxial morphine, and is less common (10%) with lipophilic opioids such as fentanyl.[14] Onset is variable and is usually localized to the face, neck, and chest areas. It is thought to be due to cephalad spread of opioid to receptor sites in the trigeminal nucleus. Although the pruritus is not mediated by histamine release, histamine-1 receptor antagonists (e.g. chlorpheniramine) can be helpful, but cause sedation. Small doses of opioid receptor antagonists such as naloxone (<2 mcg/kg/h) and naltrexone (6–9 mg) are the most effective at reversing pruritus without reversing analgesia.[46]

A high concentration of 5-HT_3 receptors is found in the dorsal horn of the spinal cord and the spinal tract of the trigeminal nerve in the medulla, and it has been suggested that an interaction between opioids and 5-HT_3 receptors may play a role in the generation of neuraxial opioid-induced pruritus. Prophylactic treatment with a single intravenous (IV) bolus of 4–8 mg of the 5-HT_3 receptor antagonist ondansetron provides a significant decrease in the incidence and the intensity score of pruritus after neuraxial opioid administration, particularly when morphine is used.[47]

Nausea and vomiting

This occurs in 20–50% of patients receiving neuraxial opioids, and is commoner in females and with intrathecal morphine. It is thought to be due to cephalad spread of the opioid to the area postrema where it acts as a partial dopamine-2 receptor agonist in the chemoreceptor trigger zone.[22,23]

Urinary retention

This occurs in approximately 30–40% of cases of neuraxial opioid use[14] and is more common with spinal morphine. Stimulation of opioid receptors in the sacral spinal cord causes inhibition of sacral parasympathetic outflow. Ureteric and bladder sphincter tone is increased and detrusor relaxation is inhibited.[23]

Respiratory depression

The incidence of respiratory depression with neuraxial opioids is similar to that found with parenterally administered opioids.[48] This is a μ-receptor response causing reduced sensitivity of the chemosensitive neurons in the respiratory centre in the medulla to carbon dioxide. The normal compensatory increase in minute ventilation when arterial carbon dioxide rises fails to occur, but the response to hypoxia is less affected. In theory, if the hypoxic stimulus is also removed by supplementary oxygen, then respiratory depression may be potentiated. Medullary generation of the respiratory rhythm is also inhibited at the pre-Botzinger complex, causing a decreased respiratory rate.[23] Respiratory depression can occur early or late with neuraxial opiate administration.

Early respiratory depression, occurring within 2 hours, is due to systemic absorption of opioid and is therefore less common after intrathecal administration and after administration of hydrophilic opioids such as morphine, but commoner after epidural administration of lipophilic opioids (e.g. sufentanil and fentanyl).[49]

Delayed respiratory depression occurring at 6–12 hours is seen after intrathecal administration of hydrophilic opioids such as morphine and is caused by cephalad spread of the opioid in the CSF to the respiratory centre. Delayed respiratory depression is uncommon with lipophilic opioids as they bind rapidly to spinal opioid receptors, removing most of the drug from the CSF before significant cephalad spread can occur.

Respiratory depression is a potentially life-threatening complication of neuraxial opioids and appropriate monitoring is mandatory (Table 17.3).[14,26,28,41,48,49,53,61,69,77,78,80,96,98]

The American Society of Anesthesiologists published guidelines in 2009[50] which recommend the following:

1. Patient identification

   All patients should have a focused history and examination to identify risk factors for increased susceptibility to respiratory depression (including sleep apnoea, diabetes, obesity, current medications) before administering neuraxial opioids.

2. Drug selection

   The duration of monitoring should be appropriate to the drug, whether delivered by single injection or continuous epidural. Lipophilic opioids such as fentanyl and sufentanil are safer than hydrophilic drugs such as morphine. Diamorphine is rarely available outside the United Kingdom.

Table 17.3 Lipophilicity of neuraxial opioids and time of peak respiratory depression risk (clinically observed ranges)[14, 26, 28, 41, 48, 49, 53, 61, 69, 77, 78, 80, 96, 98]

Intrathecal opioid	Onset of analgesia (minutes)	Duration of analgesia (hours)	Maximum risk of respiratory depression (hours)
Morphine (hydrophilic)	60–120	15–24	5–12
Fentanyl/ sufentanil (lipophilic)	10	1–5	<0.5
Diamorphine (lipophilic)	5–10	11–14	8–12

Data from various sources (see references).

3. Dose selection

   Administer the lowest effective dose of neuraxial opioids. Simultaneous administration parenteral opioids, sedatives, hypnotics, magnesium requires increased intensity and duration of monitoring.

4. Detection of respiratory depression

   Monitoring of patients receiving neuraxial opioids should include depth of respiration, oxygenation (with pulse oximetry when appropriate), and level of consciousness. These observations can be assessed in the sleeping patient, unless there are any concerning signs in which case the patient should be woken to allow evaluation of level of consciousness.

Individual groups of agents require specific recommendations:

1. Neuraxial lipophilic opioids via single injection (e.g. fentanyl):
   - Monitor for a minimum of 2 hours following injection.
   - Repeated monitoring should be performed for the first 20 minutes after administration, followed by monitoring at least every hour until 2 hours have passed.
   - Once 2 hours have passed, the clinical condition of the patients will dictate the frequency of monitoring.
2. Neuraxial lipophilic opioids via continuous infusion or patient-controlled epidural analgesia (PCEA):
   - Perform monitoring for the duration of the infusion.
   - Continual monitoring should occur for the first 20 minutes after the infusion has begun, and continued at least every hour until 12 hours have passed.
   - During the period of 12–24 hours of infusion, the monitoring should be repeated at least every 2 hours.
   - After 24 hours, repeat monitoring at least once every 4 hours.
   - Once the infusion or PCEA of lipophilic opioids has finished the frequency of monitoring will be dictated by the patient's condition and other medications.
3. Neuraxial hydrophilic opioids (e.g. morphine, not including sustained- or extended-release epidural morphine) via single injection:
   - Monitor the patient for at least 24 hours after administration.
   - Patient monitoring should be repeated at least hourly for the first 12 hours and then at least every 2 hours for the 12–24-hour period.
   - Once 24 hours have passed, the patient's clinical condition and other medications should dictate the frequency of monitoring.
4. Continuous infusion or PCEA with neuraxial hydrophilic opioids:
   - The patient should be monitored throughout the duration of the infusion.
   - The frequency of monitoring should be hourly for the first 12 hours and then at least every other hour for the next 12 hours.
   - Once 24 hours have passed, repeat the monitoring at least every 4 hours.

- Once the infusion or PCEA has stopped, the patient's condition and administration of other medications should dictate the frequency of monitoring.

5. Respiratory depression—management and treatment:

- If patients have altered level of consciousness, respiratory depression, or hypoxaemia, administer supplemental oxygen and continue until the situation has resolved.
- Supplemental oxygen should not be used routinely as it may increase the duration of apnoeic episodes, or limit the detection of transient apnoea and hypoventilation.
- If respiratory depression persists or recurs, IV access should remain.
- All patients with any degree of respiratory depression following the neuraxial administration of opioids should have reversal agents readily available.
- If severe respiratory depression occurs, resuscitation should be initiated rapidly and effectively.

In theory, a drug which acts on the κ-opioid receptor should provide analgesia without respiratory depression, and butorphanol has been studied as a likely candidate. Butorphanol is a μ-receptor antagonist and κ-receptor agonist and therefore could be predicted to reduce the side effects of epidural opioids without lessening the analgesic effect.[51,52] However, clinical studies comparing postsurgical pain found that the addition of epidural butorphanol to a bupivacaine/fentanyl mix did not result in additional analgesia or reduce side effects. Studies in obstetric patients for labour analgesia and CD found no significant reduction in pain scores but less pruritus, nausea, and vomiting (reduced μ-receptor effect, as predicted). However, there was an increased incidence of somnolence[51–53] (an unwanted κ-receptor agonist effect) associated with the butorphanol group. The role of this type of agent remains unclear.

Opioid adjuvants: individual agents

For a summary of opioid adjuvants see Table 17.4.[58,62,63,67,74]

Morphine

Pharmacology

Morphine is a naturally occurring, hydrophilic phenanthrene derivative. It was the first opioid administered neuraxially for labour analgesia[54] and is the most widely studied adjuvant. Early studies showed significant analgesic synergy[55,56] between morphine and local anaesthetic, with the local anaesthetic potentiating the antinociceptive effects of morphine by enhancing the morphine binding to the κ-opioid receptor.

Morphine is a weak base (pKa 8.0). Its half-life is 3–4 hours with up to 70% metabolized in the liver to morphine-3-glucuronide, (which affects arousal and is possibly a μ-receptor antagonist) and to morphine 6-glucuronide, which is 13 times more potent than morphine and has a similar duration of action. Both these metabolites are excreted in the urine and accumulate in renal failure.[22,23]

Lipophilicity and binding: onset and duration

Because morphine is poorly lipid-soluble (lipophobic), it is slow to bind to the dorsal horn receptors, taking 15 minutes to work intrathecally and 30 minutes epidurally. However, its longer duration of action, (~12–24 hours), means that a single dose of epidural or spinal morphine will improve the quality of pain relief for the first stage of labour and is more effective than a single dose of fentanyl at providing postoperative pain relief.[14]

Doses: intrathecal/epidural

Both intrathecal and epidural morphine have a ceiling analgesic effect; at doses greater than 100 mcg (intrathecal) and 3.75 mg (epidural) there is minimal additional analgesic benefit, but increased incidence of adverse effects, particularly pruritus.[57]

Side effects

Intrathecal and epidural morphine are associated with a high incidence of dose-related nausea, vomiting, pruritus, urinary retention, sedation, and delayed respiratory depression when compared to fentanyl. These effects can occur even at very low doses.[58]

Sustained- or extended-release epidural morphine

Extended-release epidural morphine (EREM) by single bolus injection can extend effective postoperative analgesia for up to 48 hours and was approved by the US Food and Drug Administration (FDA) in 2004.

In a randomized controlled trial (RCT) of 70 women for elective CD using a combined spinal–epidural (CSE) technique, patients received an intrathecal injection of bupivacaine 12 mg and fentanyl 10 mcg and a single-dose epidural bolus of either conventional morphine 4 mg or EREM 10 mg. Significantly improved pain scores at rest and during activity were found in those women receiving EREM, with a decrease in supplemental opioid medication usage for 48 hours post CD. (In milligram-morphine equivalents, median and interquartile range from 17 (22) to 10 (17) mg with EREM compared to conventional epidural morphine ($P = 0.037$).[59])

In 2009, Hartrick and Hartrick compared the adverse effects of EREM ($N = 801$) to IV opioids and standard epidural morphine.[60] EREM doses of 15 mg or greater were associated with a trend towards a higher incidence of hypoventilation (odds ratio 0.48; 95% confidence interval (CI) 0.21–1.09; $P = 0.081$; number-needed-to-treat (NNT) = 14) compared with placebo. The incidence of pruritus was significantly higher for all EREM doses compared with both placebo ($P = 0.004$) and standard epidural morphine ($P = 0.03$). Vomiting was also increased with EREM doses of 15 mg or greater compared with placebo (odds ratio 0.40; 95% CI 0.18–0.89; $P = 0.02$; NNT = 5). For these reasons, EREM has not been widely embraced by the obstetric anaesthetic community.

If EREM is used, then monitoring at least once every hour should be performed during the first 12 hours after administration, and at least once every 2 hours for the next 12 hours (i.e. from 12 to 24 hours).[50]

After 24 hours, monitoring should be performed at least once every 4 hours for a minimum of 48 hours.[50]

Fentanyl

The profiles of fentanyl and sufentanil are very similar except for their relative potency.

Pharmacology

Fentanyl is a phenylpiperidine derivative. It is a lipophilic opioid, which acts as an adjunct to local anaesthetics to increase

Table 17.4 Summary of opioid adjuvants[58, 62, 63, 67, 74]

Opioid	Epidural clinical dose range and optimal doses	Intrathecal dose	Epidural onset (mean, minutes)	Intrathecal onset (mean, minutes)	Epidural duration (mean, hours)	Intrathecal duration (mean, hours)	Advantages	Disadvantages
Sustained-release morphine	*10 mg–15 mg* *('optimal'10 mg)*	N/A	5	N/A	48	N/A	Longest duration	Increased pruritus compared to standard morphine, more hypoventilation and vomiting at doses >15 mg
Diamorphine	*2.5–5 mg*	*0.25–0.4 mg* (minimum dose to prevent supplementation at CD 0.4 mg)	10	5	12–20	12–20	Long duration	Rapid onset Long duration
Morphine	*3–5 mg* *('optimal '3.75 mg)*	*50–500 mcg* *('optimal' 100 mcg)*	30	15	12–24	12–24	Long duration	Nausea, vomiting, pruritus, sedation, late respiratory depression
Fentanyl	*33–124 mcg* *('optimal' 50–100 mcg)* Labour: ED_{50} 124 mcg (alone) Labour: ED_{95} 50 mcg (with Bupivacaine) CD ED_{95} 92 mcg	*10–25 mcg* Labour: ED_{95} (alone) 17.4 mcg Labour: (with bupivacaine) 10–15 mcg CD: (with bupivacaine) 25 mcg	10	5	2–4	2–4	Rapid onset	Short duration pruritus, early respiratory depression
Sufentanil	*25–60 mcg* Labour: ED_{50} (alone) 21 mcg Labour: ED_{95} (with bupivacaine) 8 mcg CD: (with bupivacaine) 10–20 mcg	*2.5–20 mcg* Labour: ED_{95} 8–10 mcg Labour: (with bupivacaine) 'optimal' 1.5–2 mcg CD: (with bupivacaine) 2.5–20 mcg 'optimal' 5 mcg	2–3	4–6	1–3	1–3	Very rapid onset	Short duration
Pethidine (Meperidine)	*10–20 mg*	25–50 mg	10	5	4–8	4–8	Rapid onset	Minimal postoperative analgesia Nausea and vomiting

CD, caesarean delivery; ED_{50}, effective dose required for desired effect in 50% of people receiving the drug; ED_{95}, effective dose required for desired effect in 95% of people receiving the drug.

Data from various sources (see references).

the duration and intensity of spinal anaesthesia[54,61–64] without intensifying motor and sympathetic block[65,66] or prolonging recovery.[67,68]

Lipophilicity/binding: onset and duration

Fentanyl has a pKa of 8.4 and is approximately 800 times more lipid-soluble than morphine. It binds rapidly to dorsal horn receptors in the spinal cord and has a corresponding rapid onset of action (5 minutes intrathecally, 10 minutes epidurally). This is advantageous for labour analgesia and emergency CD and also means that cephalad spread and delayed respiratory depression are rare. Its duration of action is short (2–4 hours intrathecally and epidurally) due to redistribution and systemic absorption, so it does not provide clinically useful postoperative analgesia.[14]

Doses

For labour analgesia, intrathecal fentanyl is effective as a sole agent, in which context it has been shown to have a median effective dose of 14 mcg (95% CI 13–15 mcg), and a ceiling effect at 25 mcg.[69]

The effective epidural dose is 100 mcg, which can be used to improve an inadequate block without prolonging recovery time,[67,68] but larger doses do not prolong the duration of analgesia in any clinically significant way.[57]

Side effects: intrathecal/epidural

Intrathecal fentanyl has been shown to decrease intraoperative nausea and vomiting,[61–64] and while respiratory depression has been described, it is unlikely with doses less than 25 mcg. Intrathecal fentanyl produces a dose-dependent incidence of pruritus in approximately 50% of patients.[67] Urinary retention is far less common with lipophilic opioid use than with morphine, and the incidence of urinary retention is not increased by the addition of intrathecal fentanyl to hyperbaric bupivacaine.[65,70]

As an adjuvant to low-dose local anaesthetic epidural solutions for labour, fentanyl can potentiate analgesia, but epidural bolus doses may result in early respiratory depression due to systemic absorption. There has been considerable controversy in the literature about the site of action of epidurally administered lipophilic opioids, with conflicting evidence suggesting that the analgesic action of epidural fentanyl may be entirely due to its action in the brain following systemic absorption rather than at spinal receptors. Ginosar et al. clarified the situation in 2003 by comparing a continuous infusion of epidural fentanyl given as a sole agent with bolus epidural fentanyl administration.[71] This human volunteer study showed that after a 100 mcg fentanyl epidural bolus, fentanyl plasma levels reached a maximum of 0.47 ng/mL (standard deviation (SD) ± 0.39 ng/mL) at 45 minutes after injection and this was accompanied by *segmental* analgesia, suggesting relevant opioid binding in the spinal cord. When fentanyl was administered by infusion at a rate of 100 mcg/h the maximum plasma concentration was 0.80 ng/mL (SD ± 0.24 ng/mL) at 180 minutes after injection, and this was accompanied by non-segmental analgesia, suggesting relevant opioid binding in the brain.

The authors speculated that administration of the bolus dose of fentanyl might create a large concentration gradient of drug between the epidural space and CSF, thereby enabling a higher concentration of drug to access the spinal sites, which might not be achieved with the lower concentration gradient at infusion doses.

The same authors have shown that in labouring women, the required dose of epidural bupivacaine can be reduced by a factor of three when co-administered with an epidural fentanyl infusion as compared with an IV fentanyl infusion.[72] This is accounted for by the supra-additive, or synergistic, effect of the two drugs; an otherwise insignificant analgesic effect by a spinal mechanism may become predominant if epidural fentanyl is infused jointly with a local anaesthetic. This study used a technique known as 'minimum local anaesthetic concentration' (MLAC), whereby the efficacy of an adjuvant, and the reduction in dose of local anaesthetic that can be achieved can be measured.[73] This technique involves systematic evaluation of dose–response pharmacodynamics and allows the median effective concentration (EC_{50}) and median effective dose (ED_{50}) to be established for local anaesthetics. This is analogous to the minimum alveolar concentration (MAC) for inhalational anaesthetics and is an accurate way of quantifying the local anaesthetic-sparing properties of adjuvants. It has been used widely in the clinical context of epidurals in labour.

Using this tool, Lyons and co-workers demonstrated that the MLAC of epidural bupivacaine can be reduced by 31–72% in a linear, dose-dependent manner by the addition of 2–4 mcg of fentanyl per mL of local anaesthetic solution.[74] The first woman in each fentanyl group received an arbitrarily chosen concentration of bupivacaine based on estimations of MLAC from preceding studies. If this produced an effective outcome (using a 100 mm visual analogue pain score (VAPS) where VAPS was <10 mm within 30 minutes), the next patient in the series received a predefined reduction of 0.01% weight/volume concentration of local anaesthetic but at the same volume and with the same dose of fentanyl. An ineffective response (VAPS ≥ 10 mm within 30 min) resulted in the next patient in the series receiving an increase in concentration of local anaesthetic by the same predefined interval. This process of sequential allocation of local anaesthetic dose continued until the concentration administered was the EC_{50} or MLAC.

Sufentanil

Pharmacology

Like fentanyl, sufentanil is a synthetic phenylpiperidine derivative. It is five to seven times more potent than fentanyl. Sufentanil has a terminal elimination half-life of 150 minutes, so accumulation is unlikely.

Lipophilicity/binding: onset and duration

Sufentanil is 1600 times more lipid-soluble than morphine[14] with a consequent very fast onset time of 2–3 minutes intrathecally, and 4–6 minutes epidurally. Its short duration of action (1–3 hours intrathecally and epidurally) means it has no useful clinical postoperative analgesic effect, and its main indication is to improve the quality of pain relief during the second stage of labour via administration as an epidural bolus or in combination with local anaesthetic agents intrathecally for CD. The use of sufentanil has been shown to be an independent significant predictor of effective analgesia in labour when used as an adjunct with epidural bupivacaine, levobupivacaine, and ropivacaine[75] and MLAC studies show that the EC_{50} of bupivacaine is reduced by 91% by the addition of sufentanil 1.5 mcg/mL.[76]

Doses: intrathecal/epidural

Doses of 2.5–5 mcg are recommended for intrathecal use and 25–50 mcg for epidural bolus use.[39]

Side effects: intrathecal/epidural

Its rapid onset time means there is a corresponding increased risk of early respiratory depression after an epidural bolus because of systemic absorption, but with a low risk of cephalad spread leading to less delayed respiratory depression. There are case reports of rapid-onset life-threatening respiratory depression occurring 5–15 minutes after intrathecal sufentanil 10–15 mcg[26,77–79] including during intrathecal use for labour analgesia.[79] However, during CD significant sedation or respiratory depression has not been reported.[53,61–63] Neurotoxicity has not been reported with clinical doses of 1.5 mcg/kg of intrathecal sufentanil, but animal studies have noted histopathological changes with doses of 7.5 mg/kg.[81]

Alfentanil

Pharmacology

Alfentanil is a lipid-soluble, synthetic phenylpiperidine derivative and a μ-receptor agonist.

Lipophilicity/binding: onset and duration

It has a pKa of 6.5 so at a pH of 7.4, 89% is present in the unionized form and able to cross lipid membranes.[23] This is why it has a faster onset of action than fentanyl, despite having lower lipid-solubility.

Dose

It is rarely used in obstetrics because of its short duration of action. Intrathecal alfentanil alone provides analgesia for 40 minutes.[82] In an epidural infusion study used at 30 mcg/kg/h, analgesia was inadequate for late first stage and second stage of labour in 30% of patients.[83]

Side effects

Neonatal hypotonia following delivery has been reported.[84]

Pethidine (meperidine)

Pharmacology

Pethidine is a lipophilic phenylpiperidine derivative, which is a combined μ-receptor and κ-receptor agonist.[85] Pethidine is the only opioid that has local anaesthetic actions, and it also has anticholinergic and stimulant effects,[22,23] which in high concentrations may cause seizures and hallucinations.[86]

Lipophilicity/binding: onset and duration

Pethidine is ten times more lipid-soluble than morphine and therefore has a faster onset (5 minutes intrathecally, 10 minutes epidurally) and shorter duration (4–8 hours intrathecally and epidurally) of action than morphine.[87] Its active metabolite norpethidine is less lipid-soluble and can accumulate in the fetus.

Doses: Intrathecal/epidural

When used as a single agent, intrathecal pethidine 10–20 mg produces analgesia in 2–12 minutes, which can last for up to 3 hours[87] and 1 mg/kg produces surgical anaesthesia.[86,88]

When used as an adjunct to local anaesthetics for CD, the addition of 25 mg pethidine intrathecally provides better blood pressure stability and a lower incidence of side effects than 5 mg bupivacaine alone, with rapid motor recovery and prolonged postoperative analgesia.[4,89] When given via the epidural route as a sole agent in labour, pethidine 25 mg provides analgesia for 50–160 minutes,[27] but opioid side effects restrict its clinical use. Doses of 50 mg given via the epidural route to non-labouring parturients resulted in no maternal haemodynamic change, but did show some local anaesthetic effects.[90]

Side effects: intrathecal/epidural

Intrathecal pethidine has a narrow therapeutic window. Respiratory depression, nausea and vomiting,[91] pruritus, bradycardia, and urinary retention can occur with doses as low as 0.5 mg/kg.[92] The incidence of nausea and vomiting was as high as 76% in one study,[86] so its use is not recommended. Epidural pethidine 10 mg reduces the shivering side effect of epidural analgesia, probably by agonist action at the κ-receptor.[85,89,93,94]

Diamorphine

Pharmacology

Diamorphine is a diacetylated semisynthetic morphine derivative with no affinity for opioid receptors.[23] It is a pro-drug, which, when administered intrathecally, diffuses across the dura more easily than morphine but more slowly than fentanyl, leading to relatively rapid clearance from the CSF. Its low pKa (7.6) means that only 37% is in its unionized form and able to diffuse onto the opioid receptors on the dorsal horn at physiological pH. Esterase metabolism in the spinal cord converts diamorphine to metabolites (6-momoacetyl morphine and morphine), which are water-soluble μ-receptor agonists with their own pharmacological effects.

Lipophilicity/binding: onset and duration

Diamorphine is 280 times more lipid-soluble than morphine and therefore has a rapid onset (<10 minutes) of analgesia and is less likely to cause delayed respiratory depression.

Doses: intrathecal/epidural

Diamorphine 0.3–0.4 mg intrathecally or 2.5–5.0 mg epidurally both effectively reduce the need for supplemental analgesia after CD.

A RCT comparing diamorphine 0.25 mg intrathecally with 5 mg epidurally as an adjunct to intrathecal bupivacaine 10 mg in 50 patients for CD using a CSE technique showed that the quality and duration of postoperative analgesia was similar in both groups (mean of 14 hours) but that the intrathecal route had significantly less nausea and vomiting than the epidural route (24% vs 4%; $P < 0.05$).[41] This is due to systemic absorption of diamorphine from the epidural space into the bloodstream and transportation to the chemoreceptor trigger zone. The degree of pruritus was 80–88% in both groups. The addition of 5 mg of diamorphine to epidural bupivacaine 0.25% significantly improves analgesia and reduces motor block in labour compared to bupivacaine alone.[95] For postoperative pain after CD, epidural diamorphine 3 mg provides significantly longer analgesia than 10 mg intramuscular morphine (mean 11 vs 6.5 hours), but more patients in the diamorphine group required catheterization and had nausea and vomiting. There was no evidence of respiratory depression on overnight pulse oximetry.[96]

Side effects

The National Institute of Health and Care Excellence (NICE) 2011 guidelines for CD[97] recommend diamorphine (0.3–0.4 mg intrathecally, or 2.5–5 mg epidurally). Both morphine and diamorphine are effective adjuvants for intra- and postoperative analgesia for

CD by the intrathecal and epidural route, but diamorphine has fewer side effects, particularly delayed respiratory depression and nausea and vomiting[98] and is therefore recommended.

The availability and use of diamorphine is limited outside the United Kingdom.

Non-opioid adjuvants

In addition to opioids, drugs from other pharmacological classes may produce spinal analgesia and have been used as adjuvants in neuraxial analgesia.

These include vasoconstrictors, agonists at the α-adrenergic, serotonergic, cholinergic, and GABA receptors, and antagonists at the NMDA receptor.

Epinephrine

Pharmacology/mechanism of action

Epinephrine works as an adjuvant to neuraxial local anaesthetics by two mechanisms, local vasoconstriction, and as a direct α_2 adrenoceptor agonist with a specific spinal analgesic action.

Vasoconstriction of epidural veins reduces vascular absorption of local anaesthetic and maintains a higher concentration at the nerve roots for a longer period, which prolongs the duration of blockade and reduces the risk of toxicity.

The efficacy of epinephrine as a vasoconstrictor adjunct depends upon the lipid solubility of the local anaesthetic used. The addition of epinephrine to epidural lidocaine decreases systemic absorption by approximately 30%.[81,82] Bupivacaine has higher lipid solubility than lidocaine, so there is less systemic absorption from the epidural space in the first instance. Consequently the addition of epinephrine to epidural bupivacaine only decreases systemic absorption by around 10–20%,[99,100] and it is less effective at prolonging the duration of blockade when compared to lidocaine.

Epidural/intrathecal use

In labouring patients, the addition of epinephrine increases the duration of epidural bupivacaine analgesia and decreases the local anaesthetic requirement,[101–104] and can be specifically shown to reduce the MLAC of epidural bupivacaine.[105] The addition of 1:300,000 epinephrine to spinal bupivacaine and sufentanil prolongs the duration of analgesia from 100 min to 140 min.[106]

Despite these advantages, the use of epinephrine for labour analgesia is now uncommon, partly because of the potential tocolytic effects due to β_2 adrenergic actions on the myometrium, which can lead to prolonged labour.[107]

There is also a theoretical concern that neuraxial adrenaline/epinephrine could cause spinal artery vasoconstriction but there is no conclusive evidence for this. If used, the dose should be kept to a minimum of 1–1.25 mcg/mL.

Systemic side effects

Epinephrine is detected in plasma after neuraxial administration and may cause dose-related sympathomimetic effects. Tachycardia and hypertension could be clinically significant in cardiac patients, pre-eclamptic patients, or patients taking tricyclic antidepressants and monoamine oxidase inhibitors. The addition of epinephrine also prolongs the time until voiding of urine,[70,108,109] and increases the incidence of nausea and vomiting.[63]

Special circumstances/specific uses of epinephrine

'Test dose'

Historically, an epidural test dose 45 mg of lidocaine with 15 mcg of epinephrine was advocated to identify accidental intravascular injection by the occurrence of tachycardia and palpitations if the catheter had been placed or migrated intravascularly.[110] A review article in 2006 examined the efficacy of test doses and concluded that, in the pregnant population, the injection of epinephrine had low sensitivity for the clinical detection of intravascular injection. It included studies that looked at the injection of 10–15 mcg of epinephrine alone and the injection of a combination of bupivacaine 12.5 mg + epinephrine 12.5 mcg and found that both had low sensitivity for the clinical detection of intravascular injection (95% CI for sensitivity 78–100 for epinephrine alone) and (95% CI for sensitivity 75–100 for bupivacaine and epinephrine combined).[111]

For the detection of intravascular catheter misplacement in pregnant women, the injection of epinephrine has a low positive predictive value (<80) and may also have significant side effects (e.g. decreased uteroplacental blood flow after epidural or IV injection). The injection of epinephrine in labour is therefore unjustified, but could be considered if the epidural is performed for CD where a larger dose of local anaesthetic is anticipated.

'Rapid top-up for operative delivery'

In practice, the main use of epinephrine on the delivery suite is as an additive to local anaesthetics in order to rapidly top-up a labour epidural for emergency CD. A 2011 meta-analysis of 11 RCTs including 779 parturients has confirmed that lidocaine 2% with epinephrine ± fentanyl gives the most rapid onset of block.[112] In one RCT, the combination of lidocaine–bicarbonate–epinephrine (concentrations 1.8%, 0.76%, and 1:200,000) reduced the median time to extend a labour epidural block for CD (sensory block to T4 for cold, T5 for touch) to 7 minutes, compared with 14 minutes for levobupivacaine 0.5% alone.[113] In all the trials included in the meta-analysis by Hillyard et al., solutions containing lidocaine and epinephrine, with or without fentanyl, showed median onset times of under 15 minutes, making epidural top-up for CD a realistic option in all but the most urgent emergency situations.

Neostigmine

Pharmacology/mechanism of action

Neostigmine is a quaternary amine, which acts by inhibiting acetylcholinesterase. This prevents the breakdown of acetylcholine so that more is available at the neuromuscular junction.[14] Neostigmine does not cross the blood–brain barrier.[22] It is a cholinesterase inhibitor which produces analgesia by increasing the concentration of acetylcholine adjacent to the muscarinic and nicotinic receptors in the superficial layers of the dorsal horn of the spinal cord.[58] This mechanism of analgesia does not produce motor or sympathetic blockade.[114] Although it has been shown to produce analgesia on its own,[114] it is most useful as an adjuvant rather than a sole agent.

Intrathecal neostigmine

Both animal and human studies show that intrathecal neostigmine does not affect spinal cord blood flow and does not induce any significant toxic effect in the spinal cord.[115–117] In animal studies it reduces the risk of hypotension induced by spinal local anaesthetic.[118,119]

Intrathecal neostigmine increases the analgesia from systemically administered opioids and neuraxial administered α_2-adrenoceptor agonists. However, with doses larger than 200 mcg, there are significant systemic effects ranging from severe nausea and vomiting to motor blockade, sedation, and hypertension.[120] This high incidence of nausea and vomiting precludes intrathecal use clinically.[14]

Epidural neostigmine

When administered epidurally neostigmine also enhances the duration and intensity of analgesia from systemic and neuraxial α_2-adrenoceptor agonists, opioids and local anaesthetics. Unlike intrathecal neostigmine, epidural neostigmine is not associated with an increased risk of nausea and vomiting.

The effective epidural dose for postoperative pain is 50–100 mcg, but the reduction in pain scores and opioid consumption is equivalent to that achieved by administration of simple analgesics (e.g. oral non-steroidal anti-inflammatory drugs).[121] Low-concentration epidural neostigmine given continuously in non-obstetric patients has a local anaesthetic-sparing effect similar to opioids, but without nausea and vomiting.[122]

For reliable analgesia via the epidural route in early labour, at least 300–500 mcg of neostigmine is required, and then only in combination with other drugs (sufentanil, clonidine, local anaesthetic). When used in this way, neostigmine may have a local anaesthetic-sparing effect similar to fentanyl and sufentanil[106] and also an opioid-sparing effect.[123,124]

Doses greater than 100 mcg have been associated with sedation[14] but neostigmine does not cause respiratory depression or pruritus either alone or increase the risk of these side effects when used in combination with neuraxial opioids. In an editorial in 2009, Eisenach considered the case for replacing epidural lipid-soluble opioids with neostigmine in view of its lack of respiratory depression and pruritus.[121] However, the safety and efficacy of epidural neostigmine in the postoperative period has not been widely studied, and there are some unusual drug interactions (e.g. the combination of systemic opioid and intrathecal neostigmine is additive for analgesia but synergistic for nausea[122]). While it is assumed that epidural neostigmine enhances analgesia from epidural or systemic drugs by its cholinergic action in the spinal cord, there are no studies with systemically administered controls to specifically test this assumption[121].

There are also theoretical concerns about the effect of neostigmine on the fetus. Stimulation of spinal cholinergic receptors can increase sympathetic nervous system activity[124], which may decrease the perfusion to the uteroplacental unit. Also, systemic absorption of neostigmine could result in stimulation of myometrial activity[124] or if enough is transferred to the fetus, fetal bradycardia.[125] However, a small observational study of 12 women showed that a neostigmine epidural bolus of 40–80 mcg did not induce contractions, alter FHR or cause nausea in non-labouring women.[124] In the same study, 40 healthy labouring women were randomized to receive bupivacaine 1.25 mg/mL alone or with neostigmine 4 mcg/mL by PCEA. Epidural neostigmine infusion reduced bupivacaine requirement by 19% in all patients and 25% in those with greater than 4 hours of treatment ($P < 0.05$ for both) but might have contributed to the incidence of mild sedation. Mode of delivery, incidence of maternal nausea, incidence of FHR abnormality, and Apgar scores were similar between groups. Larger studies are required to provide more information before neostigmine can be recommended for clinical use.

Clonidine

Pharmacology/mechanism of action

Clonidine hydrochloride, an imidazoline derivative[126] is a centrally acting partial α_2-adrenoceptor agonist with an affinity for α_2 receptors 200 times that for α_1 receptors.[14]

Clonidine binds to postsynaptic G-protein coupled inhibitory α_2 receptors, in the laminae of the dorsal horn of the spinal cord thereby inhibiting adenylate cyclase and reducing intracellular cAMP formation.[127] This reduces excitation via sodium and potassium channels and inhibits calcium channels. Within the spinal cord, α_2 receptor stimulation augments endogenous opioid release and modulates descending noradrenergic pathways involved in spinal nociceptive processing. This produces a dose-dependent analgesia not antagonized by opioid antagonists which is limited to the body regions innervated by the spinal segments where analgesic concentrations of clonidine are present.[126]

In mice, nociceptive responses induced by intrathecal substance P are inhibited in a dose-dependent manner by intrathecal clonidine,[5] indicating a synergistic effect of clonidine at the δ-opioid receptor, but not μ- or κ-opioid receptors.

Within the brainstem, α_2-receptor stimulation in the lateral reticular nucleus reduces central sympathetic outflow and causes a decrease in peripheral resistance, renal vascular resistance, heart rate, and blood pressure. It also stimulates α_2 receptors in the locus coeruleus,[128] which is responsible for vigilance and sympathetic tone,[129,130] producing sedation and ventilatory abnormalities that are usually mild[126] and have only been reported with bolus doses that are significantly larger than those used in the obstetric population.

When used via the subarachnoid or epidural route, clonidine provides prolonged analgesia without causing respiratory depression or sensory–motor blockade and exhibits synergism with concurrently administered neuraxial opioids.[23]

Intrathecal clonidine

For CD with spinal anaesthesia, intrathecal clonidine 30–60 mcg increases the duration of sensory block by 30%, delays the onset of postoperative pain, and reduces overall postoperative opioid requirements.[57]

Epidural clonidine

Epidural clonidine 75 mcg has been shown to prolong labour analgesia, reduce local anaesthetic requirements, and reduce the number of top-ups for breakthrough pain without an increase in side effects when used in combination with either bupivacaine or ropivacaine.[131] Clonidine has been shown to reduce the MLAC of epidural bupivacaine.[105] However, there remains serious concern regarding unacceptable levels of hypotension.

Side effects

At epidural doses above 100 mcg, there is evidence of maternal hypotension, bradycardia, sedation, and FHR abnormalities. This is thought to be due to vascular absorption of clonidine via the epidural veins. Systemic concentrations of 0.5–2.0 ng/mL are readily achieved, and these are associated with a hypotensive effect mediated by the CNS.[126] These cardiovascular effects are usually seen within 15–30 minutes of epidural administration and last for up to 3 hours.

It has been suggested that clonidine may mask the increase in heart rate associated with hypovolaemia.[132] Consequently, in the United States, an FDA 'black box warning' recommends that the neuraxial administration of clonidine is avoided in the obstetric population because of this risk of hypotension and bradycardia.[126] The FDA states that 'there are no adequate controlled clinical trials evaluating the safety, efficacy, and dosing of clonidine in obstetric settings. Because maternal perfusion of the placenta is critically dependent on blood pressure, use of clonidine as an analgesic during labour and delivery is not indicated'. In the presence of such a warning, clonidine should be used with caution and only when other methods of rescuing the epidural have failed.

Neostigmine and clonidine combinations

The situation with neostigmine and clonidine is further complicated by a trial in 2009, which studied the use of both agents together.[133] This was a RCT during labour in which initial intrathecal analgesia with ropivacaine and sufentanil was supplemented 15 minutes later by an epidural bolus containing clonidine 500 mcg and neostigmine 75 mcg Compared with placebo, this combination resulted in a longer initial duration of pain relief and a lower subsequent local anaesthetic requirement for maintenance of labour analgesia. There was no clinically significant hypotension and no sedation using this combination, which is difficult to achieve when using clonidine or neostigmine as single adjuvants. This study was the subject of an editorial by Paech[134] in which the risk:benefit ratio of the use of multiple neuraxial drugs was questioned, with emphasis on the dose limitations of clonidine and the limited safety data of neostigmine. Paech cautions that 'in addition to safety and efficacy, data on more definitive outcome measures are required to define the potential benefits, before these adjuvants are accepted for routine use in obstetric anaesthesia and analgesia'.

Ketamine

Pharmacology/mechanism of action

Ketamine is a phencyclidine derivative, which acts as a non-competitive NMDA receptor antagonist.[22] NMDA receptors are activated by glutamate, which is the major excitatory neurotransmitter in the CNS. Ketamine blocks activation of the ligand gated channel and reduces NMDA receptor-mediated responses[23] leading to inhibition of excitatory pathways. The channels controlled by NMDA receptors are highly permeable to Ca^{2+} and are blocked by Mg^{2+}. Ketamine is lipid-soluble and freely crosses the blood–brain barrier.

When used neuraxially, ketamine blocks NMDA receptors located on secondary afferent neurons in the dorsal horn of the spinal cord, reducing the transmission of nociceptive information in the spinal pathways.[135] In high doses it may have additional minor analgesic effects by binding opioid μ-receptors and modulating descending inhibitory pathways through inhibition of reuptake of neurotransmitters[14].

Intrathecal ketamine

Early animal studies suggested that intrathecal ketamine has local anaesthetic properties[136–138] and might provide anaesthesia without hypotension. However, when the animals were killed, their spinal cords showed vacuoles indicating neural death, so human studies on intrathecal ketamine have rarely been undertaken. The finding that ketamine can induce apoptosis when used in high doses or for prolonged periods in animal studies has caused concern from the FDA and National Institutes of Health about potential human neurotoxicity.[139] Even with the availability of a preservative-free formulation for 20 years, these concerns remain.

Previous studies have shown ketamine to be a useful neuraxial adjunct for surgery. Bion demonstrated that intrathecal ketamine in doses above 50 mg provided satisfactory rapid onset (1.7 minutes) surgical anaesthesia lasting 45–90 minutes for lower limb surgery in war field conditions.[140] For ethical reasons, such a study could probably not have been conducted other than in the setting of war conditions.

There are no studies of intrathecal ketamine in obstetrics.

Epidural ketamine

In a small prospective RCT of non-obstetric abdominal surgical cases, epidural ketamine 1 mg/kg plus morphine 50 mcg/kg produced more rapid postoperative analgesia (median 11 vs 25 minutes) and more prolonged analgesia (median 19 vs 12 hours) than the group which received only morphine.[141] The ketamine group had higher sedation scores in the first 2 hours, there was no respiratory depression or hallucinations, and the incidence of pruritus, nausea, and vomiting was the same in both groups. There are no studies of epidural ketamine in obstetrics.

Due to unresolved safety concerns, the use of neuraxial ketamine cannot be recommended, despite early hopes that it would provide anaesthesia without hypotension.

Midazolam

Pharmacology/mechanism of action

Midazolam is a benzodiazepine, which acts by enhancing presynaptic inhibition through benzodiazepine binding sites in the $GABA_A$ receptor in the spinal cord.[142] $GABA_A$ receptors are ligand-gated receptors located throughout the CNS, but the substantia gelatinosa of the dorsal horn of the spinal cord contains a particularly high density of $GABA_A$ receptors. GABA is the major inhibitory neurotransmitter of the CNS. GABA binding results in a change of receptor configuration, opening chloride ion channels and resulting in hyperpolarization of the neuron and reduced action potential propagation. Benzodiazepines have their own binding site on the $GABA_A$ receptor and the effect of binding is to increase the frequency of chloride channel opening, which enhances the effects of GABA.

There are limited studies assessing the clinical safety of neuraxial midazolam.[14] The most serious side effect reported in animal studies is neurotoxicity, but this has been attributed to the effects of injection of an acidic solution.[142,143] Midazolam has a pH of 3.5 and its structure depends on the surrounding pH. At pH 3.5 its di-asinine ring is open, resulting in an ionized molecule, which is water-soluble.[23] When the surrounding pH is greater than 4, the ring structure closes so that it is no longer ionized and therefore becomes lipid-soluble. Its pKa is 6.5 so that at physiological pH 89% is present in an unionized form and available to cross lipid membranes. The pH of CSF does not decrease below 7.0 when adding midazolam in the amounts used in clinical practice and no adverse reactions have been reported when using epidural[144] or intrathecally administered midazolam.[145]

Intrathecal midazolam

Midazolam in intrathecal doses up to 2 mg has not been shown to cause any neurological deficit in humans. In a study of 100 patients scheduled for elective non-obstetric surgery, the addition of preservative-free midazolam 2 mg to bupivacaine intrathecally resulted in prolonged sensory block (mean 90 vs 115 minutes) without prolongation of motor block, while effective analgesia was prolonged from mean 121 to 221 minutes.[145] Sedation scores were the same for both groups.

To resolve the conflicting evidence from animal studies, Tucker followed up 574 non-obstetric patients for a month after intrathecal midazolam, evaluating 18 risk factors for neurotoxicity.[146] This large cohort study compared two groups of patients who received intrathecal anaesthesia with or without intrathecal midazolam, evaluating the presence of neurological symptoms in the period following intrathecal administration. They showed that intrathecal midazolam in doses up to 2 mg did not increase the occurrence of neurological or urological symptoms, whereas age greater than 70 years and accidental venous puncture involve relative risks of 8.72 and 8.07 respectively.

In a prospective RCT of 124 patients for elective CD, Prakash and colleagues compared 1 mg and 2 mg intrathecal midazolam as an adjunct to subarachnoid block with 10 mg intrathecal bupivacaine.[147] Postoperative analgesia was significantly prolonged (mean 6.1 ± 1 hours vs 3.8 ± 0.5 hours; P = 0.001) and supplemental diclofenac analgesic requirements were significantly decreased (mean 93 ± 29 mg vs 145 ± 12 mg) by the addition of 2 mg midazolam compared to bupivacaine alone, but not by 1 mg. Both 1 mg and 2 mg doses significantly reduced the incidence of postoperative nausea and vomiting. No significant difference in sedation score was seen between groups, and no neurological complications were noted.

Intrathecal midazolam 2 mg therefore appears to prolong spinal anaesthesia, decrease postoperative analgesia requirements, and reduce the incidence of nausea and vomiting, although more evidence is required to ensure that there are no short- or long-term neurological side effects.

Epidural midazolam

Nishiyama compared postoperative thoracic epidural bupivacaine as a 6 mL 0.25% bolus with the same solution containing 0.05 mg/kg midazolam in 30 non-obstetric cases.[148] The area of analgesia was significantly larger in the midazolam group 10 and 30 minutes after administration and involved the entire spinal area and the head and face 10 minutes after administration. Sedation and amnesia were significantly greater in the midazolam group. Sedation and amnesia are probably due to the action of midazolam on benzodiazepine-GABA$_A$ receptors in the CNS, as the dose used resulted in a high enough systemic midazolam concentration to induce these effects.[149]

When midazolam is given as part of a continuous epidural infusion for postoperative pain after gastrectomy, those patients receiving 10 mg or 20 mg of midazolam, as part of a 40 mL infusion of epidural bupivacaine over 12 hours, had better analgesia as measured by the frequency of rescue analgesia compared to those receiving plain bupivacaine.[150] The midazolam groups also had increased early sedation (mean 120 minutes) and amnesia compared to the plain bupivacaine groups.

There are no studies of epidural midazolam use in obstetrics.

Droperidol

Pharmacology/mechanism of action

Droperidol is an antiemetic drug, which acts as an α_2 adrenoreceptor agonist, dopamine receptor antagonist, and 5-HT$_3$ receptor antagonist.[5] Theoretically, a drug active at these receptors could reduce the required dose of neuraxial opioids and improve the quality regional analgesia and anaesthesia.

Intrathecal droperidol

The only intrathecal use appears to be in chronic pain patients with intractable nausea, in which intrathecal droperidol 5–300 mcg/day was a safe and effective antiemetic to use along with opioid analgesics,[151] but there is no experience of its use in obstetrics.

Epidural droperidol

Naji studied 40 patients for hip replacement receiving 4 mg epidural morphine with or without 2.5 mg droperidol for postoperative analgesia. The droperidol group had significantly less pruritus, nausea and vomiting, and hypotension, but there was no difference in mean pain scores over 24 hours.[152]

An RCT in obstetric patients compared the addition of epidural or IV droperidol 2.5 mg to epidural morphine 5 mg for postoperative pain after CD.[153] This study found no difference between the groups with respect to pain, pruritus, or satisfaction, but the incidence and severity of nausea and vomiting was significantly lower in the group that received IV droperidol, as would be expected for an antiemetic drug. This effect was not seen in the epidural droperidol group.

The addition of epidural droperidol 2.5 mg to epidural sufentanil for postoperative pain has been studied in a RCT of 40 orthopaedic patients.[154] The incidence of nausea, vomiting, and pruritus associated with epidural sufentanil was significantly decreased by epidural droperidol, but sedation was increased and the duration of analgesia after sufentanil and droperidol was significantly shorter than after sufentanil and placebo. The addition of epidural droperidol therefore appeared to significantly reduce the side effects of epidural sufentanil while diminishing the duration of analgesia, which would limit its clinical usefulness.

Dexamethasone

Pharmacology/mechanism of action

Dexamethasone is a potent steroid with anti-inflammatory, immunosuppressive, and antiemetic actions.

Intrathecal dexamethasone

In an RCT involving 120 women, 8 mg intrathecal dexamethasone significantly decreased postoperative nausea and vomiting and improved patient satisfaction after CD compared to intrathecal morphine alone[155] This trial did not however, compare the antiemesis achieved with intrathecal dexamethasone to that achieved with IV dexamethasone.

Epidural dexamethasone

An RCT in non-obstetric patients showed that the epidural administration of dexamethasone 5 mg has opioid-sparing effects with lower VAPS scores after laparoscopic cholecystectomy compared with epidural bupivacaine alone or epidural bupivacaine with IV dexamethasone. This would suggest a specific neuraxial analgesic effect of the dexamethasone, the mechanism for which is unknown.[156]

A similar small trial in non-obstetric abdominal surgical cases showed that the addition of 4 mg of epidural dexamethasone to 10 mL 0.25% bupivacaine significantly improved postoperative analgesia, as measured by VAPS scores and a reduction in analgesic consumption, as well as providing significant antiemesis.[157] The analgesia produced was equivalent to the addition of 50 mcg fentanyl to the bupivacaine, again suggesting a specific analgesic effect of dexamethasone.

Maternal pyrexia has been reported in association with labour epidurals, and may be due to altered maternal thermoregulation and production of inflammatory mediators.[158–161] Maternal pyrexia may be an independent risk factor for adverse neonatal outcomes.[162,163] Following vaginal delivery, a history of epidural analgesia may be associated with a higher maternal interleukin (IL)-6 level.[164] In an RCT of 60 parturients, those receiving epidural dexamethasone 0.2 mg/mL in addition to epidural bupivacaine/fentanyl had similar pain scores and block levels to those receiving bupivacaine/fentanyl PCEA alone. The patients in the dexamethasone group did not have a rise in temperature or IL-6 levels which did occur in the control group.[164]

Side effects

Epidural dexamethasone may be associated with increased blood glucose levels, adhesive arachnoiditis, and a reduced threshold for infections including epidural abscess and meningitis.[165]

More information regarding the incidence of side effects is required before neuraxial dexamethasone can be recommended for routine clinical use.

Magnesium sulphate

Pharmacology/mechanism of action

Magnesium is a non-competitive NMDA receptor antagonist. It produces voltage-dependent membrane receptor block, preventing calcium influx. This interferes with the gating of calcium channels, transmembrane ion flux, and regulation of adenyl cyclase and will therefore affect neuronal activity, neurotransmitter release, and modulation of pain.[135,166] This can prevent induction of central sensitization due to peripheral nociceptive stimulation, abolish hypersensitivity, and may prevent post-injury pain.[167,168]

Older studies of neuraxial magnesium investigated 50 mg either as an intrathecal or epidural dose with variable results,[169,170] but two more recent prospective RCTs in obstetric patients have confirmed the analgesic effects of adding 500 mg epidural magnesium to both epidural bupivacaine with morphine[170] and with fentanyl.[171]

Intrathecal magnesium

In a recent systematic review involving 1145 patients, Albrecht et al. examined 18 trials of neuraxial magnesium published since 2002 in an attempt to define its analgesic efficacy and safety.[172] Five of the included trials examined intrathecal use in obstetric patients.[167,173–176] The meta-analysis shows that the time to first analgesic request increased by 11.1% after intrathecal magnesium administration. Although this confirms a modest improvement in pain relief for these patients, Albrecht warns that the risk of neurotoxicity has not been well defined.

Epidural magnesium

In Albrecht et al.'s systematic review,[172] only one of the trials examined epidural use in obstetric patients.[171] The review showed that overall, the time to first analgesic request increased by 72.2% after epidural magnesium administration with doses of between 50 and 100 mg.

In an RCT which was not included in the systematic review, Sun et al. demonstrated in 200 parturients that the addition of magnesium sulphate 500 mg to 0.1% epidural bupivacaine 10 mL and morphine 1.5 mg for postoperative pain relief after CD produced significantly ($P < 0.001$) lower VAPS scores at rest and on movement, increased time to first analgesia request, increased satisfaction ($P < 0.001$), and less shivering ($P < 0.02$) compared to bupivacaine alone or bupivacaine with just morphine at 6, 24 and 36 hours postoperatively.[170]

Similarly, in a prospective RCT of 90 parturients undergoing elective CD under CSE, Yousef showed that the addition of 500 mg $MgSO_4$ to 10 mL 0.25% epidural bupivacaine with 100 mcg of fentanyl following a spinal dose of 2 mL intrathecal 0.5% bupivacaine resulted in significantly later onset of postoperative pain and reduced postoperative analgesic requirement ($P < 0.05$) compared to the control group which received 10 mL N saline instead of magnesium.[171] The magnesium group had greater motor block and muscle relaxation ($P < 0.05$) and less shivering. There was no significant difference in the incidence of hypotension, nausea and vomiting, and duration of motor blockade between the groups.

Side effects

Animal studies have reported clinical and histological evidence of neurological complications with similar weight-adjusted doses,[177] and two case reports have described patients suffering from disorientation and continuous periumbilical burning pain following the injection of magnesium into the neuraxis.[178,179]

Surprisingly, only four of the 18 trials reviewed by Albrecht et al. appear to have been monitored for signs of temporary (headaches, back and leg pain, temporary nerve injury) or permanent (paraplegia, quadriplegia, peripheral nerve injuries) neurological complications, and only one of the six that involved obstetric patients (and which used 50 mg intrathecal magnesium) records having done so.[176] This corresponds to just 140 patients, and of these, only one case of a 4-day persistent headache was recorded, which was treated conservatively.

In the RCT by Sun et al.,[170] which was not included in Albrecht et al.'s systematic review, although 200 patients were studied, the authors state that the trial was not designed or powered to look for neurotoxicity.

The safety of neuraxial magnesium remains undefined.

Sodium bicarbonate

Pharmacology/mechanism of action

Sodium bicarbonate can be used to speed up the onset of action of epidural lidocaine. Unlike every other adjuvant drug, sodium bicarbonate has no intrinsic analgesic activity, and it acts by raising the pH of the injectate. Lidocaine is a weak base, pKa 7.9, and in solution the ionized and unionized fractions exist in equilibrium depending on the pH, the more alkaline the solution, the greater the unionized fraction. Although it is the ionized form which blocks the membrane sodium channel, only the unionized form is lipid-soluble and able to diffuse from the epidural space across the lipid neural membrane to the receptor site. The speed of onset of epidural lidocaine block is therefore determined by the pH of the injected drug solution and alkalinization by the addition of 1 mL of 8.4% $NaHCO_3$ per 10 mL of lidocaine results in a more rapid onset of neural blockade.[14] This is useful when rapid epidural top up for urgent CD is required.

Spinals work so quickly that there is no justification for using intrathecal bicarbonate.

Epidural bicarbonate

As previously mentioned, in a prospective double-blinded RCT, Allam et al. showed using a sequential analysis technique that a lidocaine–bicarbonate–adrenaline mixture (final concentrations 1.8%, 0.76%, and 1:200,000, respectively) halved the time taken to top up the epidural to T5 to touch and T4 for cold for urgent CD from a mean of 14 minutes with plain levobupivacaine to 7 minutes with the mixture. Intraoperative maternal sedation was greater with lidocaine–bicarbonate–adrenaline but this difference was not statistically significant (P = 0.07).[113]

New agents

Several drugs are currently under evaluation as potential neuraxial adjuvants, including adenosine, calcium channel blockers, non-steroidal anti-inflammatory agents, calcitonin, and cannabinoid receptor agonists.[14] There is as yet no information regarding their efficacy or safety.

Conclusion

A variety of chemical compounds and drugs from several classes have been considered as neuraxial adjuvants in order to improve analgesia and anaesthesia in obstetrics. Robust data for safety is still lacking with many of these agents, and obstetric anaesthetists are rightly cautious in adopting new theoretical interventions until safety for both mother and fetus is well established by good evidence. In worldwide practice, opioid adjuvants are universally accepted as beneficial, and well-established monitoring regimens are in place to ensure safety. All other agents, with the exceptions of epinephrine and bicarbonate, although interesting, remain controversial and cannot be recommended for use in routine obstetric clinical practice.

References

1. *The Concise Oxford Dictionary of Current English* (12th ed). Oxford: Oxford University Press; 2011.
2. Fan SZ, Susetio L, Wang YP, *et al.* Low dose of intrathecal hyperbaric bupivacaine combined with epidural lidocaine for cesarean section: a balance block technique. *Anesth Analg* 1994; 78:474–7.
3. Yu SC, Ngan Kee WD, Kwan AS. Addition of meperidine to bupivacaine for spinal anaesthesia for Caesarean section. *Br J Anaesth* 2002; 88(3):379–83.
4. Atalay C, Aksoy M, Aksoy AN, *et al.* Combining intrathecal bupivacaine and meperidine during caesarean section to prevent spinal anaesthesia-induced hypotension and other side-effects. *J Int Med Res* 2010; 38:1626–36.
5. Solomon RE, Gebhart GF. Synergistic antinociceptive interactions among drugs administered to the spinal cord. *Anaesth Analg* 1994; 78:1164–72.
6. Malmberg AB, Yaksh TL. Isobolographic and dose-response analyses of the interactions between intrathecal mu and delta agonists: effects of naltrindole and its benzofuran analog (NTB). *J Pharmacol Exp Ther* 1992; 263:264–75.
7. Wilcox GL, Carlsson KH, Jochim A, *et al.* Mutual potentiation of antinociceptive effects of morphine and clonidine on motor and sensory responses in rat spinal cord. *Brain Res* 1987; 405:84–93.
8. Monasky MS, Zinsmeister AR, Stevens CW, *et al.* Interaction of intrathecal morphine and ST-91 on antinociception in the rat: dose-response analysis, antagonism and clearance. *J Pharmacol Exp Ther* 1990; 254:383–92.
9. Parlow JL, Money P, Chan PS, *et al.* Addition of opioids alters the density and spread of intrathecal local anaesthetics. An in vitro study. *Can J Anaesth* 1999; 16:66–70.
10. Jayacarr A, Carp I. Progesterone-mediated potentiation of spinal sufentanil in rats. *Anaesth Analg* 1993:76:745–50.
11. Hodgson PS, Liu SS. New developments in spinal anaesthesia. *Anesthesiol Clin North Am* 2000; 18(2):235–49.
12. Andrade R, Aghajanian GK. Opiate and a2-adrenoceptor-induced hyperpolarisation of locus cereleus neurons in brain slices: reversal by cyclic adenosine 3'5'-monophosphate analogues. *J Neurosci* 1985; 5:2359–64.
13. Surprenant A, North RA. M-Opioid receptors and a-adrenoceptors coexist on myenteric but not on submucous neurons. *Neuroscience* 1985:16:425–30.
14. Kangure N. Adjuvant agents in neuraxial blockade. *Anaesthesia Tutorial of the Week 230.* [Online] http://e-safe-anaesthesia.org/e_library/03/Neuraxial_adjuvants_TOTW_230_2011.pdf
15. Wahlen BM, Roewer N, Kranke P. Use of local anaesthetics and adjuncts for spinal and epidural anaesthesia and analgesia at German and Austrian University Hospitals: an online survey to assess current standard practice. *BMC Anesthesiol* 2010; 10:4.
16. Proceedings of the 30th Annual Congress of the European Society of Regional Anaesthesia, Dresden, Germany, 2011.
17. Stamer UM, Wiese R, Stuber F, *et al.* Change in anaesthetic practice for Caesarean section in Germany. *Acta Anaesthesiol Scand* 2005; 49:170–6.
18. Rawal N, Allvin R. Epidural and intrathecal opioids for postoperative pain management in Europe—a 17-nation questionnaire study of selected hospitals. Euro Pain Study Group on Acute Pain. *Acta Anaesthesiol Scand* 1996; 40(9):1119–26.
19. Burnstein R, Buckland R, Pickett JA. A survey of epidural analgesia for labour in the United Kingdom. *Anaesthesia* 1999; 54:634–40.
20. Carson D, Binning A, Thomson M. Epidural analgesia in Scotland: a survey of extradural opioid practice. *Health Bull (Edinb)* 1996; 54:51–62.
21. Reisine T. Opiate receptors. *Neuropharmacology* 1995; 34:463–72.
22. Rang HP, Dale MM, Ritter JM, *et al. Rang and Dale's Pharmacology* (7th ed). Edinburgh: Churchill Livingstone; 2011.
23. Peck TE, Hill SA, Williams M. *Pharmacology for Anaesthesia and Intensive Care* (3rd ed). Cambridge: Cambridge University Press; 2008.
24. Sutters KA, Miaskowski C, Taiwo YO, *et al.* Analgesic synergy and improved motor function produced by combinations of mu-delta and mu-kappa-opioids. *Brain Res* 1990; 530:290–4.
25. Rawal N, Van Zundert A, Holmstrom B. Combined spinal epidural technique. *Reg Anesth* 1997:22:406–23.
26. Lu JK, Manullang TR, Staples MH, *et al.* Maternal respiratory arrests, severe hypotension, and fetal distress after administration of intrathecal, sufentanil, and bupivacaine after intravenous fentanyl. *Anesthesiology* 1997: 87:170–2.
27. Skoldebrand A, Garle M, Gustafsson LL, *et al.* Extradural pethidine with and without adrenaline during labour: wide variation in effect. *Br J Anaesth* 1982; 54(4):415–20.
28. Herman NL, Choi KC, Affleck PJ, *et al.* Analgesia, pruritus, and ventilation exhibit a dose-response relationship in parturients receiving intrathecal fentanyl during labor. *Anesth Analg* 1999; 89:378–83.
29. Stocks GM, Hallworth SP, Fernando R, *et al.* Minimum local analgesic dose of intrathecal bupivacaine in labor and the effect of intrathecal fentanyl. *Anesthesiology* 2001; 94:593–8.
30. Dahl JB, Jeppesen IS, Jorgensen H, *et al.* Intraoperative and postoperative analgesic efficacy and adverse effects of intrathecal opioids in patients undergoing cesarean section with spinal anesthesia: a qualitative and quantitative systematic review of randomized controlled trials. *Anesthesiology* 1999; 91(6):1919–27.

31. Camann W, Abouleish A, Eisenach J, *et al.* Intrathecal sufentanil and epidural bupivacaine for labor analgesia: dose-response of individual agents and in combination. *Reg Anesth Pain Med* 1998; 23:457–62.
32. Van de Velde M, Dreelinck R, Dubois J, *et al.* Determination of the full dose-response relation of intrathecal bupivacaine, levobupivacaine, and ropivacaine, combined with sufentanil, for labor analgesia. *Anesthesiology* 2007; 106:149–56.
33. Courtney MA, Bader AM, Hartwell B, *et al.* Perioperative analgesia with subarachnoid sufentanil administration. *Reg Anesth* 1992; 17:274–8.
34. Palmer CM, Emerson S, Volgoropolous D, *et al.* Dose-response relationship of intrathecal morphine for postcesarean analgesia. *Anesthesiology* 1999; 90:437–44.
35. Saravanan S, Robinson AP, Qayoum Dar A, *et al.* Minimum dose of intrathecal diamorphine required to prevent intraoperative supplementation of spinal anaesthesia for Caesarean section. *Br J Anaesth* 2003; 91:368–72.
36. Grass JA, Sakima NT, Schmidt R, *et al.* A randomized, double-blind, dose-response comparison of epidural fentanyl versus sufentanil analgesia after cesarean section. *Anesth Analg* 1997; 85:365–71.
37. Capogna G, Camorcia M, Columb MO. Minimum analgesic doses of fentanyl and sufentanil for epidural analgesia in the first stage of labor. *Anesth Analg* 2003; 96:1178–82.
38. Herman NL, Sheu KL, Van Decar TK, *et al.* Determination of the analgesic dose-response relationship for epidural fentanyl and sufentanil with bupivacaine 0.125% in laboring patients. *J Clin Anesth* 1998; 10:670–7.
39. Rosen MA, Dailey PA, Hughes SC, *et al.* Epidural sufentanil for postoperative analgesia after cesarean section. *Anesthesiology* 1988; 68:448–54.
40. Palmer CM, Nogami WM, Van Maren G, *et al.* Postcesarean epidural morphine: a dose-response study. *Anesth Analg* 2000; 90(4):887–91.
41. Hallworth SP, Fernando R, Bell R, *et al.* Comparison of intrathecal and epidural diamorphine for elective caesarean section using a combined spinal-epidural technique. *Br J Anaesth* 1999; 82:228–32.
42. Hill DA, McCarthy G, Bali IM. Epidural infusion of alfentanil or diamorphine with bupivacaine in labour—a dose finding study. *Anaesthesia* 1995; 50:415–19.
43. Lowson SM, Eggers KA, Warwick JP, *et al.* Epidural infusions of bupivacaine and diamorphine in labour. *Anaesthesia* 1995; 50:420–2.
44. Kotake Y, Matsumoto M, Kimiaki A, *et al.* Additional droperidol, not buporphanol, augments epidural fentanyl analgesia following anorectal surgery. *J Clin Anaesth* 2000; 12:9–13.
45. Capogna G. Effect of epidural analgesia on the fetal heart rate. *Eur J Obstet Gynecol Reprod Biol* 98; 2:160–4.
46. Hindle A. Intrathecal opioids in the management of acute post-operative pain. *CEACCP* 2008; 8(3):81–5.
47. Kumar K, Indu S. Neuraxial opioid-induced pruritus: an update. *J Anaesthesiol Clin Pharmacol* 2013; 29(3):303–7.
48. Etches RC, Sandler AN, Daley MD. Respiratory depression and spinal opioids. *Can J Anaesth* 1989; 36(2):165–85.
49. Kotob HI, Hand CW, Moore RA, *et al.* Intrathecal morphine and heroin in humans: six-hour drug levels in spinal fluid and plasma. *Anesth Analg* 1986; 65(7):718–22.
50. Horlocker TT, Burton AW, Connis RT, *et al.* American Society of Anesthesiologists Task Force on Neuraxial Opioids. Practice guidelines for the prevention, detection, and management of respiratory depression associated with neuraxial opioid administration. *Anesthesiology* 2009; 110:218–30.
51. Wittels B, Glosten B, Faure EA, *et al.* Opioid antagonist adjuncts to epidural morphine for postcesarean analgesia: maternal out- comes. *Anesth Analg* 1993; 77:925–32.
52. Lawhorn CD, McNitt JD, Fibuch EE, *et al.* Epidural morphine with butorphanol for postoperative analgesia after cesarean delivery. *Anesth Analg* 1991; 72:53–7.
53. Hunt CO, Naulty JS, Bader AM, *et al.* Perioperative analgesia with subarachnoid fentanyl-bupivacaine for caesarean delivery. *Anesthesiology* 1989; 71:535–40.
54. Baraka A, Noueihid R, Hajj S. Intrathecal injection of morphine for obstetric analgesia. *Anesthesiology* 1981; 54:136–40.
55. Åkerman B, Arweström E, Post C. Local anesthetics potentiate spinal morphine antinociception. *Anesth Analg* 1988 67:943–8.
56. Maves, Timothy J, Gebhart GF. Antinociceptive synergy between intrathecal morphine and lidocaine during visceral and somatic nociception in the rat. *Anaesthesiology* 1992; 76(1): 91–9.
57. McDonnell N, Keating M, Muchatuta N, *et al.* Analgesia after caesarean delivery. *Anaesth Intensive Care* 2009; 37: 539–51.
58. Grant GJ. Neuraxial analgesia and anaesthesia for labor and delivery: drugs. *UpToDate®* October 2012 (updated 2015). [Online] http://www.uptodate.com/contents/neuraxial-analgesia-and-anesthesia-for-labor-and-delivery-drugs
59. Carvalho B, Roland LM, Chu LF, *et al.* Single-dose, extended-release epidural morphine (DepoDur) compared to conventional epidural morphine for post-cesarean pain. *Anesth Analg* 2007; 105(1):176–83.
60. Hartrick CT, Hartrick K. Drug profile: extended release epidural morphine: review and safety analysis. *Expert Rev Neurother* 2008; 8:1641–8.
61. Dahlgren G, Hultstrand C, Jakobsson J, *et al.* Intrathecal sufentanil, fentanyl, or placebo added to bupivacaine for caesarean section. *Anesth Analg* 1997; 85:1288–93.
62. Palmer CM, Voulgaropoulos D, Alves D. Subarachnoid fentanyl augments lidocaine spinal anaesthesia for caesarean delivery. *Reg Anesth* 1995; 20:389–94.
63. Randalls B, Broadway JW, Browne DA, *et al.* Comparison of four subarachnoid solutions in a needle-through-needle technique for elective caesarean section. *Br J Anaesth* 1991; 66:314–18.
64. Cooper DW, Lindsay SL, Ryall DM, *et al.* Does Intrathecal fentanyl produce acute cross-tolerance to iv morphine? *Br J Anaesth* 1997; 78:311–13.
65. Ben-David B, Solomon E, Levin H, *et al.* Intrathecal fentanyl with small-dose dilute bupivacaine: better anesthesia without prolonging recovery. *Anesth Analg* 1997 85:560–5.
66. Ben-David B, Frankel R, Arzumonov T, *et al.* Minidose bupivacaine-fentanyl spinal anaesthesia for surgical repair of hip fracture in the aged. *Anesthesiology* 2000; 92:6–10.
67. Chilvers CR, Vaghadia H, Mitchell GWE, *et al.* Small dose hypobaric lidocaine-fentanyl spinal anaesthesia for short duration outpatient laparoscopy. II: optimal fentanyl dose. *Anesth Analg* 1997; 84:55–70.
68. Grace D, Lee PH. Anaesthesia and adverse effects after intrathecal pethidine hydrochloride for urological surgery. *Anaesthesia* 1995; 50:1036–40.
69. Palmer CM, Cork RC, Hays R, *et al.* The dose-response relation of intrathecal fentanyl for labor analgesia. *Anesthesiology* 1998; 88:355–61.
70. Liu S, Chiu AA, Carpenter RL, *et al.* Fentanyl prolongs lidocaine spinal anesthesia without prolonging recovery. *Anesth Analg* 1995; 80:730–4.
71. Ginosar Y, Riley ET, Angst MS. The site of action of epidural fentanyl in humans: the difference between infusion and bolus administration. *Anesth Analg* 2003; 97:1428–38.
72. Ginosar Y, Columb MO, Cohen SE, *et al.* The site of action of epidural fentanyl infusions in the presence of local anesthetics: a minimum local analgesic concentration infusion study in nulliparous labor. *Anesth Analg* 2003; 97:1439–45.
73. Columb M, Gall I. Minimum local anaesthetic concentration of local anaesthetics. *CEACCP* 2010; 10(4):114–16.
74. Lyons G, Columb MO, Hawthorne L, *et al.* Epidural pain relief in labour: bupivacaine sparing by epidural fentanyl is dose dependent. *Br J Anaesth* 1997; 78:493–7.
75. Buyse I, Stockman W, Columb M, *et al.* Effect of sufentanil on minimum local analgesic concentrations of epidural bupivacaine, ropivacaine and levobupivacaine in nullipara in early labour. *Int J Obstet Anesth* 2007; 16:22–8.
76. Polley LS, Columb MO, Wagner DS, *et al.* Dose-dependent reduction of the minimum local analgesic concentration (MLAC)

of bupivacaine by sufentanil for epidural analgesia in labor. *Anesthesiology* 1998; 89:626–32.
77. Hays RL, Palmer CM. Respiratory depression after intrathecal sufentanil during labor. *Anesthesiology* 1994; 81:511–12.
78. Ferouz F, Norris MC, Leighton BL. Risk of respiratory arrest after intrathecal sufentanil. *Anesth Analg* 1997; 85:1088–90.
79. Auroy Y, Narchi P, Messiag A, *et al.* Serious complications related to regional anesthesia: results of a prospective survey in France. *Anesthesiology* 1997; 87(3):479–86.
80. Lu JK, Schafer PG, Gardner TL, *et al.* The dose-response pharmacology of intrathecal sufentanil in female volunteers. *Anesth Analg* 1997; 85:372–9.
81. Rawal, N, Nuutinen L, Raj PP, *et al.* Behavioral and histopathologic effects following intrathecal administration of butorphanol, sufentanil, and nalbuphine in sheep. *Anesthesiology* 1991; 75(6):1025–34.
82. Hughes DA, Hill DA. Intrathecal alfentanil with and without bupivacaine for analgesia in labour. *Anaesthesia* 2000; 55:1116–21.
83. Heytens L, Cammu H, Camu F. Extradural analgesia during labor using alfentanil. *Br J Anaesthesia* 1987; 59; 331–7.
84. Redfern N, Bower S, Bullock RE, *et al.* Alfentanil for caesarean section complicated by severe aortic stenosis: a case report. *Br J Anaesth* 1987; 59(10):1309–12.
85. Davoudi M, Mousavi-Bahar SH, Farhanchi A. Intrathecal meperidine for prevention of shivering during transurethral resection of prostate. *Urol J* 2007; 4:212–16.
86. Booth JV, Lindsay DR, Olufolabi AJ, *et al.* Subarachnoid meperidine (Pethidine) causes significant nausea and vomiting during labor. The Duke Women's Anesthesia Research Group. *Anaesthesiology* 2000; 93:418–21.
87. Honet JE, Arkoosh VA, Norris MC, *et al.* Comparison among intrathecal fentanyl, meperidine, and sufentanil for labor analgesia. *Anesth Analg* 1992; 75:734–9.
88. Lui AC, Polis TZ, Cicutti NJ. Densities of cerebrospinal fluid and spinal anaesthetic solutions in surgical patients at body temperature. *Can J Anaesth* 1998; 45:297–303.
89. Roy JD, Girard M, Drolet P. Intrathecal meperidine decreases shivering during cesarean delivery under spinal anesthesia. *Anesth Analg* 2004; 98:230–4.
90. Khaw KS, Ngan Kee WD, Critchley LA. Epidural meperidine does not cause haemodynamic changes in the term parturient. *Can J Anaesth* 2000; 47:155–9.
91. Kafle SK. Intrathecal meperidine for elective Caesarean section: a comparison with lidocaine. *Can J Anaesth* 1993; 40:718–21.
92. Hansen D, Hansen S. The effects of three graded doses of meperidine for spinal anesthesia in African men. *Anesth Analg* 1999; 88(4):827–30.
93. Kurz M, Belani KG, Sessler DI, *et al.* Naloxone, meperidine, and shivering. Anesthesiology 1993; 79:1193–201.
94. Wang JJ, Ho ST, Lee SC, *et al.* A comparison among nalbuphine, meperidine, and placebo for treating postanesthetic shivering. *Anesth Analg* 1999; 88:686–9.
95. McGrady EM, Brownhill DK, Davis AG. Epidural diamorphine and bupivacaine in labour. *Anaesthesia* 1989; 44(5):400–3.
96. Stevens JD, Braithwaite P, Corke CF, *et al.* Double-blind comparison of epidural diamorphine and intramuscular morphine after elective caesarean section, with computerised analysis of continuous pulse oximetry. *Anaesthesia* 1991; 46(4):256–9.
97. National Institute of Clinical Excellence. *Caesarean Section.* Clinical Guideline 132. London: NICE; 2011 (reviewed 2014). http://guidance.nice.org.uk/CG132
98. Husaini SW, Russell IF. Intrathecal diamorphine compared with morphine for post-operative analgesia after caesarean section under spinal anaesthesia. *Br J Anaesth* 1998; 81:135–9.
99. Grice SC, Eisenach JC, Dewan DM. Labor analgesia with epidural bupivacaine plus fentanyl: enhancement with epinephrine and inhibition with 2-chloroprocaine. *Anesthesiology* 1990; 72:623–8.
100. Abboud TK, Sheik-ol-Eslam A, Yanagi T, *et al.* Safety and efficacy of epinephrine added to bupivacaine for lumbar epidural analgesia in obstetrics. *Anesth Analg* 1985; 64:585–91.
101. Okutomi T, Mochizuki J, Amano K, *et al.* Effect of epidural epinephrine infusion with bupivacaine on labor pain and mother-fetus outcome in humans. *Reg Anesth Pain Med* 2000; 25:228–34.
102. Eisenach JC, Grice SC, Dewan DM. Epinephrine enhances analgesia produced by epidural bupivacaine during labor. *Anesth Analg* 1987; 66:447–51.
103. Polley LS, Columb MO, Naughton NN, *et al.* Effect of epidural epinephrine on the minimum local analgesic concentration of epidural bupivacaine in labor. *Anesth Analg* 2002; 96:1123–8.
104. Sakaguchi Y, Sakura S, Shinzawa M, *et al.* Does adrenaline improve epidural bupivacaine and fentanyl analgesia after abdominal surgery? *Anaesth Intensive Care* 2000; 28:522–6.
105. Columb MO. Clinical trials: up-down sequential allocation. In Reynolds F (ed) *Obstetric Anaesthesia: Millennium Update.* London: Springer-Verlag; 2000:157–65
106. Gautier PE, Debry F, Fanard L, *et al.* Ambulatory combined spinal epidural analgesia for labor. Influence of epinephrine on bupivacaine-sufentanil combination. *Reg Anesth* 1997; 22:143–9.
107. Connelly NR, Freiman JP, Lucas T, *et al.* Addition of epinephrine to epidural bupivacaine infusions following initiation of labor analgesia with epidural fentanyl. *J Clin Anesth* 2011; 23(4):265–9.
108. Yaksh TL. Spinal opiates. A review of their effect on spinal function with emphasis on pain processing. *Acta Anaesthesiol Scand* 1987; 84:25–35.
109. Lu JK, Schafer PG, Garner TL, *et al.* The dose-response pharmacology of intrathecal sufentanil in female volunteers. *Anesth Analg* 1997; 85:372–9.
110. Moore DC, Batra MS. The components of an effective test dose prior to epidural block. *Anesthesiology* 1981; 55:693–6.
111. Guay J. The epidural test dose: a review. *Anesth Analg* 2006; 102(3):921–9.
112. Hillyard SG, Bate TE, Corcoran TB, *et al.* Extending epidural analgesia for emergency Caesarean section: a meta-analysis. *Br J Anaesth* 2011; 107(5):668–78.
113. Allam J, Malhotra S, Hemingway C, *et al.* Epidural lidocaine-bicarbonate-adrenaline vs levobupivacaine for emergency Caesarean section: a randomised controlled trial. *Anaesthesia* 2008; 63(3):243–9.
114. Yaksh TL, Dirksen R, Harty GJ. Antinociceptive effects of intrathecally injected cholinomimetic drugs in rat and cat. *Eur J Pharm* 1985; 117:81–8.
115. Wong CA, Slavenas P. The incidence of transient radicular irritation after spinal anesthesia in obstetric patients. *Reg Anesth Pain Med* 1999; 24:55–8.
116. Aouad MT, Siddik SS, Jalbout MI, *et al.* Does pregnancy protect against intrathecal lidocaine-induced transient neurologic symptoms? *Anesth Analg* 2001; 92:401–4.
117. Philip J, Sharma SK, Gottumukkala VN, *et al.* Transient neurologic symptoms after spinal anesthesia with lidocaine in obstetric patients. *Anesth Analg* 2001; 92:405–9.
118. Carp H, Jayaram A, Morrow, D. Intrathecal cholinergic agonists lessen bupivacaine spinal-block-induced hypotension. *Anesth Analg* 1994; 79:112–16.
119. Hood DD, Eisenach JC, Tong C, *et al.* Cardiorespiratory and spinal cord blood flow effects of intrathecal neostigmine methylsulfate, clonidine, and their combination in sheep. *Anesthesiology* 1995; 82:428–35.
120. Hood DD, Eisenach JC, Tuttle R. Phase I safety assessment of intrathecal neostigmine in humans. *Anesthesiology* 1995; 82:331–43.
121. Eisenach, JC. Epidural neostigmine: will it replace lipid soluble opioids for postoperative and labor analgesia? *Anesth Analg* 2009; 109:293–5.
122. Chia YY, Chang TH, Liu K, *et al.* The efficacy of thoracic epidural neostigmine infusion after thoracotomy. *Anesth Analg* 2006; 102:201–8.

123. Roelants F, Lavand'homme PM, Mercier-Fuzier V. Epidural administration of neostigmine and clonidine to induce labor analgesia: evaluation of efficacy and local anesthetic-sparing effect. *Anesthesiology* 2005; 102:1205–10.
124. Ross VH, Pan PH, Owen MD, *et al.* Neostigmine decreases bupivacaine use by patient-controlled analgesia during labor: a randomized controlled study. *Anesth Analg* 2009; 109:524–31.
125. Clark RB, Brown MA, Lattin DL. Neostigmine, atropine and glycopyrrolate: does neostigmine cross the placenta? *Anaesthesiology* 1996; 84:450–3.
126. Catapres (Clonidine Hydrochloride USP) Boehringer Ingelheim International GmbH 2009 accessdata.fda.gov
127. Wolff M, Heugel P, Hempelmann G, *et al.* Clonidine reduces the excitability of spinal dorsal horn neurones. *Br J Anaesth* 2007; 98(3):353–61.
128. Batra YK, Sondekoppa VR, Nidhi BP, *et al.* Intrathecal clonidine decreases propofol sedation requirements during spinal anaesthesia in infants. *Pediatr Anesth* 2010; 20:625–32.
129. James CE, Marc DK, Walter K. Alpha sub 2-adrenergic agonists for regional anesthesia: a clinical review of clonidine (1984–1995). *Anesthesiology* 1996; 85:655–74.
130. Nelson LE, Lu J, Guo T, *et al.* The alpha2-adrenoceptor agonist dexmedetomidine converges on an endogenous sleep-promoting pathway to exert its sedative effects. *Anesthesiology* 2003; 98:428–36.
131. Landau R, Schiffer E, Morales M, *et al.* The dose sparing effect of clonidine added to ropivacaine for labor epidural analgesia. *Anesth Analg* 2001; 93:1560–4.
132. Brichant JF, Bonhomme V, Mikulski M, *et al.* Admixture of clonidine to epidural bupivacaine for analgesia during labor: effect of varying clonidine doses. *Anesthesiology* 1994; 81:A1136.
133. Van de Velde M, Berends N, Kumar A, *et al.* Effects of epidural clonidine and neostigmine following intrathecal labour analgesia: a randomised, double-blind, placebo-controlled trial. *Int J Obstetric Anesth* 2009: 3:207–14.
134. Paech M, Pan P. New recipes for neuraxial labor analgesia: simple fare or gourmet combos? *Int J Obstet Anesth* 2009; 18(3):201–3.
135. Wolf CJ, Thompson SW. The induction and maintenance of central sensitization is dependent on *N*-methyl-d-aspartic acid receptor activation: implications for the treatment of post-injury pain and hypersensitivity states. *Pain* 1991; 44:293–9.
136. Iida H, Dohi S, Tanahashi T, *et al.* Spinal conduction block by intrathecal ketamine in dogs. *Anesth Analg* 1997; 85:106–10.
137. Dowdy EG, Kaya K, Gocho Y. Some pharmacological similarities of ketamine, lidocaine and procaine. *Anesth Analg* 1973; 52:839–42.
138. Crisp T, Perrotti JM, Smith DL, *et al.* The local monoaminergic dependency of spinal ketamine. *Eur J Pharmacol* 1991; 194:167–72.
139. Green SM, Cote CJ. Ketamine and neurotoxicity: clinical perspectives and implications for emergency medicine. *Ann Emerg Med* 2009; 54(2):181–90.
140. Bion JF. Intrathecal ketamine for war surgery. A preliminary study under field conditions. *Anaesthesia* 1984; 39:1023–8.
141. Subramaniam K, Subramaniam B, Pawar D, *et al.* Evaluation of the safety and efficacy of epidural ketamine combined with morphine for postoperative analgesia after major upper abdominal surgery. *J Clin Anesth* 2001; 13(5):339–44.
142. Schofield PR, Darlison MG, Fujira N, *et al.* Sequence and functional expression of the GABA A receptor shows a ligand gated receptor super-family. *Nature* 1987; 328:221–7.
143. Bozkurt P, Tunali Y, Kaya G, *et al.* Histological changes following epidural injection of midazolam in the neonatal rabbit. *Paediatr Anaesth* 1997; 7:385–9.
144. Nishiyama T, Matsukawa T, Hanaoka K. Effects of adding midazolam on the postoperative epidural analgesia with two different doses of bupivacaine. *J Clin Anaesth* 2002; 14:92–7.
145. Shadangi BK, Garg R, Pandey R, *et al.* Effects of intrathecal midazolam in spinal anaesthesia: a prospective randomized case control study. *Singapore Med J* 2011; 52(6):432–5.
146. Tucker A, Lai C, Nadeson R, *et al.* Intrathecal midazolam. A cohort study investigating safety. *Anesth Analg* 2004; 98(6):1512–20.
147. Prakash S, Joshi N, Gogia AR, *et al.* Analgesic efficacy of two doses of intrathecal midazolam with bupivacaine in patients undergoing cesarean delivery. *Reg Anesth Pain Med* 2006; 31:221–6.
148. Nishiyama T. The post-operative analgesic action of midazolam following epidural administration. *Eur J Anaesthesiol* 1995; 12:369–74.
149. Nishiyama T, Hanaoka K. Midazolam concentrations in serum and cerebrospinal fluid after epidural administration in dogs. *Br J Anaesth* 1998; 80:812.
150. Nishiyama T, Yokoyama T, Hanaoka K. Midazolam improves postoperative epidural analgesia with continuous infusion of local anaesthetics. *Can J Anaesthesia* 1998; 45(6):551–5.
151. Ahmad-Sabry MH, Shareghi G. Long-term use of intrathecal droperidol as an excellent antiemetic in nonmalignant pain—a retrospective study. *Middle East J Anesthesiol* 2012; 21(6):857–62.
152. Naji P, Farschtschian M, Wilder-Smith OH, *et al.* Epidural droperidol and morphine for postoperative pain. *Anesth Analg* 1990; 70:583–8.
153. Sanansilp V, Areewatana S, Tonsukchai N. Droperidol and the side effects of epidural morphine after cesarean section. *Anesth Analg* 1998; 86:532–7.
154. Wilder-Smith CH, Wilder-Smith OH, Farschtschian M, *et al.* Epidural droperidol reduces the side effects and duration of analgesia of epidural sufentanil. *Anesth Analg* 1994; 79:98–104.
155. Abdel-Aleem M, Osman A, Morsy K. Effect of coadministration of dexamethasone with intrathecal morphine on postoperative outcomes after caesarean delivery. *Int J Gynaecol Obstet* 2012; 116(2):158–61.
156. Thomas S, Beevi S. Epidural dexamethasone reduces postoperative pain and analgesic requirements. *Can J Anaesth* 2006; 53(9):899–905.
157. Khafagy HF, Refaat AI, El-Sabae HH, *et al.* Efficacy of epidural dexamethasone versus fentanyl on postoperative analgesia. *J Anesth* 2010; 24(4):531–6.
158. Fusi L, Steer PJ, Maresh MJ, *et al.* Maternal pyrexia associated with the use of epidural analgesia in labour. *Lancet* 1989; 1(8649):1250–2.
159. Lieberman E, Lang JM, Frigoletto F, *et al.* Epidural analgesia, intrapartum fever, and neonatal sepsis evaluation. *Pediatrics* 1997; 99(3):415–19.
160. Goetzl L, Rivers J, Zighelboim I, *et al.* Intrapartum epidural analgesia and maternal temperature regulation. *Obstet Gynecol* 2007; 109(3):687–90.
161. Goetzl L, Evans T, Rivers J, *et al.* Elevated maternal and fetal serum interleukin-6 levels are associated with epidural fever. *Am J Obstet Gynecol* 2002; 187(4):834–8.
162. Lieberman E, Lang J, Richardson DK, *et al.* Intrapartum maternal fever and neonatal outcome. *Pediatrics* 2000; 105:8–13.
163. Impey L, Greenwood C, MacQuillan K, *et al.* Fever in labour and neonatal encephalopathy: a prospective cohort study. *BJOG* 2001; 108(6):594–7.
164. DeJongh RF, Bosmans EP, Puylaert MJ, *et al.* The influence of anaesthetic techniques and type of delivery on peripartum serum interleukin-6 concentrations. *Acta Anaesthesiol Scand* 1997; 41(7):853–60.
165. Wang LZ, Hu X, Liu X, *et al.* Influence of epidural dexamethasone on maternal temperature and serum cytokine concentration after labor epidural analgesia. *Int J Gynaecol Obstet* 2011; 113(1):40–3.
166. Fawcett WJ, Haxby EJ, Male DA. Magnesium: physiology and pharmacology. *Br J Anaesth* 1999; 83:302–20.
167. Buvanendran A, McCarthy RJ, Kroin JS, *et al.* Intrathecal magnesium prolongs fentanyl analgesia: a prospective randomised controlled trial. *Anesth Analg* 2002; 95:661–6.
168. McCarthy CL, Sinha A, Katz JA. A qualitative systematic review of the role of NMDA receptor antagonists in preventive analgesia. *Anesth Analg* 2004; 98:1385–400.

169. Bilir A, Gulec S, Erkan A, *et al.* Epidural magnesium reduces post-operative analgesic requirement. *Br J Anaesth* 2007; 98:519–23.
170. Sun J, Wu X, Xu X, *et al.* A comparison of epidural magnesium and/or morphine with bupivacaine for postoperative analgesia after caesarean section. *Int J Obstet Anesth* 2012; 21(4):310–16.
171. Yousef AA, Amr YM. The effect of adding magnesium sulphate to epidural bupivacaine and fentanyl in elective caesarean section using combined spinal-epidural anaesthesia: a prospective double blind randomised study. *Int J Obstet Anesth* 2010; 19(4):401–4.
172. Albrecht E, Kirkham KR, Liu SS, *et al.* The analgesic efficacy and safety of neuraxial magnesium sulphate: a quantitative review. *Anaesthesia* 2013; 68(2):190–202.
173. Ghrab BE, Maatoug M, Kallel N, *et al.* Does combination of intrathecal magnesium sulfate and morphine improve post-caesarean section analgesia? *Ann Fr Anesth Reanim* 2009; 28:454–9.
174. Malleeswaran S, Panda N, Mathew P, *et al.* A randomised study of magnesium sulphate as an adjuvant to intrathecal bupivacaine in patients with mild preeclampsia undergoing caesarean section. *Int J Obstet Anesth* 2010; 19:161–6.
175. Shoeibi G, Sadegi M, Firozian A, *et al.* The additional effect of magnesium sulfate to lidocaine in spinal anesthesia for cesarean section. *Int J Pharmacol* 2007; 3:425–7.
176. Unlugenc H, Ozalevli M, Gunduz M, *et al.* Comparison of intrathecal magnesium, fentanyl, or placebo combined with bupivacaine 0.5% for parturients undergoing elective caesarean delivery. *Acta Anaesthesiol Scand* 2009; 53:346–53.
177. Saeki H, Matsumoto M, Kaneko S, *et al.* Is intrathecal magnesium sulfate safe and protective against ischemic spinal cord injury in rabbits? *Anesth Analg* 2004; 99:1805–12.
178. Goodman EJ, Haas AJ, Kantor GS. Inadvertent administration of magnesium sulphate through epidural catheter: report and analysis of a drug error. *Int J Obstet Anesth* 2006; 15:63–67.
179. Dror A, Henriksen E. Accidental epidural magnesium sulphate injection. *Anesth Analg* 1987; 66:1020–1.

CHAPTER 18

Alternative neural blocks for labour analgesia

Outi Palomäki and Petri Volmanen

Introduction

Although neuraxial analgesia, either epidural or spinal, is the most effective,[1] widely examined, and most often used method for pain relief during labour, alternatives are necessary due to the variety of parturients' wishes, unavailability of the anaesthetist, or rapidity of required delivery. Globally, the majority of labouring women in the world do not have the choice of epidural analgesia.[2] Some parturients may also prefer less invasive methods of analgesia as well as wishing to stay mobile and in an upright position for as long as possible. In situations where neuraxial analgesia is contraindicated, due, for example, to a low platelet count, it is possible to block the distal parts of the pain pathways transvaginally.

This chapter deals with four alternative regional analgesia techniques. The paracervical and pudendal blocks are usually administered by an obstetrician, and the two others, the sympathetic and paravertebral blocks, may be administered by an anaesthetist.

Paracervical block

Although epidural, spinal, and/or a combination of these forms of analgesia are the most effective and most widely used pain relief methods during labour, the paracervical block (PCB) has remained as an alternative method used by obstetricians.

Labour pain has both visceral and somatic components. In the first stage of labour, visceral pain predominates, arising from the uterine contractions, mechanical distension of the lower uterine segment, and from cervical dilatation. Stretching and distention of the lower segments of the uterus and the cervix stimulate mechanoreceptors, with uterine contractions causing myometrial ischaemia. Pain impulses from this area are transmitted by afferent nerves to the dorsal root ganglia in the spinal cord from T10 through L1. The object of the PCB is to block pain transmission at the paracervical ganglion, which lies posterior and lateral to the cervicouterine junction. Later in labour, at the end of the first stage and during the second stage, the descent of the presenting fetal part produces distension and traction on pelvic structures. The transmission of these painful perineal stimuli are conducted via the pudendal nerve though the anterior rami of S2 through S4, and cannot be blocked by PCB.[3–5]

The pathways of labour pain, the injection sites of PCB, as well as pudendal block (PB) are shown in Figure 18.1.

Paracervical block technique

PCB is administered transvaginally by an obstetrician when the presenting part has descended well into the pelvis, the cervix is in the active phase of dilatation, and the contractions are frequent and painful. During injection the mother lies supine with her knees flexed and hips fully abducted. To avoid aortocaval compression, left lateral tilt is recommended. After giving the injection on one side, the mother turns to a lateral position for the next one or two contractions. At the end of this, the same procedure is repeated on the other side. Continuous cardiotocography (CTG) monitoring during the procedure is recommended.

The obstetrician palpates the cervix and then inserts her/his index and middle fingers to the lateral vaginal fornix, and the needle is placed along the fingers into contact with the vaginal epithelium. The injecting needle should be kept strictly tangential to the presenting fetal part.[6] The injection technique is shown in Figure 18.2.

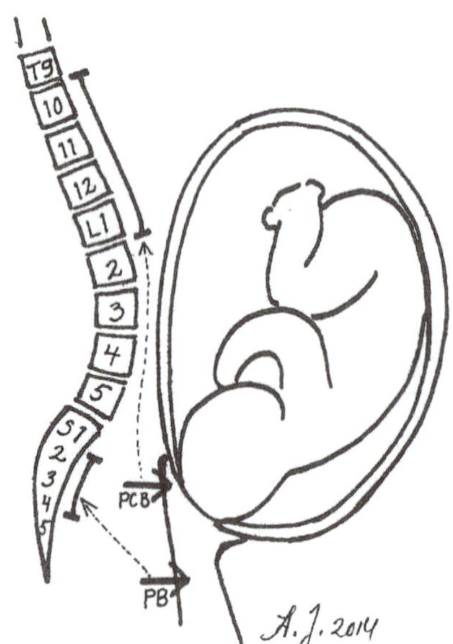

Figure 18.1 Paracervical and pudendal blocks (sagittal view).
PCB, paracervical block (transvaginal); PB, pudendal block (transvaginal); arrow, site of injection; dotted line, pain pathway; solid line, effect site.
With permission from Dr Anne Jyrkiäinen.

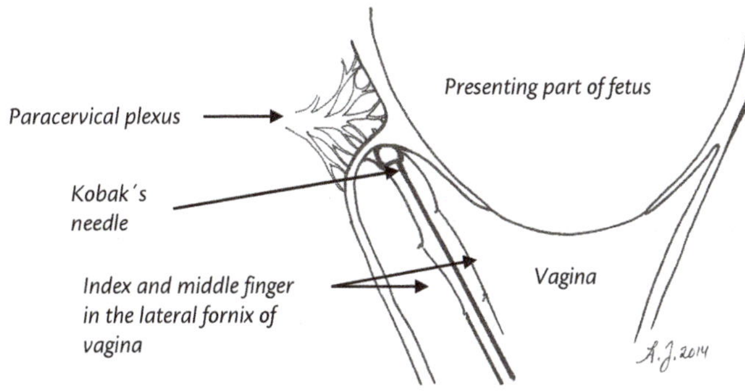

Figure 18.2 Injection technique of paracervical block (frontal view).
With permission from Dr Anne Jyrkiäinen.

The instrument used for the procedure, a Kobak needle, was originally introduced in 1960 by Kobak and Sadove.[7] It has a round-tipped sheath that can be introduced to the injection site safely and without injury to the mother or fetus. After placement of the rounded tip at the injection site, the needle is advanced in the sheath, from which it is possible to control and limit the depth of needle penetration. In the original instrument this limit was 15–20 mm, but with the modern version of the needle used in obstetric practice, the injection depth has been limited to 3 mm for safety reasons.[8] With a Kobak needle it is possible to penetrate the endopelvic fascia just under the vaginal epithelium and to inject the analgesic drug into the base of the broad ligament, thereby blocking the afferent nerves and visceral pain.[8,9] After careful aspiration the analgesic agent is injected at two different points—3 and 9 o'clock or 4 and 8 o'clock—with the operator facing the patient who is the lithotomy position. Another possibility is to inject a quarter of the total drug volume at each of these four sites. In some studies, four-site administration has been shown to be more effective and reliable than two-site injection.[10] In any method, it is essential to aspirate at every injection site. It has been shown in X-ray studies, that both 3 and 9 o'clock and 4 and 8 o'clock positions are equal in effectiveness as drug dispersion is identical in the base of the broad ligament space.[9] When carrying out the block to the patient's left-sided fornix, the operator sits on the parturient's right side, and palpates the fornix with the right hand while aspirating and injecting with the left hand. While waiting for the next contraction, the operator moves to the left side of the patient and changes hands. With this technique, the needle's course is naturally tangential to the fetal head.

Excluding the oldest studies which were performed using deep injection techniques and high doses of local anaesthetic agent, the most widely used and studied drug in PCB, especially in European delivery units, is 0.25% racemic bupivacaine, 10 mL[11–20] but even a 0.125% solution of bupivacaine 10 mL has been showed to be effective.[17]

There are two studies in which racemic bupivacaine and levobupivacaine, the S (-)-enantiomer of racemic bupivacaine, were used.[21,22] No differences were observed in safety profiles as examined with incidence of CTG—pathology or neonatal outcome—and the analgesic effect was equal with both drugs using similar doses of drug. In a few studies, amino amides other than bupivacaine, such as mepivacaine,[23–25] lidocaine,[25,26] or prilocaine,[25] have been used for PCB at total doses of 200–300 mg, 100–200 mg, and 200 mg, respectively. In the United States, some early studies with the amino ester 1–2% 2-chloroprocaine have been published.[27–29] The main problem with this local anaesthetic is the short duration of pain relief. In two studies comparing chloroprocaine to bupivacaine,[30,31] bupivacaine was determined to be the drug of choice for PCB due to its longer-lasting analgesia (mean ± standard deviation (SD); 66.8 ± 28.7 minutes vs 35.4 ± 10.2 minutes).[31]

The analgesic effect of paracervical block

Paracervical block compared to other pain relief methods

PCB has been compared to other pain relief methods, such as epidural analgesia, single-shot spinal analgesia, and intramuscular meperidine in a few small series.

In a study of 62 women, parturients were offered a choice between PCB and epidural analgesia. Thirty-nine women chose PCB for pain relief while 23 chose epidural analgesia.[12] Bupivacaine was the drug of choice for both pain relief methods with a total dose of 25 mg (10 mL of 0.25% solution) for PCB and 30 mg (6 mL of 0.5% solution) for epidural block. PCB was given by an obstetrician using two 5 mL injections, and epidural analgesia was administered by an anaesthetist using an initial bolus of 4 mL followed by a further 2 mL, 10 minutes later. Pain intensity was assessed on a linear scale of 0–10. Pain score values decreased significantly within 5 minutes in the PCB group and within 30 minutes in the epidural group. Although PCB had a rapid onset of pain relief, the analgesic effect at 30, 45, and 60 minutes after analgesia was significantly better in the epidural group. In another study, the pain relief method was randomized for 44 parturients using similar doses of bupivacaine as in the study above.[19] The main objective in that study was to compare the haemodynamic effects of PCB and epidural analgesia, but a maternal overall assessment on the efficacy of pain relief was also estimated on a 4-point scale. Excellent or good pain relief was achieved in 87% of cases in the epidural group and in 67% of cases in the PCB group (not significant, $P = 0.14$). Two parturients in the PCB group and none in the epidural group graded the pain relief as poor.

In a study by Junttila et al., among 104 multiparous women who were randomized to receive either PCB (with 10 mL of 0.25% racemic bupivacaine) or a single-shot spinal anaesthetic (with 2.5 mg hyperbaric racemic bupivacaine +2.5 mcg sufentanil), median pain scores were found to decrease from the baseline significantly in both groups, but the decrease was greater in the spinal group. The need for subsequent analgesia was more common in the PCB group, whereas shivering and pruritus occurred more often in the spinal group. There were no differences between the groups with regards to progress of labour, CTG findings, or neonatal outcome.[20]

In a double-blind, randomized study, PCB with 12 mL 0.25% racemic bupivacaine was compared with a 75 mg intramuscular injection of meperidine. Pain score data was available from 99 patients out of a total of 117 study patients. The analgesic effect was estimated by the parturient and recorded by the midwife every 20 minutes for up to 2 hours. A 4-point scale was used (full/acceptable/slight/no pain relief). The pain relief during the first hour after administration of the analgesia was rated as full or acceptable in 78% of the parturients in the PCB group and 31% in the meperidine group. The average pain relief in the PCB group stayed significantly higher than in the meperidine group for up to 60 minutes after administration of the drugs. The difference between groups was no longer statistically significant at 80 minutes after administration, although 50% of women in the PCB group and 20% in the meperidine group still experienced the pain relief as being either full or acceptable. During the study period, there was a learning curve for the five doctors involved in the study, with pain relief being complete or acceptable in 68% of women during the first half of the study compared to 85% in the latter half.[32]

Rating the effect of paracervical block

Verbal rating scores (VRS) and visual analogue scales (VAS) have been used as pain rating methods in studies on PCB only. Table 18.1 summarizes pain relief results by rating method.

Among the studies using a VRS, the study by Jägerhorn stands out with better rates (excellent or good in 94% of 204 PCBs) than the others. In this study, all PCBs were administered by the same obstetrician.[6]

The pain relief effect from a PCB has been statistically significant compared to baseline up to the beginning of the second stage of labour,[16] for up to 120 minutes in another study,[17] or for 90 minutes after PCB in a third study.[22] In a study by Jensen et al., the pain relief effect was full or acceptable in 62% of parturients 60 minutes after PCB, while 50%, 30%, and 26% found the pain relief to be full or acceptable at 80, 100, and 120 minutes after PCB respectively.[32] Since the median of the length of the delivery has found to be about 2 hours after PCB including the second stage,[12,14,15,32] it seems probable that a single PCB is sufficient for many parturients until the end of the first stage, but some women will need a second injection or another method of pain relief method to get them through the second stage of labour.

In a study of 341 women receiving PCB in the first stage of labour, pain relief was reported to be good if the VAS score had dropped by more than 50% from the baseline 30 minutes after PCB. Parturients who had delivered before the 30-minute time limit or who were already fully dilated were excluded from the analysis. Among these patients, good pain relief was achieved in 47% of the cases. In 23% of cases, the pain score had dropped to less than 20% from the baseline. Twelve per cent of parturients needed a subsequent epidural or spinal analgesia. Primiparity, a high pain score before PCB, and PCB given by a specialist obstetrician compared to a trainee obstetrician were found to be associated with better pain relief in a logistic regression analysis.[22]

Summarizing the findings from the above studies and from our own clinical experience, it appears that the effect of PCB is, on average, moderate and more variable than the effect of neuraxial analgesia. The findings that a single obstetrician or specialized obstetrician administering the block had a greater chance of success in terms of PCB and achieved lower pain scores demonstrates the importance of educational aspects. Patient selection also plays an important role. In clinical practice, it appears that the primiparae whose labour progresses rapidly, benefit from PCB the most. In other cases in which poor pain relief is achieved after a PCB, the next step is to administer a more efficient analgesic method straight away, neuraxial analgesia being the most common alternative.

Table 18.1 Studies on the analgesic effect of paracervical block with 25 mg bupivacaine

Verbal rating score (VRS)	N	Excellent/ good (%)	Moderate (%)	Poor (%)		
Jägerhorn[6]	204	94	NR[a]	6		
Puolakka et al.[11]	38	76	12	12		
Ranta et al.[16]	248	62	25	13		
Manninen et al.[19]	21	67	5	2		
Visual analogue scale (VAS)	**N**	**VAS before**	**VAS at 15/30 min**	**VAS at 60 min**	**VAS at 90/ 120min**	**VAS until 2nd stage**
Ranta et al.[16]	248	8.0	NR/5.0[b]	NR	NR	6.0[c]
Nieminen and Puolakka[17]	52	8.7	NR/4.7[c]	5.2[c]	5.8[c]/7.1[d]	NR
Palomäki et al.[22]	341	8.0	3.4[c]/4.3[c]	5.3[c]	7.1[c]	NR

[a]NR = not reported.

[b]$P < 0.0001$.

[c]$P < 0.001$.

[d]$P < 0.01$.

Data from various sources (see references).

Safety of paracervical block

Safety studies during labour

In the oldest studies on PCB from the 1960s and early 1970s, 20 mL mepivacaine (1–1.5%), lidocaine (1–1.5%), or bupivacaine (0.25–0.5%) was used, and the depth of the needle injection was up to 20 mm.[33] In these initial studies, major complications such as a high prevalence of fetal bradycardia and even fetal death were reported.[33–35] On the other hand, a study with 500 PCBs and a 1.2% incidence of transient fetal bradycardia was also published during the same decade.[10]

In 1975, Jägerhorn studied the spread of the anaesthetic agent in paracervical tissue. He used serial X-rays in a case study of 20 women undergoing termination of pregnancy between 14 and 19 weeks' gestation. He also introduced an improved technique, in which an injection depth of no more than 3 mm together with a low dose and concentration of local anaesthetic was used. With this lower injection depth of 2–3 mm no intravenous spread of contrast medium was noticed in X-rays of any patient. There is also practically no risk for injection directly into the nerve plexuses of the pelvic wall, lower uterine segment, or fetal head. In a clinical series including the parturients presented in the same article, maternal side effects were also absent.[6]

Table 18.2 is a meta-analysis of PCB studies with a relevant sample size (N > 50), in which a superficial puncture technique and low-dose administration of analgesic agent were used. CTG analysis of the study patients, criteria for fetal bradycardia, as well as fetal outcome are clearly described. Among 1566 PCBs, the bradycardia frequency was 2.8%. Among these cases, there was no need for interventions, and neonatal outcome was good. The frequency of fetal bradycardia after intrathecal analgesia has been quoted as being 5–7.3%, is transient, and does not result in the need for caesarean delivery.[36,37] One theory, which could explain the appearance of fetal bradycardia in some subjects after different pain relief methods, proposes that the onset of pain relief rapidly

Table 18.2 Rate, duration, and associated interventions of post-PCB bradycardia

Study	PCBs N	Rate of bradycardia		Duration of bradycardia (min)	Intervention due to bradycardia	Depth of injection (mm)
		N	%			
Jägerhorn[6a]	204	2	1.0	Transient[d]	No	3
Meis et al.[39a]	53	0	0	–	–	3
Jensen et al.[32a]	55	2	3.6	6–9[e]	No	3
Carlsson et al.[13b]	469	9	1.9	6.5 ± 1.7[f]	No	3
Ranta et al.[16a]	248	5	2.0	4–12[e]	No	3
Nieminen and Puolakka[17b]	97	12	12.4	Mild, transient[d]	No	3–4
Palomäki et al.[21c]	440	14	3.2	2–8[e]	No	3–4
All	1566	44	2.8			

[a]PCB with 0.25% bupivacaine.

[b]PCB with 0.25% or 0.125% bupivacaine.

[c]PCB with 0.25% bupivacaine or 0.25% levobupivacaine.

[d]Only verbal description.

[e]Range.

[f]Median ± SD.

Data from various sources (see references).

attenuates maternal catecholamines. When the plasma concentration of circulating beta-adrenergic agonists decrease, there is a predominance of alpha activity leading to an intensification in uterine contractions inducing fetal heart rate deceleration.[38]

The exact cause of fetal bradycardia is not clear; vasoconstriction of the uterine arteries, increased uterine activity, a direct effect on the fetal myocardium via circulation, or a combination of these have all been proposed as explanations.[11,13,15]

Neonatal safety studies

Fetal oxygenation measured by fetal oximetry was studied in a prospective study in which 20 healthy parturients were enrolled in PCB or epidural groups according to their own preferences and clinical situation. No change was seen in maternal oxygen saturation between groups. In the PCB group, fetal oxygen saturation was slightly elevated compared to the baseline, while in the epidural group fetal oxygen saturation values remained at baseline or slightly below. This difference was statistically significant ($P = 0.009$), but the finding was not thought to be clinically important by the authors.[18]

Levy et al.[26] prospectively studied the effect of PCB on neonatal umbilical artery pH values using linear regression analysis. They found no statistically significant association between PCB use and umbilical artery pH at birth. Comparing PCB to any other pain relief method, Carlsson et al.[13] found that 469 PCB cases had significantly fewer low Apgar scores than 1013 other cases who delivered vaginally following other methods of analgesia or indeed no analgesia at all. The incidence of 1-minute Apgar scores of 7 or less was 1.7% and 8.4% in PCB and other vaginal deliveries groups, respectively, and 0.6% and 2.0% for 5-minute Apgar scores. Meis et al. reported similar findings in a smaller study comparing neonates after PCB to those who did not receive any form of regional analgesia. The PCB group showed slightly, but statistically significant higher 1-minute Apgar scores and umbilical artery and vein pH values.[39] In a study comparing PCB to intramuscular opioid (meperidine), signs of asphyxia (pH ≤ 7.15, 1-minute Apgar score ≤ 7) were significantly more frequent in the opioid group than in the PCB group.[32] In two studies comparing PCB and epidural analgesia, no statistical difference in umbilical artery pH levels or Apgar scores were found.[12,18]

In most studies on PCB, chronic maternal illness such as diabetes or hypertensive disorders, pre- or postmaturity, signs of fetal distress before pain relief, intrauterine growth restriction, or meconium-stained amniotic fluid are exclusion criteria, therefore the method cannot be recommended for high-risk patients.[6,13,16,17,21,32,39] In one study, however, 785 risk patients were allowed to receive PCB. Among these parturients, prematurity, postmaturity, cigarette use, pre-eclampsia, or oxytocin use combined with PCB were not associated with low 5-minute Apgar scores.[25]

Neurobehavioural responses have been studied in a few series including neonates born after PCB and those without any neuraxial analgesia. The groups were compared in terms of neurobehavioural responses from 0–3 hours up to 1–5 days after birth, with the investigators blinded as to the analgesic method during labour. No statistically significant differences were found in neurobehavioural scores after delivery between the groups of neonates.[14,39,40]

Haemodynamic effects of paracervical block

One study from the 1980s used radiolabelled xenon washout to measure intervillous blood flow before and after PCB. The blood flow was shown to have stayed constant, even in three cases of post-PCB bradycardia where the flow changes were minimal.[11]

In later studies, the haemodynamic effects of PCB have been examined in three small studies using Doppler ultrasonography. Fetal and maternal blood flow was measured before and after PCB. In two studies, both with 12 patients, the maternal uterine artery pulsatility indices (PIs) did not change,[15,21] whereas in one study, which randomized 44 primiparous parturients to receive either

PCB or epidural labour analgesia, the maternal uterine artery PI increased after PCB while they remained unchanged after epidural analgesia.[19]

In two studies, no differences in fetal umbilical circulation were found after PCB in a total of 60 cases.[19,21] In a third study, the PI values in the umbilical artery were not affected if the CTG stayed normal after PCB. However, in two cases, in which post-PCB bradycardia developed, a marked increase in the PI of the umbilical artery was seen. The velocity waveforms of blood flow retuned to baseline when the CTG pattern normalized.[15]

Uterine activity after paracervical block

In some clinical PCB trials, the contractility of the uterus has been measured using an intrauterine pressure catheter. In one study with high-dose administration of local anaesthetic, a significant correlation between post PCB fetal bradycardia and uterine activity was found. In 11 out of 14 cases of bradycardia, an increase of uterine contractility of 100 Montevideo units was found, and in three cases there was no change in uterine activity.[41] In another study, intrauterine measurement was used in 52 cases, and a mean increase of 29 Montevideo units was found among parturients.[21] In a third study with 51 parturients, no statistically significant change in uterine activity was found.[42] In all these studies, bupivacaine was used as the analgesic agent.

Impact on the method of delivery

In some studies, PCB has been compared to other pain relief methods. The rate of spontaneous vaginal delivery has been higher in a group receiving PCB compared to intramuscular opioid[32] or epidural analgesia.[20] In the study by Carlsson et al. the incidence of normal vaginal birth was significantly higher in the PCB group compared to the group with any other pain relief method (88.7% vs 76.5%, $P < 0.001$).[13]

In the two biggest studies examining PCB alone, the spontaneous delivery rates have been as high as 91% and 96% and the caesarean delivery rate 4% and 0.25% respectively, with none of the indications for operative delivery being due to any complication of PCB.[16,21] Once again, this probably reflects patient selection for this type of pain relief (i.e. parturients with a rapid progression of labour).

Maternal complications

Maternal complications after PCB are rare. In all the studies referred to above, there were no maternal complications. A theoretical risk for systemic toxicity of an anaesthetic agent could occur if aspiration is not performed properly and the injection is intravascular. Insertion of the needle too deeply could result in nerve plexus trauma. Haematomas in the paracervical or parametrial area and laceration at the injection site are also possible maternal complications. In the studies reviewed above, with a total study material of 2995 PCBs, there were no maternal complications reported.

Conclusion

PCB provides an alternative pain relief method for parturients without some of the disadvantages typical of neuraxial analgesia, such as an increased risk for assisted vaginal birth, longer second stage of labour, occiput posterior presentation of fetus at delivery, hypotension, fever, postdural puncture headache, or pruritus.[1,43–49] PCB is easily available in the labour room with a minimal need for preparation or cost, its effect is rapid, and it does not interfere with the normal progress of labour or spontaneous delivery.[13,16,21] It can be used as an option for term parturients with uncomplicated pregnancy by experienced obstetricians with knowledge of the appropriate anatomy, correct technique, and clinical skills.

Pudendal block

PB is another method of providing labour analgesia, which is usually performed by an obstetrician. It is used for pain relief during the second stage of labour for spontaneous or vacuum deliveries and during repair of perineal tears. It can be combined with first-stage PCB analgesia and is especially helpful for multiparas with severe perineal pain during the final stage of delivery.[7]

Technique of pudendal block

Labour pain during the second stage and delivery is transmitted to the central nervous system via the pudendal nerve and the sacral spinal nerve roots S2–4.[50] The nerve block procedure is conducted with the mother adopting a similar position to that used for PCB with a similar Kobak needle.[51] The landmark for the site of injection, however, is the ischial spine, which can be palpated on each side of the birth canal. Two different injection techniques have been described: in the first, after injecting an initial dose into the mucosa over the tip of the ischial spine, the remainder of the dose is injected behind the ligament. Careful aspiration before injection is essential. The other technique aims to block the nerve at two different levels—on the dorsal and anterior sides of the ischial spine. If 1% lidocaine is used, the first 1 mL is injected into the mucosa, and the next 3 mL is infiltrated into the sacrospinous ligament. Then the tip of the needle is advanced behind the ligament until a decrease of resistance is felt when a further 3 mL is injected in this area. After drawing the needle back into the introducer, it is turned to the anterior side of the ischial spine, and the final 3 mL of drug is injected here under the mucosa to block the more distal part of the pudendal nerve.[52] The procedure is repeated on the other side to achieve bilateral analgesia. The palpating and injecting hands can be changed at this stage, if the operator is comfortable interchanging hands. When this form of analgesia is given for an episiotomy and its repair, a unilateral injection is sufficient. The injection site of PB is shown in Figure 18.3.

Doses of 7–10 mL of solution containing 1.0% lidocaine without epinephrine to each side gives a fast block onset.[53,54] If a PB is given for episiotomy repair, bupivacaine, ropivacaine, or levobupivacaine in equivalent doses should be used because of their longer-lasting pain relief effects and the decreased need for additional analgesics.[55]

PB has traditionally been administered with a Kobak needle, palpating the injection site using the fingers. The technique can benefit from other methods, however, such as nerve stimulation or ultrasound. A motor response to a 0.5–0.6 mA electronic nerve stimulator in the anal sphincter, vulva constrictor muscle, or movement of the clitoris should confirm close contact between the pudendal nerve or the right tissue plain in which the three tributaries of the nerve lie.[55] Ultrasound-assisted techniques for PB has been reported for non-obstetric indications.[56]

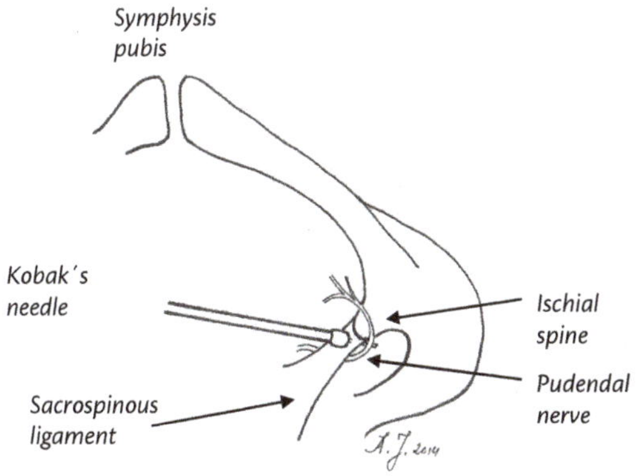

Figure 18.3 Injection site of pudendal block (horizontal view).
With permission from Dr Anne Jyrkiäinen.

Analgesic effect of pudendal block

Wilds used a spinal needle and 10 mL of 1–2% procaine or 1% hexylcaine for each side with a transvaginal technique noting an 84% success rate for analgesia.[50] One failure out of 24 blocks has been reported in testing the perineal anaesthesia by pinpricking 10 minutes after injection using a transvaginal technique with lidocaine.[54] Up to 50% uni- or bilateral failures have been reported, however, making it understandable that a perineal infiltration with local anaesthetic may often be needed along with the PB.[57,58]

The transperineal technique has been employed when PB is used to provide anaesthesia for suturing lacerations and episiotomy wounds. This block has been noted to provide analgesia and reduce the need for pain medications for up to 48 hours when 15 mL of 0.5% bupivacaine is injected unilaterally after delivery.[55]

Complications of pudendal block

Some complications for PB have been described as case reports in the literature; these are haematoma, infection, and fetal local anaesthetic toxicity.[59–61] Nerve injury is another potential complication. In clinical use, these complications are rare. Occasionally the nerve block extends to include the sciatic nerve with a subsequent transient motor block in the lower extremity.

Paravertebral techniques for labour analgesia

Afferent pain impulses from the uterine cervix travel via the lumbar sympathetic ganglia at L2–3 and enter the dorsal root of the spine at T10–L1 through the rami communicantes lying adjacent to the vertebral discs. The use of the paravertebral techniques for the treatment of labour pain began after Cleland's experiments showing that uterine pain impulses could be blocked paravertebrally were first published in 1933.[62] By the end of the 1950s a number of large case series showing the analgesic effect of lumbar sympathetic block (LSB) were published. With the increasing popularity of epidural analgesia, LSB has disappeared from use as a method of labour analgesia in most places. Thoracic paravertebral block (PVB) for labour analgesia has been increasingly used in Petrozavodsk and Arkhangelsk in Russia.[63] Paravertebral techniques are still frequently used, however, in the treatment of chronic pain and for anaesthesia and analgesia, for example, in thoracic surgery.[64,65]

Technique of sympathetic and paravertebral blocks

The LSB provides the opportunity to block pain impulses at the sympathetic trunk. The intended location for local anaesthetic is in the retroperitoneum anterolateral to the vertebra and separated by the psoas muscle and fascia from the lumbar plexus. According to the classical blind technique suggested by Bonica, the lumbar sympathetic trunk is accessed with a needle sited 8 cm laterally from the top of the L3 spinous process at a right angle to the longitudinal axis and is directed medially at a 60° angle to the plane of the back with the parturient in a sitting position. The needle is advanced to 7 cm, at which point the stylet is removed and a loss-of-resistance (LOR) syringe attached. A LOR at 9–12 cm distance should signal that the anterior border of the psoas muscle has been reached.[66] Datta and Pai noted, however, that the LOR technique gives a position anterior to the ganglion. They advocated an extraforaminal paradiscal technique in order to avoid injury to the nerve as well as contact with the lumbar vessels.[67] This method requires fluoroscopy, however, making it impractical in the delivery suite.

Visualization of the lumbar paravertebral anatomy has been noted as being feasible utilizing an ultrasound technique with curved-array transducers operating at low frequencies (3.5–5 MHz). It has been reported for needle placement in the lumbar sympathetic chain in treating chronic pain syndromes, but not for labour analgesia to date.[68] Pain impulses can also be blocked at a higher level by inserting local anaesthetic into paravertebral space at T11–12 levels.[62,69] A volume of 10 mL of 0.25–0.5% bupivacaine with epinephrine has been used for each side, although larger volumes up to 25 mL for each side have also been employed.[69–72] Needle sizes of 16–22 G have been employed with or without catheters to be left in place for further doses.

The injection and effect sites of thoracic PVB and LSB are shown in Figure 18.4.

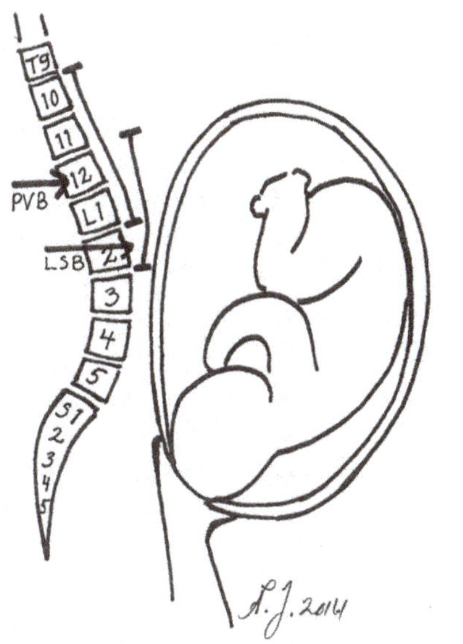

Figure 18.4 Thoracic paravertebral and lumbar sympathetic blocks (sagittal view).
PVB, paravertebral block (thoracic); LSB, lumbar sympathetic block; arrow, site of injection; solid line, effect site.
With permission from Dr Anne Jyrkiäinen.

Analgesic effect of sympathetic and paravertebral blocks

The reported failure rates have been low (0–5%) with LSB, which is surprising considering the difficult anatomic location and blind method.[70,71] The mean pain score was reduced from 7 to 4 for the first 30 minutes after the block using 10 mL 0.5% bupivacaine with epinephrine and 25 mcg fentanyl for each side with no difference from a control group which received epidural analgesia. However, subsequently the pain scores began to increase in the group receiving LSB.[70] With bupivacaine, the duration of the analgesic effect of single injections has been reported as mean (± SD) of 283 (± 103) minutes.[71] Leighton et al. noted a shorter labour when LSB was employed compared with epidural analgesia.[70] With the currently available data, no conclusion on the analgesic effects of thoracic PVB can be drawn. However, case reports suggest 3–4 hours of analgesia for the first stage of labour after paravertebral injections of bupivacaine 0.25-0.5% with epinephrine.[69] LSB and thoracic PVB do not provide analgesia for the second stage of labour unless the block is extended to the sacral somatic roots and plexuses. Therefore, a PB should be included in the transitional phase with these methods.

Complications of sympathetic and paravertebral blocks

The correct placement of the needle tip for LSB is paramount as the aorta and vena cava as well as kidneys are in close proximity to the sympathetic chain. The roots of the spinal nerves are the target for the thoracic PVB and the anatomic space for LSB communicates with the nerve roots.

With LSB, psoas muscle injections at the L2 level and intravascular injections have been noted with frequencies of 7.4% and 6.8%, respectively, even when the advancement of the needle is guided by a fluoroscopy.[73] The likelihood of the tip of the needle remaining in the psoas muscle is higher if a lower lumbar vertebra is chosen for the block level. The sensitivity of an aspiration test for intravascular injection has been shown to be only 40.7% in a non-obstetric situation.[73]

The reported complications of LSB include sensory and motor block, hypotension, dural puncture, subdural block, and haematoma.[74–79] Thoracic PVB is also associated with risk of pneumothorax.[80] It is not advisable to use paravertebral techniques in those parturients with a tendency to bleed, such as those using low-molecular-weight heparins.[70,81]

Conclusion

Alternative methods of analgesia are necessary, as many women cannot, for various reasons, benefit from neuraxial blocks. Blocking the pain pathways distally with PCB and PB is a practical and effective way with a low risk of side effects or complications. LSB and PVC are interesting methods used quite early on during the history of labour analgesia, but abandoned later with the rising popularity of epidural anaesthesia.

References

1. Jones L, Othman M, Dowswell T, *et al.* Pain management for women in labour: an overview of systematic reviews. *Cochrane Database Syst Rev* 2012; 3:CD009234.
2. Torri A. The role of social, economic, and religious factors in the availability of neuraxial labor analgesia worldwide. *Curr Anesthesiol Rep* 2013; 3:250–5.
3. Hawkins JL. Epidural analgesia for labor and delivery. *N Engl J Med* 2010; 362(16):1503–10.
4. Eltzschig HK, Lieberman ES, Camann WR. Regional anesthesia and analgesia for labor and delivery. *N Engl J Med* 2003; 348(4):319–32.
5. Lowe NK. The nature of labor pain. *Am J Obstet Gynecol* 2002; 186(5 Suppl Nature):S16–24.
6. Jägerhorn M. Paracervical block in obstetrics. An improved injection method. A clinical and radiological study. *Acta Obstet Gynecol Scand* 1975; 54(1):9–27.
7. Kobak AJ, Sadove MS. Transvaginal regional anesthesia simplified by a new instrument. *Obstet Gynecol* 1960; 15:387–90.
8. Kobak AJ, Sadove MS. Paracervical block: a transvaginal regional pain relief. *Obstet Gynecol* 1962; 19:418–19.
9. Kobak AJ, Sadove MS, Mazeros WT. Anatomic studies of transvaginal regional anesthesia. Roentgenographic visualization of neural pathways. *Obstet Gynecol* 1962; 19:302–10.
10. Saloheimo AM. Paracervical block anesthesia in labor. *Acta Obstet Gynecol Scand* 1968; 47(Suppl 5):3–21.
11. Puolakka J, Jouppila R, Jouppila P, *et al.* Maternal and fetal effects of low-dosage bupivacaine paracervical block. *J Perinat Med* 1984; 12(2):75–84.
12. Grenman S, Erkkola R, Kanto J, *et al.* Epidural and paracervical blockades in obstetrics. Catecholamines, arginine vasopressin and analgesic effect. *Acta Obstet Gynecol Scand* 1986; 65(7):699–704.
13. Carlsson BM, Johansson M, Westin B. Fetal heart rate pattern before and after paracervical anesthesia. A prospective study. *Acta Obstet Gynecol Scand* 1987; 66(5):391–5.
14. Kangas-Saarela T, Jouppila R, Puolakka J, *et al.* The effect of bupivacaine paracervical block on the neurobehavioural responses of newborn infants. *Acta Anaesthesiol Scand* 1988; 32(7):566–70.
15. Räsänen J, Jouppila P. Does a paracervical block with bupivacaine change vascular resistance in uterine and umbilical arteries? *J Perinat Med* 1994; 22(4):301–8.
16. Ranta P, Jouppila P, Spalding M, *et al.* Paracervical block—a viable alternative for labor pain relief? *Acta Obstet Gynecol Scand* 1995; 74(2):122–6.
17. Nieminen K, Puolakka J. Effective obstetric paracervical block with reduced dose of bupivacaine. A prospective randomized double-blind study comparing 25 mg (0.25%) and 12.5 mg (0.125%) of bupivacaine. *Acta Obstet Gynecol Scand* 1997; 76(1):50–4.
18. Kaita TM, Nikkola EM, Rantala MI, *et al.* Fetal oxygen saturation during epidural and paracervical analgesia. *Acta Obstet Gynecol Scand* 2000; 79(5):336–40.
19. Manninen T, Aantaa R, Salonen M, *et al.* A comparison of the hemodynamic effects of paracervical block and epidural anesthesia for labor analgesia. *Acta Anaesthesiol Scand* 2000; 44(4):441–5.
20. Junttila EK, Karjalainen PK, Ohtonen PP, *et al.* A comparison of paracervical block with single-shot spinal for labour analgesia in multiparous women: a randomised controlled trial. *Int J Obstet Anesth* 2009; 18(1):15–21.
21. Palomäki O, Huhtala H, Kirkinen P. A comparative study of the safety of 0.25% levobupivacaine and 0.25% racemic bupivacaine for paracervical block in the first stage of labor. *Acta Obstet Gynecol Scand* 2005; 84(10):956–61.
22. Palomäki O, Huhtala H, Kirkinen P. What determines the analgesic effect of paracervical block? *Acta Obstet Gynecol Scand* 2005; 84(10):962–6.
23. Rogers RE. Fetal bradycardia associated with paracervical block anesthesia in labor. *Am J Obstet Gynecol* 1970; 106(6):913–6.
24. Goins JR. Experience with mepivacaine paracervical block in an obstetric private practice. *Am J Obstet Gynecol* 1992; 167(2):342–4; discussion 344–5.
25. Day TW. Community use of paracervical block in labor. *J Fam Pract* 1989; 28(5):545–50.

26. Levy BT, Bergus GR, Hartz A, *et al.* Is paracervical block safe and effective? A prospective study of its association with neonatal umbilical artery pH values. *J Fam Pract* 1999; 48(10):778–84.
27. Arnold NI. Paracervical block with low doses of chloroprocaine. Fetal and maternal effects. *JAMA* 1975; 231(1):56–7.
28. Weiss RR, Nathanson HG, Tehrani MR, *et al.* Paracervical block with 2-chloroprocaine. *Anesth Analg* 1977; 56(5):709–16.
29. Strauss RG, Dase D, Doering PL. Prolonging paracervical block anesthesia: addition of dextran to 2-chloroprocaine. *Am J Obstet Gynecol* 1979; 133(8):891–3.
30. Nesheim BI. Which local anesthetic is best suited for paracervical blocks? *Acta Obstet Gynecol Scand* 1983; 62(3):261–4.
31. Belfrage P, Floberg J. Obstetrical paracervical block with chloroprocaine or bupivacaine. A comparison. *Acta Obstet Gynecol Scand* 1983; 62(3):245–7.
32. Jensen F, Qvist I, Brocks V, *et al.* Submucous paracervical blockade compared with intramuscular meperidine as analgesia during labor: a double-blind study. *Obstet Gynecol* 1984; 64(5):724–7.
33. Teramo K. Effects of obstetrical paracervical blockade on the fetus. *Acta Obstet Gynecol Scand Suppl* 1971; 16:1–55.
34. Nyirjesy I, Hawks BL, Hebert JE, *et al.* Hazards of the use of paracervical block anesthesia in obstetrics. *Am J Obst Gynecol* 1963; 87(2):231–5.
35. Rosefsky JB, Petersiel ME. Perinatal deaths associated with mepivacaine paracervical-block anesthesia in labor. *N Engl J Med* 1968; 278(10):530–3.
36. Mardirosoff C, Dumont L, Boulvain M, *et al.* Fetal bradycardia due to intrathecal opioids for labour analgesia: a systematic review. *BJOG* 2002; 109(3):274–81.
37. Palmer CM, Maciulla JE, Cork RC, *et al.* The incidence of fetal heart rate changes after intrathecal fentanyl labor analgesia. *Anesth Analg* 1999; 88(3):577–81.
38. Beilin Y. An update on obstetric anesthesia. *Semin Cardiothorac Vasc Anesth* 2010; 14(1):64–5.
39. Meis PJ, Reisner LS, Payne TF, *et al.* Bupivacaine paracervical block. Effects on the fetus and neonate. *Obstet Gynecol* 1978; 52(5):545–8.
40. Nesheim BI, Lindbaek E, Storm-Mathisen I, *et al.* Neurobehavioral response of infants after paracervical block during labour. *Acta Obstet Gynecol Scand* 1979; 58(1):41–4.
41. Achiron R, Rojansky N, Zakut H. Fetal heart rate and uterine activity following paracervical block. *Clin Exp Obstet Gynecol* 1987; 14(1):52–6.
42. Read JA, Miller FC. The bupivacaine paracervical block in labor and its effect on quantitative uterine activity. *Obstet Gynecol* 1979; 53(2):166–70.
43. American College of Obstetrics and Gynecology. ACOG practice bulletin. Obstetric analgesia and anesthesia. Number 36, July 2002. American College of Obstetrics and Gynecology. *Int J Gynaecol Obstet* 2002; 78(3):321–35.
44. Anim-Somuah M, Smyth RM, Jones L. Epidural versus non-epidural or no analgesia in labour. *Cochrane Database Syst Rev* 2011;12:CD000331.
45. Eriksen LM, Nohr EA, Kjaergaard H. Mode of delivery after epidural analgesia in a cohort of low-risk nulliparas. *Birth* 2011; 38(4):317–26.
46. Poignant M, Hjelmstedt A, Ekeus C. Indications for operative delivery between 1999–2010 and induction of labor and epidural analgesia on the risk of operative delivery—a population based Swedish register study. *Sex Reprod Healthc* 2012; 3(4):129–34.
47. Robinson CA, Macones GA, Roth NW, *et al.* Does station of the fetal head at epidural placement affect the position of the fetal vertex at delivery? *Am J Obstet Gynecol* 1996; 175(4 Pt 1):991–4.
48. Lieberman E, Davidson K, Lee-Parritz A, *et al.* Changes in fetal position during labor and their association with epidural analgesia. *Obstet Gynecol* 2005; 105(5 Pt 1):974–82.
49. Osborne C, Ecker JL, Gauvreau K, *et al.* Maternal temperature elevation and occiput posterior position at birth among low-risk women receiving epidural analgesia. *J Midwifery Womens Health* 2011; 56(5):446–51.
50. Wilds PL. Transvaginal pudendal-nerve block; an improved anatomic approach. *Obstet Gynecol* 1956; 8(4):385–92.
51. Kobak AJ, Evans EF, Johnson GR. Transvaginal pudendal nerve block; a simple procedure for effective anesthesia in operative vaginal delivery. *Am J Obstet Gynecol* 1956; 71(5):981–9.
52. Cunningham FG, Leveno KJ, Bloom SL, *et al.* Obstetrical anesthesia. In *Williams Obstetrics* (23rd ed). New York: The McGraw-Hill Companies, Inc.; 2010:444–63.
53. Davis JE, Frudenfeld JC, Frudenfeld K, *et al.* The combined paracervical-pudendal block anesthesia for labor and delivery. A review of 2,100 private cases. *Am J Obstet Gynecol* 1964; 89:366–76.
54. Zador G, Lindmark G, Nilsson BA. Pudendal block in normal vaginal deliveries. Clinical efficacy, lidocaine concentrations in maternal and foetal blood, foetal and maternal acid-base values and influence on uterine activity. *Acta Obstet Gynecol Scand Suppl* 1974; 34:51–64.
55. Aissaoui Y, Bruyere R, Mustapha H, *et al.* A randomized controlled trial of pudendal nerve block for pain relief after episiotomy. *Anesth Analg* 2008; 107(2):625–9.
56. Peng PW, Tumber PS. Ultrasound-guided interventional procedures for patients with chronic pelvic pain—a description of techniques and review of literature. *Pain Physician* 2008; 11(2):215–24.
57. Scudamore JH, Yates MJ. Pudendal block—a misnomer? *Lancet* 1966; 1(7427):23–4.
58. Arulkumaran S. Ingemarsson I, Hamlett JD, *et al.* Pudendal block: an obstetric procedure that needs critical evaluation. *Asia-Oceania J Obstet Gynaecol* 1987; 13(1):37–41.
59. Kurzel RB, Au AH, Rooholamini SA. Retroperitoneal hematoma as a complication of pudendal block—diagnosis made by computed tomography. *West J Med* 1996; 164(6):523–5.
60. Bozynski ME, Rubarth LB, Patel JA. Lidocaine toxicity after maternal pudendal anesthesia in a term infant with fetal distress. *Am J Perinatol* 1987; 4(2):164–6.
61. Svancarek W, Chirino O, Schaefer G Jr, *et al.* Retropsoas and subgluteal abscesses following paracervical and pudendal anesthesia. *JAMA* 1977; 237(9):892–4.
62. Cleland JGP. Paravertebral anaesthesia in obstetrics: experimental and clinical basis. *Surg Gynecol Obstet* 1933; 57:51–62.
63. Antipin E. *Sravnitelnaya Otsenka Effektivnosti i Bezopasnosti Epiduralnoi Analgezii i Paravertebralnoi Blokadi v Rodah* [*Comparative Efficacy and Safety of Epidural Analgesia and Paravertebral Blocks in Childbirth*] PhD thesis, St. Petersburg, 2009. http://www.dissercat.com/content/sravnitelnaya-otsenka-effektivnosti-i-bezopasnosti-epiduralnoi-analgezii-i-paravertebralnoi-
64. Peng P, Castano E. Survey of chronic pain practice by anesthesiologists in Canada. *Can J Anesth* 2005; 52(4)383–9.
65. Davies RG, Myles PS, Graham JM. A comparison of the analgesic efficacy and side-effects of paravertebral vs epidural blockade for thoracotomy—a systematic review and meta-analysis of randomized trials. *Br J Anaesth* 2006; 96:418–26.
66. Bonica JJ, McDonald JS. Other regional analgesic/anesthetic techniques. In Bonica JJ, McDonald JS (eds) *Principles and Practice of Obstetric Analgesia and Anesthesia* (2nd ed). Baltimore, MD: Williams & Wilkins, 1995:497–537.
67. Datta S, Pai U. Paradiscal extraforaminal technique for lumbar sympathetic block: report of a proposed new technique utilizing a cadaver study. *Pain Physician* 2004; 7(1):53–7.
68. Kirvelä O, Svedström E, Lundbom N. Ultrasonic guidance of lumbar sympathetic and celiac plexus block: a new technique. *Reg Anesth* 1992; 17(1):43–6.
69. Nair V, Richard H. Bilateral paravertebral block: a satisfactory alternative for labour analgesia. *Can J Anaesth* 2001; 48(2):179–84.
70. Leighton BL, Halpern SH, Wilson DB. Lumbar sympathetic blocks speed early and second stage induced labor in nulliparous women. *Anesthesiology* 1999; 90(4):1039–46.

71. Meguiar RV, Wheeler AS. Lumbar sympathetic block with bupivacaine: analgesia for labor. *Anesth Analg* 1978; 57(4):486–92.
72. LaSalvia LA, Copit PS, Kondon VE. Evaluation of paravertebral lumbar sympathetic block in labor. *Am J Obstet Gynecol* 1959; 78:1212–18.
73. Hong JH, Kim AR, Lee MY, *et al.* A prospective evaluation of psoas muscle and intravascular injection in lumbar sympathetic ganglion block. *Anesth Analg* 2010; 111(3):802–7.
74. Riekse JM. Terminal obstetrical anesthesia by means of lumbar sympathetic paravertebral block. *Am J Obstet Gynecol* 1959; 78(2):411–14.
75. Sugar RG. A new complication due to the lumbar sympathetic block? *Anesthesiology* 1988; 69(5):803.
76. Collucci J, Derasari M, Kirkpatrick AF. Complications of blinded lumbar sympathetic blocks. *Reg Anesth* 1992; 17(2):114–15.
77. Haynsworth RF Jr, Noe CE, Fassy LR. Intralymphatic injection: another complication of lumbar sympathetic block. *Anesthesiology* 1994; 80(2):460–2.
78. Wheatley JK, Motamedi F, Hammonds WD. Page kidney resulting from massive subcapsular hematoma. Complication of lumbar sympathetic nerve block. *Urology* 1984; 24(4):361–3.
79. Aida S, Takahashi H, Shimoji K. Renal subcapsular hematoma after lumbar plexus block. *Anesthesiology* 1996; 84:452–5.
80. Richardson J, Lönnqvist PA, Naja Z. Bilateral thoracic paravertebral block: potential and practice. *Br J Anaesth* 2011; 106(2):164–71.
81. Boezaart AP, Lucas SD, Elliott CE. Paravertebral block: cervical, thoracic, lumbar, and sacral. *Curr Opin Anaesthesiol* 2009; 22(5):637–43.

CHAPTER 19

Prevention and management of breakthrough pain during neuraxial labour analgesia

Jessica Bauerle and Mieke A. Soens

Introduction

Neuraxial analgesia is considered the gold standard for pain relief in labour. When compared to other options for labour analgesia, such as intravenous opioids or inhaled anaesthetics, neuraxial analgesia is associated with consistently lower pain scores and side effects.[1,2]

While, fortunately, the majority of epidural catheters placed for labour provide satisfactory analgesia, they also sometimes fail. In this chapter, we review potential causes of failure and strategies that can be used to prevent problems and rescue poorly functioning catheters.

Incidence and characteristics of breakthrough pain during neuraxial labour analgesia

The incidence of breakthrough pain during neuraxial labour analgesia has been reported to be 0.9–25%.[3–5] This wide variation is mostly dependent on the definition of breakthrough pain used. Some studies define failure rate as the need to replace the epidural catheter, while others assess pain relief by using visual analogue scale scores.

Recurrent episodes of breakthrough pain in labour lead to decreased maternal satisfaction and identifying those patients at high risk for breakthrough pain is beneficial as it allows the anaesthetic provider to adjust his/her anaesthetic regimen accordingly. Additionally, breakthrough pain and a frequent need for supplemental medication can be a sign of a suboptimal functioning catheter, which may fail to provide adequate anaesthesia should obstetric intervention be required.

The risk of failed analgesia and the potential need for replacement should be discussed with the patient during the pre-anaesthetic evaluation.

Risk factors for breakthrough pain

Obstetric-related risk factors

Certain obstetric factors are associated with a higher incidence of breakthrough pain (Table 19.1). Often, these factors have in common that they are associated with more severe pain. Hess and colleagues[6] performed a prospective observational study, looking at nearly 2000 parturients who received epidural analgesia during labour. The authors found that nulliparity, increased fetal weight, and epidural placement at earlier cervical dilation were risk factors for the development of breakthrough pain in labour. Also, a prolonged labour course, abnormal fetal presentation (e.g. occiput posterior), and dysfunctional labour ultimately requiring caesarean or instrumental delivery have all been associated with an increased need for repeated supplementation.[5–8] Another important consideration is that pain intensity increases as labour progresses. The median local anaesthetic concentration[9] required to achieve adequate epidural analgesia in late labour is approximately three times that required during early labour.[9] As such, an unpredictably rapid labour course can also be a cause of breakthrough pain.[5]

Maternal risk factors

Maternal obesity has been associated with a significantly increased rate of epidural catheter failure.[10] Melzack et al.[11] studied the influence of physical variables on the severity of labour pain using the McGill Pain Questionnaire and reported a positive correlation between body mass index (BMI) and severity of labour pain. Maternal obesity is also linked with an increased incidence of fetal macrosomia, which is a known risk factor for more painful contractions and complicated labour. In addition, maternal obesity significantly increases the degree of difficulty of epidural insertion, as well as the risk for subsequent epidural

Table 19.1 Risk factors for breakthrough pain

Obstetric factors	Nulliparity
	Increased fetal weight
	Abnormal fetal presentation
	Dysfunctional labour
	Rapidly progressing labour course
Maternal factors	Obesity
	Chronic low back pain/history of lumbar spine surgery

catheter migration.[5,12,13] Hamilton et al.[14] demonstrated that epidural catheters not fixed at the skin could move 1–2.5 cm inward when the patient's posture was changed from the sitting to the lateral recumbent position, with the greatest change seen in patients with a BMI greater than 30. Therefore it may be prudent to place the parturient in the lateral position before securing the catheter to the skin.[15]

Chronic low back pain and/or a history of lumbar spine surgery also increase the risk of inadequate epidural analgesia. Benzon and colleagues[16] compared the onset of lumbar epidural anaesthesia in patients with low back pain and/or radicular pain, with patients without back pain. They found that the patients with back pain and/or radicular pain had a significantly delayed onset of sensory block. In particular, the nerve roots that were involved in the lumbar radicular pathology or those adjacent to them, as determined by myelogram and electromyography, were blocked 10–70 minutes after the contralateral unaffected nerve roots.

Also, patients with prior back surgery have an increased risk of epidural failure. The epidural space may be difficult to find and the spread of local anaesthetic may be patchy due to instrumentation (arthrodesis, Harrington rods, etc.), bone graft material, or scar tissue. However, despite these possible difficulties, a success rate of 91% has been reported for epidural anaesthesia in patients with prior lumbar spine surgery.[17]

Neuraxial technique-related risk factors

Initial placement

Patient position

One possible reason for inadequate analgesia after epidural placement is intravascular placement or migration of the epidural catheter. The incidence of intravascular placement has been reported to be 1–10%. The pregnant patient is at increased risk for accidental epidural vein cannulation because inferior vena cava compression by the enlarged uterus results in dilation of collateral veins in the epidural space.[18] A systematic review of randomized controlled trials that evaluated strategies to avoid epidural vein cannulation in obstetric patients found that placement of the epidural catheter with the patient in the lateral recumbent position compared with the sitting position may decrease the incidence of intravascular placement of catheters (5.1% versus 9.5%).[19] One possible explanation is that the sitting position is associated with an increased epidural venous pressure and therefore an increased risk of vessel puncture. However, an anaesthetist unaccustomed to using the lateral recumbent position is more likely to encounter difficulty in identification of the midline, which may in turn be associated with a greater risk for blood vessel puncture and accidental dural puncture compared to an operator that has experience with the lateral position.[20] Indeed, many practitioners prefer the patient in the sitting position for administration of neuraxial analgesia, because it allows better identification of anatomical landmarks and is often found to be technically easier.

Loss of resistance to air or saline

The loss-of-resistance (LOR) technique to identify the epidural space utilizes either air or saline. It has been suggested that LOR to air may lead to a higher incidence of patchy blocks by introducing pockets of air and therefore not allowing optimal spread of local anaesthetic. Beilin et al.[21] conducted a prospective randomized study comparing 2 mL of air versus 2 mL of saline for a LOR technique. They found that the LOR to air group had higher pain scores overall and were more likely to need supplemental medication than the saline group. Another study evaluating nearly 3000 patients that allowed experienced anaesthetists to use the technique they were most comfortable with, also found that LOR to air was associated with more recurrent breakthrough pain than LOR to saline.[22] These findings were confirmed in other studies.[23,24] In contrast, others believe that LOR with saline dilutes the local anaesthetic in the epidural space and may lead to a less potent local anaesthetic effect.[25] Some providers inject large amounts of saline to distend the epidural space prior to catheter insertion, as this technique may reduce the risk of epidural vein cannulation.[19] Also, Segal and colleagues[26] found no significant difference between LOR to air versus saline in a retrospective study, in which operators used their preferred technique. They suggested that success rates are better when anaesthetists use the technique they are most comfortable with. Nevertheless, the majority of evidence suggests improved quality of epidural analgesia when a LOR technique with saline is used instead of air.

Conventional epidural technique versus combined spinal–epidural technique

Several retrospective studies have found that the incidence of failure of catheters, inserted as part of a combined spinal–epidural (CSE) technique, was significantly lower than that of catheters inserted with a conventional epidural technique.[4,27] In a retrospective analysis of 19,253 deliveries, Pan and colleagues[27] found that CSE was associated with a significantly lower failure rate than epidural (10% versus 14%), with failure defined as inadequate analgesia or no sensory block after adequate dosing at any time after initial placement, inadvertent dural puncture, intravenous epidural catheter, or any other situation requiring replacement of the epidural catheter. Another recent randomized controlled study comparing epidural analgesia and CSE analgesia for labour found that patients in the CSE group reported faster onset and better analgesia during the first stage of labour. Also, the need for epidural top-up boluses during the course of labour was significantly less in the CSE group than in the conventional epidural group.[28] Several aspects of the CSE technique could contribute to the improved subsequent functioning of the epidural catheter. For example, more accurate midline placing of the epidural catheter in the posterior epidural space, after confirmation provided by cerebrospinal fluid flow during the spinal component, and/or presence of a dural hole, which may increase subarachnoid transfer of epidurally administered medications. Cappiello and colleagues[29] demonstrated that performing a CSE with a 25 G spinal needle without injecting spinal medication, that is, 'dural puncture epidural' (DPE) is associated with faster onset, improved sacral spread, and less unilateral blocks when compared to the traditional epidural technique. However, Thomas et al.[30] did not find a benefit of DPE over conventional epidural analgesia, when they used a 27 G spinal needle.

A Cochrane review of 27 trials involving 3274 women, comparing traditional dose epidural, low-dose epidural, and CSE techniques, found little difference between low-dose epidural and CSE in terms of the maternal satisfaction, mobility in labour, headaches, caesarean delivery, or fetal adverse effects. However, CSEs had a slightly faster onset of effective pain relief, although more women had pruritus compared to low-dose epidurals.[31]

Nevertheless, the NAP 3 study of the Royal College of Anaesthetists raised some concerns about the safety of CSE. It was found to have a relatively high incidence of complications. While CSE represented less than 6% of all central neuraxial blocks performed in this study, they were associated with 13–14% of major complications, which is unexpected and should be borne in mind.[32]

Epidural catheter

Multi-orifice versus single-orifice catheters

It has been suggested that epidural catheter characteristics, such as number of ports, affects the quality of the epidural block. However, studies directly comparing these two types of epidural catheters yield conflicting results. Single-holed, open-ended (uniport) and three-holed, closed-ended (multiport) catheters are commonly used. Many studies have found that multiport catheters have been associated with reduced incidence of inadequate analgesia, since local anaesthetic distribution may be enhanced.[33–37] For example, Michael et al.[36] found a 33% incidence of unsatisfactory block with single-orifice catheters compared to only 14% when multi-orifice catheters were used. Segal and colleagues[35] evaluated 872 parturients undergoing epidural analgesia for labour and found that multi-hole catheters were associated with fewer incomplete blocks (unilateral block or unblocked segments) and a reduced need for catheter replacement. Collier and Gatt[37] also found that multi-orifice catheters were associated with superior blocks. However, a more recent study comparing an open-ended flexible, soft uniport catheter with a stiffer multiport catheter in 2612 patients found a decreased incidence of paraesthesias and intravascular placements when soft uniport catheters were used, without a reduction in the quality of analgesia.[38]

Length of the catheter into the epidural space

Several studies have looked at the optimal distance that epidural catheters should be threaded into the epidural space. Catheters that are inserted shorter distances (2–5 cm) are less likely to result in unilateral sensory analgesia, but are more likely to be dislodged. However, catheters inserted longer distances (7–8 cm) into the epidural space are more likely to be intravascular or result in unilateral blocks.[39,40] Bromage[41] recommended inserting single-orifice catheters 3–4 cm into the epidural space. For multi-orifice catheters, however, Beilin and colleagues[40] recommended an optimal distance of 5 cm. Conversely, D'Angelo et al.[39] suggested that the length of epidural catheter insertion should vary with the anticipated duration and mode of delivery. They recommended 2 cm when rapid labour is anticipated and 6 cm when prolonged labour or caesarean delivery is likely. The practicalities of varying the insertion length of the epidural catheter during different stages of labour, however, are unknown.

Table 19.2 Neuraxial technique-related risk factors

Patient position	Lateral position may decrease incidence of intravenous cannulation
Loss of resistance (LOR)	LOR to air compared to saline may be associated with higher incidence of patchy blocks and more breakthrough pain in labour
Combined spinal–epidural (CSE) vs conventional epidural	CSE has been associated with lower epidural catheter failure rates; however, there is no difference in maternal satisfaction
Epidural catheter	Multi-orifice catheters have been associated with superior blocks compared to single-orifice catheters. However, no reduction in quality of analgesia with newer soft uniport catheters The suggested optimal length in the epidural space is 3–5 cm

Drugs

Local anaesthetics

Choice

One of the most commonly used local anaesthetics for labour neuraxial analgesia is bupivacaine, because of its long duration of action and limited placental transfer. Bupivacaine is an amide local anaesthetic that exists as a racemic mixture of both the laevorotatory and dextrorotatory enantiomers. Some of the concerns with bupivacaine, such as cardiotoxicity and neurotoxicity, especially at higher concentrations, have been mainly attributed to the dextrorotatory form. Therefore two new long-acting local anaesthetics have been developed: ropivacaine and levobupivacaine. These are both pure laevorotatory forms and may therefore have some advantages over bupivacaine. Several studies have compared bupivacaine, ropivacaine, and levobupivacaine in terms of central nervous system and cardiac toxicity. In animal models, the convulsive doses of ropivacaine and levobupivacaine were found to be 1.5–2.5 times larger than for bupivacaine.[42–44] Ropivacaine has also been shown to produce fewer myocardial depression changes and conduction changes than bupivacaine.[45] Several animal studies demonstrated that the fatal dose was larger for ropivacaine than for bupivacaine.[42,46] Also, most animal studies found that it is easier to resuscitate an animal from a toxic dose of ropivacaine than from bupivacaine.[47,48]

However, to correctly interpret systemic toxicity data, the relative potency of the different drugs should be taken into account. The median effective concentration (EC_{50}) or minimal local anaesthetic concentration (MLAC) can be used to determine different potencies of local anaesthetics (see Chapter 16). Using this method, the analgesic potency of ropivacaine was found to be approximately 60% that of bupivacaine.[50,51] However, some argue that the complete dose–response curve of both drugs is unknown, and it is possible that the EC_{95} (effective concentration for 95% of the population) is not that different, despite the fact that the EC_{50} of bupivacaine is less than that of ropivacaine.

Several studies have compared the analgesic efficacy of epidural infusions of levobupivacaine, bupivacaine, and ropivacaine in labour. No significant differences were found in obstetric outcomes, nor were there any differences in overall maternal satisfaction or need for supplemental boluses of local anaesthetic.[52–55]

Concentration

Different concentrations of local anaesthetic solutions with or without adjuvants have been tested. The concentration of the epidural mixture has been trending downwards in attempts to reduce toxicity and side effects such as hypotension and motor blockade. Typically, bupivacaine concentrations of maintenance bupivacaine/opioid solutions range from 0.05% to 0.125%. Chestnut and colleagues[56] conducted a study comparing bupivacaine 0.125% with bupivacaine 0.0625% with fentanyl 2 mcg/mL and found no significant difference in pain scores throughout labour. Furthermore, the higher concentration of bupivacaine was associated with significantly more motor blockade. Similarly, Hess et al.[57], compared two concentrations of bupivacaine, 0.125% and 0.0625%, both with fentanyl 2 mcg/mL, administered at 8–12 mL/h, and bupivacaine 0.04% with fentanyl 1.7 mcg/mL and epinephrine 1.7 mcg/mL, administered at 15 mL/h. They found that there were more interventions for breakthrough pain in the two low-concentration groups, but more interventions for hypotension and motor blockade in the high-concentration group. A meta-analysis of studies comparing low concentrations versus high concentrations of local anaesthetic for labour found that high concentrations (bupivacaine > 0.1% or ropivacaine > 0.17%) were associated with more assisted vaginal deliveries, possibly because of the increased motor blockade. It is therefore recommended to use lower concentrations of local anaesthetic.[58] Capogna et al.[50] estimated MLACs of epidural bupivacaine and ropivacaine for women in the first stage of labour. For bupivacaine, the MLAC was 0.093% and for ropivacaine 0.156%. Another study comparing the relative potencies of levobupivacaine with racemic bupivacaine reported the MLAC of racemic bupivacaine to be 0.081% and of levobupivacaine to be 0.083%.[59]

Mode of epidural drug delivery

The mode of delivery of local anaesthetic solutions has also been shown to affect the quality of epidural analgesia for labour. Several studies have found that administration of maintenance epidural solutions through mandatory intermittent boluses rather than continuous infusions, results in lower local anaesthetic consumption, decreased need for manual top-up boluses by the anaesthetist, and higher patient satisfaction (see Chapter 15).[60–65] Furthermore, patient-controlled epidural analgesia (PCEA) allows the patient to adjust the dose of epidural medication according to individual needs and as labour progresses. A meta-analysis of randomized controlled trials that compared PCEA versus continuous infusion for labour analgesia demonstrated that patients who receive PCEA experience less breakthrough pain requiring anaesthetic intervention, need lower total doses of local anaesthetic, and have less motor block than those patients receiving a continuous epidural infusion.[66] However, the optimal PCEA regimen is still a subject of some debate. Initial studies favoured PCEA regimens without a continuous background infusion.[67,68] However, Ferrante et al.[69] investigated whether a continuous background infusion in addition to patient-controlled demand boluses is advantageous when compared to PCEA without continuous background infusion. The authors found that a continuous background infusion of 33% of the maximal hourly demand dose in addition to PCEA resulted in a decreased need for physician-administered supplemental local anaesthetic when compared to PCEA alone or PCEA with lower rates of background continuous infusion. A systematic review of studies comparing PCEA with continuous-infusion techniques for labour concluded that PCEA is associated with fewer patients requiring unscheduled clinician top-ups and lower dose requirements for local anaesthetics. In addition, fewer patients experience motor block.[70]

Opioids

Traditionally, epidural labour analgesia was most often maintained with local anaesthetic alone, but most anaesthetists currently use a combination of a low-dose, long-acting amide-type local anaesthetic with a lipid-soluble opioid. The addition of small doses of opioids to local anaesthetics has been shown to be associated with a local anaesthetic-sparing effect. Chestnut and colleagues[56] demonstrated that the combination of 2 mcg/mL of fentanyl with 0.0625% bupivacaine for epidural analgesia provided equivalent analgesia to 0.125% plain bupivacaine, with significantly less motor block in the fentanyl-bupivacaine group. Furthermore, the hourly and total doses of local anaesthetic were found to be significantly less when opioids were combined with local anaesthetic versus local anaesthetic alone. In addition, epidural analgesia is frequently associated with sacral sparing, resulting in persistent perineal pain or pressure. In such cases, the epidural administration of a lipid-soluble opioid (e.g. 50–100 mcg fentanyl) can often improve analgesia. Adding an opioid can also be particularly helpful when the patient is experiencing back pain because the fetus is in the occiput posterior position.[71] Of the lipid-soluble opioids, fentanyl is found more often in umbilical artery blood samples when compared to sufentanil, but this does not seem to be of clinical significance, as neonatal outcomes are good after maintenance epidural analgesia with either drug.[72]

Prevention of breakthrough pain

There is no better example of the saying 'Prevention is better than cure' than in the delivery suite, with respect to epidurals for analgesia during labour. The identification of risk factors for breakthrough pain during labour analgesia may prompt the anaesthetic provider to adjust his/her anaesthetic plan, for example, choice of CSE technique in high-risk patients or increasing the concentration of local anaesthetic in patients with rapidly progressing labours. Despite this, it is inevitable that some epidural catheters will fail to provide adequate analgesia. Therefore, it is important to discuss the risk for failed anaesthesia and the potential need to place a second epidural catheter with the patient during the pre-anaesthetic evaluation, before placement of the first epidural catheter.

In addition, after placement of an epidural catheter, regular epidural evaluation to identify problems is necessary, not only in terms of providing adequate maternal analgesia and hence satisfaction, but also in anticipation of using the epidural catheter for other potential obstetric interventions. A poorly functioning catheter will not only cause maternal dissatisfaction, but may also make another anaesthetic procedure necessary in potentially stressful circumstances. Regular epidural review will also improve communication with the obstetric and midwifery team and highlight important details which may alter epidural management, for example, failure to progress in labour or the presence of a non-reassuring fetal heart rate tracing, both of which need a good working epidural in preparation for potential surgical interventions and so lowering the threshold for replacing a less than ideal epidural catheter.

Management of breakthrough pain during neuraxial labour analgesia

When breakthrough pain occurs, despite preventative efforts, it should be managed promptly and aggressively, with the goal to restore adequate analgesia within a maximum of 60 minutes (Figure 19.1).

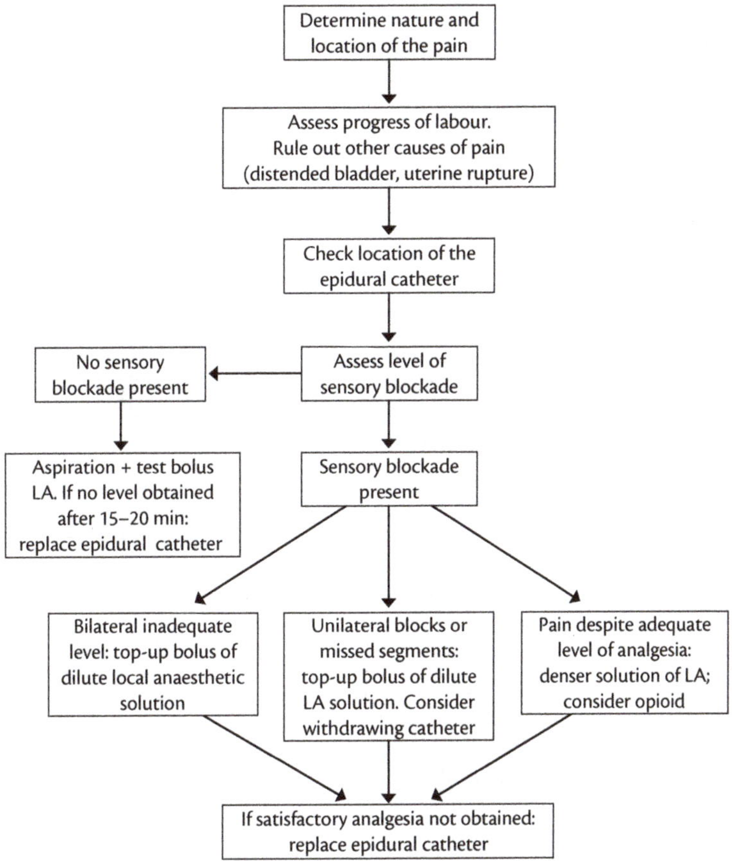

Figure 19.1 Management algorithm for breakthrough pain during neuraxial labour analgesia.

Firstly, the nature and location of the pain should be determined and the progress of labour evaluated, including the cervical dilation and rate of progression, as this may affect pain intensity which could increase local anaesthetic requirements. Although rare, other underlying obstetric causes that could lead to breakthrough pain, such as uterine rupture or placental abruption, should be ruled out. Bladder distension can also be a cause of breakthrough pain.

Secondly, the location of the epidural catheter should be examined to make sure that it still remains in the epidural space.

Subsequently, the extent of neural blockade can be assessed by loss of sensation to cold, sharp pinprick, or light touch. There has been some discussion as to which modality is preferred. In general, block to cold sensation is usually at a higher level than to sharp pinprick[73] and block to light touch is usually lower than the block to both pinprick and cold.[74] Adequate analgesia for the first stage of labour requires blockade of the T10–L1 segments. Sacral blockade is needed for the second stage of labour.

During testing, one of the following situations can be encountered:

1. *No sensory blockade:* the complete absence of sensory block, despite appropriate dosing, usually means that the epidural catheter is not in the epidural space. However, intravascular migration is also possible. After careful aspiration, a test dose can be administered. If there is no sensory block, the epidural catheter should be replaced.
2. *Bilateral inadequate level of analgesia:* if the extent of sensory blockade is inadequate to cover the required segments, a top-up bolus of a dilute local anaesthetic solution (e.g. bupivacaine 0.0625–0.125%) should be given. Larger volumes (10–15 mL) of a dilute local anaesthetic solution are often preferred in this case, over more concentrated solutions, as this allows for a better spread of analgesia.
3. *Unilateral blocks or missed segments:* asymmetric blocks or patchy blocks are usually caused by uneven spread of drug solutions. This can be due to unfavourable positioning of the epidural catheter tip or due to the presence of an anatomic barrier, such as fibrous septa, limiting the free flow of local anaesthetic solution. Some reports have suggested the presence of a dorsal median connective tissue band as a possible cause of unilateral blocks, although this is generally thought to be rare and has been attributed to an artefact of how the epidural space was studied.[75] A paramedian position for an epidural catheter is thought to be a more common cause of asymmetric block than anatomic barriers to solution spread. Hogan[76] evaluated epidural catheter tip positions by computed tomography in patients with normal functioning epidural analgesia and found that catheter tips were often situated lateral to the dura close to the intervertebral foramen. As mentioned previously (see 'Length of the Catheter into the Epidural Space', some studies have suggested that threading the catheter no more than 5 cm in the epidural space leads to fewer one-sided blocks, perhaps because these catheters are less likely to be sited laterally or even worse, exit the epidural space along the course of a nerve root.[18,40]

Different management strategies have been proposed for unilateral or patchy blocks. Some authors advocate pulling the epidural catheter 1–2 cm before administering a bolus of local anaesthetic.[39] However, Beilin and colleagues[77] performed a study in which they randomly assigned patients with breakthrough pain to receive either 5 mL of bupivacaine 0.25% after withdrawing the epidural catheter 1 cm or without withdrawal of the epidural catheter. In both groups about 75% of women were successfully treated with this first intervention. For the 25% of women that were not comfortable 15 minutes after this first intervention, a cross-over was performed, in which the catheter was withdrawn 1 cm and an additional 5 mL of 0.25% bupivacaine was administered to the initial local-anaesthetic-only group, whereas 5 mL 0.25% bupivacaine was given to the initial catheter manipulation group, without further withdrawal of the epidural catheter. All patients were comfortable after the second intervention. While this study does not reject the benefits of catheter withdrawal in certain patients, it does suggest that most women can be effectively treated with the administration of a bolus of local anaesthetic without withdrawal of the epidural catheter. Indeed, the injection of a large volume of local anaesthetic (e.g. 10 mL of bupivacaine 0.0625–0.125%) can often overcome a variety of catheter positions and non-uniform spread of local anaesthetic solution in the epidural space.[71,76] If analgesia cannot be rescued, however, the epidural catheter should be replaced.

The importance of maternal position during labour epidural analgesia is subject to some debate. While several studies have suggested that the lateral position is associated with a faster onset and increased spread and duration of anaesthesia on the dependent side compared to the upper side during the initial bolus injection, most authors think that this is of only minor clinical significance.[71,78,79] Others, however, advocate a modified supine position as this may result in more equal spread of local anaesthetic and better pain relief.[80]

4. *Breakthrough pain despite an adequate extent of sensory blockade:* if the patient experiences breakthrough pain despite a bilateral adequate level of analgesia (T10–L1), a more concentrated solution of local anaesthetic may be needed. Labour may be advancing quicker than expected and local anaesthetic requirements may be rapidly increasing. Furthermore, the patient may be experiencing dysfunctional labour or abnormal fetal presentation, both of which are associated with increased pain.[6,7,81] Also, the administration of a lipid-soluble opioid (e.g. 50–100 mcg fentanyl) can often improve analgesia, particularly if the patient is experiencing back pain because the fetus is in the occiput posterior position, or in case of persistent perineal pain or pressure.[71] Clonidine is another drug which has been used in such circumstances, although less commonly than fentanyl.

While the above-mentioned measures will often succeed in restoring adequate analgesia it is important to assess the results in a timely fashion. If satisfactory analgesia is not obtained, the epidural catheter should be replaced.

If, despite epidural replacement, the block is still less than ideal, a CSE technique should be performed. This will result in rapid analgesia as the intrathecal route is more reliable than the epidural one and is important as, by now, the patient would have been in pain for several hours during all the previous epidural manoeuvres.

References

1. Tveit TO, Seiler S, Halvorsen A, Rosland JH. Labour analgesia: a randomised, controlled trial comparing intravenous remifentanil and epidural analgesia with ropivacaine and fentanyl. *Eur J Anaesthesiol* 2012; 29:129–36.
2. Klomp T, van Poppel M, Jones L, Lazet J, Di Nisio M, Lagro-Janssen AL. Inhaled analgesia for pain management in labour. *Cochrane Database Syst Rev* 2012; 9:CD009351.
3. Paech MJ, Godkin R, Webster S. Complications of obstetric epidural analgesia and anaesthesia: a prospective analysis of 10,995 cases. *Int J Obstet Anesth* 1998; 7:5–11.
4. Eappen S, Blinn A, Segal S. Incidence of epidural catheter replacement in parturients: a retrospective chart review. *Int J Obstet Anesth* 1998; 7:220–5.
5. Agaram R, Douglas MJ, McTaggart RA, Gunka V. Inadequate pain relief with labor epidurals: a multivariate analysis of associated factors. *Int J Obstet Anesth* 2009; 18:10–14.
6. Hess PE, Pratt SD, Lucas TP, *et al.* Predictors of breakthrough pain during labor epidural analgesia. *Anesth Analg* 2001; 93:414–18.
7. Le Coq G, Ducot B, Benhamou D. Risk factors of inadequate pain relief during epidural analgesia for labour and delivery. *Can J Anaesth* 1998; 45:719–23.
8. Panni MK, Segal S. Local anesthetic requirements are greater in dystocia than in normal labor. *Anesthesiology* 2003; 98:957–63.
9. Capogna G, Celleno D, Lyons G, Columb M, Fusco P. Minimum local analgesic concentration of extradural bupivacaine increases with progression of labour. *Br J Anaesth* 1998; 80:11–13.
10. Hood DD, Dewan DM. Anesthetic and obstetric outcome in morbidly obese parturients. *Anesthesiology* 1993; 79:1210–18.
11. Melzack R, Kinch R, Dobkin P, Lebrun M, Taenzer P. Severity of labour pain: influence of physical as well as psychologic variables. *Can Med Assoc J* 1984; 130:579–84.
12. Faheem M, Sarwar N. Sliding of the skin over subcutaneous tissue is another important factor in epidural catheter migration. *Can J Anaesth* 2002; 49:634.
13. Iwama H, Katayama T. Back skin movement also causes 'walking' epidural catheter. *J Clin Anesth* 1999; 11:140–1.
14. Hamilton CL, Riley ET, Cohen SE. Changes in the position of epidural catheters associated with patient movement. *Anesthesiology* 1997; 86:778–84; discussion 29A.
15. Soens MA, Birnbach DJ, Ranasinghe JS, van Zundert A. Obstetric anesthesia for the obese and morbidly obese patient: an ounce of prevention is worth more than a pound of treatment. *Acta Anaesthesiol Scand* 2008; 52:6–19.
16. Benzon HT, Braunschweig R, Molloy RE. Delayed onset of epidural anesthesia in patients with back pain. *Anesth Analg* 1981; 60:874–7.
17. Sharrock NE, Urquhart B, Mineo R. Extradural anaesthesia in patients with previous lumbar spine surgery. *Br J Anaesth* 1990; 65:237–9.
18. Arendt K, Segal S. Why epidurals do not always work. *Rev Obstet Gynecol* 2008; 1:49–55.
19. Mhyre JM, Greenfield ML, Tsen LC, Polley LS. A systematic review of randomized controlled trials that evaluate strategies to avoid epidural vein cannulation during obstetric epidural catheter placement. *Anesth Analg* 2009; 108:1232–42.
20. Stone PA, Kilpatrick AW, Thorburn J. Posture and epidural catheter insertion. The relationship between skill, experience and maternal posture on the outcome of epidural catheter insertion. *Anaesthesia* 1990; 45:920–3.
21. Beilin Y, Arnold I, Telfeyan C, Bernstein HH, Hossain S. Quality of analgesia when air versus saline is used for identification of the epidural space in the parturient. *Reg Anesth Pain Med* 2000; 25:596–9.

22. Leo S, Lim Y, Sia AT. Analgesic efficacy using loss of resistance to air vs. saline in combined spinal epidural technique for labour analgesia. *Anaesth Intensive Care* 2008; 36:701–6.
23. Evron S, Sessler D, Sadan O, Boaz M, Glezerman M, Ezri T. Identification of the epidural space: loss of resistance with air, lidocaine, or the combination of air and lidocaine. *Anesth Analg* 2004; 99:245–50.
24. Valentine SJ, Jarvis AP, Shutt LE. Comparative study of the effects of air or saline to identify the extradural space. *Br J Anaesth* 1991; 66:224–7.
25. Sanford CL 2nd, Rodriguez RE, Schmidt J, Austin PN. Evidence for using air or fluid when identifying the epidural space. *AANA J* 2013; 81:23–8.
26. Segal S, Arendt KW. A retrospective effectiveness study of loss of resistance to air or saline for identification of the epidural space. *Anesth Analg* 2010; 110:558–63.
27. Pan PH, Bogard TD, Owen MD. Incidence and characteristics of failures in obstetric neuraxial analgesia and anesthesia: a retrospective analysis of 19,259 deliveries. *Int J Obstet Anesth* 2004; 13:227–33.
28. Gambling D, Berkowitz J, Farrell TR, Pue A, Shay D. A randomized controlled comparison of epidural analgesia and combined spinal-epidural analgesia in a private practice setting: pain scores during first and second stages of labor and at delivery. *Anesth Analg* 2013; 116:636–43.
29. Cappiello E, O'Rourke N, Segal S, Tsen LC. A randomized trial of dural puncture epidural technique compared with the standard epidural technique for labor analgesia. *Anesth Analg* 2008; 107:1646–51.
30. Thomas JA, Pan PH, Harris LC, Owen MD, D'Angelo R. Dural puncture with a 27-gauge Whitacre needle as part of a combined spinal-epidural technique does not improve labor epidural catheter function. *Anesthesiology* 2005; 103:1046–51.
31. Simmons SW, Taghizadeh N, Dennis AT, Hughes D, Cyna AM. Combined spinal-epidural versus epidural analgesia in labour. *Cochrane Database Syst Rev* 2012; 10:CD003401.
32. Cook TM, Counsell D, Wildsmith JA, Royal College of Anaesthetists Third National Audit Project. Major complications of central neuraxial block: report on the Third National Audit Project of the Royal College of Anaesthetists. *Br J Anaesth* 2009; 102:179–90.
33. Dickson MA, Moores C, McClure JH. Comparison of single, end-holed and multi-orifice extradural catheters when used for continuous infusion of local anaesthetic during labour. *Br J Anaesth* 1997; 79:297–300.
34. D'Angelo R, Foss ML, Livesay CH. A comparison of multiport and uniport epidural catheters in laboring patients. *Anesth Analg* 1997; 84:1276–9.
35. Segal S, Eappen S, Datta S. Superiority of multi-orifice over single-orifice epidural catheters for labor analgesia and cesarean delivery. *J Clin Anesth* 1997; 9:109–12.
36. Michael S, Richmond MN, Birks RJ. A comparison between open-end (single hole) and closed-end (three lateral holes) epidural catheters. Complications and quality of sensory blockade. *Anaesthesia* 1989; 44:578–80.
37. Collier CB, Gatt SP. Epidural catheters for obstetrics. Terminal hole or lateral eyes? *Reg Anesth* 1994; 19:378–85.
38. Jaime F, Mandell GL, Vallejo MC, Ramanathan S. Uniport soft-tip, open-ended catheters versus multiport firm-tipped close-ended catheters for epidural labor analgesia: a quality assurance study. *J Clin Anesth* 2000; 12:89–93.
39. D'Angelo R, Berkebile BL, Gerancher JC. Prospective examination of epidural catheter insertion. *Anesthesiology* 1996; 84:88–93.
40. Beilin Y, Bernstein HH, Zucker-Pinchoff B. The optimal distance that a multiorifice epidural catheter should be threaded into the epidural space. *Anesth Analg* 1995; 81:301–4.
41. Bromage PR. Continuous epidural anesthesia. In Bromage PR (ed) *Epidural Analgesia*. Philadelphia, PA: WB Saunders; 1978:215–57.
42. Santos AC, Arthur GR, Wlody D, De Armas P, Morishima HO, Finster M. Comparative systemic toxicity of ropivacaine and bupivacaine in nonpregnant and pregnant ewes. *Anesthesiology* 1995; 82:734–40; discussion 27A.
43. Dony P, Dewinde V, Vanderick B, *et al.* The comparative toxicity of ropivacaine and bupivacaine at equipotent doses in rats. *Anesth Analg* 2000; 91:1489–92.
44. Groban L. Central nervous system and cardiac effects from long-acting amide local anesthetic toxicity in the intact animal model. *Reg Anesth Pain Med* 2003; 28:3–11.
45. Moller R, Covino BG. Cardiac electrophysiologic properties of bupivacaine and lidocaine compared with those of ropivacaine, a new amide local anesthetic. *Anesthesiology* 1990; 72:322–9.
46. Feldman HS, Arthur GR, Covino BG. Comparative systemic toxicity of convulsant and supraconvulsant doses of intravenous ropivacaine, bupivacaine, and lidocaine in the conscious dog. *Anesth Analg* 1989; 69:794–801.
47. Groban L, Deal DD, Vernon JC, James RL, Butterworth J. Cardiac resuscitation after incremental overdosage with lidocaine, bupivacaine, levobupivacaine, and ropivacaine in anesthetized dogs. *Anesth Analg* 2001; 92:37–43.
48. Ohmura S, Kawada M, Ohta T, Yamamoto K, Kobayashi T. Systemic toxicity and resuscitation in bupivacaine-, levobupivacaine-, or ropivacaine-infused rats. *Anesth Analg* 2001; 93:743–8.
49. Dixon WJ, Massey FJ. *Introduction to Statistical Analysis* (4th ed). New York: McGraw Hill, 1983.
50. Capogna G, Celleno D, Fusco P, Lyons G, Columb M. Relative potencies of bupivacaine and ropivacaine for analgesia in labour. *Br J Anaesth* 1999; 82:371–3.
51. Polley LS, Columb MO, Naughton NN, Wagner DS, van de Ven CJ. Relative analgesic potencies of ropivacaine and bupivacaine for epidural analgesia in labor: implications for therapeutic indexes. *Anesthesiology* 1999; 90:944–50.
52. Halpern SH, Breen TW, Campbell DC, *et al.* A multicenter, randomized, controlled trial comparing bupivacaine with ropivacaine for labor analgesia. *Anesthesiology* 2003; 98:1431–5.
53. Atienzar MC, Palanca JM, Torres F, Borras R, Gil S, Esteve I. A randomized comparison of levobupivacaine, bupivacaine and ropivacaine with fentanyl, for labor analgesia. *Int J Obstet Anesth* 2008; 17:106–11.
54. Lee BB, Ngan Kee WD, Ng FF, Lau TK, Wong EL. Epidural infusions of ropivacaine and bupivacaine for labor analgesia: a randomized, double-blind study of obstetric outcome. *Anesth Analg* 2004; 98:1145–52.
55. Beilin Y, Guinn NR, Bernstein HH, Zahn J, Hossain S, Bodian CA. Local anesthetics and mode of delivery: bupivacaine versus ropivacaine versus levobupivacaine. *Anesth Analg* 2007; 105:756–63.
56. Chestnut DH, Owen CL, Bates JN, Ostman LG, Choi WW, Geiger MW. Continuous infusion epidural analgesia during labor: a randomized, double-blind comparison of 0.0625% bupivacaine/0.0002% fentanyl versus 0.125% bupivacaine. *Anesthesiology* 1988; 68:754–9.
57. Hess PE, Pratt SD, Oriol NE. An analysis of the need for anesthetic interventions with differing concentrations of labor epidural bupivacaine: an observational study. *Int J Obstet Anesth* 2006; 15:195–200.
58. Sultan P, Murphy C, Halpern S, Carvalho B. The effect of low concentrations versus high concentrations of local anesthetics for labour analgesia on obstetric and anesthetic outcomes: a meta-analysis. *Can J Anaesth* 2013; 60:840–54.
59. Lyons G, Columb M, Wilson RC, Johnson RV. Epidural pain relief in labour: potencies of levobupivacaine and racemic bupivacaine. *Br J Anaesth* 1998; 81:899–901.
60. Wong CA, Ratliff JT, Sullivan JT, Scavone BM, Toledo P, McCarthy RJ. A randomized comparison of programmed intermittent epidural bolus with continuous epidural infusion for labor analgesia. *Anesth Analg* 2006; 102:904–9.
61. Chua SM, Sia AT. Automated intermittent epidural boluses improve analgesia induced by intrathecal fentanyl during labour. *Can J Anaesth* 2004; 51:581–5.
62. Fettes PD, Moore CS, Whiteside JB, McLeod GA, Wildsmith JA. Intermittent vs continuous administration of epidural ropivacaine

with fentanyl for analgesia during labour. *Br J Anaesth* 2006; 97:359–64.

63. Sia AT, Lim Y, Ocampo C. A comparison of a basal infusion with automated mandatory boluses in parturient-controlled epidural analgesia during labor. *Anesth Analg* 2007; 104:673–8.
64. Lim Y, Sia AT, Ocampo C. Automated regular boluses for epidural analgesia: a comparison with continuous infusion. *Int J Obstet Anesth* 2005; 14:305–9.
65. Leo S, Ocampo CE, Lim Y, Sia AT. A randomized comparison of automated intermittent mandatory boluses with a basal infusion in combination with patient-controlled epidural analgesia for labor and delivery. *Int J Obstet Anesth* 2010; 19:357–64.
66. van der Vyver M, Halpern S, Joseph G. Patient-controlled epidural analgesia versus continuous infusion for labour analgesia: a meta-analysis. *Br J Anaesth* 2002; 89:459–65.
67. Boselli E, Debon R, Cimino Y, Rimmele T, Allaouchiche B, Chassard D. Background infusion is not beneficial during labor patient-controlled analgesia with 0.1% ropivacaine plus 0.5 microg/ml sufentanil. *Anesthesiology* 2004; 100:968–72.
68. Petry J, Vercauteren M, Van Mol I, Van Houwe P, Adriaensen HA. Epidural PCA with bupivacaine 0.125%, sufentanil 0.75 microgram and epinephrine 1/800.000 for labor analgesia: is a background infusion beneficial? *Acta Anaesthesiol Belg* 2000; 51:163–6.
69. Ferrante FM, Rosinia FA, Gordon C, Datta S. The role of continuous background infusions in patient-controlled epidural analgesia for labor and delivery. *Anesth Analg* 1994; 79:80–4.
70. Halpern S. Recent advances in patient-controlled epidural analgesia for labour. *Curr Opin Anaesthesiol* 2005; 18:247–51.
71. Wong CA. Epidural and spinal analgesia/anesthesia for labor and vaginal delivery. In Chestnut DH, Wong CA, Tsen LC, *et al.* (eds) *Chestnut's Obstetric Anesthesia: Principles and Practice* (5th ed). Philadelphia, PA: Elsevier; 2014:457–517.
72. Loftus JR, Hill H, Cohen SE. Placental transfer and neonatal effects of epidural sufentanil and fentanyl administered with bupivacaine during labor. *Anesthesiology* 1995; 83:300–8.
73. Camorcia M, Capogna G. Sensory assessment of epidural block for Caesarean section: a systematic comparison of pinprick, cold and touch sensation. *Eur J Anaesthesiol* 2006; 23:611–17.
74. Russell IF. A comparison of cold, pinprick and touch for assessing the level of spinal block at caesarean section. *Int J Obstet Anesth* 2004; 13:146–52.
75. Hogan QH. Lumbar epidural anatomy. A new look by cryomicrotome section. *Anesthesiology* 1991; 75:767–75.
76. Hogan Q. Epidural catheter tip position and distribution of injectate evaluated by computed tomography. *Anesthesiology* 1999; 90:964–70.
77. Beilin Y, Zahn J, Bernstein HH, Zucker-Pinchoff B, Zenzen WJ, Andres LA. Treatment of incomplete analgesia after placement of an epidural catheter and administration of local anesthetic for women in labor. *Anesthesiology* 1998; 88:1502–6.
78. Apostolou GA, Zarmakoupis PK, Mastrokostopoulos GT. Spread of epidural anesthesia and the lateral position. *Anesth Analg* 1981; 60:584–6.
79. Husemeyer RP, White DC. Lumbar extradural injection pressures in pregnant women. An investigation of relationships between rate of infection, injection pressures and extent of analgesia. *Br J Anaesth* 1980; 52:55–60.
80. Soetens FM, Meeuwis HC, Van der Donck AG, De Vel MA, Schijven MP, Van Zundert AA. Influence of maternal position during epidural labor analgesia. *Int J Obstet Anesth* 2003; 12:98–101.
81. Temple JL, Bradshaw HB, Wood E, Berkley KJ. Effects of hypogastric neurectomy on escape responses to uterine distention in the rat. *Pain* 1999; Suppl 6:S13–20.

PART 6

Anaesthesia for caesarean delivery

CHAPTER 20

Neuraxial anaesthesia for caesarean delivery

Sarah L. Armstrong, Michelle Walters, Katherine Cheesman, and Geraldine O'Sullivan†

Introduction

Caesarean delivery (CD) rates continue to increase worldwide. The reasons for this trend are multifactorial and include maternal, obstetric, fetal, medicolegal, and social factors. Significant variation exists in practice between different countries. In 2009, the World Health Organization (WHO) reported that 47.4 of 100 live births in Brazil were born by CD, compared to only 14.3/100 in the Netherlands (Figure 20.1).[1]

There is also a significant variation in the CD rate at local levels. Maternity statistics from National Health Service (NHS) hospitals in England 2012–2013 report a national average CD rate of 25.5% (including both planned and emergency CD). During the same time frame, the rates from different regions within England varied from 15% to 35%.[2] Diverse local population characteristics and different thresholds for performing emergency CD may account for this.[3]

Planned CD (compared to emergency CD) accounts for approximately 40% of all CDs in England.[2] A large proportion of these are repeat CDs or CDs for fetal breech position. Factors contributing to the rising CD rate include an increase in multiple gestation secondary to assisted reproduction, advancing maternal age, maternal obesity, patient preferences, improved operative safety, and changing practice amongst professionals. Evidence-based practice, a culture of litigation, and a risk-averse society may have led to a decrease in planned vaginal breech deliveries and vaginal births after previous CD.[4,5] In addition, there is an increasing demand for 'maternal request' CD in the absence of any medical indications, a controversial topic that has recently been addressed in national guidelines.[6,7]

The rising CD rate has wider implications and complications. The financial cost to the healthcare provider is greater than after a vaginal delivery and the hospital stay tends to be longer.[7] Maternal complications such as infection, haemorrhage, and thrombosis may occur and in subsequent pregnancies there is an increased risk of abnormal placental implantation and uterine rupture.[3,7] Neonatal morbidity and mortality may be increased, for example, neonatal respiratory distress syndrome and admissions to the neonatal intensive care unit.[8]

The upsurge in CD caseload has increased the demands on obstetric, anaesthetic, and midwifery staff. The increasing complexity of these cases (e.g. raised body mass index (BMI), placenta praevia, and multiple gestation) requires regular senior medical input on the delivery suite.[9]

Classification of caesarean delivery

CDs are classified by the degree of urgency caused by the presence or absence of fetal or maternal compromise. The traditional simple classification of 'elective' or 'emergency' was unhelpful, as this did not highlight the range of urgencies within and this could potentially lead to communication problems and high levels of stress on the labour ward. In 2010, the Royal College of Obstetricians and Gynaecologists (RCOG) and the Royal College of Anaesthetists (RCoA) produced a 'Good Practice' guideline, with a recommendation to universally accept a classification based on Lucas et al.'s 4-point classification with the addition of the colour-coded continuum scale proposed by Dupis.[10–12] This classification helps to reinforce the idea of a clearly communicated 'continuum of risk', but also allows for clearly defined categories for the purpose of audit. It allows all providers to understand the urgency and can help to highlight specific cases that require immediate delivery (category 1).

The 'emergency' caesarean delivery: how urgent is 'urgent'?

The maximal safe time to delivery from fetal distress to fetal compromise is unknown; the '30-minute rule' that is often quoted is not based on clinical trials and originates from early animal studies.[13,14] More confusing is when to 'start' and 'stop the clock'. The Association of Anaesthetists of Great Britain and Ireland (AAGBI) and the Obstetric Anaesthetists' Association (OAA) have together stated that in emergency cases the time from informing the anaesthetist to the start of operative delivery should not exceed 30 minutes, whereas the RCOG starts the clock from the time the decision to proceed to CD is made and ending at delivery of the baby—the decision to delivery interval (DDI), again aiming to achieve delivery within 30 minutes.

How feasible is this time scale and how necessary is it? The UK National Sentinel Caesarean Section Audit measured CD rates and assessed the quality of care given to woman having emergency CDs in England and Wales and included 99% of births between 1 May and 31 July 2000. There were 17,780 singleton births in this

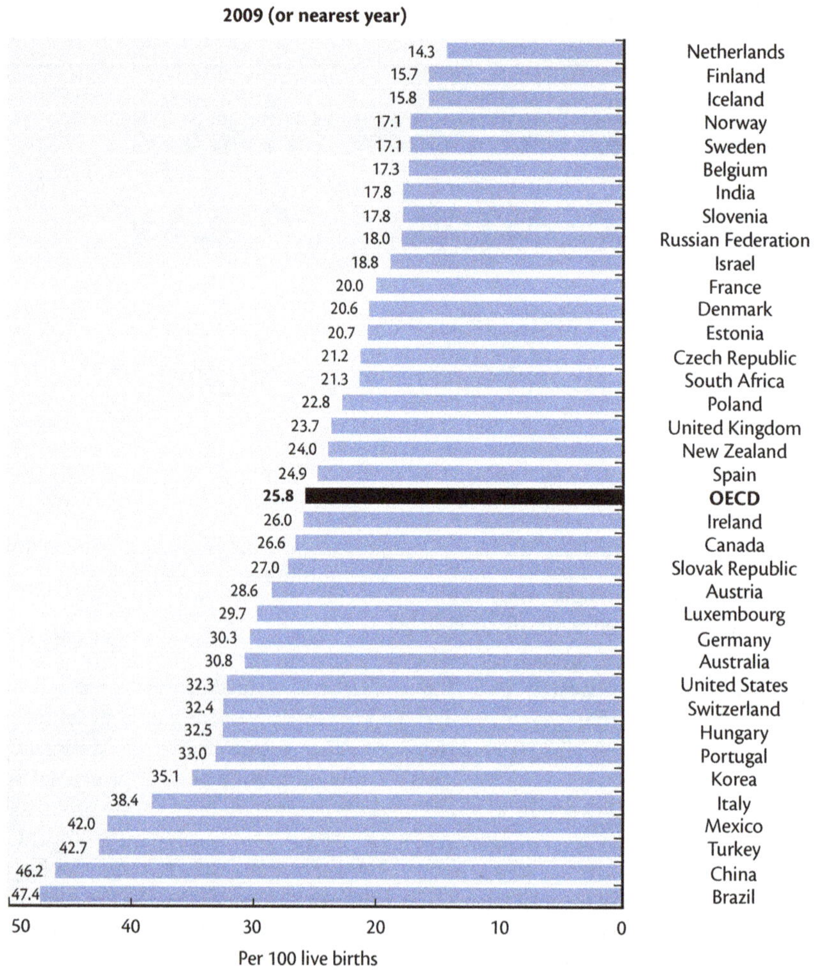

Figure 20.1 Caesarean deliveries worldwide per 100 live births in 2009. OECD, Organisation for Economic Co-operation and Development.
From OECD (2011). *Health at a Glance 2011: OECD Indicators*, OECD Publishing. http://dx.doi.org/10.1787/health_glance-2011-en

audit.[15] The perceived urgency was classified as category 1 for 26% (n = 4622), category 2 for 51.3% (n = 9122), and category 3 for 20.8% (n = 3689). Seven per cent of all CDs were delivered within 15 minutes and 22% within 30 minutes of the decision to deliver. Overall, 46% (n = 2137) of women with category 1 urgency, 16% (n = 1422), with category 2 and 9% (n = 330) with category 3 were delivered within 30 minutes.

Further analysis of this data looked at the association between DDI and neonatal outcomes (Apgar scores of <7 and <5 at 5 minutes and stillbirths).[16] The audit found that while prolonged DDIs of greater than 75 minutes were associated with poorer maternal and neonatal outcomes, reducing DDIs to less than 30 minutes neither improved nor worsened maternal or neonatal outcome (adjustment was made for clinical factors). While this research would suggest extending the clinically significant threshold from 30 to 75 minutes, the authors felt that to avoid complacency it would seem prudent to keep the '30-minute DDI' as a benchmark but add the '75 minute DDI' as an audit standard that all emergency CDs should occur within this time. In 2011, the National Institute for Health and Care Excellence (NICE) in the United Kingdom incorporated this into its CD guidelines recommending that 30 minutes be the audit standard DDI for category 1 CD and that 75 minutes the audit standard for category 2 CD. It was stressed that these times are for audit to examine the efficiency of the delivery team and not to judge performance in individual cases.[7] In certain situations such as a persistent bradycardia associated with a vasa praevia or ruptured uterus a delivery time of less than 10 minutes is warranted as well as appreciating that undue haste itself in surgery and anaesthesia can lead to maternal and neonatal harm.[17,18]

Human factors during emergency caesarean delivery

One must consider the processes required to achieve safe prompt CD and meet audit standards. Human factors such as communication and situational awareness need to be highlighted; 87% of CDs are predictable and early assessment by obstetrician or midwife can identify women who are at greater risk of CD who can then be referred promptly to the anaesthetic team (Box 20.1).[19] Anaesthetists should themselves be proactive by attending the delivery suite ward rounds and frequently reviewing high-risk mothers. High-risk women should be counselled that there might be a potential need for operative delivery and may be advised to have an early epidural for labour analgesia that could be extended to cover surgery.

Box 20.1 High-risk pregnancies that anaesthetists should be aware of

- Multiple pregnancy
- Breech/malpresentation
- Meconium-stained liquor
- Slow progress
- Oxytocin infusion in labour
- Fetal distress—pathological cardiotocograph (CTG)
- Intrauterine growth retardation (IUGR)
- Prematurity less than 36 weeks
- Antepartum haemorrhage (APH)
- Previous caesarean delivery (CD)
- Pregnancy-induced hypertension
- BMI higher than 35
- Diabetes
- Trial of labour after caesarean (TOLAC).

Practical issues such as the time it takes to move the woman to the operating theatre is critical; if more than 10 minutes elapses it is considerably less likely that the baby would be delivered within 30 or 40 minutes.[17] This rapid transfer can be distressing for women who may feel they have lost control of the situation as well as being concerned about their baby's well-being. This may be heightened by language barriers or cultural differences. Education and teamwork are vital.

Units should design guidelines that result in the shortest safely achievable DDI and it is the recommendation of the RCOG and AAGBI that formal drills be run for 'emergency CDs' with in-house teaching programmes to 'test' local channels of communication.

Advantages of neuraxial anaesthesia over general anaesthesia

Neuraxial anaesthesia is the safest and preferred method of anaesthesia for both planned and emergency CD and has significant advantages over general anaesthesia (see Chapter 22). In the United Kingdom, the RCoA recommends that 95% of planned CD and 85% of emergency CDs be performed under neuraxial anaesthesia.[20] Pregnant women are susceptible to increased morbidity and mortality from the risks of general anaesthesia including failed intubation, failed ventilation, awareness, hypoxia, and pulmonary aspiration of gastric contents.[21–23] The advantages of neuraxial anaesthesia are summarized in Box 20.2.

The Confidential Enquiry into Maternal Deaths in the United Kingdom in the triennium 2006–2008 identified two deaths directly caused by general anaesthesia for CD: one failed intubation and one aspiration on emergence.[24]

Patients in whom general anaesthesia had previously been preferable, for instance, high-risk parturients with significant cardiac co-morbidities, are increasingly being considered for regional techniques with modifications to improve haemodynamic stability.[20]

Box 20.2 Advantages of neuraxial anaesthesia for caesarean delivery

- Reduced risk of dental damage, failed intubation, failed ventilation, and hypoxia
- Reduced risk of pulmonary aspiration of gastric contents
- Removes risk of 'awareness' during general anaesthesia (see the 5th National Audit Project of the RCoA with the AAGBI—'NAP5: Accidental awareness during general anaesthesia in the United Kingdom'—results discussed in Chapter 22)
- Improved postoperative pain relief
- Reduced vomiting and postoperative ileus incidence
- Reduced thromboembolism incidence
- Ability to have birth partner present
- Alert mother and baby, improved bonding and breastfeeding
- Increased patient satisfaction.

For these reasons, current obstetric anaesthetic practice minimizes the use of general anaesthesia whenever possible. In the last decade, many European countries have completed national surveys examining their obstetric anaesthetic practice. In the south of England the use of neuraxial anaesthesia for planned CD has increased from 69% in 1992 to 95% in 2002. Spinal anaesthesia was used in 87% of cases and 1.3% of these converted to general anaesthesia during planned CD.[25] Similarly, in 2005, Benhamou reported that 99% of planned CDs in French obstetric units were carried out under neuraxial anaesthesia.[26] Likewise, both German and Polish surveys identify spinal anaesthesia as the most common anaesthetic technique for CD.[27,28]

Neuraxial anaesthesia for emergency CD has also increased although rates vary; of the 97,000 category 1 and 2 CDs that took place within NHS hospitals in the United Kingdom in 2011–2012, two-thirds were performed under neuraxial anaesthesia. For category 1 delivery, rates vary between 54% and 72%.[29,30] This may be due to a number of reasons: an increase in epidurals for labour, an increased incidence of epidurals particularly in high-risk patients, and greater awareness of the risks of airway complications during general anaesthesia. There have been improvements in understanding from the obstetric team regarding the benefits of a neuraxial technique and therefore reduced pressure on anaesthetists to rapidly perform a general anaesthetic.

Women without labour epidurals will need to be rapidly assessed and the use of general or neuraxial anaesthesia will depend on the urgency of the situation, although a general anaesthetic will usually provide the quickest onset of anaesthesia. Retrospective and simulation studies indicate that spinal anaesthesia is only marginally slower than general anaesthesia, the limiting factor being the unpredictability of the time to achieve an adequate neuraxial anaesthetic block.[31] Many situations, including a prolapsed cord, do not exclude the use of a neuraxial technique, which in emergency situations may be the safest option (see 'Rapid Sequence Spinal' section later in the chapter).

Contraindications to neuraxial anaesthesia

See Box 20.3.

Patient refusal

(See also Chapter 29.)

- Patients undergoing neuraxial anaesthesia must consent to the procedure.
- Any woman with ability to consent is entitled to refuse treatment even if it would benefit her own or her baby's health.[7]

Cardiovascular instability

(See also Chapter 23 and Chapter 35.)

- The sympatholytic effects of neuraxial anaesthesia reduce blood pressure, systemic vascular resistance, and venous return.
- The response to pre-existing hypovolaemia, inferior vena cava compression, or hypovolaemia (e.g. during major haemorrhage) is exaggerated as neuraxial anaesthesia prevents compensatory vasoconstriction.[32]
- Women with congenital or acquired cardiac disease resulting in fixed cardiac output states (aortic stenosis, hypertrophic obstructive cardiomyopathy) may decompensate following spinal neuraxial anaesthesia.[33]

Infection

(See also Chapter 28.)

- Epidural abscess, meningitis, encephalitis, or adhesive arachnoiditis after neuraxial anaesthesia are rare but potentially devastating.
- It is suggested that neuraxial anaesthesia is avoided in patients with active untreated systemic infection, but consider single-shot techniques (no indwelling epidural catheter) on an individual basis if clinically responding to antimicrobial therapy.
- Active superficial skin infection (e.g. herpes zoster) at the site of injection may cause colonization of indwelling epidural catheters and spread inwards to epidural and intrathecal spaces.[34]

Central nervous system or spinal pathology

(See also Chapter 45.)

- Neuraxial anaesthesia is contraindicated in patients with raised intracranial pressure.

Box 20.3 Contraindications to neuraxial anaesthesia

- Patient refusal
- Anticoagulant drug therapy—see Table 20.1
- Uncorrected coagulopathy, international normalized ratio 1.4 or higher
- Thrombocytopenia—see Table 20.1
- Haemodynamic compromise
- Active local skin infection, untreated systemic sepsis
- CNS or spinal pathology precluding neuraxial anaesthesia.

- There is no evidence to support or refute central neuraxial anaesthesia in patients with pre-existing neurological disease. Each case should be analysed individually with neurological or neurosurgical input and a risk:benefit assessment performed. Any pre-existing neurology requires robust documentation.
- Women who have had spinal surgery may prove a technical challenge. There is an increased risk of accidental dural puncture, and scarring of the epidural space may prevent the normal expected spread of local anaesthetic solution. The posterior elements of the vertebral column are usually still intact and spinal anaesthesia is often possible.[35] There is also the devastating potential complication of infection of scoliosis rods.

Coagulopathy, low platelets, and anticoagulant drug therapy

(See also Chapter 28 and Chapter 48.)

- In the obstetric population, spinal cord or nerve root compression due to spinal or epidural haematoma has been estimated at 1/168,000.[36] Reported cases usually occur in conjunction with coagulopathy or anticoagulation therapy (see Table 20.1).
- The thrombotic tendency of parturients combined with an increase in procoagulant risk factors (e.g. raised BMI, antiphospholipid syndrome, and assisted fertility) has led to larger numbers of antenatal patients on anticoagulant medication.
- Reduced platelet counts may occur in idiopathic thrombocytopenia (ITP), gestational thrombocytopenia, and pre-eclampsia.

Table 20.1 Relative risks related to neuraxial blockade in obstetric patients with abnormalities of coagulation or anticoagulation therapy

Risk factor	Normal risk	Increased risk	High risk
LMWH prophylactic dose	>12 h	6–12 h	<6 h
LMWH treatment dose	>24 h	12–24 h	6–12 h
Unfractionated heparin infusion	4 h after stopping and aPTTr ≤ 1.4		
Unfractionated heparin bolus dose	>4 h	<4 h	
Warfarin	INR ≤ 1.4	INR 1.4–1.7	INR 1.7–2.0
Pre-eclampsia	Platelets > 100 × 10^9/L within 6 h of block	Platelets 75–100 × 10^9/L (stable) and normal coagulation tests	Decreasing platelet count 75–100 × 10^9/L, abnormal coagulation tests, HELLP syndrome
Idiopathic or gestational thrombocytopenia	Platelets > 75 × 10^9/L within 24 h of block	Platelets 50–75 × 10^9/L	Platelets 20–50 × 10^9/L

aPTTr, activated partial thromboplastin time ratio; HELLP, haemolysis, elevated liver enzyme levels, and low platelet count; INR, international normalized ratio; LMWH, low molecular weight heparin.

Reproduced with permission from *Regional Anaesthesia in Patients with Abnormalities in Coagulation*, A guidance document produced by a Joint Working Party of the AAGBI, OAA, RA-UK, 2011.

In ITP and gestational thrombocytopenia, the platelet number rather than function is limited, and if stable and tested daily, levels above 75 × 10^9/L are considered adequate for neuraxial blockade if the count is not decreasing. Pre-eclampsia can affect platelet function and is a dynamic pathological process. In some cases, 6-hourly platelet counts and clotting studies may need to be done if neuraxial blockade is being considered. Decreasing trends would be considered a higher risk procedure and individual risk:benefit assessments should be made.[37]

- Coagulopathy may develop following other obstetric conditions such as cholestasis, intrauterine death, or placental abruption. Coagulation tests and platelet counts should be checked according to the clinical picture.

Preoperative assessment

Pregnant women are generally healthy with minimal co-morbidities, however with the increasing age of the maternal population, obesity, and the potential for unexpected events, baseline assessment of all women is important. High-risk women should be seen antenatally by both anaesthetist and obstetrician and birth plans fully discussed and documented. Routine anaesthetic assessment should be undertaken in all cases and modified for the obstetric patient as shown in Box 20.4. Preoperative assessment should not missed in the case of emergency CD. In cases of severe fetal distress, this assessment should be done simultaneously with other tasks such as obtaining intravenous (IV) access, transferring and positioning the patient as well as establishing monitoring.

Nil by mouth during labour

The policy of no food during labour was adopted universally following Mendelson's paper on pulmonary aspiration in 1946.[38] In the United Kingdom, there are currently no nationally recommended guidelines on eating/drinking during labour. Deaths from aspiration in obstetric patients are now extremely rare, an outcome that owes more to the widespread use of neuraxial analgesia/anaesthesia rather than to nil-by-mouth policies.

Box 20.4 Preoperative anaesthetic assessment

- Anaesthetic history
- Past medical/surgical history
- Obstetric history
- Current medication and allergies
- Airway assessment
- Confirm position of placenta
- Recent haemoglobin and platelet count
- Valid group and screen or cross match for women at increased risk of blood loss of more than 1000 mL
- Prescription of preoperative antacid medication
- Fasting guidelines
- Consent for neuraxial anaesthesia.

Although many women do not feel like eating in labour, some may find the nil-by-mouth restriction unpleasant, particularly those with an effective epidural who are pain free. A large randomized controlled trial of more than 2400 low-risk women showed that eating a low-fat, low-residue diet during labour does not affect obstetric (mode of delivery and labour duration) or neonatal outcome.[39]

Women with risk factors for aspiration (morbidly obese, difficult airway) or women who have increased risk for operative delivery (Figure 20.2) may have their oral intake restricted to clear fluids but this should be determined on a case-by-case basis. Low-risk women, who have not had opioid analgesia, can probably be allowed a light diet during labour.

Antacid prophylaxis and fasting times

Pregnancy increases the risk of pulmonary aspiration of gastric contents and subsequent development of aspiration pneumonitis.[38] Although awake during surgery, women undergoing neuraxial anaesthesia remain at risk due to the ever-present possibility of conversion to general anaesthesia. All patients undergoing planned CD should have an adequate period of fasting to minimize the volume of gastric contents and receive pharmacological antacid therapy to increase the pH of gastric contents.[7]

Current preoperative United Kingdom and European fasting guidelines recommend stopping solids 6 hours preoperatively with only water being consumed up to 2 hours before.[40] Some institutions advocate unrestricted sips of water until surgery.[41]

A 2010 Cochrane review looked at interventions during CD for reducing the risk of lung damage from inhaling gastric contents under general anaesthesia.[42] While the risk of aspiration is difficult to estimate due to the need for a vast sample size, studies have looked at surrogate markers such as gastric pH and volume. The review found that the quality of the evidence was poor, but the findings suggest that the combination of antacids plus an H_2 antagonist was more effective than no intervention, and superior to antacids alone in preventing low gastric pH at CD. Therefore, it seems sensible to administer oral ranitidine (150 mg 6-hourly) during labour in women at high risk of requiring a CD. In the event of an unexpected emergency CD, a slow IV injection of 50 mg ranitidine can be administered (if time allows), but this is unlikely to be effective before general anaesthesia is induced. However, due to the timescale of onset of action of both oral and IV ranitidine an oral antacid such as sodium citrate 0.3M 30 mL should also be administered, in theatre, immediately before general anaesthesia.

The H_2 antagonist ranitidine is used to neutralize stomach acid. The dose 150 mg orally is effective in 90–120 minutes and administered the night before surgery and repeated in the morning on the day of surgery. The prokinetic agent metoclopramide 10 mg is administered orally in the morning on the day of surgery to facilitate gastric emptying.[7] Proton pump inhibitors (PPIs) such as omeprazole may be of use in the elective situation to reduce gastric pH.[43,44] However, a meta-analysis comparing the ability of H_2 antagonists and PPIs to achieve appropriate gastric PH and volume showed that premedication with H_2 antagonists was more effective than PPIs in achieving a low gastric volume with a high pH.[45] Metoclopramide may have some benefits as it a prokinetic agent that increases gastric emptying and increases lower oesophageal tone as well as acting as an antiemetic.[46] However, young

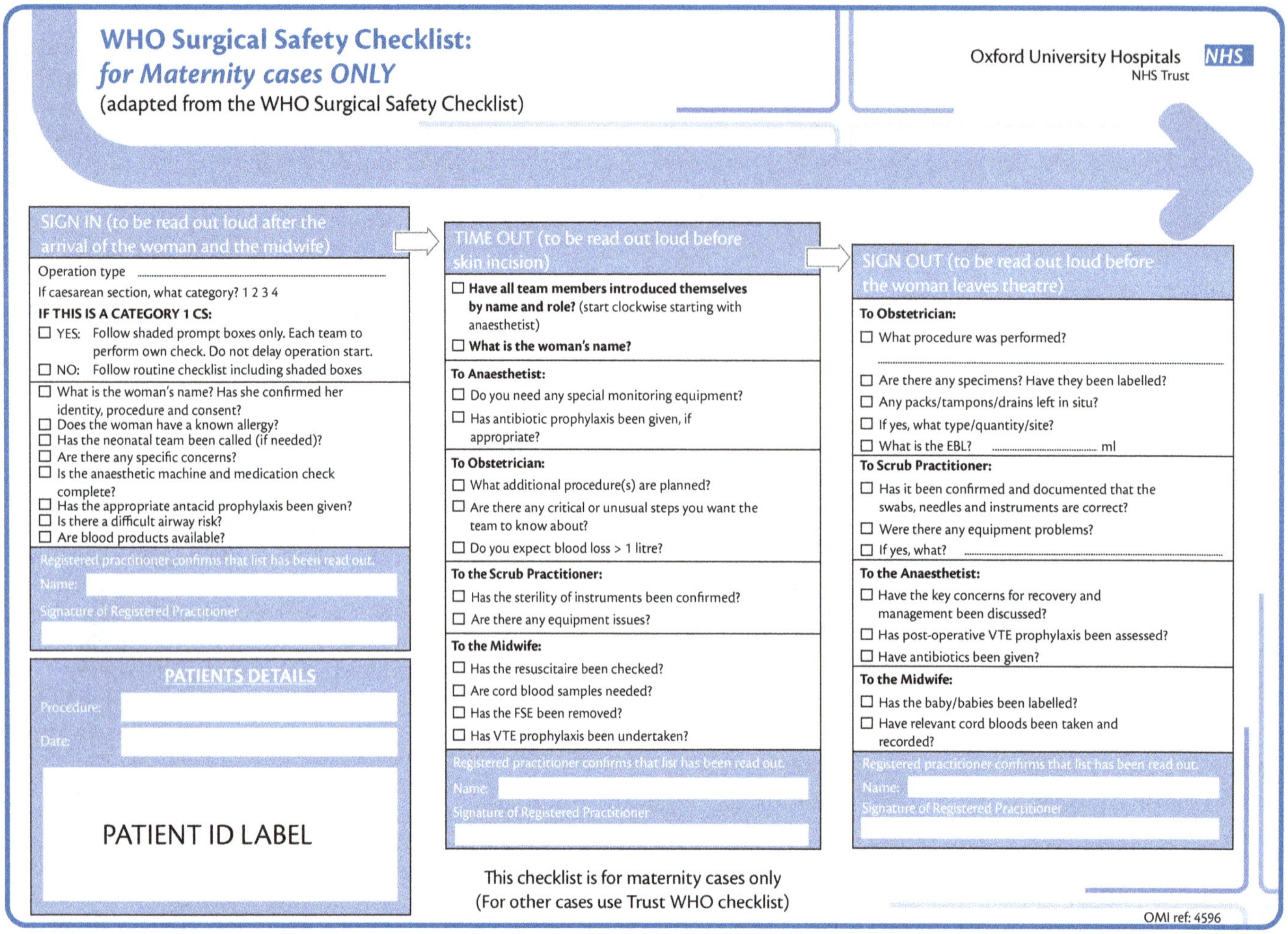

WHO Surgical Safety Checklist:
for Maternity cases ONLY
(adapted from the WHO Surgical Safety Checklist)

Oxford University Hospitals NHS
NHS Trust

SIGN IN (to be read out loud after the arrival of the woman and the midwife)

Operation type ....
If caesarean section, what category? 1 2 3 4
IF THIS IS A CATEGORY 1 CS:
☐ YES: Follow shaded prompt boxes only. Each team to perform own check. Do not delay operation start.
☐ NO: Follow routine checklist including shaded boxes
☐ What is the woman's name? Has she confirmed her identity, procedure and consent?
☐ Does the woman have a known allergy?
☐ Has the neonatal team been called (if needed)?
☐ Are there any specific concerns?
☐ Is the anaesthetic machine and medication check complete?
☐ Has the appropriate antacid prophylaxis been given?
☐ Is there a difficult airway risk?
☐ Are blood products available?
Registered practitioner confirms that list has been read out.
Name:
Signature of Registered Practitioner

PATIENTS DETAILS
Procedure:
Date:
PATIENT ID LABEL

TIME OUT (to be read out loud before skin incision)

☐ **Have all team members introduced themselves by name and role?** (start clockwise starting with anaesthetist)
☐ **What is the woman's name?**
To Anaesthetist:
☐ Do you need any special monitoring equipment?
☐ Has antibiotic prophylaxis been given, if appropriate?
To Obstetrician:
☐ What additional procedure(s) are planned?
☐ Are there any critical or unusual steps you want the team to know about?
☐ Do you expect blood loss > 1 litre?
To the Scrub Practitioner:
☐ Has the sterility of instruments been confirmed?
☐ Are there any equipment issues?
To the Midwife:
☐ Has the resuscitaire been checked?
☐ Are cord blood samples needed?
☐ Has the FSE been removed?
☐ Has VTE prophylaxis been undertaken?
Registered practitioner confirms that list has been read out.
Name:
Signature of Registered Practitioner

This checklist is for maternity cases only
(For other cases use Trust WHO checklist)

SIGN OUT (to be read out loud before the woman leaves theatre)

To Obstetrician:
☐ What procedure was performed?
....
☐ Are there any specimens? Have they been labelled?
☐ Any packs/tampons/drains left in situ?
☐ If yes, what type/quantity/site?
☐ What is the EBL? .... ml
To Scrub Practitioner:
☐ Has it been confirmed and documented that the swabs, needles and instruments are correct?
☐ Were there any equipment problems?
☐ If yes, what? ....
To the Anaesthetist:
☐ Have the key concerns for recovery and management been discussed?
☐ Has post-operative VTE prophylaxis been assessed?
☐ Have antibiotics been given?
To the Midwife:
☐ Has the baby/babies been labelled?
☐ Have relevant cord bloods been taken and recorded?
Registered practitioner confirms that list has been read out.
Name:
Signature of Registered Practitioner

OMI ref: 4596

Figure 20.2 WHO Surgical Safety Checklist.
Reprinted with permission from *WHO Surgical Safety Checklist* (first edition), 2008. Adapted for obstetric surgery by Oxford University Hospitals NHS Trust.

patients as in obstetrics, have a higher incidence of oculogyric crisis with metoclopramide.

Consent for neuraxial anaesthesia

The consent process is a two-way dynamic discussion of treatment options and potential complications of treatment (see Chapter 29). Information shared should respect the right of the woman to express birth preferences and take into account her culture and views. Concerns are acknowledged and explored and questions answered.[47] Ideally this is carried out at the pre-admission clinic prior to the day of surgery if an elective CD. Information is also available for mothers via leaflets and the Internet.[48]

Consenting for neuraxial anaesthesia may include explanation of the following side effects and risks:

- Pruritus (itching), shivering, nausea, and vomiting
- Hypotension
- Postdural puncture headache (PDPH): 1/100–200
- Block failure
- Permanent injury from nerve damage or infection: 1/66,000 (spinal); 1/166,000 (epidural)[49]
- Expected sensations of pushing, pulling, and pressure
- Treatment options if pain or discomfort experienced
- Conversion to general anaesthesia if required
- Short-term bruising to back at puncture site
- Urinary catheter to prevent bladder over-distension
- Rectal suppositories for postoperative analgesia
- Options for postoperative analgesia.

Neuraxial anaesthesia technique

Neuraxial anaesthesia for CD can be performed using the following techniques:

- Single-shot spinal anaesthesia (SSS)
- Combined spinal–epidural anaesthesia (CSE)
- Low-dose or sequential CSE anaesthesia
- Epidural anaesthesia
- Continuous spinal anaesthesia.

The choice of technique will depend on local institutional guidelines, anaesthetist experience, surgical technique, clinical judgement, and individual patient requirements. A sample procedural checklist for neuraxial anaesthesia for CD is shown in Box 20.5. Busy elective operating lists with quick turnaround times may require a neuraxial anaesthetic technique with a more rapid speed of onset. Whichever technique is used, the neuraxial block must spread sufficiently to provide anaesthesia lasting the duration of surgery and minimize perioperative discomfort. Proactive therapies are necessary to reduce side effects, in particular avoiding hypotension leading to maternal nausea and vomiting, uteroplacental hypoperfusion, and neonatal compromise.[26]

The popularity of epidural analgesia during labour means that many women presenting for unplanned CD have an epidural already in place. Anaesthesia can take longer to establish so in a true emergency (e.g. prolapsed cord or massive placental abruption), a spinal or general anaesthetic might be the technique of choice.

Box 20.5 Procedure for neuraxial anaesthesia for caesarean delivery

- Communication with team members
- Patient preparation, discussion, and consent
- Ensure antacid prophylaxis
- Confirm group and save/cross-match if required
- Check equipment and prepare medication (including emergency)
- Transfer patient
- WHO checklist—sign in
- Mandatory monitoring (electrocardiogram, non-invasive blood pressure, SpO_2)
- CTG monitoring if appropriate
- Large-bore IV access
- Consider supplemental oxygen if fetal compromise
- Fluid infusion
- Aseptic technique
- Neuraxial blockade
- Tilt (uterine displacement)—table tilt or wedge
- Urinary catheter—bladder emptying
- Testing for block adequacy
- Antibiotics prior to skin incision
- WHO surgical checklist 'time out' before skin incision
- Oxytocin at delivery to encourage uterine contraction and minimize blood loss
- Postoperative analgesia and thromboprophylaxis
- Complete anaesthetic documentation
- WHO surgical checklist "sign out" before leaving operating theatre
- Handover to recovery staff
- Follow-up within 24 hours

WHO surgical safety checklist

The worldwide implementation of the WHO surgical safety checklist has reduced death rates and complications during surgery and is now established in safe theatre practice in the United Kingdom following an alert from the National Patient Safety Agency in 2009.[50,51]

The checklist has changed practice by prompting checking of routine interventions and improving team communication and dynamics. The original version can be adapted for use according to specialty requirements and is successfully being used in obstetrics for planned and emergency CD (Figure 20.2).

The components of the checklist are read out aloud while the woman is awake.

Initially there was concern that the patient may suffer unnecessary anxiety as a result of the checklist. A questionnaire-based study found that, on the contrary, patients experienced lower levels of anxiety and were reassured by its use.[52]

Aseptic technique

Serious central nervous system (CNS) infections (vertebral canal abscess, meningitis) are rare in the obstetric population; however, potentially devastating morbidity and mortality can occur[49] (see Chapter 28). Although firm evidence is lacking for some of the components of the aseptic technique, the potential consequences from CNS infection warrants thorough attempts to reduce this risk.[53]

A series of precautions are recommended to reduce the risk of infection. These include:

- removal of jewellery, clean short fingernails, and complying with the 'bare below the elbows' policy[54]
- pre-procedural hand washing with an alcohol-based antiseptic solution
- wearing single-use sterile gloves, hat and mask, and a sterile surgical gown. It should be noted that this recommendation is common in the United Kingdom and Australia but not worldwide[55,56]
- skin disinfection with 0.5% chlorhexidine in alcohol
- maintaining a sterile field and performing the procedure with an aseptic technique using sterile equipment
- application of a sterile dressing and regular inspection
- safe disposal of sharps

Skin disinfection

Skin disinfection is performed with an alcohol-based chlorhexidine solution. Chlorhexidine is superior to iodine in onset time, its efficacy in eradicating skin flora, and in duration of action and is recommended for disinfection by the RCoA in the United Kingdom and the American Society of Anesthesiologists. Currently chlorhexidine is available as 0.5% chlorhexidine with ethanol or 2% chlorhexidine in isopropyl alcohol.[57] Malhotra et al. compared the application of a single spray of 0.5% chlorhexidine spray with double spraying.[58] The single spray rendered skin sterile and a further spray was considered unnecessary. The original application should be thorough and allowed to dry properly.[58] Given that a single application of 0.5% chlorhexidine effectively disinfects the skin there is currently no evidence to support the use of the 2% solution for neuraxial procedures.[59]

Excessive use of chlorhexidine is not without risk. It is a known neurotoxic agent and epidural injection of chlorhexidine solution or contamination of equipment used in central neuraxial block procedures has been implicated in causing severe adhesive arachnoiditis.[60] Precautions should be taken to prevent accidental contamination of any equipment with the antiseptic. The antiseptic should not be poured or applied in the vicinity of block equipment.[61] This can be avoided by using spray compared to liquid from a bottle and spraying the patient's back before the anaesthetic pack is opened. Colourless solutions should be avoided to prevent being mistaken for saline.[59] After application the antiseptic fluid should be allowed to dry in order for it to exert its effect and to prevent contaminating gloves when palpating the skin. Gloves should be checked for contamination and changed if necessary.[59] (See also Chapter 28.)

Antibiotics

Up to 8% of women are known to suffer from a wound, urinary, or endometrial infection after CD and antibiotic prophylaxis is routinely administered to prevent these postoperative infective complications. Recent guidance suggests this risk of infection can be reduced by administering maternal IV antibiotics prior to skin incision without causing undue harm to the baby.[7] Nonetheless, the use of co-amoxiclav has been discouraged due to an increased risk of necrotizing enterocolitis in the neonate, particularly in preterm deliveries or in women with premature rupture of membranes.[62,63] The current recommendation is to use cephalosporins despite deficient data on the safety profile of these in neonates.[64]

Identifying the correct vertebral interspace

In the majority of people the spinal cord tapers and ends at the level of the L1/2 interspace (Figure 20.3). In a small but significant proportion of the population the position of the conus medullaris varies and may extend down to L3. Accidental insertion of a needle into the spinal cord can result in permanent neurological injury and most anaesthetists opt to perform neuraxial anaesthesia at the L3/4 interspace or below.[65]

Tuffier's line is a radiological line and anatomical landmark used to orientate the anaesthetist. A virtual line is drawn between the patients' iliac crests and generally this crosses the spinous process of the fourth lumbar vertebra. The L3/4 interspace is palpated one space above Tuffier's line and L4/5 one below. Radiologically this line is neither affected by the position of the patient nor BMI (Figure 20.4).

Palpation and estimation of the intervertebral space using Tuffier's line are inaccurate even when performed by experienced anaesthetists. Broadbent et al. demonstrated that in over 50% of cases the interspace identified on magnetic resonance imaging (MRI) was one space higher than previously estimated on palpation and only a third of anaesthetists correctly located a specific vertebral level.[66] These discrepancies were more likely to occur in obese patients. A decade later, Lee at al. published a similar assessment of vertebral level accuracy, this time using ultrasound scanning.[67] Only 14% of ultrasound findings correlated with the findings on clinical palpation. It is apparent that what is palpated on the patient's back does not correspond to Tuffier's line as seen on ultrasound or MRI. Palpation often identifies a line that may be up to three spaces higher than anticipated.[68]

In addition to identifying the iliac crests and correct vertebral level, ultrasound has been shown to accurately calculate the distance from skin to epidural space, identify the best point and angle of needle insertion, and reduce risk of failed or traumatic lumbar punctures and epidural catheterizations[69] (see Chapter 54).

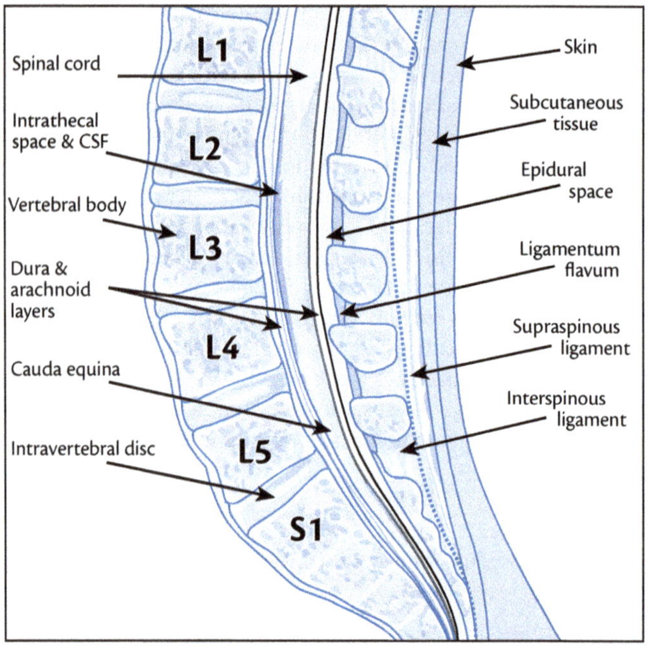

Figure 20.3 The spinal cord generally tapers and ends at the conus medullaris at L1/2. Nerve roots known as the cauda equine continue to S2 and are surrounded by cerebrospinal fluid (CSF) within the intrathecal space.

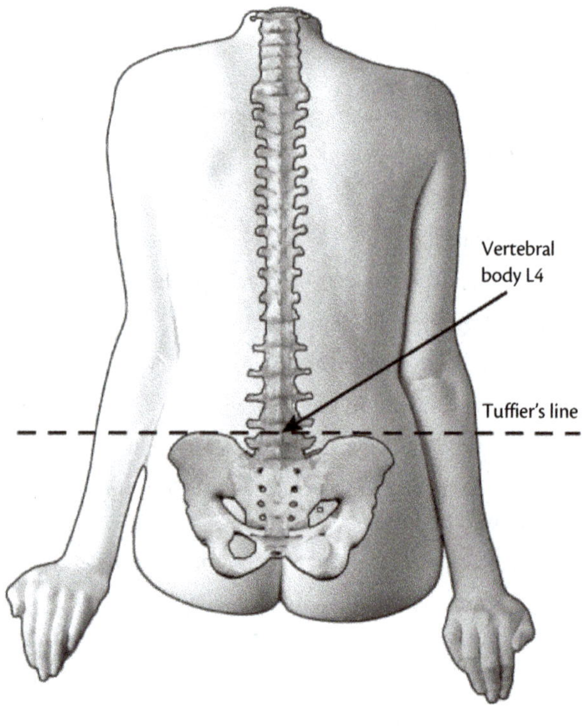

Figure 20.4 Tuffier's line is drawn between the highest points of the iliac crests and intersects L4.

Block testing

Pain or discomfort during CD is the leading cause of complaint against obstetric anaesthetists.[70] Prior to surgery it is necessary to perform an assessment of the neuraxial block to confirm block adequacy and so avoid intraoperative pain (see Chapter 21). Autonomic innervation of the abdominal viscera and peritoneum is conveyed by splanchnic nerves that descend from the thoracolumbar sympathetic trunk and spinal cord from levels as high as T5. A sensory block from sacral dermatomes to at least T4 is considered necessary for CD.

The different modalities used to test the block include temperature, pinprick, light touch, and presence of motor block. Depending on the modality used to test, the block detected may vary by several dermatomes. In the United Kingdom, practice is variable, the majority of obstetric anaesthetists aiming for a sensory block to cold up to a level of T4.[71] Nevertheless, Russell suggests that testing for an adequate block to light touch to T5 (without intrathecal opioids) or T6 (with intrathecal opioids) is the necessary standard of care.[72]

The stimulus used to test the block height is also considered to be very important. Ethyl chloride is the most common method used in the United Kingdom to test for both touch and cold;[71] however, the application (full force spray versus passive drop of the liquid) will vary according to the operator. A newer device, the Neuropen® monofilament (Owen Mumford, Oxford, UK) assesses response to touch and is not operator dependent. The Neuropen® has been well validated as accurate test of touch. Walsh et al. compared both equipment methods to assess neuraxial block to touch.[73] Findings between both were equivalent to within one dermatome; however, occasional wide individual differences were found. The height of block detected by the Neuropen® was lower than that of ethyl chloride. Despite a block to touch lower than T5, no increase in intraoperative discomfort was noted, raising the possibility that the gold standard block to touch to T5 is stimulus dependent or requires further validation.[73]

Findings from testing the block should be documented on the anaesthetic chart and include mode of testing, laterality (left or right side) and relevant timings. The use of dermatome maps is encouraged to standardize documentation.[74]

Effects of positioning

Women are either positioned sitting or lateral for neuraxial anaesthesia. Choice of position depends on patient circumstances, preference of the anaesthetist, and baricity of the local anaesthetic agent. Anaesthetists should be competent with both positions. The sitting position is more widely used and helps to locate the midline and interspace, particularly in obese patients.[75] The lateral position is preferential in emergency CD to minimize disturbances to uteroplacental blood flow with a distressed fetus.[76] However, as the sitting position may help locate the midline making neuraxial anaesthesia quicker it may be beneficial in an emergency situation.[77]

Studies investigating the influence of posture on block adequacy and incidence of hypotension vary in design, making comparisons difficult.[78] Anaesthetists may perceive increased difficulty in the position they have less experience in. Spinal or CSE anaesthesia initiated with hyperbaric bupivacaine in the lateral position may take longer to perform, however this is offset by a faster onset sensory block. Studies comparing positions using epidural anaesthesia report a higher incidence of hypotension in patients in the lateral position.[77,79] Procedural delays occurring in the sitting position (e.g. due to difficulty inserting the epidural catheter), may lead to a shorter effective duration of anaesthesia due to sacral pooling.[75] It has been hypothesized that due to a lower venous hydrostatic pressure the epidural venous plexus is less engorged and 'bloody taps' are less likely in the lateral position.[80,81]

When lying supine, all women require left uterine displacement to reduce aortocaval compression. A wedge can be applied under the right hip or the table tilted a minimum of 15° to the left. Even with these manoeuvres it is important to remember there will still be an element of aortocaval compression.[82]

The use of the head-elevated ramp position using blankets or commercially available pillows may be beneficial once anaesthesia has been established. The time of adequate surgical anaesthesia may be delayed but the incidence of hypotension following spinal anaesthesia may be reduced.[83,84] Cheesman et al. looked at 60 women undergoing elective CD under CSE and randomized them to one of three head positions following a CSE: horizontal with a small pillow under the head; head-elevated ramped position with the torso on a special elevation pillow; head-elevated ramped position, after initially being positioned horizontally (giving time for the block to be established). The authors measured the block height and time to onset of adequate block as well as maternal comfort and need for epidural supplementation. They found no significant difference in the time to establish an adequate height of block and that the women found the head-elevated positions more comfortable. However, the need for epidural supplementation was greater in the intervention groups.[83] The ramped position is useful if conversion to emergency general anaesthesia is needed as it provides optimal airway position for intubation. The arms should not be folded across the chest as this may impede airway access particularly in the obese patient.

Temperature control

Intrathecal and epidural anaesthesia for CD can cause significant decreases in core body temperature.[85] This is most likely due to the onset of sympathetic block and a mixing of warm blood in the body core with the cooler blood in the lower limbs.[86] Horn et al. evaluated whether newborns develop hypothermia during intraoperative bonding while positioned on their mothers' chests and investigated the effects of active forced air-warming of the mothers and babies during a 20-minute intraoperative bonding period.[87] They found a decreased incidence of neonatal hypothermia, an increase in the maternal core temperature and increase in the mean skin temperatures of both mother and infant, Maternal thermal comfort was improved, and maternal perioperative shivering reduced.

There is good evidence in non-obstetric patients that hypothermia leads to increased wound infection rates, length of hospital stay, and blood loss, all of which are highly relevant to obstetric practice.[88,89] Temperature management for CD is challenging due to limited body surface available for warming, peripheral vasodilatation, and exposure of the peritoneum. As the risk for major postpartum haemorrhage is greater in emergency CD, active temperature management is important; however, only 16% of UK maternity units routinely actively manage patient temperature.

The majority only initiate active warming after blood loss of over 1 L, prolonged surgery, or measured patient hypothermia.[90]

As with non-obstetric surgery, temperature should be recorded at the start of the operation, every 30 minutes until the end of the operation, and continued into the recovery period.[7]

There are limited numbers of studies that have investigated active patient warming during elective CD; the most consistently effective method of warming patients is by fluid warming either by an in-line device or by infusing fluids taken from a warming cabinet maintained at 41°C.[90,91]

There is weak evidence for maintaining theatre temperature above 21°C.[92] However, there is some evidence of benefit for higher theatre temperatures improving core temperature of premature infants delivered by CD.[93] This needs to be balanced with the environmental comfort of the surgical team.[92]

Intravenous fluids

Prior to neuraxial blockade, large-bore IV access is established to allow rapid administration of medication and fluids. Counteracting the sympathetic-mediated spinal-induced hypotension requires a combination of strategies including the administration of IV fluids. Co-loading with fluid while performing the neuraxial anaesthetic reduces vasopressor requirements and limits hypotension.[94,95] A Cochrane review identified colloid fluids to be more effective than crystalloids, regardless of timing and rate of administration; however, colloids are used with caution in daily clinical practice due to an increasingly adverse side effect profile that includes anaphylaxis, coagulation abnormalities, and renal impairment.[96] (See also Chapter 23.)

Spinal anaesthesia

Spinal anaesthesia is the technique of choice worldwide for elective CDs and emergencies where there is not an epidural already in place. Over the last 50 years the development of small-gauge pencil-point needles such as the Sprotte® and Whitacre needles has enabled a widespread change in practice in providing anaesthesia for CD.[97] Whereas previously epidural or general anaesthesia were favoured, spinal anaesthesia has been the predominant technique for planned CD since the 1990s. By the new millennium, anaesthetic departments in the United Kingdom were performing up to 95% of planned CD under neuraxial anaesthesia and up to 87% of these were single-shot spinal techniques.[25,98] Compared to epidural anaesthesia, spinal anaesthesia is simple, cheap, has a rapid onset, and provides a more effective and denser block with less breakthrough pain.[99] The use of smaller, non-cutting pencil-point needles has reduced the incidence of PDPH from up to 25% to 0.5–1%.[100] The advantages and disadvantages of spinal anaesthesia are summarized in Table 20.2.

Local anaesthetic dose for spinal anaesthesia

The most commonly used local anaesthetic in obstetric spinal anaesthesia is hyperbaric (heavy) bupivacaine. Europeans and North Americans tend to use the 0.5% and 0.75% concentrations respectively. Effects are dose dependent and therefore in Europe larger volumes are used than in the United States but with the same effect. Diluting the local anaesthetic to increase the volume will not affect the intensity or the height of the block.[101,102]

Table 20.2 Advantages and disadvantages of spinal anaesthesia

Advantages	Disadvantages
Single injection	Limited duration, no ability to extend block
Quick to perform	Rapid-onset sympathetic blockade leading to hypotension
Endpoint with visualization of CSF	
Rapid-onset surgical anaesthesia	
Dense, predictable anaesthesia	
Less breakthrough pain, less likely to require supplemental analgesia	
Reduced incidence PDPH	
More cost-effective	
Only small amount local anaesthetic used, reduced toxicity risk	
Predictable recovery	

Bupivacaine in dextrose or glucose 8% is a hyperbaric solution with a density greater than cerebrospinal fluid (CSF). Compared to isobaric or hypobaric bupivacaine, the hyperbaric formulation produces a more predictable and reliable block with a lower incidence of spinal-induced hypotension.[103] The baricity of the solution can be used to manipulate block height, for example, a head-down position encourages the block to spread in a cephalad direction if hyperbaric bupivacaine is used.

A key consideration with spinal anaesthesia is the dose-dependent incidence of hypotension. Without preventative measures (such as fluid and vasopressor administration) this can occur in up to three-quarters of women and result in maternal and neonatal morbidity.[104]

A spinal block to cold to dermatome T4 and light touch to T6 are considered necessary predictors for a painless CD.[72] There is controversy over the dose of local anaesthetic required to achieve this block and which lasts for the duration of a CD. Textbooks recommend 12–15 mg of hyperbaric bupivacaine in combination with an opioid; however, in contemporary practice a conventional dose is usually 10–12.5 mg and a low dose is considered less than 8 mg.[105]

Ginosar et al. carried out logistic regression analysis to determine the effective dose in 95% of subjects (ED_{95}) of intrathecal hyperbaric bupivacaine with 10 mcg fentanyl and 200 mcg morphine for planned CD.[106] Block success was defined as a bilateral sensory block to pinprick at T6 level within 10 minutes of intrathecal injection with no subsequent requirement to supplement the block during surgery. The ED_{95} was 11.2 mg hyperbaric bupivacaine. A subsequent study of intrathecal plain (hypobaric) bupivacaine calculated the ED_{95} at 13 mg.[107] Despite fluid administration and preloading, the patients in these studies with 'conventional' doses experienced significant hypotension with systolic blood pressures dropping 20–30% from baseline. Compared to the non-pregnant population, pregnant women require reduced doses of intrathecal anaesthetic as the gravid uterus compresses the inferior vena cava causing epidural vein engorgement and a relative reduction in the volume of the dural sac.

Once sited, apart from repositioning the patient and taking advantage of the baricity of hyperbaric bupivacaine, there is no facility to extend or manipulate the spinal anaesthetic block. Inadequate or failed block, perioperative discomfort, or prolonged surgery will require the use of Entonox®, IV analgesic supplementation, or conversion to general anaesthesia. This situation is a risk factor for both maternal morbidity and mortality and may result in dissatisfaction. In the United Kingdom, the recommended conversion rate from regional to general anaesthesia during planned CD is less than 1%.[72]

Intrathecal dose adjustments according to patient characteristics

The literature suggests that no patient variables affect block level or merit a dose alteration when using conventional intrathecal doses. Norris injected a relatively large dose (15 mg) of hyperbaric bupivacaine into 52 women and found no correlation of the sensory spread with age, height, weight, BMI, or vertebral column length.[108]

Harten et al. compared a fixed dose regimen (hyperbaric bupivacaine 12 mg with diamorphine 0.4 mg) with smaller doses adjusted to the patient's height and weight (median dose hyperbaric bupivacaine 9.5 mg with diamorphine 0.4 mg) and found no significant difference in block adequacy; however, the adjusted-dose group were less likely to have a high block spreading to cervical dermatomes and suffered less hypotension.[109]

In Caravalho's dose–response study of morbidly obese patients (BMI > 40) no dose reduction was found necessary. Lower doses (<10 mg hyperbaric bupivacaine) were able to attain the necessary block but were seldom adequate for the duration of surgery. Large confidence intervals suggests that those at the extreme end of the BMI scale demonstrate greater variability in response and a CSE technique rather than a single-shot spinal would be more suitable due to the unpredictability.[107]

Results from optimal dose-finding studies may not be generalizable or comparable.[26] Obstetric patients are a heterogeneous population and practice varies widely both between institutions and countries. Western women are taller and have a larger body weight compared to Asian women and raised BMI can result in a technically challenging surgical procedure, requiring a denser and longer-acting anaesthetic block.

Anaesthetists vary in practice and experience and perform neuraxial anaesthesia with the patient in different positions, with the needle orifice in different directions, and injecting at different lumbar interspaces with variable speed.[110] Opioids are usually added to the intrathecal local anaesthetic; however, the dose and type is variable and polymorphism in the mu-opioid receptor might cause populations of different genetic profiles to respond differently. Surgical technique, for example, incision site, application of fundal pressure, and exteriorization of the uterus can influence anaesthetic requirements. Patient expectations and pain thresholds vary individually. It is therefore clear that many factors need to be considered when selecting the optimal intrathecal dose and anaesthetic technique, and what works well in one institution may be different in another.[26]

Rapid sequence spinal for category 1 caesarean delivery

Kinsella and Scrutton described the 'rapid sequence spinal' in order to dramatically minimize anaesthetic time in the face of category 1 CD. The principles consist of a 'no-touch' spinal technique (only sterile gloves and skin prepared with a single wipe of chlorhexidine solution) with preoxygenation occurring during the attempt. Other components of the technique include consideration of omission of the spinal opioid, limiting spinal attempts to just one, allowing the start of surgery before full establishment of the spinal block, and being prepared for conversion to general anaesthesia if there are delays or problems.

Their case series of 25 rapid sequence spinals for category 1 CD demonstrated a technique that provided an anaesthetic block that was adequate to start surgery in 6–8 minutes. The authors stress that this technique should not be used by novices and not for cases where the spinal is predicted to be difficult or if the woman is not compliant. Staff teamwork is crucial, for example, in siting the cannula, attaching monitoring, and ensuring equipment is ready for general anaesthesia. There are no large trials validating this technique and it has been criticized primarily for compromising sterility, although while the wearing of a sterile gown is considered necessary in the United Kingdom and Australia, it is not common practice in the United States, Canada, and many parts of Europe.[55,56]

Epidural anaesthesia

Epidural anaesthesia was the mainstay neuraxial technique for CD prior to the introduction of small-gauge pencil-point spinal needles. It is now used infrequently for planned CD as the slow-onset incremental block limits use in current high-turnover planned CD lists. Epidural anaesthesia remains frequently used in emergency CD due to the rising number of woman having epidurals sited for labour analgesia subsequently requiring CD. Disadvantages of the epidural anaesthetic include a less dense block compared to spinals with increased rates of block failure or missed segments which may potentially put women at risk of perioperative discomfort.[99] The OAA epidural information leaflet states that 1 in 8–10 epidurals are not adequate for CD and require conversion to spinal or general anaesthesia (http://www.oaa-anaes.ac.uk).

However, there are some desirable components to the technique. The gradual onset sympathetic block may be more haemodynamically stable and beneficial in patients with cardiovascular morbidity.[33,111–113] The presence of the epidural catheter also allows perioperative top-ups or can be used to prolong the block in lengthy procedures. Nevertheless these advantages have now been combined with the advantages of spinals in CSE procedures and has further eliminated the need for stand-alone epidural anaesthesia for elective CD. The advantages and disadvantages of epidural anaesthesia are summarized in Table 20.3.

Topping-up a labour epidural for emergency caesarean delivery

The practice of 'topping-up' in the delivery room is contentious; the desire for rapid onset of surgical anaesthesia must be balanced with safety, but as any adverse outcome can be blamed on delays it is understandable that 80.5% of anaesthetists working on UK units initiate the top-up in the delivery room.[114] Once the top-up has started, the anaesthetist must not leave the patient under any circumstances and monitoring should be established as soon as is practical. Many anaesthetists give a 5 mL 'test dose' in the room and then give the full dose when in the safety of the operating theatre. Top-up of an existing epidural should lead to adequate

Table 20.3 Advantages and disadvantages of epidural anaesthesia

Advantages	Disadvantages
Titratable level of anaesthesia	Longer time to insert than spinal
Haemodynamic stability	Potential for catheter to be intravenous or intrathecal
Ability to prolong block	Administration and onset takes longer
Epidural postoperative analgesia	Less dense, less reliable, missed segments more likely, variable sacral spread
Labour analgesia epidurals can be 'topped-up' to provide anaesthesia for emergency CD	Large volumes of local anaesthetic required, systemic absorption increased, with potential for local anaesthetic toxicity

anaesthesia for CD within 10–12 minutes.[115] The properties of the local anaesthetic drug combinations often used for epidural top-ups for CD are summarized in Table 20.4.

Local anaesthetic agents used for epidural anaesthesia

- Lidocaine 2% with 1:200,000 epinephrine
- Bupivacaine 0.5%
- Levobupivacaine 0.5%
- Ropivacaine 0.75%
- 2-Chloroprocaine 3%.

Compared to the intrathecal space, the epidural space is larger. Greater volumes of local anaesthetic are required to achieve adequate block height and nerve root penetration. The volume of local anaesthetic necessary is usually 15–25 mL.

Engorged epidural venous plexuses mean that systemic absorption is more likely and may put the patient at risk of local anaesthetic toxicity or opioid-induced respiratory depression.

There is controversy over the superiority of various regimens for urgent top-up of a previously sited epidural for surgical delivery. The ideal agent should provide a rapid, predictable onset, require little preparation, provide cardiovascular stability, and have a low risk of intraoperative failure. Lidocaine, plain racemic bupivacaine, the single isomer levobupivacaine, and ropivacaine have been frequently studied when topping-up epidurals in labour for emergency CD. Hillyard et al.'s 2011 meta-analysis could not find evidence to support any one particular epidural top-up solution and highlighted the need for a large multicentre trial due to the heterogeneity of studies.[115]

Lidocaine 2%

Lidocaine 2% with epinephrine produces the fastest onset of surgical block to T4 within 7–11 minutes.[116–119] Concentrations of less than 2% can result in inadequate surgical anaesthesia and are not recommended.[120] The pKa of 7.7 means it is less ionized and therefore has a faster onset of action. The large dose (20–25 mL) given necessitates the co-administration with epinephrine to minimize systemic adsorption (0.1 mL of 1:1000 or 1 mL of 1:10,000) added to the 20 mL 2% lidocaine solution which produces a 1:200,000 = 5 mcg/ mL epinephrine solution). Epinephrine itself can also affect block as it acts both as a vasoconstrictor, limiting absorption and increasing block density, and as an independent analgesic via alpha-adrenergic blockade. These doses of epinephrine given epidurally do not appear to reduce uterine or fetal umbilical blood flow.[121] It is an easy solution to prepare in an emergency and can remain stable for up to 6 hours if kept in a fridge and protected from light. There does not appear any significant difference in the need for intraoperative supplementation when compared with bupivacaine 0.5%.[115]

Commercial preparations of lidocaine are acidic, alkalinization of lidocaine towards its pKa value increases the unionized fraction of drug thereby increasing the amount of lipid-soluble base available to cross the neuronal membrane and theoretically increase the speed of onset. Adding 2 mL of sodium bicarbonate (8.4%) to the 20 mL lidocaine/epinephrine mixture can increase the onset of block to T4 to within 5.2–7 minutes.[116] The drawback of this technique is the additional preparation time required which may offset

Table 20.4 Drugs used for epidural anaesthesia for caesarean delivery

Drug combination	Epidural dose range (mg)	Speed of onset (min)	Duration (min)	Special considerations
2% lidocaine + NaHCO3 + 5 mcg/ mL epinephrine	300–500	5.2–7	75–100	Delay in preparing mixture Potential for drug error
2% lidocaine + 5 mcg/mL epinephrine	300–500	7–11	75–100	Easy to mix Stable for 6 h Potential for drug error
Bupivacaine 0.5% or L-bupivacaine 0.5%	75–125	7.5–15	120–180	Stable at room temperature Mixing unnecessary Intraoperative failure more frequent
Ropivacaine 0.75%	75–125	7.5–15	120–180	less dense motor block Reduced intraoperative supplementation vs bupivacaine or L-bupivacaine
2-chloroprocaine, 3%	450–750	2–10	40–50	Unavailable in the UK Short duration of action

the benefit of speed of onset and the additional steps increase the risk of a drug error.[117]

Levobupivacaine/bupivacaine 0.5%

Levobupivacaine (L-bupivacaine) and bupivacaine have similar potencies, providing anaesthesia to T4 in 7.5–15 minutes. Both drugs can cause cardiovascular and CNS toxicity, but higher doses of L-bupivacaine are required to cause ventricular arrhythmias.[122,123] They have the same pKa of 8.2 which means they are more ionized than lidocaine and therefore have a slower onset of action than lidocaine (pKa 7.7). In the United Kingdom, 65% of anaesthetic departments have used bupivacaine or L-bupivacaine as their main agent for emergency CD either as a sole agent or combined with lidocaine 2%.[114] L-bupivacaine and bupivacaine are stable at room temperature and easily prepared.[117] Hillyard's meta-analysis showed that block onset requires 4.5 minutes longer that the lidocaine/epinephrine mixture but a similar incidence of need for intraoperative supplementation.[115] There was a higher incidence of intraoperative supplementation with L-bupivacaine and bupivacaine when compared to ropivacaine 0.75%.

Ropivacaine 0.75%

Ropivacaine has a similar structure to bupivacaine and the same pKa but is less lipid-soluble so penetrates the myelin sheath less readily and produces a reduced blockade of motor fibres. Ropivacaine 0.75% has similar onset time to bupivacaine when topping-up for an epidural for emergency CD requiring around 4.5 minutes longer than a lidocaine/epinephrine mixture.[124,125] The potency ratio of ropivacaine to bupivacaine has been reported to be between 1:1 and 1:2,[126,127] so a more concentrated preparation of 0.75% would account for its superiority with a reduced need for intraoperative supplementation when compared to levobupivacaine and bupivacaine and less cardiotoxicity.[115]

2-Chloroprocaine 3%

2-Chlorprocaine (2-CP) 3% is an ester local anaesthetic is not currently licensed for use in Europe but widely used in the United States. Due to high lipid-solubility it has a rapid onset of action of 6–12 minutes making it an ideal solution for emergency CD. It is hydrolysed by plasma pseudocholinesterase more rapidly than the hepatic metabolism of the amide local anaesthetics. The half-life of 2-CP in maternal plasma is less than 60 seconds therefore an unexpected IV injection would be rapidly metabolized making 2-CP extremely safe. A dose of 15–20 mL (up to 25 mL) of 3% 2-CP will provide rapid anaesthesia within 10 minutes, but its duration of action is short and will require a top-up of 10 mL after 30 minutes or there will be a rapid onset of patient discomfort, which may be difficult to control. The short duration of action may be beneficial in reducing the recovery room stay and shortening time to mobilization. 2-CP may act as a mu-receptor antagonist thereby interfering with the quality and duration of pain relief produced by epidural morphine or fentanyl and additional epidural or IV opioids may be required.[128] Unlike the amide local anaesthetics there is no fetal ion trapping so it may become the local anaesthetic of choice for delivery when the fetus is acidotic.

Opioid adjuvants in epidural top-ups

Opioids such as fentanyl (50–100 mcg) and sufentanil (10–20 mcg) are commonly added to improve the quality of anaesthesia. Malhotra and Yentis compared epidural top-up of 20 mL levobupivacaine 0.5% with or without fentanyl 75 mcg and found no difference in the speed of onset of block or the need for intraoperative supplementation.[129] Since these patients already had an epidural in labour and were being prepared for emergency CD, it was thought that the fentanyl in the labour epidural solution may have already saturated spinal opioid receptors. Interestingly, those receiving additional epidural fentanyl had a significantly higher proportion of nausea and vomiting.

Both morphine and diamorphine (2.5–3 mg) are frequently administered epidurally for postoperative CD analgesia. Pruritus and nausea and vomiting are common side effects. (See also Chapter 17 and Chapter 24.)

Rates of conversion to general anaesthesia

Unfortunately failure to convert a labour epidural to provide adequate anaesthesia for emergency CD can vary from 3% to 25%.[130] Guidance from the RCoA in the United Kingdom suggests that for planned CD the conversion rate from neuraxial anaesthesia to general anaesthesia should be less than 1% for elective CD and less than 5% for emergency CD.[131]

There are a number of factors which are thought to influence the success rates of epidural top-ups. An increasing number of unscheduled clinician-administered boluses during labour to maintain effective analgesics is a risk factor for failed epidural anaesthesia and even a single clinician top-up is an independent risk factor for failure.[132,133] The urgency of CD is also a predictor with Kinsella reporting a 25% (18/72) failure and conversion to general anaesthesia in category 1 CDs compared to a 7% (35/505) for category 2 CDs.[30] Fetal heart rate (FHR) abnormalities have not been shown to be an independent risk factor for failed conversion of epidural anaesthesia.[133]

The rate of conversion from epidural analgesia to general anaesthesia was found to be significantly increased when a non-obstetric anaesthetist was managing the anaesthetic compared to an obstetric anaesthetist (7.2% vs 1.6%).[132,134] This may be due to a number of factors including teamwork, communication, familiarity with the delivery suite operating theatre, as well as the ability to determine the urgency of the CD and to assess the quality of the labour epidural analgesia. There may be higher numbers of maternal requests for general anaesthesia, particularly in certain ethnic minorities.

A high BMI does not appear to be an independent risk factor for unsuccessful top-up but this may be due to a low tolerance for a poorly functioning labour epidural in obese mothers because of the high incidence of operative delivery and the desire to prevent a general anaesthetic.[135]

The different effects of general and neuraxial anaesthesia on the fetus also require further evaluation. Drugs used in general anaesthesia may have effects on the developing fetal brain and neuraxial anaesthesia has traditionally been considered more preferable for both mother and neonate. Nevertheless it is important to note that neuraxial anaesthesia is not entirely benign for the fetus. Spinal-induced hypotension, impaired uteroplacental perfusion, and ephedrine use have been associated with fetal umbilical artery acidosis and in recent years the vasopressor of choice has moved towards phenylephrine, which has improved fetal acid–base status compared to ephedrine.[136,137] (See also Chapter 21 and Chapter 23.)

Combined spinal–epidural anaesthesia

The CSE is a procedure combining both a spinal and an epidural block. Although considered more complex and time-consuming to perform than either block alone, a CSE offers significant advantages and is a popular technique for planned CD. The advantages and disadvantages of the CSE technique are summarized in Table 20.5.

The spinal component of the CSE enables a rapid onset dense and predictable block, whereas the additional epidural catheter enables intraoperative supplementation, block prolongation and postoperative analgesic administration. Conversion rates to general anaesthesia may be reduced when compared to stand alone spinal or epidural anaesthetics for CD.[138,139] Additionally, the presence of the epidural catheter allows the subarachnoid dose to be lowered or an incremental technique to be used. These techniques are associated with improved haemodynamic stability, reduced nausea and vomiting, and quicker recovery and are discussed further below.[140,141]

Made up of two components, the CSE procedure is seen as a more complex, lengthy and costly procedure. All complications of both spinals and epidurals may occur, including PDPH.

Technical difficulties are said to be more common with CSE than with either block alone.[75,142] The spinal component may fail if the long narrow-gauge spinal needle is displaced during the needle through needle technique (see below). If not advanced far enough to pierce the dura, fluid (epidural saline) seen in the hub of the spinal needle may be mistaken for CSF and any injection of the local anaesthetic mixture into this space will naturally fail to produce a block.[75]

The epidural catheter is usually inserted after the intrathecal injection. At this time there may already be an ascending subarachnoid block and paraesthesia or warning signs of nerve irritation while threading of the epidural catheter can theoretically be masked.[75] Also, the presence of the subarachnoid block doesn't allow for testing of the epidural catheter, so there is potential for a misplaced epidural catheter to go unnoticed until it is required perioperatively. On the other hand, it has been argued that the epidural catheter is more likely to be in the correct position when sited as part of the CSE procedure.[143]

If difficulties are encountered inserting the epidural catheter (e.g. intravascular catheter or severe paraesthesia) and the patient is in the sitting position for a prolonged length of time then a (spinal) saddle block (lumbosacral anaesthesia) may occur with hyperbaric bupivacaine.[144] This can often be remedied by repositioning the patient in a head-down position after completion of the CSE procedure, or by administering a local anaesthetic epidural top-up or epidural volume extension (EVE), as discussed in a later section in this chapter.

It has been suggested that the CSE procedure and ensuing pressure rise (from negative to atmospheric) within the epidural space could affect the flow of injected local anaesthetic within the intrathecal space and increase cephalad block spread in the CSE technique as compared to a single-shot spinal technique in elective CD.[145] Subsequent studies have not been able to replicate these findings and found that intrathecal dose requirements are the same for both single-shot spinal and CSE.[146]

Table 20.5 Advantages and disadvantages of CSE

Advantages	Disadvantages
Rapid-onset dense predictable block from spinal component	Increased failure rate of spinal component by: ◆ Wrong identification of saline for CSF ◆ Spinal needle movement ◆ Failure to obtain CSF if insertion has been paramedian
Epidural catheter *in situ* for increased flexibility: ◆ Prolong anaesthesia ◆ Perioperative supplementation ◆ Rescue inadequate block ◆ Epidural volume extension (EVE) ◆ Reduce conversion rate to general anaesthetic	Untested epidural catheter, may be intrathecal or incorrect position Paraesthesia on threading epidural catheter may be masked by ascending subarachnoid block
Epidural catheter may be used for postoperative analgesia	Risk of saddle block if delayed epidural catheter placement
Possibility to reduce intrathecal dose and perform incremental block with increased haemodynamic stability	Patient at risk of complications from both spinal and epidural procedures, e.g. postdural puncture headache

Needle-through-needle technique

A CSE can be performed either using a needle-through-needle technique using the same vertebral interspace or as two separate procedures in different vertebral interspaces—the double-spaced technique. Some centres report a higher failure rate of the spinal component with the needle through-needle-technique, however it remains the more commonly used method.[147]

With the needle-through-needle technique the epidural space is identified by a loss of resistance using a 16–18 G epidural needle and a spinal needle is subsequently passed through the epidural needle to pierce the dura. The operator may sense a dural 'click' or 'pop' during dural puncture, although the long and narrow (27–29 G) spinal needle sometimes make this difficult to feel which may contribute to the higher failure rate of the spinal component. CSF is then observed flowing through the spinal needle and an intrathecal dose of local anaesthetic and opioid is administered. During the intrathecal injection the epidural needle acts as the introducer to the spinal needle, however the spinal needle can be difficult to anchor unless specific CSE locking kits are used (see below).[148] Relatively large forces are required for the spinal fluid injection and the poorly anchored spinal needle may be subject to manual displacement which can also result in failure of the technique.[75] An alternative method when using the needle-through-needle technique is to advance the spinal needle slowly through the Tuohy needle without the spinal stillette/introducer. CSF will be seen as soon as the needle tip pierces the dura and the likelihood of advancing the spinal needle too far and causing paraesthesia may be reduced.

Standard epidural needles can be used for CSE but a longer spinal needle is needed compared to those used when performing single-shot spinals. CSE-specific commercial packs exist that may feature an epidural needle with a small hole in the greater curvature of the Huber tip to facilitate direct passage of the spinal needle through the dura and reduce friction between both needles.

Following injection the spinal needle is withdrawn and the epidural catheter is threaded through the epidural needle.

Double-space technique

The double-space technique is less popular and is made up of two separate procedures at different vertebral interspaces. If the epidural catheter is sited first then there is a theoretical risk of the spinal needle subsequently causing trauma to the catheter. Maternal satisfaction is reduced with this technique due to the need for two separate injections; however, this method allows the placement of the epidural catheter in an unhurried fashion compared to the needle-through-needle technique and if the catheter is intravascular, it can be replaced which is not the case in the latter technique. The double-space technique may also have a lower failure rate and therefore a lower conversion rate to general anaesthesia.[149]

Low-dose combined spinal–epidural

Low-dose CSE is a modified approach to anaesthesia for CD. The aim is to reduce the incidence of spinal-induced hypotension while still maintaining adequate anaesthesia. No exact definition exists for a 'low dose'. The ED_{95} of hyperbaric bupivacaine with opioid to produce a successful block without intraoperative discomfort is 11.0 ± 0.95 mg.[150] It would make sense to define a dose below this value as a 'low dose'; however, the literature tends to refer to 'low dose' as less than 8 mg hyperbaric bupivacaine.[105,151] The advantages of low-dose CSEs are summarized in Table 20.6.

The main advantage of low-dose anaesthesia is the reduction in spinal-induced hypotension. Adverse consequences of hypotension can be mild (e.g. maternal nausea and vomiting) or more serious such as circulatory collapse and cardiac arrest in already compromised patients who cannot tolerate a sudden sympathetic block.[150] Uteroplacental hypoperfusion secondary to spinal-induced hypotension can also lead to fetal acidosis and hypoxia. Reynolds and Seed carried out a meta-analysis of umbilical artery acid–base status in over 2000 subjects and found cord pH to be significantly lower and base-deficit significantly higher with spinal anaesthesia compared to epidural or general anaesthesia. Larger doses of ephedrine were administered in the spinal group.[136]

Table 20.6 Advantages and disadvantages of low-dose combined spinal epidural anaesthesia

Advantages	Disadvantages
Less sympathetic block therefore less hypotension and preserved uteroplacental perfusion	Risk of inadequate anaesthesia and perioperative discomfort, litigation potential
Reduced vasopressor requirements	Less dense block
Reduced nausea and vomiting	Faster block regression
Quicker recovery from motor block	Increased supplementation required
Safer technique in patients with respiratory or cardiovascular morbidity	Specialized technique—degree of experience necessary
Facility to extend or prolong block with epidural catheter	Pruritus may occur if using increased opioid instead of local anaesthetic
Administer postoperative pain relief with epidural catheter	Maternal satisfaction may be low if discomfort experienced

Studies lowering the dose of intrathecal anaesthetic have consistently demonstrated a reduction in the incidence of hypotension. Leo et al. compared 7, 8, and 9 mg hyperbaric bupivacaine in combination with intrathecal morphine and reported hypotension requiring vasopressor use in 30% versus 70% in the 7 mg and 9 mg groups respectively. No patient had inadequate anaesthesia.[152] Similarly, Van de Velde et al. compared 6.5 mg hyperbaric bupivacaine with 9.5 mg in combination with sufentanil.[140] A significant decrease in the systolic blood pressure greater than 20% from baseline was found in 16% versus 68% in the 6.5 mg and 9.5 mg groups respectively. A systematic review by Arzola and Wieczorek reported a risk reduction (RR) in hypotension with doses less than 8 mg to be RR 0.78.[105] It is now widely acknowledged that low doses of spinal anaesthetic are associated with less hypotension with reduced sympathetic blockade. In keeping with this, the block is also of shorter duration and the patient is at increased risk of perioperative discomfort. Subsequently low-dose techniques are only recommended for use as a part of a CSE technique where the epidural catheter can be used to top-up a regressing block, prevent discomfort, and prolong the duration of anaesthesia. Opioids are added to the intrathecal injection to intensify the sensory block without adding to the sympatholytic effect.

Opponents of low-dose spinal anaesthesia argue that current strategies to limit hypotension are much improved and therefore intrathecal dose reductions are unnecessary and put the patient at risk of intraoperative discomfort. Indeed, with tailored fluid administration and phenylephrine infusion regimens blood pressure can be maintained at near baseline values.[153] However, excessive vasopressor use has been associated with maternal morbidity.[154] Phenylephrine infusions reduce cardiac output in healthy elective parturients, but this has not yet been associated with any detrimental maternal or fetal effects.[155] It is unknown what the impact of reducing maternal cardiac output is on a compromised fetus in a high-risk pregnancy. Low-dose CSE techniques may counteract the haemodynamic derangement in the first instance and avoid effects of excessive vasopressor use.[140] Apart from the reduction in hypotension and nausea and vomiting, further advantages of a low-dose CSE may include faster recovery from motor blockade and discharge from the post-anaesthetic care unit.[156]

The lower intrathecal dose requires modification of standard techniques to provide an anaesthetic block adequate for the duration of surgery and to prevent intraoperative discomfort. Arzola and Wieczorek calculated the risk of intraoperative analgesic supplementation in low-dose anaesthetic techniques to be more than three times higher than in conventional dose groups.[105] This meta-analysis excluded studies that used mixed interventions such EVE or pre-emptive epidural top-up and advocates of low-dose anaesthesia emphasize that it is these interventions that are integral to improving outcomes.[157] Nevertheless, the increased risk of intraoperative discomfort and potential for complaint and litigation is a valid concern and has limited the widespread use of low doses.[158]

Modifications for low-dose CSE may include an initial steep Trendelenburg position and/or EVE to improve the spread of the small spinal dose and obtain a satisfactory sensory block level.

Hyperbaric bupivacaine is recommended. The resulting block is less dense and a block to touch may not be detected. A shorter duration of effective anaesthesia necessitates prudent time keeping, checking for block regression, and pre-emptive epidural top-up to avoid intraoperative discomfort.[157] Experience with the technique and good communication between patient, anaesthetist, and obstetrician has been associated with good outcomes,[55] but above all the dose reduction must not be at expense of patient discomfort.

Low-dose sequential or incremental combined spinal–epidural

Low-dose incremental or sequential CSE comprises an intrathecal injection of a small dose of local anaesthetic (4–8 mg hyperbaric bupivacaine), with or without a dose of opioid, followed by gradual epidural top-ups. The resulting initial sensory block is deliberately not adequate for proceeding with surgery and further incremental boluses of epidural local anaesthetic are administered until satisfactory anaesthesia is achieved.

The aim of this technique is to avoid any haemodynamic instability caused by a rapid onset spinal block and may be beneficial in women with severe cardiac or respiratory morbidity in whom it is desirable to avoid sudden precipitant drops in blood pressure or changes to systemic vascular resistance and cardiac output.

Traditionally these high-risk CDs have been carried out under general anaesthesia following a modified rapid sequence induction. The sequential CSE may provide a safe alternative in appropriate circumstances.[33]

A low-dose sequential CSE is also useful when the dose of spinal is in question, for example, in patients with very short stature or in the morbidly obese parturients. In short women, a small spinal dose can be used and then if block height not achieved, the epidural is used. In the very obese woman, a standard spinal dose may result in a high block and necessitate a general anaesthetic, which one has tried to avoid in the first place. A smaller spinal dose in these challenging patients may produce the requisite block height but if surgery is prolonged, then the epidural can be brought into play.

Stand-alone epidurals are also used for incremental anaesthesia but compared to sequential CSE are more likely to be associated with inadequate anaesthesia.

Epidural volume extension

EVE is occasionally used in low-dose CSE to increase block height after intrathecal injection. In studies, 5–10 mL saline is injected either through the epidural catheter into the extradural space or directly through the epidural needle after the spinal injection.[144] Evidence suggests this causes compression of the dural sac and cephalad spread of intrathecal local anaesthetic. EVE may work if given within 20 minutes of the spinal injection but is unlikely to have an effect afterwards as the local anaesthetic becomes fixed at its site of action and block regression commences. Effects should last up to 30 minutes.[159]

Blumgart et al. injected 10 mL saline or 10 mL 0.5% bupivacaine into the epidural space in pregnant patients undergoing planned CD under CSE and demonstrated an extension in sensory block height of up to four dermatomes and significantly faster onset compared to a control group who received no EVE.[160] Since there was no significant difference between the bupivacaine and saline groups they concluded that the block spread was a volume effect and using bupivacaine for EVE had no advantage over saline. Myelographic studies in non-pregnant patients undergoing CSE anaesthesia for elective surgery have shown a 75% reduction in subarachnoid space diameter together with cephalad spread of intrathecal contrast after 10 mL epidural saline injection.[161] Beale et al. found that the median effective dose (ED_{50}) of hyperbaric bupivacaine for CD could not be significantly reduced with the addition of 7 mL of saline during EVE; however, if sustaining a block to a minimum of 45 minutes were to be removed from the study criteria then the ED_{50} could have been significantly lower in the EVE group. This confirms the ability of EVE to increase intrathecal local anaesthetic spread to an adequate block height but acknowledges that the duration of this block is reduced.[162] Loubert et al. did not demonstrate any increase in sensory block height after using 5 mL saline EVE (in the sitting position, via the epidural needle immediately after the spinal injection) following a low-dose CSE technique.[144]

Continuous spinal anaesthesia

Continuous spinal anaesthesia involves using a microcatheter (28 G) or small-gauge catheter into the intrathecal space to provide analgesia and anaesthesia. Theoretically this technique offers many advantages—an accurate, continuous, titratable, dense spinal block of rapid onset and the ability to use low doses and minimize haemodynamic instability. However, the technique remains underutilized due to unavailability and unfamiliarity with the necessary equipment, technical difficulty, high failure rates, and an increase in PDPH rates.[163,164] In addition there are currently no randomized studies and a lack of consensus regarding choice and dose of local anaesthetic in continuous spinal anaesthesia. The advantages and disadvantages of continuous spinal anaesthesia are summarized in Table 20.7.

In the early 1990s, Rigler et al. reported a small case series of cauda equina syndrome and permanent neurological injury following the use of 28–32 G spinal microcatheters with hyperbaric 5% lidocaine in general surgical and orthopaedic patients.[165] It was hypothesized that the narrow internal diameter of the microcatheters encouraged slow laminar flow of local anaesthetic resulting in nerve roots being exposed to very high concentrations as opposed to a more widespread distribution of the solution

Table 20.7 Advantages and disadvantages of continuous spinal anaesthesia

Advantages	Disadvantages
Rapid onset	Lack of available equipment
Titratable dense block, haemodynamic stability	Technical insertion difficulties, high failure rate
Continuous	Increased risk of postdural puncture headache
Advantages in women after spinal surgery with scarred epidural space	Risk of being mistaken for epidural catheter and dosing errors
	Care required when dosing, calculation of catheter dead-space needed

throughout the CSF.[165] The US Food and Drug Administration subsequently withdrew licensing of catheters smaller than 24 G.

A subsequent study of 28 G catheters for continuous labour analgesia found no incidence of permanent neurological injury. However, the primary medication administered was an opioid, with bupivacaine added only for breakthrough pain.[164] More recently in Spain, Alonso et al. trialled 22–24 G spinal catheters for women undergoing planned CD but concluded that the unacceptably high failure rate (20%) and PDPH rate (29%) currently limited the use of this technique in the obstetric population.[163]

A UK study of 24 G microcatheters (Spinocath® B. Braun, Melsungen AG, Germany) in high-risk parturients for elective CD found it a useful technique to maintain haemodynamic stability. Only one procedure failed but nearly 25% of women required IV analgesic supplementation in the intraoperative period and 9% of patients experienced PDPH.[166]

At present the complications of continuous spinal techniques outweigh the potential benefits and in most circumstances using a CSE is more appropriate. However, possible useful indications include patients with previous spinal surgery and scarring of the epidural space (restricting epidural local anaesthetic flow), high-risk cardiac patients, and those in whom epidural placement is difficult or more likely to fail, for example, in morbid obesity.[167]

More commonly a continuous spinal is encountered as a result of inadvertent dural tap with an epidural needle or after a 'catheter tap' while threading the epidural catheter epidurally. Following an inadvertent dural tap, the 18–20 G epidural catheter can subsequently be deliberately inserted into the intrathecal space and used as a spinal catheter. The practice of leaving the epidural catheter in the intrathecal space may reduce the requirement for an epidural blood patch should a PDPH arise following the dural tap.[168] While providing excellent anaesthesia, care must be taken not to mistake the spinal catheter for an epidural one and putting the patient at risk of a high block or total spinal anaesthesia after inadvertent large volume injection. It is important to remember the epidural catheter and filter has more than 1 mL of dead-space so a continuous spinal catheter should be flushed with 2 mL of saline after each bolus dose.[167]

Although spinal catheters placed after accidental dural puncture may work well in labour, they are often problematic when attempting to use them for CD. There is the dead-space issue raised previously. In addition, the spread of the local anaesthetic depends on which orifice the local anaesthetic exits from. This varies depending on the pressure used to inject—a large pressure will force the injectate through the distal holes with further spread, less force will result in exit through the proximal holes with less spread. As a result, the spinal catheter top-up for CD is not reliable and many operators would prefer to abandon the spinal catheter and perform a single-shot spinal with more consistency instead.

Adjuvants

The addition of adjuvants to the intrathecal local anaesthetic injection can prolong anaesthesia and increase the time until additional analgesia is required. Safety data on several potential agents (e.g. neostigmine, midazolam, and magnesium) is lacking and these should not be used in routine clinical practice until further evidence is available.[169] (See also Chapter 17.)

Intrauterine resuscitation

Obstetricians use antepartum fetal assessment to make decisions about the timing and method of delivery. This is important for anaesthetists, as lack of familiarity with fetal assessment tools and their significance can lead to poor communication delaying delivery or a suboptimal choice of anaesthetic technique. Fetal assessment and decisions related to it may also have significant medicolegal implications[170] (see Chapter 6).

When electronic FHR monitoring shows suspicious or pathological traces, it may be possible to instigate intrauterine neonatal resuscitation measures with the aim to reverse any hypoxia that might lead to further deterioration. It should start as soon as the obstetrician/midwife makes the diagnosis of fetal compromise and continued into the operating theatre. Any resultant improvement in FHR may eliminate the need for an operative delivery or allow time for neuraxial anaesthesia for a vaginal or CD. Thurlow and Kinsella provide a good acronym for fetal resuscitation, 'SPOILT' (see Box 20.6).[171]

1. Discontinuing oxytocin: uterine blood flow is minimal at the peak of uterine contractions, which may lead to disruption of gas exchange. In normal conditions the fetus has adaptive mechanisms to compensate for this but when there is excessive uterine activity and insufficient time between contractions, fetal hypoxia and acidaemia can occur. Excessive contractions can be the result of iatrogenic oxytocin or prostaglandin and are associated with prolonged decelerations, bradycardias, or late decelerations; therefore stopping the oxytocin is warranted. Reduction in uterine activity does not happen immediately and may warrant use of a tocolytic drug.[172]
2. Position change: the first action should be to move the mother into the left or right lateral position to avoid aortocaval compression, so maximizing venous return, cardiac output, and ultimately uteroplacental perfusion.
3. Oxygen supplementation: intuitively the obvious way to improve oxygenation of the fetus would be to administer supplemental oxygen to the mother, but the data supporting its benefits to the fetus have been inconsistent. Early studies showed that maternal oxygen reduced late decelerations within

Box 20.6 'SPOILT'—intrauterine resuscitation

1. Syntocinon® off
2. Position full left lateral
3. Oxygen
4. IV infusion of 1 L crystalloid
5. Low blood pressure: IV vasopressor
6. Tocolysis: terbutaline 250 mcg (SC), glyceryl trinitrate 400 mcg (metered aerosol doses)

a few minutes,[173] but then this may only be beneficial if given for a short period of time and may precipitate fetal acidosis if given for extended periods.[174] Maternal oxygen administration during labour has gone out of vogue since the 2003 Cochrane meta-analysis which concluded that there was not sufficient evidence that maternal oxygen administration improved fetal oxygenation in labour, although most of the studies in this review excluded women with non-reassuring FHR patterns.[175] The recent use of fetal pulse oximetry has been used to determine the effects of maternal oxygenation during labour; administration of 100% oxygen (using a non-rebreathing facemask) has been shown to improve fetal oxygen saturation, with the greatest increase seen in those fetuses with an initial fetal oxygen saturation of less than 40%.[176,177] However, these studies have been too small to show any difference in neonatal outcome. Studies by Khaw et al. and Noh et al. have reported that high inspired oxygen fraction can cause an increase in oxygen free radical activity in maternal blood and that lipid peroxidation levels and antioxidant capacity in umbilical venous blood were higher in patients delivering by planned CD.[178,179] They suggested that both the mother and fetus are exposed to higher oxidative stress during CD. Clearly this is a balance of risks and it would seem sensible to give oxygen if maternal saturations were less than 95% and on balance oxygen should be given at high flow for a short period of time to see if there is improvement in fetal status.

4. Increased IV hydration: as oxygenation of the fetus is highly dependent on uterine blood flow and placenta perfusion, an optimal intravascular volume is necessary. Fluid restriction policies may result in maternal dehydration, which may be precipitated in women in prolonged labour. A bolus of 1000 mL of lactated Ringer's solution over 20 minutes significantly increases fetal oxygen saturation, which can last for more than 30 minutes.[176,180] Boluses of IV crystalloids also appear to have a mild tocolytic effect thought to be mediated by atrial natriuretic peptide release by distention of the atrium as well as some benefits due to reduced blood viscosity.[176] Caution should be observed in giving repeated boluses of IV fluids in pre-eclamptic woman and those on corticosteroids and beta-mimetic agents as these women are at increased risk of pulmonary oedema.
5. Avoidance of hypotension: similar to increasing intravascular volume by fluid, maintenance of blood pressure and placental blood flow is vital. Initiation of neuraxial blockade can result in hypotension, particularly if the woman is dehydrated. Vasopressors, such as phenylephrine, should be used to maintain blood pressure and placental perfusion.
6. Administration of tocolytics: excessive contractions can cause placental hypoperfusion. It can occur with or without the administration of synthetic oxytocin but it is important to exclude underlying serious pathology such as an abruption. Administration of a tocolytic agent can decrease the uterine activity and improve the FHR allowing labour to continue or to allow time for staff utilization, that is, getting a second anaesthetist/obstetrician or opening a second operating theatre.[181] The optimal tocolytic agent has not been found and individual departments should have protocols for their preferred drugs. Beta-agonists drugs such as terbutaline 250 mcg administered subcutaneously or IV salbutamol 100 mcg is the most commonly used drug for this purpose in the United Kingdom. Ritodrine is no longer recommended due to its high side effect profile. Glycerol trinitrate, although not licensed as a tocolytic, has a fast onset of action and can be given as a 400 mcg metered dose sublingually or 100–400 mcg IV. Maternal hypotension is a major side effect but can be treated easily with vasopressors.[182] Magnesium sulphate (4 g IV over 20 minutes) can also provide emergency tocolysis.[183]

A woman with a poorly working labour epidural requiring emergency caesarean delivery

Complications during CD such as pain and discomfort that may necessitate conversion to general anaesthesia can often be predicted with knowledge of how the epidural worked during labour—a golden rule should be that a poorly working labour epidural should not be used to top-up for a surgical delivery. This again emphasizes the importance of regular ward rounds and assurance that all labour epidurals are working effectively, a poorly working labour epidural should be removed and replaced.

A dilemma occurs when a top-up has been given and there is no or only a partially adequate block. Perhaps the best option is to do a sequential epidural top-up (injecting small doses, e.g. 5 mL of local anaesthetic epidurally, assessing the block height after a few minutes). If after 10 mL of local anaesthetic there is no cephalad spread and the patient is still feeling her contractions or the block is not bilateral, the epidural should be abandoned and an alternative method used. If time allows, manipulation of an epidural (i.e. by withdrawing the catheter 1 cm) can improve successful conversion to surgical anaesthesia in up 80% of poorly working epidurals.[133]

The concern is that performing an intrathecal injection following a long-standing epidural could result in a high spinal. This may occur in a number of ways; the large volume within the epidural space could cause sac compression resulting in a higher intrathecal block. Alternatively, a high spinal may arise from diffusing local anaesthetic in the epidural space or leakage of it into the CSF via the hole in the dural sac.[184–186] In some units, it is standard practice to remove a poorly functioning epidural and use a CSE or a single-shot spinal technique. Furst looked retrospectively at 1393 operative deliveries in a 2-year period; 672 (48%) received epidural blockade, of these 32 (5%) were identified as providing inadequate anaesthesia and an alternate mode required.[186] Twenty-seven of these 32 patients (84%) received subsequent spinal block, while the rest underwent induction of general anaesthesia. Of those patients who received both epidural and subarachnoid anaesthesia, three cases of high spinal anaesthesia were recorded making an incidence of 11%. They found the incidence in the same population having spinal anaesthesia alone (i.e. those that did not have an *in situ* epidural) was 0.2%. During the data collection period they did not have a standard dose of intrathecal bupivacaine; the mean dose used was approximately 12.0 mg of heavy bupivacaine, this did not differ greatly in patients in whom high spinal anaesthesia did or did not occur. In their discussion they recommended that a reduced dose of local anaesthesia is used (20% less) and allowing the local anaesthesia to 'set' for 60–90 seconds prior to placing the patient supine. However, this runs the risk of a low block. Other units use a standard intrathecal dose with no incidence of high block. High blocks can be avoided with the an Oxford pillow technique where the head is ramped much higher than the shoulders or tilting the table head-up once the desired block height is achieved.

At present there are no studies to recommend the safest intrathecal dose of bupivacaine following an inadequate labour epidural. Many would advocate the use of a CSE technique with reduced dose of intrathecal local anaesthetic and then using the epidural catheter component to titrate to achieve an adequate block. Full resuscitation facilities should be available to manage a high spinal block or provide a rapid and safe conversion to general anaesthesia. (See also Chapter 21.)

Table 20.8 Troubleshooting neuraxial blockade for caesarean delivery

Spinal-induced hypotension	*Causes* ◆ Rapid cephalic spread of anaesthesia ◆ Drop in systemic vascular resistance ◆ Sympathetic blockade ◆ Aortocaval compression
	Consequences ◆ Maternal nausea and vomiting, dizziness ◆ Loss of consciousness or death if limited cardiovascular reserve or pre-existing morbidity ◆ Reduced uteroplacental perfusion ◆ Fetal compromise and asphyxia ◆ Neonatal acidosis, poor outcome
	Management ◆ Multimodal approach, aim to keep systolic blood pressure within 10% of baseline ◆ Left lateral positioning and uterine displacement ◆ Crystalloid or colloid pre- and/or co-loading ◆ Low-dose CSE or incremental anaesthesia, epidural volume extension ◆ Vasopressor use, e.g. phenylephrine (α-adrenergic receptor agonist) bolus 50–100 mcg or infusion 25–100 mcg/min
Intraoperative nausea and vomiting	*Causes* ◆ Multifactorial ◆ Stimulation of area postrema in chemoreceptor trigger zone ◆ Stimulation of vomiting zone in medullary lateral reticular formation ◆ Vagal input from exteriorization of uterus, organ manipulation, visceral pain, peritoneal stimulation ◆ Cerebral hypoperfusion secondary to spinal-induced hypotension, bleeding or aortocaval compression ◆ Dopaminergic, muscarinic, tryptaminergic, histaminic, and opioid receptor stimulation ◆ IV opioids ◆ Entonox® ◆ Uterotonic agents: ergometrine (dopaminergic and serotoninergic stimulation), oxytocin (hypotension via nitric oxide and atrial natriuretic peptide release), and carboprost (prostaglandin F_2-α gastrointestinal tract stimulation)
	Consequences ◆ Maternal discomfort and reduced maternal satisfaction ◆ Pulmonary aspiration ◆ Difficult operating conditions
	Management ◆ Prevention and prompt treatment of hypotension ◆ Use of neuraxial opioids (analgesic, improve block quality, anxiolytic, dose-sparing) ◆ Reduce surgical stimuli ◆ Cautious use of uterotonic agents ◆ Pharmacological antiemetic prophylaxis not routine ◆ Antiemetics to treat existing nausea and vomiting (e.g. metoclopramide, antihistamines, 5-HT_3 antagonists)—used in practice; however, not enough data available to support efficacy

continued

Table 20.8 Continued

Pruritus	*Cause* ◆ Caused by neuraxial opioids, exact mechanism unclear, likely interaction between diamorphine and 5-HT_3 receptors in spinal cord and medulla ◆ Particularly common following intrathecal or epidural morphine ◆ Always exclude allergic reaction
	Management ◆ Serotonin 5-HT_3 antagonists, e.g. ondansetron, reduce incidence of severe pruritus and number of patients requiring treatment ◆ Opioid antagonists, e.g. naloxone (50–100 mcg), disadvantage is antanalgesic effect and patient should be warned ◆ Propofol (subhypnotic doses)—conflicting evidence of efficacy ◆ Antihistamines (e.g. chlorpheniramine) unlikely to be of use as neuraxial opioid-induced pruritus is not related to histamine release
Managing a high block	*Cause* ◆ Individual variation in response ◆ Anatomical abnormalities ◆ Subdural injection ◆ Intrathecal administration of epidural intended solution
	Features ◆ Weak upper limb function and hand paraesthesia ◆ Altered voice ◆ intercostal muscle paralysis ◆ Respiratory failure (total spinal) ◆ Profound hypotension and bradycardia ◆ Loss of consciousness
	Management ◆ Reassurance, explanation of events to patient, their partner, and team ◆ Change in position, head-up tilt ◆ Supplemental oxygen ◆ Circulatory support with fluids and vasopressors ◆ General anaesthesia and endotracheal intubation if required
Intraoperative discomfort	*Causes* ◆ Inadequate neuraxial anaesthesia, block failure ◆ Prolonged surgery, neuraxial block regression ◆ Increased surgical stimulation, e.g. uterine exteriorization ◆ Different patient expectations
	Actions ◆ Temporarily stop surgery ◆ Communicate with patient to establish nature of pain or discomfort ◆ Assess level of sensory block ◆ Reassure and offer prompt management ◆ Document events
	Management Will depend on timing (i.e. at incision, during delivery, skin closure, etc.), degree of discomfort and patient preference: ◆ Reassurance ◆ IV opioid analgesia, e.g. fentanyl, alfentanil, remifentanil ◆ Epidural top-up with local anaesthesia and/or opioid ◆ Entonox® ◆ Local anaesthetic infiltration of surgical field but beware of local anaesthetic toxicity if epidural top-up has been given as maximum doses may already have been achieved ◆ Repeatedly offer general anaesthesia as alternative strategy ◆ General anaesthesia ◆ Documentation of events ◆ Follow-up

continued

Table 20.8 Continued

Failed regional technique	*Causes* ◆ Injection into the wrong space, e.g. following a false loss of resistance or needle displacement ◆ Anatomical deviations, e.g. scoliosis, presence of an epidural or dural septum or distorted anatomy following back surgery ◆ Technical difficulty due to patient positioning, patient discomfort, obesity or anaesthetic inexperience
	Action ◆ Sensory block testing and identification if any block present ◆ Seek help if necessary ◆ Devise an alternate strategy ◆ Explain events and plan to the patient ◆ Document
	Management Alternative management will depend on the difficulty previously encountered, the patient, and any current degree of anaesthesia. For elective CD there is no urgency and plan B should not compromise patient safety. Consider: ◆ Repeating the procedure ◆ Alternative regional technique, e.g. CSE—particularly useful if patient has existing partial block and incremental anaesthesia will avoid a high block ◆ General anaesthesia

Troubleshooting

See Table 20.8.

Recovery

Following CD, specific observations are carried out to monitor recovery from anaesthesia, manage postoperative discomfort, and check for obstetric complications such as uterine atony and postpartum haemorrhage.

Basic observations such as blood pressure, heart rate, respiratory rate, urine output, and pain and sedation scores should be carried out half-hourly for 2 hours and hourly for 4 hours provided all is well.[7] Most obstetric units now record observations on 'early warning score' charts to guide midwifery and nursing staff when to seek help should any observations deviate from the norm. (See Figure 35.3 in Chapter 35 for an example of an early warning chart used in obstetrics.)

Due to the potential risks of delayed respiratory depression, it is recommended that following intrathecal diamorphine or morphine the woman should be monitored as above for 12 or 24 hours respectively.[7] Women with pre-existing comorbidities or perioperative anaesthetic or obstetric complications may be at increased risk and a more intensively monitored environment such as an obstetric high dependency unit may be appropriate.

Pregnancy and surgery increase the risk of venous thromboembolism and each woman should undergo a risk assessment for thrombosis. The method of thromboprophylaxis required may include hydration, early mobilization, graduated stockings, pneumatic compression devices, and/or low-molecular-weight heparin.

All women who undergo CD should have a follow-up within 24 hours by anaesthetic staff to check for signs or symptoms of complications from neuraxial blockade such as PDPH or epidural haematoma. It is also an opportunity to assess maternal satisfaction, answer questions, or explain any untoward events that may have occurred, for example, perioperative discomfort or the need for a general anaesthetic compared to neuraxial block.

Enhanced recovery

Increasingly popular is the concept known as 'enhanced recovery'. Well established in other specialities (e.g. orthopaedics), the programme has yet to become widespread in obstetric services.[187]

A recent UK survey found that only 6% of maternity departments had an enhanced recovery programme, were implementing one, or considering doing so and a French questionnaire found that although the concept is feasible, the majority of patients remain hospitalized for more than 72 hours.[188,189]

The principle underpinning enhanced recovery is that right from the point of booking a planned CD the woman enters a pathway designed to minimize physical and emotional stress responses and encourage a swift recovery to normality postoperatively. Multidisciplinary staff and the patient themselves have proactive roles in delivering this service. With regard to CD, this may include preoperative education on analgesia and breastfeeding, an increasing awareness of 'what to expect', and haemoglobin optimization. Starvation times should be kept to a minimum, preoperative antibiotics administered, neuraxial opioids used for postoperative analgesia, surgery kept as minimally invasive as possible (smallest possible incision and avoidance of postoperative drains), and thromboprophylaxis undertaken. Following surgery, the patient should be allowed to eat and drink, the urinary catheter removed once anaesthesia has worn off to allow early mobilization, and regular analgesia commenced. If all postoperative observations are satisfactory with mother and baby, the length of hospital stay may be able to be reduced from 3–4 nights to 1–2 nights. Implementation and success of enhanced recovery relies on regular follow-up and support from community healthcare professionals and a safety net for when problems are encountered.[190]

Conclusion

CD should be a safe and rewarding experience for the parturient. While neuraxial or general anaesthesia are both acceptable, neuraxial anaesthesia is preferable in order to minimize the risks of a general anaesthetic and to allow the mother to participate in the birth. While this is possible in the majority of elective CDs with a range of techniques being successfully employed, there is still debate as to the optimal neuraxial technique in the emergency situation. Guidelines for obstetric units should strive to organize services to minimize the time taken to deliver the baby while maximizing the analgesia, safety, and positive experience for the mother.

References

1. Organisation for Economic Co-operation and Development. *Health at a Glance 2011: OECD Indicators*. Paris: OECD; 2011.
2. Hospital Episode Statistics. *NHS Maternity Statistics - 2013–2014*. 2013 [Online] http://www.hscic.gov.uk/pubs/maternity1213
3. Bragg F, Cromwell DA, Edozien LC, *et al*. Variation in rates of caesarean section among English NHS trusts after accounting for maternal and clinical risk: cross sectional study. *BMJ* 2010; 341:c5065.
4. Hehir MP, O'Connor HD, Kent EM, *et al*. Changes in vaginal breech delivery rates in a single large metropolitan area. *Am J Obstet Gynecol* 2012; 206(6):498.e1–4.
5. Black C, Kaye JA, Jick H. Cesarean delivery in the United Kingdom: time trends in the general practice research database. *Obstet Gynecol* 2005; 106(1):151–5.
6. D'Souza R, Arulkumaran S. To 'C' or not to 'C'? Caesarean delivery upon maternal request: a review of facts, figures and guidelines. *J Perinat Med* 2013; 41(1):5–15.
7. National Institute for Health and Care Excellence. *Caesarean Section*. Clinical Guideline 132. London: National Institute for Health and Care Excellence; 2011 (reviewed 2014).
8. MacDorman MF, Declercq E, Menacker F, *et al*. Neonatal mortality for primary cesarean and vaginal births to low-risk women: application of an 'intention-to-treat' model. *Birth* 2008; 35(1):3–8.
9. O'Sullivan G. *Statement on Emergency Caesarean Section Rates*. London: Royal College of Obstetricians and Gynaecologists; 2013. http://www.rcog.org.uk/news/rcog-statement-emergency-caesarean-section-rates.
10. Royal College of Obstetricians and Gynaecologists. *Classification of Urgency of Caesarean Section—A Continuum of Risk*. Good Practice No. 11. London: Royal College of Obstetricians and Gynaecologist; 2011. http://www.rcog.org.uk/files/rcog-corp/GoodPractice11ClassificationofUrgency.pdf
11. Lucas DN, Yentis SM, Kinsella SM, *et al*. Urgency of caesarean section: a new classification. *J R Soc Med* 2000; 93(7):346–50.
12. Dupuis O, Sayegh I, Decullier E, *et al*. Red, orange and green caesarean sections: a new communication tool for on-call obstetricians. *Eur J Obstet Gynecol Reprod Biol* 2008; 140(2):206–11.
13. Windle WF. Brain damage at birth. Functional and structural modifications with time. *JAMA* 1968; 206(9):1967–72.
14. Myers RE. Four patterns of perinatal brain damage and their conditions of occurrence in primates. *Adv Neurol* 1975; 10:223–34.
15. Thomas J, Paranjothy S, Royal College of Obstetricians and Gynaecologists Clinical Effectiveness Support Unit. *The National Sentinel Caesarean Section Audit Report*. London: RCOG Press; 2001.
16. Thomas J, Paranjothy S, James D. National cross sectional survey to determine whether the decision to delivery interval is critical in emergency caesarean section. *BMJ* 2004; 328(7441):665.
17. Tuffnell DJ, Wilkinson K, Beresford N. Interval between decision and delivery by caesarean section-are current standards achievable? Observational case series. *BMJ* 2001; 322(7298):1330–3.
18. MacKenzie IZ, Cooke I. What is a reasonable time from decision-to-delivery by caesarean section? Evidence from 415 deliveries. *BJOG* 2002; 109(5):498–504.
19. Morgan BM, Magni V, Goroszenuik T. Anaesthesia for emergency caesarean section. *Br J Obstet Gynaecol* 1990; 97(5):420–4.
20. Purva M, Russell I, Kinsella M. Caesarean section anaesthesia: a technique and failure rate. In *Raising the Standard: A Compendium of Audit Recipes*. London: Royal College of Anaesthetists; 2012:220–1.
21. Mhyre JM, Riesner MN, Polley LS, *et al*. A series of anesthesia-related maternal deaths in Michigan, 1985–2003. *Anesthesiology* 2007; 106(6):1096–104.
22. Hawkins JL, Koonin LM, Palmer SK, *et al*. Anesthesia-related deaths during obstetric delivery in the united states, 1979–1990. *Anesthesiology* 1997; 86(2):277–84.
23. Paech MJ, Scott KL, Clavisi O, *et al*. A prospective study of awareness and recall associated with general anaesthesia for caesarean section. *Int J Obstet Anesth* 2008; 17(4):298–303.
24. Cantwell R, Clutton-Brock T, Cooper G, *et al*. Saving Mothers' Lives: Reviewing maternal deaths to make motherhood safer: 2006–2008. The eighth report of the confidential enquiries into maternal deaths in the United Kingdom. *BJOG* 2011; 118 Suppl 1:1–203.
25. Jenkins JG, Khan MM. Anaesthesia for caesarean section: a survey in a UK region from 1992 to 2002. *Anaesthesia* 2003; 58(11):1114–18.
26. Benhamou D, Wong C. Neuraxial anesthesia for cesarean delivery: what criteria define the 'optimal' technique? *Anesth Analg* 2009; 109(5):1370–3.
27. Marcus HE, Behrend A, Schier R, *et al*. [Anesthesiological management of caesarean sections: nationwide survey in germany]. *Anaesthesist* 2011; 60(10):916–28.
28. Furmanik J. [A survey of anaesthesia for caesarean section in poland]. *Anestezjol Intens Ter* 2010; 42(2):65–9.
29. Rafi MA, Arfeen Z, Misra U. Conversion of regional to general anaesthesia at caesarean section: Increasing the use of regional anaesthesia through continuous prospective audit. *Int J Obstet Anesth* 2010; 19(2):179–82.
30. Kinsella SM. A prospective audit of regional anaesthesia failure in 5080 caesarean sections. *Anaesthesia* 2008; 63(8):822–32.
31. Kathirgamanathan A, Douglas MJ, Tyler J, *et al*. Speed of spinal vs general anaesthesia for category-1 caesarean section: a simulation and clinical observation-based study. *Anaesthesia* 2013; 68(7):753–9.
32. Pollard JB. Common mechanisms and strategies for prevention and treatment of cardiac arrest during epidural anesthesia. *J Clin Anesth* 2002; 14(1):52–6.
33. Hamlyn EL, Douglass CA, Plaat F, *et al*. Low-dose sequential combined spinal-epidural: an anaesthetic technique for caesarean section in patients with significant cardiac disease. *Int J Obstet Anesth* 2005; 14(4):355–61.
34. Wedel DJ, Horlocker TT. Regional anesthesia in the febrile or infected patient. *Reg Anesth Pain Med* 2006; 31(4):324–33.
35. Neal JM, Bernards CM, Hadzic A, *et al*. ASRA practice advisory on neurologic complications in regional anesthesia and pain medicine. *Reg Anesth Pain Med* 2008; 33(5):404–15.
36. Ruppen W, Derry S, McQuay H, *et al*. Incidence of epidural hematoma, infection, and neurologic injury in obstetric patients with epidural analgesia/anesthesia. *Anesthesiology* 2006; 105(2):394–9.
37. Regional Anaesthesia UK. Regional anaesthesia and patients with abnormalities of coagulation: The Association of Anaesthetists of Great Britain & Ireland the Obstetric Anaesthetists' Association Regional Anaesthesia UK. *Anaesthesia* 2013; 68(9):966–72.
38. Mendelson CL. The aspiration of stomach contents into the lungs during obstetric anesthesia. *Am J Obstet Gynecol* 1946; 52:191–205.
39. O'Sullivan G, Liu B, Hart D, *et al*. Effect of food intake during labour on obstetric outcome: randomised controlled trial. *BMJ* 2009; 338:b784.
40. Association of Anaesthetists of Great Britain and Ireland. *Preoperative Assessment and Patient Preparation: The Role of the Anaesthetist*. AAGBI Safety Guideline. London: AAGBI; 2010. http://www.aagbi.org/sites/default/files/preop2010.pdf
41. Levy DM, Webster VL. Unrestricted sips of water before caesarean section. *Br J Anaesth* 2004; 92(6):910.

42. Paranjothy S, Griffiths JD, Broughton HK, *et al.* Interventions at caesarean section for reducing the risk of aspiration pneumonitis. *Cochrane Database Syst Rev* 2014; 2:CD004943.
43. Ewart MC, Yau G, Gin T, *et al.* A comparison of the effects of omeprazole and ranitidine on gastric secretion in women undergoing elective caesarean section. *Anaesthesia* 1990; 45(7):527–30.
44. Escolano F, Castaño J, López R, *et al.* Effects of omeprazole, ranitidine, famotidine and placebo on gastric secretion in patients undergoing elective surgery. *Br J Anaesth* 1992; 69(4):404–6.
45. Clark K, Lam LT, Gibson S, *et al.* The effect of ranitidine versus proton pump inhibitors on gastric secretions: a meta-analysis of randomised control trials. *Anaesthesia* 2009; 64(6):652–7.
46. Murphy DF, Nally B, Gardiner J, *et al.* Effect of metoclopramide on gastric emptying before elective and emergency caesarean section. *Br J Anaesth* 1984; 56(10):1113–6.
47. General Medical Council. *Consent Guidance: Patients and Doctors Making Decisions Together.* [Online] http://www.gmc-uk.org/guidance/ethical_guidance/consent_guidance_index.asp
48. Obstetric Anaesthetists' Association. *Your Anaesthetic for Caesarean Section.* London: OAA; 2009. http://www.labourpains.com/ui/content/content.aspx?ID=330
49. Cook TM, Counsell D, Wildsmith JAW. Major complications of central neuraxial block: report on the third national audit project of the Royal College of Anaesthetists. *Br J Anaesth* 2009; 102(2):179–90.
50. World Health Organization. *WHO Guidelines for Safe Surgery 2009: Safe Surgery Saves Lives.* [Online] http://www.who.int/patientsafety/safesurgery/tools_resources/9789241598552/en/
51. de Vries EN, Prins HA, Crolla RM, *et al.* Effect of a comprehensive surgical safety system on patient outcomes. *N Engl J Med* 2010; 363(20):1928–37.
52. Kearns RJ, Uppal V, Bonner J, *et al.* The introduction of a surgical safety checklist in a tertiary referral obstetric centre. *BMJ Qual Saf* 2011; 20(9):818–22.
53. Hebl JR. The importance and implications of aseptic techniques during regional anesthesia. *Reg Anesth Pain Med* 2006; 31(4):311–23.
54. Department of Health (DOH). *Uniforms and Workwear: An Evidence Base for Developing Local Policy.* London: DOH; 2007. http://webarchive.nationalarchives.gov.uk/20130107105354/http://www.dh.gov.uk/prod_consum_dh/groups/dh_digitalassets/documents/digitalasset/dh_078435.pdf
55. Benhamou D, Bouaziz H, Chassard D, *et al.* Anaesthetic practices for scheduled caesarean delivery: a 2005 French national survey. *Eur J Anaesthesiol* 2009; 26(8):694–700.
56. Hurford DM, De Zoysa N. Rapid sequence spinal anaesthesia—a survey of current use. *Anaesthesia* 2012; 67(11):1284–5.
57. Checketts MR. Wash & go—but with what? Skin antiseptic solutions for central neuraxial block. *Anaesthesia* 2012; 67(8):819–22.
58. Malhotra S, Dharmadasa A, Yentis SM. One vs two applications of chlorhexidine/ethanol for disinfecting the skin: Implications for regional anaesthesia. *Anaesthesia* 2011; 66(7):574–8.
59. Bogod D. The sting in the tail: antiseptics and the neuraxis revisited. *Anaesthesia* 2012; 67(12):1305–9.
60. Killeen T, Kamat A, Walsh D, *et al.* Severe adhesive arachnoiditis resulting in progressive paraplegia following obstetric spinal anaesthesia: a case report and review. *Anaesthesia* 2012; 67(12):1386–94.
61. Evans L, Cunningham M, Tilakaratna P. Chlorhexidine droplet splash from a skin preparation gallipot: effect of height of pouring. *Anaesthesia* 2013; 68(12):1243–6.
62. Kenyon S, Pike K, Jones DR, *et al.* Childhood outcomes after prescription of antibiotics to pregnant women with spontaneous preterm labour: 7-year follow-up of the ORACLE II trial. *Lancet* 2008; 372(9646):1319–27.
63. Kenyon SL, Taylor DJ, Tarnow-Mordi W, *et al.* Broad-spectrum antibiotics for preterm, prelabour rupture of fetal membranes: The ORACLE I randomised trial. ORACLE collaborative group. *Lancet* 2001; 357(9261):979–88.
64. McIlmoyle K, Young S. Antibiotic timing at caesarean section. *Int J Obstet Anesth* 2012; 21(3):283–4.
65. Reynolds F. Damage to the conus medullaris following spinal anaesthesia. *Anaesthesia* 2001; 56(3):238–47.
66. Broadbent CR, Maxwell WB, Ferrie R, *et al.* Ability of anaesthetists to identify a marked lumbar interspace. *Anaesthesia* 2000; 55(11):1122–6.
67. Lee AJ, Ranasinghe JS, Chehade JM, *et al.* Ultrasound assessment of the vertebral level of the intercristal line in pregnancy. *Anesth Analg* 2011; 113(3):559–64.
68. Margarido CB, Mikhael R, Arzola C, *et al.* The intercristal line determined by palpation is not a reliable anatomical landmark for neuraxial anesthesia. *Can J Anaesth* 2011; 58(3):262–6.
69. Shaikh F, Brzezinski J, Alexander S, *et al.* Ultrasound imaging for lumbar punctures and epidural catheterisations: systematic review and meta-analysis. *BMJ* 2013; 346:f1720.
70. Bogod D. Medicolegal implications. In Reynolds F (ed) *Regional Anaesthesia in Obstetrics: A Millennium Update.* London: Springer-Verlag; 2000:371–80.
71. Husain T, Liu YM, Fernando R, *et al.* How UK obstetric anaesthetists assess neuraxial anaesthesia for caesarean delivery: national surveys of practice conducted in 2004 and 2010. *Int J Obstet Anesth* 2013; 22(4):298–302.
72. Russell IF. At caesarean section under regional anaesthesia, it is essential to test sensory block with light touch before allowing surgery to start. *Int J Obstet Anesth* 2006; 15(4):294–7.
73. Walsh P, Columb M, Russell R. A comparison of a neuropen monofilament and ethyl chloride for assessing loss of touch sensation during combined spinal-epidural anaesthesia for caesarean section. *Int J Obstet Anesth* 2010; 19(4):365–72.
74. Yentis SM. Height of confusion: assessing regional blocks before caesarean section. *Int J Obstet Anesth* 2006; 15(1):2–6.
75. Cook TM. Combined spinal-epidural techniques. *Anaesthesia* 2000; 55(1):42–64.
76. Yun EM, Marx GF, Santos AC. The effects of maternal position during induction of combined spinal-epidural anesthesia for cesarean delivery. *Anesth Analg* 1998; 87(3):614–8.
77. Inglis A, Daniel M, McGrady E. Maternal position during induction of spinal anaesthesia for caesarean section. A comparison of right lateral and sitting positions. *Anaesthesia* 1995; 50(4):363–5.
78. Rucklidge MW, Paech MJ, Yentis SM. A comparison of the lateral, oxford and sitting positions for performing combined spinal-epidural anaesthesia for elective caesarean section. *Anaesthesia* 2005; 60(6):535–40.
79. Patel M, Samsoon G, Swami A, Morgan B. Posture and the spread of hyperbaric bupivacaine in parturients using the combined spinal epidural technique. *Can J Anaesth* 1993; 40(10):943–6.
80. Mhyre JM, Greenfield ML, Tsen LC, *et al.* A systematic review of randomized controlled trials that evaluate strategies to avoid epidural vein cannulation during obstetric epidural catheter placement. *Anesth Analg* 2009; 108(4):1232–42.
81. Bahar M, Chanimov M, Cohen ML, *et al.* Lateral recumbent head-down posture for epidural catheter insertion reduces intravascular injection. *Can J Anaesth* 2001; 48(1):48–53.
82. Kinsella SM, Lohmann G. Supine hypotensive syndrome. *Obstet Gynecol* 1994; 83(5 Pt 1):774–88.
83. Cheesman K, Massey S, Preston R, *et al.* Effects of a head elevated ramped position during elective caesarean delivery after combined spinal-epidural anaesthesia. *Int J Obstet Anesth* 2014; 23(2):106–12.
84. Loke GP, Chan EH, Sia AT. The effect of 10 degrees head-up tilt in the right lateral position on the systemic blood pressure after subarachnoid block for caesarean section. *Anaesthesia* 2002; 57(2):169–72.
85. Saito T, Sessler DI, Fujita K, *et al.* Thermoregulatory effects of spinal and epidural anesthesia during cesarean delivery. *Reg Anesth Pain Med* 1998; 23(4):418–23.

86. Matsukawa T, Sessler DI, Sessler AM, *et al.* Heat flow and distribution during induction of general anesthesia. *Anesthesiology* 1995; 82(3):662–73.
87. Horn EP, Bein B, Steinfath M, *et al.* The incidence and prevention of hypothermia in newborn bonding after cesarean delivery: a randomized controlled trial. *Anesth Analg* 2014; 118(5):997–1002.
88. Flores-Maldonado A, Medina-Escobedo CE, Ríos-Rodríguez HM, *et al.* Mild perioperative hypothermia and the risk of wound infection. *Arch Med Res* 2001; 32(3):227–31.
89. Kurz A, Sessler DI, Lenhardt R. Perioperative normothermia to reduce the incidence of surgical-wound infection and shorten hospitalization. Study of wound infection and temperature group. *N Engl J Med* 1996; 334(19):1209–15.
90. Woolnough M, Allam J, Hemingway C, *et al.* Intra-operative fluid warming in elective caesarean section: a blinded randomised controlled trial. *Int J Obstet Anesth* 2009; 18(4):346–51.
91. Yokoyama K, Suzuki M, Shimada Y, *et al.* Effect of administration of pre-warmed intravenous fluids on the frequency of hypothermia following spinal anesthesia for cesarean delivery. *J Clin Anesth* 2009; 21(4):242–8.
92. National Institute for Health and Care Excellence. *Caesarean Section.* Clinical Guideline 132. London: NICE; 2011 (reviewed 2014).
93. Kent AL, Williams J. Increasing ambient operating theatre temperature and wrapping in polyethylene improves admission temperature in premature infants. *J Paediatr Child Health* 2008; 44(6):325–31.
94. Dyer RA, Farina Z, Joubert IA, *et al.* Crystalloid preload versus rapid crystalloid administration after induction of spinal anaesthesia (coload) for elective caesarean section. *Anaesth Intensive Care* 2004; 32(3):351–7.
95. Banerjee A, Stocche RM, Angle P, *et al.* Preload or coload for spinal anesthesia for elective cesarean delivery: a meta-analysis. *Can J Anaesth* 2010; 57(1):24–31.
96. Cyna AM, Andrew M, Emmett RS, *et al.* Techniques for preventing hypotension during spinal anaesthesia for caesarean section. *Cochrane Database Syst Rev* 2006; 4:CD002251.
97. Calthorpe N. The history of spinal needles: getting to the point. *Anaesthesia* 2004; 59(12):1231–41.
98. Shibli KU, Russell IF. A survey of anaesthetic techniques used for caesarean section in the UK in 1997. *Int J Obstet Anesth* 2000; 9(3):160–7.
99. Riley ET, Cohen SE, Macario A, *et al.* Spinal versus epidural anesthesia for cesarean section: a comparison of time efficiency, costs, charges, and complications. *Anesth Analg* 1995; 80(4):709–12.
100. Turnbull DK, Shepherd DB. Post-dural puncture headache: pathogenesis, prevention and treatment. *Br J Anaesth* 2003; 91(5):718–29.
101. Lanz E, Schmitz D. [No effect of injection volume on sensory and motor blockade in isobaric spinal anesthesia]. *Reg Anaesth* 1990; 13(7):153–8.
102. Russell IF. Spinal anesthesia for cesarean delivery with dilute solutions of plain bupivacaine: the relationship between infused volume and spread. *Reg Anesth* 1991; 16(3):130–6.
103. Vercauteren MP, Coppejans HC, Hoffmann VL, *et al.* Small-dose hyperbaric versus plain bupivacaine during spinal anesthesia for cesarean section. *Anesth Analg* 1998; 86(5):989–93.
104. Rout CC, Rocke DA, Levin J, *et al.* A reevaluation of the role of crystalloid preload in the prevention of hypotension associated with spinal anesthesia for elective cesarean section. *Anesthesiology* 1993; 79(2):262–9.
105. Arzola C, Wieczorek PM. Efficacy of low-dose bupivacaine in spinal anaesthesia for caesarean delivery: systematic review and meta-analysis. *Br J Anaesth* 2011; 107(3):308–18.
106. Ginosar Y, Mirikatani E, Drover DR, *et al.* ED50 and ED95 of intrathecal hyperbaric bupivacaine coadministered with opioids for cesarean delivery. *Anesthesiology* 2004; 100(3):676–82.
107. Carvalho B, Durbin M, Drover DR, *et al.* The ED50 and ED95 of intrathecal isobaric bupivacaine with opioids for cesarean delivery. *Anesthesiology* 2005; 103(3):606–12.
108. Norris MC. Patient variables and the subarachnoid spread of hyperbaric bupivacaine in the term parturient. *Anesthesiology* 1990; 72(3):478–82.
109. Harten JM, Boyne I, Hannah P, *et al.* Effects of a height and weight adjusted dose of local anaesthetic for spinal anaesthesia for elective caesarean section. *Anaesthesia* 2005; 60(4):348–53.
110. James KS, Stott SM, McGrady EM, *et al.* Spinal anaesthesia for caesarean section: effect of Sprotte needle orientation. *Br J Anaesth* 1996; 77(2):150–2.
111. Brian JE, Seifen AB, Clark RB, *et al.* Aortic stenosis, cesarean delivery, and epidural anesthesia. *J Clin Anesth* 1993; 5(2):154–7.
112. Brighouse D. Anaesthesia for caesarean section in patients with aortic stenosis: the case for regional anaesthesia. *Anaesthesia* 1998; 53(2):107–9.
113. Ghai B, Mohan V, Khetarpal M, *et al.* Epidural anesthesia for cesarean section in a patient with eisenmenger's syndrome. *Int J Obstet Anesth* 2002; 11(1):44–7.
114. Regan KJ, O'Sullivan G. The extension of epidural blockade for emergency caesarean section: a survey of current UK practice. *Anaesthesia* 2008; 63(2):136–42.
115. Hillyard SG, Bate TE, Corcoran TB, *et al.* Extending epidural analgesia for emergency caesarean section: a meta-analysis. *Br J Anaesth* 2011; 107(5):668–78.
116. Lam DT, Ngan Kee WD, Khaw KS. Extension of epidural blockade in labour for emergency caesarean section using 2% lidocaine with epinephrine and fentanyl, with or without alkalinisation. *Anaesthesia* 2001; 56(8):790–4.
117. Lucas DN, Borra PJ, Yentis SM. Epidural top-up solutions for emergency caesarean section: a comparison of preparation times. *Br J Anaesth* 2000; 84(4):494–6.
118. Goring-Morris J, Russell IF. A randomised comparison of 0.5% bupivacaine with a lidocaine/epinephrine/fentanyl mixture for epidural top-up for emergency caesarean section after 'low dose' epidural for labour. *Int J Obstet Anesth* 2006; 15(2):109–14.
119. Ng K, Parsons J, Cyna AM, *et al.* Spinal versus epidural anaesthesia for caesarean section. *Cochrane Database Syst Rev* 2004(2):CD003765.
120. Sakura S, Sumi M, Kushizaki H, *et al.* Concentration of lidocaine affects intensity of sensory block during lumbar epidural anesthesia. *Anesth Analg* 1999; 88(1):123–7.
121. Marcus MA, Gogarten W, Vertommen JD, *et al.* Haemodynamic effects of repeated epidural test-doses of adrenaline in the chronic maternal-fetal sheep preparation. *Eur J Anaesthesiol* 1998; 15(3):320–3.
122. Lyons G, Columb M, Wilson RC, *et al.* Epidural pain relief in labour: potencies of levobupivacaine and racemic bupivacaine. *Br J Anaesth* 1998; 81(6):899–901.
123. Bader AM, Tsen LC, Camann WR, *et al.* Clinical effects and maternal and fetal plasma concentrations of 0.5% epidural levobupivacaine versus bupivacaine for cesarean delivery. *Anesthesiology* 1999; 90(6):1596–601.
124. Sanders RD, Mallory S, Lucas DN, *et al.* Extending low-dose epidural analgesia for emergency caesarean section using ropivacaine 0.75%. *Anaesthesia* 2004; 59(10):988–92.
125. Sng BL, Pay LL, Sia AT. Comparison of 2% lignocaine with adrenaline and fentanyl, 0.75% ropivacaine and 0.5% levobupivacaine for extension of epidural analgesia for urgent caesarean section after low dose epidural infusion during labour. *Anaesth Intensive Care* 2008; 36(5):659–64.
126. Crosby E, Sandler A, Finucane B, *et al.* Comparison of epidural anaesthesia with ropivacaine 0.5% and bupivacaine 0.5% for caesarean section. *Can J Anaesth* 1998; 45(11):1066–71.
127. Polley LS, Columb MO, Naughton NN, *et al.* Relative analgesic potencies of levobupivacaine and ropivacaine for epidural analgesia in labor. *Anesthesiology* 2003; 99(6):1354–8.

128. Camann WR, Hartigan PM, Gilbertson LI, *et al.* Chloroprocaine antagonism of epidural opioid analgesia: a receptor-specific phenomenon? *Anesthesiology* 1990; 73(5):860–3.
129. Malhotra S, Yentis SM. Extending low-dose epidural analgesia in labour for emergency caesarean section—a comparison of levobupivacaine with or without fentanyl. *Anaesthesia* 2007; 62(7):667–71.
130. Bauer ME, Kountanis JA, Tsen LC, *et al.* Risk factors for failed conversion of labor epidural analgesia to cesarean delivery anesthesia: a systematic review and meta-analysis of observational trials. *Int J Obstet Anesth* 2012; 21(4):294–309.
131. Kinsella M. Obstetric services. In Kinsella M (ed) *Raising the Standards: A Compendium of Audit Recipes.* London: Royal College of Anaesthetists; 2012:151–76.
132. Campbell DC, Tran T. Conversion of epidural labour analgesia to epidural anesthesia for intrapartum cesarean delivery. *Can J Anaesth* 2009; 56(1):19–26.
133. Halpern SH, Soliman A, Yee J, *et al.* Conversion of epidural labour analgesia to anaesthesia for caesarean section: a prospective study of the incidence and determinants of failure. *Br J Anaesth* 2009; 102(2):240–3.
134. Riley ET, Papasin J. Epidural catheter function during labor predicts anesthetic efficacy for subsequent cesarean delivery. *Int J Obstet Anesth* 2002; 11(2):81–4.
135. Pan PH, Bogard TD, Owen MD. Incidence and characteristics of failures in obstetric neuraxial analgesia and anesthesia: a retrospective analysis of 19,259 deliveries. *Int J Obstet Anesth* 2004; 13(4):227–33.
136. Reynolds F, Seed PT. Anaesthesia for caesarean section and neonatal acid-base status: a meta-analysis. *Anaesthesia* 2005; 60(7):636–53.
137. Lee A, Ngan Kee WD, Gin T. A quantitative, systematic review of randomized controlled trials of ephedrine versus phenylephrine for the management of hypotension during spinal anesthesia for cesarean delivery. *Anesth Analg* 2002; 94(4):920–6.
138. Viira DJ, Courtman S, Coghill J. Technical difficulties and complication rates associated with the use of combined spinal-epidural anaesthesia for caesarean section. *Int J Obstet Anesth* 2008; 17(1):86–7.
139. Ranasinghe JS, Steadman J, Toyama T, *et al.* Combined spinal epidural anaesthesia is better than spinal or epidural alone for caesarean delivery. *Br J Anaesth* 2003; 91(2):299–300.
140. Van de Velde M, Van Schoubroeck D, Jani J, *et al.* Combined spinal-epidural anesthesia for cesarean delivery: dose-dependent effects of hyperbaric bupivacaine on maternal hemodynamics. *Anesth Analg* 2006; 103(1):187–90.
141. Choi DH, Ahn HJ, Kim JA. Combined low-dose spinal-epidural anesthesia versus single-shot spinal anesthesia for elective cesarean delivery. *Int J Obstet Anesth* 2006; 15(1):13–17.
142. Blanshard HJ, Cook TM. Use of combined spinal-epidural by obstetric anaesthetists. *Anaesthesia* 2004; 59(9):922–3.
143. Norris MC. Are combined spinal-epidural catheters reliable? *Int J Obstet Anesth* 2000; 9(1):3–6.
144. Loubert C, O'Brien PJ, Fernando R, *et al.* Epidural volume extension in combined spinal epidural anaesthesia for elective caesarean section: a randomised controlled trial. *Anaesthesia* 2011; 66(5):341–7.
145. Ithnin F, Lim Y, Sia AT, *et al.* Combined spinal epidural causes higher level of block than equivalent single-shot spinal anesthesia in elective cesarean patients. *Anesth Analg* 2006; 102(2):577–80.
146. Horstman DJ, Riley ET, Carvalho B. A randomized trial of maximum cephalad sensory blockade with single-shot spinal compared with combined spinal-epidural techniques for cesarean delivery. *Anesth Analg* 2009; 108(1):240–5.
147. Lyons G, Macdonald R, Mikl B. Combined epidural/spinal anaesthesia for caesarean section. Through the needle or in separate spaces? *Anaesthesia* 1992; 47(3):199–201.
148. Stocks GM, Hallworth SP, Fernando R. Evaluation of a spinal needle locking device for use with the combined spinal epidural technique. *Anaesthesia* 2000; 55(12):1185–8.
149. Sadashivaiah J, Wilson R, McLure H, *et al.* Double-space combined spinal-epidural technique for elective caesarean section: a review of 10 years' experience in a UK teaching maternity unit. *Int J Obstet Anesth* 2010; 19(2):183–7.
150. Ginosar Y. Mini-dose single-shot spinal anesthesia for cesarean delivery: for whom the bell-shaped curve tolls. *Int J Obstet Anesth* 2012; 21(3):207–11.
151. Rucklidge MW, Paech MJ. Limiting the dose of local anaesthetic for caesarean section under spinal anaesthesia—has the limbo bar been set too low? *Anaesthesia* 2012; 67(4):347–51.
152. Leo S, Sng BL, Lim Y, *et al.* A randomized comparison of low doses of hyperbaric bupivacaine in combined spinal-epidural anesthesia for cesarean delivery. *Anesth Analg* 2009; 109(5):1600–5.
153. Ngan Kee WD, Khaw KS, Ng FF. Comparison of phenylephrine infusion regimens for maintaining maternal blood pressure during spinal anaesthesia for caesarean section. *Br J Anaesth* 2004; 92(4):469–74.
154. Newell CP, Seller C, Vizhi M, *et al.* Case report: spontaneous coronary artery dissection during elective caesarean section under spinal anaesthesia. *Anaesthesia* 2011; 66(7):615–19.
155. Stewart A, Fernando R, McDonald S, *et al.* The dose-dependent effects of phenylephrine for elective cesarean delivery under spinal anesthesia. *Anesth Analg* 2010; 111(5):1230–7.
156. Teoh WH, Thomas E, Tan HM. Ultra-low dose combined spinal-epidural anesthesia with intrathecal bupivacaine 3.75 mg for cesarean delivery: a randomized controlled trial. *Int J Obstet Anesth* 2006; 15(4):273–8.
157. Van de Velde M, Berends N, Spitz B, *et al.* Low-dose combined spinal-epidural anaesthesia vs. conventional epidural anaesthesia for caesarean section in pre-eclampsia: a retrospective analysis. *Eur J Anaesthesiol* 2004; 21(6):454–9.
158. Szypula K, Ashpole KJ, Bogod D, *et al.* Litigation related to regional anaesthesia: an analysis of claims against the NHS in England 1995–2007. *Anaesthesia* 2010; 65(5):443–52.
159. McNaught AF, Stocks GM. Epidural volume extension and low-dose sequential combined spinal-epidural blockade: two ways to reduce spinal dose requirement for caesarean section. *Int J Obstet Anesth* 2007; 16(4):346–53.
160. Blumgart CH, Ryall D, Dennison B, *et al.* Mechanism of extension of spinal anaesthesia by extradural injection of local anaesthetic. *Br J Anaesth* 1992; 69(5):457–60.
161. Takiguchi T, Okano T, Egawa H, *et al.* The effect of epidural saline injection on analgesic level during combined spinal and epidural anesthesia assessed clinically and myelographically. *Anesth Analg* 1997; 85(5):1097–100.
162. Beale N, Evans B, Plaat F, *et al.* Effect of epidural volume extension on dose requirement of intrathecal hyperbaric bupivacaine at caesarean section. *Br J Anaesth* 2005; 95(4):500–3.
163. Alonso E, Gilsanz F, Gredilla E, *et al.* Observational study of continuous spinal anesthesia with the catheter-over-needle technique for cesarean delivery. *Int J Obstet Anesth* 2009; 18(2):137–41.
164. Arkoosh VA, Palmer CM, Yun EM, *et al.* A randomized, double-masked, multicenter comparison of the safety of continuous intrathecal labor analgesia using a 28-gauge catheter versus continuous epidural labor analgesia. *Anesthesiology* 2008; 108(2):286–98.
165. Rigler ML, Drasner K, Krejcie TC, *et al.* Cauda equina syndrome after continuous spinal anesthesia. *Anesth Analg* 1991; 72(3):275–81.
166. Dresner M, Pinder A. Anaesthesia for caesarean section in women with complex cardiac disease: 34 cases using the Braun Spinocath spinal catheter. *Int J Obstet Anesth* 2009; 18(2):131–6.
167. Palmer CM. Continuous spinal anesthesia and analgesia in obstetrics. *Anesth Analg* 2010; 111(6):1476–9.

168. Heesen M, Klöhr S, Rossaint R, *et al.* Insertion of an intrathecal catheter following accidental dural puncture: a meta-analysis. *Int J Obstet Anesth* 2013; 22(1):26–30.
169. Deer TR, Prager J, Levy R, *et al.* Polyanalgesic consensus conference 2012: Recommendations for the management of pain by intrathecal (intraspinal) drug delivery: report of an interdisciplinary expert panel. *Neuromodulation* 2012; 15(5):436–64.
170. Moaveni DM, Birnbach DJ, Ranasinghe JS, *et al.* Fetal assessment for anesthesiologists: are you evaluating the other patient? *Anesth Analg* 2013; 116(6):1278–92.
171. Thurlow JA, Kinsella SM. Intrauterine resuscitation: active management of fetal distress. *Int J Obstet Anesth* 2002; 11(2):105–16.
172. Ingemarsson I, Arulkumaran S, Ratnam SS. Single injection of terbutaline in term labor. II. Effect on uterine activity. *Am J Obstet Gynecol* 1985; 153(8):865–9.
173. Khazin AF, Hon EH, Hehre FW. Effects of maternal hyperoxia on the fetus. I. Oxygen tension. *Am J Obstet Gynecol* 1971; 109(4):628–37.
174. Thorp JA, Trobough T, Evans R, *et al.* The effect of maternal oxygen administration during the second stage of labor on umbilical cord blood gas values: a randomized controlled prospective trial. *Am J Obstet Gynecol* 1995; 172(2 Pt 1):465–74.
175. Fawole B, Hofmeyr GJ. Maternal oxygen administration for fetal distress. *Cochrane Database Syst Rev* 2003; 4:CD000136.
176. Simpson KR, James DC. Efficacy of intrauterine resuscitation techniques in improving fetal oxygen status during labor. *Obstet Gynecol* 2005; 105(6):1362–8.
177. Haydon ML, Gorenberg DM, Nageotte MP, *et al.* The effect of maternal oxygen administration on fetal pulse oximetry during labor in fetuses with nonreassuring fetal heart rate patterns. *Am J Obstet Gynecol* 2006; 195(3):735–8.
178. Noh EJ, Kim YH, Cho MK, *et al.* Comparison of oxidative stress markers in umbilical cord blood after vaginal and cesarean delivery. *Obstet Gynecol Sci* 2014; 57(2):109–14.
179. Khaw KS, Wang CC, Ngan Kee WD, *et al.* Supplementary oxygen for emergency caesarean section under regional anaesthesia. *Br J Anaesth* 2009; 102(1):90–6.
180. Cheek TG, Samuels P, Miller F, *et al.* Normal saline i.v. fluid load decreases uterine activity in active labour. *Br J Anaesth* 1996; 77(5):632–5.
181. Hofmeyr GJ, Kulier R. Operative versus conservative management for 'fetal distress' in labour. *Cochrane Database Syst Rev* 2000; 2:CD001065.
182. Pullen KM, Riley ET, Waller SA, *et al.* Randomized comparison of intravenous terbutaline vs nitroglycerin for acute intrapartum fetal resuscitation. *Am J Obstet Gynecol* 2007; 197(4):414.e1–6.
183. Visser AA, Prinsloo ST, Giesteira MV. Suppression of uterine activity with salbutamol before caesarean section. *S Afr Med J* 1979; 56(25):1093–8.
184. Stone PA, Thorburn J, Lamb KS. Complications of spinal anaesthesia following extradural block for caesarean section. *Br J Anaesth* 1989; 62(3):335–7.
185. Beck GN, Griffiths AG. Failed extradural anaesthesia for caesarean section. Complication of subsequent spinal block. *Anaesthesia* 1992; 47(8):690–2.
186. Furst SR, Reisner LS. Risk of high spinal anesthesia following failed epidural block for cesarean delivery. *J Clin Anesth* 1995; 7(1):71–4.
187. Vickers R, Das B. Enhanced recovery in obstetrics. *Int J Obstet Anesth* 2013; 22(4):349.
188. Aluri S, Wrench IJ. Enhanced recovery from obstetric surgery: a UK survey of practice. *Int J Obstet Anesth* 2014; 23(2):157–60.
189. Jacques V, Vial F, Lerintiu M, *et al.* [Enhanced recovery following uncomplicated elective caesarean section in France: a survey of national practice]. *Ann Fr Anesth Reanim* 2013; 32(3):142–8.
190. Lucas DN, Gough KL. Enhanced recovery in obstetrics—a new frontier? *Int J Obstet Anesth* 2013; 22(2):92–5.

CHAPTER 21

Intraoperative management of inadequate neuraxial anaesthesia

Tauqeer Husain and Roshan Fernando

Introduction

Neuraxial anaesthesia (NA), in the form of neuraxial blockade, is increasingly seen as the preferred method of anaesthesia for elective and emergency caesarean delivery (CD). Within the United Kingdom, a number of studies have shown NA rates for CD of approximately 80%, or more (Figure 21.1). Shibli and Russell[1] conducted a prospective survey of 129 maternity hospitals, obtaining data on anaesthesia for 60,455 CDs. They found that 78% were performed under NA, with 47% under single-shot spinal, 22% epidural, and 9% with combined spinal–epidural (CSE). In elective procedures, NA was used in 87% of cases, whilst 72% of emergencies were performed under NA. The National Sentinel Caesarean Section Audit Report,[2] presented the findings of an audit of CD rates in England, Wales, and Northern Ireland between 2000 and 2001. It found that 77% of emergency and 91% of elective CDs were performed with NA. Rafi et al. demonstrated the use of continuous prospective audit increased the NA rates in both elective and emergency CD. In their study, NA rates for elective CDs increased from 95.3% to 98.2%, whilst rates in emergency deliveries increased from 82.3% to 85.7%, between 2004 and 2007.[3]

However, the increasing use of NA for CD is not just limited to the United Kingdom. Similar rates of NA use for CDs have been demonstrated in other European countries, such as France,[4,5] Germany,[6,7] and Belgium,[8] and further afield, in the United States,[9] Israel,[10] the West Indies,[11] and Nigeria.[12]

Many factors have driven the increasing use of NA in obstetric surgery. Most markedly, there has been an appreciation of the prominent role of general anaesthesia (GA) in the causes of anaesthetic mortality and morbidity in obstetrics. The MBRRACE-UK project (Mothers and Babies: Reducing Risk through Audits and Confidential Enquiries across the UK; formerly the Centre for Maternal and Child Enquires (CMACE), and the Confidential Enquiry into Maternal and Child Health) publishes triennial reports on the results of what has become the longest running audit in medicine. In the first report, covering 1952–54,[13] 49 deaths were attributed to anaesthesia, and there were at least 20 more where anaesthesia was thought to be contributory. By the 2009–12 report, published in 2014,[14] only four deaths were directly related to anaesthesia. It has been suggested that this trend of decreasing anaesthetic mortality (anaesthesia being 30 times safer than it was in the 1960s) is at least partly due to the increasing use of NA, since the 1960s.[15,16]

The predominant causes of anaesthetic death, as shown in previous reports, have either been related to failed oxygenation during intubation, or aspiration of gastric contents causing early asphyxia or late respiratory failure.

Medicolegal implications of inadequate anaesthesia

Whilst the use of NA over GA undoubtedly provides a favourable balance of risks and benefits for most pregnant women, the employment of NA does not abolish risk altogether. Along with the risk of morbidity from the actual neuraxial procedure, the risk of failed NA and potential conversion to GA also exists. A prospective audit of over 5000 CDs in a single UK hospital showed a GA conversion rate of 0.8% for elective and 4.9% for emergency cases.[17] In a US retrospective analysis of nearly 20,000 deliveries, over a 3-year period, the rate of conversion from spinal anaesthesia was 1.2%, while 4.3% of GAs occurred after conversion of epidural anaesthesia.[18]

The risk of inadequate NA has medicolegal and clinical consequences. The American Society of Anesthesiologists' Closed Claims Database (which collects detailed case summaries from malpractice insurance organization claim files) found that of the 1541 claims made between 1985 and 1990, 12% involved obstetrics, and 33% of these were associated with NA.[19] Eight per cent of obstetric claims involved pain during anaesthesia, resulting in a median payment of $17,000 (ranging from $5000 to $305,000). In a more recent study, 13% of perioperative claims made between 1990 and 2003 were related to obstetric anaesthesia.[20] The median litigation payment was $222,000, although these claims were not exclusively related to intraoperative pain. A study of the Canadian Medical Protective Association closed claims between 1990 and 1997 demonstrated 13 obstetric claims out of 61.[21] Pain during anaesthesia made up 15% (2/13) of obstetric claims. Within the United Kingdom, the Clinical Negligence Scheme for Trusts (which handles all clinical negligence claims against Nation Health Service bodies) managed 841 cases relating to any form of anaesthesia, between 1995 and 2007.[22] Of these, 245 (29%) were

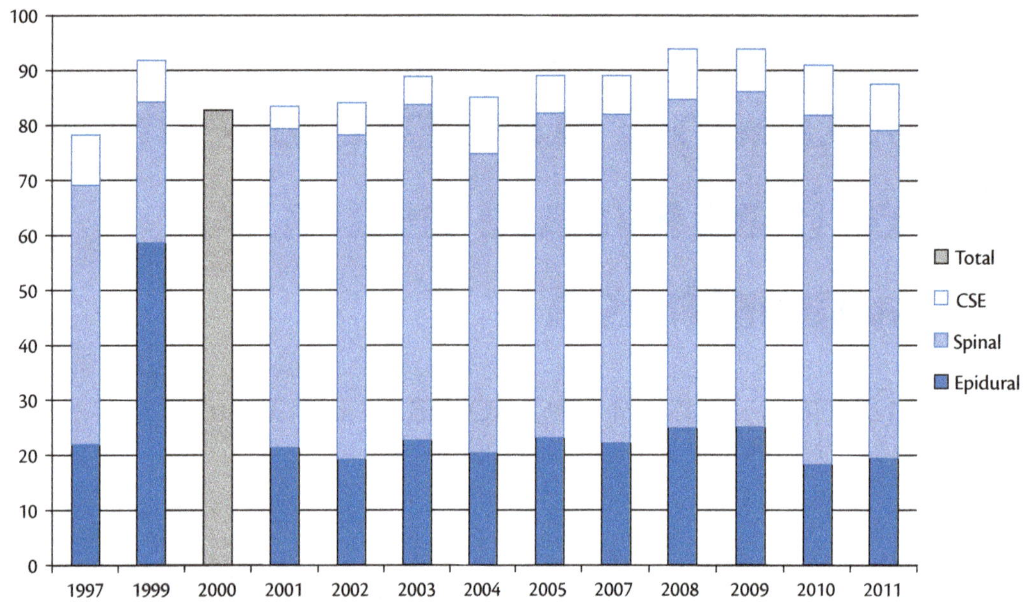

Figure 21.1 Neuraxial anaesthesia use in the UK between 1997 and 2011.

Data from Shibli KU, Russell IF, A survey of anaesthetic techniques used for caesarean section in the UK in 1997, *International Journal of Obstetric Anesthesia*, volume 9, pp. 160–7, Copyright © 2000 Elsevier and OAA National obstetric anaesthetic database (http://www.oaa-anaes.ac.uk/content.asp?ContentID=241).

classified as relating to obstetric anaesthesia. The total value of claims was £7.5 million. An examination of litigation specifically related to NA within the same period demonstrated that 186 out of 366 claims were associated with obstetric anaesthesia.[23] Of the 326 neuraxial claims, inadequate block with resulting pain accounted for 24 claims. Fifty-seven of the obstetric claims (31%) were due to inadequate block, resulting in pain during CD or labour.

Epidural anaesthesia

Risk factors for failed conversion of epidural analgesia to anaesthesia

Epidural analgesia in labour has become increasingly popular, not just for the excellent pain relief that is normally provided in labour, but also for the ability to convert labour analgesia to operative anaesthesia by the addition of higher concentrations of local anaesthetic (LA) and opioid. Reported rates of failed epidural conversion (defined as failure to induce adequate anaesthesia or to provide adequate anaesthesia throughout the procedure, requiring analgesic supplementation, an alternative regional technique or GA) for CD, varies between 7.1% and 24%.[17,18] A number of factors that may predict the risk of failed epidural conversion have been identified (Box 21.1).

Box 21.1 Factors associated with an increased risk of failed epidural conversion

- Supplementary clinician boluses in labour
- Non-obstetric anaesthetist providing care
- Urgency of caesarean delivery
- High maternal weight or height.

Clinician boluses in labour

The likelihood of successful epidural anaesthesia is related to the effectiveness of epidural labour analgesia. This has most commonly been represented by the requirement of clinician-initiated boluses to manage breakthrough pain during labour. Riley and Papasin investigated the clinical factors associated with catheter failure in a retrospective case note review of 246 patients that had continuous epidural infusions of 0.0625% bupivacaine with 0.33 mcg/mL sufentanil, for labour analgesia.[24] The authors found that failure to obtain adequate surgical anaesthesia correlated to the number of times the patient required extra clinician boluses during labour. Successful catheters required a mean (range) of 1 (0–8) clinician boluses, while the unsuccessful catheters required a mean (range) of 3 (0–10) clinician top-ups. They concluded that although additional clinician boluses had classically been attributed to 'especially painful' labours, it is equally probable that this actually reflects suboptimal catheter placement in the epidural space. Further studies have demonstrated a correlation between the need for any,[25] or more than one additional labour bolus,[26] and an increased risk of inadequate epidural anaesthesia. With this in mind, it would be reasonable to consider a patient requiring multiple clinician boluses in labour to be at high risk of failed epidural anaesthesia, if CD were required. It may therefore be prudent to have a low threshold to replace the epidural catheter in a patient where analgesia is not adequately maintained without additional clinician interventions. Additional caution should be used when patient-controlled epidural analgesia is used, as the need for additional boluses may not be as readily evident, necessitating increased vigilance and more frequent reviews.

Obstetric anaesthesia specialists

It has also been hypothesized that anaesthetists who have undergone specialist training, or are specialists, in obstetric anaesthesia may have a higher success rate at managing epidural anaesthesia.

This may be the result of them having more confidence and patience in waiting for an epidural to provide adequate anaesthesia, or in them being more likely to actively manage a suboptimal epidural by withdrawing the catheter or giving additional LA.[25] Specialists may, therefore, be less likely to convert to an alternate method of anaesthesia. These differences may result in different clinical decision-making, which may allow less time for adequate epidural block to work before it is abandoned for an alternative method. Riley and Papasin showed that non-specialists have a failed epidural anaesthesia rate of almost four times that of obstetric anaesthesia specialists, in one study.[24] However, this has not been consistently found in other studies.[26,27]

Maternal size

It has also been argued that increased maternal weight may be a risk factor for failed epidural anaesthesia; the suggestion being that maternal obesity may result in increased catheter displacement as the distance between the skin and the epidural space changes with patient movement.[24] This, again, has not been consistently demonstrated in the literature. Interestingly, Halpern et al.[26] identified increased maternal height, but not body mass index (BMI), as a factor leading to failed epidural anaesthesia. The authors hypothesized that the lack of difference in failure rate between patients with a BMI higher than 35 compared to those with a BMI lower than 35 might be due to a low tolerance of suboptimal labour analgesia by anaesthetists in this high-risk group, and therefore early replacement of inadequate epidural catheters in labour.

Local anaesthetic solutions for epidural anaesthesia

Local anaesthetic

The characteristics of LAs used to 'top-up' epidural analgesia for operative anaesthesia are numerous. High on the list of desired features are the onset and duration of anaesthesia. Epidural conversion from analgesia to anaesthesia is most commonly needed in urgent or emergency cases. In the most extreme situations, delayed anaesthesia maybe associated with maternal or fetal mortality. In such a scenario, a rapid onset of epidural anaesthesia is needed to avoid the alternatives, general or spinal anaesthesia. Additionally, the quality and duration of anaesthesia are clearly important to avoid breakthrough pain, supplementation and potential conversion to GA during the procedure.

Hillyard et al.[28] performed a meta-analysis to find if significant differences in time of onset and incidence of intraoperative supplementation exist between three LA solutions (0.5% bupivacaine or levobupivacaine (Bup/Levo), 0.2% lidocaine + 1:200 000 epinephrine ± fentanyl (LE ± F), and 0.75% ropivacaine (Ropi)) used for epidural top-up in labouring women undergoing non-elective CD. Analysis indicated that the time of onset of anaesthesia was significantly reduced by over 1.5 minutes with LE ± F, compared to either Bup/Levo or Ropi (Figure 21.2). By excluding studies with markedly different protocols, the heterogeneity of the meta-analysis was reduced, and the mean difference in onset time was further increased to 4.5 minutes. Intraoperative supplementation of anaesthesia was significantly increased with the use of Bup/Levo. The increased risk of supplementation was highest when Bup/Levo was compared to Ropi (Figure 21.3).

There are several limitations to the Hillyard et al. meta-analysis.[28] The addition of bicarbonate and opioids were not included and this is discussed in a later section. Another limitation of the meta-analysis is that it did not consider the use of 2-chloroprocaine for top-up epidural anaesthesia. As an ester-linked LA, it is rapidly hydrolysed by plasma cholinesterases to inactive metabolites, has a maternal plasma mean half-life of 3.1 ± 1. 6 minutes, after epidural anaesthesia,[29] and an approximate duration of action of 40–50 minutes. Chloroprocaine also has a rapid onset of action. Compared to 0.5% bupivacaine, 3% chloroprocaine resulted in significantly shorter injection-to-anaesthesia and injection-to-delivery times when *de novo* epidural anaesthesia was administered for CD.[30] When 3% chloroprocaine has been compared to lidocaine with epinephrine for CD, onset of block has been equal,[31] or significantly faster with chloroprocaine, and a non-significant increase in the need for supplemental analgesia has been noted in the lidocaine group.[32] Additionally, when administered via a *de novo* epidural in order to provide anaesthesia for CD, 3% 2-chloroprocaine was found to cause similar incidences of maternal and fetal side effects to 2% lidocaine and 0.75% bupivacaine.[33]

Some studies have found that the rapid onset of anaesthesia accompanying administration of chloroprocaine is associated with greater maternal hypotension, when compared to 0.5% bupivacaine.[30] However, the hypotension was not associated with adverse maternal or fetal effects when corrected rapidly. The use of chloroprocaine has also been associated with cases of neurological damage after epidural or inadvertent intrathecal administration.[34,35] Sodium bisulphite, a preservative contained within earlier commercially available preparations, was implicated in the pathogenesis of this neurotoxicity,[36] and has led to the development of bisulphite-free preparations. However, some work has questioned whether neurotoxicity might occur as a direct effect of the anaesthetic, rather than the preservative.[37] Furthermore,

Study or subgroup	LE±F Mean (min)	LE±F SD (min)	LE±F Total	Bup/levo or Ropi Mean (min)	Bup/levo or Ropi SD (min)	Bup/levo or Ropi Total	Weight	Mean difference i.v. fixed, 95% CI (min)
Balaji and colleagues	10	3.33	50	15	5.83	50	15.9%	−5.00 (−6.86, −3.14)
Goring-Morris and Russell	10.8	7.5	30	14.5	8.125	36	3.9%	−3.70 (−7.47, 0.07)
Lucas and colleagues	10	5	30	14	4.75	30	9.0%	−4.00 (−6.47, −1.53)
Sng and colleagues	9.5	2.33	30	10	2.5	30	36.8%	−0.50 (−1.72, 0.72)
Sng and colleagues	9.5	2.33	30	10	2.66	30	34.4%	−0.50 (−1.77, 0.77)
Total (95% CI)			170			176	100.0%	−1.66 (−2.40, −0.91)

Heterogeneity: $X^2 = 23.63$, df = 4 ($P < 0.0001$); $I^2 = 83\%$
Test for overall effect: $Z = 4.37$ ($P < 0.0001$)

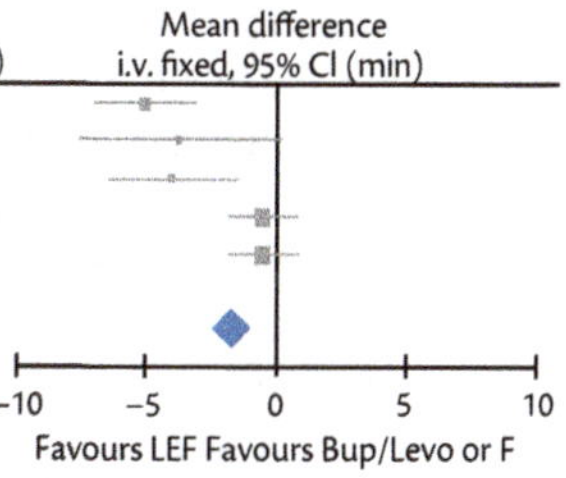

Figure 21.2 The onset time of a block suitable to allow surgery, comparing LE+F (2% lidocaine, epinephrine, and fentanyl) top-up solutions with either Bup/Levo (0.5% bupivacaine, 0.5% levobupivacaine), or Ropi (0.75% ropivacaine) solutions.

Hillyard S *et al.*, Extending epidural analgesia for emergency Caesarean section: a meta-analysis. *British Journal of Anaesthesia*, 2011 volume 107, issue 5, pp. 668–78, by permission of Oxford University Press.

Study or subgroup	Bup/Levo Events	Bup/Levo Total	LE±F or Ropi Events	LE±F or Ropi Total	Weight	Risk ratio M–H, fixed, 95% CI
6.1.1 LEF						
Balaji and colleagues	9	45	4	44	21.3%	2.20 (0.73, 6.62)
Goring-Morris and Russell	5	34	2	27	11.4%	1.99 (0.42, 9.45)
Lucas and colleagues	6	26	6	28	30.4%	1.08 (0.40, 2.92)
Sng and colleagues	3	30	2	30	10.5%	1.50 (0.27, 8.34)
Subtotal (95% CI)		135		129	73.8%	1.60 (0.86, 2.98)
Total events	23		14			
Heterogeneity: $X^2 = 1.01$, df = 3 ($P = 0.80$); $I^2 = 0\%$						
Test for overall effect: $Z = 1.50$ ($P = 0.13$)						
6.1.2 Ropi						
Hillyard and colleagues	4	31	1	27	5.6%	3.48 (0.41, 29.31)
Sanders and colleagues	9	21	2	23	10.0%	4.93 (1.20, 20.26)
Sng and colleagues	3	30	2	30	10.5%	1.50 (0.27, 8.34)
Subtotal (95% CI)		82		80	26.2%	3.24 (1.26, 8.33)
Total events	16		5			
Heterogeneity: $X^2 = 1.12$, df = 2 ($P = 0.57$); $I^2 = 0\%$						
Test for overall effect: $Z = 2.44$ ($P = 0.01$)						
Total (95% CI)		217		209	100.0%	2.03 (1.22, 3.39)
Total events	39		19			
Heterogeneity: $X^2 = 3.57$, df = 6 ($P = 0.73$); $I^2 = 0\%$						
Test for overall effect: $Z = 2.72$ ($P = 0.007$)						

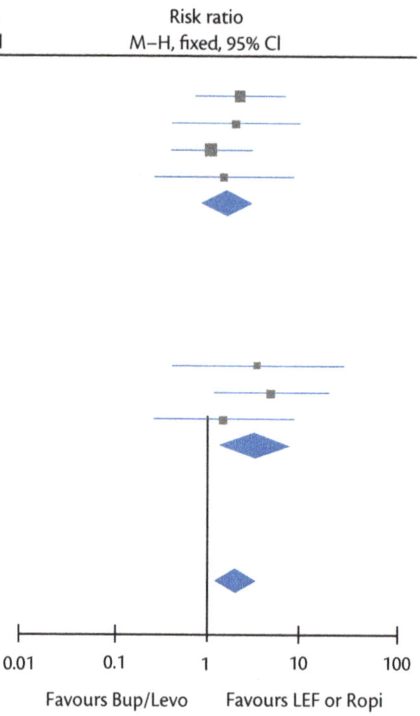

Figure 21.3 The need for intraoperative supplementation, comparing Bup/Levo (0.5% bupivacaine or 0.5% levobupivacaine) top-up solutions to LE+F (2% lidocaine, epinephrine, and fentanyl), or Ropi (0.75% ropivacaine) solutions.

Hillyard S *et al.*, Extending epidural analgesia for emergency Caesarean section: a meta-analysis. *British Journal of Anaesthesia*, 2011 volume 107, issue 5, pp. 668–78, by permission of Oxford University Press.

2-chloroprocaine has also been implicated in the antagonism of opioid receptors, resulting in a decreased duration of epidural morphine analgesia following CD.[38] Finally, although it is licensed for use in anaesthesia for short surgical procedures in parts of Europe, 2-chloroprocaine is not currently licensed in some countries, such as the United Kingdom.

As well as the type of LA solution used for epidural anaesthesia, it is also worth considering ways in which LA solutions may be modified to enhance desirable characteristics.

Opioids

The addition of a lipophilic opioid to epidural LA solution has been demonstrated to decrease the likelihood of pain during elective surgery.[39] However, this has not been supported by the meta-analysis of epidural anaesthesia for emergency CD, by Hillyard et al.[28] Although the addition of 50–75 mcg of fentanyl to the LA solution decreased the mean onset time to anaesthesia by 2 minutes, no difference in intraoperative supplementation was seen. The authors suggested that the difference observed in emergency situations may be due to the fact that opioids used in labour analgesic LA solutions may have already produced a near-maximal effect. However, these findings were generated from pooling only two trials with conflicting results.

Unlike other countries where it is not available commercially, most obstetric units in the United Kingdom use diamorphine as the opioid of choice for neuraxial anaesthesia. Indeed, the National Institute of Health and Care Excellence (NICE) has made the evidence-based recommendation that women should be offered intrathecal or epidural diamorphine, in order to reduce the need for postoperative supplemental analgesia.[40] Caranza et al. showed that administration of 3 mg epidural diamorphine at the end of CD, followed by a further 3 mg bolus at the first request for supplemental analgesia, supplied equivalent post-caesarean analgesia to 0.2 mg intrathecal morphine.[41] Hallworth et al. found that 0.25 mg diamorphine produced the same duration and quality of postoperative analgesia as 5 mg epidural diamorphine.[42] The NICE guidance recommends 0.3–0.4 mg intrathecal or 2.5–5 mg epidural diamorphine as suitable doses.[40] However, the guidance does not make any reference to the dose required to reduce intraoperative pain. In a dose finding study of women undergoing elective CD under CSE using an intrathecal dose of 0.5% 12.5 mg hyperbaric bupivacaine and diamorphine, the effective dose in 95% of subjects (ED_{95}) of diamorphine required to prevent intraoperative supplementation was 0.39 mg.[43] Although the time until the first request for supplemental postoperative analgesia increased with higher doses, so did the incidence of nausea, vomiting, and pruritus.

Alkalinization

A further limitation of the meta-analysis by Hillyard et al.[28] is that it did not consider the use of alkalinizing agents in epidural top-up solutions. LAs are weak bases. Therefore, an increase in pH would increase the extraneural amount of the lipophilic, unionized form of the LA, which diffuses through the nerve cell membrane to block nerve impulses. Since the addition of sodium bicarbonate has been found to potentiate the effect of LA on peripheral nerves *in vitro*,[44] alkalinization of LA may enhance the depth of epidural anaesthesia. The addition of 2 mL 8.4% sodium bicarbonate to either 2% lidocaine alone,[45] or in combination with 0.5% bupivacaine,[46] has been shown to significantly speed up the onset of action, and improve pain threshold and density of motor block. Furthermore, Allam et al. compared pH-adjusted 1.8% lidocaine and 1 in 200,000 epinephrine to 0.5% levobupivacaine for conversion of epidurals for emergency CD.[47] The authors found that the median onset of a block to touch to T5 was reduced from 14 minutes with levobupivacaine, to 7 minutes with the pH-adjusted lidocaine/epinephrine solution.

Temperature

Similar to alkalinization, warming LA increases the proportion of uncharged molecules available to cross the neural cell membrane. The use of epidural LA solution warmed to body temperature (37–38°C) has been demonstrated to produce a more rapid onset of anaesthesia for elective CD,[48] and faster onset and improved visual analogue scores in epidural labour analgesia.[49] However, currently this practice would involve storing LA outside the conditions recommended by manufacturers, which many clinicians may be reluctant to do.

Single solutions versus multiple drug mixtures

Although the addition of drugs, such as epinephrine and sodium bicarbonate, speed up the onset of epidural anaesthesia, there are concerns over the time delays that may result from drug mixing. Lucas et al. compared the time taken to prepare three solutions commonly used for epidural top-up in CD: (a) 0.5% bupivacaine 20 mL, (b) 2% lidocaine 20 mL with 1:200,000 epinephrine, and (c) 0.5% bupivacaine 10 mL and 2% lidocaine 10 mL with 1:200,000 epinephrine and 8.4% sodium bicarbonate 2 mL.[50] They found that preparing bupivacaine by itself took half the time required for lidocaine/epinephrine, which in turn took half the time needed to prepare the bupivacaine/lidocaine/epinephrine/bicarbonate solution. The increased time required to prepare complex solutions led the authors to conclude that if they were prepared immediately before administration, any reduction in onset time may be offset by the additional preparation time. Additionally, the speed of onset is most important in the context of fetal distress. It may be argued that there is increased potential for drug errors when mixing complex solutions in stressful, emergency situations, when compared to single-solution LA.

Some anaesthetists may prepare epidural top-up solutions in advance, in order to minimize delays and potential errors when mixing multiple drugs. The solutions are then often stored for up to 24 hours before use. Robinson et al. investigated the stability of pH-adjusted solutions containing bupivacaine, lidocaine, and epinephrine, which had been stored at room temperature for 24 hours.[51] They found that epinephrine was chemically unstable in solutions which had been alkalinized with sodium bicarbonate, but concentrations did not change in non-alkalinized solutions. Additionally, although none of the solutions demonstrated a decrease in LA concentration, the pH in all the solutions decreased with storage at room temperature. In a subsequent study, Tuleu et al. found that the epinephrine concentration in a pH-adjusted lidocaine–epinephrine solution fell by 30% after 6 hours of storage at room temperature, unprotected from light.[52] It has therefore been concluded that epinephrine should not be used with pH-adjusted solutions of LA that are to be stored, but should be added immediately before administration.[51]

Concerns also exist over the use of preservative-containing drugs within the epidural solutions. Epinephrine is sensitive to oxidative degradation and is combined with sulphites, which are preferentially oxidized, to prolong its shelf-life.[52] Sulphite preservatives have also been implicated in various reports of chronic adhesive arachnoiditis (CAA; a progressive inflammation of the arachnoid mater) after administration into the epidural space.[53,54] However, in the context of epidural anaesthesia, epinephrine is usually diluted as a dose of either 0.1 mL of 1 in 1000, or 1 mL of 1 in 10,000, in 20 mL LA solution. Additionally, the exact relationship between neuraxial sulphites and CAA remains unclear, with reports of intrathecal sulphite administration resulting in no neurological complications.[55] Alkalinization of LA solution is normally performed using 8.4% sodium bicarbonate. This is done using preservative-free solutions, as there is also a worry of neurological injury related to EDTA within alternative preparations of sodium bicarbonate.[56]

Although the risk of neurotoxicity related to neuraxial preservatives is uncertain, it would appear a sensible precaution to avoid the use of preservative-containing drugs with epidural LA solutions. If preservative-containing drugs must be administered (as in the case of epinephrine), maximal dilution of the drug should be used.

In summary, although there is no single LA solution of choice for minimizing the risk of failed epidural anaesthesia, the evidence suggests that bupivacaine or levobupivacaine 0.5% has a slower onset of anaesthesia and lower quality of block, compared to lidocaine with epinephrine or ropivacaine. Ropivacaine 0.75% may offer the lowest risk of intraoperative supplementation, whilst 2% lignocaine with epinephrine produces the fastest onset of anaesthesia. Chloroprocaine may be considered in situations where rapid conversion of epidural analgesia to anaesthesia is required, although concerns over neurotoxicity, opioid antagonism, and availability may limit its use. Lipophilic opioids, such as fentanyl, may be considered to speed the onset of anaesthesia, whilst alkalization with preservative-free 8.4% sodium bicarbonate may also be employed to enhance onset and quality of anaesthesia. Warming LA solution may increase the speed of onset.

Spinal anaesthesia

When considering the management of failed spinal anaesthesia for CD, the first step must be to consider the causes, and therefore ways to minimize the risk of pre- or intraoperative anaesthetic failure.

Causes of inadequate spinal anaesthesia

The causes of inadequate or failed spinal anaesthesia are not always clear. In a review of mechanisms of failed spinal anaesthesia, Fettes et al. described five phases of an individual intrathecal anaesthetic.[57] Each phase contains a variety of factors which might render the intrathecal anaesthetic inadequate (Box 21.2).[57]

Assuming lumbar puncture is adequately performed, a major determinate of successful intrathecal anaesthesia is the choice of an effective dose of anaesthetic. Although, it is important to appreciate that within the clinical range normally used, changes of dose have small effect on the spread of the block, but a more significant association on the duration of anaesthesia.[58]

Local anaesthetic dose for spinal anaesthesia

The choice of LA dose administered can be represented by the proportion of the population where a given effect is produced.

Common descriptions of this include the effective dose in 50% and 90% of the population (ED_{50} and ED_{90}).

Carvalho et al.[59] found the ED_{50} and ED_{90} values for intrathecal 'isobaric' bupivacaine (actually hypobaric in relation to cerebrospinal fluid) with fentanyl and morphine were 7.25 and 13.0 mg, respectively, for overall anaesthetic success. Success was defined as a bilateral T6 sensory block to pinprick within 10 minutes, and no additional epidural intraoperative supplementation. Using a similar methodology, the same group also found that the equivalent values for hyperbaric bupivacaine with fentanyl and morphine were 7.6 and 11.2 mg, respectively.[60] In a study using levobupivacaine with sufentanil and morphine, the ED_{50} and ED_{90} values for operative success (defined as T6 sensory block to pinprick, and no epidural supplementation intraoperatively) were 6.2 and 12.9 mg, respectively.[61] A number of studies that have examined dosing for intrathecal anaesthesia have found little correlation between successful induction of anaesthesia (i.e. establishment of a given sensory level by a predetermined time) and operative success. This would further support the suggestion that an intrathecal dose may have a greater effect on the duration of anaesthesia, and so an adequate block at incision is not always indicative of operative success.

However, the doses stated above may be considered by some to be unnecessarily high. It has been argued that although the primary goal of intrathecal anaesthesia is to allow a painless CD to take place, this should be done while also avoiding maternal and neonatal side effects. The use of lower doses in spinal anaesthesia aims to decrease maternal hypotension, nausea, and vomiting, allow earlier discharge from post-anaesthesia care units, and improve maternal satisfaction.[62] On the other hand, this approach may also increase the risk of failed anaesthesia, increase the need for intraoperative supplementation, or conversion to GA.

A systematic review and meta-analysis by Arzola and Wieczorek,[63] compared the efficacy of 'low'-dose spinal bupivacaine with 'conventional' dose for CD. The authors defined a 'low' dose as 8 mg of bupivacaine or less, whilst a 'conventional' dose was greater than 8 mg. They found that low-dose spinal anaesthesia was associated with a lower risk of hypotension (relative risk (RR) = 0.78) and nausea/vomiting (RR = 0.71), but a significantly higher need for intraoperative analgesic supplementation (RR = 3.76). Additionally, the only cases where conversion to GA were required occurred in two out of 21 participants in the low-dose group.

The ideal dose of intrathecal LA for CD is a balance between the need to avoid patient discomfort, and to minimize maternal side effects. If successful operative anaesthesia is the primary goal, it is advisable to consider the use of 'conventional' dose anaesthetic techniques, complemented by strategies to minimize maternal side effects. If low-dose spinal anaesthesia is used, it would be better to do this as part of a CSE technique.[64,65]

Box 21.2 Causes of inadequate spinal anaesthesia

Failed lumbar puncture

- Positioning: maximal separation of lumbar laminae and spines by flexion of whole spine, hips, and knees
- Needle insertion: knowledge of spinal anatomy and landmarks; adequate insertion level and angle
- Pseudo-successful lumbar puncture: aspiration of injected LA solution after failed epidural top-up; congenital arachnoid cysts (Tarlov cysts).

Errors in preparation and injection of solution

- Dose selection
- Loss of injectate: leakage from the syringe–hub interface
- Misplaced injection, for example, into epidural space.

Inadequate spread of drugs in cerebrospinal fluid

- Anatomical abnormalities: curvature abnormalities; spinal stenosis; previous vertebral canal surgery; intrathecal chemotherapy
- Solution density.

Failure of drug action

- Errors in identification of LA
- Chemical incompatibility
- Inactive LA solution
- LA resistance: very rare, reports tend to be anecdotal.

Failure of subsequent management

- Testing block
- Catheter and combined techniques.

Data from Fettes PDW, Jansson J-R, Wildsmith JAW. Failed spinal anaesthesia: mechanisms, management, and prevention. *British Journal of Anaesthesia*, volume 102, pp. 739–48. Copyright 2009.

Testing the adequacy of neuraxial blockade prior to operative delivery

Checking to ensure adequacy of a neuraxial block prior to surgery must be considered gold standard practice within obstetric anaesthesia. However, methods of assessment vary widely. Historically, some anaesthetists have used a technique of ensuring that the right dose of drug is injected in to the right place with complete confidence.[66] The assessment of sensory block has more recently been variably assessed by loss of pinprick,[59,61,50] cold,[46] and light touch sensation.[67]

In a prospective observational study, Russell examined the difference in level of analgesia (defined as loss of sharp pinprick sensation) and anaesthesia (loss of touch sensation), and the relationship between the level of anaesthesia and occurrence of pain in women undergoing CD under NA without opioids.[68] He found that the levels of analgesia at delivery that were associated with pain varied from T1 to T9, and that the corresponding range of anaesthesia was T4 to T10. Of the women who experienced pain, 25% had a level of analgesia at T3–T4. No women that experienced pain had a level of anaesthesia above T5. He concluded that assessing readiness for surgery by testing level of analgesia (i.e. loss of pinprick sensation) may be misleading, and that in the absence of neuraxial opioid, a level of anaesthesia up to and including T5 is required to prevent intraoperative pain. In a subsequent study, Russell assessed pinprick, cold, and touch modalities in 102 women undergoing CD under spinal anaesthesia including intrathecal diamorphine.[69] The findings indicated that there was a median difference of approximately two dermatomes between the level of block by pinprick or cold, and touch, and that there was no constant relationship between these levels of block. Additionally, using 100 mcg/mL diamorphine in 0.5% bupivacaine, no patient experienced intraoperative pain when anaesthesia provided a loss of touch sensation including T6 or above.

In a study of sensory testing and variability for spinal anaesthesia, Kocarev et al. compared cold (ethyl chloride), sharp (calibrated Neuropen®), pressure (standardized monofilament), and light touch (Neuropen® stroking, monofilament stroking, and cotton wool).[70] The median differences between the four modalities were significant, while multiple comparisons of medians showed no significant difference between the tests of light touch. The authors also noted the cost of each method of testing. When cost was also factored into the evaluation, they suggested that testing light touch with cotton wool appeared to be the cheapest method of testing. Additionally, as well as being more expensive, ethyl chloride spray, Neurotip® and monofilament use did not appear to offer any advantages. The distributions of data for each sensory test are displayed as violin plots (Figure 21.4). These show the least dermatomal spread in the tests with least variability, such as the tests of light touch. Additionally, tests that stimulate more than one sensory modality are represented by a bimodal distribution. This can be observed in the violin plot of cold sensation. Ethyl chloride spray causes stimulation which is conducted by cold-specific Aδ fibres. However, nociceptor C fibres may participate in the transmission of painful cold sensation, while the contact of the spray with skin would illicit stimulation via Aβ fibres.

There are currently no formal guidelines for the assessment of NA prior to CD. The available evidence has led to some expert opinion suggesting that intraoperative failure of NA in the absence of an assessed loss of touch sensation may result in difficulties for the anaesthetist, if litigation were to be pursued.[71] However, it should be considered that clinical conduct may not mirror expert opinion in this matter. A national survey of obstetric anaesthesia practice in the United Kingdom demonstrated that only 60% of all respondents assessed light touch prior to starting surgery, compared to 92% who assess cold.[72] Where only a single sensory modality was assessed, this went down to 26% for light touch and 69% for cold. Furthermore, only 26% of respondents ensured a block to light touch up to T5 prior to delivery. If this is to be considered the requirement to reduce the risk of intraoperative pain, it seems inconceivable that 74% of obstetric anaesthetists in the United Kingdom expose their patients to NA which may result in painful CD. The difference between the evidence and the practice may be explained by the variable course of visceral pain fibres to the upper thoracic cord, and may be why a patient with an apparently 'low' block experiences no intraoperative discomfort.[73] Alternatively, it may be that although the anaesthetist is targeting a particular level of block, they may actually inadvertently be achieving a higher level. This may be because the level of anaesthesia has continued to ascend between testing, and when

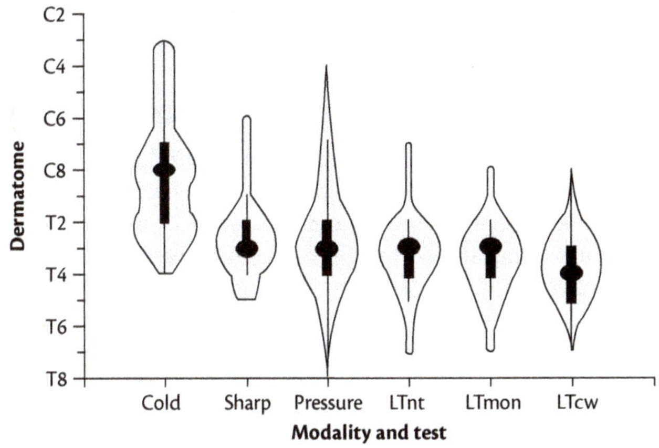

Figure 21.4 Violin plot, demonstrating density of data for each sensory test. Dot, median value; thick line, upper and lower quartiles; whiskers extend to 1.5 times the interquartile range. LTnt, light touch Neurotip®; LTmon, light touch monofilament; LTcw, light touch cotton wool.

Reprinted from *International Journal of Obstetric Anesthesia*, volume 19, issue 3, M. Kocarev, E. Watkins, H. McLure, M. Columb, G. Lyons, Sensory testing of spinal anaesthesia for caesarean section: differential block and variability, pp. 261–265, Copyright (2010), with permission from Elsevier.

the procedure begins, or due to variability or inaccuracies with the actual assessment of the block.

Congreve et al. found in a survey of anaesthetists that identification of the T5 dermatomal level showed marked inaccuracy.[74] Of the 73 anaesthetists surveyed, only 63% identified the dermatome correctly on an anatomical picture. There is also a marked variability when considering the true upper level of NA. In a study of his practice, compared to anaesthetic trainees, Yentis found that he consistently recorded higher levels of anaesthesia compared to the trainees, for the same block.[75] The differences were explained by the fact that most trainees recorded the level of anaesthesia to be where the patient first experienced any sensation from the cold or light touch stimulus. It was argued that the true upper level of anaesthesia should actually be where sensory perception returns completely to normal. Finally, it is clear that in describing NA nomenclature may also vary. Where one anaesthetist may consider the perception of sensation at T4 to be 'a block to T4', another may refer to this as 'the upper level of block being T5'.[76]

In summary, there remains much debate as to what should be considered the gold standard for adequate NA for CD. The variable nature of the assessment of neuraxial blocks, along with the differences between expert opinion and actual clinical practice, makes the evaluation of evidence difficult. Until the presentation of high-quality prospective evidence to the contrary, it might be simpler to follow the suggestion that a documented block up to and including T5 to light touch may be the best way to avoid intraoperative pain during CD. On the other hand, due to the inconsistencies and difficulties with the assessment of light touch, particularly concerning what constitutes a complete absence of touch, compared to other modalities, anaesthetists may choose to vary their method of testing according to their own clinical experience. Either way, care should be taken when checking the block to ensure the assessment is performed with an adequate and consistent degree of accuracy. Whatever modality is chosen it is important to record the first dermatomal level where initial change in that modality occurs and the dermatomal level in which complete absence of sensation of that modality occurs.

Managing inadequate neuraxial anaesthesia

Although very few formal, evidence-based guidelines exist for the management of inadequate NA in obstetrics, it is clear that management depends on the clinical context of the situation. Decision-making should take into account when inadequacy of NA is recognized in relation to the beginning of surgery, and to delivery. Additionally, consideration must be given to how urgently delivery needs to occur. Because of the numerous factors affecting the decision-making process, as well as concerns for maternal and fetal well-being, recognition of inadequate NA can prove to be a particularly stressful time for the anaesthetists, but is one which necessitates rapid formulation of a clear plan of management.

Before the start of surgery

Neuraxial anaesthetic techniques for CD can take the form of a single-shot spinal, CSE, epidural top-up, or rarely a *de novo* epidural. However, when NA has been identified as being inadequate before the start of surgery, this is broadly a failure of either spinal or epidural anaesthesia. A decision must then be made regarding whether there is sufficient time to attempt an alternative NA technique (Figure 21.5). This usually means the use of spinal anaesthesia after a previously failed spinal, or after a failed epidural top-up. A CSE may be of particular benefit in this situation, as it allows reduction of the spinal dose administered in order to manage the apparent increased risk of a high spinal block. The epidural catheter can therefore be used if the spinal component proves to be inadequate. If it is not possible to provide alternate NA, GA must be provided.

The use of spinal anaesthesia after failed epidural anaesthesia is a controversial issue. Case reports describe spinal administration of LA after failed epidural anaesthesia resulting in an unintentionally high spinal block, and the need for emergency intubation and ventilation.[77,78] The apparent unpredictable nature of spinal anaesthesia after epidural injection has even lead to some suggesting that 'the rule should be to avoid spinal anaesthesia in pregnant women who already have an epidural block or in whom an epidural block has been attempted'.[79] However, some institutions routinely perform spinal anaesthesia after inadequate epidural block, and have reported low complication rates when using both reduced,[80] and normal doses of spinal LA.[81] The role of spinal anaesthesia after failed epidural injection remain unclear, as does the spinal dose that should be used to avoid unintended high blocks. The use of a low-dose spinal component of a CSE technique with the fallback of the epidural should the block still be too low, is valuable in this situation.

There have been many hypotheses to explain the possible risk of high block.[82] The most commonly cited, and most intuitive, is that there is expansion of the dural sac by the epidural injection of LA, which causes compression of the intrathecal compartment, and results in greater spread of spinal anaesthetic. Alternative theories include leakage of epidural LA into the intrathecal space via the dural puncture, uncovering of subclinical epidural anaesthesia by the spinal dose, or incremental continuing spread of intrathecal LA.

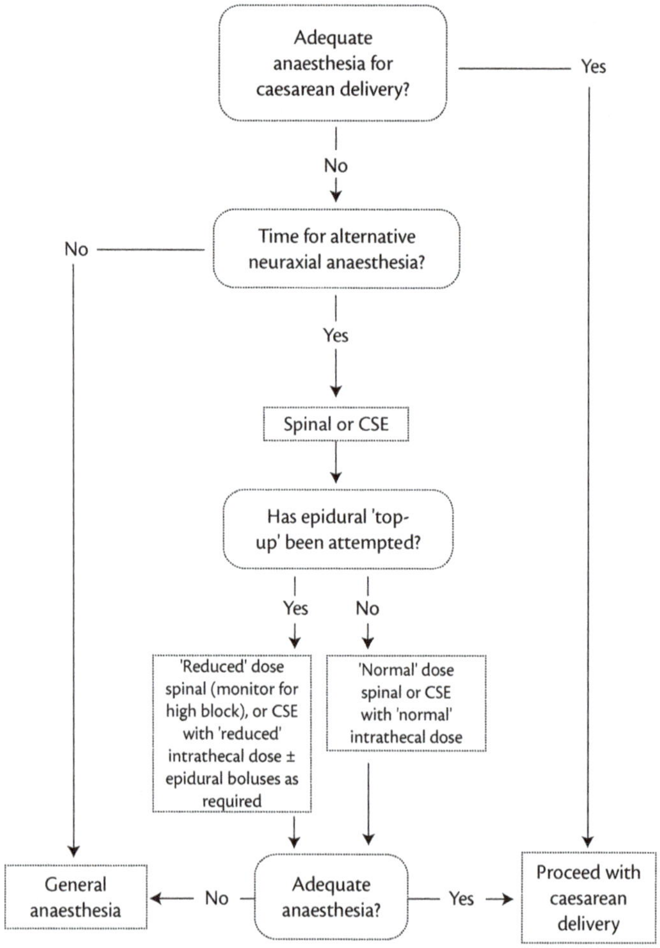

Figure 21.5 Management of inadequate neuraxial anaesthesia before the start of surgery.
With permission of Sunderland Royal Hospital.

Advocates of a reduced spinal dose (typically a reduction of 20–30%)[80] after failed epidural anaesthesia cite the fact that epidural volume extension (EVE) has been demonstrated in both pregnant[83] and non-pregnant[84] patients to cause a median dermatomal level rise. Since EVE acts as a volume effect in reverse (i.e. spinal, then epidural), it seems reasonable that compression of the dural sac preceding a normal dose of spinal LA might result in a high block. However, some studies have questioned the effect of EVE on LA sparing[85] and level of sensory block.[86] This has led to those in favour of normal spinal doses arguing that there is a lack of prospective, randomized evidence, and that reducing the dose of spinal LA exposes the patient to the risk of a second inadequate block, the risks of a second procedure, and possibly of a subsequent GA.

At a national obstetric anaesthetic conference, having heard the arguments for and against reduced spinal doses after failed epidural anaesthesia, 60% of delegates voted for the use of normal spinal doses.[81] It would therefore seem reasonable to perform a normal dose of spinal when an epidural has failed prior to surgery. However, if a normal spinal dose is to be used, care must be taken to minimize high spinal effects, with the careful use of positioning (head-up after the desired block level reached), intravenous (IV) fluid, and vasopressors in order to reduce maternal and fetal risk.

The use of repeat spinal LA after failed spinal anaesthesia appears far less controversial, which may be due to the differing causes of failure in spinal anaesthesia, compared to epidurals. Whilst there are isolated case reports of repeat spinals with 'normal' doses being successfully used,[87] a retrospective study of 1197 women undergoing CD under spinal, using 12 mg 0.5% heavy bupivacaine, found that there was a failure rate of 1.5%.[88] When spinal anaesthesia was repeated in these women, using 9 mg of the same LA, 33% experienced either hypotension, bradycardia, or both. Additionally, 5.5% of women experienced a 'high block', whilst the failure rate for the second spinal injection was also 5.5%.

The dosing for spinal anaesthesia after either failure of previous NA remains a balance between the need to provide adequate anaesthesia, and therefore avoid the need for an additional GA, and the need to avoid potentially life-threatening complications to either maternal or fetal health. An alternative, if time allows, may be to use a CSE. This allows a lower dose of spinal to be injected, in order to avoid excessive hypotension or high block, but also the relative security of an epidural catheter, so that further epidural LA may be given if required to pre-empt, or in response to intraoperative discomfort.

Intraoperatively: before delivery

Once surgery has been commenced, management of inadequate NA has classically been divided into those measures that can be undertaken prior to delivery, and those that are undertaken after delivery. One reason for this could be concern that some interventions may result in a delay in delivery of the fetus (e.g. obtaining, drawing up, and titrating IV analgesia). In situations of an emergency CD, this may add to fetal morbidity and mortality. A more probable reason for the restricted range of management options available to anaesthetists before delivery may be concerns over unintentional neonatal side effects from maternal drug administration (Figure 21.6).

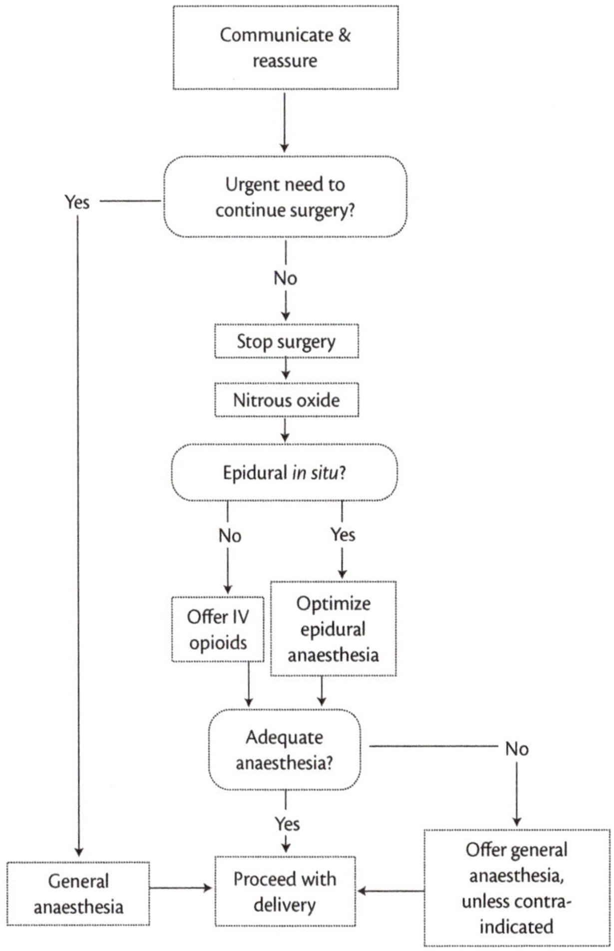

Figure 21.6 Management of inadequate neuraxial anaesthesia before delivery.
With permission of Sunderland Royal Hospital.

Extrapolating from the use of IV opioids in labour, it is clear that the use of IV fentanyl-based patient-controlled analgesia (PCA) during labour can result in lower Apgar scores at 1 minute, and increased rates of naloxone use and active resuscitation.[89] However, it may not be altogether accurate to base operative management on labour data. Firstly, the overall dose of IV fentanyl used (940 mcg) is far higher than would be expected to be used for operative supplementation. Furthermore, although active resuscitation and naloxone were more commonly used, this may just be a product of bias on the part of the unblinded clinicians that were caring for the neonates. And finally, although Apgar scores at 1 minute were significantly different, the effect was short lived, and not present at 5 minutes.

Looking specifically at the use of IV opioid analgesia intraoperatively, data is conflicting. Studies comparing the effects of IV and intrathecal sufentanil[90] and fentanyl[91] found no differences in Apgar scores where opioids were administered intravenously, compared to controls. Indeed, in a study designed to assess the safety of premedication doses of IV midazolam with fentanyl in women having elective CD, there were no significant differences in Apgar scores, arterial cord blood gases, nor newborn neurobehavioural scores compared to controls receiving saline.[92] However, the use of the ultra-short-acting opioid, remifentanil, during elective CD under GA, has been associated with significantly lower Apgar scores at 1 and 5 minutes, and lower umbilical vein pH (although this remained within the normal range).[93] Alfentanil may allow a better compromise between the depth of analgesia and length of action, compared to other IV opioids. An *in vitro* study of alfentanil pharmacokinetics suggested that it is rapidly transferred across the human placenta, with transfer occurring within 5 minutes and peaking at approximately 30 minutes.[94] However, alfentanil did not accumulate in placental tissue, and was readily washed out. Purdie et al. assessed the use and safety of an alfentanil PCA device to relieve visceral pain during elective CD.[95] There were similar incidences of sedation and nausea and respiratory changes between the PCA users and the non-PCA users. Only 2 out of 24 women used the PCA before cord clamping. However, in this small group, the Apgar scores and umbilical venous pH were similar to those observed in all the neonates.

Considering the conflicting evidence regarding neonatal side effects, it would seem sensible to attempt to avoid IV supplementation with either opioid analgesia or anxiolytics, such as midazolam, before umbilical cord clamping. If pre-delivery supplementation is to be used, short-acting opioids should be considered, and the personnel and equipment required to perform neonatal resuscitation should be immediately on hand.

Avoiding IV supplementation before delivery leaves a limited number of options available in the event of inadequate NA.

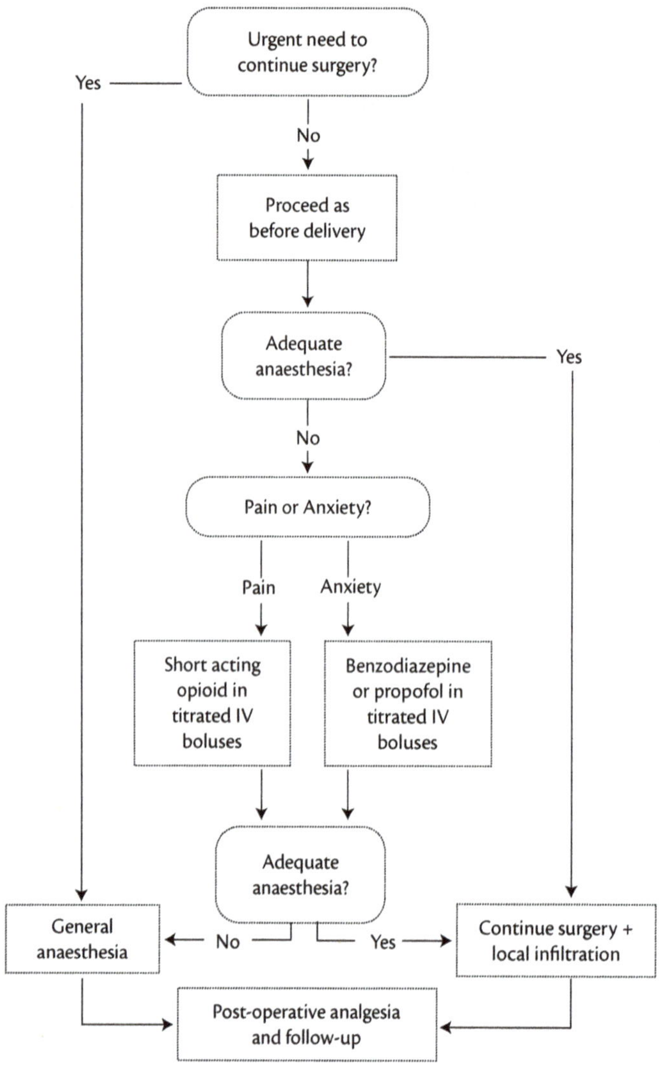

Figure 21.7 Management of inadequate neuraxial anaesthesia after delivery.
With permission of Sunderland Royal Hospital.

Importantly, a clear pre- and intraoperative explanation of the causes of any residual sensation may reassure some patients.[96] Not only might this help recruit the birth partner to distract the woman from the sensations, but also may allow discussion of a management plan that is acceptable to both the patient and clinician. Some authors recommend playing music in the background, to help relaxation and distraction.[97] However, a review of the use of music during CD found that the magnitude of improvement in maternal heart rate and satisfaction scores were low, and that the methodological quality of some studies were questionable.[98] It would therefore appear wise not to rely on musical distraction as the sole means of managing inadequate NA.

Fifty per cent nitrous oxide has long been used for labour analgesia,[99,100] and its anaesthetic-sparing effects during CD under GA.[101] Its use in situations of inadequate NA therefore seems intuitive, due to its easy availability on anaesthetic machines, the ease of administration, and the familiarity that most pregnant women have with it. However, nitrous oxide use is not without its disadvantages. Acute side effects that may be experienced include dose-dependent depression in ventilatory function and control of upper airway patency, dysphoria, and vomiting. Additionally, although it can be effective in minor procedures, it is generally less effective in severely painful procedures.[102] As a result, the use of nitrous oxide should only be considered a short-term solution, allowing time for either GA to be induced, or delivery of the fetus followed by a more definitive form of management.

Every effort should also be made to optimize pre-existing epidural anaesthesia, if a catheter has been maintained *in situ*. The use of faster-acting LA, such as 2% lidocaine with 1 in 200,000 epinephrine, and epidural opioids are ideal, although care must be taken to avoid administering doses above the upper safe limit. Furthermore, unless there is a specific contraindication to GA, this option should always be discussed with the patient, regardless of when the NA has become inadequate, along with the risks and benefits in the specific situation.

Intraoperatively: after delivery

If inadequate NA becomes apparent after delivery, more management options are generally available, as concerns over fetal transfer of drug are removed (Figure 21.7). Also, any concerns about the need to rapidly deliver the baby have also been resolved. However, the approach to management should mirror what has already been described, namely reassurance, communication, the use of nitrous oxide as a temporary analgesic, optimization of epidural anaesthesia, if an epidural catheter is *in situ*, and consideration of GA. Where possible, surgery should be halted until definitive management of the inadequate anaesthesia has occurred. This is clearly not possible in emergent situations, such as maternal haemorrhage, where the transition to GA will need to be done rapidly, but safely.

In a retrospective case notes review of 2471 women undergoing CD under NA, Garry and Davies examined the causes and management of inadequate NA.[103] Sixty-five women received GA, whilst 175 required some form of supplementation at some point during the procedure. Common post-delivery causes of supplementation or conversion to GA included pain on uterine exteriorization, bleeding, and prolonged surgery. Types of supplementation included nitrous oxide, short-acting opioids such as alfentanil or fentanyl, nitrous oxide and opioids in combination, or alternatives such as morphine, ketamine, midazolam, or propofol. Only 13 of the patients requiring supplementation also received a GA. However, the review did not present data regarding maternal or fetal side effects of IV supplementation with opioids or anxiolytics, such as benzodiazepines.

In situations where pain is the main complaint, supplementary agents of choice should undoubtedly have an analgesic effect. Short-acting opioids, such as fentanyl or alfentanil, provide the balance between a rapid onset of action, ease of titration and avoidance of side effects, such as respiratory depression. Ketamine provides a good alternative to opioid analgesia for mild to moderate pain. Although little prospective evidence is available regarding the effectiveness of ketamine at supplementing intraoperatively inadequate NA, in combination with spinal bupivacaine, 0.15 mg/kg IV ketamine has been associated with significantly lower postoperative pain scores from 60 minutes, and reduced postoperative analgesia usage up to day 2.[104] However, ketamine use is also associated with unpleasant emergence phenomenon, which may be unacceptable to the patient. Additionally, ketamine should be avoided in patients with hypertension.

If pain is localized within the surgical field, supplementation of NA with local infiltration by the surgeon should also be considered. However, many obstetricians are untrained at administering local infiltration, and perform this rarely, due to the relative reliability of NA. Therefore, it is likely that infiltration will not be effective. Surgical administration of LA within the peritoneal cavity has also been advocated where peritoneal stimulation is the major source of discomfort.[105] If supplemental LA administration is considered, attention should be given to avoiding toxic doses, when combined with NA administered within the last 4 hours.

Exteriorization of the uterus was regularly done in the past but this is no longer advocated unless there is a definite surgical indication, for example, if there is a lateral tear to optimize surgical repair. Warning should be given by the surgeon as peritoneal tugging at this time will cause discomfort particularly if done under epidural top-up.

Garry and Davies found that a cause of conversion to GA or need for supplementation was maternal anxiety, or the dislike of paraesthesia associated with established NA.[103] In cases where anxiety is the primary cause of maternal distress, and is not associated with pain, an anxiolytic may be considered. Titrated dosing of a benzodiazepine, such as midazolam, is familiar to most anaesthetists, although some have suggested that diazepam may be superior to midazolam, as it produces less amnesia during the birth period.[104] Propofol, as an alternative anxiolytic, allows for a shorter duration of action, but at the expense of greater cardiovascular side effects. Care should be taken when administering such drugs, due to the risk of respiratory and cardiovascular depression, and the potential for central nervous depression, regurgitation, and aspiration. Furthermore, if maternal distress is associated with pain, analgesia or anaesthesia should be considered the solution, rather than anxiolysis.

When all possibilities in optimizing pre-existing NA and supplementation have been unsuccessful, the only remaining option should be GA. Where possible, induction should be preceded by clear communication with the patient, partner, and surgeons, a temporary halt of surgical manipulation, adequate antacid premedication, and pre-oxygenation prior to rapid sequence induction. Once anaesthesia has been induced, endotracheal intubation has been performed, and the patient is being adequately ventilated and anaesthetized, attention should be given to intra- and postoperative analgesia, as discussed in the chapters covering GA for CD (Chapter 22) and postoperative analgesia after CD (Chapter 24).

Postoperative care

Undoubtedly, childbirth can be stressful for the parents, especially if unexpected events occur. In some cases, childbirth can be such a traumatic experience, as to precipitate, in extreme cases, post-traumatic stress disorder (PTSD). A survey of pain during labour, by Melzack,[106] found that 60% of primiparous, and 45% of multiparous women had severe or extremely severe pain during labour, whilst most reported that labour was the most intense pain they had ever experienced. A traumatic event, during which the patient feels threatened by death or serious injury, and has feelings of fear or helplessness, is the first diagnostic criteria of PTSD. It is therefore important for clinicians to be aware of when women perceive their experience of childbirth as traumatic, the risk factors for development of post-delivery complications, such as PTSD, and their impact within this.

A number of risk factors for the development of PTSD after child birth have been described. These include having a more negative experience than expected,[107] unplanned CD, obstetric or pregnancy complications,[108] and experiencing intense pain or distress during labour.[109] It is easy to see that any of these factors could be experienced during inadequate anaesthesia for CD. However, management of the spectrum from traumatic childbirth to PTSD is less well described, with limited evidence relating to the management of women with PTSD after childbirth. There is some consensus with non-childbirth-related literature that debriefing and counselling are inconclusively effective, whilst cognitive behavioural therapy may improve PTSD status.[110] That said, it has also been suggested that offering women an opportunity to discuss their experience and to differentiate this from a formal debrief, may also be appropriate.[111]

Considering all the above, it would seem reasonable to perform a postoperative visit to the patient, in the days following delivery. Not only does this give the anaesthetist a chance to review for complications of NA, but also allows an opportunity to explain the possible reasons for, and the management of, the inadequate NA. Additionally, the patient will have the opportunity to gain answers to any questions that they may still have, in a more relaxed environment. Furthermore, arrangements can be made at this point, if further discussion is required regarding the childbirth experience. Documentation should also be meticulous, as this not only supplies a record of events for subsequent discussion of the experience, but also supplies the basis of a medicolegal defence, if required.

Conclusion

NA is the preferred method of providing anaesthesia for CD. This has been primarily driven by the prominent role of GA in the morbidity and mortality related to anaesthesia in obstetrics. However, the effects of failed NA, both to the short- and long-term health of the woman, and also the medicolegal consequences, mean that clinicians need to have ways of predicting such situations. Careful choice of LA, neuraxial technique, and recognition of risk factors can reduce the risk of inadequate NA. Furthermore, if NA were to fail, clinicians need to have strategies for effective management of intraoperative pain or anxiety, whilst minimizing the risk to both the mother and newborn. Management options, such as repeating or attempting another neuraxial technique, IV analgesic, or conversion to GA could all be considered, depending on the individual situation.

References

1. Shibli KU, Russell IF. A survey of anaesthetic techniques used for caesarean section in the UK in 1997. *Int J Obstet Anesth* 2000; 9:160–7.
2. Thomas J, Paranjothy S, Royal College of Obstetricians and Gynaecologists Clinical Effectiveness Support Unit. *National Sentinel Caesarean Section Audit Report*. London: RCOG Press; 2001.
3. Rafi M, Arfeen Z, Misra U. Conversion of regional to general anaesthesia at caesarean section: increasing the use of regional anaesthesia through continuous prospective audit. *Int J Obstet Anesth* 2010; 19:179–82.
4. Clergue F, Auroy Y, Péquignot F. French Survey of Anesthesia in 1996. *Anesthesiology* 1999; 9:1509–20.
5. Benhamou D, Bouaziz H, Chassard D, *et al.* Anaesthetic practices for scheduled caesarean delivery: a 2005 French national survey. *Eur J Anaesth* 2009; 26:694–700.
6. Marcus HE, Behrend A, Schier R, *et al.* Anesthesiological management of caesarean sections: nationwide survey in Germany. *Anaesthesist* 2011; 60:916–28.
7. Stamer UM, Wiese R, Stüber F, *et al.* Change in anaesthetic practice for Caesarean section in Germany. *Acta Anaesthesiol Scand* 2005; 49:170–6.
8. Van Houwe P, Heytens L, Vercruysse P. A survey of obstetric practice in Flanders. *Acta Anaesthesiol Belg* 2006; 57:29–37
9. Bucklin B, Hawkins J, Anderson J. Obstetric anesthesia workforce survey. *Anesthesiology* 2003; (3):645–53.
10. Weiniger CF, Ivri S, Ioscovich A, *et al.* Obstetric anesthesia units in Israel: a national questionnaire-based survey. *Int J Obstet Anesth* 2010; 19:410–16.
11. Crawford-Sykes A, Scarlett M, Hambleton IR, *et al.* Anaesthesia for operative deliveries at the University Hospital of the West Indies: a change of practice. *West Indian Med J* 2005; 54:187–91.
12. Okafor UV, Ezegwui HU, Ekwazi K. Trends of different forms of anaesthesia for caesarean section in South-eastern Nigeria. *J Obstet Gynaecol* 2009; 29:392–5.
13. Ministry of Health. *Report on Confidential Enquiries into Maternal Deaths in England and Wales, 1952–54*. Reports on Public Health and Medical Subjects No. 97. London: HMSO; 1957.
14. Knight M, Kenyon S, Brocklehurst P, *et al. Saving Lives, Improving Mothers' Care - Lessons Learned to Inform Future Maternity Care from the UK and Ireland Confidential Enquiries into Maternal Deaths and Morbidity 2009–12*. Oxford: National Perinatal Epidemiology Unit, University of Oxford; 2014.
15. Ngan Kee WD. Confidential Enquiries into Maternal Deaths: 50 years of closing the loop. *Br J Anaesth* 2005; 94:413–16.
16. Cooper GM, McClure JH. Maternal deaths from anaesthesia. An extract from Why Mothers Die 2000-2002, the Confidential Enquiries into Maternal Deaths in the United Kingdom: Chapter 9: A naesthesia. *Br J Anaesth* 2005; 94:417–23.
17. Kinsella SM. A prospective audit of regional anaesthesia failure in 5080 Caesarean sections. *Anaesthesia* 2008; 63:822–32.
18. Pan PH, Bogard TD, Owen MD. Incidence and characteristics of failures in obstetric neuraxial analgesia and anesthesia: a retrospective analysis of 19,259 deliveries. *Int J Obstet Anesth* 2004; 13:227–33.
19. Chadwick H, Posner K, Caplan R, *et al.* A comparison of obstetric and nonobstetric anesthesia malpractice claims. *Anesthesiology* 1991; 74:242–9.
20. Davies JM, Posner KL, Lee LA, *et al.* Liability associated with obstetric anesthesia. *Anesthesiology* 2009; 110:131–9.
21. Peng P, Smedstad K. Litigation in Canada against anesthesiologists practicing regional anaesthesia. A review of closed claims. *Can J Anaesth* 2000; 105–12.
22. Cook TM, Bland L, Mihai R, *et al.* Litigation related to anaesthesia: an analysis of claims against the NHS in England 1995–2007. *Anaesthesia* 2009; 64:706–18.
23. Szypula K, Ashpole KJ, Bogod D, *et al.* Litigation related to regional anaesthesia: an analysis of claims against the NHS in England 1995–2007. *Anaesthesia* 2010; 65:443–52.
24. Riley ET, Papasin J. Epidural catheter function during labor predicts anesthetic efficacy for subsequent cesarean delivery. *Int J Obstet Anesth* 2002; 11:81–4.
25. Campbell DC, Tran T. Conversion of epidural labour analgesia to epidural anesthesia for intrapartum Cesarean delivery. *Can J Anaesth* 2009; 56:19–26.
26. Halpern SH, Soliman A, Yee J, Angle P, *et al.* Conversion of epidural labour analgesia to anaesthesia for Caesarean section: a prospective study of the incidence and determinants of failure. *Br J Anaesth* 2009; 102:240–3.
27. Tortosa JC. Efficacy of augmentation of epidural analgesia for Caesarean section. *Br J Anaesth* 2003; 91:532–5.
28. Hillyard SG, Bate TE, Corcoran TB, Paech MJ, *et al.* Extending epidural analgesia for emergency Caesarean section: a meta-analysis. *Br J Anaesth* 2011; 107:668–78.
29. Huhnert BR, Kuhnert PM, Philipson EH, *et al.* The half-life of 2-chloroprocaine. *Anesth Analg* 1986; 65:273–8.
30. Francis JM, Dewan DM, Floyd HM, *et al.* Chloroprocaine vs. bupivacaine for lumbar epidural analgesia for elective Cesarean section. *Anesthesiology* 1980; 52:488–91.
31. Bjornestad E, Iverson OL, Raeder J. Similar onset tie of 2-chloroprocaine and lidocaine + epinephrine for epidural anesthesia for elective Cesarean section. *Acta Anaesthesiol Scand* 2006; 50:358–63.
32. Gaiser RR, Cheek TG, Gutsche BB. Epidural lidocaine versus 2-chloroprocaine for fetal distress requiring urgent Cesarean section. *Int J Obstet Anesth* 1994; 3:208–10.
33. Abboud TK, Kim KC, Noueihed R, *et al.* Epidural bupivacaine, chloroprocaine, or lidocaine for Cesarean section—maternal and neonatal effects. *Anesth Analg* 1983; 62:914–19.
34. Reisner LS, Hockman BN, Plummer MH. Persistent neurologic deficit and adhesive arachnoiditis following intrathecal 2-chloroprocaine injection. *Anesth Analg* 1980; 59:452–4.
35. Moore DC, Spierdijk J, vanKleef JD, *et al.* Chloroprocaine neurotoxicity: four additional cases. *Anesth Analg* 1982; 61:155–9.

36. Wang BC, Hillman DE, Spielholz NI, *et al.* Chronic neurological deficits and Nescaine-CE—an effect of the anesthetic, 2-chloroprocaine, or the antioxidant, sodium bisulfite? *Anesth Analg* 1984; 63:445–7.
37. Taniguchi M, Bollen AW, Drasner K. Sodium bisulfite. Scapegoat for chloroprocaine neurotoxicity? *Anesthesiology* 2004; 100:85–91.
38. Eisenach JC, Schlairet TJ, Dobson CE 2nd, *et al.* Effect of prior anesthetic solution on epidural morphine analgesia. *Anesth Analg* 1991; 73:119–23.
39. Curatolo M, Petersen-Felix S, Scaramozzino P, *et al.* Epidural fentanyl, adrenaline and clonidine as adjuvants to local anaesthetics for surgical analgesia: meta-analyses of analgesia and side effects. *Acta Anaesthesiol Scand* 1998; 42:910–20.
40. National Institute for Health and Clinical Excellence. *Caesarean Section.* Clinical Guideline 132. London: NICE. http://guidance.nice.org.uk/CG132
41. Caranza R, Jeyapalan I, Buggy DJ. Central neuraxial opioid analgesia after caesarean section: comparison of epidural diamorphine and intrathecal morphine. *Int J Obstet Anesth* 1999; 8:90–3.
42. Hallworth SP, Fernando R, Bell R, *et al.* Comparison of intrathecal and epidural diamorphine for elective caesarean section using a combined spinal-epidural technique. *Br J Anaesth* 1999; 82:228–32.
43. Saravanan S, Robinson AP, Qayoum Dar A, *et al.* Minimum dose of intrathecal diamorphine required to prevent intraoperative supplementation of spinal anaesthesia for Caesarean section. *Br J Anaesth* 2003; 91:368–72.
44. Wong K, Strichartz GR, Raymond SA. On the mechanisms of potentiation of local anesthetics by bicarbonate buffer. *Anesth Analg* 1993; 76:131–43.
45. Curatolo M, Petersen-Felix S. Adding sodium bicarbonate to lidocaine enhances the depth of epidural blockade. *Anesth Analg* 1998; 86:341–7.
46. Fernando R, Jones H. Comparison of plain and alkalinized local anaesthetic mixtures of lignocaine and bupivacaine for elective extradural caesarean section. *Br J Anaesth* 1991; 67:699–703.
47. Allam J, Malhotra S, Hemingway C, *et al.* Epidural lidocaine-bicarbonate-adrenaline vs levobupivacaine for emergency Caesarean section: a randomised controlled trial. *Anaesthesia* 2008; 63:243–9.
48. Clark V, McGrady E. Speed of onset of sensory block for elective extradural Caesarean section: choice of agent and temperature of injectate. *Br J Anaesth* 1994; 72:221–3.
49. Sviggum HP, Yacoubian S, Liu X, *et al.* The effect of bupivacaine with fentanyl temperature on initiation and maintenance of labor epidural analgesia: a randomized controlled study. *Int J Obstet Anesth* 2015; 24(1):15–21.
50. Luca DN, Borra PJ, Yentis SM. Epidural top-up solutions for emergency Caesarean section: a comparison of preparation times. *Br J Anaesth* 2000; 84:494–6.
51. Robinson J, Fernando R, Sun Wai WYS, *et al.* Chemical stability of bupivacaine, lidocaine and epinephrine in pH-adjusted solutions. *Anaesthesia* 2000; 55:853–8.
52. Tuleu C, Allam J, Gill H, *et al.* Short term stability of pH-adjusted lidocaine-adrenaline epidural solution used for emergency caesarean section. *Int J Obstet Anesth* 2008; 17:118–122.
52. MacPherson RD. Pharmaceutics for the anaesthetist. *Anaesthesia* 2001; 56:965–979.
53. Ploteau S, de Kersaint-Gilly A, Boog G. Medullar adhesive arachnoiditis: a late complication after obstetrical epidural analgesia. *Gynecol Obstet Fertil* 2004; 32:961–4.
54. Rice I, Wee MYK, Thomson K. Obstetric epidurals and chronic adhesive arachnoiditis. *Br J Anaesth* 2004; 92:109–20.
55. Taguchi H, Oishi K, Sakamoto S, *et al.* Intrathecal betamethasone for cancer patients in the lower half of the body: a study of its analgesic efficacy and safety. *Br J Anaesth* 2007; 98:385–9.
56. Wang BC, Li D, Hiller JM, *et al.* Lumbar subarachnoid ethylenediaminetetraacetate induces hindlimb tetanic contractions in rats: prevention by $CaCl_2$ pretreatment—observation of spinal nerve root degeneration. *Anesth Analg* 1992; 75:895–9.
57. Fettes PDW, Jansson JR, Wildsmith JAW. Failed spinal anaesthesia: mechanisms, management, and prevention. *Br J Anaesth* 2009; 102:739–48.
58. Hocking G, Wildsmith JAW. Intrathecal drug spread. *Br J Anaesth* 2004; 93:568–78.
59. Carvalho B, Durbin M, Drover DR, *et al.* The ED50 and ED95 of intrathecal isobaric bupivacaine with opioids for cesarean delivery. *Anesthesiology* 2005; 103:606–12.
60. Ginosar Y, Mirikatani E, Drover DR, *et al.* ED50 and ED95 of intrathecal hyperbaric bupivacaine coadministered with opioids for cesarean delivery. *Anesthesiology* 2004; 100:676–82.
61. Bouvet L, Da-Col X, Chassard D, *et al.* ED_{50} and ED_{95} of intrathecal levobupivacaine with opioids for Caesarean delivery. *Br J Anaesth* 2011; 106:215–20.
62. Ben-David B, Miller G, Gavriel R, *et al.* Low-dose bupivacaine-fentanyl spinal anesthesia for cesarean delivery. *Reg Anesth Pain Med* 2000; 25:235–9.
63. Arzola C, Wieczorek PM. Efficacy of low-dose bupivacaine in spinal anaesthesia for Caesarean delivery: systematic review and meta-analysis. *Br J Anaesth* 2011; 107:308–18.
64. Van de Velde M, Van Schoubroeck D, Jani J, *et al.* Combined spinal epidural anesthesia for cesarean section: dose dependent effects of hyperbaric bupivacaine on maternal hemodynamics. *Anesth Analg* 2006; 103:187–90.
65. Roofthooft E, Van de Velde M. Low-dose spinal anaesthesia for caesarean section to prevent spinal-induced hypotension. *Curr Opin Anesthesiol* 2008; 21:259–62.
66. Wildsmith JAW. Caesarean section demands a block to ... ? Sacred cows and Shibboleths. *R Coll Anaesth Bull* 2004; 26:1316–17.
67. Saravanan S. Minimum dose of intrathecal diamorphine required to prevent intraoperative supplementation of spinal anaesthesia for Caesarean section. *Br J Anaesth* 2003; 91:368–72.
68. Russell IF. Levels of anaesthesia and intraoperative pain at caesarean section under regional block. *Int J Obstet Anesth* 1995; 4:71–7.
69. Russell IF. A comparison of cold, pinprick and touch for assessing the level of spinal block at caesarean section. *Int J Obstet Anesth* 2004; 13:146–52.
70. Kocarev M, Watkins E, McLure H, *et al.* Sensory testing of spinal anaesthesia for caesarean section: differential block and variability. *Int J Obstet Anesth* 2010; 19:261–5.
71. Russell IF. Assessing the block for caesarean section. *Int J Obstet Anesth* 2001; 10:83–5.
72. Husain T, Liu YM, Fernando R, *et al.* How UK obstetric anaesthetists assess neuraxial anaesthesia for caesarean delivery: national surveys of practice conducted in 2004 and 2010. *Int J Obstet Anesth* 2013; 22(4):298–302.
73. Bourne TM, deMelo AE, Bastianpillai BA, *et al.* A survey of how British obstetric anaesthetists test regional anaesthesia before caesarean section. *Anaesthesia* 1997; 52:901–3.
74. Congreve K, Scrutton M, Laxton C, *et al.* Where is T5? A survey of anaesthetists. *Anaesthesia* 2006;61:453–5.
75. Yentis SM. Is my T2 your T2 too? *Int J Obstet Anesth* 2005; 14:S12.
76. Russell IF. Testing regional anaesthesia before caesarean section. *Anaesthesia* 1998; 53:93–4.
77. Stone PA, Thorburn J, Lamb KSR. Complications of spinal anaesthesia following extradural block for caesarean section. *Br J Anaesth* 1989; 62:335–7.
78. Mets B, Broccoli E, Brown AR. Is spinal anesthesia after failed epidural anesthesia contraindicated for cesarean section? *Anesth Analg* 1993; 77:629–31.
79. Gupta A. Spinal anesthesia after failed epidural anesthesia. *Anesth Analg* 1996; 82:214–22.
80. Waters J, Leivers D, Hullander M. Response to spinal anesthesia after inadequate epidural anesthesia. *Anesth Analg* 1994; 78:1033–4.
81. Adams TJ, Peter EA, Douglas MJ. Is spinal anesthesia contraindicated after failed epidural anesthesia. *Anesth Analg* 1995; 81:659.

82. Wilson MJA, Stock GM. When using spinal anaesthesia for caesarean section after the epidural has failed, the normal dose of spinal anaesthetic should be used. *Int J Obstet Anesth* 2005; 14:53–7.
83. Blumgart CH, Ryall D, Dennison B, *et al.* Mechanism of extension of spinal anaesthesia by extradural injection of local anaesthetic. *Br J Anaesth* 1992; 69:457–60.
84. Mardirosoff C, Dumont L, Lemedioni P, *et al.* Sensory block extension during combined spinal and epidural. *Reg Anesth Pain Med* 1998; 23:92–5.
85. Beale N, Evans B, Plaat F, *et al.* Effects of epidural extension on dose requirement of intrathecal hyperbaric bupivacaine at caesarean section. *Br J Anaesth* 2005; 95:500–3.
86. Loubert C, O'Brien PJ, Fernando R, *et al.* Epidural volume extension in combined spinal epidural anaesthesia for elective caesarean section: a randomised controlled trial. *Anaesthesia* 2011; 66:341–7.
87. Deshpande S, Idriz R. Repeat dose after an inadequate spinal block. *Anaesthesia* 1996; 51:892.
88. Pokharel A. study of failed spinal anesthesia undergoing caesarean section and its management. *Postgrad Med J NAMS* 2013; 11:11–15.
89. Halpern SH, Muir H, Breen TW, *et al.* A multicenter randomized controlled trial comparing patient-controlled epidural with intravenous analgesia for pain relief in labor. *Anesth Anal* 2004; 99:1532–8.
90. Wang LZ, Zhang YF, Tang BL, *et al.* Effects of intrathecal and i.v. small-dose sufentanil on the median effective dose of intrathecal bupivacaine for caesarean section. *Br J Anaesth* 2007; 98:792–6.
91. Siddik-Sayyid SM, Aouad MT, Jalbout MI, *et al.* Intrathecal versus intravenous fentanyl for supplementation of subarachnoid block during cesarean delivery. *Anesth Analg* 2002; 95:209–13.
92. Frölich MA, Burchfield DJ, Euliano TY, *et al.* A single dose of fentanyl and midazolam prior to Cesarean section have no adverse neonatal effects. *Can J Anaesth* 2006; 53:79–85.
93. Draisci G, Valente A, Suppa E, *et al.* Remifentanil for cesarean section under general anesthesia: effects on maternal stress hormone secretion and neonatal well-being: a randomized trial. *Int J Obstet Anesth* 2008; 17:130–6.
94. Zakowski MI, Ham A, Grant G. Transfer and uptake of alfentanil in the human placenta during in vitro perfusion. *Anesth Analg* 1994; 79:1089–93.
95. Purdie NL, Kenny GNC, McGrady EM. Patient controlled administration of intravenous alfetanil during elective Caesarean section under subarachnoid anaesthesia. *Int J Obstet Anesth* 2003; 12:169–72.
96. Portnoy D, Vadhera RB. Mechanisms and management of an incomplete epidural block for cesarean section. *Anesthesiol Clin North Am* 2003; 21:39–57.
97. McKay RSF, Morrison LMM, McClure FH. Epidural anesthesia. In VanZundert A, Osthemer GW (eds). *Pain Relief and Anesthesia in Obstetrics*. New York: Churchill Livingstone; 1996:441–60.
98. Laopaiboon M, Lumbiganon P, Martis R, *et al.* Music during caesarean section under regional anaesthesia for improving maternal and infant outcomes. *Cochrane Database Syst Rev* 2009; 2:CD006914.
99. Marx GF, Katsnelson T. The introduction of nitrous oxide analgesia into obstetrics. *Obstet Gynecol* 1992; 80:715–18.
100. Rosen MA. Nitrous oxide for relief of labor pain: a systematic review. *Am J Obstet Gynecol* 2002; 186:S110–26.
101. Gambling DR, Sharma SK, White PF, *et al.* Use of sevoflurane during elective cesarean birth: a comparison with isoflurane and spinal anesthesia. *Anesth Analg* 1995; 81:90–5.
102. Tobias JD. Applications of nitrous oxide for procedural sedation in the pediatric population. *Pediatr Emerg Care* 2013; 29:245–65.
103. Garry M, Davies S. Failure of regional blockade for caesarean section. *Int J Obstet Anesth* 2002; 11:9–12.
104. Menkiti ID, Desalu I, Kushimo OT. Low-dose intravenous ketamine improves postoperative analgesia after caesarean delivery with spinal bupivacaine in African parturients. *Int J Obstet Anesth* 2012; 21:217–21.
105. Mets BA. In response to Gupta, Spinal anesthesia after failed epidural anesthesia. *Anesth Analg* 1996; 82:214–15.
106. Melzack R. Labour pain as a model of acute pain [editorial]. *Pain* 1993; 53:117–20.
107. Verreault N, Da Costa D, Marchand A, *et al.* PTSD following childbirth: a prospective study of incidence and risk factors in Canadian women. *J Psychosom Res* 2012; 73:257–63.
108. Stamrood CA, Paarlberg KM, Huis In 't Veld EM, *et al.* Posttraumatic stress following childbirth in homelike- and hospital settings. *J Psychosom Obstet Gynaecol* 2011; 32:88–97.
109. Andersen LB, Melvaer LB, Videbech P, *et al.* Risk factors for developing post-traumatic stress disorder following childbirth: a systematic review. *Acta Obstet Gynecol Scand* 2012; 91:1261–72.
110. Lapp LK, Agbokou C, Peretti CS, *et al.* Management of post traumatic stress disorder after childbirth: a review. *J Psychosom Obstet Gynaecol* 2010; 31:113–22.
111. Rowan C, Bick D, Bastos MH. Postnatal debriefing interventions to prevent maternal mental health problems after birth: exploring the gap between evidence and UK policy and practice. *Worldviews Evid Based Nurs* 2007; 4:97–105.

CHAPTER 22

General anaesthesia for caesarean delivery

David M. Levy and Ieva Saule

Introduction

In this chapter we shall review key aspects of the history of general anaesthesia (GA) and rapid sequence induction (RSI) for caesarean delivery (CD), and make comparisons with the latest concepts. The indications and contraindications to GA will be outlined and the following discussed: preoperative assessment, positioning, monitoring, intravenous (IV) access, preoxygenation, and airway management. Anaesthetic pharmacology will be summarized with a focus on neuromuscular blockade (NMB). Specific GA issues in the management of pre-eclampsia and haemorrhage will be detailed.

History of rapid sequence induction

Inhalation anaesthesia by facemask was used until a technique of IV induction, NMB, and tracheal intubation for CD was described by Hamer Hodges et al. in 1959.[1] Compared with anaesthetic techniques in which women received trichloroethylene, cyclopropane, or diethyl ether, the regimen of thiopental, succinylcholine, and nitrous oxide/oxygen resulted in the shortest times to babies' sustained respiration and crying. Certain elements of contemporary RSI were absent: cricoid pressure wasn't applied (Sellick had yet to describe his manoeuvre) and there was a period of bag and mask ventilation between induction and intubation. The novel use of succinylcholine for CD was advocated on the grounds that its rapid maternal offset reduced the chance of neonatal curarization compared with the only two alternative neuromuscular blocking drugs, gallamine and tubocurarine. The notion that recovery from succinylcholine might conceivably be advantageous for the woman in the event of airway problems did not appear to have been considered.

The salient characteristics of RSI were set out by Stept and Safar in 1970:[2]

- Preoxygenation
- Predetermined doses of thiopental and succinylcholine
- Cricoid pressure
- Avoidance of ventilation by bag and mask
- Tracheal intubation.

It has been noted that the number of maternal deaths attributable to anaesthesia in the Confidential Enquiries into Maternal Deaths in the United Kingdom virtually doubled in the period corresponding to the widespread replacement of mask and ether by RSI in the early 1960s.[3] Scott highlighted the apparent increased incidence of death due to Mendelson's syndrome and failed intubation secondary to succinylcholine and RSI.[4]

A rigorous Canadian evidence-based clinical update has analysed, in non-obstetric practice, the components of RSI. No evidence was found for decreased incidence of aspiration with RSI—the primary reason for continuing to practise the technique.[5] Despite a conspicuous lack of supportive evidence, the technique is endorsed for CD by the UK National Institute for Health and Care Excellence (NICE).[6]

Indications and contraindications to general anaesthesia

The most recent (2012) UK data from the Obstetric Anaesthetists' Association (OAA) National Obstetric Anaesthesia Database (http://www.oaa-anaes.ac.uk) revealed a median CD rate of 25.2% (range 13.4–51.3%). GA was induced in 10594 recorded cases (7.6% of CD), of which 43.1% represented conversions from neuraxial anaesthesia. These data are broadly in line with published surveys from elsewhere.

In the United Kingdom, the degree of urgency of CD is classified according to the presence of fetal or maternal compromise.[7] Category 1 denotes an immediate threat to life of woman or fetus. Category 2 indicates maternal or fetal compromise but no immediate threat to life. Category 3 describes a requirement for expedited delivery by CD in the absence of maternal or fetal compromise. Category 4 CD means that delivery can be planned to suit the woman and maternity services. The only absolute contraindication to GA is maternal refusal. GA is ideally avoided if there is predicted airway difficulty or malignant hyperthermia susceptibility. In morbid obesity, awake fibreoptic intubation can be considered (see Chapter 26 and Chapter 39). The UK Royal College of Anaesthetists has published a 'proposed standard or target for best practice'.[8] GA should be used in fewer than 5% of category 4 CD, and in fewer than 15% of Categories 1–3 combined. Fewer than half of category 1 CD should require GA. The most common indications for GA are listed in Box 22.1.

Placental abruption with significant haemorrhage is a contraindication to neuraxial anaesthesia on account of the very real risk of maternal cardiovascular collapse secondary to sympathetic blockade and not infrequent disseminated intravascular

Box 22.1 Common indications for general anaesthesia in obstetrics

- Category 1 CD for women without a working labour epidural
- Contraindications to a neuraxial technique, for example:
  - lumbar spinal abnormality (e.g. instrumented fusion)
  - coagulopathy
  - hypovolaemia
  - local sepsis
  - cardiac disease (e.g. aortic stenosis) in which abrupt sympathetic blockade would risk decompensation
- Failed neuraxial technique: uncontrollable breakthrough pain at CD
- Maternal refusal of neuraxial technique.

coagulopathy. In contrast, *elective* CD for placenta praevia, when surgery is started with a normal circulating blood volume, is not necessarily a contraindication to a neuraxial block. It is important to plan for major haemorrhage and ensure large-gauge vascular access and availability of rapid infusion devices to keep up with blood loss and maintain intravascular volume. Homologous blood must be available in theatre and, ideally, the facility for intraoperative cell salvage provided.

Although traditionally regarded as an absolute indication for GA, umbilical cord prolapse does not mandate GA. Provided that the fetus is continuously monitored and signs of compromise are not observed, a labour epidural can be topped up or spinal anaesthesia instituted in a left-lateral position.

Preparation for general anaesthesia

Preoperative assessment

The conduct of maternal preoperative assessment differs in elective and emergency settings.

Women scheduled for elective CD should ideally be reviewed before the day of surgery either on a ward or pre-assessment suite. Past medical and anaesthetic history, drug allergies and intolerances, gestation, parity, and placental site should be noted. Careful assessment of the airway is essential. Antacid premedication should be prescribed (see 'Aspiration prophylaxis: antacids'). Recent blood antibody screen (to determine ABO and Rhesus D types and detect other red cell antibodies that could haemolyse transfused red cells) and availability of matched blood must be reviewed in association with recent maternal haemoglobin concentration and platelet count. Although NICE advises that pregnant women who are healthy and have uncomplicated pregnancies do not require routine grouping and saving of serum or cross-matching of blood before CD, confirmation of a recent 'group and save' remains routine practice in many units. However, cross-matched blood must be available for women with anaemia, coagulopathy, or abnormal placentation.[6] A preoperative visit should include full informed consent and explanation of the respective risks and benefits of RSI, blood transfusion, patient-controlled analgesia, rectal medication, and transversus abdominis plane (TAP) blocks if applicable.

In an emergency, there can be a significant time limitation and assessment is often necessarily brief and limited to the following:

- Co-morbidities and anaesthetic history
- Drug allergies
- Fasting status
- Airway assessment: a minimum assessment comprises evaluation of mouth opening, Mallampati score, mandibular protrusion, neck extension, and a check for loose dentition.
- Evaluation of haemodynamic status (pallor, heart rate, and blood pressure) and respiratory rate.

A swift explanation of the procedure is offered and verbal consent elicited. Translators should ideally be employed for foreign language speakers or women with hearing impairment. Use of family members to translate can lead to omission of important and sensitive clinical information.

Consent

In the United Kingdom, for a woman to give valid consent she must have capacity, which is presumed unless there is an impairment of, or disturbance in, the functioning of her mind. Labour pain, opioid medication, or anxiety can diminish capacity. Women must be appropriately informed, and give consent voluntarily. Current practice in the United Kingdom entails discussion with the woman and provision of written information leaflets, but no separate written consent for anaesthesia. Information about anaesthesia should be offered well in advance of an elective procedure, before the preoperative meeting with the anaesthetist. New information should not be imparted after the woman has arrived in theatre.

In an emergency, the consent process is much more concise. In our experience, women will typically indicate just how much information they would like to receive. Risks will be explained and issues explored in detail only in response to an explicit request for more information. Risks and benefits discussed should be carefully documented. A pregnant woman with capacity can refuse any procedure, even if refusal jeopardizes her own life or that of the fetus. GA can be induced in a woman judged to lack capacity if it is deemed to be in her best interests (i.e. to save her life, but not that of the fetus). These issues are explored in detail in Chapter 29.

Aspiration prophylaxis: antacids

Changes in gastrointestinal physiology in pregnancy have been reviewed in Chapter 2. The numerous factors that potentially increase the chances of pulmonary aspiration of gastric contents are summarized in Figure 22.1. Decreased lower oesophageal sphincter tone and increased intra-abdominal pressure secondary to the gravid uterus predispose to reflux in a majority of women. Although gastric emptying is not delayed in pregnancy, administration of opioids in labour causes gastric stasis. In Mendelson's classic series[9] published in 1946, nitrous oxide and ether anaesthesia by facemask for operative delivery was complicated by aspiration in 66 women from 44,016 maternities (0.15%) between 1932 and 1945. The only two deaths were from airway obstruction by solid, undigested food, in two of five women who aspirated solid

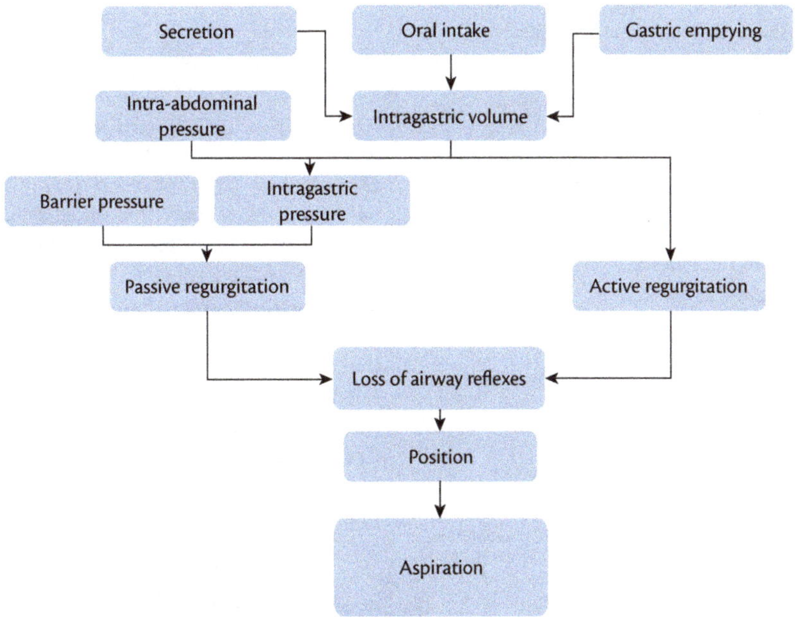

Figure 22.1 Factors contributing to pulmonary aspiration of gastric contents.
Reproduced with permission from Dr James Eldridge.

material. In those who aspirated liquid, a syndrome of dyspnoea, cyanosis, and tachycardia was observed. Recovery after 24–36 hours was universal—many decades before respiratory intensive therapy became available. Respiratory failure secondary to aspiration pneumonitis during anaesthesia became synonymous with Mendelson's syndrome, and its prevention a cornerstone of anaesthetic practice.

Prolonged fasting is distressing and can affect maternal and fetal physiology adversely by causing dehydration and ketosis. In the United Kingdom, women are typically allowed to consume a low-residue diet during labour unless they have identifiable risk factors for CD, in which case ranitidine 150 mg should be prescribed 6-hourly. Recommended fasting times before elective surgery are *2 hours for fluid* and *6 hours for food*, although every pregnant woman from late in the second trimester is deemed to have a 'full' stomach, despite notional fasting times. The risk and potential severity of the consequences of aspiration are increased if emergency GA is required in a parturient who has recently consumed solid food. Emptying the stomach before induction of anaesthesia is extremely unpleasant and rarely practised in the United Kingdom. Most obstetric units in the United Kingdom administer non-particulate antacid such as 0.3 M sodium citrate (30 mL) before all GA CDs. Ranitidine is the H_2-receptor antagonist of choice in most UK hospitals and should be prescribed for 12 and 2 hours before the anticipated time of an elective operation. Proton pump inhibitors are acceptable alternative agents. A non-particulate antacid, H_2-receptor antagonist, and/or metoclopramide are recommended in practice guidelines published by the American Society of Anesthesiologists.[10]

The risk of aspiration is high not only during induction but also emergence from GA. The eighth report of the Confidential Enquiries into Maternal Deaths in the United Kingdom[11] has suggested that consideration should be given for a gentle 'in and out' insertion of a wide-bore orogastric tube before extubation in women with a known full stomach (e.g. recent ingestion of a meal).

Location of induction

In the United Kingdom, most anaesthetic procedures are performed in an anaesthetic room—an area separate from but adjacent to the operating theatre. However, obstetric anaesthesia is an exception. GA should be induced in the operating theatre, to avoid the risks related to transporting and repositioning the woman. Monitoring will be uninterrupted, and the induction–delivery interval minimized. The woman's abdomen usually can be prepared and draped during preoxygenation. The anaesthetist can allow surgery to start as soon as the airway has been secured and ventilation of the lungs confirmed.

Process of general anaesthesia

The key steps in RSI of GA for CD are detailed in Box 22.2. Waveform capnography, the most sensitive indicator of tracheal tube position, has arguably contributed most to maternal safety over the last 30 years by allowing identification of oesophageal intubation. Given that mean maternal arterial CO_2 tension is 3.87 (standard deviation ± 0.24) kPa at 38 weeks' gestation, end-tidal CO_2 should be maintained below 4 kPa in order to maintain the gradient for fetal CO_2 elimination.[12] It has been shown that 100% oxygen in the maintenance inspired anaesthetic gas mixture increases fetal oxygenation, although it remains uncertain whether clinical outcome for the neonate is improved. Isoprostane, generated during free radical oxidation of arachidonic acid in membrane phospholipids, is a highly specific marker for *in vivo* oxidative stress. No differences were found in isoprostane concentrations resulting from 30%, 50%, or 100% oxygen in equivalent minimum alveolar concentrations of sevoflurane and nitrous oxide during elective CD under GA.[13]

The WHO's patient safety culture should be adopted in every obstetric operating environment. Team briefing, sign in, time out, sign out, and debriefing should be observed. A locally adapted sign in/time out and sign out checklist should be articulated and completed before embarking upon every case (see Figure 20.2 in Chapter 20).

Box 22.2 Key steps in rapid sequence induction of general anaesthesia for caesarean delivery

- WHO surgical safety checklist
- Left lateral table tilt to reduce aortocaval compression in association with (~25°) head-up ('reverse Trendelenburg') position to ensure stomach is below the level of the head
- Graduated compression stockings fitted, and (if used) pneumatic calf-compression system functional
- Large gauge IV access secured and patency verified
- Suction device immediately available and suction system working
- Physiological monitoring systems functioning
- Preoxygenation (denitrogenation)
- IV antimicrobial prophylaxis—ideally should be administered before skin incision
- IV induction of anaesthesia: precalculated doses of (traditionally) thiopental 7 mg/kg (maximum 500 mg) and succinylcholine (maximum 150 mg)
- Application of cricoid pressure (still taught to UK trainees) 10 N awake, increased to 30 N on loss of consciousness
- Intubation of the trachea with a cuffed tube, usually one size smaller than in the non-pregnant population (i.e. 7.0 mm internal diameter)
- Delivery of volatile agent (initially with overpressure) in nitrous oxide or air and oxygen
- Permission to obstetrician to start surgery
- After delivery: oxytocic agent, IV opioid, and antiemetic
- Emergence and tracheal extubation: woman positioned semi-recumbent/upright and awake

Intravenous access

Large-gauge IV access (16 or 14 G) is desirable for all parturients undergoing CD, to allow rapid blood transfusion if required. In women at significant risk of major obstetric haemorrhage, *two* cannulae are required. In parturients with poor peripheral venous access (e.g. morbidly obese women or IV drug users), central venous access might be necessary. A Vascath™ or Swan–Ganz sheath (7 Fr) should be inserted under ultrasound guidance into an internal jugular vein if a woman's peripheral venous access is inadequate and there is a high risk of major haemorrhage. Use of the humeral intraosseous route (EZ-IO® driver, Vidacare, San Antonio, TX, USA) (see Chapter 35) has been described in obstetric haemorrhage.[14] Familiarity with the device is essential before an obstetric anaesthetist contemplates its use in an emergency.

Positioning

When positioning a parturient on the operating table the anaesthetist must consider three key issues: avoidance of aortocaval compression, optimal conditions for securing the airway, and care of pressure points to avoid soft tissue and nerve damage.

Aortocaval compression

Compression of the aorta and/or inferior vena cava by the pregnant uterus can lead to supine hypotension in the second half of pregnancy. A 15° lateral tilt of the theatre table is generally recommended to minimize maternal hypotension. A Cochrane review examined maternal position during CD and its effects on maternal and neonatal outcome. Most studies had very small numbers and authors concluded that there was limited evidence to support or disprove the value of left or right lateral tilt, head-up or head-down positions, or use of manual displacement of the uterus.[15] When applying operating table tilt the anaesthetist has to ensure that side supports are fitted and belts secure the parturient's legs to prevent the woman falling.

In the event of maternal cardiac arrest, UK Resuscitation Council adult life support guidelines[16] recommend manual uterine displacement combined with up to 30° left tilt of the operating table to provide optimal conditions for restoration of maternal cardiac output.

Positioning for intubation

The incidence of difficult and failed intubation is higher in the obstetric as opposed to general population on account of pregnancy-induced soft tissue changes as well as the circumstances under which GA is often performed (see Box 26.3 in Chapter 26). Weight gain during pregnancy and development of airway oedema in labour or secondary to pre-eclampsia can alter airway anatomy. Changes in Mallampati score in labour and pregnancy are discussed in Chapter 26. Pregnancy-induced breast enlargement can make insertion of the laryngoscope particularly difficult; left lateral tilt and cricoid pressure complicate positioning for intubation.

The neck is extended at the atlanto-occipital joint until the external auditory meatus is in a horizontal plane with the sternal notch ('sniffing the morning air'). Ramping of shoulders and upper back by using folded blankets can help to align the neck to allow optimal laryngeal visualization (see Chapter 39 for further information and illustrations). In obese women, a reverse Trendelenburg position is all the more important in order to increase the functional residual capacity (FRC) and delay the onset of hypoxaemia after induction of anaesthesia. A number of devices and pillows such as the Oxford Head Elevating Laryngoscopy Pillow (HELP™, Alma Medical, Oxford) are available to assist with achieving the ramped position.

Pressure points

Avoidance of soft tissue, nerve, and eye damage is as important as in any speciality. The eyes should be closed and the lids taped, with careful attention to ensure no wires or tubing are in contact. Soft tissues and nerves should be protected by padding and careful positioning. The arms should not be abducted beyond 90°; the ulnar nerve must be protected at the elbow.

Monitoring

Maternal monitoring

The following monitoring modalities are essential:

- Electrocardiogram (ECG)
- Non-invasive blood pressure (NIBP)

- Peripheral arterial oxygen saturation (SpO_2)
- Gas analysis: capnography/oxygraphy/vapour concentration
- Airway pressure
- Peripheral nerve stimulator.

Means of measuring temperature (e.g. oesophageal thermistor) must be available for a case in which major haemorrhage is anticipated.

Electroencephalography-based depth of anaesthesia monitors are used by only a very small fraction (2%) of anaesthetists and are unavailable in one-third of UK hospitals.[17]

Direct arterial pressure monitoring (an arterial line) should be considered before induction of GA in the following conditions:

- Severe pre-eclampsia (to help ensure that the pressor response to laryngoscopy is obtunded—see 'General anaesthesia and pre-eclampsia')
- Morbid obesity where NIBP measurement is unreliable
- Sepsis
- Anticipated major haemorrhage (e.g. placenta praevia)
- Any systemic illness—when postoperative critical care is anticipated.

Measurement of cardiac output may be useful in women with haemodynamic instability attributable to critical illness or cardiac disease. However, there is no evidence of clinical utility of minimally invasive cardiac output monitors utilizing oesophageal Doppler velocimetry or arterial pulse waveform analysis at CD. None of the various devices has been formally validated in pregnancy.[18] The only evidence is from case reports, such as a Canadian description of data derived from a NICOM® thoracic bioreactance monitor in a woman with aortic stenosis.[19]

A real-time non-invasive haemoglobin (SpHb) monitor (the Masimo Rainbow SET® Pulse co-oximeter) has been evaluated at elective CD[20] and in five women undergoing caesarean hysterectomy.[21] A significant correlation was found between laboratory haemoglobin values and SpHb measurements, although median SpHb values were higher than laboratory Hb values. The HemoCue® point-of-care photometric cuvette system (which requires a drop of blood) provides a more accurate approximation of laboratory haemoglobin measurement.[22]

Maternal bladder catheterization is necessary at every CD to prevent surgical injury to the bladder. Urine output can therefore be measured.

Fetal monitoring

In emergency cases, fetal heart rate monitoring should be by continuous cardiotocography or intermittent Doppler ultrasound during preparation for induction of GA. Change in the fetal status (e.g. in response to intrauterine resuscitation) can influence anaesthetic management. Resolution of a fetal bradycardia might allow a change of plan from GA to neuraxial block.

Preoxygenation

Replacement of the nitrogen in the FRC of the lungs by oxygen is essential before inducing GA. The progressive reduction in FRC during pregnancy (further reduced by morbid obesity and multiple gestation) and increased oxygen consumption by the fetoplacental unit mean that arterial oxygen desaturation following apnoea is predictably accelerated.[23] Preoxygenation should be undertaken with the woman in a head-up position,[24] and the process guided by oxygraphy, as opposed to a predetermined number of breaths or duration of tidal breathing. Care should be taken to eliminate any leak between the woman's face and the face mask, to avoid entrainment of room air and impairment of the (exponential) denitrogenation process. The target end-tidal oxygen concentration is 90%.

In obstetric practice, 100% oxygen should be administered. The argument in non-obstetric anaesthesia for lower fractional inspired oxygen concentrations (in the interests of prevention of atelectasis) is outweighed by the FRC reduction/increase in oxygen consumption.[25] Following preoxygenation, time to arterial oxygen desaturation during apnoea is shorter after succinylcholine compared with rocuronium. This phenomenon is explicable by the additional skeletal muscle oxygen consumption incurred by fasciculations[26,27] (Figure 22.2).

Airway management

Laryngoscopy and intubation

The following devices can prove invaluable aids to successful intubation:

- McCoy 'levering' laryngoscope (with hinged tip)
- Polio Macintosh blade (mounted at 135° to the handle)
- A short-handled laryngoscope is particularly useful in obese women with large breasts
- Gum-elastic bougie.

In obstetric practice, a tracheal tube one size smaller than that typically used for adult females (i.e. 7.0 mm internal diameter) is recommended.

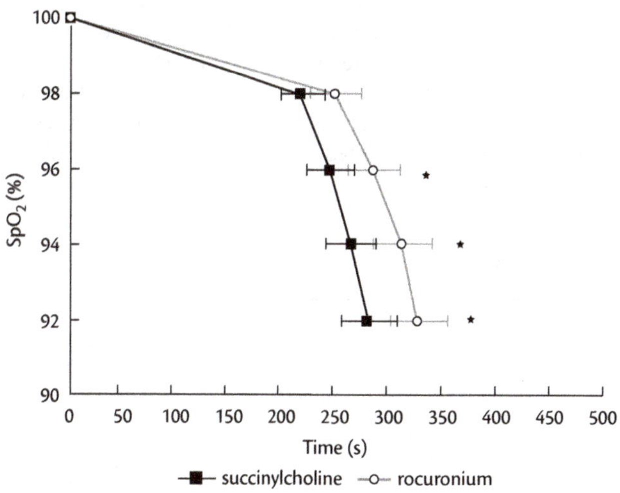

Figure 22.2 Decrement in peripheral arterial oxygen saturation (SpO_2) after succinylcholine or rocuronium. Mean (95% confidence interval) times for decrease in SpO_2 to 98%, 96%, 94%, and 92% in patients with body mass index 25–30 kg/m^2 receiving succinylcholine or rocuronium after 3 minutes' pre-oxygenation.

*$P < 0.05$.

Reproduced with permission from L. Tang, S. Li, S. Huang, H. Ma, Z. Wang., Desaturation following rapid sequence induction using succinylcholine vs. rocuronium in overweight patients, *Acta Anaesthesiologica Scandinavica*, Volume 55, Issue 2, pp. 203–208, Copyright © 2011 John Wiley & Sons.

Some authors advocate video laryngoscopy as the laryngoscopic technique of first choice, as opposed to a rescue strategy.[28] In an emergency situation, it is important to use the equipment that is most familiar to the individual anaesthetist. An emergency CD is not the right time to try out a laryngoscope for the first time. Trainees should be encouraged to familiarize themselves with various laryngoscopes in the high-fidelity simulator and in the elective setting before use in obstetrics.

Failed intubation

Every anaesthetist should have a rehearsed plan for a difficult or failed intubation. The UK incidence at CD has been reported at around 1/300 in most series. The most commonly used rescue airway in the United Kingdom appears to be the original (marketed as Classic™) laryngeal mask airway (LMA).[29] 'Secondary' tracheal intubation via LMA and exchange catheter is not recommended at emergency CD (see the UK Difficult Airway Society website, http://www.das.uk.com/).

Management of unanticipated difficult tracheal intubation is focused on 'oxygenation without aspiration'[30] and prevention of airway trauma, which can insidiously precipitate a 'can't ventilate' scenario on account of airway oedema.

Harmer's system (Table 22.1) for grading the clinical urgency to proceed with surgery remains most useful in aiding decision-making as regards whether or not to discontinue anaesthesia in the event of failure to intubate the trachea at CD.[31]

Supraglottic airway devices

Many reports have accrued of successful use of supraglottic devices as rescue airways. Mushambi and Pandey have reviewed in detail the findings of the UK National Audit Project 4 (NAP4)[32] (see Chapter 26). Details of major airway management complications (death, brain damage, emergency surgical airway, and unanticipated intensive care unit admission) in the course of anaesthesia were collected from all UK National Health Service hospitals over 1 year. There were four obstetric cases, all of whom survived. In one, an Intubating LMA® Airway (ILMA®) was used successfully. In contrast, the concurrent UK Confidential Enquiries into Maternal Deaths[11] highlighted a case of oesophageal intubation through an ILMA®.

The LMA Classic™ has been studied at elective CD in 1067 fasted Korean women of low body mass index (BMI) who received succinylcholine 1.5 mg/kg for NMB.[33] There were no data on the frequency with which cricoid pressure was relaxed or removed to facilitate LMA insertion. No instances of regurgitation or aspiration were reported. The second-generation LMA ProSeal™ (PLMA; see Figure 26.5 in Chapter 26) was studied in 3000 elective CD cases in Jordan.[34] The PLMA provides an improved seal for positive pressure ventilation, separation of the respiratory and gastrointestinal tracts, and venting of gas or liquid via a drain port. All women had BMI < 30 kg.m^{-2} and were given rocuronium 0.9 mg/kg; cricoid pressure was applied. A 14 Fr orogastric tube was preloaded on the PLMA—its distal tip extended 10 cm beyond the drain port and was guided into the oesophagus with the aid of Magill forceps before subsequent 'railroading' of the PLMA (during which cricoid force was released). The only incidence of regurgitation was during fundal pressure, at delivery of the neonate. Gastric contents reached the mouth, but not the lungs. As indicated in Figure 22.1, intragastric pressure is an important factor in the overall risk of aspiration. In an accompanying editorial, Paech concluded that there is now, arguably, clinical equipoise between tracheal intubation and use of an LMA after RSI with cricoid pressure.[35] A Chinese study examined the LMA Supreme™, a disposable version of the PLMA, in 700 fasted women with BMI less than 35 kg/m^2 with no history of gastro-oesophageal reflux.[36] Again, rocuronium was used for NMB and there was no clinical evidence of regurgitation or aspiration. Habib[37] has commented that the Supreme™ might be considered for slim, fasted parturients with no reflux scheduled for elective CD. Insertion of an LMA at an early stage after failed tracheal intubation might reduce the trauma of repeated intubation attempts whilst providing adequate oxygenation and ventilation.[37] In a review of the array of new supraglottic airways,[38] it was pointed out that a distinction must be made between clinical evidence relating to efficacy, and safety of performance. Although small clinical evaluations can determine the efficacy of particular devices in absolute and relative terms, safety evaluations (e.g. ventilation failure rates or the risk of aspiration) may need many thousands of cases before concerns are identified. In reality, this means that the risk profile of a new device is unlikely to be established until several years after introduction.

Table 22.1 Suggested actions in the event of failed tracheal intubation, according to five graded maternal/fetal clinical scenarios

Grade	Scenario	Action
Grade 1	Woman's life depends upon the completion of surgery (e.g. cardiac arrest, massive haemorrhage)	No alternative but to continue with maintenance of GA to facilitate haemostasis
Grade 2	Maternal pathology makes alternative neuraxial techniques unsuitable (e.g. decompensated heart disease, coagulopathy)	Either continue GA if supraglottic airway securely placed or discontinue anaesthesia and proceed to awake fibreoptic intubation
Grade 3	Sudden and severe fetal compromise not recovering between contractions (e.g. placental abruption, prolapsed cord)	Although abandoning GA could lead to fetal demise, maternal well-being is paramount. Unless airway is secure with a supraglottic airway, awakening the woman and institution of a neuraxial technique is appropriate
Grade 4	Long-standing fetal compromise of varying severity (e.g. showing good recovery between contractions)	GA should be abandoned: in a majority of cases the fetus will be delivered under neuraxial anaesthesia without detriment
Grade 5	Elective procedure	Woman should be woken up and awake fibreoptic intubation or neuraxial anaesthesia instituted

Reprinted from *International Journal of Obstetric Anesthesia*, Volume 6, Issue 1, M. Harmer, Difficult and failed intubation in obstetrics, pp. 25–31, Copyright (1997), with permission from Elsevier.

Videolaryngoscopes and fibreoptic intubation

Examples of current videolaryngoscopes are illustrated in Chapter 26. McGuire and Younger have explained the distinctions between rigid indirect laryngoscopes and optical stylets.[39] Awake fibreoptic intubation is the gold standard for management of the anticipated difficult airway. NAP4 pointed out that a flexible fibrescope may have several roles in the obstetric setting, and that anaesthetic departments should provide a service where the skills and equipment are available to deliver awake fibreoptic intubation whenever it is indicated. The Ambu® aScope™ is a single-use flexible intubation scope that is suitable for an obstetric theatre that might be distant from a hospital's main theatre complex. Following a difficult or failed intubation the anaesthetist must remember to inform the woman afterwards and impart verbal and written information about the airway difficulty and its importance for future anaesthetics. It should be emphasized that the woman must impart this information to future anaesthetists.

Cricoid pressure

Cricoid pressure can distort the view at laryngoscopy especially if applied with left lateral tilt of the operating table, for which the assistant has not accounted (NB The term cricoid 'pressure' is strictly incorrect—force (measured in Newtons, N) is applied, rather than pressure (force per unit area)). Priebe has summarized the case against continued use of cricoid pressure.[40] A 30 N force can cause complete loss of the glottic view;[41] the risk of occlusion of the cricoid ring and airway obstruction is greater in females.[42] Although a Canadian study concluded that cricoid pressure applied by trained assistants did not increase the rate of failed intubation in elective non-obstetric patients,[43] a risk:benefit analysis of cricoid pressure in the emergency department questioned its universal application, and recommended immediate consideration of its removal in the event of difficult intubation or ventilation.[44] Anaesthetic assistants' training is of crucial importance.[45] The anaesthetist must be assured that the assistant can discern individual patients' cricoid cartilages and apply the appropriate level of pressure.

Intravenous anaesthetics and analgesics

Induction agents

Ninety-three per cent of UK consultants who responded to an OAA survey in 2011 used thiopental for induction of GA for CD.[46] The motion 'Propofol should be the induction agent of choice for caesarean section under general anaesthesia' was debated in 2003.[47] Although a majority opposed the motion before and after the debate, the arguments highlighted minimal evidence upon which to reject propofol as a reasonable alternative in the event of non-availability of thiopental. There is a lack of clarity as to what constitute truly equipotent doses of thiopental and propofol. Reynolds has stressed that all anaesthetic agents cross the placenta readily. Even if drug concentrations are high in umbilical venous blood, these are not the concentrations in the blood reaching the fetal brain.[48] GA and the developing fetal brain is discussed in a later section.

The following should be done to minimize harm to the fetus:

- Maintenance of maternal oxygenation
- Maintenance of normocapnia for pregnancy
- Aortocaval compression minimized
- Uterine incision–delivery interval minimized
- Obligatory presence of a neonatologist to offer neonatal ventilatory support.

Opioids

Remifentanil or alfentanil are necessary adjuncts to any IV induction agent at RSI for women in whom a hypertensive response to intubation is particularly undesirable (see 'General anaesthesia and pre-eclampsia'). A review of studies evaluating remifentanil at CD concluded that remifentanil reduced the maternal circulatory response to intubation and surgery, although the incidence of brief neonatal respiratory depression was increased compared to an opioid-free induction regimen.[49] In women with cardiac disease, the chosen anaesthetic regimen should not depart from whatever would be judged best for a non-pregnant woman with similar cardiovascular compromise.[50] An opioid-based cardiac anaesthetic regimen should not be avoided on account of fetal concerns, provided that a neonatologist is present in anticipation of neonatal respiratory depression

Total intravenous anaesthesia

A propofol-remifentanil total intravenous anaesthetic regimen has been described,[51] which might prove useful when volatile agents are contraindicated (e.g. malignant hyperthermia susceptibility). A 0.5 mcg/kg remifentanil bolus was followed by an infusion at 0.20 mcg/kg/min and an induction dose of propofol (blood concentration of 5 mcg/mL by target-controlled IV infusion) reduced to 2.5 mcg/mL after the trachea was intubated. Mean arterial blood pressure remained stable. Cord umbilical artery pH was universally greater than 7.20, although 1-minute Apgar scores ranged from 1 to 9 and a brief period of bag-mask ventilation was required in half of the neonates.

Volatile agents

Historically, it was not possible to discern the respective effects on the fetus of GA and asphyxia, and the contribution of supine maternal position to impaired uteroplacental perfusion was not appreciated. Forty years ago, Crawford advocated maintenance of anaesthesia with only N_2O and O_2. He regarded uterine relaxation as the only indication for halothane.[52] Moir demonstrated improved Apgar scores with a N_2O/O_2 50:50 mixture with halothane 0.5% (inspired) compared to N_2O/O_2 70:30 without halothane.[53] He concluded that it was the higher fractional inspired oxygen concentration permitted by the use of halothane that was responsible for the improved neonatal condition. Whereas two of 50 women who received unsupplemented N_2O/O_2 had clear recall, halothane ensured lack of awareness and did not cause increased blood loss. Moir's paper was reproduced as a *British Journal of Anaesthesia* 'citation classic' in 1998.[54] Uterine relaxation conferred by a volatile agent might actually improve fetal compromise to which uterine hyperstimulation has been contributory.[55] A maternal stress response to excessively light GA might compromise uteroplacental blood flow.

In the recent survey of UK practice, 85% of respondents still used nitrous oxide and sevoflurane was the most popular vapour for maintenance.[46] Compared with isoflurane, sevoflurane[56] and desflurane[57] offer the advantage of more rapid approximation of alveolar to inspired tensions as the effect of the IV induction dose declines. However, maternal recovery was not demonstrably faster with either of the newer agents (sevoflurane was compared with isoflurane; desflurane with enflurane). Isoflurane is an entirely satisfactory agent for maintenance, provided attention is paid to end-tidal vapour concentration during the phase of overpressure after IV induction. Desflurane is contraindicated in the hypertensive disorders on account of the risk of sympathetic activation during rapid increases in inspired tension.[58]

End-tidal vapour concentration must be monitored to avoid awareness. Data support maintenance of end-tidal vapour concentration greater than 0.75 MAC (in addition to 50% N_2O) to maintain bispectral index (BIS) values less than 60 for 'adequate' depth of anaesthesia at CD.[59] BIS values have been compared between women presenting for elective CD and a group requiring CD who had previously laboured for a mean duration of 5.4 hours.[60] A fixed anaesthetic regimen was administered: induction with thiopental 4 mg/kg and maintenance with sevoflurane (end-tidal concentration 1.0%) and nitrous oxide 50%. Baseline BIS mean values were similar between the groups. After induction, from the time of tracheal intubation until 10 minutes after delivery of the neonate, BIS values were significantly greater in the elective group. In addition, more IV postoperative analgesia was self-administered by women who had undergone elective CD. The authors' explanation was that labour pain might induce release of β-endorphin by the pituitary. This study provides insufficient justification upon which to decrease vapour concentrations in women who have been labouring.

Inhalation agent monitoring is now universally available in the developed world, and the incidence of awareness should be negligible. In a prospective Australasian survey of over 1000 CDs, 70% of women were interviewed about awareness and dreaming. In the two cases of definite explicit awareness, administered drug doses were manifestly insufficient (in one case water was administered without the intended diluted thiopental). BIS or entropy monitoring was used in one-third of cases.[61]

The Fifth National Audit Project (NAP5) of the Royal College of Anaesthetists of Great Britain and Ireland was published in 2014 and looked at 3 million GAs delivered over 1 year in public hospitals in these countries.[62] NAP5 reported an overall incidence of awareness during GA of 1/19,000, much lower than previously reported. However, as previously recognized, the incidence was considerably higher in the obstetric population (1/670). Most cases were at caesarean delivery—at induction or an early stage of surgery. A key message was to 'mind the gap' between waning concentrations of intravenous induction agent and attainment of adequate vapour tension following traditional RSI.

Inhalation induction

There is neither historical nor contemporary evidence upon which to declare inhalation induction with sevoflurane as inherently unsafe. Sevoflurane causes minimal airway irritation and has been used successfully for inhalation induction of anaesthesia for CD in the absence of vascular access and in acute severe asthma. The smooth, rapid onset and lack of coughing or vomiting suggest that the technique does not necessarily cause an increased risk of aspiration. Tidal breathing of 8% sevoflurane in N_2O/O_2 66:33 can induce anaesthesia as rapidly as an IV bolus.[63] The following approach is suggested:

- 20–30° head-up tilt
- Breathing system primed with sevoflurane 8% in N_2O/O_2 (2:1)
- Tidal respiration
- Avoid cricoid pressure
- IV cannulation after loss of consciousness
- NMB, tracheal intubation.

Uterine tone

Maintenance of uterine tone is crucial in reducing intraoperative blood loss. A dose-dependent reduction in uterine muscle contractility has been shown *in vitro* with sevoflurane and desflurane[64]—a finding that agrees with earlier studies of halothane, enflurane, and isoflurane. However, myometrial responsiveness to Syntocinon® at different end-tidal volatile tensions has never been studied *in vivo*. Whereas recent work has found that adequate uterine tone can be attained with small bolus doses (0.5–3 IU) of Syntocinon® in patients undergoing elective CD under spinal anaesthesia, there is no evidence to support reducing the magnitude of the bolus dose from 5 IU in GA cases.[65]

Neuromuscular blockade

There are many diverse risks associated with the administration of succinylcholine, including anaphylaxis, increased masseter tone, malignant hyperthermia, hyperkalaemia, vagal arrest, myotonic crisis, and myalgia. Belief that spontaneous recovery will necessarily be sufficiently rapid to allow retrieval of a failed ventilation scenario is incorrect.[66]

Rocuronium is licensed for CD at 0.6 mg/kg. In its original evaluation for CD, conditions for tracheal intubation were good or excellent at 90 seconds or disappearance of the third twitch of a train of four (TOF) only after the thiopental dose had been increased from 4 to 6 mg/kg.[67] Mean duration of NMB (time to reappearance of the second TOF twitch) was 32.7 minutes. The ratio of umbilical venous:maternal venous rocuronium concentrations was 0.16, similar to other fully ionized and water-soluble quaternary ammonium compounds.

A comparison of rocuronium 0.6 mg/kg and succinylcholine 1.0 mg/kg for non-obstetric RSI found that intubation scores were superior after succinylcholine—although limb movement/coughing in response to intubation rather than inferior conditions for laryngoscopy (jaw relaxation/resistance to the blade) or vocal cord adduction/movement accounted for the difference.[68] The median time to completion of intubation was shorter after succinylcholine than rocuronium 0.6 mg/kg.

There is a body of evidence that rocuronium becomes an increasingly acceptable alternative to succinylcholine for RSI as doses are increased to 0.9 mg/kg or greater.[69] The onset time of rocuronium is inversely related to the intubating dose; histamine release remains insignificant after rocuronium 1.2 mg/kg.[70] The duration of action of this dose (at least an hour until sufficient spontaneous recovery for evoked reversal with neostigmine) precluded its use at CD until the advent of sugammadex.

The incidence of anaphylaxis to different neuromuscular blocking drugs varies according to geographical location. A recent analysis from Western Australia found that rocuronium and succinylcholine were responsible for 56% and 21%, respectively, of cases of anaphylaxis to neuromuscular blocking drugs. The study estimated the number of patients exposed to neuromuscular blocking drugs from ampoule sales data.[71]

Reversal of rocuronium with sugammadex

Sugammadex is a cyclodextrin that can chelate or encapsulate rocuronium and (to a lesser extent) vecuronium. Sugammadex has a dose-dependent speed of onset. Unlike neostigmine, there is neither acetylcholinesterase inhibition nor simultaneous requirement for (antimuscarinic) anticholinergic agents.

Reversal of rocuronium 0.6 mg/kg with sugammadex at 2–4 mg/kg has been studied at CD.[72] In an evaluation of rocuronium 1.2 mg/kg at CD, tracheal intubation was undertaken at 60 seconds. Intubating conditions were 'excellent' in two-thirds and 'good' in one-third of women. The three neonates who were admitted for neonatal intensive care were all delivered after intervention for pre-existing fetal compromise. Umbilical cord venous blood was not sampled for rocuronium assay. All women received sugammadex 4 mg/kg at the end of surgery.[73]

It might be expected that the mass of rocuronium transferred across the placenta will be broadly proportional to the maternal dose. It is uncertain whether the fraction of 1.2 mg/kg transferred in the event of prolonged surgical delivery would impair neonatal respiratory effort. Emergency reversal of rocuronium 1.2 mg/kg with sugammadex 16 mg/kg has not been reported in obstetrics. Figure 22.3 represents data from two subjects recruited to a non-obstetric study which found that spontaneous recovery of succinylcholine 1.0 mg/kg to TOF greater than 0.9 was slower than recovery evoked by sugammadex 16 mg/kg 3 minutes after rocuronium 1.2 mg/kg.[74]

Role of rocuronium/sugammadex after failed intubation

When the original failed intubation drill was conceived in the mid 1970s,[75] GA was undertaken for a much greater proportion of CD and succinylcholine was used for NMB almost exclusively. The key principle of the drill[30] was that in the event of failed intubation, either a woman could be allowed to wake up and a neuraxial technique used, or surgery could proceed with facemask and spontaneous ventilation. Nowadays, the indications for the vast majority of GA CD are immediate threat to life of the mother or fetus, or failure of neuraxial blockade.

If maternal compromise is life-threatening (e.g. massive haemorrhage), surgery must proceed to secure haemostasis, even if a definitive airway (tracheal tube) has not been secured and there is difficulty ventilating the lungs effectively. The usefulness of the emergency reversal dose of sugammadex is therefore limited. Moreover, sustained profound rocuronium blockade might be expected to offer conditions for airway management that are superior to those offered by succinylcholine. The period of initial recovery from succinylcholine increases maternal oxygen consumption and, as muscle tone increases and the patient begins to move, can make ventilation of the lungs difficult on account of decreased thoracic compliance. There is a distinct possibility of retching/vomiting and a heightened risk of aspiration of gastric contents. Proceeding to rapid reversal of profound rocuronium blockade in the event of 'can't intubate, can't ventilate' at category 1 CD would be more likely if fetal as opposed to maternal compromise was the indication for operation (see Table 22.1).

Data on placental transfer of sugammadex are sparse, and limited to animals. The manufacturer has indicated that less than 2–6% is transferred in rat and rabbit populations. There is no information about placental transfer of the sugammadex–rocuronium complex. However, adverse fetal effects of sugammadex-encapsulated rocuronium are unlikely.

General anaesthesia and the developing fetal brain

There is accumulating evidence from primate studies that neurotoxicity (a pathological increase in apoptosis—programmed cell death) can follow fetal exposure to general anaesthetics.[76] However, the induction dose of ketamine administered to pregnant Rhesus macaque females at 120 days' gestation (full term 165 days) in one prominent study was 10 mg/kg, which was followed by a continuous infusion at 10–85 mg/kg/h for 5 hours.[77] The relative dose of GA transferred to a human fetus at CD, particularly in an emergency case with impaired uteroplacental perfusion, would be inevitably smaller by many orders of magnitude. Concerns about the impact of GAs on the developing fetal brain should therefore be focused on *in utero* fetal surgical procedures (see Chapter 7), where volatile agents might be administered at high doses many weeks before term to facilitate uterine relaxation, for significant durations.

Postoperative analgesia

IV opioids such as morphine or diamorphine should be administered after delivery of the neonate, supplemented by IV paracetamol 1 g and a non-steroidal inflammatory drug (NSAID) such as diclofenac, provided there are no contraindications. Armstrong and Stocks describe detailed strategies for postoperative analgesia, including wound infiltration and TAP blocks, in Chapter 24.

General anaesthesia and obstetric haemorrhage

If there are signs of significant blood loss such as pallor and tachycardia—which can develop before significant hypotension—the approach to IV induction of anaesthesia must be particularly careful. Options include decreasing the dose of thiopental or using ketamine (1.5–2 mg/kg) or etomidate (0.2–0.3 mg/kg). The sympathomimetic effect of ketamine is a contradiction to its use in hypertensive disorders of pregnancy. It is uncertain whether concern about etomidate-induced adrenal insufficiency[78] is warranted in obstetric haemorrhage. Although there is little evidence that small doses of volatile agents in the presence of Syntocinon® exacerbate uterine atony, substitution of volatile agent by IV agent(s) (e.g. increments of ketamine 50 mg) for maintenance of anaesthesia might be considered. NSAIDs are absolutely contraindicated in women whose kidneys might have sustained hypoperfusion secondary to haemorrhage. The risk of acute kidney injury will be compounded by pre-eclampsia.

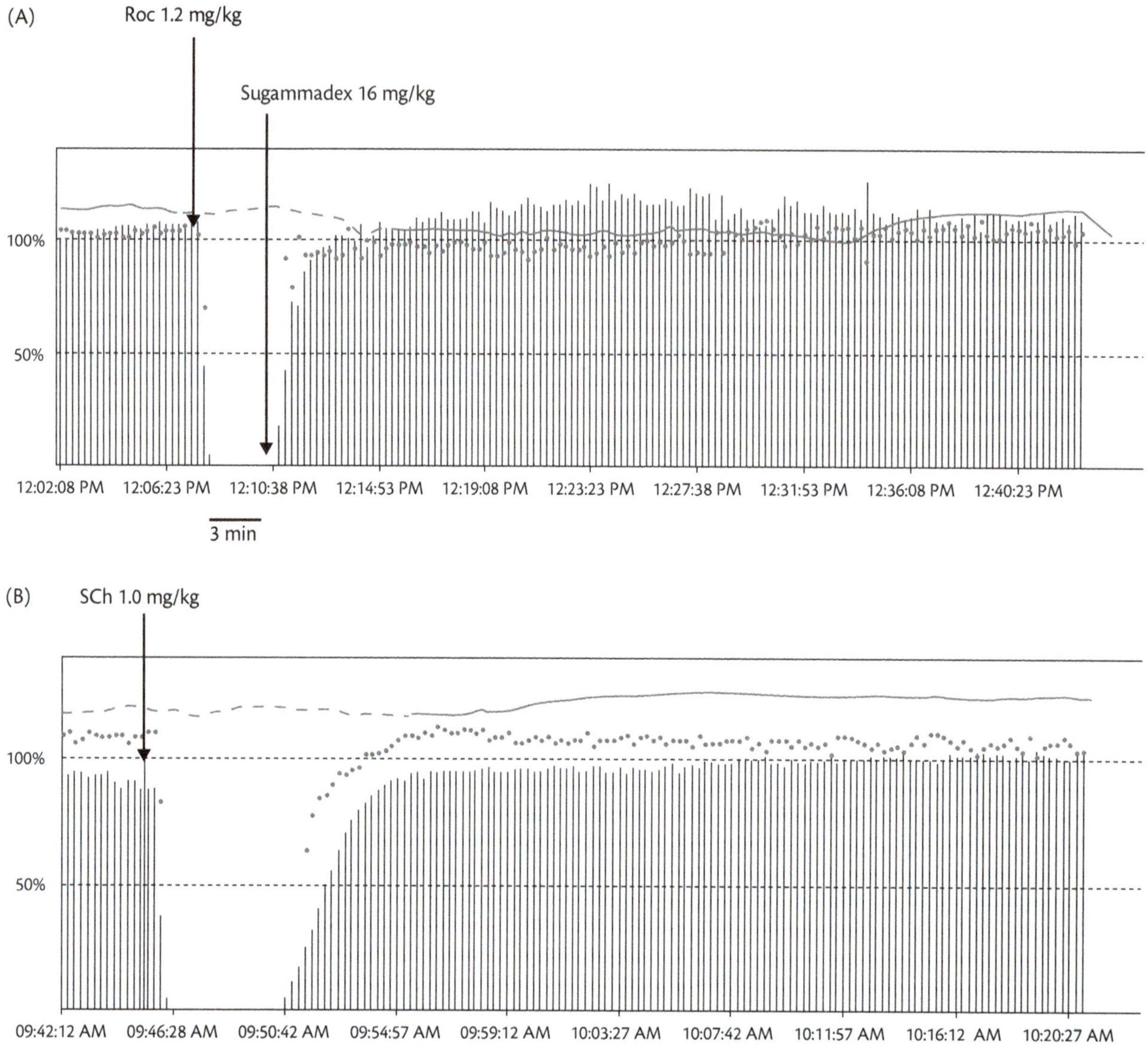

Figure 22.3 Acceleromyographic comparison of onset and offset of neuromuscular blockade with Succinylcholine and a rocuronium/sugammadex combination. (A) Recovery of the train-of-four (TOF) ratio after administration of rocuronium 1.2 mg/kg followed 3 minutes later by sugammadex 16 mg/kg. Recovery to first twitch height (T1) 90% and TOF ratio 0.94 took 110 seconds. The onset–offset time with this sequence (i.e. the time from the end of the injection of rocuronium to T1 recovery to 90%) was 4 minutes 47 seconds. (B) Effects of administering 1.0 mg/kg succinylcholine with spontaneous recovery to T1 90% after 9 minutes 23 seconds.

General anaesthesia and pre-eclampsia

There are very few comparative studies of anaesthetic techniques in women with pre-eclampsia. A study that randomized pre-eclamptic women with a 'non-reassuring' fetal heart trace to spinal or GA found that 1-minute Apgar scores were lower after GA—explicable by the transient, reversible effects of residual anaesthetic agents. However, GA was associated with increased mean umbilical cord arterial pH compared with the spinal group.[79] When uteroplacental perfusion is compromised, GA might predispose to a better neonatal acid–base outcome compared to spinal anaesthesia.

In pre-eclampsia, obtunding the dangerously exaggerated maternal hypertensive response to laryngoscopy and tracheal intubation is of critical importance. A death described in the 'Pre-eclampsia and eclampsia' chapter of the 2003–2005 UK Confidential Enquiries was attributable to lack of supplementation of a 'standard' GA induction regimen.[80] A woman suffered prolonged systolic hypertension secondary to difficult intubation, and was subsequently found to have sustained a massive intracranial haemorrhage. The ED_{95} for remifentanil in women with severe pre-eclampsia has been defined as 1.34 mcg/kg (the 'effective' dose was defined as that which prevented systolic arterial pressure increasing to > 160 mmHg for > 1 minute). Women were pretreated with a loading dose of magnesium sulphate and received thiopental 5 mg/kg.[81] Alfentanil 10 mcg/kg (1 mg maximum) is a suitable alternative.

Although the duration of action of all non-depolarizing neuromuscular blocking agents is significantly prolonged by therapeutic serum concentrations of magnesium, the onset and duration of succinylcholine is unaffected.[82]

A population-based study of 303,862 Taiwanese women identified an increased risk of stroke over a 1–6-year follow-up period following GA (compared to neuraxial anaesthesia) for CD in the presence of pre-eclampsia.[83] Speculative mechanisms include the neuroendocrine stress response to CD, increased incidence of thromboembolism after GA, and endothelial cell dysfunction mediated by nitrous oxide. There was no increased risk of stroke associated with GA in women without pre-eclampsia.

Before extubation, additional antihypertensive therapy (e.g. labetalol in 10–20 mg increments) should be considered in order to avert a dangerous pressor response.

Any woman whose larynx is noted to be swollen at laryngoscopy for GA, or in whom intubation is traumatic, will be at particular risk of laryngeal oedema. Postoperative care must therefore be undertaken in a critical care area with an anaesthetist immediately available. Midwives should be vigilant for the development of stridor, which signifies airway obstruction and a possible need for re-intubation.

Antibacterial prophylaxis

A further analysis of the Taiwanese population in which incidence of stroke was studied revealed an increased 30-day surgical site infection rate when GA was compared with neuraxial anaesthesia (odds ratio of infection 3.7).[84] It is unclear if this difference reflected greater immunosuppression and impairment of host defences associated with GA or vasodilatation and better surgical site tissue oxygenation mediated by neuraxial anaesthesia.

The recent UK NICE guideline suggests administration of antibiotics with efficacy against endometritis, urinary tract infections, and wound infections.[6] Although NICE in the United Kingdom and the American College of Obstetricians and Gynaecologists[85] recommend that antibiotic administration should precede skin incision, administration after delivery in a category 1 emergency is more realistic.

Conclusion

In many obstetric units, the regimen for GA for CD has changed little in 50 years—apart from use of increased doses of volatile agents. Thiopental can be replaced with propofol; the rocuronium/sugammadex combination is an acceptable alternative to succinylcholine. Diverse new devices have been developed to aid conventional tracheal intubation and offer an alternative means of airway management in the event of difficulty.

Recognition of the importance of human factors and universal implementation of the WHO surgical safety checklist have the potential to make a significant contribution to the safety of women undergoing CD under GA around the world.

References

1. Hamer Hodges RJ, Bennett JR, Tunstall ME, *et al.* General anaesthesia for operative obstetrics. *Br J Anaesth* 1959; 31:152–63.
2. Stept W, Safar P. Rapid induction/intubation for prevention of gastric-content aspiration. *Anesth Analg* 1970; 49:633–6.
3. Morgan M. Anaesthetic contribution to maternal mortality. *Br J Anaesth* 1987; 59:842–55.
4. Scott DB. Awareness during Caesarean section. *Anaesthesia* 1991; 46:693–4.
5. Neilipovitz DT, Crosby ET. Evidence-based clinical update. No evidence for decreased incidence of aspiration after rapid sequence induction. *Can J Anesth* 2007; 54:748–64.
6. National Institute for Health and Clinical Excellence. *Caesarean Section.* Clinical Guideline 132. London: NICE; 2011. http://www.nice.org.uk/guidance/cg132
7. Royal College of Obstetricians and Gynaecologists, The Royal College of Anaesthetists. *Classification of Urgency of Caesarean Section—A Continuum of Risk.* Good Practice No. 11, April 2010. http://www.oaa-anaes.ac.uk/assets/_managed/editor/File/RCoA/Good%20Practice%2011%20CS%20FINAL.pdf
8. The Royal College of Anaesthetists. Chapter 8.8: Caesarean section anaesthesia: technique and failure rate. In *Raising the Standard: A Compendium of Audit Recipes.* 2012. [Online] http://www.rcoa.ac.uk/system/files/CSQ-ARB-2012_1.pdf
9. Mendelson CL. The aspiration of stomach contents into the lungs during obstetric anesthesia. *Am J Obstet Gynecol* 1946; 52:191–205.
10. American Society of Anesthesiologists Task Force on Obstetric Anesthesia. Practice guidelines for obstetric anesthesia: an updated report by the American Society of Anesthesiologists Task Force. *Anesthesiology* 2007; 106:843–63.
11. Centre for Maternal and Child Enquiries (CMACE). Saving Mothers' Lives: reviewing maternal deaths to make motherhood safer: 2006–8. The Eighth Report on Confidential Enquiries into Maternal Deaths in the United Kingdom. *BJOG* 2011; 118 Suppl 1:1–203. http://onlinelibrary.wiley.com/doi/10.1111/j.1471-0528.2010.02847.x/pdf
12. Templeton A, Kelman GR. Maternal blood gases, (PA_{O2}–Pa_{O2}), physiological shunt and *VD/VT* in normal pregnancy. *Br J Anaesth* 1976; 48:1001–4.
13. Khaw KS, Ngan Kee WD, Chu CY. Effects of different inspired oxygen fractions on lipid peroxidation during general anaesthesia for elective Caesarean section. *Br J Anaesth* 2010; 105:355–60.
14. Chatterjee DJ, Bukunola B, Samuels TL. Resuscitation in massive obstetric haemorrhage using an intraosseous needle. *Anaesthesia* 2011; 66:306–10.
15. Cluver C, Novikova N, Hofmeyr GJ, *et al.* Maternal position during caesarean section for preventing maternal and neonatal complications. *Cochrane Database Syst Rev* 2010; 6:CD007623.
16. Resuscitation Council (UK). *Resuscitation Guidelines 2010.* [Online] http://www.resus.org.uk/pages/guide.htm
17. Pandit JJ, Cook TM. National Institute for Clinical Excellence guidance on measuring depth of anaesthesia: limitations of EEG-based technology. *Br J Anaesth* 2013; 110:325–8.
18. Armstrong S, Fernando R, Columb M. Minimally- and non-invasive assessment of maternal cardiac output: go with the flow! *Int J Obstet Anesth* 2011; 20:330–40.
19. Fanning N, Balki M, Sermer, M, *et al.* Noninvasive cardiac output monitoring during general anesthesia for Cesarean delivery in a patient with severe aortic stenosis. *Can J Anesth* 2011; 58:837–41.
20. Butwick A, Hilton G, Carvalho B. Non-invasive haemoglobin measurements in patients undergoing elective Caesarean section. *Br J Anaesth* 2012; 108:271–2.
21. Butwick AJ, Hilton G, Riley ET, *et al.* Non-invasive measurement of hemoglobin during cesarean hysterectomy: a case series. *Int J Obstet Anesth* 2011; 20:240–65.
22. Skelton VA, Wijayasinghe N, Sharafudeen S, *et al.* Evaluation of point-of-care haemoglobin measuring devices: a comparison of Radical-7™ Pulse CO-Oximetry, HemoCue® and laboratory haemoglobin measurements in obstetric patients. *Anaesthesia* 2013; 68:40–5.
23. McClelland SH, Bogod DG, Hardman JG. Pre-oxygenation in pregnancy: an investigation using physiological modelling. *Anaesthesia* 2008; 63:259–63.
24. Hignett R, Fernando R, McGlennan A, *et al.* A randomized crossover study to determine the effect of a 30° head-up versus a supine

position on the functional residual capacity of term parturients. *Anesth Analg* 2011; 113:1098–102.

25. Lumb AB. Editorial. Just a little oxygen to breathe as you go off to sleep … is it always a good idea? *Br J Anaesth* 2007; 99:769–71.
26. Taha SK, El-Khatib MF, Baraka AS, *et al.* Effect of suxamethonium vs rocuronium on onset of oxygen desaturation during apnoea following rapid sequence induction. *Anaesthesia* 2010; 65:358–61.
27. Tang L, Li S, Huang S, *et al.* Desaturation following rapid sequence induction using succinylcholine vs. rocuronium in overweight patients. *Acta Anaesth Scand* 2011; 55:203–8.
28. Mhyre JM, Healy D. Focused review: the unanticipated difficult intubation in obstetrics. *Anesth Analg* 2011; 112:648–52.
29. Quinn AC, Milne D, Columb M, *et al.* Failed tracheal intubation in obstetric anaesthesia: 2 yr national case–control study in the UK. *Br J Anaesth* 2013; 110:74–80.
30. Tunstall ME, Sheikh A. Failed intubation protocol: oxygenation without aspiration. *Clin Anaesth* 1986; 4:171–87.
31. Harmer M. Difficult and failed intubation in obstetrics. *Int J Obstet Anesth* 1997; 6:25–31.
32. Cook TM, Woodall N, Frerk C, *et al. 4th National Audit Project: Major Complications of Airway Management in the UK.* London: Royal College of Anaesthetists; 2011. http://www.rcoa.ac.uk/nap4
33. Han T-H, Brimacombe J, Lee EJ, *et al.* The laryngeal mask airway is effective (and probably safe) in selected healthy parturients for elective Cesarean section: a prospective study of 1067 cases. *Can J Anesth* 2001; 48:1117–21.
34. Halaseh BK, Sukkar ZF, Hassan LH, *et al.* The use of the ProSeal laryngeal mask airway in caesarean section—experience in 3000 cases. *Anaesth Intensive Care* 2010; 38:1023–8.
35. Paech MJ. 'Pregnant women having cesarean delivery under general anaesthesia should have a rapid sequence induction with cricoid pressure and be intubated'. Can this 'holy cow' be sent packing? *Anaesth Intensive Care* 2010; 38:989–91.
36. Yao WY, Li SY, Sng BL, *et al.* The LMA Supreme™ in 700 parturients undergoing Cesarean delivery: an observational study. *Can J Anesth* 2012; 59:648–54.
37. Habib AS. Is it time to revisit tracheal intubation for Cesarean delivery? *Can J Anesth* 2012; 59:642–7.
38. Cook T, Howes B. Supraglottic airway devices: recent advances. *Contin Educ Anaesth Crit Care Pain* 2011; 11:56–61.
39. McGuire BE, Younger RA. Rigid indirect laryngoscopy and optical stylets. *Contin Educ Anaesth Crit Care Pain* 2010; 10:148–51.
40. Priebe HJ. Cricoid pressure: an alternative view. *Semin Anesth Perioper Med Pain* 2005; 24:120–6.
41. Haslam N, Parker L, Duggan JE. Effect of cricoid pressure on the view at laryngoscopy. *Anaesthesia* 2005; 60:41–7.
42. Palmer JH MacG, Ball DR. The effect of cricoid pressure on the cricoid cartilage and vocal cords: an endoscopic study in anaesthetised patients. *Anaesthesia* 2000; 55:263–8.
43. Turgeon AF, Nicole PC, Trépanier CA, *et al.* Cricoid pressure does not increase the rate of failed intubation by direct laryngoscopy in adults. *Anesthesiology* 2005; 102:315–19.
44. Ellis DY, Harris T, Zideman D. Cricoid pressure in emergency department rapid sequence tracheal intubations: a risk benefit analysis. *Ann Emerg Med* 2007; 50:653–65.
45. Meek T, Gittins N, Duggan JE. Cricoid pressure: knowledge and performance amongst anaesthetic assistants. *Anaesthesia* 1999; 54:59–62.
46. Murdoch H, Scrutton M, Laxton CH. Choice of anaesthetic agents for caesarean section: a UK survey of current practice. *Int J Obstet Anesth* 2013; 22:31–5.
47. Duggal K, Russell R. Propofol should be the induction agent of choice for caesarean section under general anaesthesia. *Int J Obstet Anesth* 2003; 12:275–9.
48. Reynolds F. Anaesthesia for Caesarean section: no need for nightmares. *Anaesthesia* 1986; 41:652.
49. Heesen M, Klöhr S, Hofmann T, *et al.* Maternal and foetal effects of remifentanil for general anaesthesia in parturients undergoing caesarean section: a systematic review and meta-analysis. *Acta Anaesth Scand* 2013; 57:29–36.
50. de Souza DG, Doar LH, Mehta SH, *et al.* Aspiration prophylaxis and rapid sequence induction for elective cesarean delivery: time to reassess old dogma? *Anesth Analg* 2010; 110:1503–5.
51. Van de Velde M, Teunkens A, Kuypers M, *et al.* General anaesthesia with target controlled infusion of propofol for planned Caesarean section: maternal and neonatal effects of a remifentanil-based technique. *Int J Obstet Anesth* 2004; 13:153–8.
52. Crawford JS. The place of halothane in obstetrics. *Br J Anaesth* 1962; 34:386–90.
53. Moir DD. Anaesthesia for Caesarean section. An evaluation of a method using low concentrations of halothane and 50% of oxygen. *Br J Anaesth* 1970; 42:136–42.
54. Reynolds F. Commentary on reference 51. *Br J Anaesth* 1998; 80:688–9.
55. Crawford JS. Editorial. Fetal well-being and maternal awareness. *Br J Anaesth* 1988; 61:247–9.
56. Gambling DR, Sharma SK, White PF, *et al.* Use of sevoflurane during elective Cesarean birth; a comparison with isoflurane and spinal anesthesia. *Anesth Analg* 1995; 81:90–5.
57. Abboud TK, Zhu J, Richardson E, *et al.* Desflurane: a new volatile anesthetic for cesarean section. *Acta Anaesth Scand* 1995; 39:723–6.
58. Ebert TJ, Muzi M. Sympathetic hyperactivity during desflurane anesthesia in healthy volunteers. A comparison with isoflurane. *Anesthesiology* 1993; 79:444–53.
59. Chin KJ, Yeo SW. A BIS-guided study of sevoflurane requirements for adequate depth of anaesthesia in Caesarean section. *Anaesthesia* 2004; 59:1064–8.
60. Yoo KY, Jeong CW, Kang MW, *et al.* Bispectral index values during sevoflurane-nitrous oxide general anesthesia in women undergoing cesarean delivery: a comparison between women with and without prior labor. *Anesth Analg* 2008; 106:1827–32.
61. Paech MJ, Scott KL, Clavisi O, *et al.* A prospective study of awareness and recall associated with general anaesthesia for caesarean section. *Int J Obstet Anesth* 2008; 17:298–303.
62. The Royal College of Anaesthetists, Royal College of Anaesthetists of Great Britain and Ireland. *Report and Findings of the 5th National Audit Project: Accidental Awareness during General Anaesthesia in the United Kingdom and Ireland.* London: The Royal College of Anaesthetists. http://www.nationalauditprojects.org.uk/NAP5home#pt
63. Levy DM. Inhalational induction of anaesthesia for caesarean section: not to be sniffed at? *Int J Obstet Anesth* 2002; 11:235–7.
64. Turner RJ, Lambros M, Kenway L, *et al.* The in-vitro effects of sevoflurane and desflurane on the contractility of pregnant human uterine muscle. *Int J Obstet Anesth* 2002; 11:246–51.
65. Butwick AJ, Coleman L, Cohen SE. Minimum effective bolus dose of oxytocin during elective Caesarean delivery *Br J Anaesth* 2010; 104:338–43.
66. Levy DM. Traditional rapid sequence induction is an outmoded technique for caesarean section and should be modified. *Int J Obstet Anesth* 2006; 15:227–9.
67. Abouleish E, Abboud T, Lechevalier T, *et al.* Rocuronium (Org 9426) for Caesarean section. *Br J Anaesth* 1994; 73:336–41.
68. Sluga M, Ummenhofer W, Studer W, *et al.* Rocuronium versus succinylcholine for rapid sequence induction of anaesthesia and endotracheal intubation: a prospective, randomised trial in emergent cases. *Anesth Analg* 2005; 101:1356–61.
69. Kopman AF. Rocuronium versus succinylcholine for rapid tracheal intubation. *Anesth Analg* 2006; 102:1912.
70. Levy JH, Davis GK, Duggan J, *et al.* Determination of the hemodynamics and histamine release of rocuronium (Org 9426) when administered in increased doses under N2O/O2-sufentanil anesthesia. *Anesth Analg* 1994; 78:318–21.

71. Sadleir PHM, Clarke RC, Bunning DL, *et al.* Anaphylaxis to neuromuscular blocking drugs: incidence and cross-reactivity in Western Australia from 2002 to 2011. *Br J Anaesth* 2013; 110:981–7.
72. Pühringer FK, Kristen P, Rex C. Sugammadex reversal of rocuronium-induced neuromuscular block in Caesarean section patients: a series of seven cases. *Br J Anaesth* 2010; 105:657–60.
73. Williamson RM, Mallaiah S, Barclay P. Rocuronium and sugammadex for rapid sequence induction of obstetric general anaesthesia. *Acta Anaesth Scand* 2011; 55:694–9.
74. Lee C; Jahr JS, Candiotti, KA. Reversal of profound neuromuscular block by sugammadex administered three minutes after rocuronium: a comparison with spontaneous recovery from succinylcholine *Anesthesiology* 2009; 110:1020–5.
75. Tunstall ME. Failed intubation drill. *Anaesthesia* 1976; 31:850.
76. Sanders RD, Hassel J, Davidson AJ, *et al.* Impact of anaesthetics and surgery on neurodevelopment: an update. *Br J Anaesth* 2013; 110 (S1):i53–72.
77. Brambrink AM, Evers AS, Avidan MS, *et al.* Ketamine-induced neuroapoptosis in the fetal and neonatal Rhesus macaque brain. *Anesthesiology* 2012; 116:372–84.
78. Legrand M, Plaud B. Etomidate and general anesthesia: the butterfly effect? *Anesth Analg* 2013; 117:1267–9.
79. Dyer RA, Els I, Farbas J, *et al.* Prospective, randomized trial comparing general with spinal anaesthesia for Cesarean delivery in preeclamptic patients with a nonreassuring fetal heart trace. *Anesthesiology* 2003; 99:561–9.
80. Lewis G (ed). *The Confidential Enquiry into Maternal and Child Health (CEMACH). Saving Mothers' Lives: Reviewing Maternal Deaths to Make Motherhood Safer—2003-2005.* The Seventh Report on Confidential Enquiries into Maternal Deaths in the United Kingdom. London: CEMACH; 2007.
81. Yoo KY, Kang DH, Jeong H, *et al.* A dose-response study of remifentanil for attenuation of the hypertensive response to laryngoscopy and tracheal intubation in severely preeclamptic women undergoing caesarean delivery under general anaesthesia. *Int J Obstet Anesth* 2013; 22:10–18.
82. Dean C, Douglas J. Magnesium and the obstetric anaesthetist. *Int J Obstet Anesth* 2013; 22:52–63.
83. Huang CJ, Fan YC, Tsai PS. Differential impacts of modes of anaesthesia on the risk of stroke among preeclamptic women who undergo Caesarean delivery: a population-based study. *Br J Anaesth* 2010; 105:818–26.
84. Tsai PS, Hsu CS, Fan YC. General anaesthesia is associated with increased risk of surgical site infection after Caesarean delivery compared with neuraxial anaesthesia: a population-based study. *Br J Anaesth* 2011; 107:757–61.
85. Camann W, Tuomala R. Antibiotic prophylaxis for cesarean delivery: always before skin incision! *Int J Obstet Anesth* 2011;20:1–2.

CHAPTER 23

The aetiology and management of hypotension during spinal anaesthesia for caesarean delivery

Robert A. Dyer, Michelle J. Arcache, and Eldrid Langesaeter

Background

The benefits of neuraxial anaesthesia in obstetrics were first recognized in July 1900, when the obstetrician Oscar Kreis administered spinal cocaine to six parturients in labour. Cleland's classic experiments on anaesthetized dogs provided the anatomical basis for neuraxial anaesthesia in obstetrics in 1933.[1] However, these pain relief methods in obstetrics were initially to fall into disrepute, since inadequate training and monitoring led to a high morbidity and mortality; an editorial points out that the mortality after spinal anaesthesia (SA) was 1/1000 surgical patients prior to 1944, and as high as 1/139 in obstetrics.[2]

As understanding of maternal and fetal physiology developed, outcomes improved. Of particular importance was the early work on aortocaval compression in the third trimester.[3] A major advance in SA in obstetrics was the introduction of atraumatic pencil-point needles by Hart and Whitacre in 1951, which reduced the incidence of significant postdural puncture headache to less than 1%.[4]

Since the first Confidential Enquiry into Maternal Deaths was performed (1952–1954), the decreasing mortality associated with obstetric anaesthesia in the United Kingdom has been due both to the adoption of SA for caesarean delivery (CD) as the preferred method, and to safer general anaesthesia. Although recent literature reports a lower incidence of failed intubation[5] than an earlier study (1/250),[6] this complication continues to contribute significantly to maternal deaths.[7,8] The development of obstetric anaesthesia as a subspecialty, and the introduction of strict supervision of junior anaesthetists have also influenced obstetric anaesthesia safety.

In the United States, general anaesthesia for CD was shown to be associated with a 16.7 times higher case fatality rate than neuraxial anaesthesia for the period 1985–1990.[9] More recently, the case fatality rate for general anaesthesia has decreased, and the fatality rate has increased from 2.5 (1991–1996) to 3.8 (1997–2002) per million neuraxial anaesthetics, so that the risk ratio for general versus neuraxial anaesthesia has decreased during this period from 6.7 to 1.7.[10] This shows that SA does have an associated morbidity and mortality, although mortality is rare.

The Eighth Report on Confidential Enquiries into Maternal Deaths in the United Kingdom, published in 2011, showed that mortality as a direct result of anaesthesia remains low. For the triennium 2003–2005 there were only 6/132 deaths directly attributable to anaesthesia and in 2006–2008, there were 7/107 deaths. On analysis of the seven deaths, it was felt that substandard care was delivered to six (86%) of the women, with half of them receiving 'major' substandard care which significantly contributed to the death of the mother; different treatment may well have altered the outcome.[11]

South Africa is the only country with predominantly limited resources in which an extensive audit of maternal mortality has been in progress for many years. During the triennium 2005–2007, the report of the National Committee for the Confidential Enquiries into Maternal Deaths showed that there were 74 direct anaesthesia deaths, of which 53 were associated with spinal and 18 with general anaesthesia. For the triennium 2008–2010, 73/92(79%) of direct anaesthesia deaths were associated with SA.[12] Two-thirds of these fatalities were due to poor management of spinal hypotension or high motor block, and most were assessed as avoidable. This shows the importance of the provision of detailed recommendations for the management of haemodynamic instability during SA for CD. Such recommendations, as well as ongoing research into this important subject, should contribute to improved maternal and neonatal safety and greater maternal comfort during and after the procedure.

Haemodynamic consequences of spinal anaesthesia

Haemodynamic instability during single-shot SA for CD is the result, first and foremost, of the effects of SA in a pregnant patient predisposed to aortocaval compression.

The splanchnic vasculature provides a major reservoir for venous return in the parturient. This blood returns to the inferior vena cava via the hepatic vein, above the level of potential aortocaval compression. During a state of hypovolaemia, typically after blood loss in obstetrics, the transmural pressure of the compliant splanchnic veins is predominantly above zero,[13] due to activation of the sympathetic nervous system. The sympathectomy associated with SA would inhibit these compensatory changes, resulting in a marked decrease in venous return, due to a precipitous decrease in mean circulatory filling pressure. This may result in cardiovascular collapse. SA is thus absolutely contraindicated in this situation.

Even in the healthy parturient with her expanded blood volume, SA for CD is associated with hypotension, due to a combination of increased venous capacitance and decreased systemic vascular resistance (SVR). Since uterine blood flow is pressure dependent, hypotension results in a decrease in uterine blood flow and potential compromise to fetal oxygenation. Hypotension is commonly associated with unpleasant symptoms such as maternal nausea and vomiting, and cardiovascular collapse may rarely occur.

The definition of hypotension varies considerably between practitioners. A literature search examined 63 publications between 1999 and 2009. The two commonest definitions were a decrease in systolic blood pressure below 80% of baseline and a systolic blood pressure below 100 mmHg, or simply a decrease of 20% from baseline.[14]

Predicting hypotension in the individual case remains difficult, although the use of a supine stress test,[15] preoperative positional blood pressure change,[16] correlation between baseline heart rate (HR) and vasopressor requirements,[17] or preoperative assessment of sympathovagal balance by analysing HR variability may be useful.[18–20] Intraoperative assessment tools have included maternal symptoms, non-invasive measures such as HR and manual or oscillometric blood pressure readings, as well as central venous pressure and cardiac output (CO) measurements, including non-invasive, minimally invasive, and invasive methods.[21,22] Short-term neonatal outcome has most commonly been assessed by umbilical arterial and venous blood gas values and Apgar scores.[23]

Potential haemodynamic responses to SA are:

- hypotension and increase in HR
- hypotension and bradycardia
- persistent refractory hypotension
- high motor block with cardiorespiratory failure

These responses will be influenced by:

- aortocaval compression
- baricity and dose of local anaesthetic and opioid employed
- rational use of fluids
- goal-directed use of vasopressors.

This chapter will describe these scenarios and the mechanisms involved, and conclude with a management strategy for each one. Special considerations apply in the management of SA for patients with severe pre-eclampsia and cardiac disease.

Haemodynamic effects of aortocaval compression and spinal anaesthesia

Aortocaval compression

The association between arterial hypotension and the supine position in late pregnancy was first recognized by the Swedish obstetrician Gideon Ahltorp in 1931, as described in a review of the subject.[24] The correct aetiology was described in 1951, and classic case reports alerted anaesthetists to the importance of avoiding this complication.[25] Early studies demonstrated both vena caval and aortic compression in late pregnancy. The methodology included the measurement of right heart filling and inferior vena caval pressures, CO, differences in brachial arterial and femoral arterial pressures in the supine and the lateral or lateral tilt position, and abdominal angiography.[3] Aortic compression, shown by a decrease in femoral artery pressure, occurs earlier in pregnancy than inferior vena caval compression, as indicated by a decreased femoral artery pressure in the supine position.[26] Whilst CO may be reduced in the supine position, most women respond with compensatory increases in SVR and HR. The result is that less than 20% of women experience arterial hypotension and the 'supine hypotensive syndrome', and the quoted incidence varies greatly between studies.[24] However, the fetus may be subjected to diminished intervillous blood flow because of a rise in uterine vascular resistance secondary to aortic compression. Fetal bradycardia has been shown to occur when hypotension occurs with the mother in the supine position,[27] and HR decelerations can be reversed by turning the mother into the lateral position.

Positioning during spinal anaesthesia

During SA for CD, CO has been shown to be greatly improved by a change from the supine to the left lateral position.[28] Umbilical venous and arterial saturation was demonstrated to improve during SA in patients receiving lateral tilt.[29] A recent investigation suggests that CO is 5% higher if the patient is tilted by more than 15°.[30] However, as much as 34° of lateral tilt may be necessary to completely eliminate the effects of aortocaval compression,[31] and some investigators have recommended the performance of SA for CD in the lateral or modified lateral position.[32] It may be that the position of the parturient prior to tilting is important. One investigation showed that when women were tilted from a previous fully supine position, there was evidence of aortocaval compression. However, if they were tilted from a previously fully left lateral position, there was no evidence of aortocaval compression.[33] Interestingly, in the only published study comparing hypotension during CD in multiple gestation pregnancy with singleton pregnancy, there were no differences detectable in haemodynamic instability.[34] However, aortocaval compression may be of greater concern in patients with multiple or a large singleton pregnancy.

The effects of maternal position on the human fetal circulation have been studied using umbilical artery scanning with real-time Doppler signals during epidural anaesthesia. The results showed a higher umbilical artery vascular resistance in the supine position.[35]

Effects of spinal anaesthesia

The typical response: hypotension and an increased heart rate

During SA, sympathetic blockade diminishes the compensatory mechanisms and results in a high incidence of clinically significant hypotension. An early study of intermittent CO measurement during SA for CD, using indicator dilution, showed that SA was associated with a significant depression of CO in 10/12 patients.[28] A further study employing intermittent suprasternal Doppler flow measurements, showed that SA employing a median dose of 11 mg hyperbaric bupivacaine was associated with a decrease in CO of greater than 1 L/min in 9/16 patients.[36] By contrast, a further investigation employing lower doses of local anaesthetic

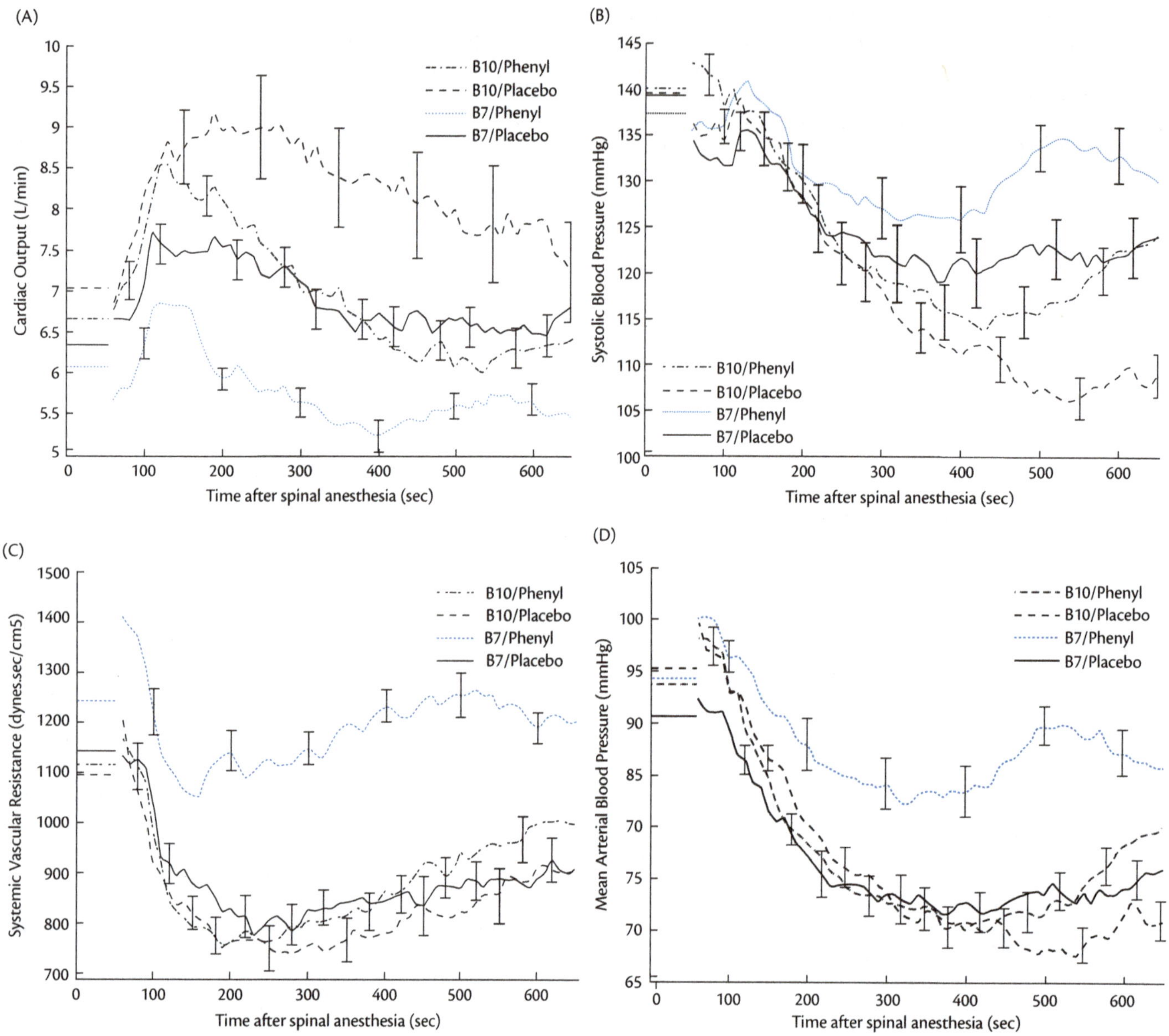

Figure 23.1 Mean differences in haemodynamic variables between the four treatment groups. (A) Cardiac output. (B) Systolic blood pressure. (C) Systemic vascular resistance. (D) Mean arterial pressure. Baseline is marked on the y-axis. Standard error (SE) for each group is marked as error bars.

Reproduced with permission from Langesæter, Eldrid; Rosseland, Leiv Arne, Continuous Invasive Blood Pressure and Cardiac Output Monitoring during Cesarean Delivery: A Randomized, Double-blind Comparison of Low-dose versus High-dose Spinal Anesthesia with Intravenous Phenylephrine or Placebo Infusion, *Anesthesiology*, Volume 109, Issue 5, pp. 856–63, Copyright © 2008 Wolters Kluwer Health, Inc.

(7 mg and 10 mg hypobaric bupivacaine) in conjunction with subarachnoid sufentanil, demonstrated a marked decrease in SVR and an *increase* in CO following SA, using pulse waveform analysis[37] (Figure 23.1).

Another study, employing both pulse waveform analysis and bioimpedance changes in the same patient, confirmed that the typical response to SA for elective CD is a decrease in SVR, which causes hypotension and a partially compensatory increase in CO, mediated by increases in both stroke volume (SV) and HR.[38] The important difference in findings between the old studies[28,36] and the more recent studies[37,38] is the methods applied. The older studies using intermittent measurements of CO 5, 10, and 15 minutes after SA, would not be able to detect the initial effects of SA as shown in the two more recent studies using continuous monitoring of CO. In addition, the modern practice of using lower doses of spinal bupivacaine, together with the recognition of the importance of patient positioning and the judicious use of fluids and vasopressors, may contribute to more stable haemodynamics once SA is established. In most women, the baroreceptor response is well preserved soon after induction of SA, despite sympathetic blockade. In the non-obstetric population, sympathovagal balance usually does not alter to complete vagal dominance during the sympathetic block associated with SA, and sinus bradycardia is therefore infrequent.[39]

Hypotension and bradycardia

Sudden severe bradycardia may occur in approximately 7% of patients,[40] and occasional cardiac arrest has been described.[41–44]

In many of the cases describing cardiac arrest, high doses of local anaesthetics were used, some with inadvertent spinal placement of an intended epidural top-up. The cause of the profound vagal activity that occurs in a small proportion of women is unknown, but it may be triggered by several different causes such as aortocaval compression, high block, emotional stress, peritoneal manipulation, or sudden haemorrhage.[45] Reflex phenomena such as the pacemaker stretch reflex,[46] Bezold–Jarisch reflex (BJR),[47] and the 'reverse' Bainbridge reflex[48,49] may be causatory, but there is no strong evidence to support this theory.

The BJR was initially described as a chemoreflex: precipitous bradycardia followed the injection of toxic steroidal alkaloids into dogs' coronary arteries. More recently, it has been postulated that there may be mechanical stretching during contraction of the poorly filled left ventricle, which results from a sudden decrease in venous return following induction of SA for CD, or in severe hypovolaemia. This may result in increased afferent input into the vasomotor centre via C-fibres in the inferoposterior wall of the left ventricle. This is followed by profound bradycardia and peripheral vasodilatation. A review supports the possibility of the involvement of the BJR in acute bradycardia during neuraxial anaesthesia, but states that there is probably more than one physiological precipitating factor or mechanism.[50] The Bainbridge reflex was described in 1915. An infusion of saline into anaesthetized dogs produced tachycardia, on the basis of activation of stretch receptors in the atria. The 'reverse' Bainbridge reflex has been proposed to explain slowing of the HR when venous return decreases.[49] Whatever the mechanism, the final common efferent pathway is the vagus nerve, and the result is occasional profound bradycardia.

Persistent refractory hypotension

Having ensured adequate uterine displacement, hypotension resistant to vasopressors should raise the suspicion that either an error has been made concerning the volume status of the patient, or there is undiagnosed cardiac pathology. In low-resourced areas,[51] the diagnosis of valvular heart disease and cardiomyopathy may be missed in patients presenting close to term.

High motor block

This scenario is fortunately rare, of the order of 1/3000.[44] The doses are not mentioned in this study. If the currently recommended doses of spinal local anaesthetic and details of technique are employed, this incidence is likely to be much lower. Therefore, when teaching SA for CD, it should be emphasized that cardiovascular instability requires immediate treatment, and is by far the more common scenario than high spinal block.[52] SA for CD is associated with a reduction in respiratory function of approximately 25%, which may impair cough strength in some patients.[53,54] High motor block results in increasing dyspnoea and weak respiratory effort, followed by apnoea. Concomitant sympathetic block may result in cardiovascular collapse.

Overall, maternal and fetal morbidity have been greatly reduced by the recognition of the effects and the avoidance of aortocaval compression during SA for CD. However, an editorial discusses the relative contribution of the venous and arterial circulation to spinal hypotension during CD.[55] The point is made that despite careful attention to fluid management and positioning in order to minimize aortocaval compression, significant hypotension still occurs in a large percentage of patients, due to the effects of SA on the *arterial* circulation. This thought-provoking editorial suggests that there is a 'lesson' to be learned 'from pre-eclampsia', in that one would expect greater haemodynamic instability in these patients if intravascular depletion and decreased venous return were the predominant contributor to spinal hypotension. Research employing continuous pulse waveform analysis (previously discussed) supports the contention that spinal hypotension is usually in large part due to effects on the *arterial* circulation during SA for elective CD.

Baricity, dose, and volume of spinal local anaesthetic, and combination with an opioid

Currently, most anaesthetists employ hyperbaric bupivacaine for SA for CD. In support of this practice, a randomized trial suggested that isobaric and hypobaric solutions were associated with more motor block, as well as more hypotension and a higher number of cervical level blocks than hyperbaric bupivacaine, if SA was performed in the sitting position.[56] A study comparing the effects of 7 and 10 mg hypobaric bupivacaine, with and without a prophylactic phenylephrine infusion during elective CD, showed that greater haemodynamic instability occurred in the higher-dose group (Figure 23.1).[37]

Since the early adoption of 0.5% bupivacaine for SA for CD, interest has focused on the optimal local anaesthetic/opioid combination and dose to achieve the goals of effective surgical anaesthesia and postoperative analgesia, with minimal maternal and neonatal side effects. This is particularly important in view of the fact that maternal pain is the commonest reason for failure of technique, particularly if the uterus is exteriorized. Pain is also the most commonly cited anaesthetic cause of litigation in obstetric practice.[57] Despite several studies on dose response and efficacy, currently there seems no advantage of either levobupivacaine or ropivacaine over bupivacaine. Most anaesthetists employ hyperbaric 0.5% bupivacaine in a dose of 7.5–15.0 mg (1.5–3.0 mL). The incidence of visceral pain has been shown to be related to the dose of spinal bupivacaine. The use of less than 10 mg alone or 8 mg in combination with an opioid is considered 'low dose'. Some investigators have examined the lower dose range, with a view to reducing side effects such as hypotension, nausea and vomiting, and prolonged motor blockade. In a comparative study of three different doses of hyperbaric bupivacaine, the use of 7.5 mg of bupivacaine was advocated in the interests of haemodynamic stability; however, many patients rated analgesia as poor.[58] Furthermore, a study employing a suprasternal Doppler flow technique was unable to demonstrate improved haemodynamic stability when comparing the initiation of SA for CD with a standard local anaesthetic dose versus a smaller dose as part of a combined spinal–epidural (CSE) technique.[59]

The addition of various doses of different intrathecal opioids may allow the reduction of the local anaesthetic dose, with an equivalent success rate and less severe side effects. Adequate surgical anaesthesia has been reported in parturients receiving only 5 mg hyperbaric bupivacaine, to which 25 mcg fentanyl was added, with less hypotension, and less nausea and vomiting than the group receiving 10 mg of bupivacaine only.[60] Other investigators reported that 8 mg of bupivacaine was sufficient if 10 mcg fentanyl was added.[61] All studies suggest that a combination of local anaesthetic and opioid allows for a reduction in local anaesthetic dose. Most studies investigating low local anaesthetic doses have employed hyperbaric bupivacaine, which allows the use of positioning to manipulate dermatomal spread. In this regard, low-dose (6.6 mg) hyperbaric bupivacaine has been shown to produce more reliable cephalad spread of anaesthesia, with less hypotension and nausea, than the hypobaric solution.[62]

When the effects of low-dose SA are studied, a CSE technique is often employed, since this allows for epidural supplementation should analgesia be inadequate. It should be noted that the interpretation of the results of these studies may, however, be influenced by the fact that single-shot SA may result in less sensorimotor anaesthesia than an identical dose administered as part of a CSE technique for elective CD.[63]

One recent investigation into the dose–response relationship for intrathecal hyperbaric bupivacaine co-administered with intrathecal fentanyl and morphine, demonstrated an ED_{50} of 7.6 mg and an ED_{95} of 11.2 mg for bupivacaine.[64] In addition, a recent meta-analysis suggests that if less than 8 mg bupivacaine is employed, there is an increased requirement for intraoperative analgesic supplementation (risk ratio 3.76; 95% confidence interval (CI) 2.38–5.92).[65] There is good evidence that a dose of less than 10 mg should also not be used in morbidly obese patients, since the ED_{95} was estimated at 15 and 12 mg respectively in two papers.[66,67] In view of the fact that the patient's experience of pain is by far the most important outcome, low-dose single-shot SA can no longer be recommended, and such low doses should only be administered as part of a CSE technique.[68]

In summary, surgical anaesthesia during single-shot SA should not be compromised due to concerns about the management of cardiovascular instability.[65,69] A dose of no less than 8 mg hyperbaric bupivacaine combined with an opioid, or 10 mg of hyperbaric bupivacaine alone, would seem appropriate. If doses lower than these are envisaged, SA should only be performed as part of a CSE technique. The use of a long-acting opioid as part of a single-shot SA technique depends upon facilities available for postoperative monitoring. Having selected the optimal combination of local anaesthetic and opioid for SA in this manner, with a view to attaining ideal surgical anaesthesia and a minimal requirement for intraoperative supplementation of analgesia, haemodynamic instability will still occur in a significant percentage of patients, despite positioning the mother in left lateral tilt. This requires careful attention to fluid and vasopressor therapy.

Fluid management

Considerable controversy exists as to the most appropriate IV fluid regimen for SA for elective CD. Widespread use of crystalloid preload was initiated by the demonstration of improvements in uterine blood flow in pregnant ewes in response to rapid fluid administration after SA-induced hypotension.[70] The rationale for 'preload' was that SA-induced venodilatation results in a decrease in SV which more than offsets the increase due to afterload reduction, and thus CO may decrease precipitously. Early promising results[71,72] may have been due to the inclusion of patients in labour, an inadequate understanding of the importance of prevention of aortocaval compression, and other aspects of study design such as blinding, randomization, and local anaesthetic dose. Patients in labour may be less susceptible to hypotension during CD, possibly due to autotransfusion during contractions.[73]

A qualitative systematic review evaluated the efficacy of increasing blood volume in reducing the incidence of hypotension during elective SA for CD.[74] Secondary outcomes were maternal nausea, vasopressor use, and umbilical cord pH and Apgar scores. The studies fell into four categories: large versus small volumes of crystalloid, colloid versus crystalloid, different colloid regimens, and mechanical methods for increasing blood volume (total N = 1504). Crystalloid solutions were ineffective as a preload. Of the nine studies examining crystalloids, only three showed a significant reduction in the incidence of hypotension in the group receiving a higher volume of preload.[71,75,76] There were considerable differences in the study protocols, which probably accounts for the heterogeneity of the results.[74] Colloids were effective in reducing, but not eliminating, hypotension in all but one of a total of 23 randomized controlled trials. Of the seven studies comparing crystalloid and colloid (albumin, hetastarch, gelatin, pentastarch, or dextran), five showed a decreased incidence of hypotension in the colloid relative to the crystalloid group.[77–81] Only one study showed a better neonatal outcome in the colloid group.[79] A limitation of the results was the variability in the volumes of colloids chosen in the studies, as well as differing definitions of hypotension and ephedrine protocols. Due to variation in study design, it was also not possible to determine whether prophylactic fluid administration affected vasopressor requirements. Some small studies have shown that wrapping the legs consistently reduced the incidence of hypotension compared with leg elevation or controls.[82] However, this is not a method that is easy to apply in routine clinical practice.

The latest update of the Cochrane Database in this field includes 75 studies with only eight trials reporting adequate allocation concealment methods, and blinding was reported in 28 trials. This review is in general agreement with findings from the above-mentioned systematic review,[74] reporting that 'Crystalloids were more effective than no fluids (relative risk 0.78, 95% confidence interval 0.60 to 1.00; one trial, 140 women, sequential analysis) and colloids were more effective than crystalloids (relative risk 0.68, 95% confidence interval 0.52 to 0.89; 11 trials, 698 women) in preventing hypotension following SA at CD. No differences were detected for different doses, rates or methods of administering colloids or crystalloids'.[83] Despite the proven advantages of colloids in terms of reducing hypotension, colloids have not been uniformly adopted for fluid management for elective CD. This is partly because of their expense, as well as the risk of anaphylactic reactions, albeit very low with most available solutions.

Many studies have therefore investigated the timing of administration of crystalloid. The relevance of the duration and timing of infusion of a crystalloid preload prior to SA for CD, has been evaluated.[84] This study demonstrated that there was no difference in the incidence of hypotension whether 20 mL/kg of crystalloid was given over 10 or 20 minutes prior to induction of SA. Central venous pressure increases were greater, but increases in HR were less, and HR returned to baseline in a shorter period in the 10-minute group than in the 20-minute group, suggesting a benefit in administering the fluid closer to the time of induction of SA. In a subsequent investigation, the authors hypothesized that in order for a fluid bolus to effectively reduce post-spinal hypotension, the administration of the fluid should produce a sustained increase in CO. Patients were preloaded with 1.5 L Ringer's lactate, or 0.5 L or 1.0 L hydroxyethyl starch. CO and blood volume were assessed before and 30 minutes after fluid loading, using a non-invasive pulse spectrophotometric technique for detecting indocyanine green. All groups had an increase in blood volume after fluid loading, but only 28% of the Ringer's lactate solution remained in the intravascular space after 30 minutes, compared with 100% of the hydroxyethyl starch solution. CO was only increased in the hydroxyethyl starch groups, and only in the 1.0 L hydroxyethyl starch group was spinal hypotension statistically and clinically significantly reduced, with an incidence of 17%, versus 75% in the Ringer's and 58% in the 0.5 L hydroxyethyl starch group.[81]

In the non-obstetric population, a sustained rise in CO has been demonstrated in a group of patients given lactated Ringer's solution after the initiation of SA.[85] A kinetic analysis of an IV infusion of Ringer's solution as preload suggested that a rapid fluid load given over 2 minutes after induction of both spinal and general anaesthesia for non-obstetric surgery, might prevent hypotension caused by central hypovolaemia.[86] These findings prompted a study of crystalloid administration after initiation of SA for CD ('co-load' or co-hydration), to overcome the problem of rapid redistribution of crystalloid fluid. The co-load group (20 mL/kg) required a lower median dose of ephedrine for the treatment of maternal hypotension prior to delivery.[87] Subsequent to this study, crystalloid co-loading has been employed in combination with phenylephrine infusion, in an attempt to obtain optimal haemodynamic stability during SA for CD.[88] Patients receiving rapid co-loading in combination with phenylephrine had an almost zero incidence of hypotension, which was an improvement on the use of phenylephrine infusions alone. This paper forms the basis for current practice, with the reservation that most practitioners use lower doses of phenylephrine than in this investigation (see 'Vasopressor Use').

Several studies have also examined the optimal volume and timing of colloid administration. In this regard, a pentastarch preload of 10 mL/kg has been found to be more effective than 5 mL/kg at preventing hypotension following SA.[89] As might be expected, colloid co-loading with 6% hydroxyethyl starch was found to be similarly effective in reducing hypotension compared with preloading.[90] Similar results were shown using hetastarch.[91] There was no difference in CO or vasopressor requirements in women randomized to colloid or crystalloid co-load.[92] However, interpretation is difficult, since a prophylactic phenylephrine infusion was used. There have been no studies comparing crystalloid co-load with colloid preload.[93]

In summary:

- Crystalloid preload is not effective.[76]
- Preload with crystalloid or colloid increases CO but this does not reduce the incidence of arterial hypotension.[94,95]
- Crystalloid co-load is partially effective and superior to crystalloid preload, however the benefit most likely depends on the volume of fluid infused (higher volume best) and the rapid administration of the fluid over the first 5–10 minutes after induction of SA, timed with the onset of the sympathectomy.[96,97]
- Colloid co-load is as effective as colloid preload.[98]
- Colloid co-load is equally effective—and possibly more effective—than crystalloid co-load.[92,97]

To conclude, colloids are more effective than crystalloids in preventing hypotension during SA for elective CD, particularly in women who have a positive preoperative supine stress test.[15] Routine use of colloids is not uniformly accepted in view of the expense, the potential for anaphylactic reactions, and the efficacy of rapid, high-volume crystalloid co-loading,[97] in combination with appropriate use of vasopressors.

Vasopressor use

Fluids alone are inadequate to treat spinal hypotension in 40–60% of cases.[99] The most commonly used vasopressors worldwide are ephedrine and phenylephrine; this discussion is therefore limited to the intravenous administration of these agents, since prophylactic intramuscular administration may cause hypertension[100] or inadequate reduction of hypotensive episodes,[101] depending on the exact timing. The choice of vasopressor should be based upon a knowledge of the maternal haemodynamic effects of the agent, efficacy (preferably rapid onset and short duration), maternal and fetal side effects.

Ephedrine is a slow onset and relatively long-acting, non-catecholamine, direct-acting β-receptor agonist, with indirect α-effects via norepinephrine release. However, the exact mechanism of action remains controversial; one study in a rat model suggested mainly indirect effects via norepinephrine release,[102] and another supported direct α-effects.[103] In either case, the fact that the uteroplacental circulation is relatively devoid of sympathetic innervation, suggests a resistance to uterine arterial vasoconstrictive effects of this agent.[102] In support of this finding, ephedrine has been found to cause relatively more femoral than uterine artery vasoconstriction in pregnant ewes.[104] The vasodilatory effects of increased nitric oxide synthase activity in the uterine artery endothelium of pregnant ewes[105] suggests that ephedrine might preferentially shunt blood to the uterus in pregnancy.[99] A dose response meta-analysis of prophylactic IV ephedrine for the prevention of spinal hypotension, suggested a dose of 12 mg as a balance between benefit as a vasopressor and risk of causing hypertension.[106] Clinical disadvantages in terms of haemodynamic effects include a low efficacy for vasopressor effect,[106] the development of tachyphylaxis to the pressor effects,[107] and tachycardia and arrhythmias.[108] The rapid onset α_1 agonist phenylephrine may be more effective for the reduction of nausea and vomiting during SA.[109]

The basis for the long-established use of ephedrine as a first-line drug for the management of spinal hypotension in obstetrics was a paper showing reductions of uterine blood flow in pregnant ewes following administration of α-agonists.[110] However an elegant subsequent study comparing pregnant with non-pregnant ewes, has shown that the pregnant uterine artery is less responsive to α_1 agonist stimulation than the non-pregnant artery.[111] In the human haemochorial placental system, flow is very dependent upon pressure in the uterine arteries; thus phenylephrine maintains flow by its predominant effect on the systemic arterial pressure, while causing relatively little uterine arterial constriction.

One of the further chief objections to ephedrine is the fetal acidosis associated with its use. The decreased umbilical arterial pH and increased base deficit have been attributed to an ephedrine-generated increase in fetal metabolic rate, evidenced by an increase in an umbilical arteriovenous PCO_2 difference in patients receiving ephedrine when compared with phenylephrine.[109] Ephedrine also increases fetal catecholamine concentrations.[112] Transplacental transfer of ephedrine is more efficient than that of phenylephrine. When large doses are used (median dose 60 mg ephedrine and 1.3 mg phenylephrine by infusion), umbilical arterial pH is lower (7.25 vs 7.34), and base deficit and lactate significantly higher (4.8 vs 1.9, and 4.2 vs 2.2 mmol/L respectively) in the ephedrine group.[113] Some neonates may have a genetic predisposition to fetal acidosis, based upon their β_2 adrenoreceptor haplotype.[114] Overall, both ephedrine and phenylephrine have been demonstrated to be safe for the fetus when used in healthy pregnant women in normal clinical doses.[115]. Minor increases in fetal metabolic rate may even be beneficial to the normal fetus; one investigation showed that neonatal respiratory rates were higher in patients randomized to placebo than the β-agonist terbutaline prior to elective CD. Neonates in the treated group also had lower airways resistance and higher pulmonary compliance.[116]

In the only published paper involving non-elective CDs, there were no significant differences in fetal acid–base status after randomization to phenylephrine or ephedrine.[117] It is, however, possible that in compromised infants already at risk of acidosis and intrapartum hypoxia, large doses of ephedrine may have a clinically deleterious effect, particularly by virtue of increased fetal oxygen consumption.

Phenylephrine is a potent direct-acting α_1 agonist which has a rapid onset and is shorter acting by virtue of metabolism by monoamine oxidase. Two excellent reviews discuss the overall effects of phenylephrine on the human circulation, and specifically during obstetric SA.[118,119] A study comparing infusions of phenylephrine and ephedrine suggested a potency ratio of 81.2 (95% CI 73.0–89.7).[120] The time to peak pressor effect has been studied employing beat-by-beat finger arterial pressure. Phenylephrine has a significantly shorter time to peak effect than ephedrine (median 27 vs 78 seconds, P-value = 0.006).[121] A further study employing the LiDCO pulse waveform analysis system showed that baseline MAP was restored in approximately 40 and 90 seconds by phenylephrine and ephedrine IV boluses respectively.[38] Two investigations employing non-invasive blood pressure monitoring have examined the ED_{95} and ED_{90}, respectively, of bolus phenylephrine, using up-down sequential allocation. The ED_{95} of phenylephrine has been found to be 137 and 159 mcg for preventing hypotension and nausea, respectively.[122] However, the authors comment that a bolus of 120 mcg was effective and safe in all of the 50 patients. Another investigation estimated the ED_{90} of phenylephrine to be approximately 150 mcg for the prevention of hypotension.[123] In view of the finding of a 75% increase in SVR after a bolus of 80 mcg phenylephrine,[37] the estimated ED_{90} and ED_{95} are too high for recommendation in routine clinical practice.

Overall, the selection and method of administration of a vasopressor to prevent hypotension should therefore be based on the efficacy in preventing *maternal symptoms*, and the maternal *haemodynamic changes in response to SA*.[124]

There are few available data comparing maternal CO responses to ephedrine and phenylephrine during SA for elective CD. Three published investigations have employed intermittent suprasternal Doppler flow measurements. In the first study, comparing bolus doses of the vasopressors, overall CO changes were not different between groups; however, bradycardia in the phenylephrine group was treated with atropine, which make the results difficult to interpret.[125] The primary outcome variable in this study was umbilical artery pH, and not maternal haemodynamic changes. Two further studies, employing infusions of vasopressors, suggested that phenylephrine may depress maternal CO.[126,127] Two studies employing beat-by-beat CO changes using the LiDCO monitor, have demonstrated the effects of phenylephrine on CO during elective CD.[37,38] In the latter investigation, the haemodynamic effects of boluses of phenylephrine (80 mcg) and ephedrine (10 mg), were studied using minimally invasive CO monitoring (both LiDCO*plus* and transthoracic bioimpedance measurements).[38] Vasopressor was administered in response to a 20% decrease in mean arterial pressure, at which point SVR had decreased by 35% and HR and CO had increased from baseline pre-SA values (~12% and 20% respectively). Figure 23.2 shows that phenylephrine reduced CO and HR to values approximating pre-SA baseline measurements, by reversing the SA-induced decrease in SVR and increase in CO. The study suggested that HR could guide phenylephrine dosing, in that HR correlated strongly with CO. In most cases, simply titrating phenylephrine to maintain the baseline HR will thus restore blood pressure and CO. When this typical response to SA is observed, it is not logical to use ephedrine to further increase CO, which in most cases is already elevated as a response to SA. A further disadvantage of ephedrine is that the peak pressor effect occurs later than in the case of phenylephrine (Figure 23.2).

Several investigators have examined the advantages of bolus versus infusion or a combination of these methods of administration of phenylephrine.[88,128,129] A comparison of a prophylactic infusion of 100 mcg/min phenylephrine with the administration of 100 mcg boluses in response to a decrease in blood pressure to less than 80% of baseline, showed a greater number of hypotensive episodes in the latter group, with no benefit in terms of cord blood gases. The prophylaxis group received approximately three times the dose of phenylephrine.[128] A subsequent investigation, using phenylephrine infusions to control blood pressure at 80%, 90%, or 100% of baseline values, suggested that tight control of blood pressure was associated with a lower incidence of nausea and vomiting, and a significantly higher umbilical arterial pH, which was, however, not clinically relevant.[129] A closed-loop feedback computer-controlled infusion has been used to maintain baseline blood pressure, using an on–off algorithm for a phenylephrine infusion at 100 mcg/min.[130] No patients were symptomatic, and umbilical arterial pH was above 7.2 in all 53 cases. Hypertension occurred in 38% of patients. Closed-loop feedback computer-controlled phenylephrine infusion has been shown to provide better arterial pressure control with fewer interventions required than with manual controlled infusion.[131] This is, however, not a readily practicable method in most units. The well-preserved cord gas values after high-dose phenylephrine,[129] suggest that phenylephrine is effective in sustaining uterine blood flow during SA by its effects on uterine artery perfusion pressure.

Initiation of a phenylephrine infusion immediately after induction of SA, rather than treating established hypotension, may be beneficial.[128] This was supported by a study in which 120 healthy women were randomized to a low-dose phenylephrine infusion (0.15 mcg/kg/min), an initial bolus of phenylephrine (50 mcg), or treatment of hypotension with phenylephrine (50 mcg).[132] In a further study using a suprasternal Doppler flow technique to measure changes in CO, three different phenylephrine infusion rates (25, 50, or 100 mcg/min) were administered after crystalloid preload in 75 patients.[127] An infusion rate of 100 mcg/min resulted in a clinically significant reduction in both HR and CO. Larger

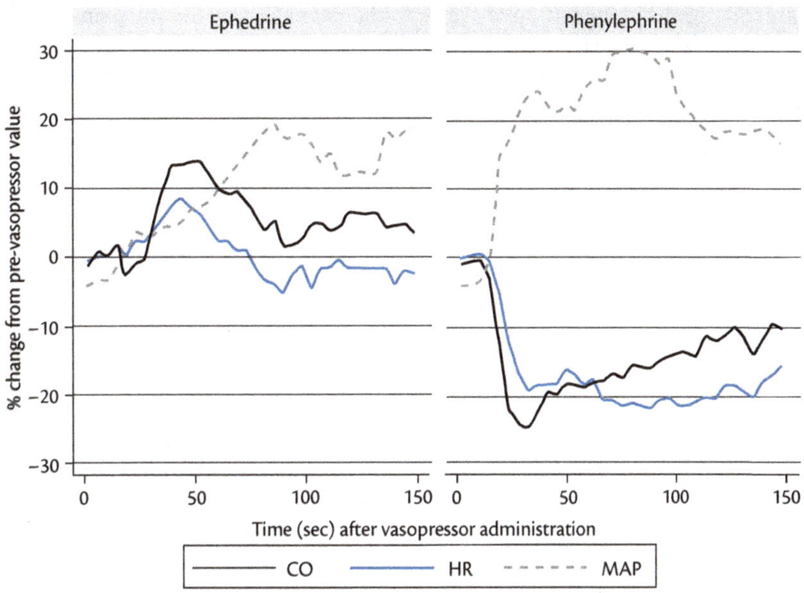

Figure 23.2 Percentage changes, from pre-vasopressor values, in cardiac output (CO, as measured by LiDCO*plus* monitor), heart rate (HR) and mean arterial pressure (MAP) following the administration of vasopressor. Note that pre-vasopressor CO was 22% higher than baseline pre-spinal anaesthesia CO.

Reproduced with permission from Dyer, Robert A.; Reed, Anthony R., Hemodynamic Effects of Ephedrine, Phenylephrine, and the Coadministration of Phenylephrine with Oxytocin during Spinal Anesthesia for Elective Cesarean Delivery, *Anesthesiology*, Volume 111, Issue 4, pp. 689–929, Copyright © 2009 Wolters Kluwer Health, Inc.

total doses of phenylephrine were required to maintain equivalent control of the blood pressure when the infusion rate was 100 mcg/min, suggesting a dose-related decrease in venous return. A further investigation compared placebo with four different fixed rates of phenylephrine infusion (25, 50, 75, and 100 mcg/min) in combination with a crystalloid co-load, using non-invasive blood pressure measurements in 101 patients.[133] There was no hypotension in the high-dose infusion group (100 mcg/min), but the incidence of hypertension in this group was 82%, and 32% of the patients developed bradycardia. There were no differences in the mean changes in systolic blood pressure when comparing the 50 and 100 cg/min groups. None of the patients in the 50 mcg/min group developed bradycardia, suggesting that the lower dose range of phenylephrine should be used. The authors also suggested that variable rate infusions would be more effective. The studies reviewed above provide valuable information on the dosing of phenylephrine when administered by bolus or infusion. However, research protocols follow a strict setup. Interpatient variability in response to SA and vasopressors require that treatment is guided both by the individual response and published recommendations.

Combinations of ephedrine and phenylephrine have also been studied. Phenylephrine added to an infusion of ephedrine halved the incidence of hypotension and increased umbilical cord pH,[134] but there is no apparent benefit over phenylephrine alone. In a study employing varying proportions of the two vasopressors by infusion, increasing proportions of ephedrine resulted in less favourable haemodynamic control as assessed by HR and blood pressure, and decreasing umbilical arterial pH and base excess.[135]

Overall, the studies confirm the finding from research pioneered by Ngan Kee et al.[108] that phenylephrine is the first line drug for the prevention or treatment of spinal hypotension. A potential disadvantage of *prophylactic* administration of phenylephrine is that the individual response, particularly in terms of HR, may be difficult to interpret. Many investigations suggest that the dose should be tailored to prevent hypertension and bradycardia. A review on vasopressor use during CD points out that the increase in blood pressure due to excessive doses of phenylephrine, is to some extent limited by a baroreceptor-mediated slowing of the HR.[136] Blocking the vagus nerve by the use of anticholinergic agents in this situation may therefore result in dangerous hypertension, as shown in two case reports.[136–138] This practice should thus be avoided.[139] In addition, administration of glycopyrrolate prior to induction of SA for CD, does not reduce the severity of hypotension, or vasopressor requirements.[140]

Despite documentation and recommendations for the use of phenylephrine and co-load,[88] a recent survey of practice amongst obstetric anaesthetists showed that the use of preload and ephedrine for prevention and treatment of spinal hypotension is still common practice.[141] This apparent reluctance of obstetric anaesthetists to change practice in response to convincing evidence from randomized trials, is highlighted in an editorial.[142]

In summary:

- *Hypotension and an increased HR is the typical response.* This response reflects a decrease in SVR, and a partial compensatory increase in CO, via an increase in HR and SV. Therefore, appropriate management is left lateral tilt, rapid crystalloid or colloid co-load, and the administration of IV phenylephrine. Given that this haemodynamic response is so common, good practice is to administer the vasopressor prophylactically. Since the haemodynamic response varies between patients, it is also reasonable to administer phenylephrine in immediate response to an increase in the HR. Current evidence is that the best approach is to titrate the rate of phenylephrine administration in order to maintain the baseline *HR*, since this restores SVR, CO, and blood pressure to baseline values. The initial dose should be a 50 mcg bolus, followed by intermittent 50 mcg boluses or infusion (25–50 mcg/min), or both as required. There is no evidence to support the use of anticholinergic agents in the setting of a normal or raised blood pressure and a decreased HR in response to phenylephrine. This can cause tachycardia and hypertension.

- *Hypotension and bradycardia.* Since the final common pathway is the vagus nerve, anticholinergics should be administered, preferably atropine 0.5 mg if bradycardia is severe, together with attention to maternal position and accelerated fluid administration. Ephedrine may also be used in conjunction with anticholinergic agents, but theoretically it may worsen bradycardia if the BJR is involved, since β_1 agonist-induced mechanical stretch of an empty left ventricle may initiate the reflex.
- *Persistent refractory hypotension.* Since a possible misdiagnosis has been made with respect to fluid balance or underlying cardiac pathology, adequate uterine displacement should be ensured, larger doses of vasopressor and/or small bolus doses of positive inotropes such as adrenaline (10 mcg) may then be necessary, together with close attention to fluid balance.
- *High motor block.* This results in increasing dyspnoea and weak respiratory effort, followed by apnoea. Concomitant sympathetic block may result in cardiovascular collapse, requiring full cardiopulmonary resuscitation.

Special considerations in pre-eclampsia

When one considers the cardiovascular pathophysiology of severe pre-eclampsia, including decreased intravascular volume and markedly raised SVR,[143] there has been an understandable caution as regards neuraxial anaesthesia in these patients, due to the theoretical possibility of precipitous hypotension, decreased CO, and associated placental hypoperfusion. Epidural anaesthesia for labour has been found to be associated with remarkable haemodynamic stability, as demonstrated by the use of pulmonary artery catheterization, in patients with severe pre-eclampsia who were receiving magnesium therapy.[144] SA has only recently been recognized to have a place in operative management in pre-eclampsia. In 1995, three groups of patients with severe pre-eclampsia were randomized to receive epidural, CSE, or general anaesthesia for CD, with similar haemodynamic stability (as assessed by HR and blood pressure) and fetal outcome in each group. Patients with non-reassuring fetal heart traces were excluded from this study.[145] Subsequently an editorial highlighted a study which showed that haemodynamic stability was equivalent in patients receiving spinal or epidural anaesthesia for non-emergency CD.[146,147] Fluid requirements were, however, higher in the spinal group. Despite the gradually emerging evidence that SA was safe in pre-eclampsia, at least one editorial called for caution, and stressed the value of epidural anaesthesia.[148] In a randomized multicentre study, SA was associated with a higher incidence of hypotension and a higher ephedrine requirement than epidural anaesthesia for CD for pre-eclampsia, but these differences were not of clinical significance.[149]

Early investigations showed that withdrawal of sympathetic activity, both by SA and by autonomic ganglion blockade, has less effect in pre-eclamptic women than in healthy pregnant and non-pregnant women.[150,151] More recently, several authors have confirmed that SA for CD in severe pre-eclampsia is associated with less hypotension and/or vasopressor requirements than in healthy parturients.[152–155] One such study used a control group consisting of healthy patients having a preterm CD, in whom the neonatal weights were similar to those in the pre-eclampsia group. This ensured that observed differences in blood pressure were not due to varying degrees of aortocaval compression in the two groups, as might have been the case in a previous study by the same authors.[153]

There are no definitive data on fluid management during SA for CD in patients with severe pre-eclampsia. Mean central venous pressure has been shown to increase significantly after a preload of 1 L of crystalloid, but returned to normal shortly after induction of anaesthesia.[156] Atrial natriuretic peptide release after a crystalloid preload is exaggerated in patients with pre-eclampsia relative to healthy parturients, and this may aid in the adaptation of maternal circulation to a volume load at elective CD.[157]

There are limited CO data in the setting of SA for CD in severe pre-eclampsia. Owing to a significant incidence of complications using the pulmonary artery catheter, the research focus has moved to non-invasive technologies. In only a few studies has CO been monitored during SA for CD. Whole-body impedance cardiography was used in a study to evaluate maternal CO changes in ten pre-eclamptic women, of whom six had severe disease, undergoing CD with SA.[158] After recovery from SA, stroke index and cardiac index in the pre-eclamptic group were significantly lower than pre-surgery levels. By contrast, using the LiDCO*plus* monitor in 15 women with severe pre-eclampsia, CO was shown to be stable during SA, suggesting that SA is well tolerated in these patients.[159] The main effect was a modest afterload reduction. On first principles this is desirable in severe pre-eclampsia, since SVR is often raised. This suggests that vasopressor therapy during SA should be conservative in patients with severe pre-eclampsia, and a modest lowering of blood pressure should be allowed before treatment is initiated. There are no randomized trials comparing the maternal or fetal effects of phenylephrine and ephedrine in this patient population. In this study, phenylephrine 50 mcg effectively raised SVR in cases in whom hypotension required treatment.

Detailed investigations employing transthoracic echocardiography have shown that the cardiac abnormality in patients with severe pre-eclampsia is diastolic dysfunction.[160,161] This work confirms and clarifies earlier findings using pulmonary artery catheterization.[162] Inotropy is usually well preserved or increased, and an 'inovasoconstrictor' state is accepted as the usual response in severe disease. Early-onset disease may be associated with greater myocardial impairment,[163,164] as well as a higher SVR at an early stage.[165] The resistance to hypotension during neuraxial anaesthesia may thus be due to a combination of factors. Firstly, there is an imbalance between pro- and anti-angiogenic factors in pre-eclampsia, due to vascular endothelial damage caused by the release of proteins derived from the placenta.[166,167] This results in vasoconstriction. Secondly, the increased inotropic state of the myocardium[161] results in adequate compensation for any decrease in SVR induced by SA. In complicated cases with established pulmonary oedema and hypoxia, neuraxial anaesthesia may be relatively contraindicated. There are no good data in these cases concerning the concomitant development of systolic hypofunction. An interesting laboratory study postulates that there may be a link between peripartum cardiomyopathy and severe pre-eclampsia. Peripartum cardiomyopathy may be due to an imbalance of angiogenesis in pregnancy, and markedly raised levels of soluble tyrosine kinase in severe pre-eclampsia may also be associated with antiangiogenic effects, with resultant systolic hypofunction.[168]

Neuraxial anaesthesia in patients with cardiac disease

Due to improved cardiac surgical techniques and follow-up, more patients with congenital heart disease reach fertile age.[169] Increasing numbers of women with congenital and acquired heart disease require operative delivery. Pregnant women with cardiac disease should be managed by a multidisciplinary team including an obstetrician, a cardiologist, and an anaesthesiologist.[148–150] Patients at high risk for cardiac instability should have a planned delivery at a tertiary centre with specialized cardiac services, including options like the intra-aortic balloon pump, and high-quality critical care.

Several case reports describe the use of titrated neuraxial anaesthesia in high-risk patients with cardiac disease.[170,171] Favourable outcomes have also been documented in case series using neuraxial anaesthesia for elective CD in high-risk patients,[172–174] despite recommendations to the contrary.[175]

One of these papers describes the management of ten pregnancies in nine women with pulmonary hypertension, all delivered by an elective CD, using an epidural or a CSE technique with perioperative CO monitoring, including admission to a critical care unit postpartum. This paper highlights the importance of antepartum treatment, an early elective CD using neuraxial anaesthesia, and postoperative monitoring in a critical care unit.[173] Another survey from the United Kingdom described continuous spinal anaesthesia in 34 women with congenital or acquired cardiac disease. Patients had continuous invasive arterial monitoring. Using a mean dose of spinal bupivacaine of approximately 10 mg, the mean dose of phenylephrine required was 550 mcg, and 18% had transient symptomatic hypotension with no adverse effects.[172] A third survey from Norway reported favourable outcomes in moderate- and high-risk patients receiving SA or CSE, with spinal bupivacaine doses of 8–10 mg (combined with opioids).[174] One patient with severe peripartum cardiomyopathy (ejection fraction 15%, HR 150) had continuous spinal anaesthesia. The anaesthesia was well tolerated by all patients. The patients were monitored with continuous arterial blood pressure and pulse waveform-derived CO. Haemodynamic changes were prevented and treated with carefully titrated phenylephrine infusion and boluses.

Anaesthetists should understand both the cardiovascular pathophysiology and potential risks of neuraxial anaesthesia in the individual patient. A favourable outcome is dependent upon careful haemodynamic monitoring and close control of fluid balance. Patients with high risk for morbidity and mortality during pregnancy are those with Eisenmenger's syndrome, pulmonary hypertension, severe aortic and mitral stenosis, hypertrophic obstructive cardiomyopathy (HOCM), and poor ventricular function with New York Heart Association (NYHA) functional class greater than II independent of underlying cause.[176]

The same principles as described above in healthy patients can be applied in cardiac compromised women. These are the avoidance of aortocaval compression, the use of judicious doses and volumes of combinations of spinal local anaesthetic and opioids, co-loading, and the use of phenylephrine to counteract the initial vasodilatation and avoid tachycardia. A focus on the maternal circulation, both in terms of pressure *and* flow is mandatory in high-risk patients.[177]

In summary:

- Pregnant women with cardiac disease should be managed by a dedicated multidisciplinary team, and high-risk patients should have a planned elective delivery during daytime hours in a tertiary centre with specialized expertise in the peripartum management of these patients.
- A suggested approach to prevent haemodynamic instability and tachycardia during neuraxial anaesthesia in pregnant women with moderate and high-risk cardiac disease, is as follows:
  - Position: cardiac compromised pregnant women are more vulnerable to aortocaval compression and must be placed in left lateral tilt.
  - Monitoring: an arterial line is mandatory to detect rapid haemodynamic changes, and minimally invasive CO-monitoring is recommended. A pulmonary artery catheter may be indicated postoperatively in women with severe pulmonary hypertension in need of controlled ventilation.
  - Titrated anaesthesia:
    - Single-shot spinal, CSE, epidural, or continuous spinal anaesthesia should be chosen according to the specific lesion and NYHA classification. NYHA class III–IV patients with severe ventricular failure are especially vulnerable to rapid haemodynamic changes and tachycardia, and continuous spinal anaesthesia is recommended with small titrated doses of IV phenylephrine to counteract vasodilatation. In cases with moderate/severe mitral or aortic stenosis or HOCM, single-shot spinal (or CSE) anaesthesia may be tolerated, with co-load and initial more aggressive use of phenylephrine to compensate for the SA-induced induced vasodilatation.
    - General anaesthesia still has a significant role to play, especially in complex urgent or emergency cases.
  - Small titrated doses of oxytocin (0.1 IU) should be used, to avoid haemodynamic instability.
  - Postoperative monitoring is crucial to ensure a negative fluid balance during the first 72 hours after delivery.

Conclusion

An improved understanding of maternal physiology, and of the haemodynamic changes associated with SA for CD, has made single-shot SA a safer and more comfortable experience for millions of mothers.

Key recommendations are as follows:

- Appropriate case selection (SA contraindicated in hypovolaemia).
- Left lateral tilt greater than 15°.
- Reducing the dose of spinal local anaesthetic reduces the incidence and severity of hypotension. However, the primary consideration is adequate maternal anaesthesia, and the dose of a single-shot spinal local anaesthetic should be not less than 10 mg bupivacaine alone or 8 mg with opioid. It can be reduced if CSE anaesthesia is used. There is no convincing evidence that the dose should be reduced in obese patients.

- Combination of crystalloid co-load 20 mL/kg (or occasionally colloid preload), and phenylephrine to prevent hypotension.
- The appropriate use of vasopressors and/or anticholinergics (see 'Vasopressor use').
- Co-morbidities:
  - In pre-eclampsia, single-shot SA is recommended, using at least as high a dose as employed in healthy term patients, if there is no epidural catheter in place.
  - CSE, and to a limited extent continuous spinal anaesthesia, appear to have a significant role to play in the management of CD in patients with cardiac disease.

Prevention is better than cure, but should spinal hypotension occur, rapid intervention is essential, based upon the exact clinical scenario and individual haemodynamic response. Thus future research in healthy patients should include the prediction and prevention of patients at risk of hypotension; for example, the development of a simple test of sympathovagal balance would be useful. In addition, for research purposes, haemodynamic monitoring during CD should be continuous—either minimally invasive, which allows for CO monitoring, or non-invasive, in which case beat-by-beat blood pressure can be measured. This would inform clinicians as to how to reduce the incidence and severity of hypotension.

The incidence of obesity is increasing in the pregnant population, and more work is required on the haemodynamic effects of SA and the correct doses of spinal local anaesthetic in women with a high body mass index. In patients with cardiac disease, the increasing sophistication of transthoracic echocardiography allows for more accurate preoperative diagnosis, which can be followed by the intraoperative use of minimally invasive monitors and reduction of spinal hypotension by careful titration of vasopressors. Further echocardiographic investigation of the haemodynamics of patients with complicated severe pre-eclampsia could identify patients with both diastolic and systolic dysfunction, and who are therefore at high risk of spinal hypotension.

References

1. Cleland JG. Paravertebral anaesthesia in obstetrics: experimental and clinical basis. *Surg Gynecol Obstet* 1933; 57:51–62.
2. Gogarten W. Spinal anaesthesia for obstetrics. *Best Pract Res Clin Anaesthesiol* 2003; 17(3):377–92.
3. Marx G. Aortocaval compression syndrome: its 50-year history. *Int J Obstet Anesth* 1992; 1:60–4.
4. Hart JR, Whitacre RG. Pencil-point needle in prevention of post spinal headache. *JAMA* 1951; 147:657–8.
5. McKeen DM, George RB, O'Connell CM, *et al.* Difficult and failed intubation: Incident rates and maternal, obstetrical, and anesthetic predictors. *Can J Anaesth* 2011; 58(6):514–24.
6. Hawthorne L, Wilson R, Lyons G, *et al.* Failed intubation revisited: 17-yr experience in a teaching maternity unit. *Br J Anaesth* 1996; 76(5):680–4.
7. Cooper GM, McClure JH. Maternal deaths from anaesthesia. An extract from Why Mothers Die 2000-2002, the Confidential Enquiries into Maternal Deaths in the United Kingdom: Chapter 9: A naesthesia. *Br J Anaesth* 2005; 94(4):417–23.
8. Cooper GM, McClure JH. Anaesthesia chapter from Saving mothers' lives; reviewing maternal deaths to make pregnancy safer. *Br J Anaesth* 2008; 100(1):17–22.
9. Hawkins JL, Koonin LM, Palmer SK, *et al.* Anesthesia-related deaths during obstetric delivery in the United States, 1979–1990. *Anesthesiology* 1997; 86(2):277–84.
10. Hawkins JL, Chang J, Palmer SK, *et al.* Anesthesia-related maternal mortality in the United States: 1979–2002. *Obstet Gynecol* 2011; 117(1):69–74.
11. Centre for Maternal and Child Enquiries (CMACE). Saving Mothers' Lives: reviewing maternal deaths to make motherhood safer: 2006–08. The Eighth Report on Confidential Enquiries into Maternal Deaths in the United Kingdom. *BJOG* 2011; 118 Suppl 1:1–203.
12. Rout CC, Farina Z. Anaesthesia-related maternal deaths in South Africa. *South Afr J Anaesth Analg* 2012; 18:279–301.
13. Gelman S. Venous function and central venous pressure: a physiologic story. *Anesthesiology* 2008; 108(4):735–48.
14. Klohr S, Roth R, Hofmann T, *et al.* Definitions of hypotension after spinal anaesthesia for caesarean section: literature search and application to parturients. *Acta Anaesthesiol Scand* 2010; 54(8):909–21.
15. Dahlgren G, Granath F, Wessel H, *et al.* Prediction of hypotension during spinal anesthesia for Cesarean section and its relation to the effect of crystalloid or colloid preload. *Int J Obstet Anesth* 2007; 16(2):128–34.
16. Jeon Y, Hwang J, Kim M, *et al.* Positional blood pressure change and the risk of hypotension during spinal anesthesia for cesarean delivery: an observational study. *Anesth Analg* 2010; 111:712–15.
17. Frolich MA, Caton D. Baseline heart rate may predict hypotension after spinal anesthesia in prehydrated obstetrical patients. *Can J Anaesth* 2002; 49(2):185–9.
18. Hanss R, Bein B, Ledowski T, *et al.* Heart rate variability predicts severe hypotension after spinal anesthesia for elective cesarean delivery. *Anesthesiology* 2005; 102(6):1086–93.
19. Hanss R, Bein B, Francksen H, *et al.* Heart rate variability-guided prophylactic treatment of severe hypotension after subarachnoid block for elective cesarean delivery. *Anesthesiology* 2006; 104(4):635–43.
20. Chamchad D, Arkoosh VA, Horrow JC, *et al.* Using heart rate variability to stratify risk of obstetric patients undergoing spinal anesthesia. *Anesth Analg* 2004; 99(6):1818–21.
21. Armstrong S, Fernando R, Columb M. Minimally- and non-invasive assessment of maternal cardiac output: go with the flow! *Int J Obstet Anesth* 2011; 20(4):330–40.
22. Dyer RA, James M. Hemodynamic monitoring in obstetric anesthesia. *Anesthesiology* 2008; 109(5):765–7.
23. Reynolds F, Seed PT. Anaesthesia for Caesarean section and neonatal acid-base status: a meta-analysis. *Anaesthesia* 2005; 60(7):636–53.
24. Kinsella SM, Lohmann G. Supine hypotensive syndrome. *Obstet Gynecol* 1994; 83(5 Pt 1):774–88.
25. Holmes F. The supine hypotensive syndrome. Its importance to the anaesthetist. *Anaesthesia* 1960; 15:298–306.
26. Marx GF, Husain FJ, Shiau HF. Brachial and femoral blood pressures during the prenatal period. *Am J Obstet Gynecol* 1980; 136(1):11–13.
27. Reed NE, Teteris NJ, Essig GF. Inferior vena caval obstruction syndrome with electrocardiographically documented fetal bradycardia. Report of a case. *Obstet Gynecol* 1970; 36(3):462–4.
28. Ueland K, Gills RE, Hansen JM. Maternal cardiovascular dynamics. I. Cesarean section under subarachnoid block anesthesia. *Am J Obstet Gynecol* 1968; 100(1):42–54.
29. Ansari I, Wallace G, Clemetson CA, *et al.* Tilt caesarean section. *J Obstet Gynaecol Br Commonw* 1970; 77(8):713–21.
30. Lee SW, Khaw KS, Ngan Kee WD, *et al.* Haemodynamic effects from aortocaval compression at different angles of lateral tilt in non-labouring term pregnant women. *Br J Anaesth* 2012; 109(6):950–6.
31. Kinsella SM, Whitwam JG, Spencer JA. Reducing aortocaval compression: how much tilt is enough? *BMJ* 1992; 305(6853):539–40.
32. Stoneham MD, Eldridge J, Popat M, *et al.* Oxford positioning technique improves haemodynamic stability and predictability of block

height of spinal anaesthesia for elective caesarean section. *Int J Obstet Anesth* 1999; 8(4):242–8.
33. Kundra P, Velraj J, Amirthalingam U, *et al.* Effect of positioning from supine and left lateral positions to left lateral tilt on maternal blood flow velocities and waveforms in full-term parturients. *Anaesthesia* 2012; 67(8):889–93.
34. Ngan Kee WD, Khaw KS, Ng FF, *et al.* A prospective comparison of vasopressor requirement and hemodynamic changes during spinal anesthesia for cesarean delivery in patients with multiple gestation versus singleton pregnancy. *Anesth Analg* 2007; 104(2):407–11.
35. Marx GF, Patel S, Berman JA, *et al.* Umbilical blood flow velocity waveforms in different maternal positions and with epidural analgesia. *Obstet Gynecol* 1986; 68(1):61–4.
36. Robson SC, Boys RJ, Rodeck C, *et al.* Maternal and fetal haemodynamic effects of spinal and extradural anaesthesia for elective caesarean section. *Br J Anaesth* 1992; 68(1):54–9.
37. Langesaeter E, Rosseland LA, Stubhaug A. Continuous invasive blood pressure and cardiac output monitoring during cesarean delivery: a randomized, double-blind comparison of low-dose versus high-dose spinal anesthesia with intravenous phenylephrine or placebo infusion. *Anesthesiology* 2008; 109(5):856–63.
38. Dyer RA, Reed AR, van Dyk D, *et al.* Hemodynamic effects of ephedrine, phenylephrine, and the coadministration of phenylephrine with oxytocin during spinal anesthesia for elective cesarean delivery. *Anesthesiology* 2009; 111(4):753–65.
39. Introna R, Yodlowski E, Pruett J, *et al.* Sympathovagal effects of spinal anesthesia assessed by heart rate variability analysis. *Anesth Analg* 1995; 80(2):315–21.
40. Shen CL, Ho YY, Hung YC, *et al.* Arrhythmias during spinal anesthesia for Cesarean section. *Can J Anaesth* 2000; 47(5):393–7.
41. Caplan RA, Ward RJ, Posner K, *et al.* Unexpected cardiac arrest during spinal anesthesia: a closed claims analysis of predisposing factors. *Anesthesiology* 1988; 68(1):5–11.
42. Mhyre JM, Riesner MN, Polley LS, *et al.* A series of anesthesia-related maternal deaths in Michigan, 1985–2003. *Anesthesiology* 2007; 106(6):1096–104.
43. Scull TJ, Carli F. Cardiac arrest after Caesarean section under subarachnoid block. *Br J Anaesth* 1996; 77(2):274–6.
44. Scott DB, Tunstall ME. Serious complications associated with epidural/spinal blockade in obstetrics: a two-year prospective study. *Int J Obstet Anesth* 1995; 4(3):133–9.
45. Stienstra R. Mechanisms behind and treatment of sudden, unexpected circulatory collapse during central neuraxis blockade. *Acta Anaesthesiol Scand* 2000; 44(8):965–71.
46. Pathak CL. Autoregulation of chronotropic response of the heart through pacemaker stretch. *Cardiology* 1973; 58(1):45–64.
47. Kinsella SM, Tuckey JP. Perioperative bradycardia and asystole: relationship to vasovagal syncope and the Bezold-Jarisch reflex. *Br J Anaesth* 2001; 86(6):859–68.
48. Sear JW. Role of cardiac reflexes in the control of heart rate: what does the anesthesiologist need to know? *Anesth Analg* 2012; 114(3):491–3.
49. Crystal GJ, Salem MR. The Bainbridge and the 'reverse' Bainbridge reflexes: history, physiology, and clinical relevance. *Anesth Analg* 2012; 114(3):520–32.
50. Campagna JA, Carter C. Clinical relevance of the Bezold-Jarisch reflex. *Anesthesiology* 2003; 98(5):1250–60.
51. Dyer RA, Reed AR, James MF. Obstetric anaesthesia in low-resource settings. *Best Pract Res Clin Obstet Gynaecol* 2010; 24(3):401–12.
52. Dyer RA, Rout CC, Kruger AM, *et al.* Prevention and treatment of cardiovascular instability during spinal anaesthesia for caesarean section. *S Afr Med J* 2004; 94(5):367–72.
53. Kelly MC, Fitzpatrick KT, Hill DA. Respiratory effects of spinal anaesthesia for caesarean section. *Anaesthesia* 1996; 51(12):1120–2.
54. Ungern-Sternberg BS, Regli A, Bucher E, *et al.* Impact of spinal anaesthesia and obesity on maternal respiratory function during elective Caesarean section. *Anaesthesia* 2004; 59(8):743–9.
55. Sharwood-Smith G, Drummond GB. Hypotension in obstetric spinal anaesthesia: a lesson from pre-eclampsia. *Br J Anaesth* 2009; 102(3):291–4.
56. Hallworth SP, Fernando R, Columb MO, *et al.* The effect of posture and baricity on the spread of intrathecal bupivacaine for elective cesarean delivery. *Anesth Analg* 2005; 100(4):1159–65.
57. Bogod D. Medico-legal implications. In Reynolds F (ed) *Regional Anaesthesia in Obstetrics: A Millennium Update.* London: Springer Verlag; 2000:375–7.
58. Kiran S, Singal NK. A comparative study of three different doses of 0.5% hyperbaric bupivacaine for spinal anaesthesia in elective caesarean section. *Int J Obstet Anesth* 2002; 11(3):185–9.
59. Bray JK, Fernando R, Patel NP, *et al.* Suprasternal Doppler estimation of cardiac output: standard versus sequential combined spinal epidural anesthesia for cesarean delivery. *Anesth Analg* 2006; 103(4):959–64.
60. Ben David B, Miller G, Gavriel R, *et al.* Low-dose bupivacaine-fentanyl spinal anesthesia for cesarean delivery. *Reg Anesth Pain Med* 2000; 25(3):235–9.
61. Choi DH, Ahn HJ, Kim MH. Bupivacaine-sparing effect of fentanyl in spinal anesthesia for cesarean delivery. *Reg Anesth Pain Med* 2000; 25(3):240–5.
62. Vercauteren MP, Coppejans HC, Hoffmann VL, *et al.* Small-dose hyperbaric versus plain bupivacaine during spinal anesthesia for cesarean section. *Anesth Analg* 1998; 86(5):989–93.
63. Ithnin F, Lim Y, Sia AT, *et al.* Combined spinal epidural causes higher level of block than equivalent single-shot spinal anesthesia in elective cesarean patients. *Anesth Analg* 2006; 102(2):577–80.
64. Ginosar Y, Mirikatani E, Drover DR *et al.* ED50 and ED95 of intrathecal hyperbaric bupivacaine coadministered with opioids for cesarean delivery. *Anesthesiology* 2004; 100:676–82.
65. Arzola C, Wieczorek PM. Efficacy of low-dose bupivacaine in spinal anaesthesia for Caesarean delivery: systematic review and meta-analysis. *Br J Anaesth* 2011; 107(3):308–18.
66. Carvalho B, Collins J, Drover DR, *et al.* ED(50) and ED(95) of intrathecal bupivacaine in morbidly obese patients undergoing cesarean delivery. *Anesthesiology* 2011; 114(3):529–35.
67. Lee Y, Balki M, Parkes R, *et al.* Dose requirement of intrathecal bupivacaine for cesarean delivery is similar in obese and normal weight women. *Rev Bras Anestesiol* 2009; 59(6):674–83.
68. Roofthooft E, Van de Velde M. Low-dose spinal anaesthesia for Caesarean section to prevent spinal-induced hypotension. *Curr Opin Anaesthesiol* 2008; 21(3):259–62
69. Dyer RA, Joubert IA. Low-dose spinal anaesthesia for caesarean section. *Curr Opin Anaesthesiol* 2004; 17(4):301–8.
70. Greiss FC, Crandell DL. Therapy for hypotension induced by spinal anesthesia during pregnancy: observations on gravid ewes. *JAMA* 1965; 191:793–6.
71. Marx GF, Cosmi EV, Wollman SB. Biochemical status and clinical condition of mother and infant at cesarean section. *Anesth Analg* 1969; 48(6):986–94.
72. Wollman SB, Marx GF. Acute hydration for prevention of hypotension of spinal anesthesia in parturients. *Anesthesiology* 1968; 29(2):374–80.
73. Clark RB. Hypotension and Caesarean section. *Br J Anaesth* 2008; 101(6):882–3.
74. Morgan PJ, Halpern SH, Tarshis J. The effects of an increase of central blood volume before spinal anesthesia for cesarean delivery: a qualitative systematic review. *Anesth Analg* 2001; 92(4):997–1005.
75. Clark RB, Thompson DS, Thompson CH. Prevention of spinal hypotension associated with Cesarean section. *Anesthesiology* 1976; 45(6):670–4.
76. Rout CC, Rocke DA, Levin J, *et al.* A reevaluation of the role of crystalloid preload in the prevention of hypotension associated with spinal anesthesia for elective cesarean section. *Anesthesiology* 1993; 79(2):262–9.

77. French GW, White JB, Howell SJ, *et al.* Comparison of pentastarch and Hartmann's solution for volume preloading in spinal anaesthesia for elective caesarean section. *Br J Anaesth* 1999; 83(3):475–7.
78. Lin CS, Lin TY, Huang CH, *et al.* Prevention of hypotension after spinal anesthesia for cesarean section: dextran 40 versus lactated Ringer's solution. *Acta Anaesthesiol Sin* 1999; 37(2):55–9.
79. Mathru M, Rao TL, Kartha RK, *et al.* Intravenous albumin administration for prevention of spinal hypotension during cesarean section. *Anesth Analg* 1980; 59(9):655–8.
80. Riley ET, Cohen SE, Rubenstein AJ, *et al.* Prevention of hypotension after spinal anesthesia for cesarean section: six percent hetastarch versus lactated Ringer's solution. *Anesth Analg* 1995; 81(4):838–42.
81. Ueyama H, He YL, Tanigami H, *et al.* Effects of crystalloid and colloid preload on blood volume in the parturient undergoing spinal anesthesia for elective Cesarean section. *Anesthesiology* 1999; 91(6):1571–6.
82. Rout CC, Rocke DA, Gouws E. Leg elevation and wrapping in the prevention of hypotension following spinal anaesthesia for elective caesarean section. *Anaesthesia* 1993; 48(4):304–8.
83. Cyna AM, Andrew M, Emmett RS, *et al.* Techniques for preventing hypotension during spinal anaesthesia for caesarean section. *Cochrane Database Syst Rev* 2006; 4:CD002251.
84. Rout CC, Akoojee SS, Rocke DA, *et al.* Rapid administration of crystalloid preload does not decrease the incidence of hypotension after spinal anaesthesia for elective caesarean section. *Br J Anaesth* 1992; 68(4):394–7.
85. Kamenik M, Paver-Erzen V. The effects of lactated Ringer's solution infusion on cardiac output changes after spinal anesthesia. *Anesth Analg* 2001; 92(3):710–14.
86. Ewaldsson CA, Hahn RG. Kinetics and extravascular retention of acetated ringer's solution during isoflurane or propofol anesthesia for thyroid surgery. *Anesthesiology* 2005; 103(3):460–9.
87. Dyer RA, Farina Z, Joubert IA, *et al.* Crystalloid preload versus rapid crystalloid administration after induction of spinal anaesthesia (coload) for elective caesarean section. *Anaesth Intensive Care* 2004; 32(3):351–7.
88. Ngan Kee WD, Khaw KS, Ng FF. Prevention of hypotension during spinal anesthesia for cesarean delivery: an effective technique using combination phenylephrine infusion and crystalloid cohydration. *Anesthesiology* 2005; 103(4):744–50.
89. Davies P, French GW. A randomised trial comparing 5 mL/kg and 10 mL/kg of pentastarch as a volume preload before spinal anaesthesia for elective caesarean section. *Int J Obstet Anesth* 2006; 15(4):279–83.
90. Nishikawa K, Yokoyama N, Saito S, *et al.* Comparison of effects of rapid colloid loading before and after spinal anesthesia on maternal hemodynamics and neonatal outcomes in cesarean section. *J Clin Monit Comput* 2007; 21(2):125–9.
91. Carvalho B, Mercier FJ, Riley ET, *et al.* Hetastarch co-loading is as effective as pre-loading for the prevention of hypotension following spinal anesthesia for cesarean delivery. *Int J Obstet Anesth* 2009; 18(2):150–5.
92. McDonald S, Fernando R, Ashpole K, *et al.* Maternal cardiac output changes after crystalloid or colloid coload following spinal anesthesia for elective cesarean delivery: a randomized controlled trial. *Anesth Analg* 2011; 113(4):803–10.
93. Loubert C. Fluid and vasopressor management for Cesarean delivery under spinal anesthesia: continuing professional development. *Can J Anesth* 2012; 59(6):604–19.
94. Tamilselvan P, Fernando R, Bray J, *et al.* The effects of crystalloid and colloid preload on cardiac output in the parturient undergoing planned cesarean delivery under spinal anesthesia: a randomized trial. *Anesth Analg* 2009; 109(6):1916–21.
95. Teoh WH, Sia AT. Colloid preload versus coload for spinal anesthesia for cesarean delivery: the effects on maternal cardiac output. *Anesth Analg* 2009; 108(5):1592–8.
96. Mercier FJ. Fluid loading for cesarean delivery under spinal anesthesia: have we studied all the options? *Anesth Analg* 2011; 113(4):677–80.
97. Mercier FJ. Cesarean delivery fluid management. *Curr Opin Anaesthesiol* 2012; 25(3):286–91.
98. Banerjee A, Stocche RM, Angle P, *et al.* Preload or coload for spinal anesthesia for elective Cesarean delivery: a meta-analysis. *Can J Anaesth* 2010; 57(1):24–31.
99. Macarthur A, Riley ET. Obstetric anesthesia controversies: vasopressor choice for postspinal hypotension during cesarean delivery. *Int Anesthesiol Clin* 2007; 45(1):115–32.
100. Rout CC, Rocke DA, Brijball R, *et al.* Prophylactic intramuscular ephedrine prior to caesarean section. *Anaesth Intensive Care* 1992; 20(4):448–52.
101. Ayorinde BT, Buczkowski P, Brown J, *et al.* Evaluation of pre-emptive intramuscular phenylephrine and ephedrine for reduction of spinal anaesthesia-induced hypotension during Caesarean section. *Br J Anaesth* 2001; 86(3):372–6.
102. Kobayashi S, Endou M, Sakuraya F, *et al.* The sympathomimetic actions of l-ephedrine and d-pseudoephedrine: direct receptor activation or norepinephrine release? *Anesth Analg* 2003; 97(5):1239–45.
103. Liles JT, Dabisch PA, Hude KE, *et al.* Pressor responses to ephedrine are mediated by a direct mechanism in the rat. *J Pharmacol Exp Ther* 2006; 316(1):95–105.
104. Tong C, Eisenach JC. The vascular mechanism of ephedrine's beneficial effect on uterine perfusion during pregnancy. *Anesthesiology* 1992; 76(5):792–8.
105. Li P, Tong C, Eisenach JC. Pregnancy and ephedrine increase the release of nitric oxide in ovine uterine arteries. *Anesth Analg* 1996; 82(2):288–93.
106. Ngan Kee WD, Khaw KS, Lee BB, *et al.* A dose-response study of prophylactic intravenous ephedrine for the prevention of hypotension during spinal anesthesia for cesarean delivery. *Anesth Analg* 2000; 90(6):1390–5.
107. Persky AM, Berry NS, Pollack GM, *et al.* Modelling the cardiovascular effects of ephedrine. *Br J Clin Pharmacol* 2004; 57(5):552–62.
108. Ngan Kee WD, Khaw KS. Vasopressors in obstetrics: what should we be using? *Curr Opin Anaesthesiol* 2006; 19(3):238–43.
109. Cooper DW, Carpenter M, Mowbray P, *et al.* Fetal and maternal effects of phenylephrine and ephedrine during spinal anesthesia for cesarean delivery. *Anesthesiology* 2002; 97(6):1582–90.
110. Ralston DH, Shnider SM, DeLorimier AA. Effects of equipotent ephedrine, metaraminol, mephentermine, and methoxamine on uterine blood flow in the pregnant ewe. *Anesthesiology* 1974; 40(4):354–70.
111. Magness RR, Rosenfeld CR. Systemic and uterine responses to alpha-adrenergic stimulation in pregnant and nonpregnant ewes. *Am J Obstet Gynecol* 1986; 155(4):897–904.
112. LaPorta RF, Arthur GR, Datta S. Phenylephrine in treating maternal hypotension due to spinal anaesthesia for caesarean delivery: effects on neonatal catecholamine concentrations, acid base status and Apgar scores. *Acta Anaesthesiol Scand* 1995; 39(7):901–5.
113. Ngan Kee WD, Khaw KS, Tan PE, *et al.* Placental transfer and fetal metabolic effects of phenylephrine and ephedrine during spinal anesthesia for cesarean delivery. *Anesthesiology* 2009; 111(3):506–12.
114. Landau R, Liu SK, Blouin JL, *et al.* The effect of maternal and fetal beta2-adrenoceptor and nitric oxide synthase genotype on vasopressor requirement and fetal acid-base status during spinal anesthesia for cesarean delivery. *Anesth Analg* 2011; 112(6):1432–7.
115. Lee A, Ngan Kee WD, Gin T. A quantitative, systematic review of randomized controlled trials of ephedrine versus phenylephrine for the management of hypotension during spinal anesthesia for cesarean delivery. *Anesth Analg* 2002; 94(4):920–6.
116. Eisler G, Hjertberg R, Lagercrantz H. Randomised controlled trial of effect of terbutaline before elective caesarean section on postnatal respiration and glucose homeostasis. *Arch Dis Child Fetal Neonatal Ed* 1999; 80(2):F88–92.
117. Ngan Kee WD, Khaw KS, Lau TK, *et al.* Randomised double-blinded comparison of phenylephrine vs ephedrine

for maintaining blood pressure during spinal anaesthesia for non-elective Caesarean section. *Anaesthesia* 2008; 63(12):1319–26.
118. Habib AS. A review of the impact of phenylephrine administration on maternal hemodynamics and maternal and neonatal outcomes in women undergoing cesarean delivery under spinal anesthesia. *Anesth Analg* 2012; 114(2):377–90.
119. Thiele RH, Nemergut EC, Lynch C, III. The clinical implications of isolated alpha(1) adrenergic stimulation. *Anesth Analg* 2011; 113(2):297–304.
120. Saravanan S, Kocarev M, Wilson RC, *et al.* Equivalent dose of ephedrine and phenylephrine in the prevention of post-spinal hypotension in Caesarean section. *Br J Anaesth* 2006; 96(1):95–9.
121. Thomas DG, Gardner S. Comparison of time to peak pressor effect of phenylephrine and ephedrine during spinal anaesthesia for caesarean section. *Int J Obstet Anesth* 2004; 13(S1), O02.
122. Tanaka M, Balki M, Parkes RK, *et al.* ED95 of phenylephrine to prevent spinal-induced hypotension and/or nausea at elective cesarean delivery. *Int J Obstet Anesth* 2009; 18(2):125–30.
123. George RB, McKeen D, Chaplin AC, *et al.* Up-down determination of the ED(90) of oxytocin infusions for the prevention of postpartum uterine atony in parturients undergoing Cesarean delivery. *Can J Anaesth* 2010; 57(6):578–82.
124. Langesaeter E, Dyer RA. Maternal haemodynamic changes during spinal anaesthesia for caesarean section. *Curr Opin Anaesthesiol* 2011; 24(3):242–8.
125. Thomas DG, Robson SC, Redfern N, *et al.* Randomized trial of bolus phenylephrine or ephedrine for maintenance of arterial pressure during spinal anaesthesia for Caesarean section. *Br J Anaesth* 1996; 76(1):61–5.
126. Ashpole KJ, Tamilselvan P, Fernando R, *et al.* Maternal cardiac output changes occurring with phenylephrine and ephedrine infusions after spinal anaesthesia for caesarean section. *Anesthesiology* 2005; 102 Suppl 1:A5:744–50.
127. Stewart A, Fernando R, McDonald S, *et al.* The dose-dependent effects of phenylephrine for elective cesarean delivery under spinal anesthesia. *Anesth Analg* 2010; 111(5):1230–7.
128. Ngan Kee WD, Khaw KS, Ng FF, *et al.* Prophylactic phenylephrine infusion for preventing hypotension during spinal anesthesia for cesarean delivery. *Anesth Analg* 2004; 98(3):815–21.
129. Ngan Kee WD, Khaw KS, Ng FF. Comparison of phenylephrine infusion regimens for maintaining maternal blood pressure during spinal anaesthesia for Caesarean section. *Br J Anaesth* 2004; 92(4):469–74.
130. Ngan Kee WD, Tam YH, Khaw KS, *et al.* Closed-loop feedback computer-controlled infusion of phenylephrine for maintaining blood pressure during spinal anaesthesia for caesarean section: a preliminary descriptive study. *Anaesthesia* 2007; 62(12):1251–6.
131. Ngan Kee WD, Khaw KS, Ng FF, *et al.* Randomized comparison of closed-loop feedback computer-controlled with manual-controlled infusion of phenylephrine for maintaining arterial pressure during spinal anaesthesia for caesarean delivery. *Br J Anaesth* 2013; 110(1):59–65.
132. das Neves JF, Monteiro GA, de Almeida JR, *et al.* Phenylephrine for blood pressure control in elective cesarean section: therapeutic versus prophylactic doses. *Rev Bras Anestesiol* 2010; 60(4):391–8.
133. Allen TK, George RB, White WD, *et al.* A double-blind, placebo-controlled trial of four fixed rate infusion regimens of phenylephrine for hemodynamic support during spinal anesthesia for cesarean delivery. *Anesth Analg* 2010; 111(5):1221–9.
134. Mercier FJ, Riley ET, Frederickson WL, *et al.* Phenylephrine added to prophylactic ephedrine infusion during spinal anesthesia for elective cesarean section. *Anesthesiology* 2001; 95(3):668–74.
135. Ngan Kee WD, Lee A, Khaw KS, *et al.* A randomized double-blinded comparison of phenylephrine and ephedrine infusion combinations to maintain blood pressure during spinal anesthesia for cesarean delivery: the effects on fetal acid-base status and hemodynamic control. *Anesth Analg* 2008; 107(4):1295–302.
136. Cooper DW. Caesarean delivery vasopressor management. *Curr Opin Anaesthesiol* 2012; 25(3):300–8.
137. Newell CP, Seller C, Vizhi M, *et al.* Case report: spontaneous coronary artery dissection during elective caesarean section under spinal anaesthesia. *Anaesthesia* 2011; 66(7):615–19.
138. Zdanowicz JA, Utz AC, Bernasconi I, *et al.* 'Broken heart' after cesarean delivery. Case report and review of literature. *Arch Gynecol Obstet* 2011; 283(4):687–94.
139. Ngan Kee WD, Lee SW, Khaw KS, *et al.* Haemodynamic effects of glycopyrrolate pre-treatment before phenylephrine infusion during spinal anaesthesia for caesarean delivery. *Int J Obstet Anesth* 2013; 22(3):179–87.
140. Yentis SM, Jenkins CS, Lucas DN, *et al.* The effect of prophylactic glycopyrrolate on maternal haemodynamics following spinal anaesthesia for elective caesarean section. *Int J Obstet Anesth* 2000; 9(3):156–9.
141. Allen TK, Muir HA, George RB, *et al.* A survey of the management of spinal-induced hypotension for scheduled cesarean delivery. *Int J Obstet Anesth* 2009; 18(4):356–61.
142. Smiley RM. Burden of proof. *Anesthesiology* 2009; 111(3):470–2.
143. Young P, Johanson R. Haemodynamic, invasive and echocardiographic monitoring in the hypertensive parturient. *Best Pract Res Clin Obstet Gynaecol* 2001; 15(4):605–22.
144. Newsome LR, Bramwell RS, Curling PE. Severe preeclampsia: hemodynamic effects of lumbar epidural anesthesia. *Anesth Analg* 1986; 65(1):31–6.
145. Wallace DH, Leveno KJ, Cunningham FG, *et al.* Randomized comparison of general and regional anesthesia for cesarean delivery in pregnancies complicated by severe preeclampsia. *Obstet Gynecol* 1995; 86(2):193–9.
146. Hood DD, Curry R. Spinal versus epidural anesthesia for cesarean section in severely preeclamptic patients: a retrospective survey. *Anesthesiology* 1999; 90(5):1276–82.
147. Santos AC. Spinal anesthesia in severely preeclamptic women: when is it safe? *Anesthesiology* 1999; 90(5):1252–4.
148. Howell P. Spinal anesthesia in severe preeclampsia: Time for reappraisal or time for caution? *Int J Obstet Anesth* 2001; 7:217–19.
149. Visalyaputra S, Rodanant O, Somboonviboon W, *et al.* Spinal versus epidural anesthesia for cesarean delivery in severe preeclampsia: a prospective randomized, multicenter study. *Anesth Analg* 2005; 101(3):862–8.
150. Assali NS, Prystowsky H. Studies on autonomic blockade. II. Observations on the nature of blood pressure fall with high selective spinal anesthesia in pregnant women. *J Clin Invest* 1950; 29(10):1367–75.
151. Assali NS, Prystowsky H. Studies on autonomic blockade. I. Comparison between the effects of tetraethylammonium chloride (TEAC) and high selective spinal anesthesia on blood pressure of normal and toxemic pregnancy. *J Clin Invest* 1950; 29(10):1354–66.
152. Aya AG, Mangin R, Vialles N, *et al.* Patients with severe preeclampsia experience less hypotension during spinal anesthesia for elective cesarean delivery than healthy parturients: a prospective cohort comparison. *Anesth Analg* 2003; 97(3):867–72.
153. Aya AG, Vialles N, Tanoubi I, *et al.* Spinal anesthesia-induced hypotension: a risk comparison between patients with severe preeclampsia and healthy women undergoing preterm cesarean delivery. *Anesth Analg* 2005; 101(3):869–75.
154. Clark VA, Sharwood-Smith GH, Stewart AV. Ephedrine requirements are reduced during spinal anaesthesia for caesarean section in preeclampsia. *Int J Obstet Anesth* 2005; 14(1):9–13.
155. Sharwood-Smith G, Clark V, Watson E. Regional anesthesia for cesarean section in severe preeclampsia. *Int J Obstet Anesth* 1999; 8:85–9.
156. Karinen J, Rasanen J, Alahuhta S, *et al.* Maternal and uteroplacental haemodynamic state in pre-eclamptic patients during spinal anaesthesia for Caesarean section. *Br J Anaesth* 1996; 76(5):616–20.

157. Pouta A, Karinen J, Vuolteenaho O, *et al.* Pre-eclampsia: the effect of intravenous fluid preload on atrial natriuretic peptide secretion during caesarean section under spinal anaesthesia. *Acta Anaesthesiol Scand* 1996; 40(10):1203–9.
158. Tihtonen K, Koobi T, Yli-Hankala A, *et al.* Maternal haemodynamics in pre-eclampsia compared with normal pregnancy during caesarean delivery. *BJOG* 2006; 113(6):657–63.
159. Dyer RA, Piercy JL, Reed AR, *et al.* Hemodynamic changes associated with spinal anesthesia for cesarean delivery in severe preeclampsia. *Anesthesiology* 2008; 108(5):802–11.
160. Dennis AT. Transthoracic echocardiography in obstetric anaesthesia and obstetric critical illness. *Int J Obstet Anesth* 2011; 20(2):160–8.
161. Dennis AT, Castro J, Carr C, *et al.* Haemodynamics in women with untreated pre-eclampsia. *Anaesthesia* 2012; 67(10):1105–18.
162. Visser W, Wallenburg HC. Central hemodynamic observations in untreated preeclamptic patients. *Hypertension* 1991; 17(6 Pt 2):1072–7.
163. Melchiorre K, Thilaganathan B. Maternal cardiac function in preeclampsia. *Curr Opin Obstet Gynecol* 2011; 23(6):440–7.
164. Melchiorre K, Sutherland GR, Watt-Coote I, *et al.* Severe myocardial impairment and chamber dysfunction in preterm preeclampsia. *Hypertens Pregnancy* 2012; 31(4):454–71.
165. Valensise H, Vasapollo B, Gagliardi G, *et al.* Early and late preeclampsia: two different maternal hemodynamic states in the latent phase of the disease. *Hypertension* 2008; 52(5):873–80.
166. Chaiworapongsa T, Espinoza J, Gotsch F, *et al.* The maternal plasma soluble vascular endothelial growth factor receptor-1 concentration is elevated in SGA and the magnitude of the increase relates to Doppler abnormalities in the maternal and fetal circulation. *J Matern Fetal Neonatal Med* 2008; 21(1):25–40.
167. Romero R, Nien JK, Espinoza J, *et al.* A longitudinal study of angiogenic (placental growth factor) and anti-angiogenic (soluble endoglin and soluble vascular endothelial growth factor receptor-1) factors in normal pregnancy and patients destined to develop preeclampsia and deliver a small for gestational age neonate. *J Matern Fetal Neonatal Med* 2008; 21(1):9–23.
168. Patten IS, Rana S, Shahul S, *et al.* Cardiac angiogenic imbalance leads to peripartum cardiomyopathy. *Nature* 2012; 485(7398):333–8.
169. Fernandes SM, Arendt KW, Landzberg MJ, *et al.* Pregnant women with congenital heart disease: cardiac, anesthetic and obstetrical implications. *Expert Rev Cardiovasc Ther* 2010; 8(3):439–48.
170. Hamlyn EL, Douglass CA, Plaat F, *et al.* Low-dose sequential combined spinal-epidural: an anaesthetic technique for caesarean section in patients with significant cardiac disease. *Int J Obstet Anesth* 2005; 14(4):355–61.
171. Pirlet M, Baird M, Pryn S, *et al.* Low dose combined spinal-epidural anaesthesia for caesarean section in a patient with peripartum cardiomyopathy. *Int J Obstet Anesth* 2000; 9(3):189–92.
172. Dresner M, Pinder A. Anaesthesia for caesarean section in women with complex cardiac disease: 34 cases using the Braun Spinocath spinal catheter. *Int J Obstet Anesth* 2009; 18(2):131–6.
173. Kiely DG, Condliffe R, Webster V, *et al.* Improved survival in pregnancy and pulmonary hypertension using a multiprofessional approach. *BJOG* 2010; 117(5):565–74.
174. Langesaeter E, Dragsund M, Rosseland LA. Regional anaesthesia for a Caesarean section in women with cardiac disease: a prospective study. *Acta Anaesthesiol Scand* 2010; 54(1):46–54.
175. Gomar C, Errando CL. Neuroaxial anaesthesia in obstetrical patients with cardiac disease. *Curr Opin Anaesthesiol* 2005; 18(5):507–12.
176. Siu SC, Sermer M, Colman JM, *et al.* Prospective multicenter study of pregnancy outcomes in women with heart disease. *Circulation* 2001; 104(5):515–21.
177. Armstrong S, Fernando R, Columb M. Minimally- and non-invasive assessment of maternal cardiac output: go with the flow! *Int J Obstet Anesth* 2011; 20(4):330–40.

CHAPTER 24

Postoperative analgesia after caesarean delivery

Sarah L. Armstrong and Gary M. Stocks

Introduction

In 1985, the World Health Organization stated that there was no justification for any region to have caesarean delivery (CD) rates higher than 10–15%, but it is recognized that in many countries around the world CD rates continue to escalate.[1] It is estimated that 18.5 million CDs are performed yearly worldwide with some South American countries reporting CD rates as high as 45% and many countries in Europe quoting rates of between 20% and 30%.[2] Postoperative pain after CD is therefore a problem affecting many millions of women each year.

Providing good quality postoperative analgesia is important not only for humanitarian reasons. It is well documented that effective pain relief after any type of surgery leads to earlier mobilization, fewer pulmonary and cardiac complications, a reduced risk of deep vein thrombosis, an earlier return of gastrointestinal function, and faster recovery.[3] Specifically for mothers after CD there are further benefits. Poor analgesia can impair the ability to look after the newborn infant and pain and/or anxiety can reduce effective breastfeeding. Furthermore inadequate treatment of acute pain can lead to chronic pain.[4] In a multicentre, prospective study of 1288 women hospitalized after CD or vaginal delivery, 10.9% experienced severe pain and women with severe acute postpartum pain had a 2.5-fold increased risk of persistent pain and a 3.0-fold increased risk of depression 8 weeks after delivery.[5]

Quite apart from the advantages of good pain relief for mothers we must increasingly respond to maternal demands and expectations. What do women think are the most important aspects of a good quality anaesthetic? Using written questionnaires Carvalho et al. asked patients to rank various anaesthetic outcomes and showed that pain during and after CD were the two most feared outcomes with minor side effects such as shivering and itching thought to be of only moderate concern.[6]

Both anaesthetists and patients therefore appreciate the importance of effective postoperative analgesia but there is evidence to suggest that provision of analgesia may not be as good as it could be. There are several ways to objectively measure pain intensity. One way is to use a visual analogue pain scale (VAPS) score, which is a unidimensional measure of pain intensity. When using a numerical VAPS score where 'no pain' is given a score of 0 and 'worst pain imaginable' scores 10, then by convention a VAPS score of greater than 3/10 is regarded as moderate to severe pain. Dolin et al. reviewed studies examining the incidence of pain (VAPS score > 3) after major surgery including CD and reported an incidence of 20.9% in patients with epidural analgesia, 35.8% for patient-controlled analgesia (PCA), and 67.2% for intramuscular (IM) analgesia.[7] Results from a US national survey suggest that a patient has a 50–71% chance of experiencing moderate to severe pain after surgery.[8] For CD there is little definitive evidence regarding achievable parameters in best practice.[9] Good practice guidelines from the United Kingdom have in the past suggested that over 90% of women after CD should have a worst pain score of less than 3/10,[10] but Wrench et al., using a multimodal analgesic approach for CD, reported that only 37.9% of their patients achieved a pain score of 3 or less and suggested, along with others, that this target was unachievable.[11] Subsequently the target for best practice has been revised, aspiring to 95% of women being 'satisfied' with analgesia the day after CD, but it would appear that there is still room for improvement.

A better understanding of the neurophysiology of pain transmission and pharmacology of analgesics has led to the realization that postoperative pain relief is best provided by using a variety of different analgesic techniques and drugs as part of a multimodal approach. This chapter will first look at the physiological basis for pain after CD before examining and evaluating the methods used for managing pain such as neuraxial, systemic, and regional techniques.

Pain pathways

Anatomy and physiology of pain transmission

In a healthy individual, pain is a complex sensory experience associated with actual or potential tissue damage. Noxious inputs stimulate the unspecialized, peripheral nociceptors which transmit signals to the dorsal horn of the spinal cord via small unmyelinated C fibres and medium A delta fibres[12] At the molecular level, pain stimulates the release of many mediators from keratinocytes and blood vessels in the dermis, including prostaglandins, substance P, and calcitonin gene-related peptide (CGRP) which depolarize nociceptive fibres and cause neurotransmitter release from the nerve itself into the periphery. This phenomenon, called axon reflex, causes vasodilation and inflammation. It results in a positive feedback loop that begins to recruit silent nociceptors and pain fibres in close proximity to the initially activated nerve.[12]

Pain fibres synapse with their secondary fibres at the superficial laminae (Rexed's I and II) of the dorsal horn where neuropeptides such as tachykinins (substance P and neurokinin A) and glutamate are released at the presynaptic level. Opioid receptors and their ligands are present on the superficial dorsal horn, particularly on Rexed's lamina II (substantia gelatinosa).

The current nomenclature (approved by the International Union of Pharmacology) for identification of the opioid receptors is that of MOP, KOP, DOP, and NOP receptors. Opioids have both presynaptic (indirect) and postsynaptic (direct) facilitatory and inhibitory actions on synaptic transmission in many regions of the nervous system via G-protein coupled receptors. These effector systems can be divided into two categories: short-term effectors involving potassium and calcium channels and longer-term effects involving second messengers such as cyclic adenosine monophosphate (cAMP). Spinal opioids exert their analgesic effects by reducing neurotransmitter release at the presynaptic level, and by hyperpolarizing the membrane of dorsal horn neurons at the postsynaptic level.[13]

Opioid receptor activation can inhibit the release of CGRP, glutamate, and substance P from nerves, thereby preventing the forward-feeding mechanism of pain that typically results in sensitization at the site of injury.[14] These injury-induced neuromodifications (which may include microglial cell activation) can be perceived as allodynia (pain due to a stimulus which does not normally provoke pain) or hyperalgesia (an increased response to a normally painful stimulus). Moreover, peripheral sensitization drives the repeated release of molecular mediators at the dorsal horn, causing secondary hyperalgesia.

Descending pathways from the somatosensory cortex also modulate the perception of pain. Opioids exerting their effect at the supraspinal level promote descending pain modulation by increasing the release of inhibitory gamma-aminobutyric acid (GABA) from the periaqueductal grey and rostral ventral medulla.[15] This opioid disinhibition activates descending inhibitory pathways and increases the concentrations of serotonin and norepinephrine at the presynaptic level thereby modulating pain signals at the spinal cord.

Pain pathways after caesarean delivery

Post-CD pain has both somatic and visceral components. Somatic pain arises from cutaneous and deep nociceptors within the abdominal wound which are transmitted within the anterior divisions of the spinal segmental nerves, usually T10–L1. These nerve fibres run laterally in the abdominal wall between the layers of the transversus abdominis and internal oblique muscles.[16] Visceral uterine nociceptive stimuli return via afferent nerve fibres that ascend through the inferior hypogastric plexus and enter the spinal cord via the T10–L1 spinal nerves.[17,18]

An ideal post-CD analgesic regimen would be one that is cost-effective and simple to implement providing high-quality pain relief despite wide interpatient variability with a low incidence of side effects and complications. This ideal regimen would not interfere with the maternal care of the newborn or breastfeeding, with minimal drug transfer into the breast milk. Achieving these goals requires a multimodal approach.[19,20]

Multimodal analgesia

An appreciation of the complexity of the neurophysiology of pain transmission and the numerous potential sites of action for analgesics to work has resulted in many different ways of providing analgesia after CD. Approaches can be divided into opioid-based techniques using intrathecal, epidural, or systemic routes with or without the use of adjuvant agents, wound infiltration, and nerve blocks and the use of oral analgesics such as paracetamol and non-steroidal anti-inflammatory drugs (NSAIDs). It is unlikely that utilization of one method alone will be effective and so the concept of multimodal analgesia is now well established in clinical practice. This is a technique intended to improve analgesia and to reduce the incidence of unpleasant opioid-related side effects. It is achieved by combining analgesics which work by different mechanisms and at different sites in the nervous system and results in an additive or even synergistic effect whilst at the same time reducing side effects (Figure 24.1). For CD, many of the techniques described in this chapter should be used as part of a multimodal approach to analgesia. A growing number of studies seem to support a multimodal approach for post-CD analgesia.[20] For example, NSAID medications combined with intravenous (IV) patient-controlled morphine administration may decrease nausea and sedation in patients when compared with those using patient-controlled morphine alone.[21] However, only NSAIDs (in combination with morphine) reduce pain intensity and the incidence of morphine-related side effects. Neither paracetamol nor the selective COX-2 inhibitors have been shown to affect the incidence of opioid-induced nausea, vomiting, or sedation when used in combination with these agents. Different classes of analgesics with different routes of administration (i.e. IV versus epidural methods) are used to produce fewer side effects such as sedation, nausea, vomiting, pruritus, and constipation, and also improve pain relief.

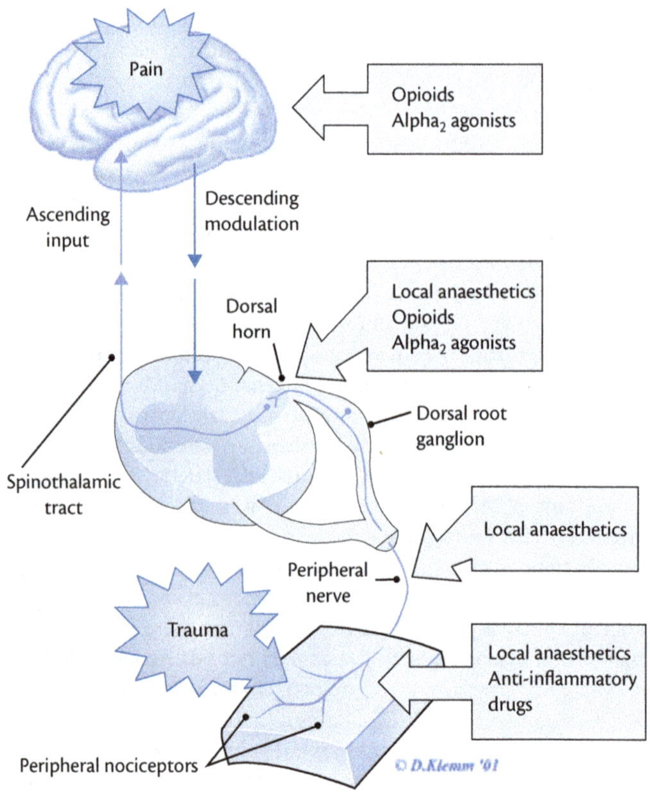

Figure 24.1 Multimodal analgesia.
Reproduced with permission from Henrik Kehlet and Jørgen Dahl. The Value of "Multimodal" or "Balanced Analgesia" in Postoperative Pain Treatment. *Anesthesia & Analgesia*, Volume 77, Issue 5, pp. 1048–1056, Copyright © 1993 Wolters Kluwer Health, Inc.

Neuraxial techniques for postoperative pain relief

Benefits

Most CDs are performed using spinal, epidural, or combined spinal–epidural (CSE) anaesthesia techniques. Data from the United Kingdom shows that neuraxial anaesthesia is used for 94.9% of elective and 86.7% of emergent CDs.[22] The safety benefits of neuraxial anaesthesia over general anaesthesia in the pregnant patient are well documented, and neuraxial opioid administration augments intraoperative anaesthesia and optimizes postoperative analgesia.[23,24]

In the non-obstetric population, the MASTER (Multicentre Australian Study of Epidural Anaesthesia and Analgesia in Major Surgery) trial was the largest prospective study to date comparing epidural and intravenous patient-controlled opioid analgesia (PCA) for postoperative analgesia. The study used random sampling to evaluate mortality and major morbidity outcomes in high-risk patients undergoing non-obstetric surgery.[25] Of the seven predefined major morbidity complications assessed in this study, respiratory failure was the only outcome with a lower incidence in the epidural infusion group than in the PCA group.

Administration of subarachnoid or epidural opioids to parturients, however, offers several advantages when recovering from CD. These include excellent postoperative analgesia with a decrease in total dose of opioid required, a low level of sedation, minimal accumulation of the drug in breast milk and facilitation of early ambulation. Neuraxial analgesic techniques appear more likely to reduce perioperative morbidity in high-risk obstetric patients than systemic analgesic techniques. The benefits include a lower rate of perioperative cardiovascular complications, a lowered incidence of pulmonary infections and pulmonary embolism, a faster return of gastrointestinal function, fewer coagulation disturbances, and reduction in inflammatory and stress responses to surgery.[26] Potency, onset, duration of action, and side effects vary depending on the opioid used and the route of its administration with pruritus, nausea, and vomiting being the most common side effects of these agents, resulting in a decrease in maternal satisfaction.

Pharmacology of neuraxial opioids

Neuraxial opioids have the advantage of producing analgesia without motor or sympathetic blockade. Opioids, especially diamorphine and preservative-free morphine, are central to many neuraxial post-CD analgesic regimens. They appear to act principally on MOP receptors in the substantia gelatinosa of the dorsal horn by suppressing the release of excitatory neuropeptides from C fibres.[27] Lipid solubility of the individual drug determines the degree of uptake from the cerebrospinal fluid (CSF) by the dorsal horn. Lipid soluble drugs like fentanyl or sufentanil have better direct diffusion into neural tissue as well as greater delivery to the dorsal horn by spinal segmental arteries. Highly soluble fentanyl, for instance, has a relatively rapid uptake into the lipid-rich dorsal horn and consequently has a rapid onset of action but a short duration. Studies that measure 24-hour opioid consumption confirm its limitations for adequate postoperative analgesia.[28] Conversely, lipid-insoluble opioids, such as morphine, are retained in the CSF, providing a longer supply to the spinal cord and consequently a slower onset, but longer duration of analgesia after the administration of a single dose.[29] As morphine resides for a longer period of time in the CSF it may spread rostrally, from which complications such as respiratory depression may arise.[30]

Lipophilicity, as assessed by octanol:buffer distribution coefficient, correlates with the meningeal permeability coefficient but in a non-linear fashion. After a drug is deposited in the epidural space but before it reaches the spinal cord, it must first cross a hydrophilic zone (extracellular and intracellular fluids) and then a hydrophobic zone (cell membrane lipids) of the arachnoid membrane.[29] Lipophilic drugs (i.e. those with high octanol:buffer partition coefficients, e.g. fentanyl and sufentanil) readily dissolve in the lipophilic component of arachnoid mater and can cross the region easily. Conversely, they penetrate the hydrophilic zone with difficulty creating the rate-limiting factor in their diffusion through the arachnoid membrane. Drugs with intermediate lipophilicity move more readily between the lipid and the aqueous zones, and their meningeal permeability coefficients are correspondingly greater (e.g. alfentanil, hydromorphone, and pethidine).[29] These physical and chemical properties of the opioids will also determine vascular permeability. Lipophilic opioids such as fentanyl and sufentanil move more easily to the intravascular compartment than to the subarachnoid compartment. In this way spinal cord concentrations of an opioid following epidural administration are the result of the net difference between the rate of uptake and distribution to the vascular and subarachnoid spaces. These differences explain why morphine, despite having a meningeal permeability coefficient similar to fentanyl and sufentanil, which are well below the optimal range of meningeal penetration, is a useful agent for epidural analgesia.

There has been some debate in the past concerning the site of action of epidurally administered opioids with some studies suggesting that epidural fentanyl produces analgesia by systemic absorption and redistribution to the brain rather than by acting through a spinal mechanism. It would appear that the site of action depends on firstly whether the epidural fentanyl is given as a bolus or infusion, and secondly whether it is co-administered with local anaesthetic. Several studies have shown that when given as a bolus, epidural fentanyl has a spinal effect but when given as an infusion, without local anaesthetic, others have shown a systemic mechanism of action.[31–33] This is probably because low concentrations of lipophilic opioid are subject to rapid vascular uptake. However, when given as an infusion in the presence of epidural bupivacaine fentanyl appears to act spinally rather than systemically. Ginosar et al. performed a prospective, randomized, double-blinded study in which women in active labour received epidural bupivacaine until pain free. The women were then randomized to receive either IV or epidural fentanyl infusions. It was found that an equivalent dose of fentanyl was more than three times as potent when administered epidurally than by the IV route, suggesting a predominantly spinal mechanism of opioid action.[34]

Intrathecal opioids

Intrathecal morphine

Morphine is highly ionized and hydrophilic and does not penetrate lipid-rich tissues as rapidly as fentanyl. Morphine remains within the CSF for a prolonged period of time, spreading rostrally and reaching the trigeminal nerve distribution 3 hours after intrathecal injection in healthy volunteers.[35] Morphine requires 45–60 minutes to achieve a peak effect, and the duration of analgesia is 14-36 hours. This duration may be dose dependent.

A variety of intrathecal morphine doses have been investigated. Palmer et al. studied patients receiving intrathecal doses from 25 to 500 mcg and found a ceiling effect with doses greater than 75 mcg, as measured by patient-controlled IV morphine consumption with no clear dose–response relationship demonstrated using doses greater than 100 mcg.[36] Higher doses conferred no additional analgesic benefit but caused a dose-dependent increase in side effects, particularly pruritus. It was also noted that despite high doses of intrathecal morphine, most parturients continued to administer additional opioid analgesia at a low but constant rate, possibly explaining the interaction between spinal and supraspinal sites of action. Yang et al. administered 100 or 250 mcg of morphine as a component of spinal anaesthesia to 60 women undergoing elective CD. Women also received 20 mcg of intrathecal fentanyl and perioperative and postoperative NSAIDs routinely. There was no significant difference between the small and larger-dose morphine groups in pain relief, as measured by a VAPS.[37] In a systematic review of intrathecal opioid usage in patients undergoing CD, Dahl et al. reported a median time to first analgesic request of 27 hours (range 11–29 hours) and recommended an intrathecal dose of 100 mcg.

Adverse effects of intrathecal morphine have been reported widely and include pruritus, nausea and vomiting, urinary retention, and early or delayed respiratory depression. The most common side effect, pruritus, increased in severity as morphine doses increased. If a morphine dose of 100 mcg is used, it is estimated that 43% of women will experience pruritus, and 12% will experience nausea and vomiting.[30]

Intrathecal diamorphine

Diamorphine (3,6-diacetylmorphine, also known as morphine diacetate) is a semi-synthetic opioid produced by acetylation of morphine. The administration of neuraxial diamorphine for the treatment of pain relief after CD is a common practice in the United Kingdom even though it is not licensed for intrathecal use.[38] In contrast, in the rest of the world diamorphine is unavailable for clinical use. Diamorphine has many of the ideal physicochemical properties to provide good pain relief during and after surgery with the potential to decrease side effects. The intermediate lipid solubility of diamorphine (oil/water partition coefficient 280), increases permeability to both hydrophobic and hydrophilic tissue compartments when compared either with morphine or fentanyl. Diamorphine undergoes metabolism within spinal cord tissue, generating active compounds (6-acetyl morphine and morphine) which increases the analgesic effects. These metabolites are less lipid soluble than the parent drug, which limits their back diffusion into the CSF. Other important physicochemical characteristics of diamorphine are lower PKa (PKa 7.8), low protein binding (40%), and a high unionized fraction (27%) that increases the bioavailability for opioid receptors within the spinal cord and increases clearance from CSF, decreasing the potential for serious side effects such as respiratory depression.[39]

These physicochemical properties explain why intrathecal diamorphine is effective for both intraoperative and postoperative analgesia. Cowan et al. randomized 74 parturients undergoing elective CD to receive either 20 mcg fentanyl or 300 mcg diamorphine intrathecally with hyperbaric bupivacaine.[40] They found no difference in intraoperative analgesia requirements between the groups but also demonstrated reduced VAPS score 12 hours postoperatively in the diamorphine group compared to only 1 hour in the fentanyl group. They found no difference in pruritus postoperatively between the opioid groups. In a study of 200 women undergoing CD, Saravanan et al. concluded that the effective dose $(ED)_{95}$ for intrathecal diamorphine to prevent intraoperative supplementation was 0.4 mg and that this provided a mean time interval to first request for analgesia of 601 minutes.[41]

There have been other studies looking at intrathecal diamorphine doses for pain relief after CD. Skilton et al. and Kelly et al. looked at doses up to 0.375 mg and found improved analgesia (as determined by the amount of rescue analgesia required) as the dose increased without a ceiling effect.[42,43] Stacey et al. randomly allocated 40 women undergoing elective CD to receive either 0.5 mg or 1 mg of intrathecal diamorphine.[44] They found the time to request for rescue analgesia was significantly longer and 24-hour morphine consumption was significantly lower in the 1 mg group (45% using no opioids postoperatively at all) and that pain scores in this group tended to be lower. Minor side effects were found to be present in both groups but the incidence did not differ between groups. In the United Kingdom, the National Institute for Health and Care Excellence (NICE) recommends women should be offered diamorphine (0.3–0.4 mg intrathecally) for intra- and postoperative analgesia.[45]

Alternative intrathecal opioids

Other less commonly used intrathecal opioids include pethidine (meperidine), buprenorphine, and nalbuphine. Pethidine is the only member of the opioid family with local anaesthetic-like effects and it has a tendency to sometimes result in motor block. It has historically been used as a sole spinal drug for CD.[46]

Fentanyl is arguably one of the most commonly administered intrathecal opioids worldwide. Its relatively high lipid solubility results in a greater restriction of segmental activity and rapid onset of action when compared to morphine. Although intrathecal fentanyl offers a relatively short duration of analgesia, it is shown to improve intraoperative analgesia, especially during uterine exteriorization, and provides the patient with a better postoperative transition to other pain medications during recovery from intrathecal anaesthesia. The short duration of action of fentanyl generally makes it an unfavourable sole choice intraoperatively to provide post-CD analgesia but one study has suggested intrathecal fentanyl may also offer a longer-term analgesic benefit when administered alongside a local anaesthetic at the time of CD.[47] In many units, intrathecal fentanyl is combined with intrathecal preservative-free morphine to give superior intraoperative analgesia combined with the benefits of analgesia extending into the second postoperative day. In contrast to morphine, intrathecal fentanyl does not appear to predispose the patient to nausea and vomiting following CD and causes less severe pruritus and respiratory depression.[30,48] Sufentanil is a thienyl derivative of fentanyl but has higher potency due to greater lipid solubility. Intrathecal sufentanil offers some theoretical advantages over fentanyl including faster onset, reduced rostral spread, and a lower level of placental transfer. Several studies have been performed comparing fentanyl and sufentanil for analgesia for CD and have found them to be equivalent but those women in the sufentanil groups experienced more pruritus. Again, the short duration of action of intrathecal sufentanil prevents routine use for postoperative analgesia for CD.[49–51]

Epidural opioids

When anaesthesia for CD is provided by using an epidural top-up or a CSE technique then the epidural catheter provides another useful route to administer neuraxial opioids and a number of different opioids are used in this way

Epidural morphine

Epidural morphine is most commonly administered as a single bolus dose. Because of its low lipid solubility it has a relatively slow onset of action with its peak analgesic effect occurring after 60–90 minutes. However, its duration of action has been shown to provide pain relief for approximately 24 hours.[52] A recent systematic review of ten studies comparing analgesia efficacy and/or adverse effects of a single bolus dose of epidural morphine versus systemic opioids after elective CD proved that a single bolus of epidural morphine provides better analgesia than parenteral opioids but with an effect limited to the first postoperative day after CD and with an increase in side effects.[53]

A range of doses have been investigated. Palmer et al. performed a dose–response study looking at varying doses of epidural morphine between 0 and 5 mg for post-CD pain and found a ceiling effect in terms of analgesia. They found no difference in cumulative systemic morphine use above 3.75 mg used epidurally while 3 mg of morphine epidurally appeared equivalent to 100 mcg intrathecally and was found to provide analgesia for 12–24 hours.[36,54] Based on this study and a systematic review, the general practice is to use 3 mg of preservative-free morphine in the epidural space.[53]

Due to its prolonged analgesic effects, epidural morphine can be administered as an intermittent bolus or as a continuous infusion. It appears that some clinical advantages exist using continuous epidural morphine infusions over intermittent bolus for epidural analgesia. Studies in the non-obstetric population evaluating morphine's cephalad migration after a lumbar epidural bolus suggest that respiratory depression may occur as a result of significant amount of the drug reaching the respiratory centre in the brainstem after the administration of a bolus dose in the lumbar epidural area.[29,55] In fact, large-scale studies suggest that respiratory depression requiring treatment may be higher with intermittent bolus than with continuous infusions.[56,57] When mean doses between 7 and 13 mg/day were utilized in the intermittent bolus group and mean doses of 6–14 mg/day were used in the continuous infusion group, the incidence of respiratory depression was different. In the bolus study group, the incidence of respiratory depression was 1/500.[56] In contrast, in the continuous infusion group, the incidence was 1/1500. Based on these data, in the non-obstetric population the maximum risk of respiratory depression within the 95% confidence intervals are 1/100 versus 1/5000 respectively. Moreover, the concurrent use of parenteral opioids for breakthrough pain, a practice which has been discouraged when intermittent dosing of epidural morphine is used, may be administered without an increased risk of delayed respiratory depression even on the surgical wards.[56]

Interestingly, the quality of analgesia appears to be more complete when utilizing continuous infusions compared with an intermittent bolus. A study in the non-obstetric population evaluating the quality of analgesia produced by epidural morphine administered either as bolus doses or via continuous infusion demonstrated that patients who received continuous infusion of epidural morphine experienced a higher quality of analgesia than those who received intermittent bolus injections.[58] Based on apparent greater clinical efficacy and a lower incidence of respiratory depression it would appear that patients would derive a greater benefit from receiving epidural morphine via a continuous infusion.

Epidural diamorphine

Diamorphine is commonly administered epidurally in the United Kingdom because its high lipid solubility provides rapid onset of action and its main metabolite (morphine) provides a prolonged duration of action. Doses have been used in the range of 2.5–5 mg and have demonstrated prolonged duration of analgesia with 5 mg doses expected to provide analgesia for a mean duration of 14 hours.[39,59] However smaller epidural doses are associated with a lower incidence of nausea and vomiting suggesting that 3 mg is the optimum dose of diamorphine to administer epidurally.[59–61]

Single-dose extended-release epidural morphine

The goal of current postoperative pain research and development is to find a medication that can work locally to give long-lasting pain relief at the site of surgical focus with as little negative impact as possible. Single-dose, extended-release epidural morphine (EREM) (DepoDur®, Endo Pharmaceuticals, Chadds Ford, PA) is a recently developed drug that delivers conventional morphine sulphate using DepoFoam® (SkypePharma, San Diego, CA) technology. DepoFoam® is a revolutionary drug delivery system containing multivesicular lipid particles comprised of non-concentric aqueous chambers that fully encapsulate the active drug. These naturally occurring lipids are broken down by erosion and reorganization, resulting in a locally contained morphine depository for up to 48 hours after a single administration.[62]

Clinical studies within the obstetric population show EREM's postoperative analgesia consistently extending into the second day with no significant side effects. This is of notable benefit as a single dose of neuraxial morphine would lose its efficacy in this time frame and peak post-CD pain levels are not typically reached until 24–48 hours following surgery.[63] When an EREM dosage of 10 mg was compared to that of a standard 4 mg dose of epidural morphine, the supplemental opioid dose usage during the 24–48 hours postoperatively was significantly decreased by 60% in patients receiving EREM. Additionally, no significant differences in the occurrence of nausea, pruritus, sedation, respiratory depression, or hypoxic events were observed between these two groups.

Clinical trials have demonstrated the efficacy of EREM for postoperative pain relief following hip arthroplasty and elective CD.[64,65] Recent pharmacokinetic data obtained by Gambling et al. have described the effective use of EREM in a controlled, dose-ranging study of 114 patients following lower abdominal surgery.[66] The authors observed that the best balance of maximum analgesia with the lowest occurrence of side effects was achieved by administration of 15 mg of EREM and as such recommended that a multimodal pain management approach—such as the addition of a NSAID to the regimen—could further reduce the dose required to provide effective analgesia and reduce concomitantly the occurrence of adverse side effects.

While the prolonged analgesic effect during the first 48 hours using EREM is quite attractive, this advantage must be weighed against the potential disadvantages. One of these includes the instability of the formulation in the presence of local anaesthetics. Local anaesthetics other than a test dose cannot be administered immediately before or after the administration of EREM which has obvious implications when topping-up an existing epidural for CD. An in-line epidural filter cannot be used due to the viscosity of the preparation. No clinical studies have evaluated the safety of administration of EREM into the intrathecal space. In cases of accidental intrathecal injection, in post-marketing experience there were signs of prolonged respiratory depression requiring naloxone administration or ventilatory support. In terms of safety, there is the need for prolonged monitoring of patients following its administration, and the cost of the formulation may be prohibitive.[67] In September 2009, the US Food and Drug Administration (FDA) approved safety labelling revisions for EREM to emphasize the need for individualized dosing adjustments, as well as the need for monitoring capabilities, resuscitative equipment, and opioid antagonist availability. When EREM is given correctly in the epidural space, monitoring should be continued for up to 48 hours.

Alternative epidural opioids

The quality of analgesia experienced after hydromorphone administration appears to be similar to that produced by morphine.[68] Based on unpublished clinical observations, a ratio of 5:1 between morphine and hydromorphone has been utilized when administering the drug in a bolus form, and a ratio of 3:1 has been recommended for continuous infusions. Hydromorphone appears to have a faster onset and shorter duration of action than morphine with a lower incidence of pruritus.

Fentanyl, which has a high octanol:buffer coefficient, appears to undergo preferential vascular absorption rather than meningeal penetration after epidural administration. In fact, the value of utilizing fentanyl for epidural analgesia is controversial. Several studies have demonstrated that the quality of analgesia, the incidence of side effects, daily fentanyl utilization, and plasma levels after 24 hours of infusion are similar between patients receiving either epidural or IV therapy after non-obstetric surgery and at CD.[69–72]

Sevarino et al. performed a double-blinded randomized study on 40 American Society of Anesthesiologists (ASA) I/II women undergoing elective CD under lidocaine epidural anaesthesia who received after delivery either saline or 100 mcg fentanyl through the epidural catheter.[73] All patients were provided with an IV pethidine PCA postoperatively and it was noted that no differences in PCA use were recorded between the groups. The authors concluded that a single bolus of epidural fentanyl does not provide an advantage for postoperative pain relief in this patient population.

Patient-controlled epidural analgesia

The first study of patient-controlled epidural analgesia (PCEA) following CD, by Parker and White, described it as a safe, effective alternative to IV PCA with less opioid use and more rapid recovery.[74] In a follow-up study, the same investigators found that the efficacy of PCEA was not improved by adding a background infusion.[75] PCEA has been compared with IM opioid analgesia where it was found that PCEA pethidine resulted in better analgesia, earlier ambulation, and improved ability to care for the neonate.[76] PCEA has been shown to provide improved quality pain relief when compared with patient-controlled IV fentanyl, morphine, or pethidine, although no difference was found when epidural hydromorphone was also infused.[68,74,76–78] PCEA without a background infusion can provide adequate analgesia after CD, using either fentanyl or pethidine.[76,79] PCEA has been repeatedly shown to reduce opioid requirements and could potentially be an excellent method of postoperative pain relief for CD.[20,80,81] The combination of local anaesthetics and opioids in PCEA postoperatively for CD appears to have the benefit of achieving postoperative analgesia without significant motor blockade. This is extremely important to allow the mother to take care of her baby. However, the overall popularity of the technique is limited. The requirement for prolonged epidural catheterization can result in failures and interfere with thromboprophylactic low-molecular-weight heparin (LMWH) administration and removal of the urinary catheter. Furthermore, carrying an epidural infusion pump can be cumbersome whilst ambulating and caring for a newborn. In addition, Vercauteren et al. considered the cost-effectiveness of PCEA by randomizing 53 women for elective or semi-urgent CD to receive either PCEA with bupivacaine and sufentanil or intrathecal bupivacaine and morphine. They found that in the PCEA group patients had lower VAPS scores both at rest and during mobilization. Manpower and drug costs were equal in both groups. The total cost per head was more expensive in the PCEA group mainly as a result of the more costly equipment required.[82]

Intrathecal and epidural opioids compared

When a CSE is used to provide anaesthesia for CD, longer-acting opioids could be administered either intrathecally with the initial spinal injection of local anaesthetic or epidurally towards the end of the operation. When an opioid is administered intrathecally, the analgesic effects and side effects such as respiratory depression, pruritus, and nausea and vomiting are caused by the drug gaining access to the spinal cord and brainstem via the CSF. In contrast, when an opioid is administered epidurally, a small proportion of the dose crosses the meningeal layer whilst the remainder gains access to the central nervous system via IV absorption through the epidural venous plexus, potentially leading to side effects. The rate of dural transfer of an opioid has been shown to be inversely proportional to the molecular weight of the drug with the exception of fentanyl which has a much higher rate of transfer possibly due to its linear molecular shape.[83] Deciding whether to administer an opioid intrathecally or epidurally therefore needs to balance the benefits of analgesia and the occurrence of side effects and is complicated by an incomplete understanding of equivalent intrathecal and epidural doses and the different physicochemical properties of various opioids.

There are, however, several studies in the literature comparing the use of epidural and intrathecal opioids for post-CD analgesia. Sarvela et al. performed a double-blinded, randomized controlled trial comparing 3 mg epidural morphine with either 100 mcg or 200 mcg intrathecal morphine and found no significant differences in pain scores. However, rescue analgesia was requested more frequently in the 100 mcg group suggesting this dose was less effective for post-CD analgesia and perhaps unsurprisingly this group were shown to have less pruritus.[84] When Bloor et al. compared intrathecal diamorphine 0.3 mg with 3.0 mg epidural diamorphine they demonstrated that the duration and quality of analgesia was comparable in the two groups but the incidence of pruritus was higher and more severe in the intrathecal group.[61] In contrast, Hallworth et al. showed a high incidence of pruritus in both groups but more nausea and vomiting in the epidural group when comparing intrathecal diamorphine 0.25 mg with diamorphine 5 mg epidurally.[39] Again, duration and quality of analgesia were similar. It would appear that in terms of analgesic efficacy there is little to choose between the two routes; however, intrathecal and epidural opioids can result in significant levels of pruritus and larger epidural opioid doses produce more nausea and vomiting.

Side effects of neuraxial opioids

There are certain side effects associated with neuraxial blockade although it is widely accepted that the benefits outweigh the risks. The main adverse effects are that of respiratory depression, nausea and vomiting, pruritus, and urinary retention and these appear to be associated with the degree of rostral migration of the opioid in the CSF. The timing for the appearance of these side effects varies between lipophilic and hydrophilic opioids after epidural administration. Morphine's rostral migration is a phenomenon which is dose dependent and follows a predictable time course.[55] Lipophilic opioids also exhibit rostral migration, but on a less predictable timescale than morphine.

Respiratory depression

Although rare, respiratory depression is a serious concern when considering the use of neuraxial opioids. It is thought to occur through depression of the brainstem respiratory centres through either direct or indirect mechanisms.[52,85,86] Respiratory depression is an uncommon but potentially serious side effect, though the incidence in the obstetric population is difficult to determine. Lipophilic opioids such as fentanyl may cause early-onset respiratory depression due to significant vascular uptake, rostral spread within the CSF, and possibly direct transit in epidural veins although the incidence of this occurrence in obstetric patients is unknown.[86,87] Respiratory depression has been described after administration of epidural fentanyl 90–100 mcg for CD.[88] In a study by Arai et al., intrathecal fentanyl 20 mcg in combination with bupivacaine was not shown to cause a reduction in peak expiratory flow rate, or vital capacity despite improving the quality of anaesthesia.[89] These opioids have a relatively low incidence of late-onset respiratory depression in contrast to the biphasic pattern of respiratory depression seen with neuraxial morphine.[90] Abouleish et al. studied 856 parturients who received 200 mcg of intrathecal morphine during CD and found respiratory depression, as defined by SpO_2 less than 85% or respiratory rate of less than 10 breaths per minute, in eight patients (0.93%), all of whom were markedly obese.[91] It should be noted, however, that smaller dosages of intrathecal morphine (75 mcg) therapy may result in a reduced duration of analgesia and may therefore require an increased need for supplemental analgesics. Also, due to the variability in patient response to intrathecal morphine, some patients may additionally experience inadequate postoperative analgesia and/or opioid-related side effects. Systemic vascular absorption may lead to early-onset respiratory depression (30–90 minutes after administration) followed by rostral spread within the CSF and slow penetration into the brainstem causing delayed respiratory depression up to 18 hours after neuraxial morphine administration.[27,35] As noted previously, EREM has not been reported in small studies looking at post-CD analgesia but has been reported when used in larger doses in the non-obstetric population.[63–66] The physiological changes of pregnancy, specifically the higher respiratory rate associated with elevated progesterone levels, may provide a greater margin of safety in comparison to other patient populations.

Respiratory depression from neuraxial opioids can be prevented by the identification of high-risk patients such as those who are obese or have coexisting disease such as sleep apnoea. Caution should be particularly exercised in those women receiving sedative drugs or pre-eclamptic women receiving magnesium therapy. Several studies have demonstrated that there is a ceiling effect for analgesia and thus caution should be exercised to limit the dose used in clinical practice.[30,36,54] The ASA has formulated guidelines to address the prevention, detection, and management of respiratory depression associated with neuraxial opioid administration in non-obstetric patients but there are no specific guidelines for the parturient.[92] All patients should ideally be monitored for level of consciousness, oxygenation, and adequacy of ventilation for the duration of the opioid action and it has been suggested that vigilant hourly assessments are probably adequate in low-risk patients as long as there is anaesthetic support immediately available to manage the complications of respiratory depression. The guidelines recommend that the lowest efficacious dose of neuraxial opioids should be administered to minimize the risk of respiratory depression and that parenteral opioids or hypnotics should be carefully administered in the presence of neuraxial opioids. If there is concomitant administration of neuraxial opioids and parenteral opioids, sedatives, hypnotics, or magnesium, this requires increased monitoring (e.g. intensity, duration, or additional methods). Patients receiving EREM should be monitored for 48 hours.

Nausea and vomiting

Nausea and vomiting are common complaints during and after CD and the causes may be multifactorial including hypotension, increased vagal activity, surgical manipulation, and the use of uterotonic agents.[93] In addition, neuraxial opioids may increase the risk of postoperative nausea and vomiting either from rostral spread of the opioids in the CSF to the brainstem or from vascular uptake and subsequent effects on the chemoreceptor trigger zone and vomiting centre.[35,94] There have been multiple studies looking at regimens to reduce postoperative nausea and vomiting after CD in those patients who have received neuraxial opioids. However, the ability to interpret comparative data in these studies is hindered by the lack of standardization of nausea and vomiting outcome measures and lack of risk stratification or predictive models for postoperative nausea and vomiting in these groups of patients.[95]

Pruritus

Pruritus is another regular complaint from patients receiving neuraxial opioids for CD with one study reviewing almost 5000

CDs in patients receiving epidural morphine 2–5 mg reporting pruritus in 58%.[96] Approximately 40% of patients receiving epidural morphine request treatment for pruritus.[96–98] The incidence and severity is more common after increasing opioid dose and intrathecal administration although patients who have received intrathecal opioids rank pain and nausea and vomiting as more undesirable than pruritus.[6,99]

Urinary retention

The non-specific definition of urinary retention post CD makes an assessment of the potential effects of neuraxial opioids on urinary function difficult. The mechanisms by which neuraxial opioids affect specific components of micturition are not fully understood although spinal and supraspinal sites of action are likely to be involved. Other risk factors for post-CD urinary retention include low body mass index and multiparity.[100] One observational study investigating the effects of epidural morphine and methadone in 120 women undergoing CD found a higher rate of urinary retention and catheterization in the morphine group (57% and 50% respectively).[101] Currently there is a relative lack of research in this area.

Reactivation of oral herpes simplex

Neuraxial morphine administration has also been linked to reactivation of oral herpes simplex. In a study of women with a past history of oral herpes simplex, reactivation occurred in 38% receiving intrathecal morphine compared with 16% of those receiving IV morphine.[102]

Local anaesthetics

Transversus abdominis plane block

The transversus abdominis plane (TAP) block is performed by introducing local anaesthetic into the plane between the fascia of the transversus abdominis muscle and the internal oblique muscle. It is possible to block the sensory nerves of the anterior abdominal wall before they leave this plane and pierce the musculature to innervate the anterior abdominal wall (Figure 24.2). It has a high margin of safety and is technically simple to perform, especially under ultrasound guidance but despite this, TAP blocks remain overwhelmingly underutilized in both the obstetric and non-obstetric populations. Duration of action is dependent on the type of local anaesthetic used and if prolonged analgesia is needed, a catheter for continuous infusion can also be placed using ultrasound imaging.

There are a number of studies in the literature looking at TAP blocks for analgesia after CD. Baaj et al. randomized 40 women to receive either local anaesthetic or saline TAP blocks in addition to a hypobaric bupivacaine spinal block for elective CD.[103] A significant reduction in 24-hour morphine requirement was observed in the local anaesthetic TAP block group versus controls (26 vs 63 mg). Although the authors reported lower postoperative nausea and vomiting, lower 24-hour VAPS scores, and higher satisfaction in the local anaesthetic TAP block group, no statistical measures were reported.[104] McDonnell et al. randomized 50 women to receive either bilateral TAP blocks with 0.75% ropivacaine or saline placebo.[105] They found that the median time to first morphine request was extended from 90 to 220 minutes in the TAP block group. The TAP block group were also found to have lower morphine requirements in the first 48 hours postoperatively and a corresponding reduction in sedation and nausea. However, not all studies have confirmed this finding. Belavy et al. performed a similar study which showed a decrease in postoperative IV opioids use between groups but no difference in pain scores whereas Costello et al. found no difference between groups in either opioid use, satisfaction, or pain scores with the additional TAP block.[106,107] McMorrow et al. compared the TAP block to intrathecal morphine for analgesia post CD. They randomized 80 patients to one of four groups (n = 20 in each arm) to receive (in

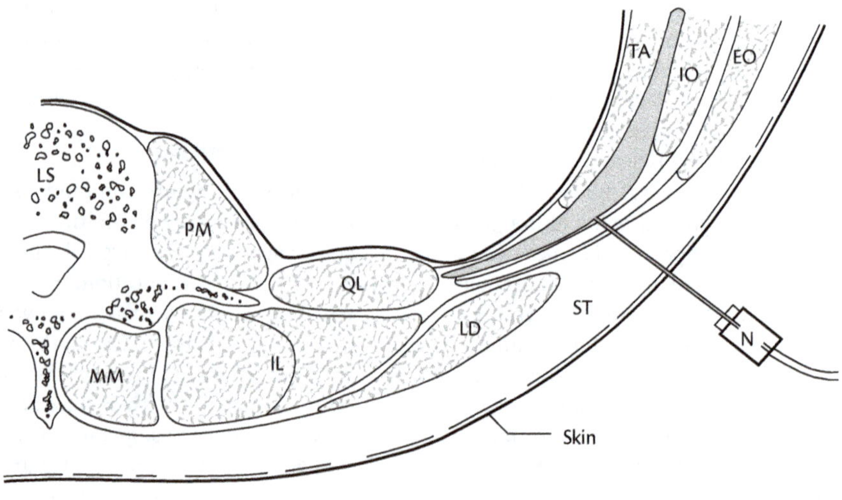

Figure 24.2 Transversus abdominis plane block. Line drawing of a transverse section through the abdominal wall at the level of the lumbar triangle of Petit (TOP). The floor of the triangle is composed, from superficial to deep, of the fascial extensions of external oblique, internal oblique, and transversus abdominis, respectively, and the peritoneum. The needle is inserted through the triangle, using the loss-of-resistance technique. The needle is shown in the transversus abdominis plane, and the fascial layers have separated as a result of the injection of local anaesthetic.
EO, external oblique; IL, longissimus iliocostalis; IO, internal oblique; LD, latissimus dorsi; LS, lumbar spine; pm, psoas major; MM, multifidus muscle; QL, quadratus lumborum; ST, subcutaneous tissue; TA, transversus abdominis.

addition to spinal anaesthesia) either spinal morphine 100 mcg, or saline and a postoperative bilateral TAP block with either 2 mg/kg bupivacaine or saline.[108] Pain on movement and early morphine consumption were lowest in the groups receiving spinal morphine and they found no incremental benefits of TAP block when intrathecal morphine was used. They also reported similar overall patient satisfaction among groups despite more frequent pruritus in the intrathecal morphine group. In a study by Singh et al., 60 women having CD under spinal anesthesia were randomized to receive ultrasound-guided TAP blocks using either high-dose ropivacaine (3 mg/kg), low-dose ropivacaine (1.5 mg/kg), or placebo. Patients received intrathecal 0.75% bupivacaine 10–12 mg, fentanyl 10 mcg, and morphine 150 mcg, and standard multimodal analgesia.[109] The primary outcome was the difference in pain with movement using a numeric rating scale at 24 hours. They found that neither high- nor low-dose TAP blocks as part of a multimodal analgesia regimen including intrathecal morphine improved pain scores with movement at 24 hours after CD when compared to placebo TAP blocks. They found that high-dose TAP blocks may improve pain scores up to 12 hours after CD.

In response to these varying studies, Abdallah et al. performed a systematic review and meta-analysis looking at TAP blocks for postoperative analgesia after CD performed under intrathecal anaesthesia.[110] They looked at five trials including 312 patients and concluded that TAP blocks provide superior analgesia compared with placebo and can reduce the first 24-hour morphine consumption in the setting of a multimodal analgesic regimen that excludes morphine.

Few studies have compared TAP blocks to epidural anaesthesia. Kadam and Moran performed a retrospective matched case–control study on 30 patients comparing continuous TAP block catheters to thoracic epidural analgesia in the non-pregnant population.[111] There were no appreciable differences in patient satisfaction between the two groups over a 3-day follow-up period. The TAP group was found to require a significantly higher amount of supplemental fentanyl for breakthrough pain over the study period. There was a higher therapeutic failure rate and rate of hypotension seen in the thoracic epidural group.

Tap blocks are not without their limitations. In non-obstetric patients, complications include visceral perforation, peritoneal injection, femoral nerve palsies, and local anaesthetic toxicity.[112] From these conflicting studies it would seem reasonable to conclude that TAP blocks should currently not be used in preference to neuraxial opioids for post-CD analgesia and should probably be reserved for a parturient undergoing general anaesthesia or where neuraxial opioids have not been used either because they are contraindicated or unavailable.

Wound infiltration

There has been recent interest in wound infiltration using both local anaesthetic and NSAIDs. Results after general abdominal surgery are mixed, probably due to differences in the site of catheter placement, the drugs used, and the outcome with continuous versus bolus techniques. A Cochrane review in 2009 looked at 20 studies involving local anaesthetic wound infiltration during CD and found that:

- local anaesthetic infiltration and abdominal nerve blocks as adjuncts to regional and general anaesthesia are of benefit by reducing opioid consumption
- NSAIDs as an adjuvant in the local anaesthetic mixture may confer additional pain relief.[113]

Lavand'homme et al. found that diclofenac alone via a wound infusion catheter decreases 48-hour morphine requirements compared with ropivacaine infusion or IV diclofenac, suggesting that diclofenac may have peripheral analgesic properties in addition to its systemic effects.[114] Further studies are required to assess local anaesthetic infusions and NSAIDs on outcomes beyond analgesic efficacy such as wound healing and the formation of adhesions.

Systemic opioid analgesia

In developed countries, most women will receive neuraxial opioids for post-CD pain relief. Large reviews indicate that the neuraxial approach provides superior analgesia over systemic administration but many patients will require additional systemic analgesics to further improve pain relief and to limit side effects.[30,115] Also patients who receive general anaesthesia will usually require systemic analgesics.

Patient-controlled analgesia

PCA, which permits the patient to self-administer small doses of IV opioid analgesic at frequent intervals, often provides effective and sustained analgesia after major surgery. However, when neuraxial opioids are used, studies have shown that IV PCA is not usually required. Pain scores equivalent to mild to moderate pain are achieved using an average of only 5 mg PCA morphine in 24 hours and 15% and 32% of patients required no morphine at all when intrathecal diamorphine was used.[116,117] However, for those patients who receive no neuraxial opioids such as in CD under general anaesthesia and in whom potent analgesia via the IV route is required, different opioids can be delivered utilizing a PCA pump, including fentanyl, morphine, and hydromorphone. When comparing IV PCA with IM administration of opioid most studies conclude that the IV PCA route is preferable resulting in better analgesia, earlier ambulation, less sedation, and greater patient satisfaction regardless of which opioid is used.[118,119]

When deciding which opioid to use for PCA, most experience is reported using morphine. In a study by Howell et al. comparing PCA fentanyl with PCA morphine post CD, both analgesic solutions provided effective pain relief for a mean of 37 hours postoperatively with high levels of patient satisfaction and no differences in VAPS scores between groups.[120] However, more patients in the fentanyl group required supplementary boluses or alterations to the PCA settings and one patient in this group had to be removed from the study due to inadequate analgesia. The authors concluded that morphine PCA should be used in preference to fentanyl PCA for routine use after CD.[120] Pethidine has also been used for PCA but its use is now discouraged because of concerns about accumulation of the metabolite norpethidine in the neonate which may affect neurobehavioural scores.[121]

PCA is associated with all the usual opioid-related side effects, including potentially lethal respiratory depression, so close monitoring including continuous pulse oximetry and frequent nursing assessments is recommended.

Common oral opioids and combinations

Once patients are tolerating an oral diet, analgesics are given via the oral route as a convenient 'step-down' after primary management with neuraxial or IV opioids as part of a multimodal regimen.

Common regimens used worldwide include:

- hydrocodone (dihydrocodeine) + paracetamol
- oxycodone + paracetamol
- hydromorphone
- oxycodone
- oral morphine.

There are a number of studies looking at these regimens in the literature. Davis et al. performed a randomized controlled trial comparing IV patient-controlled morphine with oral oxycodone–paracetamol after CD.[122] They assessed pain at 6 and 24 hours after delivery and found that the oral group experienced less pain at both time intervals. They also found that this group had less nausea and drowsiness at 6 hours but slightly more nausea at 24 hours. Another study by Jakobi et al. assessed patient satisfaction with oral analgesia following CD and found that it provided satisfactory pain relief, was easily administered and was substantially less expensive compared to IV methods of analgesia.[123]

Codeine

Codeine (3-methylmorphine) is a naturally occurring opioid, which is also synthesized synthetically and used for analgesia, antitussive, antidiarrhoeal, sedative, and hypnotic properties. It is used to treat mild-to-moderate pain and is marketed both as a single-ingredient drug and in combination preparations with paracetamol (as co-codamol) and NSAIDs such as aspirin and ibuprofen. Common side effects include drowsiness and constipation. Codeine is metabolized to codeine-6-glucoronide (C6G) by uridine diphosphate glucoronosyl transferase in the liver.[124] About 5% of codeine is metabolized by cytochrome P450 (CYP)-2D6 and the current evidence suggests that C6G is the primary active compound. About 0.5–2% of the population are 'extensive metabolizers' having multiple copies of the gene for CYP2D6 and producing high levels of CYP2D6 which metabolize drugs through that pathway more quickly.

CYP2D6 has been implicated in the toxicity and death of neonates when codeine is administered to lactating mothers, particularly those who are 'ultrafast metabolizers' and as a result, codeine phosphate has been withdrawn from use in many maternity units.[125,126]

Tramadol

Tramadol is a synthetic, centrally acting analgesic, acting as a weak serotonin and norepinephrine re-uptake inhibitor, as well as a weak MOP receptor agonist. It is indicated for moderate to severe pain. It is supplied as 50 mg tablets (immediate release) and 100 mg, 200 mg, and 300 mg tablets (extended release). Side effects may include nausea/vomiting, dizziness, and constipation, amongst others. There is an increased risk of seizure in those with history of epilepsy. It should be avoided in those with anaphylactoid reactions to codeine and used with caution in those on medications that affect serotonin (risk of serotonin syndrome). There have been case reports suggesting a neonatal withdrawal including seizure activity after maternal antenatal use of tramadol but this appears rare and associated with long-term, high-dose maternal use.[127] Dosage adjustments should be made in those with renal or hepatic impairment and in those with advanced age. In severe impairment, it should be avoided. A randomized clinical trial by Ollé Fortuny et al. compared tramadol to ketorolac for postoperative pain after abdominal hysterectomy.[128] Seventy-six women were enrolled for this study and two treatment groups were formed: the TRA (tramadol) group received 100 mg of tramadol orally, while the KET (ketorolac) group received 30 mg of ketorolac IV every 6 hours. During the first 12 hours after surgery, the 100 mg dose of tramadol was shown to be more effective for pain relief compared to the 30 mg ketorolac every 6 hours. There was, however, increased incidence of postoperative vomiting in the TRA group. Epidural tramadol was evaluated in women undergoing CD with epidural anaesthesia.[47] Addition of tramadol 50 mg to 2% lidocaine with adrenaline extended the mean (SD) duration of postoperative analgesia from 2.46 (±0.45) to 15.39 (±0.54).

Methadone

Methadone is a MOP receptor agonist more commonly used to treat opioid dependency. However, there is interest in methadone administration as an analgesic and possibly as a preventative of chronic wound pain. Shahrkai et al. performed a prospective randomized double-blinded study on 102 elective CD patients who all received spinal anaesthesia followed by a single IM dose of pethidine 50 mg in the recovery room.[129] They were then randomized to receive either 0.7 mL/kg pethidine every 6 hours or 0.07 mg/kg methadone orally every 6 hours. There was no statistical difference found in terms of analgesia, patient satisfaction, or requirements for breakthrough pain relief between the two groups. In a retrospective case–control study of parturients undergoing general anaesthesia for CD and multimodal analgesia, Russell et al. compared 25 women who had received a single IV bolus of methadone (mean dose 14 mg) at the time of delivery with 50 matched controls.[130] Women in the methadone group had lower pain scores, lower IV PCA opioid consumption, and were less likely to require IV opioid supplementation. Further work is needed in this area.

Paracetamol and non-steroidal anti-inflammatory drugs

Paracetamol

Paracetamol inhibits cyclooxygenase-2 (COX-2) resulting in decreased production of prostaglandin E_2 and the activation of descending serotonergic pathways. In the general surgical population, it has been shown to have a useful opioid-sparing effect by reducing postoperative IV PCA morphine consumption.[131,132] In patients receiving PCA morphine after CD, Alhashemi et al. compared the effects of IV paracetamol with those of oral ibuprofen with respect to pain control and morphine requirements.[133] They measured both VAPS scores and patient satisfaction. VAPS scores were found to decrease similarly in both groups over time; however, there were no differences between groups at any time. Patient satisfaction was high in both groups. They concluded that IV paracetamol was a reasonable adjunct to IV PCA morphine. There have been surprisingly few trials looking at paracetamol alone after CD. Munishankar et al. compared oral paracetamol, diclofenac, and the combination of these for pain relief after CD in a double-blind randomized controlled trial of paracetamol.[134]

Patients given the combination of diclofenac and paracetamol required 38% less morphine than patients given paracetamol alone. Morphine use in patients given diclofenac alone was not significantly different from morphine use in the other two groups. Nauta et al. performed a systematic review of randomized trials comparing a combination of codeine–paracetamol versus NSAIDs in the treatment of postoperative abdominal pain.[135] They found that none of the studies showed the codeine–paracetamol to be superior to NSAIDs in controlling post-laparotomy pain and that fewer adverse effects were reported in the NSAID group. There are currently no similar studies that have been performed in obstetric patients.

Diclofenac sodium

NSAIDS are now widely established as a basic analgesic in the management of severe postoperative pain both in the general postoperative setting and post CD where they have been shown to potentiate opioid effect, decrease opioid consumption, and reduce side effects. They seem to be particularly effective against the visceral pain originating from the uterus and wound site and complement the somatic pain relief provided by opioids. They are usually used immediately post CD and then continued regularly for at least 48 hours postoperatively. They are thought to work by inhibiting COX, an enzyme which converts arachidonic acid to prostaglandins and thromboxane. NSAIDS are associated with side effects such as increased bleeding, renal impairment, gastrointestinal bleeding, and acute bronchospasm and should be used with caution in at-risk patients. Diclofenac sodium is commonly used to treat pain, inflammatory disorders, dysmenorrhea, endometriosis, and mild-to-moderate postoperative or post-traumatic pain. As with similar NSAIDs it predisposes to gastrointestinal bleeding but is amongst the better tolerated NSAIDs. As well as inhibiting COX there is some evidence that diclofenac inhibits lipoxygenase pathways, thus reducing leukotriene formation and may also inhibit phospholipase A_2. These actions may explain the high potency of diclofenac—it has a wide variety of effects including anti-inflammatory, antipyretic, and analgesic actions.[136] Approximately half of the diclofenac dose is metabolized during first-pass hepatic metabolism. Sixty per cent is excreted renally, with 1% remaining unchanged in the urine.

Diclofenac has been shown in a number of studies to have a significant opioid sparing effect. When given in the recommended dose of 150 mg daily, opioid consumption can be reduced by 35–40%.[137,138] So-called high-dose diclofenac (rectal diclofenac 200 mg daily) has also been shown to be morphine sparing without increased side effects and has been adopted by many units because of the simplicity of administration.[139] Diclofenac has been shown previously to confer significant pain relief when used in combination with paracetamol. Mitra et al. compared this combination with a diclofenac–tramadol combination when considering pain relief after CD in a randomized double-blinded parallel-group controlled trial involving 204 parturients.[140] They found both combinations to provide satisfactory postoperative pain relief after CD. The diclofenac–tramadol combination was overall more efficacious but associated with a higher incidence of postoperative nausea.

Available recent data indicate that the cardiovascular risk with diclofenac is similar to that of the selective COX-2 inhibitors and as a result is now contraindicated in those with ischaemic heart disease, peripheral arterial disease, cerebrovascular disease, or established congestive heart failure (New York Heart Association classification II–IV) and this applies to all systemic formulations including suppositories.[141] As a result, many units have switched to ibuprofen as the preferred NSAID for use after CD in doses of up to 2.4 g daily.

Ketorolac

Ketorolac is a NSAID indicated for short-term use (5 days or less due to gastric ulceration, bleeding, and perforation risk) in managing moderate-to-severe acute pain. Routes of administration are oral, IV, or IM. When given by the IV route, usual adult dosing is 15–30 mg IV every 6 hours, with a maximum of 120 mg in 24 hours. Side effects and adverse effects are similar to other NSAIDs.

Ketorolac has been evaluated as a perioperative analgesic, as it appears to have greater potency (similar to opioids) than other NSAIDs and an opioid-sparing effect. El-Tahan et al. studied the effect of preoperative ketorolac for CD, randomly assigning 90 patients to receive either IV ketorolac bolus at 15 mg prior to induction followed by infusion at 7.5 mg/h, or saline placebo.[142] The results showed, in part, that 15.6% of patients in the ketorolac group requested postoperative tramadol for analgesia, compared with 31.1% in the control group. The conclusion was that prophylactic ketorolac improved analgesia after CD. A randomized, controlled trial by Lowder et al. compared ketorolac with placebo after CD in 44 patients.[143] The ketorolac group was found to have significantly reduced morphine IV PCA requirements at 24 hours compared to the control group. It was concluded that ketorolac reduced opioid usage and postoperative pain. Another study was performed by Tzeng and Mok to determine the analgesic effect from a combination of ketorolac and low-dose epidural morphine after CD.[144] Ninety patients were enrolled in the study and randomized to three groups to receive postoperatively either (a) epidural morphine 2 mg and IV placebo, (b) epidural morphine 2 mg and IM ketorolac 30 mg, or (c) epidural saline placebo and IM ketorolac 30 mg. Group (b) had significant superior pain relief compared to the other two groups. The addition of ketorolac was thought to enhance the analgesic effect of low-dose epidural morphine.

Cyclooxygenase-2 inhibitors

These drugs work by selectively inhibiting the COX-2 enzyme, which is involved in prostaglandin synthesis as part of the inflammatory response pathway. COX-2-specific inhibition both reduces the risk of gastrointestinal adverse events and lacks effect on platelet aggregation, in comparison to non-selective COX inhibitors (that block both the COX-1 and COX-2 enzyme), such as naproxen or ibuprofen. A number of COX-2 inhibitors have been withdrawn from the market because of concerns over serious cardiovascular events including valdecoxib and parecoxib.[145] Carvalho et al. randomized patients undergoing CD under spinal anaesthesia with intrathecal morphine 0.1 mg into two groups to receive either valdecoxib 20 mg or placebo. They were unable to demonstrate any significant analgesic effect of this COX-2 inhibitor.[146]

Celecoxib is a COX-2 inhibitor that is still available but it carries a FDA black box warning for possible increased risk of serious cardiovascular and gastrointestinal adverse events.

It is supplied as 50 mg, 100 mg, 200 mg, and 400 mg capsules and is metabolized hepatically, thus dosage adjustments must be made in those with impairment in hepatic function. It should be used with great caution in those with renal insufficiency, as NSAIDs may decrease renal perfusion. Celecoxib has been used in the perioperative period as an adjuvant analgesic and a Cochrane review evaluated the efficacy of a single dose of oral celecoxib for postoperative pain.[147] Eight trials were included. A 200 mg dose of celecoxib was as effective as 600/650 mg of aspirin and 1000 mg of paracetamol for relieving postoperative pain. A dose of 400 mg was as effective as 400 mg of ibuprofen. Adverse event rates were similar with celecoxib and placebo. The conclusion of the study was that a single dose of celecoxib was effective for postoperative pain relief. A 400 mg dose was recommended for acute pain. However, in the obstetric population there is little published work. Lee et al. evaluated a 200 mg oral dose compared to placebo and demonstrated no analgesic benefit whilst Fong et al. reported some analgesic benefit after CD with a 400 mg dose.[148,149] Because of concerns about the cardiovascular side effects of these drugs, currently there is very little evidence to support their use for post-CD pain relief.

Patient-controlled oral analgesia

One of the disadvantages of IV PCA is that once the opioid PCA is discontinued, patients are no longer in charge of their own analgesia and must traditionally rely on nursing staff to administer medication. This has led to increased interest in patient-controlled oral analgesia (PCOA) programmes using short-acting oral medications for postoperative pain relief. This is gaining particular interest in the United Kingdom as part of enhanced recovery pathways in both obstetric and non-obstetric surgery. CD patients are often given a supply of three types of oral analgesia—paracetamol, ibuprofen, and a opioid-based oral analgesic in hospital with written instructions discussing how and when to take the medication and reinforcing the importance of regular administration to prevent breakthrough pain. Early PCOA studies suggest the benefits of PCOA are similar to IV PCA—that of improved pain control and increased patient satisfaction.[150,151] It is also a simple, low-cost system of analgesia delivery that teaches patients how and when to take pain medication before they are sent home. Further research and controlled trials are necessary to validate its role in the obstetric population.

Conclusion

Failure to treat acute postoperative pain after CD can have adverse physical and psychological consequences for the patient and the potential to progress to a persistent, chronic pain state. The mainstay of postoperative analgesia for CD encompasses a multimodal regimen based on neuraxial opioids. This provides excellent postoperative analgesia with a decrease in total dose of parenteral opioid, low level of sedation, early ambulation, early return of bowel function, and better maternal–infant bonding with minimal accumulation of the drug in breast milk. However, neuraxial opioids may have side effects and complications; the most serious of which is delayed respiratory depression and these patients must be monitored appropriately postoperatively. Oral analgesia continues to have an important role in the subsequent step-down management of post-CD pain.

References

1. Anonymous. Appropriate technology for birth. *Lancet* 1985; 2(8452):436–7.
2. Gibbons L, Belizán JM, Lauer JA, *et al. The Global Numbers and Costs of Additionally Needed and Unnecessary Caesarean Sections Performed per Year: Overuse as a Barrier to Universal Coverage.* World Health Report (2010) Background Paper, 30. Geneva: World Health Organization; 2010. http://www.who.int/healthsystems/topics/financing/healthreport/30C-sectioncosts.pdf
3. Kehlet H. Multimodal approach to control postoperative pathophysiology and rehabilitation. *Br J Anaesth* 1997; 78(5):606–17.
4. Macrae WA. Chronic post-surgical pain: 10 years on. *Br J Anaesth* 2008; 101(1):77–86.
5. Eisenach JC, Pan P, Smiley RM, *et al.* Severity of acute pain after childbirth, but not type of delivery, predicts persistent pain and postpartum depression. *Pain* 2008; 140(1):87–94.
6. Carvalho B, Cohen SE, Lipman SS, *et al.* Patient preferences for anesthesia outcomes associated with cesarean delivery. *Anesth Analg* 2005; 101(4):1182–7.
7. Dolin SJ, Cashman JN, Bland JM. Effectiveness of acute postoperative pain management: I. Evidence from published data. *Br J Anaesth* 2002; 89(3):409–23.
8. Apfelbaum JL, Chen C, Mehta SS, *et al.* Postoperative pain experience: results from a national survey suggest postoperative pain continues to be undermanaged. *Anesth Analg* 2003; 97(2): 534–40.
9. Lucas N, Pickering E, Plaat F. Pain relief after caesarean section. In Colvin JR, Peden CJ (eds) *Raising the Standard: A Compendium of Audit Recipes* (3rd ed). London: Royal College of Anaesthetists; 2012:226–7.
10. Pickering E, Holdcroft A. Pain relief after caesarean section. In Kinsella M (ed) *Raising the Standard: A Compendium of Audit Recipes* (2nd ed). London: Royal College of Anaesthetists; 2006:168–9.
11. Noblet J, Plaat F. Raising the standard ... to unachievable heights? *Anaesthesia* 2010; 65(1):88–9.
12. Merskey H, Bogduk N (eds). *IASP Task Force on Taxonomy, Classification of Chronic Pain* (2nd ed). Seattle, WA: IASP Press; 1994.
13. Gourlay GK, Cherry DA, Cousins MJ. Cephalad migration of morphine in CSF following lumbar epidural administration in patients with cancer pain. *Pain* 1985; 23(4):317–26.
14. Julius D, Basbaum AI. Molecular mechanisms of nociception. *Nature* 2001; 413(6852):203–10.
15. Devor M. Neurobiology of normal and pathophysiological pain. In Aronoff GM (ed) *Evaluation and Treatment of Chronic Pain.* Baltimore, MD: Williams and Wilkins; 1998:11–27.
16. Moore KA, Kohno T, Karchewski LA, *et al.* Partial peripheral nerve injury promotes a selective loss of GABAergic inhibition in the superficial dorsal horn of the spinal cord. *J Neurosci* 2002; 22(15):6724–31.
17. McDonnell NJ, Keating ML, Muchatuta NA, *et al.* Analgesia after caesarean delivery. *Anaesth Intensive Care* 2009; 37(4):539–51.
18. Tingaker BK, Irestedt L. Changes in uterine innervation in pregnancy and during labour. *Curr Opin Anaesthesiol* 2010; 23(3):300–3.
19. Lavand'homme P. Postcesarean analgesia: effective strategies and association with chronic pain. *Curr Opin Anaesthesiol* 2006; 19(3):244–8.
20. Pan PH. Post cesarean delivery pain management: multimodal approach. *Int J Obstet Anesth* 2006; 15(3):185–8.
21. Elia N, Lysakowski C, Tramer MR. Does multimodal analgesia with acetaminophen, nonsteroidal antiinflammatory drugs, or selective cyclooxygenase-2 inhibitors and patient-controlled analgesia morphine offer advantages over morphine alone? Meta-analyses of randomized trials. *Anesthesiology* 2005; 103(6):1296–304.
22. Jenkins JG, Khan MM. Anaesthesia for Caesarean section: a survey in a UK region from 1992 to 2002; *Anaesthesia* 2003; 58(11):1114–18.

23. Hawkins JL, Koonin LM, Palmer SK, *et al.* Anesthesia-related deaths during obstetric delivery in the United States, 1979–1990. *Anesthesiology* 1997; 86(2):277–84.
24. Reynolds F. Labour analgesia and the baby: good news is no news. *Int J Obstet Anesth* 2011; 20(1):38–50.
25. Rigg JR, Jamrozik K, Myles PS, *et al.* Epidural anaesthesia and analgesia and outcome of major surgery: a randomised trial. *Lancet* 2002; 359(9314):1276–82.
26. Guay J. The benefits of adding epidural analgesia to general anesthesia: a metaanalysis. *J Anesth* 2006; 20(4):335–40.
27. Cousins MJ, Mather LE. Intrathecal and epidural administration of opioids. *Anesthesiology* 1984; 61(3):276–310.
28. Belzarena SD. Clinical effects of intrathecally administered fentanyl in patients undergoing cesarean section. *Anesth Analg* 1992; 74(5):653–7.
29. Bernards CM, Hill HF. Physical and chemical properties of drug molecules governing their diffusion through the spinal meninges. *Anesthesiology* 1992; 77(4):750–6.
30. Dahl JB, Jeppesen IS, Jørgensen H, *et al.* Intraoperative and postoperative analgesic efficacy and adverse effects of intrathecal opioids in patients undergoing cesarean section with spinal anesthesia: a qualitative and quantitative systematic review of randomized controlled trials. *Anesthesiology* 1999; 91(6):1919–27.
31. Polley LS, Columb MO, Naughton NN, *et al.* Effect of intravenous versus epidural fentanyl on the minimum local analgesic concentration of epidural bupivacaine in labor. *Anesthesiology* 2000; 93(1):122–8.
32. Cohen S, Pantuck CB, Amar D, *et al.* The primary action of epidural fentanyl after cesarean delivery is via a spinal mechanism. *Anesth Analg* 2002; 94(3):674–9
33. Ginosar Y, Columb MO, Cohen SE, *et al.* The site of action of epidural fentanyl infusions in the presence of local anesthetics: a minimum local analgesic concentration infusion study in nulliparous labor. *Anesth Analg* 2003; 97(5):1439–45.
34. Ginosar Y, Riley ET, Angst MS. The site of action of epidural fentanyl in humans: the difference between infusion and bolus administration. *Anesth Analg* 2003; 97(5):1428–38.
35. Bromage PR, Camporesi EM, Durant PA, *et al.* Rostral spread of epidural morphine. *Anesthesiology* 1982; 56(6):431–6.
36. Palmer CM, Emerson S, Volgoropolous D, *et al.* Dose-response relationship of intrathecal morphine for postcesarean analgesia. *Anesthesiology* 1999; 90(2):437–44.
37. Yang T, Breen TW, Archer D, *et al.* Comparison of 0.25 mg and 0.1 mg intrathecal morphine for analgesia after Cesarean section. *Can J Anaesth* 1999; 46(9):856–60.
38. Giovannelli M, Bedforth N, Aitkenhead A. Survey of intrathecal opioid usage in the UK. *Eur J Anaesthesiol* 2008; 25(2):118–22.
39. Hallworth SP, Fernando R, Bell R, *et al.* Comparison of intrathecal and epidural diamorphine for elective caesarean section using a combined spinal-epidural technique. *Br J Anaesth* 1999; 82(2):228–32.
40. Cowan CM, Kendall JB, Barclay PM, *et al.* Comparison of intrathecal fentanyl and diamorphine in addition to bupivacaine for caesarean section under spinal anaesthesia. *Br J Anaesth* 2002; 89(3):452–8.
41. Saravanan S, Robinson AP, Qayoum Dar A, *et al.* Minimum dose of intrathecal diamorphine required to prevent intraoperative supplementation of spinal anaesthesia for Caesarean section. *Br J Anaesth* 2003; 91(3):368–72.
42. Skilton RW, Kinsella SM, Smith A, *et al.* Dose response study of subarachnoid diamorphine for analgesia after elective caesarean section. *Int J Obstet Anesth* 1999; 8(4):231–5.
43. Kelly MC, Carabine UA, Mirakhur RK. Intrathecal diamorphine for analgesia after caesarean section. A dose finding study and assessment of side-effects. *Anaesthesia* 1998; 53(3):231–7.
44. Stacey R, Jones R, Kar G, *et al.* High-dose intrathecal diamorphine for analgesia after Caesarean section. *Anaesthesia* 2001; 56(1):54–60.
45. National Institute of Health and Care Excellence. *Caesarean Section.* Clinical Guideline 132. London: NICE; 2011.
46. Kafl SK. Intrathecal meperidine for elective caesarean section: a comparison with lidocaine. *Can J Anaesth* 1993; 40(8):718–21.
47. Siddik-Sayyid SM, Aouad MT, Jalbout MI, *et al.* Intrathecal versus intravenous fentanyl for supplementation of subarachnoid block during cesarean delivery. *Anesth Analg* 2002; 95(1):209–13.
48. Horlocker TT, Burton AW, Connis RT, *et al.* Practice guidelines for the prevention, detection, and management of respiratory depression associated with neuraxial opioid administration. *Anesthesiology* 2009; 110(2):218–30.
49. Lee JH, Chung KH, Lee JY, *et al.* Comparison of fentanyl and sufentanil added to 0.5% hyperbaric bupivacaine for spinal anesthesia in patients undergoing cesarean section. *Korean J Anesthesiol* 2011; 60(2):103–8.
50. Ngiam SK, Chong JL. The addition of intrathecal sufentanil and fentanyl to bupivacaine for caesarean section. *Singapore Med J* 1998; 39(7):290–4.
51. Dahlgren G, Hultstrand C, Jakobsson J, *et al.* Intrathecal sufentanil, fentanyl, or placebo added to bupivacaine for cesarean section. *Anesth Analg* 1997; 85(6):1288–93.
52. Bernards CM. Recent insights into the pharmacokinetics of spinal opioids and the relevance to opioid selection. *Curr Opin Anaesthesiol* 2004; 17(5):441–7.
53. Bonnet MP, Mignon A, Mazoit JX, *et al.* Analgesic efficacy and adverse effects of epidural morphine compared to parenteral opioids after elective caesarean section: a systematic review. *Eur J Pain* 2010; 14(9):894.e1–9.
54. Palmer CM, Nogami WM, Van Maren G, *et al.* Postcesarean epidural morphine: a dose-response study. *Anesth Analg* 2000; 90(4):887–91.
55. Thomas DA, Williams GM, Iwata K, *et al.* The medullary dorsal horn. A site of action of morphine in producing facial scratching in monkeys. *Anesthesiology* 1993; 79(3):548–54.
56. Ready LB, Loper KA, Nessly M, *et al.* Postoperative epidural morphine is safe on surgical wards. *Anesthesiology* 1991; 75(3):452–6.
57. de Leon-Casasola OA, Parker B, Lema MJ, *et al.* Postoperative epidural bupivacaine-morphine therapy. Experience with 4,227 surgical cancer patients. *Anesthesiology* 1994; 81(2):368–75.
58. Rauck RL, Raj PP, Knarr DC, *et al.* Comparison of the efficacy of epidural morphine given by intermittent injection or continuous infusion for the management of postoperative pain. *Reg Anesth* 1994; 19(5):316–24.
59. Roulson CJ, Bennett J, Shaw M, *et al.* Effect of extradural diamorphine on analgesia after caesarean section under subarachnoid block. *Br J Anaesth* 1993; 71(6):810–3.
60. Eskander WF, Harvey PB, Kestin IG. Subarachnoid diamorphine compared with extradural diamorphine for postoperative pain relief following elective caesarean section. *Int J Obstet Anesth* 1994; 3:173.
61. Bloor GK, Thompson M, Chung N. A randomised, double-blind comparison of subarachnoid and epidural diamorphine for elective caesarean section using a combined spinal-epidural technique. *Int J Obstet Anesth* 2000; 9(4):233–7.
62. Sumida S, Lesley MR, Hanna MN, *et al.* Meta-analysis of the effect of extended-release epidural morphine versus intravenous patient-controlled analgesia on respiratory depression. *J Opioid Manag* 2009; 5(5):301–5.
63. Carvalho B, Roland LM, Chu LF, *et al.* Single-dose, extended-release epidural morphine (DepoDur) compared to conventional epidural morphine for post-cesarean pain. *Anesth Analg* 2007; 105(1):176–83.
64. Hartrick CT, Hartrick KA. Extended-release epidural morphine (DepoDur): review and safety analysis. *Expert Rev Neurother* 2008; 8(11):1641–8.
65. Carvalho B, Riley E, Cohen SE, *et al.* Single-dose, sustained-release epidural morphine in the management of postoperative pain after elective cesarean delivery: results of a multicenter randomized controlled study. *Anesth Analg* 2005; 100(4):1150–8.
66. Gambling DR, Hughes TL, Manvelian GZ. Extended-release epidural morphine (DepoDur) following epidural bupivacaine in patients

undergoing lower abdominal surgery: a randomized controlled pharmacokinetic study. *Reg Anesth Pain Med* 2009; 34(4):316–25.
67. Atkinson Ralls L, Drover DR, Clavijo CF, *et al.* Prior epidural lidocaine alters the pharmacokinetics and drug effects of extended-release epidural morphine (DepoDur(R)) after cesarean delivery. *Anesth Analg* 2011; 113(2):251–8.
68. Chaplan SR, Duncan SR, Brodsky JB, *et al.* Morphine and hydromorphone epidural analgesia. A prospective, randomized comparison. *Anesthesiology* 1992; 77(6):1090–4.
69. Glass PS, Estok P, Ginsberg B, *et al.* Use of patient-controlled analgesia to compare the efficacy of epidural to intravenous fentanyl administration. *Anesth Analg* 1992; 74(3):345–51.
70. Loper KA, Ready LB, Downey M, *et al.* Epidural and intravenous fentanyl infusions are clinically equivalent after knee surgery. *Anesth Analg* 1990; 70(1):72–5.
71. Sandler AN, Stringer D, Panos L, *et al.* A randomized, double-blind comparison of lumbar epidural and intravenous fentanyl infusions for postthoracotomy pain relief. Analgesic, pharmacokinetic, and respiratory effects. *Anesthesiology* 1992; 77(4):626–34.
72. Ellis DJ, Millar WL, Reisner LS. A randomized double-blind comparison of epidural versus intravenous fentanyl infusion for analgesia after cesarean section. *Anesthesiology* 1990; 72(6):981–6.
73. Sevarino FB, McFarlane C, Sinatra RS. Epidural fentanyl does not influence intravenous PCA requirements in the post-caesarean patient. *Can J Anaesth* 1991; 38(4 Pt 1):450–3.
74. Parker RK, White PF. Epidural patient-controlled analgesia: an alternative to intravenous patient-controlled analgesia for pain relief after cesarean delivery. *Anesth Analg* 1992; 75(2):245–51.
75. Parker RK, Sawaki Y, White PF. Epidural patient-controlled analgesia: influence of bupivacaine and hydromorphone basal infusion on pain control after cesarean delivery. *Anesth Analg* 1992; 75(5):740–6.
76. Yarnell RW, Polis T, Reid GN, *et al.* Patient-controlled analgesia with epidural meperidine after elective cesarean section. *Reg Anesth* 1992; 17(6):329–33.
77. Cooper DW, Saleh U, Taylor M, *et al.* Patient-controlled analgesia: epidural fentanyl and i.v. morphine compared after caesarean section. *Br J Anaesth* 1999; 82(3):366–70.
78. Paech MJ, Moore JS, Evans SF. Meperidine for patient-controlled analgesia after cesarean section. Intravenous versus epidural administration. *Anesthesiology* 1994; 80(6):1268–76.
79. Yu PY, Gambling DR. A comparative study of patient-controlled epidural fentanyl and single dose epidural morphine for post-caesarean analgesia. *Can J Anaesth* 1993; 40(5 Pt 1):416–20.
80. Gadsden J, Hart S, Santos AC. Post-cesarean delivery analgesia. *Anesth Analg* 2005; 101(5 Suppl):S62–9.
81. Parris-Piper T. Post caesarean delivery pain management: do not dismiss pethidine. *Int J Obstet Anesth* 2008; 17(1):95–6.
82. Vercauteren M, Vereecken K, La Malfa M, *et al.* Cost-effectiveness of analgesia after Caesarean section. A comparison of intrathecal morphine and epidural PCA. *Acta Anaesthesiol Scand* 2002; 46(1):85–9.
83. Moore RA, Bullingham RE, McQuay HJ, *et al.* Dural permeability to narcotics: in vitro determination and application to extradural administration. *Br J Anaesth* 1982; 54(10):1117–28.
84. Sarvela J, Halonen P, Soikkeli A, *et al.* A double-blinded, randomized comparison of intrathecal and epidural morphine for elective cesarean delivery. *Anesth Analg* 2002; 95(2):436–40.
85. Gourlay GK, Murphy TM, Plummer JL, *et al.* Pharmacokinetics of fentanyl in lumbar and cervical CSF following lumbar epidural and intravenous administration. *Pain* 1989; 38(3):253–9.
86. Negre I, Gueneron JP, Ecoffey C, *et al.* Ventilatory response to carbon dioxide after intramuscular and epidural fentanyl. *Anesth Analg* 1987; 66(8):707–10.
87. Cohen SE, Labaille T, Benhamou D, *et al.* Respiratory effects of epidural sufentanil after cesarean section. *Anesth Analg* 1992; 74(5):677–82.
88. Brockway MS, Noble DW, Sharwood-Smith GH, *et al.* Profound respiratory depression after extradural fentanyl. *Br J Anaesth* 1990; 64(2):243–5.
89. Arai YC, Ogata J, Fukunaga K, *et al.* The effect of intrathecal fentanyl added to hyperbaric bupivacaine on maternal respiratory function during Cesarean section. *Acta Anaesthesiol Scand* 2006; 50(3):364–7.
90. Kafer ER, Brown JT, Scott D, *et al.* Biphasic depression of ventilatory responses to CO2 following epidural morphine. *Anesthesiology* 1983; 58(5):418–27.
91. Abouleish E, Rawal N, Rashad MN. The addition of 0.2 mg subarachnoid morphine to hyperbaric bupivacaine for cesarean delivery: a prospective study of 856 cases. *Reg Anesth* 1991; 16(3):137–40.
92. Horlocker TT, Burton AW, Connis RT, *et al.* Practice guidelines for the prevention, detection, and management of respiratory depression associated with neuraxial opioid administration. *Anesthesiology* 2009; 110(2):218–30.
93. Balki M, Carvalho JC. Intraoperative nausea and vomiting during cesarean section under regional anesthesia. *Int J Obstet Anesth* 2005; 14(3):230–41.
94. Chaney MA. Side effects of intrathecal and epidural opioids. *Can J Anaesth* 1995; 42(10):891–903.
95. Carvalho B, Butwick AJ. Postoperative analgesia: epidural and spinal techniques. In Chestnut DH (ed) *Chestnut's Obstetric Anesthesia: Principles and Practice.* Philadelphia, PA: Elsevier; 2013:594–620.
96. Fuller JG, McMorland GH, Douglas MJ, *et al.* Epidural morphine for analgesia after caesarean section: a report of 4880 patients. *Can J Anaesth* 1990; 37(6):636–40.
97. Kendrick WD, Woods AM, Daly MY, *et al.* Naloxone versus nalbuphine infusion for prophylaxis of epidural morphine-induced pruritus. *Anesth Analg* 1996; 82(3):641–7.
98. Cohen SE, Ratner EF, Kreitzman TR, *et al.* Nalbuphine is better than naloxone for treatment of side effects after epidural morphine. *Anesth Analg* 1992; 75(5):747–52.
99. Slappendel R, Weber EW, Benraad B, *et al.* Itching after intrathecal morphine. Incidence and treatment. *Eur J AnaesthesioL* 2000; 17(10):616–21.
100. Liang CC, Chang SD, Chang YL, *et al.* Postpartum urinary retention after cesarean delivery. *Int J Gynaecol Obstet* 2007; 99(3):229–32.
101. Evron S, Samueloff A, Simon A, *et al.* Urinary function during epidural analgesia with methadone and morphine in post-cesarean section patients. *Pain* 1985; 23(2):135–44.
102. Davies PW, Vallejo MC, Shannon KT, *et al.* Oral herpes simplex reactivation after intrathecal morphine: a prospective randomized trial in an obstetric population. *Anesth Analg* 2005; 100(5):1472–6.
103. Baaj JM, Alsatli RA, Majaj HA, *et al.* Efficacy of ultrasound-guided transversus abdominis plane (TAP) block for postcesarean section delivery analgesia—a double-blind, placebo-controlled, randomized study. *Middle East J Anesthesiol* 2010; 20(6):821–6.
104. Young MJ, Gorlin AW, Modest VE, *et al.* Clinical implications of the transversus abdominis plane block in adults. *Anesthesiol Res Pract* 2012; 2012:731645.
105. McDonnell JG, Curley G, Carney J, *et al.* The analgesic efficacy of transversus abdominis plane block after cesarean delivery: a randomized controlled trial. *Anesth Analg* 2008; 106(1):186–91.
106. Belavy D, Cowlishaw PJ, Howes M, *et al.* Ultrasound-guided transversus abdominis plane block for analgesia after Caesarean delivery. *Br J Anaesth* 2009; 103(5):726–30.
107. Costello JF, Moore AR, Wieczorek PM, *et al.* The transversus abdominis plane block, when used as part of a multimodal regimen inclusive of intrathecal morphine, does not improve analgesia after cesarean delivery. *Reg Anesth Pain Med* 2009; 34(6):586–9.
108. McMorrow RC, Ni Mhuircheartaigh RJ, Ahmed KA, *et al.* Comparison of transversus abdominis plane block vs spinal morphine for pain relief after Caesarean section. *Br J Anaesth* 2011; 106(5):706–12.
109. Singh S, Dhir S, Marmai K, *et al.* Efficacy of ultrasound-guided transversus abdominis plane blocks for post-cesarean delivery analgesia: a double-blind, dose-comparison, placebo-controlled randomized trial. *Int J Obstet Anesth* 2013; 22(3):188–93.

110. Abdallah FW, Adham AM, Chan VW, *et al.* Analgesic benefits of preincisional transversus abdominis plane block for abdominal aortic aneurysm repair. *J Cardiothorac Vasc Anesth* 2013; 27(3):536–8.
111. Kadam VR, Moran JL. Epidural infusions versus transversus abdominis plane (TAP) block infusions: retrospective study. *J Anesth* 2011; 25(5):786–7.
112. Farooq, M, Carey M. A case of liver trauma with a blunt regional anesthesia needle while performing transversus abdominis plane block. *Reg Anesth Pain Med* 2008; 33(3):274–5.
113. Bamigboye AA, Hofmeyr GJ. Local anaesthetic wound infiltration and abdominal nerves block during caesarean section for postoperative pain relief. *Cochrane Database Syst Rev* 2009; 3:CD006954.
114. Lavand'homme PM, Roelants F, Waterloos H, *et al.* Postoperative analgesic effects of continuous wound infiltration with diclofenac after elective cesarean delivery. *Anesthesiology* 2007; 106(6):1220–5.
115. Block BM, Liu SS, Rowlingson AJ, *et al.* Efficacy of postoperative epidural analgesia: a meta-analysis. *JAMA* 2003; 290(18):2455–63.
116. Graham, D, Russell IF. A double-blind assessment of the analgesic sparing effect of intrathecal diamorphine (0.3 mg) with spinal anaesthesia for elective caesarean section. *Int J Obstet Anesth* 1997; 6(4):224–30.
117. Husaini SW, Russell IF. Intrathecal diamorphine compared with morphine for postoperative analgesia after caesarean section under spinal anaesthesia. *Br J Anaesth* 1998; 81(2):135–9.
118. Ballantyne JC, Carr DB, Chalmers TC, *et al.* Postoperative patient-controlled analgesia: meta-analyses of initial randomized control trials. *J Clin Anesth* 1993; 5(3):182–93.
119. Hudcova J, McNicol E, Quah C, *et al.* Patient controlled opioid analgesia versus conventional opioid analgesia for postoperative pain. *Cochrane Database Syst Rev* 2006; 4: CD003348.
120. Howell PR, Gambling DR, Pavy T, *et al.* Patient-controlled analgesia following caesarean section under general anaesthesia: a comparison of fentanyl with morphine. *Can J Anaesth* 1995; 42(1):41–5.
121. Goetzl LM; ACOG Committee on Practice Bulletins-Obstetrics. ACOG Practice Bulletin. Clinical Management Guidelines for Obstetrician-Gynecologists Number 36, July 2002. Obstetric analgesia and anesthesia. *Obstet Gynecol* 2002; 100:177–91.
122. Davis KM, Esposito MA, Meyer BA. Oral analgesia compared with intravenous patient-controlled analgesia for pain after cesarean delivery: a randomized controlled trial. *Am J Obstet Gynecol* 2006; 194(4):967–71.
123. Jakobi P, Weiner Z, Solt I, *et al.* Oral analgesia in the treatment of post-cesarean pain. *Eur J Obstet Gynecol Reprod Biol* 2000; 93(1):61–4.
124. Armstrong SC, Cozza KL. Pharmacokinetic drug interactions of morphine, codeine, and their derivatives: theory and clinical reality, Part II. *Psychosomatics* 2003; 44(6):515–20.
125. Koren G, Cairns J, Chitayat D, *et al.* Pharmacogenetics of morphine poisoning in a breastfed neonate of a codeine-prescribed mother. *Lancet* 2006; 368(9536):704.
126. Willmann S, Edginton AN, Coboeken K, *et al.* Risk to the breast-fed neonate from codeine treatment to the mother: a quantitative mechanistic modeling study. *Clin Pharmacol Ther* 2009; 86(6):634–43.
127. O'Mara K, Gal P, Davanzo C. Treatment of neonatal withdrawal with clonidine after long-term, high-dose maternal use of tramadol. *Ann Pharmacother* 2010; 44(7–8):1342–4.
128. Ollé Fortuny G, Opisso Julia L, Oferil Riera F, *et al.* Ketorolac versus tramadol: comparative study of analgesic efficacy in the postoperative pain in abdominal hysterectomy. *Rev Esp Anestesiol Reanim* 2000; 47(4):162–7.
129. Shahraki AD, Jabalameli M, Ghaedi S. Pain relief after cesarean section: oral methadone vs. intramuscular pethidine. *J Res Med Sci* 2012; 17(2):143–7.
130. Russell T, Mitchell C, Paech MJ, *et al.* Efficacy and safety of intraoperative intravenous methadone during general anaesthesia for caesarean delivery: a retrospective case-control study. *Int J Obstet Anesth* 2013; 22(1):47–51.
131. Schug SA, Sidebotham DA, McGuinnety M, *et al.* Acetaminophen as an adjunct to morphine by patient-controlled analgesia in the management of acute postoperative pain. *Anesth Analg* 1998; 87(2):368–72.
132. Moore A, Collins S, Carroll D, *et al.* Paracetamol with and without codeine in acute pain: a quantitative systematic review. *Pain* 1997; 70(2–3):193–201.
133. Alhashemi JA, Alotaibi QA, Mashaat MS, *et al.* Intravenous acetaminophen vs oral ibuprofen in combination with morphine PCIA after Cesarean delivery. *Can J Anaesth* 2006; 53(12):1200–6.
134. Munishankar B, Fettes P, Moore C, *et al.* A double-blind randomised controlled trial of paracetamol, diclofenac or the combination for pain relief after caesarean section. *Int J Obstet Anesth* 2008; 17(1):9–14.
135. Nauta M, Landsmeer ML, Koren G. Codeine-acetaminophen versus nonsteroidal anti-inflammatory drugs in the treatment of post-abdominal surgery pain: a systematic review of randomized trials. *Am J Surg* 2009; 198(2):256–61.
136. Scholer DW, Ku EC, Boettcher I, *et al.* Pharmacology of diclofenac sodium. *Am J Med* 1986; 80(4B):34–8.
137. Olofsson CI, Legeby MH, Nygårds EB, *et al.* Diclofenac in the treatment of pain after caesarean delivery. An opioid-saving strategy. *Eur J Obstet Gynecol Reprod Biol* 2000; 88(2):143–6.
138. Rorarius MG, Suominen P, Baer GA, *et al.* Diclofenac and ketoprofen for pain treatment after elective caesarean section. *Br J Anaesth* 1993; 70(3):293–7.
139. Dahl V, Hagen IE, Sveen AM, *et al.* High-dose diclofenac for postoperative analgesia after elective caesarean section in regional anaesthesia. *Int J Obstet Anesth* 2002; 11(2):91–4.
140. Mitra S, Khandelwal P, Sehgal A. Diclofenac-tramadol vs. diclofenac-acetaminophen combinations for pain relief after caesarean section. *Acta Anaesthesiol Scand* 2012; 56(6):706–11.
141. Coxib and traditional NSAID Trialists' (CNT) Collaboration, Bhala N, Emberson J, *et al.* Vascular and upper gastrointestinal effects of non-steroidal anti-inflammatory drugs: meta-analyses of individual participant data from randomised trials. *Lancet* 2013; 382(9894):769–79.
142. El-Tahan MR, Warda OM, Yasseen AM, *et al.* A randomized study of the effects of preoperative ketorolac on general anaesthesia for caesarean section. *Int J Obstet Anesth* 2007; 16(3):214–20.
143. Lowder JL, Shackelford DP, Holbert D, *et al.* A randomized, controlled trial to compare ketorolac tromethamine versus placebo after cesarean section to reduce pain and narcotic usage. *Am J Obstet Gynecol* 2003; 189(6):1559–62.
144. Tzeng JI, Mok MS. Combination of intramuscular Ketorolac and low dose epidural morphine for the relief of post-caesarean pain. *Ann Acad Med Singapore* 1994; 23(6 Suppl):10–3.
145. Aldington S, Shirtcliffe P, Weatherall M, *et al.* Increased risk of cardiovascular events with parecoxib/valdecoxib: a systematic review and meta-analysis. *N Z Med J* 2005; 118(1226):U1755.
146. Carvalho B, Chu L, Fuller A, *et al.* Valdecoxib for postoperative pain management after cesarean delivery: a randomized, double-blind, placebo-controlled study. *Anesth Analg* 2006; 103(3):664–70.
147. Derry S, Barden J, McQuay HJ, *et al.* Single dose oral celecoxib for acute postoperative pain in adults. *Cochrane Database Syst Rev* 2008; 4:CD004233.
148. Lee LH, Irwin MG, Lim J, *et al.* The effect of celecoxib on intrathecal morphine-induced pruritus in patients undergoing Caesarean section. *Anaesthesia* 2004; 59(9):876–80.
149. Fong WP, Yang LC, Wu JI, *et al.* Does celecoxib have pre-emptive analgesic effect after Caesarean section surgery? *Br J Anaesth* 2008; 100(6):861–2.
150. Striebel HW, Römer M, Kopf A, *et al.* Patient controlled oral analgesia with morphine. *Can J Anaesth* 1996; 43(7):749–53.
151. Striebel HW, Scheitza W, Philippi W, *et al.* Quantifying oral analgesic consumption using a novel method and comparison with patient-controlled intravenous analgesic consumption. *Anesth Analg* 1998; 86(5):1051–3.

CHAPTER 25

Persistent pain after caesarean delivery and vaginal birth

Patricia Lavand'homme and Fabienne Roelants

Introduction

Acute pain following surgical intervention is one of the most frequent reasons for patients to seek medical care with some suffering chronic pain and long-lasting disabilities. Among the 20% of the US and European population who report chronic non-cancer pain, the majority are female.[1] Studies on sex-gender differences show that females have a higher incidence of severe pain, which is more anatomically diffuse and longer lasting compared to males[2] with the prevalence of visceral pain being more frequent in females. The abdomen (47%) and the perineal region (38%) are often mentioned as sites for persistent postsurgical pain (PPSP) by patients attending pain clinics.[3]

Few studies have examined long-term health outcomes for women after pregnancy.[4] Although childbirth may be considered a natural process, some deliveries need instrumentation and/or surgical intervention. Since caesarean delivery is one of the most common surgical procedures performed, the assessment of persistent pain after childbirth is therefore of significant interest[5] especially since the majority of women will not spontaneously consult a health professional about their chronic pain.[6] Furthermore, the prevention of chronic pain post surgery is currently a challenge for clinicians as an indicator of the quality of healthcare.

This chapter will review the different persistent pain symptoms, which are seen after vaginal and caesarean delivery, their prevalence, and nature. The possible risk factors as well as some preventive and therapeutic measures will also be discussed

The definition of persistent pain after childbirth

If we superimpose the definition of persistent pain after childbirth on that of PPSP,[7] persistent pain after childbirth (vaginal delivery or caesarean delivery) is defined as:

- new pain that has developed after childbirth
- pain that lasts at least 2 months after delivery
- other causes for the pain having been excluded (e.g. infection, malignancy) as well as pain from a condition pre-existing to *or* developing during the pregnancy.

There are some limitations to the application of the definition of PPSP to persistent pain after childbirth. Firstly, so far, few studies designed to find the prevalence of persistent pain after childbirth have met this definition because the majority of them did not exclude pre-existing pain. Secondly, the time frame of 2 months usually considered for PPSP has been strongly debated because the exact duration of the inflammatory process caused by tissue injury still remains undetermined. Actually, some authors consider persistent pain as pain still present beyond 3–6 months (often > 6 months) after tissue damage.[8] Finally, as observed in the context of PPSP, the prevalence of persistent pain after childbirth shows some variability caused by the differences in study design including the criteria used to define patients suffering chronic pain, for example, pain intensity, frequency, and impact on the quality of life.

Outcome of common pain syndromes reported during pregnancy

Chronic pain conditions may exist before pregnancy, as it is not uncommon for women of childbearing age to suffer from chronic pelvic pain, backache, and headaches.

Pelvic pain of visceral origin

Epidemiological data show that 15% of women of reproductive age report chronic pelvic pain defined as non-cyclic pelvic pain of at least 6 months' duration, of sufficient severity to cause functional disability or to lead to medical care.[9] Chronic pelvic pain before pregnancy, that is, pain at ovulation, dysmenorrhea, or level of cramps during a menstrual period, and suspicion of endometriosis or interstitial cystitis can predispose to preterm delivery[10] and often persists after delivery.[11]

Pelvic girdle pain and back pain

Pain may also develop during pregnancy and then persist after delivery. Sacroiliac joint and pelvic girdle pain are frequently reported as well as back pain.[12,13] However, symptoms may greatly vary and individuals are affected to different degrees. The prevalence of low back pain episodes may reach 72–77% during pregnancy.[14] Pelvic girdle pain is also common with an incidence rate of 18–56%. The most frequent complaints are located around the sacroiliac joints (76.6%) and the pubic symphysis (57.2%).[13] The pain usually starts in the first trimester of the first pregnancy and worsens with subsequent pregnancies. As with low back pain, the cause of pelvic girdle pain during pregnancy remains unclear. A large cohort follow-up study in Norway reported the presence of pelvic girdle pain in more than 55% of women during pregnancy with the onset of pain around 17 weeks of gestation.[15] Within 6 months after delivery, 78% of these women had recovered, while 18.5% reported persistent pain at one or two pelvic locations with severe persistent pelvic girdle pain syndrome affecting 0.5% of the women.[15] The recovery rates were lower if women experienced a high level of pain severity at 30 weeks of gestation and 'emotional distress' (as defined in the original paper) during pregnancy.[15] A recent study among women continuing to work during their pregnancy has shown a 43% prevalence of pelvic girdle pain at 12 weeks postpartum.[17] Although the occurrence of back pain or pelvic girdle pain does not affect the outcome of pregnancy, their persistence is often associated with postpartum absence from work, which represents an important socioeconomic problem. Finally, results from a prospective observational cohort have highlighted an incidence of 21% of persistent low back pain developed during pregnancy 2 years after delivery. Patients with persistent low back pain were older, had an earlier onset of severe low back pain symptoms during their pregnancy, and had a higher weight gain, that is, a lower weight loss (inability to reduce weight to their pre-pregnant level) after delivery.[18]

New postdelivery backache is a very frequent complaint expressed by 28–49% of women at 6 months postpartum and by 10–15% at 12 months and later.[19,20] In a prospective study regarding health outcome after delivery, primigravida women who had a caesarean delivery were more likely to report back pain at 6 and 12 months postpartum than women who had a spontaneous vaginal delivery.[20] That finding, however, was not observed in another prospective study showing a prevalence of 11% of back pain at 2 years whatever the mode of delivery.[21] A possible relationship between the use of epidural analgesia during labour and postpartum backache has been questioned but numerous studies do not confirm an increased risk of low back pain after epidural use.[22] According to Breen et al.,[19] the incidence of back pain at 2 months postpartum was unrelated to the use of epidural analgesia and unrelated to the mode of delivery. Predictive factors for back pain included pain during the pregnancy and higher body mass index. Thompson et al.[23] found no statistically significant difference between the use of epidurals or not during labour and backache at 8, 16, and 24 weeks after delivery.

Headaches

Headaches, either primary (migraine, tension headache) or secondary (postdural puncture headache, pregnancy-related hypertensive disorders, intracranial pathology), are frequently reported in the peripartum period making headache one of the most common reason for seeking medical care during the puerperium.[24,25] Primary headaches represent 75% of the postpartum headaches and are 20 times more frequent than postdural puncture headaches. While migraine headaches generally improve during the pregnancy due to a rapid increase of oestrogens, a high rate of migraine recurrence occurs after delivery.

Approximately 30% of mothers experience severe headaches within the first week of delivery.[25] In a large survey questioning women's health after delivery, the incidence increased from 5.7% up to 25.4% between hospital stay and 18 months postpartum.[20] Interestingly, breastfeeding until 6 months postpartum seems to be a protective factor as it significantly reduces migraine recurrence. In a prospective study dedicated to persistent pain after childbirth, Eisenach et al.[26] reported a headache incidence at 6 months of 18% after vaginal delivery and 0% after caesarean delivery. A history of headaches prior to pregnancy seemed to be the most relevant risk factor to present with headaches during the pregnancy and at 8 weeks postpartum.[25] Other risk factors for postpartum headaches include analgesic use surrounding pregnancy, multiparity, shorter pushing during the second stage of labour, and increasing maternal age.[25] Patients who have headaches during their pregnancy are nearly four times more likely to report headaches shortly after delivery and are three times more likely to experience headaches if they receive needle-based neuraxial anaesthesia for delivery pain treatment. However, the presence of headaches during pregnancy or shortly after delivery does not predict persistent headaches at 8 weeks after childbirth.[25]

Key points

- Pelvic pain of visceral origin before pregnancy might predispose to preterm delivery and often persists after childbirth.
- Pelvic girdle pain can start around 17 weeks of pregnancy; its prevalence is 18–56% during pregnancy with an incidence of 18.5% of persistent pain at 6 months postdelivery. Low back pain: 72–75% during pregnancy and 21% persisting 2 years after delivery. Predictive risk factors include older patients, large weight gain, and early onset of severe low back pain during pregnancy.
- Postpartum headaches: primary headaches in 75% of the cases. Usually, migraine headaches improve during the pregnancy but with a high rate of recurrence after delivery (30% within the first week).

Prevalence and characteristics of persistent perineal pain after vaginal delivery

In a large prospective multicentre study, severe acute perineal pain within 36 hours postpartum was present in 10.9% of the women after vaginal delivery while persistent pain at 8 weeks postpartum affected 10% of the women.[27] Patients experiencing severe acute pain after childbirth had a 2.5-fold increased risk of persistent pain and 3.0-fold risk of postpartum depression at 8 weeks postpartum compared with women having mild pain after delivery. In another prospective study, the degree of perineal trauma was responsible for the immediate intensity of pain (from 24 hours until day 7 postpartum), but by 6 weeks postpartum the incidence of perineal pain (around 9%) did not differ among the patients.[28] Therefore, the degree of tissue injury after vaginal birth appears to be independent of the risk to develop persistent pain.[27,28] Studies assessing persistent pain after vaginal delivery have found 2–10% of women with pain at 6 months and later after delivery, almost exclusively in mothers who had an assisted vaginal birth.[21,29,30] The prospective Pain After Delivery (PAD) study reported a much lower prevalence with less than 1% of persistent pain at 1 year.[26]

Two observations, however, need mentioning. First, the nature of persistent pain after vaginal delivery is poorly characterized perhaps because pain complaints localized to perineal areas that are related to sexual function, defaecation, and urination are often considered taboo.[9,31] A survey aimed to determine the prevalence and characteristics of postpartum-onset genital or pelvic pain found 9% of women continuing to experience pain triggered by both sexual and non-sexual activities at 12 months after delivery, with none receiving treatment.[31] Among these women, 90% reported genital pain and 50% pelvic pain, which began at delivery. A survey assessing postpartum sexual dysfunction after delivery demonstrated that 27.6% of women present with late dyspareunia defined as pain during intercourse at 1 year after childbirth.[32] There was no relation between late postpartum dyspareunia and the mode of vaginal delivery, that is, spontaneous versus instrumental delivery, perineal lacerations or episiotomy. Recent publications suggest that women consult specialists in urology or pain medicine because of severe perineal pain and the interval between birth and the consultation is often long (mean interval from genital tract trauma (i.e. childbirth or surgery) to consultation for pain: 8 months, range 3 months to 20 years).[33,34] Difficult labour with a prolonged second stage and assisted vaginal delivery with/without episiotomy are frequently mentioned as the triggering event. Prospective studies also report the presence of deep abdominal, pelvic, and even buttock/leg pain associated with pain in the genital area.[21,26] Secondly, persistent pain after vaginal delivery might be worse than PPSP after caesarean delivery. Slowly resolving inflammatory reaction and scar tissue formation in the perineum, sometimes associated with deep pelvic pain, causes chronic lower genital tract pain, which may have a major impact on daily life. Indeed, around 11–15% of women complain that such persistent pain interferes significantly with their daily life.[35,36] Women not only mention dyspareunia but also complain when walking or sitting. Genital pain is often described as severe pain (i.e. visual analogue scale score ≥6 out of 10) in both intensity (5.6 ± 1.6) and unpleasantness (5.9 ± 1.9).[31] Retrospective data report intense, unbearable pain in 30% of women after vaginal delivery versus similar pain severity in 10% of women at 1 year after caesarean delivery.[30] In the PAD study, persistent pain at 2 months after childbirth is described as constant daily pain in 60% of women who had a vaginal delivery versus 36% of women who experienced caesarean delivery.[27] At 6 months, average worst pain severity was significantly higher after vaginal delivery (pain scores of 4.5 ± 2.7 out of 10 with 73% of these women taking analgesics) than after caesarean delivery (pain scores of 1.8 ± 1.0 out of 10 with 0% analgesics intake).[26] Finally, although the incidence of pain at 12 months was extremely low, it is worth noting that all the women who had pain underwent a vaginal delivery.[26]

Key points

- Incidence of perineal pain after vaginal delivery: 10.9% at 24–48 hours; 1–10% at 2–6 months; less than 1% at 1 year
- The degree of perineal trauma:
  - is responsible for the immediate intensity of the pain (from 24 hours to 7 days after delivery)
  - does not seem to be associated with persistent pain (at 2 months and later)
- Dyspareunia (incidence: 9–27% at 12 months after delivery) is not associated with:
  - mode of vaginal delivery (spontaneous, instrumental delivery)
  - presence of lacerations or episiotomy.

Prevalence and characteristics of persistent pain after caesarean delivery

A majority of studies investigating chronic pain after caesarean delivery are retrospective, including the small original study from Nikolajsen et al.[37] and the large survey 'Listening to Mother II'.[29] These studies report a prevalence after 6 months of approximately 18% of women who complain of pain following their caesarean delivery.[29,30,37] However, the prevalence of disabling pain with a negative impact on the mother's quality of life and on the mother–child relationship is consistently approximately 6% among retrospective studies.[38] Prospective studies are scarce but include a large cohort of patients. Their strength relies on the fact that they focus on 'new' pain related to the surgery and have excluded pre-existing pain. A Canadian study following 917 women with a breech presentation found a persistent pain incidence of 20% at 2 years after caesarean delivery, which reduced to 10% when the pain was restricted to the abdominal wall and within the abdominal cavity but, excluding backache and headache.[21] An Australian cohort survey examining long-term health outcomes after childbirth among 1507 nulliparae reported a similar prevalence of persistent pain in the long term, that is, 8% at 18 months including 1.8% scar pain.[20] Questioning 1228 women, the US PAD study from Eisenach et al.[26] shows an even lower incidence of persistent pain after delivery, as low as 1.8% (95% confidence interval (CI) 1.4–5.3%) at 6 months and 0.3% (95% CI 0.3–1.2%) at 12 months. This study only considered pain that began at delivery and that was not already present before pregnancy nor developed during pregnancy, such as back pain or pelvic girdle pain. Finally, a prospective Australian cohort study including 426 women reports persistent pain at the abdominal wound in 4.2% of women at 12 months after caesarean delivery, with only 1.1% of patients reporting mild constant daily pain.[39] By comparison, the first large study aimed to assess the prevalence of chronic postsurgical pain in a general population reported a prevalence of 18.3% moderate to severe pain in the area of surgery 3–36 months after the procedure.[40] In this survey, 62% of patients had local pain in the area of surgery before surgery. When excluding all these patients from the analysis, 6.2% of patients were left with chronic postsurgical pain. According to a recent meta-analysis, the incidence of persistent pain after gynaecologic surgery (hysterectomy for benign causes) is around 13.7%.[41] By contrast, the very low prevalence of persistent pain observed after childbirth in Eisenach et al.'s[26] and Liu et al.'s studies[39] is intriguing. However, only those subjects who reported pain at 2 months after delivery were followed-up at 6 months, and similarly, only those who reported pain at 6 months were contacted at 12 months.[5] Such follow-up assumes that chronic postsurgical pain is a continuum from acute postoperative pain, an assumption which may be far from the reality. Indeed, other surgical procedures suggest that persistent postsurgical pain may develop later, that is, within the first months as found after inguinal hernia repair and thoracotomy.[42] A recent study assessing persistent pain and sensory disturbances after surgery for breast cancer demonstrated that persistent pain is not static but seems to fluctuate considerably over time.[43] Therefore, the PAD study might have missed some patients who developed neuropathic pain later than within the first 2 months after surgery. Similarly, very little is known about the evolution of visceral pain and deep abdominal pain resulting from a uterine scar or pelvic adherences should not be excluded (Table 25.1).

Table 25.1 Prevalence of pain after caesarean delivery compared with other surgical procedures

	Severe acute pain (<36 hours)	Sub-acute pain (at 2 months)	Persistent pain (>6 months)	Neuropathic component in persistent pain
Caesarean delivery	17%	9% (9–16%)	0.3–1.8% (4–10%)	53–60%
Hysterectomy (non-malignant)	–	–	4.8% (13.7%)	19%
Inguinal hernia	–	14%	7% (2.5–19%)	31–45%
All procedures (general adult population)	30%	–	6.2% (18.3%)	24.5%

Percentages in brackets are found in retrospective studies; other percentages were determined in prospective studies and/or concern new pain directly related to the surgical procedure.

References are in the text.

The nature of persistent postsurgical pain is still unclear in many cases because inflammatory mechanisms play an important role even in the development of neuropathic pain.[8] Recent arguments are in favour of a predominant neuropathic origin as there is a strong association between sensory disturbances such as hypoesthesia and hyperesthesia and the presence and the intensity of chronic postsurgical pain;[40] some surgical procedures appear to carry a higher risk than others.[41] After caesarean delivery, pain may result from nerve entrapment, caesarean scar problems, or pelvic adhesions.[44] In other words, scar pain (i.e. neuropathic pain) and deep intra-abdominal pain (i.e. visceral pain) may develop and even coexist. Retrospective studies usually mention pain as located at the site of (or very close to) the surgical incision.[29,30,37] In the prospective studies, deep intra-abdominal pain and pelvic pain are also reported although pain in the area of incision seems to dominate.[21,26] A Pfannenstiel incision is commonly used for caesarean delivery; its advantages include a low incidence of incisional hernia and an aesthetic scar. However, the risk of ilio-inguinal and ilio-hypogastric nerve entrapment related to the technique is real; up to 32% of women who have undergone obstetric or gynaecologic procedures with a Pfannenstiel incision report PPSP at incision site up to 2 years after surgery (7% suffering severe pain).[45] Few studies have used adequate screening tools to characterize abdominal pain after caesarean delivery. Bollag et al.[46] have found persistent pain as predominantly neuropathic in 56%, 50%, and 26% of the patients at 3, 6, and 12 months after caesarean delivery, respectively. The French study 'EDONIS',[47,48] a prospective epidemiological study, aimed to assess the prevalence and possible neuropathic character of postsurgical pain mentions a 6-month cumulative incidence of persistent pain after caesarean delivery of approximately 20%, with an established neuropathic origin in 61% of the cases. It is interesting to note that the reported pain intensity was generally low (pain score > 3/10 in only 2% of the patients). The low intensity of neuropathic pain diagnosed after caesarean delivery is intriguing. According to the EDONIS results, neuropathic pain following other procedures (e.g. breast surgery, thoracotomy, and varicose vein surgery) is perceived as much more painful.[47,48] Furthermore, in the literature, chronic pain of neuropathic origin is usually associated with higher pain intensity (average pain scores of approximately 7–8/10) than non-neuropathic chronic pain.[49] In other published studies as well, more than 85% of patients with persistent pain at 6 months after caesarean delivery rated their pain as low (average pain score of 2/10),[21,26,30,39] including the affective descriptors associated with the pain experience.[46]

As previously highlighted, childbirth may cause persistent pain located in the pelvic area and/or the deep abdomen. Chronic pelvic pain is a common gynaecological problem which concerns 15–24% of women of reproductive age.[9,50] Chronic pelvic pain is defined by the American College of Obstetricians and Gynecologists as non-cyclic pelvic pain localized in the lower abdomen, anatomical pelvis, lumbosacral back, or buttocks, present for at least 6 months, and which is of sufficient severity to cause functional disability or lead to medical care.[9] According to the prospective studies published to date, persistent pelvic pain and deep abdominal pain may occur independent of the type of delivery, that is, vaginal or caesarean delivery. In the PAD study, among the few women reporting persistent pain at 6 months after childbirth, 53% mention a pelvic pain location and 24% a deep intra-abdominal pain, whatever the type of delivery.[26] Two other large surveys which have examined persistent health problems after childbirth report a 6–10% incidence of persistent pelvic and deep intra-abdominal pain at 12 months and later after either vaginal or caesarean delivery.[20,21] Not surprisingly, in women undergoing a laparoscopy for diagnostic investigation of chronic pelvic pain, among risk factors like pelvic inflammatory diseases and endometriosis, a history of caesarean delivery may be found as the aetiology in 67% of the cases (odds ratio (OR) 3.7).[51] Otherwise, previous caesarean delivery is also an established risk factor for PPSP after hysterectomy for a benign indication (OR 1.5).[50]

Key points

- Persistent pain after caesarean delivery is uncommon (incidence at 6 months and later, 0.3–1.8%) compared to the rate of PPSP observed after other surgical procedures in a general adult population (average incidence 6.2–18%).
- Although visceral pain, that is, pelvic pain and deep intra-abdominal pain, is also reported after caesarean delivery, the nature of persistent pain is neuropathic (abdominal wall pain) in more than 50% of the cases with a very low intensity which contrasts with the severity of neuropathic pain usually reported by the patients after other surgical procedures.
- A history of caesarean delivery is a risk factor for the development of chronic pelvic pain as well as for PPSP after hysterectomy for non-malignant indication.

Risk factors for persistent pain after childbirth

Predictive factors for PPSP can be surgery specific, that is, related to tissue trauma, or patient specific.[8] Some studies have tried to predict the risk factors for severe acute pain after delivery, either by vaginal or caesarean delivery. Principal predictors for severe acute postdelivery pain revealed in the PAD study were history

Table 25.2 Risk factors involved in the development of acute and persistent pain after childbirth

	Incidence (%)	Risk factors
Severe acute pain (< 36h postpartum)	CD: 17 VD: 10	History of pain during pregnancy Intensity of menstruation pain Tissue damage caused by delivery Presence of mechanical hyperalgesia surrounding the scar (central sensitization caused by a previous CD)
Pain at 8 weeks	CD: 9.2 VD: 10	Severity of acute postpartum pain, i.e. individual pain response to injury
Pain at 6 months	CD and VD: 1.8	Not identified (small sample size)
Pain at 12 months	CD and VD: 0.3	Not identified (small sample size)

CD, caesarean delivery; VD, vaginal delivery.

Data from Eisenach JC *et al.*, Severity of acute pain after childbirth, but not type of delivery, predicts persistent pain and postpartum depression, *Pain*, Volume 140, pp. 87–94, Copyright © 2008 Elsevier and Bollag L *et al.*, Effect of transversus abdominis plane block with and without clonidine on post-cesarean delivery wound hyperalgesia and pain, *Regional Anesthesia and Pain Medicine*, volume 37, pp. 508–514, Copyright © 2012 Wolters Kluwer Health.

of pain during the pregnancy (relative risk 0.70), pain during menstruation (relative risk 0.44), and giving birth by caesarean delivery (relative risk 1.08).[27] Regarding chronic pain, the low incidence of persistent pain found in prospective studies make further analysis of the potential risk factors difficult (Table 25.2).[26]

Surgery- and tissue damage-specific risk factors

Mode of delivery: caesarean versus vaginal delivery, spontaneous versus assisted vaginal delivery

As the rate of caesarean delivery is increasing worldwide for both medical indications and maternal choice, an important debate is now arising over the relationship of the method of delivery to maternal postpartum physical health.[29,44] Three large prospective studies published to date did not find differences in maternal pain outcomes at 12 months and beyond postpartum between caesarean and vaginal delivery.[20,21,26] In the context of vaginal childbirth, the degree of tissue injury appears to be independent of the risk of persistent pain as the extent of perineal trauma was responsible for the immediate intensity of pain (from 24 hours until day 7 postpartum), but by 6–8 weeks postpartum, the incidence of perineal pain did not differ among the patients.[27,28] Finally, retrospective studies indicate no correlation between the mode of birth and persistent pain including late dyspareunia at 12 months after delivery.[31,32,35]

Elective versus emergency caesarean delivery

One might hypothesize that having an unplanned caesarean delivery could increase the risk of reporting persistent pain as the risk of abdominal wall nerve injury may be higher during emergency procedures.[45] Furthermore, the depth of anaesthesia provided by either general anaesthesia or epidural anaesthesia, two techniques commonly used in cases of non-elective caesarean delivery, might be less effective to prevent nociceptive inputs to reach and to sensitize the central nervous system than spinal anaesthesia usually used in elective procedures.[52] Although an earlier study by Nikolajsen et al.[37] found that patients with persistent pain had more often undergone the procedure under general anaesthesia than spinal anaesthesia (37% versus 17.1% persistent pain at 10 months), a recent prospective study did not find an apparent increase in incidence of persistent pain associated with general versus neuraxial anaesthesia.[39] Furthermore, no published study so far either retrospective[35,36] or prospective[39] mentions emergency caesarean delivery as a significant risk factor for persistent pain by comparison with an elective procedure. Interestingly a trial of vaginal birth has not been associated with an increased risk of developing persistent pain after previous caesarean delivery.[35,36]

Extent of tissue damage during caesarean delivery

Surgical factors such as operative technique have also been investigated. Closure of the parietal peritoneum is currently debated as this technique not only seems to increase acute postpartum pain but also to enhance the risk of persistent discomfort at 8 months after surgery.[53] The type of incision (i.e. vertical or Pfannenstiel incision) only has an impact on acute pain and does not affect persistent pain.[35,36] Most of the procedures are performed via a Pfannenstiel incision which carries a risk of injury of the lower abdominal wall nerves, with a risk of developing chronic neuropathic pain.[45] Neuropathic pain is frequently involved in persistent pain after caesarean delivery but the reported pain intensity is surprisingly low by comparison with that of neuropathic pain observed in other PPSP. It is worth noting that, not all lesions in the somatosensory system lead to neuropathic pain.[42] Persistent sensory dysfunction can be highlighted in pain-free postsurgical patients (e.g. 20% after hernia repair[54]). Individual related co-factors such as poor capacity of nerve regeneration, decreased pain tolerance related to altered endogenous pain processes, and particular psychological profile play a major role in the development of persistent neuropathic pain after a peripheral nerve lesion.[55]

Patient-specific risk factors for persistent pain after childbirth

The fact that the degree of tissue trauma by itself (e.g. caesarean delivery versus vaginal delivery, and peripheral nerve damage) is not a risk factor to develop persistent pain suggests that some individuals may be predisposed to the development of persistent pain. To support this, the recent literature on PPSP, specifically the research on the transition from acute to chronic postsurgical pain, has moved from general risk factors such as gender, age, obesity, and so on to more individualized risk factors.[42,56–58] This view is confirmed by recent studies aiming to develop a risk index for the prediction of chronic postsurgical pain.[59]

Severe early postpartum pain as an individual risk factor

Poorly relieved acute pain is commonly mentioned as a striking risk factor for PPSP and severe acute pain is involved in the transition from acute to chronic pain.[4,8] It is still unclear why acute pain severity may increase the risk for PPSP: the risk may be due either to an increased individual susceptibility to develop both acute and chronic pain condition or to the fact that inadequately managed postoperative pain itself enhances the risk to develop persistent pain. Whatever the mode of delivery, several retrospective studies mention that patients with persistent pain recalled severe acute postpartum pain.[35,37,60] However, all of these studies may suffer major recall bias. Otherwise, the conclusions of two prospective studies, the PAD study and the study from Liu et al.,[39] do not support that finding. Severe acute postpartum pain concerns 17% and 13% of women within the first 36 hours of caesarean and vaginal delivery respectively, and caesarean delivery is associated with a 32.5% increase in acute pain scores by comparison with vaginal delivery.[27] However, acute pain severity, independent of the type of delivery, only predicted an 2.5-fold increase in the risk of persistent pain at 2 months (incidence 10%) but not later (incidence 0.3–1.8%).[26,27]

Pre-existing chronic pain condition as an individual risk factor

Preoperative pain found in more than 50% of patients undergoing surgery,[40,61] either at the operative site or elsewhere, is one of the most consistent patient-related factors for both severe postoperative pain and PPSP.[4,58,59] Both the presence of a chronic pain condition and the potential regular intake of analgesics may contribute to sensitize the central nervous system and so may favour pain chronicity after tissue injury.[62] All the retrospective studies on chronic pain after childbirth mention the presence of pain elsewhere as a major risk factor for the development of persistent pain after delivery with an OR even superior to that related to the recall of intense acute postdelivery pain (OR 2.5 vs 1.3).[60] In the initial study from Nikolajsen et al.,[37] the occurrence of pain problems elsewhere was reported by 63% of the patients with persistent pain (versus 19% in patients without pain). Kainu et al.[35] also mention chronic pain after childbirth as significantly more common in women with previous pain or any chronic disease (22% versus 12%). In the study by Paterson et al.,[31] only a history of non-genital chronic pain was significantly correlated with persistent postpartum-onset genital pain. The large prospective study, the PAD study,[26] mentions pain history predictors such as pain during pregnancy and pain ratings during menstruation as risk factors for postpartum pain at 24 hours but not later. It is noteworthy that the very low incidence of pain at 6 months later precluded further statistical analysis. Beyond the aforementioned findings, clinical observations show that patients reporting pelvic pain often suffer from more than one pain, that raises the question of potential alterations of endogenous pain modulatory mechanisms rather than only local organ-based mechanisms.[9]

Hyperalgesia, central sensitization, and altered endogenous pain processing as individual risk factors

Nociceptive inputs from injured tissues trigger a prolonged and usually reversible increased state of nervous system hyperexcitability referred to as central sensitization.[63] This amplification of neural signalling within the central nervous system elicits pain hypersensitivity, which translates into clinical hyperalgesia, mainly evoked by mechanical stimuli. Sustained central sensitization is thought to be one of the mechanisms underlying the development of persistent pain after injury. Secondary hyperalgesia (i.e. mechanical hypersensitivity in uninjured tissues surrounding the wound) has caught particular attention as a surrogate measure of central sensitization after surgery.[64,65] The extent of secondary hyperalgesia may correlate with the risk for PPSP as demonstrated after major abdominal surgery. However, all individuals presenting with secondary mechanical hyperalgesia at 24–48 hours after surgery will not develop PPSP.[42] In humans, clinical data on the incidence, extent, and duration of postoperative secondary hyperalgesia are scarce as this objective parameter is rarely assessed.[62] Moreover, the correlation between postoperative secondary hyperalgesia and the risk of persistent pain is even less frequently investigated. After caesarean delivery with a Pfannenstiel incision, 10–30% of the patients presented with secondary mechanical hyperalgesia surrounding the wound within the first 48 hours[46,66] while less than 15% of the patients reported persistent pain at 3 months and later. In a different study, at 6 weeks postdelivery, the incidence of persistent pain was 16% but that of secondary mechanical hyperalgesia was only 8%.[67] The prospective study from Liu et al.[39] shows that a history of previous caesarean delivery is not a risk factor for persistent pain. Ortner et al.[68] were the first to assess the presence of hyperalgesia surrounding the scar of a previous caesarean delivery in women who came to undergo repeat caesarean delivery. Scar hyperalgesia was present in 41% of the women, at 22 months and later after a previous caesarean section. These women had overall higher acute postoperative pain scores for both somatic pain and visceral cramping pain. Although the later study did not examine the development of persistent pain, it demonstrates that pre-existing hyperalgesia (i.e. a sign of central sensitization) correlated with enhanced acute postoperative pain. Similar findings also exist with hysterectomy where preoperative pain sensitization as reflected by cutaneous and vaginal hypersensitivity was associated with acute pain severity but less predictive to persistent pain.[69]

The preoperative assessment of pain sensitivity may predict to some extent the degree of postoperative pain and the probability to develop persistent pain.[70] Nociceptive signals from damaged tissues undergo a central modulation leading to either attenuation or enhancement of pain. Recent interesting developments have focused on dynamic test paradigms—in contrast with static tests like pain threshold—designed to measure endogenous pain processing and to depict individuals' pain modulation capacity.[57,71] Inter-individual differences in the modulation of endogenous pain perception and modulation place patients at more or less risk to present with severe acute pain or chronic pain.[56] As a consequence, the mechanisms involved in central sensitization, which result from the balance between endogenous inhibitory and excitatory processes, may differ among patients. Although human studies are still scarce, they seem to indicate that patients who display central hyperexcitability or impaired endogenous modulation would be more prone to have a poor outcome after a surgical procedure as found after thoracotomy[72] or major abdominal surgery.[73] Hyperexcitability of endogenous pain processes can be assessed by temporal summation, a surrogate measure of wind-up pain, defined as increased pain from repetitive tactile stimulation.[74] The presence of a positive temporal summation is highly suggestive of an altered central nociceptive processing. As a matter of fact, the presence of a preoperative temporal summation has been associated with enhanced postoperative pain after thoracotomy,[75] abdominal surgery,[76] and also caesarean delivery.[68] In the later study, the authors also found a positive correlation between the presence of a preoperative scar hyperalgesia and a preoperative positive mechanical temporal summation in women undergoing a repeat caesarean delivery.[68] It is important to note that, beyond its association with postoperative pain intensity, temporal summation might also be predictive of a risk for persistent pain after surgery or trauma as it predicted a poor outcome after spine injury.[77] Also, after herniorrhaphy, mechanical temporal summation was found in 51% of PPSP patients but only in 15% (and at low intensity) in pain-free patients.[54,78] Studies aiming to assess the function of endogenous pain processes during pregnancy and in the immediate postpartum period are currently ongoing.[79]

Psychosocial vulnerability as individual risk factors

Mental health has an important impact on the patient's willingness to recover. Psychological mechanisms of pain processing (emotion and when pain is perceived as a threat) already known to play a role in chronic pain conditions have recently attracted interest in trauma and perioperative conditions.[42] Obviously, there is a vulnerable population who present with a reduced ability to cope with pain, to anticipate pain, and to control pain when confronted with it. Pain hypervigilance[80] and catastrophization are currently investigated as important mental states to predict both severe postoperative pain and PPSP. In the context of childbirth, their impact may extend beyond the trauma period as, for example, catastrophization not only plays a role in the experience of pain during labour and delivery but also compromises social functioning and recovery after delivery.[81,82] A novel emergent concept is the relation between persistent pain and post-traumatic stress symptoms, and emotional numbing, observed after some trauma or surgical procedures.[42,58] Traumatic birth experiences may be associated with postpartum psychological impairment that could favour persistent pain. As an example, late postpartum dyspareunia seems to be linked more with the mother's experience of childbirth (low satisfaction with delivery) than with perineal trauma.[32]

Genetic predisposition as an individual risk factor

Over the last few years, major developments in genomic research have shown how genetic variability may affect not only the response to medications including analgesics but also may account for the side effects of the medication. An actual challenge would be to find 'pain genes' allowing to identify individuals with an increased vulnerability to pain and genes which confer an increased risk of developing intense acute pain and chronic pain after tissue injury.[42,58,83] To date, a few reports have identified polymorphisms in human genes associated with some chronic pain conditions. However, none of these genes have been identified as specific markers for the generation of persistent pain after surgery or tissue trauma related to childbirth.[84] Persistent pain after childbirth like PPSP is multifaceted, characterized by multiple sensory-discriminative, affective-emotive, and cognitive variables. By consequence, translating pharmacogenetics into clinical practice is and will remain particularly challenging.[42,58] Nevertheless, several investigators are currently assessing pain modulation tests in combination with genetics to predict an individual's risk of developing persistent pain after tissue trauma.[79,83]

Key points

- The extent of tissue damage, that is, mode of delivery, influences intensity of acute postpartum pain within the first week but not later.
- Other risk factors such as elective versus emergency caesarean delivery, trial of vaginal birth, or history of previous caesarean delivery have not been associated with an increased risk of developing persistent pain.
- An individual's pain response seems to be the most relevant factor in the development of persistent pain.
- In retrospective studies, patient-specific risk factors, for example, pre-existing chronic pain conditions or pain elsewhere as well as severity of immediate postpartum pain, were predictive of an increased risk of persistent pain after childbirth.
- Psychosocial vulnerability and genetic factors might be involved but further studies are needed.

Does childbirth have a protective mechanism against pain?

Lower incidence of persistent pain after delivery, independent of the degree of tissue injury, by comparison with common surgical procedures, questions whether it might not be due to protective biological or psychosocial factors occurring during the puerperium.[26] Some experimental data support that hypothesis by demonstrating a reversal of hypersensitivity induced by peripheral nerve injury in rats during the postpartum period but not during the pregnancy itself.[85] First, endogenous oxytocin might exert protective effects by spinal inhibitory modulation of pain transmission and/or central modulation of the negative emotional experience related to pain at the supraspinal level (i.e. in the amygdale).[85] Increased postpartum oxytocin levels have been associated with elevated mood and decreased anxiety.[86] Second, the puerperium also seems to alter endogenous pain processes in favour of an inhibitory balance as the density of spinal noradrenergic inhibitory fibres increases following nerve injury in the postpartum period.[87]

Prevention and management of persistent pain after childbirth

Although the prevalence of persistent pain after childbirth seems to be low, for the women who suffer persistent pain, this significantly affects their quality of life and also interferes with the mother–child bonding relationship. It is interesting to point out that a majority of women do not consult a health professional even if they feel that they need advice.[6] Furthermore, there is still a lack of education regarding pain relief in the postpartum period. There may be inadequate analgesic intake during the breastfeeding period for which both the caregivers and the mothers must take responsibility.

As 'prevention is better than cure', the evidence favours a preventive approach. However, very few studies have been designed to examine the possibility that PPSP can be prevented or attenuated.[58] In the context of obstetrics, peripartum administration of intravenous magnesium sulphate,[67] ketamine,[88] oral gabapentin,[89] and spinal clonidine[66] have failed to prevent the development of persistent pain after caesarean delivery. It is worth noting that these preventive treatments have been administered to all the women without any attempt of individualization which might explain the lack of effect observed.[42]

In a more practical way, the extent of tissue injury during childbirth (e.g. a nerve injury) accounts for the intensity of acute postpartum pain and might cause persistent pain in predisposed patients. Consequently, as a first-line preventive measure, the obstetrician should ensure the least traumatic delivery possible. More importantly, obstetricians and all care providers should offer any patient the opportunity to contact them in case of any postpartum problem. If dealing with pain postpartum, the patients might be directed as soon as possible to an obstetric anaesthetist in the first instance, then if pain persists, to a pain specialist.[90] After tissue injury, the subacute pain period remains a grey zone which however might play an important role in the chronicity of the pain.[42] Finally, it should be pointed out that the use of systemic analgesics is restricted in breastfeeding women due to the concerns about the excretion of drugs in the breast milk and hence the potential toxicity for the infant. Therefore, if indicated, local analgesic treatments will be preferable, for example, scar infiltration of the abdominal wall,[91] intravaginal injection,[33] or pudendal block,[92] using a combination of corticosteroids and local anaesthetics. Beyond their diagnostic value, these nerve blocks may provide long-term pain relief in some patients. In case of intractable persistent pain caused by a nerve entrapment, the surgical neurectomy may represent an effective solution.[90,91]

Conclusion

Excluding pre-existing pain or pain which developed during pregnancy, prospective studies show a surprisingly low prevalence of persistent pain after childbirth, much lower than the prevalence reported in retrospective studies and that of PPSP in a general population for similar procedures. The nature of persistent pain itself remains poorly characterized, particularly after vaginal delivery, and seems predominantly neuropathic after caesarean delivery but with a lower intensity than usually reported for chronic neuropathic pain. Finally, the fact that the type of delivery and the degree of tissue trauma do not seem to impact on the risk to develop persistent pain seems to suggest that individual factors may place people at risk for persistent pain, and furthermore, that protective mechanisms may occur during the peripartum as demonstrated in experimental studies.

References

1. Breivik H, Collett B, Ventafridda V, *et al.* Survey of chronic pain in Europe: prevalence, impact on daily life, and treatment. *Eur J Pain* 2006; 10:287–333.
2. Hurley RW, Adams MC. Sex, gender, and pain: an overview of a complex field. *Anesth Analg* 2008; 107:309–17.
3. Crombie IK, Davies HT, Macrae WA. Cut and thrust: antecedent surgery and trauma among patients attending a chronic pain clinic. *Pain* 1998; 76:167–71.
4. Kehlet H, Jensen TS, Woolf CJ. Persistent postsurgical pain: risk factors and prevention. *Lancet* 2006; 367:1618–25.
5. Flood P, Wong CA. Chronic pain secondary to childbirth: does it exist? *Anesthesiology* 2013; 118:16–18.
6. Schytt E, Lindmark G, Waldenstrom U. Physical symptoms after childbirth: prevalence and associations with self-rated health. *BJOG* 2005; 112:210–17.
7. Macrae WA. Chronic post-surgical pain: 10 years on. *Br J Anaesth* 2008; 101:77–86.
8. Schug S, Pogatzki-Zahn E. Chronic pain after surgery or injury. *Pain Clin Updates* 2011; XIX:1–5.
9. Wesselmann U. Chronic pelvic and urogenital pain syndromes. *Pain Clin Updates* 2008; XVI:1–4.
10. Bayram C, Osmanagaoglu MA, Aran T, *et al.* The effect of chronic pelvic pain scoring on pre-term delivery rate. *J Obstet Gynaecol* 2013; 33:32–7.
11. Driul L, Bertozzi S, Londero AP, *et al.* Risk factors for chronic pelvic pain in a cohort of primipara and secondipara at one year after delivery: association of chronic pelvic pain with autoimmune pathologies. *Minerva Ginecol* 2012; 63:181–7.
12. Mogren IM, Pohjanen AI. Low back pain and pelvic pain during pregnancy: prevalence and risk factors. *Spine* 2005; 30:983–91.
13. Rost CC, Jacqueline J, Kaiser A, *et al.* Pelvic pain during pregnancy: a descriptive study of signs and symptoms of 870 patients in primary care. *Spine* 2004; 29:2567–72.
14. Mogren IM. BMI, pain and hyper-mobility are determinants of long-term outcome for women with low back pain and pelvic pain during pregnancy. *Eur Spine J* 2006; 15:1093–102.
15. Bjelland EK, Stuge B, Engdahl B, *et al.* The effect of emotional distress on persistent pelvic girdle pain after delivery: a longitudinal population study. *BJOG* 2013; 120:32–40.
16. Albert H, Godskesen M, Westergaard J. Evaluation of clinical tests used in classification procedures in pregnancy-related pelvic joint pain. *Eur Spine J* 2000; 9:161–6.
17. Stomp-van den Berg SG, Hendriksen IJ, Bruinvels DJ, *et al.* Predictors for postpartum pelvic girdle pain in working women: the Mom@Work cohort study. *Pain* 2012; 153:2370–9.
18. To WW, Wong MW. Factors associated with back pain symptoms in pregnancy and the persistence of pain 2 years after pregnancy. *Acta Obstet Gynecol Scand* 2003; 82:1086–91.
19. Breen TW, Ransil BJ, Groves PA, *et al.* Factors associated with back pain after childbirth. *Anesthesiology* 1994; 81:29–34.
20. Woolhouse H, Perlen S, Gartland D, *et al.* Physical health and recovery in the first 18 months postpartum: does cesarean section reduce long-term morbidity? *Birth* 2012; 39:221–9.
21. Hannah ME, Whyte H, Hannah WJ, *et al.* Maternal outcomes at 2 years after planned cesarean section versus planned vaginal birth for breech presentation at term: the international randomized Term Breech Trial. *Am J Obstet Gynecol* 2004; 191:917–27.
22. Macarthur A, Macarthur C, Weeks S, Epidural anaesthesia and low back pain after delivery: a prospective cohort study. *BMJ* 1995; 311:1336–9.
23. Thompson JF, Roberts CL, Currie M, *et al.* Prevalence and persistence of health problems after childbirth: associations with parity and method of birth. *Birth* 2002; 29:83–94.
24. Gennaro S, Bloch JR. Postpartum health in mothers of term and preterm infants. *Women Health* 2005; 41:99–112.
25. Turner DP, Smitherman TA, Eisenach JC, *et al.* Predictors of headache before, during, and after pregnancy: a cohort study. *Headache* 2012; 52:348–62.
26. Eisenach JC, Pan P, Smiley RM, *et al.* Resolution of pain after childbirth. *Anesthesiology* 2013; 118:143–51.
27. Eisenach JC, Pan PH, Smiley R, *et al.* Severity of acute pain after childbirth, but not type of delivery, predicts persistent pain and postpartum depression. *Pain* 2008; 140:87–94.
28. Macarthur AJ, Macarthur C. Incidence, severity, and determinants of perineal pain after vaginal delivery: a prospective cohort study. *Am J Obstet Gynecol* 2004; 191:1199–204.
29. Declercq E, Cunningham DK, Johnson C, *et al.* Mothers' reports of postpartum pain associated with vaginal and cesarean deliveries: results of a national survey. *Birth* 2008; 35:16–24.

30. Kainu JP, Sarvela J, Tiippana E, *et al.* Persistent pain after caesarean section and vaginal birth: a cohort study. *Int J Obstet Anesth* 2010; 19(1):4–9.
31. Paterson LQ, Davis SN, Khalife S, *et al.* Persistent genital and pelvic pain after childbirth. *J Sex Med* 2009; 6:215–21.
32. Fauconnier A, Goltzene A, Issartel F, *et al.* Late post-partum dyspareunia: does delivery play a role? *Prg Urol* 2012; 22:225–32.
33. Doumouchtsis SK, Boama V, Gorti M, *et al.* Prospective evaluation of combined local bupivacaine and steroid injections for the management of chronic vaginal and perineal pain. *Arch Gynecol Obstet* 2011; 284:681–5.
34. Vancaillie T, Eggermont J, Amstrong G, *et al.* Response to pudendal nerve block in women with pudendal neuralgia. *Pain Med* 2012; 13:596–603.
35. Kainu JP, Sarvela J, Tiippana E, *et al.* Persistent pain after caesarean section and vaginal birth: a cohort study. *Int J Obstet Anesth* 2010; 19:4–9.
36. Declercq E, Cunningham DK, Johnson C, *et al.* Mothers' reports of postpartum pain associated with vaginal and cesarean deliveries: results of a national survey. *Birth* 2008; 35:16–24.
37. Nikolajsen L, Sorensen HC, Jensen TS, *et al.* Chronic pain following Caesarean section. *Acta Anaesthesiol Scand* 2004; 48:111–16.
38. Vermelis JM, Wassen MM, Fiddelers AA, *et al.* Prevalence and predictors of chronic pain after labor and delivery. *Curr Opin Anaesthesiol* 2010; 23:295–9.
39. Liu TT, Raju A, Boesel T, *et al.* Chronic pain after caesarean delivery: an Australian cohort. *Anaesth Intensive Care* 2013; 41:496–500.
40. Johansen A, Romundstad L, Nielsen CS, *et al.* Persistent postsurgical pain in a general population: prevalence and predictors in the Tromso study. *Pain* 2012; 153:1390–6.
41. Haroutiunian S, Nikolajsen L, Finnerup NB, *et al.* The neuropathic component in persistent postsurgical pain: a systematic literature review. *Pain* 2013; 154:95–102.
42. Lavand'homme P. The progression from acute to chronic pain. *Curr Opin Anaesthesiol* 2011; 24:545–50.
43. Mejdahl MK, Andersen KG, Gartner R, *et al.* Persistent pain and sensory disturbances after treatment for breast cancer: six year nationwide follow-up study. *BMJ* 2013; 346:f1865.
44. Silver R. Delivery after previous Cesarean: long-term maternal outcomes. *Semin Perinatol* 2010; 34:258–66.
45. Loos MJ, Scheltinga MR, Mulders LG, *et al.* The Pfannenstiel incision as a source of chronic pain. *Obstet Gynecol* 2008; 111:839–46.
46. Bollag L, Richebe P, Siaulys M, *et al.* Effect of transversus abdominis plane block with and without clonidine on post-cesarean delivery wound hyperalgesia and pain. *Reg Anesth Pain Med* 2012; 37:508–14.
47. Dualé C, Schoeffler P, Ouchchane L, *et al.* T271 EDONIS—Epidemiologic study of postsurgical neuropathic pain. *Eur J Pain Suppl* 2012; 5:S56–7.
48. Duale C, Ouchchane L, Schoeffler P, *et al.* Neuropathic aspects of persistent postsurgical pain: a French multicenter survey with a 6-month prospective follow-up. *J Pain* 2014; 15:24 e21–4 e20.
49. Torrance N, Smith BH, Bennett MI, *et al.* The epidemiology of chronic pain of predominantly neuropathic origin. Results from a general population survey. *J Pain* 2006; 7:281–9.
50. Brandsborg B. Pain following hysterectomy: epidemiological and clinical aspects. *Dan Med J* 2012; 59:B4374.
51. Almeida EC, Nogueira AA, Candido dos Reis FJ, *et al.* section as a cause of chronic pelvic pain. *Int J Gynaecol Obstet* 2002; 79:101–4.
52. Lavand'homme P. Chronic pain after vaginal and cesarean delivery: a reality questioning our daily practice of obstetric anesthesia. *Int J Obstet Anesth* 2010; 19:1–2.
53. Shahin AY, Osman AM. Parietal peritoneal closure and persistent postcesarean pain. *Int J Gynaecol Obstet* 2009; 104:135–9.
54. Aasvang EK, Kehlet H. Persistent sensory dysfunction in pain-free herniotomy. *Acta Anaesthesiol Scand* 2010; 54:291–8.
55. Taylor KS, Anastakis DJ, Davis KD. Chronic pain and sensorimotor deficits following peripheral nerve injury. *Pain* 2010; 151:582–91.
56. Edwards RR. Individual differences in endogenous pain modulation as a risk factor for chronic pain. *Neurology* 2005; 65:437–43.
57. Yarnitsky D. Conditioned pain modulation (the diffuse noxious inhibitory control-like effect): its relevance for acute and chronic pain states. *Curr Opin Anaesthesiol* 2010; 23:611–15.
58. Katz J, Seltzer Z. Transition from acute to chronic postsurgical pain: risk factors and protective factors. *Expert Rev Neurother* 2009; 9:723–44.
59. Althaus A, Hinrichs-Rocker A, Chapman R, *et al.* Development of a risk index for the prediction of chronic post-surgical pain. *Eur J Pain* 2012; 16:901–10.
60. Sng BL, Sia AT, Quek K, *et al.* Incidence and risk factors for chronic pain after caesarean section under spinal anaesthesia. *Anaesth Intensive Care* 2009; 37:748–52.
61. Fletcher D, Fermanian C, Mardaye A, *et al.* A patient-based national survey on postoperative pain management in France reveals significant achievements and persistent challenges. *Pain* 2008; 137:441–51.
62. Steyaert A, De Kock M: Chronic postsurgical pain. *Curr Opin Anaesthesiol* 2012; 25:584–8.
63. Woolf CJ. Central sensitization: implications for the diagnosis and treatment of pain. *Pain* 2011; 152:S2–15.
64. Eisenach JC. Preventing chronic pain after surgery: who, how, and when? *Reg Anesth Pain Med* 2006; 31:1–3.
65. De Kock M. Expanding our horizons: transition of acute postoperative pain to persistent pain and establishment of chronic postsurgical pain services. *Anesthesiology* 2009; 111:461–3.
66. Lavand'homme PM, Roelants F, Waterloos H, *et al.* An evaluation of the postoperative antihyperalgesic and analgesic effects of intrathecal clonidine administered during elective cesarean delivery. *Anesth Analg* 2008; 107:948–55.
67. Paech MJ, Magann EF, Doherty DA, *et al.* Does magnesium sulfate reduce the short- and long-term requirements for pain relief after caesarean delivery? A double-blind placebo-controlled trial. *Am J Obstet Gynecol* 2006; 194:1596–602.
68. Ortner CM, Granot M, Richebe P, *et al.* Preoperative scar hyperalgesia is associated with post-operative pain in women undergoing a repeat Caesarean delivery. *Eur J Pain* 2013; 17:111–23.
69. Brandsborg B, Dueholm M, Kehlet H, *et al.* Mechanosensitivity before and after hysterectomy: a prospective study on the prediction of acute and chronic postoperative pain. *Br J Anaesth* 2011; 107:940–7.
70. Abrishami A, Chan J, Chung F, *et al.* Preoperative pain sensitivity and its correlation with postoperative pain and analgesic consumption: a qualitative systematic review. *Anesthesiology* 2011; 114:445–57.
71. Granot M. Can we predict persistent postoperative pain by testing preoperative experimental pain? *Curr Opin Anaesthesiol* 2009; 22:425–30.
72. Yarnitsky D, Crispel Y, Eisenberg E, *et al.* Prediction of chronic post-operative pain: pre-operative DNIC testing identifies patients at risk. *Pain* 2008; 138:22–8.
73. Wilder-Smith OH, Schreyer T, Scheffer GJ, *et al.* Patients with chronic pain after abdominal surgery show less preoperative endogenous pain inhibition and more postoperative hyperalgesia: a pilot study. *J Pain Palliat Care Pharmacother* 2010; 24:119–28.
74. Eide PK. Wind-up and the NMDA receptor complex from a clinical perspective. *Eur J Pain* 2000, 4:5–15.
75. Weissman-Fogel I, Granovsky Y, Crispel Y, *et al.* Enhanced presurgical pain temporal summation response predicts post-thoracotomy pain intensity during the acute postoperative phase. *J Pain* 2009; 10:628–36.
76. Stubhaug A, Breivik H, Eide PK, *et al.* Mapping of punctuate hyperalgesia around a surgical incision demonstrates that ketamine is a powerful suppressor of central sensitization to pain following surgery. *Acta Anaesthesiol Scand* 1997; 41:1124–32.
77. Sterling M. Differential development of sensory hypersensitivity and a measure of spinal cord hyperexcitability following whiplash injury. *Pain* 2010; 150:501–6.

78. Aasvang EK, Brandsborg B, Jensen TS, *et al.* Heterogeneous sensory processing in persistent postherniotomy pain. *Pain* 2010; 150:237–42.
79. Landau R, Kraft JC, Flint LY, *et al.* experimental paradigm for the prediction of Post-Operative Pain (PPOP). *J Vis Exp* 2010; 35:1671.
80. Lautenbacher S, Huber C, Schofer D, *et al.* Attentional and emotional mechanisms related to pain as predictors of chronic postoperative pain: a comparison with other psychological and physiological predictors. *Pain* 2010; 151:722–31.
81. Ferber SG, Granot M, Zimmer EZ. Catastrophizing labor pain compromises later maternity adjustments. *Am J Obstet Gynecol* 2005; 192:826–31.
82. Flink I, Mroczek M, Sullivan M, *et al.* Pain in childbirth and postpartum recovery—the role of catastrophizing. *Eur J Pain* 2009; 13:312–16.
83. Landau R, Kraft JC. Pharmacogenetics in obstetric anesthesia. *Curr Opin Anaesthesiol* 2010; 23:323–9.
84. Sia AT, Sng BL, Lim EC, *et al.* The influence of ATP-binding cassette sub-family B member -1 (ABCB1) genetic polymorphisms on acute and chronic pain after intrathecal morphine for caesarean section: a prospective cohort study. *Int J Obstet Anesth* 2010; 19:254–60.
85. Gutierrez S, Liu B, Hayashida K, *et al.* Reversal of peripheral nerve injury-induced hypersensitivity in the postpartum period: role of spinal oxytocin. *Anesthesiology* 2013; 118:152–9.
86. Lee H-J, Macbeth A, Pagani J, *et al.* Oxytocin: the great facilitator of life. *Prog Neurobiol* 2009; 88:127–51.
87. Gutierrez S, Hayashida K, Eisenach JC. The puerperium alters spinal cord plasticity following peripheral nerve injury. *Neuroscience* 2013; 228:301–8.
88. Bauchat JR, Higgins N, Wojciechowski KG, *et al.* Low-dose ketamine with multimodal postcesarean delivery analgesia: a randomized controlled trial. *Int J Obstet Anesth* 2011; 20:3–9.
89. Short J, Downey K, Bernstein P, *et al.* A single preoperative dose of gabapentin does not improve postcesarean delivery pain management: a randomized, double-blind, placebo-controlled dose-finding trial. *Anesth Analg* 2012; 115:1336–42.
90. Ducic I, Moxley M, Al-Attar A. Algorithm for treatment of postoperative incisional groin pain after cesarean delivery or hysterectomy. *Obstet Gynecol* 2006; 108:27–31.
91. Loos MJ, Scheltinga MR, Roumen RM. Surgical management of inguinal neuralgia after a low transverse Pfannenstiel incision. *Ann Surg* 2008; 248:880–5.
92. Vancaillie T, Eggermont J, Armstrong G, *et al.* Response to pudendal nerve block in women with pudendal neuralgia. *Pain Med* 2012; 13:596–603.

PART 7

Anaesthetic complications

CHAPTER 26

Management of the difficult airway

Mary C. Mushambi and Rajesh Pandey

Introduction

Over the past four decades, mortality primarily due to anaesthesia has declined from 1/2500 to 1/5000,[1] but the causes of death during anaesthesia have remained the same. Inadequate airway management is one of the four leading causes of anaesthetic-related deaths and the factors contributing to this are human error, inadequate communication, substandard care, lack of supervision and organizational issues.[2,3]

In the United Kingdom, the Confidential Enquiry into Maternal Deaths (CEMD) has been publishing reports continuously for the last six decades. The numbers of direct deaths from anaesthesia have declined from 30–50 deaths in each triennium until 1981 to seven deaths in the 2006–2008 triennium. Mortality is usually associated with general anaesthesia (GA) and only a minority of deaths are associated with neuraxial anaesthesia. The major causes of death from GA are either failure to oxygenate the lungs at the time of intubation or aspiration of gastric contents.[4] The rates of caesarean delivery (CD) in the United Kingdom have increased over the last four decades (3.4% to 21% of all maternities) but the rate of direct deaths due to anaesthesia for CD has declined from 36 (1964–1966) to 1 (2000–2002) per 100,000 CDs. There has been a significant decrease in the rate of GA for CD from 77% in 1982 to 44% in1992 to 10% in 2001.[5,6] According to the National Obstetric Anaesthetic Database (NOAD), 91% of all CDs are performed under neuraxial anaesthesia[7] and the Royal College of Anaesthetists' audit recipe suggests that greater than 95% of elective CDs should be performed under neuraxial anaesthesia.[8] In the latest Centre for Maternal and Child Enquiries (CMACE) report, two of seven anaesthetic deaths were a result of failure to ventilate and the recommendation was that effective management of failed tracheal intubation is a core anaesthetic skill which should be taught and rehearsed regularly [4] and the use of simulation for teaching and rehearsing failed intubation drills is strongly recommended.

The four obstetric cases reported to the 4th National Audit Project (NAP4) were associated with failed tracheal intubation during emergency CD.[9] The learning points and recommendations of the audit are summarized in Box 26.1.

Definitions

Several attempts have been made to define the difficult airway. The practice guidelines of the American Society of Anesthesiologists (ASA) define a *difficult airway* as the clinical situation in which a conventionally trained anaesthesiologist experiences difficulties with face mask ventilation of the lungs, difficulty with tracheal intubation and ventilation, or both.[10]

The two main objectives of airway management during GA are *maintaining oxygenation* and *ventilation of the lungs*, which can be achieved either by mask ventilation or by means of an airway device (supraglottic airway device (SAD) or tracheal tube). Therefore an alternative method of defining a difficult airway is based on the stage of airway management when difficulty is encountered.

The ASA defined *difficult mask ventilation* as a clinical situation that develops when it is not possible for the anaesthetist to provide adequate face mask ventilation as a result of one or more of the following problems: inadequate mask seal, excessive gas leak, or excessive resistance to ingress or egress of gas.[10] They described the signs of inadequate face mask ventilation as:

- absent or inadequate chest movement or breath sounds
- gastric air entry or dilatation
- decreasing or inadequate oxygen saturation
- decreasing or inadequate expired carbon dioxide
- haemodynamic changes associated with hypoxaemia or hypercapnia.

A four-point scale to grade difficulty in performing mask ventilation was proposed by Han and colleagues and modified by Kherterpal:[11,12]

- Grade 1—ventilation is possible with mask alone
- Grade 2—ventilation achieved with an oropharyngeal airway or muscle relaxant (neuromuscular blockade (NMB))
- Grade 3—difficult mask ventilation requiring additional manual assistance ± NMB
- Grade 4—ventilation is not possible with a mask.

Box 26.1 Learning points and recommendations of the 4th National Audit Project (NAP4) on major complications of airway management in the United Kingdom

Learning points

1. Physiological changes in pregnancy, active labour, and isolated location increase the complexity of management of airway complications when they occur
2. All theatre personnel (obstetricians, midwives, and ODPs) should be aware of the considerable difficulty in managing airway complications in obstetric patients
3. Three of four parturients were obese and had complex obstetric, medical, and anaesthetic issues
4. While preparing failed intubation strategies, it should be recognized that it is not always possible to wake the patient
5. Decisions regarding management of complex patients require multidisciplinary collaboration when forming initial and back-up plans.

Recommendations

1. Obstetric anaesthetists should maintain airway skills which include management of difficult and failed tracheal intubation and CICV[a]
2. Obstetric anaesthetists should be competent in the use the second-generation SADs[b] which give better protection against aspiration and facilitate ventilation and/or intubation
3. Anaesthetic departments should ensure airway skills and equipment are available whenever awake fibreoptic intubation is indicated
4. Recovery staff including midwives should be trained and be competent to recover patients following an anaesthetic.

[a] Can't intubate, can't ventilate.
[b] Supraglottic airway devices.

Grades 3 and 4 are most likely to alter a future anaesthetic plan hence these should be documented in the patient's notes. However, the degree of difficult mask ventilation is also dependent on the skill and experience of the anaesthetist. The incidence of difficult mask ventilation is 1.4–5% and impossible mask ventilation is 0.07–0.16%.[12,13]

The laryngeal mask airway (LMA) has an established role as a routine airway device and also as a rescue device in a difficult airway. A *difficult LMA* is when the LMA is unable to provide adequate airway patency, oxygenation, and ventilation despite correct selection of the laryngeal mask size and provision of optimal airway opening manoeuvres when inserted. The signs of inadequate ventilation are similar to those with difficult mask ventilation.

Difficult laryngoscopy is the inability to visualize any portion of the vocal cords after multiple attempts at conventional laryngoscopy. A definition of difficult laryngoscopy was proposed by Cormack and Lehane (CL),[14] and this has been adopted by anaesthetists worldwide. They classified the view obtained at direct laryngoscopy using a Macintosh blade into four grades (Figure 26.1).

Subsequently, the CL classification has been modified to include a subdivided grade 2 (2a and 2b).[15] An easy grade 2a is where part of the vocal cords can be seen and a difficult grade 2b is where only the arytenoids are visible. In 2000, Cook proposed another more practical modification of the CL classification and graded the degree of difficulty into easy, restricted and difficult[16] (Table 26.1).

Difficult tracheal intubation is considered if more than three attempts are required or it takes longer than 10 minutes to intubate a patient in the presence or absence of tracheal pathology[10] and *failed intubation* occurs when placement of the endotracheal tube fails after multiple intubation attempts. A more appropriate definition reflecting events occurring in clinical practise is definition suggested by the Canadian Task Force[17] which is when an experienced laryngoscopist, using direct laryngoscopy (i) requires more than two attempts with same blade or a change in the blade, (ii) requires an adjunct to a direct laryngoscope such as a bougie, or (iii) uses an alternative device/technique following failed intubation with direct laryngoscopy. A UK national study aimed at estimating rate of failed intubation in obstetrics defined an *obstetric failed intubation* as failure to achieve tracheal intubation during a rapid sequence induction (RSI) for obstetric anaesthesia, thereby initiating a failed intubation drill.[18]

Incidence of difficult tracheal intubation

Approximately 2.9 million GAs are administered in the United Kingdom every year with tracheal tubes being used in 38% of patients.[9] Of the airway deaths reported to the NAP4, 13% were associated with difficult tracheal intubation.[9] The incidence of failed tracheal intubation is quoted to be 1/300–800[19–21] for all types of emergency surgery (Table 26.2).

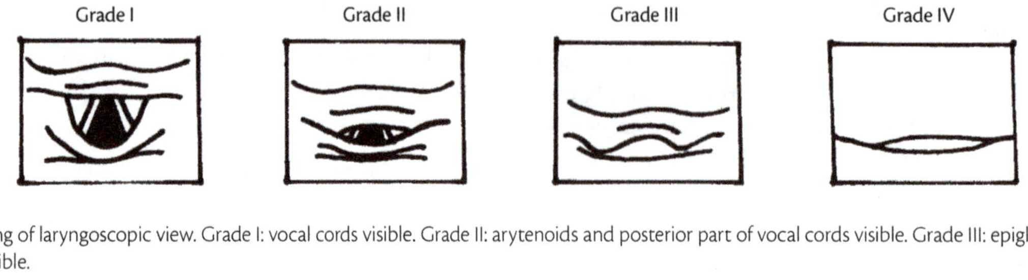

Figure 26.1 Grading of laryngoscopic view. Grade I: vocal cords visible. Grade II: arytenoids and posterior part of vocal cords visible. Grade III: epiglottis visible. Grade IV: epiglottis not visible.

Table 26.1 Classification of laryngeal grade: Cormack and Lehane classification and new classification of view at laryngoscopy

Cormack and Lehane classification	**Grade 1**	**Grade 2**		**Grade 3**		**Grade 4**
Modification	**Grade 1**	**Grade 2A**	**Grade 2B**	**Grade 3A**	**Grade 3B**	**Grade 4**
Laryngeal views	Most of cords visible	Posterior cord visible	Only arytenoids visible	Epiglottis visible and liftable	Epiglottis adherent to pharynx	No laryngeal structures seen
Method of intubation	Direct		Indirect		Specialist	
New grading	Easy		Restricted		Difficult	

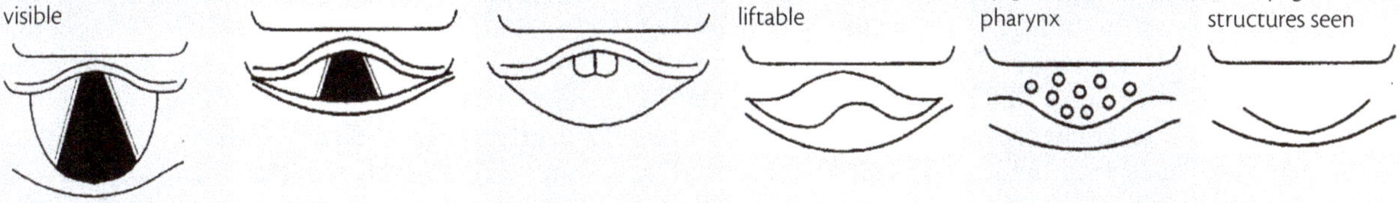

Reproduced with permission from TM Cook, A new practical classification of laryngeal view, *Anaesthesia*, Volume 55, Issue 3, pp. 74–279, Copyright © 2002 John Wiley and Sons.

Since 1985, the incidence of failed intubation in the obstetric patient has largely remained the same at 1/225–300.[18,19,22–27] These studies are summarized in Table 26.3. However, there is a wide variation in the sample size and the experience of anaesthetists in these studies. One study looked at the incidence of failed intubation over a 6-year period in the same maternity unit[22] and another study looked at a wider region including 13 maternity units over 1 year.[25] Despite this, all the studies have shown similar results. The exceptions to this are two studies, one by McKeen[27] (1/1300) and the second by Djabatey[26] (no case of failed intubation), who have shown improvement in the incidence of failed intubation. This improvement has been attributed to the fact that these studies took place in very busy maternity units where there was good antenatal anaesthetic consultation, anaesthetists who were experienced in GA for obstetrics, experienced anaesthetic assistance, and a high epidural rate (80% in the McKeen study[27]). Two studies have demonstrated a relationship between failed intubation and increasing age and obesity.[18,27] A UK national study conducted in 2008–2010 reflects obstetric practice in clinical environments with diverse settings.[18] The incidence of failed intubation in this study was 1/224. With an increase in the prevalence of obesity, rate of CD, and an ageing maternal population, providing safe obstetric anaesthetic care will no doubt continue to be challenging in the future.

Assessment and prediction of the difficult airway

> Poor airway assessment contributes to poor outcome; this is either due to omission, incomplete assessment or failure to alter the airway management techniques in response to findings at the assessment. (NAP4[9])

Table 26.2 Incidences of failed intubation[19–21]

General population	1/2000–3000
Obstetric population	1/225–1300
In all emergencies	1/300–800

Data from various sources (see references).

Assessment is one of the first steps in managing an airway. However, failure to assess the obstetric airway correctly is a consistent finding in many studies.[9,26] Airway assessment allows the anaesthetist to choose the most appropriate and safest management technique (with backup plans) together with any extra equipment, and anaesthetic and surgical help that may be required.

When to assess

The airway should be assessed as early as possible in the pregnancy. Ideally, every maternity healthcare professional should be able to identify and understand the consequences of a difficult airway. In the antenatal period, this is usually a midwife or obstetrician, but because of their lack of knowledge and experience, some patients with a difficult airway may not be identified.

Table 26.3 Incidence of difficult and failed tracheal intubation in obstetric practice

Study	**Total GAs**	**Difficult intubation**	**Failed intubation**	
Lyons (1985)[22]	2331	NR	8	(1/291)
Hawthorne et al. (1996)[19]	5802	NR	23	(1/250)
Barnardo and Jenkins (2000)[23]	8970	NR	36	(1/249)
Rahman and Jenkins (2005)[24]	4768	NR	20	(1/238)
McDonnell et al. (2009)[25]	1086	36 (1/30)	4	(1/272)
Djabatey and Barclay (2009)[26]	3530	23 (1/156)	0	
McKeen et al. (2011)[27]	2633	123 (1/21)	2	(1/1316)
Quinn et al. (2013)[18]	12800	NR	57	(1/224)

NR = not recorded.

Data from various sources (see references).

This can be addressed by ensuring that an anaesthetic referral system is in place. In the United Kingdom, only 30% of hospitals operate a formal anaesthetic clinic whereas the remainder have an ad hoc referral arrangement.[28] A referral checklist (Box 26.2) to identify diseases associated with difficult intubation may increase early identification by non-anaesthetists. Any patient with a body mass index (BMI) higher than 40 at booking should be assessed in the antenatal anaesthetic clinic.[29] Studies have shown an increase in the Mallampati scores with increasing gestation and at different stages of labour.[30–32] Another study demonstrated an increase in Mallampati score at the end of pregnancy but no further changes were noted during labour.[33] The authors attributed their findings to the difference in the amounts of fluids given during labour when compared with previous studies (554 vs 2500 mL in Kodali et al. study[31]) and they postulated that a low-fluid regimen policy might provide better Mallampati scores during labour probably by reducing neck oedema. It is recommended that the airway should be assessed as pregnancy progresses as well as during labour because of these changes in Mallampati scores.

Box 26.2 Airway related pre-assessment checklist for referral to anaesthetists in the antenatal period in order to identify potential airway problems

1. Previous history of difficult or failed intubation
2. High body mass index > 40
3. Head and neck pathology:
    - Previous radiotherapy
    - Tumours
    - Trauma/burns
    - Previous surgery
4. Musculoskeletal diseases:
    - Rheumatoid arthritis
    - Ankylosing spondylitis
    - Kyphoscoliosis
    - Cervical spine abnormalities
5. History of obstructive sleep apnoea
6. Congenital abnormalities such as:
    - Pierre Robins
    - Treacher Collins
    - Downs
    - Goldenhar
    - Achondroplasia
    - Klippel–Feil
7. Endocrine disorders:
    - Acromegaly
    - Diabetes
8. Autoimmune disorders:
    - Scleroderma.

How to assess

History, clinical examination, bedside tests, and investigations form the main components of assessing an airway. A good clinical history should include a review of the patient's notes with an emphasis on detecting previous airway difficulties. The presence of conditions such as morbid obesity, tumours of the neck, tumours or infection of the airway, cervical spine immobility, trauma, and congenital malformations of the upper airway are associated with potential airway difficulty. Risk factors for difficult mask ventilation include increased BMI, increased age, history of snoring, obstructive sleep apnoea, lack of teeth, Mallampati class III or IV, and airway tumours. Hence the history should also exclude symptoms suggesting airway pathology such as snoring, obstructive sleep apnoea, dyspnoea, dysphonia, dysphagia, and hoarseness of voice.

Several bedside tests have been described to predict a difficult airway. An ideal bedside test is one that is easy, quick to perform, has very low interobserver variability, and is highly sensitive (ability to detect difficult intubation) and specific (ability to detect easy intubations) with very low false-positive and false-negative values. Unfortunately all the bedside tests have high sensitivity, but low specificity values and moderate interobserver variability. Because of these limitations, when used individually, the tests have a poor positive predictive value (PPV).

Table 26.4 shows a list of simple bedside tests. A single abnormal finding should act as a cautionary sign for GA. However, it is recommended that an alternative anaesthetic plan including awake intubation should be considered if abnormal findings are present.

Mouth opening is assessed with the mouth maximally opened and measuring the inter-incisor gap. Normal adults are capable of inserting at least three fingers which corresponds to a mouth opening of between 4 and 6 cm.[34] An inter-incisor gap of greater than 3 cm allows insertion of a standard Macintosh blade. If mouth opening is less than 4 cm, it suggests an increased risk factor for difficult intubation and if it is less than 3 cm, it suggests significant temporomandibular joint dysfunction.[35]

Mandibular subluxation assesses the temporomandibular joint mobility. This is assessed by asking the patient to push the lower jaw in front of the upper jaw. If the lower incisors can be moved in front of the upper ones, the trachea is more likely to be easy to intubate but if they cannot, it is more likely to be difficult.[36] The classification is as follows:

- Class A: the lower incisors can be protruded in front of the upper incisors
- Class B: the lower incisors can be advanced to be in line with upper incisors only.
- Class C: the lower incisors cannot be protruded to reach the level of the upper incisors.

Table 26.4 Suggested list of simple bedside tests to perform in the obstetric patient[18,19,22–27]

Airway component to be assessed	Normal findings
Mouth opening	Inter-incisor gap ≥ 4cm
	Or 3 finger breadths
Pharyngeal view	Uvula visible when tongue protruded, patient in sitting position (Mallampati ≤ II)
Temporomandibular joint movement	Protrusion of the lower jaw in front of upper jaw
Thyromental distance	>6.5 cm
Neck mobility	Flexion—can touch chin to chest
	Extension—can extend the neck
Weight	BMI < 30 or weight < 90 kg
(No snoring/obstructive sleep apnoea)	
Obvious airway compromise or pathology	
Upper airway tumours	
Stridor	
Voice changes	
Oedema (pregnancy-induced hypertension)	

In 1983, Mallampati[37] evaluated a simple grading system of classifying the *pharyngeal view* obtained with patients sitting upright, head in the neutral position, and asking them to open the mouth and protrude the tongue out maximally. He hypothesized that an increase in the size of the tongue made laryngoscopy difficult. Depending on the visibility of the faucial pillars, soft palate, and the uvula, the view obtained was classified into three grades. This was modified in 1985 when class IV was added when the soft palate was not visible[38] (Figure 26.2). According to the authors, patients with a modified Mallampati score of class III or IV were at risk of a difficult intubation. In 1998, Ezri et al.[39] added a further class zero where the epiglottis is seen, the incidence of class zero was 1% and it was concluded that this was a good predictor of grade I laryngoscopy. However, anecdotal case reports have suggested that laryngoscopy may be difficult in patients with class zero view and this was attributed to a large epiglottis.[40]

A good range of *neck movements* is needed to achieve the optimum intubating position. The patient is asked to touch the chin to the chest and extend the neck maximally. A sternomental distance of less than 12.5 cm,[41] thyromental distance of 6.5 cm or less, and restricted neck movements caused by cervical spine immobility are associated with difficult laryngoscopy.

In spite of the use of several bedside predictors and their association with predicting airway difficulty it is hard to recommend a single test because of lack of good evidence. Although the Mallampati score is used commonly by anaesthetists, it has a low sensitivity and high interobserver variability.[42] A meta-analysis of 55 studies found only 35% of patients with Mallampati score III and IV had difficult intubation. As a stand-alone test of a difficult laryngoscopy or tracheal intubation, it has a low PPV but this is improved if it is combined with other tests such as the thyromental distance and jaw protrusion.[43–45] The ASA Task Force practice guidelines recommend the use of several airway features for prediction and management of difficult airway.[10] Therefore in summary, multiple abnormal tests predicting difficult intubation are better than any single test.

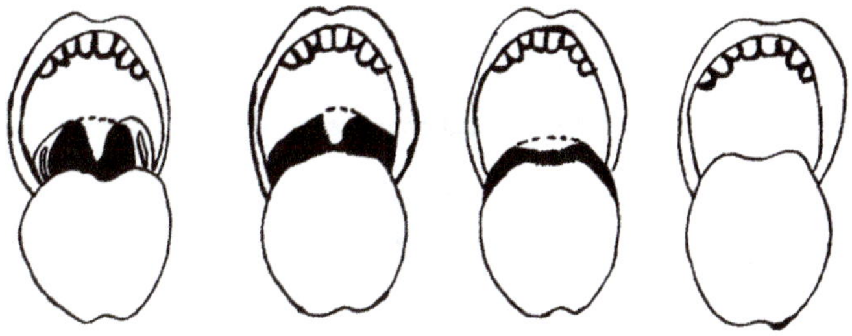

Figure 26.2 Classification of the pharyngeal structures as seen when conducting the Mallampati test. Class 1: pharyngeal pillars, soft palate, uvula visible. Class II: soft palate and uvula visible. Class III: only soft palate visible. Class IV: soft palate not visible.
Reproduced with permission from G. L. T. Samsoon, J. R. B. Young, Difficult tracheal intubation: a retrospective study, *Anaesthesia*, Volume 42, Issue 5, pp. 487–490, Copyright © 1987 John Wiley and Sons.

Communication and documentation

Depending on the severity of the difficulty the anaesthetist should formulate an airway and anaesthetic management plan, discuss the risks and alternatives with the patient and their partners, and document them in the notes. There are many reports on poor documentation of preoperative airway assessment of pregnant women.[18,19,26] Good communication and documentation are extremely important to ensure details of the management plan are available to the team and anaesthetists involved in the final care of the patient. If airway problems are identified antenatally, these patients should be encouraged to have an early epidural which should be reviewed regularly when in labour to ensure that the epidural is functioning well to reduce the chances of requiring a GA. One of the key contributing factors for mortality from inadequate airway management is inadequate, or lack of, communication.[1,46]

Causes of difficult tracheal intubation in obstetric practice

The reasons for difficult airway and intubation in obstetrics can be divided into anatomical and physiological changes, training, and situational factors and these are summarized in Box 26.3.

Anatomical and physiological changes

Airway oedema

During pregnancy, there is an increase in total body water leading to engorgement and swelling of the nasal mucosa, tongue, pharynx, larynx, and trachea. An increased incidence of Mallampati

Box 26.3 Causes of difficult airway and tracheal intubation in obstetric practice

Anatomical and physiological changes

- ↑ airway oedema and engorgement
- ↑ weight and breasts enlargement
- ↓ FRC
- ↑ oxygen requirements
- ↓ lower oesophageal pressure and ↑ risk of aspiration
- ↓ gastric emptying during labour.

Training issues

- ↓ clinical experience of trainees
- ↓ number of general anaesthetic cases for CD per trainee
- ↓ number of CD under general anaesthetic
- ↓ use of STP and suxamethonium for RSI in non-obstetric patients.

Situational issues

- Emergency situation and time pressure to deliver the baby
- Application of cricoid pressure on a tilted table
- Remote location of the delivery suite
- Lack of communication with senior staff and between the delivery suite team members.

CD, caesarean delivery; FRC, functional residual capacity; RSI, rapid sequence induction; STP, thiopentone.

score (class III/IV) has been demonstrated from the eighth month of pregnancy and these changes persist until 48 hours after delivery.[32,47] Laryngeal oedema especially in pre-eclamptic women presenting with hoarseness may compromise the airway, therefore a wide selection of tracheal tubes down to 5.5 mm internal diameter should be available when inducing GA in these patients.[48] Engorgement of blood vessels of the airway increases the risks of mucosal bleeding especially if the nasal route is used for fibreoptic intubation and the oral route is therefore the preferred choice.

Increased weight gain and breast enlargement

Weight gain during pregnancy is due to the growing fetus, increase in maternal fluid volume, and soft tissue. On average, a pregnant woman gains 20 kg during pregnancy of which 3.5 kg is due to storage of fat.[49] Enlargement of the breasts make laryngoscopy difficult. Use of the short-handled laryngoscope or polio blade may overcome this difficulty.

Obesity in pregnancy is defined as a BMI of greater than 30 kg/m^2 at booking. The prevalence of maternal obesity in England has increased from 7% (1990) to 16% (2007).[50] One in 1000 pregnant women have a BMI of greater than 50 and have a higher CD rate of 50% compared with 22%. The incidence of failed intubation in obese patients is 15%[51] and for every 1 kg/m^2 there is a 7% increased risk of failed intubation.[18] Airway complications are attributed to difficult mask ventilation, short and thick neck, large tongue, and large breasts which make laryngoscopy and intubation difficult. Obesity increases the risk of regurgitation and aspiration because of hiatus hernia and increased gastric reflux and increased gastric volume.[52]

Effect of the gravid uterus

Enlargement of the uterus displaces the diaphragm cephalad and affects the lung volumes and capacities. A decrease in functional residual capacity (FRC) and increase in oxygen demand decreases overall oxygen reserve. The FRC decreases by 20% in the sitting position and 25% in the recumbent position. As a result, the time taken to desaturate following apnoea is considerably faster in pregnant patients (173 seconds) compared with the non-pregnant patients (243 seconds) and is unaffected by change to a head-up position (pregnant 153 seconds vs non-pregnant 331 seconds).[53]

An increased risk of regurgitation and aspiration is caused by the displacement of the stomach by the gravid uterus and relaxation of the lower oesophageal sphincter. Labour is associated with delayed gastric emptying which is further exacerbated with the use of opioids. All patients should be considered at risk of aspiration during pregnancy.

Training issues

There has been a considerable reduction in the sum total of all clinical experience gained by trainees because of the introduction of the European Working Time Directive (EWTD). The number of CD performed under GA has reduced over the past few decades[54] and as a result, the number of GAs for CD performed by trainees is decreasing. There is a perceived lack of skill (and especially self-confidence) in mask ventilation because trainees favour the use of SADs. Many trainees have received very little training in the classic RSI using thiopentone and suxamethonium as many senior anaesthetists are choosing to use modified RSI using alternate induction agents and muscle relaxants in non-obstetric patients.[55] The infrequency of difficult and failed intubation means that most trainees would never see a case during their obstetric module.

Situational issues

The majority of cases of difficult or failed intubations in obstetrics occur during emergencies[9] and the risk of aspiration is further compounded if the mother has recently eaten. The added pressure of delivering the baby quickly means that a relatively inexperienced practitioner in a stressful environment may feel rushed with the preoperative assessment; this compounded with suboptimal positioning and inadequate preoxygenation contribute to increased risk of failure. Incorrect application of cricoid pressure on a tilted table may impair the view at laryngoscopy and make intubation difficult. Some delivery suites in the United Kingdom, are located in separate buildings or isolated from the main operating theatres. Due to the remote location, help in the form of senior anaesthetists and specialists (e.g. ear, nose, and throat (ENT) specialists), trained assistants, and equipment may not be easily accessible for anaesthetists in the delivery suite. Lack of awareness of difficulties faced during difficult intubation amongst non-anaesthetic staff in the delivery suite is of major concern.[9] In the United Kingdom where electronic patient records are not routine practice in all hospitals, handheld notes are vital if patients are admitted as an emergency or at another hospital.

Optimum airway management in the pregnant patient

Airway management and tracheal intubation in the pregnant patient require careful planning, preparation, and an optimal technique in order to reduce morbidity and mortality associated with the airway.

Planning and preparation

Communication

Good communication between the members of the delivery suite team is essential to ensure patient safety. Anaesthetists are encouraged to attend ward rounds with the obstetricians in order to identify high-risk women. Team briefing should be carried out daily to identify problems and allow time to plan any airway strategies. Good communication must occur between anaesthetists and obstetricians if there is a patient in labour with a potentially difficult airway. If there is fetal distress, this should be identified and communicated early so that an epidural top-up or *de novo* spinal can be used, thereby avoiding the 'crash' GA. A World Health Organization checklist should be carried out on every patient.[56] Junior anaesthetic staff should have appropriate supervision for their level of experience and should know who and how to call for help if this is required urgently.

Training

Because trainees are undertaking fewer obstetric cases under GA,[57] all elective cases under GA should be used to teach RSI in the pregnant patient. The teaching of simulated failed intubation drills should involve obstetricians, midwives, and operating department practitioners (ODPs) in order to improve communication and non-technical skills between the team.[58,59] ODPs should be trained in the correct application of cricoid pressure. ODPs and recovery staff should also be trained to the same national standard as staff in the general theatres.

Anaesthetic equipment

The obstetric theatre should be equipped to the same standard as the general theatres and monitoring should comply with the Association of Anaesthetists of Great Britain and Ireland (AAGBI) standards.[60] Equipment should include basic airway equipment and equipment for the difficult airway (Box 26.4). The standardization of the contents of difficult intubation trolleys was a recommendation of NAP4.[9] The layout of the difficult intubation trolley in plans A, B, C, and D of the Difficult Airway Society (DAS) unanticipated difficult airway guidelines may help the anaesthetist and assistant to progress through the Failed intubation guidelines during an unanticipated difficult airway[61] and avoid fixation on one aspect of patient care to the detriment of other more clinically important areas.[62] Figure 26.3 is an example of a similarly designed difficult intubation trolley. The multiple use bougie with a coudé tip (gum elastic bougie) is traditionally the most commonly used adjunct to facilitate intubation in the United Kingdom.[63,64] With increasing concern regarding cross-infection,[65] single-use bougies are now widely used. However, studies have shown that single-use plastic bougies are associated with lower success rates[64] and more trauma.[66]

Box 26.4 Airway equipment for the obstetric theatres

Routine equipment

1. Masks of various sizes
2. Oropharyngeal airways of different sizes
3. Wide selection of tracheal tubes (including size 7 or less)
4. Macintosh laryngoscopes with standard and long blades
5. Short handle Macintosh laryngoscopes
6. McCoy laryngoscope with sizes 3 and 4 blades
7. Bougies
8. Intubating stylet
9. A video laryngoscope
10. Magill forceps.

Equipment for the unanticipated difficult airway

1. Laryngeal mask airways (LMAs) including second-generation SADs (e.g. The LMA ProSeal™, Supreme™ LMA, or i-gel®)
2. Equipment for 'can't intubate can't oxygenate':
    - Narrow-bore kink-resistant cannulae and a high-pressure ventilating system such as the Manujet® (VBM)
    - Large-bore cannulae (Quicktrach® or Melker® cricothyroid cannulae)
    - Surgical cricothyroidotomy set and tracheostomy tube
3. Fibreoptic scope
4. Equipment for awake fibreoptic intubation:
    - Equipment to apply local anaesthetic to the upper airway such as the mucosal atomizer device (MAD®), or oxygen tubing, three-way tap, and cannula for the Mackenzie technique
    - Re-enforced or intubating LMA tracheal tubes
    - Epidural catheter
    - Berman airway or 'Safe Bite' to prevent the patient biting on the fibreoptic scope
    - Local anaesthetics such as 4% lignocaine, 2% lignocaine gel (Instillagel®), 5% lignocaine/0.5% phenylephrine mixture.

Video laryngoscopes have been shown to improve the grade of laryngoscopy at intubation compared with the standard Macintosh laryngoscope.[67–76] They should be available for the management of a difficult airway on the delivery suite. Figure 26.4 shows some examples of video laryngoscopes that are available. These can be classified into 'channelled video laryngoscopes' such as the Airtraq® and the Pentax Airway Scope® (AWS), and the 'non-channelled video laryngoscopes' such as the Glidescope®, C-Mac® and McGrath MAC®.

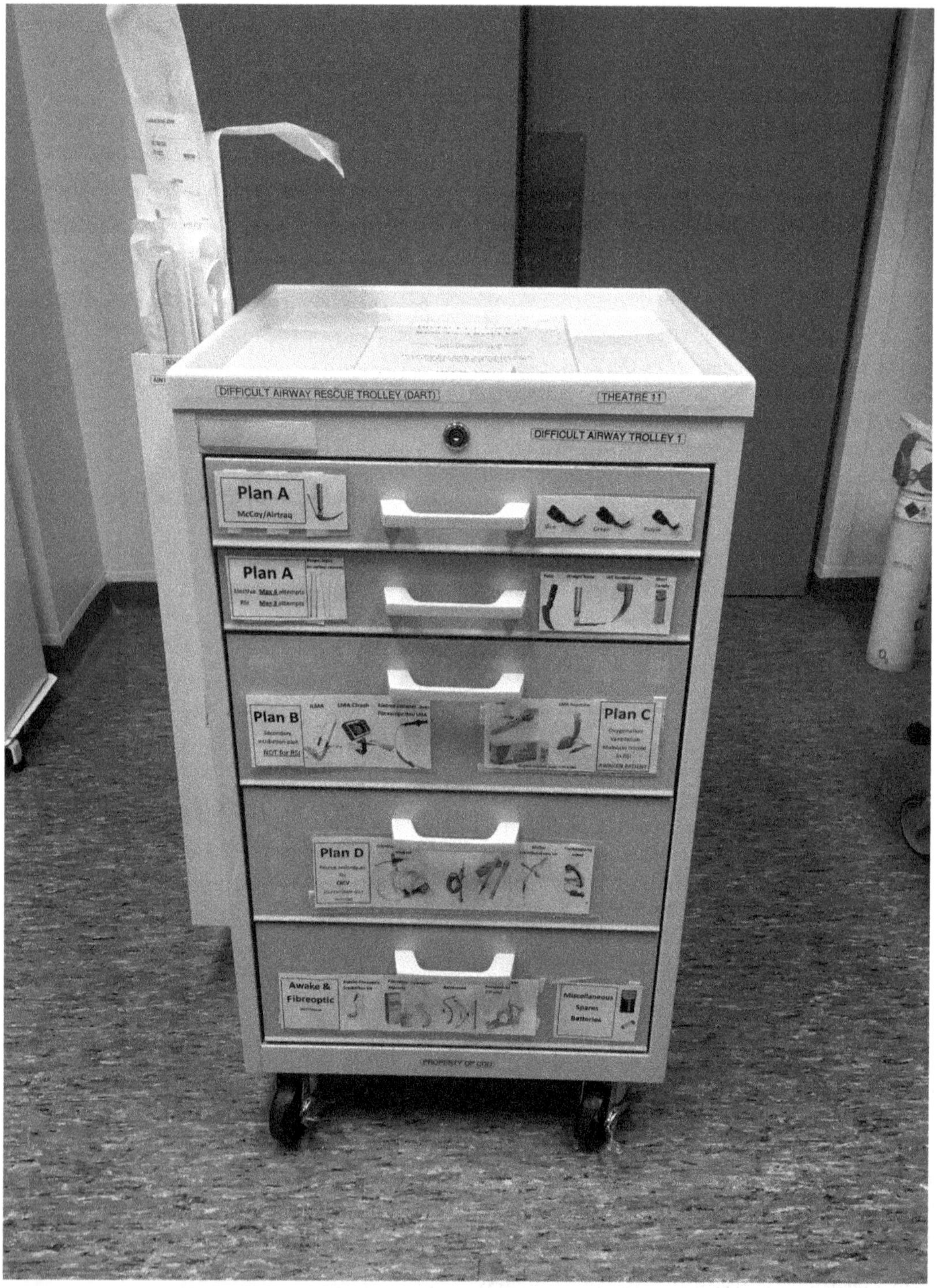

Figure 26.3 An example of a difficult intubation trolley. The drawers are arranged according to layout plan A, B, C, and D of the DAS unanticipated difficult airway guidelines in order to help the anaesthetist and anaesthetic assistant to progress through the DAS guidelines during an unanticipated difficult airway.

The Airtraq® is a single-use laryngoscope with a guiding channel which acts as a conduit for the tracheal tube. The second channel has an optical system which transfers the image from the illuminated tip to the viewfinder. The laryngoscope has the option of a wireless video system.

The Pentax airway scope is a reusable, rigid, portable video laryngoscope that combines a camera, LCD screen, and a disposable blade. The blade has a side channel for tracheal tube placement.

The McGrath MAC® is a reusable laryngoscope with an integral display monitor mounted on the handle of the laryngoscope. It uses disposable blades.

The C-Mac® is a reusable laryngoscope which resembles a Macintosh laryngoscope but with an integral video camera. The camera projects

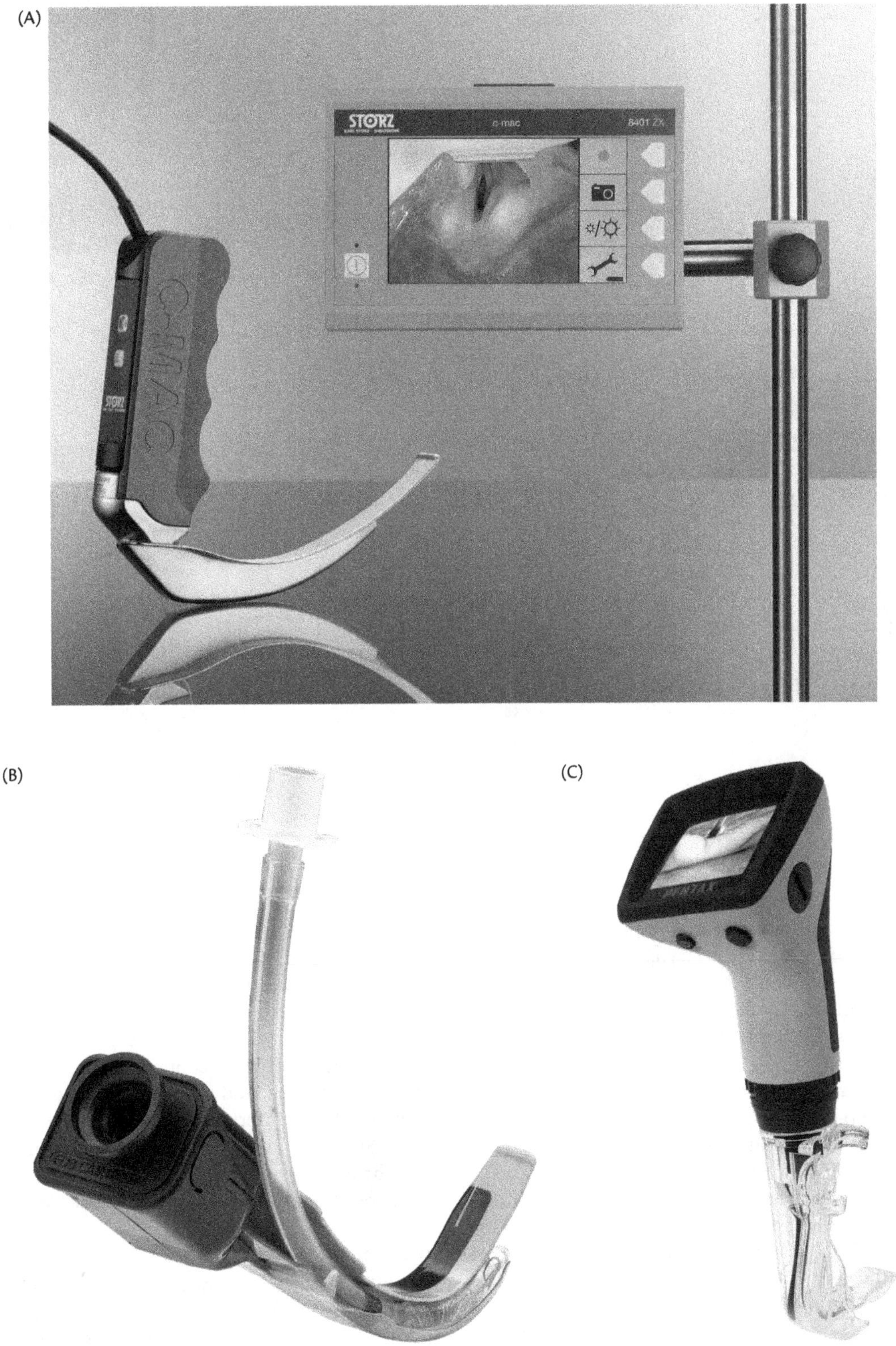

Figure 26.4 Some of the types of video laryngoscopes available: (A) C-Mac®. (B) Airtraq®. (C) Pentax airway scope®. (D) Venner AP Advance®. (E) McGrath MAC®.
(A) © Storz; (B) Image courtesy of Prodol Meditec; (C) Image courtesy of Pentax Medical; (E) Image courtesy of Aircraft Medical (McGRATH® MAC).

(D)

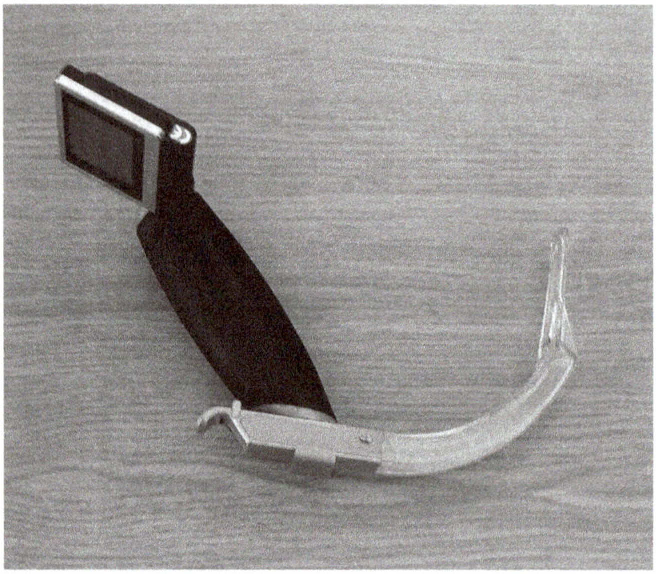

(E)

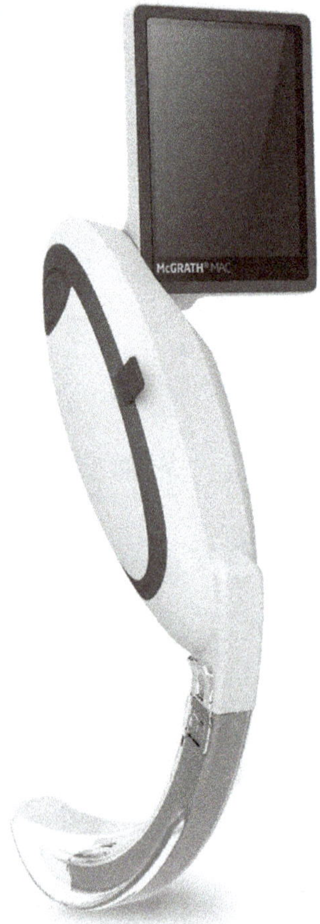

Figure 26.4 Continued

the image onto a portable screen. It may be used with a D-blade for a difficult intubation and a bougie may be required for this.

The Glidescope® is a reusable video laryngoscope with a video camera at the tip of the reusable baton. The camera is connected by a cable to a separate display monitor. The baton fits into different sizes of single-use blades. A stylet or bougie is required to facilitate intubation.

The Venner AP Advance® video laryngoscope is a new laryngoscope which has two types of disposable blades, the conventional size 3 and 4 Macintosh for standard laryngoscopy and the difficult airway blade which is angulated and has a guiding channel.[77] King Vision® video laryngoscope is another new video laryngoscope which has two types of disposable blades depending on the preferred technique. It has a standard blade that requires a stylet to direct the endotracheal tube and a channelled blade where one can guide the tube with the blade.

Most video laryngoscopes have been shown to improve laryngoscopy grades but an adequate view of the glottis does not always translate into quick intubation. This is because a good view of the glottis on the screen does not guarantee easy passage of the tracheal tube into the larynx, as hand–eye coordination may be impaired by the indirect view.

At least one type of a SAD including a second-generation SAD such as the LMA ProSeal™, Supreme™ LMA, or i-gel® (Figure 26.5) should be available.

The LMA ProSeal™ is a reusable LMA with a better oropharyngeal seal (10 cm higher than the classic LMA (cLMA)) and a drain tube which forms a more effective seal with the gastrointestinal tract thereby decreasing aspiration risk. The drainage tube can be used to pass an orogastric tube for aspiration.[78]

The i-gel® has a gastric channel which allow early recognition of regurgitation of gastric contents and passage of a drainage tube, an epiglottic ridge, and a built-in bite block (a ridged flattened stem) which aids insertion and reduces the risk of axial rotation.

The Supreme™ LMA is a single-use second-generation LMA with the features of the LMA ProSeal™ and intubating LMA.

A fibreoptic scope should be readily available on the delivery suite.[9]

Reducing the risk of aspiration

Fasting guidelines for women undergoing elective surgery should be the same as in the non-pregnant patient. However, fasting guidelines for women in labour is less uniform. Oral intake of a light diet during labour increases gastric contents, incidence of vomiting, and volume of vomit significantly compared with those taking only sips of water.[79] However, in 2007 the National Institute of Health and Clinical Excellence (now the National Institute of Health and Care Excellence (NICE)) published guidelines which classify women into low aspiration risk (LAR) for those with uncomplicated labour and high aspiration risk (HAR) for those who develop risks factors making GA more likely or who

(A) (B) (C)

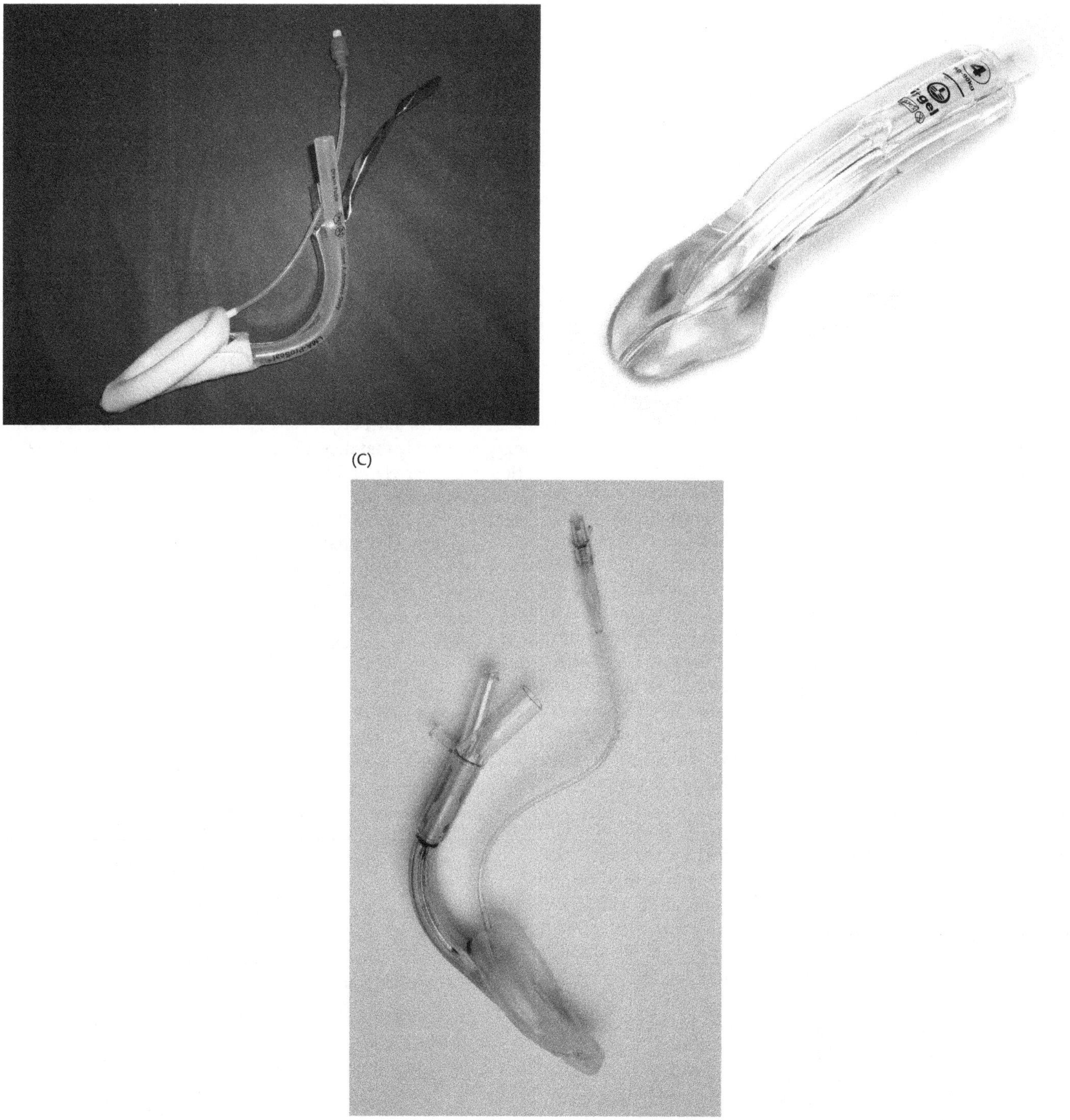

Figure 26.5 Second-generation laryngeal mask airways: (A) The LMA ProSeal™ (showing the optional Introducer), (B) i-gel®, and (C) Supreme™ LMA.
(A) Image courtesy of Intersurgical Ltd; (B) Image courtesy of Teleflex Incorporated.

received opioids. It is recommended that women in the LAR group receive a light diet while women in the HAR receive liquids only.[80] However, recent evidence shows that prediction of those women who may require a GA is inaccurate.[81] Women who undergo GA for CD are at risk of aspiration at induction and at extubation. To reduce aspiration risk at tracheal extubation, an orogastric tube passed after induction of anaesthesia should be considered in any women with a history of recent food ingestion. This was highlighted in the only case of aspiration and death in the 2006–2008 CEMD report in which the patient aspirated at extubation and an orogastric tube had not been used.[82]

Pharmacological agents should be used routinely to neutralize acid in the stomach. A recent Cochrane review suggested that compared with no treatment or placebo, antacids, histamine 2 receptor (H_2) antagonists and proton pump antagonists reduced the risk of an intragastric pH of less than 2.5 at intubation.[83] However, for women in labour, proton pump antagonists are less effective compared with H_2 antagonists and antacids alone.[84]

Women undergoing elective surgery should receive an H_2 antagonist administered the night before and 2 hours prior to anaesthesia (with or without a prokinetic drug such as metoclopramide) followed by an antacid immediately prior to the GA. High-risk women in labour should receive 6-hourly oral H_2 antagonist and antacid immediately prior to GA. However, mothers who have not received an H_2 antagonist in labour should be given an antacid to cover induction and intravenous H_2 antagonists to cover tracheal extubation.

General anaesthetic techniques

As well having correct equipment available and appropriate choice of induction agents and muscle relaxants, an optimum RSI requires (a) good position, (b) effective preoxygenation, (c) correct application of cricoid pressure, and (d) optimum laryngoscopy.

Positioning

Good position is essential to optimize laryngoscopy views. Jackson described the method of laryngoscopy in which the head was elevated and neck extended [85] and in 1936, Magill suggested the term 'sniffing position'.[86] Bannister and colleague used X-rays to investigate which positions gave the best alignment of the mouth, pharyngeal and laryngeal axes and concluded that cervical flexion and atlanto-axial extension provided the best alignment.[87] However, Adnet questioned Bannister's conclusion and used magnetic resonance imaging to show that the sniffing position did not align the three axes in normal awake volunteers.[88,89] They also demonstrated that the 'sniffing position' did not provide a better view of the glottis than with simple extension except in patients with morbid obesity and reduced cervical mobility.[90] Therefore although the sniffing position is generally advocated for providing the best alignment of the three axes at laryngoscopy, there is evidence that this may not always be the case in all patients and other factors may need to be considered.[91]

Sitting patients in a 30° head-up position increases FRC and decreases the restriction caused by large breasts. Other methods which have been shown to improve laryngoscopic view especially in the obese patient is the 'ramped' position in which the patient's upper body and head are elevated to create a horizontal alignment between the external auditory meatus and the sternal notch. Collins and colleagues demonstrated that the 'ramped' position was superior to the standard 'sniffing position' for direct laryngoscopy in morbidly obese patients.[92] The ramped position can also be achieved using commercial devices such as the Oxford H.E.L.P (Head Elevating Laryngoscopy Pillow)[93,94] (see Figure 39.3 in Chapter 39). In patients with braided hair or knotted scarves, these should be undone or removed as they may limit neck extension.[95]

Preoxygenation

An end-tidal O_2 of 0.9 is regarded as the gold standard[96] for optimal preoxygenation. As a result of reduced FRC and increased oxygen consumption, oxygen reserves in the pregnant woman are rapidly depleted following apnoea. A useful concept is the 'safe duration of apnoea' also termed duration of apnoea without desaturation (DAWD). This is defined as the interval between the onset of apnoea and the moment when SpO_2 reaches a value of less than 90%. In healthy non-pregnant adults, DAWD is typically 6.9 minutes after inhaling 100% oxygen.[97] The DAWD is shorter in pregnant women (2 minutes). In non-pregnant subjects, the efficacy of preoxygenation in obese and non-obese subjects is improved by positioning the subject in a head-up position compared with the supine position.[98–100] However, in contrast with obese patients, the head-up position has not been found to confer any advantages in the pregnant women probably because parturients and morbidly obese patients have different fat distributions, and the gravid uterus significantly impairs diaphragmatic excursion, irrespective of position.[101] Leaks around the face mask during preoxygenation which reduce the efficacy of preoxygenation, have been reported in up to 22% of preoxygenation sessions.[102] The effect of fresh gas flow rates on DAWD has also been investigated. Russell and colleagues showed that flow rates of 10 L/min or more for 3 minutes provided optimal preoxygenation in the pregnant patient but this optimization was not improved by increasing the flow from 10 to 15 L/min.[102] Thus a tight fit must be achieved between mask and the patient's face and sufficient gas flow of at least 10 L/min must be provided. Air in the lungs is replaced with oxygen at a rate that depends directly on alveolar minute ventilation and inversely on FRC. In normal adults, to obtain 95% gas exchange, that is FEO_2 greater than 90%, approximately five half times are required and this equates to 2.9 minutes.[101] Hence it is recommended that tidal volume breathing for a minimum of 3 minutes is the most reliable if time allows. However, in emergency situations where time is crucial, the 'fast technique' which involves asking the patient to take deep or vital capacity breaths has been proposed. It has been shown that 8 deep breaths are as effective as 3 minutes of tidal slow breaths and that 4 deep breaths are ineffective[103] although more recent work has recommended 12 deep breaths as being more effective than 8 deep breaths.[104] The use of 10 cmH_2O of positive end-expiratory pressure (PEEP) has been advocated in obese subjects to prolong safe apnoea time.[105,106] However, this may not translate to the pregnant woman where the gravid uterus limits the ability of PEEP to increase FRC. Insufflation of 5L/min oxygen using nasal canulae has also been tried to improve safe apnoea time in obese patients[107] and may be used in obstetrics, particularly in the obese parturient. Apnoeic mass oxygen transfer can be used to delay the onset of desaturation provided the oxygen mask is kept on with a good seal and a patent airway.[108] Therefore, in summary, effective preoxygenation in pregnant patients should be as follows:

- Tidal breathing 10 L/min for 3 minutes with tightly fitting face mask
- In emergency situation with insufficient time for full preoxygenation, 8–12 deep breaths of 10 L/min with tightly fitting face mask.

Cricoid pressure

Cricoid pressure which was first described by Sellick in 1961[109] is aimed at occluding the upper oesophageal sphincter by applying pressure on the cricoid cartilage to prevent regurgitation and aspiration of gastric contents. However, there is controversy regarding the benefit, the technique, the timing, and the method of applying cricoid pressure.[110–113] One prospective study demonstrated that cricoid pressure did not have an effect on preventing regurgitation or reducing mortality.[111] However, this study was not randomized and the possibility of bias could not be excluded. In an editorial to accompany this paper, Vanner stated that cricoid pressure is probably effective in preventing regurgitation at induction of anaesthesia in patients at risk but randomized controlled trials are awaited to confirm this. Although cricoid pressure can improve laryngoscopy view, it can also make the view worse in some patients. Insertion of a laryngeal mask is made more difficult, and ventilation with a face mask is more likely to be obstructed the more cricoid force is applied. It is therefore important that cricoid pressure is released or reduced if intubation or ventilation with a mask is difficult. In the United Kingdom, there is universal agreement amongst anaesthetists to use cricoid pressure during RSI[114] whereas in France, cricoid pressure is used by only 66% of anaesthetists during GA for CD. [115] The amount of force applied is crucial. Too much force (e.g. >45 N) is associated with airway obstruction[116,117] and insufficient force may not protect the patient from regurgitation. In a study in cadavers, 20 N of cricoid force prevented regurgitation with oesophageal pressures of 25 mmHg and 30 N prevented regurgitation with oesophageal pressures of 40 mmHg.[118] Therefore 30 N of cricoid force may replace the function of the upper oesophageal sphincter (UOS) which has a normal functioning pressure of 40 mmHg.[119] Average gastric pressures are 11 mmHg at emergency CDs and below 25 mmHg in 99% of patients.[120] This suggests that the optimum cricoid force in anaesthetized patients should be 30 N.[121,122] The timing of cricoid pressure is important because too much force in the conscious patient will be uncomfortable and can cause retching and vomiting and increase the risk of oesophageal rupture.[123] Thiopentone causes a rapid reduction in the UOS pressure which starts before loss of consciousness.[119] Therefore ideally cricoid pressure should be applied in the awake patient before loss of consciousness as described originally by Sellick.[109] Awake subjects tolerate up to 20 N cricoid pressure without discomfort.[124]

Incorrectly applied cricoid pressure may lead to inability to ventilate the lungs or a poor view of the glottis at laryngoscopy[125] and females are at a higher risk of airway occlusion.[116] If cricoid pressure is applied correctly, it may improve the laryngoscopy grade and does not increase the rate of failed intubation in elective cases.[126,127] There is debate as which hand to use and on which side of the patient to stand while applying cricoid pressure. The force applied by the left hand (non-dominant hand) with the ODP standing on the left side of the patient tends to be lower than that applied by the right hand (dominant hand) and that inadequate or excessive force is more frequent with the left hand.[122] When prolonged cricoid pressure is required, for example, in a failed intubation scenario, incorrect cricoid force is applied more with the left hand than with the right hand.[122] There is no proven benefit in a two-handed technique[128–131] and there is no difference in the incidence of airway obstruction when cricoid pressure is applied in the supine or lateral tilt position.[132] The use of cricoid pressure did not affect the success or duration of intubation when using the Airtraq® video laryngoscope.[133] In a patient with a nasogastric tube, it is not necessary to remove the tube but it should be left open to atmospheric pressure.[134,135]

Therefore in summary, evidence supports:

- applying a force of less than 20 N (10 N should be adequate[135]) cricoid pressure in the conscious patient and 30 N after loss of consciousness
- using one hand and preferably the right hand (dominant hand), applied at 90° to the tilt of the table by a trained assistant[122]
- adjusting or releasing cricoid pressure during a difficult airway and/or intubation.

Optimal laryngoscopy

With correct positioning, optimal preoxygenation, correct choice of drugs, correct application of cricoid pressure, and correct choice of laryngoscope, the first attempt at intubation should result in successful tracheal intubation in the majority of patients. A short-handle or Polio blades are helpful in patients with enlarged breasts. A size 3 Macintosh blade is the standard but size 4 should be selected if deemed necessary in larger women. A McCoy blade (size 3 or 4) may help to lift the epiglottis and should be considered early. If the glottis is partially visible, the tracheal introducer (bougie) is useful but should be used carefully to avoid causing trauma. External laryngeal manipulation consisting of applying backwards, upwards, and rightward pressure on the thyroid cartilage (BURP) and optimal external laryngeal manipulation (OELM) may be used to improve laryngeal view.[136,137] However, it is important to clarify that the two manoeuvres (BURP and OELM) differ from cricoid pressure and the need for cricoid pressure may preclude the use of these manoeuvres. There is now a large amount of data to show that the laryngeal views obtained using video laryngoscopes are significantly better than those using conventional Macintosh laryngoscopy. This has been shown in patients with normal airways, predicted difficult airways, and restricted cervical spine mobility.[67–77] Video laryngoscopes have been used with success in obstetrics.[133,138–140] As a result, video laryngoscopes are becoming accepted as a rescue strategy and should be considered early should the first attempt at intubation fail. Smaller endotracheal tubes (<7 mm internal diameter) should be used routinely especially in patients with airway oedema.

Table 26.5 summarizes the ideal technique in order to optimize airway management and reduce the chance of either a difficult airway or a failed intubation.

Management of the anticipated difficult airway

Management of anticipated difficult airway and tracheal intubation in the pregnancy entails early recognition in the antenatal period and multidisciplinary discussion on the mode of delivery and an airway management strategy.

Antenatal management

Assessment

Any pregnant woman with a suspected or known difficult airway should be referred in the antenatal period to the anaesthetic team. The time of referral to the anaesthetic team should allow sufficient time to obtain previous notes and investigations and carry out any further investigations. Depending on the severity of the difficult airway, an airway and anaesthetic management strategy should be identified and documented in the notes.

Plan

If a difficult airway is anticipated, the anaesthetist should liaise with the obstetrician to decide on the mode of delivery to ensure safe

Table 26.5 Optimum GA to reduce the risks of difficult airway or failed intubation the obstetric patient

Staff	Multidisciplinary team briefing/WHO check
	Trained ODP staff
Fasting	Nil by mouth for elective cases
	Oral fluids only for HAR and light diet for LAR in labour
Premedication	H_2 antagonist/antacid ± prokinetics
Equipment	Full AAGBI standard monitoring
	Electric operating table capable of taking >160 kg on a tilt
	Airway equipment (Box 26.3)
	Suction
Position	Slight head-up and optimize head and neck position
	Ramping in obese patient (external auditory meatus is aligned horizontally with the sternal notch)
	15° left lateral tilt
Pre-oxygenation	End-tidal oxygen of >90%
	3 minutes' tidal breathing or 8–12 vital capacity breaths of 100% oxygen, 10 L/min with tight-fitting mask
	Maintain mask on face and maintain a clear airway to allow apnoeic mass oxygen transfer
	+/– use of insufflation of 5L of oxygen via nasal canuale
Drugs	Correct doses of induction agent and muscle relaxant
Cricoid pressure	At 90° to the tilted table
	10 N with induction agent and 30 N at loss of consciousness
Optimal laryngoscopy	Correct choice of laryngoscope
	Availability of an alternate laryngoscope
	Appropriate use of a bougie
Confirm intubation	Confirm correct placement of the tracheal tube (visual/chest movement/auscultation and end-tidal CO_2 measurement)
	Maintenance of a balanced anaesthetic technique with volatile agents, muscle relaxants, and analgesia
Extubation	Consider insertion and aspiration of orogastric tube where necessary
	Suction under direct vision and insert bite block
	Use of peripheral nerve stimulator
	Use of reversal agents
	Extubate awake
	Position—left lateral or head-up
Recovery	Monitoring and appropriately trained staff

HAR, high aspiration risk; LAR, low aspiration risk.

outcome for both mother and baby. The decision for vaginal birth will mean that an unscheduled operative procedure may occur with all the potential for a failed intubation. Elective CD allows the opportunity for timed planned delivery. The risks and benefits of management options should be clearly explained to the patient and partner. Neuraxial anaesthesia should be strongly recommended.

Communication

Communication with the multidisciplinary team regarding a management plan for the patient with a known difficult airway is essential in order to ensure a safe outcome for both mother and baby.[144] The theatre team should be given sufficient notice to ensure that appropriate equipment and trained staff are available. Backup plans are necessary to recruit additional senior anaesthetic staff when necessary.

Management options

Airway management of a patient with anticipated difficult airway depends on whether the elected mode of delivery is a planned vaginal delivery or elective CD. A suggested algorithm in Figure 26.6 summarizes pathways that could be followed. These are not the only approaches as patient co-morbidity and different situations vary significantly and will influence the final decision.

Planned vaginal delivery

When vaginal delivery is planned, the type of labour analgesia and anaesthetic management for unanticipated operative delivery should be documented in the notes. The best way to circumvent a difficult airway or a failed intubation is to avoid GA by siting an epidural early in labour and active management to ensure a good working epidural block which can be used confidently for any operative procedure. However, the risks of a failed regional, high or total spinal blockade, and inadvertent intravenous injection should be considered. It may be advisable therefore that regional block in such a patient should be carried out by a very experienced anaesthetist. Approximately 5% of women who have epidural analgesia for labour and require topping up for operative delivery need conversion to GA[141] and this should be anticipated. The patient should receive regular antacid prophylaxis during labour and oral intake should be restricted in case a GA is required. There should be a plan for the administration of a GA should this be required and this could entail either the use of awake fibreoptic intubation or awake intubation using other rigid airway devices.[142–146] An awake tracheostomy or cricothyroid cannula may be considered before inducing GA in patients with a severe difficult airway.

Planned elective caesarean delivery

Ideally, an elective CD in a patient with known difficult airway should be carried out under neuraxial anaesthesia. The choice of anaesthesia can be either a single-shot spinal, epidural, combined spinal–epidural (CSE), or continuous spinal catheter[147] anaesthetic. Despite meticulous technique, these techniques may fail to produce adequate anaesthesia for surgery and plans should be in place if this should happen. For this reason, a CSE may be preferable to a single-shot spinal or epidural because of its added flexibility should a top-up be required. However, even a CSE may fail as reported in a woman who had both failed CSE and failed intubation.[148] A backup plan such as an awake intubation or the use of a SAD should be in place for when neuraxial anaesthesia fails or serious complications of regional block occur.

Awake intubation using the fibreoptic scope or other airway devices is an alternative plan for elective CD when regional block is contraindicated, when regional anaesthesia fails, or when serious complications occur.

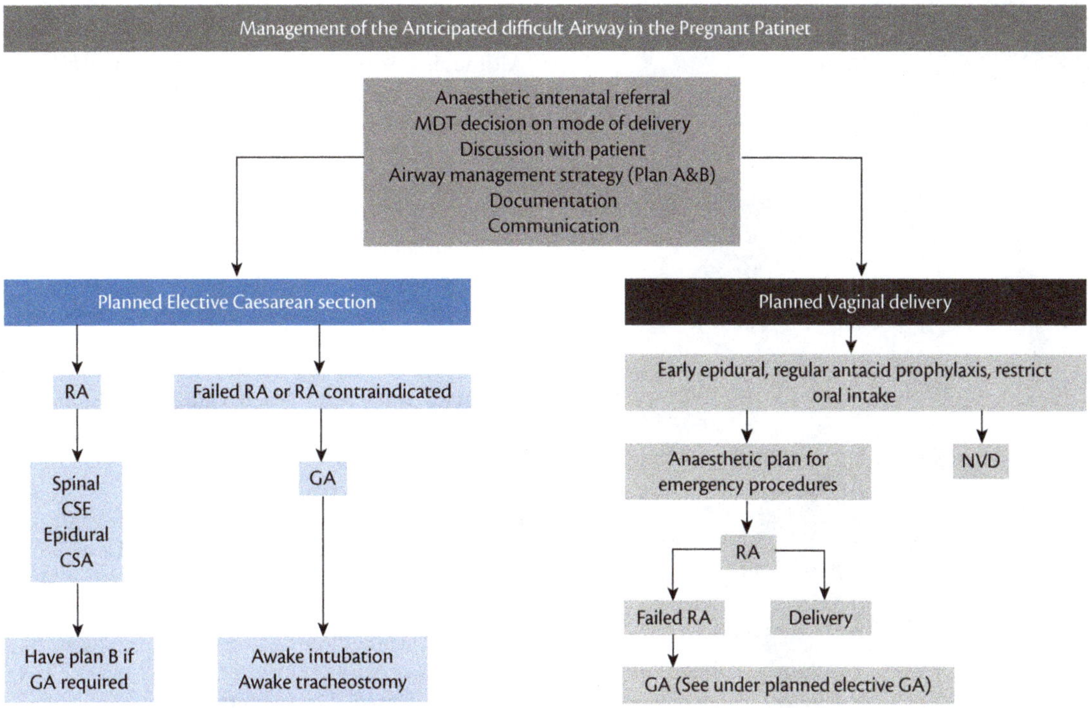

MDT-Multidisciplinary team, GA-General anaesthetic, NVD-Normal vaginal delivery, CSE-Combined spinal epidural, CSA-Continuous spinal anaesthetic, RA-Regional anaesthetic

Figure 26.6 A suggested algorithm for the management of the anticipated difficult airway in the pregnant patient.
This article was published in *Chestnut's Obstetric Anesthesia, Principles and Practice*, Chestnut DH *et al.*, Copyright Elsevier (2014).

Local anaesthetic infiltration as the sole anaesthetic for CD is an option but this is seldom carried out in the United Kingdom because of lack of experience. The majority of obstetricians are neither familiar nor proficient with this technique. Large volumes of local anaesthetic are required with the possibility of toxicity especially when the maximum dose of local anaesthetic may already have been reached with previously attempted central neuraxial blockade.

Awake intubation techniques

Intubation may be performed by awake fibreoptic intubation, awake intubation via a SAD such as an intubating LMA[143,144] or an LMA[142] or intubation using rigid laryngoscopes such as the Macintosh, a video laryngoscope[146] or the Bullard laryngoscope.[145] The classic and more conventional way for awake intubation is to use a flexible fibreoptic scope.

Awake fibreoptic intubation

Preparation

Consent: the patient should be well informed of the need for the awake intubation. The procedure should be explained and informed consent obtained.

Fasting: for an elective procedure, the patient should be starved for 6 hours as normal practice.

Premedication: premedication should include an H_2 antagonist and 30 mL of 0.3 M sodium citrate immediately prior to starting sedation. An antisialogogue—glycopyrrolate 200 mcg intravenously—should be administered as soon as an intravenous cannula has been inserted.

Team: two experienced anaesthetists are required, one to perform the endoscopy and the other to monitor and administer sedation. An experienced ODP is essential. Neonatologists should be made aware in advance of the use of sedation and its potential effects on the neonate.

Equipment—the following equipment should be available:

- full monitoring
- fibreoptic scope with camera and monitor
- an airway adjunct to stop the patient biting and damaging the fibreoptic scope, such as the Berman airway (Figure 26.7)
- equipment to apply local anaesthetic to the upper airway, for example, mucosal atomizing device or cannula, oxygen tubing, and three-way tap for the Mackenzie technique[149] (Figure 26.8)
- epidural catheter fed through the working channel of the scope for administration of local anaesthetic
- tracheal tube size 6–7 mm (re-enforced or intubating LMA tracheal tube are recommended)
- syringe pump for administration of drugs by infusion.

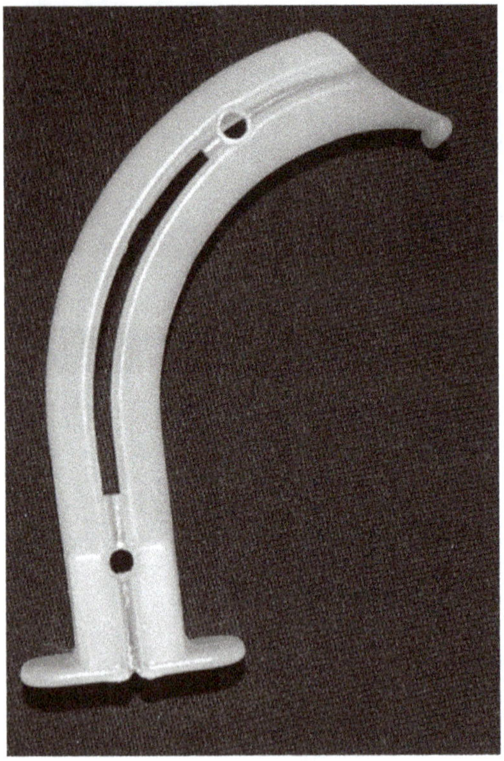

Figure 26.7 The Berman airway used to protect the fibreoptic scope during awake fibreoptic intubation.

Performance of intubation

Conscious sedation

Although it is possible to carry out awake fibreoptic intubation with local anaesthetic alone,[150] it is more comfortable for the patient to receive some form of sedation/analgesia using midazolam, fentanyl, alfentanil, remifentanil, or propofol. Midazolam 0.5–1 mg is useful to ensure a degree of amnesia. Remifentanil is gaining popularity as it provides the best analgesia for the mother with conscious and cooperative sedation and suppression of the gag reflex which gives good intubating conditions. Infusion rates of 0.05–0.175 mcg/kg/min[151] or target-controlled infusion (TCI) of up to 3 ng/mL have been used in non-obstetric patients. TCI with propofol has been used for awake fibreoptic intubation in obstetrics when a target concentration of 0.8–1.2 mcg/mL was used successfully combined with midazolam 1 mg and topical anaesthesia.[152] A recent extensive review on conscious sedation for awake fibreoptic intubation by Johnston and Rai, recommended remifentanil TCI (effect-site concentration 3–5 ng/mL) in conjunction with midazolam 1–2 mg or with propofol TCI (effect-site concentration 0.5–0.8 mcg/mL).[153] Excessive sedation should be avoided as it makes the larynx incompetent and increases the likelihood of aspiration. Antagonists such as flumazenil and naloxone should be readily available. Oxygen should be administered. Dexmedetomidine, which has found favour for sedation in critical care, has been enthusiastically advocated for awake fibreoptic intubation on the grounds of its ability to

(A)

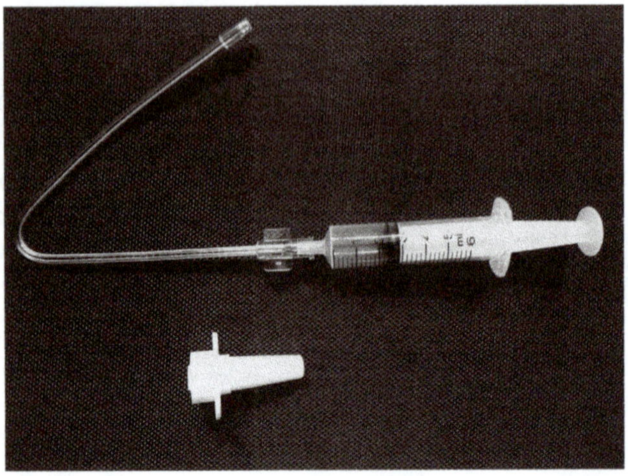

(B)

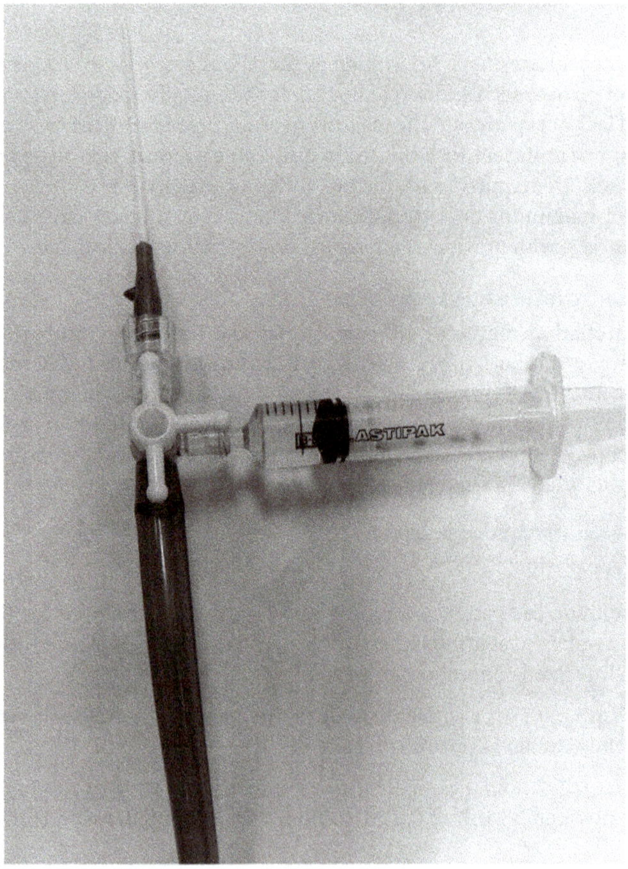

Figure 26.8 Two methods for applying local anaesthetic to the upper airway during awake fibreoptic intubation. (A) LMA MADgic™ (Mucosal Atomising Device). (B) Oxygen tubing, three-way tap, and a cannula for the Mackenzie technique. Image courtesy of Teleflex Incorporated.

provide profound sedation without causing respiratory depression. However, experience of its use in the United Kingdom either in the general or the obstetric population is limited. There is some evidence in case reports of its use in obstetrics.[154,155]

Topical anaesthesia

Concern has been raised in the use of topical airway anaesthesia in patients at risk of regurgitation and aspiration. However, Ovassapian et al. showed that provided sedation was not excessive, there was no evidence that there is increased risk of regurgitation and aspiration.[156]

The nose, mouth, and pharynx may be anaesthetized by direct spray using a device such as the commercially produced mucosal atomizing device (MAD®) (Figure 26.8A) or the Mackenzie technique which uses a size 18 or 20 G cannula attached by a three-way tap to oxygen tubing which is connected to 2 L/min oxygen supply[149] (Figure 26.8B). The patient may also be asked to gargle using 6 mL of 2% lignocaine gel (Instillagel®). The remainder of the airway can be anaesthetized using one of three techniques: spray as you go (SAYGO), nerve blocks, and nebulized lignocaine:

- SAYGO: this involves dripping local anaesthetic into the airway via an epidural catheter fed through the working channel of the fibreoptic scope. Aliquots of 1–2 mL of 4% lignocaine are injected into the supraglottic, glottis, and subglottic area.
- Nerve blocks: this is seldom carried out. It involves blocking the lingual branch of the glossopharyngeal nerve which supplies the base of the tongue. Injection is made into the base of the anterior tonsillar pillar with 2 mL of 1% lignocaine. The second nerve block is the internal branch of the superior laryngeal nerve which is performed by locating the greater cornu of the hyoid bone and injecting 2–3 mL of 1% lidocaine into the thyrohyoid membrane. This is followed by transtracheal injection of 2–3 mL of 2% lignocaine through the cricothyroid membrane using a cannula.
- Nebulized lignocaine: nebulized 4% lignocaine (4–6 mL) anaesthetizes the nose, mouth, pharynx, larynx, and trachea. However, when used alone, it is not fully effective and requires supplementation with the SAYGO technique.

In general, the total dose of lignocaine for awake fibreoptic intubation exceeds the normal recommended dose of 200 mg. This is because a large proportion is swallowed and because of the high first-pass metabolism, toxic blood concentrations are not reached when using doses up to 9 mg/kg in non-pregnant patients.[157,158] However, this may need to be reduced in the pregnant patient because of the increased vascularity of the upper airway.

Route of intubation

The oral intubation is the preferred route of intubation because of the risks of nasal bleeding from the congested nasal and airway mucosa. Occasionally, this route is not possible due to oral or temporomandibular joint pathology or trismus and the nasal route must be used and if so, the type of vasoconstrictor should be considered carefully.[159] Cocaine is a very effective vasoconstrictor but it is associated with reduced placental blood flow and placental abruption and therefore is best avoided during pregnancy.[160,161] Phenylephrine 0.5%/lignocaine 5% combination and xylometazoline hydrochloride 0.1% spray are safer alternatives. Vasoconstrictors should be used with care in pre-eclamptic patients as they may cause hypertension.

Position

It is important that aortocaval compression is avoided during the procedure by positioning the patient in either the sitting posture or with left lateral tilt.

Intubation

A small size tracheal tube such as size 6–7 should be used to reduce the chance of impingement on the arytenoids. The design of the tip of the tube may also make a difference and the intubating LMA tracheal tube with a Huber tip is the least likely to impinge. When the trachea is intubated, the cuff should be inflated and the position of the tube confirmed before the patient is anaesthetized.

Management of unanticipated difficult intubation

The unanticipated difficult intubation in the pregnant patient presents problems different from those in the non-pregnant patient (Box 26.5).

If tracheal intubation fails after the first attempt despite reducing or removing cricoid pressure, external laryngeal manipulation, adjustment of head and neck position and use of a bougie if appropriate, then gentle mask ventilation is recommended to oxygenate the lungs, assess the ease of ventilation and provide time to prepare equipment for the second intubation strategy.[162–165] However care should be taken to avoid insufflation of the stomach. A second attempt at intubation should be with an alternative laryngoscope with cricoid pressure removed. In order to avoid bleeding and airway oedema, the number of attempts to intubate should be limited to a maximum of two as excessive attempts at airway manipulation may convert a 'can't intubate, can oxygenate' scenario to a 'can't intubate, can't oxygenate' scenario. If

Box 26.5 Factors to consider during unanticipated difficult intubation in the pregnant patient

1. Physiological changes which accelerate the onset of hypoxaemia—may need mask ventilation between attempts at intubation
2. Risk of upper airway oedema and bleeding—avoid excess multiple attempts, avoid the use of nasopharyngeal airway
3. Enlarged breasts which obstruct the insertion of the laryngoscope—use short-handle laryngoscope
4. Remote site which means that help make take a while to arrive—call for help earlier
5. The presence of a fetus which confounds the decision of when to wake the mother up or continue with the surgery—an advance multidisciplinary decision is recommended
6. Application of fundal pressure may exacerbate the risk of regurgitation and aspiration if anaesthesia is continued using a supraglottic airway device—ask obstetrician to avoid or minimize during delivery of baby
7. Choice of anaesthesia to minimize uterine relaxation—be prepared for postdelivery haemorrhage.

Box 26.6 Proceed with surgery?

Factors to consider		WAKE	⟵	⟶	PROCEED
Before induction	**Maternal condition**	• No compromise	• Mild acute compromise	• Haemorrhage responsive to resuscitation	• Hypovolaemia requiring corrective surgery • Critical cardiac or respiratory compromise, cardiac arrest
	Fetal condition	• No compromise	• Compromise corrected with intrauterine resuscitation pH < 7.2 but > 7.15	• Continuing fetal heart rate abnormality despite intrauterine resuscitation pH < 7.15	• Sustained bradycardia • Fetal haemorrhage • Suspected uterine rupture
	Anaesthetist	• Novice	• Junior trainee	• Senior trainee	• Consultant / specialist
	Obesity	• Supermorbid	• Morbid	• Obese	• Normal
	Surgical factors	• Complex surgery or major haemorrhage anticipated	• Multiple uterine scars • Some surgical difficulties expected	• Single uterine scar	• No risk factors
	Aspiration risk	• Recent food	• No recent food • In labour • Opioids given • Antacids not given	• No recent food • In labour • Opioids not given • Antacids given	• Fasted • Not in labour • Antacids given
	Alternative anaesthesia • **regional** • **securing airway awake**	• No anticipated difficulty	• Predicted difficulty	• Relatively contraindicated	• Absolutely contraindicated or has failed • Surgery started
After failed intubation	**Airway device / ventilation**	• Difficult facemask ventilation • Front-of-neck	• Adequate facemask ventilation	• First generation supraglottic airway device	• Second generation supraglottic airway device
	Airway hazards	• Laryngeal oedema • Stridor	• Bleeding • Trauma	• Secretions	• None evident

Criteria to be used in the decision to wake or proceed following failed tracheal intubation. In any individual patient, some factors may suggest waking and others proceeding. The final decision will depend on the anaesthetist's clinical judgement.

Reproduced from Mushambi MC, Kinsella SM, Popat M., et al. Obstetric Anaesthetists' Association and Difficult Airway Society guidelines for the management of difficult and failed intubation in obstetrics. *Anaesthesia* 2015; 70: 1286–1306, copyright © 2015 The authors. Anaesthesia published by John Wiley & Sons Ltd on behalf of Association of Anaesthetists of Great Britain and Ireland.

intubation fails after the second attempt, the anaesthetist should declare a failed intubation, communicate this to the obstetrician and theatre team and help urgently summoned. Help should be sought from senior anaesthetists including a consultant, a senior obstetrician and an additional ODP.

The decision needs to be made whether to proceed or to wake the patient. This decision is complicated because of the two lives at risk and ideally this decision should be made with the team prior to the administration of GA. The new OAA/DAS obstetric airway guidelines[166] propose a list of factors to be considered to help with this decision making and is shown in Box 26.6. The table demonstrates clearly that the decision to wake the mother or proceed with surgery is influenced by multiple factors relating to the woman, fetus, staff and clinical situation and this information is available prior to the induction of GA. Factors relating to the rescue device and airway patency are only available once failed intubation has occurred.

Failed intubation algorithm

Traditionally, the teaching has been to awaken the woman if failed intubation occurs, in order to avoid continuing with an unprotected airway. However in a recent article, 8 anaesthetists describe continuing GA with cLMA for non-urgent cases (category 3 and 4)[18]. This is in contrast with previous publications in which anaesthetists tended to wake patients up during a failed intubation.[19,23] This change of practice may be as a result of increased experience in the use of SAD in the non-pregnant patients and publications of the use of supraglottic airway devices for elective Caesarean delivery.[167–169] Traditionally, SADs are used for elective surgery when the patient is considered at low risk of regurgitation

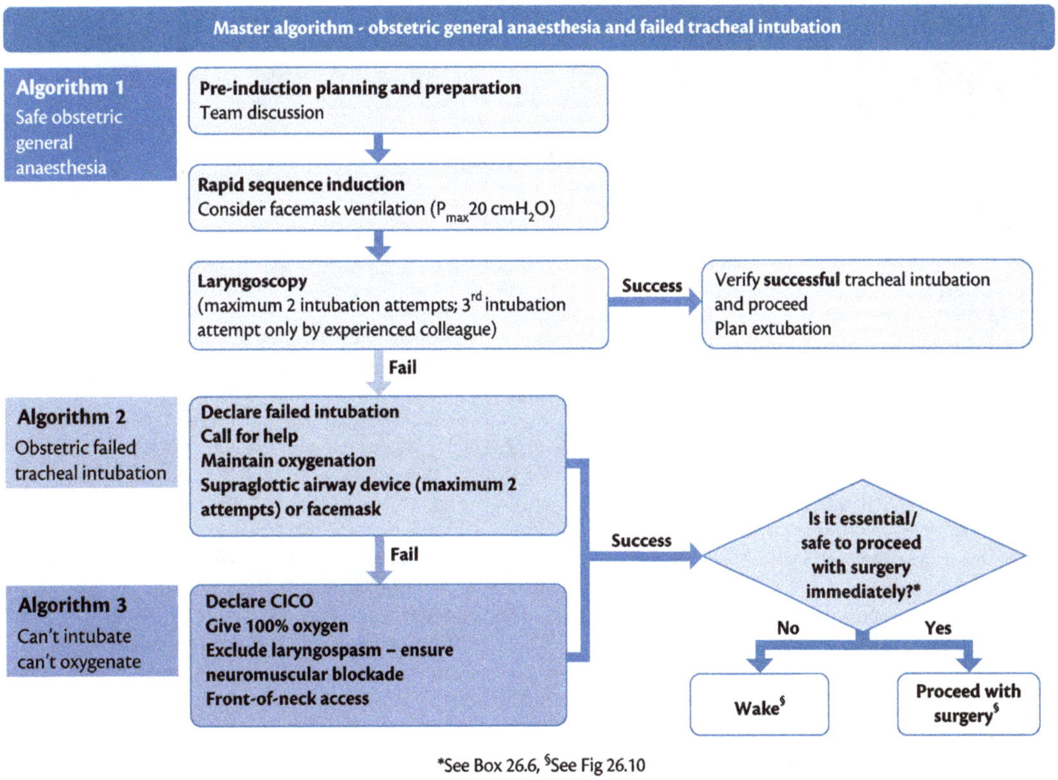

Figure 26.9 Obstetric Anaesthetists' Association/Difficult Airway Society: Master algorithm—Obstetric general anaesthesia and failed tracheal intubation with permission from OAA.

Reproduced from Mushambi MC, Kinsella SM, Popat M., et al. Obstetric Anaesthetists' Association and Difficult Airway Society guidelines for the management of difficult and failed intubation in obstetrics. *Anaesthesia* 2015; 70: 1286–1306, copyright © 2015 The authors. *Anaesthesia* published by John Wiley & Sons Ltd on behalf of Association of Anaesthetists of Great Britain and Ireland.

and aspiration. As a result, the use of SADs for Caesarean deliveries had been limited to failed intubations.[170–176] In 2001, Han evaluated the use of classic LMAs in 1,067 elective Caesarean sections and recommended it for experienced users and selected patients.[168] However in an editorial following this publication, Preston argued that the use of SAD in selected patients in this study should not be accepted as safe for airway management in the pregnant patient who is at risk of aspiration.[177] The conclusion in this editorial was that the SAD is acceptable as an emergency rescue device for airway management in the parturient but not as the sole chosen airway device. The UKOSS survey showed that the commonest airway rescue device was the cLMA with 39 out of 57 cases using it.[18] The choice of the cLMA over other types of SADs such as the second generation SADs in this survey is likely to be related to experience and familiarity with the cLMA. The LMA ProSeal™ and Supreme LMA have also been evaluated in selected patients for elective Caesarean section with no adverse effects.[167,169]

In the past, several failed intubations algorithms for the pregnant patient have been described[166,180–185] and in 2004 DAS published guidelines for the management of unanticipated difficult intubation in the non-pregnant patient[186] and these have recently been updated.[187] However it is only recently that the OAA and DAS published the obstetric specific airway guidelines which are based around four algorithms and two tables.[166] The master algorithms Figure 26.9, gives a composite overview of three specific algorithms that deal with induction of general anaesthesia, failed intubation and can't intubate can't oxygenate situation.

Oxygenation of the patient following a failed intubation should be with the use of either a face mask with or without simple adjuncts such as an oropharyngeal airway or the use of a supraglottic airway device. A nasopharyngeal airway should be avoided because of the risk of epistaxis which may then worsen the situation. If an oropharyngeal airway fails, this is followed by two person mask ventilation technique and then a removal of cricoid pressure. If a supraglottic airway is used, a second generation supraglottic airway device such as LMA ProSeal™, LMA Supreme, i-gel® is recommended. It is necessary to remove cricoid pressure during insertion of the supraglottic device. If ventilation and oxygenation fails, the anaesthetist should declare a can't intubate, can't oxygenate situation and ensure muscle paralysis before proceeding to a front-of-the-neck access.

Front-of-neck access is a rescue technique which is used when there is increasing hypoxaemia and inability to ventilate the lungs and the three options for oxygenating the patient are:

(i) Cricothyroidotomy with a narrow bore non-kinking cannula and oxygenation with a high pressure system (eg. Manujet®)

(ii) Cricothyroidotomy with large bore cannula and ventilation of lungs using normal anaesthetic circuit.

(iii) Surgical cricothyrodotomy or tracheostomy with ventilation using normal anaesthetic circuit.

Narrow bore cricothyroidotomy has the advantage of being quick and simple to perform but has a high failure rate particularly in

Management after failed tracheal intubation

Wake

- Maintain oxygenation
- Maintain cricoid pressure if not impeding ventilation
- Either maintain head-up position or turn left lateral recumbent
- If rocuronium used, reverse with sugammadex
- Assess neuromuscular blockade and manage awareness if paralysis is prolonged
- Anticipate laryngospasm / can't intubate, can't oxygenate

After waking

- Review urgency of surgery with obstetric team
- Intrauterine fetal resuscitation as appropriate
- For repeat anaesthesia, manage with two anaesthetists
- Anaesthetic options:
  - Regional anaesthesia preferably inserted in lateral position
  - Secure airway awake before repeat general anaesthesia

Proceed with surgery

- Maintain anaesthesia
- Maintain ventilation -consider merits of:
  - controlled or spontaneous ventilation
  - paralysis with rocuronium if sugammadex available
- Anticipate laryngospasm/ can't intubate, can't oxygenate
- Minimise aspiration risk:
  - Maintain cricoid pressure until delivery (if not impeding ventilation)
  - after delivery maintain vigilance and reapply cricoid pressure if signs of regurgitation
  - empty stomach with gastric drain tube if using second generation supraglotticairway device
  - minimise fundal pressure
  - **administer H_2 receptor blocker i.v. if not already given**
- Senior obstetrician to operate
- Inform neonatal team about failed intubation
- Consider total intravenous anaesthesia

Figure 26.10 OAA/DAS obstetric airway guidelines—Management after failed tracheal intubation.[166]
Reproduced from Mushambi MC, Kinsella SM, Popat M., et al. Obstetric Anaesthetists' Association and Difficult Airway Society guidelines for the management of difficult and failed intubation in obstetrics. *Anaesthesia* 2015; 70: 1286–1306, copyright © 2015 The authors. Anaesthesia published by John Wiley & Sons Ltd on behalf of Association of Anaesthetists of Great Britain and Ireland.

the obese patient.[9] It only provides a temporary airway and is associated with complications such as barotrauma from the high pressure ventilating system. Large bore cannulae have a higher success rate but are associated with more complications at insertion such as haemorrhage and damage to neck structures. These may be inserted using the Seldinger technique. The use of surgical cricothyroidotomy using a scalpel, bougie and tube technique is now recommended by the new 2015 DAS Unanticipated difficult airway guidelines.[187] Tracheostomy requires an ENT surgeon and may not be practical because most labour wards in the UK are sited remotely from the central operating department.

How to proceed with general anaesthesia or awaken the patient

Should a decision be made to either continue with general anaesthesia to allow surgery to continue or awaken the patient, Table 2 of the OAA/DAS obstetric guidelines (Figure 26.10) provides information on positioning, mode of anaesthesia and ventilation and prevention of aspiration and awareness. The choice of airway will depend on what has already been used as a rescue airway strategy and this could be mask ± oropharyngeal airway (less preferable) or a SAD (preferably a second generation SAD). Further attempts to intubate the trachea are discouraged as this may lead to loss of airway from airway trauma and oedema. Intubation of the trachea in this situation should only be considered if the patient requires admission to the ITU for further ventilation of the lungs. In this situation, the SAD may be used to facilitate fibreoptic laryngoscopy to achieve tracheal intubation. However, only an anaesthetist skilled in fibreoptic intubation skills should undertake this task. A ventilation- exchange bougie such as the Aintree Intubating Catheter (AIC) may be used to facilitate intubation and removal of the SAD if prolonged intubation is anticipated.[188] The AIC is loaded onto the fibreoptic scope and placed into the trachea under direct vision. The SAD is then removed and an endotracheal tube is railroaded over the AIC and passed into the trachea using the AIC as a bougie. This task should again only be carried out by an anaesthetist who is trained and experienced in its use as its misuse has been associated with significant morbidity and mortality. A tracheostomy may be an alternative choice of airway. Uterine relaxation from the inevitable use of higher inspired concentrations of a volatile agent may cause postpartum haemorrhage. The choice of agent depends on the anaesthetist's experience, but sevoflurane offers an advantage in being less irritant to the airway. Measures should be taken to prevent postpartum haemorrhage such the use of an oxytocin infusion. At delivery, the surgeons should be warned about minimising fundal pressure to avoid reflux, regurgitation and the risk of aspiration.

Tracheal extubation and recovery

In the NAP4 report, 28% of the reported cases were airway complications at emergence and in the recovery period emphasizing that both these periods are high risk for airway complications.[9] Some of the recommendations of NAP4 were that patients at high risk of airway problems at emergence require specific extubation and re-intubation plans; recovery staff should be trained to an agreed standard in all hospital sites and this must include prevention, early recognition, and management of airway obstruction; and the use of capnograph in the recovery area especially in high-risk cases. In the 2006–2008 CMACE report,[4] one mother died from aspiration of gastric contents on emergence from a GA following emergency CD. She had had a full meal shortly before

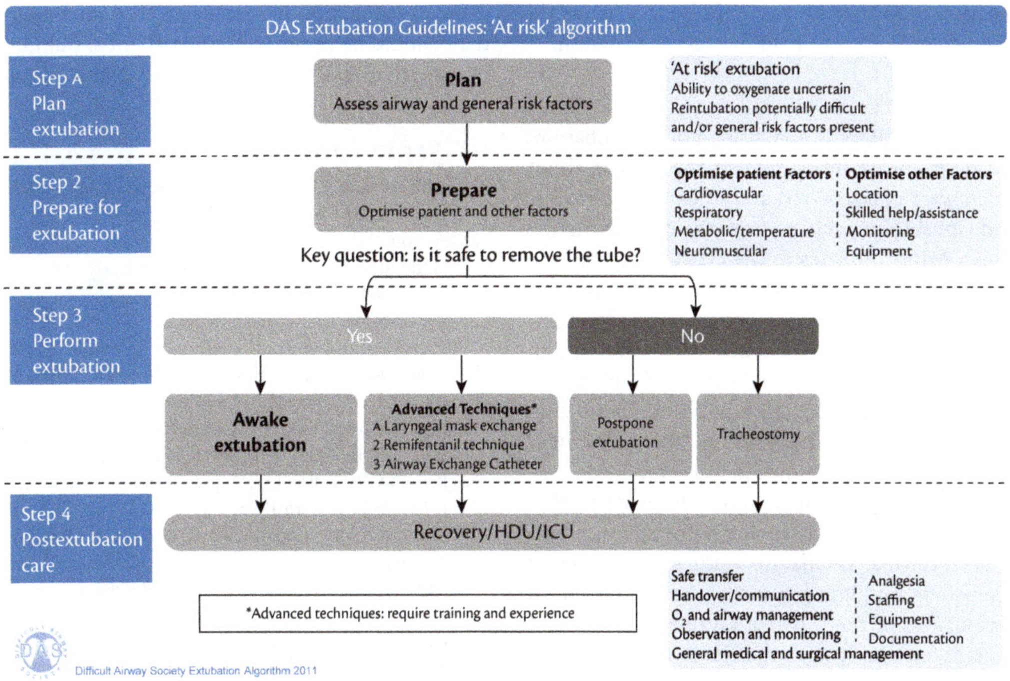

Figure 26.11 The Difficult Airway Society extubation guidelines—'at-risk' patient.

Reproduced with permission from V. Mitchell *et al.* Difficult Airway Society Guidelines for the management of tracheal extubation, *Anaesthesia*, Volume 67, Issue 3, pp. 318–30, Copyright © 2012 John Wiley and Sons.

the decision for an emergency (category 1) CD and an orogastric tube was not used. In a series of anaesthesia-related deaths from Michigan, United States,[189] five of eight anaesthesia related deaths, occurred from obstruction or hypoventilation during emergence and recovery. Inadequate postoperative monitoring was recognized in five patients and in two of these continuous pulse oximetry was not used. In a paper by McDonnell and colleagues, regurgitation of gastric contents occurred in 8/1095 patients (0.7%); four episodes were at induction, five at extubation (one patient regurgitated at induction and extubation), and two of these cases were elective.[25]

DAS has recently published guidelines for the management of extubation[190] and these may be used for both the pregnant or recently pregnant patient (Figure 26.11).

The guidelines describe four steps of the extubation process:

1. *Planning extubation*: the risk factors such as known difficult airway, risk of aspiration, airway oedema, obesity, obstructive sleep apnoea, and any special medical conditions which may have an impact on the airway at extubation should be identified and included in the decision-making of how to extubate the trachea.
2. *Preparing for extubation*: this requires optimizing the patient and the environment for extubation. Equipment, monitoring, and skilled assistance should be available and the location for extubation should be chosen according to the patient's risk factors. In cases where there are concerns about airway oedema (e.g. in pre-eclampsia), tracheal extubation can be delayed until the swelling has subsided and a leak around the tracheal tube is present.
3. *Performing extubation*: because of the nature of increased aspiration risk, obstetric patients are in the 'at-risk' category of the algorithm. If the patient has a difficult airway, this should be taken into account whether the trachea is extubated awake, delayed, or a tracheostomy is required prior to extubation. The advanced techniques in the algorithm are unlikely to apply in the obstetric patient who is at high risk of aspiration. Oropharyngeal suction should occur under direct vision and with the patient in a deep plane of anaesthesia. The use of a bite block can prevent occlusion of the airway if the patient bites down on the tube. NMB should be checked with a peripheral nerve stimulator and antagonized and the patient's lungs pre-oxygenated. Traditionally, all obstetric patients underwent awake tracheal extubation and in the left lateral head-down position. There is a general trend towards extubating patients awake but in the head-up position, especially the obese patient.
4. *Post-extubation care:* after extubation, the patient should be given oxygen and safely transferred to the recovery ward where full monitoring should be used and the patient looked after by trained recovery staff.

Post-failed intubation/difficult airway management plan

The team

Difficult airway or failed intubation can be very stressful to the staff involved in the management of the patient. The psychological impact of a failed intubation and the aftermath on the staff should not be underestimated. It is vital that all members of staff are supported and a mentor assigned if necessary. Debriefing of the team at a time to suit all staff but preferably within a few hours of the incident is recommended as it may help allay anxiety and provide reassurance to the staff. Another aim is to provide and record information and to gain feedback while the details are still fresh.[191]

The patient

Following management of difficult airway or failed intubation, the patient should be followed up to inform the patient about the difficulties which were encountered and to carry out a clinical review to exclude morbidities arising from the difficult airway management process. Minor injuries to the airway may include dental damage, minor bruises to the lips, and sore throat. Serious morbidities include damage to the larynx (oedema or perforation) and perforation of the pharynx or oesophagus. Perforation might present with pyrexia, retrosternal pain, and surgical emphysema. This can be associated with high mortality and therefore if suspected, urgent review by the ENT specialist and early treatment with antibiotics and nil by mouth regimen is recommended.[192]

Reviewing the patient is a good opportunity to explain what happened, express regret, and provide apologies for any morbidities that may have been caused. The nature of the problem should be explained to the patient and it is paramount for the patient to understand the seriousness of the problem and that they should convey this to clinicians, especially anaesthetists, in the future. The possibility of awareness should be explored as there is an increased incidence in the obstetric patient with a difficult airway.[193]

Documentation

The patient's case notes should have the full documentation of the incident and any discussions with the patient. A summary of airway management should be fully documented on the anaesthetic chart. The airway management information should state what the difficulty was (e.g. difficulty with mask ventilation), direct laryngoscopy or tracheal intubation, grade of laryngoscopy, how the airway was managed, airway equipment or adjuncts used, and any advice about management in the future if appropriate (e.g. recommend an awake fibreoptic intubation).

Communication regarding the airway problem should be in the form of a medical alert bracelet, documentation in the notes, a letter to the general practitioner, and a copy of the letter should be given to the patient to present to the clinicians at future. An example of a form which can be used is available on the DAS website.[194]

Conclusion

Management of difficult airway in obstetrics still remains challenging. Over the past 6 decades, increasing use of neuraxial anaesthesia has helped to decrease the mortality and morbidity associated with anaesthesia. However, the incidence of difficult airway in obstetrics remains largely unchanged. This may be due to lack of training opportunities, and increase in maternal obesity and age with the associated comorbidities. Early referral to the anaesthetist for antenatal planning and preparation, involvement of multidisciplinary teams, use of skills drills and simulation, availability of advanced airway management devices, and the skills to use the devices can be helpful in managing both unanticipated and anticipated difficult intubation. During a failed or difficult intubation, the primary goal is to maintain maternal and fetal oxygenation and the decision-making whether to proceed or wake the patient during a failed intubation should involve the senior anaesthetist and obstetrician. Extubation remains a high-risk period and therefore requires careful planning and preparation. When a failed or difficult intubation has occurred, full documentation of the incident should be performed, the patient should be followed up, and documentation to inform future anaesthetists put into place.

References

1. Aitkenhead AR. Injuries associated with anaesthesia. A global perspective. *Br J Anaesth* 2005; 95 (1):95–109.
2. Arbous MS, Grobbee DE, van Kleef JW, *et al.* Mortality associated with anaesthesia: a qualitative analysis to identify risk factors. *Anaesthesia* 2001; 56(12):1141–53.
3. Kawashima Y, Takahashi S, Suzuki M, *et al.* Anesthesia-related mortality and morbidity over a 5-year period in 2,363,038 patients in Japan. *Acta Anaesthesiol Scand* 2003; 47(7):809–17.
4. Centre for Maternal and Child Enquiries (CMACE). Saving mothers lives. Reviewing maternal deaths to make motherhood safer: 2006–2008. *BJOG* 2011; 118 Suppl 1: 1–203.
5. Brown GW, Russell IF. A survey of anaesthesia for Caesarean section. *Int J Obstet Anesth* 1995; 4:214–18.
6. Thomas J, Paranjothy S, Royal College of Obstetricians and Gynaecologists Clinical Effectiveness Support Unit. *The National Sentinel Caesarean Section Audit Report.* London: RCOG Press; 2001.
7. Obstetric Anaesthetists' Association. *National Obstetric Anaesthesia Database.* [Online] http://www.oaa-anaes.ac.uk/ui/content/content.aspx?id=131
8. Colvin JR, Peden J (eds). *Raising the Standard: A Compendium of Audit Recipes* (3rd ed). London: The Royal College of Anaesthetists; 2012.
9. Cook TM, Woodall N, Frerk C (eds). *4th National Audit Project: Major Complications of Airway Management in the UK.* London: Royal College of Anaesthetists; 2011. http://www.rcoa.ac.uk/nap4.
10. American Society of Anesthesiologists Task Force on Management of the Difficult Airway. Practice guidelines for management of the difficult airway: an updated report by the American Society of Anesthesiologists Task Force on Management of the Difficult Airway. *Anesthesiology* 2003; 98:1269 –77.
11. Han R, Tremper KK, Kheterpal S, *et al.* Grading scale for mask ventilation. *Anesthesiology* 2004; 101(1):267.
12. Kherterpal S, Han R, Tremper KK, *et al.* Incidence and prediction of difficult and impossible mask ventilation. *Anesthesiology* 2006; 105:885–91.
13. Langeron O, Massa E, Huraux C, *et al.* Prediction of difficult mask ventilation. *Anesthesiology* 2000; 92:1217–18.
14. Cormack RS, Lehane J. Difficult tracheal intubation in obstetrics. *Anaesthesia* 1984; 39:1105–11.
15. Yentis SM, Lee DJH. Evaluation of an improved scoring system for the grading of direct laryngoscopy. *Anaesthesia* 1998; 53:1041–4.
16. Cook TM. A new practical classification of laryngeal view. *Anaesthesia* 2000; 55: 260–87.
17. Crosby ET, Cooper RM, Douglas MJ, *et al.* The unanticipated difficult airway with recommendations for management. *Can J Anaesth* 1998; 45:757–76.
18. Quinn AC, Milne D, Columb M, *et al.* Failed tracheal intubation in obstetric anaesthesia: 2 yr national case–control study in the UK. *Br J Anaesth* 2013; 110(1): 74–80.
19. Hawthorne L, Wilson R, Lyons G, *et al.* Failed intubation revisited: 17-yr experience in a teaching maternity unit. *Br J Anaesth* 1996; 76:680–4.
20. Rose DK, Cohen MM. The incidence of airway problem depends on the definition used. *Can J Anaesth* 1996; 43:30–4.
21. Rocke DA, Murray WB, Rout CC, *et al.* Relative risk analysis of factors associated with difficult intubation in obstetric anesthesia. *Anesthesiology* 1992; 77:67–73.
22. Lyons G. Failed intubation: six years' experience in a teaching maternity unit. *Anaesthesia* 1985; 40:759–62.
23. Barnardo PD, Jenkins JG. Failed tracheal intubation in obstetrics: a 6-year review in a UK region. *Anaesthesia* 2000; 55:690–4.

24. Rahman K, Jenkins JG. Failed tracheal intubation in obstetrics: no more frequent but still managed badly. *Anaesthesia* 2005; 60:168–71.
25. McDonnell NJ, Paech MJ, Clavisi OM, *et al.* Difficult and failed intubation in obstetric anaesthesia: an observational study of airway management and complications associated with general anaesthesia for caesarean section. *Int J Obstet Anesth* 2008; 17(4):292–7.
26. Djabatey EA, Barclay PM. Difficult and failed intubation in 3430 obstetric general anaesthetics. *Anaesthesia* 2009; 64:1168–71.
27. McKeen DM, George RB, O'Connell CM, *et al.* Difficult and failed intubation: Incident rates and maternal, obstetrical and anesthetic predictors. *Can J Anaesth* 2011; 58:514–24.
28. Rai MR, Lua SH, Popat M, *et al.* Antenatal anaesthetic assessment of high-risk pregnancy: a survey of UK practice. *Int J Obstet Anesth* 2005; 14:219–22.
29. Centre for Maternal and Child Enquiries, Royal College of Obstetricians and Gynaecologists. *Joint Guideline: Management of Women with Obesity in Pregnancy.* London: RCOG/CMACE; 2010.
30. Hayes I, Rathore R, Enohumah K, *et al.* Prevalence of factors associated with difficult intubation in early and late pregnancy: a prospective observational study. *Anaesthesia* 2011; 66:234–5.
31. Kodali BS, Chandrasekhar S, Bulich LN, *et al.* Airway changes during labor and delivery. *Anesthesiology* 2008; 108:357–62.
32. Pilkington, F. Carli, M. J. Dakin, *et al.* Increase in Mallampati score during pregnancy. *Br J Anaesth* 1995; 74: 638–42.
33. Chassard D, Le Quang D. Mallampati score during pregnancy. *Br J Anaesth* 2012; 108 Suppl 2:ii200.
34. Finucane BT, Tsui BCH, Santora A. Evaluation of the airway. In *Principles of Airway Management* (4th ed). New York: Springer Science Media; 2011:27–58.
35. El-Ganzouri AR, McCarthy RJ, Tuman KT, *et al.* Pre-operative airway assessment: predictive value of a multivariate risk index. *Anesth Analg* 1996; 82:1197–204.
36. Calder I, Calder J, Crockard HA. Difficult direct laryngoscopy in patients with cervical spinal disease. *Anaesthesia* 1995; 50:756–63.
37. Mallampati SR. Clinical sign to predict difficult tracheal intubation (hypothesis). *Can Anaesth Soc J* 1983; 30:316–17.
38. Samsoon GL, Young JRB. Difficult tracheal intubation: a retrospective study. *Anaesthesia* 1987; 42:487–90.
39. Ezri T, Cohen Y, Geva D, *et al.* Pharyngoscopic views. *Anesth Analg* 1998; 87:748.
40. Grover VK, Mahajan R, Tomar M. Class zero airway and laryngoscopy. *Anaesth Analg* 2003 96(3):911.
41. Savva D. Prediction of difficult tracheal intubation. *Br J Anaesth* 1994; 73:149–53.
42. Wilson ME, John R. Problems with the Mallampati sign. *Anaesthesia* 1990; 45:486–502.
43. Lundstrom LH, Vester-Andersen M, Moller AM, *et al*, Anaesthesia database, poor prognostic value of the MMS, a meta-analysis involving a 177088 patients. *Br J Anaesth* 2011; 107:659–67.
44. Frerk CM. Predicting difficult intubation. *Anaesthesia* 1991; 46:1005–8.
45. Lewis M, Keramati S, Benumof JL, *et al.* What is the best way to determine oropharyngeal classification and mandibular space length to predict difficult laryngoscopy? *Anesthesiology* 1994; 81:69–75.
46. Gannon K. Mortality associated with anaesthesia. *Anaesthesia* 1991; 46:962–6.
47. Boutonnet M, FaitotV, Katz A, *et al.* Mallampati class changes during pregnancy, labour, and after delivery: can these be predicted? *Br J Anaesth* 2010; 104(1): 67–70.
48. Brock-Utne JG, Downing JW, Seedat F. Laryngeal oedema associated with pre-eclamptic toxaemia. *Anaesthesia* 1977; 32:556–8.
49. Hytten FE. Weight gain in pregnancy. In Hytten F, Chamberlain G (eds) *Clinical Physiology in Obstetrics.* Oxford: Blackwell Scientific Publications; 1991:173–203.
50. Heslehurst N, Rankin J, Wilkinson JR, *et al.* A nationally representative study of maternal obesity in England, UK: trends in incidence and demographic inequalities in 619 323 births, 1989-2007. *Int J Obes* 2010; 34:420–8.
51. Juvin P, Lavaut E, Dupont H, *et al.* Difficult tracheal intubation is more common in obese than lean patients. *Anesth Analg* 2003; 97:595–600.
52. Roberts RB, Shirley MA. Reducing the risk of acid aspiration during Caesarean section. *Anesth Analg* 1974; 53: 859–68.
53. Baraka AS. Preoxygenation during pregnancy in the head-up versus the supine position. *Anesthesiology* 2006; 104:1110–15.
54. Searle RD, Lyons G. Vanishing experience in training for obstetric general anaesthesia: an observational study. *Int J Obstet Anaesth* 2008; 17(3):233–7.
55. Koerber JP, Roberts GEW, Whitaker R, *et al.* Variation in rapid sequence induction techniques: current practice in wales. *Anaesthesia* 2009; 64:54–9.
56. Haynes AB, Weiser TG, *et al.* The safe surgery saves lives study group. A surgical safety checklist to reduce morbidity and mortality in a global population. *N Engl J Med* 2009; 360:491–9.
57. Johnson RV, Lyons GR, Wilson RC, *et al.* Training in obstetric general anaesthesia: a vanishing art? *Anaesthesia* 2000; 55:163–83.
58. Mercer SJ, Whittle CL, Mahoney PF. Lessons from the battlefield: human factors in defence anaesthesia. *Br J Anaesth* 2010; 105:9–20.
59. National Health Service Litigation Authority. *Clinical Negligence Scheme for Trusts 2011/12: Maternity.* London: NHS Litigation Authority.
60. Association of Anaesthetists of Great Britain and Ireland. *Recommendations for Standards of Monitoring During Anaesthesia and Recovery* (4th ed). London: Association of Anaesthetists of Great Britain and Ireland; 2007.
61. Thompson C, Webster S, Pachucki M. Improving the difficult airway trolley: Aiming to diminish fixation errors in anaesthetist and empower anaesthetic assistants in the management of the unanticipated difficult airway. In *Difficult Airway Society ASM 2010*, Cheltenham. Abstract 73A.
62. Bromiley M. Have you ever made a mistake? *R Coll Anaesth Bull* 2008; 48:2442–5.
63. Nolan JP, Wilson ME. An evaluation of the gum elastic bougie. Intubation times and incidence of sore throat. *Anaesthesia* 1992; 47:878–81.
64. Marfin AG, Hames KC, Pandit JJ, *et al.* Comparison of the single-use bougie and the multiple-use gum elastic bougie for tracheal intubation in simulated grade 3 difficult laryngoscopy. *Anaesthesia* 2003; 58:511–12.
65. Cupitt JM. Microbial contamination of gum-elastic bougies. *Anaesthesia* 2000; 55:466–8.
66. Arndt GA, Cambray AJ, Tomasson J. Intubation bougie dissection of tracheal mucosa and intratracheal airway obstruction. *Anesth Analg* 2008; 107(2):603–4.
67. Maharaj CH, Costello JF, McDonnell JG, *et al.* Evaluation of the Airtraq and Macintosh laryngoscopes in patients at increased risk for difficult tracheal intubation. *Anaesthesia* 2008; 63:182–8.
68. Malin E, De Montblanch J, Ynineb Y, *et al.* Performance of the Airtraq laryngoscope after failed conventional tracheal intubation: a case series. *Acta Anaesthesiol Scand* 2009; 53:858–63.
69. Frova G. Do videolaryngoscopes have a new role in the SIAARTI difficult airway management algorithm? *Minerva Anesthesiol* 2010; 76:637–40.
70. Sun DA, Warriner CB, Parsons DG, *et al.* The Glidescope video laryngoscope: randomised clinical trial in 200 patients. *Br J Anaesth* 2005; 94:381–4.
71. Ndoko SK, AmathieuR, Tual L, *et al.* Tracheal intubation of morbidly obese patients: a randomized trial comparing performance of Macintosh and Airtraq laryngoscopes. *Br J Anaesth* 2008; 100:263–8.
72. Jungbauer A, Schumann M, Brunkhorst V, *et al.* Expected difficult tracheal intubation: a prospective comparison of direct laryngoscopy and videolaryngoscopy in 200 patients. *Br J Anaesth* 2009; 102:546–50.
73. Bathory I, Frascarolo P, Kern C, *et al.* Evaluation of the Glidescope for tracheal intubation in patients with cervical spine immobilisation by semi-rigid collar. *Anaesthesia* 2009; 64:1337–41.

74. Suzuki A, Toyama Y, Kastumi N, *et al.* The Pentax -AWS rigid indirect video laryngoscope: clinical assessment of performance in 320 cases. *Anaesthesia* 2008; 63:641–7.
75. Cunningham V, Chrystie P, Erskine J. The new McGrarth MAC3 Videolaryngoscope. A case series. In *Difficult Airway Society ASM 2011*, Nottingham. Abstract 108.
76. Campbell M, Vincent V, Ong C, *et al.* Clinical experience with the Venner AP Advance laryngoscope in 35 patients. In *Difficult Airway Society ASM 2011*, Nottingham. Abstract 94.
77. Burdett E, Ross-Anderson DJ, Makepeace J, *et al.* Randomised controlled trial of the A.P. Advance, McGrath and Macintosh laryngoscopes in normal and difficult intubation scenarios: a manikin study. *Br J Anaesth* 2011; 107:983–8.
78. Keller C, Brimacombe J, Kleinsasser A, *et al.* Does the Proseal laryngeal mask airway prevent aspiration of regurgitated fluid? *Anesth Analg* 2000; 91:1017–20.
79. Crutton MJL, Metcalfe GA, Lowy C, *et al.* eating in labour. A randomized controlled trial assessing the risks and benefits. *Anaesthesia* 1999; 54:329–34.
80. National Institute of Health and Clinical Excellence. *Intrapartum Care: Care of Healthy Women and their Babies During Childbirth.* Clinical Guideline 55. London: NICE; 2007.
81. Vickers RJ, Reddy MS. General anaesthesia in the obstetric patient: can we predict who will require it. *Int J Obstet Anaesth* 2009; 18:S38.
82. McClure J, Cooper G in Centre for Maternal and Child Enquiries (CMACE), Saving mothers lives. Reviewing maternal deaths to make motherhood safer: 2006–2008. *Br J Obstet Gynaecol* 2011; 118 Suppl. 1:104.
83. Paranjothy S, Griffiths JD, Broughton HK, *et al.* Interventions at caesarean section for reducing the risk of aspiration pneumonitis. *Cochrane Database Syst Rev* 2010; 1:CD004943.
84. YauG, Kan AF, Gin T, *et al.* A comparison of omeprazole and ranitidine for prophylaxis against aspiration pneumonitis in emergency Caesarean section. *Anaesthesia* 1992; 47:101–4.
85. Jackson C. The technique of insertion of intra-tracheal insufflation tubes. *Surg Gynecol Obstet* 1913; 17:507–9.
86. Magill IW. Endotracheal anaesthesia. *Am J Surg* 1936; 34:450–5.
87. Bannister FB, MacBeth RB. Direct laryngoscopy and tracheal intubation. *Lancet* 1944; 2:651–4.
88. Adnet F, Borron SW, Lopostolle F, *et al.* The three axes alignment theory and the 'sniffing position': perpetuation of anatomic myth? *Anesthesiology* 1999; 91:1964–5.
89. Adnet F, Borron SW, Dumas JL, *et al.* Study of the 'sniffing position' by magnetic resonance imaging. *Anesthesiology* 2001; 94:83–6.
90. Adnet F, Baillard C, Borron SW, *et al.* Randomised study comparing the sniffing position' with simple head extension for laryngoscopic view in elective surgery patients. *Anesthesiology* 2001; 95:836–41.
91. Cooper RM. Laryngoscopy—its past and future. *Can J Anesth* 2004; 51:21–5.
92. Collins JS, Lemmens HJ, Brodsky JB, *et al.* Laryngosocpy and morbid obesity: a comparison of the 'sniff' and 'ramped' positions. *Obes Surg* 2004; 14(9):1171–5.
93. Hood E, Mitchell E, Norman A. Improvement in view at laryngoscopy in an obese patient using the Oxford H.E.L.P. pillow. In *Difficult Airway Society ASM 2011*, Nottingham. Abstract 107.
94. Cattano D, Cavallone L. Airway management and patient positioning: a clinical perspective. *Anesthesiol News*, 2011; 2011:17–22.
95. Chikungwa MT. Popular hair style—an anaesthetic nightmare. *Anaesthesia* 2000; 55:305–6.
96. Rassam S, Stacey M, Morris S. How do you pre-oxygenate your patient? *Int J Obstet Anaesth* 2005; 14:79.
97. Edmark L, Kostova-Aherdan K, Enlund M, *et al.* Optimal oxygen concentration during induction of general anaesthesia. *Anesthesiology* 2003; 98:28–33.
98. Bakara AS, Hanna MT, Jabbour SI, *et al.* Preoxygenation of pregnant and non-pregnant women in the headup versus supine position. *Anesth Analg* 1992; 75:757–9.
99. Altematt FR, Munoz HR, Delfine AE, *et al.* Pre-oxygenation in the obese patient: effects of position on tolerance to apnea. *Br J Anaesth* 2005; 95:706–9.
100. Dixon BJ, Dixon JB, Carden JR, *et al.* Preoxygenation is more effective in the 25 degrees head up position than in the supine position in the severely obese patients: a randomised controlled study. *Anesthesiology* 2005; 102:1110–15.
101. Tanoubi I, Donati F. Optimising preoxygenation in adults. *Can J Anaesth* 2009; 56:449–66.
102. Russell EC, Wrench I, Feats M, *et al.* Pre-oxygenation in pregnancy: the effect of fresh gas flow rates within a circle breathing system. *Anaesthesia* 2008; 63:833–6.
103. Chiron B, Laffon M, Ferrandiere M, *et al.* Standard preoxygenation technique versus two rapid techniques in pregnant patients. *Int J Obstet Anaesth* 2004; 13:11–14.
104. Baraz R, Collis RE. Preoxygenation in the obstetric and non-obstetric population: effectiveness of a new technique. *Int J Obstet Anaesth* 2009; 18:S12.
105. Gander S, Frascaralo P, Suter, *et al.* Positive airway pressure during induction of general anaesthesia increases duration of non-hypoxic apnea in morbidly obese patients. *Anesth Analg* 2005; 100:580–4.
106. Cressey DM, Berthound MC, Reilly CS. Effectiveness of continuous positive airway pressure to enhance preoxygenation in morbidly obese women. *Anaesthesia* 2001; 56:680–4.
107. Baraka AS, Taha SK, Siddik-Sayyid SM, *et al.* Supplementation of pre-oxygenation in morbidly obese patients using nasopharyngeal oxygen insufflation. *Anaesthesia* 2007; 62:769–73.
108. Sirian R, Wills J. Physiology of apnoea and the benefits of pre-oxygenation. *CEACCP* 2009; 9:105–8.
109. Sellick BA. Cricoid pressure to control regurgitation of stomach contents during induction of anaesthesia. *Lancet* 1961; 2:404–6.
110. Benhamou D, Vanner R. Controversies in obstetric anaesthesia. Cricoid is unnecessary in obstetric general anaesthesia. *Int J Obstet Anaesth* 1995; 4:30–33.
111. Fenton PM, Reynolds F. Life saving or ineffective? An observational study of the use of cricoid pressure and maternal outcome in an African setting. *Int J Obstet Anaesth* 2009; 18:106–10.
112. Vanner R. Cricoid pressure. *Int J Obstet Anaesth* 2009; 18:103–5.
113. Priebe H-J. Cricoid pressure: an alternate view. *Sem Anaesth Periop Med Pain* 2005; 24:120–6.
114. Morris J, Cook TM. Rapid sequence induction: a national survey of practice. *Anaesthesia* 2001; 56:1090–115.
115. Benhamou D, Bouaziz H, Chassard D, *et al.* Anaesthesia practices for scheduled Caesarean delivery: a 2005 French national survey. *Eur J Anaesth* 2009; 26:694–700.
116. Palmer JHM, Ball DR. The effect of cricoid pressure on the cricoid cartilage and vocal cords: an endoscopic study in anaesthetized patients. *Anaesthesia* 2000; 55:263–8.
117. Hartsilver EL, Vanner RG. Airway obstruction with cricoid pressure. *Anaesthesia* 2000; 55:208–11.
118. Vanner RG, Dwyer JP, Pryle BJ, *et al.* Upper oesophageal pressure and the effect of cricoid pressure. *Anaesthesia* 1992; 47:95–100.
119. Vanner RG, Pryle BJ, O'Dwyer JP, *et al.* Upper oesophageal sphincter pressure and the iv induction of anaesthesia. *Anaesth Analg* 1992; 47:371–5.
120. Hartsilver EL, Vanner RG, Bewley J, *et al.* Gastric pressure during caesarean sections under general anaesthesia. *Br J Anaesth* 1999; 54:752–4.
121. Vanner RG, Asai T. Safe use of cricoid pressure. *Anaesthesia* 1999; 54:1–3.
122. Cook TM, Godfrey I, Rockett M, *et al.* Cricoid pressure: which hand? *Anaesthesia* 2000; 55:648–53.

123. Ralph SJ, Wareham CA. Rupture of oesophagus during cricoid pressure. *Anaesthesia* 1991; 46:40–1.
124. Vanner RG. Tolerance of cricoid pressure by conscious volunteers. *Int J Obstet Anaesth* 1992; 1:195–8.
125. Haslam N, Parket L, Duggan JE. Effect of cricoid pressure on the view at laryngoscopy. *Anaesthesia* 2005; 60:41–7.
126. Meleki A, Zahedi H. The effect of cricoid pressure on glottis view improvement at laryngoscopy. *Eur J Anaesth* 2012; 29:232.
127. Turgeon AF, Nicole PC, Trepanier CA, *et al.* Cricoid pressure does not increase the rate of failed intubation by direct laryngoscopy in adults. *Anesthesiology* 2005; 102:315–19.
128. Vanner RG, Clarke P, Moore WJ, *et al.* The effect of cricoid pressure and neck support on the view at laryngoscopy. *Anaesthesia* 1997; 52:896–900.
129. Cook TM. Cricoid pressure: one hand or two? *Anaesthesia* 1996; 51:365–8.
130. Yentis SM. The effect of single-handed and bimanual cricoid pressure on the view at laryngoscopy. *Anaesthesia* 1997; 52:332–5.
131. Hashemi SJ, Jabalameli M., Mazoochi M. Which cricoid pressure technique is better in order to laryngoscopy view and intubation time? *Eur J Anaesth* 2005; 22:68.
132. Hocking G, Roberts FL, Thew ME. Airway obstruction with cricoid pressure and lateral tilt. *Anaesthesia* 2001; 56:825–8.
133. Riad W, Ansari T. Effect of cricoid pressure on the laryngoscopic view by Airtraq in elective Caesarean sections: a pilot study. *Eur J Anaesth* 2009; 26:981–2.
134. Vanner RG, Pryle BJ. Regurgitation and oesophageal rupture with cricoid pressure: a cadaver study. *Anaesthesia* 1992; 47:732–5.
135. Vanner RG. Mechanism of regurgitation and its prevention with cricoid pressure. *Int J Obstet Anaesth* 1993; 2:207–15.
136. Knill RL. Difficult laryngoscopy made easy with a BURP. *Can J Anaesth* 1992; 40:279–82.
137. Benemof JL, Copper SD. Quantitative improvement in laryngoscopic view by optimal external laryngeal manipulation. *J Clin Anesth* 1996; 8:136–40.
138. Dhonneur G, Ndoko S, Amathieu R, *et al.* Tracheal intubation using the Airtraq in morbid obese patients undergoing emergency cesarean delivery. *Anesthesiology* 2007; 106:629–30.
139. Turkstra TP, Armstrong PM, Jones PM, *et al.* Glidescope use in the obstetric patient. *Int J Obstet Anaesth* 2010; 19:123–4.
140. Gray K, Lucas N, Robinson PN, *et al.* A case series of successful videolaryngoscopic intubation in obstetric patients. *Int J Obstet Anaesth* 2009; 18:512.
141. Bauer ME, Kountanis JA, Tsen LC, *et al.* Risk factors for failed conversion of labor epidural analgesia to caesarean delivery anesthesia: a systematic review and met-analysis of observational trials. *Int J Obstet Anaesth* 2012; 21:294–309.
142. Godley M, Reddy AR. Use of LMA for awake intubation for Caesarean section. *Can J Anaesth* 1996; 43:299–302.
143. Shung J, Avidan MS, Ing R, *et al.* Awake intubation of the difficult airway with the intubating laryngeal mask airway. *Anaesthesia* 1998; 53:645–9.
144. Delger SM, Dowling RD, Sucherman DR, *et al.* Awake intubation using an Intubating laryngeal mask airway in a parturient with spinal bifida. *Int J Obstet Anaesth* 2005; 14:77–8.
145. Cohn AI, Hart RT, McGraw SR, *et al.* The Bullard laryngoscope for emergency airway management in a morbidly obese parturient. *Anesth Analg* 1995; 81: 872–3.
146. Suzuki A, Toyama Y, Iwasaki H., *et al* Airtraq for awake tracheal intubation. *Anaesthesia* 2007; 62:746–7.
147. Syed N, Kuchi N, Stone, J, *et al.* Management of multiple Caesarean sections in a parturient with Conradi Hunermann syndrome. *Int J Obstet Anaesth* 2009; 18:S53.
148. Hawksworth CR, Purdie J. Failed combined spinal epidural then failed intubation at an elective caesarean section. *Hosp Med* 1998; 59:173.
149. Mackenzie I.A new method of drug application to the nasal passage. *Anaesthesia* 1998; 53:309–10.
150. Broomhead CJ, Davies W, Higgins D. Awake fibreoptic intubation for caesarean section. *Int J Obstet Anaesth* 1995; 4:172–4.
151. Puchner CV, Egger P, Puhringer F, *et al.* Evaluation of remifentanil as a single drug for awake fibreoptic intubation. *Acta Anesth Scand* 2002; 46:350–4.
152. Popat M, Russell R. Awake fibreoptic intubation following previous failed intubation.*Int J Obstet Anaesth* 2001; 10:332–3
153. Johnston KD, Rai M. Conscious sedation for awake fibreoptic intubation: a review of the literature. *Can J Anesth* 2013; 60:584–99.
154. Neumann MM, Davio MB, Macknet MR, *et al.* Dexmedetomidine for awake fibreoptic intubation in a parturient with spinal muscular atrophy type III for Caesarean delivery. *Int J Obstet Anaesth* 2009; 18:403–7.
155. Shah TH, Badve MS, Olajide KO, *et al.* Dexmedetomidine for awake fibreoptic intubation of a parturient with Klippel-Feil syndrome, type I Arnold Chiari malformation and status post released tethered spinal cord presenting for repeat caesarean section. *Clin Pract* 2011; 1:e57.
156. Ovassapian A, Krejcie TC, Yelich SJ, *et al.* Awake fibreoptic intubation in the patient at high risk of aspiration. *Br J Anaesth* 1989; 62:13–16.
157. Efthimou J, Higenbottam T, Holt D, *et al.* Plasma concentrations oflignocaine during fibreoptic bronchoscopy. *Thorax* 1982; 37:68–71.
158. Williams K, Barker G, Harwwood R, *et al.* Plasma lidocaine levels during local anaesthesia of the airway. *Anaesthesia* 2003; 58: 506–12.
159. Arendt KW, Khan K, Curry TB, *et al.* Topical vasoconstrictor use for nasal intubation during pregnancy complicated by cardiomyopathy and pre-eclampsia. *Int J Obstet Anaesth* 2011; 20:246–9.
160. Woods JR, Plessinger MA, Clark KE. Effect of cocaine on uterine blood flow andfetal oxygenation. *JAMA* 1987; 257:957–61.
161. Addis A, Moretti ME, Ahmed Syed F, *et al.* Fetal effect of cocaine: an updated meta-analysis. *Reprod Toxicol* 2001; 15:341–69.
162. Baraka AS, Taha SK, Aouad MT, *et al.* Preoxygenation: comparison of maximal breathing and tidal volume breathing techniques. *Anesthesiology* 1999; 91:612–16.
163. Chiron B, Laffon M, Ferrandiere M, *et al.* Standard preoxygenation technique versus two rapid techniques in pregnant patients. *Int J Obstet Anaesth* 2004; 13:11–14.
164. Crosby E. The difficult airway in obstetric anesthesia. In Hagberg CA (ed) *Benumof's Airway Management: Principles and Practice* (2nd ed). Philadelphia, PA: Mosby Elsevier; 2007:834–58.
165. Munnur U, Suresh MS. Difficult airway management in the pregnant patient. In Bucklin BA, Gambling DR, Wlody D (eds) *A Practical Approach to Obstetric Anaesthesia*. Philadelphia, PA: Lippincott Williams & Wilkins; 2009:209–22.
166. Mushambi MC, Kinsella SM, Popat M, *et al.* Obstetric Anaesthetists' Association and Difficult Airway Society guidelines for the management of difficult and failed tracheal intubation in obstetrics. *Anaesthesia* 2015; 70: 1286–306.
167. Halaseh BK, Sukkar ZFL, Hassan HAJ, *et al.* The use of ProSeal laryngeal mask airway in caesarean section—experience in 3,000 caesareans. *Anaesth Intensive Care* 2010; 38:1023–8.
168. Han TH, Brimacombe J, Lee E-J, *et al.* The laryngeal mask airway is effective (and probably safe) in selected healthy parturients for elective Cesarean section: a prospective study of 1067 cases. *Can J Anaesth* 2001; 48:1117–21.
169. Yao WY, Li SY, Sng BL, *et al.* The LMA supreme in 700 parturients undergoing cesarean delivery: an observational study. *Can J Anaesth* 2012; 59(7):648–54.
170. Anderson KJ, Quinlan MJ, Popat M, *et al.* Failed intubation in a parturient with spina bifida. *Int J Obstet Anaesth* 2000; 9:64–8.
171. Sharma B, Sahai C, Sood J, *et al.* The Proseal laryngeal mask airway in two failed obstetric intubation scenarios. *Int J Obstet Anaesth* 2006; 15:338–9.

172. Berger M, Corso RM, Piraccini E. The i-gel® in failed obstetric tracheal intubation. *Anaesth Intensive Care* 2011; 39:136–7.
173. Bailey SG, Kitching AJ. The laryngeal mask airway in failed obstetric intubation. *Int J Obstet Anaesth* 2005; 14:270–1.
174. Keller C, Brimacombe J, Lirk P, *et al.* Failed obstetric tracheal intubation and postoperative respiratory support with the Proseal laryngeal mask. *Anesth Analg* 2004; 98:1467–70.
175. Awan R, Nolan J, Cook TM. Use of the Proseal LMA for airway maintenance during emergency Caesarean section after failed intubation, *Br J Anaesth* 2004; 92:144–6.
176. Vaida SJ, Gaitini LA, Cook TM, *et al.* Another case of use of Proseal laryngeal mask airway in a difficult obstetric airway. *Br J Anaesth* 2004; 92:905.
177. Preston R. The evolving role of the laryngeal mask airway in obstetric. *Can J Anaesth* 2001; 48:1061–5.
178. Rees GAD, Willis BA. Resuscitation in late pregnancy. *Anaesthesia* 1988; 43:347–9.
179. Lindsay SL, Hanson GC. Cardiac arrest in near term pregnancy. *Anaesthesia* 1987; 42:1074–7.
180. Nair A, Alderson JD. Failed intubation drill in obstetrics. *Int J Obstet Anaesth* 2006; 15:172–4.
181. Mhyre J, Healy D. The unanticipated difficult intubation in obstetrics. *Anesth Analg* 2011; 112:648–52.
182. Ezri T, Szmuk P, Evron S, *et al.* Difficult airway in obstetric anesthesia: a review. *Obstet Gynecol Surv* 2001; 56:631–41.
183. Berkow LC. Strategies for airway management. *Best Pract Res Clin Anaesthesiol* 2004; 18:531–48.
184. Kuczkowski KM, Reisner LS, Benumof JL. Airway problems and new solutions for the obstetric patient. *J Clin Anaesth* 2003; 15:552–63.
185. Vasdev GM, Harrison BA, Keegan MT, *et al.* Management of the difficult and failed airway in obstetric anesthesia. *J Anesth* 2008; 22:38–48.
186. Henderson JJ, Popat MT, Latto IP, *et al.* Difficult Airway Society guidelines for the management of the unanticipated difficult intubation. *Anaesthesia* 2004; 59:675–94.
187. Frerk C, Mitchell VS, McNarry AF, *et al.* Difficult Airway Society 2015 guidelines for management of unanticipated difficult intubation in adults. *British Journal of Anaesthesia* 2015; 115: 827–48.
188. Atherton DPL, O'Sullivan E, Lowe D, *et al.* A ventilation-exchange bougie for fibreoptic intubation with a laryngeal mask airway. *Anaesthesia* 1996; 51:1123–6.
189. Mhyre JM, Reisner MN, Polley LS, *et al.* A series of anesthesia-related maternal deaths in Michigan 1985–2003. *Anesthesiology* 2007; 106:1096–104.
190. Popat M, Mitchell V, Dravid R, *et al.* Difficult Airway Society guidelines for the management of tracheal extubation. *Anaesthesia* 2012; 67:318–40.
191. The Association of Anaesthetists of Great Britain and Ireland. *Catastrophes in Anaesthetic Practice—Dealing with the Aftermath.* London: The Association of Anaesthetists of Great Britain and Ireland; 2005.
192. Domino KB, Posner KL, Caplan RA, *et al.* Airway injury during anesthesia. A closed claim analysis. *Anaesthesiology* 1999; 91:1703–11.
193. Errando CL, Sigl JC, Robles M, *et al.* Awareness with recall during general anaesthesia: a prospective observational evaluation of 4001 patients. *Br J Anaesth* 2008; 101(2):178–85.
194. Difficult Airway Society. *Airway Alert Form.* [Online] http://www.das.uk.com/guidelines/downloads.html

CHAPTER 27

Postdural puncture headache

Michael J. Paech and Patchareya Nivatpumin

Introduction

In obstetric anaesthesia, postdural puncture headache (PDPH) is an important potential complication of neuraxial anaesthesia and analgesia or diagnostic lumbar puncture, and follows both spinal techniques and unintentional (also termed accidental or inadvertent) dura and arachnoid mater (hereafter 'dural') puncture during epidural needle or catheter insertion. Pregnant women appear a high-risk population for PDPH because of their gender, age, and, arguably, hormonal status. The headache and associated symptoms can cause considerable suffering and dissatisfaction, usually prolong hospital stay, and sometimes persist for weeks or months. This has implications for healthcare costs, subsequent loss of productivity, and litigation, making correct diagnosis and effective early management vital.

Pathophysiology of postdural puncture headache

PDPH is initiated by loss of cerebrospinal fluid (CSF) and the subsequent changes in intracranial CSF volume when the head is elevated or the body erect.[1,2] Normal CSF formation, largely by ependymal cells of the choroid plexuses in the ventricles, is 450–500 mL/day (approximately 0.35 mL/min) in adults. A volume of 150 mL is located within the cerebral ventricles (~25 mL) and subarachnoid spaces (~125 mL). Absorption into the venous circulation occurs via cranial and spinal arachnoid villi, but if CSF efflux through a dural hole exceeds replacement, CSF pressure dynamics alter significantly with changes in body position. On assuming an upright position, redistribution causes low intracranial pressure (ICP) and this may precipitate headache, not only after dural puncture but also among patients with spontaneous intracranial hypotension, which follows spontaneous CSF leak.[2–4]

One possible explanation for pain (and some associated symptoms and complications) is loss of buoyancy when the head is elevated, leading to brain descent, traction on cranial nerves, meninges, and intracranial and meningeal veins. This pathology can be seen as pachymeningeal enhancement on cranial magnetic resonance imaging (MRI), although tonsillar descent or change in intracranial structure position is not necessarily evident.[1,5] Dilatation of the anterior internal vertebral venous plexus and spinal hygromas appears common.[5] A further plausible explanation for headache is the compensatory cerebral vasodilatation seen on imaging.[2,5] This is thought to be mediated by adenosine receptors in response to reduced ICP and the theory is supported by the changes that occur during induced hypercapnia or hypocapnia that maintain the intracranial volume; and by the immediate reduction in cerebral blood flow that follows an epidural blood patch (EBP).[6]

The individual's predisposition to headache varies, with several postulated explanations. CSF substance P concentrations have been implicated,[7,8] as have differences in CSF loss secondary to orifice occlusion by the intrinsic elastic recoil of the dura mater. The histological and anatomical characteristics of the dura mater vary, even within different areas of adjacent dura within an individual.[9] Differences in baseline ICP and cerebrovascular responses may also be relevant,[10,11] with patients having lower baseline ICP possibly more susceptible. Higher levels of oestrogen in women alter cerebral vessel tone responsiveness and possibly increase vascular distension in response to CSF hypotension.[11]

Incidence of postdural puncture headache

The incidence of PDPH is largely determined by physical factors such as the size and configuration of the meningeal perforation, which influences the volume of CSF loss until the breach has healed; and patient factors that determine the subsequent response to changes in CSF compartment dynamics. *In vitro* studies of CSF loss associated with various needles and human observational or randomized trials show that the characteristics of the needle are critical determinants of risk, with higher rates of PDPH after use of larger gauge (G) spinal, and possibly also epidural, needles (Table 27.1).

A meta-analysis of obstetric studies found an incidence of PDPH of 1.5–11% from spinal needles and 52% after unintentional puncture by an epidural needle.[12] The incidence following use of small-gauge pencil-point needles is as low as 0.4–0.5%[13,14] compared with 80–100% after puncture by a 16–17 G Tuohy epidural needle.[15–17]

Risk factors for postdural puncture headache

Needle characteristics

For spinal-induced PDPH, the relevance of needle gauge and tip configuration is well recognized.[18,19] A larger-diameter needle with a traumatic tip results in more CSF loss and a cadaver study found a fivefold increase in the volume lost after puncture by the same-gauge Quincke versus Whitacre needle and a sixfold greater loss from a 22 G versus 25 G spinal needle of the same design.[18] Clinical observations confirm that the lowest risk is conferred by smaller-gauge needles of pencil-point or non-cutting bevel design (Whitacre, Sprotte, or other atraumatic needle tip).[13,14,20–23]

Table 27.1 The incidence of PDPH associated with different needles used in obstetric anaesthesia

Needle characteristics	Incidence (%) and references
Spinal needle	
24 G Sprotte	0.7–4[20–22]
25 G Quincke	7–9[20,21]
25 G Whitacre	2.5–3[13,21,23]
26 G Atraucan	5[21]
27 G Quincke	3.5–8[20]
27 G Whitacre	0–0.5[13,14]
29 G Whitacre	0[14]
Epidural needle	
16–18 G Tuohy	52–100[12,15–17,27,28]
18 G Sprotte	55[17]

G, gauge.
Data from various sources (see references).

Meta-analysis shows a threefold reduction in the risk of severe PDPH (odds ratio (OR) 0.26; 95% confidence interval (CI) 0.11–0.62) compared with cutting needles.[19] The relative risk of developing PDPH from a 27 G pencil-point needle compared with a 27 G Quincke needle is 0.38 (95% CI 0.19–0.75).[24]

Despite the frequency of PDPH after epidural needle dura penetration (50–90%), the contribution of needle size and design (and thus the characteristics of the meningeal perforation) is unclear because of the absence of randomized trials. Low levels of evidence from studies in which PDPH was a secondary outcome suggest that smaller-gauge epidural needles reduce risk.[17,25–27] However, there was no difference in either the severity of PDPH or the need for repeat EBP after puncture by 16, 17, or 18 G Tuohy needles in a prospective trial with an open choice of needle gauge (unpublished data).[28] The incidence of PDPH from an 18 G Sprotte tip epidural needle is lower than that from a 17 G Tuohy needle.[17]

Needle bevel orientation

Electron microscopy shows that the lumbar dura mater consists of collagen fibre bundles oriented in various directions, plus elastic fibres arranged mainly longitudinal to the long axis of the spine.[29] Consequently, inserting a cutting-edge spinal needle with the bevel parallel to the longitudinal axis is thought to decrease the tendency of a dural hole to remain open under tension when the patient is erect, reducing the PDPH risk (OR 0.29; 95% CI 0.17–0.50).[30] On this basis, some have advocated epidural needle insertion with the bevel facing laterally, but subsequent needle rotation to facilitate catheter placement has been condemned by others, because it could tear the dura mater, which can lie close to the ligamentum flava in the posterior epidural space.[31]

Reinsertion of the needle stylet

Reinserting the stylet of a large (21 G) spinal needle prior to its withdrawal from the subarachnoid space may reduce the risk of PDPH, perhaps by avoiding strands of arachnoid mater being pulled into the dural defect and prolonging the duration of CSF leak.[32] This is of little relevance to obstetric practice, in which smaller-gauge needles should always be used.

Direction of needle approach

It has been suggested that approaching the dura at an angle creates a tissue flap and valvular closure of the meningeal hole, reducing the risk of PDPH, but a cadaver study found no difference in CSF loss through holes made at a 30° versus 90° puncture angle[18] and clinical studies report no advantage from a paramedian approach.[33]

Multiple needle insertions

Repeated needle passes during unsuccessful attempts to locate the subarachnoid space may result in multiple dural holes, increasing CSF loss, and the risk of PDPH.[34]

Neuraxial technique: combined spinal–epidural versus epidural only

A needle-through-needle combined spinal–epidural (CSE) technique provides a secure conduit for spinal needle puncture. Although it might be anticipated that PDPH rates would be higher after CSE than epidural-only approaches, given a deliberate dural puncture, it has been suggested that the risk of unintentional puncture is lower because the operator is more cautious, using CSF efflux from the spinal needle to confirm correct epidural needle-tip location. A large obstetric observational study involving small-gauge needles and meta-analysis both indicate that CSE and epidural-only techniques are associated with similar rates of PDPH and EBP.[16,35]

Operator experience

During epidural techniques, operator inexperience (and possibly fatigue) is associated with increased risk of unintentional dural puncture.[36]

Epidural loss of resistance with air or saline

A loss-of-resistance technique using normal saline has been advocated on the basis that saline allows continuous advancement of the epidural needle and on entry into the epidural space, saline pushes the dura away from the needle tip. A large quasi-randomized non-obstetric study by a single operator found no difference in the rate of dural puncture between saline and air, but a higher incidence of PDPH due to subarachnoid injection of air. Intracranial pneumocephalus may be visible on brain computed tomography (CT) scans and the ensuing headache is of earlier onset but shorter duration than typical PDPH.[37] A meta-analysis of five trials found no difference in the risk of headache between use of saline or air.[38]

Ultrasound-guided epidural insertion

Although the incidence of PDPH was a secondary outcome, randomized trials comparing an ultrasound-guided pre-scan to a conventional landmark-guided epidural insertion report no difference in PDPH risk.[38]

Patient age

Observational studies indicate that patient age is an important risk factor, with young children and the geriatric population very resistant to PDPH.[39] Pregnant women appear at high risk, with possible explanations being different dural elasticity, vascular responsiveness, and lower epidural space compliance (greater tamponade of CSF loss) compared with older populations.

Patient gender

Non-pregnant females are at greater risk of PDPH than males (OR 0.55; 95% CI 0.44–0.67).[40] Possible explanations include oestrogen-influenced differences in cerebral vasodilatory responses and nociceptive processing; and in pregnancy the effects of further hormonal changes, although it is not known whether pregnancy per se confers an additional risk.

Patient history

Patients with a history of previous PDPH appear at greater risk of developing PDPH following a subsequent spinal technique.[41] Those who suffer from migraine are also postulated to be at greater risk, because of their vascular responsiveness.

Body habitus and anatomy

Although women with an epidural space located at the shallowest depth beneath the skin (2–3 cm) or those with abnormal ligamentous anatomy might be at increased risk, logistic regression of a large obstetric anaesthetic database identified only one significant factor, namely increasing depth to the epidural space.[42] Retrospective data suggest that parturients of body mass index (BMI) greater than 35 kg/m^2 are less likely to develop PDPH after unintentional dural puncture with a 17–18 G epidural needle, although conflicting data also exist.[43–45] A postulated explanation is that higher intra-abdominal pressure limits CSF loss from smaller breaches of the meninges.[43,46]

Pushing during labour

Retrospective data suggest an increased incidence of PDPH and EBP among women who bear down in the second stage of labour after unintentional dural puncture with a 17 G epidural needle.[47] It was suggested this was due to increased CSF loss, but a prospective study after 22 G Quincke needle spinal anaesthesia did not confirm that bearing down was a risk.[48] There are no prospective studies associated with use of small-gauge pencil-point needles or after unintentional dural puncture.

Features of postdural puncture headache

Symptoms

The pathognomonic feature of PDPH is its postural or orthostatic component, such that it is precipitated or exacerbated by erect postures and relieved by recumbency, although paradoxical (reverse) postural headache can occur.[49] Pain is located in a bifrontal and/or occipital distribution, and in almost 50% of cases is accompanied by shoulder or neck stiffness.[25,50] The characteristics are a throbbing or dull headache of mild to excruciating intensity. Lybecker et al. graded the severity from mild to severe based on interference with activities and related symptoms,[50] defining PDPH as moderate if it confined the patient to bed at times. Severe PDPH rendered the patient incapable or reluctant to raise their head or to stand and was always associated with other symptoms. Paech et al. defined a severe PDPH as one which prevented normal ambulation and care of the neonate.[15] Approximately half the obstetric cases after unintentional dural puncture meet this latter definition.[15,25]

Most associated symptoms appear consequent to low ICP or nerve traction, with neck stiffness due to irritation of upper cervical nerves. Nausea is also common, whereas ocular symptoms such as diplopia and photophobia are rare.[50] Most case reports describe an abducens (sixth) cranial nerve palsy, due to its long intracranial route from the pons across the petrous bone.[51–53] Diplopia usually presents a few days after dural puncture but may outlast, by several weeks, the resolution of PDPH[51,53] and can be resolved by an EBP.[54,55]

Hearing loss is demonstrable after spinal anaesthesia with (inappropriately) large-gauge needles[56] and is due to reduced pressure transmitted to the cochlear aqueduct through the inner ear, causing an endolymphatic hydrops that affects hair cell position. Auditory symptoms or tinnitus are associated with PDPH in 10% of patients.[50]

A variety of other neurological complications may be caused by dural puncture, so imaging should always be considered as a means of excluding concurrent intracerebral pathology.[57]

Diagnosis of postdural puncture headache

The International Headache Society introduced the International Classification of Headache Disorders. In its third edition (ICHD-3), diagnostic criteria for postdural (post-lumbar) puncture headache were provided[58] (Box 27.1).

The diagnostic key is headache or neck pain, occurring hours to days after dural puncture, and resolving when supine or exacerbated when upright. Supporting features of low ICP may or may not be present on MRI. A sitting epigastric pressure test to raise abdominal pressure and momentarily relieve headache has been

Box 27.1 ICHD-3 diagnostic criteria for postdural puncture headache

Description

Headache occurring within 5 days of a lumbar puncture, caused by cerebrospinal fluid (CSF) leakage through the dural puncture. It is usually accompanied by neck stiffness and/or subjective hearing symptoms. It remits spontaneously after 2 weeks, or after sealing of the leak with autologous epidural lumbar patch.

Diagnostic criteria

A. Any headache fulfilling criterion C

B. Dural puncture has been performed

C. Headache has developed within 5 days of the dural puncture

D. Not better accounted for by another ICHD-3 diagnosis

ICHD-3, The International Headache Society's *International Classification of Headache* Disorders, 3rd edition, 2013.

described but has low sensitivity and is not widely used.[25] Given that PDPH is principally a clinical diagnosis and that it is associated with potentially life-threatening pathologies, the myriad of causes of postpartum headache need to be excluded from the differential diagnosis.[59,60] Atypical presentations of apparent PDPH warrant investigation,[57] by reviewing the patient's history, repeating a physical examination, especially neurological, and sometimes by blood tests and brain imaging. Symptoms can be mimicked by preeclampsia; tension, migraine, and sinus headache; muscular pain; sleep deprivation; and caffeine withdrawal. Rarely the differential includes meningitis,[61,62] cerebral tumour,[63] arteriovenous malformation,[64] neurocysticercosis,[65] or a number of complications directly related to dural puncture.

Onset of postdural puncture headache

In approximately 85% of cases, PDPH begins within 48 hours of dural puncture.[15,50] Onset as early as 20 minutes after spinal anaesthesia with a 27 G Whitacre needle has been reported, [66] although immediate or rapid onset is typical following intrathecal injection of even only a few millilitres of air.[37,67] The ICHD-3 criterion is onset within 5 days, but delayed onset, 12 days after epidural analgesia for labour, has been described.[68]

Duration of postdural puncture headache

The duration of PDPH varies considerably. Symptom severity and duration tends to be greater after epidural needle dural puncture, making interpretation of the literature, including about interventions such as EBP, more difficult. Post-spinal headache usually lasts 1–12 days (mean 5 days).[50] Pneumoencephalus may cause severe headache of shorter duration (lasting hours to a maximum of 3–5 days) compared with headache from CSF loss.[37] Post-epidural PDPH frequently lasts at least 4–6 days and at least 10% of women will remain symptomatic after a month.[16] Surveys suggest that women with PDPH are more likely to develop chronic headache (not necessarily postural), with reported incidences of almost 30% at 18 months [69] and almost 20% at 3–6 years.[70]

Low ICP headache is a rare condition (incidence 2–5/100,000) which is thought to be precipitated by a spontaneous dural tear and CSF leak somewhere in the neuraxis.[3,4,71] This type of headache can be of gradual onset and very persistent, such that it is often treated conservatively for 2–3 weeks after presentation and may persist for months, despite treatment with an EBP. Nevertheless the response to a non-targeted lumbar EBP is good, with two-thirds of patients experiencing relief. If repeatedly unsuccessful, blood patching or fibrin glue administration at the site of a leak located by radionucleotide cisternography may be required. Of note, an EBP can effectively resolve long-standing PDPH up to years later.[72]

Serious complications associated with postdural puncture headache

Although individually very rare, many pathologies warrant consideration in the differential diagnosis of PDPH or occur concurrently with PDPH after dural puncture. Cranial nerves other than ocular nerves may be involved[73] and severe upper limb or back pain has been successfully treated by an EBP.[74,75] Due to traction on intracerebral vessels, especially cortical bridging veins, subdural haematoma appears to be the most frequently reported of the rare serious neurological complications.[76] Extremely rare but potentially fatal cerebral tonsillar[77] or uncal brain herniation has been described.[78]

Although a direct relationship is difficult to establish, some patients with PDPH present with other neurological events, such as cortical vein thrombosis,[53,79] posterior reversible leucoencephalopathy,[80] generalized tonic–clonic seizures,[81,82] subarachnoid or intracerebral haemorrhage,[83] ischaemic stroke,[84] and acute psychiatric illness.[85]

Prevention of postdural puncture headache

No intervention is very effective in preventing PDPH after unintentional dural puncture and the evidence supporting some measures is too weak to permit firm recommendations (Figure 27.1).[86] The lack of efficacy of some widely advocated therapies has been demonstrated with high (e.g. hydration) or moderate (e.g. caffeine) levels of evidence. For others (e.g. oral opioids) there is no supporting evidence (Table 27.2).

Bed rest, manipulation of posture, or abdominal binders

It was thought that bed rest for 24 hours might decrease CSF hydrostatic pressure and reduce CSF leak, this has proven ineffective for obstetric patients after spinal anaesthesia.[87] A Cochrane review of studies comparing bed rest with early ambulation found no significant difference in the incidence (OR 1.21; 95% CI 0.94–1.55) or severity (OR 1.10; 95% CI 0.79–1.53) of PDPH.[87] An abdominal binder increases intra-abdominal and epidural pressure, which theoretically might help tamponade CSF loss, but is unsupported and has been abandoned because of the impracticalities.

Fluid intake

There is no apparent relationship between PDPH and the volume of oral fluid ingested.[88] Administering intravenous (IV) fluid or encouraging additional oral intake, with the hope of maximizing CSF production, does not prevent PDPH (OR 1.00; 95% CI 0.44–2.25)[87] and makes management more difficult.

Intrathecal saline

A small non-randomized study[89] of patients who experienced an unintentional dural puncture suggested that either immediate injection of intrathecal saline 10 mL through the epidural needle, or later injection through an intrathecal catheter prior to removal, might decrease the incidence of PDPH and need for EBP. This has not been confirmed by larger series or randomized trials and severe radicular pain and paraesthesia have been reported,[90] so this approach cannot be recommended.

Intrathecal insertion of an epidural catheter

Deliberate subarachnoid placement of the epidural catheter at the time of dural puncture is a useful analgesic management option and several case series suggest it lowers the risk of PDPH after catheter removal.[91–94] The rationale is that the presence of a catheter mechanically obstructs CSF loss when bearing down during childbirth and promotes an inflammatory response that aids puncture closure, although the latter supposition is based on an animal study involving weeks, not days, of catheterization. Initial opinions that the intrathecal catheter should be retained for more than 24 hours have not been supported by larger case series.[92,93] An updated meta-analysis of nine studies found no significant reduction in PDPH (RR 0.82; 95% CI 0.067–1.01) but a significantly lower risk of EBP (RR 0.64; 95% CI 0.49–0.84)[94] (Figure 27.2). Since then, a retrospective analysis of accidental dural punctures with 18 G needles, followed by intrathecal catheterization for at least 24 hours and post-delivery intrathecal saline infusion, found a reduction in PDPH from 62% to 42% (OR 2.3; 95% CI 1.04–4.86) and a reduced need for EBPs.[95] If there is a benefit, it is probably modest, because the best quality but underpowered

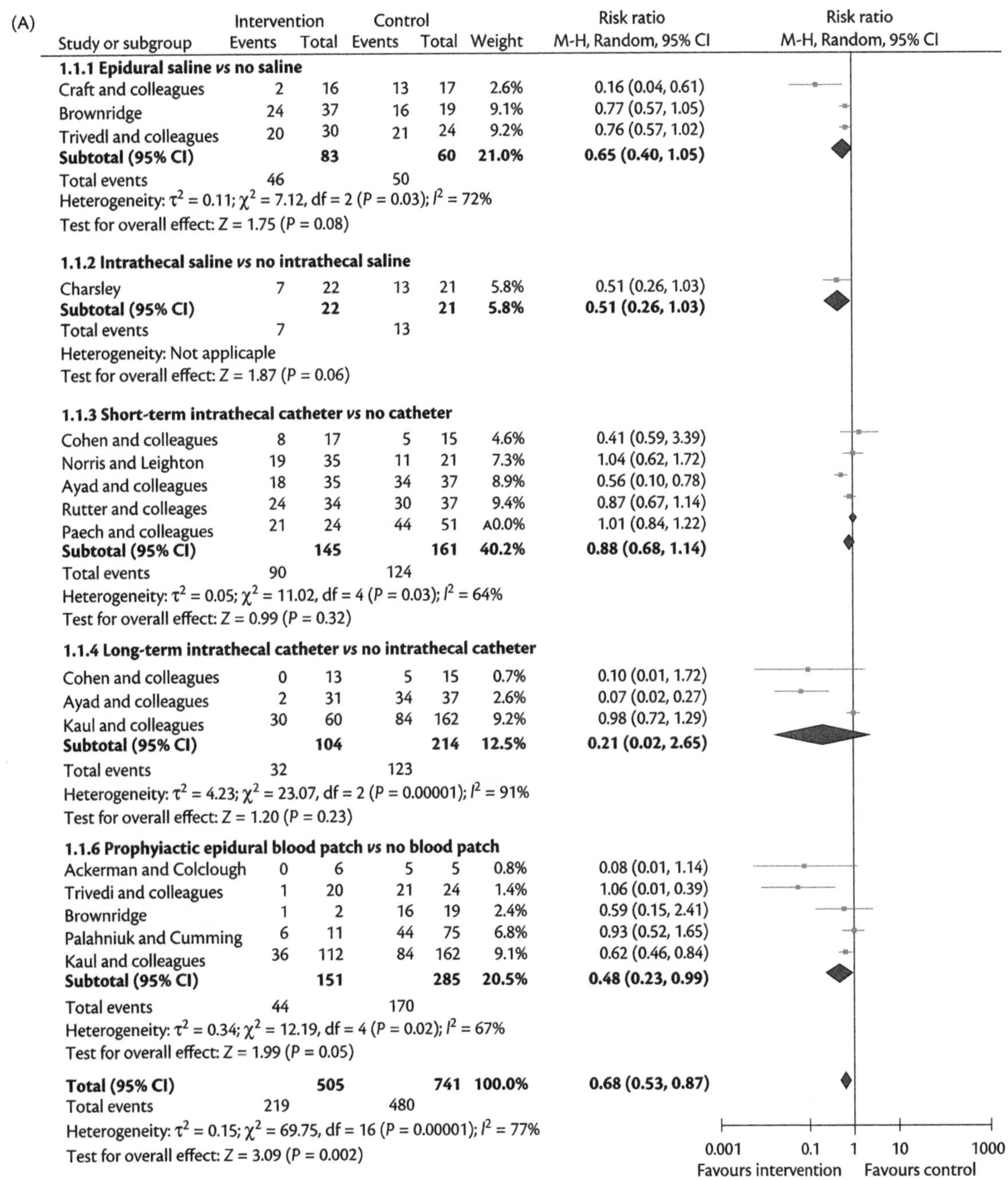

Figure 27.1 Forest plots for risk ratio of PDPH after various interventions. (A) PDPH non-randomized controlled trials for headache. (B) PDPH randomized controlled trials for headache.

RR, relative risk. RR <1 favours the intervention.

Reproduced with permission from C. C. Apfel *et al.*, Prevention of postdural puncture headache after accidental dural puncture: a quantitative systematic review, *British Journal of Anaesthesia*, Volume 105, Issue 3, p. 86, Copyright © 2010 Oxford University Press.

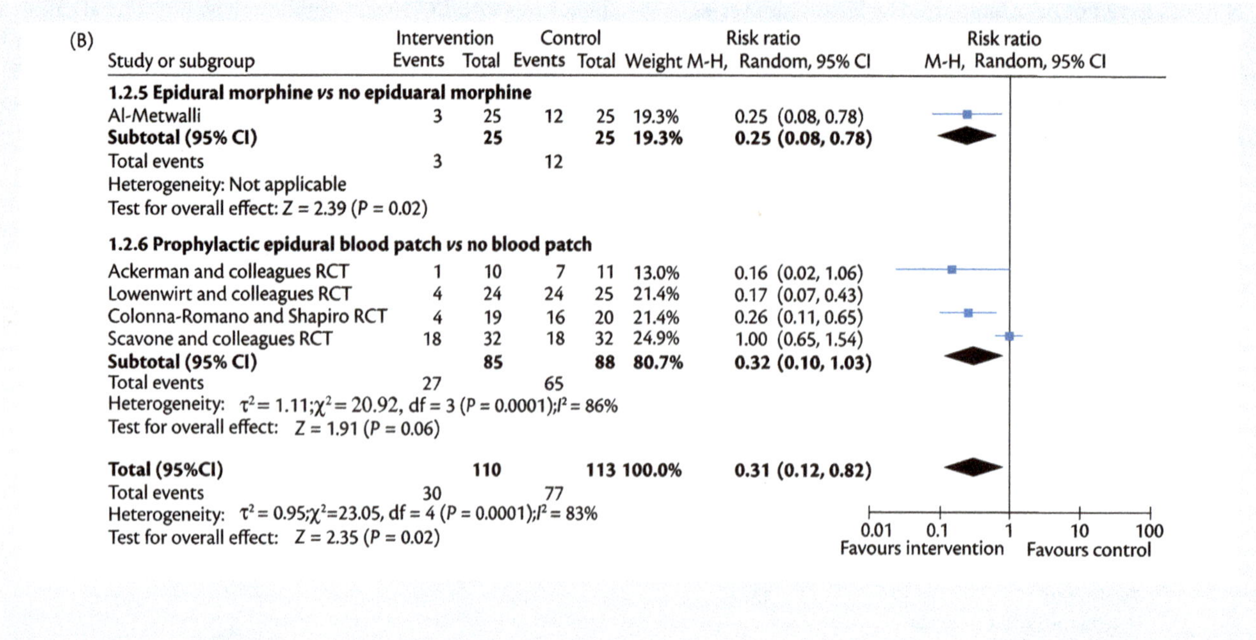

Figure 27.1 Continued

Table 27.2 Best levels of evidence[a] and grade of recommendation supporting various prophylactic measures against development of PDPH

Treatment	Post-spinal	Recommendation	Post-epidural	Recommendation
Avoiding pushing during labour and delivery	2b[48]	B for NOT recommended	4[47]	C
Bed rest, manipulation of posture or abdominal binders	1[87]	A for NOT recommended	N/A	
Fluid intake	1[87]	A for NOT recommended	N/A	
Intrathecal saline			3[89]	C
Spinal catheter (epidural catheter intrathecal)			2b[94]	B
Oral non-opioid and opioid analgesics	N/A		N/A	
Epidural morphine	N/A		2b[103]	B
Subarachnoid morphine	2b[102]	B for NOT recommended	N/A	
Caffeine and cerebral vasocontrictors	3[97]	B for NOT recommended	N/A	
Triptans	4[101]	C	N/A	
Cosyntropin	N/A		2b[104]	B
Epidural blood patch			1[114]	B for NOT recommended
Epidural saline or colloid			1[86]	B for NOT recommended

Grades of recommendation A = consistent level 1 studies. B = consistent level 2 or 3 studies or extrapolations from level 1 studies. C = level 4 studies or extrapolations from level 2 or 3 studies. D = level 5 evidence or troubling inconsistent or inconclusive studies of any level.

[a]Center for Evidence-based Medicine Levels of Evidence. Accessed 16 November 2012 at http://www.cebm.net/index.aspx?o=1025

N/A, not available.

Data from various sources (see references).

study, a quasi-randomized trial in obstetric patients,[27] found no reduction in PDPH or EBP associated with intrathecal catheter placement.

Cerebral vasoconstrictors (caffeine and triptans)

Caffeine is a central adenosine receptor antagonist while the triptans are 5-hydroxytriptamine-1_D and -1_B agonists, and aminophylline a phosphodiesterase inhibitor and adenosine receptor antagonist. These drugs cause vasoconstriction of cranial and basilar arteries. Low-quality investigation of IV caffeine sodium benzoate 500 mg suggested PDPH after non-obstetric spinal anaesthesia was less severe,[96] but multidose oral caffeine 75–150 mg combined with paracetamol (acetaminophen) 500 mg, started prior to spinal anaesthesia and repeated regularly for 3 days after, is ineffective.[97] A review concluded that caffeine is insufficiently supported to warrant prophylaxis against PDPH.[98] Caffeine is often poorly tolerated due to insomnia and agitation and it may be a risk factor in postpartum seizures.[99]

IV aminophylline appears of no value.[100] Subcutaneous sumatriptan and oral frovatriptan, which has a longer half-life, are effective for migraine headache. A small open study indicates frovatriptan might have promise, but this has not been tested in a high-quality trial or an obstetric setting.[101]

Neuraxial morphine

A small randomized trial found no effect of subarachnoid morphine,[102] but a blinded study among parturients suffering unintentional puncture with a 17 G epidural needle reported a significantly reduced incidence of PDPH and EBP if epidural morphine 3 mg was given after delivery and again 24 hours postpartum.[103] This therapy requires validation in larger trials and may not always be an appropriate strategy because of the potential side effects and monitoring requirements.

Intravenous cosyntropin (tetracosactide) or dexamethasone

A single, small randomized trial in obstetric patients suffering an unintentional dural puncture found that IV cosyntropin 1 mg reduced the incidence of PDPH from 69% to 33% and the need for an EBP from 40% to 31%.[104] The authors postulated that cosyntropin, a synthetic derivative of adrenocorticotrophic hormone (ACTH) that retains full activity, increases CSF volume through unspecified mechanisms. While encouraging, this finding requires confirmation. Studies of IV dexamethasone are conflicting, with the largest randomized trial reporting that dexamethasone increased the incidence and severity of headache on the first postoperative day and had no effect thereafter.[105]

Prophylactic epidural blood patch

Injection of 15–20 mL of blood into the epidural space markedly increases subarachnoid pressure for 15 minutes[106] and sustains this rise in CSF pressure compared to very transient increases after epidural saline or dextran.[107] Epidural injection of blood also induces cranial vasoconstriction, immediately returning the elevated cerebral blood flow that is associated with reduction of CSF volume to normal.[6] The mass effect of blood distributed along the epidural space is also thought to prevent CSF loss from, and promote healing of, the meningeal perforation.[108,109]

Prior to catheter removal, administration of autologous blood through a re-sited epidural catheter is a popular prophylactic approach in some countries but rarely used in others.[110,111] A number of low-quality studies with inadequate blinding describe good efficacy from a prophylactic epidural blood patch (PEBP) compared with no intervention, symptomatic expectant treatment (bed rest, oral fluid, and analgesics) or epidural saline. The two randomized trials, only one of which used a sham PEBP as the comparator, found conflicting results after accidental dural puncture. One found a clinically relevant reduction in the incidence and severity of PDPH after PEBP (from 80% to 18%).[112] The study including a sham PEBP to reduce bias found that the incidence of PDPH and therapeutic EBP did not differ between groups, although the duration of PDPH was shorter.[113] Prior to the positive study,[112] a meta-analysis of randomized trials[86] had shown no benefit (Figure 27.1) and both a Cochrane systematic and a focused review had concluded that there was insufficient evidence to recommend the routine use of a PEBP.[114,115]

Study or Subgroup	ITC Events	ITC Total	Control Events	Control Total	Weight	Risk Ratio M-H, Random, 95% CI
Ayad[13]	20	66	34	37	10.6%	0.33 [0.23, 0.48]
Cohen[12]	8	30	5	15	3.8%	0.80 [0.32, 2.03]
Kaul[11]	30	60	84	162	12.3%	0.96 [0.72, 1.29]
Norris[12]	19	35	11	21	8.3%	1.04 [0.62, 1.72]
Paech[15]	21	24	44	51	14.4%	1.01 [0.84, 1.22]
Russell[18]	38	57	36	58	12.7%	1.07 [0.82, 1.41]
Rutter[14]	24	34	30	37	12.8%	0.87 [0.67, 1.14]
Spiegel[10]	71	102	42	52	14.4%	0.86 [0.72, 1.04]
Walters[17]	27	61	24	37	10.8%	0.68 [0.47, 0.99]
Total (95% CI)		469		470	100.0%	0.82 [0.67, 1.01]
Total events	258		310			

Heterogeneity: $Tau^2 = 0.07$; $Chi^2 = 33.98$, df = 8 ($P < 0.0001$); $I^2 = 76\%$
Test for overall effect: $Z = 1.85$ ($P = 0.06$)

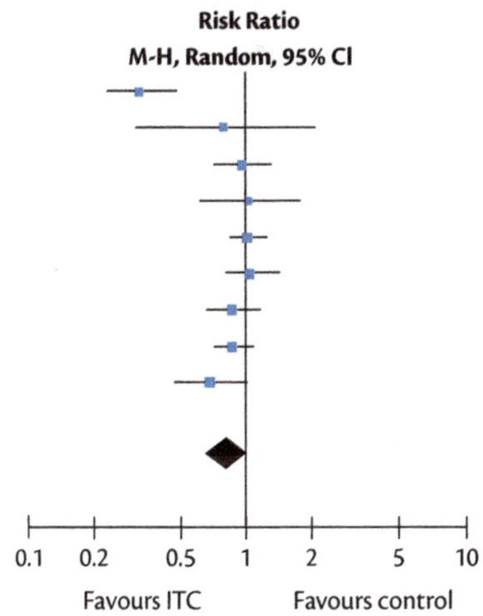

Figure 27.2 Forest plot for risk ratio of PDPH after intrathecal catheter placement.
RR, relative risk. RR < 1 favours the intervention.
Reprinted from *International Journal of Obstetric Anesthesia*, Volume 22, issue 1, M. Heesen *et al.*, Insertion of an intrathecal catheter following accidental dural puncture: a meta-analysis, pp. 26–30, Copyright (2013), with permission from Elsevier.

Epidural saline or colloid

Infusing saline into the epidural space causes a very brief pressure increase of a few centimetres of water[116] and the possibility that this might translate to a clinical effect resulted in clinical studies investigating prophylaxis with either intermittent boluses of normal saline (40–60 mL) or a continuous infusion. Meta-analysis shows a non-significant relative risk reduction in PDPH (RR 0.65; 95% CI 0.40–1.05)[86] (Figure 27.1). Case reports describe severe interscapular or neck pain or intraocular haemorrhage during saline infusion.[116,117] Low-quality studies have evaluated Dextran 40 (20 mL) as an alternative injectate, but neither efficacy nor safety has been established.[118]

Treatment of postdural puncture headache

Symptomatic versus interventional management

Although headache usually resolves spontaneously within days to weeks, the high frequency of moderate to severe and functionally disabling headache[15,25] makes relief an imperative. Regular counselling and psychological support is an essential component of management irrespective of whether an expectant or interventional approach is planned. While awaiting spontaneous resolution, PDPH is traditionally managed with supine bed rest, fluid hydration, and analgesic drugs. This approach increases the length of hospital stay and number of emergency room visits post discharge,[119] and unfortunately symptomatic relief has proven very disappointing. Most drugs have either analgesic or cerebral vasoconstrictor properties, for example, non-opioid and opioid analgesics, caffeine, theophylline, triptans, ergot alkaloids, gabapentinoids, adrenocorticotrophic hormone, and steroids. The evidence base supporting these various drug therapies is very poor.[120,121]

The longest established and best supported therapy is an EBP.[114] Although an invasive procedure, EBP has withstood the test of time because it shows inconsistent but generally moderate to high efficacy[122,123] and symptoms resolve rapidly (Table 27.3).

Pharmacological treatments

Oral non-opioid and opioid analgesics

Oral opioids presumably improve mood and provide sedation, but there are no data supporting relief of PDPH.

Epidural morphine

Case reports suggest that epidural morphine 3.5–4.5 mg can relieve PDPH after spinal anaesthesia[124] but there are no evaluations after unintentional dural puncture or clinical studies on which to base a positive recommendation.

Table 27.3 Best levels of evidence[a] and grade of recommendation supporting various treatments of PDPH

Treatment	Post-spinal	Recommendation	Post-epidural	Recommendation
Oral non-opioid and opioid analgesics	N/A		N/A	
Epidural morphine	4[124]	C	N/A	
Caffeine	2b[125]	C	2b[125]	C
Theophylline	2b[126]	C	N/A	
Triptans	2b[127]	C for NOT recommended	2b[130]	C for NOT recommended
Ergot alkaloid	4[130]	C	N/A	
Gabapentin Pregabalin	2b[132] 2b[133]	C C	N/A	
Adrenocorticotrophic hormone	2b[136]	C for NOT recommended	2b[136]	C for NOT recommended
Hydrocortisone	2b[137,138]	B	N/A	
Occipital nerve block	2b[140]	C	N/A	
Acupuncture			4[141]	C
Epidural saline or colloid	3[142]	C	3[142,144]	C
Epidural fibrin glue	4[150]	C	N/A	
Epidural blood patch	2b[123]	B	3[114]	C

Grades of recommendation A = consistent level 1 studies. B = consistent level 2 or 3 studies or extrapolations from level 1 studies. C = level 4 studies or extrapolations from level 2 or 3 studies. D = level 5 evidence or troubling inconsistent or inconclusive studies of any level.

[a]Center for Evidence-based Medicine Levels of Evidence. Accessed 16 November 2012 at http://www.cebm.net/index.aspx?o=1025

N/A, not available.

Data from various sources (see references).

Caffeine

Caffeine 500 mg IV was proposed several decades ago as an appropriate treatment for post-spinal PDPH, but appears to have, at best, low efficacy.[38,121] For example, a randomized controlled trial of single-dose oral caffeine 300 mg versus placebo for parturients suffering from PDPH due to 26 G spinal or 17 G epidural needles found that pain was reduced 4 hours after treatment but that the effect was short-lived and EBP requirement unchanged.[125] Therapeutic doses cause problematic excitatory side effects, with case reports describing dizziness, flushing, jitteriness,[125] insomnia,[99] and an association with convulsions.[99] Adverse effects in the newborn are well documented[126] and maternal ingestion of large quantities when breastfeeding may contribute to irritability and poor sleeping patterns in the infant.[127]

Theophylline

Theophylline is a methylxanthine causing cerebral vasoconstriction. A pilot study suggested that theophylline might be effective against post-spinal PDPH and IV theophylline 200 mg showed efficacy but it is not clear whether the study was randomized or blinded and there was no patient follow-up.[128] Until larger randomized trials are conducted there is insufficient evidence or safety data to support this treatment.

Triptans

The triptans are serotonin agonists that are considered the most effective cerebral vasoconstrictors for treatment of acute migraine. Their side effects include injection site reactions, nausea, vomiting, pressure and heat sensations, flushing, fatigue, tingling, and coronary vasoconstriction (making coronary artery disease or co-administration with other vasoconstrictors a contraindication). A small case series suggested possible efficacy but the only randomized, double-blind trial for PDPH, while probably underpowered, found no improvement in severe PDPH after a single dose of subcutaneous sumatriptan 6 mg.[129]

Ergot alkaloids

Methylergonovine maleate (methergine) is an ergot alkaloid derivative with activity at serotonin, dopamine and noradrenaline receptors. Side effects are nausea and vomiting, numbness and tingling of digits, muscle pain, coronary and peripheral vasoconstriction, hypertension, and rarely acute vasospasm. Despite some efficacy in treating migraine, there are several contraindications. A dose of 0.25 mg three times a day was reported to be effective for obstetric patients with spinal-induced PDPH, with only one of 25 patients requiring an EBP.[130] However the combination of oral ergotamine and caffeine is less effective than oral gabapentin,[131] so the ergot drugs are not recommended.

Gabapentinoids

Gabapentin and pregabalin are analogues of gamma-aminobutyricacid (GABA) and are effective against acute, neuropathic and inflammatory pain. Small, non-obstetric, placebo-controlled randomized trials in patients with post-spinal PDPH found gabapentin 300 mg every 8 hours for 4 days significantly reduced headache intensity, with side effects such as somnolence, ataxia, light-headedness and visual disturbance;[132] or was more effective and less nauseating than oral ergotamine 1 mg and caffeine 100 mg.[131] Pregabalin may be effective in the same population based on a case report and a randomized, single-blinded study (150 mg/day for 3 days, then 300 mg/day for 2 days, versus placebo).[133] Its side effects are short-lived dizziness and somnolence.

One unit reported encouraging improvement in PDPH from obstetric epidural dural puncture when gabapentin was titrated against sedation[134] but currently the evidence-base is poor. Data on breast milk transfer is limited and potential effects on the developing brain have been raised based on adverse effects in rodent models. Thus gabapentinoids appear the most promising of the symptomatic treatments, but further evaluation is required.

Adrenocorticotrophic hormone and cosyntropin

It has been postulated that ACTH or cosyntropin (1-24 corticotropin or tetracosactin) may reduce the severity of PDPH due to anti-inflammatory, salt and water retention and ß-endorphin enhancing properties.[135,136] Potential side effects include hypersensitivity reactions, flushing, malaise and dyspnoea; and postpartum seizures have occurred contemporaneously.[82] Open studies indicated successful relief of PDPH after single doses of intramuscular ACTH or cosyntropin (1.5 units/kg IV infusion over 30 minutes),[135] but a small, randomized, double-blind trial in obstetric patients found no effect of Synacthen® Depot 1 mg (equivalent to ACTH 100 units) intramuscularly on the severity of headache or requirement for EBP.[136] Based on this evidence, these agents cannot be supported.

Intravenous hydrocortisone

Although beneficial actions are speculative, possibly through suppression of algogenic inflammatory mediators, steroids may be effective against low ICP headache. Efficacy against post-spinal PDPH has been found in obstetric and non-obstetric small, randomized, double-blind trials, with IV hydrocortisone 100 mg every 8 hours for 48 hours reducing headache severity within 6 hours compared with conventional symptomatic treatment.[137,138] There were no apparent side effects, but very low rates of blood patching indicate that external validity and efficacy after unintentional dural puncture need to be established.

Non-pharmacological treatments

Occipital nerve block

PDPH is often experienced in the frontal and occipital regions, where the scalp is supplied by the greater and lesser occipital nerves of C2 and C3 roots. Occipital nerve block is a minimally invasive treatment for occipital neuralgia, cluster, and migraine headache. For PDPH, it has been postulated that this block might reduce central sensitization, by transiently disrupting nociceptive input to the dorsal roots and trigeminal nucleus.[139] In addition to case reports of resolution of post-spinal and post-epidural PDPH, a randomized, single-blinded trial allocated a mixed group of obstetric and non-obstetric patients with post-spinal PDPH to either greater or lesser occipital nerve blocks with lignocaine, bupivacaine, fentanyl, and clonidine or conventional expectant treatment. Occipital block reduced pain, analgesic consumption, and provided complete relief for 68% versus 8% after 1 to 2 daily injections.[140] Potential risks such as subcutaneous haematoma, local pain, or alopecia are minor. Larger randomized studies in obstetric patients and with different injectates are required, but occipital nerve block may prove to be a relatively straightforward treatment for patients who refuse an EBP.

Acupuncture

Case reports suggest acupuncture can reduce the severity of PDPH, sometimes with immediate effect,[141] but there is insufficient evidence to support this treatment.

Epidural saline

After epidural injection of saline 10–30 mL, epidural and subarachnoid space pressures increase for 3–10 minutes. Whether this is of benefit in restoring ICP and reducing headache is uncertain, because although good success was reported in treating PDPH due to 25 G spinal needles, there was no benefit for post-epidural PDPH.[142]

Epidural normal saline infusions (15–30 mL/h for 24 hours) might sustain a rise in vertebral canal pressure more effectively and are claimed to have relieved PDPH following a failed EBP.[143] For patients with spinal deformity, caudal normal saline injection is an alternative. A small observational study of male and female patients with post-spinal PDPH used 80–220 mL of caudal saline infusion up to twice per day for 1–2 days and noted that 85% improved after 3–4 sessions, with only 7% requiring an EBP, but there was no control group.[144] In practice, epidural saline infusion is limited by pressure-related adverse effects such as back, neck or ocular pain, and retinal haemorrhage has been reported.[142–145] Given the poor evidence base, this approach should only be considered for women for whom an EBP is contraindicated or has repeatedly failed.

Epidural colloids

Dextran, gelatins, and starch-based colloids show delayed reabsorption from the epidural space compared with normal saline. After lumbar puncture a small number of case reports describe the resolution of PDPH.[146,147] No immunohistochemical evidence of neurotoxic change was seen in experimental animals receiving intrathecal Dextran 40 or 3.5% colloidal solution of polygeline (Haemaccel®),[148] but some patients experience dysaesthesia or burning at the injection site. Given that the epidural colloids have not been adequately evaluated, they should only be considered when blood is contraindicated or refused; and specific informed consent would be essential.

Epidural fibrin glue

Gel-like fibrin glue has high tensile strength and successfully closes dural defects in neurosurgical patients and after removal of intrathecal catheters in cancer patients. An effective seal of a 17 G epidural needle hole was obtained in a swine model[149] and a case report described a non-pregnant patient who was suffering a post-spinal PDPH that had not responded to an EBP, but which resolved after injection of epidural fibrin glue 3 mL.[150] This epidural medium has not been tested in obstetric patients or after unintentional dural puncture, but warrants investigation.

Epidural blood patch

Compared to conservative treatment

A Cochrane review concluded that EBP is more effective than either conservative treatment or a sham procedure (OR for PDPH 0.18; 95% CI 0.04–0.76 and OR 0.04; 95% CI 0.00–0.39 respectively).[114] The best quality randomized study, involving 42 non-obstetric patients, found that EBP with 15–20 mL produced headache relief on the first and the seventh post-procedural day in 42% and 84% of participants respectively, compared with 10% and 14% of those receiving conservative treatment.[123] EBP is thought to resolve symptoms through an immediate and sustained tamponade, with the increase in intracranial CSF pressure leading to adenosine receptor inhibition, cerebral vasoconstriction, and fall in the elevated cerebral blood flow .[6,107] Animal studies show a sustained CSF pressure increase for up to 240 minutes after epidural injection of blood or fibrin glue, compared with only a few minutes after epidural saline or Dextran.[107] In humans, the increase in subarachnoid pressure is sustained for at least 15 minutes after EBP.[106] CSF accelerates coagulation and it is thought that relief is then sustained if the blood clots over the meningeal hole, preventing further CSF loss[108,151] and stimulating the fibroblastic proliferative response and collagen repair of the defect.

Contraindications to an epidural blood patch

Although relative contraindications, in a number of circumstances an EBP may present an unacceptable degree of risk. The injection of infected blood or tissue is inadvisable, precluding EBP in those with suspected or known systemic infection or skin infection at the puncture site. Injection of matched allogeneic blood into a febrile patient with severe PDPH has been described but is controversial, as the risk of creating suitable conditions for abscess formation still exists.[147,152] The risk of spinal canal haematoma may be unacceptable in those with defective haemostasis or on anticoagulant therapy. For example, patients on prophylactic low-molecular-weight heparin should not receive a neuraxial block for at least 12 hours and most consider a platelet count of less than 50,000 × 10^9/L a contraindication. Oncological seeding of the central nervous system has been raised as an issue for patients with haematological malignancy[147,153] but EBP is not contraindicated in HIV-positive patients.[154] Jehovah's Witness patients may find EBP acceptable if a continuous circuit from the venous circulation to the epidural space is used,[155] but alternative solutions are saline or colloid.

Efficacy and success of an epidural blood patch

The efficacy of an EBP is thought to depend on several factors, such as the diameter and shape of the meningeal perforation, the timing of the procedure, the technique and volume of blood used, patient response, and post-procedural management. An EBP for PDPH from 20–27 G spinal needles has a short-term success rate of 88–96%, but relief is complete in only 50–75%.[122,156] After dural puncture with a 16–18 G epidural needle in obstetric patients, partial relief from EBP occurs in more than 70% and complete relief in 30–50%.[28,157,158] After unintentional puncture in the obstetric population, recurrent headache occurs after initial success in approximately 30%, of whom 30–60% request another EBP.[157,158] The success rate of a second EBP is similar to the initial.[122,157] A third EBP is only very occasionally indicated and re-evaluation, with possibly further diagnostic investigation, should first be undertaken.[57] Back pain during injection may limit the volume of blood that can be administered .[28] Nevertheless successful EBP, performed years after dural puncture, is reported.[72,159]

A large observational study identified two risk factors for the failure of an EBP, namely penetration of the dura and arachnoid by a needle of size 20 G or less (OR 5.96: 95% CI 2.63–13.47) and performing the procedure within 4 days (OR 2.63; 95% CI 1.06–6.51).[122] The failure rate of EBP was noted to be higher in those patients who received an EBP less than 24 hours after dural puncture, compared with beyond 24 hours.[122] This finding is supported by other observational studies, including in obstetrics, where success rates within 24 hours of dural puncture are extremely low[158,160] and both partial and complete success rates of EBP performed after 48 hours are higher.[28] The advantage of delaying an EBP is that the anticoagulant effect of local anaesthetic drugs in the epidural space will have waned[161] and closure of the meningeal perforation may have commenced. Although selection bias cannot be discounted, it appears that EBP should ideally be delayed for at least 24 hours and possibly 48 hours after unintentional dural puncture, keeping in mind that delay increases the period of suffering and hospitalization.[119]

Technique and volume of blood in the epidural blood patch

To minimize the risk of a repeat dural puncture, an EBP should be performed by experienced personnel after the patient has been informed about its efficacy and complications, found to be free of relative contraindications, and has given written informed consent. The procedure should be performed under standard monitoring, due to the possibility of bradycardia and syncope.[162] The lateral position is more comfortable for the patient but a short period of sitting is usually tolerated. A full aseptic technique is obligatory and is easier if an assistant deals with the sterile venepuncture. A warning about mild (and occasionally moderate to severe) back pain during the injection of blood is mandatory, because this is experienced by 30–50% of patients, usually after at least 10 mL of blood has been administered. The risk increases as more blood is injected.[28] Injection at an interspinous space at, or a space below, the level of the dural breach is common, but is not based on outcome data and only supported by imaging that demonstrates spread of blood across multiple segments, favouring cephalad distribution.[1,109,163] Use of EBP in patients with spontaneous intracranial hypotension shows that injection of blood remote to the location of the CSF leak can be effective,[3,4,71] so the level of insertion is probably not critical. A slow rate of injection is recommended because it limits the peak neuraxial pressure, which is thought to minimize nerve root pain. Intolerable back or leg pain may necessitate termination of the procedure—20% of women do not tolerate the injection of 20 mL and 50% do not tolerate 30 mL of autologous blood.[28]

The optimum volume of blood has been addressed in two randomized trials in obstetric patients who had post-epidural PDPH. There was no difference in clinical outcome between 7.5 and 15 mL.[164] A three-arm study (15, 20, or 30 mL) found that immediate and permanent relief was more likely after 20 mL than 15 mL (OR 4.49; 95% CI 1.31–15.42), although all volumes were of similar efficacy in achieving partial or permanent relief.[28] In addition to larger volumes of blood being more poorly tolerated, linear regression shows a direct relationship between increasing EBP volumes and worsening neurological compression syndromes.[165] On this basis, injecting at least 20 mL of blood is recommended when treating PDPH after unintentional dural puncture in obstetric patients.

Post-epidural blood patch management

The lumbar CSF pressure is increased in the semi-erect or erect position, which in theory might overcome the proposed 'dural plug' effect of an EBP. Although observations suggest that outcomes after EBP are not significantly affected by patient ambulation, a small randomized trial in non-obstetric patients recommended placing patients in a supine position for 2 hours after the procedure rather than a shorter period of recumbency, because the headache was then of lesser intensity.[166] Based on anecdotes of recurrent PDPH after EBP following heavy lifting, coughing, or abdominal straining, stool softeners may be advised. Occasional cases of fever[122] mandate early observation of vital signs including temperature. Patients must be reviewed after EBP and their general or family practitioner informed, so that rare complications such as an epidural haematoma or abscess are diagnosed. The patient should be given advice about potential back pain and who to contact with post-discharge concerns.

Complications of epidural blood patch

More than half of those having an EBP experience post-procedural back, buttock, or leg pain for several days. This is usually mild but can be moderate to severe in up to a quarter of cases.[28,122] Other complications include transient bradycardia,[162] nausea, neck pain, dizziness, auditory disturbance, and fever.[122,123] Serious neurological complications have not been quantified but appear very rare. These include radicular back pain, lumbovertebral syndrome (low back pain with neurological deficit in the lower extremities), cauda equina syndrome, arachnoiditis, seizures, and subdural haematoma.[165] Adverse outcomes have resulted from cerebral ischaemia[167] and VI and VIIth cranial nerve palsies are thought to be precipitated by changes in ICP that affect neural blood supply.[168] The duration of cranial nerve palsy associated with PDPH correlates with days delayed before EBP, so early treatment of cranial nerve palsy with EBP has been recommended.[168] Although imaging suggests there is rapid reabsorption of epidural blood,[163] and success rates of subsequent epidural techniques are unaffected,[169] it appears that rarely adhesions are formed, resulting in subsequent inadequate block, possible subdural block[170] or chronic back pain due to calcification.[171]

Surgical closure of the dural tear

Surgery is the most invasive management of PDPH and may be required for the management of subdural haematoma, but meningeal repair is very rarely used and reserved for patients for whom all less invasive methods have failed to stop a chronic CSF fistula or persisting headache.

Conclusion

There is still much to be learned about the pathophysiology, risk factors (needle, technical, and patient related), natural history, diagnosis, and management of PDPH. High-level evidence supports prevention by using small-gauge, non-cutting spinal needles, but other preventative strategies against either unintentional dural puncture or PDPH are poorly supported. The absent or poor efficacy of commonly applied measures such as bed rest, hydration, cerebral vasoconstrictor therapy, epidural or intrathecal saline injection, intrathecal catheter placement, or PEBP, is noted. Validation of stronger evidence supporting epidural morphine or IV cosyntropin (tetracosactide) is required. Symptomatic treatment of PDPH is also unreliable and the limited evidence that supports a modest benefit from caffeine, gabapentinoids, or IV hydrocortisone requires substantiation.

The intervention of an EBP is highly likely to relieve post-spinal PDPH, and is effective for PDPH after unintentional dural puncture, but in the latter situation a single blood patch only completely resolves headache in a minority of cases. The mechanism of action and best methodology for EBP also requires further research, but delayed intervention and injection of approximately 20 mL of autologous blood appear appropriate.

References

1. Vakharia SB, Thomas PS, Rosenbaum AE, *et al.* Magnetic resonance imaging of cerebrospinal fluid leak and tamponade effect of blood patch in postdural puncture headache. *Anesth Analg* 1997; 84:585–90.
2. Grant R, Condon B, Hart I, *et al.* Changes in intracranial CSF volume after lumbar puncture and their relationship to post-LP headache. *J Neurol Neurosurg Psychiatry* 1991; 54:440–2.
3. Diaz JH. Treatment outcomes in spontaneous intracranial hypotension: do epidural blood patches stop the leaks? *Pain Pract* 2004; 4:295–302.
4. Madsen SA, Fomsgaard JS, Jensen R. Epidural blood patch for refractory low CSF pressure headache: a pilot study. *J Headache Pain* 2011; 12:453–7.
5. Yousry I, Förderreuther S, Moriggl B, *et al.* Cervical MR imaging in postural headache: MR signs and pathophysiological implications. *Am J Neuroradiol* 2001; 22:1239–50.
6. Boezaart AP. Effects of cerebrospinal fluid loss and epidural blood patch on cerebral blood flow in swine. *Reg Anesth Pain Med* 2001; 26:401–6.
7. Mokri B, Atkinson JL, Piepgras DG. Absent headache despite CSF volume depletion (intracranial hypotension). *Neurology* 2000; 55:1722–4.
8. Clark JW, Solomon GD, Senanayake PD, *et al.* Substance P concentration and history of headache in relation to postlumbar puncture headache: towards prevention. *J Neurol Neurosurg Psychiatry* 1996; 60:681–3.
9. Valenca MM, Amorim JA, Moura TP. Why don't all individuals who undergo dura mater/arachnoid puncture develop postdural puncture headache? *Anesth Pain Med* 2012; 1:207–9.
10. Nowaczewska M, Ksiazkiewicz B. Cerebral blood flow characteristics in patients with post-lumbar puncture headache. *J Neurol* 2012; 259:665–9.
11. Paulson PE, Minoshima S, Morrow TJ, *et al.* Gender differences in pain perception and patterns of cerebral activation during noxious heat stimulation in humans. *Pain* 1998; 76:223–9.
12. Choi PT, Galinski SE, Takeuchi L, *et al.* PDPH is a common complication of neuraxial blockade in parturients: a meta-analysis of obstetrical studies. *Can J Anaesth* 2003; 50:460–9.
13. Smith EA, Thorburn J, Duckworth RA, *et al.* A comparison of 25 G and 27 G Whitacre needles for caesarean section. *Anaesthesia* 1994; 49:859–62.
14. Van de Velde M, Teunkens A, Hanssens M, *et al.* Post dural puncture headache following combined spinal epidural or epidural anaesthesia in obstetric patients. *Anaesth Intensive Care* 2001; 29:595–9.
15. Paech M, Banks S, Gurrin L. An audit of accidental dural puncture during epidural insertion of a Tuohy needle in obstetric patients. *Int J Obstet Anesth* 2001; 10:162–7.
16. Sprigge JS, Harper SJ. Accidental dural puncture and post dural puncture headache in obstetric anesthesia: presentation and management: a 23-year survey in a district general hospital. *Anaesthesia* 2008; 63:36–43.
17. Morley-Forster PK, Singh S, Angle P, *et al.* The effect of epidural needle type on postdural puncture headache: a randomized trial. *Can J Anaesth* 2006; 53:572–8.
18. O'Connor G, Gingrich R, Moffat M. The effect of spinal needle design, size, and penetration angle on dural puncture cerebral spinal fluid loss. *Am Assoc Nurse Anesth J* 2007; 75:111–6.
19. Halpern S, Preston R. Postdural puncture headache and spinal needle design: metaanalyses. *Anesthesiology* 1994; 81:1376–83.
20. Mayer DC, Quance D, Weeks SK. Headache after spinal anesthesia for cesarean section: a comparison of the 27-gauge Quincke and 24-gauge Sprotte needles. *Anesth Analg* 1992; 75:377–80.
21. Vallejo MC, Mandell GL, Sabo DP, *et al.* Postdural puncture headache: a randomized comparison of five spinal needles in obstetric patients. *Anesth Analg* 2000; 91:916–20.
22. Devcic A, Sprung J, Patel S, *et al.* PDPH in obstetric anesthesia: comparison of 24-gauge Sprotte and 25-gauge Quincke needles and effect of subarachnoid administration of fentanyl. *Reg Anesth* 1993; 18:222–5.
23. Douglas MJ, Ward ME, Campbell DC, *et al.* Factors involved in the incidence of post-dural puncture headache with the 25 gauge Whitacre needle for obstetric anesthesia. *Int J Obstet Anesth* 1997; 6:220–3.
24. Flaatten H, Felthaus J, Kuwelker M, *et al.* Postural post-dural puncture headache. A prospective randomized study and a meta-analysis comparing two different 0.40 mm O.D. (27G) spinal needles. *Acta Anaesthesiol Scand* 2000; 44:643–7.
25. Chan TM, Ahmed E, Yentis SM, *et al.* Postpartum headaches: summary report of the National Obstetric Anaesthetic Database (NOAD) 1999. *Int J Obstet Anesth* 2003; 12:107–12.
26. Sadashivaiah J, McLure H. 18-G Tuohy needle can reduce the incidence of severe post dural puncture headache. *Anaesthesia* 2009; 64:1379–80.
27. Russell IF. A prospective controlled study of continuous spinal analgesia versus repeat epidural analgesia after accidental dural puncture in labour. *Int J Obstet Anesth* 2012; 21:7–16.
28. Paech MJ, Doherty DA, Christmas T, *et al.* The volume of blood for epidural blood patch in obstetrics: a randomized, blinded clinical trial. *Anesth Analg* 2011; 113:126–33.
29. Fink BR, Walker S. Orientation of fibers in human dorsal lumbar dura mater in relation to lumbar puncture. *Anesth Analg* 1989; 69:768–72.
30. Richman JM, Joe EM, Cohen SR, *et al.* Bevel direction and postdural puncture headache: a meta-analysis. *Neurologist* 2006; 12:224–8.
31. Cowan CM, Moore EW. A survey of epidural technique and accidental dural puncture rates among obstetric anaesthetists. *Int J Obstet Anesth* 2001; 10:11–16.
32. Strupp M, Brandt T, Muller A. Incidence of post-lumbar puncture syndrome reduced by reinserting the stylet: a randomized prospective study of 600 patients. *J Neurol* 1998; 245:589–92.
33. Mosaffa F, Karimi K, Madadi F, *et al.* Post-dural puncture headache: a comparison between median and paramedian approaches in orthopedic patients. *Anesth Pain Med* 2011; 1:66–9.
34. Seeberger MD, Kaufmann M, Staender S, *et al.* Repeated dural punctures increases the incidence of postdural puncture headache. *Anesth Analg* 1996; 82:302–5.
35. Simmons SW, Taghizadeh N, Dennis AT, *et al.* Combined spinal-epidural versus epidural analgesia in labour. *Cochrane Database Syst Rev* 2012; 10:CD003401.
36. Aya AG, Mangin R, Robert C, *et al.* Increased risk of unintentional dural puncture in night-time obstetric epidural anesthesia. *Can J Anaesth* 1999; 46:665–9.
37. Aida S, Taga K, Yamakura T, *et al.* Headache after attempted epidural block: the role of intrathecal air. *Anesthesiology* 1998; 88:76–81.
38. Bradbury C, Singh SI, Badder SR, *et al.* Prevention of post-dural puncture headache in parturients: a systematic review and meta-analysis. *Acta Anaesthesiol Scand* 2012; 57:417–30.
39. Vilming ST, Schrader H, Monstad I. The significance of age, sex and cerebrospinal fluid pressure in post-lumbar-puncture headache. *Cephalalgia* 1989; 9:99–106.
40. Wu CL, Rowlingson AJ, Cohen SR, *et al.* Gender and post-dural puncture headache. *Anesthesiology* 105:613–18.
41. Amorim JA, Valenca MM. Postdural puncture headache is a risk factor for new postdural puncture headache. *Cephalalgia* 2008; 28:5–8.
42. Hollister N, Todd C, Ball S, *et al.* Minimising the risk of accidental dural puncture with epidural analgesia in labour: a retrospective review of risk factors. *Int J Obstet Anesth* 2012; 21:236–41.
43. Faure E, Moreno R, Thisted R. Incidence of postdural puncture headache in morbidly obese parturients. *Reg Anesth* 1994; 19:361–3.

44. Peralta F, Higgins N, Chalifoux LA, *et al.* Obese parturients and the incidence of postdural puncture headache after unintentional dural puncture. *SOAP Abstracts* 2010:6. https://soap.org/2010-abstracts-list.php
45. Kovacheva VP, Bateman B, Farber M, *et al.* The incidence, risk factors, and outcome of post-dural puncture headache after dural puncture with a 17G epidural needle. *SOAP Abstracts* 2012:S-26. https://www.soap.org/2012-abstracts-list.php
46. Ranta P, Jouppila P, Spalding M, *et al.* The effect of maternal obesity on labour and labour pain. *Anaesthesia* 1995; 50:322–6.
47. Angle P, Thompson D, Halpern S, *et al.* Second stage pushing correlates with headache after unintentional dural puncture in parturients. *Can J Anaesth* 1999; 46:861–6.
48. Ravindran RS, Viegas OJ, Tasch MD, *et al.* Bearing down at the time of delivery and the incidence of spinal headache in parturients. *Anesth Analg* 1981; 60:524–6.
49. Mokri B, Aksamit AJ, Atkinson JL. Paradoxical postural headaches in cerebrospinal fluid leaks. *Cephalalgia* 2004; 24:883–7.
50. Lybecker H, Djernes M, Schmidt JF. Postdural puncture headache (PDPH): onset, duration, severity, and associated symptoms. An analysis of 75 consecutive patients with PDPH. *Acta Anaesthesiol Scand* 1995; 39:605–12.
51. Arcand G, Girard F, McCormack M, *et al.* Bilateral sixth cranial nerve palsy after unintentional dural puncture. *Can J Anaesth* 2004; 51:821–3.
52. Nishio I, Williams BA, Williams JP. Diplopia: a complication of dural puncture. *Anesthesiology* 2004; 100:58–64.
53. Fiala A, Furgler G, Baumgartner E, *et al.* Delayed subdural haematoma complicated by abducens nerve palsy and cortical vein thrombosis after obstetric epidural anaesthesia. *Br J Anesth* 2012; 108:705–6.
54. Bechard P, Perron G, Larochelle D, *et al.* Case report: epidural blood patch in the treatment of abducens palsy after a dural puncture. *Can J Anaesth* 2007; 54:146–50.
55. Mannes AJ, Shepard M, Quezado Z. Resolution of diplopia with late treatment of post-dural puncture headache and intracranial hypotension. *Can J Anaesth* 2008; 55:256–7.
56. Fog J, Wang LP, Sundberg A, *et al.* Hearing loss after spinal anesthesia is related to needle size. *Anesth Analg* 1990; 70:517–22.
57. Stella CL, Jodicke CD, How HY, *et al.* Postpartum headache: is your work-up complete? *Am J Obstet Gynecol* 2007; 196:318.e1–7.
58. Headache Classification Subcommittee of the International Headache Society (IHS). The International Classification of Headache Disorders, 3rd edition (beta version). *Cephalalgia* 2013; 33:629–808.
59. Klein AM, Loder E. Postpartum headache. *Int J Obstet Anesth* 2010; 19:422–30.
60. Goldszmidt E, Kern R, Chaput A, *et al.* The incidence and etiology of postpartum headaches: a prospective cohort study. *Can J Anaesth* 2005; 52:971–7.
61. Roberts SP, Petts HV. Meningitis after obstetric spinal anaesthesia. *Anaesthesia* 1990; 45:376–7.
62. Cohen S, Hunter CW, Sakr A, *et al.* Meningitis following intrathecal catheter placement after accidental dural puncture. *Int J Obstet Anesth* 2006; 15:171.
63. Boyd AH, Pigston PE. Postpartum headache and cerebral tumour. *Anaesthesia* 1992; 46:450–1.
64. Wark HJ. An unusual complication of an inadvertent dural tap. *Anaesthesia* 1977; 32:336–8.
65. Browne IM, Birnbach DJ. Neurocysticercosis: a new differential in the diagnosis of postdural puncture headache. *Anesth Analg* 2003; 97:580–2.
66. Lomax S, Qureshi A. Unusually early onset of post-dural puncture headache after spinal anaesthesia using a 27G Whitacre needle. *Br J Anesth* 2008; 100:707–8.
67. Laviola S, Kirvelä M, Spoto MR, *et al.* Pneumocephalus with intense headache and unilateral pupillary dilatation after accidental dural puncture during epidural anesthesia for cesarean section. *Anesth Analg* 1999; 88:582–3.
68. Reamy BV. Post-epidural headache: how late can it occur? *J Am Board Fam Med* 2009; 22:202–5.
69. Webb CA, Weyker PD, Zhang L, *et al.* Unintentional dural puncture with a Tuohy needle increases risk of chronic headache. *Anesth Analg* 2012; 115:124–32.
70. Jeskins GD, Moore PA, Cooper GM, *et al.* Long-term morbidity following dural puncture in an obstetric population. *Int J Obstet Anesth* 2001; 10:17–24.
71. Couch JR, Persson J. Treatment of spontaneous intracranial hypotension with epidural blood patch: is a complex approach necessary or better than a simple one? *Acta Anaesthesiol Scand* 2012; 56:1207–9.
72. Abouleish EI, Rashid S. Successful epidural blood patch 2 years after post-lumbar puncture headaches. *Am J Emerg Med* 1995; 13:683–4.
73. Fang JY, Lin JW, Li Q, *et al.* Trigeminal nerve and facial nerve palsy after combined spinal-epidural anesthesia for cesarean section. *J Clin Anesth* 2010; 22:56–8.
74. Schabel JE, Wang ED, Glass PS. Arm pain as an unusual presentation of postdural puncture intracranial hypotension. *Anesth Analg* 2000; 91:910–2.
75. Errando CL, Peiro CM. Postdural puncture upper back pain as an atypical presentation of postdural puncture symptoms. *Anesthesiology* 2002; 96:1019–20.
76. Zeidan A, Farhat O, Maaliki H, *et al.* Does postdural puncture headache left untreated lead to subdural hematoma? Case report and review of the literature. *Int J Obstet Anesth* 2006; 15:50–8.
77. Hart IK, Bone I, Hadley DM. Development of neurological problems after lumbar puncture. *Br Med J* 1988; 296:51–2.
78. Eerola M, Kaukinen L, Kaukinen S. Fatal brain lesion following spinal anaesthesia. Report of a case. *Acta Anaesthesiol Scand* 1981; 25:115–6.
79. Mouraux A, Gille M, Dorban S, *et al.* Cortical venous thrombosis after lumbar puncture. *J Neurol* 2002; 249:1313–15.
80. Ho CM, Chan KH. Posterior reversible encephalopathy syndrome with vasospasm in a postpartum woman after postdural puncture headache following spinal anesthesia. *Anesth Analg* 2007; 105:770–2.
81. Rice I, Mountfield J, Radhakrishnan D, *et al.* Puerperal seizures associated with post dural puncture headache. *Int J Obstet Anesth* 2003; 12:126–9.
82. Oliver CD, White SA. Unexplained fitting in three parturients suffering from postdural puncture headache. *Br J Anesth* 2002; 89:782–5.
83. Bleeker CP, Hendriks IM, Booij LH. Postpartum post-dural puncture headache: is your differential diagnosis complete? *Br J Anesth* 2004; 93:461–4.
84. Ng MD, Manikappa S. Postpartum seizure and ischaemic stroke following dural puncture and epidural blood patch. *Anaesth Intensive Care* 2012; 40:347–51.
85. Loures V, Savoldelli GL, Alberque C, *et al.* Post-dural puncture cerebrospinal fluid leak presenting as an acute psychiatric illness. *Br J Anesth* 2012; 108:529–30.
86. Apfel CC, Saxena A, Cakmakkaya OS, *et al.* Prevention of postdural puncture headache after accidental dural puncture: a quantitative systematic review. *Br J Anesth* 2010; 105:255–63.
87. Sudlow C, Warlow C. Posture and fluids for preventing post-dural puncture headache. *Cochrane Database Syst Rev* 2002; 2:CD001790.
88. Dieterich M, Brandt T. Incidence of post-lumbar puncture headache is independent of daily fluid intake. *Eur Arch Psychiatry Neurol Sci* 1988; 237:194–6.
89. Charsley MM, Abram SE. The injection of intrathecal normal saline reduces the severity of postdural puncture headache. *Reg Anesth Pain Med* 2001; 26:301–5.
90. Tsai PB, Zehnaly A, Chen BJ, *et al.* Lower extremity radicular pain after prophylactic intrathecal saline injection through a subarachnoid catheter following accidental dural puncture. *Int J Obstet Anesth* 2011; 20:262–5.

91. Ayad S, Demian Y, Narouze SN, *et al.* Subarachnoid catheter placement after wet tap for analgesia in labor: influence on the risk of headache in obstetric patients. *Reg Anesth Pain Med* 2003; 28:512–5.
92. Kaul B, Sines D, Vallejo MC, *et al.* A five year experience with post dural puncture headaches. *Anesthesiology* 2007; 107:A1762.
93. Van de Velde M, Schepers R, Berends N, *et al.* Ten years of experience with accidental dural puncture and post-dural puncture headache in a tertiary obstetric anaesthesia department. *Int J Obstet Anesth* 2008; 17:329–35.
94. Heesen M, Klöhr S, Rossaint R, *et al.* Insertion of an intrathecal catheter following accidental dural puncture: a meta-analysis. *Int J Obstet Anesth* 2013; 22:26–30.
95. Verstraete S, Walters MA, Devroe S, *et al.* Lower incidence of post-dural puncture headache with spinal catheterization after accidental dural puncture in obstetric patients. *Acta Anaesthesiol Scand* 2014; 58:1233–9.
96. Yucel A, Ozyalçin S, Talu GK, *et al.* Intravenous administration of caffeine sodium benzoate for postdural puncture headache. *Reg Anesth Pain Med* 1999; 24:51–4.
97. Esmaoglu A, Akpinar H, Ugur F. Oral multidose caffeine-paracetamol combination is not effective for the prophylaxis of postdural puncture headache. *J Clin Anesth* 2005; 17:58–61.
98. Halker RB, Demaerschalk BM, Wellik KE, *et al.* Caffeine for the prevention and treatment of postdural puncture headache: debunking the myth. *Neurologist* 2007; 13:323–7.
99. Paech M. Unexpected postpartum seizures associated with post-dural puncture headache treated with caffeine. *Int J Obstet Anesth* 1996; 5:43–6.
100. Zajac K, Zajac M, Hładki W, *et al.* [Is there any point in pharmacological prophylaxis of PDPH (post-dural puncture headache) after spinal anaesthesia for Caesarean section?] *Przeglad Lekarski* 2012; 69:19–24.
101. Bussone G, *et al.* Frovatriptan for the prevention of postdural puncture headache. *Cephalalgia* 2007; 27:809–13
102. Abboud TK, Zhu J, Reyes A, *et al.* Effect of subarachnoid morphine on the incidence of spinal headache. *Reg Anesth* 1992; 17:34–6.
103. Al-metwalli RR. Epidural morphine injections for prevention of post dural puncture headache. *Anaesthesia* 2008; 63:847–50.
104. Hakim SM. Cosyntropin for prophylaxis against postdural puncture headache after accidental dural puncture. *Anesthesiology* 2010; 113:413–20.
105. Yousefshahi F, Dahmardeh AR, Khajavi M, *et al.* Effect of dexamethasone on the frequency of postdural puncture headache after spinal anesthesia for cesarean section: a double-blind randomized clinical trial. *Acta Neurol Belg* 2012; 112:345–50.
106. Coombs DW, Hooper D. Subarachnoid pressure with epidural blood "patch". *Reg Anesth* 1979; 4:3–6.
107. Kroin JS, Nagalla SK, Buvanendran A, *et al.* The mechanisms of intracranial pressure modulation by epidural blood and other injectates in a postdural puncture rat model. *Anesth Analg* 2002; 95:423–9.
108. Rosenberg PH, Heavner JE. In vitro study of the effect of epidural blood patch on leakage through a dural puncture. *Anesth Analg* 1985; 64:501–4.
109. Szeinfeld M, Ihmeidan IH, Moser MM, *et al.* Epidural blood patch: evaluation of the volume and spread of blood injected into the epidural space. *Anesthesiology* 1986; 64:820–2.
110. Harrington BE, Schmitt AM. Meningeal (postdural) puncture headache, unintentional dural puncture, and the epidural blood patch: a national survey of United States practice. *Reg Anesth Pain Med* 2009; 34:430–7.
111. Baraz R, Collis RE. The management of accidental dural puncture during labour epidural analgesia: a survey of UK practice. *Anaesthesia* 2005; 60:673–9.
112. Stein MH, Cohen S, Mohiuddin MA, *et al.* Prophylactic vs therapeutic blood patch for obstetric patients with accidental dural puncture—a randomised controlled trial. *Anaesthesia* 2014; 69:320–6.
113. Scavone BM, Wong CA, Sullivan JT, *et al.* Efficacy of a prophylactic epidural blood patch in preventing post dural puncture headache in parturients after inadvertent dural puncture. *Anesthesiology* 2004; 101:1422–7.
114. Boonmak P, Boonmak S. Epidural blood patching for preventing and treating post-dural puncture headache. *Cochrane Database Syst Rev* 2010; 20:CD001791.
115. Agerson AN, Scavone BM. Prophylactic epidural blood patch after unintentional dural puncture for the prevention of postdural puncture headache in parturients. *Anesth Analg* 2012; 115:133–6.
116. Shah JL. Epidural pressure during infusion of saline in the parturient. *Int J Obstet Anesth* 1993; 2:190–2.
117. Clark CJ, Whitwell J. Intraocular haemorrhage after epidural injection. *Br Med J* 1961; 2:1612–3.
118. Salvador L, Carrero E, Castillo J, *et al.* Prevention of post dural puncture headache with epidural-administered dextran 40. *Reg Anesth* 1992; 17:357–8.
119. Angle P, Tang SL, Thompson D, *et al.* Expectant management of postdural puncture headache increases hospital length of stay and emergency room visits. *Can J Anaesth* 2005; 52:397–402.
120. Paech MJ. Iatrogenic headaches: giving everyone a sore head. *Int J Obstet Anesth* 2012; 21:1–3.
121. Basurto Ono X, Martínez García L, Solà I, *et al.* Drug therapy for treating post-dural puncture headache. *Cochrane Database Syst Rev* 2011; 8:CD007887.
122. Safa-Tisseront V, Thormann F, Malassiné P, *et al.* Effectiveness of epidural blood patch in the management of post-dural puncture headache. *Anesthesiology* 2001; 95:334–9.
123. van Kooten F, Oedit R, Bakker SL, *et al.* Epidural blood patch in post dural puncture headache: a randomised, observer-blind, controlled clinical trial. *J Neurol Neurosurg Psychiatry* 2008; 79:553–8.
124. Eldor J, Guedj P, Cotev S. Epidural morphine injections for the treatment of postspinal headache. *Can J Anaesth* 1990; 37:710–1.
125. Camann WR, Murray RS, Mushlin PS, *et al.* Effects of oral caffeine on postdural puncture headache. A double-blind, placebo-controlled trial. *Anesth Analg* 1990; 70:181–4.
126. Howell J, Clozel M, Aranda JV. Adverse effects of caffeine and theophylline in the newborn infant. *Semin Perinatol* 1981; 5:359–69.
127. Howard CR, Lawrence RA. Breast-feeding and drug exposure. *Obstet Gynecol Clin North Am* 1998; 25:195–217.
128. Ergün U, Say B, Ozer G, *et al.* Intravenous theophylline decreases post-dural puncture headaches. *J Clin Neurosci* 2008; 15:1102–4.
129. Connelly NR, Parker RK, Rahimi A, *et al.* Sumatriptan in patients with postdural puncture headache. *Headache* 2000; 40:316–19.
130. Hakim S, Khan RM, Maroof M, *et al.* Methylergonovine maleate (methergine) relieves postdural puncture headache in obstetric patients. *Acta Obstet Gynecol Scand* 2005; 84:100.
131. Erol DD. The analgesic and antiemetic efficacy of gabapentin or ergotamine/caffeine for the treatment of postdural puncture headache. *Adv Med Sci* 2011; 56:25–9.
132. Erol DD. The effect of gabapentin on postdural puncture headache. *Acute Pain* 2006; 8:169–73.
133. Huseyinoglu U, Huseyinoglu N, Hamurtekin E, *et al.* Effect of pregabalin on post-dural-puncture headache following spinal anesthesia and lumbar puncture. *J Clin Neurosci* 2011; 18:1365–8133.
134. Wagner Y, Storr F, Cope S. Gabapentin in the treatment of post-dural puncture headache: a case series. *Anaesth Intensive Care* 2012; 40:714–18.
135. Canovas L, Barros C, Gómez A, *et al.* Use of intravenous tetracosactin in the treatment of postdural puncture headache: our experience in forty cases. *Anesth Analg* 2002; 94:1369.
136. Rucklidge MW, Yentis SM, Paech MJ. Synacthen Depot for the treatment of postdural puncture headache. *Anaesthesia* 2004; 59:138–41.

137. Noyan Ashraf MA, Sadeghi A, Azarbakht Z, *et al.* Evaluation of intravenous hydrocortisone in reducing headache after spinal anesthesia: a double blind controlled clinical study. *Middle East J Anesthesiol* 2007; 19:415–22.
138. Alam R, Rahman A, Ershad R. Role of very short-term intravenous hydrocortisone in reducing postdural puncture headache. *J Anaesthesiol Clin Pharmacol* 2012; 28:190–3.
139. Akin Takmaz S, Unal Kantekin C, Kaymak C, *et al.* Treatment of post-dural puncture headache with bilateral greater occipital nerve block. *Headache* 2010; 50:869–72.
140. Naja Z, Al-Tannir M, El-Rajab M, *et al.* Nerve stimulator-guided occipital nerve blockade for postdural puncture headache. *Pain Pract* 2008; 9:51–8.
141. Sharma A, Cheam E. Acupuncture in the management of post-partum headache following neuraxial analgesia. *Int J Obstet Anesth* 2009; 18:417–9.
142. Bart AJ, Wheeler AS. Comparison of epidural saline placement and epidural blood placement in the treatment of post-lumbar-puncture headache. *Anesthesiology* 1978; 48:221–3.
143. Stevens RA, Jorgensen N. Successful treatment of dural puncture headache with epidural saline infusion after failure of epidural blood patch. *Acta Anaesthesiol Scand* 1988; 32:429–31.
144. Abdulla S, Abdulla W, Eckhardt R. Caudal normal saline injections for the treatment of post-dural puncture headache. *Pain Physician* 2011; 14:271–9.
145. Woods SD, Hodgson P, Walker T, *et al.* Epidural infusion and neuropraxia. *Anaesthesia* 1992; 47:720.
146. Reynvoet ME, Cosaert PA, Desmet MF, *et al.* Epidural dextran 40 patch for postdural puncture headache. *Anaesthesia* 1997; 52:886–8.
147. Vassal O, Baud MC, Bolandard F, *et al.* Epidural injection of hydroxyethyl starch in the management of postdural puncture headache. *Int J Obstet Anesth* 2013; 22:153–5.
148. Chanimov M, Berman S, Cohen ML, *et al.* Dextran 40 (Rheomacrodex) or Polygeline (Haemaccel) as an epidural patch for post dural puncture headache: a neurotoxicity study in a rat model of Dextran 40 and Polygeline injected intrathecally. *Eur J Anaesth* 2006; 23:776–80.
149. Garcia-Aguado R, Gil F, Barcia JA, *et al.* Prophylactic percutaneous sealing of lumbar postdural puncture hole with fibrin glue to prevent cerebrospinal fluid leakage in swine. *Anesth Analg* 2000; 90:894–8.
150. Crul BJ, Gerritse BM, van Dongen RT, *et al.* Epidural fibrin glue injection stops persistent postdural puncture headache. *Anesthesiology* 1999; 91:576–7.
151. Cook MA, Watkins-Pitchford JM. Epidural blood patch: a rapid coagulation response. *Anesth Analg* 1990; 70:567–8.
152. Cesur M, Alici HA, Erdem AF, *et al.* Epidural blood patch with allogeneic blood for post-dural puncture headache. *Int J Obstet Anesth* 2005; 14:261–2.
153. Miguel R, Behrmann H, Diaz AP. Postdural puncture headaches in special patient populations. *Anesth Analg* 1999; 89:264.
154. Tom DJ, Gulevich SJ, Shapiro HM, *et al.* Epidural blood patch in the HIV-positive patient. *Anesthesiology* 1992; 76:943–7.
155. Kanumilli V, Kaza R, Johnson C, *et al.* Epidural blood patch for Jehovah's Witness patient. *Anesth Analg* 1993; 77:872–3.
156. Abouleish E, Vega S, Blendinger I, *et al.* Long-term follow-up of epidural blood patch. *Anesth Analg* 1975; 54:459–63.
157. Williams EJ, Beaulieu P, Fawcett WJ, *et al.* Efficacy of epidural blood patch in the obstetric population. *Int J Obstet Anesth* 1999; 8:105–9.
158. Banks S, Paech M, Gurrin L. An audit of epidural blood patch after accidental dural puncture with a Tuohy needle in obstetric patients. *Int J Obstet Anesth* 2001; 10:172–6.
159. Klepstad P. Relief of postural post dural puncture headache by an epidural blood patch 12 months after dural puncture. *Acta Anaesthesiol Scand* 1999; 43:964–6.
160. Loeser EA, Hill GE, Bennett GM, *et al.* Time vs. success rate for epidural blood patch. *Anesthesiology* 1978; 49:147–8.
161. Kohrs R, Hoenemann CW, Feirer N, *et al.* Bupivacaine inhibits whole blood coagulation in vitro. *Reg Anesth Pain Med* 1999; 24:326–30.
162. Andrews PJ, Ackerman WE, Juneja M, *et al.* Transient bradycardia associated with extradural blood patch after inadvertent dural puncture in parturients. *Br J Anesth* 1992; 69:401–3.
163. Beards SC, Jackson A, Griffiths AG, *et al.* Magnetic resonance imaging of extradural blood patches: appearances from 30 min to 18 h. *Br J Anesth* 1993; 71:182–8.
164. Chen LK, Huang CH, Jean WH, *et al.* Effective epidural blood patch volumes for postdural puncture headache in Taiwanese women. *J Formos Med Assoc* 2007; 106:134–40.
165. Diaz JH, Weed JT. Correlation of adverse neurological outcomes with increasing volumes and delayed administration of autologous epidural blood patches for postdural puncture headaches. *Pain Pract* 2005; 5:216–22.
166. Martin R, Jourdain S, Clairoux M, *et al.* Duration of decubitus position after epidural blood patch. *Can J Anaesth* 1994; 41:23–5.
167. Mercieri M, Mercieri A, Paolini S, *et al.* Postpartum cerebral ischaemia after accidental dural puncture and epidural blood patch. *Br J Anesth* 2003; 90:98–100.
168. Perez M, Olmos M, Garrido FJ. Facial nerve paralysis after epidural blood patch. *Reg Anesth* 1993; 18:196–8.
169. Hebl JR, Horlocker TT, Chantigian RC, *et al.* Epidural anesthesia and analgesia are not impaired after dural puncture with or without epidural blood patch. *Anesth Analg* 1999; 89:390–4.
170. Collier CB. Blood patches may cause scarring in the epidural space: two case reports. *Int J Obstet Anesth* 2011; 20:347–51.
171. Willner D, Weissman C, Shamir MY. Chronic back pain secondary to a calcified epidural blood patch. *Anesthesiology* 2008; 108:535–7.

CHAPTER 28

Neurological complications of neuraxial blockade

Vibeke Moen

Introduction

Neuraxial techniques for obstetric analgesia and anaesthesia are widespread, and serious complications are extremely rare. However, no medical procedure is completely without risks, and the symptoms of severe complications might present themselves after the woman has left the delivery suite. The knowledge of possible complications to central neuraxial blockade (CNB) is therefore essential not only to anaesthetists, obstetricians, and midwives, but also to general practitioners.[1] A recent meta-analysis of studies published after 1990 estimated the incidence of persistent neurological injury following obstetric CNB as 1/260,000.[2] The Third National Audit Project of the Royal College of Anaesthetists (NAP3) prospectively estimated complications of CNB and found that obstetric CNB accounted for more than 45% of all CNBs, but only 14% of all complications.[3] More than 80% of all complications followed adult perioperative CNB. Twelve serious complications occurred in 320,425 obstetric CNBs, and the risk of permanent neurological injury was 'optimistically' estimated as 0.3/100,000, 'pessimistically' as 1.2/100,000. These numbers indicate the safety of obstetric CNB, but it should also be remembered they apply to healthy parturients. Women with severe systemic disease, neurological and haematological disorders become pregnant, and may expect the same methods for pain relief during labour and delivery. Risk factors that explain higher incidence of complications in perioperative patients might be present in these women. Some smaller studies are published regarding outcome of CNB in pregnant women with spinal pathology or haemostatic disorders, but produce statistics that are not clinically useful, due to the extremely low incidence of complications in healthy women.[4–6] Previously healthy women may also develop haemostatic disorders during labour caused by major obstetric haemorrhage, severe pre-eclampsia, or the syndrome of haemolysis, elevated liver enzymes, and low platelets (HELLP). Intravertebral spinal haematoma (SH), an otherwise rare complication of obstetric CNB, is predominantly described in these patients (Table 28.1).[7–9]

The possible injuries caused by CNB include direct trauma, cranial or spinal haematomas, and infectious complications. Arachnoiditis is a rare condition that in recent years has received renewed attention. Although the incidence of each single possible complication is extremely low, one study indicates that the majority of women wish to be informed even of unlikely events; however, this may not be feasible in emergency situations.[10] Intrinsic obstetric neuropathies, on the other hand, are not infrequent as they are reported to occur in 0.6–92/10,000 labouring women.[11] Due to the widespread use of neuraxial techniques for labour analgesia, many of the women suffering from an intrinsic obstetric neuropathy will also have received CNB, and frequently obstetricians and midwives will assume the CNB to have caused the neuropathy. The anaesthetist must therefore be familiar even with these obstetric neuropathies, particularly as there is some inconclusive evidence that obstetric neuropathies could be more frequent in women receiving neuraxial labour analgesia.[11,12] The explanation could be that the pain from impending damage to peripheral nerves would also be alleviated by the CNB along with the labour pain. Positional nerve compression in a person without neuraxial anaesthesia will induce change of position, but profound neuraxial anaesthesia may mask the experience of pain, and cause the woman to remain in an unaltered position for longer periods of time.[11,13]

Traumatic injuries

The last decades have seen an increase in the use of obstetric CNB, and this is also reflected in a related increase in insurance claims in different countries. Nerve injury has become the most frequent damaging event in obstetric anaesthesia reported in the American Society of Anesthesiologists Closed Claims Project, and a recent review of claims against the National Health Service in England revealed the same pattern.[14,15] Only surpassed by claims for intraoperative pain, nerve injury was the second most common cause for litigation in England. Fortunately, most of these nerve injuries are less severe and temporary.[15] A large prospective French study found 24 radiculopathies, accounting for an incidence of 4.7/10,000 procedures using spinal anaesthesia (SA) and 1.6/10,000 cases of epidural anaesthesia (EA). In most cases there was either paraesthesia or pain during performance of the CNB, and the symptoms of the following radiculopathy had the same topographic distribution.[16] The usual presentation of a radiculopathy was that of hypoaesthesia and in some cases also muscle weakness.[13] All were reversible, except one case following SA. The NAP3 reported permanent nerve injury following SA in two obstetric patients, accounting for an incidence of 1/67,000.[3]

More severe damage can occur when the conus medullaris or the medulla itself is damaged. Reynolds described seven cases of damage to the conus during SA in six obstetric and one female urological patient.[17] All cases of SA were believed to have been performed at the L2/3 interspace, whereas later magnetic resonance

Table 28.1 Spinal haematoma following CNB in three recent large series

		Obstetric anaesthesia			Non-obstetric anaesthesia (men and women)		
		SA	EA	CSE	SA	EA	CSE
Sweden 1990–1999[8]							
	Cases	1[a]	1[a]		7	24	
	Patients	55,000	205,000		1,210,000	245,000	
	Incidence	1/55,000	1/205,000		1/173,000	1/10,200	
UK 2006–2007[3]							
	Cases	0	0	0	0	6	0
	Patients	133,525	161,550	25,350	189,000	97,925	16,525
	Incidence					1/16,320	
Finland 2000–2009[9]							
	Cases	0	0	0	1	4	5
	Patients	66,000	144,000	101,000	775,000	185,000	89,000
	Incidence				1/775,000	1/46,250	1/17,800
Total							
	Cases	1[a]	1[a]	0	8	34	5
	Patients	254,525	510,550	126,350	2,174,000	527,925	105,525
	Incidence	1/254,525[a]	1/510,550[a]		1/271,750	1/15,527	1/21,105

The incidence of SH following SA, EA and CSE in three recent, large series. CSE was very rarely performed in Sweden during the actual period.

[a]Both obstetric patients in Sweden had severe coagulopathy due to HELLP. In one case, SA was performed for emergency caesarean delivery, and although the patient had severe haemostatic compromise, SA was preferred to GA. A small SH developed, but the patient recovered completely with conservative management. In the other case, the epidural catheter was withdrawn while the coagulopathy was deteriorating. Diagnosis was delayed, and although laminectomy was performed, the patient did not recover completely.

Data from Cook TM, Counsell D, Wildsmith JA. Major complications of central neuraxial block: report on the Third National Audit Project of the Royal College of Anaesthetists. *British Journal of Anaesthesia*. Volume 102(2), pp. 179–90. Copyright 2009. Data from Moen V, Dahlgren N, Irestedt L. Severe neurological complications after central neuraxial blockades in Sweden 1990-1999. *Anesthesiology*. Volume 101(4), pp. 950–9. Copyright 2004. Data from Pitkanen MT, Aromaa U, Cozanitis DA, Forster JG. Serious complications associated with spinal and epidural anaesthesia in Finland from 2000 to 2009. *Acta Anaesthesiologica Scandinavica*. Volume 57(5), pp. 553–64. Copyright 2013.

imaging (MRI) of the patients showed damage at levels varying from T10 to L2. None had spinal cords ending at exceptionally low levels and all had experienced pain during performance of the SA. There were three obstetric patients among the nine who experienced damage to the conus in a Swedish study and the anaesthetist thought that the block had been performed at L1/2 in only one case.[8] In all other cases, a lower level was assumed. EA was performed on eight of these patients and SA in one. Pain was experienced during performance of the CNB in all cases but one, and all patients were left with neurological deficit. A recent case of traumatic damage to the conus medullaris followed SA for caesarean delivery. The SA was reported to have been performed at the L2/3 interspace; however, the MRI accompanying the case report apparently indicates damage of the conus at the level of L1/2 (Box 28.1 and Figure 28.1).[18]

Direct trauma to the cord or conus medullaris evidently occurs even when the anaesthetist believes the CNB to be performed at a safe interspace.[17] This may be due to the spinal cord ending lower than usual, erroneous identification of the lumbar interspace, or an unfortunate combination of both these circumstances.

The cord usually terminates above the L1/2 interspace, but may extend further.[17] Results from two separate studies, one using MRI, the other in cadavers, indicate that the spinal cord terminates below L1 in 60–80% of adults, and below the lower part of L2 in 5–20% of adults.[19,20] The MRI study indicates that the conus may end as high up as the middle-third of the T12 vertebral body, or extend to the L3 vertebral body.[19] Moreover, the conus tends to end lower in women compared to men, and there are also racial differences, as the conus is reported to end at L2 or L2–3 in 32% of Africans compared to 20% of Europeans.[21,22]

The imaginary line joining the iliac crests, most often named Tuffier's line, is commonly used as an anatomical landmark for neuraxial anaesthesia.[17] When Tuffier's line is determined by palpation, it is considered to cross the spine at the L3/4 interspace (see Figure 20.4 in Chapter 20). However, Tuffier's line was originally a radiological landmark, and on imaging, Tuffier's line crosses

Box 28.1 Traumatic injury to the conus medullaris during spinal anaesthesia

A 28-year-old healthy woman at 40 weeks' gestation was admitted for urgent caesarean delivery. A senior anaesthetist performed SA in the L2/3 'where the inter-space was best palpated' using a 26 G Atraucan needle. When the needle had been introduced approximately 85 mm, the patient experienced shooting pain radiating from the lumbar region to the back of the left leg and foot. When the spinal needle was withdrawn 2–3 mm, CSF flowed freely, and the local anaesthetic was injected without causing pain. The caesarean delivery was successfully completed with good anaesthesia. On the second postoperative day the patient complained of back pain, and severe pain radiating to the left leg. The left patellar and Achilles reflexes were weak, and there was also a sensorial deficit in the left L3 and L4 dermatomes. MRI showed a hyperintense lesion in the conus medullaris. The patient was treated with methylprednisolone for 24 hours. After 2 months she had recovered completely.

On the MRI, the lesion would appear to be at the L1/2 level, not the L2/3 level (Figure 28.1). This case therefore also illustrates the difficulty of correctly determining the interspace.

Data from Erk G, Taspinar V, Akay M, Gokcil Z., Spinal hematoma as a result of spinal anesthesia for cesarean section. *Neurosciences (Riyadh, Saudi Arabia)*, volume 14, Issue 2, pp. 182–3, Copyright 2009.

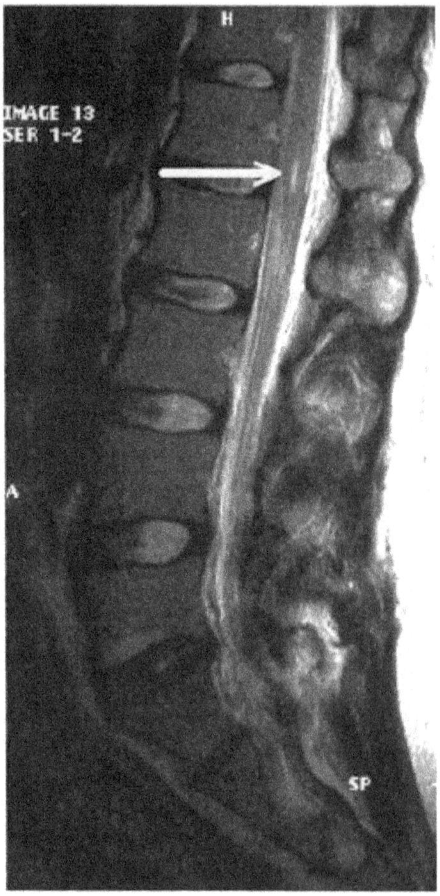

Figure 28.1 A hyperintense lesion at the conus medullaris (arrow) shown on the T2-weighted sagittal MRI scan of the patient.

Reprinted with permission from Erk G, Taşpınar V, Akay M, Gokçil Z. Spinal hematoma as a result of spinal anesthesia for cesarean section. *Neurosciences*. Volume 14, issue 2, pp. 182–3, Copyright © 2009 with special permission of *Neurosciences*.

the spine at the spinal process of L4 or at the L4/5 interspace, and therefore some authors may refer to Tuffier's line as crossing the spine at this lower level.[17,23,24] It is of course not surprising that the intercristal line determined by palpation lies higher than when it is determined on imaging, and the inaccuracy may be increased in the pregnant patient.[25] In addition to hyperlordosis and weight gain, patient positioning may also lead to inaccuracy when determining Tuffier's line in the obstetric patient when lying on her side. The width of the woman's hips compared to that of her shoulders will induce the imaginary intercristal line to cross the spine obliquely, and at a higher level.[25]

Two recent studies have assessed by ultrasound the level at which the intercristal line, determined by palpation, crossed the spine in pregnant women at term.[23,24] The results from these two studies show that Tuffier's line crossed the spine immediately above the L2–3 interspace in 27% and 35.5% respectively.

The inability even amongst experienced anaesthetists to correctly localize the interspace has been repeatedly documented.[26,27] Broadbent and colleagues found that the interspace identified was one to four interspaces higher than intended on 68% of all occasions. Similar results were found in a more recent study that used ultrasound 24–72 hours after delivery to determine the actual level of insertion of CNB in 99 obstetric patients who had received CNB during labour.[22] Ultrasound examination showed that the CNB had been performed higher than the level noted in the anaesthetic record in almost 50% of the patients, and at a lower level only in 15% of the patients. From these studies, it is apparent that SA is quite often performed at levels where many patients could still have underlying spinal cord.

A recent study found that in 29% of occasions even experienced anaesthetists perforated the dura with a 27 G Whitacre needle without experiencing the 'pop-sign' and the needle advanced further than intended.[28] The authors recommend that in addition to choosing a low interspace, anaesthetists should advance the spinal needle with an incremental rather than continuous technique. It should also be remembered that the tip of the modern atraumatic needles is also approximately 1 mm beyond the orifice compared to the older cutting edge Quincke needles, so insertion to obtain cerebrospinal fluid (CSF) is deeper and the potential for cord damage is greater.[17] Therefore, the practice of routinely performing SA in the L2/3 interspace exposes the patient to an unnecessary risk, and should be discouraged, as it is associated with a high probability of performing SA at an interspace with underlying conus.[20]

Ultrasound technology may prove a valuable tool for the safe placement of CNB, as this technique may correctly determine the midline and the interspace before performing CNB. Also, the ultrasound may predict the distance from the skin to the ligamentum flavum.[29] One study used ultrasound imaging of the spine to determine the depth of the epidural space in 61 patients requiring EA for labour analgesia.[30] The predicted depth of the epidural space correlated well with the actual needle depth, with a correlation coefficient of 0.881 (95% confidence interval (CI) 0.820–0.942). However, the use of ultrasound in an emergency situation would be difficult in all but experienced hands, and palpation of Tuffier's line will continue to be the standard technique in the future. Therefore, knowledge of anatomical details and caution particularly when performing SA are of upmost importance. For further details, see Chapter 54.

Spinal haematoma following central neuraxial blockade

The development of intravertebral SH following obstetric CNB is a very rare event. Scott and Hibbard reported one case of SH following 505,000 obstetric CNBs performed between 1982 and 1986.[31] A recent meta-analysis calculated the incidence of SH following obstetric EA as 1/562,628 in contrast to the incidence of 1/11,243 in the general surgical population.[32] Whereas the incidence of SH following SA is reported as 1/173,000 to 1/775,000 in non-obstetric patients, the rare case reports of SH following obstetric SA preclude any statistic calculation (Table 28.1).[8,13,33] Spontaneously occurring SH during pregnancy is also described.[34] The few reported cases of obstetric SH following CNB have mostly, but not exclusively, occurred in patients with compromised haemostasis due to major obstetric haemorrhage, severe pre-eclampsia, or HELLP (Table 28.1, Box 28.2, and Figure 28.2).[7,8,14,33] In rare cases, previously asymptomatic arteriovenous malformations may cause SH following CNB.[11]

The haematomas may be localized in the spinal, epidural, or in the subdural space.[35] With MRI this distinction is possible, and recent papers describe more accurately the localization. Most of the rare cases reported in the literature are reported simply as SH without further distinction of localization and are discussed as such in this section. Risk factors for the development of SH in the non-obstetric population are spinal pathology, vascular disease, anticoagulant therapy, and haemostatic disorders, including those caused by renal insufficiency.[8,32,36] The performance of CNB in women with spinal pathology or previous spinal surgery may be technically difficult or unsuccessful, and in one study neurological complications appeared to be more frequent.[4] If an obstetric patient has risk factors she should be informed of the increased risks of developing a SH but the actual quantifiable risk is difficult to define.[6] However, an individualized risk:benefit analysis should be performed in order to determine if a neuraxial block is justified.

Box 28.2 Spinal haematoma after large obstetric haemorrhage

During delivery of her first baby, a healthy 38-year-old woman had an epidural inserted for analgesia. Her coagulation status was normal, with a platelet count of 118 × 10⁹/L. The epidural catheterization was uneventful with no bloody tap, and the catheter was introduced 3 cm in the L4/5 interspace. She was delivered by ventouse extraction because of a non-reassuring fetal heart rate. The baby had an Apgar score of 0 at birth, and did not respond to resuscitation. Massive postpartum haemorrhage ensued, with severe coagulopathy. The lowest platelet count was 16 × 10⁹/L. Under general anaesthesia, ligation of the hypogastric arteries was performed, this being necessary to control haemorrhage. When the patient was extubated, 48 hours after delivery, she was paraplegic. An emergency MRI showed a haematoma extending from T3 to T5 (Figure 28.2). No surgical intervention was considered necessary, because the cord had minimal compression, and the patient recovered completely. The epidural catheter had accidentally been withdrawn during the transfers between operating theatre and intensive care units, while her coagulation was severely compromised. This manipulation of the epidural catheter was considered to have caused the haematoma.

Data from Nguyen L, Riu B, Minville V, Chassery C, Catalaa I, Samii K., Epidural hematoma after hemorrhagic shock in a parturient, *Canadian Journal of Anaesthesia*, volume 53, issue 3, pp. 252–7, copyright © 2006 Springer.

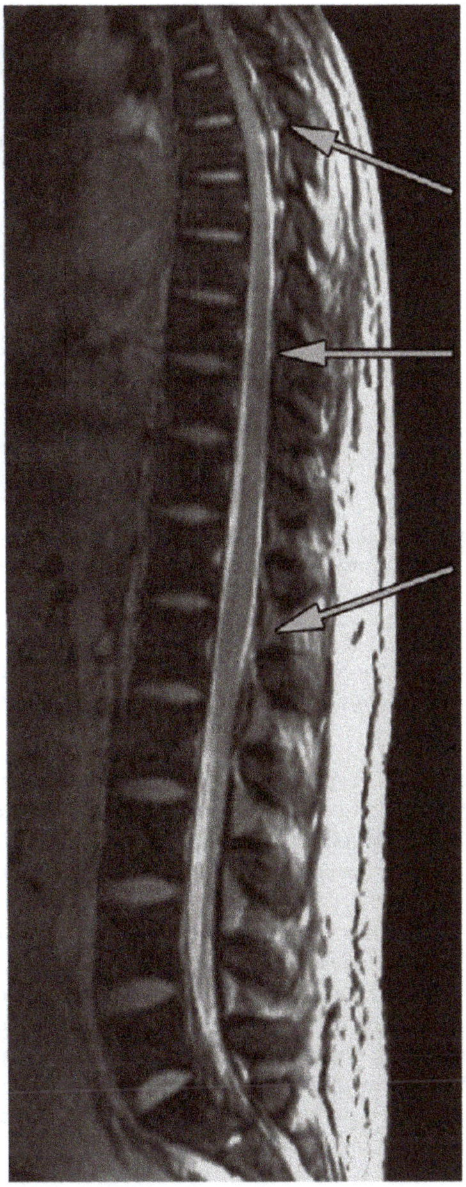

Figure 28.2 Sagittal view at the dorso-lumbar level; The arrows indicate: Hyperdense epidural collection reaching from T3 to L5 (white) in relation to the medulla (recent blood: methemoglobin) and hypodense (black) corresponding to old blood, hemosiderine at the borders of the collection.
Springer and the *Canadian Journal of Anesthesia*, volume 53, issue 3, 2006, pp. 252–7, Epidural hematoma after hemorrhagic shock in a parturient. Luc Nguyen. With kind permission from Springer Science and Business Media.

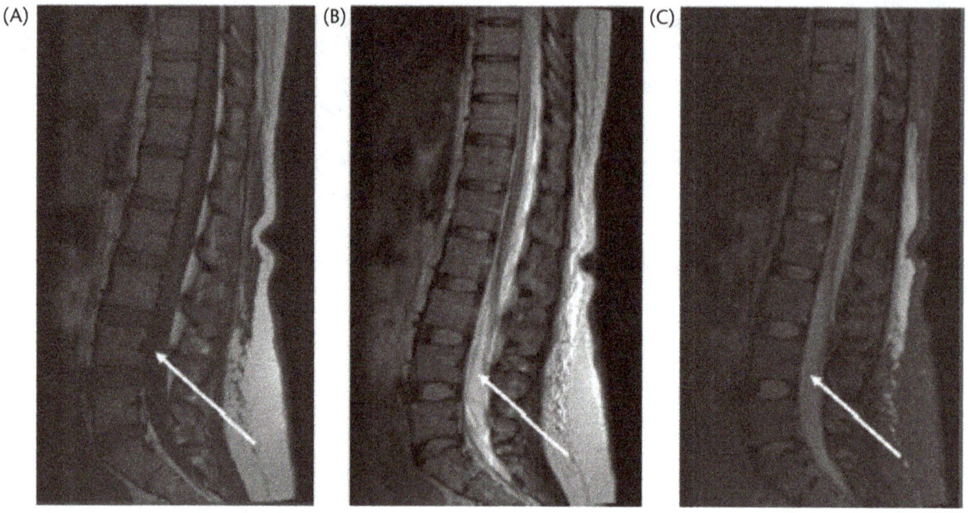

Figure 28.3 MRI images 48 hours after CSE anaesthesia, approximately 44 hours after the onset of sensorimotor symptoms. (A) Lumbar spine sagittal T1-weighted image showing haematoma up to L2–3 (arrow) which is difficult to identify due to isointensity with spinal cord and CSF. (B) Lumbar spine sagittal T2-weighted inversion recovery image with fat saturation showing heterogenous collection between L3 and L5 (arrow) in the caudal sac with compression of the cauda equina and nerve root displacement. (C) Sagittal turbo inversion-recovery image with fat saturation showing a hypointense area of the dural sac from L3 to S1 (arrow), consistent with CSF contamination with blood.

Traumatic CNB insertion has also been considered a risk factor for the development of SH. European guidelines advise considering postponing non-obstetric surgery in the case of a bloody tap, particularly when intraoperative anticoagulation is planned.[32,37] However, in obstetrics, the luxury of postponing delivery is not possible, and the discrepancy between the low incidence of SH and the frequent bloody tap when performing obstetric EA is therefore of particular interest.[38] The incidence of bloody tap, reported as varying between 1% and 12%, is influenced by the positioning of the obstetric patient during performance of the CNB.[38] A study involving 900 women reported the incidence of bloody tap when performing EA in the sitting, lateral recumbent, or lateral recumbent head-down position (25–30°) as 10.7%, 6%, and 2% respectively. Women with a body mass index above 35 kg/m^2 were excluded from this study, and a subsequent study examined the influence of position in the morbidly obese.[39] The results from this study showed that bloody tap occurred in 1.3% patients in the lateral recumbent head-down position compared to 12.9% and 12.0% in the lateral recumbent and sitting position respectively.

The lack of serious consequences of a bloody tap in obstetric patients is obvious from clinical practice. The state of hypercoagulability in the pregnant woman could limit bleeding following a bloody tap. Also, the young spine is more forgiving if there is bleeding in the spinal canal, as demonstrated by a series of MRIs performed between 30 minutes and 18 hours after blood patches in five individuals, all younger than 45 years.[40] The MRI showed extensive leakage of blood into the subcutaneous tissue in all patients. In contrast, a case report showed that an epidural infusion of local anaesthetic at a rate of 5 mL/h caused compression of the medulla in an elderly woman with severe scoliosis.[41]

Removal of the epidural catheter is as critical to the formation of a SH as the insertion of the EA. This is indicated by the fact that 30–50% of all SHs reported have occurred following catheter removal.[8,36,42] The healthy obstetric patient can develop severe coagulopathy after placement of the epidural catheter, thus becoming a high-risk patient for SH.[42] Postpartum haemorrhages resulting in coagulopathy is a contraindication to removal of an epidural catheter. Coagulopathy must be reversed before removal of the catheter, and the epidural catheter should not be removed within 12 hours of administration of thromboprophylaxis. Similarly, administration of anticoagulant must be delayed for more than 4 hours after an epidural catheter is removed.[43,44] Midwives should be aware of this, and there should be written and established routines regarding management and withdrawal of the epidural catheter.

Symptoms and diagnosis

Contrary to widespread belief, the first symptom of SH following CNB is usually not pain, but more often progressive motor blockade and sensory deficit. Bladder and bowel dysfunction may also be present.[3,7,8,11,32,36] The possibility of SH should therefore not be dismissed by the absence of pain. Interestingly, a recent review describes pain, often intense, as the presenting symptom in all 11 cases of spontaneous SH in pregnant women.[34] These differences could have pathophysiological explanations. In more slowly progressing compression, an impairment of the venous drainage reduces circulation in the medulla, with slow development of symptoms.[45,46] Abrupt interruption of circulation as caused by spontaneous SH may cause more dramatic symptoms.

Modern labour analgesia causes little or no motor impairment, therefore the greatest confounding factor in a newly delivered woman would be an obstetric neuropathy. Obstetric neuropathies, compared to SH, are common and usually unilateral. Postoperative pain relief by epidural infusion of local anaesthetics may, however, cause some motor block, thereby inducing the well-described mistake of attributing motor blockade to the local anaesthetic.

The presence of motor or sensory impairment in a newly delivered woman should generate prompt evaluation, and all anaesthetists involved in obstetric anaesthesia should be able to recognize an obstetric neuropathy.[11,47]

Computed tomography (CT) is usually more readily available, but may not provide the correct information, thus delaying diagnosis.[35] The definitive diagnosis of SH should be made by MRI, and as the MRI findings of a SH evolve over time, information regarding time perspective is important for the radiologist (Figure 28.3).[35] In the hyperacute phase (within 12 hours of haematoma formation), the oxyhaemoglobin present will produce an isointense signal on T1-weighted images, and it may also be difficult to visualize the SH on the T2-weighted images. Therefore, a negative MRI in a patient with symptoms should not definitively rule out the diagnosis of SH. Diagnostic delay caused by a negative CT scan and misinterpretation of MRI images led to permanent neurological damage described in a recent tragic case report.[35] Laminectomy is most often warranted, and the time at disposal for diagnosis and surgery is very short. For a prognosis of full restitution, a time frame of 8 hours from appearance of symptoms to definitive treatment is usually quoted.[36]

Risk factors and prevention

Coagulopathies and haemostatic disorders are the most important risk factors for SH in obstetric CNB.[7,48] Guidelines regarding thromboprophylaxis and CNB are issued by government bodies and specialist subcommittees in many countries.[37,43,49–53] The most recent guidelines issued in the United Kingdom include specific recommendations for obstetric patients, and are easily accessible also in cases of emergency (Table 28.2).[44] These guidelines also grade their recommendations according to level of risk associated with CNB.

Guidelines may differ in their recommendations, reflecting the lack of robust data assessing specific risk. Consensus relies heavily on expert opinion, and concern has been expressed regarding medicolegal implications of the guidelines.[54] However, the lack of guidelines has also been recognized as a risk factor.[3] Patient safety should therefore be expected to benefit from adherence to guidelines, with the knowledge that recommendations never can guarantee absolute safety, and all treatment must be individualized.

Thrombocytopenia and haemostatic disorders

Platelet count is not usually performed before placement of CNB in a healthy parturient, nor is it considered necessary without a history that indicates risk of abnormal bleeding.[11,44,53] Platelet count should be performed whenever coagulation abnormality is suspected, and in women receiving thromboprophylaxis, as well as in women with pre-eclampsia, placental abruption, or intrauterine fetal death.[44] Cholestasis may cause malabsorption of vitamin K, leading to coagulopathy due to a deficit in clotting factors.[44] However, thrombocytopenia may be accidentally discovered, and benign gestational thrombocytopenia accounts for 75% of thrombocytopenic cases encountered during pregnancy.[55]

Gestational thrombocytopenia typically appears in the third trimester and may be repeated in subsequent pregnancies. Platelet count can decrease up to 20% during normal pregnancy, but remains above 150×10^9/L in most of these women. However, 7% of pregnant women have platelet counts below 150×10^9/L; of these, 0.5–1% will have platelet counts below 100×10^9/L. The platelet count usually remains above 90×10^9/L, and platelet function is normal. Importantly, the fetus is not affected. The gestational thrombocytopenia is therefore usually without clinical significance, and does not preclude CNB.[56] A stable platelet count above 75×10^9/L is proposed as adequate level for CNB in healthy women in the recent UK guidelines (Table 28.2).[44,56]

Idiopathic thrombocytopenic purpura (ITP) is an autoimmune disorder that accounts for 4% of the observed cases of thrombocytopenia in pregnancy.[55] Thrombocytopenia due to ITP may predate pregnancy, may worsen during pregnancy, and the platelet count may decrease below 50×10^9/L. One study found that detection of thrombocytopenia prior to 28 weeks of gestation and platelet levels lower than 50×10^9/L were highly sensitive indicators of ITP.[55] The maternal antibodies may be transferred to the fetus, leading to fetal platelet destruction, and caesarean delivery might be chosen to reduce fetal risk. The low platelet level associated with ITP has been considered a contraindication for CNB, but small studies report CNB performed without complications.[5] Douglas suggests that patients with ITP, and no history of bleeding at that count, can receive CNB at a platelet count above 50×10^9/L, and this view is supported by Abramovitz and Beilin.[56,57] The recent UK guidelines consider relative risk of CNB 'normal' in women with ITP and platelet count above 75×10^9/L, and 'increased risk' with platelets 50–75×10^9/L (Table 28.2).[44]

Platelet count may also decrease in pre-eclampsia and HELLP, and together with gestational thrombocytopenia and ITP these conditions account for 99% of all cases of thrombocytopenia in pregnancy.[57] Thrombocytopaenia may also be caused by treatment with heparin and low-molecular-weight heparin (LMWH).[44]

The platelet function is as important as the platelet number.[44,57] In gestational thrombocytopenia and ITP the platelet function is normal, whereas thrombocytopenia in association with decreased platelet function may be present in pre-eclampsia and HELLP.[57] HELLP is associated with a significantly increased risk of bleeding, including risk of SH following CNB, but the risk of SH in pre-eclamptic women is more difficult to evaluate.[7,48,58] One epidemiological study found a significant increase in postpartum bleeding in pre-eclamptic women compared to healthy women.[59] This population-based study did not find that bleeding was correlated to the severity of pre-eclampsia. However, Davis and collaborators found that while only women with HELLP had reduced clotting strength examined with thromboelastography, platelet function was decreased in all pre-eclamptic women when measured with a platelet function analyser.[60]

The safe level of platelet count has yet to be determined, and probably also varies according to the cause of thrombocytopenia, with stability and preserved function being more important issues.[57,61] In gestational thrombocytopenia and ITP, the number of platelets is more constant and the platelet function normal, whereas the platelet count might be rapidly diminishing in pre-eclampsia and HELLP.[57] Platelet count and evaluation of coagulation by activated partial thromboplastin time (aPTT) and prothrombin time (PT), usually measured by international normalized ratio (INR), should be performed in close temporal relationship to CNB in women affected by severe pre-eclampsia and HELLP. When considering the method of anaesthesia for caesarean delivery in these patients, the indefinable risk of SH following SA must be weighed against the documented risk of lethal

Table 28.2 Relative risks related to neuraxial blocks in obstetric patients with abnormalities of coagulation

Risk factor	Normal risk	Increased risk	High risk	Very high risk
LMWH–prophylactic dose	>12 h	6–12 h	<6 h	<6 h
LMWH–therapeutic dose	>24 h	12–24 h	6–12 h	
UFH–infusion	Stopped > 4 h and APTTR ≤ 1.4			APTTR above normal range
UFH–prophylactic bolus dose	Last given > 4 h	Last given < 4 h		
NSAID + aspirin	Without LMWH	With LMWH dose 12–24 h	With LMWH dose < 12 h	
Warfarin	INR ≤ 1.4	INR 1.4–1.7	INR 1.7–2.0	INR > 2.0
General anaesthesia*	Starved, not in labour, antacids given		Full stomach or in labour	
Pre-eclampsia	Platelets > 100 × $10^9.1^{-1}$ within 6 h of block	Platelets 75–100 × $10^9.1^{-1}$ (stable) and normal coagulation tests	Platelets 75–100 × $10^9.1^{-1}$ (decreasing) and normal coagulation tests	Platelets < 75 × $10^9.1^{-1}$ or abnormal coagulation tests with indices ≥ 1.5 or HELLP syndrome
Idiopathic thrombocytopenia	Platelets > 75 × $10^9.1^{-1}$ within 24 h of block	Platelets 50–75 × $10^9.1^{-1}$	Platelets 20–50 × $10^9.1^{-1}$	Platelets < 20 × $10^9.1^{-1}$
Intra–uterine fetal death	FBC and coagulation tests normal within 6 h of block	No clinical problems but no investigation results available		With abruption or overt sepsis
Cholestasis	INR ≤ 1.4 within 24 h	No other clinical problems but no investigation results available		

LMWH, low molecular weight heparin; UFH, unfractionated heparin; APTTR, activated partial thromboplastin time; NSAID, non-steroidal anti-inflammatory drug; INR, international normalised ratio.

*Although general anaesthesia is not a risk factor per se for coagulation complications, it is included in this Table to highlight that the alternatives to regional anaesthesia are not free of risk; thus a risk-benefit comparison is required when choosing one over the other.

intracerebral haemorrhage during intubation, in addition to the well-known risks of failed intubation in this group.[44,58]

Placental abruption and intrauterine fetal death may also be complicated by coagulopathy, therefore platelets, INR, and aPTT should be determined before performance of CNB.[44]

Thromboprophylaxis

Pregnant women are at high risk of thromboembolic events, and a large number of women receive thromboprophylaxis or even therapeutic doses of anticoagulants, usually LMWH.[43] The guidelines issued by the Royal College of Obstetricians and Gynaecologists suggest that women receiving thromboprophylactic doses of LMWH discontinue their medication at the onset of labour or prior to planned delivery to allow administration of CNB during labour.[43] For women receiving high prophylactic or therapeutic doses of LMWH, the dose of heparin should be reduced to thromboprophylactic levels the day before induction of labour. CNB should not be used until at least 12 hours after the previous prophylactic dose of LMWH, and if a woman receives therapeutic doses of LMWH, CNB should not be administered for at least 24 hours after the last dose of LMWH (Table 28.2).[44] Likewise, the epidural catheter should not be removed within 12 hours of the most recent injection. Administration of LMWH should be delayed for 4 hours after SA or after an epidural catheter has been removed.[43,44] NICE guidelines also recommend aspirin 75 mg daily to women at high risk of pre-eclampsia, and some of these women may also receive LMWH. However, aspirin per se is not a contraindication to receiving neuraxial anaesthesia.[62] The recent UK guidelines recommend that CNB be delayed 12–24 hours after last dose of LMWH in these patients (Table 28.2).[44]

However, in the clinical setting, the anaesthetist will also have to consider the different risks and benefits related to EA for labour pain compared to SA for emergency caesarean delivery. Neuraxial anaesthesia is recommended for emergency caesarean delivery as it is considered safer than general anaesthesia.[44,48,63] Therefore, the lower risk of SH following SA could permit its use in patients with a degree of haemostatic disturbance that would be considered a contraindication to EA.[56] No case of SH is reported after CNB in obstetric patients receiving thromboprophylaxis with LMWH. As always, the final decision must rely on an individualized evaluation and risk:benefit analysis.

Major obstetric haemorrhage

In the obstetric patient with deteriorating coagulation, most frequently due to large obstetric haemorrhage or HELLP, haemostatic function should be monitored and INR should be interpreted with great caution.[50]

The correlation between the actual levels of vitamin K-dependent coagulation factors (II, VII, IX, and X) and PT expressed as INR are reliable indicators of adequate haemostasis only in the stable patient. The PT is most sensitive to factors II and VII, less to factor X, and does not measure the activity of factor IX at all. The half-life of factor VII is 6–8 hours, factor II has a half-life of 50–80 hours, and the half-life of factor X lies in between, at 25–60 hours. Bleeding may occur if the level of any of the clotting factors is reduced to 20–40% of its baseline. In stable conditions, an INR of 1.5 is associated with a reduction of factor VII to 40% of baseline, and is therefore considered an indicator of adequate haemostasis. In unstable conditions, however, these correlations are unreliable. The patient recovering from coagulopathy due to large obstetric haemorrhage may have an INR of 1.4, but INR will mainly reflect the increase of factor VII, as factors II and X will recover more slowly. Therefore, in these situations, an INR of 1.4 might not be associated with good haemostasis.[50] Removal of an epidural catheter should not be considered before the INR has indicated adequate haemostasis for the time necessary for all coagulation factors to reach 40% of baseline. It would therefore seem prudent to wait until the INR has been stable at 1.4 or below for 24 hours before considering removal of an epidural catheter. One case report describes a SH that occurred following major obstetric haemorrhage, and it was later discovered that the epidural catheter had been inadvertently withdrawn when severe coagulopathy was present (Box 28.2 and Figure 28.2).[42]

In summary, available data suggest that platelet level, and eventual rate of decline of platelet level, should be considered as well as platelet function before performing CNB in a woman with thrombocytopenia. Additional tests of haemostasis such as INR and aPTT should be performed in these women, and also after large obstetric bleeding, and in cases of intrauterine fetal death or placental abruption.[44] Removal of the epidural catheter is as critical with respect to SH formation as the insertion of EA. SA performed with a small-gauge atraumatic needle carries a lower risk of SH than EA.[8,44,56] Adherence to guidelines may enhance patient safety.

Cranial subdural haematoma

Cranial subdural haematoma (CSH) is a well-documented complication of accidental dural puncture as well as uncomplicated SA, and is usually considered extremely rare. Vos reported 45 cases of CSH before 1991 in the literature, and Errando and Perez-Caballero reported 57 cases from 1994 to 2010.[8,64,65] However, a Medline search discloses eight cases reported in 2012 alone, including five obstetric cases.[32,66–72] The incidence of CSH might be very low, but the large number of CNBs performed will most probably continue to cause this potentially life-threatening complication. The prevalence of obstetric patients amongst those suffering CSH after accidental dural puncture might reflect the larger proportion of obstetric EAs performed, but the presence of risk factors particular to the obstetric population cannot be ruled out.

A recent review described 25 cases of CSH following SA performed with needle sizes varying between 19 and 27 G.[73] The age of the patients varied between 20 and 88 years, and six of these patients were obstetric. The same review reported 21 patients with CSH after accidental dural puncture, of these 19 were obstetric patients. The earliest diagnosis of CSH following SA was made 6 hours after SA, the latest after 29 weeks. The time intervals were similar following accidental dural puncture. Surgery was performed in 35 patients, and of these six patients died.

Often the diagnosis was delayed, typically in a case of post-dural puncture headache (PDPH) that despite change in severity or characteristics was left without further investigation until severe neurological symptoms developed. These symptoms vary from confusion and disorientation, hemiparesis, and seizures and obviously will depend on the size and localization of the haematoma. Thus, the severity and diagnostic difficulties of CSH are not to be neglected, as illustrated by a case report published in 2011 (Box 28.3 and Figure 28.4).[74]

Box 28.3 Cranial subdural haematoma following epidural analgesia

A 43-year-old healthy woman received an uncomplicated EA for pain relief during labour. Delivery was uneventful. In the following 3 weeks, the woman developed headache, which was worse on standing. She sought medical attention for her complaints, but as she had no other symptoms beside headache, no further investigations were made. Twenty-two days after delivery, she was taken to the emergency department with disorientation and altered mental status. The Glasgow Coma Scale score was 9/15. A CT brain scan showed large bilateral chronic subdural haematomas (Figure 28.4). She was immediately transferred to the neurosurgical department. On arrival she had fixed dilated pupils. The haematomas were evacuated, but the patient never recovered consciousness, and died 24 hours later.

This case report is very scant on details; however, it is also very illustrative. Most probably, an inadvertent dural perforation occurred during performance of the EA, and the headache was interpreted as PDPH, also when symptoms changed characteristics. The case report also highlights the necessity not only for anaesthetists, but also for general practitioners and obstetricians, to correctly diagnose intracranial pathology.

Data from Demetriades AK, Sheikh MF, Minhas PS., Fatal bilateral subdural haematoma after epidural anaesthesia for pregnancy, *Archives of Gynecology and Obstetrics*, volume 284, issue 6, pp. 1597–8, Copyright © 2011 Springer.

Leakage of CSF and the consequent low intracranial pressure (ICP) are considered the cause of both PDPH and CSH.[75] The downward displacement of the brain with traction of the bridging cerebral veins is believed to cause their rupture, leading to the formation of a subdural haematoma.[70]

However, based on data from experimental studies, Grände offers an alternative explanation to the mechanisms that cause PDPH, and in extension, also to the development of CSH.[76] The subdural draining veins just inside the dura are normally collapsed, as the ICP is higher than the venous pressure. These collapsed veins prevent retrograde transmission of systemic venous pressure variations, creating a venous gate protecting the brain. Lumbar puncture (LP) causes distal opening to the atmosphere of the normally closed dural space, thereby reducing ICP. Lowering of ICP will reverse the normal subdural venous collapse, leading to venous dilation which causes pain and an increase in intracranial blood volume. The effect of these changes in pressure gradients is most evident in the upright position, explaining the typical positional severity of PDPH.[76] One study showed that bearing down after accidental dural puncture increased the incidence of PDPH.[77] This could be explained by the loss of the protective venous gate as described by Grände, thereby permitting transmission of increased venous pressure, and could also favour the development of CSH in obstetric patients. Brain size decreases by approximately 2% during pregnancy, and the ventricles increase proportionally, returning to original size 24 weeks after delivery.[78] It is not known whether this physiological variation has any impact on the hydrostatic changes that follows perforation of the dura in the obstetric patient.

An epidural blood patch as treatment for PDPH has been proposed also to prevent the development of CSH, but in several case reports the CSH occurred in patients who already had received a blood patch.[65,70,73,79] However, the above-mentioned pathophysiological mechanisms support the use of a blood patch in patients suffering from PDPH.

The diagnosis of CSH is best performed with MRI, but if only a CT scan is available, this must be contrast enhanced. A CT scan performed without contrast may be unreliable 7–21 days after all forms of subdural haematoma, because the haematoma and brain tissue have the similar radiographic density.[70] For some patients with CSH, conservative treatment has been appropriate, but craniotomy has been necessary in many of the cases described.[65,70,74,79]

Cranial nerve palsies

Focal neurological deficit due to isolated cranial nerve palsies may be present in patients who have received CNB.[12] It is believed that a dural puncture may cause low ICP leading to stretching of the cranial nerves as well as PDPH. Patients may complain of diplopia and hearing loss that may accompany or precede PDPH.[42] Diplopia is most frequently caused by stretching of the abducens nerve (cranial nerve VI). The oculomotor nerve (cranial nerve III) and the trochlear nerve (cranial nerve IV) may also be affected. The palsy is usually unilateral, but can be bilateral. Low ICP is also reflected in a decreased pressure in the perilymph within the cochlea that causes hearing impairment, typically in the low frequency area.[12] Smaller-gauge needles more rarely cause cranial nerve palsies, and blood patches may not always resolve the condition once it has become manifest.[42] Patients may suffer from chronic palsies despite a blood patch for PDPH.[8,42]

Bell's palsy is three times more common in the pregnant compared to the non-pregnant patient, and may occur even after delivery.[43] Facial nerve palsy is usually not related to CNB, but there are occasional reports of facial nerve palsy that have been considered associated with obstetric CNB.[12]

Ischaemic injury to the spinal cord

Ischaemic injury to the spinal cord is most often described following aortic surgery, but rare cases are reported in obstetric patients.[13,45,80] Prolonged hypotension may cause cord ischaemia in obstetric patients, but also aortic compression, epidurally administered vasoconstrictors, as well as vasospasm elicited by the epidural catheter are believed to have caused cord ischaemia.[81,82] The anterior lumbar spinal cord is particularly sensitive to hypoperfusion, as its blood supply depends on a single unilateral artery, the artery of Adamkiewicz.[46] A secondary blood supply arising from the internal iliac artery is described in 15% of individuals. Compression of this artery by the fetal head could cause ischaemia even in the absence of systemic hypoperfusion.[83] The anterior spinal artery syndrome arises from ischaemic damage limited to the anterior part of the cord. The symptoms are therefore characteristic, with motor deficit and dissociated sensory loss, as pain and sensation of temperature is lost, but sensation of vibration and position is preserved. MRI is the method of choice for visualizing ischaemic damage to the cord.[80] Fluids and vasoactive drugs

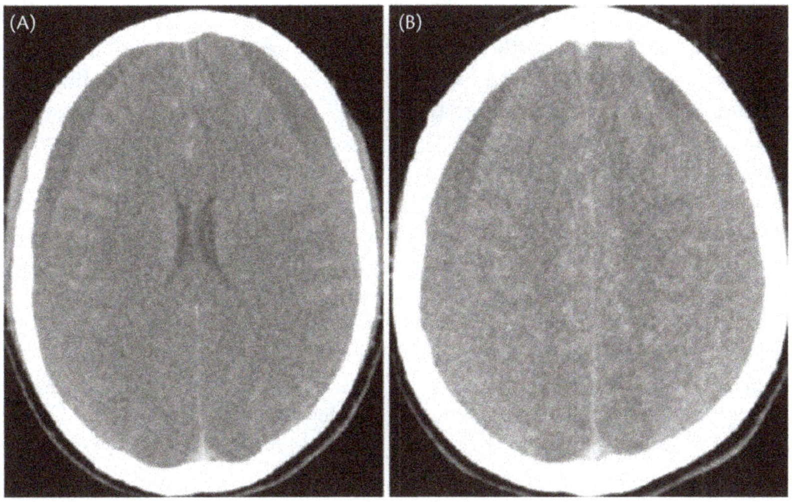

Figure 28.4 CT brain scan showing large bilateral isodense chronic subdural haematomas with (A) lateral ventricle compression, and (B) significant mass effect on brain parenchyma.

Springer and *Archives of Gynecology and Obstetrics*, volume 284, issue 6, 2011, pp. 1597–8. Fatal bilateral subdural haematoma after epidural anaesthesia for pregnancy, Demetriades AK, Sheikh MF, Minhas PS, With kind permission from Springer Science and Business Media.

should be used to restore mean arterial pressure to normal values following spinal injury, but there are no clear guidelines for specific pharmacological treatment of spinal strokes.[45] The outcome of spinal cord infarction following aortic surgery is worse than when ischaemia has other causes.[80] Some obstetric patients have recovered completely, whereas others have suffered severe damage.[13,81,82]

Infectious complications

Meningitis and epidural abscess are severe infectious complications of CNB. Their incidences are difficult to quantify, but these complications are often preventable, potentially life-threatening, and therefore of major concern. Although infectious complications are considered rare, they accounted for 46% of neuraxial complications following obstetric CNB reported in the American Society of Anesthesiologists Closed Claims Project from 1990 to 2003.[14] The incidences reported in literature vary greatly, and whereas the lowest incidences are reported in large surveys and reviews of literature, smaller studies performed in a clinical setting report higher incidences, possibly as they identify cases that easily may be lost to follow-up.[2,3,8,84–86] EA and SA cause different complications, as epidural abscess is most often caused by EA, and meningitis is most frequently a complication of SA.[8,84,87]

Epidural abscess and deep tissue infections following obstetric CNB are reported to occur in 0.2–48/100,000 cases.[86] The incidence of bacterial meningitis following obstetric CNB calculated on cases reported in surveys varies between 1/3000 and 25.5/million.[84] The number of cases reported in the literature is not in proportion to the reporting countries' population, indicating a probable under-reporting, in addition to cases of meningitis, that although unrecognized as such, have been adequately treated with antibiotics.[87] The several clusters of iatrogenic meningitis described in the literature confirm the consequences of breaches in aseptic technique.[87–89]

Bacterial meningitis

When meningitis occurs as a complication to CNB, it almost invariably follows a perforation of the dura, intended or accidental, and may therefore appropriately be renamed postdural puncture meningitis (PDPM).[87] Streptococci of the viridans group, also called α-haemolytic streptococci, are the most frequently encountered pathogens in cases of PDPM and accounted for 49% of all positive CSF cultures in Baer's comprehensive review.[87]

Viridans streptococci are part of the normal flora of the upper airways, gastrointestinal tract, and female genital tract, but are usually not found on the skin.[90] *Streptococcus salivarius* is the most frequent viridans pathogen of PDPM; other viridans streptococci encountered are *S. anginosus, S. mitis, S. mutans*, and *S. sanguinis*.[91] The viridans streptococci are facultative Gram-positive aerobic bacteria and their presence in saliva is in the magnitude of 10^9 colony forming units per millilitre of saliva.[92] Several clusters of PDPM are reported in literature, and when the origin of the pathogen has been determined, it has been found in the oral flora of the LP operator.[87–89,93,94]

Viridans streptococci lack the virulence of the bacteria causing community-acquired meningitis, *Haemophilus influenzae, Neisseria meningitides*, and *Streptococcus pneumonia*. Therefore viridans streptococci only very rarely cause spontaneously occurring meningitis, but they do cause meningitis when inoculated directly into the CSF.[87] No patient predisposition has been found in patients suffering PDPM, nor is it necessary for the development of PDPM, as the breach of defences against infection are caused mechanically.

It is noteworthy, however, that almost all cases of obstetric PDPM have been in women who were or had been in labour when they received the CNB.[84] The occurrence of meningitis could possibly be caused by bacteraemia induced by labour or bladder catheterization, or indicate that the hygienic conditions in the delivery suite are less satisfactory. However, there are no cases of maternal meningitis reported without the use of CNB, indicating that labour itself is not a risk factor for meningitis.[90] Only in one case published in 1989 was haematogenous spread of viridans streptococci considered to have caused postpartum meningitis following but unrelated to EA. *Streptococcus uberis* was found in the patient's CSF as well as in her blood, urine, and vaginal secretions.

Bacteraemia caused by brushing of teeth has also been proposed as important for the development of PDPM.[95] In one study, bacteraemia occurred following brushing of teeth in 23% of the study subjects, and the bacteraemia lasted for 60 minutes in 9% of these study participants.[96] Roughly half of the bacteria detected belonged to the viridans group. However, polymerase chain reaction (PCR) is not known to have linked any case of obstetric PDPM either to the woman's own oral flora or to her vaginal flora.

Other bacteria occasionally found in PDPM are *Staphylococcus aureus* (5%), *Pseudomonas aeruginosa* (4%), and *Enterococcus faecalis* (2%).[87] Two cases of PDPM caused by *Serratia marescens* have been described.[97] Investigation disclosed the presence of *Serratia* in multi-use bottles, once again illustrating the importance of investigation following any case of PDPM (and discouraging the use of multi-use bottles). The most recent case report of PDPM was caused by *Abiotrophia descens*.[98] *Abiotrophia* is also part of the oral flora, and the authors report that the anaesthetist might have omitted his/her mask during the performance of the blockade. One case of meningitis in an obstetric patient, reported in 2003, followed combined spinal–epidural anaesthesia (CSE), performed without the use of a mask.[99] *Neisseria meningitides* was identified as the pathogen in this case, and the meningitis was therefore considered as community-acquired meningitis, only temporarily linked with the CSE. However, symptomatic carriers of *N. meningitides* are not uncommon, indeed, they are believed to spread the infection.[100] *N. meningitides* might thus be contained in the same droplets as viridans streptococci. In this actual case, PCR was performed only for diagnosis, not for tracing bacterial origin, so no certain conclusions can be made regarding transmission. However, the case serves as a reminder of the considerable risks involved when performing CNB with inadequate aseptic technique.

In a large series of 27 cases of PDPM from India, 11 cases followed SA for caesarean delivery. The mortality was significantly higher amongst these obstetric patients, but the article does not disclose the exact number of obstetric deaths.[101] The pathogens were different from the series originating in Western countries, as 37% were diagnosed with chronic meningitis caused by tuberculosis. The authors considered that the SA might have caused rupture into the CSF of a central nervous tubercle, causing acute deterioration. There were also five cases of meningitis caused by *Aspergillus fumigatus*, and of the 22% with positive CSF culture, there were three cases of *Staphylococcus aureus*, and one case each of *Pseudomonas* and *Acinetobacter*.

The risk of PDPM also highlights one long-lasting controversy: should the dura routinely be breached during labour?[90,102] A 2012 Cochrane report did not find evidence of increased incidence of PDPM following CSE, but the low number of patients in the studies included would not be expected to reveal an increase of such a rare complication.[103] Interestingly, no case of PDPM has been reported from Scandinavian countries, where CSE is not routinely used for labour analgesia.

The oral flora of the performer of the CNB is often the most likely source of the pathogen in PDPM.[84,87] One important exception is the cluster of PDPM in Sri Lanka 2005, caused by *Aspergillus fumigatus* and responsible for the death of three women following caesarean delivery.[104] These deaths prompted a major epidemiological investigation and the most probable explanation found was *Aspergillus* contaminating syringes and needles used for SA, equipment that had been donated following the tsunami catastrophe and stored in a humid and hot environment. The onset time for *Aspergillus* to cause meningitis is long, 7–36 days in the series from Sri Lanka, making epidemiological research even more difficult.[104] *Aspergillus* is an ubiquitous fungus that will cause infection only in immunocompromised patients, and meningitis only if inoculated directly into the CSF. Meningitis from *Aspergillus* carries a high mortality rate, 50% was reported in the series from Sri Lanka. However, treatment before symptoms occur may prevent the development of meningitis, and in Sri Lanka no further deaths occurred after patients at risk were identified and treated.[104] The management of this tragedy should be a learning point, indicating the need for scrupulous investigation of hygienic procedures whenever a case of iatrogenic meningitis occurs.

Lumbar puncture and bacteraemia

Performing a LP in the presence of bacteraemia has been proposed as a possible cause of iatrogenic meningitis.[105–107] The dural puncture could cause a breach in the blood–brain barrier, thus introducing bacteria into the CSF. Bacteria lacking the virulence necessary to breach the blood–brain barrier could by this mechanism also cause meningitis. This could be of concern to the obstetric patient, as bacteraemia may be present in 1–4% of women following uncomplicated delivery, and in 8% following bladder catheterization.[84,108,109] One study found bacteraemia in 8% of women affected by chorioamnionitis, but no infectious complications developed following CNB, and only a minority received antibiotics.[110] It can be assumed that bacteraemia is probably present in many of the obstetric patients who also receive CNB, but the bacteraemia may be completely asymptomatic, and the febrile patient is not necessarily bacteraemic.[111] However, it should also be taken into account that most of these are low-grade bacteraemias. The human and animal studies correlating LP to meningitis have had high bacterial blood counts.[109] Epidemiological studies found significantly higher mortality from *Staphylococcus aureus* infection in patients with high-grade bacteraemia compared to mortality in patients with low-grade bacteraemia.[112] Data presented in a review suggested that SA may be performed in patients at risk of low-grade bacteraemia.[113] This is supported by the low incidence of infectious complications to CNB despite the probable high prevalence of low-grade bacteraemia in obstetric patients. However, patients with signs of systemic infection should be treated with antibiotics prior to administration of CNB.[3,109]

Symptoms, diagnosis, and treatment of bacterial meningitis

The symptoms of PDPM usually appear within 24 hours of the CNB, but may occur after only 8 hours, or after a delay of 8 days, probably caused by partially effective antibiotic treatment.[8,87] It is difficult to mistake the typical symptoms of bacterial meningitis when a patient presents with the classical triad of fever, altered mental status, and nuchal rigidity.[100] Intense headache and photophobia may be present together with other signs of meningeal irritation such as Kernig's sign (the inability to lift the leg without bending the knee) and Brudzinski's sign (spontaneous flexion of the hip during passive flexion of the neck). Severe meningitis will increase ICP causing altered levels of consciousness and cause pupillary abnormalities as well as seizures and focal neurological signs.

The signs and symptoms of PDPM may, however, be more subtle, probably due to the lower virulence of the infective agent.[8,87,114] All patients in a large series presented with headache and fever, but in several cases the absence of more serious symptoms led to an initial diagnosis of PDPH, often with an additional diagnosis of infection such as urinary tract infection or endometritis.[8] Therefore, meningitis should be in the differential diagnosis whenever a woman who has received CNB for labour or delivery complains of headache and also presents with fever.

LP is usually performed when meningitis is suspected, but is no longer essential for aetiological diagnosis, as this can be provided by PCR long after live bacteria have disappeared from the CSF.[93,94] Moreover, LP is not completely without its own risks as it may precipitate herniation in patients with high ICP.[76,87,115] Neither CT scan nor ophthalmoscopy are reliable methods of determining acutely increased ICP.[76,116] CT scans were performed in an outcome study regarding active management of increased ICP in community-acquired bacterial meningitis.[115] Radiological signs of brain swelling were evident only in five out of the ten patients who all had increased ICP measured with invasive monitoring. A retrospective assessment of CT scans performed in 103 patients with bacterial meningitis found that all patients with radiological signs of cerebral oedema also had clinical signs of increased ICP.[116] These studies indicate that increased ICP may be present despite normal CT scans, and that clinical signs of increased ICP, when present, are reliable indicators of increased ICP.

When LP is performed, CSF may be cloudy with increased white cell count, protein, and lactate, together with glucose content lower than plasma glucose, typical findings of bacterial meningitis.[100] Increased white cell count or C-reactive protein in blood may be delayed. Gram stain of the CSF may be done, and when suspecting PDPM, culture in broth medium will favour growth of viridans streptococci.[84] In a large proportion of PDPM (36%), the CSF culture was negative, or was not reported.[87] This may have several explanations: Viridans streptococci are usually not pathogens, so their presence might have been considered as contamination or in any case not significant.[87,117] The failure to grow might erroneously lead to the diagnosis of chemical meningitis.[84] Often antibiotics are administered prior to LP, effectively clearing the CSF within hours.[100] Finally, viridans streptococci often do not grow well on agar, so broth culture is to be preferred.[84] However, PCR may identify the pathogen in the CSF even when LP is performed after antibiotics have been given.[94]

Empirical broad-spectrum antibiotics according to national guidelines for management of community-acquired bacterial meningitis should be administered.[87] Treatment should not be delayed by the performance of diagnostic LP or CT scans.

Most of the patients with PDPM are successfully treated, but several deaths have been reported in the literature.[84,87] At least seven previously fit obstetric patients have died following PDPM, reflecting the potentially lethal nature of this condition.[87,88,104] The latest obstetric death occurred in 2009 in Ohio, United States, when the anaesthetist, omitting the use of a mask, performed SA for pain relief during labour causing lethal meningitis in a previously healthy young woman. PCR was used in the epidemiological follow-up, and the origin of the pathogen (*Streptococcus salivarius*) was traced to the anaesthetist (Box 28.4).[88] Another issue, not to be dismissed, is the increasing resistance to antibiotics, also amongst the viridans streptococci.[118] As PDPM is such a serious complication, a root/cause analysis should be done to investigate the sequence of events leading to the infection so that lessons can be learnt and preventative measures put in place.[93,94,119]

Box 28.4 Cluster of PDPM in Ohio 2009

Patient A: a 26-year-old healthy woman was admitted to the delivery suite in active labour. She received SA for labour analgesia, and delivered a healthy baby. Approximately 15 hours after receiving the SA, the patient developed fever, nausea, and severe headache, and she later became lethargic and unresponsive. She received treatment for meningitis, and recovered.

Patient B: a second healthy 30-year-old woman in active labour was admitted to the same hospital 3 hours after patient A. Patient B also received SA, performed by the same anaesthetist, and delivered a healthy baby. Approximately 13 hours after the SA she developed symptoms of meningitis. Despite adequate treatment she died 12 hours after debut of symptoms.

Blood and CSF cultures from both patients revealed *Streptococcus salivarius*.

The subsequent investigation included culture of medication vials and a review of the SA procedure protocols. Staff interviews disclosed that the anaesthetists in the hospital did not always wear masks while performing SA. Culture and analysis by PCR of medication vials revealed no evidence of contamination. Cultures performed on swabs obtained from oropharynx, buccal mucosa, and tongue from the anaesthetist that had performed the two SA resulted in no growth, as the anaesthetist had received post-exposure antibiotic prophylaxis for a presumed meningococcal meningitis. However, subsequent laboratory analysis enabled the identification of a strain of *S. salivarius* that was genetically indistinguishable from the *S. salivarius* of the two patients.

Data from Schroeder TH, Krueger WA, Neeser E, Hahn U, Unertl K, Spinal epidural abscessa rare complication after epidural analgesia for labour and delivery. *British Journal of Anaesthesia*, volume 92, pp. 896–8, Copyright © 2004 Oxford University Press.

Epidural abscess

Spontaneously occurring epidural abscess is reported with an incidence of 2/10,000 hospital admissions per year.[120] The reported incidence of deep epidural infection and epidural abscess following obstetric CNB varies between 0.2 and 48/100,000 with higher incidences reported in smaller series.[86] However, obstetric patients appear to develop epidural abscess after CNB less frequently than non-obstetric patients. The recent NAP3 reported 13 cases of epidural abscess in 312,450 perioperative CNBs, but only one case of epidural abscess occurring after 186,900 obstetric EAs (including 25,350 CSEs).[3]

The pathogens involved are most often *Staphylococcus* species both when epidural abscess occurs spontaneously or following CNB; therefore the microbial agent does not indicate route of transmission as in most cases of PDPM.[84,121] However, in one case report, genetic fingerprinting identified the anaesthetist's flora as the origin of the *S. aureus* responsible for the epidural abscess.[122] Another study could identify the origin of the *S. aureus* in the patient's own skin flora.[123] The predominant microorganism of the skin flora is *S. epidermidis* (65–69%), whereas *S. aureus* (1–2% of skin flora) is the prevalent pathogen in cases of epidural abscess complicating CNB.[124] This discrepancy would indicate that disinfectants more effectively prevent further contamination from *S. epidermidis* compared to *S. aureus*.[124]

During spontaneous epidural abscess, the bacteria reach the epidural space by haematogenous spread, whereas the catheter is believed to facilitate the introduction of bacteria from the skin in cases of epidural abscess following CNB.[125] This is supported by the results from a carefully conducted prospective study involving 205 epidurals. The study results showed that a positive culture at the catheter tip following removal was significantly correlated to positive culture of the skin near the point of entry.[125]

The development of epidural abscesses is also related to the duration of catheterization, and it is well known that the risk of superficial infection increases with the duration of catheterization.[121] Loo and collaborators recommended that the indwelling time of epidural catheters on most occasions should be limited to 24 hours in obstetric patients.[13] Studies have reported 3–4 days as median time of catheterization in patients with catheter-related epidural abscesses, but epidural abscesses has also been described after only a few hours of catheterization.[126–128]

Risk factors for the development of epidural abscess also include immunosuppression of any origin and traumatic performance of blockade.[126] The pregnant woman is often considered immunosuppressed. However, while cell-mediated immunity is decreased during pregnancy, normal humoral immunity is maintained.[3,129] The pregnant woman is therefore only more susceptible to certain intracellular organisms, such as viruses, parasites, and intracellular bacteria. This may explain the increased number of infections during pregnancy from listeria and toxoplasmosis, and the increased severity of influenza in the pregnant patient, but at the same time less frequent epidural abscesses following CNB when compared to non-obstetric patients.[3] However, diabetes is often found as a risk factor in cases of epidural abscess and one review found that 46% of the patients were diabetic.[130] In a recent series from Australia, three out of the four obstetric patients who developed an epidural abscess or deep infection following EA were affected by gestational diabetes.[86] With the exception of possible traumatic insertions, other risk factors usually associated with the development of epidural abscesses are absent in the healthy obstetric patient, thus possibly decreasing the risk of epidural abscess formation in the obstetric population.[131]

Symptoms, diagnosis, and treatment of an epidural abscess

The first symptoms of an epidural abscess usually appear 2–5 days following catheterization, but significant delay has been described in some cases.[86,126,127] A lapse of 6 weeks up to 4 months is reported.[8,121] The development of symptoms is classically described as evolving in four phases. Phase I is characterized by backache, usually at the level of the developing abscess. The symptoms progress over 2 or 3 days into phase II with the development of radicular pain. After another 3 or 4 days, sensory and motor deficits, as well as sphincter dysfunction develop, typical of phase III. The progression to the paralysis characteristic of phase IV may be rapid.[126,132] Fever and even severe signs of general infection might be present at any stage, confounding the picture. In a retrospective survey of 42 patients with catheter-related epidural abscesses, the correct diagnosis was considered initially only in 15 patients.[126]

Box 28.5 Epidural abscess after epidural analgesia for labour and delivery

A healthy woman received an epidural for pain relief during labour. The skin was disinfected with chlorhexidine 0.5% in 70% alcohol, and the anaesthetist wore a mask and sterile gloves, but not a gown, and there is no mention of a cap. The epidural insertion was uneventful, the baby was delivered 3 hours after catheter placement, and the catheter was removed approximately 6 hours after placement.

During the following days, the patient complained of back pain of increasing intensity. She had no local or systemic signs of infection, and no neurological impairment. Five days after delivery, her back pain became unbearable. White blood cell count was 10.1×10^9/L, and C-reactive protein was 26 mg/dL. A contrast-enhanced lumbar CT scan was performed, but was inconclusive. However, a median, sagittal T2-weighted MRI showed an intraspinal, ellipsoid fluid collection in the dorsal epidural space at L2/3, with compression of the dural sac (Figure 28.5). Empirical antibiotic treatment was initiated. On the following day, the patient developed a sensory deficit in the left leg, necessitating a neurosurgical intervention, with decompression and drainage of the abscess. *Staphylococcus aureus* was cultured from the abscess fluid. The patient was treated with antibiotics for 4 weeks, and recovered completely.

Epidural abscess after obstetric EA is exceptionally rare, but this case reminds us of the need for scrupulous aseptic technique. It also illustrates the limitations of CT scan, and the fact that neurosurgical intervention often is necessary.

Data from Schroeder TH, Krueger WA, Neeser E, Hahn U, Unertl K., Spinal epidural abscess – a rare complication after epidural analgesia for labour and delivery., *British Journal of Anaesthesia*, volume 92, Issue 6, pp. 896–8, Copyright 2004.

Other studies confirm the diagnostic difficulties, and the low rate of initial accurate diagnosis.[128,130] The NAP3 reported 17 cases of epidural abscesses, and local signs of infection were present in the nine patients who made complete recovery, probably leading earlier to the correct diagnosis. In seven of the eight patients who did not attain full recovery, there were no local signs of infection.[3] The diagnostic difficulties of this rare condition may be even greater in an obstetric patient (Box 28.5 and Figure 28.5).[128]

The diagnosis of an epidural abscess should be performed by MRI, but when this is unavailable, a CT myelography may be performed. However, its invasiveness carries additional risks, and the CT scan may be falsely negative.[128] Surgical treatment in addition to long-lasting antibiotic treatment is often necessary. Unfortunately, complete recovery is less probable if diagnosis and treatment is delayed until the appearance of neurological deficit.[120]

Aseptic technique for performance of central neuraxial blockade

Medical costs and patient morbidity and mortality from hospital-acquired infections are increasing. In many countries, subspecialty societies and official government bodies issue guidelines regarding the importance and methods of strict aseptic technique during performance of CNB.[133–135]

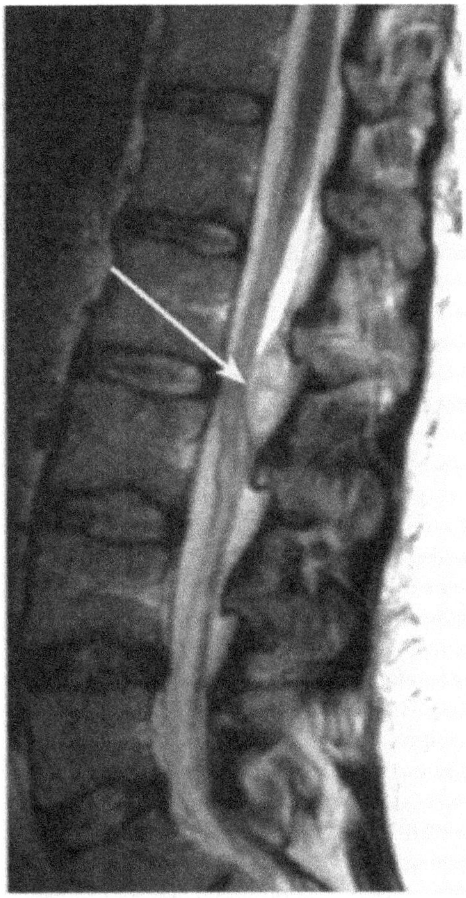

Figure 28.5 Median sagittal T2-weighted MRI showing intraspinal, ellipsoid fluid collection (arrow) in the dorsal epidural space at disc level L2–3, compressing the dural sac. Epidural abscess complicating epidural analgesia.

Reprinted with permission from Schroeder TH, Krueger WA, Neeser E, Hahn U, Unertl K. Spinal epidural abscess – a rare complication after epidural analgesia for labour and delivery. *British Journal of Anaesthesia*. Volume 92, issue 6, pp. 896–8, Copyright © 2004 Oxford University Press.

A recent observational study of residents performing EA found that their skills improved over 6 months but their breaches in aseptic technique did not diminish, despite formal education.[136] The authors concluded that their results reflected major gaps in teaching as well as understanding of aseptic technique. This conclusion is supported by another study that found that experienced physicians performed more breaches than their residents.[137]

A recent survey in the United Kingdom regarding prevention of infection in obstetric CNB revealed that although all anaesthetists used sterile gloves, and 99% wear a gown, only 91% use a mask, and 87% use a cap.[138]

The effectiveness of masks in preventing droplet spread of bacteria is well documented.[139,140] A good surgical mask has been shown to prevent the growth of oral flora on agar plates that were placed at a distance of 30 cm from the mouths of 25 speaking study participants. When the same subjects talked without the mask, bacterial growth was found on 50% of the agar plates.[139] However, until recently, the use of a mask as a preventive measure was much debated.[135] The use of masks has been questioned in the operating theatre, and one study addressing this issue found no increase in surgical wound infections when masks were omitted.[141] However, this study did not include patients undergoing orthopaedic or vascular prosthetic surgery, as viridans streptococci are well known to cause infection in these patients, the same viridans streptococci that may cause PDPM. Studies of infectious complications in surgical patients are therefore not directly applicable to the practice of neuraxial anaesthesia. The use of masks when performing CNB is now considered mandatory, and included in guidelines.[131,134,135] Nonetheless, the latest death caused by PDPM followed SA for labour analgesia, performed by an anaesthetist who omitted his/her mask, violating the previously issued guidelines.[94,133] The mask must be a good quality surgical mask, and should be changed between patients. The assistants present during preparation and performance of the CNB should also wear a mask.[90] The mask itself should never be touched.[84,124] Caps are important protective measures that should always be worn when performing CNB.[84,131] The hands should be disinfected with alcohol-based disinfectant before applying the gloves and, of course, after removal of watches and jewellery that ideally should not be worn at all during work hours.[124] The skin must be disinfected with an appropriate disinfectant and due to superior disinfectant qualities, chlorhexidine in alcohol is now considered the most appropriate agent, and is therefore widely recommended.[3,124,133,134]

Chlorhexidine is available in concentrations varying from 0.5% to 4%, but there are no substantial data in support of the use of a stronger solution than 0.5%.[143,144] The neurotoxic potential of chlorhexidine should also be considered.[109,144,145] The safety of chlorhexidine 2% is advocated by a retrospective analysis of 12,465 SAs performed in the same institution without detecting increase in neurological complications after the introduction of chlorhexidine gluconate 2% as disinfectant.[146] However, the statistical value of this study is hardly reassuring, as the result is compatible at the 95% confidence level with an incidence of one case of arachnoiditis following 4000 SAs.[144] Chlorhexidine 0.5% in alcohol is therefore the disinfectant of choice.[134] It is also advised that it should be applied twice, and left to dry after each application.[90,143] Malhotra and colleagues compared single versus repeated application of chlorhexidine gluconate 0.5% in 70% alcohol, and found no growth of bacteria following either methods.[147] These results would support the single application of chlorhexidine at least in emergency situations, when the risk of not allowing chlorhexidine to dry completely is apparent.[148]

The neurotoxic effects of chlorhexidine should also imply that great attention must be made never to contaminate any equipment that may come into contact with the central nervous system.[143] The use of chlorhexidine spray for disinfection, *before* opening the neuraxial anaesthesia pack, would appear to offer the smallest risk of contamination or risk of wrong route injection, and may also permit adequate disinfection without causing delay.[84] Reinsertion of the stylet in the spinal needle, before removing the needle from the patient, could be a critical moment both for the development of PDPM and contamination with chlorhexidine.[87] The removed stylet could have been exposed to contamination both from droplets as well as chlorhexidine, and therefore the practice of reinsertion of the stylet should be discouraged.

Chlorhexidine may also cause severe allergic reactions and these appear with increasing frequency as a large number of people are exposed to chlorhexidine in commercial products such as mouthwashes.[149] Anaphylactic reactions have been described to appear with 20–40 minutes' delay, and the condition can be of great severity. Diagnostic difficulties are increased in the anaesthetized patient undergoing surgery.[150]

Chemical meningitis and arachnoiditis

Chemical meningitis was described in older medical literature, and by 1947 more than 100 cases had been described.[151] The incidence decreased rapidly after studies had shown that chemical contamination, mainly detergents, caused chemical meningitis. Contrast media, and other substances injected into the CSF, may also cause chemical meningitis, but the complication has practically disappeared from modern anaesthetic practice, together with the disappearance of reusable needles. A wide range of systemic medications may also cause chemical meningitis.[151]

One study in neurosurgical patients, who may develop both types of meningitis, described the differences in chemical and bacterial meningitis.[152] Bacterial meningitis can be culture negative, therefore meningitis was defined as non-infectious only if the bacterial culture was negative, and the patient recovered without antibiotics. The study results showed that chemical meningitis could be excluded if the white cell count in the CSF exceeded 7500 × 10^6, and glucose levels were below 10 mg/dL. The clinical picture of chemical meningitis may resemble that of bacterial meningitis with high fever and meningeal irritation, but the patients recover without antibiotics, usually within a week. However, due to the improbability of aseptic meningitis following modern CNB, no patient with suspected meningitis can be left without antibiotic treatment.[84]

The term aseptic meningitis is sometimes used as synonym for chemical meningitis, but more often indicates meningitis of viral origin.[151] To add to the confusion, culture-negative bacterial meningitis may also be referred to as aseptic meningitis, although culture-negative bacterial meningitis is common.[100,152]

Infection or injection of neurotoxic chemical substances may lead to chronic adhesive arachnoiditis.[144,153] Two large surveys including a total of approximately 2.5 million CNB found one case of arachnoiditis each.[3,8] One patient in the United Kingdom received compensation in 2007 for a severe case of arachnoiditis considered to have been caused by chlorhexidine 0.5% in 70% alcohol contaminating the spinal needle during performance of SA for planned caesarean delivery.[144] The anaesthetic community initially questioned the causality, but when a patient in Australia received an admittedly erroneous injection of chlorhexidine into the epidural space there could be no doubt regarding the pathogenesis of the severe arachnoiditis that developed. Since then, several cases of arachnoiditis following CNB have been described, but the causality is not always apparent. However, the neurotoxic potential of chlorhexidine is recognized[144] and therefore, the anaesthetist must pay scrupulous attention not to contaminate equipment with disinfectant of any kind.

Chlorhexidine induces inflammation that transforms the pia-arachnoid into scar tissue. In severe cases, this can tether neural tissue and lead to atrophy. The MRI changes are typical and diagnostic, but presentation of symptoms in relationship to insult varies greatly, both in terms of severity and timing. Pain in the back and legs develop and sphincter dysfunction may also be present. In some of the most severe cases the patient may even become tetraplegic and develop obstructive hydrocephalus.

Transient radicular irritation

Transient pain in the lower back or buttock, irradiating to the lower extremities, has been described, typically occurring 12 hours after the resolution of uncomplicated SA.[154] The condition is not associated with motor impairment, and disappears within 5 days. Neurological examination is normal, and no long-lasting consequences are reported. Analgesic treatment may be offered with non-steroidal anti-inflammatory drugs. A Cochrane report found the syndrome to occur seven times more frequently when lidocaine was used for SA compared to all other local anaesthetics, but the complication is also described following SA with bupivacaine.[155] The report could not draw conclusions regarding incidence in the obstetric population.

Investigation and diagnosis of neurological deficits

Headache and backache are common following delivery, and urinary retention, incontinence, and fever may also result from normal labour.[11] The anaesthetist is often consulted to consider PDPH in a woman who has received CNB. The presence of fever, although possibly caused by the recent delivery, should cause a review of a possible alternative diagnosis. Meningitis will usually occur within 24 hours of CNB, and the symptoms of PDPM might not be of the severity usually seen in community-acquired meningitis.[8] Headache from meningitis is not expected to be positional as in PDPH, but the patient could suffer from the two conditions simultaneously. Nausea and vomiting may also be present in both conditions. Alterations of mental status might be difficult to appreciate, but opinions from relatives and midwives might be valuable. Signs of meningeal irritation such as nuchal rigidity and photophobia should be sought. Severe headache and visual disturbances may also be present in pre-eclampsia with impending eclampsia, and other symptoms of pre-eclampsia are not always present.[156] Migraine may also be accompanied by these symptoms, but the woman should be able to recognize the symptoms from earlier attacks. Cerebral venous thrombosis carries an incidence of 1/10,000 deliveries and may present itself with a vast variety of symptoms.[157] CSH usually presents with a delay of days or weeks following dural puncture, but may occur within 6 hours of dural puncture.[73] Headache is frequent in these two conditions, and any neurological symptom including seizures may be present. The first symptoms of an epidural abscess may be limited to fever and headache, therefore the anaesthetist should always perform inspection and palpation of the site of epidural catheterization when attending a woman with any type of complaint after CNB.[3] Backache can also be the first symptom of an epidural abscess, even preceding signs of infection.[128] An LP should be performed if PDPM is suspected, but could cause meningitis in the case of an epidural abscess. Antibiotic treatment should not be delayed by diagnostic procedures if the patient has symptoms of meningitis.

An obstetric patient who complains of focal neurology of any kind, including lower extremity motor impairment, sensorial deficit, or pain, should be examined without delay. The more severe conditions that may cause such symptoms are extremely rare, but must nonetheless be considered and excluded. The anaesthetist will often be consulted even in cases of obstetric palsies, due to the frequent administration of CNB during labour. Therefore, the anaesthetist should be familiar with their signs and symptoms, and consult a neurologist or neurosurgeon if the diagnosis of the obstetric palsy is not straightforward. Particularly when an obstetric palsy is bilateral, which is possible, a reliable clinical diagnosis must be obtained if radiological investigation is to be avoided.[11] Peripheral neuropathies, for example, affecting the lateral cutaneous nerve of the thigh, and femoral nerve are described in Chapter 45.

Neurological examination should be performed to distinguish between central and radicular lesions, indicating complications possibly related to the CNB, and plexus and peripheral nerve lesions, indicating obstetric nerve palsies.[11] The clinical investigation alone may, however, be unable to give a precise diagnosis. Examination of the paraspinous muscles may differentiate between peripheral and central nerve root injury.[11,158] The paraspinous muscles and the skin over the lower back are innervated by the posterior rami of the spinal nerves. Intact paraspinous muscles and sensitivity of the lower back suggests more distal injury, whereas the opposite indicates more central damage.[11,158] Sacral numbness without any other neurological symptom has been reported after caesarean delivery with SA.[12,159] Local anaesthetic neurotoxicity has been proposed, but the condition has also been described after EA.[12] Pressure-related compression of sacral nerves has therefore been considered responsible. Attention to positioning is advocated, and the patient can be reassured, as the numbness wears off within 8 weeks. However, all neurological symptoms must be carefully evaluated, to avoid delay in diagnosis of the more severe complications.

The first symptoms of SH are usually motor and sensorial deficits, and SH may present itself without pain, but pain on the other hand is always absent in obstetric palsies, and if present, should raise suspicion of SH or epidural abscess.[7,8,11,36] Radicular pain is typical of epidural abscess.[126]

The patient history should include information regarding previous neurological or muscular impairment. Detailed information regarding the CNB should be documented. There may be relevant information indicating the probability of an obstetric palsy with regards to duration of second stage and mode of delivery. The onset of the symptoms should be described, as the neurological deficit of obstetric palsies usually are noted immediately following delivery, but the symptoms due to SH or epidural abscess occur with latency, and will be progressive in severity. The severity of obstetric nerve palsies will not be progressive and get better with time.[11] However, in case of femoral nerve palsy, the patient might not realize her nerve injury before her leg gives way when she bends her knee getting into the car to get home. Meralgia paraesthetica may have been present before delivery, but may have gone unnoticed or may have been aggravated during delivery, and therefore noted only afterwards. In serious cases there might be paraesthesia and hyperaesthesia, but otherwise intrinsic obstetric palsies are not associated with pain. Pubic symphysis separation may cause severe pain, irradiating to the back or the hips, and may also cause walking difficulties.[11]

Even the slightest suspicion of either SH, CSH, or epidural abscess should lead to radiological diagnostic intervention without delay, as patient outcome depends entirely upon speed of surgical intervention. MRI is necessary for the diagnosis of SH and CSH, as well as epidural abscess, as a CT scan may give false-negative results.[35,70,128] MRI techniques are also best for the diagnosis of cerebral venous thrombosis, but CT angiography may also be diagnostic.[157]

Conclusion

Serious neurological complications following CNB do occur but are rare. Measures must be undertaken to prevent them at all costs. They require prompt diagnosis to prevent lasting patient harm and obstetric anaesthetists must therefore be competent in the examination of a patient presenting with neurological deficit and the ability to detect symptoms or signs of spinal/epidural space-occupying lesions and systemic infection. Appropriate consultation with medical experts from other specialities may be necessary to exclude other pathologies and urgent investigation is warranted.

References

1. Cornforth BM, Dalgleish DJ, Bromilow J, *et al.* Use of an information leaflet to improve general practitioners' knowledge of post dural puncture headache. *Int J Obstet Anaesth* 2006; 15(1):28–32.
2. Ruppen W, Derry S, McQuay H, *et al.* Incidence of epidural hematoma, infection, and neurologic injury in obstetric patients with epidural analgesia/anesthesia. *Anesthesiology* 2006; 105(2):394–9.
3. Cook TM, Counsell D, Wildsmith JA. Major complications of central neuraxial block: report on the Third National Audit Project of the Royal College of Anaesthetists. *Br J Anaesth* 2009; 102(2):179–90.
4. Hebl JR, Horlocker TT, Kopp SL, *et al.* Neuraxial blockade in patients with preexisting spinal stenosis, lumbar disk disease, or prior spine surgery: efficacy and neurologic complications. *Anesth Analg* 2010; 111(6):1511–19.
5. Deruddre S, Peyrouset O, Benhamou D. Anesthetic management of 52 deliveries in parturients with idiopathic thrombocytopenic purpura. *J Gynecol Obstet Biol Reprod (Paris)* 2007; 36(4):384–8.
6. Vercauteren M, Heytens L. Anaesthetic considerations for patients with a pre-existing neurological deficit: are neuraxial techniques safe? *Acta Anaesth Scand* 2007; 51(7):831–8.
7. Lee LA, Posner KL, Domino KB, *et al.* Injuries associated with regional anesthesia in the 1980s and 1990s: a closed claims analysis. *Anesthesiology* 2004; 101(1):143–52.
8. Moen V, Dahlgren N, Irestedt L. Severe neurological complications after central neuraxial blockades in Sweden 1990–1999. *Anesthesiology* 2004; 101(4):950–9.
9. Pitkanen MT, Aromaa U, Cozanitis DA, *et al.* Serious complications associated with spinal and epidural anaesthesia in Finland from 2000 to 2009. *Acta Anaesth Scand* 2013; 57(5):553–64.
10. Bethune L, Harper N, Lucas DN, *et al.* Complications of obstetric regional analgesia: how much information is enough? *Int J Obstet Anaesth* 2004; 13(1):30–4.
11. Wong CA. Nerve injuries after neuraxial anaesthesia and their medicolegal implications. *Best Pract Res Clin Obstet Gynaecol* 2010; 24(3):367–81.
12. Dar AQ, Robinson AP, Lyons G. Postpartum neurological symptoms following regional blockade: a prospective study with case controls. *Int J Obstet Anaesth* 2002; 11(2):85–90.
13. Loo CC, Dahlgren G, Irestedt L. Neurological complications in obstetric regional anaesthesia. *Int J Obstet Anaesth* 2000; 9(2):99–124.
14. Davies JM, Posner KL, Lee LA, *et al.* Liability associated with obstetric anesthesia: a closed claims analysis. *Anesthesiology* 2009; 110(1):131–9.
15. Szypula K, Ashpole KJ, Bogod D, *et al.* Litigation related to regional anaesthesia: an analysis of claims against the NHS in England 1995–2007. *Anaesthesia* 2010; 65(5):443–52.

16. Auroy Y, Benhamou D, Bargues L, *et al.* Major complications of regional anesthesia in France: The SOS Regional Anesthesia Hotline Service. *Anesthesiology* 2002; 97(5):1274–80.
17. Reynolds F. Damage to the conus medullaris following spinal anaesthesia. *Anaesthesia* 2001; 56(3):238–47.
18. Erk G, Taspinar V, Akay M, *et al.* Spinal hematoma as a result of spinal anesthesia for cesarean section. *Neurosciences (Riyadh)* 2009; 14(2):182–3.
19. Saifuddin A, Burnett SJ, White J. The variation of position of the conus medullaris in an adult population. A magnetic resonance imaging study. *Spine* 1998; 23(13):1452–6.
20. Reynolds F. Logic in the safe practice of spinal anaesthesia. *Anaesthesia* 2000; 55(11):1045–6.
21. Kim JT, Bahk JH, Sung J. Influence of age and sex on the position of the conus medullaris and Tuffier's line in adults. *Anesthesiology* 2003; 99(6):1359–63.
22. Schlotterbeck H, Schaeffer R, Dow WA, *et al.* Ultrasonographic control of the puncture level for lumbar neuraxial block in obstetric anaesthesia. *Br J Aneasth* 2008; 100(2):230–4.
23. Margarido CB, Mikhael R, Arzola C, *et al.* The intercristal line determined by palpation is not a reliable anatomical landmark for neuraxial anesthesia. *Can J Anaesth* 2011; 58(3):262–6.
24. Lee AJ, Ranasinghe JS, Chehade JM, *et al.* Ultrasound assessment of the vertebral level of the intercristal line in pregnancy. *Anesth Analg* 2011; 113(3):559–64.
25. Chakraverty R, Pynsent P, Isaacs K. Which spinal levels are identified by palpation of the iliac crests and the posterior superior iliac spines? *J Anat* 2007; 210(2):232–6.
26. Van Gessel EF, Forster A, Gamulin Z. Continuous spinal anesthesia: where do spinal catheters go? *Anesth Analg* 1993; 76(5):1004–7.
27. Broadbent CR, Maxwell WB, Ferrie R, *et al.* Ability of anaesthetists to identify a marked lumbar interspace. *Anaesthesia* 2000; 55(11):1122–6.
28. Kathirgamanathan A, Hawkins N. Reliability of the 'pop' sign as an indicator of dural puncture during obstetric spinal anaesthesia: a prospective observational clinical study. *Anaesthesia* 2007; 62(8):802–5.
29. Arendt KW, Segal S. Present and emerging strategies for reducing anesthesia-related maternal morbidity and mortality. *Curr Opin Anaesth* 2009; 22(3):330–5.
30. Arzola C, Davies S, Rofaeel A, *et al.* Ultrasound using the transverse approach to the lumbar spine provides reliable landmarks for labor epidurals. *Anesth Analg* 2007; 104(5):1188–92.
31. Scott DB, Hibbard BM. Serious non-fatal complications associated with extradural block in obstetric practice. *Br J Aneasth* 1990; 64(5):537–41.
32. Volk T, Wolf A, Van Aken H, *et al.* Incidence of spinal haematoma after epidural puncture: analysis from the German network for safety in regional anaesthesia. *Eur J Anaesth* 2012; 29(4):170–6.
33. Koyama S, Tomimatsu T, Kanagawa T, *et al.* Spinal subarachnoid hematoma following spinal anesthesia in a patient with HELLP syndrome. *Int J Obstet Anaesth* 2010; 19(1):87–91.
34. Wang P, Xin XT, Lan H, *et al.* Spontaneous cervical epidural hematoma during pregnancy: case report and literature review. *Eur Spine J* 2011; 20 Suppl 2:S176–9.
35. Walters MA, Van de Velde M, Wilms G. Acute intrathecal haematoma following neuraxial anaesthesia: diagnostic delay after apparently normal radiological imaging. *Int J Obstet Anaesth* 2012; 21(2):181–5.
36. Vandermeulen EP, Van Aken H, Vermylen J. Anticoagulants and spinal-epidural anesthesia. *Anesth Analg* 1994; 79(6):1165–77.
37. Gogarten W, Vandermeulen E, Van Aken H, *et al.* Regional anaesthesia and antithrombotic agents: recommendations of the European Society of Anaesthesiology. *Eur J Anaesth* 2010; 27(12):999–1015.
38. Bahar M, Chanimov M, Cohen ML, *et al.* Lateral recumbent head-down posture for epidural catheter insertion reduces intravascular injection. *Can J Anaesth* 2001; 48(1):48–53.
39. Bahar M, Chanimov M, Cohen ML, *et al.* The lateral recumbent head-down position decreases the incidence of epidural venous puncture during catheter insertion in obese parturients. *Can J Anaesth* 2004; 51(6):577–80.
40. Beards SC, Jackson A, Griffiths AG, *et al.* Magnetic resonance imaging of extradural blood patches: appearances from 30 min to 18 h. *Br J Aneasth* 1993; 71(2):182–8.
41. Jacob AK, Borowiec JC, Long TR, *et al.* Transient profound neurologic deficit associated with thoracic epidural analgesia in an elderly patient. *Anesthesiology* 2004; 101(6):1470–1.
42. Nguyen L, Riu B, Minville V, *et al.* Epidural hematoma after hemorrhagic shock in a parturient. *Can J Anaesth* 2006; 53(3):252–7.
43. Royal College of Obstetricians and Gynaecologists. *Thrombosis and Embolism During Pregnancy and the Puerperium, Reducing the Risk*. Green-top Guideline No. 37a. London: RCOG; 2015. http://www.rcog.org.uk/womens-health/clinical-guidance/reducing-risk-of-thrombosis-greentop37a
44. Membership of the Working Party, Harrop-Griffiths W, Cook T, *et al.* Regional anaesthesia and patients with abnormalities of coagulation. *Anaesthesia* 2013; 68(9):966–72.
45. Bosmia AN, Tubbs RS, Hogan E, *et al.* Blood supply to the human spinal cord. II. Imaging and pathology. *Clin Anat* 2015; 28(1):65–74.
46. Bosmia AN, Hogan E, Loukas M, *et al.* Blood supply to the human spinal cord. I. Anatomy and hemodynamics. *Clin Anat* 2015; 28(1):52–64.
47. Wong CA, Scavone BM, Dugan S, *et al.* Incidence of postpartum lumbosacral spine and lower extremity nerve injuries. *Obstet Gynecol* 2003; 101(2):279–88.
48. Moen V, Irestedt L. Neurological complications following central neuraxial blockades in obstetrics. *Curr Opin Anaesth* 2008; 21(3):275–80.
49. Butwick AJ, Carvalho B. Neuraxial anesthesia in obstetric patients receiving anticoagulant and antithrombotic drugs. *Int J Obstet Anaesth* 2010; 19(2):193–201.
50. Horlocker TT, Wedel DJ, Rowlingson JC, *et al.* Regional anesthesia in the patient receiving antithrombotic or thrombolytic therapy: American Society of Regional Anesthesia and Pain Medicine Evidence-Based Guidelines (Third Edition). *Reg Anesth Pain Med* 2010; 35(1):64–101.
51. Breivik H, Bang U, Jalonen J, *et al.* Nordic guidelines for neuraxial blocks in disturbed haemostasis from the Scandinavian Society of Anaesthesiology and Intensive Care Medicine. *Acta Anaesth Scand* 2010; 54(1):16–41.
52. Vandermeulen E, Decoster J, Dewandre PY, *et al.* Central neural blockade in patients with a drug-induced alteration of coagulation. Third edition of the Belgian Association for Regional Anaesthesia (BARA) Guidelines. *Acta Anaesthesiol Belg* 2011; 62(4):175–91.
53. Van De Velde M, Vercauteren M, Stockman W, *et al.* Recommendations and guidelines for obstetric anesthesia in Belgium Central neural blockade in patients with a drug-induced alteration of coagulation. Third edition of the Belgian Association for Regional Anaesthesia (BARA) Guidelines Regional anaesthesia and antithrombotic agents: recommendations of the European Society of Anaesthesiology. *Acta Anaesthesiol Belg* 2013; 64(3):97–104.
54. Llau JV, De Andres J, Gomar C, *et al.* Anticlotting drugs and regional anaesthetic and analgesic techniques: comparative update of the safety recommendations. *Eur J Anaesth* 2007; 24(5):387–98.
55. Kwon JY, Shin JC, Lee JW, *et al.* Predictors of idiopathic thrombocytopenic purpura in pregnant women presenting with thrombocytopenia. *Int J Gynaecol Obstet* 2007; 96(2):85–8.
56. Douglas MJ. The use of neuraxial anaesthesia in parturients with thrombocytopenia: what is an adequate platelet count? In Halpern SH, Douglas MJ (eds) *Evidence-Based Obstetric Anaesthesia* (2nd ed). Boston, MA: Blackwell; 2005:165–77.
57. Abramovitz S, Beilin Y. Thrombocytopenia, low molecular weight heparin, and obstetric anesthesia. *Anesthesiol Clin North America* 2003; 21(1):99–109.

58. Gogarten W. Preeclampsia and anaesthesia. *Curr Opin Anaesth* 2009; 22(3):347–51.
59. Eskild A, Vatten LJ. Abnormal bleeding associated with preeclampsia: a population study of 315,085 pregnancies. *Acta Obstet Gynecol Scand* 2009; 88(2):154–8.
60. Davies JR, Fernando R, Hallworth SP. Hemostatic function in healthy pregnant and preeclamptic women: an assessment using the platelet function analyzer (PFA-100) and thromboelastograph. *Anesth Analg* 2007; 104(2):416–20.
61. Douglas MJ. Platelets, the parturient and regional anesthesia. *Int J Obstet Anaesth* 2001; 10:113–20.
62. National Institute of Health and Care Excellence. *Hypertension in Pregnancy.* Clinical Guideline 107. London: NICE; 2010. http://www.nice.org.uk/guidance/CG107
63. National Institute of Health and Care Excellence. *Caesarean Section.* Clinical Guideline 132. London: NICE; 2011. https://www.nice.org.uk/guidance/cg132
64. Errando CL, Perez-Caballero P. Cranial subdural haematoma after spinal anaesthesia: perhaps not so rare complication. *Eur J Anaesth* 2010; 27(3):307–8.
65. Vos PE, de Boer WA, Wurzer JA, *et al.* Subdural hematoma after lumbar puncture: two case reports and review of the literature. *Clin Neurol Neurosurg* 1991; 93(2):127–32.
66. Barbara DW, Smith BC, Arendt KW. Images in anesthesiology: spinal subdural hematoma after labor epidural placement. *Anesthesiology* 2012; 117(1):178.
67. Bisinotto FM, Dezena RA, Fabri DC, *et al.* Intracranial subdural hematoma: a rare complication following spinal anesthesia: case report. *Rev Bras Anestesiol* 2012; 62(1):88–95.
68. Chang CH, Wu JC, Tu TH, *et al.* Intracranial subdural hematoma coexisting with improvement in spontaneous intracranial hypotension after an epidural blood patch. *J Chin Med Assoc* 2012; 75(11):610–13.
69. Fiala A, Furgler G, Baumgartner E, *et al.* Delayed subdural haematoma complicated by abducens nerve palsy and cortical vein thrombosis after obstetric epidural anaesthesia. *Br J Aneasth* 2012; 108(4):705–6.
70. Liang MY, Pagel PS. Bilateral interhemispheric subdural hematoma after inadvertent lumbar puncture in a parturient. *Can J Anaesth* 2012; 59(4):389–93.
71. Nepomuceno R, Herd A. Bilateral subdural hematoma after inadvertent dural puncture during epidural analgesia. *J Emerg Med* 2013; 44(2):e227–30.
72. Verduzco LA, Atlas SW, Riley ET. Subdural hematoma after an epidural blood patch. *Int J Obstet Anaesth* 2012; 21(2):189–92.
73. Zeidan A, Farhat O, Maaliki H, *et al.* Does postdural puncture headache left untreated lead to subdural hematoma? Case report and review of the literature. *Int J Obstet Anaesth* 2006; 15(1):50–8.
74. Demetriades AK, Sheikh MF, Minhas PS. Fatal bilateral subdural haematoma after epidural anaesthesia for pregnancy. *Arch Gynecol Obstet* 2011; 284(6):1597–8.
75. Vandam LD, Dripps RD. Long-term follow-up of patients who received 10,098 spinal anesthetics; syndrome of decreased intracranial pressure (headache and ocular and auditory difficulties). *JAMA* 1956; 161(7):586–91.
76. Grände PO. Mechanisms behind postspinal headache and brain stem compression following lumbar dural puncture—a physiological approach. *Acta Anaesth Scand* 2005; 49(5):619–26.
77. Angle P, Thompson D, Halpern S, *et al.* Second stage pushing correlates with headache after unintentional dural puncture in parturients. *Can J Anaesth* 1999; 46(9):861–6.
78. Oatridge A, Holdcroft A, Saeed N, *et al.* Change in brain size during and after pregnancy: study in healthy women and women with preeclampsia. *AJNR* 2002; 23(1):19–26.
79. Davies JM, Murphy A, Smith M, *et al.* Subdural haematoma after dural puncture headache treated by epidural blood patch. *Br J Aneasth* 2001; 86(5):720–3.
80. Novy J, Carruzzo A, Maeder P, *et al.* Spinal cord ischemia: clinical and imaging patterns, pathogenesis, and outcomes in 27 patients. *Arch Neurol* 2006; 63(8):1113–20.
81. Levy NA, Strauss H. Myelopathy following compression of abdominal aorta for postpartum hemorrhage. Report of a case. *Arch Neurol Psych* 1942; 48:85–91.
82. Ben-David B, Vaida S, Collins G, *et al.* Transient paraplegia secondary to an epidural catheter. *Anesth Analg* 1994; 79(3):598–600.
83. Reynolds F. Neurologic complications of pregnancy and neuraxial anesthesia. In Chestnut DH, Polley LS, Tsen LC, *et al.* (eds) *Obstetric Anesthesia: Principles and Practice* (4th ed). Philadelphia, PA: Elsevier Mosby; 2009:701–26.
84. Reynolds F. Neurological infections after neuraxial anesthesia. *Anesthesiol Clin* 2008; 26(1):23–52.
85. Grewal S, Hocking G, Wildsmith JA. Epidural abscesses. *Br J Aneasth* 2006; 96(3):292–302.
86. Green LK, Paech MJ. Obstetric epidural catheter-related infections at a major teaching hospital: a retrospective case series. *Int J Obstet Anaesth* 2010; 19(1):38–43.
87. Baer ET. Post-dural puncture bacterial meningitis. *Anesthesiology* 2006; 105(2):381–93.
88. Bacterial meningitis after intrapartum spinal anesthesia—New York and Ohio, 2008–2009. *MMWR* 2010; 59(3):65–9.
89. Rubin L, Sprecher H, Kabaha A, *et al.* Meningitis following spinal anesthesia: 6 cases in 5 years. *Infect Control Hosp Epidemiol* 2007; 28(10):1187–90.
90. Reynolds F. Infection as a complication of neuraxial blockade. *Int J Obstet Anaesth* 2005; 14(3):183–8.
91. Wilson M, Martin R, Walk ST, *et al.* Clinical and laboratory features of Streptococcus salivarius meningitis: a case report and literature review. *Clin Med Res* 2012; 10(1):15–25.
92. Amoroso P, Fernando A. de Ávila, Gagliardi CMO. Prevalence of different streptococci species in oral cavity of children and adolescents. *Braz J Oral Sci* 2003; 2(4):164–8.
93. Srinivasan V, Gertz RE, Jr, Shewmaker PL, *et al.* Using PCR-based detection and genotyping to trace Streptococcus salivarius meningitis outbreak strain to oral flora of radiology physician assistant. *PloS One* 2012; 7(2):e32169.
94. Shewmaker PL, Gertz RE, Jr, Kim CY, *et al.* Streptococcus salivarius meningitis case strain traced to oral flora of anesthesiologist. *J Clin Microbiol* 2010; 48(7):2589–91.
95. Hutter CD. Face masks, spinal anaesthesia and meningitis. *Anaesthesia* 2008; 63(7):781–2.
96. Lockhart PB, Brennan MT, Sasser HC, *et al.* Bacteremia associated with toothbrushing and dental extraction. *Circulation* 2008; 117(24):3118–25.
97. Hadzic A, Koluder-Cimic N, Hadzovic-Cengic M, *et al.* Serratia marcescens meningitis following spinal anaesthesia and arthroscopy. *Medicinski Arhiv* 2012; 66(3 Suppl 1):54–5.
98. Tena D, Solis S, Lainez S, *et al.* Meningitis caused by Abiotrophia defectiva: case report and literature review. *Infection* 2013; 41(2):571–4.
99. Pinder AJ, Dresner M. Meningococcal meningitis after combined spinal-epidural analgesia. *Int J Obstet Anaesth* 2003; 12(3):183–7.
100. Bhimraj A. Acute community-acquired bacterial meningitis in adults: an evidence-based review. *Cleve Clin J Med* 2012; 79(6):393–400.
101. Pandian JD, Sarada C, Radhakrishnan VV, *et al.* Iatrogenic meningitis after lumbar puncture-a preventable health hazard. *J Hosp Infect* 2004; 56(2):119–24.
102. Russell R. The dura is too vulnerable to be breached routinely in labour. *Int J Obstet Anaesth* 1999; 8(1):56–61.
103. Simmons SW, Taghizadeh N, Dennis AT, *et al.* Combined spinal-epidural versus epidural analgesia in labour. *Cochrane Database Syst Rev* 2012; 10:CD003401.
104. Rodrigo N, Perera KN, Ranwala R, *et al.* Aspergillus meningitis following spinal anaesthesia for caesarean section in Colombo, Sri Lanka. *Int J Obstet Anaesth* 2007; 16(3):256–60.

105. Petersdorf RG, Swarner DR, Garcia M. Studies on the pathogenesis of meningitis. II. Development of meningitis during pneumococcal bacteremia. *J Clin Invest* 1962; 41:320–7.
106. Carp H, Bailey S. The association between meningitis and dural puncture in bacteremic rats. *Anesthesiology* 1992; 76(5):739–42.
107. Eng RH, Seligman SJ. Lumbar puncture-induced meningitis. *JAMA* 1981; 245(14):1456–9.
108. Sullivan NM, Sutter VL, Mims MM, *et al.* Clinical aspects of bacteremia after manipulation of the genitourinary tract. *J infect Dis* 1973; 127(1):49–55.
109. Horlocker TT, Wedel DJ. Infectious complications of regional anesthesia. *Best Pract Res Clin Anaesthesiol* 2008; 22(3):451–75.
110. Bader AM, Gilbertson L, Kirz L, *et al.* Regional anesthesia in women with chorioamnionitis. *Reg Anesth* 1992; 17(2):84–6.
111. Davies JM, Thistlewood JM, Rolbin SH, *et al.* Infections and the parturient: anaesthetic considerations. *Can J Anaesth* 1988; 35(3 (Pt 1)):270–7.
112. Schonheyder HC, Gottschau A, Friland A, *et al.* Mortality rate and magnitude of Staphylococcus aureus bacteremia as assessed by a semiquantitative blood culture system. *Scand J Infect Dis* 1995; 27(1):19–21.
113. Wedel DJ, Horlocker TT. Regional anesthesia in the febrile or infected patient. *Reg Anesth Pain Med* 2006; 31(4):324–33.
114. Barnwell R, Ball V. Iatrogenic bacterial meningitis: an unmasked threat. *CJEM* 2012; 14:1–4.
115. Grande PO, Myhre EB, Nordstrom CH, *et al.* Treatment of intracranial hypertension and aspects on lumbar dural puncture in severe bacterial meningitis. *Acta Anaesth Scand* 2002; 46(3):264–70.
116. Nagra I, Wee B, Short J, *et al.* The role of cranial CT in the investigation of meningitis. *JRSM Short Rep* 2011; 2(3):20.
117. Cascio M, Heath G. Meningitis following a combined spinal-epidural technique in a labouring term parturient. *Can J Anaesth* 1996; 43(4):399–402.
118. Lyytikainen O, Rautio M, Carlson P, *et al.* Nosocomial bloodstream infections due to viridans streptococci in haematological and non-haematological patients: species distribution and antimicrobial resistance. *J Antimicrob Chemother* 2004; 53(4):631–4.
119. Veringa E, van Belkum A, Schellekens H. Iatrogenic meningitis by Streptococcus salivarius following lumbar puncture. *J Hosp Infect* 1995; 29(4):316–8.
120. Curry WT Jr, Hoh BL, Amin-Hanjani S, *et al.* Spinal epidural abscess: clinical presentation, management, and outcome. *Surg Neurol* 2005; 63(4):364–71.
121. Breivik H. Infectious complications of epidural anaesthesia and analgesia. *Curr Opin Anaesth* 1999; 12(5):573–7.
122. North JB, Brophy BP. Epidural abscess: a hazard of spinal epidural anaesthesia. *Aust N Z J Surg* 1979; 49(4):484–5.
123. Sakuragi T, Yasunaka K, Hirata K, *et al.* The source of epidural infection following epidural analgesia identified by pulsed-field gel electrophoresis. *Anesthesiology* 1998; 89(5):1254–6.
124. Hebl JR, Niesen AD. Infectious complications of regional anesthesia. *Curr Opin Anaesth* 2011; 24(5):573–80.
125. Yuan HB, Zuo Z, Yu KW, *et al.* Bacterial colonization of epidural catheters used for short-term postoperative analgesia: microbiological examination and risk factor analysis. *Anesthesiology* 2008; 108(1):130–7.
126. Kindler CH, Seeberger MD, Staender SE. Epidural abscess complicating epidural anesthesia and analgesia. An analysis of the literature. *Acta Anaesth Scand* 1998; 42(6):614–20.
127. Sarubbi FA, Vasquez JE. Spinal epidural abscess associated with the use of temporary epidural catheters: report of two cases and review. *Clin Infect Dis* 1997; 25(5):1155–8.
128. Schroeder TH, Krueger WA, Neeser E, *et al.* Spinal epidural abscess—a rare complication after epidural analgesia for labour and delivery. *Br J Aneasth* 2004; 92(6):896–8.
129. Jamieson DJ, Theiler RN, Rasmussen SA. Emerging infections and pregnancy. *Emerg Infect Dis* 2006; 12(11):1638–43.
130. Tang HJ, Lin HJ, Liu YC, *et al.* Spinal epidural abscess—experience with 46 patients and evaluation of prognostic factors. *J Infect* 2002; 45(2):76–81.
131. Hebl JR. The importance and implications of aseptic techniques during regional anesthesia. *Reg Anesth Pain Med* 2006; 31(4):311–23.
132. Heusner AP. Nontuberculous spinal epidural infections. *N Engl J Med* 1948; 239(23):845–54.
133. Infection control in anaesthesia. *Anaesthesia* 2008; 63(9):1027–36.
134. Practice advisory for the prevention, diagnosis, and management of infectious complications associated with neuraxial techniques: a report by the American Society of Anesthesiologists Task Force on infectious complications associated with neuraxial techniques. *Anesthesiology* 2010; 112(3):530–45.
135. Baer ET. Iatrogenic meningitis: the case for face masks. *Clin Infect Dis* 2000; 31(2):519–21.
136. Friedman Z, Siddiqui N, Katznelson R, *et al.* Experience is not enough: repeated breaches in epidural anesthesia aseptic technique by novice operators despite improved skill. *Anesthesiology* 2008; 108(5):914–20.
137. Guzzo JL, Seagull FJ, Bochicchio GV, *et al.* Mentors decrease compliance with best sterile practices during central venous catheter placement in the trauma resuscitation unit. *Surg Infect* 2006; 7(1):15–20.
138. McKenzie AG, Darragh K. A national survey of prevention of infection in obstetric central neuraxial blockade in the UK. Anaesthesia. 2011; 66(6):497–502.
139. Philips BJ, Fergusson S, Armstrong P, *et al.* Surgical face masks are effective in reducing bacterial contamination caused by dispersal from the upper airway. *Br J Aneasth* 1992; 69(4):407–8.
140. Schneeberger PM, Janssen M, Voss A. Alpha-hemolytic streptococci: a major pathogen of iatrogenic meningitis following lumbar puncture. Case reports and a review of the literature. *Infection* 1996; 24(1):29–33.
141. Tunevall TG, Jorbeck H. Influence of wearing masks on the density of airborne bacteria in the vicinity of the surgical wound. *Eur J Surg* 1992; 158(5):263–6.
142. Lee JJ, Parry H. Bacterial meningitis following spinal anaesthesia for caesarean section. *Br J Aneasth* 1991; 66(3):383–6.
143. Scott M, Stones J, Payne N. Antiseptic solutions for central neuraxial blockade: which concentration of chlorhexidine in alcohol should we use? *Br J Aneasth* 2009; 103(3):456.
144. Bogod D. The sting in the tail: antiseptics and the neuraxis revisited. *Anaesthesia* 2012; 67(12):1305–9.
145. Checketts MR. Wash & go—but with what? Skin antiseptic solutions for central neuraxial block. *Anaesthesia* 2012; 67(8):819–22.
146. Sviggum HP, Jacob AK, Arendt KW, *et al.* Neurologic complications after chlorhexidine antisepsis for spinal anesthesia. *Reg Anesth Pain Med* 2012; 37(2):139–44.
147. Malhotra S, Dharmadasa A, Yentis SM. One vs two applications of chlorhexidine/ethanol for disinfecting the skin: implications for regional anaesthesia. *Anaesthesia* 2011; 66(7):574–8.
148. Kinsella SM, Girgirah K, Scrutton MJ. Rapid sequence spinal anaesthesia for category-1 urgency caesarean section: a case series. *Anaesthesia* 2010; 65(7):664–9.
149. Parkes AW, Harper N, Herwadkar A, *et al.* Anaphylaxis to the chlorhexidine component of Instillagel: a case series. *Br J Aneasth* 2009; 102(1):65–8.
150. Garvey LH, Roed-Petersen J, Husum B. Anaphylactic reactions in anaesthetised patients—four cases of chlorhexidine allergy. *Acta Anaesth Scand* 2001; 45(10):1290–4.
151. Burke D, Wildsmith JA. Meningitis after spinal anaesthesia. *Br J Aneasth* 1997; 78(6):635–6.
152. Forgacs P, Geyer CA, Freidberg SR. Characterization of chemical meningitis after neurological surgery. *Clin Infect Dis* 2001; 32(2):179–85.
153. Killeen T, Kamat A, Walsh D, *et al.* Severe adhesive arachnoiditis resulting in progressive paraplegia following obstetric

spinal anaesthesia: a case report and review. *Anaesthesia* 2012; 67(12):1386–94.

154. Pollock JE. Transient neurologic symptoms: etiology, risk factors, and management. *Reg Anesth Pain Med* 2002; 27(6):581–6.
155. Zaric D, Pace NL. Transient neurologic symptoms (TNS) following spinal anaesthesia with lidocaine versus other local anaesthetics. *Cochrane Database Syst Rev* 2009; 2:CD003006.
156. Knight M. Eclampsia in the United Kingdom 2005. *BJOG* 2007; 114(9):1072–8.
157. Bousser MG, Crassard I. Cerebral venous thrombosis, pregnancy and oral contraceptives. *Thromb Res* 2012; 130 Suppl 1:S19–22.
158. Aminoff MJ. Neurological disorders and pregnancy. *Am J Obstet Gynecol* 1978; 132(3):325–35.
159. Paech MJ. Unexplained neurologic deficit after uneventful combined spinal and epidural anesthesia for cesarean delivery. *Reg Anesth* 1997; 22(5):479–82.

CHAPTER 29

Medicolegal issues

Elizabeth Combeer, Rehana Iqbal, and Steve Yentis

Introduction

Medical law covers a vast breadth of issues including individuals' rights to access healthcare, confidentiality, end-of-life decisions, and research. It also varies across different countries, though in general law is developed through two processes, legislative (Acts of Parliament) and judicial (case law, also known as common law or precedent).

Acts of Parliament (statutes) are developed following identification of a need to develop new statutory law to regulate a particular issue. Examples of such Acts that are important within the sphere of medical law are the Mental Capacity Act 2005 and the Human Tissue Act 2004.

In case law, decisions made in legal courts on a case-by-case basis set precedents in determining how future, similar cases should be decided ('similar' referring to the principles of a case, rather than the setting—for example, a case concerning the sale of defective non-medical products may inform cases concerning harm resulting from defective drugs or medical products). Prior judgements of higher (appeal) courts tend to be binding on lower courts within the same jurisdiction, and also offer guidance to cases in other common law jurisdictions. Where no case law exists that relates to a case being tried, the judiciary are, in essence, creating brand new law with their decisions.

Medical statutory and case law is reactive to the ever-changing technology and possibilities of medicine and also reflects the evolution in values held by society. The judiciary have attempted to use ethical reasoning in addition to legal principle in order to arbitrate in difficult cases that have presented brand new dilemmas to society and healthcare professionals.[1] The robustness of such ethical reasoning has been extensively debated[2] and yet has frequently been the basis on which a case has been decided, blurring the boundary between law and ethics. As previously explained, such decisions then form a precedent for future cases and so the evolution in law continues. It is for these reasons that there are no definitive answers in medical law, just an interpretation of the current position.

In this chapter we attempt to give a brief overview of some of the key areas of medical law that relate to obstetric anaesthesia and, where possible, to offer some guidance to the practising anaesthetist. The emphasis is on English law although we have attempted to be as broad as possible to allow extrapolation of the principles to other jurisdictions.

Battery

If a doctor touches a patient without her consent then a case in battery may be brought against the doctor. Battery is a civil wrong (tort) that one person may do to another and, as such, the case would be heard in a civil court; if the judge finds in favour of the claimant then compensation would be awarded. Battery, legally defined, is any form of non-consensual contact and is therefore not restricted to contact between a doctor and patient. The patient does not even have to prove that harm has occurred in order to win her case. A claim in battery may also apply where consent has been taken but is irrelevant to the procedure that actually takes place, for example, wrong-sided surgery, or where a doctor operates beyond that which they have gained consent for (e.g. in *Bartley* v *Studd* where the patient had given consent for a hysterectomy but the surgeon performed an oophorectomy in addition[3]).

Negligence

Negligence is also a tort, so a case would also be heard in a civil court. A case in negligence could be brought if a patient believes she has suffered harm during treatment as a result of substandard care. In order for a case in negligence to be successful, the patient must be able to demonstrate three things to the court. Firstly, that the doctor owed her a duty of care. In the majority of situations this is not a difficult issue to resolve: a doctor who has engaged in any form of assessment or treatment of a patient clearly has a duty of care to her. However, even when harm has occurred due to the absence of care, the duty of care is usually straightforward to prove. When a National Health Service (NHS) hospital accepts referral of a woman for obstetric care, there is the implicit undertaking that the hospital and its healthcare employees have accepted a duty of care for her. In the private healthcare setting, there is a contract between the doctor or hospital and the patient, which establishes a duty of care.

Secondly, the patient must prove that the care she received fell short of the standard that it should have been. The difficulty here is in establishing precisely what the standard for any given form of treatment or interaction between doctor and patient should be. The traditional stance is derived from the *Bolam* case: if a doctor acted in line with a 'responsible body of medical men' (even a minority), then their actions would be viewed as appropriate and legally they would not be found negligent.[4] However, case law has evolved since *Bolam*, the major change being signified in the case of *Bolitho*, in which it was ruled that a doctor's actions (and the view of said responsible body of medical men) must be 'capable of withstanding logical analysis'.[5] For example, in a case of harm resulting from failure to check an anaesthetic machine it is not enough to offer the defence that, say, 40% of anaesthetists as a whole would also not check it—the judge might reasonably conclude that whilst satisfying the *Bolam* principle, such a claim fails the *Bolitho* test in that such practice is neither reasonable nor responsible.

Finally, the patient must prove to the court that this breach in the duty of care has resulted in harm to her.

Gross negligence, manslaughter, and murder

Negligent care of a patient may rarely result in death. In such cases, a doctor may face a criminal prosecution for manslaughter if it is considered that the degree of negligence demonstrates 'such disregard for the life and safety of others as to amount to a crime ... deserving of punishment'.[6] The borderline between 'ordinary' negligence and 'gross' negligence is the subject of considerable debate. There has been concern in recent years that criminal charges of manslaughter have been brought against doctors (including anaesthetists) too readily for cases involving simple (but admittedly catastrophic) mistakes rather than what the medical profession might consider 'gross negligence'.[7]

The key case describing gross negligence unfortunately involves an anaesthetist, Dr Adomako, who took over the care of an anaesthetized patient having ophthalmic surgery. He failed to notice when the breathing circuit became disconnected. When the patient became bradycardic and hypotensive, he administered atropine but failed to respond to other alarms warning of the disconnection. Approximately 9 minutes after disconnection was thought to have occurred, the patient suffered a cardiac arrest. The disconnection was discovered during the unsuccessful resuscitation attempt.[8]

The Corporate Manslaughter and Corporate Homicide Act 2007 enables charges of manslaughter to be brought against corporate entities, for example, companies and NHS trusts, that practise gross negligence resulting in death.[9] Only a small number of convictions have resulted (three up to the end of 2012[10]) but the number of cases being brought is increasing each year. Senior managers within trusts (including doctors) are theoretically vulnerable if they are deemed to have failed sufficiently in their duty so as to constitute gross negligence.

Manslaughter is distinguished from murder by a lack of intent. It is rare for anaesthetists—especially obstetric anaesthetists—to face a murder charge, but this may occur if they are involved in end-of-life decisions in which drugs are administered that are judged to have ended the life of a patient, and where this is found to have been the intended purpose. Most such cases have involved intensivists.

Clinical guidelines

Recent years have seen a proliferation of written statements advising on or directing the delivery of healthcare. Terms used to describe these written statements include recommendations, protocols, guidance, policies, and guidelines. This is confusing and may suggest greater compliance is legally required with, for example, a protocol than a recommendation, although there is no objective support for this suggestion. The number and varying roles of agencies that are involved in the development and dissemination of guidance further compound this confusion.

A large number of agencies have developed guidelines that impact on both the provision of obstetric anaesthetic services[11] and the management of specific clinical conditions.[12] Advocates for guidelines would argue that their use minimizes unjustifiable variation in clinical practice thus improving patient safety and clinical outcomes. However, there is concern about the impact of guidelines on the use and development of clinical judgement, the quality and evidence base for their development and the legal and professional consequences of deviating from them. Although clinical practice is influenced by guidelines, there is a lack of data looking at outcomes following their introduction to support claims of improvements in quality of care.[13] Despite this, guidelines are often viewed as documented standards of care.

The courts have recognized the difficulties associated with determining the legal status of guidelines. In *Crawford* v *Board of Governors of Charing Cross Hospital*, Lord Denning stated that 'the time may come in a particular case when a new recommendation may be so well proved and so well known, and so well accepted that it should be adopted'.[14] It has been suggested that if a guideline fulfils the elements of this 'Denning Test' (i.e. that the guideline is proven, disseminated, accepted, and adopted by the profession) then there may be a greater legal requirement to comply with it.[15]

Adherence to guidelines has been used as a successful defence against negligence claims. In *Early* v *Newham* the claimant experienced a period of awareness following a failed intubation attempt. However, her claim was unsuccessful, as the anaesthetist had adhered to locally developed failed intubation guidelines.[16] The quality of the local guideline was unsuccessfully challenged as the claimant was unable to prove that the guideline was such that no responsible body of practitioners would have complied with it.[4]

It should not, however, be assumed that adherence to guidelines provides an impenetrable shield against litigation claims. In the case of *Wickline* v *The State of California*, a patient was discharged early from hospital, in accordance with guidelines, but subsequently came to harm. The court emphasized the importance of clinical judgement and the responsibilities of the physician. It recognized that clinical judgement may be contrary to guidelines and that rigid compliance with guidelines in these circumstances may not be legally defensible.[17] The importance of clinical judgement has also been emphasized in the English courts, for example, in an unsuccessful claim of negligence against clinicians for failure to follow clinical guidelines in the management of severe asthma in a pregnant patient. The courts supported the use of clinical judgement despite the existence of guidelines.[18]

There are a number of reasons why a clinician may choose to comply with or deviate from guidelines. These reasons may include a professional assessment of robustness of the evidence base for the guideline, its applicability to the current clinical situation, the existence of conflicting guidelines, and whether the particular circumstances dictate different management. Guideline compliance may also be limited by the cost of its implementation.

The precise hierarchy of authority of guidelines, where conflict exists between two guidelines advising on the management of the same issue, has yet to be tested. However, guidelines developed by national regulatory bodies such as the General Medical Council (GMC), the National Institute for Health and Care Excellence (NICE), and the Royal Colleges are likely to have greater authority than other sources. When choosing to manage patients contrary to guidelines, clear documentation of the reasons for departure from guidance, explicit consent, and an acceptable standard of care that promotes best interests would be necessary.

Autonomy and informed consent

Autonomy refers to an individual's right to 'self-govern' and make one's own decisions. Respect for autonomy (along with justice, beneficence, and non-maleficence) is one of the moral principles underpinning medical ethics,[19] and medical paternalism has given way to an era of respect for the decision-making of the patient. Consent is the process by which a doctor recognizes a patient's autonomy. For consent to be valid, adequate information must be given to the patient, she must have the capacity to make a decision (see 'Capacity and the Mental Capacity Act'), there must be adequate time to do so, and there must be freedom from coercion.

A patient can bring a case in negligence against her doctor if she develops a complication from treatment, the possibility of which was not disclosed during the consent process. If no consent took place then the claim would be brought in battery, although this would be unusual. The usual principles of negligence apply to cases concerning inadequate consent: that a duty of care exists; that there was a breach in the duty of care (the level of information disclosure was inadequate); and that harm has occurred as a direct result of the breach because, if warned, the patient would not have given consent.

It can be difficult to judge precisely how much information is 'adequate', sufficient to enable an informed decision by a patient without overburdening her with an endless list of rare or trivial possible complications. GMC guidance advises doctors to try to understand the particular patient they are caring for and the adverse outcomes they may be most concerned about when deciding what risks to discuss.[20] Patients must be advised of serious adverse outcomes (those resulting in death, permanent or long-term disability, effect on employment, or social or personal life) 'even if the likelihood is very small'. Withholding information concerning adverse outcomes for fear that it may unduly scare the patient or lead her to decline an intervention is not permitted. Patients who do not wish to be told about potential risks should still be advised of the general nature of an intervention or treatment and should be informed about any serious risks. If a patient refuses to hear even this most basic information, then she should be advised that she can change her mind at any time and the discussion should be fully documented.

The GMC guidance can be difficult to apply in practice. Obstetric anaesthetists meet many of the patients they care for in emotionally charged, emergency situations when the patient may be suffering significant pain. Limited time for discussion makes it difficult to establish the individual wishes of each patient concerning information disclosure. The *Bolam* case established that an explanation that was in line with that of colleagues would be viewed as adequate from a legal perspective.[4] However, 40 years later, *Bolitho* determined that merely providing the same standard of explanation as some of one's peers is inadequate: that standard must be 'capable of withstanding logical analysis'.[5]

As previously discussed, guidelines from professional bodies may be viewed as standards of care. The Royal College of Anaesthetists (RCoA),[21] the Association of Anaesthetists of Great Britain and Ireland (AAGBI), and the Obstetric Anaesthetists' Association (OAA) have all produced patient information leaflets explaining the risks associated with anaesthesia. The OAA, for example, has produced an information card to facilitate discussion of risks with women during the consent process for labour epidural analgesia. The OAA clearly concurs with the GMC on the need to offer maximal information to patients: adverse consequences stated on the card include the possibility of paralysis of 1 in 250,000 women.[22] Application of such a guideline may be regarded as a standard that is capable of 'withstanding logical analysis' due to the authority of the professional body from which it originates. Furthermore, as the use of the OAA information card becomes more widespread, the 'Denning Test' may be seen to apply: deviation from such a guideline might therefore require documented evidence of justification.

The case of *Chester* v *Afshar* is an interesting reflection on how important the judiciary now believe a patient's right to information is.[23] Miss Chester was not warned of the risk of cauda equina syndrome following back surgery, and it was admitted by the defendant that she should have been. However, Miss Chester admitted to the Court that she would probably have gone ahead with the surgery anyhow, thus failing to prove causality, a key component of a negligence claim. Nonetheless, the Court was so keen to compensate Miss Chester for the breach to her right of autonomy that it found in her favour.

There is no definitive way to ensure that one's method of obtaining consent will provide immunity from claims of negligence. Ensuring that practice is in line with colleagues would seem to help. Applying the guidance on consent published by professional bodies will ensure that information disclosure achieves a documented standard that should be capable of withstanding logical analysis. Ensuring that information disclosure is of a level and quality to facilitate patient autonomy is an important focus.

Capacity and the Mental Capacity Act

Testing capacity (competence) evolved through case law, as the courts were called upon to make decisions in situations where there was doubt as to whether individuals could reasonably be allowed to make up their own minds about proposed medical treatment. C[24] was a man with paranoid schizophrenia who developed a gangrenous leg. His doctors wanted to amputate his leg in his best interests, as they considered that he did not have the ability to decide for himself owing to his mental health problems. C did not want to have his leg amputated and sought an injunction against his doctors. The courts found C to be competent and a simple test of mental capacity was developed that has since been enshrined in statutory law in England and Wales in the form of the Mental Capacity Act 2005. The Act's starting point is that all persons over 16 years old should be assumed to have capacity unless shown otherwise. In order to demonstrate capacity, a patient must understand and retain the information given to her, use this information to make a decision, and then to be able to communicate that decision back to the doctor caring for her (Box 29.1).

A woman with capacity has the absolute right to determine what happens to her body in the context of agreeing to or refusing medical treatment. The right of a competent patient to refuse treatment, even if this will lead directly to her death, has been upheld in case law.[25]

The Mental Capacity Act regards capacity in the context of being situation or decision specific, rather than something one either has or has not. However, when considering the management of patients who lack capacity for a specific decision, it is useful to view them as falling into four broad categories: those who have yet

Box 29.1 Capacity testing according to the Mental Capacity Act 2005

(a) To understand the information relevant to the decision

(b) To retain that information

(c) To use or weigh that information as part of the process of making the decision

(d) To communicate his decision (whether by talking, using sign language or any other means)

to develop capacity (children); those who have never had capacity and are never likely to; those who have previously had capacity but have permanently lost it; and those who usually have capacity but have temporarily lost it. Parturients who lack capacity are most likely to fall into this fourth group as temporary loss of capacity may result from factors associated with labour. (Management of this group is discussed later in 'Patients Who Temporarily Lack Capacity, Consent in Labour, and Birth Plans'.) However, obstetric anaesthetists may also be required to provide treatment for patients from the other three categories and so the legal approach to managing the care of such women will be described here.

Children and capacity

The law concerning consent in children is important to obstetric anaesthetists because parturients may be under 16 years of age: the rate of pregnancy in girls aged 15–17 years in England and Wales is 35.5 per 1000.[26] The interpretation of law concerning children and consent has been made problematic by the fact that there is no clear statutory law that dictates a precise age at which a child assumes complete responsibility for giving or withholding consent for her own medical treatment. The Mental Capacity Act assumes competence for anyone over 16 years old, whilst the Family Law Reform Act 1969 has been interpreted as meaning that children are not able to *refuse* treatment if they are under 18 years old.[27] This interpretation has been reflected in subsequent case law.[28]

The *Gillick* case concerned the legitimacy of doctors providing sexual healthcare to girls less than 16 years without the knowledge or consent of their parents.[29] From this case stems the term 'Gillick competence', used to describe children who are under the age of 16 but who demonstrate the maturity and understanding required to give consent for their own treatment. Gillick competency is probably better referred to as Fraser competency after the judge who described the criteria for such circumstances. It is important to note that these guidelines require the doctor to decide that it is in the child's best interests, both in terms of her medical best interests and her social circumstances, to proceed with care in the absence of parental knowledge or permission. Lord Fraser stated that, occasionally, a situation might arise where 'a doctor is a better judge of the medical advice and treatment which will conduce to a girl's welfare than her parents'.[29] Thus the *Gillick* case empowers mature children to give assent to treatment thought to be in their best interests by their doctors or their parents, and it allows them to have medical treatment without their parents' knowledge

Table 29.1 Summary of consent rights according to patient age

	Child	Gillick competent child	16–17 years	18 years
Right to give consent?	No	Yes	Yes	Yes
Right to refuse treatment?	No	No	No	Yes
Parents (or those with parental responsibility) may give consent on child's behalf?	Yes	Yes	Yes	No
Doctors able to treat the patient in her best interests despite parental and patient refusal of consent?	Yes	Yes	Yes	No

or permission if that is thought by their doctor to be in their overall best interests. It does not, however, allow them to refuse treatment that is thought (by their parents or doctors) to be in their best interests and the courts have demonstrated themselves willing to compel underage children to have such treatment if they attempt to refuse.[30]

Cases tried subsequent to *Gillick* have continued to debate the precise meaning and application of its ruling. If the judiciary are unclear, then it is unsurprising that many clinicians have an indistinct grasp of how to manage consent in adolescents. The following is a summary of the current legal position (Table 29.1). Once a girl is 18 years old, she has the absolute right to accept or decline medical treatment offered to her. Over the age of 16 years, it should be assumed that a girl is competent to give consent for her own care unless there are factors that lead the clinician to decide that she lacks competence. Under the age of 16 years, the doctor must assess whether a girl is Gillick competent according to whether she displays the specifics of capacity laid down in the Mental Capacity Act (see Box 29.1). If the child appears to be competent, she may give consent for herself for medical treatment offered to her. It is good practice, where the competent child permits, to involve parents in supporting a teenager's decision-making.[31] However, there will be occasions where parents (or those with parental responsibility) may disagree with the consent given by a Gillick competent child or adolescent patient. In these situations, the parents are not legally permitted to overrule the consent of the patient. (NB Parental responsibility is held by all mothers, a father if he was married to the mother at the time of the birth, fathers who jointly registered the birth with the mother (from 1 December 2003), and fathers who have attained parental responsibility through agreement with the mother or through a court order. Parental responsibility may also be held by a legally appointed guardian, a local authority in whose care a child is or a local authority or person with an emergency protection order for a child.)

Although a Gillick competent child or girl over 16 years may give consent for her own treatment, she is not permitted to refuse treatment if this may lead to death or serious injury. A situation might arise, therefore, where the parents and doctors of a Gillick competent child wish to proceed with treatment but the child refuses. Where time permits, legal assistance should be sought to assist in resolving such disputes. However, in an emergency situation, doctors should treat in accordance with the best interests of a child under 18 years, even if this is contrary to the child's and/or the parents' wishes.

Until a child is 16 or has developed capacity, the parents (or those with parental responsibility) are entitled to give consent for them. It is obvious that discussions and explanations should involve the child as much as possible, even if she is not legally in a position to sign a consent form for herself.[32] The child benefits from time spent with a doctor who is prepared to give explanations targeted to her level of maturity. This maximizes her autonomy and allows her to develop trust in her clinicians. It is important that children should develop a relationship based on trust with those treating them in order that healthcare experiences as a child do not deter them from seeking treatment in later life. Once again, if parents refuse to give consent for treatment that clinicians believe to be in the child's best interests, then an application must be made to the Court of Protection (through the hospital lawyers) for the resolution of the dispute. In an emergency, treatment should proceed whilst this is being undertaken.

The rights of a pregnant teenager concerning consent do not alter despite the fact that she is about to give birth to her own child. However, the potential for dispute between the girl, her parents, and the healthcare professionals should be anticipated where possible. It is of paramount importance to engage young pregnant girls early in antenatal care. They are statistically more likely to come from a background associated with deprivation, abuse, lack of parental involvement, and mental health and educational problems, and are more likely to be poor antenatal attendees.[33] Their babies are significantly more at risk of prematurity, perinatal death, or death in infancy than the babies of older mothers. Ideally, specialized, multidisciplinary antenatal care (often including social care professionals) targeted to the needs of teenage women should be offered. Discussions concerning possible outcomes and the potential need for medical treatment in labour should happen during the child's pregnancy in order to avoid conflict, rushed decisions and the need to act contrary to a girl's wishes in an emergency. It is important that obstetric anaesthetists are included in such discussions.

Patients who no longer have capacity

Before the Mental Capacity Act 2005, no person could act as a proxy in giving consent to medical treatment on behalf of another adult. If treatment was considered necessary for a patient who lacked capacity, the medical team caring for her would act in her best interests. The Mental Capacity Act has sought to improve the method by which decisions are made for patients who lack capacity, to ensure that (where known) the patient's views can be included in decisions and to ensure that all people who lack capacity are represented by an advocate (whether friend, family member, or professional) when major decisions are being made on their behalf.[34] There are three ways in which this may be achieved:

1. The Mental Capacity Act requires doctors caring for a patient who lacks capacity to discuss the medical plans with family, carers, or friends who may hold key information about the patient's thoughts and beliefs before making a best interests judgement about how to proceed with treatment. In this manner, the patient's wider best interests may be respected rather than making a decision based purely on likely medical outcomes.
2. The Mental Capacity Act also reinforces the concept of Advance Decisions (previously known as Advance Directives) to detail an individual's wishes concerning future medical treatment. An Advance Decision may be made verbally or in writing. If made verbally, some form of record of the decision must be made, for example, in the hospital notes. If it is a written statement it does not need to be witnessed, unless it concerns refusal of life-sustaining treatment. However, it must be sufficiently detailed and specific to ensure that it clearly applies to the circumstances that eventuate. A patient cannot make advance requests for treatment that the clinicians do not believe to be appropriate.[35] An Advance Decision only comes in to force after the individual loses capacity and may be withdrawn at any time, verbally or in writing, until capacity is lost. Doctors are legally bound to follow the wishes laid out in an Advance Decision or they may find themselves liable for battery. However, situations may arise where there is doubt as to the validity of a decision: the circumstances in reality may differ from those described in the decision; there may have been a significant change in the individual's life; there may be doubt regarding the capacity of the individual at the time of making the decision; or a Lasting Power of Attorney (LPA; see below) might have been subsequently appointed who advises the medical team contrary to that which is stated in the decision.[36] The clinicians caring for the patient should continue to treat the patient according to her best interests until an assessment of the validity of such an Advance Decision is made. A form of Advance Decision commonly encountered in obstetric practice is a mother's birth plan, which is discussed later. Another relevant Advance Decision is that made by Jehovah's Witnesses concerning refusal of administration of blood products. Ideally, such a decision should be explored antenatally in an unhurried manner. However, it is feasible for an Advance Decision to be produced in an emergency situation when the woman herself is either unconscious or under general anaesthesia. Such circumstances are fortunately rare but should they occur, urgent consultation with the hospital lawyers is recommended; medical management should continue in the woman's best interests in the interim, with careful documentation of all aspects of her immediate care.
3. Individuals may also appoint a LPA to act as a proxy decision maker on their behalf once capacity has been lost. This appointment will be registered with the Public Guardian and may be a friend, relative, or professional adviser of the individual ('donor' of power). Unless the LPA has been given express, written permission by the donor, they may not make decisions regarding the continuation or cessation of life-sustaining treatment. Furthermore, they cannot request treatment that the medical team caring for the patient believes to be inappropriate. Before loss of capacity, the donor can revoke the decision to appoint an LPA at any time.

Patients who have never had capacity

If a woman has never had capacity she will not have been able to appoint an LPA or make an Advance Decision. However, it is still reasonable to involve her friends, carers, and relatives when decisions are made on her behalf as these people will be able to advise the clinicians about the woman's likes and dislikes.[37] In conjunction with the medical team caring for such a woman, the majority of medical decisions made on her behalf should be straightforward. However, there are situations where a woman who has never had capacity or who has permanently lost capacity (and has no Advance Decision or LPA) has no friends or relatives to support her in making appropriate medical decisions. For all but minor treatment decisions, the Mental Capacity Act requires that an Independent Mental Capacity Advocate (IMCA) be consulted. The IMCA is permitted access to the patient (and her records) in order to attempt to represent the patient's views in the decision-making process. Like family members and friends, an IMCA does not have the power to act as a proxy decision-maker.

The Court of Protection has the power to appoint a Court Appointed Deputy (CAD) to act as a proxy decision-maker for an individual who lacks capacity and who does not have an LPA (whether this is because she never had capacity to do so or because she did not exercise this right when capacitous). This may be done if there are particularly complex issues to address or if there is likely to be an ongoing requirement for decisions to be made. A member of the patient's family may be appointed as a CAD, for example, the parent of an adult with severe learning difficulties. Just like an LPA, a CAD must always act in the best interests of the individual whom they represent. The Court of Protection remains the ultimate arbiter in cases where there is dispute between family, friends, LPAs, IMCAs, CADs, and healthcare professionals about how best to proceed in medically treating an adult who lacks the capacity to make her own decisions.[38]

Patients who temporarily lack capacity, consent in labour, and birth plans

A multitude of factors encountered in labour may temporarily compromise a previously competent woman's decision-making capacity. These include pain, lack of sleep, anxiety, opioid analgesia, and physiological disturbance caused by blood loss. It is therefore important to reassess her capacity for each new decision in labour. Any healthcare professional can make this assessment of capacity, and it is decision specific: a woman who has the capacity to consent to a vaginal examination does not necessarily have the capacity to decide whether to consent to anaesthesia for caesarean delivery.

Case law has recognized that 'confusion, shock, fatigue, pain or drugs' may temporarily incapacitate a woman in labour.[39] All practising obstetric anaesthetists will be familiar with the scenario of a deeply distressed labouring woman who appears to care little about any risks explained to her when discussing epidural analgesia. It is difficult, however, to be certain of the point at which a woman crosses the line between capacity and incapacity. The AAGBI recognizes the existence of factors that contribute to difficulties in establishing capacity in a labouring woman. However, its stated opinion is that 'the compromise will need to be severe to incapacitate her'.[40] The very same case law that offered recognition of the compromise to capacity that these factors may cause also gave the warning that healthcare professionals caring for such women should be careful in assessing whether 'such factors are operating to such a degree that the ability to decide is absent'.[39] No guidance is given by either of these sources, however, on how one can be sure that a labouring woman still has capacity.

Recall of risks discussed during the consent process has been used as a surrogate indicator of capacity. Failure of recall is taken to indicate lack of capacity, as the second of the four necessary components of capacity testing according to the Mental Capacity Act is not met. Swan and Borshoff demonstrated poor recall of conversations during labour concerning risks associated with epidural analgesia. They suggested that consent should therefore take place antenatally, where possible, as this led to improved recall.[41] The use of written information has been demonstrated to improve recall of risks associated with epidural analgesia following consent in labour.[42] However, it is far from clear that actual recall is a valid indicator of capacity. Although Affleck and colleagues demonstrated poor recall of risks discussed during labour, it was comparable with recall by patients receiving information about a variety of medical treatments such as chemotherapy, ophthalmic and cosmetic surgery.[43] It was also demonstrated that the pain scores of the parturients had no significant impact on their levels of recall.

Other research has focused on the opinions of women who have recently had neuraxial blockade in labour about the level of disclosure of risks that they deem to be appropriate during the consent process. On the whole, many of these women appear to want an in-depth explanation about potential complications.[44,45] This might suggest that the women involved felt able to handle the information delivered to them, and to use it to make a reasoned decision. Jackson and colleagues asked 38 women to assess whether they had met the Mental Capacity Act's four components of capacity at the time of their decision during labour to have an epidural.[46] Over 80% of the women felt that they could 'completely agree' that they were able to communicate a decision regarding epidural analgesia but less than 30% completely agreed that they could retain information. The implication of this is that by lacking one or more of the four components constituting capacity, fewer than 30% of these women deemed themselves to have capacity (according to the Act) at the time of their decision, although a high proportion of women were still satisfied with the consent process. Once again, recall appears to be an important sticking point in deciding whether labouring women have capacity. The Mental Capacity Act does not stipulate the duration of recall necessary to demonstrate capacity, just that 'The fact that a person is able to retain the information relevant to a decision for a short period only does not prevent him from being regarded as able to make the decision'.[37] Failure to recall details of the consent process after the event should not, therefore, necessarily lead to the assumption that the woman lacked capacity at the time of decision-making. The Act requires clinicians to take into account the wishes and preferences of an incapacitous patient and to involve her in decision-making processes to the best of her ability. Therefore anaesthetists should still attempt to explain risks and benefits as far as possible to all women in labour, even those considered to have borderline capacity.

There is a lack of conclusive research to define satisfactorily a 'cut-off' at which women can be deemed as having lost capacity as a result of factors associated with labour. Perhaps the fact that a request for epidural analgesia when experiencing severe labour pains seems so reasonable that the question of whether the mother has strict legal capacity is not always addressed. Likewise, if obstetricians recommend an urgent caesarean delivery for the sake of the baby's well-being, the woman's capacity to give consent is less likely to be called into question if she acquiesces to the recommendation. Whilst the law reminds clinicians that an individual should not be deemed to lack capacity purely because her decision seems unreasonable,[48] it might seem that the opposite is true: we are ready to accept a woman as capacitous if she agrees with our recommendations. However, it should also be remembered that capacity is a decision-specific assessment. In the circumstances of a much-wanted baby's life being (potentially) at risk, a woman may retain the information regarding the risks and benefits of anaesthesia and surgical delivery for as long as it takes her to agree to this course of action. This process might require just a few seconds—the fact that she does not retain the information any longer than this should not necessarily lead to the conclusion that she lacks competence. Difficulty arises, however, when a birth plan (a form of Advance Decision) exists that has been made at a time when a woman supposedly has full capacity. Can a woman in the throes of labour request or accede to an intervention that she has previously expressly refused?

The NHS Choices website describes birth plans as 'a record of what you would like to happen during your labour and after the birth', and advises women that they should consider their wishes concerning pain relief, place and mode of delivery, and care of the baby after birth before writing one.[48] However, it reminds mothers of the 'need to be flexible and prepared to do things differently from your birth plan if complications arise with you or your baby'.

The AAGBI stresses the importance of providing information regarding anaesthesia and analgesia antenatally.[40] It may be considered that women are more able to make truly capacitous decisions about their future care at a time when their recall has been shown to be better and they are not compromised by pain, fear, fatigue, and drugs. Birth plans might therefore be viewed to represent the truly autonomous decisions of a woman about her labour. One aspect of informed consent is, however, lacking in the antenatal period. Until a woman is in labour, she has no personal experience of the pain associated with it.[49] Further, until there is evidence of fetal compromise, she has no true ability to evaluate the pros and cons of expediting delivery, for example, through the use of forceps. She therefore lacks the necessary information with which to make a valid decision.

In the event of loss of capacity in labour, a birth plan should be regarded as representing a form of Advance Decision.[40] However, birth plans vary greatly: although some are very detailed and specific about a woman's wishes, others contain merely a few statements regarding what her ideal labour would entail, and would not meet the criteria for a binding Advance Decision. It is quite possible that the woman did not intend her birth plan to be used as an Advance Decision—indeed, if she had read the guidance from the NHS Choices website she may not have been aware of the legal implications of writing such a plan. Where a woman has lost capacity, birth plans that have not been written in a manner to satisfy the requirements of an Advance Decision should be regarded as evidence of the woman's values and wishes, to be taken into account as far as possible when making decisions based on a best interests assessment.[37]

If following a birth plan entails a significant risk to the life of the mother, the plan must have been signed and witnessed and must state clearly that she would prefer death to whatever treatment has been refused. If there is risk to the baby's life then the plan must be specific enough to have included this eventuality. If it is considered that any of the circumstances of the situation could not have been reasonably anticipated by the woman at the time of writing the birth plan, this may also invalidate it for use as an Advance Decision. Obviously, no Advance Decision comes into force until its author loses capacity and so a woman who consents to treatments in labour that she had previously excluded in her birth plan is fully at liberty to change her mind in this manner so long as she has the capacity to do so.

The obstetric anaesthetist may occasionally face a birth plan in which a woman attempts to dictate her future care even if she changes her mind once in labour (the so-called Ulysses Directive).[50] A woman may state, for example, that she does not want to have epidural analgesia even if, once in labour, she begs for this method of pain relief. If written clearly, signed, and witnessed, such a directive would have the same legal footing as any other Advance Decision. However, for it to take effect, the woman must lose capacity. If she still retains capacity, then she is able to change her mind. In such circumstances, it is imperative to ensure a very thorough discussion of risks and benefits of epidural analgesia with the woman, involving her midwife and birth partner if permitted. In this way, the anaesthetist can clarify that the woman remains capacitous and that she appreciates the consequences of the decision she is currently making. This conversation should, of course, be fully documented and the AAGBI suggests that the woman should countersign the entry in the notes.[40] A woman who has been unable to meet the expectations she has made of herself in a birth plan may be upset and frustrated postnatally, and resentful of the healthcare professionals who aided her 'labouring self' to defy the wishes of her 'antenatal self'. A debrief with the woman after analgesia has been established and again after birth may help the woman reconcile the events that have occured.[50] Ideally, a woman should not even start labour without a discussion regarding the implications and limitations of a birth plan for directing future care.

Voluntariness and consent

After provision of information and capacity, the third component of valid consent is freedom from coercion. Sources of coercion that may apply to a labouring woman are her birth partner, the father of her baby, other family members, healthcare professionals, and other paid providers of maternity care such as doulas. It is important to remember the inequality in 'power' that exists between a woman in labour and the healthcare team that attend her. The healthcare team are in a familiar environment, have extensive knowledge, may be under pressure of time, may arrive in groups to see her, may remain standing, may use unfamiliar terminology, and will know the patient's name and medical details. In contrast, the labouring woman is in an unfamiliar environment, may be minimally clothed, may have little knowledge of the events that are unfolding, may be in pain or fear and may not comprehend the roles or know the names of the staff. The resolution of this disparity is more of an ethical than a legal debate and so beyond the scope of this chapter.[51] Suffice to say here that all staff should be aware of these factors and their influence on a woman's decision-making.

A woman may have spoken extensively to others concerning her wishes for labour, utilizing such discussions in the same manner as some women use birth plans.[50] In the event of her changing her mind, these individuals may attempt to exert influence on the woman in order to keep her to her prearranged plans.[50] However, a woman who retains capacity in labour is free to make her own decisions and healthcare professionals must make sure that such decisions are voluntary. In order to ensure voluntariness, the obstetric anaesthetist may need to speak alone with a labouring woman. The anaesthetist has a duty to voice any concerns that the opinion of others is interfering with the patient's right to decide her own medical management. Ultimately, consultation with the hospital legal team may be required in order to help manage a particularly persistent and intrusive third person.

Case law has demonstrated that the judiciary is prepared to find consent (or refusal of consent) invalid if it is believed that there has been excessive influence on a patient from other sources. *Re T* concerned a young woman, 34 weeks pregnant, involved in a road traffic accident.[47] She developed pneumonia and was admitted to hospital. Her condition necessitated the administration of oxygen and the use of pethidine for pain control. That night, T went into labour and a decision was made that delivery by caesarean delivery was necessary, so she was transferred to an obstetric unit. T was not a Jehovah's Witness but her mother was. During a visit from her mother, T informed a nurse that she would not accept blood products. She later stated the same to a doctor. A midwife produced a refusal form, which T signed without further discussion or clarification. After caesarean delivery of a stillborn baby, T's condition deteriorated due to a lung abscess and she was admitted to intensive care. Blood transfusion was deemed necessary but withheld because of T's documented refusal. T's father and boyfriend made a successful court application to authorize blood transfusion, arguing that T had been coerced by her mother.

There were many factors that compromised T's ability to make a valid refusal of treatment. Lord Donaldson praised her boyfriend and father for their application but stated that the hospital authorities should have taken the initiative the previous day. T was critically ill, she had a condition requiring oxygen, she had pain necessitating the use of pethidine, and she was in early labour following a car accident. In this condition, she might have been unduly receptive to her mother's religious beliefs. After her verbal refusal of consent, T signed a form refusing transfusion without further discussion of the consequences of such an action. T's refusal was therefore considered by the court to be invalid.

Enforced caesarean delivery

The topic of decision-making in labour would not be complete without a discussion of enforced caesarean delivery. Although the case of T, discussed above, revolved around overriding a woman's refusal of consent as it was deemed to be invalid, Lord Donaldson made some important statements concerning the right to refuse treatment when he made his judgment. He stated that a competent adult had the right to choose to accept or to refuse treatment, regardless of whether her reasons were 'rational, irrational, unknown or even non-existent'.[47] *Re T* set the benchmark of an adult's right to refuse treatment, even if this will lead to certain death.[24] However, Lord Donaldson made an important caveat to this right: that where a woman's decision to refuse treatment might 'lead to the death of a viable fetus.'[47]

The decision in *Re S* followed the precedent set by Lord Donaldson.[52] S was in obstructed labour with a baby in a transverse lie and an elbow presentation. She refused caesarean delivery due to her religious beliefs. A very brief court hearing (at which S was not represented) did not analyse whether S had capacity, but followed directly the precedent set in *Re T* and authorized a caesarean delivery against the woman's wishes. A number of similar cases followed.[53,54]

Re MB broke the established trend.[39] The case concerned a needle-phobic woman who was advised to have a caesarean delivery after going into labour at term with a footling breech baby. She consented to the operation and wanted her baby to be born alive but refused to have an anaesthetic that involved her feeling a needle. The Court determined that although MB would usually have capacity to make decisions by herself, her fear of needles had temporarily incapacitated her. In the judgment of the Court of Appeal, it was made clear that the interests of the fetus should play no part in a decision to force a woman to undergo a caesarean delivery against her will. In this manner, a new precedent was set that directly contradicted that made by Lord Donaldson in *Re T*. A decision based on the best interests of an incompetent woman should consider the woman's desire to have a healthy, live baby, but should not consider this from the point of view of the baby. No competent woman should be forced to have a caesarean delivery against her will.

It may be difficult, however, for medical staff to watch a woman make decisions that compromise not only her own life but also that of a viable fetus. The doctors caring for S (a different S from that referred to previously) seem to have been desperate to prove that she was incompetent in order to deliver her baby by caesarean delivery against her will. S was diagnosed with pre-eclampsia at 36 weeks' gestation.[55] She refused admission for induction despite acknowledging that her decisions might result in the death of herself and her baby. She preferred to allow nature to take its course and stated that she did not want the baby anyway. S was compulsorily admitted to a psychiatric hospital under an assessment order from which she was transferred to the delivery suite of a neighbouring hospital against her will. A court order authorizing urgent caesarean delivery was granted on the premise that S was incompetent to refuse.

This decision to permit a caesarean delivery against the wishes of S was overturned at appeal, after delivery of the baby. The Court of Appeal reiterated that no competent woman should be forced to have a caesarean delivery against her will. The fact that S had been detained under the Mental Health Act did not equate to her being incompetent to make her own decisions. Furthermore, it was determined that her doctors would not have detained S if she had not been suffering from pre-eclampsia—it was a medical rather than a psychiatric problem that caused the doctors so much concern. S was not represented in the initial hearing and so did not have the opportunity to demonstrate her capacity to the Court. If she had been, she may have convinced them in a statement that she wrote for the doctors to explain her reasoning for refusing consent for caesarean delivery. In this statement, she clearly demonstrated that she understood the risks involved in refusing a caesarean delivery, had retained the information, weighed it up, and had reached a decision that she was capable of communicating back to her doctors.[55]

The Court reiterated that a fetus has no separate legal personality from its mother and thus its health and well-being cannot take precedence over the mother's rights, including the right to refuse treatment, however 'morally repugnant' that decision may be.[55]

The Court issued guidelines about how to handle future cases.[55] These guidelines state that no court will sanction a forced caesarean delivery on a competent woman. Where a competent woman refuses consent, written notes detailing discussions with the patient should be made and a signed refusal of treatment by the patient requested. Furthermore, the requirement was made that, in future, the woman who was the focus of the case should be legally represented in order that her opinions and evidence of her capacity be made known to the court. Only cases where there is uncertainty about a woman's capacity should be referred to the courts.

The case concerning O demonstrates the current position of case law on the subject of enforced caesarean delivery. O suffered from panic attacks that prevented her from being able to submit to a caesarean delivery. Her doctors believed that the panic attacks were sufficiently disabling as to incapacitate O temporarily. A court application was made to seek authority for an operative delivery against O's wishes. The judge who heard the case ensured that O had the opportunity to have legal representation and spoke directly to O. In this conversation, it was ascertained that O wanted to have the operation and did not wish to cause harm to herself or her baby. O had the insight to recognize that her panic attacks were preventing her from exercising her autonomous decision. The court therefore authorized the hospital to perform a caesarean delivery for O on the basis that she was temporarily incapacitated by panic attacks.[56]

The message is therefore clear: even if there is a risk of harm or death to a full-term fetus, medical staff are not permitted to override the refusal of consent of a capacitous woman. If, however, there are concerns about the woman's capacity then an application should be made to the courts for adjudication. The woman must be given the opportunity of representation in order that her views are heard. In the event that any delay is likely to result in serious morbidity or death, senior doctors in conjunction with a senior midwife should document the reasons why they believe that the woman lacks the capacity to refuse. The involvement of the hospital legal team should take place in parallel.

Legal rights of a fetus

Once born, healthcare staff are obliged to provide their very best care to the baby and yet the above-mentioned cases demonstrate that whilst it remains *in utero*, their ability to provide it with care depends on the permission of the mother. It can be difficult to comprehend how the 'location' of the baby has such a profound impact on its legal status.

The moral worth of a fetus

There is no universal ethical agreement on the point at which a fetus should be attributed the same moral status as a baby or an adult human and so be offered the same protection and rights. Being genetically human may be seen as the crucial factor, and this would imply that full moral status is achieved at the time of conception.[57] Another view is that no moral rights can be attributed to the cell mass that results from conception until after set time periods, before which it cannot be certain that conception will result in the development of a unique human individual,[58] or even until after birth. Further arguments revolve around the absence or presence of sentience, the definition of 'personhood', and the concept of 'potentiality'.[59]

This brief paragraph gives just a hint of the debate that has vexed ethicists, legal experts, religious and healthcare groups, and lay people for years. Even if unanimous conclusions could be reached concerning the point at which moral protection should be afforded to human life, there remains one more important issue: the rights of the woman in whom the new life is developing. If human life is given moral (and subsequently legal) rights antenatally, there will be occasions when these rights conflict with the woman's rights to bodily autonomy. It is on the background of these enormous ethical conundrums that inconsistencies in the approach of the law to the status of the fetus have developed.

Abortion

Some form of protection of fetal life has existed in statutory law for many years. The Offences Against the Person Act 1861 made it a criminal offence for a woman to induce abortion in herself or for any other person to assist her in this process.[60] No statutory exceptions were made to this rule, although case law established that a doctor who performed an abortion in order to save the life of the mother would not be convicted of a criminal offence.[61] This exception was put on a statutory footing with the Infant Life (Preservation) Act 1929. To cause the death of a fetus that was capable of life independent from its mother (certainly from 28 weeks' gestation onwards, earlier if the prosecution could offer evidence to support their case) could result in a conviction for child destruction.

The Abortion Act of 1967 sought to clarify the law regarding when termination could be legal. According to the original statute, abortion is permissible if two doctors are in agreement that the circumstances satisfy one of two situations: that continuation of the pregnancy would result in injury to the woman's physical or mental health or that of her existing children greater than if termination occurred; or that there was a substantial risk of the baby being born with a serious mental or physical handicap. The provisions of the Infant Life Preservation Act remained and hence the 28-week limit for terminations.

The Abortion Act has since been amended by section 37 of the Human Fertilisation and Embryology Act 1990, with a reduction in the time limit on terminations on the grounds of injury to the mother's physical or mental health or that of her existing children to 24 weeks (in line with advances in survival of preterm infants). A termination is permissible at any gestation in order to prevent death of the mother, as previously, and now also at any point if there is a 'substantial risk' that the pregnancy will result in a child with mental or physical abnormalities causing it to be 'seriously handicapped'.[62] It has been noted that this Act has created an inequality in rights accorded to fetuses: a baby capable of life independent from its mother may now lawfully be killed, but only if it is disabled.[63] The extent of disability necessary for a termination to take place on these grounds has been extensively debated as the wording of the statute, like that of any other, is open to interpretation. A case was brought against West Mercia Police for their failure to investigate doctors who had permitted a termination at 28 weeks because the fetus had bilateral cleft lip and palate.[64] The Crown Prosecution Service, after hearing the evidence, decided that the doctors had acted appropriately, thus setting a precedent in case law for what may constitute being 'seriously handicapped'.

Antenatal harm

The Congenital Disabilities (Civil Liability) Act 1976 is a route of redress for any child born disabled as a result of events (including medical treatment) that occurred pre-conception, during pregnancy or at the time of birth. For a claim to be successful, it must be demonstrated that the person who caused the damage failed in their duty of care to the child's parent, even if they did not cause actual or visible harm to the parent. The Act is complicated and requires proof that the disability has come about as a direct consequence of a specific occurrence for which an identifiable individual or individuals are responsible. It may be difficult for a claimant to achieve this level of proof.

Similarly, a criminal case can be brought against an individual who causes antenatal harm to a fetus that results in the subsequent death of the baby or child. A man who stabbed his pregnant girlfriend causing damage to their fetus and its premature birth was convicted of manslaughter when the baby eventually died as a consequence.[65] The Law Lords confirmed that a charge of murder might also be brought in similar circumstances if the level of intent required to prove a case of murder was present. However, they affirmed that if the baby was stillborn as a result of such actions, there would be no case of murder or manslaughter to answer: the baby must be born alive in order to achieve the legal personality necessary to become the victim of either murder or manslaughter.

The duties of a mother

Under the terms of The Congenital Disabilities Act, a child damaged by antenatal events can bring a case in negligence against the individual who caused the damage. The one exception to this is the mother (unless the harm is caused by the mother's negligent driving).[66] Whilst a mother may have a moral responsibility to protect her unborn baby, an attempt to coerce her through the weight of the law (as has occurred in some states in the United States) can be counterproductive.[67] Harm may occur to a fetus before a woman knows she is pregnant. Criminalizing women for their behaviour in pregnancy is likely to require caregivers to report episodes of potential harm or face being complicit with a crime. This may result in a breakdown in the relationship of trust between a woman and the doctors and midwives caring for her. Women may therefore be less likely to seek healthcare in pregnancy in order to avoid such scrutiny, or may seek termination rather than continuance of pregnancy for fear that harm they have caused might be discovered.

The case of *Re F* demonstrated that the English courts were unwilling to use the force of the law to safeguard babies *in utero*.[68] A local authority attempted to make an unborn baby a ward of court as its mother, who suffered from mental health problems, was refusing all antenatal care. The application was refused on the basis that a fetus does not have legal personality in English law, that it would result in great practical problems, and that such an action puts the interests of the mother in direct conflict with those of the fetus.

Confidentiality

Medical confidentiality is governed extensively by legal, professional, and employer requirements. It consists of a negative obligation, not to disclose information, but also a positive obligation, to ensure information is kept secure and not accessed improperly (Table 29.2).[69] Maternal confidentiality requires unique considerations, as information is likely to have consequences for the fetus and father.

A duty to maintain confidentiality

The duty to maintain medical confidentiality derives from common law, which has typically focused on the public interest. For example, following a threat of disclosure of the identity of two general practitioners who had contracted HIV, the court decided that there was great public interest in maintaining medical confidentiality of people with HIV and AIDS in order that they should seek healthcare without fear of identification.[70] This interest, it was decided, outweighed the public interest in the freedom of the press to publish information that had been obtained improperly from hospital records. The decision turned on the balance of factors impacting on the public interest more than any privacy rights of the two doctors involved.

The Human Rights Act 1998 came into force in the United Kingdom in 2000. Article 8 offers legal protection to private information in the interests of the individual concerned, although it recognizes that disclosure is sometimes justified in the public interest.

When a breach of confidentiality has occurred, remedies in law would lie in negligence, equity and contract. The GMC[71] and the British Medical Association[72] have issued guidance to doctors reinforcing the duty of confidentiality and the courts are likely to place great emphasis on these when considering cases relating to breaches in confidence, as there is limited case law in this area. Negligence would require proof of harm and this tends to

Table 29.2 Challenges to maintaining confidentiality

Challenge	Example
Clinical details discussed in public settings	Curtains around bedspaces, conversations in corridors
Medical information shared with non-medical personnel (although it should be noted that these individuals have a common law duty to maintain confidentiality)[82]	Administrative staff, audit, clinical governance, adverse event analysis, chaplains, work experience students
Clinical information visible to members of public	Patient boards with detailed patient information, electronic check-in systems, openly accessible research
Portability of information	Laptops, smartphones, electronic medical records, memory sticks
Increasing subspecialization	Increased number of professionals requiring access to an individual patient's information, cross-site working with possibility for loss of patient records
Social media	Discussion of patients online
Clinical information requested by non-medical agencies	Employers, insurers, pharmaceutical companies
Educational activities	Conferences, educational meetings, journals, professional body publications

be of a financial or physical nature rather than embarrassment. Breach of contract could be applicable with private patients but no contract exists between an NHS patient and doctor. However, the NHS doctor could be found in breach of his employment contract and professional obligations, and face disciplinary proceedings from both their employer and the GMC. Claims in equity are most likely to be sought. Equitable obligations of confidence require that the information disclosed was confidential in nature and was shared in a relationship of confidence. Legal claims for alleged breach of medical confidentiality are unusual due to the difficulty in satisfying legal requirements in negligence.

A duty to disclose

The ethical duty to maintain confidentiality is not absolute and, in certain circumstances, the adverse consequences of maintaining confidentiality may override the individual patient's right to confidentiality. There are a number of situations where statutory law requires disclosure of patient information to certain authorities (Table 29.3) and situations where judgement must be used by the clinician.

The law permits disclosure where the public interest in disclosure outweighs the public interest for patients to trust their doctors.[73] Legally, information may only be disclosed if the clinician perceives there to be a real threat posed by maintaining confidentiality. Only the minimal information necessary should be disclosed and only to those with a legitimate interest.

HIV is not a notifiable disease but, in the context of maternal HIV infection, disclosure may be justifiable. Wherever possible the patient should be encouraged to share this information. However, if the patient refuses, the potential risk to the partner must be balanced against the harms to the mother. The GMC advises that, where disclosure of patient information is to take place, the patient should be informed in advance of this if it is considered possible and safe. Referral to such guidelines is essential as the courts are likely to be guided by these in the event of litigation. It is also important to seek advice from the trust legal team, Caldicott Guardian, and professional defence organizations. Ultimately, however, it is the clinician's responsibility to ensure that there are valid ethical reasons for the disclosure.

Case law has also considered occasions where a doctor might have had a duty to disclose confidential information but did not do so. For a case in negligence to be successful, the victim of harm must be someone who could reasonably have been identified as being at risk. In this manner, a duty of care (or duty to warn) is established. In *Palmer*, a health authority successfully defended itself against a claim of negligence for not acting to prevent a patient with a psychiatric disorder from committing murder, on the grounds that it did not owe a duty of care to the subsequent victim who could not have been identified in advance.[74] However, a NHS trust has accepted liability and a duty of care towards the family of a psychiatric patient who, upon release, killed his mother and himself.[75]

Table 29.3 Legally permitted breaches of confidentiality

Disclosure is mandatory	The Public Health (Control of Diseases) Act 1984
	The Births and Deaths Registration Act 1953
	The Road Traffic Accident Act 1988
	The Prevention of Terrorism Act 2005
Disclosure may be justifiable	Through patient consent
	In the public interest: ◆ Information to ensure functioning of public bodies such as the GMC ◆ Disclosure to avoid harm to the public generally or to an identifiable individual

Access to medical records

The Data Protection Act 1998 governs the processing of medical records of living persons. It applies to both manual and electronic records and the key principles relate to ensuring fair and lawful storage, handling and use.[76] Patients can apply to the courts if the terms of the Act are not met but would need to prove that harm had occurred in order to succeed in a case in negligence. Patients can apply to have access to their own medical records provided disclosure does not reveal information about a third party and will not cause serious harm to the patient or a third party.

The Access to Medical Reports Act 1988 gives individuals the right to obtain medical reports prepared for third parties (such as insurance companies or employers) before their release and the right to prevent release.

In the context of maternal confidentiality, it is common for partners to request medical information and refusal of disclosure may upset the patient and partner. GMC guidance is to obtain patient consent and discuss what information the patient would like to be shared, particularly if she is likely to lose capacity.[71]

Research, audit, teaching and publication

Secondary uses of patient information may be essential to providing effective, safe and efficient clinical care. There is a balance between the obligation to protect an individual's right to privacy and the implications of this in areas including audit, research and public health, which may be in the public interest. The National Health Service Act 2006 section 251(1) permits disclosure of medical information without patient consent for these secondary uses, but requests are conditional on fulfilling certain criteria and are overseen by the National Information Governance Board for Health and Social Care. It must be shown that disclosure is necessary, consent is not practical or possible and the data are to be used in the interests of the public and patients.

The GMC states that when using information for secondary purposes, information should be anonymized wherever possible or express permission from the patient sought.[71] Before using patient information without prior consent, one should consider the nature of the information, the purpose and extent of disclosure, the adequacy of safeguards limiting disclosure, the advice of a Caldicott Guardian who is not involved with the secondary use, and the potential harms to the individual patient.

Confidentiality and patients lacking capacity

The duty of confidentiality relating to minors is complex. Those aged 16 or over are presumed to have capacity and should be entitled to the same duty of confidentiality as capacitous adults. For those aged 15 years or under, professional discretion is required if the child refuses consent for sharing of information with those who have parental responsibility. This situation is unusual but considerations should include the competence of the child (her understanding of the implications of disclosure or non-disclosure), the promotion of the child's welfare, and the harms and benefits of disclosure. The balancing of these factors should be undertaken in much the same manner as when deciding whether a child is sufficiently mature to give consent for her own medical treatment. Ultimately, if the clinician believes that the child's best interests are served by sharing information, this is permissible even if against the child's wishes. Doctors are obliged to communicate concerns regarding child abuse to the relevant authorities even if the child concerned has asked for the information to be kept confidential.[77]

In the case of incapacity, the key legal principle is to act in the best interests of the patient. It is generally justifiable to disclose information if it is necessary for the care of the patient. The GMC recognizes the potential 'need to share personal information with a patient's relatives, friends or carers to enable you to assess the patient's best interests ... that does not mean they have a general right of access to the patient's records or to have irrelevant information about, for example, the patient's past healthcare'.[71]

The legal[78] and professional duty of confidentiality persists after death although this is not absolute. It is generally in the public interest that confidentiality of current patients is maintained following death. The GMC guidance relating to disclosure following death requires consideration of the wishes of the patient, the harms and benefits to the patient's family, whether disclosure will reveal information about the patient's family or a third party, and the purpose of the disclosure.[71]

In summary, the duty of confidentiality is not absolute. The predominant legal basis is that of public interest and the fair use of information. Sharing of information is recognized as necessary for clinical care. In situations where disclosure is necessary, the amount of information and the number of recipients should be kept to a minimum. Professional guidelines should be consulted as legal judgements are likely to refer to these in assessing the validity of a practitioner's reasons for disclosure.

Teaching

The postgraduate training of a doctor is a complex mixture of academic learning, independent delivery of care, and apprenticeship-style training. In line with the increased awareness and respect of patient autonomy by the medical profession, non-consensual examination and unnecessary procedures purely for the purposes of training are not acceptable. There is very little case law concerning medical training, and standards are derived mostly from professional guidelines. Patients should be viewed as part of a three-way partnership of learning, along with the trainer and trainee. It may be argued that the patient has a moral duty to contribute to the education of junior doctors as they have themselves benefitted from the care of fully trained doctors who have learnt their skills through the involvement of previous patients.

Consent and medical training

As with all other aspects of patient care, the importance of consent cannot be over-emphasized. The GMC stipulates that patients must be informed about the roles of the people involved in their care, the involvement of students, and their right to refuse to take part in teaching.[20] Department of Health guidance states that where a trainee or student undertakes a procedure (in which they are competent) for the purposes of patient care, it is not legally necessary to tell the patient that they are a trainee, although it is good practice.[79] However, if the trainee or student is planning on undertaking an assessment or examination that is purely for the purposes of their own education then it is important that this distinction is made clear to the patient.

Whilst knowledge can be learnt and some degree of development of manual skills can take place through simulation, ultimately, every doctor must perform every procedure in which they are to become competent on a patient for the first time. There is difficulty in deciding precisely how much information should be given to a patient regarding trainee involvement in a procedure. The AAGBI recognizes that most procedures have a number of components, that there are numerous learning points in the course of a single anaesthetic, and that it would be impractical to seek consent for every one of these learning points that involves a trainee anaesthetist.[40] It is also noted that every practitioner continues to learn with every procedure undertaken. The AAGBI offers the advice, however, that the trainer must assess the risks and benefits to the patient for each aspect of care that is to be delivered by a trainee. In minimizing the risks, the trainer must ensure that the trainee has adequate knowledge, has had the opportunity to make use of any appropriate simulation or skills based training, that there is close supervision and that there is clear purpose to teaching this particular trainee this particular skill (e.g. avoiding exposure of patients to the learning curve of a trainee attempting to develop a skill for which they have no longer-term need). In the case of certain procedures with definable risks, it will be necessary to gain specific, informed consent.[80]

Supervision of trainees

Adequate supervision of trainees is an important component of minimizing the risks to patients of being involved in the training of junior staff. It is difficult to define a precise cut-off between the areas of care delivered by the trainee that are service delivery and those that constitute training, since the two overlap significantly. Medical training involves permitting trainees to develop their independent practice with ever more distant supervision. It is important to remember that when care is being delivered by a trainee, there should be a nominated consultant supervising that trainee at all times.[81] Trainees should ensure that they do not act beyond the limits of their capabilities and consultants should ensure that they are readily available and contactable for advice or assistance. Difficulty arises where communication has broken down and a consultant is unaware of cases being performed by a trainee.

Trainees and the standard of care

When trainees are delivering patient care independently, it is important that the standard of care is that of a competent doctor working in the same post; inexperience will not be a sufficient defence against a claim in negligence. It is expected that trainee doctors should recognize the limits of their abilities and experience and call for assistance appropriately.[82]

Conclusion

The key aspects of case and statutory law that relate to obstetric anaesthesia, and their impact on practice, have been presented in this chapter. The role of professional guidelines is of increasing importance in setting a benchmark for standards of care, especially where precedent is absent. Medical law is greatly influenced by ethical values and reasoning in the development of guidelines, as the driving force for new statutory law and in judgements made in case law. The presence of the fetus adds a unique ethical and legal consideration in law relating to obstetrics and obstetric anaesthesia.

References

1. *Re A* (children) (conjoined twins: surgical separation) [2000] 4 All ER 961.
2. Keown J. Restoring moral and intellectual shape to the law after Bland. *Law Quarterly Review* 1997; 113: 481–503.
3. *Bartley* v *Studd* (1995) 2. *Medical Law Monitor*, 15 July 1997.
4. *Bolam* v *Friern Hospital Management Committee* [1957] 2 All ER 118.
5. *Bolitho* v *City and Hackney H.A.* [1998] A.C. 232 (H.L.).
6. *R* v *Bateman* (1925) 41 TLR 557.
7. Ruddy G. R v Southampton and fatal medical negligence: an anomaly or a sign of things to come? *Plymouth Law Review* 2010; 1:81–92.
8. *R* v *Adomako* [1994] 3 WLR 288, HL.
9. The Corporate Manslaughter and Corporate Homicide Act 2007 (c19) s1.
10. British Safety Council. £485,000 fine imposed in third corporate manslaughter case. 2012. [Online] https://sm.britsafe.org/%C2%A3485000-fine-imposed-third-corporate-manslaughter-case#sthash.TQlGNcZx.dpuf
11. Association of Anaesthetists of Great Britain and Ireland and Obstetric Anaesthetists' Association. *Guidelines for Obstetric Anaesthetic Services 3.* London: AAGBI; 2013.
12. Centre for Maternal and Child Enquiries and the Royal College of Obstetricians and Gynaecologists. *CMACE/RCOG Joint Guideline: Management of Women with Obesity in Pregnancy.* London: RCOG/CEMACE; 2010.
13. Grimshaw J, Freemantle N, Wallace S, *et al.* Developing and implementing clinical practice guidelines. *Qual Health Care* 1995; 4:55–64.
14. *Crawford* v *Board of Governors of Charing Cross Hospital* [1953]. *The Times* 1953:8 December.
15. Hurwitz B. Clinical guidelines: proliferation and medicolegal significance. *Qual Health Care* 1994; 3:37–44.
16. *Early* v *Newham Health Authority* [1994] 5 Med LR 214.
17. *Wickline* v *California*. Cal Repr 1986; 288:661–71.
18. *Kent* v *Griffiths* [2000] 2 All ER 474.
19. Beauchamp T, Childress J. *Principles of Biomedical Ethics.* Oxford: Oxford University Press; 2001:12.
20. General Medical Council. *Consent: Patients and Doctors Making Decisions Together.* London: General Medical Council; 2008.
21. The Royal College of Anaesthetists. *The Risks of Anaesthesia* [Online] http://www.rcoa.ac.uk/patients-and-relatives/risks
22. The Obstetric Anaesthetists' Association. *Epidural Information Card.* [website] http://www.labourpains.com/ui/content/content.aspx?id=45
23. *Chester* v *Afshar* [2004] 4 All ER 587.
24. *Re C* [1994] 1 All ER 819.
25. *B* v *NHS Hospital Trust* [2002] 2 All ER 449.
26. Department for Education. *Under-18 and Under-16 Conception Statistics.* [Online] http://www.education.gov.uk/childrenandyoungpeople/healthandwellbeing/teenagepregnancy/a0064898/under-18-and-under-16-conception-statistics
27. *Hewer* v *Bryant* [1970] 1 QB 357, at 369.
28. *Re W (A Minor) (Medical Treatment)* [1992] 4 All ER 627.
29. *Gillick* v *West Norfolk and Wisbech Area Health Authority* [1986] AC 112.
30. *Re L (medical Treatment: Gillick Competency)* [1998] 2 FLR 810.
31. General Medical Council. *0–18 Years: Guidance for Doctors.* London: General Medical Council; 2007.
32. Pearce J. Consent to treatment during childhood. *Br J Psychiatry* 1994; 165:713–16.
33. Whitworth M, Cockerill R. Antenatal management of teenage pregnancies. *Obstet Gynaecol Reprod Med* 2010; 20(11):323–8.
34. Department for Constitutional Affairs. *Mental Capacity Act 2005 Code of Practice.* London: The Stationery Office; 2007.
35. *Burke* v *United Kingdom* [2006] App 19807/06.
36. *HE* v *NHS Trust* [2003] 2 FLR 408.
37. The Mental Capacity Act 2005 (c9).
38. Taylor J. Woman with limited mental capacity can have her baby. *The Independent* 2013; 10 January. [Online] http://www.independent.co.uk/news/uk/home-news/woman-with-limited-mental-capacity-can-have-her-baby-8446477.html
39. *Re MB* [1997] 2 FLR 426.
40. Association of Anaesthetists of Great Britain and Ireland. *Consent for Anaesthesia. Revised Edition 2006.* London: Association of Anaesthetists of Great Britain and Ireland; 2006:24.
41. Swan H, Borshoff D. Informed consent—recall of risk information following epidural analgesia in labour. *Anaesth Intensive Care* 1994; 22:139–41.
42. White L, Gorton P, Wee M, *et al.* Written information for women in labour: does it improve knowledge about epidurals? *Int J Obstet Anesth* 2003; 12:93–7.
43. Affleck P, Waisel D, Cusick J, *et al.* Recall of risks following labor analgesia. *J Clin Anesth* 1998; 10:141–4.
44. Bethune L, Harper N, Lucas D, *et al.* Complications of obstetric regional analgesia: how much information is enough? *Int J Obstet Anesth* 2004; 13:30–4.
45. Kelly G, Blunt C, Moore P, *et al.* Consent for regional anaesthesia in the United Kingdom: what is material risk? *Int J Obstet Anesth* 2004; 13:71–4.
46. Jackson G, Sensky T, Reide P, *et al.* The capacity to consent to epidural analgesia in labour. *Int J Obstet Anesth* 2011; 20:269–70.
47. *Re T (adult: refusal of medical treatment)* [1992] 4 All ER 649, CA.
48. NHS Choices. *How to Make a Birth Plan.* [Online] http://www.nhs.uk/Conditions/pregnancy-and-baby/pages/how-to-make-birth-plan.aspx
49. Scott W. Ethics in obstetric anaesthesia. *Anaesthesia* 1996; 51(8):717–18.
50. Burcher P. The Ulysses contract in obstetrics: a woman's choices before and during labour. *J Med Ethics* 2013; 39:27–30.
51. Bowman D, Spicer J, Iqbal R. Voluntariness: the freedom to choose. In *Informed Consent: A Primer For Clinical Practice.* Cambridge: Cambridge University Press; 2012:56–66.
52. *Re S* [1992] 4 All ER 671.
53. *Norfolk and Norwich NHS Trust* v *W* [1996] 2 FLR 613.
54. *Tameside and Glossop Acute Services Trust* v *CH* (a patient) [1996] 1 FLR 762.
55. *St George's Healthcare NHS Trust* v *S, R V Collins and others, ex parte S* [1998] All ER 673.
56. *Bolton Hospitals NHS Trust* v O [2002] EWHC 2871.
57. Genesis 9:5–6. In *The Good News Bible.* London: Collins; 1976.
58. Jones D, Telfer B. Before I was an embryo I was a pre-embryo: or was I? *Bioethics* 1995; 9(1):32–49.
59. Harris J. *The Value of Life: An Introduction to Medical Ethics.* London: Routledge; 2002.
60. Offences Against the Person Act 1861, s58.
61. *R* v *Bourne* [1939] 1 KB 687.
62. Abortion Act 1967 (as amended by The Human Fertilisation and Embryology Act 1990), s1.
63. Brazier M, Cave E. *Medicine, Patients and the Law* (4th ed). London: Penguin; 2007:366.
64. *Jepson* v *The Chief Constable of West Mercia Police Constabulary* [2003] EWHC 3318.
65. *Attorney General's Reference (No 3 of 1994)* [1997] 3 All ER 936.
66. Congenital Disabilities (Civil Liability) Act 1976, ss1 and 2.

67. Cook M. From conception until birth: exploring the maternal duty to protect fetal health. *Wash Uni Law Q* 2002; 80:1307–40.
68. *Re F* [1989] 2 All ER 193.
69. Department of Health. *Confidentiality: NHS Code of Practice*. London: Department of Health; 2003.
70. *X* v *Y* [1988] 2 All ER 649.
71. General Medical Council. *Confidentiality: Guidance for Doctors*. London: General Medical Council; 2009.
72. British Medical Association. *Confidentiality and Disclosure of Information Toolkit*. [Online] http://www.bma.org.uk/practical-support-at-work/ethics/confidentiality-tool-kit
73. *W* v *Egdell* [1990] 1 All ER 835 CA.
74. *Palmer* v *Tees HA* [2000] PIQR 1.
75. Frean, A. Sister who saw killing wins record trauma sum. *The Times* 2001; 5 November:5.
76. Data Protection Act 1998.
77. Department of Health, Home Office, Department for Education and Employment. *Working Together to Safeguard Children: Inter-Agency Guidance to Safeguard and Promote the Welfare of Children*. London: HMSO, 2010.
78. *Nicholas Lewis* v *Secretary of State for Health & Michael Redfern* [2008] EWHC 2196 (QB).
79. Department of Health. *Reference Guide to Consent for Examination and Treatment* (2nd ed). London: Department of Health; 2009.
80. Yentis SM. The use of patients for learning and maintaining practical skills. *J R Soc Med* 2005; 98:299–302.
81. Association of Anaesthetists of Great Britain and Ireland. *Consultant: trainee Relationships: A Guide for Consultants*. London: Association of Anaesthetists of Great Britain and Ireland; 2001.
82. *Wilsher* v *Essex Area HA* 1988 AC 1074.

PART 8

Obstetric complications

CHAPTER 30

High dependency and intensive care

Philip Barclay and Helen Scholefield

Maternal critical care and recommendations from the triennial reports

The triennial Confidential Enquiries into Maternal Deaths in the United Kingdom have played a major role in the reduction of maternal mortality since the 1950s.[1] The importance of developing maternal critical care has long been recognized in reducing the significant number of deaths still associated with a substandard level of care. The 1988–90 triennial report[2] stated that every consultant obstetric unit should incorporate a properly staffed high dependency unit (HDU). The 1997–99 triennial report[3] emphasized the requirement that invasive monitoring should be available and used appropriately. The 2000–2002 report[4] focused on the need for earlier recognition of the sick parturient and to apply a higher level of care promptly before transfer to the intensive care unit (ICU). These requirements for maternal critical care formed a part of the Joint Royal Colleges Safer Childbirth document.[5]

Critical care: replacing existing divisions between the HDU and ICU

The *Comprehensive Critical Care* document published in 2000[6] reviewed adult critical care services and recommended a new approach based upon severity of illness, as it was recognized that critically ill patients should receive an equivalent level of care outside of an ICU or HDU. The existing division between high dependency and intensive care beds would then be replaced by a classification focusing on the level of care required by the individual patient, with staff numbers, skill, and expertise deployed appropriately. Four levels of care were described in *Comprehensive Critical Care* from level 0 normal ward care through to level 3 intensive care.

The original descriptions of levels of critical care excluded patient care in the delivery suite. The guidelines have since been revised and updated by the Intensive Care Society's *Level of Critical Care for Adult Patients*[7] to describe levels of critical care in terms of the type and number of organ systems requiring support (Box 30.1).

The Critical Care Information Advisory Group now agrees that these definitions can be applied to obstetrics to describe critical care given on a delivery suite.

Wheatly described specific examples of levels of care most likely to be applicable to patients on a delivery suite, which were used in the Maternal Critical Care Working Group report *Providing Equity of Critical and Maternity Care for the Critically Ill Pregnant or Recently Pregnant Woman* (Table 30.1).[8,9] For example, if a woman in labour has pre-eclampsia requiring oral labetalol with an oxytocin infusion and an epidural, that would be classified as Level 1 care. If her blood pressure control requires an intravenous infusion of labetalol with arterial monitoring, that meets the definition of basic cardiovascular support, which is Level 2 care. If she then has an eclamptic convulsion and requires a magnesium infusion to treat the eclampsia, she then requires neurological support in addition to basic cardiovascular support. Her two-organ system support now defines her as receiving Level 3 care.

The definitions of levels of care provide a standard for critical care data collection throughout the United Kingdom using the critical care minimum dataset (CCMDS), which now includes a specific code for obstetrics area [CRITICAL CARE LOCATION 07].[10] This is useful to capture activity where Level 2 and Level 3 care is delivered outside of a critical care environment. It can also be used

Box 30.1 Levels of critical care

Level 0

Care needs met on normal ward.

Level 1

At risk of their condition deteriorating or recently stepped down from higher level.

Care needs can be met on acute ward with additional support from critical care team (outreach).

Level 2

Detailed observation or intervention required, including single-organ support or postoperative care and step-down from level 3.

Level 3

Advanced respiratory support alone.

Or

Basic respiratory support plus at least two-organ system failure. Includes all complex patients requiring support for multi-organ failure.

Courtesy of The Intensive Care Society. *Levels of Critical Care for Adult Patients*. London: Intensive Care Society, 2009.

Table 30.1 Maternity examples of levels of care

Level of care	Maternity example
Level 0: normal ward care	Care of low-risk mother
Level 1: additional monitoring or intervention, or step down from higher level of care	Risk of haemorrhage: oxytocin infusion Blood pressure control: mild pre-eclampsia on oral antihypertensives/fluid restriction etc. Coexisting medical conditions: woman with medical condition such as congenital heart disease, diabetic on insulin infusion
Level 2: single-organ support	*Basic respiratory support (BRS):* 50% or more oxygen via facemask to maintain oxygen saturation Continuous positive airway pressure (CPAP), bi-level positive airway pressure (BIPAP) *Basic cardiovascular support (BCVS):* Intravenous antihypertensives, to control blood pressure in pre-eclampsia Arterial line used for pressure monitoring or sampling CVP line used for fluid management and CVP monitoring to guide therapy *Advanced cardiovascular support (ACVS):* Simultaneous use of at least two intravenous, antiarrhythmic/anti- hypertensive/vasoactive drugs, one of which must be a vasoactive drug Need to measure and treat cardiac output *Neurological support:* Magnesium infusion to control seizures (not prophylaxis) Intracranial pressure monitoring Hepatic support Management of acute fulminant hepatic failure, e.g. from HELLP syndrome or acute fatty liver, such that transplantation is being considered
Level 3: advanced respiratory support alone, or support of two or more organ systems above	*Advanced respiratory support:* Invasive mechanical ventilation *Support of two or more organ systems:* Renal support and BRS BRS/BCVS[a] and an additional organ supported

[a]BRS and BCVS occurring simultaneously during the episode count as a single organ support.

Reproduced here with permission from The Royal College of Anaesthetists. Originally published in *Providing equity of critical and maternity care for the critically ill pregnant or recently pregnant woman*, July 2011. Adapted from *International Journal of Obstetric Anesthesia*, Volume 19, issue 4 S. Wheatly, Maternal critical care: what's in a name?, pp. 353–355, Copyright (2010), with permission from Elsevier.

for funding, providing that the local critical care network accepts that care given is of an appropriate standard in terms of facilities, staff training, and competency.

How many parturients require Level 3 critical care?

Escalation and transfer to Level 3 care is a well-defined and documented event but only a very small proportion of obstetric patients go to an ICU.[11] In our own hospital, between July 2004 and November 2008, 18 of 35,276 parturients were transferred for Level 3 care: 0.51/1000 deliveries. Larger-scale audits at a regional or national scale are therefore required to produce descriptive and comparative statistics that will help us understand Level 3 intensive care requirements in this population.

Hazelgrove et al.[12] examined obstetric admissions to 14 ICUs in Southern England over a 3-year period between 1994 and 1996. There were 210 women admitted, representing 1.8% of all ICU admissions, although this varied from 0.18% to 3.18% in individual ICUs. The ICU admission rate was 1.7/1000 deliveries. The overall mortality rate for those admitted to ICU was 3.3%, with seven maternal deaths.

The main reasons for admission to the ICU were complications of hypertensive disease of pregnancy, including HELLP (haemolysis, elevated liver enzyme levels, and low platelet count) syndrome (39.5%) and major haemorrhage (33.3%). The median duration of stay on the ICU was 1 day. Seven patients were transferred from general ICUs to specialist ICUs for neurological, renal, liver, and respiratory support. Forty-five per cent of patients required intermittent positive pressure ventilation, 20% needed cardiovascular support with inotropes, 13% had pulmonary artery catheters for haemodynamic monitoring, and 3% required renal support with continuous veno-venous haemofiltration.

In 35% of patients, no ICU interventions were required and their length of stay was less than 2 days. This was more likely in those admitted with pre-eclampsia (48%) and emphasized the need to develop high dependency facilities on the delivery suite as only 50% of the patients met the criteria for Level 3 care. This would have reduced their ICU admission rate down to 0.85/1000 deliveries.

Mirghani et al.[13] examined all obstetric patients admitted to the ICU at Al-Ain hospital, Al-Ain, United Arab Emirates over a 6-year period from 1997 to 2002. Of 23,383 deliveries, 60 were admitted to the ICU, a rate of 2.6/1000 deliveries. This represented 2.4% of all ICU admissions over this period. The main reason for admission was haemorrhage (28.4%) and pre-eclampsia (25%) whilst 31.8% were admitted due to severe pre-existing medical problems including cardiovascular disease, diabetes, asthma, and chronic renal failure. There were two deaths (3.3% of all obstetric ICU admissions); one due to cerebral malaria associated with acute respiratory distress syndrome and another with suspected aspiration after a general anaesthetic for placental abruption. There were no HDU facilities available on the delivery suite of that hospital. On retrospective review of illness severity, only 47% met the criteria for Level 3 ICU care, a similar finding to that of Hazelgrove et al.[12]

The largest reported series of obstetric admissions to ICU is from the Intensive Care National Audit and Research Centre (ICNARC) Case Mix Programme, which audited all admissions in England, Wales, and Northern Ireland between 1995 and 2003.[14] Of 219,468 admissions to 159 critical care units, 1452 (0.7%) had a direct obstetric cause. An additional group of 450 (0.2%) pregnant women had a coincidental reason for their ICU admission. The main direct obstetric reasons for admission are outlined in Table 30.2—33% were due to haemorrhage and 38% due to hypertensive disorders of pregnancy.

The reasons for indirect admission were far more varied, with a total of 115 different primary reasons. The commonest reasons are shown in Table 30.3.

Table 30.2 Incidence of obstetric conditions as a direct cause of admission to ICU

Obstetric cause of direct admission	Admissions (%)	Mortality (%)
Peripartum or postpartum haemorrhage	29.1	0.6
Pre-eclampsia	18.2	2
HELLP syndrome	12.6	2.6
Eclampsia	7.4	3.5
Ectopic pregnancy	5.5	1
Intrauterine death	5	6.3
Antepartum haemorrhage	3.7	7.3
Infected retained products of conception	1.4	3.8
Amniotic fluid embolus	1.2	9.1
Septic abortion	0.9	11.1
Amnionitis	0.4	16.7
Molar pregnancy	0.2	25

The median length of stay on the ICU was 1.1 days for direct and 1.5 for coincidental admissions. The overall mortality rate for direct obstetric admissions was 2.2% compared with 6% for coincidental obstetric admissions and 19.6% for all non-obstetric female admissions in the 16–50 years age group. The lower mortality seen in the obstetric group was attributed to the lower admission threshold to ICU, change in maternal physiology, pregnancy identifying a group of patients with better health status, and the self-limiting nature of most obstetric pathology, given timely supportive care.

The ICNARC dataset specification was updated in 2006 to incorporate a number of obstetric-related fields. A further study was then carried out of all ICU admissions from 1 January to 31 December 2007 who were currently or recently pregnant.[15] Of the 38,461 admissions to the 107 ICUs who participated, 95 women were currently and 418 were recently pregnant. This was extrapolated to all 240 ICUs and compared with national pregnancy statistics, making an admission rate of 2.6/1000 deliveries. This compares with a maternal death rate in the 2006 to 2008 triennium of 0.11/1000.[16]

Of those who were currently pregnant, only 13.7% had an obstetric reason for admission, of which ectopic pregnancy, amnionitis, and pre-eclampsia were the most frequent. The commonest non-obstetric indication for admission was respiratory failure (35%), with 20% due to pneumonia and 7% due to asthma.

By contrast, 72% of those who were 'recently pregnant' had an obstetric indication for ICU admission. Peri- and postpartum haemorrhage was the commonest reason (34%) followed by hypertensive disorders of pregnancy (9%).

Table 30.3 Most common primary reasons for admission to ICU for indirect or coincidental obstetric admissions

Commonest causes of coincidental admission	Admissions (%)
Pneumonia (bacterial and 'no organism isolated')	5.1
Status epilepticus or uncontrolled seizures	4.2
Asthma attack in new or known asthmatic	3.6
Septic shock	3.6
Non-cardiogenic pulmonary oedema (ARDS)	2.4
Anaphylaxis	2.2
Pulmonary embolus (thrombus)	2.2
Septicaemia	2
Acute kidney injury, other cause	1.6
Hypovolaemic shock	1.6
Pelvic infection or abscess	1.6

Zwart et al.[17] found a similar rate of ICU admission at 2.4/1000 deliveries in the Netherlands, with a maternal mortality rate of 3.5%.

A systematic review by Pollock et al.[18] examined 40 studies published between 1990 and 2008 that covered a total of 7887 pregnant and postpartum admissions to ICUs around the world; 60% of the studies were from developed countries. The median admission rate was 2.7/1000 deliveries (interquartile range (IQR) 1.9 to 5.4). The majority of admissions were for obstetric reasons (1.9/1000). The commonest obstetric reasons for admission were hypertensive disorders of pregnancy (0.9/1000), obstetric haemorrhage (0.7/1000), and sepsis (0.2/1000). Only 25 out of 40 studies reported whether the patients were currently pregnant on admission to ICU, with a median value of 16%.

There were no differences between developed and developing countries in their overall rates of ICU admission (3.0 vs 2.7) or the reasons for admission. There was a significant difference in maternal death rates on ICU (3.4% (IQR 0–18.4) vs 14.0% (IQR 0–14.0)) respectively and severity of illness scores on admission.

How many women require high dependency care?

The maternal death rate (0.11/1000) and ICU admission rate (2.6/1000) are well defined with unequivocal end points but there is a further subset of women who develop severe illness during their pregnancy and require high dependency care.

Mantel et al.[19] looked at the progression from maternal health through to critical illness. He defined a maternal 'near miss' as a very ill parturient who would have died if her condition had not been diagnosed and she received appropriate treatment which prevented her progression to organ failure and then death at any point during pregnancy or in the first 6 weeks after delivery/termination (Table 30.4).

They applied this to a prospective audit of 13,429 deliveries in the Pretoria health region, South Africa, during 1 year. There were 147 near misses (1.1%) and 30 deaths. They found that hypovolaemia was the commonest organ dysfunction in patients with near miss (37%), whereas respiratory (53%) and renal (30%) failure were commonest in those who died. Mantel's criteria for near miss have the advantage of being both objective and readily applicable in a district general hospital.

Table 30.4 Mantel's criteria for maternal 'near miss'

	Markers
Organ system-based	
1. Cardiac dysfunction	i. Pulmonary oedema: a clinical diagnosis necessitating intravenous furosemide or intubation
	ii. Cardiac arrest
2. Vascular dysfunction	i. Hypovolaemia requiring ≥ 5 units whole blood or packed cells for resuscitation
3. Immunological dysfunction	i. Intensive care admission for sepsis
	ii. Emergency hysterectomy for sepsis
4. Respiratory dysfunction	i. Intubation and ventilation for > 60 min for any reason other than for a general anaesthetic
	ii. Oxygen saturation on pulse oximetry < 90% lasting > 60 min
	iii. $PaO_2/FiO_2 \leq 3$
5. Renal dysfunction	i. Oliguria, defined as < 400 mL/24 h, which does not respond to either careful adequate intravascular rehydration or diuresis with furosemide
	ii. Acute deterioration of urea to > 15 mmol/L or of creatinine to > 400 mmol/L
6. Liver dysfunction	i. Jaundice in the presence of pre-eclampsia
7. Metabolic dysfunction	i. Diabetic ketoacidosis
	ii. Thyroid crisis
8. Coagulation dysfunction	i. Acute thrombocytopenia requiring a platelet transfusion.
9. Cerebral dysfunction	ii. Subarachnoid or intracerebral haemorrhage.
	i. Coma in a patient lasting > 12 h
Management-based	
1. Intensive care admission	i. For any reason
2. Emergency hysterectomy	i. For any reason
3. Anaesthetic accidents	i. Severe hypotension associated with a spinal or epidural anaesthetic. Hypotension defined as a systolic pressure < 90 mmHg lasting > 60 min
	ii. Failed tracheal intubation requiring anaesthetic reversal

In 2003, a continuous, prospective Scottish Confidential Audit on Severe Maternal Morbidity (SCASMM) was started, to capture data from all obstetric units using the Mantel criteria to provide a consistent definition of near-miss events. In 2010, 385 women were reported to the audit, making a near-miss incidence of 6.5/1000 births (95% confidence interval (CI) 5.9–7.2),[20] similar to the rate of 6.4/1000 births in the 2008 report.[21] Comparing these figures with maternal death rates in Scotland over the 2008–10 triennium, the mortality/morbidity ratio was 1:85. There was a significant variation in the rates of reported maternal morbidity amongst the 18 consultant-led maternity units, from 0 to 10.6/1000. This variation is thought to be due in part to different unit characteristics, with smaller units transferring high-risk women to larger units for delivery. Much of the variation, however, is due to the individual unit's diligence in case identification.[21]

The commonest cause of severe morbidity in pregnancy in Scotland is major obstetric haemorrhage (MOH), accounting for 85% of cases, at rate of 5.5/1000 births; 80% were post-partum, and 16% of women with MOH required admission to an ICU (Table 30.5).

Mantel's definition of maternal near miss was also thought to be the most stable and epidemiologically sound criterion in a recently published systematic review by Tuncalp et al.[22] A meta-analysis of the 11 studies that used Mantel criteria showed an incidence of 4.2/1000 deliveries (95% CI 4.0–4.4).

Zeeman et al.[23] audited 483 admissions to the obstetric intermediate care unit over a 2-year period at Parkland Hospital, Dallas, Texas. The admission rate was 1.7%, 15% of whom then required transfer to an ICU. Eighty per cent of the admissions

Table 30.5 Causes of severe maternal morbidity in Scotland 2010

Category of severe maternal morbidity	Number of events	Rate per 1000 births (95% CI)
Major obstetric haemorrhage	328	5.55 (4.94–6.16)
Eclampsia	12	0.20 (0.10–0.35)
Renal or liver dysfunction	10	0.17 (0.08–0.31)
Cardiac arrest	4	0.07 (0.02–0.17)
Pulmonary oedema	3	0.05 (0.01–0.15)
Acute respiratory dysfunction	3	0.05 (0.01–0.15)
Anaesthetic problem	3	0.05 (0.01–0.15)
Cerebrovascular event	1	0.02 (0.0–0.09)
Anaphylactic shock	1	0.02 (0.0–0.09)
Septicaemic shock	1	0.02 (0.0–0.09)
Coma	0	0.00 (0.0–0.06)
Status epilepticus	0	0.00 (0.0–0.06)
Massive pulmonary embolism	0	0.00 (0.0–0.06)
Intensive care or coronary care admission	76	1.29 (1.01–1.60)

were post-partum. Two-thirds were admitted due to obstetric disorders, the commonest reason being hypertensive disorders of pregnancy (43%) and haemorrhage (18%).

Ryan et al. audited admissions to the two-bedded HDU at the Rotunda Hospital, Dublin,[24] from its inception in June 1996 to May 1998 and compared them with the rate of transfer to ICU in the 2 years before and 2 years after the unit opened. They found that 18% of the 123 admissions were antenatal. The HDU admission rate was 1.0% of all deliveries and 86% of HDU admissions were due to haemodynamic instability. There was a non-significant fall in the number of patients requiring ICU transfer after the HDU was established, from 12 (0.8/1000) in 2004–06 down to five (0.4/1000) in 2006–08 (Fisher's exact test P = 0.25).

Saravanakumar et al. analysed data for 3551 pregnant or recently pregnant women admitted to their obstetric HDU in Aberdeen between 1984 and 2007.[25] They found the admission rate had risen significantly from less than 1% in the 1980s to 5.01% at the end of the audit period, with an overall admission rate of 2.67%. The rise was thought to be due to a change in demographics, with an increasing number of women from ethnic minorities, maternal age, and Caesarean delivery rate. Obstetric-related conditions accounted for 75% of admissions and 11.3% of patients were antenatal. The commonest indication for admission was pre-eclampsia in the earlier years but this was overtaken by haemorrhage, accounting for 37.5% of admissions in 2006–07. Thirty-nine patients were transferred for ICU care in the last 4 year of the audit, a rate of 1.4/1000 deliveries.

High dependency care is required both for patients who have already met the criteria of sustaining a near miss and also for those who may do so in the future, so that they can receive appropriate monitoring and prompt treatment. There are many advantages for the parturient in keeping high dependency care within the delivery suite,[26] in terms of continuity of input from expert obstetrician and obstetric anaesthetic teams, holistic care from midwives, the ability to continuously monitor antenatal patients, and avoiding the hazards of emergency transport of the critically ill obstetric patient.[27]

What facilities for obstetric high dependency care (OHDC) are available on delivery suites in the United Kingdom? In 1994, Cordingley and Rubin surveyed lead obstetric anaesthetists in 262 UK obstetric units and received responses from 232 units.[28] They found that only 41% of units had dedicated OHDC beds, although 92% of units were able to provide temporary facilities when required; 81% of units had access to ICU on the same hospital site. The rate of transfer to ICU care in isolated units was lower than in non-isolated units (median rate of 0.92/1000 deliveries vs 1.33, P < 0.01).

Hussain et al. carried out a similar survey of OHDC facilities in 2006 and received 170 responses from 228 UK obstetric units.[29] They found that 96% of units were able to provide temporary HDU facilities, only 40% had at least one dedicated bed: almost unchanged over the past 12 years. The admission rate to HDU beds was 4.2%, considerably above the recommended figure of 1% quoted in *Safer Childbirth*[5] and similar to the 5% figure found by Saravanakumar.

Intensive care unit physiological scoring systems

Many different scores have been developed to evaluate the severity of critical illness. The Acute Physiology and Chronic Health Evaluation (APACHE) score[30] was developed from the hypothesis that the severity of critical illness can be measured by quantifying the degree of physiological disturbance using multiple variables. Due to difficulties with previous predictive scoring systems, APACHE was not designed to assist in making individual treatment decisions but instead to classify groups of patients by their severity of illness. This allowed stratification by illness severity so that the outcome from intensive care could be evaluated[31] and the success of different treatment programmes compared.[32]

The original APACHE system was complex, producing a weighted score derived from 34 possible physiological measurements. A revised version, APACHE II, was introduced in 1985[33] to produce a simpler system that was more accurate. The number of variables used in APACHE II was reduced from 34 to 12 by discarding those that were infrequently measured and by evaluating each variable's impact on patient outcome using a multivariate analysis.

The APACHE II score is calculated from the degree of physiological disturbance, with a maximum of 4 points given to each of temperature, blood pressure, respiratory rate, heart rate, oxygenation, blood pH, sodium, potassium, creatinine, haematocrit, and white blood cell count. A neurological score is derived from the 15-point Glasgow Coma Scale (GCS) score, to a maximum of 12 points. This gives a total of 60 for severity of illness. A maximum of 6 points are added for age and 5 for comorbidity, making a total of 71. For female admissions to adult ICUs reported as currently or recently pregnant, a score of 0–17 is associated with a mortality rate of 1%, rising to 85% with APACHE II scores of greater than 42.[15]

The APACHE II system was found to have a good overall ability to stratify patients due to the strong association between acute physiological derangement and risk of death during acute illness. However, there remain significant variations in death rate by disease, due to nature of the underlying disease process. It is therefore essential to combine the APACHE II score with a description of the disease so that conditions with a high mortality such as septic shock can be differentiated from those with a better prognosis such as acute asthma. The risk of mortality for an individual can be calculated using an exponential equation, which combines the APACHE II with a weighting for the diagnostic category.

The value of APACHE II in obstetric patients was questioned by Koch et al.[34] who looked at the mortality predicted by APACHE II for 22 pregnant patients admitted to the medical ICU between 1984 and 1987. Eight maternal deaths occurred (36%), with three due to pre-eclampsia, two due to amniotic fluid embolism, and two assigned to immunodeficiency. The APACHE II scores were low, with no patient having a score greater than 20 and the predicted mortality from APACHE II was therefore only 11.5% for the whole group and 13.75% for the non-survivors. The underlying disease conditions in this series such as amniotic fluid embolism and HELLP syndrome are associated with a high mortality and this may explain the underestimation. The Koch et al. paper, however, does not give details of the diagnostic category weighting used to predict mortality.

Other authors since have found that APACHE II overestimates maternal mortality. Lewinsohn et al.[35] looked at predicted mortalities in 58 obstetric patients admitted to an ICU, together with a similar group of 120 non-pregnant young women, over an 8-year period. Their pattern of admission to ITU was quite different to that reported by Koch et al., with the majority of patients being admitted due to sepsis and haemorrhagic shock. From the APACHE II scores, the predicted mortality rate in the obstetric patients was 16.6%, more than double the actual obstetric mortality rate of 4/58 (7%). By contrast, the predicted mortality rate in the non-obstetrical group was 10.1%, which was very close to the actual mortality rate of 12/120 (10%). Both obstetric and non-obstetric groups had similar mean APACHE II scores, indicating similar degrees of physiological derangement. The actual mortality for a given APACHE II score has been shown to vary considerably by ICU, with improved outcomes where there was good coordination between the intensive care staff.[36] The authors speculated that the obstetrician-intensivist performance, with good communication and open collaboration, led to better results.

The Simplified Acute Physiology Score (SAPS II) has also been used to predict mortality on admission to intensive care,[36] refined from the original SAPS using a multiple logistical regression model. It includes variables that are not used in APACHE II such as serum bilirubin and urine output. In addition, urea is substituted for creatinine and bicarbonate in place of arterial blood pH. SAPS II can be similarly used to calculate predicted mortality for obstetric patients admitted to the ICU. Scarpinato[37] used SAPS II to predict mortality for 29 obstetric patients admitted to the ICU. The SAPS II score predicted a higher mortality risk of 3% compared with the actual mortality of 0%, which was similar to Lewinsohn et al.'s findings with APACHE II.

The Mortality Probability Model (MPM II)[38] uses fewer physiological variables than APACHE II or SAPS II to estimate mortality at the time of ICU admission but includes additional information such as urine output, vasoactive drug therapy and raised prothrombin time together with computed tomography to estimate intracranial mass effect for patients with head injury.

El-Solh and Grant compared the predictive ability of APACHE II with SAPS II and the MPM II.[39] They applied the scoring systems to 93 obstetric patients admitted to the ICU between 1989 and 1995 and compared them with a control group of 96 non-obstetric female patients in the 17-41 year age group. Most admissions in the obstetric group were due to respiratory complications or emergency obstetric procedures. The observed mortality rates of each group were 10.8% and 10.4% respectively. There was no significant difference between the observed mortality and the mortality rates predicted by each scoring system. All three systems were found to be effective.

Bhagwanjee et al.[40] examined APACHE II scores in 105 women with eclampsia who were admitted to ICU in Durban, South Africa. The main indications for ICU admission were poor oxygenation, low GCS score, extreme restlessness, and laryngeal oedema. The overall mortality was 10.5% (11 patients). The APACHE II score was significantly higher in non-survivors than survivors but this was due to the contribution from the GCS score. The GCS score alone showed the same level of difference between the groups as the APACHE II, whilst the APACHE II–GCS showed no difference between the non-survivors and survivors. The number of organ systems failing was also significantly higher in non-survivors, most frequently respiratory failure. This reflects the multiorgan failure that accompanies severe eclampsia together with other complications such as HELLP syndrome.

Hazelgrove et al. measured the performance of APACHE II, APACHE III, and SAPS II scores in their study of 210 obstetric ICU admissions in Southern England.[12] Mortality ratios were assessed for each scoring system. Discrimination between survivors and non-survivors was assessed using the area under the receiver operating characteristic curve (AUC).[41] All three ICU scoring systems could accurately distinguish between survivors and non-survivors with APACHE II being the closest fit for the pregnancy population.

Harrison et al.'s study of 1902 obstetric ICU admissions using the ICNARC database[14] similarly evaluated the performance of APACHE II scores to discriminate between survivors and non-survivors using AUC values. The mortality predicted by APACHE II scores was calibrated using the mortality ratio, Hosmer–Lemeshow C statistic, and Cox regression calibration. The mean APACHE II score was 10.9, which was similar to the Acute Physiological Score as age points are only assigned above age 45 and the very severe chronic health conditions of APACHE II are rare in this population. Discrimination of the APACHE II score was good, with higher values for obstetric admissions (AUC 0.839; 95% CI 0.820–0.857) than for the control group of non-obstetric female admissions aged 16–50 years (AUC 0.812; 95% CI 0.807–0.818). The mortality predictions by APACHE II were similar to those found by Hazelgrove et al., with a mortality ratio of 0.245 for obstetric admissions compared to 0.907 for controls. The calibration plots (Figure 30.1) show how the APACHE II scores were able to predict mortality accurately in the control group but vastly overestimated mortality in the obstetric group.

Of the individual components of the APACHE II score, the GCS was the best predictor of mortality, a similar finding to Bhagwanjee's study of eclamptic patients.[40]

Rojas-Suarez et al.[42] reviewed 725 obstetric patients admitted to the ICU between 2006 and 2011. They found that APACHE II, SAPS II, and SAPS III overestimated maternal mortality whereas MPM II and MPM III were more accurate, with observed/predicted ratios of 0.89 and 1.25 respectively. They recommended that APACHE II should not be used to predict mortality in this population.

APACHE II is still popular in ICUs in the United Kingdom due to its simplicity but it has since been superseded by more accurate scoring systems: APACHE III [43] in 1991 and APACHE IV[44] in 2006. The authors of APACHE IV state that APACHE II is a useful summary measure of severity of illness but that it should no longer be used to predict mortality. APACHE IV instead uses a set of 142 variables in its mortality equation together with a more complex set of equations that require a computer to evaluate. The chart and scoring systems for APACHE II are freely available whereas APACHE III and IV are proprietary tools that have to be obtained from the developers, although the Cerner Corporation has recently made hospital mortality and length of stay algorithms available to registered users (https://apachefoundations.cernerworks.com/apachefoundations/login/auth).

APACHE IV provides ICU and hospital predictions for mortality and length of stay whilst MPM III and SAPS III only provide hospital mortality predictions. In the general adult intensive care setting, the latest versions of these ICU scoring systems have been shown to be more accurate than their predecessors.[45,46] Although newer scoring systems have better performance, the difference may not affect efficacy and choice of system depends on ease of use and local preferences.[47]

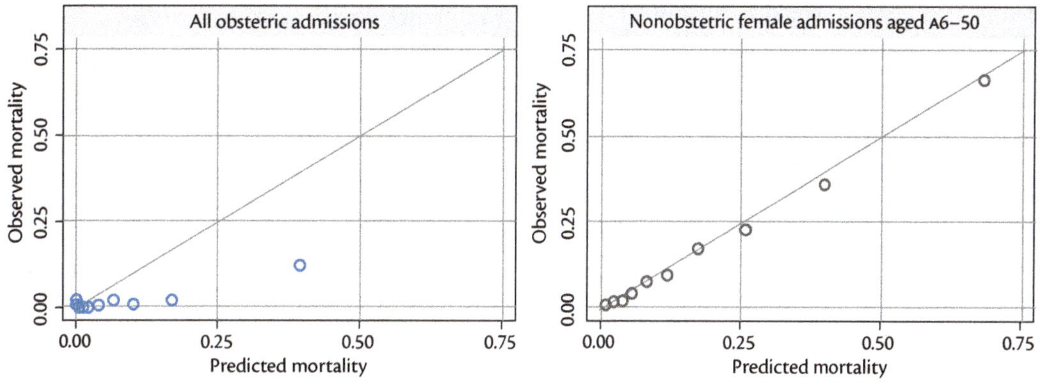

Figure 30.1 Calibration plots for APACHE II mortality probability in obstetric and non-obstetric admissions. Observed mortality is plotted against deciles of predicted mortality. Diagonal line indicates perfect calibration.

APACHE, Acute Physiology and Chronic Health Evaluation.

Physiological scoring systems may perform poorly in obstetric critical illness due to the physiological changes in pregnancy or because of the unique scoring profile of obstetric conditions such as pre-eclampsia. These issues were considered by Gopalan and Muckart, who recommended using organ failure scoring systems.[48] They avoid many of these problems as the development of multiorgan failure is a common antecedent to death in all critically ill patients: the presence of three organ systems failures for 3 or more days, regardless of any other factors is associated with 100% mortality.[49,50] Several scores have been developed to quantify this, including Sequential Organ Failure Assessment (SOFA),[51] Multiple Organ Dysfunction (MOD),[49] and Logistic Organ Dysfunction (LOD).[50] However, none of these scoring systems have yet been validated in critically ill obstetric patients.

Early warning scores

General wards

Physiological deterioration precedes critical illness and it has became clear that many patients on general wards who have had an in-hospital cardiac arrest have documented evidence of clinical deterioration before the arrest, which was not acted on appropriately by the ward nurse or junior doctor.[52] Similarly, unplanned admissions to general adult ICUs are often associated with abnormalities in patients' vital signs that have been recorded without appropriate action taken.[53] Goldhill et al. applied the APACHE II scoring system to vital signs recorded in the 24 hours prior to ICU admission.[54] They found that 80% of patients had at least one value for heart rate, respiratory rate outside of the normal range, scoring one or more APACHE II points.

A number of early warning scoring systems have been developed that are based on physiological measurements used by APACHE II, using variables that are routinely measured on the acute general ward. These include Medical Emergency Team (MET) calling criteria,[55] Patient At Risk score (PAR),[56] and Modified Early Warning Score (MEWS).[57] All of the scoring systems assign a score dependent upon the degree of deviation from normality but differ in the number of parameters measured. The MET system is a list of calling criteria whereas both PAR and MEWS assign a weighted value according to the degree of deviation from normality and generate a total score.

Goldhill et al. showed that the number of physiological abnormalities and the PAR score both predicted hospital mortality.[56] All physiological variables contributed to the need for intervention, apart from temperature.

Hillman and colleagues introduced METs[55,58] to provide urgent attention for those with patients who met the MET calling criteria. Buist et al. showed that this reduced the incidence of deaths due to cardiac arrests.[59]

Hillman then conducted a large-scale prospective study to see whether the MET system could reduce the composite incidence of cardiac arrest, unplanned ICU admission, and unexpected death.[55] In a prospective study, 23 Australian hospitals were randomized to either continue as before or to introduce the MET system. The MET system did not improve the composite or individual secondary outcomes but did lead to an increase in emergency call outs.

Subbe et al. similarly found that the introduction of a MEWS failed to improve primary or secondary outcomes when introduced in a medical admissions unit in North Wales.[60]

However, Priestley et al. found that the introduction of Critical Care Outreach teams, together with a MEWS, in an acute general hospital did decrease in-hospital mortality compared with control wards (two-level odds ratio 0.52; 95% CI 0.32–0.85).[61]

Doubts about the clinical utility of early warning systems led to concern that the choice of both parameters and cut-offs was largely based on clinical intuition rather than the use of rigorous derivation and validation methodologies.[62]

The National Institute for Health Research Service Delivery and Organisation from ICNARC commissioned Gao and co-workers to review 36 studies on early warning scores (EWSs).[63] The search strategies were then updated to include a further 11 studies published after 2004 and this was used as the basis of evidence for the National Institute of Clinical Excellence (now the National Institute of Health and Care Excellence) (NICE) review on recognition of acutely illness in hospital.[64] NICE recommended that aggregate weighted scoring systems should be used in UK hospitals. Although NICE recommended which physiological parameters should be monitored, it did not propose a standardized early warning system.

The wide variety of physiological parameters used in different early warning systems, together with the weightings given to individual parameters led to the problem that clinical staff in different hospitals or different clinical settings were unfamiliar with local systems. The Acute Medicine Task force stated that 'there is no justification for the continued use of multiple different EWSs to assess illness severity'.[65] They recommended the development of a national Early Warning Score to provide a standardize record of illness severity and urgency of need, from first assessment and throughout the patient journey. The report recognized that a key weakness in current practice was the lack of a standardized EWS embedded in the culture of the NHS, which prevent EWS being used as part of routine training and education for all staff.

The new National Early Warning Score (NEWS) developed by the Royal College of Physicians[66] used the same physiological parameters recommended in the NICE report,[64] with physiological weightings based on a published systematic review (Figure 30.2 and Figure 30.3). This compared performances from 33 warning systems when applied to a database of 9987 vital signs derived from an acute medical assessment unit, collected using the VitalPAC electronic data gathering system.[67] Only 12 of the systems reviewed showed reasonable discrimination, using an AUC method, and none achieved an AUC greater than 0.8.

The NEWS was found to achieve an AUC of 0.722 for cardiac arrest, 0.857 for unanticipated ICU admission, 0.894 for death, and 0.873 for any of the outcomes, all within 24 hours.[68] The NEWS is designed to be used for all acutely ill patients admitted to hospital apart from children or women who are currently or recently pregnant.

Maternity early warning scores

The well-recognized problem of recognizing critical illness had led to a number of obstetric units introducing EWSs, some of whose parameters were modified for obstetrics, using local clinical judgement. This practice was highlighted and put as a top ten recommendation by the *Saving Mothers Lives* report of the Confidential Enquiry, published in 2007,[11] with a number of maternal death vignettes cited where MEWS may have helped staff realize the severity of illness. The report stated that a national Modified Early Obstetric Warning Score (MEOWS) should be developed and piloted from December 2008. This has not yet happened. The subsequent Confidential Enquiry report, published in 2011, repeated the top ten recommendation that a national MEOWS should be used, although there is no further update regarding the progress of this project.

There are several challenges in validating a national MEOWS. The PAR scoring system described by Goldhill et al. was used for acutely ill general patients requiring critical care outreach with an overall mortality of 14.6%.[56] This made it possible to distinguish which physiological variables of the PAR score were able to accurately predict mortality. Similarly, Subbe et al. were able to validate their modified EWS score in an acute medical admissions unit, with a mortality of 7.9%.[69] With an mortality rate of 0.011%[16] and an ICU admission rate of 0.26%,[15] it is not feasible to use these unequivocal endpoints for validation.

Carle et al. extracted a dataset of 2240 critically ill obstetric patients in the ICNARC case mix programme captured over a 13-year period and measured the ability of nine different MEWS scores, to distinguish between survivors and non-survivors.[70] All MEWS systems performed well, with AUCs of 0.967–0.985. However, the two 'obstetric' MEWS did not offer any additional benefit, with AUC values of 0.967 and 0.985. The obstetric dataset only contains data after admission to critical care. To evaluate a MEWS properly, the authors stated that parameters should be

National Early Warning Score (NEWS)

PHYSIOLOGICAL PARAMETERS	3	2	1	0	1	2	3
Respiration Rate	≤8		9–11	12–20		21–24	≥25
Oxygen Saturations	≤91	92–93	94–95	≥96			
Any Supplemental Oxygen		Yes		No			
Temperature	≤35.0		35.1–36.0	36.1–38.0	38.1–39.0	≥39.1	
Systolic BP	≤90	91–100	101–110	111–219			≥220
Heart Rate	≤40		41–50	51–90	91–110	111–130	≥131
Level of Consciousness				A			V, P, or U

Figure 30.2 (See colour figure section). The National Early Warning Score (NEWS).

Reproduced with permission from the Royal College of Physicians. *National Early Warning Score (NEWS): Standardising the assessment of acute illness severity in the NHS*. Report of a working party.

The National Early Warning Score (NEWS) thresholds and triggers

NEW scores	Clinical risk
0	Low
Aggregate 1–4	
RED score (Individual parameter scoring 3)	Medium
Aggregate 5–6	
Aggregate 7 or more	High

Figure 30.3 (See colour figure section). The National Early Warning Score (NEWS) thresholds and triggers.

Reproduced with permission from the Royal College of Physicians. *National Early Warning Score (NEWS): Standardising the assessment of acute illness severity in the NHS*. Report of a working party. © Royal College of Physicians 2012.

examined before admission but this was unlikely to be feasible in future studies.

A maternal early warning system that is based on physiological changes in disease also has to contend with physiological adaptations that occur in each trimester of normal pregnancy, labour and the post-partum period. There remains the question as to whether a modified early warning system should be further modified according to maternal gestation.

Singh et al. examined the use of MEOWS in 676 consecutive obstetric admissions:[71] 30% of the patients triggered the MEOWS and 13% had morbidity including haemorrhage, hypertension, and suspected sepsis. The MEOWS score had a positive predictive value of 39% and negative predictive value of 98%. There were no ICU admissions, cardiorespiratory arrests, or deaths during the study, making it impossible to measure the value of MEOWS in detecting severe morbidity or mortality. The authors also acknowledge that the triggers in the MEOWS are very close to the levels that define morbidity (e.g. high systolic blood that defines hypertensive disorder) so that this becomes a self-fulfilling prophecy.

In January 2012, an All Wales Consensus paper was written with the aim of agreeing the normal/abnormal physiological parameters for an obstetric EWS and to explore alignment with the National Early Warning System.[72] They noted that the MEOWS chart described in both Confidential Enquiry reports[11,16] relied on colour-coded triggers whereas NICE guidance CG50[64] recommends an aggregated numerical scoring system. Whilst colour-coded charts are of use in triggering an intervention, an objective scoring system allows a graded response and monitoring of progression of treatment.

Many different adaptations of MEOWS were in use throughout Wales. A survey of UK obstetric anaesthetists revealed the consensus of opinion that a national EWS should be used.[73] A draft Obstetric National Early Warning scheme was produced, with scoring system and escalation policy which mirrored that used for the general NEWS. However, on further enquiry, there was feedback from the service that there was no need for a new MEOWS as even if a new tool was devised, the need for further validation would delay its introduction.[74] It was agreed that maternity units should continue to use their existing MEOWS charts and would agree local escalation guidance based on the Royal College report.[9]

The Maternal Critical Care Working Group[9] similarly recommended that a national chart should be produced as a longer-term goal.

In Liverpool Women's Hospital, a MEWS has been in regular use for a decade. The six parameters of NEWS, adjusted for physiological changes in pregnancy, are monitored, together with urine output, if the patient is catheterized or has not passed urine for 7 hours.

Recognition of the critically ill patient

The Maternal Critical Care Working Group[9] recommended that maternity services should implement the NICE guidance on care of the critically ill in hospital.[64] All admissions to hospital should have physiological observations recorded at the time of their admission or an initial assessment together with a clear monitoring plan that specifies which physiological observations should be recorded and how often. These should be recorded using an EWS or Physiological Track and Trigger system. This plan will depend upon whether the pregnancy is low- or high-risk, the reason for admission, co-morbidities and the agreed treatment plan. Table 30.6 shows the frequency of routine MEWS observations, and Table 30.7 shows the thresholds that are used to calculate weighted scores, at the Liverpool Women's Hospital.

Table 30.6 Frequency of routine MEWS observations performed at the Liverpool Women's Hospital

Condition	Frequency of observations
Lower segment caesarean delivery	½-hourly for 4 hours Hourly for 6 hours 4-hourly for 48 hours (use clinical judgement 24 hours during sleep) Daily until discharge
Other procedures under anaesthesia	½-hourly for 4 hours Hourly for 6 hours (or until discharge) 4-hourly for 24 hours
Postpartum haemorrhage	½-hourly for 4 hours (remain on CDS if possible) 4-hourly for 24 hours
Prophylactic Syntocinon®	4-hourly for 24 hours
Diastolic of 90 or over	Minimum 4-hourly until discharge or start of labour
Identified antenatal in patients (diabetes, ruptured membranes, known or suspected infection)	4-hourly (unless indicated otherwise) until discharge
Postnatal women with suspected or confirmed infection	4-hourly for a minimum of 24 hours Once daily until discharged
Medical management of miscarriage	Hourly from start of treatment until discharge
Blood transfusion	Prior to start of transfusion 15 minutes into transfusion Post transfusion *(must be done for each unit of blood transfused)*

Liverpool Women's Hospital MEWS escalation algorithm. Reproduced with permission.

Table 30.7 Thresholds and scores in the MEWS used at the Liverpool Women's Hospital

Score	3	2	1	0	1	2	3
Pulse (bpm)	<40	40–59	60–74	75–105	106–110	111–130	>130
Systolic BP (mmHg)	<80	80–90	95–140	141–150	151–199	>200	
Respiratory rate (breaths/min)	<6	6–8	9–14	15–20	21–25	26–29	>30
Temperature (°C)	<35		35–36	36.1–38	38.1–38.5		>38.5
UOC	<10 mL	<100 mL in 4 h	<50 mL in 2 h				
UO no catheter	Not PU in 10 h	Not PU in 8 h and no bladder					
CNS	Unresponsive	Voice	Alert		Confused	Agitated	
SpO_2	<88%	88–89	90–94	>95%			

A graded response strategy for patients should be agreed locally and harmonized with that used in the National Early Warning Score so that staff who also care for patients on general wards are familiar with the system. It should consist of three levels of scores:

Low risk: Total score 3–4.

Medium risk: Total score 5–6 *or* single parameter 3.

High risk: Total score ≥ 7.

CNS, central nervous system; PU, passed urine UO, urine output UOC,urine output in catheterized patient.

Liverpool Women's Hospital MEWS escalation algorithm. Reproduced with permission.

Critical care competencies

The Department of Health document *Competencies for Recognising and Responding to Acutely Ill Patients in Hospital*[75] was produced in 2009, to support the implementation of the NICE guidance about care of acutely ill patients in hospital.[64] Critical care competencies define knowledge, skills, and attitudes required for safe and effective treatment, together with a chain of response from non-clinical staff all the way through to a critical care level tertiary responder (Figure 30.4). One staff group could play several different roles in the chain, for example, the recognizer may also be the primary responder.

- *Non-clinical staff*: they may also be the 'alerter' and include the patient herself or her visitor.
- *Recorder*: takes designated physiological measurements and records observations and information. This could be a maternity support worker, healthcare assistant, or midwife.
- *Recognizer*: monitors the patient's condition, interprets designated information that has been recorded, and adjusts the frequency of observations and level of monitoring. This would typically be a midwife, recovery nurse, or other nurse in the unit or a foundation doctor.
- *Primary responder*: goes beyond just interpreting the designated information to formulate a clinical management plan, for example, starting oxygen therapy, selection of intravenous fluids, and administering a bolus of intravenous fluids. This would be a core trainee or junior specialist trainee.
- *Secondary responder*: is likely to be called when the patient fails to respond to the primary intervention and continues to 'trigger' or 're-trigger' a response. This person will assess the clinical effect of the primary intervention, diagnose the problem, refine the management plan, and initiate a secondary response and have the knowledge when to refer to critical care. This is the role of the obstetric or anaesthetic senior specialist trainee (ST 3–7).
- *Tertiary responder*: role undertaken by staff with critical care competencies including advanced airway management, resuscitation, clinical examination, and interpretation of the critically ill patient. In a maternity unit, this role is provided by consultants in anaesthesia and obstetrics.

(Reproduced here with permission from The Royal College of Anaesthetists. Originally published in Providing equity of critical and maternity care for the critically ill pregnant or recently pregnant woman, July 2011)

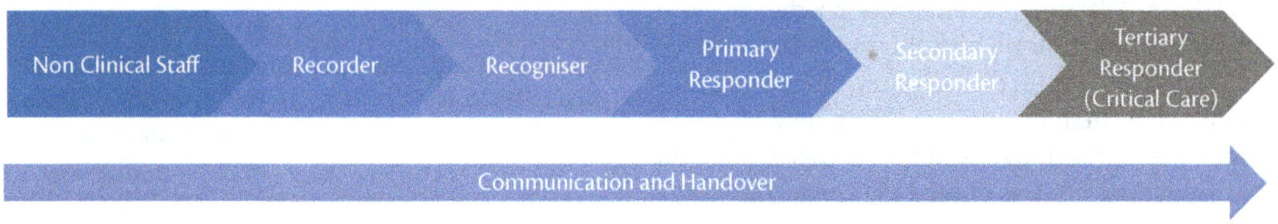

Figure 30.4 Chain of response to a critical incident.

Reproduced from Competencies for Recognising and Responding to Acutely Ill Patients in Hospital. DH, London 2008 (http://www.dh.gov.uk/en/Publicationsandstatistics/Publications/PublicationsPolicyAndGuidance/DH_096989). Crown copyright.

The competencies are mainly about clinical and technical level of care and delivery of effective patient management but are not exclusive and assume that generic competencies are in place. This assumption cannot always be taken for granted as many midwives are now 'direct entry' and gain little experience of nursing acutely ill patients during their training.

The key competency for all levels of staff is knowing when to refer to a clinician with greater knowledge and experience. The chain of response provides a tiered response but is not a fixed hierarchy—a recorder who recognizes a very sick woman should be able to access critical care expertise immediately, most straightforwardly through a 'crash call'.

The chain of response requires that staff recognize and respond to signs of deterioration in the patient. The EWS plays a part in this by providing a jointly agreed scale to measure the patient's degree of risk of further deterioration. It also allows escalation to an appropriate tier of competency. At the Liverpool Women's Hospital, patients who score an aggregate MEWS of 4 are referred to a primary responder, those with an aggregate score of 5–6 or a single parameter of 3 are referred to a secondary responder, whilst those with a score of 7 or more are referred directly to a tertiary responder. Review by the responder should be undertaken within 30 minutes, with escalation to a higher level if this does not occur (Figure 30.5).

Once escalation has occurred, a minimum of hourly MEWS observations are required to confirm that the patient has responded to the initial intervention. If the patient's score has not improved, further escalation is then required (Figure 30.5).

Implementing critical care competencies requires a system-wide approach with effective leadership and change management from board to ward. The approach required will depend upon the individual hospital's setting but may include the following elements:

- Identifying clinical and managerial leads and implementation team
- Monitoring outcomes with board-level reporting and intervention
- Critical incident analysis and peer supervision with regular multidisciplinary meetings to review severe maternal morbidity cases
- Education and training of competencies included in inducted and ongoing training plus formal performance review and development
- Appropriate resources in place
- Adapt local policies to clarify levels of authority and responsibility

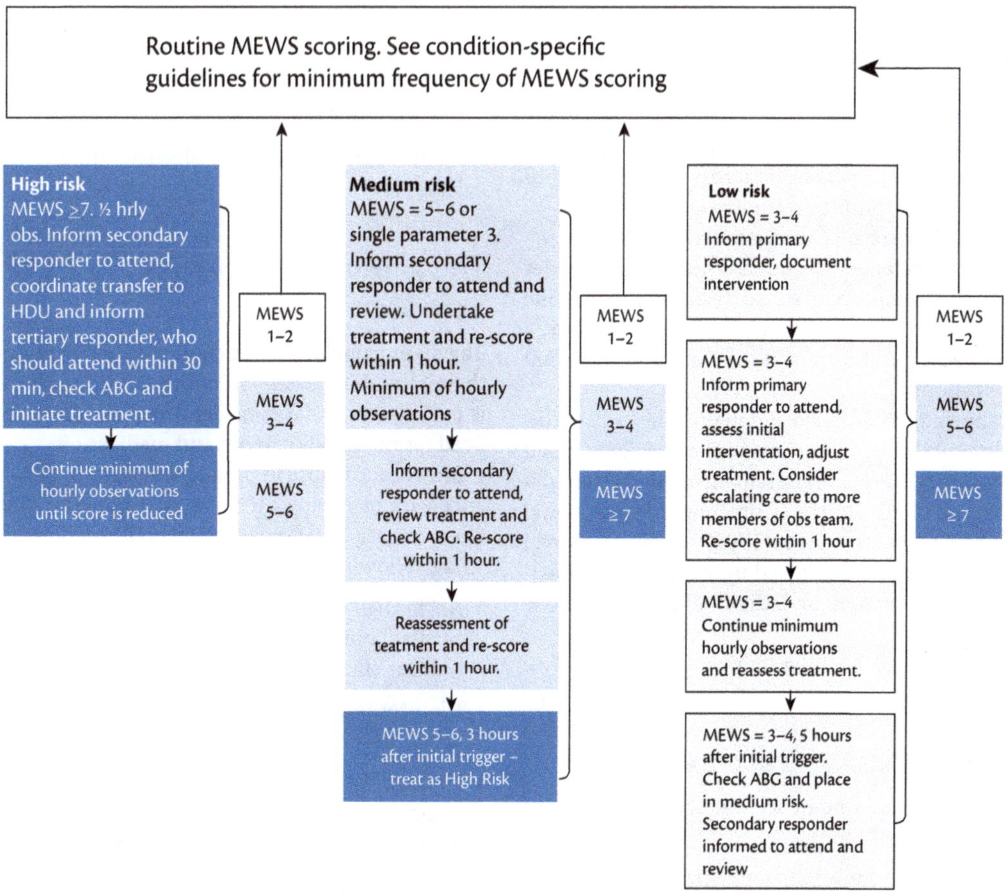

Figure 30.5 Liverpool Women's Hospital MEWS escalation algorithm.
Liverpool Women's Hospital MEWS escalation algorithm. Reproduced with permission.

- Develop team working, assertiveness, and inter-professional working relationships. All team members must have confidence in the competency of their colleagues and are ready both to challenge and to be challenged.

Workforce development

Lead professionals for maternity services have a responsibility to ensure that staff are adequately trained. There are a number of national, certified courses which will support workforce development in this area such as ALERT. Maternal critical care courses for trainee obstetricians and midwives have been developed by providers such as Leeds University (http://www.healthcare.leeds.ac.uk/study/PG/midwifery/PGC-CICBW-09/details.htm)

SCOTTIE (Scottish Core Teaching and Training in Emergencies) has been developed to provide a standardized training course in managing emergencies for all healthcare professionals who participate in the care of pregnant women. The course has been designed to cover the fundamental aspects of maternal emergencies and is suitable for all maternity-care professionals working in all care environments in Scotland (http://www.scottishmaternity.org/Courses/Introduction%20to%20The%20Courses/obstetric_emergencies.html).

REACTS (Recognition, Evaluation, Assessment, Critical Treatment and Stabilisation) has been developed to provide a standardized training course in recognizing and managing the critically ill obstetric patient for the many healthcare professionals who participate in the care of pregnant women. The course has been designed to cover the fundamental aspects of caring for critically ill women and is suitable for most maternity-care professionals working in Scotland. The Scottish Maternity REACTS course is one of the skills-based courses developed and rolled out by the Scottish Multi-professional Maternity Development Programme in support of maternity-care professionals across Scotland (http://www.scottishmaternity.org/Courses/Introduction%20to%20The%20Courses/scottish-maternity-reacts-course.htm).

The Critical Care competencies required at tertiary responder level are defined by the *C*ompetency *Ba*sed *Tr*aining programme in *I*ntensive *C*are Medicine for *E*urope (CoBaTrICE) syllabus,[76] which includes a specific section on life-threatening maternal peripartum complications.

Critical care competencies are incorporated in the core training curriculum for anaesthetic trainees as well as being included in the revalidation programme. 'Assessment of the Critically Ill Parturient' is included in the Continued Professional Development for Anaesthetists matrix (2B06)[77] from the Royal College of Anaesthetists. Level 2 is based upon both the knowledge and skills that are relevant to an individual doctor's 'whole' practice.[78]

There are several simulation training courses also available (see Chapter 53 for more details).

Transfers to and from critical care

Transfer to Level 3 care should be in accordance with Intensive Care Society guidelines:[79]

- All hospitals to have a lead consultant for critical care transfers.
- All must have systems to resuscitate, stabilize, and transport critically ill, with a plan for all critical care areas.
- Training: all staff must have appropriate training in transfer medicine.
- Equipment: all must have access to a transfer trolley, with all monitoring and equipment mounted in a suitable way to be compliant with the Comité Européen de Normalisation (CEN) 1789:2007 European Union standard for ambulances. Ideally all equipment within a region should be standardized to enable seamless transfers.
- Prior to transfer, a risk assessment must be made by a consultant or other suitably experienced member of staff, to determine the competences of staff required for the transfer.
- Patients should be resuscitated and stabilized before transfer, with pre-transfer checklists.
- Minimum standards of monitoring must be used, continuously visible to accompanying staff, with a written record of observations.
- Safety: patients secured, equipment secured, staff seated and using seat belts. If unanticipated intervention is required, the ambulance should be stopped in a safe place before administering treatment.
- Standardized documentation should be used.[79]

In addition, a clear plan is required to meet the maternal, fetal, or postnatal needs of the patient.

An intensive care transfer form must be completed for all transfers, documenting the:

- reason for transfer
- history of stabilization prior to transfer
- date and time of transfer
- identification of staff involved in the decision to transfer to HDU/ITU.

The acutely ill parturient in a general critical care area

The main principle in managing an acutely ill pregnant woman is that optimal management of the condition causing critical illness is paramount. Fetal considerations are secondary, including the need for maternal imaging and medication.

Maternal collapse in pregnancy needs to be managed in accordance with physiological changes, outlined in the Royal College of Obstetricians and Gynaecologists (RCOG) green top guideline.[80]

The following need to be considered:

- *Aortocaval compression*: after 20 weeks gestation, can reduce cardiac output by 30–40% when supine and significantly reduces efficacy of chest compressions during resuscitation.
- *Changes in lung function*: increased risk of hypoxia and make ventilation more difficult.
- *Difficult intubation risk*: this is more likely in pregnancy and critical illness due to the presence of large breasts reducing access to the laryngoscope and laryngeal oedema.
- *Increased risk of aspiration*: early intubation is required in critical illness, with the use of cricoid pressure, non-particulate antacids, and H_2 antagonists.

- *Blood pressure*: limits are different in pregnancy. A blood pressure (BP) of 90/60 mmHg is normal in healthy women whilst in pregnancy-induced hypertension, aim to keep BP <150/100 mmHg.
- *Blood loss*: high cardiac output and uterine blood flow means that large volumes can be lost quickly.
- *Hypercoagulopathy*: all parturients will require venous thromboembolism prophylaxis if prolonged immobilization and critical illness.
- *Nutrition*: need an extra 300 kcal/day plus micronutrients.

Specific points for antenatal care of a critically ill parturient

- Patients should be nursed in left lateral tilt position in third trimester.
- There is an increased risk of urinary tract infection, which requires regular mid-stream urine specimens sent to bacteriology.
- Women with pregnancy-induced hypertension tolerate fluid overload poorly—fluid management should be in accordance with NICE guidelines.[81]
- Access to a delivery set will be required for vaginal or caesarean delivery in case of urgent delivery.
- In terms of care for the fetus, antenatal steroids will be required for fetal lung maturation. A fetal monitoring surveillance plan is required with regular fetal growth ultrasound and daily fetal heart rate monitoring if no maternal perception of fetal movements after 28 weeks of gestation.

Specific points for postpartum care

- Breastfeeding should be encouraged, with consideration given to the safety of medications in breast milk.
- A diuresis is normal, as the transition occurs from maternal to non-pregnant physiology.
- Thromboprophylaxis will be required for all women, once coagulopathy has been corrected.
- Routine post-delivery checks will be required such as anti-D for rhesus-negative parturients and perineal care.

Maternity and general critical care interface

A daily review is required by the multidisciplinary team, who must include a named obstetrician and a named senior midwife. Contact telephone numbers for the team should appear on the patient's chart, together with a management plan for obstetric/midwifery care. Ongoing obstetric issues need to be discussed with the critical care team (e.g. pre-eclampsia) so that they are not overshadowed by current medical emergency.

Resources available to look after the critically ill mother

Appropriate equipment must be available within Level 2 care rooms (Box 30.2) and all electrical equipment must be kept plugged in at all times to ensure that batteries are fully charged.

Box 30.2 Equipment required in Level 2 rooms

- Wall suction and the relevant accessories
- Airway adjuncts
- Piped oxygen and oxygen masks, with high-concentration oxygen masks available
- Equipment to secure intravenous and administer fluids
- Intravenous pumps and syringe drivers
- Monitoring equipment for pulse oximetry, ECG, non-invasive blood pressure, and transducer facility for invasive monitoring
- Equipment for insertion and management of invasive monitoring
- Intravenous fluid warmer
- Forced air warming device
- Blood gas analyser, with facility to measure serum lactate
- Emergency massive haemorrhage trolley
- Emergency eclampsia box
- Transfer equipment: monitor and ventilator
- Computer terminal for access to blood results, patient administration systems, and intranet for access to local guidelines
- Resuscitation trolley with defibrillator and airway management equipment.

Maternal critical care admission criteria

Admission criteria for Level 2 care on the delivery suite

1. Escalation in care for women within the delivery suite

- Patients who require stabilization of hypertension.
- Patients who require seizure control.
- Patients with pre-existing co-morbidity, which affects daily living.
- Patients with massive blood loss (2000 mL or smaller loss associated with cardiovascular instability).
- Patients who require greater than 4 units of blood transfused.
- Patients requiring more than 40% oxygen via a fixed concentrated mask.
- Patients who show signs of severe sepsis.
- Patients who trigger a MEWS score of 7 or higher.
- Management of invasive lines.
- Patients who develop coagulopathy.

2. Step-down after Level 3 care or specialist care

This will require joint medical and midwifery judgement regarding the level of critical care required, taking into account all factors pertaining to the actual case including the patient's wishes and availability of other beds.

3. Transfer criteria for Level 2 respiratory support

If Level 2 respiratory support is thought necessary, expert advice should be sought from the on-call consultant anaesthetist. Women should be transferred for Level 2 care if any of the following are present:

- Tachypnoea with a respiratory rate greater than 20 breaths/min
- SpO_2 consistently less than 93 % on air
- PO_2 of 8.0 kPa on air
- PCO_2 of 5.0 kPa
- Pulmonary oedema confirmed by chest X-ray
- MEWS 7 or above.

Escalation to Level 3 care

Expert advice should be sought from the consultant intensivist at the receiving ICU, prior to stabilization and transfer, where further deterioration has occurred. Women requiring the following support must be transferred to Level 3:

- Mechanical ventilation
- Advanced renal support
- Multisystem organ failure
- Plasmapheresis
- Coronary care.

Safe transfer is the responsibility of the consultant anaesthetist on call.

Discharge criteria

Discharge from maternity HDU is generally appropriate when the condition that has led to the admission has been adequately treated or stabilized or when the patient no longer requires the level of monitoring and nursing provided on the maternity HDU and can be managed on the ward. This should be considered when the patient has been stabilized and no longer require close monitoring. In addition, discharge of a patient from the HDU (Level 1 or 2, to 0, or vice versa) should be considered in order to accommodate another patient. This decision must be by the consultants involved.

Critical care outreach

Critical Care Outreach developed in the United Kingdom in response to the finding that suboptimal care was often evident at the time of critical admission,[6] with increasing evidence linking this to missed opportunities for earlier intervention and poor outcome.[82]

The Critical Care Outreach service is defined by the Intensive Care Society as a multidisciplinary approach to the identification of patients at risk of developing critical illness, and those patients recovering from a period of critical illness, to enable early intervention or transfer (if appropriate) to an area suitable to care for that patient's individual needs.[83]

Outreach should be a collaboration and partnership between the critical care department and other departments to ensure a continuum of care for patients regardless of location, and should enhance the skills and understanding of all staff in the delivery of critical care. It is not a remedy for inadequate provision of a critical care bed, inadequate ward facilities for lower dependency patients, decreasing ward nursing numbers, or inexperienced trainees with lack of supervision. The outreach team should be prepared to take over or at least direct the care of critically ill patients whose admission to a critical care facility is delayed.

The majority of general hospitals in the United Kingdom have intensive care nurse-led outreach systems, supported by critical care doctors.[84] In the Liverpool Women's Hospital, the critical care outreach team is led by midwives from the HDU, supported by on-call anaesthetists and obstetricians.

Care of the critically ill parturient in different settings

The National Service Framework for Children, Young People and Maternity Services requires that consultant-led obstetric units have adequate facilities for comprehensive emergency obstetric care, including transfer to intensive care. Pathways must therefore be designed at local level to ensure that a critically ill parturient has equitable access to critical care, with arrangements taking into account local configuration, size, and complexity of maternity and critical care services.[9] These pathways should facilitate mother and baby staying together unless precluded by clinical reason.

Different models of care may include:

- designated area within the delivery suite for Level 2 care, with medical input from anaesthetists and obstetricians, staffed by suitably trained critical care midwives, supported by escalation policies to Level 3 care
- importing critical care skills onto the delivery suite using critical care outreach or other arrangement with local critical care services
- transferring women to a general Level 2 unit, with local arrangements to provide obstetric and midwifery input, whilst maintaining direct contact between mother and baby.

Monitoring in the high dependency unit

All critically ill patients in the HDU require pulse oximetry, electrocardiogram (ECG), and blood pressure monitoring. There should be a low threshold for using arterial lines in HDU, particularly where the patient is unstable or requires repeated arterial blood samples.

Central venous pressure monitoring can be used as a guide to right ventricular filling pressures. However, titrating fluid challenges against central venous pressure should be performed cautiously, due to poor correlation between right- and left-sided filling pressures, particularly in patients with pre-eclampsia.[85]

Cardiac output monitoring

Measurement of blood pressure alone gives the clinician little information about its constituent components of cardiac output and systemic vascular resistance, which is essential information in both the diagnosis and management of critical illness.

Cardiac monitoring is not routinely used at present in obstetric practice. A recent survey of tertiary referral centres found that only 22% of obstetric anaesthetists had experience of cardiac

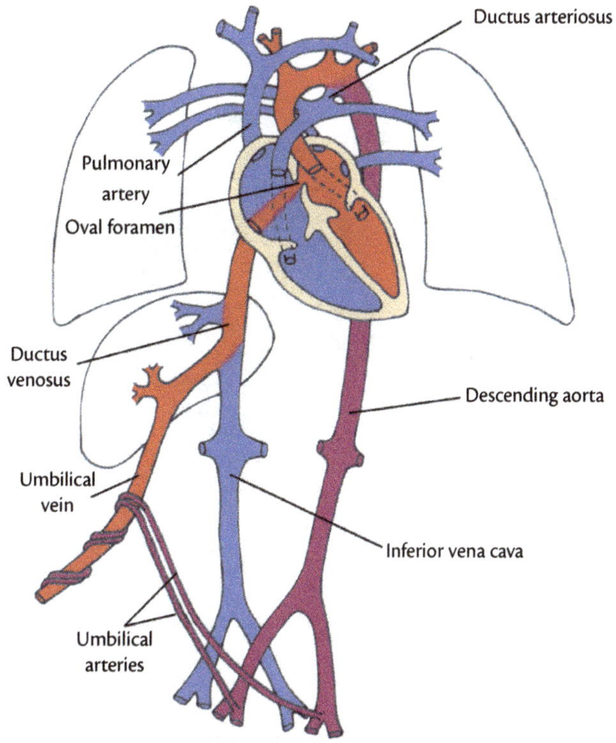

Figure 4.1 The fetal circulation before birth. Fetal circulation is characterized by three shunts: (1) ductus venosus, (2) oval foramen, and (3) ductus arteriosus. Blood flow is directed to bypass the liver in the ductus venosus. From the right atrium oxygenated blood flows through the oval foramen into the left atrium, left ventricle, and into the aorta.

PHYSIOLOGICAL PARAMETERS	3	2	1	0	1	2	3
Respiration Rate	≤8		9–11	12–20		21–24	≥25
Oxygen Saturations	≤91	92–93	94–95	≥96			
Any Supplemental Oxygen		Yes		No			
Temperature	≤35.0		35.1–36.0	36.1–38.0	38.1–39.0	≥39.1	
Systolic BP	≤90	91–100	101–110	111–219			≥220
Heart Rate	≤40		41–50	51–90	91–110	111–130	≥131
Level of Consciousness				A			V, P, or U

Figure 30.2 The National Early Warning Score (NEWS).
Reproduced with permission from the Royal College of Physicians. *National Early Warning Score (NEWS): Standardising the assessment of acute illness severity in the NHS*. Report of a working party. © Royal College of Physicians 2012.

NEW scores	Clinical risk
0	Low
Aggregate 1–4	
RED score (Individual parameter scoring 3)	Medium
Aggregate 5–6	
Aggregate 7 or more	High

Figure 30.3 The National Early Warning Score (NEWS) thresholds and triggers.
Reproduced with permission from the Royal College of Physicians. *National Early Warning Score (NEWS): Standardising the assessment of acute illness severity in the NHS*. Report of a working party. © Royal College of Physicians 2012.

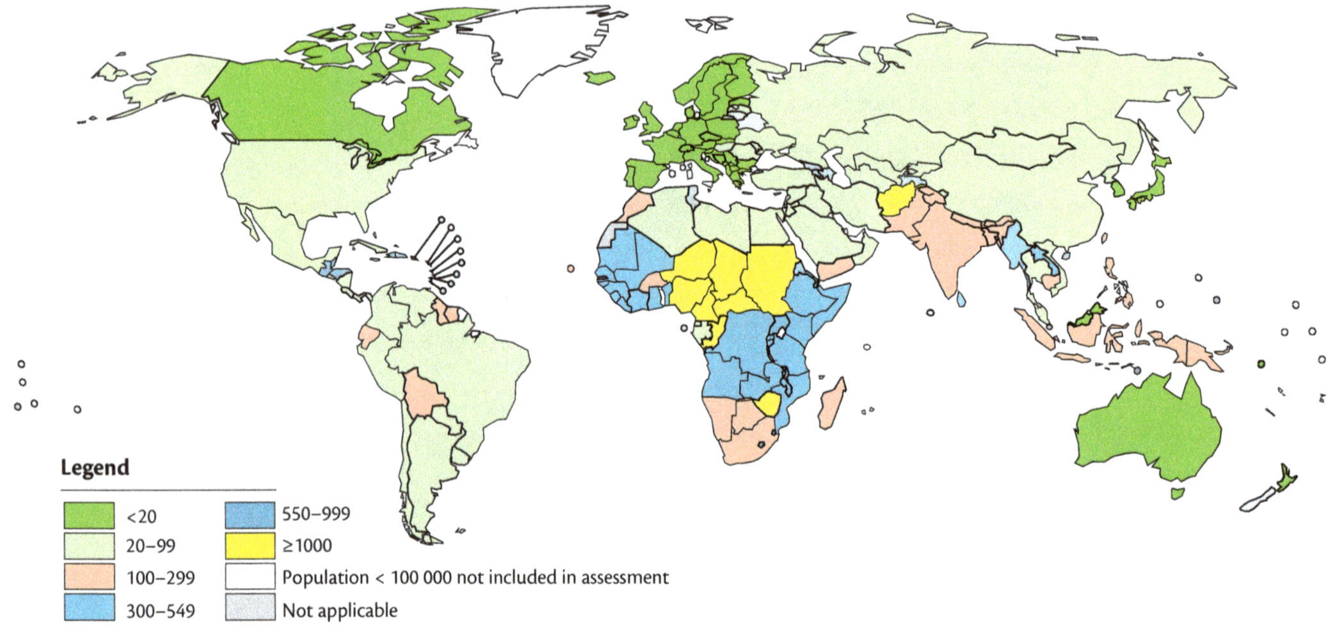

Figure 31.1 Maternal mortality ratio (per 100,000 live births) worldwide, 2010.
Reproduced with permission from WHO, *Trends in Maternal Mortality: 1990 to 2010 WHO, UNICEF, UNFPA and The World Bank estimates*, Geneva, World Health organization, Copyright © 2012.

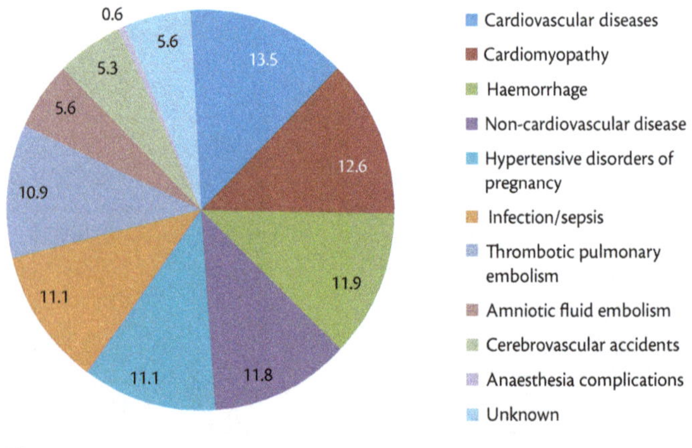

Figure 31.10 Causes of pregnancy-related deaths in the United States: 2006 to 2007.
Data from Berg CJ. From identification and review to action--maternal mortality review in the United States. *Semin Perinatol* 2012; 36:7–13, Copyright © 2012 Elsevier.

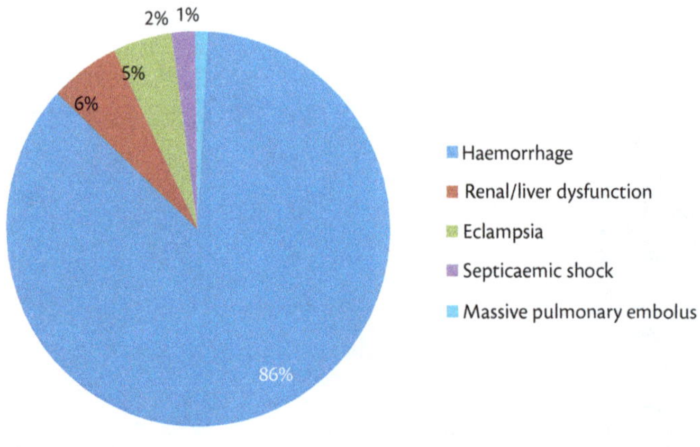

Figure 31.11 Causes of maternal morbidity (as a percentage of total) from Scottish Confidential Audit of Severe Maternal Morbidity: 2006–2008.
Data from various sources (see References).

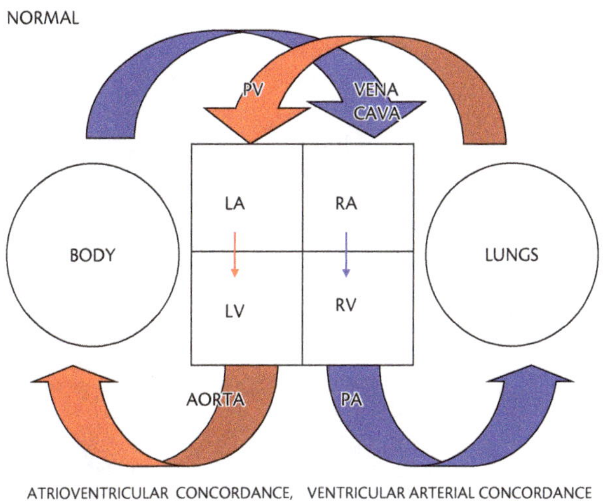

Figure 40.1 The normal configuration.
Reprinted from *International Journal of Obstetric Anesthesia*, Volume 19, edition 3, D.P. Dob, M.A. Naguib, M.A. Gatzoulis, A functional understanding of moderate to complex congenital heart disease and the impact of pregnancy. Part I: The transposition complexes, pp. 298–305, Copyright (2010), with permission from Elsevier.

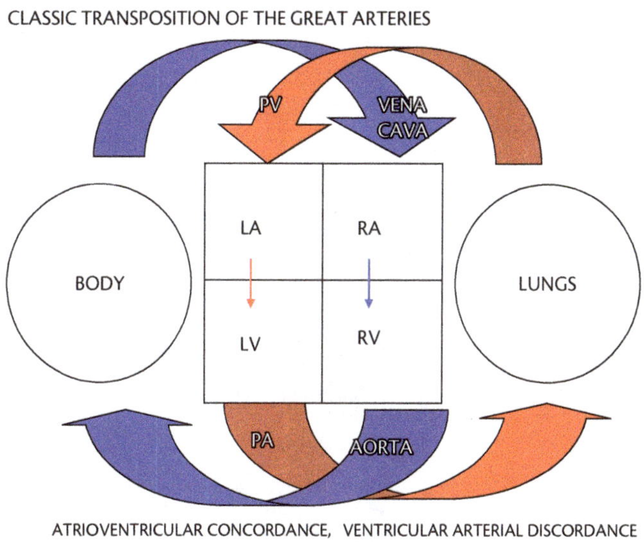

Figure 40.2 Classic transposition of the great arteries.
Reprinted from *International Journal of Obstetric Anesthesia*, Volume 19, edition 3, D.P. Dob, M.A. Naguib, M.A. Gatzoulis, A functional understanding of moderate to complex congenital heart disease and the impact of pregnancy. Part I: The transposition complexes, pp. 298–305, Copyright (2010), with permission from Elsevier.

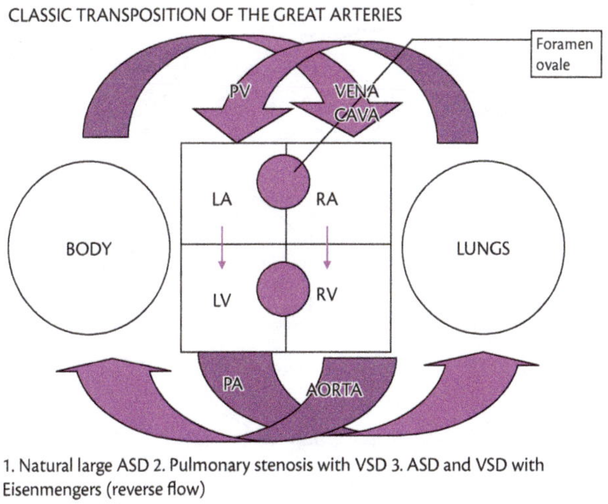

Figure 40.3 Classic transposition of the great arteries with a large shunt.
Reprinted from *International Journal of Obstetric Anesthesia*, Volume 19, edition 3, D.P. Dob, M.A. Naguib, M.A. Gatzoulis, A functional understanding of moderate to complex congenital heart disease and the impact of pregnancy. Part I: The transposition complexes, pp. 298–305, Copyright (2010), with permission from Elsevier.

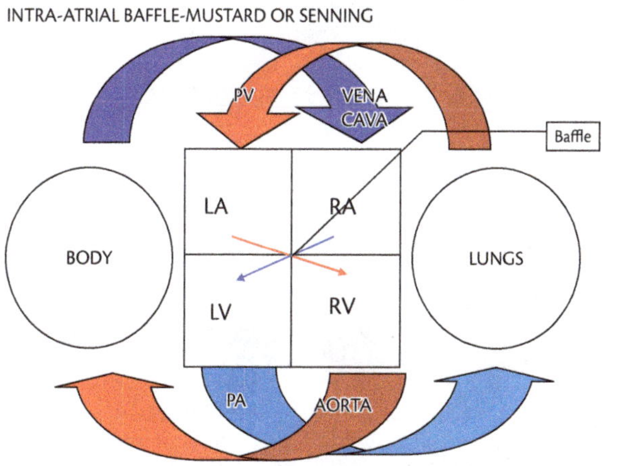

Figure 40.4 Intra-atrial baffle (Mustard or Senning atrial switch), represented by the red and blue crossed arrows.
Reprinted from *International Journal of Obstetric Anesthesia*, Volume 19, edition 3, D.P. Dob, M.A. Naguib, M.A. Gatzoulis, A functional understanding of moderate to complex congenital heart disease and the impact of pregnancy. Part I: The transposition complexes, pp. 298–305, Copyright (2010), with permission from Elsevier.

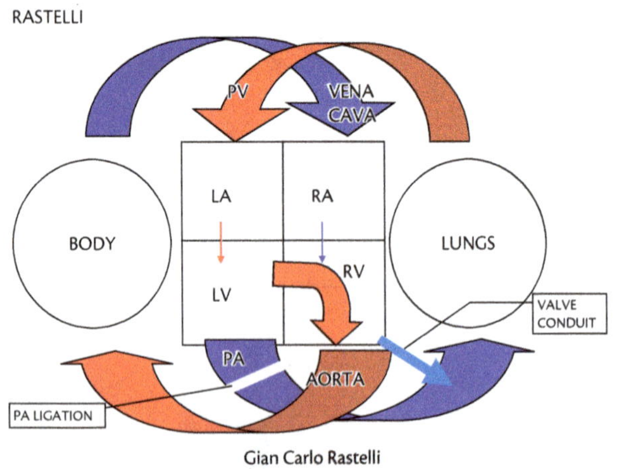

Figure 40.5 Rastelli procedure. The large red arrow represents the Dacron tunnel from the left ventricle to the aorta. The blue arrow represents the valved conduit from the right ventricle to the pulmonary artery. The pulmonary trunk is transected and sewn up.
Reprinted from *International Journal of Obstetric Anesthesia*, Volume 19, edition 3, D.P. Dob, M.A. Naguib, M.A. Gatzoulis, A functional understanding of moderate to complex congenital heart disease and the impact of pregnancy. Part I: The transposition complexes, pp. 298–305, Copyright (2010), with permission from Elsevier.

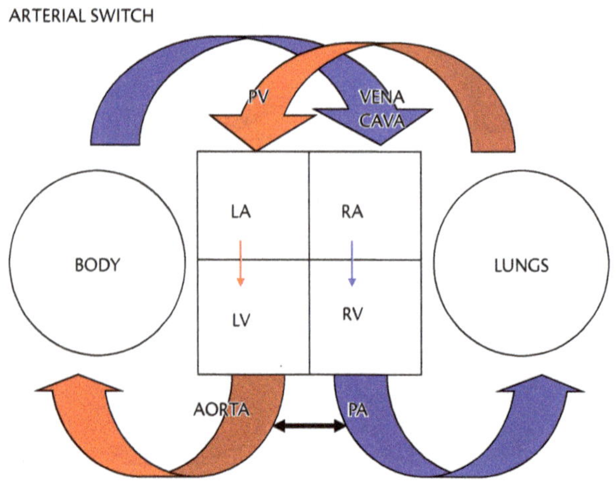

Figure 40.6 Arterial switch (Jatene) procedure. Aorta and pulmonary artery switched to the correct ventricle (represented by the black arrow). The coronary arteries are transected with a 'button' of pulmonary artery wall and re-implanted into the neo-aorta, which was the old pulmonary artery.
Reprinted from *International Journal of Obstetric Anesthesia*, Volume 19, edition 3, D.P. Dob, M.A. Naguib, M.A. Gatzoulis, A functional understanding of moderate to complex congenital heart disease and the impact of pregnancy. Part I: The transposition complexes, pp. 298–305, Copyright (2010), with permission from Elsevier.

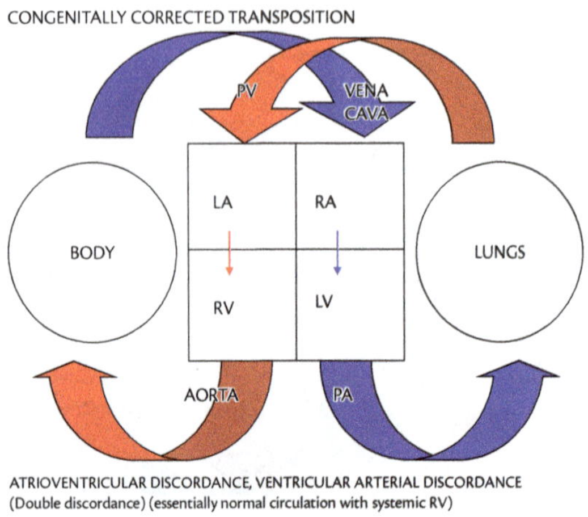

Figure 40.7 Congenitally corrected transposition of the great arteries showing double discordance.
Reprinted from *International Journal of Obstetric Anesthesia*, Volume 19, edition 3, D.P. Dob, M.A. Naguib, M.A. Gatzoulis, A functional understanding of moderate to complex congenital heart disease and the impact of pregnancy. Part I: The transposition complexes, pp. 298–305, Copyright (2010), with permission from Elsevier.

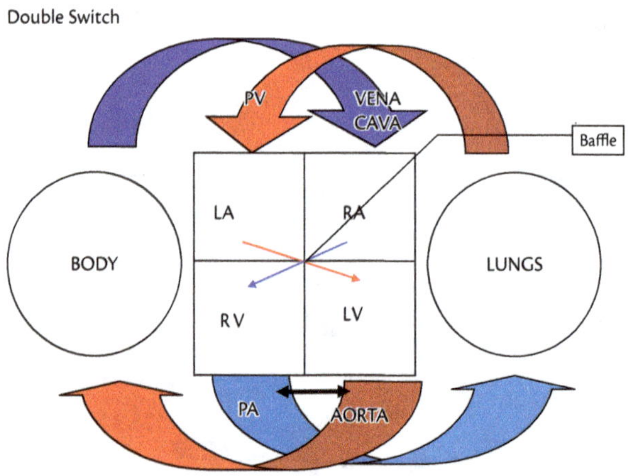

Figure 40.8 Double-switch procedure—an intra-atrial switch is combined with an arterial switch to give a near normal circulation to repair congenitally corrected transposition of the great arteries.
Reprinted from *International Journal of Obstetric Anesthesia*, Volume 19, edition 3, D.P. Dob, M.A. Naguib, M.A. Gatzoulis, A functional understanding of moderate to complex congenital heart disease and the impact of pregnancy. Part I: The transposition complexes, pp. 298–305, Copyright (2010), with permission from Elsevier.

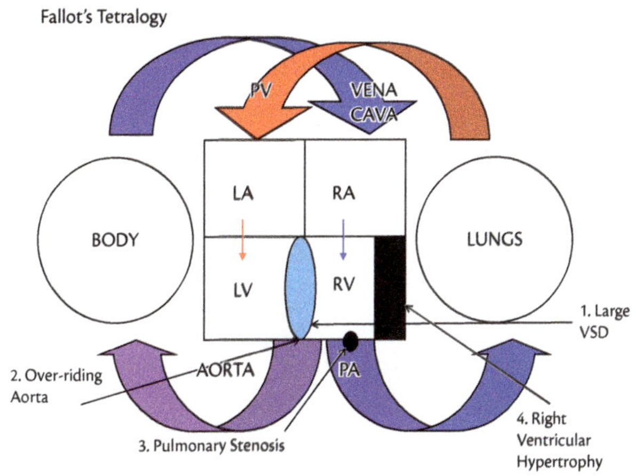

Figure 40.9 Fallot's tetralogy. The purple colour represents mixed oxygenated and de-oxygenated blood.
Reprinted from *International Journal of Obstetric Anesthesia*, Volume 19, edition 3, M.A. Naguib, D.P. Dob, M.A. Gatzoulis, A functional understanding of moderate to complex congenital heart disease and the impact of pregnancy. Part II: Tetralogy of Fallot, Eisenmenger's syndrome and the Fontan operation, pp. 306–312, Copyright (2010), with permission from Elsevier.

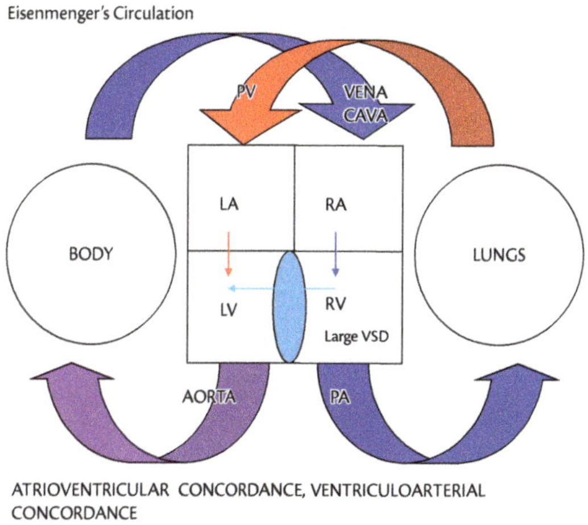

Figure 40.10 Eisenmenger's circulation. The purple colour represents mixed oxygenated and de-oxygenated blood.
Reprinted from *International Journal of Obstetric Anesthesia*, Volume 19, edition 3, M.A. Naguib, D.P. Dob, M.A. Gatzoulis, A functional understanding of moderate to complex congenital heart disease and the impact of pregnancy. Part II: Tetralogy of Fallot, Eisenmenger's syndrome and the Fontan operation, pp. 306–312, Copyright (2010), with permission from Elsevier.

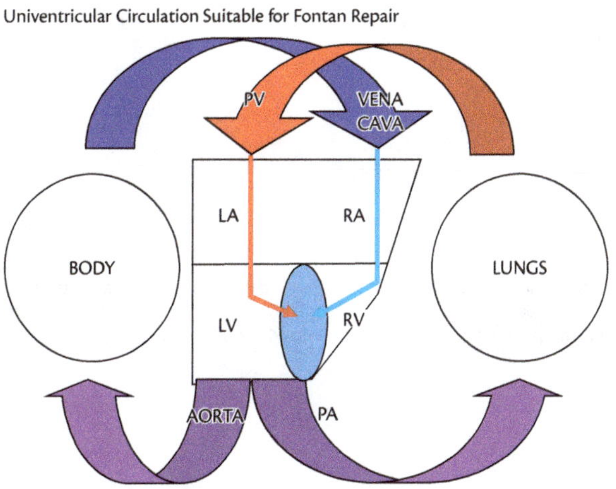

Figure 40.11 Univentricular circulation suitable for the Fontan operation. The purple colour represents mixed oxygenated and de-oxygenated blood.
Reprinted from *International Journal of Obstetric Anesthesia*, Volume 19, edition 3, M.A. Naguib, D.P. Dob, M.A. Gatzoulis, A functional understanding of moderate to complex congenital heart disease and the impact of pregnancy. Part II: Tetralogy of Fallot, Eisenmenger's syndrome and the Fontan operation, pp. 306–312, Copyright (2010), with permission from Elsevier.

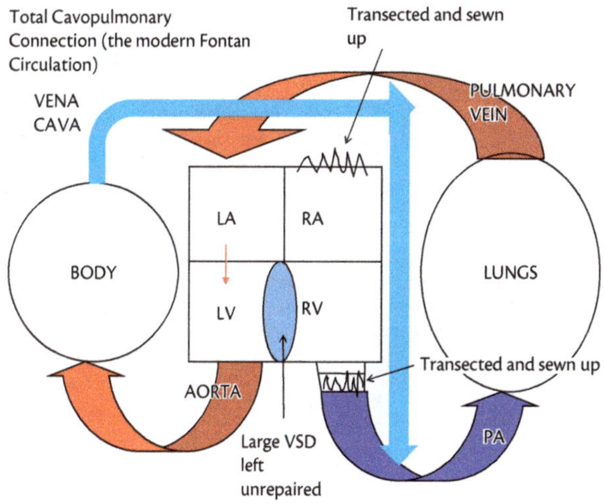

Figure 40.12 Total cavopulmonary connection (TCPC), the modern Fontan circulation.
LA = left atrium, LV = left ventricle, RA = right atrium, ASD = atrial septal defect, RV = right ventricle, VSD = ventricular septal defect, PA = pulmonary artery, PV = pulmonary veins.
Reprinted from *International Journal of Obstetric Anesthesia*, Volume 19, edition 3, M.A. Naguib, D.P. Dob, M.A. Gatzoulis, A functional understanding of moderate to complex congenital heart disease and the impact of pregnancy. Part II: Tetralogy of Fallot, Eisenmenger's syndrome and the Fontan operation, pp. 306–312, Copyright (2010), with permission from Elsevier.

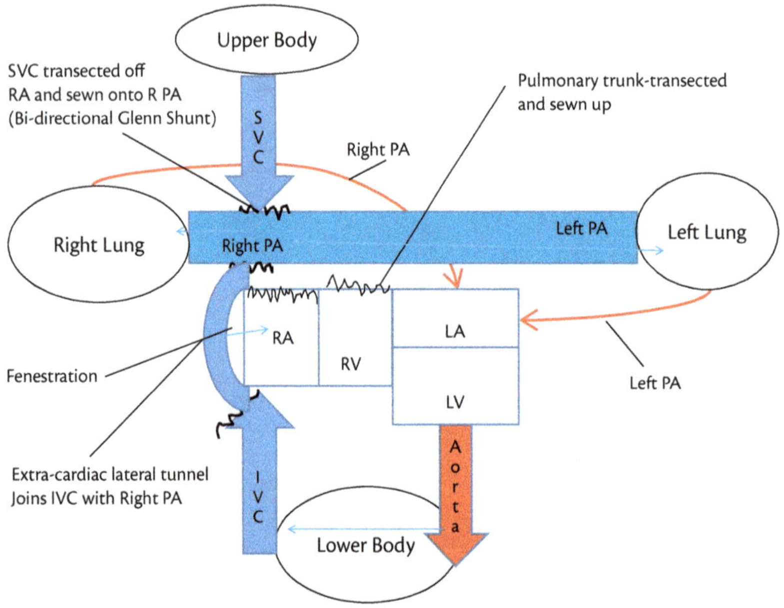

Figure 40.13 Total cavopulmonary connection (TCPC) in detail with extracardiac lateral tunnel and fenestration (the modern Fontan). The superior vena cava is transected and connected to the right pulmonary artery. This is known as a bi-directional Glenn shunt and is usually the first part of the palliation. Subsequently, the inferior vena cava is transected and connected to the underside of the pulmonary artery confluence with an extracardiac conduit. The proximal pulmonary trunk is then transected and sewn up.

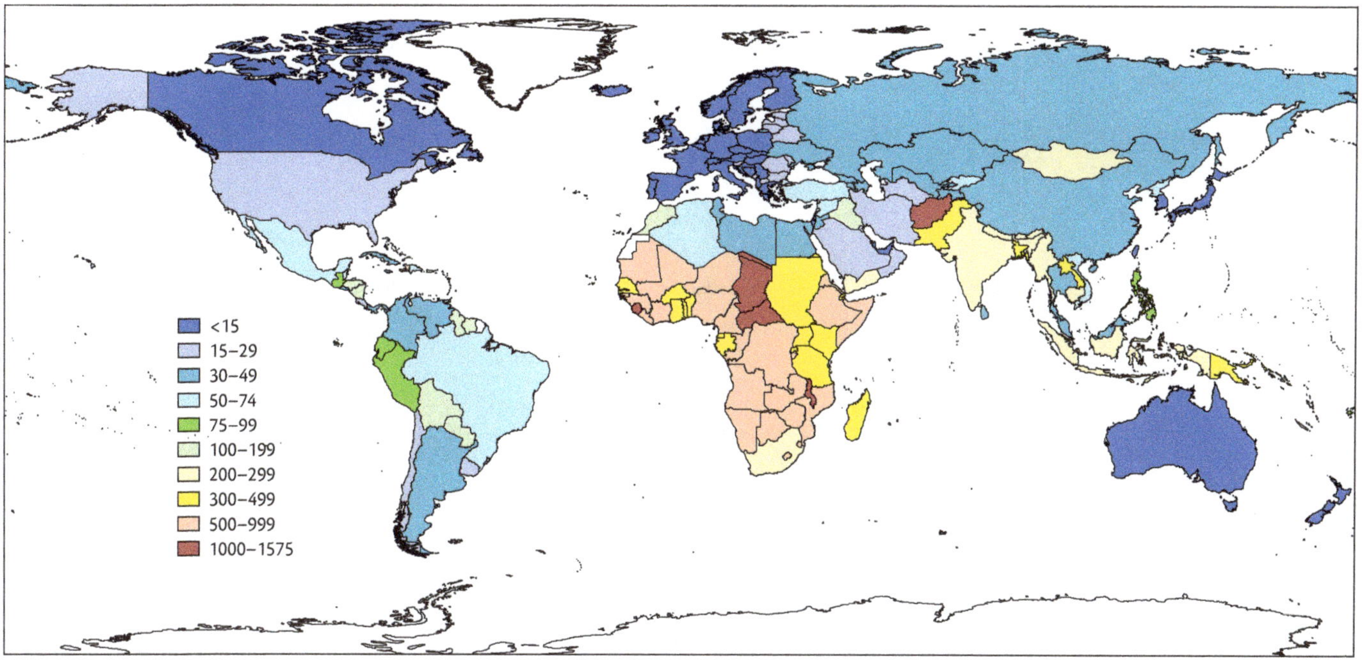

Figure 55.1 Maternal mortality ratio per 100,000 live births, 2008.
Reprinted from *The Lancet*, Volume 375, number 9726, Margaret C Hogan *et al.*, Maternal mortality for 181 countries, 1980–2008: a systematic analysis of progress towards Millennium Development Goal 5, pp. 1609–1623, Copyright (2010), with permission from Elsevier.

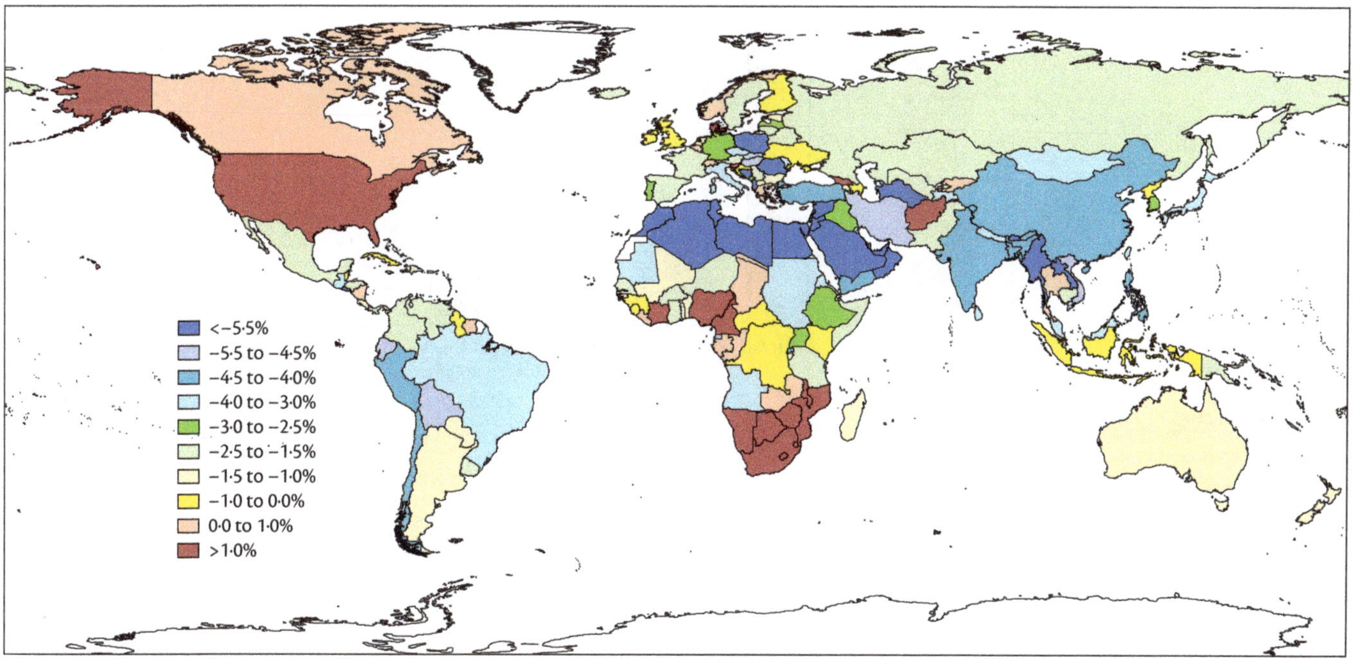

Figure 55.2 Yearly rate of decline in maternal mortality ratio, 1990–2008.
Reprinted from *The Lancet*, Volume 375, number 9726, Margaret C Hogan *et al.*, Maternal mortality for 181 countries, 1980–2008: a systematic analysis of progress towards Millennium Development Goal 5, pp. 1609–1623, Copyright (2010), with permission from Elsevier.

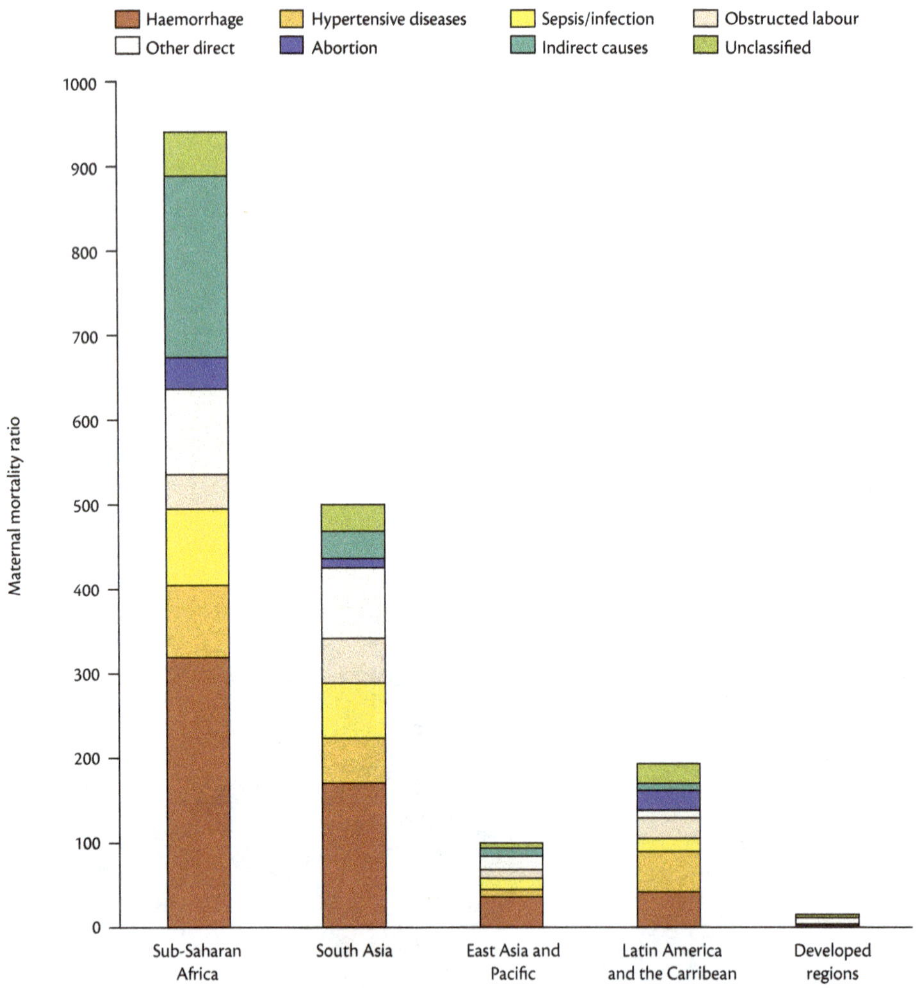

Figure 55.5 Maternal mortality ratios for 2000 by medical cause and world region.

Reprinted from *The Lancet*, Volume 368, number 9542, Ronsmans C, Graham W, Maternal survival 1. Maternal mortality: who, when, where and why, pp. 1189–1200, Copyright (2006), with permission from Elsevier.

output monitors although half those surveyed believed that they should be available in all obstetric units in the next 10 years.[86]

Pulmonary artery catheters

The pulmonary artery catheter (PAC) was first described by Swan, Ganz, and associates in 1970[87] and rapidly evolved from a research device into a clinical tool. It was widely used in adult general ICUs to measure intracardiac pressures and cardiac output and became very popular with over 2 million catheters sold worldwide in 1996.[88]

However, unequivocal proof that information from PACs improved outcome was scarce. A review of the use of PACs in obstetric critical illness questioned the lack of proven benefit from the haemodynamic information when set against the potential risk of complications such as pneumothorax, ventricular arrhythmias, air embolism, pulmonary infarction, pulmonary artery rupture, sepsis, local vascular thrombosis, intracardiac knotting, and valve damage.[89]

There are also concerns about the use of PACs in general ICUs. An observational study of 5735 critically ill adults using case-matching analysis showed that PAC use was associated with increased 30-day mortality, increased stay in ICU, and increased utilization of resources, with no apparent benefit from using the PAC.[90] The accompanying editorial in *JAMA*,[91] suggested a complete moratorium on their use until the matter was resolved but it was clear that many physicians intending to continue using PACs. A Consensus Conference held in December 1996[92] examined the risks and benefits of using PACs in different critical care scenarios. For its use in maternal critical care, no evidence was found that routine use of PACs reduced complications and mortality associated with pre-eclampsia but it was agreed that it may be of use when dealing with severe pre-eclampsia. There was also uncertainty as to whether PACs improved outcomes in patients with septic shock but it was agreed that they may be useful in patients who have not responded to initial fluid resuscitation and vasopressors. The conference did find that the PAC provided information that altered diagnosis and treatment in patients admitted with respiratory failure. The conference concluded that there should not be a moratorium on the use of PACs.

PACs remained in regular use for obstetric patients admitted to ICUs, although there was a wide variation in their use.[12] A retrospective review of PAC use in severe pre-eclampsia at the obstetric ICU at the Groote Schuur Hospital, Cape Town, South Africa, was performed between 1995 and 1997.[93] Of the 598 women admitted to the unit, 115 required pulmonary artery catheterization; 53% had renal failure, 30% pulmonary oedema, and 17% had eclampsia. Review of the ICU charts showed that the initial readings from the PAC allowed a determination of maternal fluid status that was judged to be helpful in guiding management in 93% of cases. Four per cent of patients developed complications: three cases of venous thrombosis and one case of cellulitis. There were no cases of pulmonary haemorrhage or infarction.

The initial high incidence of complications from PACs improved with better medical and nursing care, for example, pneumothorax has fallen from 6% to less than 0.1%; pulmonary infarction from 7.2% to 0–1.3% and pulmonary artery rupture from 0.1– 0.2% to less than 0.1%.[94]

By 2001, Hazelgrove et al. found that there was a wide variation amongst different ICUs in the use of PACs for haemodynamic monitoring of critically ill parturients.[12]

In 2003, a large-scale randomized, blinded study by Sandham et al. of 1994 patients showed that there was no benefit to therapy directed by PACs over standard care.[95] There was a higher incidence of pulmonary embolus in the PAC group: eight patients versus none in the standard care group.

A Cochrane review published in 2013 found that the use of PACs did not alter the mortality or length of stay in ICU or hospital and recommended that newer, less invasive haemodynamic tools needed to be validated against PACs prior to clinical use in critically ill patients.[96]

Transthoracic and transoesophageal echocardiography

Echocardiography is readily accepted by pregnant women as ultrasonography is used routinely in pregnancy in childbirth to monitor mother and fetus and has been shown to have an excellent safety profile. Cardiac output may be measured at a number of anatomical locations: the left ventricular outflow tract, ascending aorta, pulmonary artery, right ventricular outflow tract, and mitral valve. Transthoracic echocardiography (TTE) uses an ultrasound probe placed on the chest well whereas transoesophageal echocardiography (TOE) requires an ultrasound transducer to be placed within the oesophagus. Both methods allow an assessment of filling status, myocardial contraction, valvular function, and detection of pericardial effusion as well as being used for measurement of haemodynamic variables.

TTE is truly non-invasive and suitable for all obstetric patients. During pregnancy, anterior and left displacement of the heart together with an elevated diaphragm and partial lateral tilt facilitate apical and lateral views with TTE.

TOE provides clearer images and better views of the atria and septa but requires the patient to receive sedation or general anaesthesia, which makes it less suitable for routine use in the parturient. There are many case reports in the literature of its use in critically ill women with cardiac disease or emergencies.[97–104]

Haemodynamic measurements made using echocardiography have been shown to compare well to those with the gold standard of pulmonary artery thermodilution. Belfort et al.[105] showed a high correlation between ultrasound-derived measurements and PAC measurements for stroke volume, cardiac output, cardiac index, left ventricular filling pressure, pulmonary artery systolic pressure, and right atrial pressure in 11 critically ill obstetric patients. Right atrial pressure is calculated by measuring the maximum and minimum size of the inferior vena cava in inspiration and expiration. The Doppler-derived stroke volume and two-dimensional estimates of end-diastolic volume were used to calculate ejection fraction.

A subsequent study showed that results obtained from M-mode echocardiography and two-dimensional Doppler yielded similar results and proved reliable in critically ill pregnant women.[106]

Belfort et al. then conducted a subsequent study to see if these values could be used in clinical patient management of critically ill women with an indication for invasive monitoring.[107] These included oliguria unresponsive to boluses of crystalloid, severe, pregnancy-induced hypertension despite hydralazine, and patients with other cardiac conditions that put them at a high risk of developing pulmonary oedema. Fourteen patients were studied and all but two were managed without the need to proceed to pulmonary artery catheterization. Of these, one had a hypertensive cardiomyopathy whilst the other had severe asthma requiring intubation and ventilation. Of the six oliguric patients, all had pre-eclampsia and had previously received fluid challenges with crystalloid. Echocardiography excluded volume overload in all patients and none developed pulmonary oedema or required invasive monitoring. The authors concluded that a knowledge of the ejection fraction, intracardiac pressures, and cardiac output allowed a more informed decision to be made regarding whether a preferential vasodilator (e.g. calcium channel blocker or arterial vasodilator) should be used or an agent with a predominantly negative inotropic effect such a beta blocker. One patient with pre-eclampsia and oliguria had developed a coagulopathy due to placental abruption and intrauterine fetal death in which circumstances central line insertion would have been hazardous.

More recently, TTE has been used intraoperatively to guide fluid management and ensure an adequate pre-load in a patient with severe hypertrophic cardiomyopathy.[108] The authors intended to repeat the TTE on the intensive care 4 hours after surgery but this was not possible for logistic reasons, due to the lack of specialist skills to perform TTE. The consequence was that an insidious postpartum bleed was not acted on overnight, which subsequently required interventional radiology.

Recent advances in image quality, device portability, and ease of use now enable TTE to be used for obstetric applications in locations such as the delivery suite, operating theatre, and HDU.[109] The frequent absence of a 24-hour immediate TTE service has provided an incentive for clinicians to be trained in bedside TTE. This has the additional advantage that the clinician can use TTE to answer clinical questions and then perform repeated measurements to follow the response to intervention.

Echocardiography has been used in recent research to examine haemodynamic changes accompanying severe pre-eclampsia. Dennis et al. compared TTE studies of non-pregnant, healthy pregnant and women with pre-eclampsia.[110] Patients with pre-eclampsia had a predominantly raised cardiac output, due to a raised stroke volume, with only a mild increase seen in systemic vascular resistance compared with healthy parturients and reduced diastolic function. These findings support the hyperdynamic model of pre-eclampsia.

Arterial pulse waveform analysis

Arterial pulse waveform analysis methods of measuring stroke volume are attractive for the obstetric anaesthetist as they provide beat-by-beat assessment and can be used both for critical care and research in the delivery suite and operating theatre.[111] They are particularly suitable for use in the awake parturient as they only require an arterial line. This has the advantage that many critically ill patients already have an arterial line *in situ* and enables monitoring of changes in cardiac output and stroke volume on continuous basis.

Limits of agreement of up to 30% between new cardiac output monitors and gold standard devices such as PACs are regarded as acceptable.[112] Current commercially available devices that meet these criteria consist of the calibrated LiDCOplus® (LiDCO, Cambridge, United Kingdom) and PiCCOplus® (Pulsion Medical Systems, Munich, Germany) and the uncalibrated Flotrac-Vigileo® monitor (Edwards Lifesciences, Irvine, CA, United States).

The LiDCOplus® monitor uses arterial pulse power analysis to measure and monitor stroke volume from the arterial pulse pressure waveform from a standard peripheral arterial line.[113] The system can be calibrated using a lithium dilution method. LiDCOplus® has been used to study cardiac output changes during caesarean delivery.[114–116] It has also been shown to predict fluid responsiveness in mechanically ventilated patients,[117] although this is of limited value on the obstetric HDU where most patients breathe spontaneously. LiDCOplus® haemodynamic readings in patients with pre-eclampsia agreed closely with those obtained from pulmonary artery catheterization.[118]

The PiCCOplus® system uses an algorithm that analyses the systolic component of the arterial waveform.[119] Calibration is performed using transpulmonary thermodilution, which requires cannulation of both a proximal artery and a central vein. This has limited its use to intensive care settings and to date there are no studies published using PiCCOplus® in obstetric anaesthesia or maternal critical care research.

The Flotrac-Vigileo® monitor analyses waveform characteristics from a specialized transducer using a multivariate polynomial equation that does not require calibration. It has been used to monitor cardiac output changes during caesarean delivery.[120] Despite software revision, there is a poor agreement with gold standard measures of cardiac output.[121]

Doppler velocimetry may also be used to measure cardiac output. When an ultrasound beam is reflected from moving red blood cells, a change in frequency is seen that is proportional to their velocity. Aortic cross-sectional area can be estimated from nomograms or measured directly and multiplied by total flow to calculate stroke volume. Oesophageal Doppler monitoring (ODM) uses a transducer introduced under sedation or general anaesthesia.[122] ODM is recommended by NICE guidelines for fluid optimization during major surgery to reduce the need for central venous lines, hospital stay, and postoperative complications.[123] It has shown to be of benefit in many different types of surgery[124] but these do not include any obstetric procedures. It has been used to assess critically ill patients with pre-eclampsia, where it was found to underestimate cardiac output by up to 40%, although it did follow trends accurately over time.[125]

Red blood cell velocity in the aortic outflow tract can alternatively be measured using an ultrasound probe placed in the suprasternal notch (USCOM®, USCOM Pty Ltd, Coffs Harbor, NSW, Australia). This is completely non-invasive and has a steep learning curve.[126] USCOM® has been used to measure cardiac output in pregnancy[127] and to assess fluid status during caesarean delivery.[128]

Bioimpedance techniques were first described in the 1970s. Vascular blood flow within the thorax causes a change in electrical resistance, which is detected by skin electrodes. It is non-invasive and low cost but validation studies in critically ill and septic patients have shown poor results.[122]

Bioreactance measures changes in phase shift of an oscillating current passed across the thorax to produce an improved signal:noise ratio. The technique is gaining acceptance with a number of obstetric anaesthetic research studies now published.[129–131]

Aortic blood flow can also be estimated from finger arterial pressure (Portapres®, Finapres Medical Systems, Amsterdam, the Netherlands). This compares reasonably to sphygmomanometry in pregnant patients[132] but was shown to consistently underestimate stroke volume.[133] It was also found to have discrepancies when measuring changes in peripheral vascular resistance[134] or hypovolaemia,[135] making it unsuitable for regular use in obstetric clinical practice.

Table 30.8 Devices that can be used to monitor the cardiovascular system in obstetric HDU/ITU

Technology	Device	Advantages	Limitations
Pulse pressure waveform analysis	LiDCO™plus	Continuous haemodynamic data from patients with arterial lines	Calibration with Lithium dilution
	PiCCO®		Proximal artery cannulation required for calibration
	Vigileo Monitor® with FloTrac® sensor		Poor agreement and slower response than LiDCO or PiCCO
Oesophageal Doppler monitoring	CARDIOQ-ODMTM monitor	Proven value in high-risk general surgery	Requires sedation or general anaesthesia
Continuous wave Doppler ultrasound	USCOM 1A®	Steep learning curve. Non-invasive	Repeated measurements required
Bioimpedance	Oriel 4000®	Low cost, simplicity	Poor validation in critically ill patients
Bioreactance	NICOM® monitor	Low cost, simplicity	

Adapted from NHS Technology Adoption Centre. *Intraoperative Fluid Management Technologies Adoption Pack*. London: NHS Technology Adoption Centre; 2012.

Table 30.8 summarizes the devices that can be used in an obstetric patient, their mode of action, advantages, and disadvantages.

Other patient monitors used in maternal critical care

Monitoring haemoglobin

The Hemocue® (HemoCue Ltd, Sheffield, UK) gives rapid and accurate measurement of haemoglobin concentration in parturients from either venous blood or capillary blood samples.[136] This is of value in the differential diagnosis of shock but requires a clinical decision regarding the timing of measurements (see Chapter 35).

Ideally, it would be possible to continuously monitor haemoglobin in critically ill patients using a non-invasive device so that clinicians could be alerted to a fall in haemoglobin concentration before the clinical signs of shock became apparent. The Rainbow SET® Radical 7 Pulse Co-Oximeter (Masimo Corp., Irvine, CA, United States) uses a seven-wavelength spectrophotometer in place of the conventional two-wavelength pulse oximeter to give a continuous non-invasive estimation of haemoglobin concentration (SpHb). The finger probe is wrapped in an optical shield to prevent interference from outside light. Preliminary studies appeared promising, with a mean difference between haemoglobin concentrations from SpHb and arterial blood of 1 g/dL.[137] Unfortunately, subsequent publications have shown that the device is far less accurate. One study of five women undergoing caesarean hysterectomy showed a median difference of 2 g/dL in 16 out of 17 SpHb readings.[138] Another study in patients undergoing spinal surgery showed that 22% of readings disagreed with laboratory values by more than 2 g/dL.[139] Accuracy of SpHb readings were affected by finger perfusion, with increased variability in the presence of major haemorrhage. There is great potential for SpHb monitoring but the inaccuracies demonstrated in some patients mean that invasive measurement of Hb cannot be abandoned.[140]

Care bundles

Care bundles have been shown to result in a demonstrable reduction in morbidity in the acute hospital setting. Robb et al.[141] examined the impact of eight care bundles on hospital mortality within an acute hospital in North West London. Thirteen diagnoses were targeted by the care bundles, which had accounted for 1142 deaths in 2006–07. This included sepsis and heart failure bundles (available from http://www.bmj.com/content/suppl/2010/03/31/bmj.c1234.DC1). By 2007–08, the crude death rate had fallen by 174 for the targeted diagnoses. These mortality reductions were maintained over the subsequent years between 2009 and 2011.

In 2008, the 1000 Lives Plus campaign was introduced in Wales with the aim of reducing 1000 deaths in acute trusts and 50,000 adverse events. The programme succeeded, reducing mortality by an estimated 1199 lives from April 2008 to April 2010.[142]

The lessons learnt by the 1000 Lives Plus campaign have now been applied to maternity services in the Transforming Maternity Services report.[143] This focused on the need to reduce avoidable harm in two key areas in maternity: acute deterioration and venous thromboembolism. To ensure early detection of critical illness, a mini-collaborative was set up to ensure that MEWS systems were used consistently in all maternity units. One focus of the collaborative was the implementation of care bundles that enable a rapid response in a way that is owned by the clinical team responsible for patient care, without adding a significant burden of work. The Surviving Sepsis Campaign Sepsis Care bundles contain interventions that have strong evidence of improving mortality in sepsis.[144] The 1000 Lives Plus campaign enabled acute and critical care teams to implement the care bundles, with particular emphasis on the sepsis six. This is important in the management of genital tract sepsis, highlighted by a special Centre for Maternal and Child Enquiries (CMACE) emergent theme briefing[145] which showed the need for clear recognition and prompt management, clear leadership, careful documentation, prompt antibiotics, careful fluid balance, and a collaborative approach.

Improved communication is also essential in the care of the acute deteriorating parturient. Clinical teamwork often involves hurried interactions between different human beings with varying styles of communication. The SBAR (Box 30.3) system improves this, originating in the nuclear submarine service.

Box 30.3 SBAR system

S—Situation: What is happening at the present time?
B—Background: What are the circumstances leading up to this situation?
A—Assessment: What do I think the problem is?
R—Recommendation: What should we do to correct the problem?

Adapted from the SBAR Toolkit, available from the Institute for Healthcare Improvement at: http://www.ihi.org/knowledge/Pages/Tools/SBARToolkit.aspx. The SBAR Toolkit was originally developed by Michael Leonard, Doug Bonacum, and Suzanne Graham at Kaiser Permanente of Colorado.

The mini-collaborative aims to ensure that care bundles are introduced based on guidance from CMACE, NICE, and RCOG. They recommended that four care bundles are introduced:

1. Admissions bundle: within 2 hours of admission (earlier if 'unwell'), all women admitted should have a full set of observations and a plan for frequency of observations, which has been communicated to all clinical staff. This should include a DVT risk assessment and a recorded body mass index. This is in accordance with NICE CG50.[64]
2. Recognition bundle: all women should have a plan for risk assessment using MEWS, screening for sepsis if found to be at risk, and DVT risk assessment, together with communication with the clinical team.
3. Response bundle: all women should have a plan for escalation of care if their condition deteriorates, including change of frequency of observations and input from junior and senior medical staff. The cardiac arrest team needs to ensure that they have full details of how to access the maternity department. Appropriate prophylaxis should be given to all women according to their risk assessment. An acute care or critical care outreach team service should be utilized appropriately.
4. Sepsis six: within 1 hour of diagnosis, all women with suspected sepsis should receive:
    a. oxygen to achieve an oxygen saturation of greater than 94%
    b. fluid resuscitation
    c. blood cultures should be taken before antibiotic administration
    d. broad-spectrum antibiotic
    e. serum lactate and haemoglobin should be checked, ensuring haemoglobin concentration is greater than 8 g/dL
    f. urine output should be monitored hourly, using catheterization or self-void.

Care bundles represent a grouping of best practices for a disease process that individually improve care but when applied together may result in a significantly greater improvement. The 1000 Lives Plus campaign implemented care bundles for interventions such as central lines and ventilators and achieved a compliance of more than 95%. There has been an association with this very high compliance and improvements in patient outcome such as a marked reduction in the rate of central line and ventilator-related infections.

The care bundles are not intended as a comprehensive list of all actions to be taken nor are they a care pathway. The main aim is to reduce the opportunity for omission of any of the essential elements of the process. By using care bundles to implement systems for the detection and early treatment of the acutely deteriorating patient, it is possible for clinical teams to demonstrate improvements in one area without having to change everything at once.

Management of the critically ill obstetric patient

Respiratory failure

Acute respiratory distress syndrome

Acute respiratory distress syndrome (ARDS) is a process of non-hydrostatic pulmonary oedema and hypoxaemia which is diagnosed according to the North American-European Consensus Conference criteria (Table 30.9).[146]

The commonest causes of ARDS in pregnancy are haemorrhage and infection. Direct damage may occur to alveolar lung cells or indirect damage may occur due to systemic disease, leading to an acute inflammatory lung injury. The inflammatory response occurs in exudative, proliferative, and fibrotic phases, which result in progressive hypoxaemia and respiratory failure. This may then be complicated by nosocomial pneumonia, pulmonary hypertension, and ventilator-induced lung injury.

Despite recent advances in lung protective mechanical ventilation, the mortality from ARDS remains unacceptably high at around 50–60%.[147] The most frequent cause of death in ARDS is sepsis syndrome with multiorgan failure rather than irreversible respiratory failure.

The management of ARDS involved respiratory support together with identification and treatment of the precipitating

Table 30.9 North American-European Consensus Conference ARDS and acute lung injury criteria

	ARDS
Timing	Acute onset
Oxygenation	$PaO_2/FiO_2 \leq 200$ mmHg (26.7 kPa), regardless of PEEP
Chest X-ray	Bilateral infiltrates
Paw	≤ 18 mmHg, if measured or no clinical evidence of left atrial hypertension, to exclude cardiogenic pulmonary oedema
	Acute lung injury—same criteria as ARDS except
Oxygenation	$PaO_2/FiO_2 \leq 300$ mmHg (40 kPa), regardless of PEEP
PaO_2	Partial pressure of oxygen in arterial blood
FiO_2	Fraction of inspired oxygen
PaO_2/FiO_2 ratio	Normal range is 300–500 mmHg (40–66.7 kPa)
Paw	Pulmonary capillary wedge pressure, used to measure left atrial pressure

Paw, airway pressure; PEEP, positive end expiratory pressure.

Data from Bernard GR, Artigas A, Brigham KL, *et al.* Report of the American-European consensus conference on ARDS: Definitions, mechanisms, relevant outcomes and clinical trial coordination. *Intensive Care Medicine*, volume 20, issue 3, pp. 34–56. Copyright © 1994 Springer.

cause. For mild acute lung injury, oxygen therapy, physiotherapy, and diuretics to reduce extravascular lung water may suffice. More severe lung injury/ARDS will require mechanical ventilation with a protective lung strategy.

With widespread usage of pulse oximetry, arterial hypoxaemia can be readily detected and confirmed by measurement of arterial blood gas tension.

Shock

Shock is defined as acute circulatory collapse with inadequate delivery of oxygen at a tissue level. The commonest causes of shock in pregnancy are massive haemorrhage and sepsis.

The causes of shock in pregnancy can be divided into low and high cardiac output states (Table 30.10). Shock causes physiological disturbances, detectable on routine monitoring (Table 30.11). Patients with a high cardiac output shock are 'warm and dilated' with a bounding pulse and are flushed.

Patients with low cardiac output are peripherally vasoconstricted and shutdown with a low volume pulse. In hypovolaemia, a low central venous pressure will differentiate from the high pressures seen in obstructive or cardiogenic shock. However, central venous pressure is not a reliable measurement of volaemic status in previously healthy obstetric patients due to their ability to compensate for volume loss by maintaining both blood pressure and central venous pressure.

Early detection and prompt management is required as mortality increases after the first hour. Generic supportive treatment includes oxygen therapy to improve oxygen delivery, and appropriate intravenous fluids and inotropic or vasopressor drugs to maintain circulation.

It is essential to diagnose the underlying cause promptly to ensure that the correct treatment is given. Patients with cardiogenic shock require very careful intravenous fluid administration and inotropic support of blood pressure whereas patients with hypovolaemic shock due to concealed haemorrhage require aggressive fluid therapy and identification of the source of blood loss.

Sepsis and systemic inflammatory response syndrome

2001 Sepsis definitions

Sepsis was defined at the American College of Chest Physicians (ACCP) and the Society of Critical Care Medicine (SCCM) 'Consensus Conference in 1991. In 1992, the ACCP and SCCM introduced the concept of Sepsis and Systemic inflammatory Response Syndrome (SIRS), which is defined as the presence of at least two of the following quartet:

Table 30.10 Causes of shock in pregnancy

Low cardiac output: 'cold and clammy'	
Hypovolaemic	Loss of circulating blood volume with major haemorrhage or diabetic ketoacidosis
Obstructive	Embolus (pulmonary or amniotic fluid) or cardiac tamponade
Cardiogenic	Low cardiac output, e.g. after myocardial infarction
High cardiac output: 'warm and dilated'	
Early sepsis	Decreased venous return due to low systemic vascular resistance
Anaphylactic	Allergic induced vasodilation
Neurogenic	Loss of sympathetic outflow due to lesion above T6, causing vasodilation and bradycardia

Table 30.11 Signs of 'shock'

Hypotension	Systolic < 100 mmHg
Tachycardia	Pulse > 100 bpm (except neurogenic)
Tachypnoea	Respiratory rate > 30 breaths/min
Oliguria	Urine output < 30 mL/h (0.5 mL/kg/h)
Level of consciousness	Confused, agitated, or drowsy

Table 30.12 Diagnostic criteria for sepsis, where infection is documented or suspected

General	
Temperature	Fever (>38.3°C) or hypothermia (<36°C)
Heart rate	>90/min
Respiratory	Tachypnoea
Level of consciousness	Altered mental status
Circulation	Significant oedema or positive fluid balance (>20 mL/kg over 24 h)
Glucose control	Hyperglycaemia (>7.7 mmol/L), in absence of diabetes.
Inflammatory	
White cell count	>12,000 cells/μL or < 4000 cells/μL *or* normal with >10% immature forms
C-reactive protein	>2 SD above normal value
Plasma procalcitonin	>2 SD above normal value
Haemodynamic: sepsis induced hypotension	
Blood pressure	Systolic < 90 mmHg *or* mean arterial pressure < 70 *or* fall of > 40 mmHg
Organ dysfunction	
Oxygenation	PaO_2/FiO_2 < 300
Renal	Urine output < 0.5 mL/kg/h for > 2 h despite fluid resuscitation
	Creatinine rise of > 44.2 μmol/L
Clotting	International normalized ratio > 1.5 or activated partial thromboplastin time > 60 s
	Platelet count < 100,000 cells/μL
Hepatic	Bilirubin > 70 μmol/L
Gastrointestinal	Ileus
Tissue perfusion	
Acidosis	Lactate > 1 mmol/L
Clinical	Decreased capillary refill or mottling

SD, standard deviations.

With kind permission from Springer Science+Business Media: *Intensive Care Medicine, 'Surviving Sepsis Campaign: International Guidelines for Management of Severe Sepsis and Septic Shock*, 2012', 39, 2, 2013, pp. 165–228, R. P. Dellinger *et al.* © SCCM and ESICM 2013; and adapted with kind permission from Springer: Intensive Care Medicine, '2001 SCCM/ESICM/ACCP/ATS/SIS International Sepsis Definitions Conference', 29, 4, 2003, pp. 530–538, M. M. Levy *et al.*, © Springer-Verlag 2003.

1. Body temperature, greater than 38°C or less than 36°C
2. Heart rate greater than 90 bpm
3. Hyperventilation evidenced by a respiratory rate of greater than 20 breaths/min or a $PaCO_2$ of less than 32 mmHg
4. White blood cell count of greater than 12,000 cells/μL or less than 4000 cells/μL.

The 2001 SCCM/ESICM/ACCP/ATS/SIS International Sepsis Definitions Conference addressed these definitions so that they could be readily applied by clinicians.[148]

(With kind permission from Springer Science + Business Media: *Critical Care Medicine*, 2001 SCCM/ESICM/ACCP/ATS/SIS International Sepsis Definitions Conference, 2003 31(4): 1250–6. Levy M, Md F, Fink M, et al.)

Sepsis

Sepsis is the clinical syndrome defined by both the presence of infection (probable/documented) together with a systemic inflammatory response. An infection is the invasion of a normal sterile tissue fluid or body cavity by pathogenic or potentially pathogenic microorganisms. This is not a perfect definition: the colitis caused by *Clostridium difficile* is due to overgrowth in the non-sterile colon, with inflammatory effects occurring due to the cytopathic effects of the exotoxin produced by the bacteria. Thus, sepsis may occur without microbiological confirmation.

A systemic inflammatory response may be produced by a variety of infectious and non-infectious conditions (e.g. burns and acute pancreatitis). Table 30.12 shows a list of possible signs that prompt an experienced clinician to conclude that an infected patient 'looks septic'. None of these are specific to sepsis and could occur as an inflammatory response to major surgery or trauma. In many cases of early sepsis, the patients do not exhibit the classic signs or symptoms (Table 30.12) but experienced clinicians often intuitively make the correct diagnosis without any hard evidence. Once there is a clinical suspicion, the source of sepsis is then sought.

Table 30.13 Parameters of severe sepsis

Haemodynamic: sepsis-induced hypotension	
Blood pressure	Systolic < 90 mmHg or fall of > 40 mmHg
Tissue perfusion	
Acidosis	Lactate above upper limit of laboratory normal range
Organ dysfunction	
Oxygenation	PaO_2/FiO_2 < 250 in absence of pneumonia or < 200 with pneumonia
Renal	Creatinine > 176.8 μmol/L
Clotting	International normalized ratio > 1.5
	Platelet count < 100,000 cells/μL
Hepatic	Bilirubin > 34.2 μmol/L

With kind permission from Springer Science+Business Media: *Intensive Care Medicine, 'Surviving Sepsis Campaign: International Guidelines for Management of Severe Sepsis and Septic Shock*, 2012', 39, 2, 2013, pp. 165–228, R. P. Dellinger *et al.* © SCCM and ESICM 2013; and data from Springer: Intensive Care Medicine, '2001 SCCM/ESICM/ACCP/ATS/SIS International Sepsis Definitions Conference', 29, 4, 2003, pp. 530–538, M. M. Levy *et al.*, © Springer-Verlag 2003.

Severe sepsis

Severe sepsis is sepsis plus sepsis-induced organ dysfunction or tissue hypoperfusion. Organ dysfunction can be defined using the definitions in the SOFA[51] score. Dellinger et al.[144] include a table (Table 30.13) which is adapted from Levy et al.'s paper.[148]

Septic shock has developed when hypotension persists despite adequate fluid resuscitation. Severe sepsis is the leading cause of multiorgan failure, acute kidney injury, and ARDS and has a mortality of 40–60%. It is the commonest cause of death in general ICUs and the commonest cause of direct maternal death in the latest triennial Confidential Enquiry report.[4]

Goals in management of sepsis are to restore cardiac output and oxygen supply to vital tissues. This requires fluid administration, oxygen, and respiratory support, together with vasopressors to maintain blood pressure. Identification of the cause is essential to ensure that the correct antibiotics are given.

More detail of obstetric sepsis can be found in Chapter 34.

Conclusion

Outcomes from critical illness are improved if diagnosis and effective treatment is provided at the earliest opportunity. Physiological changes in pregnancy may mask the signs of impending critical illness and it is therefore essential to have robust mechanisms in place so that escalation of care occurs in a timely fashion. Obstetric anaesthetists have a prominent part to play in the multidisciplinary team that provides higher levels of care on the delivery suite.

References

1. Maresh M. Quality in obstetrics and gynaecology: the example of the enquiries into maternal mortality. *J Qual Clin Pract* 1998; 18(1):21–8.
2. Department of Health. *Report on Confidential Enquiries into Maternal Deaths in the UK 1988–90*. London: HMSO; 1994.
3. Department of Health. *Why Mothers Die. Fifth Report of the Confidential Enquiry into Maternal Death in the UK, 1997–1999*. London: RCOG Press; 2001.
4. Clutton-Brock T. Maternal deaths from anaesthesia. An extract from Why Mothers Die 2000–2002, the Confidential Enquiries into Maternal Deaths in the United Kingdom: Chapter 17: Trends in intensive care. *Br J Anaesth* 2005; 94(4):424–9.
5. Royal College of Anaesthetists, Royal College of Midwives, Royal College of Obstetricians and Gynaecologists, *et al. Safer Childbirth: Minimum Standards for the Organisation and Delivery of Care in Labour. Joint Royal Colleges Report*. London: RCOG Press; 2007.
6. Department of Health. *Comprehensive Critical Care: A Review of Adult Critical Care Services*. London: Department of Health; 2000.
7. The Intensive Care Society. *Levels of Critical Care for Adult Patients*. London: Intensive Care Society; 2009.
8. Wheatly S. Maternal critical care: what's in a name? *Int J Obstet Anesth* 2010; 19(4):353–5.
9. Maternal Critical Care Working Group. *Providing Equity of Critical and Maternity Care for the Critically Ill Pregnant or Recently Pregnant Woman*. London: The Royal College of Anaesthetists; 2011.
10. Information Standards Board for Health and Social Care. *Critical Care Minimum Dataset* (Version 8.0 ed). London: Information Standards Board for Health and Social Care; 2010.
11. Confidential Enquiry into Maternal and Child Health. *Saving Mothers Lives: Reviewing Maternal Deaths to Make Motherhood Safer 2003–2005*. London: CEMCH; 2007.
12. Hazelgrove JF, Price C, Pappachan VJ, *et al.* Multicenter study of obstetric admissions to 14 intensive care units in southern England. *Crit Care Med* 2001; 29(4):770–5.

13. Mirghani HM, Hamed M, Ezimokhai M, *et al.* Pregnancy-related admissions to the intensive care unit. *Int J Obstet Anesth* 2004; 13(2):82–5.
14. Harrison DA, Penny JA, Yentis SM, *et al.* Case mix, outcome and activity for obstetric admissions to adult, general critical care units: a secondary analysis of the ICNARC Case Mix Programme Database. *Crit Care* 2005; 9 Suppl 3:S25–37.
15. Intensive Care National Audit and Research Centre. *Female Admissions (Aged 16–50 years) to Adult, General Critical Care Units in England, Wales and Northern Ireland, Reported as 'Currently Pregnant' or 'Recently Pregnant' in 2007.* London: Intensive Care National Audit and Research Centre; 2009.
16. Cantwell R, Clutton-Brock T, Cooper G, *et al.* Saving Mothers' Lives: reviewing maternal deaths to make motherhood safer: 2006–2008. The Eighth Report of the Confidential Enquiries into Maternal Deaths in the United Kingdom. *BJOG* 2011; 118 Suppl 1:1–203.
17. Zwart JJ, Dupuis JRO, Van Roosmalen J, *et al.* Obstetric intensive care unit admission: a 2-year nationwide population-based cohort study. *Intensive Care Med* 2010; 36(2):256–63.
18. Pollock W, Rose L, Dennis CL. Pregnant and postpartum admissions to the intensive care unit: a systematic review. *Intensive Care Med* 2010; 36(9):1465–74.
19. Mantel GD, Buchmann E, Rees H, *et al.* Severe acute maternal morbidity: a pilot study of a definition for a near-miss. *BJOG* 1998; 105(9):985–90.
20. Lennox C, Marr L. *Scottish Confidential Audit of Severe Maternal Morbidity.* Scotland: Healthcare Improvement Scotland; 2012.
21. Lennox C, Marr L. *Scottish Confidential Audit of Severe Maternal Morbidity.* Scotland: Healthcare Improvement Scotland; 2008.
22. Tuncalp O, Hindin MJ, Souza JP, *et al.* The prevalence of maternal near miss: a systematic review. *BJOG* 2012; 119(6):653–61.
23. Zeeman GG, Wendel GD Jr, Cunningham FG. A blueprint for obstetric critical care. *Am J Obstet Gynecol* 2003; 188(2):532–6.
24. Ryan M, Hamilton V, Bowen M, *et al.* The role of a high-dependency unit in a regional obstetric hospital. *Anaesthesia* 2000; 55(12):1155–8.
25. Saravanakumar K, Davies L, Lewis M, *et al.* High dependency care in an obstetric setting in the UK. *Anaesthesia* 2008; 63(10):1081–6.
26. Zeeman GG. Obstetric critical care: a blueprint for improved outcomes. *Crit Care Med* 2006; 34(9 Suppl):S208–14.
27. Katz V, Hansen A. Complications in the emergency transport of pregnant women. *South Med J* 1990; 83(1):7–10.
28. Cordingley JJ, Rubin AP. A survey of facilities for high risk women in consultant obstetric units. *Int J Obstet Anesth* 1997; 6(3):156–60.
29. Hussain S, Srinivas K, Yadthore S, *et al.* Obstetric high-dependency care: a 2005–06 UK survey of practice and facilities. *Int J Obstet Anesth* 2011; 20(1):100–1.
30. Knaus WA, Zimmerman JE, Wagner DP, *et al.* APACHE-acute physiology and chronic health evaluation: a physiologically based classification system. *Crit Care Med* 1981; 9(8):591–7.
31. Knaus WA, Draper EA, Wagner DP, *et al.* Evaluating outcome from intensive care: a preliminary multihospital comparison. *Crit Care Med* 1982; 10(8):491–6.
32. Knaus WA, Le Gall JR, Wagner DP, *et al.* A comparison of intensive care in the U.S.A. and France. *Lancet* 1982; 2(8299):642–6.
33. Knaus WA, Draper EA, Wagner DP, *et al.* APACHE II: a severity of disease classification system. *Crit Care Med* 1985; 13(10):818–29.
34. Koch KA, Rodeffer HD, Sanchez-Ramos L. Critically ill obstetrical patients: outcome and predictability. *Crit Care Med* 1988; 16(4):A409.
35. Lewinsohn G, Herman A, Leonov Y, *et al.* Critically ill obstetrical patients: outcome and predictability. *Crit Care Med* 1994; 22(9):1412–14.
36. Le Gall JR, Lemeshow S, Saulnier F. A new Simplified Acute Physiology Score (SAPS II) based on a European/North American multicenter study. *JAMA* 1993; 270(24):2957–63.
37. Scarpinato L. Critically ill obstetric patients: outcome and predictability utilizing the SAPS II score in a 314 bed community hospital. *Chest* 1995; 108 Suppl 3:184S.
38. Lemeshow S, Teres D, Klar J, *et al.* Mortality probability models (MPM II) based on an international cohort of intensive care unit patients. *JAMA* 1993; 270(20):2478–86.
39. El-Solh AA, Grant BJB. A comparison of severity of illness scoring systems for critically ill obstetric patients. *Chest* 1996; 110(5):1299–304.
40. Bhagwanjee S, Paruk F, Moodley J, *et al.* Intensive care unit morbidity and mortality from eclampsia: an evaluation of the Acute Physiology and Chronic Health Evaluation II score and the Glasgow Coma Scale score. *Crit Care Med* 2000; 28(1):120–4.
41. Hanley JA, McNeil BJ. The meaning and use of the area under a receiver operating characteristic (ROC) curve. *Radiology* 1982; 143(1):29–36.
42. Rojas-Suarez J, Paternina A, Miranda J, *et al.* A comparison of severity of illness scores in critically ill obstetric patients: a six-year retrospective analysis. *Chest* 2012; 142(4):281A.
43. Knaus WA, Wagner DP, Draper EA, *et al.* The APACHE III prognostic system. Risk prediction of hospital mortality for critically ill hospitalized adults. *Chest* 1991; 100(6):1619–36.
44. Zimmerman JE, Kramer AA, McNair DS, *et al.* Acute Physiology and Chronic Health Evaluation (APACHE) IV: hospital mortality assessment for today's critically ill patients. *Crit Care Med* 2006; 34(5):1297–310.
45. Breslow MJ, Badawi O. Severity scoring in the critically ill severity scoring in the critically ill. Part 2: maximizing value from outcome prediction scoring systems. *Chest* 2012; 141(2):518–27.
46. Breslow MJ, Badawi O. Severity scoring in the critically ill. Part 1: interpretation and accuracy of outcome prediction scoring systems. *Chest* 2012; 141(1):245–52.
47. Juneja D, Singh O, Nasa P, *et al.* Comparison of newer scoring systems with the conventional scoring systems in general intensive care population. *Minerva Anestesiol* 2012; 78(2):194–200.
48. Gopalan PD, Muckart DJ. The critically ill obstetric patient: what's the score? *Int J Obstet Anesth* 2004; 13(3):144–5.
49. Marshall JC, Cook DJ, Christou NV, *et al.* Multiple Organ Dysfunction Score: a reliable descriptor of a complex clinical outcome. *Crit Care Med* 1995; 23(10):1638–52.
50. Le Gall JR, Klar J, Lemeshow S, *et al.* The logistic organ dysfunction system: a new way to assess organ dysfunction in the intensive care unit. *JAMA* 1996; 276(10):802–10.
51. Vincent JL, De Mendonça A, Cantraine F, *et al.* Use of the SOFA score to assess the incidence of organ dysfunction/failure in intensive care units: results of a multicenter, prospective study. *Crit Care Med* 1998; 26(11):1793–800.
52. Franklin C, Mathew J. Developing strategies to prevent inhospital cardiac arrest: analyzing responses of physicians and nurses in the hours before the event. *Crit Care Med* 1994; 22(2):244–7.
53. McQuillan P, Pilkington S, Allan A, *et al.* Confidential inquiry into quality of care before admission to intensive care. *BMJ* 1998; 316(7148):1853–8.
54. Goldhill DR, White SA, Sumner A. Physiological values and procedures in the 24 h before ICU admission from the ward. *Anaesthesia* 1999; 54(6):529–34.
55. Hillman K, Chen J, Cretikos M, *et al.* Introduction of the medical emergency team (MET) system: a cluster-randomised controlled trial. *Lancet* 2005; 365(9477):2091–7.
56. Goldhill DR, McNarry AF, Mandersloot G, *et al.* A physiologically-based early warning score for ward patients: the association between score and outcome. *Anaesthesia* 2005; 60(6):547–53.
57. Stenhouse C, Coates S, Tivey M, *et al.* Prospective evaluation of a modified Early Warning Score to aid earlier detection of patients developing critical illness on a general surgical ward. *Br J Anaesth* 2000; 84(5):663.
58. Lee A, Bishop G, Hillman KM, *et al.* The medical emergency team. *Anaesth Intensive Care* 1995; 23(2):183–6.
59. Buist MD, Moore GE, Bernard SA, *et al.* Effects of a medical emergency team on reduction of incidence of and mortality from unexpected cardiac arrests in hospital: preliminary study. *BMJ* 2002; 324:1–6.

60. Subbe CP, Davies RG, Williams E, *et al.* Effect of introducing the Modified Early Warning score on clinical outcomes, cardio-pulmonary arrests and intensive care utilisation in acute medical admissions. *Anaesthesia* 2003; 58(8):797–802.
61. Priestley G, Watson W, Rashidian A, *et al.* Introducing Critical Care Outreach: a ward-randomised trial of phased introduction in a general hospital. *Intensive Care Med* 2004; 30(7):1398–404.
62. Cuthbertson BH, Smith GB. A warning on early-warning scores! *Br J Anaesth* 2007; 98(6):704–6.
63. Gao H, McDonnell A, Harrison DA, *et al.* Systematic review and evaluation of physiological track and trigger warning systems for identifying at-risk patients on the ward. *Intensive Care Med* 2007; 33(4):667–79.
64. National Institute for Clinical Excellence. *Recognition of and Response to Acute Illness in Adults in Hospital.* London: NICE; 2007.
65. Royal College of Physicians. *Acute Medical Care: The Right Person, in the Right Setting—First Time.* Report of the Acute Medicine Task Force. London: RCP; 2007.
66. Royal College of Physicians. *National Early Warning Score (NEWS): Standardising the Assessment of Acute Illness Severity in the NHS.* Report of a working party. London: RCP; 2012.
67. Smith GB, Prytherch DR, Schmidt PE, *et al.* Review and performance evaluation of aggregate weighted 'track and trigger' systems. *Resuscitation* 2008; 77(2):170–9.
68. Smith GB, Prytherch DR, Meredith P, *et al.* The ability of the National Early Warning Score (NEWS) to discriminate patients at risk of early cardiac arrest, unanticipated intensive care unit admission, and death. *Resuscitation* 2013; 84(4):465–70.
69. Subbe CP, Kruger M, Rutherford P, *et al.* Validation of a modified early warning score in medical admissions. *QJM* 2001; 94(10):521–6.
70. Carle C, Johal J, Columb M, *et al.* Evaluation of modified early warning scores as a predictor of outcome in obstetric admissions to critical care units: secondary analysis of the Intensive Care National Audit and Research Centre (ICNARC) Case Mix Program (CMP) database. *Br J Anaesth* 2010; 105(5):707P.
71. Singh S, McGlennan A, England A, *et al.* A validation study of the CEMACH recommended modified early obstetric warning system (MEOWS). *Anaesthesia* 2012; 67(1):12–18.
72. Banfield P, Roberts C. *Transforming Maternity Services: All Wales Consensus Paper Obstetric Early Warning Systems Proposal Paper 1.* Cardiff: 1000 Lives Plus; 2012.
73. Swanton RD, Al-Rawi S, Wee MY. A national survey of obstetric early warning systems in the United Kingdom. *Int J Obstet Anesth* 2009; 18(3):253–7.
74. Banfield P, Roberts C. *Transforming Maternity Services: All Wales Consensus Paper Obstetric Early Warning Systems Paper 2.* Cardiff: 1000 Lives Plus; 2012.
75. Department of Health. *Competencies for Recognising and Responding to Acutely Ill Patients in Hospital.* London: DH; 2009.
76. The CoBaTrICE Collaboration. *CoBaTrICE Syllabus.* Version 1, 2006. http://www.cobatrice.org/Data/upload/images/File/About/Coba-resources/CoBaTrICE_Syllabus%28all%29_v1.0_2006.pdf
77. Royal College of Anaesthetists. *The Royal College of Anaesthetists CPD Matrix.* London: Royal College of Anaesthetists; 2013.
78. Royal College of Anaesthetists. *Continuing Professional Development: Guidance for Doctors in Anaesthesia, Intensive Care and Pain Medicine.* London: Royal College of Anaesthetists; 2013.
79. The Intensive Care Society. *Guidelines for the Transport of the Critically Ill Adult* (3rd ed). London: Intensive Care Society; 2011.
80. Royal College of Obstetricians and Gynaecologists. *Maternal Collapse in Pregnancy and the Puerperium.* Green-top Guideline No. 56. London: RCOG, 2011.
81. National Institute for Clinical Excellence. *The Management of Hypertensive Disorders in Pregnancy.* London: NICE; 2011.
82. National Confidential Enquiry into Patient Outcome and Death. *An Acute Problem? A report of the National Confidential Enquiry into Patient Outcome and Death.* London: NCEPOD, 2005.
83. The Intensive Care Society. *Guidelines for the Introduction of Outreach Services.* London: Intensive Care Society, 2002.
84. Bright D, Walker W, Bion J. Clinical review: outreach—a strategy for improving the care of the acutely ill hospitalized patient. *Crit Care* 2004; 8(1):33–40.
85. Young P, Johanson R. Haemodynamic, invasive and echocardiographic monitoring in the hypertensive parturient. *Best Pract Res Clin Obstet Gynaecol* 2001; 15(4):605–22.
86. Paech MJ, Hillyard SG. New techniques and technologies for obstetric anaesthesia. *Int J Obstet Anesth* 2012; 21(1):101–2.
87. Swan HJC, Ganz W, Forrester J, *et al.* Catheterization of the heart in man with use of a flow-directed balloon-tipped catheter. *N Engl J Med* 1970; 283(9):447–51.
88. Murdoch SD, Cohen AT, Bellamy MC. Pulmonary artery catheterization and mortality in critically ill patients. *Br J Anaesth* 2000; 85(4):611–15.
89. Nolan TE, Wakefield ML, Devoe LD. Invasive hemodynamic monitoring in obstetrics. A critical review of its indications, benefits, complications, and alternatives. *Chest* 1992; 101(5):1429–33.
90. Connors AF, Speroff T, Dawson NV, *et al.* The effectiveness of right heart catheterization in the initial care of critically III patients. *JAMA* 1996; 276(11):889.
91. Dalen JE, Bone RC. Is it time to pull the pulmonary artery catheter? *JAMA* 1996; 276(11):916–18.
92. Taylor RW, Ahrens T, Viejo A, *et al.* Pulmonary Artery Catheter Consensus Conference: consensus statement. *Crit Care Med* 1997; 25(6):910–25.
93. Gilbert WM, Towner DR, Field NT, *et al.* The safety and utility of pulmonary artery catheterization in severe preeclampsia and eclampsia. *Am J Obstet Gynecol* 2000; 182(6):1397–403.
94. Fujitani S, Baldisseri MR. Hemodynamic assessment in a pregnant and peripartum patient. *Crit Care Med* 2005; 33(10):S354–61.
95. Sandham JD, Hull RD, Brant RF, *et al.* A randomized, controlled trial of the use of pulmonary-artery catheters in high-risk surgical patients. *N Engl J Med* 2003; 348(1):5–14.
96. Rajaram SS, Desai NK, Kalra A, *et al.* Pulmonary artery catheters for adult patients in intensive care. *Cochrane Database Syst Rev* 2013; 2:CD003408.
97. Ecker JL, Solt K, Fitzsimons MG, *et al.* Case records of the Massachusetts General Hospital. Case 40-2012. A 43-year-old woman with cardiorespiratory arrest after a cesarean section. *N Engl J Med* 2012; 367(26):2528–36.
98. Ioscovich A, Elstein D. Images in anesthesia: transesophageal echocardiography during cesarean section in a Marfan's patient with aortic dissection. *Can J Anesth* 2005; 52(7):737–8.
99. James CF, Feinglass NG, Menke DM, *et al.* Massive amniotic fluid embolism: diagnosis aided by emergency transesophageal echocardiography. *Int J Obstet Anesth* 2004; 13(4):279–83.
100. Nam E, Toque Y, Quintard JM, *et al.* Use of transesophageal echocardiography to guide the anesthetic management of cesarean section in a patient with hypertrophic cardiomyopathy. *J Cardiothorac Vasc Anesth* 1999; 13(1):72–4.
101. Sentilhes L, Verspyck E, Bauer F, *et al.* Management of maternal cor triatriatum during pregnancy. *Obstet Gynecol* 2004; 104(5 Pt 2):1212–15.
102. Stanten RD, Iverson LI, Daugharty TM, *et al.* Amniotic fluid embolism causing catastrophic pulmonary vasoconstriction: diagnosis by transesophageal echocardiogram and treatment by cardiopulmonary bypass. *Obstet Gynecol* 2003; 102(3):496–8.
103. Vellayappan U, Attias MD, Shulman MS. Paradoxical embolization by amniotic fluid seen on the transesophageal echocardiography. *Anesth Analg* 2009; 108(4):1110–12.
104. Wei J, Yang HS, Tsai SK, *et al.* Emergent bedside real-time three-dimensional transesophageal echocardiography in a patient with cardiac arrest following a caesarean section. *Eur J Echocardiogr* 2011; 12(3):E16.
105. Belfort MA, Rokey R, Saade GR, *et al.* Rapid echocardiographic assessment of left and right heart hemodynamics in critically ill obstetric patients. *Am J Obstet Gynecol* 1994; 171(4):884–92.
106. Rokey R, Belfort MA, Saade GR. Quantitative echocardiographic assessment of left ventricular function in critically ill

obstetric patients: a comparative study. *Am J Obstet Gynecol* 1996; 173(4):1148–52.
107. Belfort MA, Mares A, Saade G, *et al.* Two-dimensional echocardiography and Doppler ultrasound in managing obstetric patients. *Obstet Gynecol* 1997; 90(3):326–30.
108. Ferguson EA, Paech MJ, Veltman MG. Hypertrophic cardiomyopathy and caesarean section: intraoperative use of transthoracic echocardiography. *Int J Obstet Anesth* 2006; 15(4):311–16.
109. Dennis AT. Transthoracic echocardiography in obstetric anaesthesia and obstetric critical illness. *Int J Obstet Anesth* 2011; 20(2):160–8.
110. Dennis AT, Castro J, Carr C, *et al.* Haemodynamics in women with untreated pre-eclampsia. *Anaesthesia* 2012; 67(10):1105–18.
111. Dyer RA, James MF. Maternal hemodynamic monitoring in obstetric anesthesia. *Anesthesiology* 2008; 109(5):765–7.
112. Critchley LAH, Critchley JAJH. A meta-analysis of studies using bias and precision statistics to compare cardiac output measurement techniques. *J Clin Monit Comput* 1999; 15(2):85–91.
113. Rhodes A, Sunderland R. Arterial pulse power analysis: the LiDCO plus system. In Pinsky M, Payen D (eds) *Functional Hemodynamic Monitoring.* Berlin: Springer; 2005:183–92.
114. Daniel N, Barclay P, Sieunarine R, *et al.* Effects of crystalloid preload and spinal anaesthesia for caesarean section on maternal haemodynamics using LiDCOplus system. *Int J Obstet Anesth* 2007; 16 Suppl 1:S9.
115. Langesaeter E, Rosseland LA, Stubhaug A. Hemodynamic effects of oxytocin during cesarean delivery. *Int J Gynaecol Obstet* 2006; 95(1):46–7.
116. Langesaeter E, Rosseland LA, Stubhaug A. Continuous invasive blood pressure and cardiac output monitoring during cesarean delivery: a randomized, double-blind comparison of low-dose versus high-dose spinal anesthesia with intravenous phenylephrine or placebo infusion. *Anesthesiology* 2008; 109(5):856–63.
117. Belloni L, Pisano A, Natale A, *et al.* Assessment of fluid-responsiveness parameters for off-pump coronary artery bypass surgery: a comparison among LiDCO, transesophageal echochardiography, and pulmonary artery catheter. *J Cardiothorac Vasc Anesth* 2008; 22(2):243–8.
118. Dyer RA, Piercy JL, Reed AR, *et al.* Comparison between pulse waveform analysis and thermodilution cardiac output determination in patients with severe pre-eclampsia. *Br J Anaesth* 2011; 106(1):77–81.
119. Litton E, Morgan M. The PiCCO monitor: a review. *Anaesth Intensive Care* 2012; 40(3):393–409.
120. Auler Junior JOC, Torres MLA, Cardoso MM, *et al.* Clinical evaluation of the Flotrac/Vigileo® system for continuous cardiac output monitoring in patients undergoing regional anesthesia for elective cesarean section: a pilot study. *Clinics* 2010; 65:793–8.
121. Compton FD, Zukunft B, Hoffmann C, *et al.* Performance of a minimally invasive uncalibrated cardiac output monitoring system (Flotrac™/Vigileo™) in haemodynamically unstable patients. *Br J Anaesth* 2008; 100(4):451–6.
122. Armstrong S, Fernando R, Columb M. Minimally- and non-invasive assessment of maternal cardiac output: go with the flow! *Int J Obstet Anesth* 2011; 20(4):330–40.
123. Department of Health. *Innovation Health and Wealth.* London: Department of Health; 2011.
124. NHS Technology Adoption Centre. *Intraoperative Fluid Management Technologies Adoption Pack.* London: NHS Technology Adoption Centre; 2012.
125. Penny JA, Anthony J, Shennan AH, *et al.* A comparison of hemodynamic data derived by pulmonary artery flotation catheter and the esophageal Doppler monitor in preeclampsia. *Am J Obstet Gynecol* 2000; 183(3):658–61.
126. Dey I, Sprivulis P. Emergency physicians can reliably assess emergency department patient cardiac output using the USCOM continuous wave Doppler cardiac output monitor. *Emerg Med Aust* 2005; 17(3):193–9.
127. Kager CCM, Dekker GA, Stam MC. Measurement of cardiac output in normal pregnancy by a non-invasive two-dimensional independent Doppler device. *Aust N Z J Obstet Gynaecol* 2009; 49(2):142–4.
128. Teoh WH, Sia AT. Colloid preload versus coload for spinal anesthesia for cesarean delivery: the effects on maternal cardiac output. *Anesth Analg* 2009; 108(5):1592–8.
129. Doherty A, Ohashi Y, Downey K, *et al.* Phenylephrine infusion versus bolus regimens during cesarean delivery under spinal anesthesia: a double-blind randomized clinical trial to assess hemodynamic changes. *Anesth Analg* 2012; 115(6):1343–50.
130. Fanning N, Balki M, Sermer M, *et al.* Noninvasive cardiac output monitoring during general anesthesia for Cesarean delivery in a patient with severe aortic stenosis. *Can J Anaesth* 2011; 58(9):837–41.
131. Ohashi Y, Ibrahim H, Furtado L, *et al.* Non-invasive hemodynamic assessment of non-pregnant, healthy pregnant and preeclamptic women using bioreactance. [corrected]. *Rev Bras Anestesiol* 2010; 60(6):603–13.
132. Hehenkamp WJ, Rang S, van Goudoever J, *et al.* Comparison of Portapres with standard sphygmomanometry in pregnancy. *Hypertens Pregnancy* 2002; 21(1):65–76.
133. Carlin A, Alfirevic Z. Physiological changes of pregnancy and monitoring. *Best Pract Res Clin Obstet Gynaecol* 2008; 22(5):801–23.
134. Dyson KS, Shoemaker JK, Arbeille P, *et al.* Modelflow estimates of cardiac output compared with Doppler ultrasound during acute changes in vascular resistance in women. *Exp Physiol* 2010; 95(4):561–8.
135. Reisner AT, Xu D, Ryan KL, *et al.* Monitoring non-invasive cardiac output and stroke volume during experimental human hypovolaemia and resuscitation. *Br J Anaesth* 2011; 106(1):23–30.
136. Richards NA, Boyce H, Yentis SM. Estimation of blood haemoglobin concentration using the HemoCue® during caesarean section: the effect of sampling site. *Int J Obstet Anesth* 2010; 19(1):67–70.
137. Macknet M, Allard M, Applegate R, *et al.* The accuracy of noninvasive and continuous total hemoglobin measurement by pulse CO-oximetry in human subjects undergoing hemodilution. *Anesth Analg* 2010; 111(6):1424–6.
138. Butwick AJ, Hilton G, Riley ET, *et al.* Non-invasive measurement of hemoglobin during cesarean hysterectomy: a case series. *Int J Obstet Anesth* 2011; 20(3):240–5.
139. Miller RD, Ward TA, Shiboski SC, *et al.* A comparison of three methods of hemoglobin monitoring in patients undergoing spine surgery. *Anesth Analg* 2011; 112(4):858–63.
140. Stocks G. Monitoring transfusion requirements in major obstetric haemorrhage: out with the old and in with the new? *Int J Obstet Anesth* 2011; 20(4):275–8.
141. Robb E, Jarman B, Suntharalingam G, *et al.* Using care bundles to reduce in-hospital mortality: quantitative survey. *BMJ* 2010; 340:861–6.
142. 1000 Lives Plus. *Two years to make a difference in Welsh Healthcare 2008–2010.* Cardiff: 1000 Lives Plus; 2011.
143. Banfield P, Roberts C. *Transforming Maternity Services* (17 ed). Cardiff: 1000 Lives Plus; 2011.
144. Dellinger RP, Levy MM, Rhodes A, *et al.* Surviving Sepsis Campaign: international guidelines for management of severe sepsis and septic shock: 2012. *Crit Care Med* 2013; 41(2):580–637.
145. Centre for Maternal and Child Enquiries. *CMACE Emergent Theme Briefing #1: Genital Tract Sepsis.* London: Centre for Maternal and Child Enquiries; 2010.
146. Bernard GR, Artigas A, Brigham KL, *et al.* Report of the American-European consensus conference on ARDS: definitions, mechanisms, relevant outcomes and clinical trial coordination. *Intensive Care Med* 1994; 20(3):225–32.
147. Del Sorbo L, Slutsky A. Acute respiratory distress syndrome and multiple organ failure. *Curr Opin Crit Care* 2011; 17:1–6.
148. Levy MM, Fink MP, Marshall JC, *et al.* 2001 SCCM/ESICM/ACCP/ATS/SIS International Sepsis Definitions Conference. *Crit Care Med* 2003; 31(4):1250–6.

CHAPTER 31

Maternal mortality and morbidity

Suni Halder and Steve Yentis

Introduction

Anaesthetists are acutely involved in the prevention of maternal mortality and morbidity. First, they have an important role in promoting and improving safety in a wide variety of clinical areas, and particularly in the delivery suite, where high-risk cases are all too common. Second, anaesthetists have skills and knowledge that are very relevant to resuscitation of critically ill obstetric patients, whether in the delivery suite, critical care units, or elsewhere. And third, anaesthesia itself is an important potential cause of maternal death; until relatively recently, anaesthesia consistently featured as a major direct cause of mortality in the United Kingdom's Confidential Enquiries into Maternal Deaths (CEMD; see later in this chapter), and the potential for anaesthesia to cause significant maternal morbidity, if not mortality, must never be forgotten.

As for anaesthesia outside obstetrics, where improving standards have led to large reductions in perioperative mortality such that much emphasis is now placed on morbidity, so it is with obstetrics. Thus, in developed countries at least, the numbers of maternal deaths have fallen to the point where some have argued that continuing to focus on death is now less productive than concentrating on morbidity.[1–7] However, maternal mortality continues to be an important outcome measure in developed countries, as well as worldwide, for a number of reasons: first, it ought to be a relatively easy outcome to record on an individual patient basis—there usually being little disagreement about when death has occurred—although counting *all* deaths within a region or country may not always be straightforward. Second, there are agreed national and international definitions for maternal death statistics that allow comparisons between countries and regions.[8–11] Third, such figures are generally accepted as being valid markers of the quality of the underlying healthcare infrastructure including education, resources, staffing levels and skill, sanitation, and family planning.[11–15] Fourth, regular or continuous analysis of trends in maternal mortality statistics allows changes to be detected that might otherwise go unnoticed.[13,17–19]

Maternal morbidity is much harder to define than mortality, although attempts have been made to monitor morbidity in the same way as for mortality, with some systems successfully providing useful feedback as part of an overall regional or national risk management strategy (discussed in more detail below). In practical terms, healthcare workers (including obstetric anaesthetists) are much more likely to encounter morbidity on the delivery suite than mortality.

Maternal mortality

Definitions

As in so many other areas of healthcare, the use of standardized definitions is crucial when comparing maternal mortality figures between regions or countries.

International definitions

The following definitions are those used by the World Health Organization (WHO) and classified by the Tenth Revision of the International Classification of Diseases, Injuries and Causes of Death (ICD-10):[8]

- *Maternal death*: death of a women while pregnant or within 42 days of termination of pregnancy, irrespective of the duration and site of pregnancy, from any cause related to or aggravated by the pregnancy or its management but not from accidental or incidental causes.[8]
- *Pregnancy-related death*: death of a woman while pregnant or within 42 days of termination of pregnancy, irrespective of the cause of death.[8]
- *Maternal mortality ratio (MMR)*: direct and indirect maternal deaths, but not late maternal deaths, per 100,000 live births.[8]

UK definitions

Because of the importance of the CEMD over the last 50 years, it is important to be aware of the definitions used in this audit even though they differ somewhat from those used internationally:[10,11]

- *Direct maternal death*: death resulting from obstetric complications of the pregnant state (pregnancy, labour, and puerperium), from interventions, omissions, incorrect treatment, or from a chain of events resulting from any of the above.[10,11]
- *Indirect maternal death*: death resulting from previous existing disease, or disease that developed during pregnancy and which was not the result of direct obstetric causes, but which was aggravated by the physiological effects of pregnancy.[10,11]
- *Late maternal death*: death occurring between 42 days and 1 year after abortion, miscarriage, or delivery that is the result of direct or indirect maternal causes.[10,11]
- *Coincidental death*: death from unrelated causes which happen to occur in pregnancy or the puerperium.[10] (NB the ICD-10 refers to these deaths as 'fortuitous', as did previous reports from the CEMD; however, the latter changed the term to 'coincidental' because of widespread confusion between 'fortuitous'

(which means 'by chance') and 'fortunate' (which means 'lucky')).

- *Maternal mortality rate*: direct and indirect maternal deaths, but not late maternal deaths, per 100,000 maternities (pregnancies resulting in a live birth or stillbirth at greater than 20 weeks' gestational age).[10,11]

It should be noted that the international maternal mortality *ratio* and the CEMD's maternal mortality *rate* differ in two important respects: first, the former uses data only from death certificates for its numerator, whilst CEMD's numerator includes all deaths related to pregnancy, even those not noted on death certificates, by cross-checking death certificate data against other national registries and the Office for National Statistics (ONS); this has occurred since the mid 1990s. Second, the international MMR has as its denominator all *live births*, whereas the CEMDs' denominator is *maternities*, which includes live births and stillbirths. This has led to confusion (not helped by the similarity in the statistics' names) between the two figures, most recently the suggestion that maternal mortality in the United Kingdom was considerably higher than it actually was.

The CEMD's classification and definition system itself may give rise to some anomalies. For example, all cardiac deaths are included in figures on indirect deaths even though peripartum cardiomyopathy could be considered a 'complication of the pregnant state'. Similarly, an anaesthetic death arising from failed intubation at caesarean delivery would be a direct maternal death, whereas death from failed intubation in a pregnant woman undergoing appendicectomy would, strictly speaking, classify as an indirect death since the reason for the intervention was not related to pregnancy but the intubation was adversely affected by her pregnant state.

Methods of estimation of maternal mortality

If comprehensive records of deaths and causes of deaths exist then accurate maternal mortality statistics could, theoretically, be obtained easily. However, there are very few countries in the world where this occurs. The United Kingdom is thought to have one of the most comprehensive and accurate systems to estimate maternal mortality through the CEMD, especially via its cross-linking process to ascertain all deaths. In developed countries, the process is aided by having relatively accurate death certification services. Countries' civil registration systems whereby routine birth and death data are recorded historically provide the largest data pool used to calculate international maternal mortality rates. Only one-third of countries are known to have complete civil registration data.[13] However, even in developed countries there may be inaccuracies; for example, a recent record-linkage study from Italy suggested considerable under-reporting of maternal deaths, with only a third of actual deaths accounted for in official (death certificate) figures.[20] This problem has been shown to exist in other countries, including the United States.[21] In the developing world, death certification systems are much less robust to start with, so that other methods (e.g. surveys,[22] censuses,[23] and verbal autopsies[24]) have to be used to estimate the number of maternal deaths. WHO is trying to improve the system for identifying maternal deaths by adding a checkbox on death certificates for recording a woman's pregnancy status, and by the publication of a new guide to reduce errors in coding for maternal death.[9,25] It should be noted that a failure in reporting or obtaining the correct number of deaths would always result in an underestimation rather than overestimation. Furthermore, if a country cannot provide basic maternal healthcare needs for its population, it may well be unlikely to be able to provide accurate mortality statistics. This can be due to a number of factors, including not recording maternal deaths because of the unknown pregnancy status of women of childbearing age; further, in some developing countries medical certification of cause of death does not exist.[13] Attempts to improve matters include the RAMOS (reproductive age mortality survey) method, which triangulates multiple sources of information and can be applied in local languages to improve reporting accuracy.[26] Using regression models, new global and regional estimates of maternal mortality can be developed at regular intervals.[13]

The global picture: developing countries

WHO produces statistics on the annual estimates of MMR from 194 countries (Figure 31.1). The most recent world estimate of the overall MMR is around 210/100,000 live births. By the defined WHO regions of the world, the MMR is highest in sub-Saharan Africa (500/100,000), followed by South Asia (220/100,000), Oceania, excluding Japan, Australia and New Zealand (200/100,000), and the Caribbean (190/100,000). The MMR is relatively low in developed countries (16/100,000). These figures hide wide variations even within countries, as major discrepancies can exist between remote and urban areas as well as between affluent and poorer members of the population.

The majority of maternal deaths—over 99%—still occur in the developing world. In sub-Saharan Africa, there is an exceptionally high mortality rate, thought to be related to poor infrastructure and medical provision combined with a high fertility rate and poor compliance with contraception.[13–15] In the developing world as a whole, a 15-year-old woman has a 1/150 chance of mortality, whereas in the developed world the chance of mortality is 1/3800.[15] In Sub-Saharan Africa, when a women is of reproductive age she has a 1/10 chance of death as a result of pregnancy or delivery

There has been an encouraging downward trend in deaths overall: from 1990 to 2010 there has been a decline in maternal mortality of 47%, a fall of 3% per year. In 1990 there were an estimated 540,000 maternal deaths worldwide; this number has been reduced to 287,000 by 2010. This reduction has occurred despite the improvements in reporting within developing countries.[13] A worrying statistic, however, is that around one-third of these deaths occurred in just two countries: 19% of total global maternal deaths occurred in India and 14% occurred in Nigeria.[13] This is a very high death toll, with around one death every 2 minutes. However, it should be noted that over the period from 1990 to 2010, the MMR has incrementally decreased in India from 600 in 1990 to 200 in 2010, giving an average annual 5.9% decrease in MMR; in Nigeria the MMR has reduced from 1100 in 1990 to 630 in 2010, giving an average annual 2.6% decrease in MMR.[13] In India it is thought that the large number of maternal deaths is due to the vast overall population as opposed to an extremely high MMR.

To address worldwide health issues including maternal mortality, the United Nations (UN) set up some Millennium Development Goals (MDGs) in September 2000. These were goals that UN member states agreed to try to achieve by 2015.[27–29] The

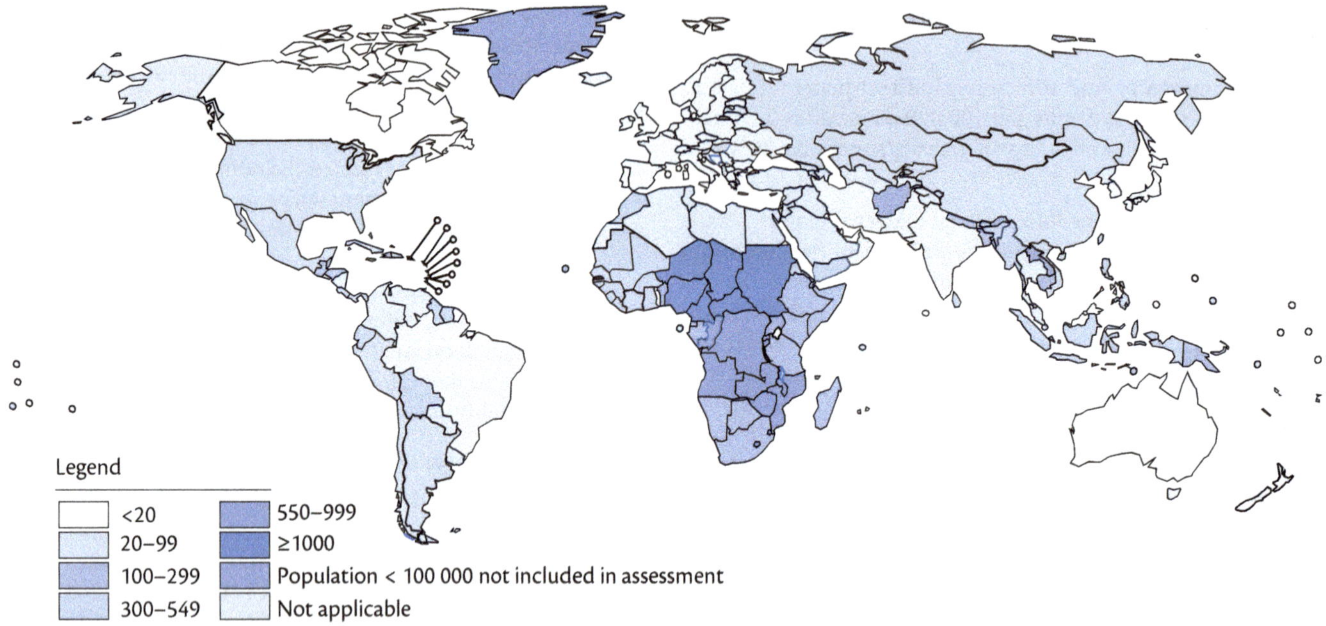

Figure 31.1 (See colour figure section). Maternal mortality ratio (per 100,000 live births) worldwide, 2010.
Reproduced with permission from WHO, *Trends in Maternal Mortality: 1990 to 2010 WHO, UNICEF, UNFPA and The World Bank estimates*, Geneva, World Health organization, Copyright © 2012.

bold overview was to 'improve maternal health', with two targets being to 'reduce by three-quarters, between 1990 and 2015, the maternal mortality ratio' and achieve, by 2015, 'universal access to reproductive health'. Despite the significant decline in death rate discussed above, maternal mortality by 2010 has only achieved half the required target reduction of MMR between 1990 and 2015. Globally, overall, a figure of 3.1% reduction per year was obtained; this is, however, far from the 5.5% per year required to obtain the MDG.[13,29,30] Encouraging data reveal that ten countries have already reached the target: Estonia (95% reduction), Maldives (93%), Belarus (88%), Romania (84%), Bhutan (82%), Equatorial Guinea (81%), Islamic Republic of Iran (81%), Lithuania (78%), Nepal (78%), and Vietnam (76%).[13] The reasons for the improvement made in some countries include improvement in healthcare systems, increased female education, and easier physical access to health facilities.[13]

In the developing world, there is a strong correlation between maternal and newborn mortality, with 3 million newborn and 2.5 million stillborn deaths each year.[31,32] Worldwide, the proportion of women attending antenatal care has increased secondary to the MDGs, with 81% of women seen once during the antenatal period in 2009, compared with 64% in 1990.[13] This proportion in 2009, however, reduces to 55% of women when the recommended minimum of four antenatal appointments is taken into account. The proportion of deliveries attended by skilled personnel, a key determinant to reduce maternal and perinatal mortality, is currently above 90% in only three of the six WHO regions. Overall, worldwide in 1990, 55% of women were attended by skilled personnel, this number increasing to 65% by 2009.[12,13] Alarmingly, in some regions, such as sub-Saharan Africa, the attendance rate is less than 50%.[13] As one might expect, the highest mortality rate is among women from poorer and more rural areas.

The major complications that cause maternal mortality in the developing world include severe bleeding, infections, high blood pressure, obstructed labour,[33,34] and unsafe abortion.[27,35-40] Worldwide, unsafe abortion, defined by WHO as 'a procedure for terminating an unintended pregnancy either by individuals without the necessary skills or in an environment that does not conform to minimum medical standards, or both', [35] accounts for a large proportion, around 13% of maternal deaths worldwide. The prevalence of unsafe abortion is highest in South America, with 30 or more unsafe abortions per 100 live births. Other deaths in the developing world can be attributed to malaria and human immunodeficiency viral (HIV) infection. In some Southern African countries such as Botswana, Lesotho, Namibia, South Africa, and Swaziland, the MMR increased from 1990 to 2000, mainly due to a HIV epidemic. This increase in MMR was reduced in the 2000s by the availability of antiretrovirals in these countries, with all five countries preventing mother-to-child transmission to 80% of pregnant women living with HIV.[13] It should be noted that without adequate laboratory facilities, deaths resulting from sepsis would be underestimated.[41] As haemorrhage is a major cause of death in the developing world, pre-existing severe anaemia secondary to poor diet, haemoglobinopathy, or parasitic infection with malaria can all increase the risk of mortality.[42] Many of the causes of maternal death in the developing world are preventable.[18,43] For all the MDGs to be reached, factors in the developing world such as poverty, lack of information and transport, inadequate services, and cultural practices all need to be addressed.[13,16,44–50] This is highlighted in a study of a religious group in the United States whose members, even though they were in a good state of health, refused modern obstetric and medical care because of their beliefs, leading to a maternal mortality rate similar to that in the developing world.[51] When obstetric anaesthetic services are provided in the developing world they tend to be less well funded, with fewer staff and equipment resources.[52–54] This leads to a greater incidence of maternal death due to inexperience and a lack of education, especially relating to the anaesthetic management of high-risk patients who may have severe untreated co-morbidities and present with hypovolaemic or septic shock.[55,56] Caesarean delivery is a common surgical procedure in the developing world, especially in Africa.[57,58] However, airway problems secondary to general anaesthesia are also a common cause of mortality, as is the lack of availability of blood products.[59–62]

South Africa Confidential Enquiry

The South African Confidential Enquiry analysing maternal deaths has been in operation since 1997, with the first report published in 1999, reviewing deaths during 1998 only. Since then, subsequent reports have looked at triennia. The latest triennial report, 'Saving Mothers 2008–2010', was published in 2012.[63] Data on institutional MMR, perinatal mortality rate, stillbirth rate, and early neonatal death rate per district are given in the report. Information about maternal deaths is confidentially reported to the National Committee for Confidential Enquiries into Maternal Deaths (NCCEMD) Secretariat and entered on the Maternal Morbidity and Mortality Audit System (MaMMAS) database, where data are collated and reports are produced. The general annual trend of maternal mortality since the Enquiry started is upwards, with 676 maternal deaths reported in 1998, 1173 maternal deaths reported in 2004, and 1643 maternal deaths reported in 2010. This increase is thought to be due to the greater proportion of cases reported and also the number of women dying.[63] In the latest triennial report, the MMR has increased overall to 176/100,000 live births, compared with 152/100,000 live births in 2005–2007. The major causes of maternal death in the latest (2008–2010) report include non-pregnancy related infections (40.5%, mainly due to HIV infection complicated with tuberculosis (TB) and/or pneumocystis pneumonia), obstetric haemorrhage (14.1%), complications of hypertension in pregnancy (14.0%), pregnancy-related sepsis (9.1%, including puerperal sepsis and septic miscarriage), and medical and surgical disorders (8.8%). These five account for 86.5% of all maternal deaths.[63] HIV infection is the most common contributing factor to maternal death in South Africa. Almost 80% of women who died in pregnancy, childbirth, or the puerperium were tested for HIV infection throughout South Africa. Of these women, 70% were infected with HIV. The majority of pregnant women with the acquired immunodeficiency syndrome (AIDS) (67%) had respiratory complications, namely TB (26.9%), pneumocystis pneumonia (13.3%), and other non-specified pneumonia (26.7%). The majority of emergency events occurred in the antenatal period (52%), whereas the majority of the women (61%) died postnatally.[63] Anaemia was a common factor, with 42.9% of women who died having a haemoglobin concentration lower than 10 g/dL.[63] Obstetric haemorrhage was the most common avoidable cause of maternal death. Postpartum haemorrhage during or after caesarean delivery accounted for 26.2% of deaths due to obstetric haemorrhage. The largest number of deaths due to haemorrhage were associated with caesarean delivery occurring at district hospitals but the numbers at regional and tertiary hospitals were also reported and caused concern. Resuscitation was poorly carried out in 22.3% of cases.[63] The 2008–2010 report made specific recommendations for the management of non-pregnancy-related infections, complications of hypertension in pregnancy, and obstetric haemorrhage. These included widespread screening for and treatment of HIV infection; recognition and protocols for immediate treatment of severe hypertension, imminent eclampsia, eclampsia, and the haemolysis, elevated liver enzymes, low platelets (HELLP) syndrome (including availability of magnesium sulphate, antihypertensives, and monitoring); and prevention of anaemia and safe management of labour.[63]

The global picture: developed countries

The United Kingdom: Confidential Enquiries into maternal deaths

The most recent Confidential Enquiry, Saving Lives Improving Mothers' Care (MBRRACE-UK) report,[11] covering the years 2009-2012, describes a significant reduction in maternal mortality rate from 11 per 100,000 maternities in 2006-2008 to 10 per 100, 000 maternities. (See Table 31.1).

Following the trend of the previous report, indirect deaths i.e. of women with pre- existing disease are twice as frequent (6.87 per 100,00 maternities) as those who die directly as a result of their pregnancy (3.25 per 100,000 maternities) possibly owing to better

Table 31.1 Rolling three year average Direct and Indirect maternal mortality rates per 100,000 maternities; UK 2003–12

3-year period	Total UK maternities	Direct deaths			Indirect deaths			Total Direct and Indirect deaths		
		n	Rate	95% CI	n	Rate	95% CI	n	Rate	95% CI
2003–05	2 114 004	132	6.24	5.26–7.41	163	7.71	6.61–8.99	295	13.95	12.45–15.64
2004–06	2 165 909	118	5.45	4.55–6.53	154	7.11	6.07–8.33	272	12.56	11.15–14.14
2005–07	2 220 979	113	5.09	4.23–6.12	146	6.57	5.59–7.73	259	11.66	10.32–13.17
2006–08	2 291 493	107	4.67	3.86–5.64	154	6.72	5.74–7.87	261	11.39	10.09–12.86
2007–09	2 331 835	101	4.33	3.53–5.26	153	6.56	5.56–7.69	254	10.89	9.59–12.32
2008–10	2 366 082	89	3.76	3.02–4.63	172	7.27	6.22–8.44	261	11.03	9.73–12.45
2009–11	2 379 014	83	3.49	2.78–4.32	170	7.15	6.11–8.30	253	10.63	9.36–12.03
2010–12	2 401 624	78	3.25	2.57–4.05	165	6.87	5.86–8.00	243	10.12	8.89–11.47

CMACE, MBRRACE-UK, Office for National Statistics, National Records Scotland, Northern Ireland Statistics and Research Agency.

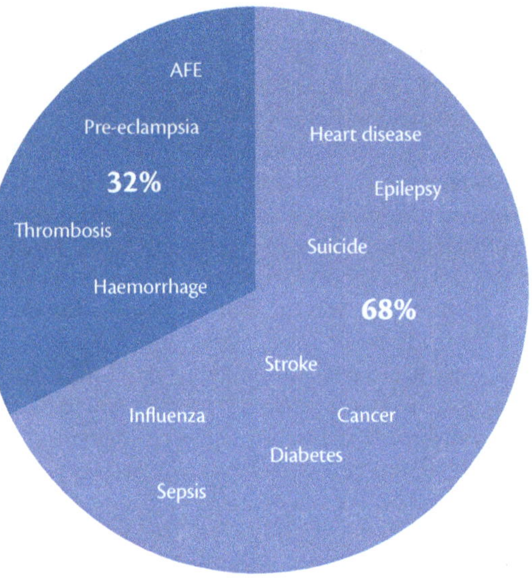

Figure 31.2 Causes of maternal death 2009–2012. Direct deaths are in dark blue. Indirect deaths are in light blue.

Reproduced with permission from Knight M, Kenyon S, Brocklehurst P, Neilson J, Shakespeare J, Kurinczuk JJ (Eds.) on behalf of MBRRACEUK. Saving Lives, Improving Mothers' Care - Lessons learned to inform future maternity care from the UK and Ireland Confidential Enquiries into Maternal Deaths and Morbidity 2009–12. Oxford: National Perinatal Epidemiology Unit, University of Oxford 2014. © 2014 National Perinatal Epidemiology Unit, University of Oxford.

management of 'direct' obstetric conditions and/or an increase in co-morbidities and risk factors over this period, in particular obesity[66] and increasing maternal age. (Figures 31.2 and 31.3).

CEMD: direct deaths

Sepsis

An increase in the number of deaths related to sepsis was noted during the collection and reporting process of the 2006-2008 CEMD report,[10] and this led CMACE to the unusual step of releasing an interim statement.[67] The final report for 2006-2008 revealed sepsis to be the leading direct cause of maternal death, with 26 deaths during this period (maternal mortality rate 1.13/100,000 maternities), compared with 18 deaths (maternal mortality rate 0.85/100,000 maternities) in the previous triennium. This increase reflects a generally increasing trend over the last 20 years and follows a dramatic fall in the rate in the 1950s that is thought to be related to the introduction of antibiotics, better general healthcare, and sanitation, the Abortion Act of 1968, and increased awareness due to the CEMD process itself.

In the 2006-2008 CEMD report, genital tract sepsis due to group A streptococcal disease was the predominant cause; however, other pathogens were also isolated.[68] Nine women died following caesarean delivery, highlighting the need for timely administration of antibiotics.[69] A lack of recognition of severe sepsis and absent or late involvement of senior medical staff and multidisciplinary critical care were highlighted. The CEMD report also emphasized the sometimes very atypical or non-specific histories and symptoms with which women with sepsis may present, the risk of rapid decompensation when their physiological reserves are exhausted, and the need for prompt treatment according to internationally accepted sepsis guidelines including early broad spectrum antibiotics, careful fluid resuscitation, and circulatory support if required.

Although not specific to sepsis, the 2006–2008 CEMD report[10] highlighted the usefulness of early warning scores, raised in the 2003–2005 report,[65] in monitoring mothers' physiological variables over time and aiding the detection of gradual deterioration, with triggers for seeking medical input (and at an appropriate level of seniority). Such modified early obstetric warning scores (MEOWS)[70] are an extension of the concept of early warning scores (EWS) used in general hospital wards and a national EWS has recently been developed by the Royal College of Physicians.[71] A specific national MEOWS is less well developed although the process of developing such a system based on proper evaluation/ evidence is underway .

In the recent MBRRACE-UK report,[11] sepsis was no longer the leading cause of maternal mortality but was still responsible for a

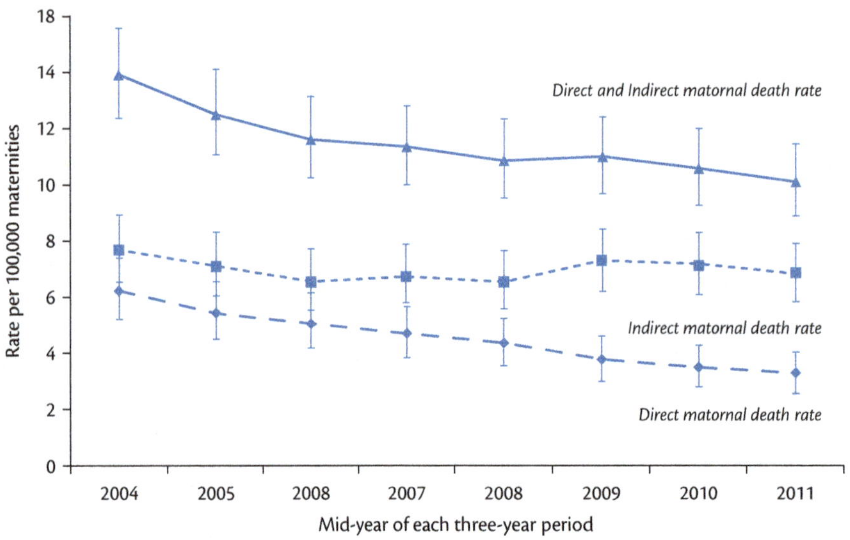

Figure 31.3 Direct and Indirect maternal mortality rates per 100 000 maternities; rolling three year average rates 2003–12.

Reproduced with permission from Knight M, Kenyon S, Brocklehurst P, Neilson J, Shakespeare J, Kurinczuk JJ (Eds.) on behalf of MBRRACEUK. Saving Lives, Improving Mothers' Care - Lessons learned to inform future maternity care from the UK and Ireland Confidential Enquiries into Maternal Deaths and Morbidity 2009–12. Oxford: National Perinatal Epidemiology Unit, University of Oxford 2014. © 2014 National Perinatal Epidemiology Unit, University of Oxford.

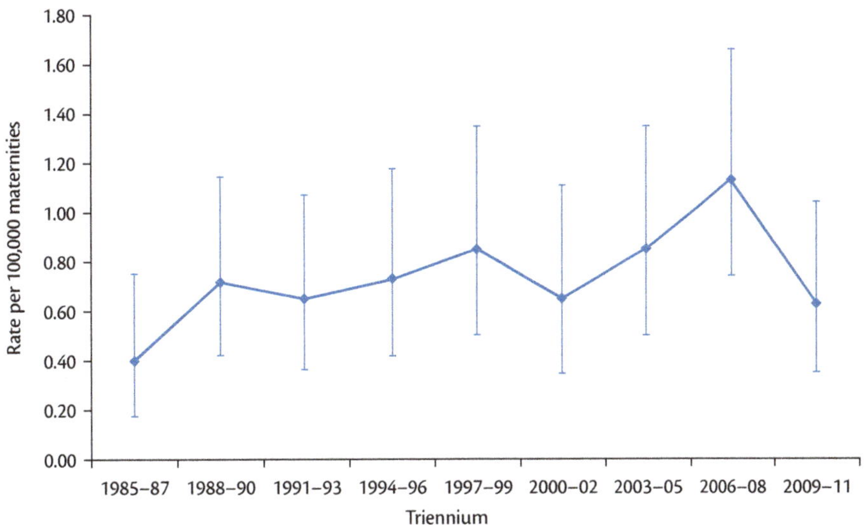

Figure 31.4 Maternal mortality rates per 100,000 maternities in the United Kingdom due to sepsis: 1985–2008.

Reproduced with permission from Knight M, Kenyon S, Brocklehurst P, Neilson J, Shakespeare J, Kurinczuk JJ (Eds.) on behalf of MBRRACEUK. Saving Lives, Improving Mothers' Care - Lessons learned to inform future maternity care from the UK and Ireland Confidential Enquiries into Maternal Deaths and Morbidity 2009–12. Oxford: National Perinatal Epidemiology Unit, University of Oxford 2014. © 2014 National Perinatal Epidemiology Unit, University of Oxford.

quarter of the deaths. One in 11 maternal deaths was due to influenza and increasing the immunisation rates for seasonal flu is seen as a priority for health services.

Thromboembolism

Thromboembolism is once again the commonest cause of direct maternal death with 56 women dying from this condition in the recent MBRRACE-UK report.[11] The reduction in the number of deaths from thromboembolism previously seen is evidence of the success of both the CEMD and the use of national guidelines on thromboprophylaxis. In the 2006-2008 CEMD report, the number of deaths from this cause was the lowest reported in 20 years, with the most dramatic reduction between 2003–2005 (41 deaths; 1.94/100,000 maternities) and 2006–2008 (18 deaths; 0.79/100,000 maternities). The publication of national guidelines on thromboprophylaxis for caesarean delivery in 1995,[72] and for pregnancy/labour/vaginal delivery in 2004,[73] was followed in each case by a reduction in the number of deaths in the following triennium (Figure 31.5).

In the 2006–2008 report, 16 deaths were from pulmonary embolism and two were from cerebral venous thrombosis. The reduced mortality was mainly seen in the antenatal period and in women delivering vaginally. The main risk factor still appears to be obesity, with 14 of the 18 women having a body mass index (BMI) exceeding 25 kg/m^2. Guidance on thromboprophylactic dosing in obesity was published by CMACE and the Royal College of Obstetricians and Gynaecologists in 2009.[74] At the time of publication, the effect of this guidance is still yet to be seen. Substandard care, present in over half of the deaths, included inadequate risk assessment and thromboprophylaxis as well as failure to investigate and treat women when they presented with often classic symptoms of deep vein thrombosis and/or pulmonary embolism.

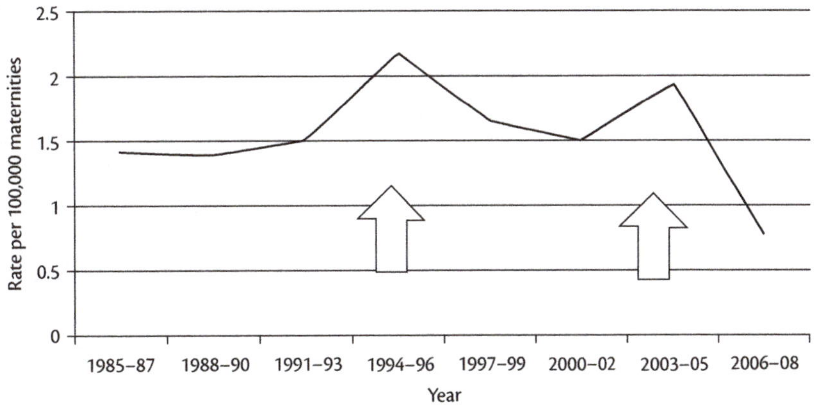

Figure 31.5 Maternal mortality rates per 100,000 maternities in the United Kingdom due to thrombosis and thromboembolism: 1985–2008. Publication of national guidelines on thromboprophylaxis for obstetrics and gynaecology in 1995 and thromboprophylaxis during pregnancy, labour and after vaginal delivery in 2004 are shown by the vertical arrows.

Reproduced from Confidential Enquiry on Maternal and Child Health, Saving mothers iives: reviewing maternal deaths to make motherhood safer 2006–2008, *BJOG: An International Journal of Obstetrics and Gynaecology*, 118, pp. 1–203, Copyright 2011, with permission from Centre for Maternal and Child Enquiries (CMACE), BJOG, and Wiley.

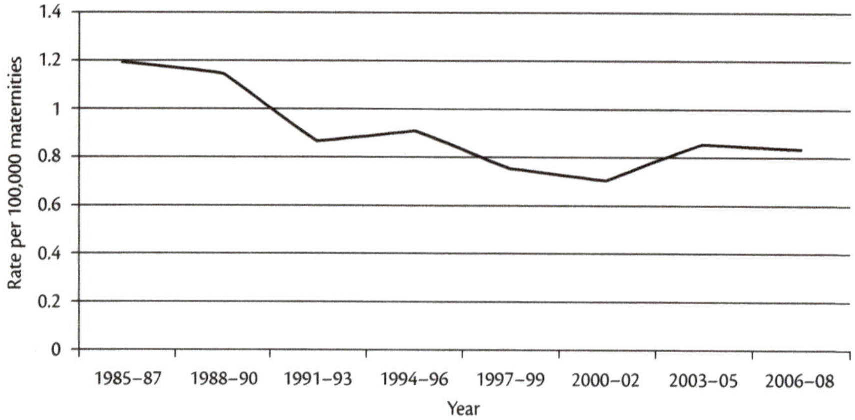

Figure 31.6 Maternal mortality rates per 100,000 maternities in the United Kingdom due to pre-eclampsia and eclampsia: 1985–2008.

Data from Lewis G (editor) Centre for Maternal and Child Enquiries (CMACE). Saving Mothers' Lives: reviewing maternal deaths to make motherhood safer: 2006–08. The Eighth Report on Confidential Enquiries into Maternal Deaths in the United Kingdom, *BJOG: An International Journal of Obstetrics and Gynaecology*, volume 118, supplement s1, pp. 1–203, Copyright © 2011 RCOG.

Pre-eclampsia and eclampsia

In 2003, deaths from acute fatty liver of pregnancy (AFLP) have been included in those from pre-eclamptic toxaemia (PET)/eclampsia, on the basis that they may be part of the same spectrum of disease. The total number of deaths from these combined conditions has remained approximately constant between 1997–1999 (20) and 2006–2008 (22), with four and three deaths, respectively, from AFLP.

Over the previous 30-year period there has been an overall reduction in the death rate from pre-eclampsia and eclampsia (Figure 31.6). The likely reason for the decreasing trend is thought to be earlier recognition and treatment of hypertensive disorders in pregnancy. In the 2006–2008 report,[10] nine deaths occurred secondary to intracranial haemorrhage and four from anoxia following cardiac arrest after an eclamptic seizure. The report emphasizes the importance of severe headache and epigastric pain as warning signs, and of systolic pressure, not just diastolic pressure, as a target for more intensive treatment. Substandard care was noted in 20 out of the 22 deaths; in 14 cases, this was classified as major. The predominance of intracranial bleed and absence of pulmonary complications as the cause of death reflects a continuation of the trend whereby pulmonary oedema and acute lung injury (considered now to be related to excessive administration of intravenous fluids in order to prevent renal injury) was the most common cause of death in women with PET/eclampsia 20–30 years ago but is uncommon now. NICE released guidelines for management of hypertension in pregnancy in 2010,[75] and figures from the most recent MBRRACE report[11] indicate that the mortality rate from hypertensive disease in pregnancy in 2009–2012 is the lowest since the Confidential Enquiries began in 1952. This is a major achievement and is thought to reflect adherence to protocols and guidelines on recognition and timely treatment of the condition.

Amniotic Fluid Embolism

Numbers of deaths due to amniotic fluid embolism (AFE) have remained small but consistent over the last 30 years (Figure 31.7); in the 2006–2008 CEMD report there were 13 deaths due to AFE, compared with 17 in the previous triennium.[10,65] The MBRRACE report[11] from 2009–2012 identified 11 women from the United Kingdom and Ireland who died from AFE. Evidence from elsewhere[76] suggests that AFE should no longer be considered an

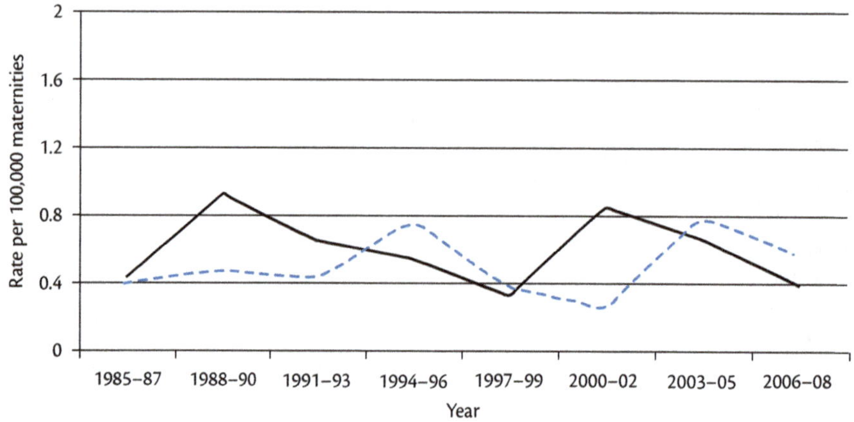

Figure 31.7 Maternal mortality rates per 100,000 maternities in the United Kingdom due to haemorrhage (black solid line) and amniotic fluid embolism (blue dashed line): 1985–2008.

Data from Lewis G (editor) Centre for Maternal and Child Enquiries (CMACE). Saving Mothers' Lives: reviewing maternal deaths to make motherhood safer: 2006–08. The Eighth Report on Confidential Enquiries into Maternal Deaths in the United Kingdom, *BJOG: An International Journal of Obstetrics and Gynaecology*, volume 118, supplement s1, pp. 1–203, Copyright © 2011 RCOG.

invariably fatal condition. There was substandard care in many cases, mostly related to the general management of critically ill obstetric patients (communication/referral/transfer) and failure to deliver by perimortem caesarean delivery quickly enough, although it is uncertain whether these women would have survived even had care not been substandard.

Haemorrhage

The death rate from haemorrhage fell dramatically between the 1950s and the 1970s, possibly owing to better recognition of high-risk mothers and their elective admission to hospital for delivery, better resuscitation before transfer to hospital if bleeding occurred at home or in smaller units, better management of coagulopathy, and earlier hysterectomy. In the last 30 years the mortality from haemorrhage has stayed relatively constant, reflecting early recognition and active treatment (Figure 31.7). In the 2006–2008 CEMD report, there were nine maternal deaths from haemorrhage (0.39/100,000 maternities), reduced from 14 in the previous report.[10,65] Worryingly, six of these women were assessed as receiving substandard care, in particular a lack of postoperative observations/monitoring and/or a failure to act on them, with the assessors judging that different management could have altered the outcome in six cases. The importance of diagnosing and treating antenatal anaemia was highlighted,[42] as was the requirement for effective multidisciplinary team-working with senior clinical involvement in cases of massive obstetric haemorrhage. Reassuringly, it was noted that the management of expected major haemorrhage in patients with placenta accreta had improved from the previous triennium.[65] Recommendations were made that patients with known major risks of haemorrhage should be delivered in maternity units with access to critical care, cell salvage, and interventional radiology.

In the MBRRACE-UK report[11] there were 17 deaths in the United Kingdom and Ireland accounting for 10% of maternal deaths in 2009-2012 and responsible also for significant maternal morbidity. There is a continuing trend toward increasing incidence of postpartum haemorrrhage.

Anaesthesia

In the 1970s to 1980s, anaesthesia was the third most common direct cause of maternal death. The dramatic decline in the number of deaths related to anaesthesia is rightly seen as a major achievement of the specialty, and of the CEMD itself (Figure 31.8). The factors that have contributed to the fall in anaesthetic deaths are thought to be the emergence of obstetric anaesthesia as a consultant-led subspeciality, the provision of dedicated anaesthetic cover for delivery suite especially out of hours, the increased use of neuraxial anaesthesia over general anaesthesia for caesarean delivery and other procedures, and better standards of monitoring, anaesthetic assistance, equipment, and general anaesthetic safety. It should be noted, however, that the impressive results shown in Figure 31.8 do not demonstrate the even more impressive improvement in safety associated with caesarean delivery. Since the caesarean delivery rate has increased so markedly over the years, the actual mortality rate due to anaesthesia has fallen from 36/100,000 caesarean deliveries in 1964–1966, to 6/100,000 in 1982–1984, and just 1/100,000 in 2000–2002.[77]

Factors that have been associated with substandard care over the years have included inadequate assistance for the anaesthetist, a lack of dedicated anaesthetic cover, inadequate antacid prophylaxis, a lack of referral to senior staff and to critical care services, inadequate antenatal referral of high-risk cases to anaesthetists, and inadequate airway management including failure to recognize oesophageal intubation and persistence with attempts

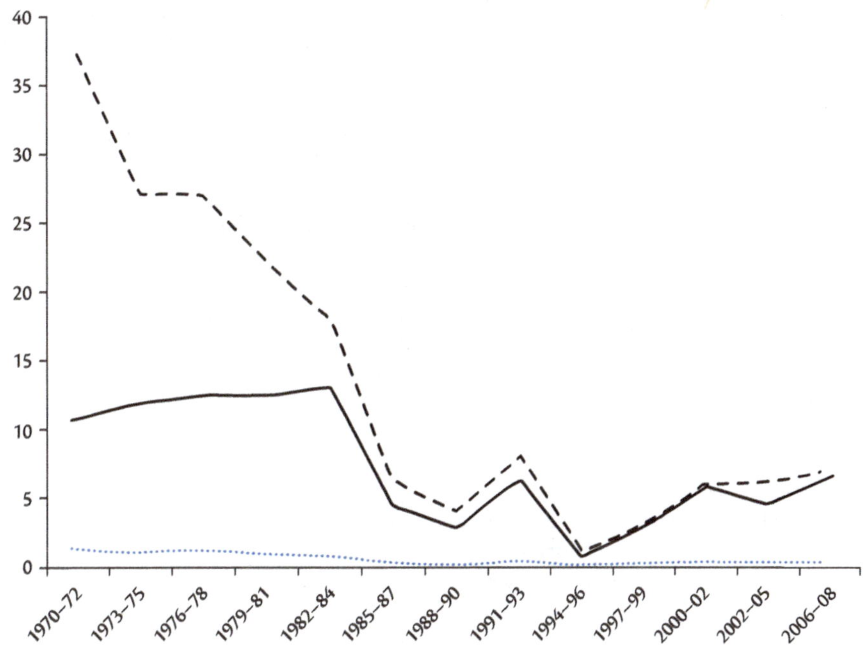

Figure 31.8 Maternal mortality due to anaesthesia in the CEMD over the last 40 years. Dashed line = number of deaths; solid line = proportion of direct deaths; dotted line = rate per 100,000 maternities.

Data from Lewis G (editor) Centre for Maternal and Child Enquiries (CMACE). Saving Mothers' Lives: reviewing maternal deaths to make motherhood safer: 2006–08. The Eighth Report on Confidential Enquiries into Maternal Deaths in the United Kingdom, *BJOG: An International Journal of Obstetrics and Gynaecology*, volume 118, supplement s1, pp. 1–203, Copyright © 2011 RCOG.

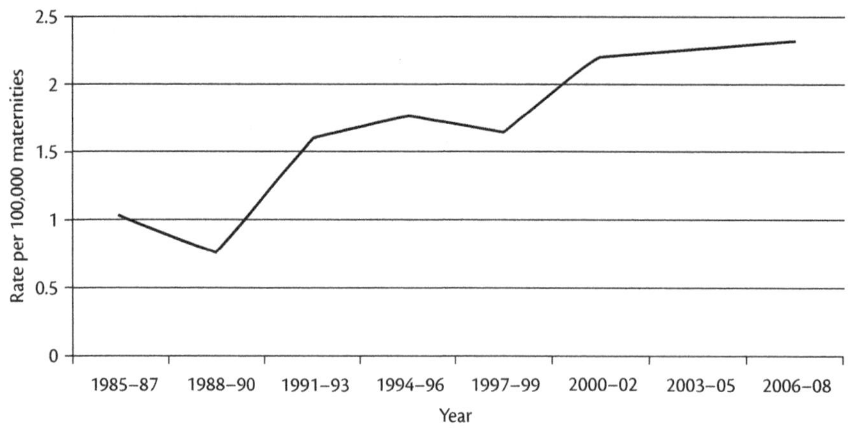

Figure 31.9 Maternal mortality rates per 100,000 maternities in the United Kingdom due to cardiac disease: 1985–2008.

Data from Lewis G (editor) Centre for Maternal and Child Enquiries (CMACE). Saving Mothers' Lives: reviewing maternal deaths to make motherhood safer: 2006–08. The Eighth Report on Confidential Enquiries into Maternal Deaths in the United Kingdom, *BJOG: An International Journal of Obstetrics and Gynaecology*, volume 118, supplement s1, pp. 1–203, Copyright © 2011 RCOG.

at tracheal intubation instead of using alternative methods of oxygenation. Many of these have been addressed over the years through training and provision of adequate resources, though the same lessons continue to be highlighted, even in recent reports, with anaesthesia continuing to contribute to maternal deaths even if not their direct cause. Other factors include the provision of anaesthetic care out of hours largely with relatively junior staff, and the increase in maternal age, obesity, and other morbidity.

Because the actual number of deaths directly due to anaesthesia has fallen to such low levels, it is difficult to extrapolate too much from discussion of individual cases, although as stated above, the same points tend to be raised each triennium. In the 2006–2008 CEMD report,[10] there were seven deaths directly due to anaesthesia, making it the seventh leading cause of direct maternal death. Six deaths were thought to involve substandard care, although the outcome was judged as being affected by this in only three. Two of the deaths were airway related; in one of these a working epidural was not topped up for caesarean delivery. Four deaths occurred postoperatively, one from opioid toxicity thought to be associated with patient-controlled analgesia, one possibly associated with incompatible blood transfusion, one associated with substance abuse, and one from aspiration of gastric contents. One death was attributed to acute haemorrhagic leucoencephalitis, a rare condition, that followed spinal anaesthesia. Eighteen further deaths had some anaesthetic contribution, with 12 deaths noted as involving anaesthetists and intensivists too late. Key learning points included improvements in communication, human factors and non-technical skill awareness, maintenance of airway and life support skills, and adequate topping-up of effective epidurals, if clinically appropriate, to avoid general anaesthesia and the need for tracheal intubation for emergency caesarean delivery.

In the 2009–2012 MBRRACE-UK report[11], there were 4 deaths directly attributable to anaesthesia. Two deaths occurred after accidental dural puncture (ADP) resulting in a subdural haematoma in one patient and a cerebral vein thrombosis in the other and highlight the need for hospital follow up and primary care notification after ADP. Two patients also died following periods of hypoventilation during or following general anaesthesia, highlighting the need for vigilance and high standards of perioperative and post operative care.

CEMD: indirect deaths

Cardiac disease

The spectrum of cardiac disease in the CEMD reports has changed over the years, reflecting changing patterns of disease generally. In the 1960s to the 1980s, the majority of deaths (70–85%) were from acquired disease, usually rheumatic heart disease, with congenital conditions a minority. By the mid to late 1980s, the deaths were approximately equally split between acquired and congenital, but this changed back over subsequent reports such that acquired disease again accounts for the majority of deaths (60–80% in the most recent two triennia). Rheumatic heart disease features only rarely in recent reports (there were no deaths from this cause in 2006–2008), most acquired disease consisting of myocardial infarction and cardiomyopathy. Over the last 30 years the number of deaths secondary to cardiac disease has increased (Figure 31.9). This is thought to reflect the increasing age at which women are becoming pregnant, with concomitant risk factors such as obesity and smoking, and advancements in surgical treatment of congenital cardiac disease in early life.

In the 2006–2008 CEMD report, cardiac disease was the leading overall cause of maternal mortality, with 53 deaths (a mortality rate of 2.31 per 100,000 maternities).[10] The main causes were sudden adult death syndrome (SADS), myocardial infarction, thoracic aortic dissection, and cardiomyopathy. Death from SADS is assumed to be due to idiopathic arrhythmias leading to sudden cardiac death. Half of the deaths were in obese patients with a BMI greater than 30 kg/m^2. Substandard care was noted in 51% of cases, including inappropriate diagnosis/investigation of symptoms such as chest pain, especially where other risk factors such as obesity, hypertension, and smoking were known.

The 2009–2012 MBRRACE-UK report[11] has also found that cardiac disease remains the single largest cause of indirect maternal deaths.

Psychiatric disease

Deaths from suicide have only been analysed and discussed separately in the CEMD reports since the 1993–1997 report, and the discussion of deaths from psychiatric causes has widened to include deaths associated with substance abuse, including alcohol. It became clear from cross-linking with the ONS that many deaths from suicide were missed from previous reports, leading to a sudden increase in the number of cases in 2000–2002, due to better case ascertainment. A particular feature that arose from more detailed analysis of maternal death from suicide is the high incidence of violent death (e.g. jumping from buildings) compared with non-pregnant women, in whom medication overdose is the main cause of self-inflicted death. The analysis and discussion of psychiatric disease, including the influence of substance abuse and other indicators of vulnerability, including domestic violence, demonstrates the importance of the CEMD in commenting on and influencing the social aspects of healthcare in pregnancy.

In the 2006–2008 CEMD report, there were 67 deaths associated with psychiatric causes, including suicide, drug overdose, medical conditions associated with the psychiatric condition, and accidents.[10] Areas of substandard care relate to service provision in general rather than to specific areas in which anaesthetists might be involved.

Other Indirect Causes

This description includes a varying number of deaths from causes too uncommon to warrant their own chapter in the CEMD reports. In the 2006-2008 report,[10] there were 88 such deaths, 36 involving the central nervous system, and 18 involving the respiratory or metabolic/endocrine/immune systems. Over the years, subarachnoid haemorrhage and epilepsy have been consistently highlighted. Care was judged to have been substandard in 51 cases, in 28 of them serious enough to have influenced the outcome.

Other relevant lessons from the CEMD

Critical care

Over 50% of women reported in each CEMD report have been admitted to a critical care unit. Review of Intensive Care National Audit and Research Centre (ICNARC) data has revealed that 11.4% of women between 16 and 50 years old admitted to critical care units are obstetric patients, of whom 80% were reported as 'recently pregnant' rather than 'currently pregnant'.[10] The most common pregnancy-related diagnosis, accounting for 34% of admissions, was haemorrhage, with sepsis being another major cause. Lessons highlighted from CEMD reports include the importance of providing critical care support early to severely unwell women—including before formal admission to the intensive care unit (ICU)—and early protocol-driven multidisciplinary management of severe sepsis and severe obstetric haemorrhage, including guidelines for the rate and composition of fluid administration.[10] The role of simulation in improving the management of life-threatening obstetric emergencies was also highlighted.

Obesity

This is an increasing problem in developed countries. In 2007, 24% of women in the United Kingdom were classified as obese, compared with 16% noted in 1993. Forty per cent of women who died in the 2006–2008 report were obese.[10] Obesity was associated with an increased risk of cardiac disease (61%) and thromboembolism (78%). The risks of gestational diabetes, pre-eclampsia, and ICU admission are all increased in obese patients.[66]

Age

There is a recognized associated between increasing maternal age and the risk of pregnancy-associated death. In the triennium of 1985–1987, there were 35 deaths in the age range 35–39 years and 13 in the over 40s; in the 2006–2009 CEMD report these numbers have increased to 71 and 24, respectively.[10]

Emergency care

Deaths in women who presented several times to emergency departments led to the highlighting of emergency medicine as an area of focus in recent CEMD reports.[10,65] In the 2006–2008 CEMD report, 27 women died in emergency departments, the majority having cardiac arrests before arrival to hospital.[10] The need for perimortem caesarean delivery in these cases was again highlighted, as was the need for pregnancy tests for all women of childbearing age and review of frequent attenders by senior clinicians. A lack of input from appropriately trained senior doctors in high-risk emergency cases was also highlighted. Key learning points were the development of clear guidelines to aid junior staff to escalate calling for senior help early and appropriately.

Other national schemes (in developed countries) for reporting maternal mortality

Many other developed countries have attempted to establish their own systems for analysing maternal deaths, including the United States,[17,78–87] France,[88,89] Australia,[90,91] and Canada.[17,92]

United States of America

In the United States, maternal death counts from 1900 were collated by the National Center for Health Statistics (NCHS); MMR data was produced by the NCHS from 1915.[78] In 1915, the US MMR was reported as 600 deaths per 100,000 live births, this number reduced to 10 by 1980.[78] The accuracy of this data was limited as the system at that stage relied on death certification data, not on surveillance. Also, the death certification process was the responsibility of individual states, with considerable variation. In 1987, the Centers for Disease Control and Prevention (CDC) partnered with the State Health Department and the American College of Obstetrics and Gynecology to form the Pregnancy Mortality Surveillance System (PMSS).[85] The PMSS recommended active voluntary surveillance systems for maternal deaths with death certificates and matching live birth or fetal death certificates for all pregnancy-associated deaths. Each state thus collates its own data through maternal mortality review committees and forwards this summated information to the CDC, where epidemiologists review the data to identify all pregnancy-related deaths. In the United States, two systems collect information on women who die from maternal complications. The National Vital Statistics System (NVSS) reports on maternal mortality and publishes this maternal mortality data for the United States, to be used for comparisons with other countries. The PMSS conducts voluntary epidemiologic surveillance of pregnancy-related deaths collated by the CDC, including clinical information. Even with the resources available, a number of maternal deaths are still not reported, leading to underestimation.[21] To improve the detection of pregnancy-related deaths, state death certificates now include a specific question or tick box about the pregnancy status at the time of death.[93] In the period between the 1980s and 1990s, the MMR ranged between 6.6 and 8.4 per 100,000 live births. For the period between 2006 and 2007, the MMR was 15.1 deaths per 100,000 live births. The increase in MMR over this period has been attributed to improvement of identification of cases and the use of ICD-10 classifications[8] for coding of US death certificates, increasing the criteria whereby death could be linked with pregnancy.[86,94] Maternal obesity, increasing age, and co-morbidities have also increased the MMR. Causes of maternal mortality in the United States during the period from 2006 to 2007 are listed

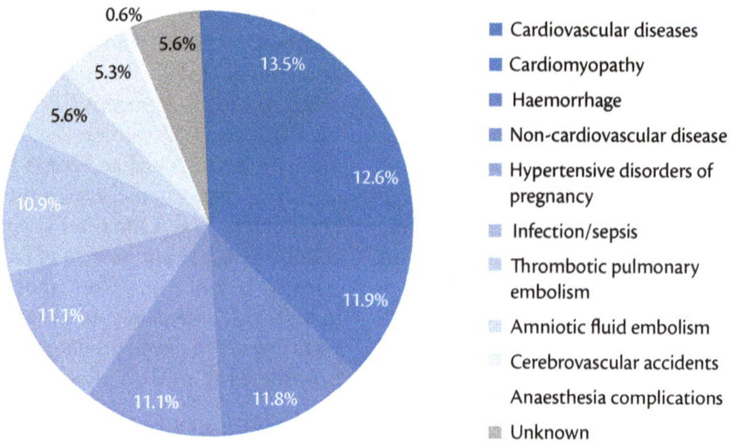

Figure 31.10 (See colour figure section). Causes of pregnancy-related deaths in the United States: 2006 to 2007.
Data from Berg CJ. From identification and review to action--maternal mortality review in the United States. *Semin Perinatol* 2012; 36:7–13, Copyright © 2012 Elsevier.

in Figure 31.10. These figures show that in the United States, cardiac disease features as the leading cause of death. Sepsis is also an important cause of death; however, there is a greater proportion of deaths from haemorrhage compared with UK data.[10,84] As with UK data, it can be seen that in recent years the numbers of indirect deaths in the United States are on the increase: there has been a rise from 6.1% in 1995 to 25.5% in 2005.[79–83,95-100] In the United States, there still exist significant racial disparities, with 15.1 deaths per 100,000 live births for white women, 34.8 deaths per 100,000 live births for black women, and 15.7 deaths per 100,000 live births for women of other races.[84] The strongest factors in the United States that appear to cause maternal deaths in varying racial groups are medical co-morbidities, deficient medical care, and poor social circumstances.

Australia

A triennial confidential enquiry into maternal deaths has occurred in Australia since 1964.[91] The Australian enquiry involves several levels of reporting and review. Initially, maternal deaths are notified to the local State and Territory Maternal Mortality Committees (STMMC) by doctors, midwives, hospitals, public health departments, and through the coroner and postmortem investigations. Maternal deaths are further ascertained from death certificates from perinatal and hospital morbidity collections and the Australian Bureau of Statistics. Every separate STMMC is responsible for conducting confidential death enquiries to determine primary and contributory causes of each maternal death. Regional variation in roles and responsibilities of each the STMMC occurs. Some STMMCs perform root cause analysis of maternal deaths while others do not. A national report on maternal deaths is prepared on a triennial basis on behalf of the Australian Institute of Health and Welfare (AIHW) by the National Perinatal Statistics Unit (NPSU), with expert input from the National Advisory Committee on Maternal Mortality (NACMM). The NACMM comprises of members from STCMM, professional medical colleges, patients, indigenous Aboriginal representation, National Health and Medical Research Council (NHMRC), Australian Commission on Safety and Quality in Healthcare (ACSQH), and other stakeholders.[101] A subcommittee reviews all anonymous maternal death data, ensuring consistency. It provides information so a clinical commentary can be produced from the data collected, allowing identification of substandard care and flagging areas that require protocol and guideline development. Case review has shown around 50% of the maternal deaths in Australia are potentially preventable. The MMR has been relatively static in Australia for over 30 years with no sustained improvement. The period 1973–1999 revealed 646 maternal deaths, including 397 (61.5%) direct deaths and 249 (38.5%) indirect deaths.[102] The MMR was 9.8 deaths per 100,000 maternities during this period, having declined from 12.7 in 1973–1975 to 6.2 in 1991–1993. The leading causes of all maternal deaths during 1973–1999 were cardiovascular disease (15.3%), haemorrhage (11.8%), pulmonary thromboembolism (11.3%), hypertensive disorders of pregnancy (9.9%), AFE (7.4%), and infection (6.7%).[102] The main direct causes of death remained unchanged during the period 1973–1999, with pulmonary embolism accounting for nearly 20% deaths. Indirect deaths were dominated by cardiovascular disease, which accounted for an average of 40% of maternal deaths per triennium.[102] In the 2003-2005 triennial report, published in 2008, the MMR was 8.4/100,000 maternities, with a total of 65 deaths (29 direct (44.6%) and 36 indirect (55.4%) deaths). The main direct causes of maternal death were AFE (27.6%), hypertensive disorders of pregnancy (17.2%), and thrombosis and thromboembolism (17.2%). Significant indirect causes were cardiac conditions (27.8%), psychiatric causes (16.7%), and infection (11.1%). The MMR for Aboriginal and Torres Strait Islander women at 21.5/100,000 maternities was more than two and a half times that of other non-indigenous women at 7.9/100,000 maternities.[91] Recommendation from the 2008 report revealed that the current data collection process did not provide enough quality and sufficient information on clinical pathways and management to inform recommendations on practice and policy.

Canada

The Public Health Agency of Canada produces a Canadian Perinatal Health Report that has 29 healthcare indicators, including maternal mortality. The Public Health Agency of Canada works with the Canadian Perinatal Surveillance System (CPSS) to collate maternal mortality data. The 2008 report is the fifth report that the CPSS has produced.[103] The CPSS collaborates with Statistics Canada, the Canadian Institute for Health Information, healthcare organizations, provincial and territorial governments, patient groups, and university delegates. Within the CPSS the Maternal Health Study Group assesses the maternal mortality. MMRs for the CPSS are calculated using National Vital Statistics (NVS) data from death certificate information. The NVS data are collated locally within provinces to ensure accuracy and can be used to verify inpatient maternal mortality data. According to CPSS data, the MMR in Canada has increased significantly over 30 years from 3.4/100,000 in 1984–1986 and 1990–1992 to 5.5/100,000 live births in 2002–2004.[103] The CPSS recognized in its 2008 report that as the data were obtained from death certificates, the MMR was an underestimation; in the future it is intended to include data from coroner/medical examiners, medical death review teams, and inpatient statistics.[103] One non-governmental group has looked at trends in maternal mortality in Canada using a combination of NVS and inpatient data and found a very different trend from the CPSS data,[104] with maternal mortality rates in the period 1981–2007 increasing significantly from 4.5/100,000 in 1981–1983 to 4.7/100,000 in 1996–1998, and 7.2/100,000 live births in 2005–2007.[104] The most common causes of maternal death were cardiac disease, postpartum haemorrhage, and hypertensive disorders of pregnancy.[104] Maternal mortality rates from inpatient data were higher but did not increase over time.[104] The non-governmental group revealed that provincial maternal mortality rates from NVS data showed varying degrees of under-ascertainment (12–70%) compared with inpatient data.[104] Recently, the Public Health Agency of Canada has started to publish data on maternal mortality based solely on inpatient data placed in biennial cohorts.[105] This has revealed that during the 10 years from 1996 to 2010, MMR fell from 11.9/100,000 deliveries in 2000–2002 to 6.8/100,000 deliveries in 2004–2006, rising to 7.8/100,000 deliveries in 2008–2010. The most common causes of death from 2002 to 2010 were cardiac disease (25.7%), postpartum haemorrhage (13.0%), hypertensive disorders of pregnancy (13%), and venous thromboembolism or AFE (11.5%).[105] The striking message when reading through the Canadian national reports on maternal mortality is that although they give information on statistics, they do not give information on strategies for prevention of the maternal deaths or information on the major lessons learnt.

France

In France, the national confidential enquiry into maternal deaths (ENCMM) and its committee (CNEMM) collect all data on maternal deaths in the country. Two assessors (one obstetrician and one anaesthetist) gather information on patients after being informed of the maternal deaths by the epidemiological centre on medical causes of deaths (CépiDC); they gather information by the means of a detailed and specific questionnaire. The anonymous files are then reviewed by a committee at the CNEMM. Maternal mortality rates and ratios are then calculated, looking at specific causes of death and identifying substandard care.[89,106] The MMR from France has been relatively stable over the previous 15 years: in 1999 it was 7.4/100,000, from 2001 to 2006 it was 8.0/100,000, and from 2003 to 2004 it was 7.0/100,000.[107] From 1996 to 2006, 729 maternal deaths were included in the confidential enquiry process, of which 553 were reviewed by the CNEMM. Direct causes formed the majority of maternal deaths (73%): haemorrhage (22%), AFE (12%), venous thromboembolism (10%), and complications of pregnancy-associated hypertension (10%). Fifty per cent of maternal deaths were assessed by the CNEMM as being preventable, mainly from haemorrhage and sepsis.[106]

Maternal morbidity

Healthcare staff are much more likely to encounter pregnant women suffering morbidity than maternal deaths, and as numbers of deaths have declined there has been increased emphasis on examining cases of morbidity in order to learn lessons and improve the care of obstetric patients. Although morbidity is more common, however, it is much more difficult to obtain accurate data about the spectrum of conditions encountered and their incidence, although attempts to do so are ongoing.[108]

Methods of estimation of maternal morbidity

In developing countries, attention is rightly focused on preventing maternal mortality as the major priority, though the importance of severe morbidity should not be forgotten. Severe maternal morbidity occurs in around 1% of maternities in the United States compared with 3.01–9.05% in some developing settings.[3] However, collecting data on morbidity in such environments is usually considered too difficult or not as urgent compared with mortality. In developed countries, the identification of severe maternal morbidity has emerged as a complement to the investigation of maternal deaths, the assumption being that conditions causing morbidity may ultimately lead to maternal deaths.[5,10,108]

The main difficulties with collecting and analysing maternal morbidity data are first, establishing a system for reliable reporting and second, setting definitions that are meaningful and reproducible—and ideally, widely accepted, so that systems in different regions/countries can compare their findings, as for mortality data. As far as reporting systems are concerned, their strength is also their weakness: the potentially large numbers involved (that can give rise to more robust data with narrower confidence intervals than those describing small numbers) can make it difficult to capture all the cases, especially where the healthcare/communication infrastructure is itself less reliable. Difficulties in standardizing definitions for morbidity have led to a more fragmented approach to morbidity studies than for mortality.

Definitions

Initially, reports on maternal morbidity focused on admission to the ICU as a proxy measure of morbidity.[109–113] However, admission rates to ICU vary widely between units and especially in different countries, depending on case mix, admission criteria, and availability of ICU resources. This led to attempts to define maternal morbidity in terms of specific organ dysfunction.

In 1998, Mantel et al. referred to severe acute maternal morbidity as the concept of maternal 'near-miss', defining this as 'a women with severe organ dysfunction or organ failure'.[113] There were specified defined criteria for each organ dysfunction. A maternal 'near-miss' was noted as an event where a pregnant woman comes close to death, but does not die. In 2004, Brace et al. referred to severe maternal morbidity using 14 categories that were a combination of organ dysfunction, diagnosis and management strategies. An example would be renal dysfunction secondary to massive obstetric haemorrhage leading to ICU admission.[114,115] In 2005, Wen et al. proposed their definition for severe maternal morbidity, consisting of one or more of: venous thromboembolism; eclampsia; pulmonary, cardiac, or central nervous system complications of anaesthesia; cerebrovascular disorders in the puerperium (including intracranial venous sinus thrombosis); uterine rupture; adult respiratory distress syndrome; pulmonary oedema; myocardial infarction; acute kidney injury after labour and delivery; cardiac arrest/failure or cerebral anoxia after obstetric surgery; severe postpartum haemorrhage requiring hysterectomy or transfusion; and the need for assisted ventilation. With definitions becoming increasingly complicated, Zhang et al. tried to simplify the definition for severe maternal morbidity in 2005 by relating it to the commonest causes of maternal morbidity based on defined criteria for pre-eclampsia, severe obstetric haemorrhage and sepsis.

In 2005, WHO established five factors with respect to maternal death during pregnancy, childbirth and the first week postpartum. The five factors were admission to the ICU, blood transfusion, hysterectomy, eclampsia, or cardiac and renal complications. It was assumed that combinations of these factors indicated severe maternal morbidity and could be considered maternal near-misses.[116] In 2011, WHO defined a maternal near-miss case as 'a woman who nearly died but survived a complication that occurred during pregnancy, childbirth or within 42 days of termination of pregnancy'.[116–120] To allow the identification of near-misses and maternal deaths, WHO has produced a set of signs of organ dysfunction, describing inclusion criteria for dysfunction of the cardiovascular, respiratory, renal, coagulation, hepatic, neurological, and uterine systems (Table 31.2).[119,121,122]

Table 31.2 Inclusion criteria of organ dysfunction from WHO 'near-miss' assessment of severe maternal morbidity

Organ dysfunction	Criteria
Cardiovascular	Shock
	Cardiac arrest
	Severe hypoperfusion (lactate > 5 mmol/L or > 45 mg/dL)
	Severe acidosis (pH < 7.1)
	Use of continuous vasoactive drugs
Respiratory	Acute cyanosis
	Gasping
	Severe tachypnoea (respiratory rate > 40 breaths/min)
	Severe bradypnoea (respiratory rate < 6 breaths/min)
	Severe hypoxaemia (O_2 saturation < 90% for ≥ 60min or PAO_2/FIO_2 < 200)
	Intubation and ventilation not related to anaesthesia
Renal	Oliguria non responsive to fluids or diuretics
	Severe acute azotaemia (creatinine > 300 μmol/ml or > 3.5 mg/dL)
	Dialysis for acute kidney injury
Coagulation/ haematological	Failure to form clots
	Severe acute thrombocytopenia (<50 × 10^6/L)
	Massive transfusion of blood or red cells (≥5 units)
Hepatic	Jaundice in the presence of pre-eclampsia
	Severe acute hyperbilirubinaemia (bilirubin > 100 μmol/L or > 6.0 mg/dL)
Neurological	Prolonged unconsciousness or coma (lasting > 12 h)
	Stroke
	Uncontrollable fit/status epilepticus
	Global paralysis
Uterine	Hysterectomy due to uterine infection or haemorrhage

Data from Cecatti JG, Souza JP, Oliveira Neto AF, *et al.*, Pre-validation of the WHO organ dysfunction based criteria for identification of maternal near miss. *Reprod Health* 2011; 8:22–29, Copyright © 2011 Springer Science+Business Media.

Morbidity studies

In general, there are three broad approaches to studying maternal morbidity: individual 'one-off' studies in single units or areas/regions, usually involving admissions to critical care units; continuous surveillance of morbidity across regions/countries; or specific reporting of individual rare events/conditions.

Single studies

There have been many studies based in a single unit or small groups of units within single cities; of more interest in global terms are those attempting to broaden the scope of study by including units across wider regions. Some of these are described below.

Netherlands Assessment of Severe Maternal Morbidity

In 2008, Zwart et al. reviewed cases of severe maternal morbidity collected over a 2-year period in 98 maternity units, covering a population of around 371,000.[123] Severe maternal morbidity had an incidence of 7.1/1000 deliveries, ICU admission 2.4/1000 deliveries, eclampsia 6.2/1000 deliveries, uterine rupture 6.1/1000, and major obstetric haemorrhage 4.5/1000. Immigrant women had the highest risk, with a 1.3-fold increased risk compared with western women. Substandard care was noted in 62% of cases.[123]

European Audit of Severe Maternal Morbidity

In 2005, Zhang et al. conducted a study looking at morbidity data from nine European countries.[124] Severe maternal morbidity was defined using criteria based on three common causes of morbidity of pregnancy: severe haemorrhage, pre-eclampsia (including eclampsia and HELLP), and sepsis. Data were gathered prospectively for the majority of cases; however, French data were retrospective. Overall differences between countries were mainly attributed to differences in haemorrhage data, which ranged from 8.8/1000 deliveries in Finland to 0.7/1000 deliveries in Austria. This was thought to reflect differences in the age of the women giving birth and in the care that was provided. It was noted that around 25% of women with severe maternal morbidity were admitted to ICU, with a great variation in regions (e.g. 25% admission rates in some regions (Belgium, France, Italy, and the United Kingdom), and 50% in others (e.g. Austria)). The conclusions were that using standardized definitions and a population-based approach, severe maternal morbidity was more common than previously thought and ICU admission was not a good surrogate marker.[124]

English Audit of ICU admissions

Hazelgrove et al. conducted a multicentre study involving 14 ICUs in Southern England.[125] Retrospective analysis was performed over a 2-year period from 1994 to 1996. Data revealed that 1.84% of admissions to ICUs during the period were from pregnant or postpartum patients. The majority of admissions were due to complications of postpartum haemorrhage (33.3%) and hypertensive disorders of pregnancy (39.5%); the overall mortality rate in these patients was 3.3%, and 35.7% of patients had an ICU stay shorter than 2 days. The study concluded that obstetric admissions required minimal interventions and had low associated mortality rates.[125]

Ongoing surveillance studies

ICNARC Case Mix Programme

The Intensive Care National Audit and Research Centre (ICNARC) was established in 1994 and established a system that identifies key indicators in the management of adults who require critical care management.[126] It involves voluntary data collection from currently 82% of ICUs in England, Wales, and Northern Ireland. In 2006, the Royal College of Anaesthetists, Royal College of Obstetricians and Gynaecologists, and Obstetric Anaesthetists' Association jointly commissioned ICNARC to include new fields into its electronic data collection form to include 'currently pregnant' and 'recently pregnant'. The first report was produced in 2009 and reviewed data from 2007 on level 3 obstetric critical care admissions.[127] The incidence of such patients admitted to critical care areas was 260 per 100,000 maternities, higher than the deaths for that period noted from the CEMD (13.95/100,000).[10] During 2007, obstetric patients represented of 11.4% of ICU admissions in females aged 16–50 years. Of these, 18.5% were classified as 'currently pregnant' and 81.5% as 'recently pregnant'. The majority (86%) of 'currently pregnant' women were admitted with non-obstetric related problems, the most common of these (20%) being pneumonia. In the 'recently pregnant' group, most patients (61%) were admitted secondary to obstetric reasons, most commonly (34%) postpartum haemorrhage. The 'recently pregnant' and 'currently pregnant' patients had a much lower critical care unit mortality compared with age-matched controls (2% vs 11%, respectively) and overall in-hospital admission (8 days vs 11 days, respectively).

Scottish Confidential Audit of Severe Maternal Morbidity

In Scotland, an audit of specified severe maternal morbidities has been running in all consultant (attending) led maternity units since 2003, covering a population of around 60,000 births per annum. Data collection is entirely voluntary, but it is hoped that most of the data available is collected. A designated coordinator within each unit identifies cases and sends completed datasets to the Reproductive Health Programme of NHS Quality Improvement Scotland. The data are then analysed and an annual report is produced. Collated morbidity data are based on work originally conducted in South Africa,[113] which looked at 14 variables associated with morbidity including major haemorrhage, eclampsia, renal/liver dysfunction, cardiac arrest, pulmonary oedema, respiratory dysfunction, coma, cerebrovascular disease, status epilepticus, anaphylaxis, septic shock, anaesthetic problems, pulmonary embolism, and ICU/coronary care unit admission (additional information on interventional radiology has also been collected from January 2010). Two particular areas of interest are major obstetric haemorrhage and eclampsia. Detailed information for each case of major haemorrhage and eclampsia are gathered and discussed by risk management teams locally. Following analysis, reports are sent to the Reproductive Health Programme. There is a lag time of around 2 years from collection of data to production of reports.[128] The consistent use of the same auditing tools and case definitions have allowed the identification of changes in numbers and rates of certain morbidities, compliance with national guidelines and changes in clinical management. The Scottish Confidential Audit of Severe Maternal Morbidity (SCASMM) has also disseminated information through anecdotal vignettes and produced data on clinical use of resources within Scotland. From January 2009, SCASMM has also collected sociodemographic data. This has revealed that deprivation, obesity, smoking, and substance misuse are all factors linked with increased maternal morbidity.

Figure 31.11 shows SCASMM data for 2006–2008.[128–130] Comparisons between Figure 31.11 and Figure 31.2 shows how morbidity and mortality data vary for presumably similar populations receiving similar levels of care—albeit with the SCASMM population forming part of the population covered by the CEMD data. Such comparisons demonstrate how studies of morbidity can complement those of mortality, and the difference between conditions that are common but rarely fatal, and those that are rare but with a high mortality rate.

Exploration of two particular conditions, haemorrhage and eclampsia, illustrates how the data from SCASMM can be used.

SCASMM Haemorrhage Data

The collection of morbidity data for the audit allows review of all cases of massive haemorrhage, ideally at the local level to

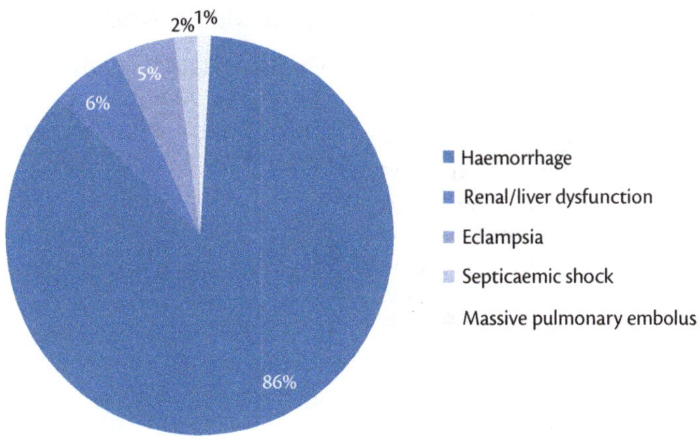

Figure 31.11 (See colour figure section). Causes of maternal morbidity (as a percentage of total) from Scottish Confidential Audit of Severe Maternal Morbidity: 2006–2008.

Data from various sources (see references).[129–31]

assess whether local guidelines are being followed. Data can be obtained on exact medical therapy given and surgical interventions received, including interventional radiological procedures. During the period 2006–2008, risk factors for massive obstetric haemorrhage included previous caesarean delivery (16%) and delivery by emergency caesarean delivery (46%), with 21% of those emergency caesarean deliveries taking place at full dilatation. There was an increase in conservative surgical techniques (intrauterine balloon tamponade and uterine brace sutures). The standard of care was assessed as being high in 64% of cases, but direct obstetric consultant involvement only occurred in 78%, thought to reflect the number of massive obstetric haemorrhage cases occurring out of hours.[128–130]

SCASMM eclampsia data

The reported incidence of eclampsia has stayed relatively constant during 2006–2008: in 2008 the rate of admission to ICU for eclampsia was 1.5/1000 live births. It was noted that few of the cases presented with classical prodromal signs and symptoms. Appropriate care was assessed as being present in only 41% of cases, with a consultant obstetrician present in fewer than half. Recommendations for protocol-driven pathways and senior early involvement were made.[128–130]

South Africa Audit of Severe Maternal Morbidity

In the Pretorian region of South Africa, four hospitals combine to form the Pretoria Academic Complex. They have performed audits looking at severe acute maternal morbidity since 1997,[113,131] with morbidity and maternal deaths identified at daily audit meetings using specific organ dysfunction criteria to define 'near-misses'. Since 2006, data have been recorded electronically using the MaMMAS software developed by the local research team.[132] The audits over the years highlighted that severe complications of obstetric haemorrhage, hypertension in pregnancy, non-pregnancy related sepsis, and pregnancy-related sepsis are increasing. The increase in prevalence of HIV-infected pregnant women is known to be the cause of increased non-pregnancy sepsis.[133] However, the increase in severe complications due to obstetric haemorrhage and hypertension was a cause for concern, leading to the implementation of new guidelines for managing obstetric haemorrhage and hypertension in all maternity facilities within the Pretoria Academic Complex.

Brazilian Audit of Severe Maternal Morbidity

In 2009, Brazil set up a multicentre, cross-sectional study in 27 obstetric units in different geographical regions.[121,134,135] The population of the cross-sectional component consists of women surviving either potentially life-threatening conditions (severe maternal complications) or life-threatening conditions (the maternal near-miss criteria) and maternal deaths. The definitions used are in accordance with the new WHO definition and criteria. A study to validate the WHO definition of a 'near-miss' was conducted and revealed that maternal near-miss criteria were associated with maternal deaths (positive likelihood ratio 106.8 (95% confidence interval (CI) 99.56–114.6)). In the same study a maternal severity index (MSI) model was also developed and found to be able to describe the relationship between life-threatening conditions and mortality (area under the ROC curve: 0.95 (95% CI 0.91–0.99)).[120]

Canadian Perinatal Surveillance System

The CPSS has collected yearly morbidity data since 1995.[103] Morbidity data are extracted from the Canadian Institute for Health Information and the Discharge Abstract Database from inpatient hospital admissions. A panel from the Maternal Health Study Group selects specific conditions deemed indicative of severe maternal morbidity including eclampsia, pulmonary oedema, and severe obstetric haemorrhage requiring blood transfusion.[92] Of note, the audit has revealed that the majority of maternal morbidity in Canada occurs in previously healthy women and that having a pre-existing co-morbidity did not increase the likelihood of developing severe maternal morbidity.[136]

Surveillance of rare events

UKOSS

The UK Obstetric Surveillance System (UKOSS) was established in 2005 to study rare disorders of pregnancy, based on a successful paediatric surveillance system that has been running in the United Kingdom for over 25 years. Reporters (anaesthetists, midwives, and obstetricians) in all consultant-led maternity units within the United Kingdom are contacted monthly to indicate on a card the number of women who have any of the morbidity conditions under study. If there are no cases the units are requested to confirm this as a 'nil report', hence UKOSS provides an active negative surveillance system. This allows exact numbers to be obtained and produces the denominator population to allow calculation of disease incidences.[137] As with the CEMD, clinicians are sent data collection forms for further details when a case is identified. Details on control patients are also requested.

The UKOSS programme has led to the publication of several reports including on peripartum hysterectomy,[138] eclampsia,[139,140] acute fatty liver,[141] antenatal pulmonary embolism,[141] tuberculosis,[143] gastroschisis, extreme obesity,[66,144] therapies for peripartum haemorrhage,[145] multiple repeat caesarean delivery,[146] pregnancy in renal transplant recipients,[147] myocardial infarction,[148] uterine rupture,[149] risk factors for progression from severe maternal morbidity to death,[150] and H1N1 influenza in pregnancy.[151–154] Ongoing topics at the time of writing include adrenal tumours in pregnancy, AFE,[76,155] anaphylaxis in pregnancy, cardiac arrest in pregnancy, massive transfusion in major obstetric haemorrhage, pituitary tumours, stage 5 chronic kidney disease, advanced maternal age and pregnancy outcomes in women with artificial heart valves.[156]

Amniotic Fluid Embolism Registry

The original AFE registry was established in the United States by Clarke[157] and a similar registry based in the United Kingdom was set up in 1996 by Tuffnell.[158] This project was incorporated into the UKOSS study of AFE. The incidence of AFE thought to be around 2/100,000 deliveries.[76]

Obstetric Anaesthetists' Association UK Registry

This project ran from 1996 to 2003 collecting data voluntarily reported on women who had severe co-morbidities requiring anaesthetic input. Cardiorespiratory disease was the initial topic studied, with a smaller report on neurological disease following.[71,94,106] The project was subsequently superseded by UKOSS.

Common themes in maternal mortality and morbidity studies

Some common themes arise out of the mortality and morbidity studies and surveillance systems outlined above, that have relevance to every health system. Some have particular relevance to obstetric anaesthetists:

Resources

A lack of adequate numbers of trained staff and essential equipment and drugs is a common theme in developing countries,[10,11,14] and attempts to improve this is a constant priority of all programmes to improve maternal health worldwide.[10,11,14,16,49] Such attempts are considerably hampered where there is poor underlying infrastructure, both locally (e.g. communication networks, availability of blood products, and intensive care facilities) and nationally. The diversion of resources away from public health issues in favour of other programmes (e.g. arms development) may also be a problem in some countries. Concerns about resources and their allocation are also increasingly common in developed countries in the current economic climate, albeit at a different level. Recent events in Mid-Staffordshire in the United Kingdom have highlighted the hazards of putting financially-based targets above basic patient care, and although not focusing on maternity care, obstetric anaesthetists will recognize the concerns raised in the aftermath of the final report.[159,160]

Training/education

A lack of knowledge and skill in healthcare staff is one of the leading potentially avoidable causes for poor management leading to morbidity and ultimately to mortality.[10,11] Remedies include the institution and maintenance of proper training programmes, especially in developing countries, with education of the women themselves as well as all staff who may come into contact with pregnant women, and those responsible for managing services. A lack of resources for effective training and education is a particular problem, and increasingly one that is not confined to developing countries.

Simulation is increasingly accepted as an important tool in medical/paramedical training and its use in obstetrics has been highlighted (and indeed, recommended) in recent CEMD reports. Training programmes based on simulation are often expensive in terms of equipment and staff, though it is likely that their uptake will continue to increase in developed countries.

Antenatal screening/referral

Many of the reports on morbidity and mortality throughout the world define at-risk groups during (or before) pregnancy, and stress the importance of identifying these groups in advance. For example, in response to the high number of maternal deaths in immigrants in the 2003–2005 CEMD report who were late or non-attenders for antenatal care and subsequently presented late to delivery suites with serious co-morbidities, the report recommended that all immigrants should be screened with a full medical history and examination at booking or as soon as possible after.[65] Similarly, routine antenatal screening for psychiatric problems was improved throughout the United Kingdom following the 2000–2002 CEMD report,[77] and the importance of detecting antenatal anaemia has been noted by several reports.[27,42,161–165] Indeed, the provision of good antenatal care is one of the aims highlighted in programmes to improve maternal mortality in developing countries, as noted above.[11]

A particular area of antenatal care of relevance to anaesthetists is the appropriate referral of women for anaesthetic assessment, either early in pregnancy in known high-risk cases, later in pregnancy when complications occur, or pre-delivery in women who become acutely unwell. This problem is not limited to anaesthesia: the CEMD reports repeatedly comment on late or absent involvement of specialists, especially of adequate seniority, in the care of high-risk parturients.[10,11] In some cases, failure to obtain early referral occurs at community level (e.g. the general practitioner), or even with the woman herself; in the 2006–2008 CEMD report, 41 of the women who died had no antenatal care, of whom the majority were late bookers or poor attenders for care and six had concealed pregnancies.[10]

The same concerns apply to pre-conception counselling and support for women with known significant co-morbidities.

Recognition of severe illness

When pregnant women, especially those who are healthy beforehand, deteriorate, it may be difficult to detect this, since their compensatory mechanisms often maintain basic observations such as blood pressure and pulse rate until a very rapid decline. This is consistently highlighted in the various mortality and morbidity reports, and has led to the interest in early warning scores in maternity care, as recommended by recent CEMD reports.[10,11,68,70,166,167]

Human factors

The place of human factors in acute medicine, both as an important factor in adverse outcomes and as a focus for training,[168,169] is now well established, and the environment of maternity care is one where such factors are particularly pertinent, with several disciplines working together and the mother (and partner/family) supposedly at the centre of her care.[170] A common and consistent theme in mortality and morbidity reports is of poor team working, with inadequate communication between staff of different disciplines, and between staff and patients, absent or late involvement of senior help, insufficient use of protocols and guidelines to guide care (especially for rare disorders or emergencies), and a general absence of a risk management culture. In the United Kingdom, increased emphasis on such factors over the last decade, the use of simulator training (especially multidisciplinary)[10,11] and the use of financial incentives such as provided by the Clinical Negligence Scheme for Trusts (whereby premiums paid by hospital trusts are reduced if there are appropriate aspects of good risk management in place) has raised awareness of these issues.[171] In developing countries some of these initiatives may be seen as luxuries; however, even simple ones such as the WHO surgical safety checklist may improve outcomes.[172,173]

Conclusion

The death of a parturient is a catastrophe for the family she leaves behind and a hugely stressful event for the local healthcare team. This impact should not be lost when viewing regional, national, or global figures, when such an event may be merely one of many. Investigating and monitoring maternal mortality and morbidity beyond analysis of individual cases locally requires great effort and both financial and political commitment, but few, if anyone, involved in maternity care would doubt its importance. The fact that maternity care is often seen as a surrogate for the provision of healthcare in general reinforces the need to continue to support all initiatives that aim to improve the health of pregnant women. Anaesthetists have been central to achieving enormous improvements in maternal outcomes as charted by the CEMD reports, and continue to have a central role in maintaining this improvement despite increasing challenges locally/regionally, as well as assisting other disciplines and those in other healthcare systems around the world.

References

1. Pattinson RC, Buchmann E, Mantel G, *et al.* Can enquiries into severe acute maternal morbidity act as a surrogate for maternal death enquiries? *BJOG* 2003; 110:889–93.
2. Pattinson RC, Hall M. Near misses: a useful adjunct to maternal death enquiries. *Br Med Bull* 2003; 67:231–43.
3. Wilson RE, Salihu HM. The paradox of obstetric "near misses": converting maternal mortality into morbidity. *Int J Fertil Womens Med* 2007; 52:121–7.
4. Reichenheim ME, Zylbersztajn F, Moraes CL, *et al.* Severe acute obstetric morbidity (near-miss): a review of the relative use of its diagnostic indicators. *Arch Gynecol Obstet* 2009; 280:337–43.
5. Lawn JE, Kinney M, Lee AC, *et al.* Reducing intrapartum-related deaths and disability: can the health system deliver? *Int J Gynecol Obstet* 2009; 107 Suppl 1:S123–40, S40–2.
6. Callaghan WM, Mackay AP, Berg CJ. Identification of severe maternal morbidity during delivery hospitalizations, United States, 1991–2003. *Am J Obstet Gynecol* 2008; 199:133 e1–8.
7. Harmer M. Maternal mortality—is it still relevant? *Anaesthesia* 1997; 52:99–100.
8. World Health Organization. *International Statistical Classification of Diseases and Related Health Problems: 10th Revision.* Geneva: WHO; 1992.
9. World Health Organization. *Application of ICD-10 to Deaths during Pregnancy, Childbirth and the Peurperium: ICD Maternal Mortality (ICD-MM).* Geneva: WHO; 2012.
10. Centre for Maternal and Child Enquiries (CMACE). Saving Mothers' Lives: reviewing maternal deaths to make motherhood safer: 2006–08. The Eighth Report on Confidential Enquiries into Maternal Deaths in the United Kingdom. *BJOG* 2011; 118 Suppl 1:1–203.
11. Knight M, Kenyon S, Brocklehurst P et al. Saving Lives, Improving Mothers' Care. (MBRRACE-UK) 2014. Healthcare Quality Improvement Partnership
12. Department of Making Pregnancy Safer, World Health Organization. *Ensuring Skilled Care for Every Birth.* Geneva: WHO; 2006.
13. World Health Organization. *Trends in Maternal Mortality: 1990 to 2010. WHO, UNICEF, UNFPA and The World Bank estimates.* Geneva: WHO; 2012.
14. Mathers CD, Fat DM, Inoue M, *et al.* Counting the dead and what they died from: an assessment of the global status of cause of death data. *Bull World Health Organ* 2005; 83:171–7.
15. Patton GC, Coffey C, Sawyer SM, *et al.* Global patterns of mortality in young people: a systematic analysis of population health data. *Lancet* 2009; 374:881–92.
16. Campbell OM, Graham WJ. Strategies for reducing maternal mortality: getting on with what works. *Lancet* 2006; 368:1284–99.
17. Hoyert DL, Danel I, Tully P. Maternal mortality, United States and Canada, 1982–1997. *Birth* 2000; 27:4–11.
18. Hill K, Thomas K, AbouZahr C, *et al.* Estimates of maternal mortality worldwide between 1990 and 2005: an assessment of available data. *Lancet* 2007; 370:1311–19.
19. Jokhio A, Winter H, Cheng KK, *et al.* Strategies for reducing maternal mortality. *Lancet* 2006; 368:2122.
20. Donati S, Senatore S, Ronconi A. Maternal mortality in Italy: a record-linkage study. *BJOG* 2011; 118:872–9.
21. Deneux-Tharaux C, Berg C, Bouvier-Colle MH, *et al.* Underreporting of pregnancy-related mortality in the United States and Europe. *Obstet Gynecol* 2005; 106:684–92.
22. Hill K, El Arifeen S, Koenig M, *et al.* How should we measure maternal mortality in the developing world? A comparison of household deaths and sibling history approaches. *Bull World Health Organ* 2006; 84:173–80.
23. Stanton C, Hobcraft J, Hill K, *et al.* Every death counts: measurement of maternal mortality via a census. *Bull World Health Organ* 2001; 79:657–64.
24. Chandramohan D, Setel P, Quigley M. Effect of misclassification of causes of death in verbal autopsy: can it be adjusted? *Int J Epidemiol* 2001; 30:509–14.
25. World Health Organization. *International Statistical Classification of Diseases and Related Health Problems: Tenth Revision* (4th ed). Geneva: WHO; 2010.
26. Geynisman J, Latimer A, Ofosu A, *et al.* Improving maternal mortality reporting at the community level with a 4-question modified reproductive age mortality survey (RAMOS). *Int J Gynecol Obstet* 2011; 114:29–32.
27. Khan KS, Wojdyla D, Say L, Gulmezoglu AM, *et al.* WHO analysis of causes of maternal death: a systematic review. *Lancet* 2006; 367:1066–74.
28. van den Broek NR and Falconer AD. Maternal mortality and Millennium Development Goal 5. *Br Med Bull* 2011; 99:25–38.
29. Hogan MC, Foreman KJ, Naghavi M, *et al.* Maternal mortality for 181 countries, 1980–2008: a systematic analysis of progress towards Millennium Development Goal 5. *Lancet* 2010; 375:1609–23.
30. Lozano R, Wang H, Foreman KJ, *et al.* Progress towards Millennium Development Goals 4 and 5 on maternal and child mortality: an updated systematic analysis. *Lancet* 2011; 378:1139–65.
31. Blencowe H, Cousens S, Oestergaard MZ, *et al.* National, regional, and worldwide estimates of preterm birth rates in the year 2010 with time trends since 1990 for selected countries: a systematic analysis and implications. *Lancet* 2012; 379:2162–72.
32. Cousens S, Blencowe H, Stanton C, *et al.* National, regional, and worldwide estimates of stillbirth rates in 2009 with trends since 1995: a systematic analysis. *Lancet* 2011; 377:1319–30.
33. Neilson JP, Lavender T, Quenby S, *et al.* Obstructed labour. *Br Med Bull* 2003; 67:191–204.
34. Wall LL. Obstetric vesicovaginal fistula as an international public-health problem. *Lancet* 2006; 368:1201–9.
35. Department of Reproductive Health and Research, World Health Organization. *Unsafe Abortion: Global and Regional Estimates of the Incidence of Unsafe Abortion and Associated Mortality in 2008.* Geneva: WHO; 2011.
36. Gupta SD, Khanna A, Gupta R, *et al.* Maternal mortality ratio and predictors of maternal deaths in selected desert districts in Rajasthan a community-based survey and case control study. *Women's Health Issues* 2010; 20:80–5.
37. Sedgh G, Henshaw S, Singh S, *et al.* Induced abortion: estimated rates and trends worldwide. *Lancet* 2007; 370:1338–45.
38. Shah I, Ahman E. Unsafe abortion in 2008: global and regional levels and trends. *Reprod Health Matters* 2010; 18:90–101.
39. Grimes DA, Benson J, Singh S, *et al.* Unsafe abortion: the preventable pandemic. *Lancet* 2006; 368:1908–19.
40. Bhutta ZA, Cabral S, Chan CW, *et al.* Reducing maternal, newborn, and infant mortality globally: an integrated action agenda. *Int J Gynecol Obstet* 2012; 119 Suppl 1: S13–17.
41. Costello A, Azad K, Barnett S. An alternative strategy to reduce maternal mortality. *Lancet* 2006; 368:1477–9.

42. van den Broek N. Anaemia and micronutrient deficiencies. *Br Med Bull* 2003; 67:149–60.
43. Schuitemaker NW, Gravenhorst JB, Van Geijn HP, *et al.* Maternal mortality and its prevention. *Eur J Obstet Gynecol Reprod Biol* 1991; 42 Suppl: S31–5.
44. Thaddeus S, Maine D. Too far to walk: maternal mortality in context. *Soc Sci Med.* 1994; 38:1091–110.
45. Kilpatrick SJ, Crabtree KE, Kemp A, *et al.* Preventability of maternal deaths: comparison between Zambian and American referral hospitals. *Obstet Gynecol* 2002; 100:321–6.
46. Paxton A, Bailey P, Lobis S, *et al.* Global patterns in availability of emergency obstetric care. *Int J Gynecol Obstet* 2006; 93:300–7.
47. Bailey P, Paxton A, Lobis S, *et al.* The availability of life-saving obstetric services in developing countries: an in-depth look at the signal functions for emergency obstetric care. *Int J Gynecol Obstet* 2006; 93:285–91.
48. Paxton A, Bailey P, Lobis S. The United Nations Process Indicators for emergency obstetric care: reflections based on a decade of experience. *Int J Gynecol Obstet* 2006; 95:192–208.
49. Bullough C, Meda N, Makowiecka K, *et al.* Current strategies for the reduction of maternal mortality. *BJOG* 2005; 112:1180–8.
50. Ariff S, Soofi SB, Sadiq K, *et al.* Evaluation of health workforce competence in maternal and neonatal issues in public health sector of Pakistan: an Assessment of their training needs. *BMC Health Serv Res.* 2010; 10:319.
51. Kaunitz AM, Spence C, Danielson TS, *et al.* Perinatal and maternal mortality in a religious group avoiding obstetric care. *Am J Obstet Gynecol* 1984; 150:826–31.
52. Rout C. Maternal mortality and anaesthesia in Africa: a South African perspective. *Int J Obstet Anesth* 2002; 11:77–80.
53. Tumwebaze J. Lamula's story. *Anaesthesia* 2007; 62 Suppl 1:4.
54. Fawcus SR, van Coeverden de Groot HA, *et al.* A 50-year audit of maternal mortality in the Peninsula Maternal and Neonatal Service, Cape Town (1953–2002). *BJOG* 2005; 112:1257–63.
55. Hodges SC, Mijumbi C, Okello M, *et al.* Anaesthesia services in developing countries: defining the problems. *Anaesthesia* 2007; 62:4–11.
56. Clyburn P, Morris S, Hall J. Anaesthesia and safe motherhood. *Anaesthesia* 2007; 62 Suppl 1:21–5.
57. McKenzie AG. Operative obstetric mortality at Harare Central Hospital 1992–1994: an anaesthetic view. *Int J Obstet Anesth* 1998; 7:237–41.
58. Betran AP, Merialdi M, Lauer JA, *et al.* Rates of caesarean section: analysis of global, regional and national estimates. *Paediatr Perinat Epidemiol* 2007; 21:98–113.
59. Enohumah KO, Imarengiaye CO. Factors associated with anaesthesia-related maternal mortality in a tertiary hospital in Nigeria. *Acta Anaesth Scand* 2006; 50:206–10.
60. Ouro-Bang'na Maman AF, Tomta K, *et al.* Deaths associated with anaesthesia in Togo, West Africa. *Trop Doct* 2005; 35:220–2.
61. Hansen D, Gausi SC, Merikebu M. Anaesthesia in Malawi: complications and deaths. *Trop Doct* 2000; 30:146–9.
62. Cruz JR. Reduction of maternal mortality: the need for voluntary blood donors. *Int J Gynecol Obstet* 2007; 98:291–3.
63. Department of Health. *The Fifth Report on Confidential Enquires into Maternal Deaths in South Africa. 2008–2010.* Pretoria: Department of Health; 2012.
64. Yentis SM. From CEMD to CEMACH to CMACE to …? Where now for the confidential enquiries into maternal deaths? *Anaesthesia* 2011; 66:859–60.
65. Lewis G (ed). *The Confidential Enquiry into Maternal and Child Health (CEMACH): Saving Mother's Lives: Reviewing Maternal Deaths to Make Motherhood Safer, 2003–2005. The Seventh Report of the Confidential Enquiries into Maternal Deaths in the United Kingdom.* London: CEMACH; 2007.
66. Knight M, Kurinczuk JJ, Spark P, *et al.* Extreme obesity in pregnancy in the United Kingdom. *Obstet Gynecol* 2010; 115:989–97.
67. Centre for Maternal and Child Enquiries. *CEMACH Emergent Theme Briefing No.1: Genital Tract Sepsis.* [Online] http://www.hqip.org.uk/assets/NCAPOP-Library/CMACE-Reports/13.-September-2010-Emergent-Theme-Briefing-Genital-Tract-Septis-2006-2008.pdf
68. Loughnan BA, Grover M, Nielsen PB. Maternal death due to extended spectrum beta-lactamase-producing E. coli: a warning for the future? *Int J Obstet Anesth* 2010; 19:327–30.
69. Sullivan SA, Smith T, Chang E, *et al.* Administration of cefazolin prior to skin incision is superior to cefazolin at cord clamping in preventing postcesarean infectious morbidity: a randomized, controlled trial. *Am J Obstet Gynecol* 2007; 196:455.e1–5.
70. Singh S, McGlennan A, England A, *et al.* A validation study of the CEMACH recommended modified early obstetric warning system (MEOWS). *Anaesthesia* 2012; 67:12–8.
71. Royal College of Physicians. *National Early Warning Score (NEWS): Standardising the Assessment of Acute Illness Severity in the NHS.* London: Royal College Press; 2012.
72. Royal College of Obstetricians and Gynaecologists. *Thromboprophylaxis in Obstetrics and Gynaecology.* London: RCOG Press; 1995.
73. Royal College of Obstetricians and Gynaecologists. *Thromboprophylaxis During Pregnancy, Labour and after Vaginal Delivery.* Green-top Guideline No. 37. London: RCOG Press; 2004.
74. Royal College of Obstetricians and Gynaecologists. *Reducing the risk of Thrombosis and Embolism During Pregnancy and the Peurperium.* London: RCOG Press; 2009.
75. National Institute of Health and Care Excellence. *Hypertension in Pregnancy: The Management of Hypertensive Disorders During Pregnancy.* London: NICE; 2010.
76. Knight M, Tuffnell D, Brocklehurst P, *et al.* Incidence and risk factors for amniotic-fluid embolism. *Obstet Gynecol* 2010; 115:910–17.
77. Lewis G (ed). *The Confidential Enquiry into Maternal and Child Health (CEMACH): Saving Mother's Lives: Reviewing Maternal Deaths to Make Motherhood Safer, 2000–2002.* The Sixth Report of the Confidential Enquiries into Maternal Deaths in the United Kingdom. London: CEMACH; 2004.
78. Hoyert DL. Maternal mortality and related concepts. *Vital Health Stat 3* 2007; 33:1–13.
79. Hoyert DL, Arias E, Smith BL, *et al.* Deaths: final data for 1999. *Natl Vital Stat Rep* 2001; 49:1–113.
80. Hoyert DL, Heron MP, Murphy SL, *et al.* Deaths: final data for 2003. *Natl Vital Stat Rep* 2006; 54:1–120.
81. Hoyert DL, Kochanek KD, Murphy SL. Deaths: final data for 1997. *Natl Vital Stat Rep* 1999; 47:1–104.
82. Hoyert DL, Kung HC, Smith BL. Deaths: preliminary data for 2003. *Natl Vital Stat Rep* 2005; 53:1–48.
83. Kung HC, Hoyert DL, Xu J, *et al.* Deaths: final data for 2005. *Natl Vital Stat Rep* 2008; 56:1–120.
84. Berg CJ. From identification and review to action—maternal mortality review in the United States. *Semin Perinatol* 2012; 36:7–13.
85. Berg CJ, Callaghan WM, Syverson C, *et al.* Pregnancy-related mortality in the United States, 1998 to 2005. *Obstet Gynecol* 2010; 116:1302–9.
86. Berg CJ, Chang J, Callaghan WM, *et al.* Pregnancy-related mortality in the United States, 1991-1997. *Obstet Gynecol* 2003; 101:289–96.
87. Berg CJ, Harper MA, Atkinson SM, *et al.* Preventability of pregnancy-related deaths: results of a state-wide review. *Obstet Gynecol* 2005; 106:1228–34.
88. Bouvier-Colle MH, Ould El Joud D, *et al.* Evaluation of the quality of care for severe obstetrical haemorrhage in three French regions. *BJOG* 2001; 108:898–903.
89. Bouvier-Colle MH, Varnoux N, Breart G. Maternal deaths and substandard care: the results of a confidential survey in France. Medical Experts Committee. *Eur J Obstet Gynecol Reprod Biol* 1995; 58:3–7.
90. King JF, Slaytor EK, Sullivan EA. Maternal deaths in Australia, 1997–1999. *Med J Aust* 2004; 181:413–14.
91. Sullivan EA, Ford JB, Chambers G, *et al.* Maternal mortality in Australia, 1973–1996. *Aust N Z J Obstet Gynaecol* 2004; 44:452–7.

92. Allen VM, Campbell M, Carson G, *et al.* Maternal mortality and severe maternal morbidity surveillance in Canada. *J Obstet Gynaecol Can* 2010; 32:1140–6.
93. MacKay AP, Rochat R, Smith JC, *et al.* The check box: determining pregnancy status to improve maternal mortality surveillance. *Am J Prev Med* 2000; 19:35–9.
94. Mac KAP, Berg CJ, Liu X, *et al.* Changes in pregnancy mortality ascertainment: United States, 1999–2005. *Obstet Gynecol* 2011; 118:104–10.
95. Arias E, Anderson RN, Kung HC, *et al.* Deaths: final data for 2001. *Natl Vital Stat Rep* 2003; 52:1–115.
96. Peters KD, Kochanek KD, Murphy SL. Deaths: final data for 1996. *Natl Vital Stat Rep* 1998; 47:1–100.
97. Murphy SL. Deaths: final data for 1998. *Natl Vital Stat Rep* 2000; 48:1–105.
98. Minino AM, Arias E, Kochanek KD, *et al.* Deaths: final data for 2000. *Natl Vital Stat Rep* 2002; 50:1–119.
99. Minino AM, Heron MP, Murphy SL, *et al.* Deaths: final data for 2004. *Natl Vital Stat Rep* 2007; 55:1–119.
100. Kochanek KD, Murphy SL, Anderson RN, *et al.* Deaths: final data for 2002. *Natl Vital Stat Rep* 2004; 53:1–115.
101. Sullivan EA, Hall B, King JF. *Maternal Deaths in Australia 2003–2005.* Sydney: AIHW National Perinatal Statistics Unit, 2008.
102. Slaytor ES, Sullivan EA, King JF. *Maternal Deaths in Australia 1997–1999.* Sydney: AIHW National Perinatal Statistics, 2004.
103. Public Health Agency of Canada. *Canadian Perinatal Health Report, 2008 Edition.* Ottawa: Public Health Agency of Canada, 2008.
104. Lisonkova S, Bartholomew S, Rouleau J, *et al.* Temporal trends in maternal mortality in Canada I: estimates based on vital statistics data. *J Obstet Gynaecol Can* 2011; 33:1011–19.
105. Public Health Agency of Canada. *Maternal Mortality in Canada.* 2013. [Online] http://www.phac-aspc.gc.ca/rhs-ssg/maternal-maternelle/mortality-mortalite/index-eng.php#tbl2
106. Bouvier-Colle MH, Saucedo M, Deneux-Tharaux C. The confidential enquiries into maternal deaths, 1996–2006 in France: what consequences for the obstetrical care? *J Gynecol Obstet Biol Reprod (Paris)* 2011; 40:87–102.
107. Bouvier-Colle MH, Mohangoo AD, Gissler M, *et al.* What about the mothers? An analysis of maternal mortality and morbidity in perinatal health surveillance systems in Europe. *BJOG* 2012; 119:880–9.
108. Tuncalp O, Hindin MJ, Souza JP, *et al.* The prevalence of maternal near miss: a systematic review. *BJOG* 2012; 119:653–61.
109. Kilpatrick SJ, Matthay MA. Obstetric patients requiring critical care. A five-year review. *Chest* 1992; 101:1407–12.
110. Wheatley E, Farkas A, Watson D. Obstetric admissions to an intensive therapy unit. *Int J Obstet Anesth* 1996; 5:221–4.
111. Baskett TF, Sternadel J. Maternal intensive care and near-miss mortality in obstetrics. *Br J Obstet Gynaecol* 1998; 105:981–4.
112. Mahutte NG, Murphy-Kaulbeck L, Le Q, *et al.* Obstetric admissions to the intensive care unit. *Obstet Gynecol* 1999; 94:263–6.
113. Mantel GD, Buchmann E, Rees H, *et al.* Severe acute maternal morbidity: a pilot study of a definition for a near-miss. *Br J Obstet Gynaecol* 1998; 105:985–90.
114. Brace V, Penney G, Hall M. Quantifying severe maternal morbidity: a Scottish population study. *BJOG* 2004; 111:481–4.
115. Penney G, Brace V. Near miss audit in obstetrics. *Curr Opin Obstet Gynecol* 2007; 19:145–50.
116. Souza JP, Cecatti JG, Faundes A, *et al.* Maternal near miss and maternal death in the World Health Organization's 2005 global survey on maternal and perinatal health. *Bull World Health Organ* 2010; 88:113–19.
117. Say L, Pattinson RC, Gulmezoglu AM. WHO systematic review of maternal morbidity and mortality: the prevalence of severe acute maternal morbidity (near miss). *Reprod Health* 2004; 1:3.
118. Say L, Souza JP, Pattinson RC. Maternal near miss—towards a standard tool for monitoring quality of maternal health care. *Best Pract Res Clin Obstet Gynaecol* 2009; 23:287–96.
119. Pattinson R, Say L, Souza JP, *et al.* WHO maternal death and near-miss classifications. *Bull World Health Organ* 2009; 87:734.
120. Souza JP, Cecatti JG, Haddad SM, *et al.* The WHO maternal near-miss approach and the maternal severity index model (MSI): tools for assessing the management of severe maternal morbidity. *PloS One* 2012; 7:e44129.
121. Cecatti JG, Souza JP, Oliveira Neto AF, *et al.* Pre-validation of the WHO organ dysfunction based criteria for identification of maternal near miss. *Reprod Health.* 2011; 8:22.
122. Department of Reproductive Health and Research, World Health Organization. *Evaluating the Quality of Care for Severe Pregnancy Complications: The WHO Near-Miss Approach for Maternal Health.* Geneva: WHO; 2011.
123. Zwart JJ, Richters JM, Ory F, *et al.* Severe maternal morbidity during pregnancy, delivery and puerperium in the Netherlands: a nationwide population-based study of 371,000 pregnancies. *BJOG* 2008; 115:842–50.
124. Zhang WH, Alexander S, Bouvier-Colle MH, *et al.* Incidence of severe pre-eclampsia, postpartum haemorrhage and sepsis as a surrogate marker for severe maternal morbidity in a European population-based study: the MOMS-B survey. *BJOG* 2005; 112:89–96.
125. Hazelgrove JF, Price C, Pappachan VJ, *et al.* Multicenter study of obstetric admissions to 14 intensive care units in southern England. *Crit Care Med* 2001; 29:770–5.
126. Harrison DA, Parry GJ, Carpenter JR, *et al.* A new risk prediction model for critical care: the Intensive Care National Audit & Research Centre (ICNARC) model. *Crit Care Med* 2007; 35:1091–8.
127. ICNARC. *Female Admissions (Aged 16–50 Years) to Adult, General Critical Care Units in England, Wales and Northern Ireland, Reported as "Currently Pregnant" or "Recently Pregnant".* 2009. [Online] http://www.oaa-anaes.ac.uk/assets/_managed/editor/File/Reports/ICNARC_obs_report_Oct2009.pdf
128. Lennox C, Marr L. *Scottish Confidential Audit of Severe Maternal Morbidity: 6th Annual Report (Data from 2008).* Edinburgh: Reproductive Health Programme, *Healthcare Improvement Scotland*; 2012.
129. Lennox C, Marr L. *Scottish Confidential Audit of Severe Maternal Morbidity: 4th Annual Report (Data from 2006).* Edinburgh: Reproductive Health Programme, Healthcare Improvement Scotland; 2010.
130. Marr L. *Scottish Confidential Audit of Severe Maternal Morbidity: 5th Annual Report (Data from 2007).* Edinburgh: Reproductive Health Programme, Healthcare Improvement Scotland; 2011.
131. Vandecruys HI, Pattinson RC, Macdonald AP, *et al.* Severe acute maternal morbidity and mortality in the Pretoria Academic Complex: changing patterns over 4 years. *Eur J Obstet Gynecol Reprod Biol* 2002; 102:6–10.
132. Pattinson RC, Say L, Makin JD, *et al.* Critical incident audit and feedback to improve perinatal and maternal mortality and morbidity. *Cochrane Database Syst Rev* 2005; 4:CD002961.
133. Moodley J, Pattinson RC, Baxter C, *et al.* Strengthening HIV services for pregnant women: an opportunity to reduce maternal mortality rates in Southern Africa/sub-Saharan Africa. *BJOG* 2011; 118:219–25.
134. Cecatti JG, Souza JP, Parpinelli MA, *et al.* Brazilian network for the surveillance of maternal potentially life threatening morbidity and maternal near-miss and a multidimensional evaluation of their long term consequences. *Reprod Health* 2009; 6:15.
135. Haddad SM, Cecatti JG, Parpinelli MA, *et al.* From planning to practice: building the national network for the Surveillance of Severe Maternal Morbidity. *BMC Public Health* 2011; 11:283.
136. Wen SW, Huang L, Liston R, *et al.* Severe maternal morbidity in Canada, 1991–2001. *CMAJ* 2005; 173:759–64.
137. Knight M, Kurinczuk JJ, Tuffnell D, *et al.* The UK Obstetric Surveillance System for rare disorders of pregnancy. *BJOG* 2005; 112:263–5.

138. Knight M. Peripartum hysterectomy in the UK: management and outcomes of the associated haemorrhage. *BJOG* 2007; 114:1380–7.
139. Knight M. Eclampsia in the United Kingdom 2005. *BJOG* 2007; 114:1072–8.
140. Kayem G, Kurinczuk JJ, Spark P, *et al.* Maternal and obstetric factors associated with delayed postpartum eclampsia: a national study population. *Acta Obstet Gynecol Scand* 2011; 90:1017–23.
141. Knight M, Nelson-Piercy C, Kurinczuk JJ, *et al.* A prospective national study of acute fatty liver of pregnancy in the UK. *Gut* 2008; 57:951–6.
142. Knight M. Antenatal pulmonary embolism: risk factors, management and outcomes. *BJOG* 2008; 115:453–61.
143. Knight M, Kurinczuk JJ, Nelson-Piercy C, *et al.* Tuberculosis in pregnancy in the UK. *BJOG* 2009; 116:584–8.
144. Homer CS, Kurinczuk JJ, Spark P, *et al.* Planned vaginal delivery or planned caesarean delivery in women with extreme obesity. *BJOG* 2011; 118:480–7.
145. Kayem G, Kurinczuk JJ, Alfirevic Z, *et al.* Specific second-line therapies for postpartum haemorrhage: a national cohort study. *BJOG* 2011; 118:856–64.
146. Knight M, Kurinczuk JJ, Spark P, *et al.* Cesarean delivery and peripartum hysterectomy. *Obstet Gynecol* 2008; 111:97–105.
147. Sibanda N, Briggs JD, Davison JM, *et al.* Pregnancy after organ transplantation: a report from the UK Transplant pregnancy registry. *Transplantation* 2007; 83:1301–7.
148. Bush N, Nelson-Piercy C, Spark P, *et al.* Myocardial infarction in pregnancy and postpartum in the UK. *Eur J Prevent Cardiol* 2013; 20:12–20.
149. Fitzpatrick KE, Kurinczuk JJ, Alfirevic Z, *et al.* Uterine rupture by intended mode of delivery in the UK: a national case-control study. *PLoS Med* 2012; 9:e1001184.
150. Kayem G, Kurinczuk J, Lewis G, *et al.* Risk factors for progression from severe maternal morbidity to death: a national cohort study. *PloS One* 2011; 6:e29077.
151. Knight M, Pierce M, Seppelt I, *et al.* Critical illness with AH1N1v influenza in pregnancy: a comparison of two population-based cohorts. *BJOG* 2011; 118:232–9.
152. Pierce M, Kurinczuk JJ, Spark P, *et al.* Perinatal outcomes after maternal 2009/H1N1 infection: national cohort study. *BMJ* 2011; 342:d3214.
153. Yates L, Pierce M, Stephens S, *et al.* Influenza A/H1N1v in pregnancy: an investigation of the characteristics and management of affected women and the relationship to pregnancy outcomes for mother and infant. *Health Technol Assess* 2010; 14:109–82.
154. Knight M, McClymont C, Fitzpatrick K, *et al. United Kingdom Obstetric Surveillance System (UKOSS) Annual Report 2012.* Oxford: National Perinatal Epidemiology Unit; 2012.
155. Knight M, Berg C, Brocklehurst P, *et al.* Amniotic fluid embolism incidence, risk factors and outcomes: a review and recommendations. *BMC Pregnancy Childbirth* 2012; 12:7.
156. UKOSS. *UK Obstetric Surveillance System.* [Online] https://www.npeu.ox.ac.uk/ukoss
157. Clark SL, Hankins GD, Dudley DA, *et al.* Amniotic fluid embolism: analysis of the national registry. *Am J Obstet Gynecol* 1995; 172:1158–67.
158. Tuffnell DJ. United Kingdom amniotic fluid embolism register. *BJOG* 2005; 112:1625–9.
159. Royal College of Obstetricians and Gynaecologists. *RCOG Statement on Findings of the Final Report of the Francis Inquiry.* 2013. [Online] http://www.rcog.org.uk/news/rcog-statement-findings-final-report-francis-inquiry
160. Royal College of Midwives. *Royal College of Midwives Comments on Francis Report.* 2013. [Online] http://www.rcm.org.uk/college/about/media-centre/press-releases/royal-college-of-midwives-comments-on-francis-report-06-2-13/
161. Kavatkar AN, Sahasrabudhe NS, Jadhav MV, *et al.* Autopsy study of maternal deaths. *Int J Gynecol Obstet* 2003; 81:1–8.
162. Kagu MB, Kawuwa MB, Gadzama GB. Anaemia in pregnancy: a cross-sectional study of pregnant women in a Sahelian tertiary hospital in Northeastern Nigeria. *J Obstet Gynaecol* 2007; 27:676–9.
163. McClure EM, Goldenberg RL, Dent AE, *et al.* A systematic review of the impact of malaria prevention in pregnancy on low birth weight and maternal anemia. *Int J Gynecol Obstet* 2013; 121(2):103–9.
164. Yi SW, Han YJ, Ohrr H. Anemia before pregnancy and risk of preterm birth, low birth weight and small-for-gestational-age birth in Korean women. *Eur J Clin Nutr* 2013; 67(4):337–42.
165. Stephansson O, Dickman PW, Johansson A, *et al.* Maternal hemoglobin concentration during pregnancy and risk of stillbirth. *JAMA* 2000; 284:2611–17.
166. McGlennan AP, Sherratt K. Charting change on the labour ward. *Anaesthesia* 2013; 68:338–42.
167. Carle C, Alexander P, Columb M, *et al.* Design and internal validation of an obstetric early warning score: secondary analysis of the Intensive Care National Audit and Research Centre Case Mix Programme database. *Anaesthesia* 2013; 68:354–67.
168. Toff NJ. Human factors in anaesthesia: lessons from aviation. *Br J Anaesth* 2010; 105:21–5.
169. Hardman JG, Moppett IK. To err is human. *Br J Anaesth* 2010; 105:1–3.
170. Flin R, Patey R, Glavin R, *et al.* Anaesthetists' non-technical skills. *Br J Anaesth* 2010; 105:38–44.
171. Impey P. Achieving level three of the Clinical Negligence Scheme. *J Perioper Pract* 2006; 16:204–8.
172. World Health Organization. *Surgical Safety Checklist.* Geneva: WHO; 2008.
173. Kearns RJ, Uppal V, Bonner J, *et al.* The introduction of a surgical safety checklist in a tertiary referral obstetric centre. *BMJ Qual Saf* 2011; 20:818–22.

CHAPTER 32

Problems in early pregnancy

W. Colin Duncan

Normal pregnancy

The establishment of pregnancy: basic physiology

After menstruation, the follicular phase of the ovarian cycle is associated with growth and selection of a dominant follicle and increasing oestradiol secretion. High oestradiol, signifying a mature follicle, induces a luteinizing hormone (LH) surge that causes ovulation. After ovulation the cells of the dominant follicle form the corpus luteum (CL) that produces large amount of progesterone. Progesterone prepares the endometrial lining to support a pregnancy and promotes uterine quiescence. The CL has a limited lifespan and will lose its functional and structural integrity in a process known as luteolysis after 14 days.[1] It is this loss of progesterone support that induces menstruation.

A woman ovulates 2 weeks before her menstrual period. If her cycle is 28 days in duration she will ovulate on day 14, and if she has a regular 35-day cycle she will ovulate on day 21.

Shortly after ovulation the oocyte enters the Fallopian tube where fertilization occurs. The embryo will continue to the uterine cavity where implantation occurs approximately 7 days after ovulation.[2] The implanting blastocyst secretes rapidly increasing amounts of human chorionic gonadotropin (hCG). It can be detected in the urine in sensitive pregnancy tests 1 or 2 days before the expected date of menstruation. Exponentially increasing hCG acts on the CL to rescue it from luteolysis to maintain progesterone secretion, prevent menstruation, and support the early conceptus. The CL supports the pregnancy for approximately 8 weeks when the early placental tissue becomes the main source of progesterone support.[3]

In the first few weeks of pregnancy, serum concentrations of hCG will normally double every 48 hours.

It is relatively common for positive pregnancy tests to occur around the time of the expected period but for menstruation to occur as expected or 1 or 2 days later. This transiently positive hCG is a result of pregnancy failure during the early stages of implantation and it is known as a biochemical pregnancy. This is one of the pitfalls of carrying out pregnancy testing prior to the anticipated date of menstruation. More commonly women delay taking a pregnancy test after a missed period. This is because women have premenstrual symptoms in the early stages of pregnancy and may believe that menstruation is about to occur.

Key points in normal development

The gestational age is calculated from the last menstrual period (LMP) rather than the time of conception.

When a patient is 6 weeks pregnant, they have conceived 4 weeks previously. This is important as it sometimes causes the patient some confusion as it assumes a 28-day cycle. If a woman has a 35-day cycle 7 weeks after her LMP she may only be 6 weeks pregnant based on the size of the fetus.

A transvaginal ultrasound scan (TVS) can detect an early gestational sac, the first sign of pregnancy, around 5 weeks' gestation. A few days later, a round yolk sac can be seen within the gestational sac and the embryonic fetus, which is associated with the yolk sac, can be identified after 5.5 weeks' gestation (Figure 32.1). The heartbeat may be visible as early as 6 weeks' gestation. As there is a time when the pregnancy test is positive but no definitive gestational sac can be seen in the uterus, a 'discriminatory zone' has been defined.[4] This is the concentration of serum hCG that should be associated with scan evidence of an intrauterine pregnancy.

A normal pregnancy with serum hCG concentrations of greater than 1500 IU/L should be able to be confirmed as intrauterine on ultrasound scan.

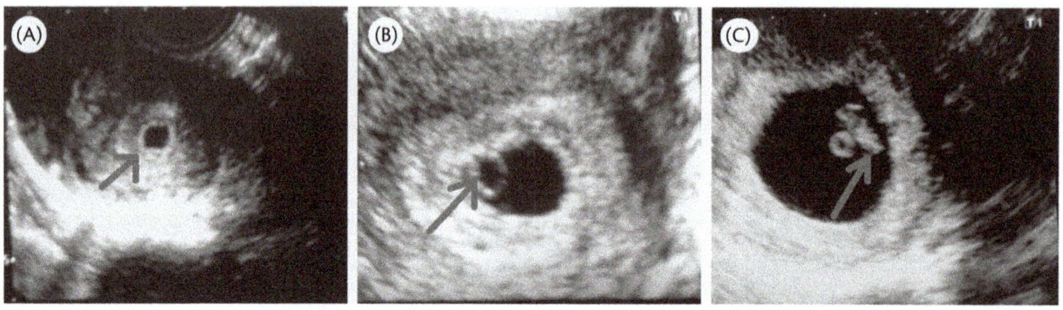

Figure 32.1 Intrauterine scan findings in a normal pregnancy. (A) Early pregnancy sac at 5 weeks' gestation (arrow). (B) Before 6 weeks' gestation the yolk sac is visible (arrow). (C) Pregnancy at 7 weeks' gestation with yolk sac and fetal pole (arrow).

Assisted reproduction and pregnancy

Infertility affects one in seven couples in the United Kingdom[5] and the number of pregnancies that result from assisted conception is increasing. In the United Kingdom, approximately 1.5% of births are a result of *in vitro* fertilization (IVF) while in Denmark it is three times higher.[6] As the length of ovarian stimulation and timing of embryo transfer varies, the gestation should be calculated as 2 weeks more than the date of oocyte collection, which corresponds to ovulation in a natural cycle. It is more complicated after frozen embryo replacement or egg donation. Generally the timing of 'ovulation', for gestational calculation, will be between 2 and 5 days before transfer.

During assisted conception, the ability of the CL to produce normal levels of progesterone may be impaired. That means that women will usually take progesterone supplementation in the form of vaginal pessaries twice daily.[7] The highly vascular CL secretes angiogenic and vascular permeability molecules such as vascular endothelial growth factor.[1] After IVF there are multiple CL and the markedly increased capillary permeability can cause loss of fluid from the vascular space. Ovarian hyperstimulation syndrome occurs in 2–4% of IVF cycles with ascites, pleural effusions, and hypercoagulability and, as hCG stimulates CL, it worsens in early pregnancy. Management involves heparin thromboprophylaxis, intravenous volume expansion, and consideration of paracentesis.[8]

Assessment of early pregnancy

The diagnostic tools

Early pregnancy problems can present in disparate ways to multiple health professionals when a woman is unaware of her pregnancy. There should be a high suspicion of the possibility of pregnancy in all women of reproductive age and a low threshold for urinary pregnancy testing. Increased awareness of ectopic pregnancy (EP) in women and healthcare providers is associated with earlier and more accurate diagnosis and timely management.[4,9]

The greatest assessment tool is the awareness of the possibility of pregnancy and knowledge of early pregnancy problems.

Similarly, an awareness that acute medical, gynaecological, or surgical conditions not related to pregnancy, such as urinary tract infection, ovarian torsion, or appendicitis, may also occur in pregnancy is also essential. It is fundamentally important to assess the woman clinically and not to rely entirely on the results of investigations to manage the patient. For example, ruptured ectopic pregnancies can occur when there is a negative pregnancy test,[10] or very low levels of hCG, and in acute situations delaying management to facilitate ultrasound scanning may adversely affect outcomes.

The possibility of an ongoing intrauterine pregnancy should not preclude clinically necessary investigations, such as a chest X-ray or diagnostic laparoscopy.

A pelvic ultrasound scan is the mainstay in the assessment of early pregnancy problems (Figure 32.1). It allows systematic assessment of uterine abnormalities, intrauterine contents, ovarian cysts, adnexal masses, and free fluid in the pelvis.[11] While transvaginal ultrasonography is the gold standard for early pregnancy assessment, transabdominal scanning may also be appropriate and is particularly useful where there is pelvic pathology such as fibroids and large ovarian cysts.[9] The other key investigative tool is the measurement of serum hCG concentrations. Quantification of hCG is required in the assessment of pregnancies of unknown location, ectopic pregnancies, or suspected gestational trophoblastic disease.

Serum hCG assessment is not useful in the diagnosis of viability when it is known that the pregnancy is intrauterine in location.

Problems in early pregnancy

Early pregnancy assessment units

The mainstay of the investigation and management of problems in early pregnancy is a dedicated outpatient early pregnancy assessment unit (EPAU). This provides a comprehensive service that improves and streamlines care and reduces the need for admission to hospital. The dedicated staff ensure sensitive discussion and empowers women to make informed decisions about their care and treatment. Many EPAUs offer a 7-day service with direct patient access through a self-referral appointment system.

Women generally attend the EPAU with vaginal bleeding and/or lower abdominal pain that may be central or unilateral in nature. They may present with altered pregnancy symptoms, such as loss of breast tenderness or excessive vomiting. In addition, some women are routinely seen because of a past history of recurrent miscarriage or EP. After clinical assessment, the most appropriate investigation is often a pelvic ultrasound scan.

Ongoing pregnancy

Ultrasonography may reveal an ongoing pregnancy with an intrauterine gestational sac with a yolk sac and fetal pole with fetal heart motion (Figure 32.1). Further scans are not indicated unless the bleeding worsens or persists for more than 14 days.[9] One in three women will experience per vaginal (PV) bleeding in early pregnancy. As around 60% of women with light bleeding will have an ongoing pregnancy[12] women are often initially reassured by the EPAU staff and advised to observe the bleeding for 24 hours.

The CL is maintained in early pregnancy and this may result in an enlarged or cystic ovary on the side of ovulation that may cause unilateral pain, particularly at the time of the luteo-placental shift when it begins to regress. In addition, as the CL causes increased vascular permeability, there is often a small accumulation of fluid in the pelvis that can be detected by ultrasonography. As luteal cysts are transient, and are required to maintain pregnancy, their management is usually conservative in the clinically stable patient.

It is not uncommon for women to experience bleeding or unilateral abdominal pain in a normal ongoing pregnancy.

Adjacent to an ongoing pregnancy there may be a haematoma or a second sac that represents a non-viable twin gestation. The patient would be expected to experience further PV bleeding as the abnormality resolves. There is no good management strategy that can be used in a threatened miscarriage to reduce the risk of subsequent miscarriage. While both rest and progesterone supplementation can reduce the amount of bleeding there is no good quality evidence from adequately powered trials that they change the outcome of the pregnancy.[13,14] However, there is widespread use of progesterone supplementation internationally and in the United Kingdom there is an increasing expectation among patients for progesterone supplementation to be prescribed and its use is becoming more common.[9]

There is an unmet need for the safety and efficacy of this progesterone supplementation to prevent miscarriage to be robustly assessed.

Although the pregnancy is ongoing, there may be concerns about the scan findings. There may be a mismatch of the gestational sac and fetal size, a slow or irregular fetal heart rate, an irregular gestational sac, or the presence of cystic areas or 'bumps' associated with the developing placenta.[15,16] These may increase the chance of future miscarriage and management usually involves a repeat ultrasound scan.

A further ultrasound scan, where required, should routinely be arranged at least 1 week from the previous scan.

Miscarriage

Miscarriage is common, occurring in 10–20% of clinical pregnancies, with the risk increasing as a woman ages. Before the age of 30, one in ten pregnancies will end in miscarriage while at the age of 35, the change of miscarriage is 20%. This has increased to approximately 40% at the age of 40 and in women over the age of 45, 80% of pregnancies miscarry.[17]

Women usually present with PV bleeding that is often associated with cramping lower abdominal pain, which is usually central but may be unilateral and radiate to the back. Miscarriage can be diagnosed on clinical assessment when confirmed products of conception have been passed or the cervical os is open on vaginal examination (VE). It is striking, however, how much a woman can bleed and continue to have a viable pregnancy. Tissue trapped in the cervix during miscarriage can cause cervical shock and resuscitation involves VE and removal of tissue from the cervix. Cervical shock is due to dilatation of the cervix and an autonomic response resulting in bradycardia and hypotension, common with dilatation of many organs with smooth muscle (e.g. anus and oesophagus). Apart from the surgical treatment, resuscitation may require oxygen, fluids, glycopyrrolate, and vasopressors. General anaesthesia is performed as neuraxial anaesthesia is contraindicated in the face of sympathetic block.

A single ultrasound scan can diagnose miscarriage if there is irregular pregnancy tissue within the cavity consistent with retained products of conception. The diagnosis of miscarriage on one scan where there is an intrauterine gestation sac depends on rigorous criteria with clear national guidelines.[9,18] This is because of the variability of scan measurements between observers[19] and the absolute necessity to ensure that a viable pregnancy is not misdiagnosed[20] (Box 32.1).

Box 32.1 The diagnosis of miscarriage

Transvaginal scan shows fetal pole with no identifiable heartbeat

- If the crown–rump measurement is ≥7 mm, and a second observer has confirmed this measurement, a miscarriage can be diagnosed.
- If the measurement is <7 mm, a second scan is required a minimum of 7 days after the first to make the diagnosis.

Transvaginal scan VS shows gestational sac with no fetal pole

- If the mean gestational sac diameter is <25 mm, a second scan is required a minimum of 7 days later.
- If the mean diameter is ≥25 mm, a miscarriage can be diagnosed after a second opinion on the scan.
- A third scan may be required if there is significant change before a definitive diagnosis can be made.

Once a miscarriage is diagnosed there are three main management options with regards to pregnancy tissue that remains within the uterine cavity. The first is expectant management and in around 40% of cases a complete miscarriage will occur within 7 days.[18] Miscarriage can take much longer when the pregnancy sac is intact and it may be useful to review the patient after 14 days if the miscarriage has not occurred. After miscarriage it is not necessary to repeat the ultrasound scan to confirm completion if the pain and bleeding resolve normally. Women, however, may be advised to take a urinary pregnancy test after 3 weeks and return if it is positive.

There is no evidence that expectant management is associated with an increased risk of infection or adverse effects on future fertility.

The second strategy is medical management using single-dose vaginal or sublingual administration of the prostaglandin E analogue misoprostol.[18] This is increasingly used in an outpatient setting to allow the miscarriage to complete at home with review or repeat the following day if PV bleeding has not started. There may be a role for repeated misoprostol and/or pre-treatment with the progesterone antagonist mifepristone and this is popular in some units.[21] The side effects include pain, vomiting, and diarrhoea and women are routinely provided with pain relief and antiemetics. The success rate for completion of miscarriage varies from study to study but it is generally over 80% although bleeding may persist for up to 21 days.[18] Like expectant management there is no need for routine scan follow-up although a post miscarriage pregnancy test is recommended.[9]

The third option is surgical management of miscarriage and this is preferred if women favour that option, or if there is persistent excessive bleeding or haemodynamic instability. It can be done by manual vacuum aspiration under local anaesthetic in an outpatient clinic setting but more commonly it is done as a day case in theatre under general anaesthesia.[22] Vaginal or sublingual misoprostol is frequently used to ripen the cervix to facilitate cervical dilatation for suction curette insertion and reduce the risk of trauma and haemorrhage.[18] Women may continue to bleed for up to 2 weeks after surgical management of miscarriage. In the absence of reflux, women usually have a short general anaesthetic for this with propofol and a laryngeal mask plus a short-acting opiate and antiemetic. If there is reflux, a rapid sequence induction with endotracheal tube is required.

There is an increased incidence of infection after surgical management and there should be a low threshold for antibiotic use if there is increasing pain, bleeding, and discharge after the procedure. There is not enough evidence to suggest routine antibiotic prophylaxis is beneficial but the clinical indications for antibiotics should be reviewed in each case and routine screening for *Chlamydia trachomatis* should be considered.[18]

In the presence of sepsis, delaying the procedure for 12 hours to allow intravenous antibiotic initiation is recommended if the patient is stable.

In addition to infection, the risks associated with surgical evacuation of the uterus include significant haemorrhage during or immediately after the procedure. Although in the first trimester of pregnancy the oxytocin responsiveness of the uterus is poor there is a role for bolus oxytocin as well as bimanual compression in the management of haemorrhage.[23] Another immediate risk is uterine perforation, with an incidence of 1/1000, which is usually recognized immediately and often requires laparoscopic assessment because of the risk of intraperitoneal bleeding. The risk of Asherman's syndrome, associated with intrauterine adhesions and subsequent amenorrhoea and infertility,[24] is difficult to quantify although it occurs more frequently than perforation.

Miscarriage can be a very distressing experience and the psychological impact, sense of bereavement, and feelings of depression and anxiety should not be underestimated.

In the United Kingdom, the Association of Early Pregnancy Units and the Miscarriage Association have championed a change in the key terminology of miscarriage. It is now recommended that 'miscarriage' is used rather than 'spontaneous abortion' and that 'surgical management of miscarriage' is preferred to 'evacuation of retained products of conception'.

Women should be reassured that after a miscarriage they are not at increased risk of miscarriage in subsequent pregnancies.

Recurrent miscarriage

While most miscarriage is sporadic and associated with genetic or structural defects, some couples, however, do experience recurrent miscarriage. Recurrent miscarriage is defined as the loss of three or more consecutive pregnancies and it affects 1% of couples.[17] As this is greater than would be expected by chance there must be factors increasing the likelihood of miscarriage in some of these couples. After three consecutive losses the chance of subsequent miscarriage is increased to approximately 40%.

Advancing age is a risk factor for recurrent miscarriage, as both maternal and paternal age increase the chance of miscarriage, as does obesity. There is an association with antiphospholipid syndrome and investigation of recurrent miscarriage should involve testing for inherited and acquired thrombophilias[25] as aspirin and low-dose heparin can reduce the miscarriage rate by 50% in these cases. Parental or fetal karyotyping can identify balanced translocations that may suggest preimplantation genetic diagnosis or gamete donation. The uterine structure is assessed as congenital uterine abnormalities, including uterine septum and cervical weakness, may be amenable to surgery.

Although treatment with progesterone, corticosteroids, or metformin has been advocated, and randomized studied are underway, there is insufficient evidence to recommend their use at present.

Most couples, however, have unexplained recurrent miscarriage and although empirical treatment has not been shown to be effective, their prognosis for a good outcome in future pregnancy is excellent.[17] The value of psychological support and serial ultrasound scans during pregnancy in recurrent miscarriage has been demonstrated in several non-randomized studies although the mechanism is unclear.[26]

Ectopic pregnancy

One of the primary roles of EPAUs is the timely diagnosis and management of EP. Approximately 1 in every 80 pregnancies and 4% of cases seen in the EPAU is an EP, occurring when the blastocyst implants outside the normal uterine cavity, generally in the Fallopian tube. In the United Kingdom, EP is the leading cause of maternal mortality in the first trimester because of its association with tubal rupture and massive intraperitoneal haemorrhage (Figure 32.2). The chance of dying of an EP is 1 in 3000[4] and 9% of deaths directly related to pregnancy are a result of EP.[27]

There is a long list of factors that are associated with an increased risk of EP.[4] These may cause adhesions around or affect the structure and/or function of the Fallopian tube (Box 32.2). These should be considered along with symptoms in the appraisal of the risk of EP and the need for urgent clinical assessment.[28]

There is a fourfold risk of EP in heavy smokers and in those conceiving during IVF treatment.

More than half of women diagnosed with an EP do not have identifiable risk factors or evidence of pre-existing tubal damage.

Some women present acutely in early pregnancy with shock, pallor, abdominal pain associated with rebound, cervical excitation on VE, and referred pain to the shoulders, and the clinical diagnosis facilitates timely surgery. The diagnosis is clear when a woman presents. Such an acute presentation is unusual and one-third of patients with an EP have no clinical signs and up to 10% have no symptoms. The classical symptoms of EP are unilateral abdominal pain associated with PV bleeding presenting between 5 and

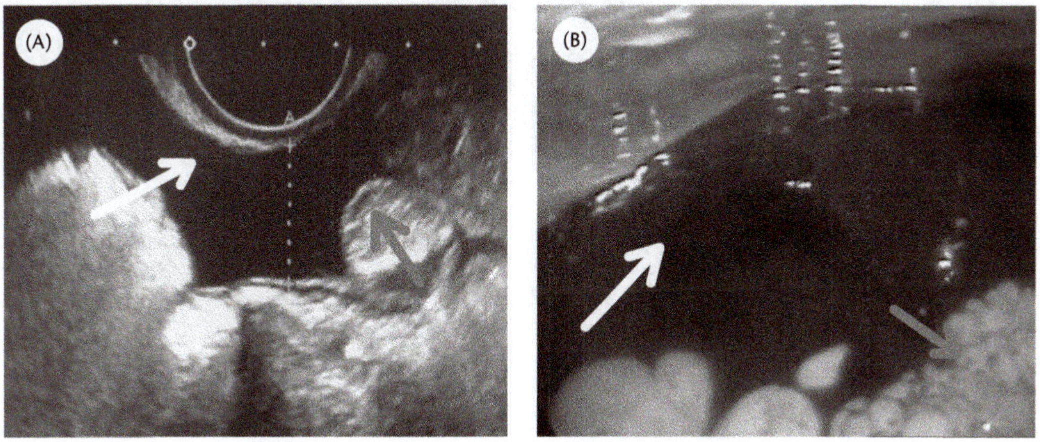

Figure 32.2 Haemoperitoneum in ruptured ectopic pregnancy. (A) Transvaginal scan and (B) laparoscopy of ruptured actopic pregnancy showing intraperitoneal blood (white arrows) surrounding the bowel/omentum (black arrows).

Box 32.2 Risk factors for ectopic pregnancy

Prior Fallopian tube damage with scarring

- Past pelvic inflammatory disease
- Past chlamydia/gonorrhoea
- Previous appendicitis or abdominal surgery
- Previous pelvic surgery
- Documented tubal disease or tubal surgery
- Endometriosis
- Sterilization and reversal of sterilization.

Functional alterations in the Fallopian tube

- Smoking
- Age over 35
- Hormonal contraceptive failure.

Additional risk factors

- Infertility
- Infertility treatment including IVF
- Previous ectopic pregnancy
- Conception with intrauterine contraceptive device in place.

8 weeks of gestation although gastrointestinal upset and central cramping pain are common.

Most women with symptoms of an EP will not have an EP.

A TVS showing an empty uterus with an adnexal mass has a sensitivity of 90% and specificity of 95% in the diagnosis of EP.[29] Typically the adnexal mass is separate from, medial, and superior to the ovary (Figure 32.3), usually on the same side as the CL, and may contain a small gestational sac surrounded by a hyperechoic ring. Free fluid, particularly when it surrounds the ovary, is suggestive of intraperitoneal bleeding.[30] One of the pitfalls is the presence of an intrauterine pseudo-sac in some EPs that mimics a gestational sac although it is transient, midline rather than eccentric, and is not surrounded by a hyperechoic decidual reaction.

However, in up to 50% of women with an EP the diagnosis is not made on first attendance and they are labelled as having a pregnancy of unknown location (PUL). The 2006–08 Centre for Maternal and Child Enquiries (CMACE) report into maternal deaths highlighted that PUL is not a diagnosis and every PUL is a potential EP.[27]

The mainstay of investigation of a PUL is measurement of serum hCG concentrations that is repeated 48 hours later.

If the hCG rises by more than 63% it is likely that there is a developing intrauterine pregnancy although an EP has not been excluded and emergency contact details are provided should her symptoms deteriorate.[9] An ultrasound should be arranged in 7 to 14 days' time, or earlier if symptoms worsen or continue and a predicted doubling of hCG every 2 days would predict a level of 1500 IU/L or higher. A decline in hCG by more than 20% suggests a spontaneous miscarriage although as an EP has not been excluded, further serial monitoring of hCG concentrations are often required.[4] If the fall is greater than 50%, then all that may be required is a urinary pregnancy test 2 weeks later.[9]

In a tubal EP, serial hCG patterns are variable although usually they rise at a slower rate than a viable intrauterine pregnancy or fall slower than a complete miscarriage. Often more than two hCG samples are required to assist in making the diagnosis and one pattern suggestive of an EP is a rise after an initial fall in hCG concentrations. When the pattern of serial hCG assessment is consistent with an EP, a repeat ultrasound scan may now identify an adnexal mass although when absent an EP should be assumed and a management strategy clearly documented.

There is sometimes a role for a diagnostic laparoscopy in the assessment of a PUL. It is particularly valuable when on first attendance there has been minimal bleeding, the ultrasound scan is inconclusive, and serum hCG is well within the discriminatory zone. An endometrial biopsy with urgent histology looking for the presence chorionic villi may also have a diagnostic role in a chronic PUL with static hCG.

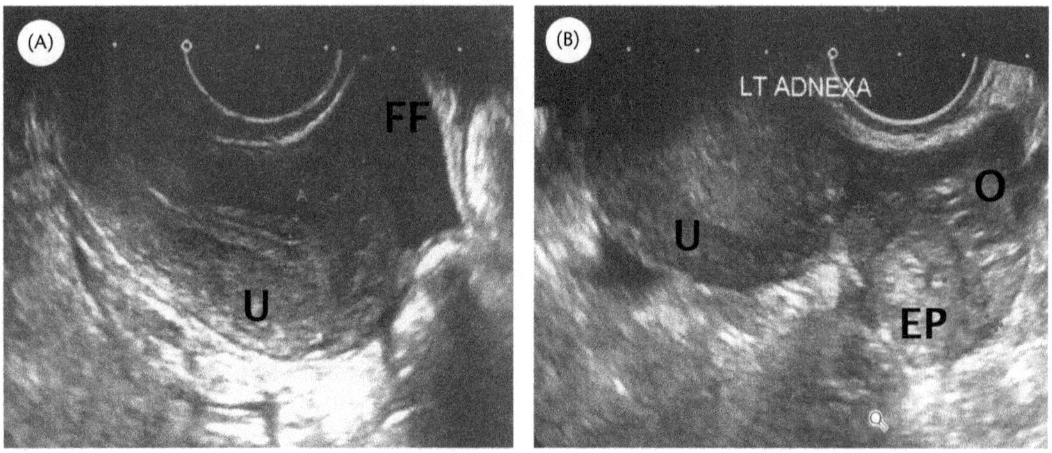

Figure 32.3 Ultrasonography of a tubal ectopic pregnancy. (A) Uterus (U) with a normal endometrial echo (measurement A) with free fluid (FF). (B) In the left adnexa next to the uterus (U) and medial to the ovary (O) is the adnexal mass (measurement A) representing the ectopic pregnancy (EP).

Once diagnosed, an EP can be managed surgically, medically, or expectantly depending on past history, clinical presentation, results of investigations, and patient preference.[31]

Surgical management is required if there is significant pain, clinical or sonographic evidence of tubal rupture, or a large EP. This includes the presence of moderate free fluid particularly if it is around the ovary,[30] an adnexal mass of 35 mm or larger, the presence of a fetal pole with evidence of cardiac activity, or hCG concentrations generally higher than 3000 IU/L and certainly greater than 5000 IU/L.[9,32]

The standard surgical treatment is laparoscopic in nature, although in the presence of haemodynamic instability the treatment should be the one that prevents further blood loss most quickly, and this might be laparotomy.[32] The operation of choice is a salpingectomy rather than a salpingotomy which has a similar future intrauterine pregnancy rate but an increased risk of subsequent EP.[31] However, if the contralateral tube is absent or visibly damaged, a salpingostomy is recommended[32] after which hCG concentrations are measured as up to one in five women will have residual trophoblast that requires further management.[9]

Medical treatment involves intramuscular methotrexate that is generally administered as a single dose of 50 mg/m² body surface area.

Methotrexate is particularly suited to women with minimal symptoms and hCG concentrations less than 1500 IU/L (Box 32.3).[4,32] Although it is commonly used up to hCG concentrations of 3000 IU/L, and can be used up to 5000 IU/L, it becomes less cost-effective and more likely to fail with increasing hCG concentrations. Methotrexate use is increasing and the proportion of EPs treated medically is now approaching that of those treated surgically. Women should abstain from alcohol and strong sunlight for 7 days, and avoid pregnancy in the 3 months after methotrexate treatment.

Box 32.3 Criteria to assess suitability for medical management of ectopic pregnancy

Clinical features

- Clinically stable with minimal pain.

Scan features

- Adnexal mass < 35 mm diameter
- No more than minimal free fluid
- No fetal cardiac activity within the EP.

Serum hCG concentrations

- Ideally hCG < 3000 IU/L
- No significant anaemia
- Normal renal and liver function.

Patient features

- Prefers medical option
- Able to attend prolonged follow-up
- No active peptic ulcer disease
- No concurrent potentially nephrotoxic or hepatotoxic medication.

Side effects of methotrexate include some lower abdominal discomfort and bloating and transient elevation of liver function tests. After methotrexate, serum hCG is routinely measured 4 and 7 days later and once or twice weekly thereafter until negative. Although a fall by day 4 is a useful predictor of future success[33] the main initial assessment of success is a fall in hCG concentrations from day 4 to day 7 of greater than 15%.[32] If this fall has not occurred, further management, generally a repeat injection of methotrexate, is indicated. Around 15% of patients will require a repeat dose and 10% will require surgery, although this is generally for failure of the hCG to adequately fall rather than acute tubal rupture.[9,32,34]

As some EPs will resolve spontaneously without risk to the patient there is a role for expectant management with serial hCG assessment in some cases. This is most effective if the initial hCG level is low (< 1000 IU/L) and is consistently falling,[9,32] particularly if this is associated with a low serum progesterone concentration.[4] The follow-up regimen mirrors that of medical management and it is successful in up to 80% of suitable patients with the others requiring medical or surgical intervention.

After an EP, the risk of a future EP is increased to around 18% and an early location scan in any future pregnancy is indicated.

That risk will fall to approximately 5% if the next pregnancy is intrauterine and triple if the next pregnancy is also an EP.[4] With regards to fertility, if the tube is removed or blocked as a result of the EP there will be a reduction in fertility. Fertility on the month where the egg is released on the damaged side will be reduced so it will take longer to become pregnant although most women will achieve a pregnancy before referral to an infertility clinic is indicated.

A very important, and difficult to diagnose, EP is a heterotopic pregnancy that is the coexistence of an EP with an intrauterine pregnancy. It occurs in 1/40,000 spontaneous pregnancies although the incidence is increased after IVF.[35] As serial hCG assessment is not useful, the diagnosis is generally scan based and the key elements are clinical suspicion and not delaying surgical management because of the coexisting intrauterine pregnancy. As medical management is not possible, and expectant management cannot be monitored, treatment is surgical.

Although 98% of ectopic pregnancies are in the Fallopian tube, the 2% in other sites cause management difficulties.[36] Implantation can occur in the cervix, caesarean delivery scar, ovary, peritoneal cavity, and interstitial portion of the Fallopian tube. In these cases, the EP can progress further and become increasingly vascularized before rupture with an increased risk of catastrophic intraperitoneal bleeding. The standard investigative pathways can diagnose these unusual ectopic pregnancies but surgical management is more complex and the risk of hysterectomy is increased.[36] As they are rare, intervention is individualized and although this may involve surgery, direct injection of drugs into the EP to interrupt its growth, or embolization, systemic methotrexate, with one or more repeated doses as an inpatient, is the most common initial strategy in the stable patient. The increased risk of future EP is difficult to quantify but an early location scan is indicated in subsequent pregnancy.

Recommendation on future mode of delivery will depend on the site of the EP, nature of surgery, and the risk of uterine rupture during labour.

Anaesthesia for EPs can be challenging as there may be significant blood loss into the peritoneum. Large-bore intravenous access should be secured and blood available. A rapid sequence induction is indicated. The surgeon should be scrubbed ready to start the procedure before the patient is anaesthetized as suxamethonium will cause paralysis of the rectus muscles and resultant loss of tamponade with subsequent bleeding. Profound hypotension may ensue, so rapid surgical access to the source of bleeding, and ligation of the appropriate vessels is indicated. Cell salvage is an underused technique in this area and should be considered.

Hyperemesis gravidarum

Seventy per cent of women experience nausea and vomiting in pregnancy and hyperemesis affects up to 2% of pregnant women. This is an extreme form of persistent vomiting associated with dehydration, ketonuria, and a loss of 5% of pre-pregnancy weight.[37] It is important that other causes of nausea and vomiting, such as urinary tract infection, diabetic ketoacidosis, hyperparathyroidism, cholecystitis, or small bowel obstruction, are considered. Severe cases can have electrolyte imbalance, vitamin deficiency, thyroid and liver dysfunction, and coagulation defects. Management is often supportive (Box 32.4) and symptoms usually peak around 9 weeks' gestation and subside in the second trimester.[38] Although there are links with reduced birthweight, women should be reassured about fetal development.[38]

Box 32.4 Management of hyperemesis gravidarum

Lifestyle

- Ginger
- Small frequent light meals.

Fluid and electrolyte replacement

- Avoid dextrose-containing fluids
- Potassium replacement usually required.

Antiemetic therapy

- Regular prescription
- Intramuscular or intravenous initially with oral or rectal maintenance
- Combination drugs may be required:
  - First line: one or two of prochlorperazine, cyclizine, or metoclopramide
  - Second line: addition of ondansetron
  - Third line: glucocorticoids.

Nutrition

- Nil by mouth progressing to frequent small intake
- Clear fluids initially
- Dietetic involvement
- Total parental or enteral nutrition in extreme cases.

Additional treatment

- Vitamin supplementation (thiamine)
- Thromboprophylaxis.

Molar pregnancy

Gestational trophoblastic disease (GTD) is a group of disorders consisting of complete and partial molar pregnancies and malignant conditions such as invasive mole and choriocarcinoma. Overall, the incidence of GTD in the United Kingdom is approximately 1/750 live births.[39] The incidence of GTD increases with age progressively over the age of 40 and women from Asia have double the risk of GTD than non-Asian women.

There is an effective supraregional registration programme for GTD in the United Kingdom and monitoring and treatment is managed nationally.

Complete moles are diploid but both sets of chromosomes are paternal in origin resulting either from duplication of the male pronuclei (75%) or dispermic fertilization (25%) with loss of the female pronuclei.[39] Paternally imprinted genes regulate placental development and there is no evidence of fetal tissue. Partial moles are generally triploid with two sets of paternal chromosomes as a result of dispermic fertilization and there is usually evidence of fetal tissue.

Although GTD can present with hyperemesis, hyperthyroidism, early pre-eclampsia, large uterine size, or metastasis, most molar pregnancies present in the first trimester of pregnancy with irregular vaginal bleeding.[40] Although ultrasound examination can suggest the diagnosis at presentation (Figure 32.4), definitive diagnosis is made by histological examination of the products of conception when suspicion has been raised.[39]

The recommendation that tissue from all failed pregnancies is examined for molar change is difficult to achieve in practice, but products from repeat evacuations should undergo histological assessment.

Suction curettage is the method of choice for the evacuation of molar pregnancy except in partial moles with a fetus over 14 weeks in size where medical evacuation of the uterus may be required. Surgical expertise is important because of the increased risk of excessive bleeding and the need to completely empty the uterus. As well as histological analysis, tissue may need to be sent, with paired parental blood samples if possible, for cytogenetic analysis. Although there is a theoretical risk of trophoblast embolization after prolonged prostaglandin use, preparation of the cervix immediately prior to evacuation is safe although the use of an oxytocic prior to evacuation is not recommended.[39]

Follow-up of GTD is by serial monitoring of hCG for 6 months from the evacuation of the uterus or from normalization of hCG, when this has taken more than 56 days. Follow-up is arranged through supraregional centres. Women should be advised not to conceive until their follow-up is complete although hormonal contraception before hCG has normalized may slow resolution. The need for chemotherapy following a complete mole is 15% and following a partial mole is 0.5% and there is an excellent cure rate even with metastatic disease. The risk of further GTD is 1 in 80 and hCG monitoring is required after any subsequent pregnancy.[39,40]

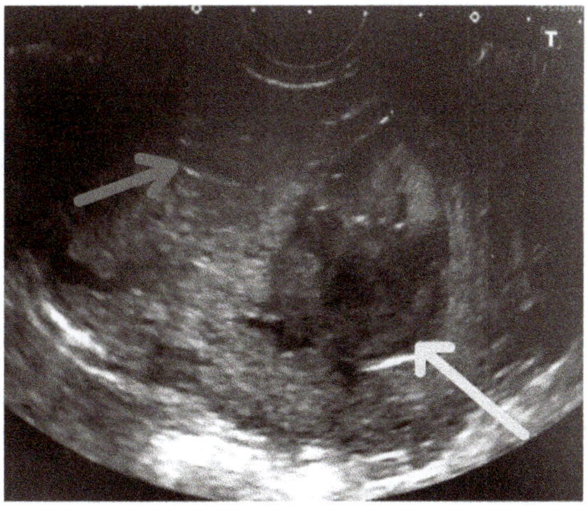

Figure 32.4 Ultrasound features suggestive of a molar pregnancy. Inside the uterus (white arrow) there is irregular cystic pregnancy tissue (black arrow) with no clear pregnancy sac, yolk sac or fetal pole suggestive of a complete mole.

Important issues in early pregnancy care

Quality care provision

The CMACE enquires into maternal death highlight the need for clear documentation, communication and management planning, and the success of EPAUs. The biggest challenge in reducing morbidity and mortality associated with early pregnancy problems is increasing the access of disadvantaged women and minority ethnic groups to timely care.[27]

Anti-D administration

As rhesus isoimmunization can occur after early pregnancy problems, there are some circumstances where women who are rhesus negative require anti-D prophylaxis.[41] All women who have a surgical procedure to manage an EP or miscarriage should be offered anti-D at a dose of 50 mcg (250 IU) as soon as possible but within 72 hours. In the first trimester of pregnancy, a Kleihauer test is not needed to quantify fetomaternal haemorrhage and anti-D is not required for threatened, incomplete, or complete miscarriage. Anti-D may not be required after the medical management of miscarriage or EP but guidelines differ[9,41] and prophylaxis is often given.

Sensitive disposal of pregnancy tissue

It is important that there are clear pathways for the appropriate disposal of tissue from pregnancy losses whether or not fetal tissue can be identified.[42] In recognition of the sensitivity around early pregnancy loss it is no longer considered acceptable for pregnancy tissue to be disposed of by clinical waste incineration. In the United Kingdom, the minimum standard is collective disposal in a crematorium or collective burial where such disposal is not available. Women may decline this disposal and are free to make alternative arrangements if they wish.

Guidelines

There are excellent national guidelines available in the United Kingdom for the assessment and management of early pregnancy problems (Box 32.5).

Box 32.5 Guidelines relevant to early pregnancy problems

- National Institute for Health and Clinical Excellence. NICE Clinical Guideline 154: *Ectopic Pregnancy and Miscarriage.*
- Royal College of Obstetricians and Gynaecologists. Green-top Guideline 17: *The Investigation and Treatment of Couples with Recurrent First-trimester and Second-trimester Miscarriage.*
- Royal College of Obstetricians and Gynaecologists. Green-top Guideline 21: *The Management of Tubal Pregnancy.*
- Royal College of Obstetricians and Gynaecologists. Green-top Guideline 22: *The Use of Anti-D Immunoglobulin for Rhesus D Prophylaxis.*
- Royal College of Obstetricians and Gynaecologists. Green-top Guideline 25: *The Management of Early Pregnancy Loss.*
- Royal College of Obstetricians and Gynaecologists. Green-top Guideline 38: *The Management of Gestational Trophoblastic Disease.*

Conclusion

The management of early pregnancy problems involves an awareness of normal pregnancy and early pregnancy problems, and their investigation and treatment which may be surgical or medical. The multidisciplinary team involved in the care of women with these problems includes primary care, radiographers, midwives, nurses, gynaecologists, and reproductive medicine specialists. The anaesthetist is also a key member of the team as they often have to provide anaesthesia for evacuation of the products of conception or ectopic pregnancies in women who may be hypovolaemic and an understanding of the physiology and pathology surrounding their care is therefore essential.

References

1. Duncan WC, Myers M, Dickinson RE, *et al.* Luteal development and luteolysis in the primate corpus luteum. *Animal Reprod* 2009; 6:34–46.
2. Diedrich K, Fauser BC, Devroey P, *et al.* The role of the endometrium and embryo in human implantation. *Hum Reprod Update* 2007; 13:365–77.
3. Csapo AI, Pulkkinen M. Indispensability of the human corpus luteum in the maintenance of early pregnancy. Luteectomy evidence. *Obstet Gynecol Surv* 1978; 33:69–81.
4. Sivalingam VN, Duncan WC, Kirk E, *et al.* Diagnosis and management of ectopic pregnancy. *J Fam Plann Reprod Health Care* 2011; 37:231–40.
5. Templeton A. Infertility and the establishment of pregnancy—overview. *Br Med Bull* 2000; 56:577–87.
6. Nyboe Andersen A, Erb K. Register data on Assisted Reproductive Technology (ART) in Europe including a detailed description of ART in Denmark. *Int J Androl* 2006; 29:12–16.
7. van der Linden M, Buckingham K, Farquhar C, *et al.* Luteal phase support for assisted reproduction cycles. *Cochrane Database Syst Rev* 2011; 10:CD009154.
8. Royal College of Obstetricians and Gynaecologists. *The Management of Ovarian Hyperstimulation Syndrome.* Green-top Guideline 5. London: RCOG; 2006.
9. National Institute for Health and Clinical Excellence. *Ectopic Pregnancy and Miscarriage.* Clinical Guideline 154. London: NICE; 2012.

10. Grynberg M, Teyssedre J, Andre C, *et al.* Rupture of ectopic pregnancy with negative serum beta-hCG leading to hemorrhagic shock. *Obstet Gynecol* 2009; 113:537–9.
11. Kirk E, Bourne T. Diagnosis of ectopic pregnancy with ultrasound. *Best Pract Res Clin Obstet Gynaecol* 2009; 23:501–8.
12. Bottomley C, Van Belle V, Kirk E, *et al.* Accurate prediction of pregnancy viability by means of a simple scoring system. *Hum Reprod* 2013; 28:68–76.
13. Wahabi HA, Fayed AA, Esmaeil SA, *et al.* Progestogen for treating threatened miscarriage. *Cochrane Database Syst Rev* 2011; 12:CD005943.
14. Walch KT, Huber JC. Progesterone for recurrent miscarriage: truth and deceptions. *Best Pract Res Clin Obstet Gynaecol* 2008; 22:375–89.
15. Nyberg DA, Laing FC, Filly RA. Threatened abortion: sonographic distinction of normal and abnormal gestation sacs. *Radiology* 1986; 158:397–400.
16. Harris RD, Couto C, Karpovsky C, *et al.* The chorionic bump: a first-trimester pregnancy sonographic finding associated with a guarded prognosis. *J Ultrasound Med* 2006; 25:757–63.
17. Royal College of Obstetricians and Gynaecologists. *The Investigation and Treatment of Couples with Recurrent First-trimester and Second-trimester Miscarriage*. Green-top Guideline 17. London: RCOG; 2011.
18. Royal College of Obstetricians and Gynaecologists. *The Management of Early Pregnancy Loss*. Green-top Guideline 25. London: RCOG; 2006.
19. Pexsters A, Luts J, Van Schoubroeck D, *et al.* Clinical implications of intra- and interobserver reproducibility of transvaginal sonographic measurement of gestational sac and crown-rump length at 6–9 weeks' gestation. *Ultrasound Obstet Gynecol* 2011; 38:510–15.
20. Abdallah Y, Daemen A, Kirk E, *et al.* Limitations of current definitions of miscarriage using mean gestational sac diameter and crown-rump length measurements: a multicenter observational study. *Ultrasound Obstet Gynecol* 2011; 38:497–502.
21. Neilson JP, Gyte GM, Hickey M, *et al.* Medical treatments for incomplete miscarriage (less than 24 weeks). *Cochrane Database Syst Rev* 2010; 1:CD007223.
22. Forna F, Gülmezoglu AM. Surgical procedures to evacuate incomplete abortion. *Cochrane Database Syst Rev* 2001; 1:CD001993.
23. Ali PB, Smith G. The effect of syntocinon on blood loss during first trimester suction curettage. *Anaesthesia* 1996; 51:483–5.
24. Yu D, Wong YM, Cheong Y, *et al.* Asherman syndrome—one century later. *Fertil Steril* 2008; 89:759–79.
25. Rai R, Regan L. Recurrent miscarriage. *Lancet* 2006; 368:601–11.
26. Clifford K, Rai R, Regan L. Future pregnancy outcome in unexplained recurrent first trimester miscarriage. *Hum Reprod* 1997; 12:387–9.
27. Centre for Maternal and Child Enquiries (CMACE). Saving Mothers' Lives: reviewing maternal deaths to make motherhood safer: 2006–08. The Eighth Report on Confidential Enquiries into Maternal Deaths in the United Kingdom. *BJOG* 2011; 118 Suppl 1:1–203.
28. Crochet JR, Bastian LA, Chireau MV. Does this woman have an ectopic pregnancy?: the rational clinical examination systematic review. *JAMA* 2013; 309:1722–9.
29. Condous G, Okaro E, Khalid A, *et al.* The accuracy of transvaginal ultrasonography for the diagnosis of ectopic pregnancy prior to surgery. *Hum Reprod* 2005; 20:1404–9.
30. Popowski T, Huchon C, Toret-Labeeuw F, *et al.* Hemoperitoneum assessment in ectopic pregnancy. *Int J Gynaecol Obstet* 2012; 116:97–100.
31. Hajenius PJ, Mol F, Mol BW, *et al.* Interventions for tubal ectopic pregnancy. *Cochrane Database Syst Rev* 2007; 1:CD000324.
32. Royal College of Obstetricians and Gynaecologists. *The Management of Tubal Pregnancy*. Green-top Guideline 21. London: RCOG; 2010.
33. Skubisz M, Dutton P, Duncan WC, *et al.* Using a decline in serum hCG between days 0-4 to predict ectopic pregnancy treatment success after single-dose methotrexate: a retrospective cohort study. *BMC Pregnancy Childbirth* 2013; 13:30.
34. Lipscomb GH. Medical management of ectopic pregnancy. *Clin Obstet Gynecol* 2012; 55:424–32.
35. Talbot K, Simpson R, Price N, *et al.* Heterotopic pregnancy. *J Obstet Gynaecol* 2011; 31:7–12.
36. Chetty M, Elson J. Treating non-tubal ectopic pregnancy. *Best Pract Res Clin Obstet Gynaecol* 2009; 23:529–38.
37. Jarvis S, Nelson-Piercy C. Management of nausea and vomiting in pregnancy. *BMJ* 2011; 342:d3606.
38. Wegrzyniak LJ, Repke JT, Ural SH. Treatment of hyperemesis gravidarum. *Rev Obstet Gynecol* 2012; 5:78–84.
39. Royal College of Obstetricians and Gynaecologists. *The Management of Gestational Trophoblastic Disease*. Green-top Guideline 38. London: RCOG; 2010.
40. Sebire NJ, Seckl MJ. Gestational trophoblastic disease: current management of hydatidiform mole. *BMJ* 2008; 337:a1193.
41. Royal College of Obstetricians and Gynaecologists. *The Use of Anti-D Immunoglobulin for Rhesus D Prophylaxis*. Green-top Guideline 22. London: RCOG; 2011.
42. Cameron MJ, Penney GC. Are national recommendations regarding examination and disposal of products of miscarriage being followed? A need for revised guidelines? *Hum Reprod* 2005; 20: 531–5.

CHAPTER 33

Prematurity, multiple gestation, and abnormal presentation

Oonagh Keag and E. Sarah Cooper

Preterm labour and delivery

Preterm labour is defined as the onset of regular contractions accompanied by cervical change prior to 37 completed weeks of gestation. Preterm delivery is defined by the World Health Organization as delivery between 20 and 37 weeks of gestation.

In high-income countries, the incidence of preterm birth is estimated at 6–10% of all births[1] and has remained unchanged over the last four decades despite intensive antenatal care programmes aimed at high-risk groups, the widespread use of pharmacological agents to inhibit preterm birth (tocolytics), and a series of other preventive and therapeutic interventions.

Prematurity remains a leading cause of neonatal morbidity and mortality in developed countries, accounting for 60–80% of deaths of infants without congenital anomalies.[2] Survival rates continue to improve with advances in neonatal intensive care but are very much dependent on gestational age and birth weight with smaller and earlier gestation infants carrying a higher risk of long-term morbidity or mortality. Mortality increases from about 2% for infants born at 32 weeks of gestation to more than 90% for those born at 23 weeks of gestation.[3]

Short-term morbidities associated with preterm delivery include respiratory distress syndrome, intraventricular haemorrhage, periventricular leucomalacia (brain injury involving necrosis of white matter around fluid-filled areas), necrotizing enterocolitis, bronchopulmonary dysplasia, sepsis, and patent ductus arteriosus. Long-term morbidities include cerebral palsy, mental retardation, and retinopathy of prematurity. Cerebral palsy is defined as a non-progressive motor disorder and complicates approximately two per 1000 of all live births. Causes may be attributed to antenatal, intrapartum (10% of cases), or postnatal events, though in many cases there is no identifiable cause. The relative risk for a preterm infant developing cerebral palsy is nearly 40 times that for term infants. Approximately 8–10% of surviving newborns weighing less than 1000 g at birth will develop cerebral palsy. These infants also have substantially higher rates of mental retardation and visual disabilities, as well as neurobehavioral dysfunction and poor school performance.[2,4]

Preterm birth may have huge psychosocial and emotional effects on the family, as well as being costly for health services.

Aetiology

About two-thirds of preterm births result from spontaneous preterm labour or preterm premature rupture of the membranes (PPROM), with the remainder iatrogenic due to medical interventions for maternal or fetal indications such as pre-eclampsia or severe intrauterine growth restriction.[2] One in five preterm births is associated with multiple pregnancy, and these have been greatly increased by assisted reproduction techniques.[5]

The pathophysiology of preterm labour is poorly understood, but infection is thought to play a major role, present in 40% of preterm deliveries. Infection is often subclinical and can occur spontaneously within the amniotic sac or can originate in another system such as the urinary or genital tract and cause intrauterine infection or spontaneous PPROM and subsequent chorioamnionitis. Organisms that have been associated with histological chorioamnionitis include *Ureaplasma urealyticum, Mycoplasma hominis, Gardnerella vaginalis*, peptostreptococci, and *Bacteroides* species.[6] Positive amniotic fluid cultures increase the risks of neonatal sepsis, respiratory distress syndrome, chronic lung disease, periventricular leucomalacia, intraventricular haemorrhage, and cerebral palsy.[7–9]

The presence of subclinical infection is associated with increased production of various cytokines in the amniotic fluid particularly tumour necrosis factor alpha, interleukin (IL)-1β, -6, and -8, with subsequent activation and production of prostaglandins $F2_{\alpha}$ and E_2 resulting in uterine contractions. It is thought that the micro-organisms gain access to the amniotic fluid and fetus by ascending from the vagina through the cervix and into the choriodecidual space during pregnancy.[10]

Bacterial vaginosis is a common condition where due to pH imbalance there is overgrowth of certain vaginal commensal bacteria causing a malodorous off-white vaginal discharge. This condition is associated with preterm labour and if discovered during pregnancy should be treated with a course of metronidazole.

Chlamydia trachomatis infection has also been associated with preterm delivery, and in Scotland, women under the age of 25 are routinely screened for this at the antenatal booking appointment using first-void urine or a self-taken low vaginal swab. Women and their partners are treated as necessary, usually with azithromycin. Contact tracing is arranged and repeat testing ('test of cure') performed.

Urinary tract infections (UTIs) during pregnancy increase the risk of pyelonephritis, and are associated with preterm labour. It has been suggested that as many as 40% of preterm births may be attributable to untreated UTIs.[11] For this reason, any pregnant woman with symptoms or urinalysis suggestive of a UTI must be treated promptly with appropriate antibiotics.

Aside from infection and multiple pregnancy, there are other predisposing factors for preterm labour. These can be divided into

Table 33.1 Causes of preterm labour

Maternal factors	Fetal factors	Obstetric factors
Past history of preterm labour	Genetic abnormalities	Recurrent antepartum haemorrhage
Uterine abnormalities	Fetal death	Cervical incompetence
Trauma	Multiple pregnancy	Abnormal placentation
Abdominal surgery		Preterm premature rupture of membranes
Acute or chronic systemic disease		Polyhydramnios
Age < 17 or > 35 years		
Low socioeconomic status		
Low prepregnancy BMI		
Smoking or substance misuse		
Working hours > 35/week		
High-stress jobs		

various categories, as seen in Table 33.1. Maternal factors include a past history of preterm labour, uterine abnormalities such as bicornuate uterus, trauma, abdominal surgery during the pregnancy, or acute or chronic systemic disease. Other risk factors in this category include extremes of age (<17 or >35 years), low socioeconomic status, low prepregnancy body mass index (BMI), tobacco use, and substance misuse. Observational studies of working conditions, for example, long working hours (>35 hours/week) and high-stress jobs, have had conflicting results but despite many confounding factors, these conditions are thought to be associated with an increased risk of preterm labour.[2] Fetal factors predisposing the woman to preterm labour include intrauterine growth restriction, genetic abnormalities, and fetal death. Obstetric factors include persistent bleeding throughout the pregnancy, incompetent cervix (this could be secondary to previous large loop excision of the transformation zone treatment for abnormal smears), abnormal placentation, PPROM, and polyhydramnios.[12–14]

It is important to note that PPROM does not always lead to premature labour, but occasionally labour is induced or expedited if there are concerns for maternal or fetal well-being. Close monitoring of these patients in the form of maternal temperature, white cell count, C-reactive protein, and high vaginal swabs is essential to make an informed decision of when to intervene. These patients are also prescribed prophylactic antibiotics.[15] Guidelines produced by the Royal College of Obstetricians and Gynaecologists (RCOG) recommend that erythromycin should be given for 10 days following the diagnosis of PPROM.[16] A meta-analysis of 22 trials has shown the use of antibiotics following PPROM is associated with a statistically significant reduction in chorioamnionitis, in the numbers of babies born within 48 hours, and a reduction in neonatal infection.[17] In the presence of Group B *Streptococcus* infection, penicillin should be administered 4-hourly.

Cervical cerclage

For those patients with a history of three or more previous midtrimester losses or preterm births, the RCOG recommends 'history-indicated' cervical cerclage. This is a transvaginal cervical suture inserted electively at 12–14 weeks as a prophylactic measure. For patients with a history of one or more midtrimester losses or preterm deliveries, transvaginal scans can be arranged to assess the cervical length between 14 and 24 weeks' gestation. If there is evidence of shortening of the cervix, that is, if the cervix is 25 mm or less, 'ultrasound-indicated' cervical cerclage may be offered to prevent preterm labour. In women with a previous failed transvaginal cerclage, insertion of a transabdominal cerclage via laparotomy or laparoscopy may be considered and this may be performed preconceptually or in early pregnancy. 'Rescue cerclage' may be indicated as a salvage measure in the case of premature cervical dilatation with exposed fetal membranes in the vagina. The decision to insert a rescue cerclage will depend on the presentation and the gestation of the pregnancy, as it poses the risk of severe preterm delivery and neonatal mortality and morbidity. Rescue cerclage may delay delivery by a further 5 weeks on average compared with expectant management alone, but the risk of cerclage failure increases with cervical dilatation. Cervical cerclage is not recommended in multiple pregnancy.[18] Other contraindications to cervical cerclage include active preterm labour, evidence of chorioamnionitis, continuing vaginal bleeding, and PPROM.

Anaesthesia for cervical cerclage

Both general and spinal anaesthesia are appropriate for cervical cerclage. Many women are understandably anxious due to their poor obstetric history and therefore opt for general anaesthesia (GA). As these operations are carried out in the first trimester, a laryngeal mask can be used unless there is a contraindication. Most anaesthetists would use a total intravenous technique although there is no reason why an inhalational technique is not acceptable or safe as none of the agents are teratogenic. Other women prefer to be awake and the procedure can be done with a low-dose spinal technique (2.0 mL 0.5% heavy bupivacaine). Postoperative pain is not severe and intrathecal opiates are not indicated.

If a mini-laparotomy is performed for an abdominal approach to cervical cerclage, a GA is indicated with muscle paralysis to facilitate the surgery which is often challenging for the obstetrician. At the end of the procedure, some units use a non-steroidal anti-inflammatory drug (NSAID), indomethacin 100 mg, two doses at 12-hourly intervals, to prevent premature labour. NSAIDs are cyclooxygenase (COX) inhibitors and prevent prostaglandins synthesis, thus preventing uterine contractions. The woman is confined to bed for a further period and therefore anticoagulation should also be prescribed.

Diagnosis of preterm labour

For any woman admitted with suspected preterm labour, the accuracy of the expected date of delivery should be re-checked especially at extremes of gestational age below 24 weeks. Clinically, the diagnosis of preterm labour is made when there are regular painful, palpable contractions, lasting longer than 30 seconds, accompanied by evidence of a change in the position, consistency, length, and/or dilatation of the cervix. This is determined by sterile speculum examination initially if there is suspected rupture of membranes, followed by digital vaginal examination if there is a strong suspicion that the woman may be in labour.[19]

When preterm labour is established, a diagnostic workup should include the assessment of any risk factors that could be modified together with a complete medical history, a thorough physical examination, ultrasound assessment of fetal growth, morphology, well-being and presentation, together with infectious screening (high vaginal swab, midstream sample of urine) and blood screening (white cell count, C-reactive protein). Fetal heart rate monitoring should be commenced and any acute causes of preterm labour excluded such as placental abruption or sepsis.

In uncertain cases when membranes are intact, fetal fibronectin (FFN) testing may be performed. FFN is a glycoprotein found in high concentrations in the placenta and amniotic fluid. FFN is detectable in the cervicovaginal secretion in about 4% of pregnant women after 20 gestational weeks, possibly reflecting transudation of amniotic fluid or disruption of the choriodecidual interface.[20] FFN is most sensitive when measured before 34 weeks' gestation with a sensitivity of predicting preterm birth ranging from 21 to 94% (median 80%).[21] If FFN is absent (negative test result), the risk of preterm delivery within 1 or 2 weeks is less than 1%, and the patient can be reassured.[22]

Management

Once the diagnosis of preterm labour is established, the woman must be admitted to an obstetric unit with facilities for resuscitating and managing a preterm infant. In some cases, depending on the gestational age and if time allows, an *in utero* transfer is required. If delivery is thought to occur within the next few days, corticosteroids should be administered to the mother. A Cochrane review of 21 studies (3885 women and 4269 infants) showed that treatment of women at risk of preterm birth with a single course of antenatal corticosteroids reduced the risk of neonatal death by 31% (95% confidence interval (CI) 19–42%), respiratory distress syndrome by 44% (95% CI 31–57%), and intraventricular haemorrhage by 46% (95% CI 31–67%). Antenatal corticosteroid use is also associated with a reduction in necrotizing enterocolitis, respiratory support, intensive care admissions, and systemic infections in the first 48 hours of life compared with no treatment or treatment with placebo.[23] The recommended dose is two doses of betamethasone 12 mg, 24 hours apart or four doses of dexamethasone 6 mg, 12 hours apart by intramuscular injection. Antenatal corticosteroids have been shown to have effect if administered between 24 and 34 + 6 weeks gestation. The decision to administer corticosteroids between 23 and 23 + 6 weeks should be made at a senior obstetric level in conjunction with the parents and the neonatologists after a full discussion of survival rates and a sonographic measurement of estimated fetal weight. The evidence shows that a single course of antenatal corticosteroids does not appear to be associated with any significant short-term maternal or fetal adverse effects.[24]

As mentioned above, if the membranes have ruptured, antibiotics are recommended. Randomized controlled trials and a meta-analysis have concluded that antibiotics prolong pregnancy and reduce maternal and neonatal morbidity.[15, 25] There is insufficient evidence that antibiotics are useful when the membranes are intact.[26]

The gestation at which delivery should be considered following PPROM remains a contentious issue. A balance must be struck between the neonatal morbidity risk (mainly respiratory) of immediate delivery and the increasing risk of chorioamnionitis with expectant management. Randomized controlled trials are in progress but the current RCOG guideline recommends consideration of delivery at 34 weeks' gestation.[16]

Tocolysis

Tocolysis is a method of suppressing uterine contractions to prolong pregnancy. This is particularly important in women at very early gestations or in women who require transfer to a tertiary obstetric unit with appropriate neonatal facilities. However, it may not always be appropriate to prolong pregnancy, for example, in the presence of intrauterine infection or placental abruption where prolonging pregnancy could be hazardous to the mother or her baby. A systematic review has shown that tocolytic drugs are associated with prolonging pregnancy for up to 7 days but with no significant effect on preterm birth and no clear effect on perinatal or neonatal mortality or morbidity.[27] RCOG guidelines state that they should be considered to allow time to complete a course of corticosteroids or an *in utero* transfer.[28] There is insufficient evidence to support the use of tocolytic drugs in multiple pregnancy or in cases of PPROM.

A range of tocolytic agents have been used to inhibit preterm labour and postpone preterm birth (and are the topics of Cochrane systematic reviews) including nitric oxide donors glyceryl trinitrate,[29] calcium channel blockers (commonly nifedipine),[30] betamimetics,[31] magnesium sulphate,[32] COX inhibitors,[33] and oxytocin receptor antagonists (atosiban).

The popularity of the betamimetics, ritodrine and terbutaline, for tocolysis has declined in recent years and ritodrine has been withdrawn from UK and US markets. In the United Kingdom, terbutaline is only indicated for external cephalic version (ECV) or when the uterus is hypertonic usually as a result of Syntocinon® (oxytocin) overstimulation. In addition to its beta-2 effects on smooth muscle causing bronchial and uterine relaxation, it also causes vasodilatation and hypotension. Beta-1 effects include tachycardia and arrhythmias which limit its usefulness. Life-threatening pulmonary oedema has also been reported.

According to the RCOG guidelines, atosiban and nifedipine have comparable effectiveness in delaying preterm birth for up to 7 days. These both have fewer side effects and nifedipine has the advantage of oral administration and low cost. The use of multiple tocolytic drugs is associated with a higher risk of adverse effects and so should be avoided.[34] A recent systematic review and meta-analysis looked at data from 95 randomized controlled trials and found that prostaglandin inhibitors and calcium channel blockers had the highest probability of delaying delivery and improving neonatal and maternal outcomes.[35] Table 33.2 displays the different tocolytics available, their mode of action, contraindications, and salient maternal and neonatal side effects.

Magnesium sulphate

For women in suspected preterm labour under 30 weeks' gestation, a 2011 RCOG Scientific Impact Paper[36] has recommended the use of magnesium sulphate as neuroprotection for reduction of the incidence of cerebral palsy and motor deficits. A loading dose of 4 g is recommended, followed by an infusion of 1 g per hour for 24 hours or until delivery, whichever occurs soonest. Side effects include facial flushing, chest pain, palpitations, nausea, transient hypotension, sedation, and blurred vision.[37,38] These may be exaggerated if the woman is also taking calcium channel antagonists. Absolute contraindications to the use of magnesium sulphate include myasthenia gravis and heart block. Relative contraindications include underlying renal disease and recent myocardial infarction. Pulmonary oedema has been reported in

Table 33.2 Properties and side effects of tocolytics

Tocolytic	Mode of action	Contraindications	Maternal side effects	Fetal or neonatal side effects
Terbutaline	Beta-agonist	Cardiac arrhythmias	Tachycardia, tremor, cardiac arrhythmias, pulmonary oedema, myocardial ischaemia	Fetal tachycardia, hyperinsulinaemia, hypoglycaemia
Nifedipine	Calcium channel blocker	Cardiac disease, hypotension. Caution if concomitantly with magnesium sulphate	Flushing, headache, dizziness, nausea, hypotension	
Atosiban	Oxytocin antagonist		Nausea, headache, dizziness, tachycardia	
Magnesium sulphate	Myosin light chain inhibitor	Myasthenia gravis	Flushing, lethargy, headache, muscle weakness, diplopia, pulmonary oedema, cardiac arrest	Lethargy, hypotonia, respiratory depression
Indomethacin	NSAID	Late pregnancy, hepatic or renal impairment	Nausea, reflux	Constriction of ductus arteriosus, pulmonary hypertension, impaired renal function, intraventricular haemorrhage

approximately 1% of women treated with magnesium sulphate. Because of the potential risk of fluid overload, periodic assessment of fluid intake and output is essential.[39] Magnesium can fortuitously cause uterine relaxation, useful if there is also premature labour.

Delivery

The method of delivery of the preterm infant depends on the aetiology of the preterm labour, the gestation, and presentation and the decision should be made in conjunction with the parents and the neonatology team. Often in iatrogenic cases, for example, if delivery is indicated for severe intrauterine growth restriction, induction of labour is not possible either due to malpresentation or the presence of features of fetal distress on cardiotocographic (CTG) monitoring. In such cases, a caesarean delivery would be the most appropriate method of safe delivery of the preterm infant.

In established spontaneous preterm labour where the presentation of the fetus is cephalic, and there are no concerns about fetal heart rate monitoring, the woman is encouraged to deliver vaginally. It must be noted though, that preterm infants, and especially very early preterm infants, are more vulnerable to trauma during delivery than fetuses at term. They are far more likely to suffer soft tissue damage, neurological injury, and traumatic intracranial haemorrhage than term infants.[39] For this reason, the fetal heart rate should be monitored closely and special care should be taken not to traumatize these infants, for example, by avoiding the use of ventouse and fetal scalp electrodes where at all possible, especially under 34 weeks' gestation. Forceps are also generally avoided but in the past were used to protect the fetal skull from sudden decompression when exiting the genital tract. In the incidence of suspected fetal distress, fetal blood sampling is not used as the preterm fetus has more fragile skull bones, and is less able to cope with acidosis and so immediate delivery is indicated.

Analgesia and anaesthesia for preterm delivery

As with a woman labouring at term, women in established preterm labour may also request an epidural. During preterm labour, an epidural is advantageous in providing a relaxed pelvic floor and perineum to facilitate a smooth controlled delivery of the more vulnerable preterm vertex, and in inhibiting inappropriate maternal expulsive efforts prior to complete cervical dilatation. In addition, it is thought that epidural analgesia decreases maternal concentrations of catecholamines and in some patients it may improve uteroplacental perfusion.[40]

If a caesarean is indicated, and as long as there were no contraindications, neuraxial anaesthesia is the technique of choice. The drugs used in GA cross the placenta and may further depress the already compromised preterm infant.[41] Pre-eclampsia is one of the commonest causes of premature delivery and GA in these patients can be even more hazardous due to the hypertensive response to laryngoscopy which can result in myocardial ischaemia or cerebral haemorrhage, and potential difficult intubation due to laryngeal oedema. Further, if magnesium has been used as a prophylaxis against eclampsia prior to GA, as it is a calcium antagonist, it prevents release of acetyl choline at the neuromuscular junction and has the potential for prolonged neuromuscular blockade. If muscle relaxants are used, a smaller dose is required and neuromuscular monitoring performed particularly when reversal is attempted. Prolonged neuromuscular block may be exacerbated by combining magnesium with nifedipine.[42]

A spinal or combined spinal–epidural (CSE) can be used for most operative deliveries where the fetus is premature. A larger dose of local anaesthetic is necessary to achieve the desired block height. This is due to the smaller fetus causing less uterine compression of the vena cava and engorgement of the epidural blood vessels. The subarachnoid and epidural spaces have thus larger volumes than with the term fetus and require more volume of local anaesthetic to spread to the appropriate height. Magnesium can cause vasodilatation and if neuraxial anaesthesia is employed, hypotension may occur and should be prevented with suitable vasopressors.

Key points

- Preterm labour is a common cause of neonatal morbidity and mortality.

- Transfer to a neonatal unit with appropriate facilities is key.
- Tocolysis may be useful to enable transfer or administration of corticosteroids.
- Chorioamnionitis is a significant complication and antibiotic prophylaxis is essential.
- Neuraxial anaesthesia is generally preferred where possible.
- Local anaesthetic requirements are increased.

Multiple gestation

The incidence of multiple pregnancy is rising, mainly as a result of increasing assisted reproduction techniques including *in vitro* fertilization. Currently, the rate of twins is about 1/67 births, triplets 1/5000, and quadruplets 1:360,000.[43] This chapter will focus mainly on twin pregnancy. Triplets and higher-order multiples are generally delivered by elective caesarean delivery.

Twin pregnancies are described according to the number of ova originally fertilized (zygosity) and the number of placentae (chorionicity). Two-thirds of twin pregnancies are dizygotic, where two separate ova are fertilized by two separate sperm resulting in two separate gestational sacs with two placentas—they are dichorionic and diamniotic. These twins may be of different sex. Monozygotic twins result from the division of a single embryo; therefore, these twins are genetically identical. The chorionicity will depend on the stage at which the embryo separates and this is demonstrated in Figure 33.1.[44] Monozygotic twins can be diamniotic dichorionic, diamniotic monochorionic, monoamniotic monochorionic (1% of pregnancies), or, if the separation occurs later after 12 days, conjoined twins. The rate of dichorionic twins is 1/80, and the rate of monochorionic twins is 4/1000.

Diagnosis

The diagnosis of multiple pregnancy and determination of chorionicity is best determined by ultrasound scan in the first trimester. Those scans with a 'lambda' or 'twin-peak' sign at the membrane insertion are dichorionic. Those with a dividing membrane thicker than 2 mm are often dichorionic or indeed if there are different sex fetuses, they are dichorionic.[45]

Management of twin pregnancy

Twin pregnancies are high-risk pregnancies requiring consultant-led antenatal care which should include regular growth scans. The RCOG has produced Study Group guidelines outlining the careplan each woman with twin pregnancy should follow.[46] The first scan at 10–13 weeks should determine viability, chorionicity, and nuchal translucency to assess risk of aneuploidy. Women with a dichorionic twin pregnancy will then have a structural anomaly scan at 20–22 weeks' gestation. Following this, serial fetal growth scans will be performed from 24 weeks

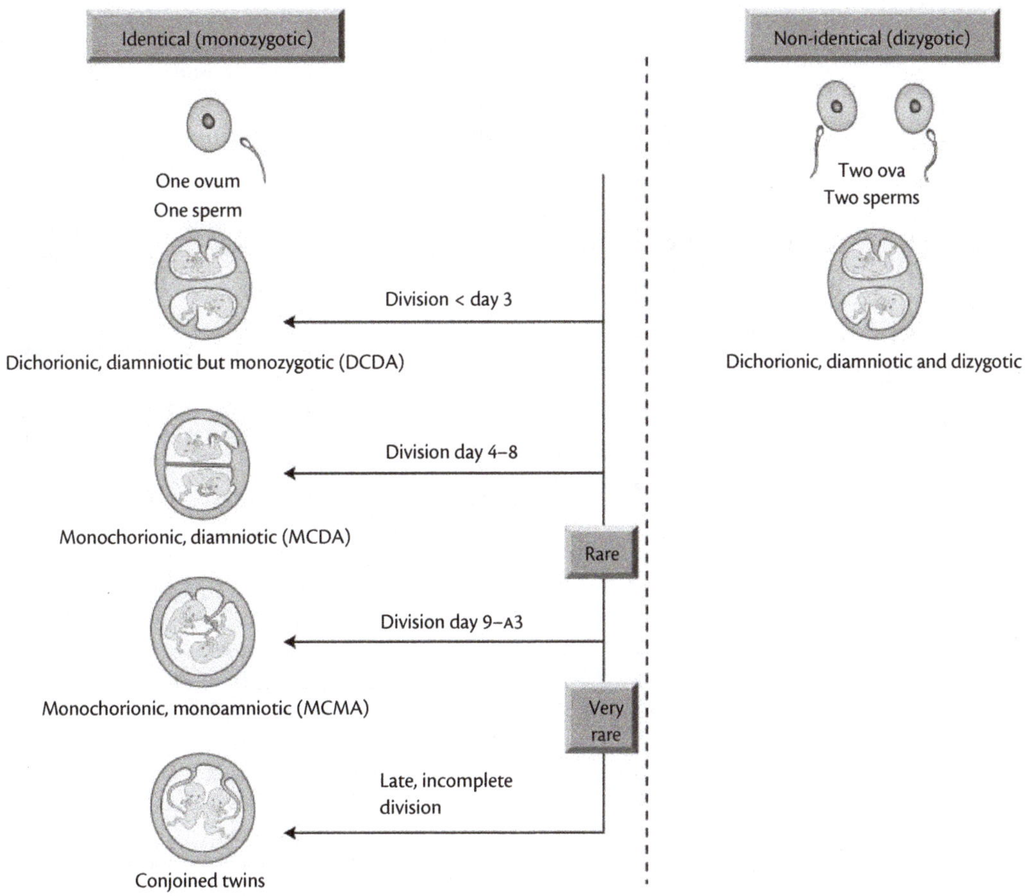

Figure 33.1 Mechanisms of twinning.

at 4-weekly intervals. Blood pressure monitoring and urinalysis should be performed at 20, 24, and 28 weeks' gestation and fortnightly thereafter. Elective delivery is recommended at 37–38 completed weeks' gestation.

For monochorionic twin pregnancies, monitoring is more frequent due to an increased risk of complications. Following the initial scan at 10–13 weeks' gestation, ultrasound surveillance begins at 16 weeks' gestation and 2-weekly thereafter, to highlight any growth discordance or twin-to-twin transfusion syndrome (TTTS; see 'Complications of Monochorionic Twin Pregnancy'). The structural anomaly scan at 20–22 weeks will also include a fetal echocardiogram. As with dichorionic twins, blood pressure monitoring and urinalysis should be performed at 20, 24, and 28 weeks of gestation and fortnightly thereafter. Elective delivery is recommended at 36–37 completed weeks of gestation in uncomplicated monochorionic twin pregnancies.

Complications

There is a higher risk of obstetric complications associated with multiple pregnancy and these can be classed as fetal or maternal, as demonstrated by Table 33.3.

Complications of monochorionic twin pregnancy

A completely separate but serious complication of monochorionic twin pregnancy is TTTS. This affects about 10–15% of monochorionic twins and left untreated has an 80% mortality rate.[47] It is caused by placental vascular anastomoses which result in transfusion of blood from the 'donor' twin to the 'recipient' twin. As a result, the donor twin becomes hypovolaemic, anaemic, and develops growth restriction and oligohydramnios. The recipient twin becomes hypervolaemic and polycythaemic with a large bladder and polyhydramnios. There may be evidence of fetal hydrops in this twin (ascites, pleural and pericardial effusions). The mother may present with a sudden increase in swelling of her abdomen or breathlessness, and urgent ultrasound is advised. Treatment options for TTTS include laser ablation of the placental anastomoses, selective feticide, serial amnioreductions, or septostomy which allows equilibration between the two amniotic sacs. In the incidence of death of a co-twin in a monochorionic pregnancy, an acute TTTS can occur, causing a high risk of death or neurological damage in the surviving twin of up to 50%.

A further complication specific to monochorionic twin pregnancy is twin reversed arterial perfusion sequence (TRAP). This occurs when one twin is acardiac but continues to be partially perfused through vascular connections from the surviving twin. This is a rare complication but one which has a high mortality for the donor twin, usually secondary to cardiac failure and prematurity. Cord ligation has been beneficial in some cases.[45]

Monochorionic monoamniotic twins carry all the risk of complications as already mentioned but with an additional risk of cord entanglement. This may hinder fetal movement and development and complicate labour. For this reason, it is recommended that all monochorionic monoamniotic twins are delivered by elective caesarean delivery at 32 weeks' gestation after corticosteroid administration.[45] Conjoined twins also pose mechanical difficulties for labour and so are delivered by elective caesarean delivery at a time to suit the entire multidisciplinary team including obstetricians, anaesthetists, and paediatric surgeons.

Table 33.3 Risks associated with multiple pregnancy

Maternal risks	Fetal risks
Hyperemesis gravidarum	Increased risk of miscarriage
Anaemia	Congenital abnormalities
Pre-eclampsia	Intrauterine growth restriction
Gestational diabetes	Preterm labour—40% of twins deliver before 37 weeks
Polyhydramnios	Increased perinatal mortality
Placenta praevia	Increased intrauterine death
Antepartum and postpartum haemorrhage	Increased risk of disability
	Increased risk of cerebral palsy

Delivery of twins

It is recommended by the RCOG that dichorionic twins are delivered at 37–38 weeks' gestation. If the presenting twin is cephalic and there are no other complications, a trial of vaginal delivery is encouraged but in some cases the mother may request elective caesarean delivery. Forty per cent of twin pregnancies have both twins in cephalic presentation at term.[43]

When a woman with twin pregnancy presents in labour or for induction of labour, an ultrasound scan should be performed to determine the lie and presentation of the twins. Intravenous access should be obtained with a large-bore cannula and a group and save sample should be taken due to the risk of postpartum haemorrhage. A Syntocinon® infusion should be prepared in advance in anticipation of uterine atony after delivery.

Fetal distress is more common when labouring with a twin pregnancy, and fetal distress in twin two is a concern, particularly after delivery of twin one.[48] For this reason, continuous monitoring is essential throughout labour. Usually the presenting twin is monitored via fetal scalp electrode and twin two is monitored abdominally. Once twin one has delivered vaginally, twin two must be 'stabilized'; this is where the midwife or obstetrician palpates the abdomen keeping the twin stable in a longitudinal lie. Vaginal examination and ultrasound will determine the presentation and station of the second twin. If fetal monitoring of the second twin remains reassuring, labour can be allowed to continue and as the twin descends into the pelvis, amniotomy can be performed. It is usual for contractions to become more infrequent after delivery of twin one and so an infusion of Syntocinon® should always be available. Providing there is no fetal distress of the second twin, there is no specified time to wait before commencing the infusion.

The management of fetal distress in twin two will depend on the presentation and station. If the presenting part is above the ischial spines or if there is transverse lie, a caesarean delivery is indicated. Caesarean delivery for twin two occurs in 10% of twin deliveries.[46] For this reason, some units choose to have mothers deliver in the operating theatre, or have a low threshold for transferring to theatre when the CTG is non-reassuring. Another option would be internal podalic version and total breech extraction. If twin two is cephalic and at the ischial spines or lower, instrumental delivery is indicated for fetal distress.

In uncomplicated monochorionic twin pregnancies, the RCOG recommends that women aim for vaginal delivery unless there is a clinical indication for caesarean delivery such as the presenting twin lying breech. Delivery should be planned for 36–37 weeks' gestation.[45] Continuous surveillance of both twins during labour is essential as there is a small risk of acute transfusion during labour. Some units deliver all monochorionic twins by planned caesarean delivery.

Analgesia and anaesthesia for twin delivery

For women opting for vaginal delivery of twins, epidural anaesthesia is strongly recommended. Twin labour and delivery can be unpredictable. Epidural anaesthesia will keep the mother comfortable during a possibly long labour and two deliveries which may require Syntocinon® augmentation, while being flexible in affording anaesthesia in cases requiring instrumental or caesarean delivery. Anaesthetists should be aware that analgesic requirements may change rapidly according to fetal monitoring and presentation, particularly once twin one is delivered. It is strongly recommended that the anaesthetist stays within the vicinity of the patient delivering twins.

Whether elective or emergency, caesarean delivery may be performed under spinal, epidural, or general anaesthesia. However, because of the increased uterine contents, both fetuses and amniotic fluid, there is a reduced dose requirement of local anaesthesia. This is because the very gravid uterus compresses the vena cava, engorging the epidural vessels and creating effectively a space-occupying lesion in the epidural space. This squeezes the local anaesthetic cephalad and if the standard doses of local anaesthetic are used, the block can rise too high and cause significant hypotension. although a recent study has challenged this.[49]

As with vaginal delivery, there is an increased risk of uterine atony and postpartum haemorrhage therefore all twin deliveries should be followed by administration of a prophylactic Syntocinon infusion. If bleeding continues, further oxytocics may be requested by the obstetrician and in some cases, Bakri or Rusch balloon insertion may be required to tamponade the bleeding. In extreme cases emergency hysterectomy may be necessary. See Chapter 35 for more details.

Key points

- Chorionicity should be determined early and antenatal care tailored accordingly.
- Twin pregnancies are high risk with many potential complications, especially when monochorionic.
- Mode of delivery will depend on the lie of the presenting twin.
- Epidural anaesthesia during labour is advised.
- Local anaesthetic requirements are reduced.
- Postpartum haemorrhage is a serious and common complication and the necessary preparations should be made in anticipation.

Abnormal presentation

The presentation of a fetus is the portion of that fetus which overlies the pelvic inlet. This can be determined via abdominal palpation of the pregnant uterus, vaginal examination, or ultrasound. The presentation may be cephalic, breech, or shoulder. Cephalic presentations can be further divided into vertex, brow, and face presentation.

The lie of the fetus refers to the direction of the fetal spine in relation to the mother's spine and can be longitudinal (in the majority of cases), transverse, or oblique. The lie of the fetus can also be classed as unstable, where it is constantly changing. The recommended method of delivery for transverse, oblique, and unstable lie is caesarean delivery. Abnormal lie and some breech presentations are associated with the risk of cord prolapse therefore all women are warned of this possibility and to present to hospital if membranes have ruptured. This obstetric emergency requires prompt delivery by caesarean delivery, usually under GA.

Abnormal cephalic presentations

The position of the fetus is determined by vaginal examination and describes the cranial sutures of the fetus in relation to the mother's pelvis, for example, the occiput or posterior fontanelle will be anterior, posterior, or transverse. Occipito-posterior (OP) positions are associated with a longer and more painful labour and delay in the second stage. Epidural anaesthesia is strongly recommended for OP labours as not only will it provide good analgesia but also anaesthesia for interventive deliveries which is common in OP presentations. Spontaneous vaginal delivery of this position occurs in one-third of primiparous and 55% of parous women,[50] but in prolonged second stage in OP or occipito-transverse positions, it may be necessary to transfer the woman to theatre for a trial of rotational instrumental delivery. If this is not successful or if the vertex is above the ischial spines, a caesarean delivery will be performed. Therefore, any neuraxial anaesthesia given for a trial of forceps in theatre should have a sufficient block to enable a caesarean delivery.

Face

Face presentation occurs in about 1/500 live births and 70–80% of these can be delivered vaginally.[51] The success of this depends on the position of the chin. Mento-anterior positions (90% of face presentations) tend to be successful whereas mento-posterior positioned babies require delivery by caesarean delivery.

Brow

This is where the head occupies a position midway between full flexion and full extension. Brow presentation occurs in between 1/1000 and 1/3500 deliveries and when persistent, requires caesarean delivery. Spontaneous flexion or extension of the neck may occur during labour, allowing vaginal delivery.[43,51]

Breech presentation

The incidence of breech presentation decreases from about 20% at 28 weeks of gestation to 3–4% at term, as most babies turn spontaneously to the cephalic presentation.[52] Persistent breech presentation is associated with abnormalities of the baby, the amniotic fluid volume, the placental localization, or the uterus (Box 33.1). One per cent of breech deliveries occur in multiple pregnancy, and these rates are rising with the increase in assisted reproduction techniques. There is higher perinatal mortality and morbidity with breech than cephalic presentation, due principally to prematurity, congenital malformations, and birth asphyxia or trauma.[53,54] Caesarean delivery for breech presentation has been suggested as a way of reducing the associated perinatal problems.[54,55]

Breech presentation can be further classified (usually by ultrasound scan) into frank or extended breech, where the legs are

Box 33.1 Fetal abnormalities associated with breech presentation

- Hydrocephalus
- Anencephaly
- Neural tube defects
- Neck masses
- Aneuploidy

flexed at the hips and extended at the knees with the buttocks presenting. This is the most common breech presentation (70% of cases); 15% of cases are flexed breeches with the legs flexed at the knees so buttocks and feet are both presenting, and 15% of cases are footling breeches where one leg is flexed and one extended.

External cephalic version

Women are given the option of ECV which aims to convert a breech to cephalic presentation. Success rates have been reported as between 30% and 80%. Spontaneous reversion to breech presentation after successful ECV occurs in less than 5%.[56,57] The highest success rates are seen with multiparous, non-white women with a relaxed uterus, where the breech is not engaged and the head is easily palpable.[58] Absolute contraindications include antepartum haemorrhage, ruptured membranes, and multiple pregnancy. Relative contraindications include intrauterine growth restriction, reduced liquor volume, and previous caesarean delivery.

The RCOG recommends tocolysis with beta-sympathomimetics at the time of ECV as it has been shown to increase the success rate. Terbutaline or salbutamol may be given subcutaneously or intravenously. The procedure should be offered from 36 weeks' gestation in nulliparous women and from 37 weeks in multiparous women. Women should be counselled that ECV has a very low complication rate, though they should also be aware of the possible complications. These include fetal bradycardia or non-reassuring CTG features which may be transient but in around 1/300 cases persist and require emergency caesarean delivery. The incidence of placental abruption during ECV is 1/1000. For these reasons, ECV should take place in a unit where monitoring is available and arrangements can be made for immediate delivery if necessary. Therefore all women having ECV should be fasted and have been given ranitidine. Women should also be advised that ECV may be painful and that the procedure can be suspended at any point. There is a higher rate of successful ECV with spinal anaesthesia but this has not been adopted by the obstetric community.[59]

Mode of delivery for breech presentation

Women who have breech presentation diagnosed, or those who have had an unsuccessful ECV, should be given information on the options of vaginal breech delivery versus planned caesarean delivery. They should be informed that planned caesarean delivery carries a reduced perinatal mortality and early neonatal morbidity for babies with a breech presentation at term compared with planned vaginal birth.

A systematic review of randomized trials including the Term Breech Trial, compared a policy of intended caesarean delivery with a policy of intended vaginal birth, and involved 2396 participants.[60] Caesarean delivery occurred in 1060/1169 (91%) of those women allocated to planned caesarean delivery and 550/1227 (45%) of those allocated to a vaginal delivery protocol. Perinatal or neonatal death (excluding fatal anomalies) or short-term neonatal morbidity was reduced with a policy of planned caesarean delivery (relative risk (RR) 0.33; 95% CI 0.19–0.56) and perinatal or neonatal death alone (excluding fatal anomalies) was reduced with a policy of planned caesarean delivery (RR 0.29; 95% CI 0.10–0.86). Although these conclusions are still somewhat disputed,[61] caesarean delivery is recommended for breech presentation. However, there is still a place for vaginal breech delivery, for example, in the case of twin two, in advanced labour where caesarean delivery would be technically difficult, or on maternal request. See Box 33.2 for factors regarded as unfavourable for vaginal breech delivery.

Caesarean delivery for breech presentation

According to the RCOG, women should be informed that planned caesarean delivery for breech presentation carries a small additional risk of serious immediate complications compared with planned vaginal birth, in terms of abdominal pain, but no there is no evidence of any additional risk to their long-term health. Spinal anaesthesia is the usual technique for caesarean delivery in breech presentation. Occasionally, abdominal delivery of the fetus may be difficult if skin and uterine incisions are insufficient, or if there are fetal abnormalities such as hydrocephalus. In certain circumstances, the obstetrician may request provision of a uterine relaxant, such as glyceryl trinitrate or terbutaline. In some cases, women who have opted for a planned caesarean delivery go into spontaneous labour. Each of these cases is managed individually and many will proceed to vaginal breech delivery if labour is too advanced.

Vaginal delivery for breech presentation

Vaginal breech delivery may occur in three different ways. The first is spontaneous breech delivery where there is no manipulation or traction other than support of the infant's body. In assisted breech delivery, the infant is delivered spontaneously as far as the umbilicus and the chest and after-coming head are

Box 33.2 Factors regarded as unfavourable for vaginal breech birth

Factors include the following:

- Other contraindications to vaginal birth (e.g. placenta praevia, compromised fetal condition)
- Clinically inadequate pelvis
- Footling or kneeling breech presentation
- Large baby (usually defined as >3800 g)
- Growth-restricted baby (usually defined as <2000 g)
- Hyperextended fetal neck in labour (diagnosed with ultrasound or X-ray where ultrasound is not available)
- Lack of presence of a clinician trained in vaginal breech delivery
- Previous caesarean section.

delivered with the assistance of the obstetrician. Total breech extraction is only really ever used for delivery of a second twin, where the obstetrician applies traction on the feet and ankles to deliver the entire body of the infant. The RCOG states that spontaneous delivery of the trunk and limbs is preferable. If there is delay in delivery of the arms, they may be delivered by sweeping them across the baby's face and downwards or by the Lovset manoeuvre (rotation of the baby to facilitate delivery of the arms). For delivery of the after-coming head, suprapubic pressure by an assistant may be used to assist flexion of the head, and the Mauriceau–Smellie–Veit manoeuvre should be considered. This involves two fingers of the right hand placed over the maxilla and two fingers of the left hand at the back of the head to flex it[52,62] (Figure 33.2). Forceps are occasionally used to facilitate delivery of the after-coming head.

If there is delay in the second stage of labour, caesarean delivery should be considered, as this would be a sign of relative fetopelvic disproportion. In cases of fetal head entrapment, Dührssen incisions to the cervix may be necessary, at the 4 and 7 o'clock positions; however, this is associated with genitourinary trauma and haemorrhage. Alternatives would be administering a smooth muscle relaxant such as glyceryl trinitrate, or performing an emergency caesarean delivery.

Anaesthesia for vaginal breech delivery

There is no evidence that epidural analgesia is essential,[52] but certainly women would be given this option during labour for vaginal breech delivery. As well as adequate pain relief, its advantages would also be the inhibition of early pushing (as pushing past a cervix which is not fully dilated has implications for fetal head entrapment), a relaxed pelvic floor and perineum for delivery, and the option of extending the block in cases requiring emergency caesarean delivery.

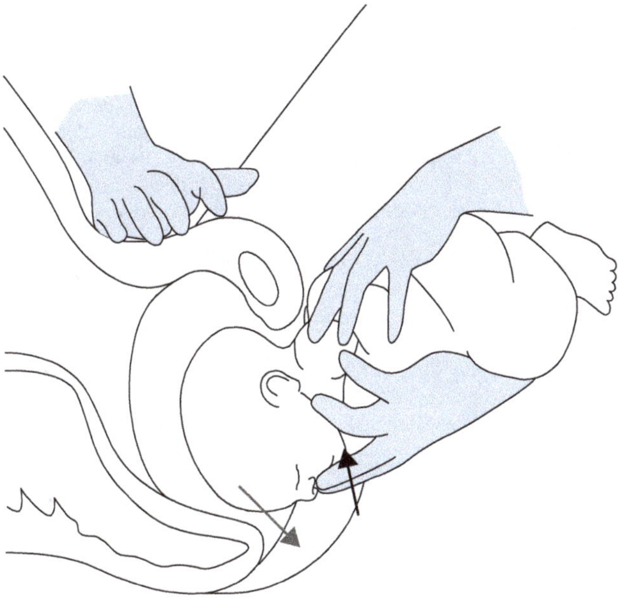

Figure 33.2 Delivery of the head by jaw flexion and shoulder traction.
Reproduced with permission from Keith Edmonds, *Textbook of Obstetrics and Gynaecology*, Eighth Edition, John Wiley & Sons, Oxford, UK, Copyright © 2012.

Other abnormal presentations

Transverse lie

Transverse lie or shoulder presentation is principally managed by performing caesarean delivery. This is most difficult if the baby is 'back-down' in which case a classical uterine incision may be made. Vaginal delivery may be possible following successful ECV or following internal podalic version and breech extraction of a second twin.

Compound presentation

Compound presentation is where an extremity (usually an upper extremity) is prolapsed alongside the main presenting fetal part and occurs in 1/400 to 1/1200 deliveries. Complications include umbilical cord prolapse in 10–20% for which immediate caesarean delivery is required, and neurological or musculoskeletal damage to the involved extremity.[51] However, labour and delivery can occur safely and manipulation of the prolapsed extremity should be avoided.

Key points

- Abnormal presentation can take many forms: abnormal cephalic presentations, breech, transverse, oblique, and compound.
- Women should be offered information on the risks and benefits on modes of delivery for breech presentation.

Conclusion

In conclusion, patients with preterm labour, multiple gestation, and pregnancies with malpresentation are all high-risk obstetric cases requiring a multidisciplinary approach using local and national guidelines. This chapter has endeavoured to highlight the important issues in each of these high-risk situations to enable safe and effective clinical care.

References

1. Lumley J. Defining the problem: the epidemiology of preterm birth. *BJOG* 2003; 110:3–7.
2. Goldenberg RL, Culhane JF, Iams, JD, *et al.* Epidemiology and causes of preterm birth. *Lancet* 2008; 371:5–84.
3. Draper ES, Manktelow B, Field DJ, *et al.* Prediction of survival for preterm births by weight and gestational age: retrospective population based study. *BMJ* 1999:319:1093–7.
4. Hack M, Taylor HG. Perinatal brain injury in preterm infants and later neurobehavioral function. *JAMA* 2000; 284:1973–4.
5. Steer PJ. The epidemiology of preterm labour – why have advances not equated to reduced incidence? *BJOG* 2006; 113 Suppl 3:1–3.
6. Goldenberg RL, Hauth JC, Andrews WW. Intrauterine infection and preterm delivery. *N Engl J Med* 2000; 342:1500–7.
7. Yoon BH, Jun JK, Romero R, *et al.* Amniotic fluid inflammatory cytokines (interleukin-6, interleukin-1beta, and tumor necrosis factor-alpha), brain white matter lesions, and cerebral palsy. *Am J Obstet Gynecol* 1997; 177:19–26.
8. Yoon BH, Romero R, Jun JK, *et al.* Amniotic fluid cytokines (interleukin-6, tumor necrosis factor-alpha, interleukin-1 beta, and interleukin-8) and the risk for the development of bronchopulmonary dysplasia. *Am J Obstet Gynecol* 1997; 177:825–30.
9. Yoon BH, Park CW, Chaiorapongsa T. Intrauterine infection and the development of cerebral palsy. *BJOG* 2003; 110 Suppl 20:124–7.

10. Taylor D, Kenyon S, Tarnow-Mordi W. Infection and preterm labour. *BJOG* 1997; 104:1338–40.
11. Cram LF, Zapata MI, Toy EC, *et al.* Genitourinary infections and their association with preterm labor. *Am Fam Physician* 2002; 65:241–8.
12. Pschirrer ER, Monga M. Risk factors for preterm labor. *Clin Obstet Gynecol* 2000; 43:727–34.
13. Iams JD, Romero R. Preterm birth. In Gabbe SG, Niebyl JR, Simpson JL (eds) *Obstetrics: Normal and Problem Pregnancies* (5th ed). Philadelphia, PA: Churchill Livingstone Elsevier; 2007:669–712.
14. Moutquin JM. Socio-economic and psychosocial factors in the management and prevention of preterm labour. *BJOG* 2003; 110:56–60.
15. Mercer BM, Miodovnik M, Thurnau GR, *et al.* Antibiotic therapy for reduction of infant morbidity after preterm premature rupture of membranes. *JAMA* 1997; 278:989–95.
16. Royal College of Obstetricians and Gynaecologists. *Preterm Premature Rupture of Membranes.* Green-top Guideline No. 44. London: RCOG; 2006.
17. Kenyon S, Boulvain M, Neilson J. Antibiotics for preterm rupture of membranes. *Cochrane Database Syst Rev* 2003; 2:CD001058.
18. Royal College of Obstetricians and Gynaecologists. *Cervical Cerclage.* Green-top Guideline No. 60. London: RCOG; 2011.
19. Di Renzo GC, Roura LC. The European Association of Perinatal Medicine-Study Group on Preterm Birth. Guidelines for the management of spontaneous preterm labor. *J Perinat Med* 2006; 34:359–66.
20. Herbst A, Nilsson C. Diagnosis of early preterm labour. *BJOG* 2006; 113:60–7.
21. Honest H, Bachmann LM, Gupta JK, *et al.* Accuracy of cervicovaginal fetal fibronectin test in predicting risk of spontaneous preterm birth: systematic review. *BMJ* 2002; 325:301.
22. Smith V, Devane D, Begley CM, *et al.* A systematic review and quality assessment of systematic reviews of fetal fibronectin and transvaginal length for predicting preterm birth. *Eur J Obstet Gynaecol Repord Biol* 2007; 133:134–42.
23. Roberts D, Dalziel SR. Antenatal corticosteroids for accelerating fetal lung maturation for women at risk of preterm birth. *Cochrane Database Syst Rev* 2006; 3:CD004454.
24. Royal College of Obstetricians and Gynaecologists. *Antenatal Corticosteroids to Reduce Neonatal Morbidity and Mortality.* Green-top Guideline No. 7. London: RCOG; 2010.
25. Kenyo SL, Taylor DJ, Tarnow-Mordi W. Broad-spectrum antibiotics for preterm, prelabour rupture of fetal membranes. The ORACLE I randomised trial. ORACLE Collaborative Group. *Lancet* 2001; 257:979–88.
26. King J, Flenady V. Antibiotics for preterm labour with intact membranes. *Cochrane Database Syst Rev* 2000; 2:CD000246.
27. Gyetvai K, Hannah ME, Hodnett ED, *et al.* Tocolytics for preterm labor: a systematic review. *Obstet Gynecol* 1999; 94:869–77.
28. Royal College of Obstetricians and Gynaecologists. *Tocolysis for Women in Preterm Labour.* Green-top Guideline No. 1B. London: RCOG; 2011.
29. Duckitt K, Thornton S. Nitric oxide donors for the treatment of preterm labour. *Cochrane Database Syst Rev* 2002; 3:CD002860.
30. King JF, Flenady VJ, Papatsonis DN, *et al.* Calcium channel blockers for inhibiting preterm labour. *Cochrane Database Syst Rev* 2003; 1:CD002255.
31. Anotayanonth S, Subhedar NV, Garner P, *et al.* Betamimetics for inhibiting preterm labour. *Cochrane Database Syst Rev* 2004; 4:CD004352.
32. Crowther CA, Hiller JE, Doyle LW. Magnesium sulphate for preventing preterm birth in threatened preterm labour. *Cochrane Database Syst Rev* 2002; 4:CD001060.
33. King J, Flenady V, Cole S, *et al.* Cyclo-oxygenase (COX) inhibitors for treating preterm labour. *Cochrane Database Syst Rev* 2005; 2:CD001992.
34. de Heus R, Mol BW, Erwich JJ, *et al.* Adverse drug reactions to tocolytic treatment for preterm labour: Prospective Cohort Study. *BMJ* 2009; 338:b744.
35. Haas DM, Caldwell DM, Kirkpatrick P, *et al.* Tocolytic therapy for preterm delivery: systematic review and network meta-analysis. *BMJ* 2012; 345:e6226.
36. Royal College of Obstetricians and Gynaecologists. *Magnesium Sulphate to Prevent Cerebral Palsy following Preterm Birth.* Scientific Impact Paper No. 29. London: RCOG; 2011.
37. Hollander DI, Nagey DA, Pupkin MJ. Magnesium sulfate and ritodrine hydrochloride: a randomized comparison. *Am J Obstet Gynecol* 1987; 156:631–7.
38. Chau AC, Gabert HA, Miller JM Jr. A prospective comparison of terbutaline and magnesium for tocolysis. *Obstet Gynecol* 1992; 80:847–51.
39. Goldenberg RL. The management of preterm labour. *ACOG* 2002; 100:1020–37.
40. Hollmen AI, Jouppila R, Jouppila P, *et al.* Effect of extradural analgesia using bupivacaine and 2-chloroprocaine on intervillous blood flow during normal labour. *Br J Anaesth* 1982; 54:837–42.
41. Rolbin SH, Cohen MM, Levinton CM, *et al.* The premature infant: anesthesia for cesarean delivery. *Anesth Analg* 1994; 78:912–17.
42. Ben-Ami M, Giladi Y, Shalev E. The combination of magnesium sulphate and nifedipine: a cause of neuromuscular blockade. *Br J Obstet Gynaecol* 1994; 101:262–3.
43. Collins S, Arulkumeran S, Hayes K, *et al.* (eds). *Oxford Handbook of Obstetrics and Gynaecology* (2nd ed). Oxford: Oxford University Press; 2008.
44. Impey L, Child T (eds). *Obstetrics and Gynaecology* (4th ed). Chichester: John Wiley & Sons; 2012.
45. Magowan BA, Owen P, Drife J (eds). *Clinical Obstetrics and Gynaecology* (2nd ed). Edinburgh: Saunders Elsevier; 2009.
46. Royal College of Obstetricians and Gynaecologists. *Consensus Views Arising from the 50th Study Group: Multiple Pregnancy.* London: RCOG; 2006.
47. Royal College of Obstetricians and Gynaecologists. *Management of Monochorionic Twin Pregnancy.* Green-top Guideline No. 51. London: RCOG; 2008.
48. Wen SW, Fung KF, Oppenheimer L, *et al.* Occurrence and predictors of cesarean delivery for the second twin after vaginal delivery of the first twin. *Obstet Gynecol* 2004; 103:413–19.
49. Ngan Kee WD, Khaw KS, Ng FF, *et al.* A Prospective comparison of vasopressor requirement and hemodynamic changes during spinal anesthesia for cesarean delivery in patients with multiple gestation versus singleton pregnancy. *Anesth Analg* 2007; 104:407–11.
50. Fitzpatrick M, McQuillan K, O'Herlihy C. Influence of persistent occiput posterior position on delivery outcome. *Obstet Gynecol* 2001; 98:1027–31.
51. Lanni S, Seeds J. Malpresentations. In Gabbe SF, Niebyl JR, Simpson JL (eds) *Obstetrics: Normal and Problem Pregnancies* (5th ed). New York: Churchill Livingstone; 2007:428–55.
52. Royal College of Obstetricians and Gynaecologists. *The Management of Breech Presentation.* Green-top Guideline No. 20b. London: RCOG; 2006.
53. Pritchard JA, MacDonald PC. Dystocia caused by abnormalities in presentation, position, or development of the fetus. In Pritchard JA, MacDonald PC (eds) *Williams Obstetrics.* Norwalk, CT: Appleton-Century-Crofts; 1980:787–96.
54. Cheng M, Hannah M. Breech delivery at term: a critical review of the literature. *Obstet Gynecol* 1993; 82:605–18.
55. Ghosh MK. Breech presentation: evolution of management. *J Reprod Med* 2005; 50:108–16.
56. Lumley J. Any room left for disagreement about assisting breech births at term? *Lancet* 2000; 356:1369–70.
57. Su M, Hannah WJ, Willan A, *et al.* Planned caesarean section decreases the risk of adverse perinatal outcome due to both

labour and delivery complications in the Term Breech Trial. *BJOG* 2004;111:1065–74.

58. Hannah ME, Hannah WJ, Hodnett ED, *et al.* Outcomes at 3 months after planned cesarean vs planned vaginal delivery for breech presentation at term: the International Randomized Term Breech Trial. *JAMA* 2002; 287:1822–31.
59. Goetzinger KR, Harper LM, Tuuli MG, *et al.* Effect of regional anesthesia on the success rate of external cephalic version: a systematic review and meta-analysis. *Obstet Gynecol* 2011; 118(5):1137–44.
60. Hofmeyr GJ, Hannah ME. Planned caesarean section for term breech delivery. *Cochrane Database Syst Rev* 2003; 2:CD000166.
61. Van Roosmalan J, Rosendaal F. There is still room for disagreement about vaginal delivery of breech infants at term. *BJOG* 2002; 109:967–9.
62. Edmonds K (ed). *Dewhurst's Textbook of Obstetrics and Gynaecology* (8th ed). Edinburgh: Wiley & Sons; 2012.

CHAPTER 34

Sepsis in obstetrics

Nuala Lucas, Colleen D. Acosta, and Marian Knight

Introduction

Sepsis in obstetrics is an important cause of maternal mortality and morbidity worldwide, accounting for 15% of all maternal deaths.[1] In the United Kingdom, the maternal mortality rate from sepsis has almost tripled in the last 25 years[2] and in the penultimate Confidential Enquiry into Maternal Death in the United Kingdom, sepsis was the leading cause of direct maternal death. There has also been an increase in the incidence and severity of sepsis morbidity in other parts of the resourced world including other European countries and the United States.[3–5] The Scottish Confidential Audit of Severe Maternal Morbidity showed a rate of septicaemic shock of 0.13/1000 maternities in the 2003–2005 triennium.[6] In a retrospective analysis covering 10 years between 1998 and 2008 and using data from the Nationwide Inpatient Sample, Bauer et al. demonstrated that of 44,999,260 hospitalizations for delivery, sepsis complicated 1/3333 (95% confidence interval (CI) 1/3151–1/3540) deliveries with severe sepsis complicating 1/10,823 (95% CI 1/10,000–1/11,792) deliveries.[5]

Sepsis in the obstetric population poses significant challenges: the physiological changes of pregnancy may mask the clinical signs of sepsis and lead to a delay in diagnosis and treatment. When sepsis occurs in the antenatal period, maternal deterioration can quickly lead to fetal compromise. Early recognition and diagnosis with rapidly instituted therapy are key to ensuring a good outcome.

History of obstetric sepsis

> There was never a time when this disease did not exist.
>
> Nathaniel Hulme, *A Treatise on the Puerperal Fever* (London, 1772)

Like all infectious diseases, the history of 'childbed fever' is a tragic one, rooted in the incomprehension of contagiousness. Historically, childbed fever referred to puerperal sepsis due to infection, primarily by Group A *Streptococcus* (GAS), contracted from aseptic, unsanitary birthing conditions. Until the recent era of antibiotics, puerperal sepsis was the leading cause of maternal mortality worldwide. In eighteenth-century England, sepsis accounted for approximately 50% of all maternal deaths.[7] During this time and up until the latter part of the nineteenth century, the concept of germs or how infection was spread was unknown or misunderstood. Hence, there was no form of antisepsis at this time. Births were attended to by midwives or accoucheurs (licensed physicians with some training in midwifery), and it was these medical professionals who unknowingly acted as vectors of transmission. As obstetrics became a more formal part of medical practice in mid-nineteenth-century Europe and America, physicians reluctantly began to accept the contagious nature of puerperal infection. Louis Pasteur and Robert Koch confirmed this several decades later with their development of germ theory. After the advent of penicillin in 1944, severe puerperal sepsis was finally relegated to the rare case study in most obstetricians' careers—until recently.

Although insufficient written accounts were made or have survived from before the seventeenth century to make an estimate of the burden of maternal sepsis, it is generally thought that the incidence was relatively rare. This is attributed to the fact that women gave birth at home and were usually attended to by another female family member.[7] In seventeenth-century Europe however, several determinants of maternal health changed, and so too did rates of childbed fever.

Seventeenth-century Europe saw the burgeoning of hospital establishments and with it the beginning of 'lying-in' hospitals. One of the first schools of midwifery and lying-in wards was established at the Hôtel Dieu Hospital in Paris in 1610.

Although viewed by impoverished women as preferable to giving birth in squalor outside of the hospital, accounts of conditions inside the hospital were appalling. As the only hospital in the city, it was severely overcrowded with often more than 2000 patients occupying its 1200 beds.[8] Most patients shared beds and it was not uncommon to find a live patient occupying a bed with another who had already died.[8] At this time, obstetricians or accoucheurs were still not recognized in the medical profession. Obstetric surgery was performed by barber-surgeons, and physicians were seen as superior to either barber-surgeons or midwives. When physicians on occasion had to visit the wards, it is said that they held sponges soaked in vinegar or perfume to their noses to block the vile stench of the sick and dying destitute.[8]

It was in these noxious wards, where mortality is estimated to have been one in four to five,[9] that conditions were rife for epidemics of childbed fever. After the establishment of the Hôtel Dieu lying-in ward in Paris, other lying-in wards and hospitals were founded throughout the eighteenth century in many European cities including Berlin, Vienna, Amsterdam, Stockholm, Copenhagen, Dublin, and London. The first documented epidemic of childbed fever occurred at the Hôtel Dieu in 1646. Subsequent epidemics followed in Paris and other European cities throughout the eighteenth and nineteenth centuries. In the 1770s, the highest annual mortality rate during an epidemic year in the London General Lying-in Hospital was 398/10,000 deliveries.[7] In the Vienna Maternity Hospital during the 1820s, the highest annual mortality rate of an epidemic year was 745/10,000, and in the Paris Maternité during the 1830s the highest annual mortality rate of an epidemic year was 880/10,000.[7] These rates compare sharply with those of poor women attended to at home by charity midwives. For example, from 1831 to 1843, the rate of mortality due to puerperal sepsis among home births attended to by the Royal Maternity Charity in London was 10/10,000 births, while the mortality rate at the London General Lying-in Hospital was over 600/10,000 births.[7] During epidemic periods, case fatality rates in lying-in hospitals could soar to over 80%. In two of the most devastating epidemics, in the Hôtel Dieu in 1746 and another in Edinburgh, the case fatality rate was 100%—every woman in the wards died.[7]

These epidemics are today widely accepted as having been caused by GAS, mainly due to the fact that puerperal fever epidemics closely correlated with other less invasive GAS infections, particularly erysipelas. In lying-in hospitals midwives, barber-surgeons or accoucheurs would carry out frequent vaginal examinations and successively deliver women without any form of antisepsis in between. In addition, because women were crowded onto the wards and often shared beds, direct transmission of GAS from one woman, with either erysipelas or puerperal fever, to their bed-partner would have been likely.

As accounts of epidemics in lying-in hospitals and towns became more frequently known, what did people think caused this illness? Physicians and midwives agreed that puerperal sepsis was in some way contagious and seasonal, peaking in the winter. Germ theory, however, was not developed until the late nineteenth century. In 1843, Oliver Wendell Holmes published the results of a scholarly review of all published reports of puerperal fever epidemics in the *New England Quarterly Journal of Medicine*. He emphasized the thesis of his work, which was:

> The disease known as puerperal fever is so far contagious as to be frequently carried from patient to patient by physicians and nurses.[10,11]

He went on to write:

> The time has come when the existence of a private pestilence in the sphere of a single physician should be looked upon not as a misfortune, but a crime; and in the knowledge of such occurrences, the duties of the practitioner in his profession, should give way to his paramount obligations to society.[10,11]

Almost at the same time, a similar story was unfolding independently in Vienna. In the 1850s, the Vienna Lying-in hospital was the largest in the world with approximately 7000 births per year.[7] Because of the large volume of patients, in 1833 the hospital was divided into two clinics which admitted patients on alternating days. In 1839, one clinic was allocated to serve as the teaching hospital for male medical students training to be obstetricians, and the other was allocated to female midwifery students. After the teaching allocation, the mortality rate of the physicians' clinic rose to three times that of the midwifery clinic (984/10,000 deliveries vs. 388/10,000 deliveries).[7] In 1846 a physician by the name of Ignaz Semmelweis was appointed as assistant to the physicians' teaching clinic. He soon realized that the mortality difference was a result of medical students and physicians going directly from postmortem dissections to examinations on the wards without washing their hands in between.

Despite dogged resistance to Holmes and Semmelweis, the climate of opinion eventually swayed in the latter half of the nineteenth century. This occurred for several reasons. Firstly, Holmes, Semmelweis and their predecessors had created enough controversy on the topic of contagion and antisepsis to begin to cast doubt in budding and open-minded obstetric practitioners. Secondly, the vehicle of transmission was eventually confirmed by the development of germ theory by Louis Pasteur in 1865 and Robert Koch in the 1870s and 1880s. Lastly, the introduction and acceptance of antisepsis in surgery and childbirth by Joseph Lister in the 1860s resulted in a remarkable decrease in puerperal morbidity and mortality that continued into the twentieth century.

At the turn of the century until the introduction of sulphonamides in 1936, rates of puerperal sepsis mortality were on average 175 per 100,000 births per year in England and Wales.[12] From 1936 to 1943, they had fallen to below 30/100,000, which is a testament to the impact of sulphonamides. By 1950, after the introduction of penicillin, the rate was four and by 1960 there was only one death per 100,000 births.[7] Between 1985 and 1987, the rate of death from puerperal sepsis in England was nearly zero (Figure 34.1).[7] This dramatic decrease in puerperal sepsis mortality was mirrored in the United States and the rest of Europe.

However, since the 1980s there has been an increase in the maternal death rate from sepsis (Figure 34.2). This was first highlighted by the UK Confidential Enquiry into Maternal Death covering the 2006–2008 triennium.[2] In this report, sepsis was noted to be the leading cause of direct maternal deaths, accounting for 29 deaths (26 'direct' deaths and a further three deaths classified as 'late direct'). This was in the context of a decline in maternal deaths from other causes, notably thromboembolic disease and haemorrhage (Figure 34.3).[2] Bauer et al. used data from the Nationwide Inpatient Sample in the United States to investigate the frequency and trends in maternal morbidity and mortality from sepsis. They found that sepsis-related death complicated 1/105,263 (95% CI 1/83,333–1/131,579) deliveries.[5]

Definitions

There is currently no universally accepted definition of sepsis in obstetric practice. Various terms are used interchangeably but there are important distinctions. 'Infection' describes a microbial phenomenon characterized by an inflammatory response to the presence of microorganisms or the invasion of normally sterile host tissue by these organisms. Bacteraemia describes the presence of viable bacteria in the blood.

The term sepsis includes illness that ranges from minor signs and symptoms through to organ dysfunction and shock. The term puerperal sepsis is still used to describe sepsis occurring after delivery and the World Health Organization (WHO) has defined it as 'infection of the genital tract occurring at any time between rupture of membranes or labour, and the 42nd day postpartum', in which two or more of the following are present (Box 34.1).[13]

A widely used definition for sepsis in the non-pregnant patient came from the American College of Chest Physicians and the Society of Critical Care Medicine (Box 34.2).[14] This was modified in 2001 by the International Sepsis Definition Forum to include alterations in physiological variables, in order to more accurately convey the clinical experience. However, because of the physiological changes of pregnancy and particularly those around the time of delivery, this definition lacks validity in obstetric patients.

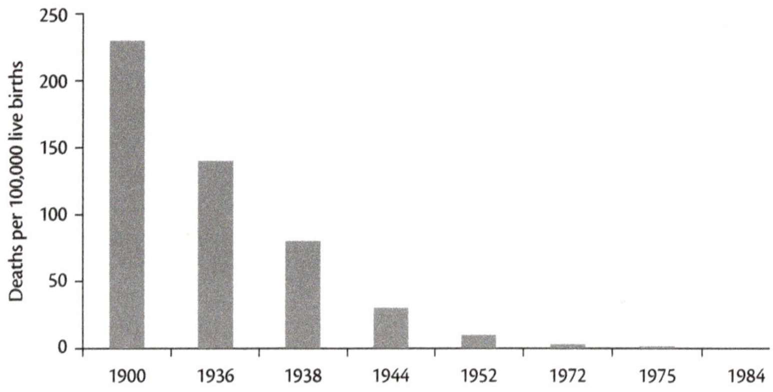

Figure 34.1 Mortality rates from puerperal sepsis in England and Wales 1900–1984.
Data from: Loudon I. The Tragedy of Childbed Fever. 1st ed. Oxford University Press, USA; 2000; and UK Confidential Enquiries 1972, 1975 and 1984.

There are various other reasons that add to the difficulty of defining sepsis in obstetric practice. Sepsis may arise in an obstetric patient at any time: before delivery, during labour, or in the postnatal period. In addition, sepsis in obstetric patients can arise from many sources and is not limited to infections arising from the genital tract. This difficulty in reaching a definition is demonstrated by the organization of cases in the UK Confidential Enquiry reports. Deaths due to group A beta-haemolytic *Streptococcus pyogenes*, as well as other infections related to pregnancy or delivery, are classified as direct deaths, whereas deaths from infections unrelated to the genital tract such as pneumococcal meningitis and HIV disease are classified as indirect maternal deaths. A new pathological classification has been proposed for future confidential enquiries.[2]

The WHO Technical Working Group has introduced the term puerperal infections as a more general term than puerperal sepsis, to include not only infections related to genital tract sepsis, but also all extragenital infections and incidental infections (Box 34.3).[13]

The immune system in pregnancy

Pregnancy has traditionally been viewed as an immunocompromised state arising as a result of the necessity not to immunologically reject the fetus, and therefore placing the mother at increased risk of infectious diseases. However, there is now a wealth of evidence to suggest that rather than being an immunosuppressed state, pregnancy presents a modified immune state whereby there may be contrasting responses to different infections, responses that are also determined by the stage of pregnancy.[15,16,17] From a logical and evolutionary perspective a successful pregnancy is key to the conservation of the species and it has been suggested by Wilson that pregnancy is a 'paradoxical immune state where foreign tissue is not only tolerated but nurtured'.[18]

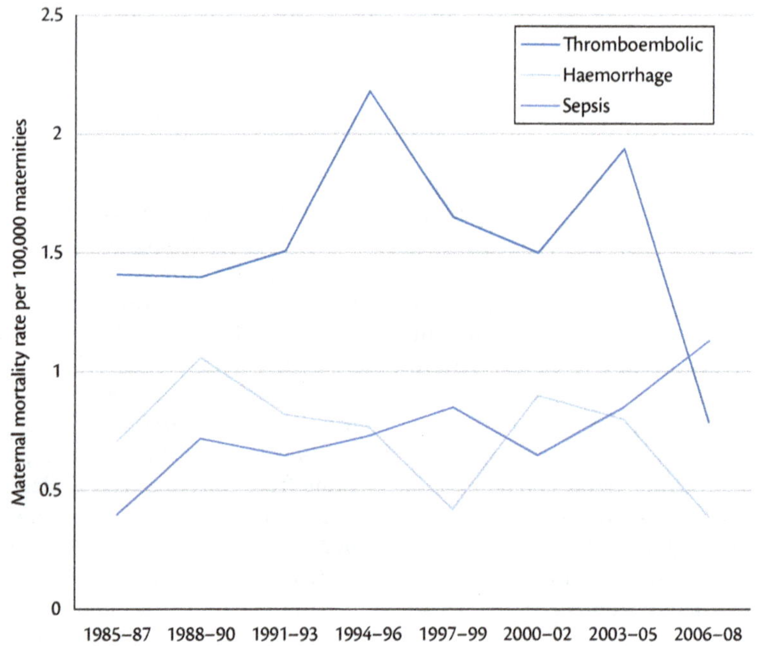

Figure 34.2 Causes of direct maternal death in the United Kingdom 1985–2008.
Reproduced from Confidential Enquiry on Maternal and Child Health, Saving mothers iives: reviewing maternal deaths to make motherhood safer 2006–2008, *BJOG: An International Journal of Obstetrics and Gynaecology*, 118, pp. 1–203, Copyright 2011, with permission from Centre for Maternal and Child Enquiries (CMACE), BJOG, and Wiley.

Box 34.1 WHO definition of puerperal sepsis

- Pelvic pain
- Fever
- Abnormal vaginal discharge
- Abnormal smell of discharge
- Delay in postpartum reduction of size of uterus.

Reprinted from *The Prevention and Management of Puerperal Infections. Report of a technical working group*, WHO, p.3 Copyright (1992).

A competent immune response is essential to protect the mother directly and the fetus indirectly. The immune response depends on either cell-mediated immunity (particularly T lymphocytes) or the humoral response (antibodies secreted by B lymphocytes and plasma cells). During pregnancy, progesterone and oestrogen reduce T-cell proliferation and there is consequently a reduction in cell-mediated immunity which might otherwise prove harmful to the fetus. The maternal immune system is therefore biased towards humoral immunity.[19] Coupled with this is the developing active immune system of the fetus, which will also modify the maternal response to infection.

Box 34.2 American College of Chest Physicians and Society of Critical Care Medicine definitions related to sepsis

Systemic inflammatory response syndrome

Systemic inflammatory response syndrome (SIRS) is a widespread inflammatory response to a variety of severe clinical insults. This syndrome is clinically recognized by the presence of two or more of the following:

- Temperature > 38°C or < 36°C
- Heart rate > 90 beats/min
- Respiratory rate > 20 breaths/min or $PaCO_2$ < 32 mmHg
- White blood cells > 12 × 10^9/dL or < 4 × 10^9/dL or > 10% immature (band) forms.

Sepsis

Sepsis is the systemic response to infection. Thus in sepsis, the clinical signs describing SIRS are present together with definitive evidence of infection.

Severe sepsis

Sepsis is considered severe when it is associated with organ dysfunction, hypoperfusion, or hypotension. The manifestations of hypoperfusion may include, but are not limited to, lactic acidosis, oliguria, or an acute alteration in mental status.

Septic shock

Septic shock is sepsis with hypotension despite adequate fluid resuscitation. It includes perfusion abnormalities such as lactic acidosis, oliguria, or an acute alteration in mental status. Patients receiving inotropic or vasopressor agents may not necessarily be hypotensive at the time that perfusion abnormalities are present.

Reprinted from *Chest*, 101, 6, Bone RC, Balk RA, Cerra FB, et al. Definitions for sepsis and organ failure and guidelines for the use of innovative therapies in sepsis. The ACCP/SCCM Consensus Conference Committee, pp. 1644–55. Copyright 1992 American College of Chest Physicians.

Box 34.3 World Health Organization definition of puerperal infections

Infections of the genitourinary system related to labour, delivery and the puerperium:

Infections related to the uterus and its associated structures (endometritis)

Infections related to the urinary tract

Infections specifically related to the birth process but not of the genitourinary system:

e.g. breast abscess

Incidental infections:

e.g. malaria, respiratory tract infections

Reprinted from *The prevention and management of puerperal infections: report of a technical working group*, Geneva, 20–22 May 1992, Technical Working Group on the Prevention and Management of Puerperal Infections (1992: Geneva, Switzerland) World Health Organization. Maternal Health and Safe Motherhood Programme, Copyright (1995) WHO.

Three distinct immunological phases have been described in pregnancy, roughly corresponding with the first, second, and third trimesters, and associated with dramatic changes in cytokine levels.[17] The combined effect of these interactions serves to explain why pregnancy women may exhibit a diverse response to infection, depending not only on the infecting organism but also on the stage of the pregnancy, for example, pregnant women living in malarial endemic areas are more susceptible to malarial infection in the first half of pregnancy and this susceptibility decreases as the pregnancy progresses.[20]

Risk factors for sepsis in obstetrics

Sepsis can arise at any time during pregnancy and the puerperium, and may develop as a result of bacteraemia (although bacteraemia does not always lead to sepsis), or as a result of local infection. Risk factors for maternal sepsis may be divided into intrinsic patient factors and obstetric factors, and these are summarized in Box 34.4. In addition, women from poor socioeconomic backgrounds are at greater risk of sepsis although the mechanisms are unclear.[21] Although none of the women who died from sepsis in the 2006–2008 UK Confidential Enquiry report were obese, obesity remains a significant risk factor for obstetric sepsis; in the 2003–2005 report, the majority of the women who died from sepsis were obese.[22] More recently in a Scottish population-based case–control study, obese women had twice the odds of uncomplicated sepsis, that is, with no diagnosis of septic shock or additional organ dysfunction (adjusted odds ratio (aOR) 2.12; 95% CI 1.14–3.89) compared with women of normal weight.[23] The same study also identified other significant risk factors as age less than 25 years (aOR 5.15; 95% CI 2.43–10.90) and multiparity (aOR for uncomplicated sepsis and severe sepsis, 6.29, 12.04 respectively). It

Box 34.4 Risk factors for sepsis in obstetrics

Obstetric factors

Amniocentesis, and other invasive intrauterine procedures

Cervical suture

Prolonged rupture of membranes

Prolonged labour with multiple (>5) vaginal examinations

Vaginal trauma

Caesarean delivery

Operative vaginal delivery

Retained products of conception after miscarriage or delivery.

Patient factors

Obesity

Impaired glucose tolerance/diabetes

Impaired immunity, for example, immunosuppressive therapy

Anaemia

Chronic comorbid conditions (renal/hepatic/cardiac disease)

Sickle cell disease

History of pelvic infection.

has been suggested that a possible explanation for sepsis associated with the identified risk factors is low serum 25-hydroxyvitamin D (25(OH)D) concentrations.[24] Vitamin D has been found to reduce the risk of sepsis through induction of antimicrobial peptides known as cathelicidin and defensins.[25] Women who are obese have lower serum 25(OH)D concentrations because of their larger body mass. It is well established that chronic comorbid conditions such as congestive heart failure, chronic liver disease, and chronic renal disease are risk factors for sepsis in the general population and Bauer et al demonstrated these associations for parturients also.[5] In the same study, systemic lupus erythematosus was also identified as a risk factor, likely as a result of the immunological effects of the disease itself but also secondary to the use of steroids and immunosuppressive medications. Although women with these conditions are a relatively small proportion of obstetric patients, the study authors suggested that the magnitude of risk associated with these conditions prompted consideration of the diagnosis and treatment of sepsis in patients with these conditions.

In patients with sickle cell disease, functional asplenia results in increased susceptibility to bacterial infection; three women whose deaths were reported in the 2006–2008 Confidential Enquiry were noted to have either sickle cell disease or sickle trait. An analysis of maternal outcomes in almost 18,000 deliveries by women with sickle cell disease found that there was a significantly higher rate of sepsis in this group (odds ratio (OR) 6.8) compared to women without sickle cell disease.[26] This risk may be further compounded by the presence of anaemia.[27] Sickle cell trait has in the past been viewed as a benign carrier state but there is now some evidence that it can be viewed as an intermediate disease phenotype.[28] A study of maternal outcomes amongst haemoglobinopathy carriers found an increased risk of bacteriuria in women with sickle cell trait.[29]

Causes of sepsis in obstetrics

The causes of sepsis in obstetrics may be divided into obstetric causes and other causes, and are summarized in Box 34.5. In early pregnancy, the commonest causes of sepsis are septic abortion and termination of pregnancy. Caesarean delivery endometritis used to be a major cause of postpartum infection with the incidence of sepsis following operative delivery once being as high as 36%.[30] Women undergoing caesarean delivery still have a 5–20-fold greater risk for infection and infectious morbidity compared with a vaginal birth.[31] A cohort study from Denmark of over 32,000 women compared the risk of postpartum infections within 30 days of delivery, following vaginal delivery, or emergency or elective caesarean delivery. The risk of postpartum infection for all women delivered by caesarean delivery was 7.6%, versus 1.6% for women who had a vaginal delivery (aOR 4.71).[32] Routine antibiotic prophylaxis at caesarean delivery was in place during the study period and therefore even with this precaution infection was five times more likely in women who delivered by caesarean delivery rather than vaginal delivery. The authors also found a nearly 50% higher risk of postpartum wound infection after emergency caesarean delivery compared to elective caesarean delivery (OR 1.49).

Smaill et al. reviewed 86 studies involving over 13,000 women.[31] They found prophylactic antibiotics in women undergoing caesarean delivery substantially reduced the incidence of febrile morbidity, wound infection, endometritis, and serious maternal

Box 34.5 Causes of sepsis in obstetrics

Obstetric causes

- Genital tract causes:
  - Chorioamnionitis
  - Endometritis
  - Septic abortion
  - Wound infection following caesarean delivery/episiotomy/vaginal tear
- Non-genital tract causes:
  - Lower urinary tract infection
  - Pyelonephritis
  - Breast infection—abscess/mastitis
  - Septic pelvic thrombophlebitis.

Non-obstetric causes

- Human immunodeficiency virus
- Pneumonia
- Tuberculosis
- Malaria.

infectious complications. The mandatory use of prophylactic antibiotics at caesarean delivery has been a recommendation for some time. However, the timing of prophylactic antibiotics has been the subject of some discussion.[33] Largely because of concerns about neonatal infection, the prevailing practice in the United Kingdom has been to use narrow-range antibiotics after cord clamping, compared to the practice of broad-spectrum pre-incision antibiotics which is standard in non-obstetric surgery. A recent meta-analysis suggests the latter approach may be more effective in reducing infections after caesarean delivery, without any detrimental effect on the neonate.[34] The American College of Obstetricians and Gynecologists recommends this strategy[35] and in the United Kingdom the National Institute for Health and Care Excellence (NICE) *Caesarean Section* guideline update has also made similar recommendations.[36] The appropriate and optimal antibiotic for prophylaxis likewise remains unclear.[37] A Cochrane review found there was no conclusive evidence of any outcome difference between cephalosporins and penicillins in regard to maternal sepsis, endometritis, fever, wound infection, urinary tract infection, and adverse effects.[38]

Septic abortion was once the leading cause of maternal death around the world and remains a significant cause of maternal mortality in the under-resourced world, largely as a result of illegal abortions. According to the WHO, an estimated 21.6 million unsafe abortions took place worldwide in 2008 with deaths from unsafe abortion accounting for 13% of all maternal deaths (as a result of sepsis and haemorrhage).[39] In the UK Confidential Enquiry into Maternal Death, eight women died as a result of infection associated with spontaneous miscarriage or therapeutic/artificial abortion. Initially infection involves the endometrium and any retained products of conception, thus removal of retained products of conception are essential in the early management. Rarely hysterectomy may be required.[40]

Chorioamnionitis may be defined as acute inflammation of the membranes and chorion of the placenta. It typically arises secondary to ascending bacterial infection in the presence of membrane rupture, although it can occur with intact membranes.[41] More rarely it occurs as result of haematogenous spread[42] or as an iatrogenic infection secondary to an invasive procedure. The incidence of chorioamnionitis varies according to different diagnostic criteria (clinical, microbiological, or histopathological). Risk factors for the development of chorioamnionitis include prolonged rupture of membranes,[43,44] multiple vaginal examinations,[43] the use of internal monitoring,[43] meconium-stained amniotic fluid,[45,46] and bacterial vaginosis.[47] Women who smoke are also at increased risk.[44] In addition to the risks of infection, chorioamnionitis is associated with significant other risks to both the mother and baby; for the mother there is an increased risk of caesarean delivery and postpartum haemorrhage, likely as a result of dysfunctional uterine activity.[48] Fetal/neonatal risks include fetal death, neonatal sepsis, intraventricular haemorrhage, and long-term disability including cerebral palsy.

It has been estimated that after vaginal delivery, mastitis and urinary tract infections are the commonest causes of infection.[49] Mastitis affects up to 20%[50] of postpartum women but is comparatively rare as a cause of postpartum sepsis. It is usually unilateral and associated with hardening of the affected breast, erythema, and severe pain. It has been estimated that one-third of women admitted with mastitis develop breast abscesses that require surgical drainage. The majority of these are caused by community-acquired methicillin-resistant *Staphylococcus aureus* (MRSA).[51,52] One of the deaths in the 2006–2008 UK Confidential Enquiry into Maternal Death occurred as a result of sepsis arising from mastitis. There are isolated case reports of toxic shock syndrome occurring as a result of mastitis.

As a result of the physiological and anatomical changes of pregnancy within the urinary tract there is increased susceptibility to urinary tract infection and urosepsis. There is renal pelvic and ureteric dilatation secondary to mechanical obstruction by the gravid uterus. Progesterone-induced smooth muscle relaxation leads to decreased peristalsis of the ureters, increased bladder capacity, and urinary stasis. Asymptomatic bacteriuria has an incidence in pregnancy of between 2% and 10% but it has been estimated that if left untreated as many as 20–40% will go on to develop pyelonephritis.[53,54] A retrospective cohort study of over half a million pregnancies in the United States found an incidence of acute antepartum pyelonephritis of 0.5%.[55] Pyelonephritis in pregnancy is associated with increased maternal and fetal morbidity, including acute kidney injury, acute respiratory distress, stillbirth, and preterm birth.[56] The presence of a urinary catheter in association with operative delivery and/or neuraxial analgesia increases the risk.[57] A Cochrane review found that antibiotic treatment compared to placebo or no treatment was effective in clearing asymptomatic bacteriuria (risk ratio (RR) 0.25; 95% CI 0.14–0.48) and that the incidence of pyelonephritis was also reduced (RR 0.23; 95% CI 0.13–0.41). Antibiotic treatment was also associated with a reduction in the incidence of low birthweight babies (RR 0.66; 95% CI 0.49–0.89) but there was no difference in preterm delivery.[58]

Postpartum ovarian vein thrombophlebitis is a rare complication of sepsis in pregnancy. The incidence varies from 1/600 to 1/2000 deliveries.[59] It occurs as a result of the hypercoagulable state of pregnancy combined with blood flow stasis and is then further compounded by vessel wall damage by direct trauma which then predisposes to infection. The right ovarian vein is involved in the majority of cases.[60] The right-sided prevalence is due to two factors: the physiological dextrorotation of the uterus during pregnancy, which compresses the ovarian vein on the right; and to the direction of postpartum blood flow, which is antegrade in the right ovarian vein and retrograde in the left ovarian vein. The symptoms of ovarian vein thrombosis usually develop within 4 weeks of delivery, most frequently within the first 4 days. Symptoms may be vague and can include abrupt onset fever, rigors, and lower abdominal pain. The differential diagnosis includes endometritis, acute appendicitis, and pyelonephritis.[61] Abdominal examination may reveal a tender elongated mass and the diagnosis may be confirmed by ultrasound, computed tomography (CT), or magnetic resonance imaging (MRI). Treatment involves broad-spectrum antibiotics and anticoagulation and may rarely require surgical intervention.[62] One study estimated a mortality of 5% if untreated.

Pneumonia as a cause of sepsis in pregnancy is associated with significant morbidity and mortality.[63] It is one of the leading causes of sepsis arising in the antepartum period. The true incidence of antepartum pneumonia is difficult to ascertain but has been estimated at 0.78–2.7/1000 deliveries.[64,65] In the United Kingdom, pneumonia is the most common reason for admission to intensive care for pregnant women;[66] in the United States, respiratory failure as a result of pneumonia is the third leading indication for intubation during pregnancy.[67] The risk of developing pneumonia appears to increase with advancing gestation with the lowest risk in the first trimester and the highest risk in the third trimester. There are various maternal risk factors associated with an increased incidence of developing pneumonia; these include co-morbidities such as cardiac disease and asthma, one study showed a fivefold increase for the risk of pneumonia in a pregnant woman with asthma. Maternal obesity is another significant risk factor.[68,69] In pregnant women who develop pneumonia, there is a higher rate of complications such as respiratory failure. Fetal outcome in pregnant women with pneumonia is significantly worsened: the fetus is vulnerable to intrauterine growth retardation and *in utero* death; preterm delivery may be required to improve maternal respiratory function.[68]

The clinical features of pneumonia can mimic the physiological changes of pregnancy and delay diagnosis and treatment leading to a poor outcome. The specific respiratory physiological changes of pregnancy predispose the parturient with pneumonia to rapid desaturation and a reduced ability to compensate for the development of a metabolic acidosis.

The differential diagnosis of pneumonia in pregnancy includes pulmonary embolus and pulmonary oedema. It is essential to remember that pregnancy does not exclude the use of chest radiography. The most common bacterial agent causing pneumonia in pregnancy is *Streptococcus* pneumoniae. The consequences of viral pneumonia in pregnancy have been particularly topical in recent years as a result of the H1N1 flu pandemic. Women in pregnancy and the puerperium are known to be at higher risk of complications of seasonal flu than the non-pregnant population. In previous flu pandemics, pregnant women had significantly higher mortality and morbidity rates and this effect was seen in the 2009 pandemic.[70,71] A UK-based case–control cohort study found that pregnant women admitted to hospital with H1N1 influenza had significantly higher rates of adverse pregnancy outcomes than uninfected pregnant women. These included three to four times higher rates of preterm birth, four to five times higher rates of stillbirth, and four to six times higher rates of neonatal death.[72]

Risk factors associated with admission to hospital with 2009/H1N1 in pregnancy include maternal obesity, asthma, multiparity, multiple pregnancy, black or other minority group ethnicity, and smoking. A delay in starting treatment with antiviral drugs, more than 2 days after the onset of symptoms, was associated with an increased risk of admission to intensive care.[70–72]

Microbiology

The genitourinary tract is colonized with a wide variety of organisms; however, not all of these will cause infection and sepsis. Pregnant women who develop sepsis are very likely to be infected with more than one organism. Analysis of the microbiological causes of deaths from sepsis (direct and indirect) over the last 20 years of the UK Confidential Enquiries is shown in Table 34.1.

Historically, although they were not characterized serologically by Rebecca Lancefield until 1933, it seems likely that GAS was the predominant cause of obstetric sepsis in the first half of the twentieth century.[73,74] Outbreaks were frequently described, particularly when scarlet fever was also prevalent. In the latter part of the twentieth century, factors such as improved antiseptic techniques, the use of antibiotics, and an increase in natural immunity lead to a decline in the virulence of this organism. Gram-negative organisms such as *Escherichia coli* then became more common sources of infection. However, over the past 20 years Gram-positive organisms, and in particular GAS infections, have again become predominant. This is consistent with the pattern of GAS infections in the general population of the developed world, where there has been a dramatic rise in the number of such infections.[75,76] The Lancefield classification of *Streptococcus* species is based on their haemolytic properties. GAS are β-haemolytic species that cause complete rupture of red blood cells in culture media leading to a clear zone around the bacteria. They have a number of factors that affect their virulence, for example, M proteins which form complexes which adhere to vascular endothelium and cause endothelial leaks and hypercoagulability leading to disseminated intravascular coagulation. Other factors that further contribute to the virulence of GAS include the production of toxins such as streptokinase, streptolysins, and exotoxins.[77] The epidemiology of GAS is of relevance in obstetric sepsis. It has been estimated that in the resourced world between 5% and 30% of the community are asymptomatic carriers of GAS, usually on the skin or in the throat. It is present in the vaginal tract of only 0.03% of pregnant women; however, postpartum women have a 20-fold increased incidence of GAS infection compared with non-pregnant women.[78] In the 2006–2008 Confidential Enquiry, the majority of the deaths were noted to occur between December and April; GAS upper respiratory tract infections are most common during winter and early spring in contrast to skin infections caused by GAS which are seen more frequently during the summer, when the skin is exposed and abrasions and insect bites are more likely to occur. In many of the women who died in the Confidential Enquiry there was a history of a recent upper respiratory tract infection and/or of contact with young children.[2] It is thought that women auto-inoculate themselves, through contamination of the perineum, and the organism then ascends leading to systemic infection. GAS is highly communicable and this has implications for identifying the source of infection and also for contacts of a parturient with GAS infection, including healthcare workers.

A major source of concern is sepsis arising as a result of extended-spectrum beta-lactamase (ESBL)-producing organisms.[79] ESBLs are enzymes that can be produced by bacteria making them resistant to third-generation cephalosporins commonly used for treatment of serious infections. The first beta-lactamase was identified in an isolate of *Escherichia coli* in 1940[80] and since then an increasing number of organisms producing ESBL have been identified. Initially ESBLs were mostly found in *Klebsiella* species in hospital, particularly intensive care patients. However, a new group of ESBLs (called CTX-M enzymes) has emerged and these have been widely detected among *Escherichia coli* bacteria.[81]

The emergence of these bacteria has been attributed to the extensive use of broad-spectrum beta-lactamase in empiric therapy and rapid plasmid-mediated distribution of resistance genes between bacterial species. Although ESBL-producing organisms occur principally in *Enterobacter* species, particularly *Escherichia coli, Klebsiella pneumoniae*, and *Proteus mirabilis* (all recognized causes of obstetric sepsis), they can occur in other members of the non-enteric organisms, such as *Acinetobacter* species.[82]

In the developing world, there are more limited data on the specific microbiological causes of obstetric sepsis. Available evidence suggests a similar pattern of bacterial causes to that in the developed world.[83] However, in recent times the HIV/AIDS pandemic

Table 34.1 Microbiological causes of maternal death identified in UK Confidential Enquiries 1991–93 to 2006–08

	1991–93	1994–96	1997–99	2000–02	2003–05	2006–08	Total
β-haemolytic *Streptococcus* Lancefield group A	1	7	3	3	8	13	**25**
Escherichia coli	2	3	6	2	7	5	**25**
Streptococcus pneumoniae		3	4	2	5	3	**17**
HIV			1	4	5	2	**11**
Staphylococcus aureus			1	3	2	4	**10**
Streptococcus unspecified	5	3					**8**
Clostridium species	1	1	1	1		1	**5**
β-haemolytic *Streptococcus* Lancefield group B		2		2	1		**5**
TB					4	2	**6**
Pseudomonas	1				3		**4**
Proteus species	2				2		**4**
Meningococcus		1	1	1			**3**
Toxoplasmosis		2	1				**3**
Enterococcus faecalis			1			1	**3**
Varicella		1	1				**2**
β-haemolytic *Streptococcus* Lancefield group C			1				**1**
β-haemolytic *Streptococcus* Lancefield group D				1			**1**
Morganella						1	**1**
Actinobacter					1		**1**
Listeria					1		**1**
Citrobacter kosseri					1		**1**
Fusobacterium necrophorum				1			**1**
Bacteroides melaminogenicus	1						**1**

Reprinted from *International Journal of Obstetric Anesthesia*, Volume 21, issue 1, D.N. Lucas, P.N. Robinson, M.R. Nel, Sepsis in obstetrics and the role of the anaesthetist, pp. 56–67, Copyright (2012), with permission from Elsevier.

Number of deaths in table may not equal actual number of deaths from reports as full microbiological data not always available.

has undoubtedly been the most important factor with regard to sepsis-related maternal morbidity and mortality in the developing world. A major WHO analysis assessing progress towards the Millennium Development Goal of reducing maternal mortality, found that in 2008 there were an estimated 342,900 maternal deaths worldwide from all causes, a 34% decline from 1980.[84] It is estimated that HIV disease accounted for 61,400 of these deaths. The impact of this disease was greatest in sub-Saharan Africa, where WHO estimates for 2008 suggest that without HIV/AIDS-related deaths, the maternal mortality ratio for sub-Saharan Africa would have been 580 maternal deaths per 100,000 live births instead of the actual figure of 640.[85]

Pregnant women with HIV/AIDS are more susceptible to sepsis and postsurgical complications. Many opportunistic infections associated with HIV/AIDS may complicate pregnancy and cause maternal mortality.[86] *Pneumocystis jirovecii* (previously *carinii*) pneumonia has a more aggressive course during pregnancy, with an increase in both morbidity and mortality.[87] The South African confidential enquiry into maternal deaths, 'Saving Mothers', found that bacterial pneumonias, bacterial sepsis, atypical pneumonia, cryptococcal meningitis, and tuberculosis (TB) are common co-morbid conditions associated with HIV/AIDS, and may be the primary causes of maternal death in that country.[88] Worldwide the most significant infection contributing to maternal mortality in HIV-infected women is TB. TB accounts for about 700,000 deaths annually in women of reproductive age,[89] and is by far the most common opportunistic infection associated with HIV in the developing world. A 5-year review of maternal mortality at a tertiary referral centre in Johannesburg found that mortality in HIV-infected women was 6.2 times greater than in HIV-negative women and that 31% of HIV-related deaths were due to TB.[90]

Postnatal care is often poor in African countries, and puerperal sepsis is a major cause of maternal mortality.[91] It has been suggested that the impact of puerperal sepsis could be significantly reduced if, following delivery, women were to remain in hospital for at least 24 hours, and/or improved arrangements were put in place for postnatal follow-up. Clinical experience suggests that HIV-infected women may be clinically well at the time of early discharge, only to be re-admitted with florid sepsis 7–10 days after delivery.[88]

Clinical presentation and diagnosis

Sepsis is a clinical diagnosis and microbiological investigations may be negative. The onset of sepsis may be insidious and non-specific, particularly given the physiological changes of pregnancy, labour, and the puerperium. There is significant overlap with the clinical features associated with the physiological changes of pregnancy (particularly around the time of delivery) and the pathophysiology of sepsis. Diagnosis can therefore be difficult, especially in the early stages. Conversely the disease process can be fulminant, overwhelming, and rapidly fatal.[92–94] The clinician must often rely on a high index of clinical suspicion rather than objective criteria. Women at risk of infection (e.g. the immunocompromised) should be identified early in pregnancy.

Initially infection may present with non-specific symptoms such as fever, malaise, and muscle ache. A careful history should aim to elicit features of localized symptoms and clarify the possible source of infection; the presenting features vary depending on the source of infection (Table 34.2). Maternal infection can rapidly affect the fetus: the uteroplacental circulation does not exhibit autoregulation, so that fetal perfusion and oxygenation is dependent on maternal oxygenation and cardiovascular stability.

Table 34.2 Symptoms and signs of sepsis

Symptoms	General	Specific
	Fever	Premature contractions
	Influenza-like symptoms	Abdominal pain
	Sore throat	Sickle cell crisis
	Diarrhoea	Atonic uterus precipitating postpartum haemorrhage
	Vomiting	
	Shortness of breath	Mastitis
	Wound infection	Vaginal discharge—profuse and/or malodorous
Signs	Pyrexia or hypothermia, < 36°C	
	Early pregnancy loss/abnormal fetal heart rate/death *in utero*	
	Tachycardia > 100 beats/min	
	Tachypnoea > 20 breaths/min	
	Elevated white cell count and neutrophilia or low white cell count/neutropenia	
	Rising C-reactive protein	
	Lactic acidosis	
	Signs of organ decompensation: hypoxaemia; hypotension; cool extremities; reduced capillary refill; oliguria	

Thus the septic woman may present with an abnormal fetal heart rate pattern or intrauterine fetal death.

Women will invariably experience some degree of pain following caesarean delivery or significant vaginal tears. However, the presence of constant, severe abdominal or perineal pain, poorly responsive to analgesics and disproportionate to that which would be anticipated, is a cause for concern, particularly when it is associated with diarrhoea, and sepsis must then always be considered in the differential diagnosis.[2] When mastitis that does not respond to conservative management within 24 hours, and the woman is becoming systemically unwell, then the breasts must be considered as a possible source of sepsis.

The onset of sepsis is characterized by a hyperdynamic circulation, reduced systemic vascular resistance secondary to arterial vasodilatation, and increased respiratory rate in association with the development of anaerobic metabolism and lactic acidosis. Therefore when sepsis develops not only can diagnosis be made more difficult because of the physiological changes of pregnancy, but in addition the combined effect of pathological processes superimposed on a state of increased physiological demand may result in a particularly severe disease burden.

Pyrexia is common in sepsis but normothermia may also be present. Hypothermia is a particularly significant finding. Swinging pyrexia suggests a persistent source of infection or inadequate treatment.[2] Although an elevated white cell count is commonly associated with sepsis, pregnancy also leads to an increase in white cell count, particularly during labour. After delivery, the white cell count usually decreases to prepregnancy levels within a week: a white cell count that fails to decrease to normal levels or conversely decreases rapidly or becomes less than 4×10^9/L may indicate severe infection. One of the most sensitive and earliest clinical signs of sepsis is tachypnoea which arises as a result of pyrexia, lactic acidosis, or cytokine-mediated effects on the respiratory centre. The overlapping physiological changes of pregnancy and clinical features of sepsis will often pose diagnostic difficulty and the existence of a suitable biomarker in this context would be particularly useful. In the intensive care community, there has been significant interest in the use of biomarkers to help establish a diagnosis of sepsis. Much of this discussion has focussed on procalcitonin. Procalcitonin is a peptide precursor of the hormone calcitonin and is produced by the parafollicular cells of the thyroid and the neuroendocrine cells of the lung and the intestine. Procalcitonin levels rise specifically in the presence of bacterial but not viral or fungal sepsis.[95] Therefore laboratory measurement of procalcitonin levels can potentially assist with diagnosis. However, meta-analyses have produced conflicting results on whether procalcitonin is an effective and useful sepsis biomarker.[96,97] A recent comprehensive review states that clinical judgement should remain the cornerstone of clinical decision-making. A more encouraging role for procalcitonin is its measurement to guide duration of antibiotic therapy.[98] Paccolat and colleagues have published work establishing procalcitonin levels during pregnancy, delivery, and postpartum.[99]

Management and the surviving sepsis campaign

Management of the septic pregnant patient follows the same principles as that of any septic patient: resuscitation, identification and treatment of the source of sepsis, management of complications such as hypotension and tissue hypoxia, and the application of organ-protection strategies. The management of sepsis arising in the antenatal period is complicated by the presence of the fetus; in this situation, maternal resuscitation is key to ensuring fetal well-being[100] and attempting early delivery in women with cardiovascular compromise due to sepsis may increase maternal and fetal mortality.[101] However, when intrauterine infection is suspected as the source of sepsis, delivery should be expedited.[102]

Early recognition of the obstetric patient with sepsis is vital to ensuring optimal outcome. As noted previously, the physiological changes of pregnancy can make early detection difficult and at the same time exacerbate the course of sepsis in an obstetric patient. The use of early warning scores was a recommendation in the 2003–2005 UK Confidential Enquiry.[22] Clear evidence of outcome benefit is, however, lacking, with one major study on the use of early warning scores and medical response teams in the non-obstetric hospital population failing to demonstrate a reduction in mortality, though this has been attributed to a possible lack of sensitivity in the criteria used for triggering clinical calls.[103] The importance of developing maternity early warning scores with appropriately sensitive parameters for use in obstetric patients has been emphasized by a retrospective review[104] and work in this area is starting to emerge. A prospective review of almost 700 obstetric admissions evaluated a maternal early warning score (MEOWS) chart adapted from the Confidential Enquiry into Maternal and Child Health report.[105] The authors looked at completed MEOWS charts for triggers and hospital notes for evidence of morbidity. Two hundred patients (30%) triggered and 86 patients (13%) had morbidity according to preset criteria, including haemorrhage (43%), hypertensive disease of pregnancy (31%), and suspected infection (20%). The MEOWS was 89% sensitive (95% CI 81–95%), 79% specific (95% CI 76–82%), with a positive predictive value of 39% (95% CI 32–46%) and a negative predictive value of 98% (95% CI 96–99%). There were no admissions to the intensive care unit (ICU), cardiorespiratory arrests, or deaths during the study period. Although these results are encouraging, the authors recognize that adjustment of the trigger parameters may lead to an improvement in positive predictive value. Another group has used data from direct obstetric admissions from the Intensive Care National Audit and Research Centre's Case Mix Programmed Database to design and validate an aggregate weighted early warning scoring system specific to the obstetric population that could be used in the ward environment.[106] Over two thousand direct obstetric admissions from the Intensive Care National Audit and Research Centre's Case Mix Programmed Database were randomly allocated to model development and a similar number allocated to validation sets. The authors analysed physiological variables collected during the first 24 hours of critical care admission and used logistic regression analysis for mortality in the model development set to create a statistically based early warning score. The statistical score was then modified to create a clinically acceptable early warning score. Again, this work produced encouraging results though the study did have some limitations. Although the dataset analysed a large number of admissions these were from admission to the ICU. Therefore it has been postulated that after multiple medical interventions have already taken place, such data may not actually be reliable enough to base an obstetric early warning score on. It is clear that this is an important area and studies such as the Oxford 4P study Pregnancy Physiology Pattern Prediction will provide further valuable information in the future.[107]

Recommendations from the Royal College of Obstetricians and Gynaecologists are that sepsis should be managed in accordance with the Surviving Sepsis Campaign guidelines.[108] This campaign, a collaboration between the European Society of Intensive Care Medicine, the Society of Critical Care Medicine, and the International Sepsis Forum, was launched as a major international health initiative in 2002 and recently updated.[109] It aimed to improve outcome in sepsis and advocated a standardized 'bundle'-based approach for management of the (non-pregnant) critically ill septic patient. A clinical care bundle is a set of interventions, usually no more than five, that when grouped and implemented together lead to better outcomes with a greater impact than if performed individually. The elements in a bundle are ideally based on high-quality or level 1 evidence such as systematic reviews of multiple, well-designed randomized controlled trials. In clinical practice, the application of these elements may not always be done consistently, leading to variations in patient care, so a bundle aims to tie the care elements together into a cohesive unit that must be strictly adhered to for every patient, every time. Lastly, all the components of a clinical care bundle must be completed in a specified time period and place ('the golden hour'). Compliance is measured in an 'all or none' approach.[110]

The Surviving Sepsis Campaign guidelines described two clinical care bundles—the resuscitation bundle and the management bundle. The Royal College of Obstetricians and Gynaecologists advocates the use of these in obstetrics.

The following care bundle, shown in Box 34.6, should be applied immediately where possible or within 6 hours and has been shown to significantly improve survival rates.[111]

Box 34.6 Surviving sepsis care bundle

To be completed within 3 hours

1. Measure lactate level.
2. Obtain blood cultures prior to administration of antibiotics.
3. Administer broad spectrum antibiotics.
4. Administer 30 mL/kg crystalloid for hypotension or lactate ≥ 4 mmol/L.

To be completed within 6 hours

5. Apply vasopressors (for hypotension that does not respond to initial fluid resuscitation) to maintain a mean arterial pressure (MAP) ≥ 65 mmHg.
6. In the event of persistent hypotension after initial fluid resuscitation [MAP <65 mm Hg] or if initial lactate was greater than or equal to 4 mmol/L, reassess volume status and tissue perfusion and document findings.
7. Remeasure lactate if initial lactate was elevated.

Reproduced with permission Dellinger RP, Levy MM, Rhodes A et al. Surviving Sepsis Campaign: International Guidelines for Management of Severe Sepsis and Septic Shock: 2012, Crit Care Med 2013; 41(2): 580–637.

Antibiotic therapy via the intravenous route and in high therapeutic doses should be started as early as possible, and preferably within 1 hour. There is overwhelming evidence that delay in starting antibiotics is associated with increased mortality[112] and this has consistently been cited as an area of substandard care in successive UK Confidential Enquiries. Causes of delay include errors in administration, prescription errors, patients awaiting senior review, and patients being transferred between departments, and strenuous efforts must be made to avoid such delays.[113] Broad-spectrum antibiotics should be used initially and two or more agents are likely to be needed.[114,115] Urgent microbiological advice should be sought as soon as possible but should also not delay starting antibiotics. The physiological changes of pregnancy, including the increased volume of distribution, which can also be increased in sepsis, can have an effect on the pharmacodynamic and pharmacokinetic profile of the drug. Some women may have impaired renal or hepatic function and serum drug levels may need to be monitored to ensure correct dosage. However, the appropriate loading dose when starting antibiotic therapy is independent of the patient's renal function and the initial loading dose is particularly important to ensure appropriate serum concentrations of drugs.[116]

Regular reassessment of antibiotic therapy should occur in relation to the patient's clinical condition. Treatment should be for a minimum of 7–10 days and it is essential that treatment is not discontinued too soon.[2,22] The 2006–2008 UK Confidential Enquiry[2] suggested a stratified approach to antibiotics in sepsis (Box 34.7); antibiotic regimens should be altered to adapt to the requirements of the local population and the particular clinical situation of the patient.

Early haemodynamic resuscitation is a key goal of therapy.[118,119] The objective is to restore adequate oxygen delivery to peripheral tissues. It is well recorded that in high-risk surgical patients with sepsis, early haemodynamic optimization before the development of organ failure reduces mortality by 23% in comparison with those optimized after the development of organ failure.[120,121] In hypotensive septic patients with a serum lactate greater than 4 mmol/L, volume resuscitation should be used initially, aiming to reach the following clinical endpoints: central venous pressure 8–12 mmHg, mean arterial pressure 65 mmHg, and a urine output of 0.5 mL/kg/h. If measurable, a central venous oxygen saturation of greater than 70% should be aimed for. There is no evidence to support one type of intravenous fluid over another[122] but it is important to note that starch solutions have been withdrawn in the light of recent evidence suggesting they are associated with increased mortality in the critically ill septic patient.[123] Vasopressor support may be considered even before optimal intravenous loading has been achieved.[124] Transfusion of red blood cells may be considered if tissue oxygen delivery still remains inadequate.[125]

Fluid management is difficult in sepsis and may be particularly so in the severely ill obstetric patient: fluid overload leading to pulmonary oedema has contributed to the deaths of some women in UK Confidential Enquiries reports.[2] There are various reasons why the obstetric patient may be vulnerable to fluid overload: the physiological changes of pregnancy are such that at term the parturient is already in a relatively volume overloaded state; co-morbidity such as pre-eclampsia may be present and uterotonic drugs that are known to predispose to fluid retention (e.g. oxytocin) or pulmonary oedema (e.g. prostaglandins) may have been used. Oesophageal Doppler monitoring to guide intravenous fluid therapy has been endorsed by NICE. [126] Although this report did not assess its use in obstetric patients, the oesophageal Doppler has successfully been used in the obstetric emergency situation.[127] A variety of other minimally and non-invasive techniques for maternal cardiac output monitoring are available[128] and it would seem likely and appropriate that these should become increasingly used in obstetric practice. Further details on these devices are available in Chapter 30.

Box 34.7 Suggested antibiotic therapy in obstetric sepsis

Where the organism is unknown and the woman is not critically ill

- Co-amoxiclav 1.2 g 8-hourly or cefuroxime 1.5 g 8-hourly or cefotaxime 1–2 g 8-hourly or 6-hourly *plus* metronidazole 500 mg 8-hourly
- In cases of allergy to penicillin and cephalosporins, use clarithromycin 500 mg 12-hourly or clindamycin 600 mg to 1.2 g 8-hourly or 6-hourly *plus* gentamicin to give Gram-negative cover, while waiting for microbiological advice

In severe sepsis or septic shock

- Piperacillin–tazobactam 4.5 g 8-hourly or ciprofloxacin 600 mg 12-hourly *plus* gentamicin 3–5 mg/kg daily in divided doses every 8 hours[a]
- A carbapenem such as meropenem 500 mg to 1 g 8-hourly ± gentamicin
- Metronidazole 500 mg 8-hourly may be considered to provide anaerobic cover
- NB If Group A streptococcal infection is suspected, clindamycin 600 mg to 1.2 g three or four times daily 8-hourly is more effective than penicillins

If there are risk factors for MRSA septicaemia, add teicoplanin 10 mg/kg 12-hourly for three doses, then 10 mg/kg 24-hourly or linezolid 600 mg 12-hourly.

[a]Gentamicin is more commonly given as a once-daily dose: studies have shown increased efficacy and reduced nephrotoxicity with this strategy.[117]

Supplemental oxygen therapy is recommended even if there is no respiratory distress. Tracheal intubation and ventilation should be considered if the level of consciousness is reduced or if there is hypoxia or progressive respiratory distress.[129]

A simplified strategy for the bundle-based approach to sepsis (the 'sepsis six'), has recently been shown to be effective in a general hospital setting (Box 34.8.[130])

In addition to starting antibiotic therapy and the strategies described above, it is essential that any septic focus is identified and removed wherever feasible. Even with effective antibiotics the woman may continue to deteriorate unless the source of infection is identified. Relevant swabs and cultures should be taken

Box 34.8 The sepsis six

The sepsis six to be delivered within 1 hour

1. Deliver high-flow oxygen
2. Take blood cultures
3. Administer empiric intravenous antibiotics
4. Measure serum lactate and send full blood count
5. Start intravenous fluid resuscitation
6. Commence accurate urine output measurement.

Daniels R, Nutbeam T, McNamara G, *et al.* The sepsis six and the severe sepsis resuscitation bundle: a prospective observational cohort study. *Emerg Med J* 2011; 28:507–12.

before antibiotic therapy is started but should not delay treatment. Where applicable, these should include placental and neonatal swabs, as well as breast milk culture in the presence of mastitis. In women with endometritis, particularly after surgical instrumentation (caesarean delivery or septic abortion) or in patients who fail to respond to antibiotic therapy, imaging with ultrasound or CT is indicated to detect abscess formation. The choice of imaging depends on the condition of the patient and the presence or absence of localizing features. Although ultrasound is more portable than other imaging modalities, the information yielded may not be as helpful and advice from radiologists will be useful. A surgical opinion should be sought as soon as possible with surgery where required.

Necrotizing fasciitis is rare but constitutes a surgical emergency. It has been described in association with caesarean delivery [131] and can present as a perineal infection after vaginal delivery.[132] It is characterized by widespread necrosis of the subcutaneous tissue and fascial layers and can progress to necrosis of muscle. It is most commonly associated with GAS infection, though a mixed bacterial flora including anaerobes is often present. In the early stages it may be difficult to distinguish between cellulitis and necrotizing fasciitis and any patient with a wound infection and signs of systemic sepsis needs careful evaluation to exclude necrotizing fasciitis. Distinguishing features include the presence of copious and malodorous discharge, dusky skin discolouration, and radiological or clinical evidence of gas in the soft tissues.[133] Markedly severe pain disproportionate to that which would be anticipated in the context of individual patients may be present initially but as the condition advances can become painless as a result of disruption in blood supply and innervation. Surgical exploration and extensive debridement is indicated and without early aggressive treatment the mortality is 100%.

Timing of delivery in the septic parturient

Traditionally it was thought that fetal outcome is entirely dependent on maternal outcome and that delivery is not mandated by the presence of maternal sepsis. However, this approach is being re-evaluated particularly in the context of care of the critically ill parturient, although there is limited data in this area. The considerations of whether there is potential benefit to the mother and fetus need to be balanced against the risks of delivery to both (including issues around fetal viability) and the method of delivery (caesarean or possibly vaginal delivery). From a maternal perspective, there seems to be some evidence that maternal respiratory function and oxygen requirements in the critically ill ventilated parturient may be improved by delivery of the fetus.[134] In a study of obstetric sepsis, worsening maternal respiratory function was the primary indication for delivery.[135] From a fetal perspective, oxygenation is dependent on maternal oxygen delivery, uterine/placental blood flow, with a relative maternal hypocapnia facilitating fetal carbon dioxide extraction. All of these factors may be adversely affected in severe sepsis. Fetal assessment with cardiotocography is indicated and may show fetal tachycardia with an absence of variability occurring as a result of maternal pyrexia. The production of endotoxins can cause uterine contractions. An editorial suggested possible criteria, shown in Box 34.9, that might be considered to indicate a need for delivery.[136]

Box 34.9 Suggested criteria indicating early delivery when sepsis present

1. Maternal rapid deterioration
2. Failure to maintain adequate blood oxygenation
3. Difficulty with mechanical ventilation due to the gravid uterus
4. Multiorgan failure
5. Fetal compromise
6. Other obstetric indications.

The same authors emphasized that such decisions must be made in discussion with the patient or her family emphasizing our current lack of firm evidence.

A further consideration in this area is the paucity of evidence on the fetal effects of drugs used in the management of maternal sepsis (antibiotics and inotropes). Decisions relating to the delivery of the baby are ultimately the responsibility of the obstetrician, though the obstetric anaesthetist may be able to advise on the timing of this decision in relation to maternal resuscitation. The key elements of maternal status, fetal status, and gestational age need to be carefully weighed to ensure optimal outcome.

Role of the anaesthetist

Anaesthetists have broad experience in all the elements (resuscitation skills, organ support techniques, and a thorough knowledge of obstetric physiology) required to care for a critically ill parturient and thus the obstetric anaesthetist may have a pivotal role in the management of the septic parturient.[137]

In UK practice, acute management and stabilization of the septic obstetric patient in the maternity unit is most often conducted by the obstetric anaesthetic team. The initial multidisciplinary 'golden hour' of immediate treatment needs to be guided by using a specially adapted sepsis bundle written for the parturient.[108] If the patient does not respond rapidly and the decision is made to escalate her care to level 3 critical care, this transfer should be carried out by an appropriately skilled doctor. Transfer of the critically septic patient requires satisfactory stabilization, rigorous en route monitoring, and close communication with the receiving unit. Lack of early and precise communication between specialties is an ongoing problem with clinicians involved with obstetric emergencies, and the anaesthetist is often best placed to communicate between the various teams involved.[2,22]

When the decision to deliver has been made, the anaesthetist then has to make a decision about whether to recommend surgery using neuraxial or general anaesthesia. It is generally agreed that neuraxial anaesthesia is relatively contraindicated in patients with severe sepsis. The biggest concerns are the hypothesized increased risk of epidural abscess or meningitis. Quantifying these risks is difficult—the white cell count increases in pregnancy and particularly during labour[138] and there is little correlation between white cell count and the presence of bacteraemia in pregnancy.[139]

Epidural abscess in association with neuraxial blockade can occur as a result of direct introduction of microorganisms on the needle, via local infection at the puncture site, contaminated fluids, or the epidural catheter acting as a foreign body and a nidus for infection in the presence of bacteraemia. Spontaneous cases unrelated to neuraxial anaesthesia are also described and while underlying medical conditions such as diabetes can increase risk, epidural abscesses have also occurred in postpartum women without risk factors and who did not receive neuraxial block.[140] The incidence in all patients admitted to hospital has been estimated at 0.2–1.2/10,000.[141] The Third National Audit Project of the Royal College of Anaesthetists found an incidence of 1/47,000 cases although the majority of reports were in perioperative patients;[142] there was only one report in an obstetric patient. Scott and Hibbard in a retrospective review found only one case in 505,000 women who received epidural anaesthesia for vaginal delivery or caesarean delivery.[143] An incidence of 3% has been quoted in patients who had epidural catheters inserted for chronic pain procedures.[144] Similarly there are several case reports in the literature of meningitis following spinal and epidural anaesthesia and also epidural blood patches,[145–147] but it is difficult to draw firm conclusions from isolated reports. Common features to these reports include difficult procedures, multiple attempts, and epidural catheters remaining *in situ* for extended periods.

In 2004, the American Society of Regional Anesthesia and Pain Medicine convened a Practice Advisory Panel on the Infectious Complications Associated with Regional Anesthesia and Pain Medicine who produced a series of practice guidelines.[148,149] They noted that all patients with local or systemic infection who require neuraxial anaesthesia should be considered at risk of central nervous system infection. The current evidence suggests that patients with evidence of systemic infection may safely receive spinal anaesthesia provided the patient has been commenced on antibiotics and has begun to show a response to treatment. Regarding epidural insertion, evidence is limited to very small studies in women with chorioamnionitis which suggest that it may be safe in similar circumstances. Only in the most unusual circumstances should central neural blockade be performed in patients with untreated systemic infection.

Two final points to consider in relation to neuraxial anaesthesia and sepsis are that a septic hypotensive patient may not tolerate the sympathetic blockade and that coagulopathy may have developed. Ultimately the decision to perform an epidural or spinal in these circumstances must be considered on a case by case basis, assessing the risk:benefit ratio for that individual.

General anaesthesia may often be indicated and once achieved this can facilitate initiating invasive vascular monitoring and inotropic support, if indicated. Decisions as to the reversal of general anaesthesia will depend on the stability of the patient. It may be safer to first transfer the sedated, intubated, ventilated patient to a more appropriate environment.

When radiological imaging (CT or MRI scanning) is required to help identify the source of sepsis, this should only occur in the stabilized patient. Early removal of the source of sepsis is recommended whenever possible and suitably cross-matched blood and blood products may be required before and during surgery.

A secondary role in this area for the anaesthetist is that of education and training in the recognition and management of obstetric sepsis. A systematic review on the effectiveness of multidisciplinary teamwork training in a simulation setting was found to be potentially effective in the prevention of errors and improved patient safety in acute obstetric emergencies.[150] Sepsis shares many features of other obstetric emergencies that simulation training is used for and would benefit from addition to an obstetric training programme.

A strategy including a mandatory rigorous annual training programme and computerized guidelines in an emergency department had a beneficial effect on the management of sepsis, as evidenced by earlier administration of antibiotics and more liberal use of intravenous fluids.[151] In the obstetric setting, anaesthetists are uniquely placed to lead on similar teaching initiatives.

The future

Sepsis is a major cause of morbidity and mortality worldwide and much work has been directed at improving the outcome of this condition. The management of sepsis in obstetric practice is likely to benefit from this work. The UK maternal death enquiry (Mothers and Babies, Reducing Risk through Audit and Confidential Enquiries across the UK, MBRRACE-UK), are currently conducting a detailed themed review of maternal sepsis and this is likely to yield further valuable information. Recommendations from the 2006–2008 UK Confidential Enquiry emphasize the importance of early recognition of and response to the septic obstetric patient in a 'back to basics' manner.

References

1. Dolea C, Stein C. *Global Burden of Maternal Sepsis in the Year 2000*. Evidence and Information for Policy (EIP), World Health Organization, Geneva, July 2003. [Online] http://www.who.int/healthinfo/statistics/bod_maternalsepsis.pdf
2. Centre for Maternal and Child Enquiries (CMACE). Saving mothers' lives: reviewing maternal deaths to make motherhood safer: 2006–2008. The Eighth Report on Confidential Enquiries into Maternal Deaths in the United Kingdom. *BJOG* 2011; 118 Suppl 1: 1–203.
3. Kramer HM, Schutte JM, Zwart JJ, *et al*. Maternal mortality and severe morbidity from sepsis in the Netherlands. *Acta Obstet Gynecol Scand* 2009; 88:647–53.
4. Bødker B, Hvidman L, Weber T, *et al*. Maternal deaths in Denmark 2002–2006. *Acta Obstet Gynecol Scand* 2009; 88:556–62.
5. Bauer ME, Bateman BT, Bauer ST, *et al*. Maternal sepsis mortality and morbidity during hospitalization for delivery: temporal trends and independent associations for severe sepsis. *Anesth Analg* 2013; 117:944–50.

6. Scottish NHS Quality Improvement Scotland. *Scottish Confidential Audit of Severe Maternal Morbidity. 6th Annual Report.* Edinburgh: NHS QIS; 2010.
7. Loudon I. *The Tragedy of Childbed Fever.* New York: Oxford University Press; 2000.
8. Radcliffe W. *Milestones in Midwifery; And, The Secret Instrument (The Birth of the Midwifery Forceps).* London: Heinemann; 1947.
9. Loudon I. Deaths in childbed from the eighteenth century to 1935. *Med Hist* 1986; 30(1):1–41.
10. Holmes OW. The contagiousness of puerperal fever. *N Engl Q J Med Surg* 1843; 1:1503–30.
11. Holmes OW. *Puerperal Fever, as a Private Pestilence.* Boston, MA: Ticknor and Fields; 1855.
12. Macfarlane A, Mugford M (eds) *Birth Counts. Statistics of Pregnancy and Childbirth* (2nd ed, Volumes 1 and 2). London: The Stationery Office; 2000.
13. World Health Organization. *The Prevention and Management of Puerperal Infections.* Report of a Technical Working Group. Geneva: Division of Family Health, Maternal Health and Safe Motherhood Programme; 1992. http://whqlibdoc.who.int/hq/1995/WHO_FHE_MSM_95.4.pdf
14. Bone RC, Balk RA, Cerra FB, *et al.* Definitions for sepsis and organ failure and guidelines for the use of innovative therapies in sepsis. The ACCP/SCCM Consensus Conference Committee. American College of Chest Physicians/Society of Critical Care Medicine. *Chest* 1992; 101:1644–55.
15. Lapinsky SE. Obstetric infections. *Crit Care Clin* 2013; 29:509–20.
16. Mor G, Cardenas I. The immune system in pregnancy: a unique complexity. *Am J Reprod Immunol* 2010; 63:425–33.
17. Mor G, Cardenas I, Abrahams V, *et al.* Inflammation and pregnancy: the role of the immune system at the implantation site. *Ann NY Acad Sci* 2011; 1221:80–7.
18. Wilson RC. Immune problems in pregnancy. In Russell IF, Lyons G (eds) *Clinical Problems in Obstetric Anaesthesia.* London: Chapman and Hall Medical; 1997:103–22.
19. Szekeres-Bartho J. Immunological relationship between the mother and the fetus. *Int Rev Immunol* 2002; 21:471–95.
20. Okoko BJ, Enwere G, Ota MO. The epidemiology and consequences of maternal malaria: a review of immunological basis. *Acta Trop* 2003; 87:193–205.
21. Maharaj D. Puerperal pyrexia: a review. Part I. *Obstet Gynecol Surv* 2007; 62:393–9.
22. Lewis G (ed). *The Confidential Enquiry into Maternal and Child Health (CEMACH). Saving Mothers Lives: Reviewing Maternal Deaths to Make Motherhood Safer 2003–2005. The Seventh Report on Confidential Enquiries into Maternal Deaths in the United Kingdom.* London: CEMACH; 2007.
23. Acosta C, Bhattacharya S, Tuffnell D, *et al.* Maternal sepsis: a Scottish population-based case–control study. *BJOG* 2012; 119:474–83.
24. Grant, W. Low vitamin D status may predict women at risk of sepsis associated with delivery. *BJOG* 2012; 119:1018–19.
25. Watkins RR, Yamshchikov AV, Lemonovich TL, *et al.* The role of vitamin D deficiency in sepsis and potential therapeutic implications. *J Infect* 2011; 63:321–6.
26. Villers MS, Jamison MG, De Castro LM, *et al.* Morbidity associated with sickle cell disease in pregnancy. *Am J Obstet Gynecol* 2008; 199:125.e1–15.
27. Dare FO, Bako AU, Ezechi OC. Puerperal sepsis: a preventable post-partum complication. *Trop Doct* 1998; 28:92–5.
28. Key NS, Derebail VK. Sickle-cell trait: novel clinical significance. *Hematology Am Soc Hematol Educ Program* 2010; 2010:418–22.
29. Tsaras G, Owusu-Ansah A, Boateng FO, *et al.* Complications associated with sickle cell trait: a brief narrative review. *Am J Med* 2009; 122:507–12.
30. Sweet RL, Ledger WJ. Puerperal infectious morbidity: a two-year review. *Am J Obstet Gynecol* 1973; 117:1093–100.
31. Smaill FM, Gyte GML. Antibiotic prophylaxis versus no prophylaxis for preventing infection after cesarean section. *Cochrane Database Syst Rev* 2010; 1:CD007482.
32. Leth RA, Moller JK, Thomsen RW, *et al.* Risk of selected postpartum infections after cesarean section compared with vaginal birth: a five-year cohort study of 32,468 women. *Acta Obstet Gynecol Scand* 2009; 88:976–83.
33. Camann W, Tuomala R. Antibiotic prophylaxis for cesarean delivery: always before skin incision! *Int J Obstet Anesth* 2011; 20:1–2.
34. Costantine MM, Rahman M, Ghulmiyah L, *et al.* Timing of perioperative antibiotics for caesarean delivery: a metaanalysis. *Am J Obstet Gynecol* 2008; 199:301.e1–6.
35. American College of Obstetricians and Gynecologists. ACOG Committee Opinion No. 465: Antimicrobial prophylaxis for caesarean delivery: timing of administration. *Obstet Gynecol* 2010; 116:791–2.
36. National Institute for Health and Care Excellence. *Caesarean Section.* Clinical Guideline 132. London: NICE; 2011 (reviewed 2014). http://guidance.nice.org.uk/CG132
37. Lamont R, Sobel J, Kusanovic J, *et al.* Current debate on the use of antibiotic prophylaxis for caesarean section. *Br J Obstet Gynaecol* 2011; 118:193–201.
38. Alfirevic Z, Gyte GML, Dou L. Different classes of antibiotics given to women routinely for preventing infection at caesarean section. *Cochrane Database Syst Rev* 2010; 10:CD008726.
39. World Health Organization. *Unsafe Abortion: Global and Regional Estimates of the Incidence of Unsafe Abortion and Associated Mortality in 2008* (6th ed). Geneva: WHO; 2011. http://whqlibdoc.who.int/publications/2011/9789241501118_eng.pdf
40. Stubblefield PG, Grimes DA. Septic abortion. *N Engl J Med* 1994; 33:310–14.
41. Tita ATN, Andrews WW. Diagnosis and management of clinical chorioamnionitis. *Clin Perinatol* 2010; 37(2):339–54.
42. Gibbs RS, Duff P. Progress in pathogenesis and management of clinical intraamniotic infection. *Am J Obstet Gynecol* 1991; 164:1317–26.
43. Soper DE, Mayhall CG, Froggatt JW. Characterization and control of intraamniotic infection in an urban teaching hospital. *Am J Obstet Gynecol* 1996; 175:304–9.
44. Rickert VI, Wiemann CM, Hankins GD, *et al.* Prevalence and risk factors of chorioamnionitis among adolescents. *Obstet Gynecol* 1998; 92:254–7.
45. Tran SH, Caughey AB, Musci TJ. Meconium-stained amniotic fluid is associated with puerperal infections. *Am J Obstet Gynecol* 2003; 189:746–50.
46. Seaward PG, Hannah ME, Myhr TL, *et al.* International Multicentre Term Prelabor Rupture of Membranes Study: evaluation of predictors of clinical chorioamnionitis and postpartum fever in patients with prelabor rupture of membranes at term. *Am J Obstet Gynecol* 1997; 177:1024–9.
47. Newton ER, Piper J, Peairs W. Bacterial vaginosis and intraamniotic infection. *Am J Obstet Gynecol* 1997; 176:672–7.
48. Mark SP, Croughan-Minihane MS, Kilpatrick SJ. Chorioamnionitis and uterine function. *Obstet Gynecol* 2000; 95:909–12.
49. Yokoe DS, Christiansen CL, Johnson R, *et al.* Epidemiology of and Surveillance for Postpartum Infectious. *Emerg Infect Dis* 2001; 7:837–41.
50. KinlayJ, O'Connell D, Kinlay S. Incidence of mastitis in breastfeeding women six months after delivery: a prospective cohort study. *Med J Aust* 1998; 169:310–12.
51. Stafford I, Hernandez J, Laibl V, *et al.* Community-acquired methicillin-resistant Staphylococcus aureus among patients with puerperal mastitis requiring hospitalization. *Obstet Gynecol* 2008; 112:533–7.
52. Lee IW, Kang L, Hsu HP, *et al.* Puerperal mastitis requiring hospitalization during a nine-year period. *Am J Obstet Gynecol* 2010; 203:332.

53. Macejko AM, Schaeffer AJ. Asymptomatic bacteriuria and symptomatic urinary tract infections during pregnancy. *Urol Clin North Am* 2007; 34:35–42
54. Gilstrap LC, Ramin SM. Urinary tract infections during pregnancy. *Obstet Gynecol Clin North Am* 2001; 28:581–91.
55. Wing DA, Fassett MJ, Getahun D. Acute pyelonephritis in pregnancy: a 18-year retrospective analysis. *Am J Obstet Gynecol* 2014; 210(3):219.e1–6.
56. Farkash E, Weintraub AY, Sergienko R, *et al.* Acute antepartum pyelonephritis in pregnancy: a critical analysis of risk factors and outcomes. *Eur J Obstet Gynecol Reprod Biol* 2012; 162:24–7.
57. Stray-Pdersen B, Blakstad M, Bergan T. Bacteriuria in the puerperium. Risk factors, screening procedures, and treatment programs. *Am J Obstet Gynecol* 990; 162:792–7.
58. Smaill FM, Vazquez JC. Antibiotics for asymptomatic bacteriuria in pregnancy. *Cochrane Database Syst Rev* 2007; 2:CD000490.
59. Khlifi A, Kebaili S, Hammami M, *et al.* Postpartum ovarian vein thrombophlebitis: report of a case and review of the literature. *North Am J Med Sci* 2010; 2:389–91.
60. Takach TJ, Cervera RD, Gregoric ID. Ovarian vein and caval thrombosis. *Tex Heart Inst J* 2005; 32:579–82
61. Dessole S, Capobianco G, Arru A, *et al.* Postpartum ovarian vein thrombosis: an unpredictable event: two case reports and review of the literature. *Arch Gynecol Obstet* 2003; 267:242–6.
62. Carr S. Surgical treatment of ovarian vein thrombosis. *Vasc Endovascular Surg.* 2007; 40:505–8.
63. Goodnight WH, Soper DE. Pneumonia in pregnancy. *Crit Care Med* 2005; 33:S390–S397.
64. Berkowitz K, LaSala A. Risk factors associated with the increasing prevalence of pneumonia during pregnancy. *Am J Obstet Gynecol* 1990; 163:981–5.
65. Munn MB, Groome LJ, Atterbury JL, *et al.* Pneumonia as a complication of pregnancy. *J Matern Fetal Med* 1999; 8:151–4
66. Intensive Care National Audit & Research Centre. *Female Admissions (Aged 16–50 years) to Adult, General Critical Care Units in England, Wales and Northern Ireland Reported as 'Currently Pregnant' or 'Recently Pregnant'.* Report from the Intensive Care National Audit & Research Centre. London: ICNARC; 2013. https://www.icnarc.org/documents/Obstetric%20admissions%20to%20critical%20care%20 2009-2012.pdf
67. Jenkins TM, Troiano NH, Graves CR, *et al.* Mechanical ventilation in an obstetric population: characteristics and delivery rates. *Am J Obstet Gynecol* 2003; 188:549–52
68. Graves CR. Pneumonia in pregnancy. *Clin Obstet Gynecol* 2010; 53:329–36.
69. Lima WS, Macfarlane JT, Colthorpe CL. Pneumonia and pregnancy. *Thorax* 2001; 56:398–405
70. Australian and New Zealand Intensive Care Influenza Investigators, Australasian Maternity Outcomes Surveillance System. Critical illness due to 2009 A/H1N1 influenza in pregnant and postpartum women: population based cohort study. *BMJ* 2010; 340:c1279.
71. Siston AM, Rasmussen SA, Honein MA, *et al.* Pandemic 2009 influenza A(H1N1) virus illness among pregnant women in the United States. *JAMA* 2010; 303:1517–25.
72. Pierce M, Kurinczuk JJ, Spark P, *et al.* Perinatal outcomes after maternal 2009/H1N1 infection: national cohort study. *BMJ* 2011; 342:d3214.
73. Drife J. Infection and maternal mortality. In Maclean AB, Regan L, Carrington D (eds) *Infection and Pregnancy.* London: RCOG Press; 2001:355–64.
74. Steer P. Puerperal sepsis. In Chamberlain G, Steer P (eds) *Turnbull's Obstetrics* (3rd ed). London: Churchill Livingstone; 2001:663–70.
75. Carapetis JR, Steer AC, Mulholland EK, *et al.* The global burden of group A streptococcal disease. *Lancet Infect Dis* 2005; 5:685–94.
76. Abouzeid H, Wu P, Mohammed N, *et al.* Group A streptococcal puerperal sepsis: the return of a potentially fatal disease. *J Obstet Gynaecol* 2005; 25:806–8.
77. Efstratiou A. Group A streptococci in the 1990s. *J Antimicrob Chemother* 2000; 45 Suppl:3–12.
78. Hamilton SM, Stevens DL, Bryant AE. Pregnancy-related group A streptococcal infections: temporal relationships between bacterial acquisition, infection onset, clinical findings, and outcome. *Clin Infect Dis* 2013; 57:870–6.
79. Loughnan BA, Grover M, Nielsen PB. Maternal death due to extended spectrum beta-lactamase-producing E. coli: a warning for the future? *Int J Obstet Anesth* 2010; 19:327–30.
80. Abraham EP, Chain E. An enzyme from bacteria able to destroy penicillin [letter]. *Nature* 1940; 146:837.
81. Public Health England. *Extended-Spectrum Beta-Lactamases (ESBLs): Guidance, Data, Analysis.* 2014. [Online] http://www.hpa.org.uk/Topics/InfectiousDiseases/InfectionsAZ/ESBLs/
82. Turner PJ. Extended-spectrum beta-lactamases. *Clin Infect Dis* 2005; 15; 41 Suppl 4:S273–5.
83. Akram S, Hossain, A, Shamsuzzaman AKM, *et al.* Aerobic bacterial pattern in puerperal sepsis. *Bangladesh J Med Microbiol* 2008; 2:22–7.
84. Hogan MC, Foreman KJ, Naghavi M, *et al.* Maternal mortality for 181 countries, 1980–2008: a systematic analysis of progress towards Millennium Development Goal 5. *Lancet* 2010; 375:1609–23.
85. World Health Authority. *Trends in Maternal Mortality 1990–2008.* [Online] http://whqlibdoc.who.int/publications/2010/9789241500265_eng.pdf
86. McIntyre J. Mothers infected with HIV. *Br Med Bull* 2003; 67:127–35.
87. Ahmad H, Mehta NJ, Manikal VM, *et al.* Pneumocystis carinii pneumonia in pregnancy. *Chest* 2001; 120:666–71.
88. National Committee for Confidential Enquiries into Maternal Deaths. *Saving Mothers 2005–2007: Fourth Report on Confidential Enquiries into Maternal Deaths in South Africa.* Pretoria: National Department of Health, 2009.
89. Mnyani C, McIntyre J. Tuberculosis in pregnancy. *BJOG* 2011; 118:226–31.
90. Black V, Brooke S, Chersich MF. Effect of human immunodeficiency virus treatment on maternal mortality at a tertiary center in South Africa: a 5-year audit. *Obstet Gynecol* 2009; 114:292–9.
91. Moodley J, Pattinson R, Baxter C, *et al.* Strengthening HIV services for pregnant women: an opportunity to reduce maternal mortality rates in Southern Africa/sub-Saharan Africa. *BJOG* 2011; 118:219–25.
92. Dombrovskiy VY, Martin AA, Sunderram J, *et al.* Rapid increase in hospitalisation and mortality rates for severe sepsis in the United States: a trend analysis from 1993 to 2003. *Crit Care Med* 2007; 35:1414–15.
93. Harrison DA, Welch CA, Eddlestone JM. The epidemiology of severe sepsis in England, Wales and Northern Ireland, 1996 to 2004: secondary analysis of a high quality database, the ICNARC Case Mix Programme database. *Crit Care* 2006; 10:R42.
94. Brun-Buisson C, Doyon F, Carlet J. Incidence, risk factors, and outcome of severe sepsis and septic shock in adults. A multi-center prospective study in intensive care units. French ICU group for Severe Sepsis. *JAMA* 1995; 274:968–74.
95. Gendrel D, Raymond J, Coste J, *et al.* Comparison of procalcitonin with C-reactive protein, interleukin 6 and interferon-alpha for differentiation of bacterial vs. viral infections. *Pediatr Infect Dis* J 1999; 18:875–81.
96. Uzzan B, Cohen R, Nicholas P, *et al.* Procalcitonin as a diagnostic test for sepsis in critically ill adults and after surgery or trauma: a systematic review and meta-analysis. *Crit Care Med* 2006; 34:1996–2003.
97. Tang BMP, Eslick GD, Craig JC, *et al.* Accuracy of procalcitonin for sepsis diagnosis in critically ill patients: systematic review and meta-analysis. *Lancet Infect Dis* 2007; 7:210–17.
98. Kive S, Adams K, Barlow G. Diagnostic and prognostic biomarkers of sepsis in critical care. *J Antimicrob Chemother* 2011; 66: Suppl 2:ii33–ii40.

99. Paccolat C, Harbarth S, Courvoisier D, *et al.* Procalcitonin levels during pregnancy, delivery and postpartum. *J Perinat Med* 2011; 39:679–83.
100. Paruk F. Infection in obstetric critical care. *Best Pract Res Clin Obstet Gynaecol* 2008; 22:865–83.
101. Sheffield JS. Sepsis and septic shock in pregnancy. *Crit Care Clin* 2004; 20:651–60.
102. Casey BM, Cox SM. Chorioamnionitis and endometritis. *Infect Dis Clin North Am* 1997; 11:203–22.
103. Hillman K, Chen J, Cretikos M, *et al.* Introduction of the medical emergency team (MET) system: a cluster-randomised controlled trial. *Lancet* 2005; 365:2091–7.
104. Lappen JR, Keene M, Lore M, *et al.* Existing models fail to predict sepsis in an obstetric population with intrauterine infection. *Am J Obstet Gynecol* 2010; 203:573.e1–5.
105. Singh S, McGlennan A, England A, *et al.* A validation study of the CEMACH recommended modified early obstetric warning system (MEOWS). *Anaesthesia* 2012; 67:12–18.
106. Carle C, Alexander P, Columb M, *et al.* Design and internal validation of an obstetric early warning score: secondary analysis of the Intensive Care National Audit and Research Centre Case Mix Programme database. *Anaesthesia* 2013; 68:354–67.
107. Oxford Biomedical Research Centre. *Biomedical Informatics and Technology — Oxford 4P Study Pregnancy Physiology Pattern Prediction.* [Online] http://oxfordbrc.nihr.ac.uk/biomedical/biomedical-research/oxford-4p-study-pregnancy-physiology-pattern-prediction
108. Royal College of Obstetricians and Anaesthetists. *Maternal Collapse in Pregnancy and the Puerperium.* Green-top Guideline No. 56. London: RCOG; 2011. http://www.rcog.org.uk/files/rcog-corp/GTG56.pdf
109. Surviving Sepsis Bundle http://www.survivingsepsis.org/sitecollectiondocuments/sscbundle.pdf (accessed January 2016)
110. Peden CJ, Rooney KD. The science of improvement as it relates to quality and safety in the ICU. *J Intensive Care Soc* 2009; 10:260–4.
111. Gao F, Melody T, Daniels R, *et al.* The impact of compliance with 6-hour and 24-hour sepsis bundles on hospital mortality in patients with severe sepsis: a prospective observational study. *Crit Care* 2005; 9:764–70.
112. Kumar A, Roberts D, Wood KE, *et al.* Duration of hypotension before initiation of effective antimicrobial therapy is the critical determinant of survival in human septic shock. *Crit Care Med* 2006 34:1589–96.
113. Zubert S, Funk DJ, Kumar A. Antibiotics in sepsis and septic shock: like everything else in life, timing is everything. *Crit Care Med* 2010; 38:1211–12.
114. Handelsman J, Maki DG, Does combination antimicrobial therapy reduce mortality in Gram-negative bacteraemia? A meta-analysis. *Lancet Infect Dis* 2004; 4:519–27.
115. Guinn DA, Abel DE, Tomlinson MW. Early goal directed therapy for sepsis during pregnancy. *Obstet Gynecol Clin North Am* 2007; 34:459–79.
116. Pea F, Viale P. Bench to bedside review: appropriate antibiotic therapy in severe sepsis and septic shock—does the dose matter? *Crit Care* 2009; 13:214.
117. Murry KR, McKinnon PS, Mitrzyk B, *et al.* Pharmacodynamic characterization of nephrotoxicity associated with once-daily aminoglycoside. *Pharmacotherapy* 1999; 19:1252–60.
118. Gattimoni L, Brazzi L, Pelosi P, *et al.* A trial of goal directed hemodynamic therapy in critically ill patients. *N Engl J Med* 1995; 333:1025–32.
119. Rivers E, Nguyen B, Havstad S, *et al.* Early Goal-Directed therapy Collaborative Group. Early goal-directed therapy in the treatment of severe sepsis and septic shock. *N Engl J Med* 2001; 345:1368–77.
120. Kern JW, Shoemaker WC. Meta-analysis of hemodynamic optimization in high-risk patients. *Crit Care Med* 2002; 30:1686–92.
121. Russell JA, Walley KR, Gordon AC, *et al.* Interaction of vasopressin infusion, corticosteroid treatment, and mortality of septic shock. *Crit Care Med* 2009; 37:811–18.
122. Perel P, Roberts I, Ker K. Colloids versus crystalloids for fluid resuscitation in critically ill patients. *Cochrane Database Syst Rev* 2013; 2:CD000567.
123. European Medicines Agency. *Hydroxyethyl-Starch Solutions (HES) Should No Longer be Used in Patients with Sepsis or Burn Injuries or in Critically Ill Patients - CMDh Endorses PRAC Recommendations.* 2013. [Online] http://www.ema.europa.eu/ema/index.jsp?curl=pages/news_and_events/news/2013/10/news_detail_001930.jsp&mid=WC0b01ac058004d5c1
124. Annane D, Vigno P, Renault A, *et al.* Norepinephrine plus dobutamine versus epinephrine alone for management of septic shock: a randomized trial. *Lancet* 2007; 370:676–84.
125. Park DW, Chun BC, Kwon SS, *et al.* Red blood cell transfusions are associated with lower mortality in patients with severe sepsis and septic shock: a propensity-matched analysis. *Crit Care Med* 2012; 40:3140–5.
126. National Institute for Health and Clinical Excellence. *Cardio Q-ODM Oesophageal Doppler Monitor.* NICE Medical Technologies 3. London: National Institute for Health and Clinical Excellence; 2011.
127. Chatterjee, DJ, Bukunola B, Samuels TL, *et al.* Resuscitation in massive obstetric haemorrhage using an intraosseous needle. *Anaesthesia* 2011; 66:306–10.
128. Armstrong S, Fernando R, Columb M. Minimally- and non-invasive assessment of maternal cardiac output: go with the flow! *Int J Obstet Anesth* 2011; 20:330–40.
129. Hayes MA, Timmins AC, Yau EHS. Elevation of systemic oxygen delivery in the treatment of critically ill patients. *N Engl J Med* 1994; 330:1712–22.
130. Daniels R, Nutbeam T, McNamara G, *et al.* The sepsis six and the severe sepsis resuscitation bundle: a prospective observational cohort study. *Emerg Med J* 2011; 28:507–12.
131. Pauzner D, Wolman I, Abramov L, *et al.* Post-cesarean-section necrotizing fasciitis: report of a case and review of the literature. *Gynecol Obstet Invest* 1994; 37:59–62.
132. Ghandi P, Singh S, Farkas A. Group B streptococcal necrotising fasciitis following normal vaginal delivery. *J Obstet Gynaecol* 2009; 29:554.
133. Gallup DG, Freedman MA, Meguiar RV, *et al.* Necrotizing fasciitis in gynecologic and obstetric patients: a surgical emergency. *Am J Obstet Gynecol* 2002; 187:305–10.
134. Tomlinson MW, Caruthers TJ, Whitty JE, *et al.* Does delivery improve maternal condition in the respiratory-compromised gravida? *Obstet Gynecol* 1998; 91:108–11.
135. Snyder CC, Barton JR, Habli M, *et al.* Severe sepsis and septic shock in pregnancy: indications for delivery and maternal and perinatal outcomes. *J Matern Fetal Neonatal Med* 2013; 26:503–6.
136. Wong SF, Chow KM, de Swiet, M. Severe acute respiratory syndrome and pregnancy. *BJOG* 2003; 110:641–2.
137. Eissa D, Carton EG, Buggy DJ. Anaesthetic management of patients with severe sepsis. *Br J Anaesth* 2010; 105:734–43.
138. Broughton-Pipkin F. Maternal physiology in obstetrics. In Chamberlain G, Steer P (eds) *Turnbull's Obstetrics* (3rd ed). London: Churchill Livingstone; 2001:71–91.
139. Blanco JD, Gibbs RS, Castaneda YS. Bacteremia in obstetrics: clinical course. *Obstet Gynecol* 1981; 58:621–5.
140. Kitching AJ, Rice ASC. Extradural abscess in the postpartum period. *Br J Anaesth* 1993; 70:703.
141. Reihsaus E, Waldbaur H, Seeling W. Spinal epidural abscess: a meta-analysis of 915 patients. *Neurosurg Rev* 2000; 23:175–204.
142. Cook TM, Counsell D, Wildsmith JAW. Major complications of central neuraxial block: report on the Third National Audit of The Royal College of Anaesthetists. *Br J Anaesth* 2009; 102:179–90.

143. Scott DB, Hibbard BM. Serious non-fatal complications associated with epidural block in obstetric practice. *Br J Anaesth* 1990; 64:537–41.
144. Strong WE. Epidural abscess associated with epidural catheterisation: A rare event? Report of two cases with markedly delayed presentation. *Anesthesiology* 1991; 74:943–6.
145. Lee JJ, Parry H. Bacterial meningitis following spinal anaesthesia for Caesarean section. *Br J Anaesth* 1991; 66:383–6.
146. Ready LB, Heifer D. Bacterial meningitis in parturients after epidural anesthesia. *Anesthesiology* 1989; 71:988–90.
147. Harding SA, Collis RE, Morgan BM. Meningitis after combined spinal-extradural anaesthesia in obstetrics. *Br J Anaesth* 1994; 73:545–7.
148. Hebl JR. The importance and implications of aseptic techniques during regional anesthesia. *Reg Anesth Pain Med* 2006; 31:311–23.
149. Wedel DJ, Horlocker TT. Regional anesthesia in the febrile or infected patient. *Reg Anesth Pain Med* 2006; 31:324–33.
150. Merién AE, van de Ven J, Mol BW, *et al.* Multidisciplinary team training in a simulation setting for acute obstetric emergencies: a systematic review. *Obstet Gynecol* 2010; 115:1021–31.
151. De Miguel-Yanes JM, Muñoz-González J, Andueza-Lillo JA, *et al.* Implementation of a bundle of actions to improve adherence to the Surviving Sepsis Campaign guidelines at the ED. *Am J Emerg Med* 2009; 27:668–74.

CHAPTER 35

Obstetric haemorrhage

Jane E. Norman and Vicki Clark

Definitions

Obstetric haemorrhage encompasses both antepartum (APH) and postpartum haemorrhage (PPH).

Antepartum haemorrhage

The Royal College of Obstetricians and Gynaecologists (RCOG) defines APH as 'bleeding from or into the genital tract, occurring from 24 weeks of pregnancy and prior to the birth of the baby'.[1] This symptom-based definition will be used throughout this chapter.

Postpartum haemorrhage

PPH is defined as loss of 500 mL or more of blood from the genital tract within 24 hours of the birth of a baby.[2] PPH can be minor (500–1000 mL) or major (more than 1000 mL). These definitions are endorsed in a World Health Organization (WHO) guideline on the management of PPH.[3] Secondary PPH is defined as abnormal or excessive bleeding from the birth canal between 24 hours and 12 weeks postnatally. The tenth revision of the International Classification of Diseases (ICD-10) code for PPH [072] is defined as 'haemorrhage after delivery of the fetus or infant' with no specific volume or time interval attached (Box 35.1).

In the Scottish Confidential Audit of Severe Maternal Morbidity (SCASMM), major obstetric haemorrhage has been defined as occurring in women with 'estimated blood loss of ≥2500 mL, or who are transfused 5 or more units of blood or receive treatment for coagulopathy (fresh frozen plasma, cryoprecipitate, platelets)'.[4]

Statistics

Major obstetric haemorrhage was reported to occur in around 3.7/1000 births in Scotland during the period 2003–2005 (95% confidence interval (CI) 3.4–4.0).[5] Most recent data from Scotland suggests that the rate of major obstetric haemorrhage has increased to 5.5/1000 births in 2010.[4] This increase has been attributed to better ascertainment rather than increased incidence, although the fact that PPH itself is increasing raises cause for concern (see later in this section). Less than 10% of major obstetric haemorrhages occur antenatally (usually due to praevia or abruption) with the remainder occurring either intrapartum (10%) or postpartum (80%).[4] These data confirm major obstetric haemorrhage to be the commonest major obstetric complication. On the background of this increasing incidence of major obstetric haemorrhage, it is reassuring that the rate of direct maternal deaths due to haemorrhage (i.e. deaths resulting from obstetric haemorrhage complications of the pregnant state (pregnancy, labour and puerperium) is stable[6] (Table 35.1). In the last 'Saving Lives, Improving Mothers' Care (MBRRACE)' report for which data is available (2009–2012), the maternal death rate due to haemorrhage was 0.49/100,000 maternities (95% CI 0.29–0.78).[6]

Worldwide rates of PPH (of which major obstetric haemorrhage occurs in a subset) are around 30–70/1000 births, and have also been found to be increasing.[7–10] Increasing rates of atonic PPH appear to be a major cause.[7,9,10] There is a significant regional variation in PPH rates, perhaps reflecting either differences in methods to measure blood loss, or a truly lower prevalence in Asian compared with European women.[11]

Major obstetric haemorrhage is the commonest reason for intensive therapy unit (ITU) admission amongst pregnant women, accounting for nearly 50% of admissions. The outcome for the baby is also compromised, with perinatal mortality rates of 55.3/1000 in the last SCASSM report.[4,12]

Risk factors for postpartum haemorrhage

Uterine atony is the commonest cause of major obstetric haemorrhage,[4] occurring in 52% of those affected. A further 18% have retained placenta/fetal membranes. Women undergoing emergency caesarean delivery are over-represented amongst those with major obstetric haemorrhage, with 44% of major obstetric haemorrhage associated with this scenario (compared to 15% of those without).

In a large population-based study of over 850,000 deliveries, the following were independent risk factors for PPH due to uterine atony that was sufficiently severe to require blood transfusion: age less than 20 or greater than 40 years, caesarean delivery, hypertensive diseases of pregnancy, polyhydramnios, chorioamnionitis,

Box 35.1 Obstetric haemorrhage—definitions

The ICD-10 codes antepartum haemorrhage by both aetiology (e.g. premature separation of the placenta (abruption placentae) [045], and placenta praevia (a condition in which the placenta is implanted in the lower part of the uterus) [044]) and by symptoms (e.g. antepartum haemorrhage not elsewhere classified [046], which specifically excludes haemorrhage in early pregnancy, placenta praevia, and abruption placentae; and intrapartum haemorrhage [067]). These definitions are important for international comparisons, but include women with pathology (placenta praevia) who are not actively bleeding.

Data from various sources (see references).

Table 35.1 Direct deaths by type of obstetric haemorrhage 1994–2012

Time period	Placental Abruption	Placental praevia	Postpartum haemorrhage		Total deaths from haemorrhage	Direct haemorrhage death rate per 100,000 maternities	
			Atony	Genital Tract Trauma		rate	CI
1994–06	4	3	5	5	17	0.77	0.45–1.24
1997–99	3	3	1	2	9	0.42	0.19–0.80
2000–02	3	4	10	1	18	0.9	0.53–1.42
2003–05	2	3	9	3	17	0.8	0.47–1.29
2006–08	2	2	3+2	(0/2)	9	0.39	0.18–0.75
2009–12†	2	1*	7**	7***	17	0.49	0.29–0.78

Reproduced from Knight M, Kenyon S, Brocklehurst P, *et al. Saving Lives, Improving Mothers' Care – Lessons Learned to Inform Future Maternity Care from the UK and Ireland Confidential Enquiries into Maternal Deaths and Morbidity 2009–12*. Oxford: National Perinatal Epidemiology Unit, University of Oxford; 2014. © 2014 National Perinatal Epidemiology Unit, University of Oxford.

†Figures for UK and Ireland. All other figures are UK only.

*One placenta praevia percreta.

**Includes one woman who had a portion of retained placenta which contributed to the bleeding, and one who also sustained vaginal tears.

***There were four ruptured uteri, two others were lower genital tract trauma, and one had trauma sustained in the form of angle extensions at caesarean section.

multiple pregnancy, retained placenta, and APH.[13] The adjusted odds of PPH were stronger after emergency compared with elective caesarean delivery, but the greatest odds of PPH were observed in association with retained placenta, leading to a 4.1 (3.1–5.5) adjusted odds of atonic PPH requiring transfusion. In another population-based study of 650,000 deliveries, extremes of age, caesarean delivery, hypertensive diseases of pregnancy, polyhydramnios, chorioamnionitis, and multiple pregnancy were also confirmed as risk factors for atonic PPH, with the presence of a large fetus, maternal diabetes, genital tract trauma, and instrumental delivery being additional risk factors.[9] The highest relative risk (RR) of haemorrhage was in women diagnosed with a morbidly adherent placenta who had a markedly higher risk of total PPH (unadjusted RR 13.14; 95% CI 11.43–15.11).[9] Other known risk factors for PPH include upright position in labour (RR 1.65; 95% CI 1.32–2.60, although there is evidence of publication bias),[14] obesity[15] and antidepressant use in pregnancy (RR 1.4–1.9-fold[16]). Elective and/or postdates induction of labour may be protective against PPH.[17] Having a mother or grandmother with PPH does not appear to confer increased risk.[18]

The association between caesarean delivery and PPH noted in both the above-mentioned large prospective studies and in Scottish data on major obstetric haemorrhage is important. Given that emergency caesarean delivery (particularly emergency caesarean at full dilatation) is a stronger risk factor than elective caesarean delivery, it is possible that the association derives from common risk factors for both (such as poor uterine contractility), rather than the process of caesarean delivery itself. The independent effect of caesarean delivery can be inferred from the few randomized trials of caesarean delivery compared with vaginal delivery, either for breech presentation[19] or in the scenario of previous caesarean delivery.[20] In the former scenario, there were no significant differences in rates of maternal PPH between the groups (with the trends favouring elective caesarean delivery).[19] A randomized trial of mode of delivery in women with a previous caesarean delivery favoured repeat elective caesarean delivery, with the risk of major haemorrhage (blood loss > 1500 mL and/or need for blood transfusion) actually being lower in the elective caesarean delivery group in women with a previous caesarean delivery (RR 0.37; 95% CI 0.17–0.80).[20]

Antenatal and intrapartum optimization

Prevention of anaemia

A major strand of antenatal optimization of major obstetric haemorrhage involves ensuring pregnant women maintain their haemoglobin concentrations during pregnancy. The National Institute of Health and Care Excellence (NICE) identifies maternal anaemia (haemoglobin of <8.5g/dL) as a possible risk factor for PPH, although it notes that the evidence is inconclusive. Regardless, women with a low haemoglobin are evidently more at risk of adverse consequences following any further blood loss. Screening for anaemia is part of good antenatal care, with NICE advising that 'Screening should take place early in pregnancy (at the booking appointment) and at 28 weeks when other blood screening tests are being performed. This allows enough time for treatment if anaemia is detected'.[21] This is a grade B recommendation. NICE further suggests that haemoglobin levels outside the normal UK range for pregnancy (that is, 11 g/100 mL at first contact and 10.5 g/100 mL at 28 weeks' gestation) should be investigated and iron supplementation considered if indicated (grade A recommendation).[21] Although routine iron supplementation reduces the risk of maternal anaemia, it is associated with adverse maternal effects without improving outcomes and is not therefore recommended. Despite these recommendations, which are not new, the recent Confidential Enquiries on Maternal Health again identified a low haemoglobin at the time of delivery as a factor in maternal haemorrhage due to atony attributed to depleted uterine myoglobin levels necessary for uterine contraction.[6] Parenteral iron preparations should be considered in women who are unable to take or are unresponsive to oral iron (see Chapter 48).

Antenatal identification of placenta praevia/accreta

Pre-delivery identification has a major role to play in optimizing outcomes in women with placenta praevia or accreta. All women with a previous caesarean delivery should have ultrasound localization of placental site performed in the third trimester because of the increased risk of placenta praevia and accreta in this scenario.[3] The risk of both praevia and accreta is proportional to the number of previous caesarean deliveries—women with three or more caesarean deliveries *and* placenta praevia in the index pregnancy have over a 50% risk of each of placenta accreta and hysterectomy, and over an 80% risk of composite maternal morbidity. Although magnetic resonance imaging is increasingly used before delivery as an adjunct to ultrasound in women with suspected placenta accreta, MRI is not 100% accurate in the diagnosis of accreta and current expert advice is that ultrasound is sufficient unless there is uncertainty.[22]

Intrapartum and immediate postpartum care

Routine management of the third stage after vaginal delivery

The mainstay of 'routine' obstetric management to prevent major obstetric haemorrhage is 'active' management of the third stage of labour. This is a package of care consisting of prophylactic administration of a uterotonic agent, early cord clamping and controlled cord traction to deliver the placenta. Active management of third stage of labour is associated with a major reduction in the risk of blood loss over 1 L (RR 0.34; 95% CI 0.14–0.87),[23] although recent evidence suggests that controlled cord traction adds little to the efficacy of the other components of active management, and can be omitted with minimal effect on major haemorrhage rates.[24] NICE indicates that 'Active management of the third stage is recommended, which includes the use of oxytocin (10 international units [IU] by intramuscular injection), followed by deferred clamping and cutting of the cord and controlled cord traction'.[25] In view of the maternal side effects of active management (nausea, vomiting, and headache), and the strong wish by some women to have a 'physiological' third stage, NICE also suggests that 'Women at low risk of postpartum haemorrhage who request physiological management of the third stage should be supported in their choice.'

Importantly, the oxytocic agent endorsed by NICE is oxytocin, 10 IU.[25] Although there is evidence that routine oxytocin–ergometrine (Syntometrine) is superior to oxytocin alone for prevention of PPH (with the odds of blood loss > 500 mL in the oxytocin–ergometrine group being 0.82 times that of the oxytocin group),[26] the side effects of combination therapy are considered to be too great to warrant routine use. Sublingual misoprostol also reduces the risk of severe PPH (compared with no treatment), but is associated with both a greater risk of severe PPH *and* a greater risk of maternal shivering and pyrexia compared with conventional injectional uterotonics, so its use is best restricted to countries where other agents are not available.[27]

Routine management of the third stage during caesarean delivery

In women undergoing caesarean delivery, 5 IU of oxytocin given slowly intravenously is recommended to prevent PPH—this dose appears as effective as a 10 IU dose but is associated with fewer side effects such as hypotension and tachycardia.[28,29] The oxytocin analogue carbetocin may reduce the requirement for further uterotonics, but does not appear to be superior to Syntocinon® in terms of prevention of PPH.[30]

Delivery of women with placenta praevia/accrete

Where placenta praevia and/or placenta accreta is identified, delivery should be by caesarean. In asymptomatic women, delivery should be deferred until at least 38 weeks of gestation for women with placenta praevia and 36–37 weeks of gestation for women with suspected placenta accreta. Delivery in both these scenarios should be conducted in units that can cope with the risk of major obstetric haemorrhage—blood transfusion and intensive care facilities should both be available. In women with placenta praevia but not accreta, the RCOG suggests that the method of anaesthesia can be a decision for an individual anaesthetist.[3] Where there is anterior placenta praevia, a strategy of inserting the operator's hand through the lower segment incision and then superiorly between the uterus and the placenta to access the fetus is likely to be safer than cutting through the placenta.

Good practice advice is that women with suspected placenta accreta should be cross-matched before delivery and the use of cell salvage considered. If the placenta is morbidly adherent, consideration should be given to leaving it *in situ* rather than risking its traumatic avulsion.[3] There is no evidence for the efficacy of methotrexate in this scenario[22] but follow-up with human chorionic gonadotropin and ultrasound may be useful in confirming regression of placental tissue. Alternatively, where there is accreta, the use of a fundal uterine incision may avoid placental incision, although the latter is preferred by some authors.[31]

Interventional radiology (IR) balloon occlusion techniques are increasingly used to prevent haemorrhage in placenta accreta. Additionally, IR-administered embolization is increasingly used therapeutically in PPH. If an obstetric patient is at high risk of haemorrhage (e.g. has placenta accreta or fibroids), then prophylactic internal iliac balloons can be inserted prior to caesarean delivery (Figure 35.1). There is some controversy regarding the efficacy of this, with some studies demonstrating a reduction in blood loss or need for hysterectomy and others showing no difference.[32] This may be due to non-standardization of the techniques applied. Further, there is substantial collateral circulation to the uterus from the ovarian artery and vaginal plexuses so that even total occlusion of the internal iliac arteries may still result in bleeding.

There is also controversy about where surgery for the bleeding obstetric patient should take place—the obstetric theatre or the IR suite. Patients with suspected placenta accreta can be managed in the IR suite but this must match theatre standards of sterility and safety. If the patient is to be looked after in the obstetric suite, then an image intensifier and a radiologically compatible theatre table must be available.

Regardless of the therapeutic strategy employed, senior obstetric and anaesthetic staff should be readily available for the delivery of all women with placenta praevia, and directly involved in the delivery of all women with suspected placenta accreta.

Resuscitation in obstetric haemorrhage

Initial management

Management of obstetric haemorrhage requires more than one attendant, so help should be requested as soon as possible. Many

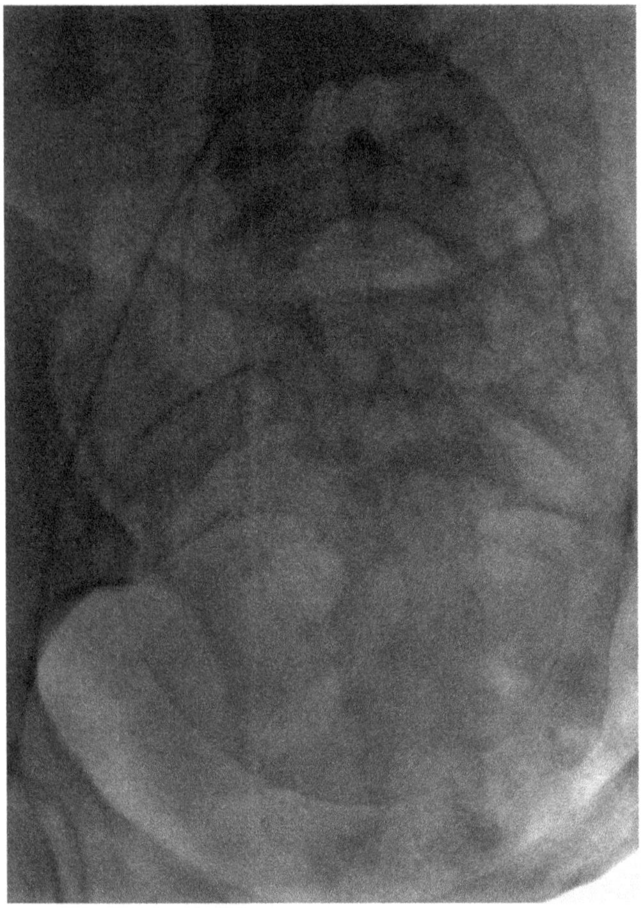

Figure 35.1 Interventional radiology bilateral internal iliac artery catheters inserted via contralateral femoral arteries prior to caesarean delivery in a case of placenta accrete. Balloons deflated.

Thanks to Dr. Hamish Ireland, Consultant Radiologist for the image of the internal iliac catheters.

hospitals have an emergency protocol in place whereby the switchboard will set off simultaneous pagers of all the relevant staff, that is, obstetricians, anaesthetists, midwives, operating department practitioners, and porters. The presence and experience of senior staff are essential in a major obstetric haemorrhage and in several CEMD reports[6,33,34] attendance of senior personnel too late in the care of such a patient and lack of continuity of care[6] have been criticized.

Assessment of the amount of blood loss can be difficult due to loss outside the hospital, on the bed linen, and floor. In some placental abruptions, blood loss may be entirely concealed. Observations of pulse rate, blood pressure, and peripheral circulation may guide assessment but often it is a 'guesstimate'. It is important to note that healthy parturients may maintain their blood pressure remarkably well until they have a lost a significant part of their (unreplaced) circulating blood volume by compensatory vasoconstriction, so pulse rate is a better indication of blood loss than blood pressure. Oliguria and poor capillary refill are other important signs, as is tachypnoea (Table 35.2). All these parameters normalize as the patient is appropriately resuscitated.

Obstetric haemorrhage should be treated, as all emergencies, along ABC lines. Most women are conscious unless hypovolaemia has compromised cerebral perfusion. Therefore the airway usually

Table 35.2 Signs of haemorrhagic shock

	Compensated	Mild	Moderate	Severe
Blood loss (mL)	<1000	1000–1500	1500–2000	>2000
Pulse rate (beats/min)	<100	100–120	120–140	>140
Systolic blood pressure	>100	<100	<80	Unrecordable
Peripheral extremities	Warm	Slightly cool	Very cool	Cold
Respiratory rate (breaths/min)	<20	20–25	25–30	>30
Urinary output (mL/h)	>30	<30	<20	Anuric
Conscious level	Normal	Agitated	Confused	Lethargic, unresponsive

does not need to be secured. A Hudson mask and high-flow oxygen should be given to maximize oxygen saturation. If the patient is antenatal, the wedged position is vital as aortocaval compression which reduces venous return, will worsen an already hypotensive situation.

Two large-bore cannulae should be inserted and appropriate blood samples sent for a full blood count, coagulation screen, biochemistry profile, and, most importantly, a group and save sample for cross-match.

From a practical point of view, both venous cannulae should be sited preferably in the same arm. Siting cannulae in different arms results in one cannula being occluded whenever the non-invasive blood pressure cuff is inflated and also reduces access for obtaining blood samples later. However, a patient who has lost significant blood may have peripherally collapsed veins and if it is only possible to gain venous access in both arms, then this should be pursued.

Many rapid infuser devices are available (e.g. the Belmont™ infusers). These can infuse at 1000 mL/min and simultaneously warm the fluids. Hypothermia should be avoided as this worsens coagulopathy.

Recently the intraosseous (IO) needle has been introduced to gain venous access when peripheral veins cannot be found (Figure 35.2).[35] This is particularly useful in the patient who is 'shut-down' or in the obese. The needle is inserted into the humerus or near the tibial tuberosity and fluids pumped into the medullary canal. The infusion rate through the IO needle can be 68–205 mL/min (without and with pressure bag)[36] and once the patient is resuscitated, conventional venous access may become easier.

Most obstetric patients should be able to withstand a degree of hypovolaemia without permanent effects. However, in previously healthy labouring women during PPH, Karpati et al. found that low systolic (<88 mmHg) and diastolic (<50 mmHg) pressures

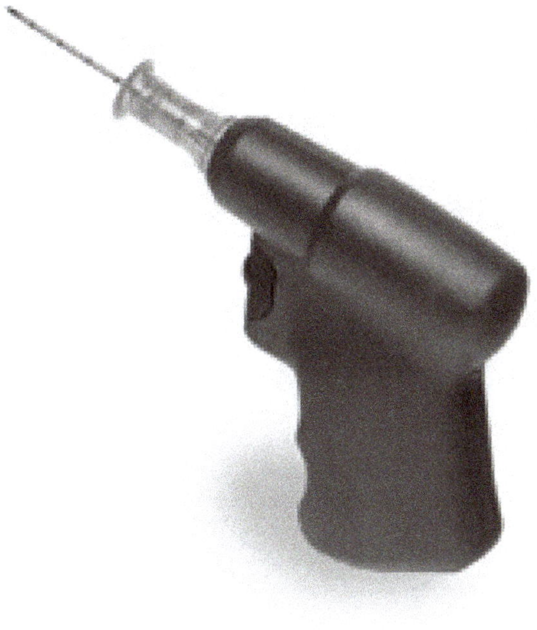

Figure 35.2 EZ IO® (intraosseous needle).
Reproduced with permission of Vidacare Corporation.

and a tachycardia of more than 115 beats/min were independent predictors of myocardial ischaemia[37] and therefore every effort should be made to maintain normotension and avoid tachycardia.

The patient who is bleeding should be resuscitated first with crystalloid fluid, for example, Hartmann's solution or saline to a maximum of 2 L. But if the patient is hypotensive, colloid is an alternative. No more than 1.5 L of colloid should be given. There is a danger of inducing pulmonary oedema and dilutional coagulopathy if large volumes of fluid are given.

Monitoring in obstetric haemorrhage

Essential monitoring includes electrocardiography, non-invasive blood pressure, and pulse oximetry. The patient should also be catheterized and placed on a Modified Early Warning Score (MEWS) chart (see Figure 35.3).

An arterial line is useful in a patient with major haemorrhage as it will give continuous blood pressure, is useful to guide inotropic support if needed, and also allows easy access for blood sampling. A central venous catheter (CVC) can also be useful to guide fluid therapy and to give inotropes. However, invasive lines are not without potential complications. Arterial spasm, thrombosis, and aneurysm formations are all well-known complications of arterial lines. CVC insertion may complicated by pneumothorax, carotid puncture, and air embolism. The risks versus the benefits should be considered before placing these lines.

Treatment of specific causes of bleeding

Management of antepartum haemorrhage

The major causes of APH include abruption and/or placenta praevia. Effective treatment of *both* of these causes of APH involves delivering the baby, and this should be undertaken in good time if the pregnancy is at term. When there is major haemorrhage, delivery by caesarean delivery is normally required in the maternal interest regardless of gestation. When bleeding is 'minor' (e.g. <500 mL), conservative treatment to enable fetal maturation or (in the case of abruption) induction of labour, may be appropriate. A detailed discussion of when it is reasonable to delay delivery in women with a preterm APH is discussed in Chapter 33. As described previously, caesarean delivery can be a challenging operation in women with massive obstetric haemorrhage, and senior assistance is advisable.

Pharmacological management of postpartum haemorrhage

Effective 'treatment' of PPH requires identification of the cause and appropriately directed therapy. Uterine atony is the single biggest cause of PPH. In the '4Ts' nomenclature, a useful method of remembering the causes of PPH, uterine atony is described as problems with 'tone'. This may be aggravated by 'tissue'—retained products of conception. Other causes include 'trauma' of the genital tract and 'thrombin' problems—coagulation defects.

Conservative therapy/examination under anaesthesia

Where uterine atony appears the likely cause of PPH, and when haemorrhage is minor, it is reasonable to attempt conservative therapy with oxytocic agents without transferring the woman to theatre. Where bleeding is heavier, regardless of the suspected cause of bleeding, transfer to theatre and examination under anaesthetic (EUA), including exploration of the uterine cavity, is wise. Any retained products of conception can then be removed. If bleeding is thought to be due to genital trauma, packing may be a useful interim measure, or an alternative to formal suturing if a repairable source of bleeding cannot be identified. The decision of which women can reasonably be managed conservatively is difficult, especially for the inexperienced clinician—PPH is a condition which can deteriorate rapidly and a low threshold both for requesting senior help *and* for transfer to theatre for EUA is advisable.

Atonic postpartum haemorrhage

Retained placental fragments can contribute to PPH—exploration of the uterine cavity is useful to determine firstly whether there are any placental fragments and secondly to remove them. Thereafter, bimanual compression of the uterus may temporarily halt the bleeding and gain some time. The evidence base for pharmacological management (in contrast to prevention) of PPH is limited. The following is based on good practice advice from the RCOG, and represent widely used strategies for the management of this condition. In order, relevant treatment strategies are: Syntocinon® 5 IU by slow intravenous administration (may be repeated); ergometrine 0.5 mg either intramuscularly or intravenously (note this can cause vomiting and is contraindicated in women with hypertension because of the risk of further amplifying hypertension and associated cerebrovascular accidents); and Syntocinon® 10 IU/h intravenously (administered as 40 IU in a 500 mL bag of crystalloid, administered at 125 mL/h).[2] Thereafter, further measures include carboprost 0.25 mg administered intramuscularly, to a total of eight doses at 15-minute intervals (there are some reports of improved outcomes with intramyometrial injection, although this is not normally recommended, and women with asthma should not be given carboprost regardless of route of administration as

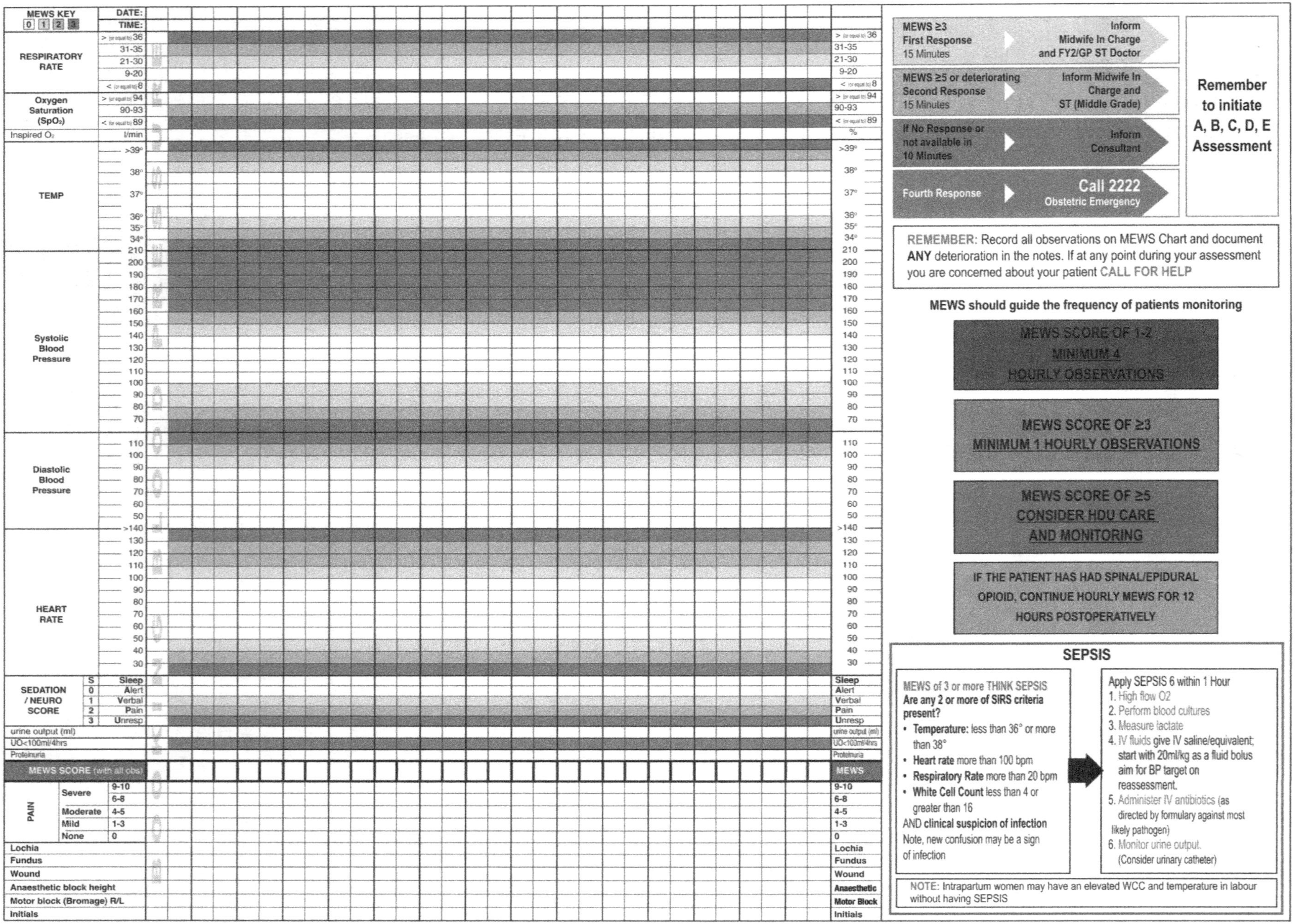

Figure 35.3 Example of a Modified Early Warning Score (MEWS) chart.

MEWS Chart

Consultant: ....
Date chart commenced: ....
This is chart number .... this admission
Booking weight .... kg BMI ....
Booking BP: ....

Attach a patient addressograph here
or
Name: ....
DOB: ....
CHI: ....

How to calculate a Maternal Early Warning Score (MEWS) in NHS Lothian

The clinical observations used to calculate a MEWS score are:

- Respiratory rate
- Oxygen saturation
- Temperature
- Systolic and diastolic blood pressure
- Heart rate
- Sedation/Neurological score (AVPU)
- Urine output

The MEWS chart is colour coded to identify when a clinical observation is outside the normal range. A MEWS of 0-3 is allocated to each parameter using the MEWS key as shown.

MEWS KEY

0 1 2 3

All the observations have to be recorded and the total score added up. **A MEWS score of 3 or more** is an alert that a patient is acutely ill or deteriorating and an appropriate response using the escalation procedure is required... MEWS should NOT replace sound clinical judgement. Immediate action and appropriate escalation should take place if there are any concerns regarding a patient's clinical condition. Staff are accountable for seeking further help if not reassured by the response and action taken.

Staff should use SBAR in all communications

Definition
- **S ituation**
- **B ackground**
- **A ssessment**
- **R ecommendations**

HOW TO ASSESS BP IN A PREGNANT PATIENT

Initial BP measurement must be manual
Appropriate sized cuff should be used
Diastolic BP reading is when the sound **disappears**
CMACE recommends treatment of hypertension if above 150/100

Systolic BP ≥160mmHg — Recheck manually
If BP still elevated – CONTACT SENIOR TRAINEE IMMEDIATELY

Diastolic BP ≥110mmHg — Recheck manually
If BP still elevated – CONTACT SENIOR TRAINEE IMMEDIATELY

When assessing the patient the following symptoms may indicate severe pre-eclampsia and require further action

Headache	Visual Disturbance	Facial Oedema	Breathlessness
Epigastric Pain	Right Upper Quadrant Pain	Vomiting	+++ Proteinuria

LOT211 MEWS Chart Version 1 Aug 2014

THIS SECTION SHOULD BE COMPLETED BY THE ANAESTHETIST IF THE PATIENT HAS HAD A SPINAL/EPIDURAL/CSE OR BY THE MIDWIFE WHO REMOVES A LABOUR EPIDURAL CATHETER.

1. Check motor block at ....(time and date) (4 hours after epidural catheter removed or spinal injection performed)
2. If motor block is Bromage 2-4, give dalteparin as per kardex
3. If Bromage is 1, withhold dalteparin and inform anaesthetist *
4. Recheck motor block 4 hours after dalteparin
5. If motor block has increased or fails to resolve or a new motor block develops, inform anaesthetist * immediately and CONSIDER EPIDURAL HAEMATOMA.

*CONTACT DETAILS OF ANAESTHETIST: ....

....

Intrathecal or Epidural Opioid

Drug:	Dose	Route	Time

IMPORTANT
IF INTRATHECAL / EPIDURAL OR PCA OPIOIDS, PLEASE ENSURE THAT RESPIRATORY RATE, SEDATION AND PAIN SCORES ARE RECORDED HOURLY FOR THE FIRST 12 HOURS AFTER INITIAL DOSE

Bromage scale
1. **unable to move feet or knees**
2. **able to move feet only**
3. **just able to move knees**
4. **full flexion of knees and feet**

Pain Assessment & Management Guidelines
How to score pain:

Acute pain: Score current pain on movement e.g. deep breathing

Pain Score:		Action:
0	NONE	Continue to assess pain with every set of observations (**must be** at least daily)
1-3	MILD	Continue to assess pain with every set of observations (**must be** at least daily)
4-5	MODERATE	Assess. Using guidelines, prescribe/give analgesia as appropriate for the patient. Review.
6-10	SEVERE	Assess. Using guidelines, prescribe/give analgesia as appropriate for the patient. Review.

Figure 35.3 Continued

it can cause bronchospasm and hypoxia with V/Q mismatch), followed where necessary by misoprostol 1000 mcg rectally.

Pharmacological measurements have little to contribute to the management of PPH caused by tissue or trauma. Treatment of 'thrombin'-related PPH is by replacement of specific clotting factors or increasing concentrations of other prothrombotic agents, and is discussed later in 'Transfusion of Blood and Blood Products'.

Surgical treatments of postpartum haemorrhage

Genital tract trauma sufficient to cause major haemorrhage should be repaired in theatre where there is good lighting and access to appropriate anaesthesia.

Surgical treatments for PPH due to uterine atony include placement of an intrauterine balloon followed by inflation to prevent bleeding by inducing tamponade (e.g. the Bakri™ balloon (Figure 35.4)), a haemostatic 'brace' suture around the uterus (e.g. the B-lynch suture), hysterectomy and either external ligation of uterine or internal iliac arteries, or use of IR to embolize the uterine artery. The frequency with which these agents were used, in a series of 323 women in Scotland in 2010 with major haemorrhage, together with their 'success' rates (in terms of hysterectomy avoided) are shown in Table 35.3.[4] It should be noted that apparently superior success rates of one strategy compared with another cannot be firmly inferred from this series, since different strategies will have been used in different clinical scenarios. However, the fact that only 5% of women treated with an intrauterine balloon went on to need hysterectomy, together with its relative ease of placement are likely to account for the more than eightfold increase in use of the balloon since 2003. There has also been a threefold increase in the use of compression sutures over this time period. A systematic review of hysterectomy-sparing treatments for PPH (balloon tamponade, uterine compression sutures, arterial embolization, and uterine devascularization or arterial ligation) demonstrated efficacies of 84–92%, with no significant difference in efficacies.[38]

Although intrauterine balloon tamponade has not been subjected to formalized randomized controlled trials, the demonstration of a reduction in the need for arterial embolization and conservative surgical procedures after its introduction supports its use.[39] It works by applying pressure greater than systemic arterial pressure to the inside of the uterus. The RCOG endorses the use of intrauterine balloon tamponade as a first-line surgical intervention in women with bleeding due to uterine atony.[2] Balloon tamponade appears equally effective in resource poor settings.[40] A variety of balloon devices are suitable, including a Foley catheter, a Bakri™ balloon (Figure 35.4), a Sengstaken–Blakemore oesophageal catheter, a condom catheter, and the Rusch balloon (see Georgiou[41] for further details on use in practice). The Rusch balloon appears to have advantages in terms of size, cost and ease of use, although the Bakri™ balloon with its opening in the uterine cavity may allow earlier detection of continued bleeding. Regardless of the balloon used, it should be kept in place for at least 4–6 hours with most publications suggesting its removal by 48 hours.

The next most commonly used treatment for PPH is the haemostatic brace suture, as described by Christopher B-Lynch in 1997[42] (Figure 35.5). Again, there have been no large randomized trials comparing the haemostatic brace suture to alternative treatments. The UK Obstetric Surveillance System (UKOSS) cohort reported outcomes of 272 women needing second-line treatment for PPH (i.e. when drug treatment and/or uterine balloon tamponade had failed): uterine compression sutures were successful in 75% of the 199 women so treated.[43] Uterine necrosis and pyometra have been reported as complications, but these can be minimized with appropriate attention to technique and the use of a suture such as polynecaperone (Monocryl®) which degrades completely over 3 weeks, losing its tensile strength.[44] Again, the use of the B-Lynch suture and/or other compression sutures is endorsed by the RCOG.[2]

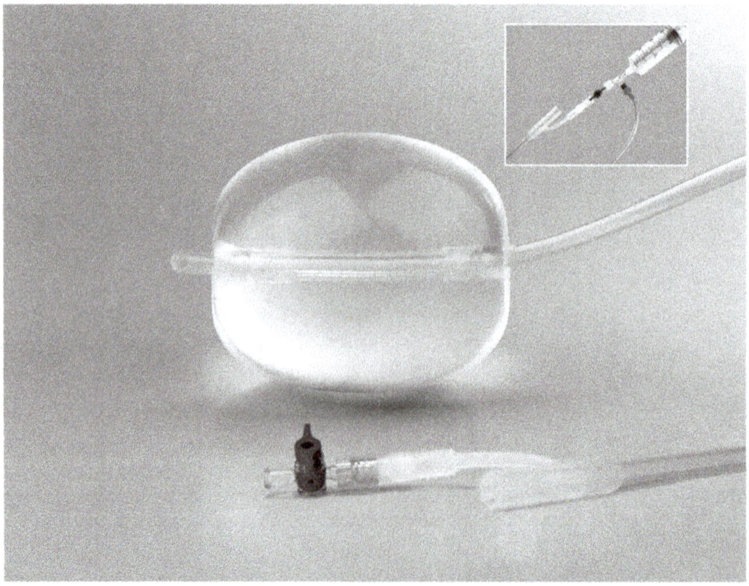

Figure 35.4 Bakri™ balloon.
Permission for use granted by Cook Medical Incorporated, Bloomington, Indiana.

Table 35.3 Frequency of use and 'efficacy' (hysterectomy avoided) of procedures used to treat major obstetric haemorrhage in Scotland in 2010

Procedure	Number	% of total	% Success rate[a]
Intrauterine balloon tamponade	81	21.5%	95%
Haemostatic brace uterine suturing (e.g. B-Lynch)	34	10.5%	82%
Hysterectomy	18	5.6%	0
Uterine artery embolization (interventional radiology)	17	5.3%	70%
Bilateral ligation of uterine or internal iliac arteries	5	1.5%	80%

[a]Hysterectomy avoided.

Lennox C, Marr L. *Scottish Confidential Audit of Severe Maternal Morbidity* © Healthcare Improvement Scotland 2014. First published July 2014. You can copy or reproduce the information in this report for use within NHS Scotland and for educational purposes. Commercial organisations must get our written permission before reproducing this report. http://www.healthcareimprovementscotland.org

The use of IR techniques is increasingly popular in the management of obstetric haemorrhage. Its use in placenta accreta has been described previously in this chapter. Bilateral uterine arterial embolization is appropriate when the uterus is thought to be the source of bleeding. Where the source of bleeding is unknown, or where it is likely to come from vaginal, cervical, or pelvic 'trauma', imaging can be useful to visualize the bleeding point, followed by embolization to the relevant vessel. Again, there are no randomized trials, and few series reporting long-term outcomes. Out of 19 women treated with embolization in the UKOSS series, 17 (89%) avoided hysterectomy.[43] These immediate success rates are similar to those from the Netherlands in a series of 114 women with arterial embolization, although 25% women ultimately underwent hysterectomy.[45] One series of 28 women with mean follow-up of 12 years, noted that all six who wished to become pregnant again did so and delivered successfully.[46] Another series demonstrated future successful pregnancy in all 16 women who wished another pregnancy after arterial embolization to treat PPH.[47]

Hysterectomy is the definitive treatment for PPH in women with uterine atony or uterine trauma. However, hysterectomy is life-saving in selected cases and should not be denied in an effort to preserve fertility. The Confidential Enquiry into Maternal and Child Health recommends that 'consider[ing] hysterectomy early' is an important component of effective management of PPH.[33] The RCOG guidelines endorse this advice, especially in cases of placenta accreta or uterine rupture, and suggest that a second consultant be involved in both the decision-making and the surgery.[2] UKOSS reviewed a series of 315 women undergoing peripartum hysterectomy in the United Kingdom.[48] The majority (53%) were performed because of uterine atony, with a further 38% performed because of placenta percreta, accreta, or increta. Eighty per cent of peripartum hysterectomies followed caesarean delivery. Complications included death (0.6%), need for intensive care unit

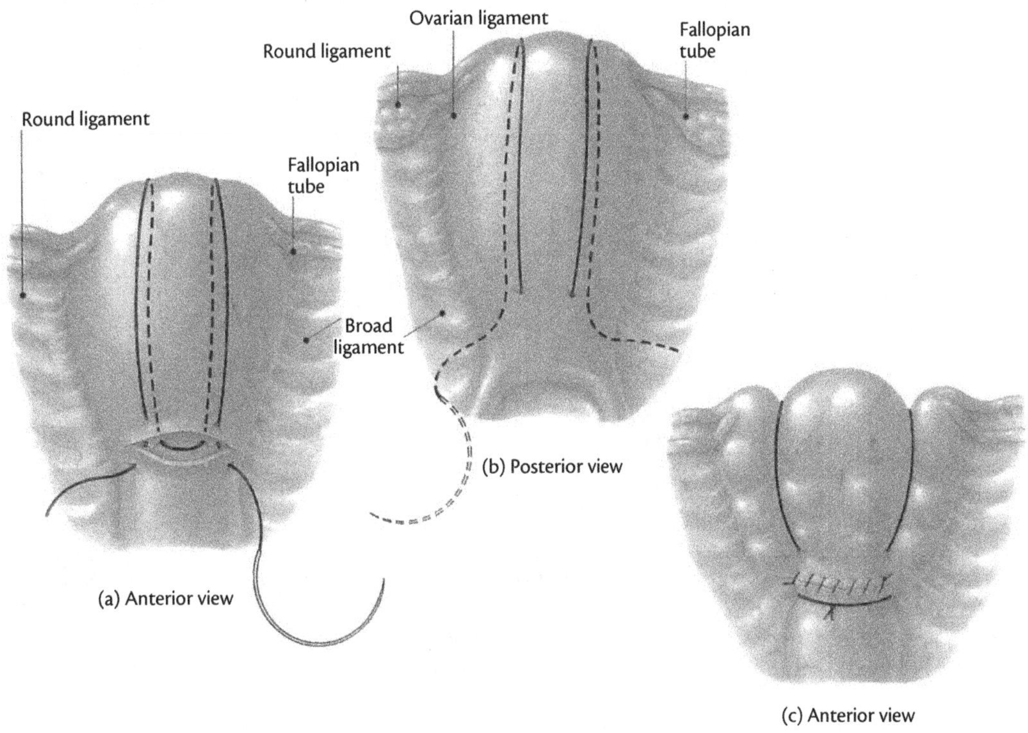

Figure 35.5 B-Lynch suture.
Reproduced from Christopher B Lynch *et al.*, 'The B-Lynch surgical technique for the control of massive postpartum haemorrhage: an alternative to hysterectomy? Five cases reported', *BJOG: An International Journal of Obstetrics & Gynaecology*, Volume 104, Issue 3, pp. 372–375, Copyright 1997, with permission from Wiley.

admission (80%), bladder damage (12%), ureteric damage (4.4%), ovary removal (5.7%), other further surgery (19.4%), and other severe morbidity (17%). There were no differences in complication rate comparing subtotal with total hysterectomy. Bladder damage was more likely in the presence of placenta accreta, and younger and multiparous women. Caesarean delivery and morbidly adherent placenta were noted as risk factors for peripartum hysterectomy in another systematic review.[49]

Transfusion of blood and blood products

The term uterus has a blood flow of approximately 750 mL/min and therefore in the event of a massive haemorrhage, all obstetric units should have immediate access to O-negative blood. Blood transfusion is, however, not without its potential hazards,[50] specifically transfusion reactions, transfusion-related lung injury, and infection. Blood should not therefore be given without due consideration.[51] Furthermore, most obstetric patients are healthy prepregnancy and have no co-morbidities. They can usually therefore tolerate relative anaemia well and a haemoglobin of 7 g/dL is acceptable to most stable postpartum women. See Figure 35.6 for the Simpson Centre for Reproductive Health transfusion algorithm for stable postpartum women.

However, in the actively bleeding parturient, it is recommended that the haemoglobin be kept between 7 and 9 g/dL by transfusion.[52] Laboratory samples for a full blood count and clotting screen are useful only for baseline purposes as in a haemorrhage, the patient may have lost several circulating blood volumes before these results are to hand which will therefore not reflect the real-time picture. Some units may have near-patient testing devices like the HemoCue® (Figure 35.7) and a thromboelastograph (Figure 35.8) which will give very rapid haemoglobin[53] and clotting status respectively. Furthermore, the thromboelastograph will indicate which blood products are required to treat any coagulopathy which may be present although the reference ranges may be different in obstetric patients.[54]

Lothian guidelines for blood transfusion in stable postpartum women

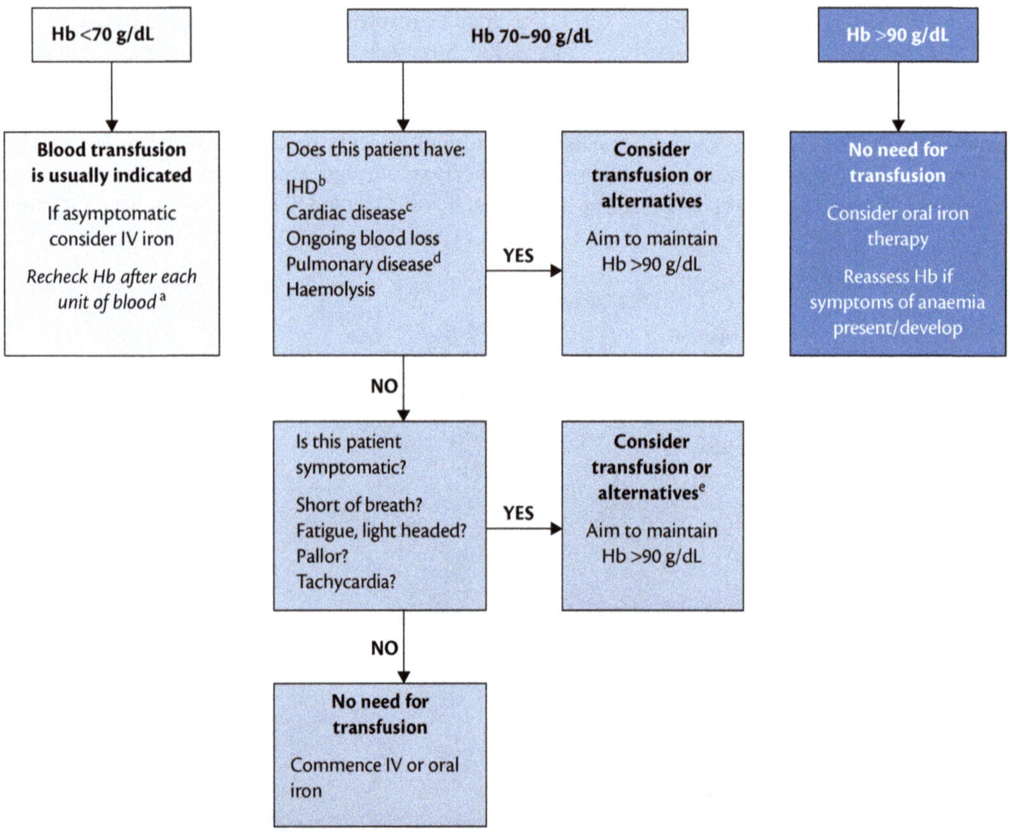

[a]*Reassessing patients between units prevents unnecessary transfusion and minimizes patient exposure to multiple blood donors.*

[b]*IHD = ischaemic heart disease.*

[c]*If cardiac disease, consider giving furosemide 20 mg per 2 units of blood.*

[d]*Pulmonary disease that causes low SpO_2 (excluding well controlled asthma) is an indication to maintain haemoglobin level >90 g/dL.*

[e]*Alternatives to blood transfusion may be oral or intravenous iron therapy.*

Figure 35.6 Lothian guidelines for blood transfusion in stable postpartum women.

© NHS Lothian; Data from Carson JL *et al.*, Transfusion triggers: a systematic review of the literature. *Transfusion Medicine Reviews*, 2002, volume 16, issue 3, pp. 187–99; and Data from Murphy MF *et al.* Guidelines for the clinical use of red cell transfusions. *British Journal of Haematology*, 2001, volume 113, issue 1, pp. 24–31.

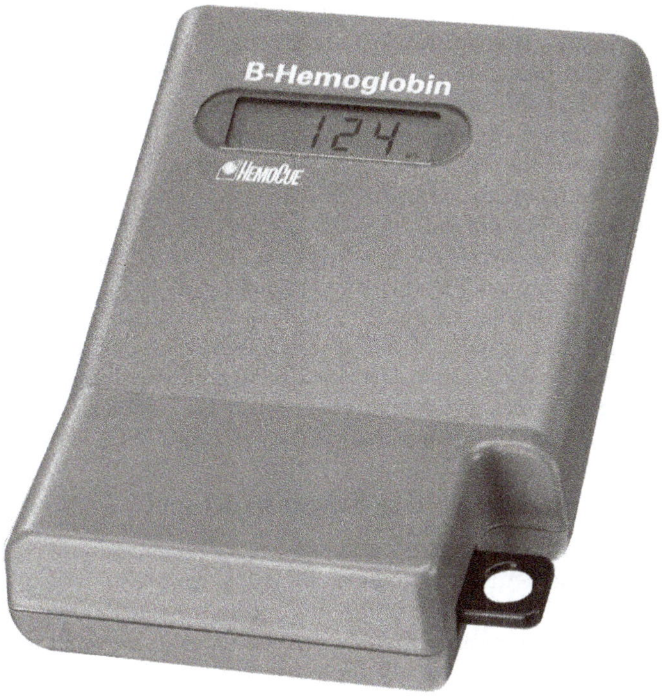

Figure 35.7 HemoCue®.
Reproduced with permission of Sylva Lindskog, Hemocue.

A more detailed explanation of the thromboelastograph and its interpretation are available in Chapter 48.

Where a thromboelastograph is not available, it has been suggested from major trauma studies[52] that the platelet count should be maintained above 50×10^9/L and prothrombin and activated prothrombin time within 1.5 times the mean control. Fibrinogen should be 1.5–2 g/L, higher than that recommended by the RCOG[55] of 1 g/L as most pregnant women have fibrinogen levels often greater than 4 g/L, so 1 g/L would seem excessively low. In fact, a fibrinogen level less than 2 g/L has a positive predictive value of 100% for severe PPH and is the only marker among those investigated to do so.[56] Fibrinogen can be given as fresh frozen plasma (FFP) 10–15 mL/kg or as cryoprecipitate (10 units). Recently there have been case reports of fibrinogen concentrate used in obstetric haemorrhage.[57] This has the advantages that it does not need to be thawed and can be given in small volumes thus reducing the volume load and the chances of pulmonary oedema.

A 1:1 transfusion ratio of blood:FFP: has been advocated following improved survival in military casualties in Iraq and Afghanistan.[58] Here the patients were aggressively treated with blood products along with early damage control surgery and avoiding the 'lethal triad' of hypothermia, acidosis, and coagulopathy. However, obstetric patients are of a different physiological milieu than soldiers, with a higher thrombotic potential than their male non-pregnant counterparts. The Association of Anaesthetists of Great Britain and Ireland (AAGBI) has currently advised against this 1:1:1 regimen in routine obstetric practice.[59]

Donor blood has been anticoagulated with acid citrate dextrose which chelates calcium, resulting in hypocalcaemia after massive transfusion. It is recommended that calcium chloride is given to maintain calcium levels above 0.9 mmol/L.[55]

Cell salvage

The collection and re-transfusion of autologous blood from surgical sites has been well established in many specialities—orthopaedics, cardiac, vascular, and hepatobiliary surgery—for decades.[60] However, there has been a reluctance to embrace it in obstetrics because of the fears of amniotic fluid embolism and rhesus isoimmunization.

The cause of amniotic fluid embolism, now re-named anaphylactoid syndrome of pregnancy[61] is unknown. It is rare, occurring in approximately 1/50,000 births but with a high mortality (20%)[62]

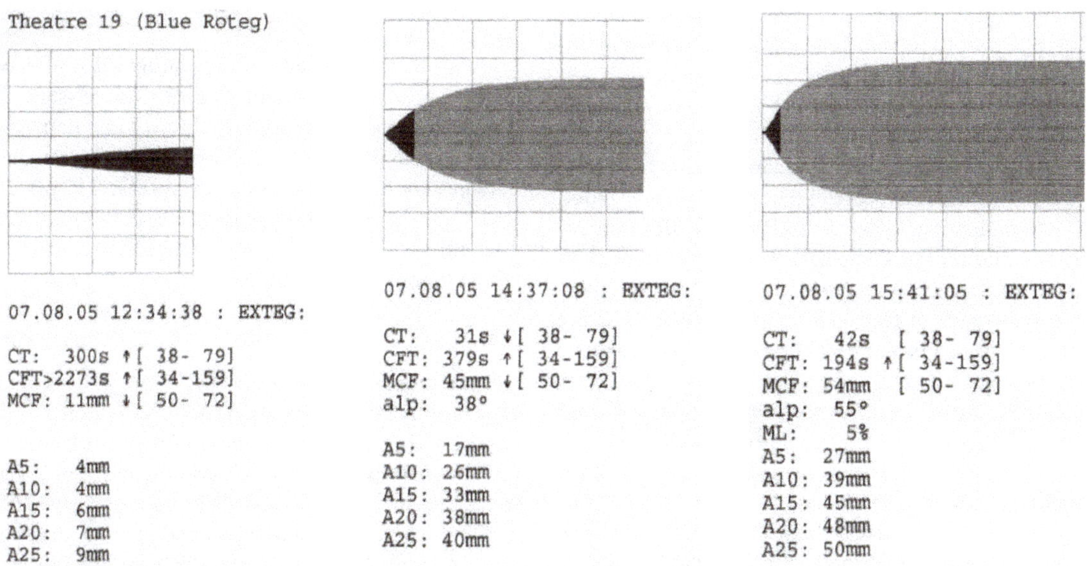

Figure 35.8 Thromboelastograph in patient with disseminated intravascular coagulation (left) and subsequent normalization following treatment with fresh frozen plasma and platelets.

and accounted for 15 deaths in the most recent Confidential Enquiry into Maternal Deaths in the United Kingdom.[6] Previously, fetal squames and other debris were thought to cause the syndrome which resulted in cardiovascular collapse, hypoxia, and coagulopathy. More recently, it is thought that there is a systemic inflammatory response which results in release of endogenous inflammatory mediators.[63]

More detail about anaphylactoid syndrome of pregnancy can be found in Chapter 38.

When cell salvage was first introduced into obstetrics, a separate suction device was used to collect amniotic fluid and another introduced post delivery to collect maternal blood.[64] The cell saver machines have integral filters and when a leucocyte depletion filter (LDF) is used as well, the salvaged blood returned to the mother has similar levels of amniotic fluid contaminants as that seen in maternal blood after a normal delivery.[65] Recently, however, some units have abandoned the two-sucker approach and aspirate amniotic fluid as well as blood into the same suction device. There appears to be no increased risk of anaphylactoid syndrome with this approach[66] and it may be that this is the way forward as in some cases (e.g. placenta praevia or anterior fibroids), most of the blood is lost before delivery.

In 2011, there were case reports of severe hypotension with salvaged blood given with a LDF.[67,68] The mechanism of this was postulated to be bradykinin release, bradykinin being a potent vasodilator. An article in 2013 suggests that interleukin 6 may be the culprit if the blood has been filtered using subatmospheric pressures applied with a 50 mL syringe.[69] But neither theory explains why hypotension does not occur in the millions of patients receiving non-autologous blood which has been filtered through the LDF.[70] If severe hypotension does occur, the filter should be removed and the salvaged blood transfused without it. A SHOT (Serious Hazards of Transfusion) report should be completed.

Using the LDF has another practical disadvantage. The rate of blood flow through the filter is severely hampered by the fine mesh and is a major drawback in replacing blood in a rapidly haemorrhaging patient. Removing the filter speeds up re-transfusion rates significantly. It should be remembered that before the introduction of filters several hundred patients were transfused salvaged blood uneventfully and continue to do so in non-obstetric settings.

The cell saver machines cannot differentiate maternal from fetal cells and there can be transfusion of fetal cells from salvaged blood back to the mother. This may give rise to Rhesus isoimmunization in Rhesus-negative mothers who have Rhesus-positive babies with problems in subsequent pregnancies if anti-D is not given. However, the transference of fetal cells in cell salvage is of the same magnitude as occurs in a normal delivery.[71] The Kleihauer test done postnatally, and after the salvaged blood has been given, will detect how much anti-D needs to be given to prevent Rhesus isoimmunization. Transference of other alloantibodies has not given rise to any clinical problems following cell salvage (J. Faulds, personal communication).

One of the problems of cell salvage is the uncertainty of which patients would benefit from the process. In the 2007 SCASMM, Peacock and Clark identified all the Scottish women in that year who had had a loss greater than 2500 mL, or required a 5-unit transfusion of blood or coagulation products.[72] It would appear that worthwhile volumes of blood could be salvaged in those with placenta praevia, accreta, and abruption, pre-eclampsia, caesarean after induction of labour, and at exploratory laparotomy. However, a definitive study has yet to be done to confirm this. If clinicians are unsure about potential blood loss, the collect-only reservoir of the cell savage system can be used without the centrifuge, the more expensive part. This can easily be activated if blood loss becomes significant.

It must be remembered that there are no coagulation products in salvaged blood and FFP, cryoprecipitate, and platelet transfusions may be required.

NICE, the AAGBI, RCOG, and MBRRACE have all recently endorsed cell salvage in obstetrics. A large randomized trial is underway which will determine the role of cell salvage in reducing blood transfusion in obstetrics (SALVO, ISRCTN66118656).

Women who refuse blood products

There are some parturients who refuse blood products due to religious beliefs.[34] They are at increased risk of dying with two such women dying in the last MBRRACE report.[6] The implications of their decisions regarding refusal of blood products should be discussed at length antenatally. The best place for this to be done is in the high-risk clinic or similar suitable environment. The partner should accompany the patient as they may have different views but must be made aware that the patient's wishes supersede theirs. Some women may request their religious advisor attend the clinic appointment also.

Haematinics must be prescribed and a full blood count should be checked at 32 and 36 weeks to ensure that their haemoglobin is optimized for delivery. Some may need intravenous iron or erythropoietin to bring the haemoglobin above 10 g/dL.[5]

Apart from impressing upon these women that they have a greater chance of dying compared to others, the exact nature of what they will accept in the event of a haemorrhage must be discussed and documented. Some adjuncts, if they have non-blood components (e.g. recombinant factor VIIa), and some techniques like cell salvage, may be acceptable. A useful chart is shown in Figure 35.9.

On admission to the delivery suite, all staff should be aware of the status of the patient. Senior medical staff should also be informed. If there is a haemorrhage, a consultant obstetrician and consultant anaesthetist should be called in a timely manner. The patient should be monitored for at least 4 hours postpartum so that any complications are diagnosed and managed early. Each hospital should have a group which liaises with organizations whose members refuse blood.

Anaesthesia in obstetric haemorrhage

Neuraxial anaesthesia is relatively contraindicated in a patient who is actively bleeding as spinal or epidural anaesthesia causes sympathetic blockade with resultant vasodilatation and removes the compensatory vasoconstriction which would naturally occur in the presence of blood loss. General anaesthesia (GA) is the technique of choice with judicious use of induction agents to avoid vasodilation and hypotension. This is offset somewhat initially by the hypertensive stimulus of laryngoscopy. The use of volatile agents for maintenance of anaesthesia used to be notoriously associated with relaxation of the uterus but since the demise of

ANAESTHETIC CHECKLIST FOR

WOMEN WHO MAY REFUSE BLOOD PRODUCTS

NHS Lothian

Patient label

	WILLING TO HAVE IF REQUIRED	REFUSE UNDER ANY CIRCUMSTANCES
Red cells		
Platelets		
Fresh frozen plasma		
Cryoprecipitate		
Fibrinogen concentrate		
Factor VIIa		
Cell saver		
Haemofiltration/dialysis		
Cardiac bypass		
Erythropoietin		

Any other information :

Signature (Patient) ____________________

Signature (Anaesthetist) ____________________

Figure 35.9 Simpson Centre for Reproductive Health checklist for women who refuse blood products.

halothane this has not clinically been a problem and up to 0.46 minimum alveolar concentration of sevoflurane and isoflurane can be given without affecting uterine tone.[73] During a haemorrhage, if the patient is hypovolaemic and hypotensive, reducing the volatile will not necessarily lessen atony and increases the risk of awareness.

Unfortunately, haemorrhage often occurs unexpectedly in obstetrics and many patients who bleed will already have a spinal or epidural *in situ*. Provided the patient is kept well-filled, and comfortable, the anaesthetist may persevere with the regional technique. However, if the operation is prolonged and outlasts the spinal, or if there is pain or discomfort, there is no choice but to provide a GA. Further, a hypovolaemic hypotensive patient will feel faint and nauseous and a GA indicated for these reasons. Inducing GA can also be advantageous as it then frees the anaesthetist to proceed with insertion of arterial and CVCs and for the staff in theatre to communicate more frankly without the need to curtail discussion to prevent alarming the patient and partner.

Unless already *in situ*, two large-bore cannulae are indicated as well as use of the rapid infuser and cell saver if available. An arterial line and CVC are indicated in a massive haemorrhage. A second dose of antibiotic is necessary if blood loss exceeds 1500 mL. Perioperative thromboelastography and HemoCue® are invaluable to guide blood and coagulation product replacement in these circumstances. If there is evidence of fibrinolysis, tranexamic acid may be considered.

There are some cases where using neuraxial anaesthesia is controversial. One of these is for placenta praevia. This can potentially cause catastrophic bleeding and theoretically a GA should be given for the reasons described above. However, if the placenta praevia is minor or posterior, bleeding is less likely and many experienced anaesthetists would use a regional technique. In a series of 350 consecutive placenta praevia cases, Parekh found that neuraxial anaesthesia even in the presence of considerable haemorrhage was not problematic and was associated with significantly less blood loss and transfusion.[74] Hong and colleagues[75] also demonstrated that epidural anaesthesia as opposed to GA resulted in less transfusion requirements in grade 4 placenta praevia patients. An alternative to epidural or single-shot spinal would be a combined spinal–epidural (CSE). This would allow longer surgical time if problems were encountered.

Another area where the choice of anaesthetic depends on anaesthetic experience is in the management of an elective caesarean with a placenta accreta. In many of these cases, internal iliac balloons are placed preoperatively. Some anaesthetists insert a CSE providing anaesthesia for insertion of the radiology catheters with the spinal component. The caesarean is then performed under epidural top-up, although if blood loss becomes excessive, conversion to a GA is advised (G. O'Sullivan, personal communication). This will work well if the bleeding from the adherent placenta is not excessive but many of these cases bleed torrentially despite the internal iliac balloons if the placenta starts to separate and the anaesthetic team may be stretched to cope with a nauseous anxious patient (and partner) rather than proceeding unhampered with resuscitation.

Patient choice should be taken into consideration when discussing anaesthetic techniques unless there is an overwhelming reason to choose one technique over another. In a case like placenta praevia and accreta, the patient and partner should understand that neuraxial anaesthesia can be initiated but GA may be necessary if complications arise. The partner's understanding that they should leave when requested must be determined from the outset.

Patients who have had a major haemorrhage will inevitably require level 3 (intensive) care. A period of ventilation will buy time for re-warming, reversing coagulopathy, and often righting fluid balance as one of the commonest causes for ITU admission is pulmonary oedema caused by over-generous fluid resuscitation in the early stages of haemorrhage.

Simulation training for management of obstetric haemorrhage

Simulation training using 'drills' is an increasingly important component of quality improvement in obstetrics. Simulation training may either focus on the individual (e.g. MOET, ALSO) or the 'team' (PROMPT). There is some (weak) evidence that drills may improve team-working and identify knowledge and performance gaps.[76]

Debriefing

The mortality and morbidity associated with major obstetric haemorrhage are considerable. Communication with the woman and her relatives is an important feature of the management of obstetric haemorrhage and appropriate management requires good team communication.

Once the immediate danger period has past, it is appropriate to conduct a formal debriefing with the woman and her relatives. This should include an accurate account of events, some explanation of 'why' this happened, 'why' any specific measures or treatments were undertaken, and 'what this means' for future health (including pregnancies). Regular morbidity reviews identify examples of good practice, and management that could be improved in the future. This should be fed back to staff who will also require some debriefing, both to help them come to terms with what has happened, and for educational purposes.

Controversies in obstetric haemorrhage

Treatment modalities in massive obstetric haemorrhage have rarely been subjected to randomized trials, and it could therefore be argued that much of the accepted treatment lacks a robust evidence base. Many 'new' techniques and drugs are introduced by enthusiasts—in the presence of a life-threatening situation is it difficult to persuade such individuals to randomize to 'no treatment'. Some new treatments are described below.

Recombinant factor VIIa

Factor VIIa is an important component of the clotting cascade—the recombinant form can be given intravenously. The RCOG advises: 'In the face of life-threatening PPH, and in consultation with a haematologist, rFVIIa may be used as an adjuvant to standard pharmacological and surgical treatments'.[2] A suggested dose is 90 mcg/kg, which may be repeated in the absence of clinical response within 15–30 minutes. Importantly, factor VIIa requires adequate concentrations of fibrinogen and platelets to be effective—consideration should be given to fibrinogen and/or platelet administration for those with fibrinogen below 1 g/L and platelets greater than 20×10^9/L. Patients who are hypothermic, hypocalcaemic, and acidotic will not respond to factor VII treatment either.[77] There have been recent reports of arterial thrombosis following the use of factor VIIa in non-obstetric patients.[78]

Tranexamic acid

Although the RCOG does not endorse the use of tranexamic acid, there is weak evidence for its efficacy in PPH[79] and considerable evidence for its use in trauma.[80] In trauma usage, a dose of 1 g is given slowly intravenously and repeated if required after 8 hours. The WOMAN trial is currently addressing the role of tranexamic acid in obstetrics.[81]

Cell salvage

The last controversy is the use of cell salvage, which is widely used, although there is no evidence it has any clinical benefit or cost-effectiveness (both in terms of reducing transfusion). A multicentre trial 'SALVO' is ongoing in the United Kingdom to address this issue, as described previously.

Conclusion

Major obstetric haemorrhage remains a significant cause of maternal mortality and morbidity. Risk factors should be identified. Prompt and effective anaesthetic and obstetric intervention (ideally as part of a multidisciplinary team) significantly improves outcomes. Management includes pharmacological and surgical techniques with frequent input from blood transfusion and intensive care services. IR is sometimes required. Research increasingly identifies effective and ineffective strategies in the treatment of this condition.

Acknowledgements

We thank Dr Hamish Ireland, Consultant Radiologist, Royal Infirmary, Edinburgh for the image of the internal iliac catheters (Figure 35.1).

References

1. Royal College of Obstetricians and Gynaecologists. *Antepartum Haemorrhage*. Green-top Guideline No. 63. London: RCOG; 2011.
2. Royal College of Obstetricians and Gynaecologists. *Prevention and Management of Postpartum Haemorrhage*. Green-top Guideline No. 52. London: RCOG; 2009.
3. Royal College of Obstetricians and Gynaecologists. *Placenta Praevia and Placenta Praevia Accreta: Diagnosis and Management*. Green-top Guideline No. 27. London: RCOG; 2011.
4. Health Improvement Scotland. *Scottish Confidential Audit of Severe Maternal Morbidity, 8th Annual Report (Data from 2010)*. Edinburgh: Health Improvement Scotland; 2012.
5. Brace V, Kernaghan D, Penney G. Learning from adverse clinical outcomes: major obstetric haemorrhage in Scotland, 2003–05. *BJOG* 2007; 114(11):1388–96.
6. Knight M, Kenyon S, Brocklehurst P, *et al*. *Saving Lives, Improving Mothers' Care - Lessons Learned to Inform Future Maternity Care from the UK and Ireland Confidential Enquiries into Maternal Deaths and Morbidity 2009-12*. Oxford: National Perinatal Epidemiology Unit, University of Oxford; 2014.
7. Knight M, Callaghan WM, Berg C, *et al*. Trends in postpartum hemorrhage in high resource countries: a review and recommendations from the International Postpartum Hemorrhage Collaborative Group. *BMC Pregnancy Childbirth* 2009; 9:55.
8. Mehrabadi A, Hutcheon JA, Lee L, *et al*. Trends in postpartum hemorrhage from 2000 to 2009: a population-based study. *BMC Pregnancy Childbirth* 2012; 12(1):108.
9. Lutomski JE, Byrne BM, Devane D, *et al*. Increasing trends in atonic postpartum haemorrhage in Ireland: an 11-year population-based cohort study. *BJOG* 2012; 119(3):306–14.
10. Callaghan WM, Kuklina EV, Berg CJ. Trends in postpartum hemorrhage: United States, 1994–2006. *Am J Obstet Gynecol* 2010; 202(4):353.e1–6.
11. Calvert C, Thomas SL, Ronsmans C, *et al*. Identifying regional variation in the prevalence of postpartum haemorrhage: a systematic review and meta-analysis. *PLoS One* 2012; 7(7):e41114.
12. Zwart JJ, Dupuis JR, Richters A, *et al*. Obstetric intensive care unit admission: a 2-year nationwide population-based cohort study. *Intensive Care Med* 2010; 36(2):256–63.
13. Bateman BT, Berman MF, Riley LE, *et al*. The epidemiology of postpartum hemorrhage in a large, nationwide sample of deliveries. *Anesth Analg* 2010; 110(5):1368–73.
14. Gupta JK, Hofmeyr GJ, Shehmar M. Position in the second stage of labour for women without epidural anaesthesia. *Cochrane Database Syst Rev* 2012; 5:CD002006.
15. Norman JE, Reynolds R. The consequences of obesity and excess weight gain in pregnancy. *Proc Nutr Soc* 2011 70:450–6.
16. Palmsten K, Hernandez-Diaz S, Huybrechts KF, *et al*. Use of antidepressants near delivery and risk of postpartum hemorrhage: cohort study of low income women in the United States. *BMJ* 2013; 347:f4877.
17. Stock SJ, Ferguson E, Duffy A, *et al*. Outcomes of elective induction of labour compared with expectant management: population based study. *BMJ* 2012; 344:e2838.
18. Sharp G, Saunders P, Greene S, *et al*. Intergenerational transmission of postpartum haemorrhage risk—analysis of two Scottish birth cohorts. *Am J Obstet Gynecol* 2014; 211(1):51.e1–7.
19. Hannah ME, Hannah WJ, Hewson SA, *et al*. Planned caesarean section versus planned vaginal birth for breech presentation at term: a randomised multicentre trial. Term Breech Trial Collaborative Group. *Lancet* 2000; 356(9239):1375–83.
20. Crowther CA, Dodd JM, Hiller JE, *et al*. Planned vaginal birth or elective repeat caesarean: patient preference restricted cohort with nested randomised trial. *PLoS Med* 2012; 9(3):e1001192.
21. National Collaborating Centre for Women's and Children's Health. *Antenatal Care: Routine Care for the Healthy Pregnant Woman*. Clinical Guideline 62. London: NICE; 2008.
22. Committee on Obstetric Practice. Committee opinion no. 529: placenta accreta. *Obstet Gynecol* 2012; 120(1):207–11.
23. Begley CM, Gyte GM, Devane D, *et al*. Active versus expectant management for women in the third stage of labour. *Cochrane Database Syst Rev* 2011; 11:CD007412.
24. Lewin S, Bosch-Capblanch X, Oliver S, *et al*. Guidance for evidence-informed policies about health systems: assessing how much confidence to place in the research evidence. *PLoS Med* 2012; 9(3):e1001187.
25. National Institute for Health and Care Excellence. *Intrapartum Care for Healthy Women and Babies*. Clinical Guideline 190. London: NICE, 2014. https://www.nice.org.uk/guidance/cg190
26. McDonald S, Abbott JM, Higgins SP. Prophylactic ergometrine-oxytocin versus oxytocin for the third stage of labour. *Cochrane Database Syst Rev* 2004; 1:CD000201.
27. Tuncalp O, Hofmeyr GJ, Gulmezoglu AM. Prostaglandins for preventing postpartum haemorrhage. *Cochrane Database Syst Rev* 2012; 8:CD000494.
28. Stephens LC, Bruessel T. Systematic review of oxytocin dosing at caesarean section. *Anaesth Intensive Care* 2012; 40(2):247–52.
29. National Institute for Clinical Excellence. *Caesarean Section*. Clinical Guideline 132. London: NICE; 2011 (reviewed 2014).
30. Su LL, Chong YS, Samuel M. Carbetocin for preventing postpartum haemorrhage. *Cochrane Database Syst Rev* 2012; 4:CD005457.
31. Oyelese Y, Smulian JC. Placenta previa, placenta accreta, and vasa previa. *Obstet Gynecol* 2006; 107(4):927–41.
32. Jeffrey A, Clark V. The anaesthetic management of caesarean section in the interventional radiology suite. *Curr Opin Anaesthesiol* 2011; 24(4):439–44.
33. Lewis, G (ed). *The Confidential Enquiry into Maternal and Child Health (CEMACH). Saving Mothers' Lives: Reviewing Maternal Deaths to Make Motherhood Safer - 2000-2002. The Sixth Report on Confidential Enquiries into Maternal Deaths in the United Kingdom*. London UK: CEMACH, 2005.
34. Lewis, G (ed). *The Confidential Enquiry into Maternal and Child Health (CEMACH). Saving Mothers' Lives: Reviewing Maternal Deaths to Make Motherhood Safer - 2003-2005. The Seventh Report on Confidential Enquiries into Maternal Deaths in the United Kingdom*. London: CEMACH; 2007.
35. Luck RP, Haines C, Mull CC. Intraosseous access. *J Emerg Med* 2010; 39(4):468–75.
36. Ngo AS, Oh JJ, Chen Y, *et al*. Intraosseous vascular access in adults using the EZ-IO in an emergency department. *Int J Emerg Med* 2009; 2(3):155–60.
37. Karpati PC, Rossignol M, Pirot M, *et al*. High incidence of myocardial ischemia during postpartum hemorrhage. *Anesthesiology* 2004; 100(1):30–6.
38. Doumouchtsis SK, Papageorghiou AT, Arulkumaran S. Systematic review of conservative management of postpartum hemorrhage: what to do when medical treatment fails. *Obstet Gynecol Surv* 2007; 62(8):540–7.
39. Laas E, Bui C, Popowski T, *et al*. Trends in the rate of invasive procedures after the addition of the intrauterine tamponade test to a protocol for management of severe postpartum hemorrhage. *Am J Obstet Gynecol* 2012; 207(4):281.e1–7.

40. Tindell K, Garfinkel R, Abu-Haydar E, *et al.* Uterine balloon tamponade for the treatment of postpartum haemorrhage in resource-poor settings: a systematic review. *BJOG* 2013; 120(1):5–14.
41. Georgiou C. Balloon tamponade in the management of postpartum haemorrhage: a review. *BJOG* 2009; 116(6):748–57.
42. B-Lynch, C, Coker A, Lawal AH, *et al.* The B-Lynch surgical technique for the control of massive postpartum haemorrhage: an alternative to hysterectomy? Five cases reported. *Br J Obstet Gynaecol* 1997; 104(3):372–5.
43. Kayem G, Kurinczuk JJ, Alfirevic Z, *et al.* Specific second-line therapies for postpartum haemorrhage: a national cohort study. *BJOG* 2011; 118(7):856–64.
44. B-Lynch, C. Partial ischemic necrosis of the uterus following a uterine brace compression suture. *BJOG* 2005; 112(1):126–7.
45. Zwart JJ, Dijk PD, van Roosmalen J. Peripartum hysterectomy and arterial embolization for major obstetric hemorrhage: a 2-year nationwide cohort study in the Netherlands. *Am J Obstet Gynecol* 2010; 202(2):150.e1–7.
46. Ornan D, White R, Pollak J, *et al.* Pelvic embolization for intractable postpartum hemorrhage: long-term follow-up and implications for fertility. *Obstet Gynecol* 2003; 102(5 Pt 1):904–10.
47. Chauleur C, Fanget C, Tourne G, *et al.* Serious primary post-partum hemorrhage, arterial embolization and future fertility: a retrospective study of 46 cases. *Hum Reprod* 2008; 23(7):1553–9.
48. Knight M. Peripartum hysterectomy in the UK: management and outcomes of the associated haemorrhage. *BJOG* 2007; 114(11):1380–7.
49. Rossi AC, Lee RH, Chmait RH. Emergency postpartum hysterectomy for uncontrolled postpartum bleeding: a systematic review. *Obstet Gynecol* 2010; 115(3):637–44.
50. Serious Hazards of Transfusion (SHOT). *Annual SHOT Report 2011*. Manchester: SHOT; 2012. http://www.shotuk.org/shot-reports/shot-annual-report-summary-2011/
51. Clark V, Waters JH. Blood transfusions: more is not necessarily better. *Int J Obstet Anesth* 2009; 18(4):299–301.
52. Rossaint R, Bouillon B, Cerny V, *et al.* Management of bleeding following major trauma: an updated European guideline. *Crit Care* 2010; 14(2):R52.
53. Yau R, Kathigamanathan T, Plaat F, *et al.* Evaluation of the HemoCue® for measuring haemoglobin concentration in the obstetric population. *Int J Obstet Anesth* 2002; 11 Suppl 1:8.
54. Armstrong S, Fernando R, Ashpole K, *et al.* Assessment of coagulation in the obstetric population using ROTEM® thromboelastometry. *Int J Obstet Anesth* 2011 Oct; 20(4):293–8.
55. Royal College of Obstetricians and Gynaecologists. *Blood Transfusion in Obstetrics*. Green-top Guideline No. 47. London: RCOG; 2008.
56. Charbit B, Mandelbrot L, Samain E, *et al.* The decrease of fibrinogen is an early predictor of the severity of postpartum hemorrhage. *J Thromb Haemost* 2007; 5(2):266–73.
57. Bell SF, Rayment R, Collins PW, *et al.* The use of fibrinogen concentrate to correct hypofibrinogenaemia rapidly during obstetric haemorrhage. *Int J Obstet Anesth* 2010; 19(2):218–23.
58. Borgman MA, Spinella PC, Perkins JG, *et al.* The ratio of blood products transfused affects mortality in patients receiving massive transfusions at a combat support hospital. *J Trauma* 2007; 63(4):805–13.
59. Association of Anaesthetists of Great Britain and Ireland. *Blood Transfusion and the Anaesthetist: Management of Massive Haemorrhage*. London: AAGBI; 2010.
60. Carless PA, Henry DA, Moxey AJ, *et al.* Cell salvage for minimising perioperative allogeneic blood transfusion. *Cochrane Database Syst Rev* 2010; 3:CD001888.
61. Benson MD. Anaphylactoid syndrome of pregnancy. *Am J Obstet Gynecol* 1996; 175(3 Pt 1):749.
62. Knight M, Tuffnell D, Brocklehurst P, *et al.* Incidence and risk factors for amniotic-fluid embolism. *Obstet Gynecol* 2010; 115(5):910–17.
63. Dildy GA, Belfort MA, Clark SL. Anaphylactoid syndrome of pregnancy (amniotic fluid embolism). In Belfort MA, Saade G, Foley M, *et al.* (eds) *Critical Care Obstetrics* (5th ed). Oxford: Wiley-Blackwell; 2010.
64. Catling SJ, Freites O, Krishnan S, *et al.* Clinical experience with cell salvage in obstetrics: 4 cases from one UK centre. *Int J Obstet Anesth* 2002; 11(2):128–34.
65. Waters JH, Biscotti C, Potter PS, *et al.* Amniotic fluid removal during cell salvage in the cesarean section patient. *Anesthesiology* 2000; 92(6):1531–6.
66. Sullivan I, Faulds J, Ralph C. Contamination of salvaged maternal blood by amniotic fluid and fetal red cells during elective Caesarean section. *Br J Anaesth* 2008; 101(2):225–9.
67. Kessack LK, Hawkins N. Severe hypotension related to cell salvaged blood transfusion in obstetrics. *Anaesthesia* 2010; 65(7):745–8.
68. Sreelakshmi TR, Eldridge J. Acute hypotension associated with leucocyte depletion filters during cell salvaged blood transfusion. *Anaesthesia* 2010; 65(7):742–4.
69. Choi ES, Ahn WS, Lee JM, *et al.* A laboratory study of the effects of processing blood through a cell salvage device and leucocyte depletion filter on levels of pro-inflammatory cytokines and bradykinin. *Anaesthesia* 2013; 68(12):1259–65.
70. Peacock L, Clark V, Catling S. Recent developments in the obstetric use of cell salvage. *Transfus Altern Transfus Med* 12012; 2(3–4):66–71.
71. Rainaldi MP, Tazzari PL, Scagliarini G, *et al.* Blood salvage during caesarean section. *Br J Anaesth* 1998; 80(2):195–8.
72. Peacock L, Clark V. Cell salvage in obstetrics: a review of data from the 2007 Scottish Confidential Audit of Severe Maternal Morbidity. *Int J Obstet Anesth* 2011; 20(2):196–8.
73. Gambling DR, Sharma SK, White PF, *et al.* Use of sevoflurane during elective cesarean birth: a comparison with isoflurane and spinal anesthesia. *Anesth Analg* 1995; 81(1):90–5.
74. Parekh N, Husaini SW, Russell IF. Caesarean section for placenta praevia: a retrospective study of anaesthetic management. *Br J Anaesth* 2000; 84(6):725–30.
75. Hong JY, Jee YS, Yoon HJ, *et al.* Comparison of general and epidural anesthesia in elective cesarean section for placenta previa totalis: maternal hemodynamics, blood loss and neonatal outcome. *Int J Obstet Anesth* 2003; 12(1):12–16.
76. Crofts JF, Winter C, Sowter MC. Practical simulation training for maternity care—where we are and where next. *BJOG* 2011; 118 Suppl 3:11–16.
77. Ahonen J. The role of recombinant activated factor VII in obstetric hemorrhage. *Curr Opin Anaesthesiol* 2012; 25(3):309–14.
78. Levi M, Levy JH, Andersen HF, *et al.* Safety of recombinant activated factor VII in randomized clinical trials. *N Engl J Med* 2010; 363(19):1791–800.
79. Novikova N, Hofmeyr GJ. Tranexamic acid for preventing postpartum haemorrhage. *Cochrane Database Syst Rev* 2010; 7:CD007872.
80. Shakur H, Roberts I, Bautista R, *et al.* Effects of tranexamic acid on death, vascular occlusive events, and blood transfusion in trauma patients with significant haemorrhage (CRASH-2): a randomised, placebo-controlled trial. *Lancet* 2010; 376(9734):23–32.
81. Shakur H, Elbourne D, Gulmezoglu M, *et al.* The WOMAN Trial (World Maternal Antifibrinolytic Trial): tranexamic acid for the treatment of postpartum haemorrhage: an international randomised, double blind placebo controlled trial. *Trials* 2010; 11:40.

CHAPTER 36

Hypertension in pregnancy

John A. Anderson, Pierre-Antoine Laloë and Derek J. Tuffnell

Introduction

Hypertensive disorders during pregnancy occur in women with pre-existing primary or secondary chronic hypertension, and in women who develop new-onset hypertension in the second half of pregnancy. Both carry risks for the woman and the baby. Although the rate of eclampsia in the United Kingdom appears to have fallen,[1] hypertension in pregnancy still caused 19 maternal deaths in the United Kingdom between 2009 and 2012 in the latest 2014 national report, 'Saving Lives, Improving Mothers' Care'.[2] Hypertensive disorders during pregnancy may also result in substantial maternal morbidity. A study reported that one-third of severe maternal morbidity was a consequence of hypertensive conditions.[3] A study from one region of the United Kingdom reported that 1 in 20 (5%) women with severe pre-eclampsia or eclampsia were admitted to intensive care.[4] Pre-eclampsia is associated with significant fetal mortality and morbidity, mostly as a result of prematurity. One in 20 perinatal deaths of deaths of infants without congenital abnormalities in the United Kingdom are associated with pre-eclampsia.[5]

Spectrum of hypertensive disease in pregnancy

Non-proteinuric hypertension

Women with normal blood pressure at the onset of pregnancy who subsequently develop hypertension without proteinuria after 20 weeks of gestation have gestational hypertension (GH). In itself, GH is less likely to cause significant morbidity than pre-eclampsia, but it pre-disposes women to the development of pre-eclampsia.

Primary or secondary chronic hypertension

There is a group of women who have pre-existing, chronic, primary or secondary hypertension prior to conception. In the United Kingdom it is likely that the majority of these women are unknown to their general practitioner, midwife, or obstetrician (though rates are estimated at 0.6–2.7%)[6] and the diagnosis of underlying chronic hypertension is revealed at final postnatal follow-up. It is therefore difficult to truly identify patients with chronic pre-existing hypertension, from hypertensive patients in the antenatal clinic with GH. For this reason, women presenting with GH prior to 20 weeks are considered to have chronic hypertension. In excess of 95% of women with chronic hypertension will not have any underlying discoverable pathology, and therefore have essential hypertension. The remainder may have associated, proven cardiovascular, renal, or endocrine disease.[7]

Rising rates of obesity and increasing maternal age in the developed world are increasing the incidence of chronic pre-existing hypertension and GH.[8] These conditions are additional risk factors for subsequently developing pre-eclampsia.[9,10]

Proteinuric hypertension

This encompasses pre-eclampsia and eclampsia; haemolysis, elevated liver enzyme levels, and low platelet count (HELLP) syndrome; and acute fatty liver of pregnancy (AFLP). They all may be considered as a continuum of the same disease at a cellular level and are more likely to result in harm than non-proteinuric hypertension. The careful management of women with moderate and severe proteinuric hypertension in the intra- and postpartum periods reflects this. It is also worth noting that HELLP and AFLP may not initially present with significant hypertension or proteinuria, though this may develop later.

Definitions

About one in ten pregnancies in the developed world are affected by hypertension in pregnancy and this includes two relatively benign conditions (chronic and gestational hypertension) and a potentially dangerous one (pre-eclampsia).[11] Considerable debate has always surrounded the definition of the hypertensive disorders of pregnancy. Consequently broad clinical definitions are used, reflecting that much overlap occurs in the phenotypic presentations of conditions of hypertension in pregnancy.

Pre-eclampsia affects up to 1 in 20 pregnancies dependent on parity[12] and is characterized by placental dysfunction, and maternal vascular, neurological, renal, and hepatic dysfunction which may lead to hypertension, stroke, seizures (eclampsia), end-organ damage, haemorrhage, placental abruption, fetal growth restriction, and both fetal and maternal death. Rarely this disease may manifest itself as HELLP and AFLP.

Clinically differentiating the more benign conditions of chronic hypertension and GH from pre-eclampsia to predict outcome has been dependent on traditional, but non-specific, clinical markers such as blood pressure, urinary protein excretion, signs, and symptoms. The difficulty in identifying women with pre-eclampsia is underlined by the knowledge that HELLP and AFLP patients may not present with hypertension in the initial stages of the disease and up to 20% of women with eclamptic seizures do not meet typical diagnostic criteria prior to their seizure event.[13] The lack of specificity makes the prediction and prevention of complications difficult.

Clinical definitions advocated by the National Institute of Health and Care Excellence (NICE)[14] have been used in an effort to provide consistency about the parameters to classify the condition in the United Kingdom. These depend upon the detection of hypertension, with or without proteinuria. However, these are crude proxy measurements of disease activity as both are signs of the condition rather than its cause or consequence. Clinically it is much more difficult to identify the more important consequences of pre-eclampsia such as cerebral oedema, glomerular damage, or basement membrane permeability.

Hypertension

Pregnancy-related hypertension is currently defined in the United Kingdom as a sustained raised blood pressure of over 140/90 mmHg, with a diastolic blood pressure of 90 mmHg on two separate occasions or a single diastolic reading of 110mmHg, in a woman who is pregnant or in the puerperium (6 weeks postnatal).[15] Current guidance divides cases into:

- *Mild hypertension:* diastolic blood pressure 90–99 mmHg, systolic blood pressure 140–149 mmHg.
- *Moderate hypertension:* diastolic blood pressure 100–109 mmHg, systolic blood pressure 150–159 mmHg.
- *Severe hypertension:* diastolic blood pressure 110 mmHg or greater, systolic blood pressure 160 mmHg or greater.[16] This definition is used in the United Kingdom and by the American Society of Hypertension and Society of Obstetricians and Gynaecologists of Canada. The Society of Obstetric Medicine of Australia and New Zealand use a level of 170/110 mmHg for severe hypertension

Significant proteinuria

Defined as 300 mg of protein excreted in 24 hours, or a urine protein:creatinine ratio greater than 30 mg/mmol.[16]

Gestational hypertension

Raised blood pressure falling within the above-mentioned categories, without proteinuria or associated biochemical abnormalities developing after 20 weeks of gestation, is described as gestational hypertension (GH) and used to be termed pregnancy-induced hypertension (PIH). Raised blood pressure prior to 20 weeks is considered to be chronic underlying hypertension.

Chronic hypertension

Chronic hypertension is hypertension that is present at the booking visit or before 20 weeks of gestation or hypertension requiring treatment when referred to maternity services. It can be primary or secondary in aetiology.

Pre-eclampsia

Pregnant women with confirmed hypertension with significant persistent proteinuria (i.e. >300 mg on 24-hour urine collection or a urinary protein:creatinine ratio greater than 30 mg/mmol) are said to have pre-eclampsia.

In the United Kingdom, severe pre-eclampsia is considered to be pre-eclampsia with severe hypertension and/or with symptoms, and/or biochemical and/or haematological impairment. The Society of Obstetricians and Gynaecologists of Canada includes gestation of onset before 34 weeks, heavy proteinuria, maternal symptoms, signs of end-organ dysfunction, abnormal laboratory tests, or signs of fetal morbidity. The American Society of Hypertension includes gestation below 35 weeks, maternal symptoms, abnormal laboratory tests, or fetal morbidity. This generates difficulty in comparisons of outcomes in different settings. Eclampsia is a convulsive condition associated with pre-eclampsia.

Epidemiology

Hypertension complicates between 6% and 12% of all pregnancies.[17] Around one in ten women will develop hypertension and over 4% pre-eclampsia in their first pregnancy[12] though most will have straightforward pregnancies and good maternal and neonatal outcomes.[1] Good care of hypertensive women in pregnancy involves minimizing risk in the antenatal period along with good surveillance and effective antenatal treatment. Timely intervention for delivery and multidisciplinary care in the face of severe disease or complications can minimize the morbidity and mortality for both mother and fetus. The hypertensive conditions of pregnancy can result in life-threatening multisystem pathology, affecting the nervous, hepatic, haematological, renal, and respiratory systems.

Maternal morbidity and mortality

An estimated 63,000 women die worldwide as a consequence of pre-eclampsia and its complications with 98% of these occurring in the developing world.[18] In the United Kingdom, pre-eclampsia accounts for the second largest number of direct maternal deaths. There were 22 deaths in the triennium 2006–2008.[2] Of these, nine died of cerebral haemorrhage, five due to cardiac arrest due to uncontrolled eclamptic seizures, three from liver failure, two from multiorgan failure while in critical care, two from complications of AFLP, and one from an intra-abdominal haemorrhage of uncertain origin. In 20 cases their care was viewed as 'substandard' by the assessors. This was usually due to a failure to manage severe hypertension. The overall mortality rate has ranged from 0.66 to 0.83/100,000 maternities. The three predominant causes of death are cerebral events, pulmonary problems, or liver disease. The lack of a reduction in cerebral deaths has led to tighter recommendations for the control of hypertension with a gradual reduction in the recommendation to treat hypertension from 170/110 mmHg to the current recommendation of treating blood pressure above 150/100 mmHg and that a systolic blood pressure above 170 mmHg should be a medical emergency. A significant success has been the reduction in pulmonary deaths. This is predominantly due to fluid restriction regimens avoiding pulmonary overload leading to adult respiratory distress syndrome. Deaths from liver disorders have remained relatively constant.

Severe pre-eclampsia

Determining the incidence of severe pre-eclampsia is difficult because of a lack of precision about exact criteria to differentiate between moderate and severe cases. In Yorkshire between 1999 and 2003, there were 1087 cases of severe pre-eclampsia in 210,631 maternities. This was a rate of 5.2/1000 maternities.[4] There were no maternal deaths in this series but 49 women (rate of 23/10,000 maternities) needed intensive care; Pulmonary oedema developed in 2.3% of cases, 0.55% of women required renal dialysis, and 4.3% of women had platelets below 50×10^9/L and an alanine aminotransferase (ALT) level over 70 IU/mL. Oliguria (defined as <80 mL/4-hour block for two consecutive blocks) occurred in 7.9% of cases.

Fetal morbidity and mortality

Hypertensive disorders also carry a risk for the baby. In the most recent UK perinatal mortality report, 1 in 20 (5%) stillbirths in infants without congenital abnormality occurred in women with pre-eclampsia.[5] The contribution of pre-eclampsia to the overall preterm birth rate is substantial; 1 in 250 (0.4%) women in their first pregnancy will give birth before 34 weeks as a consequence of pre-eclampsia[12] and 8–10% of all preterm births result from hypertensive disorders.[19] Half of women with severe pre-eclampsia give birth preterm. Small-for-gestational-age babies (mainly because of fetal growth restriction arising from placental disease) are common, with 20–25% of preterm births and 14–19% of term births in women with pre-eclampsia being less than the tenth centile of birth weight for gestation.[20]

Pathogenesis

Most research relating to the pathogenesis of hypertension in pregnancy relates to pre-eclampsia, largely because chronic hypertension, essential or otherwise, has its causes outside pregnancy, while GH on its own has a less severe impact on maternal or neonatal outcome, unless pre-eclampsia develops.

The pathogenesis of pre-eclampsia is unresolved but it is widely accepted that abnormal placentation is involved in the pathophysiology. The disease will begin to resolve following the delivery of the fetus and placenta, while pre-eclampsia can occur in the absence of fetal tissue, as occurs in a complete molar pregnancy, a condition in which pre-eclampsia is more frequent.

It has become increasingly apparent that the manifestation of pre-eclampsia in a given pregnancy is determined at the outset of pregnancy, when the trophoblast implants in the endometrium and invades to access the maternal spiral arteries arising from the myometrium. Normally the infiltration of fetal cytotrophoblasts act to trigger the maturation and remodelling of the spiral arteries from small-capacity, narrow vessels into high-capacity, wide vessels. The failure of this process is a consistent histological finding in the placentae of those pregnancies complicated by pre-eclampsia clinically. The balance of opinion is that the failure of the maturation of these spiral arteries and the subsequent placental ischaemia causes cytokines, interleukins, and growth factors to be released into the circulation, whose vasoactive properties can cause end-organ damage and lead to the clinical signs and symptoms of the disease. This would also support the observation that pre-eclampsia is an independent variable for maternal cardiovascular disease in later life.[21]

Research has been aimed at identifying these key vasoactive factors and several possible molecules have been identified. These include elements of the angiotensin pathway and tumour necrosis factor alpha. While alterations in these substances have been identified in pre-eclampsia, a definitive mode or pattern of causation has yet to be defined. This may reflect the complexity of the biochemical milieu surrounding pregnancy and pre-eclampsia and also the biochemical research difficulties in developing a valid animal model,[22] as pre-eclampsia only occurs in primates.

The most promising avenues have focused on the vascular endothelial growth factor (VEGF) family of cytokines, its receptors and variants. VEGF is one of the platelet-derived growth factor family and has several variants including VEGF-A, placental growth factor (PGF), and VEGF-B, VEGF-C, and VEGF-D. The main activities of all of these molecules are to promote the growth of blood or lymph vessels and modulate the behaviour of that growth. In the case of VEGF-A, this includes angiogenesis, lumen, and fenestration formation, while VEGF-B encourages the formation of the myocardium in the embryo. All the VEGF molecules act by activating specific, tyrosine kinase type receptors, which span the cell membrane of target cells. In pre-eclampsia, abnormal levels of VEGF have been implicated as predictive of pre-eclampsia.[23]

Soluble fms-like tyrosine kinase-1 (sFlt1) has also been implicated in the development of pre-eclampsia. This variant of the VEGF receptor (VEGFR)-1, which lacks the usual transmembrane and intracellular components, can bind to circulating VEGF and PGF, thereby reducing the free levels of these molecules and their subsequent biological activity to promote angiogenesis and placentation. Women with pre-eclampsia have increased amounts of sFlt1 and smaller amounts of circulating VEGF and PGF leading to theories that reduced levels of the former may lead to early renal manifestations of PET. *In vitro* and *in vivo* primate studies have demonstrated higher levels of sFlt-1 in hypoxic placentae.[24]

Similarly, endoglin (sEng), a version of the transforming growth factor beta co-receptor, is increased in pre-eclampsia and has been demonstrated to have some synergy with sFlt-1 in hepatic damage associated with pre-eclampsia.[25] It is becoming increasingly evident that the levels of these molecules can be elevated in women who will go on to become severely pre-eclamptic, weeks before any clinical manifestations.[26]

A hypothesized link to a longstanding observation has also been put forward as a consequence of these findings. Cigarette smokers are known to have a reduced rate of pre-eclampsia in comparison to the background population. Haemoxidase (HO)-1 is induced by the inhaled products of tobacco smoke as a probable stress response. The induction of HO-1, a stress response gene, promotes cellular protective measures, particularly against hypoxia, including the degradation of haem to biliverdin and carbon monoxide. Both biliverdin and carbon monoxide have been shown to reduce the production of sFlt1 and sEng.[27] Investigation into the possible role of statins in obstetrics to treat pre-eclampsia, via this mode of action, may reveal an effective therapy. Pilot work to assess the maternal-fetal safety and pharmacokinetic profile of pravastatin in patients at high risk of pre-eclampsia is also being studied in the United States.[28]

The mode of action of aspirin in reducing the rate of recurrence of pre-eclampsia has not been precisely elucidated but is likely to be a consequence of its selective antagonism of cyclooxygenase-1. A randomized control trial is prospectively studying the value of 81 mg daily aspirin for patients with high pre-eclampsia risk scores.[29]

Pre-eclampsia is more common in scenarios where there has been a reduced exposure time to paternal antigens prior to conception. Classically pre-eclampsia presents more commonly in first pregnancies, though extends to first pregnancies to current partners and is more common in pregnancy following *in vitro* fertilization treatment with donor sperm.

Antenatal risk assessment and risk reduction

Over 100 different methods of testing women antenatally to predict their risk of developing pre-eclampsia have been put forward over the last 60 years. These have included biochemical, physical, and epidemiological methods; however, none has proven singularly superior. It is still possible to counsel women to some extent in the preconceptual or early antenatal period regarding their risks of developing GH and most importantly pre-eclampsia.

All pregnant women in the United Kingdom will have a risk assessment performed as part of routine antenatal care, in order to identify those women at high risk of pre-eclampsia. Several risk factors are known and these have been incorporated into NICE guidance[30] and are summarized in Box 36.1.

In high-risk women, management involves increased antenatal surveillance. Clinicians should ensure women are aware of important symptoms and should have a lower threshold for investigation with symptoms or abnormalities on urinalysis or blood pressure assessment. The principal reason for this is the lack of a definitive diagnostic or screening test with sufficient positive predictive value. Whilst uterine artery Doppler does also predict women who are at increased risk, it is only appropriate in women who are already identified as at higher risk. Since all higher-risk women need aspirin, uterine artery Doppler does not alter clinical management and is therefore unwarranted in most cases.

Box 36.1 Risk factors for the development of pre-eclampsia

High risk factors

- Hypertensive disease during a previous pregnancy
- Chronic renal disease
- Autoimmune disease such as systemic lupus erythematosus or antiphospholipid syndrome
- Type 1 or type 2 diabetes
- Chronic hypertension

Moderate risk factors

- First pregnancy
- Age 40 years or older
- Pregnancy interval of greater than 10 years
- Body mass index (BMI) of 35 kg/m^2 or greater at booking visit
- Family history of pre-eclampsia
- Multiple pregnancy

National Institute for Health and Clinical Excellence (2011) CG 107 Hypertension in pregnancy: the management of hypertensive disorders during pregnancy. Manchester: NICE. Available from www.nice.org.uk/CG107 Reproduced with permission. Information accurate at time of press. For up-to-date information, please visit www.nice.org.uk.

Table 36.1 Antenatal risk factors for the development of pre-eclampsia

Risk factor	Relative risk	Confidence intervals
Antiphospholipid syndrome	9.72	4.34–21.75
Previous history of pre-eclamptic toxaemia	7.19	5.83–8.83
Pre-existing diabetes	3.56	2.54–4.99
Multiple pregnancy	2.93	2.04–4.21
Nulliparity	2.91	1.28–6.61
Family history	2.90	1.70–4.93
Raised BMI		
Before pregnancy	2.47	1.66–3.67
At booking	1.55	1.28–1.88
Age over 40	1.96	1.34–2.87
Diastolic blood pressure >80 mmHg	1.38	1.01–1.87

Adapted by permission from BMJ Publishing Group Limited., *The BMJ*, Risk factors for pre-eclampsia at antenatal booking: systematic review of controlled studies, Kirsten Duckitt, Deborah Harrington, volume 330, pp. 576–580, © 2005.

When discussing risk with individual patients, assessing the likelihood of pre-eclampsia is difficult and is more complex than a cumulative assessment of the risk factors listed above. Factors, such as family history of pre-eclampsia, can have a variable significance on risk assessment; one first-degree relative with a history of pre-eclampsia is significant, whereas two will increase these risk factors further. It is therefore possible to counsel women about their risk dependent on history and the strength of positive risk factors despite the difficulty of no definitive investigative testing. The relative risks of history factors and co-morbidities are outlined in Table 36.1.[31]

Prevention of pre-eclampsia

Antenatal aspirin

The only intervention shown to reduce the rate of pre-eclampsia is aspirin 75 mg daily. Therefore women at high risk of pre-eclampsia should be advised to take 75 mg of aspirin daily from at least 12 weeks of gestation. Although NICE recommends aspirin only from 12 weeks onwards, this is because firm evidence for its use has only been widely tested in randomized controlled trials from this gestation.[32] In theory and probably in practice it would have more effect if started as early in pregnancy as possible. Women at high risk include those with previous or current relevant obstetric history, or existing co-morbidities known to increase the risk of hypertensive disease of pregnancy.

Women who are at high risk or have a number of moderate risk factors should therefore be advised to take daily low-dose aspirin. The use of aspirin or non-steroidal anti-inflammatory drugs in obstetrics patients is not considered to increase the relative risk (RR) of complications for regional anaesthesia and requires no additional precaution.[33]

Other 'preventative therapies'

Many drugs have been put forward as effective therapies for the prevention of pre-eclampsia in at risk women. However, only aspirin is known to be effective. Despite anecdotal evidence, no robust evidence base exists for the use of nitric oxide donors,[34] progesterone,[35] diuretics,[36] fish/algal oils,[37] garlic oil,[38] antioxidants (vitamins C and E),[39] folic acid, or magnesium. Indeed, there is evidence that pharmacological doses of vitamins C and E are associated with an increased risk of adverse outcome.[40] Dietary salt reduction also has no evidence base to support it. High-dose folic acid (4 mg daily) is being studied in Canada to prospectively determine if it can lower the incidence of pre-eclampsia.[41] There were no suitable randomized control trials assessing the value of Chinese herbal medicine in pre-eclampsia in a Cochrane review, despite identification of 45 trials on the subject.[55]

Low-molecular-weight heparin (LMWH) should not be prescribed to reduce the risk of hypertension in pregnancy. However, women with conditions such as systemic lupus erythematosus and antiphospholipid syndrome, which not only carry an increased risk of pre-eclampsia, but are more likely to suffer thromboembolic disease or pregnancy loss, will be given LMWH to reduce these risks.[33]

Controversy still surrounds the use of dietary calcium supplementation antenatally to reduce the risk of hypertensive diseases in pregnancy. Trials have produced ambiguous results in varied populations making a definitive conclusion impossible. In women with a low dietary calcium intake, some preventative benefit has been seen; however, in women with good dietary calcium intake, no benefit is seen.[43] Nevertheless, the intervention is low risk, low cost, likely to be well tolerated, and holds little harm to mother and fetus. Thus, even modest benefits, would warrant the use of oral calcium supplementation. The case for its use remains to be proven.

No particular additional lifestyle advice for women at risk of, or suffering from, hypertension in pregnancy is required beyond that normally given to pregnant women regarding rest, exercise or the timing of maternity leave from work. Additional information can provide further indications to shape antenatal management.

Diagnosis of pre-eclampsia

The primary method for the diagnosis of pre-eclampsia is the measurement of the blood pressure and the assessment of the urine for proteinuria. Other clinical signs have limited specificity for pre-eclampsia. The validity of methods used to assess the blood pressure and to quantify proteinuria in order to make the diagnosis is therefore very important.

Assessment of blood pressure

Given the nationally defined thresholds for blood pressure measurement and categorization of hypertension in pregnancy, the accurate assessment of blood pressure is paramount in the screening of the pregnant population and for the diagnosis and risk assessment of hypertensive disease in pregnancy. The margin for error commonly introduced when measuring blood pressure in the pregnant and non-pregnant population has been widely documented either through mechanical or operator limitations. Strict validation protocols now exist for automatic blood pressure measuring devices for use within specific populations and clinical settings.[44] Similarly, inaccuracies introduced by operator error when using manual devices have led to the introduction of guidance for the use of manual devices.[45] Simple measures such as being aware of digit preference, where practitioners will round blood pressure readings up or down to the nearest 5 or 10 mmHg, will reduce inaccuracies. Use of standard sphygmomanometer cuffs will be inappropriate for up to a quarter of women who require a larger cuff to reduce the incidence of artificially elevated blood pressures and thus the over-diagnosis of hypertension. Similarly, use of the correct Korotkoff sounds to measure blood pressure will reduce over-diagnosis of hypertension when taking blood pressure manually. Using Korotkoff phase 5 rather than Korotkoff phase 4 will prevent over-diagnosis of diastolic hypertension, while keeping the rate of cuff deflation lower than 2–3 mmHg/s will also reduce this error.[46,47]

All women in the United Kingdom will have their blood pressure routinely monitored as part of their antenatal care. This will occur at midwifery-led appointments at home or in the community when the women first registers her pregnancy (typically just after finding out she is pregnant), and then at 16 and 25 weeks (for primigravid women), 28 (for all women), 31 (primigravidae), and then for all women at 34, 36, 38, 40, and 41 weeks of gestation. If the blood pressure readings gained at these visits are above the threshold of 140/90 mmHg as specified in the NICE guidance this will result in escalation of care, usually for a period of sustained blood pressure monitoring in an outpatient maternity day unit type setting.[48] Additional investigation will occur as per Table 36.2 dependent upon persistent increases in blood pressure and significant proteinuria.

Table 36.2 Management of gestational hypertension and pre-eclampsia

	Gestational hypertension	Pre-eclampsia
Admission to hospital	Only to control severe hypertension	Yes
Anti-hypertensive treatment	For moderate or severe hypertension to target of 80–100 mmHg diastolic and below 150 mmHg systolic	For moderate or severe hypertension to target of 80–100 mmHg diastolic and below 150 mmHg systolic
Measure blood pressure	Weekly in mild hypertension Twice-weekly in moderate hypertension Four times daily with severe hypertension until controlled	Four times daily or more if severe hypertension
Assessment of proteinuria	At each visit using automated assessment or PCR	Not necessary once diagnosis confirmed
Blood tests: Full blood count Renal function Transaminases Bilirubin Electrolytes Albumin	Not necessary with mild hypertension As a baseline with moderate hypertension but do not repeat Weekly if has had severe hypertension	Mild pre-eclampsia—twice-weekly Moderate and severe pre-eclampsia check three times a week (though more frequent if abnormal)

National Institute for Health and Clinical Excellence (2011) CG 107 Hypertension in pregnancy: the management of hypertensive disorders during pregnancy. Manchester: NICE. Available from www.nice.org.uk/CG107 Reproduced with permission. Information accurate at time of press. For up-to-date information, please visit www.nice.org.uk

Assessment of proteinuria in hypertensive disorders of pregnancy

The differentiation and diagnosis of GH and pre-eclampsia and therefore the increased likelihood of more serious complications, is dependent upon the reliable and accurate diagnosis of significant proteinuria. This has traditionally been taken at a level of greater than 300 mg excretion in a 24-hour period. This level is endorsed in international guidelines. However, the accuracy of the quantification of proteinuria is vulnerable to collection and measurement error. By its very nature, the length of time required to undertake a 24-hour collection rules it out as a bedside test and a tool for immediate assessment at first presentation to secondary care. A widely used screening test is urine dipstick analysis, but good evidence has established that significant error exists in measuring proteinuria even when experienced staff read urinalysis strips.[49] To reduce inaccuracies of proteinuria measurement, use of an automated reagent-strip reading device is recommended by NICE guidance in secondary care settings.[30] However it should be stressed that this is still insufficient for absolute confirmation of significant proteinuria and formal quantification of proteinuria should be performed. The two approaches are either a 24-hour urine protein collection or a urinary protein:creatinine ratio. There is no evidence to suggest that this is necessary in the routine screening of the whole pregnant population. Urine protein:creatinine ratio requires a single urine sample that is sent for immediate biochemical analysis which allows for faster turnaround than a 24-hour urine collection. It is now recognized that this investigation is comparable to a 24-hour urine protein measurement.[50] Results of 300 mg of protein excreted in 24 hours, or a urine protein:creatinine ratio result greater than 30 mg/mmol, indicates significant proteinuria.

Further research to improve accuracy is still needed. Similarly convincing evidence, as to where the correct thresholds lie to determine prognostic significance (and thus influence management), remains to be discovered. Once the degree of hypertension and presence and quantity of protein are confirmed, the initial treatment regimens will follow the patterns outlined in Table 36.2.

Symptoms of pre-eclampsia

The symptoms listed in Box 36.2 are commonly associated with pre-eclampsia but are by no means universal. Symptoms do not necessarily correspond with the objective severity of disease and subsequent maternal or fetal complications. Similarly, women may only have one of these symptoms and not the expected constellation. A woman with no symptoms can yet present with severe pre-eclampsia.

Box 36.2 Symptoms of pre-eclampsia

- Severe headache
- Problems with vision, such as blurring or flashing before the eyes
- Severe pain just below the ribs
- Nausea and vomiting
- Sudden swelling of the face, hands, or feet.

Antenatally it is important that all pregnant women, especially those diagnosed with hypertension, are aware of the above symptoms and their significance. They must therefore be able to seek advice from a healthcare professional 24 hours a day, or if necessary, attend secondary care obstetric services directly should these symptoms manifest themselves.

Antenatal care

Gestational hypertension

Women with GH should have a full assessment carried out in secondary care by the obstetric team. They will need ongoing follow-up and care throughout and after the pregnancy. The risk factors of developing GH and pre-eclampsia are listed in Box 36.3.

Dependent on the severity of disease, obstetric units offering care and follow-up to these women should have the capability to offer admission to hospital, treatment, regular measurement of blood pressure, facilities for accurate testing for proteinuria, and blood tests as described in Table 36.2. Most women with non-proteinuric hypertension can and should be managed as outpatients.

Women who have been treated as inpatients for severe GH, which has then been subsequently stabilized, will usually be managed on an outpatient basis with regular reviews.[51] A recommended regimen of monitoring in these patients will include blood pressure and urine checks twice weekly, with weekly blood testing. Similarly, those women presenting with mild hypertension prior to 32 weeks, and those women with hypertension and increased risk factors for pre-eclampsia (see Box 36.3), should be offered increased outpatient monitoring, with blood pressure and urine check twice per week.

There is no evidence regarding the benefit of bed-rest in women with hypertension in pregnancy.[30]

Pre-eclampsia

Women diagnosed with pre-eclampsia should usually be managed as inpatients.

The monitoring of pre-eclampsia requires regular blood pressure monitoring and relevant blood testing. Once the diagnosis of pre-eclampsia is confirmed by the presence of significant

Box 36.3 Risk factors for developing gestational hypertension and pre-eclampsia

- Nulliparity
- Age 40 years or older
- Pregnancy interval of more than 10 years
- Family history of pre-eclampsia
- Multiple pregnancy
- BMI of 35 kg/m^2 or more
- Low gestational age at presentation
- Previous history of pre-eclampsia or gestational hypertension
- Pre-existing vascular disease
- Pre-existing kidney disease.

proteinuria there is little value to the ongoing monitoring of urinary protein excretion. The blood tests include a full blood count (FBC) to assess haemoglobin levels and platelets, liver function tests to monitor enzymatic changes, and renal function tests. Clotting tests to diagnose any developing coagulopathy are appropriate if there are abnormalities of platelet levels or liver function. There is no evidence of additional value to urate assessment. The advice from NICE is summarized in Table 36.2. Ongoing monitoring of physiological and biochemical markers should be organized, a plan made for management of hypertension, along with a plan for delivery. Ideally, thresholds in blood pressure or biochemistry should be should be specified to trigger an escalation in monitoring and management, including those which would warrant an expedited delivery.

If the likelihood of premature or urgent delivery is deemed significant due to severe hypertension, defined as hypertension which is refractory to first-line antihypertensives, concerns regarding fetal growth or well-being, or if a women has significant co-morbidities, then anaesthetic pre-assessment is indicated.

Women diagnosed with pre-eclampsia should be managed with an integrated care package. Due to the unpredictable nature of pre-eclampsia and the difficulty in anticipating which women will develop complications such as severe pre-eclampsia, eclampsia, and fetal complications, women must be fully assessed on a regular basis. When women are assessed, they need to be seen by professionals experienced in the management of pre-eclampsia, who have the facilities to measure blood pressure, test for proteinuria, and blood tests

Antihypertensive treatment

The evidence available regarding the use of antihypertensives in pregnancy is limited due to a surprising lack of good quality clinical trial data relating to pregnant women, and the unwillingness of clinicians to use untried and untested newer antihypertensives. First-line treatment is labetalol. Labetalol has both non-selective β-adrenoreceptor antagonism and selective α-adrenoreceptor antagonism which together reduce systemic vascular resistance, reduce heart rates, and reduce the risk of arrthymias.[52] If commencing treatment for the first time, a graduated course of treatment should be commenced and titrated to control hypertension. A blood pressure with a systolic below 149 mmHg and between 80 and 100 mmHg diastolic should be aimed for, whilst avoiding profound and sudden drops in blood pressure. Labetalol is superior to other agents including methyldopa and other beta blockers such as atenolol in various studies demonstrating effectiveness in reducing hypertension while minimizing maternal and fetal side effects.[53–57] It also has a licence for use in pregnancy. Whilst some studies have suggested that particular drugs are associated with impaired fetal growth it is probably the lowering of blood pressure that drives this effect. Therefore it is likely that any drug which effectively lowers blood pressure will be associated with a reduction in fetal weight. A reasonable initial dosage for moderate hypertension is 200 mg orally two or three times a day.

In the more acute setting with severe hypertension, an initial dose of oral labetalol 200 mg is used when commencing antihypertensive treatment. If blood pressure has not started to fall within 20 minutes a repeat dose should be given. Rarely if a third dose fails to manage blood pressure, 50 mg of intravenous labetalol should be given. Again this should be repeated every 10–15 minutes, until the blood pressure is brought below 150/100 mmHg, but maintaining a diastolic above 80 mmHg to avoid fetal complications. Once this is achieved a labetalol infusion up to a maximum of 2 mg/min should be commenced.[30] In some settings, an arterial line for closer blood pressure monitoring and frequent blood sampling is inserted when intravenous antihypertensives are required, though this is uncommon in the United Kingdom.

If bolus doses of IV labetalol fail to bring hypertension under control then second-line treatments such as hydralazine or nifedipine can be used. In some settings nicardipine or urapadil are used. An initial dose of 10–20 mg of oral nifedipine is recommended. Note that oral nifedipine is recommended over sublingual nifedipine as the latter can cause precipitous falls in blood pressure. Modified- or slow-release preparations help reduce this phenomenon and are very useful in ante- or postnatal settings, but are less helpful in the acute situation. Rarely nifedipine can cause profound drops in blood pressure, leading to fetal compromise due to placental hypoperfusion and in severe cases this may necessitate delivery. Whilst there have been concerns about nifedipine and a possible interaction with magnesium sulphate, that does not seem to have been the case in the larger trials or in clinical practice.

Hydralazine is a very effective treatment when given intravenously. However, it is more commonly associated with profound reductions in blood pressure and tachycardia than other agents. A dose of 5 mg hydralazine can be given intravenously. Usually a fluid bolus of up to 500 mL crystalloid fluid should be given before or at the same time as the first dose of intravenous hydralazine prior to delivery. This is to avoid fetal compromise. Other agents are less commonly used in the United Kingdom but can be considered. Diazoxide 15mg intravenous is an arterial vasodilator and could be used as an alternative to hydralazine.

Nicardipine is an alternative calcium channel blocker that can be given parenterally. Intravenous nicardipine 10 mg over 5minutes may be given in severe hypertension.

Angiotensin-converting enzyme (ACE) inhibitors and angiotensin II receptor blockers are contraindicated antenatally as they are associated with congenital abnormalities. They may be considered postnatally.

In all cases it is important not to drop the maternal blood pressure precipitously. Stabilizing the maternal condition, thus preventing the secondary consequences of hypertension such as a cerebrovascular accident, remains the principal objective of treatment and supersedes any indication for delivery. A precipitous decision to delivery prior to maternal stabilization can lead to sudden physiological changes in response to anaesthesia and surgery with increased maternal and fetal complications. During administration of antihypertensive medication, ongoing critical care and fetal monitoring must be continued to track any response and modify treatment accordingly and identify any adverse outcomes for both mother and fetus.

Timing of birth

Women with chronic hypertension or GH should not be advised to have elective delivery prior to 37 weeks due to the increased risks of the complications of prematurity and increased admission to special care baby services.[5] Only women with severe hypertension above 160/110 mmHg, which is refractory to medical treatment, should be offered delivery prior to 37 weeks.[58–60] Delivery arrangements should be agreed between the woman, the obstetric team, the anaesthetic, and critical care teams in consultation with other professionals as required (cardiology, haematology, and neurology). When planning elective delivery it is important to ensure optimization of maternal blood pressure and to decide on the administration of corticosteroids with a possible 48-hour delay to optimize their effect.[61] If vaginal birth is planned, steroids are usually given before 34 weeks of gestation but if elective caesarean delivery is planned, then they are beneficial up to 38 weeks.

When women present with pre-eclampsia prior to 34 weeks, the aim should be to manage them conservatively. The blood pressure should be treated and stabilized, ideally avoiding same-day delivery, unless fetal or maternal risks from pre-eclampsia are critical. The main contraindication to delivery is the more serious consequences of prematurity in this group. However, prior to 34 weeks, women with pre-eclampsia will have hypertension increasingly refractory to antihypertensive treatment. They are also more likely to have worsening biochemical or haematological profiles or concern about fetal well-being. Even women with severe hypertension and pre-eclampsia should have their blood pressure stabilized and a plan to aim for delivery after 34 weeks as associated neonatal morbidity begins to decline. However, these decisions are multidisciplinary and must not be detrimental to the woman's well-being. The advantage of prolonging gestation is to the fetus alone.

Obstetric care plans should indicate clinical and investigation thresholds, which must be crossed to warrant elective delivery prior to 34 weeks. Mode of delivery should be agreed between the woman and obstetric team. A semi-planned caesarean delivery or induction may be offered. However, induction is less likely to result in labour and subsequent vaginal birth at earlier gestations. Before 32 weeks a caesarean delivery will probably be required. The multidisciplinary team should also be involved in decision-making, including the anaesthetic and neonatal consultants, who can provide maternal and neonatal support respectively, in the event of any associated morbidity.

Women with mild or moderate pre-eclampsia can be offered delivery from 34 weeks onwards and prior to 37 weeks, as clinically indicated by maternal or fetal condition. The neonatal risks are reduced after 34 weeks; however, they must be considered as their incidence does not drop below 10% until after the 36th week of gestation. After 37 weeks, once the diagnosis of pre-eclampsia is confirmed, obstetricians will usually advise women to deliver within 24–48 hours of confirmation of the diagnosis.

There is a 'grey' zone for women who have pre-eclampsia with mild or moderate hypertension between 34 and 37 weeks when the optimal timing of birth is not clear. Women who have pre-eclampsia with mild or moderate hypertension may progress to severe disease with its risks, but it is not clear whether these risks outweigh or should outweigh the risks of planned late preterm birth for the baby. Neonatal services are under constant pressure and planned preterm birth without clear benefit to either woman or baby would have costs. The HYPITAT study[62] in 2008 randomized women with GH and mild pre-eclampsia to induction of labour at 36 weeks versus expectant management and delivery as clinically dictated by changing symptoms. Of women who were randomized, 117 (31%) allocated to induction of labour developed poor maternal outcome (as measured by a range of composite outcomes, including severe hypertension and the development of HELLP syndrome) compared with 166 (44%) allocated to expectant monitoring (RR 0.71; 95% confidence interval (CI) 0.59–0.86; $P < 0.0001$). No cases of maternal or neonatal death were seen due to the limited size of the trial. Interestingly women randomized to induction of labour were probably less likely to require a caesarean delivery RR 0.75 (95% CI 0.55–1.04; $P = 0.085$). This is likely to be due to the decreased likelihood of these women developing more severe hypertensive disease.

Future randomized controlled trials are planned that compare policies of immediate planned birth between 34 + 0 and 36 + 6 weeks in women who have pre-eclampsia with mild or moderate hypertension with expectant management and birth for clinical progression.

Intrapartum management

Women with pre-eclampsia should receive the same basic care in labour as all women and in particular they should have one-to-one midwifery care. Additionally, blood pressure should be monitored hourly in women with mild or moderate hypertension and more frequently in women with severe hypertension. Any antenatal hypertensive medication should be continued in labour with dose titration as per the clinical picture.

Blood testing and analgesia

Haematological and biochemical testing in women with mild or moderate hypertension should be organized according to the antenatal criteria outlined in Table 36.2, even when considering neuraxial anaesthesia. This means that women with mild hypertension and no proteinuria do not need a platelet count or coagulation screen and are suitable for neuraxial anaesthesia barring other concurrent pathology or contraindication. There is evidence to avoid over-testing by only performing a thromboelastograph study if platelets are less than 100.[63]

Decision about level of care (critical care levels)

Woman with severe hypertension or severe pre-eclampsia should be managed in a critical care setting with:

- close blood pressure monitoring
- continuous heart rate monitoring
- continuous oxygen saturation monitoring
- fluid balance
- fluid restriction
- intravenous access (2 × 16 G cannulae if possible)
- haematological and biochemical testing
- continuous fetal heart rate monitoring prior to delivery

Close blood pressure monitoring does not imply invasive blood pressure monitoring, though that may be required on occasions. Generally non-invasive blood pressure monitoring with checks at frequent intervals depending on the blood pressure reading is reasonable. One possible advantage of invasive monitoring is that it can also make repeated blood sampling more patient-friendly and especially if there is concurrent thrombocytopaenia.

A multidisciplinary approach to treating pre-eclampsia and severe hypertension is crucial and critical care is a vital part of management. Obstetric and midwifery teams are often proficient in diagnosing, treating, and managing pre-eclampsia. They are also acutely aware of the complications which may arise due to the disease itself or iatrogenically, but will be unable to supply a full range of supportive care for these women. Anaesthetists on the labour ward are therefore ideally placed to offer this expertise and support to the woman and the team.

In order to manage complicated pre-eclampsia appropriately, the following recommendations are made to guide appropriate obstetric critical care support:[30]

- *Level 3 care (or intensive therapy unit (ITU) care)*—severe pre-eclampsia needing ventilatory or inotropic support or renal replacement therapy.
- *Level 2 care (or high dependency unit (HDU) care)*—step-down from Level 3 or severe pre-eclampsia with any of the following complications:
    - eclampsia
    - HELLP syndrome
    - haemorrhage (estimated blood loss greater than 1000 mL)
    - hyperkalaemia
    - severe oliguria
    - coagulation support
    - intravenous antihypertensive treatment
    - initial stabilization of severe hypertension
    - evidence of cardiac failure
    - abnormal neurological findings.
- *Level 1 care (routine delivery suite care)*—women with the following conditions:
    - Pre-eclampsia with mild or moderate hypertension
    - Ongoing conservative antenatal management of severe preterm hypertension
    - Step-down treatment after the birth.

(National Institute for Health and Clinical Excellence (2011) CG 107 Hypertension in pregnancy: the management of hypertensive disorders during pregnancy. Manchester: NICE. Available from www.nice.org.uk/CG107 Reproduced with permission. Information accurate at time of press. For up-to-date information, please visit www.nice.org.uk)

Fluid management and renal complications of pre-eclampsia

Fluid overload has been a contributory factor in deaths due to pre-eclampsia.[2] Whilst it is the case that the intravascular volume is depleted, the fact that the capillary membranes are more permeable can lead to fluid entering the tissues. This is exacerbated if there is excess fluid administration. Therefore women with pre-eclampsia should not be given volume expanders intrapartum. The one exception is if hydralazine or other potent vasodilators are the antihypertensives being used, prior to birth. The vasodilatation and drop in blood pressure can cause a reduction in placental blood flow and fetal compromise.

Where fluid management is problematic, intrapartum monitoring should include invasive arterial blood pressure but pulmonary artery flotation catheters are not recommended as there is a high reported complications rate (1/25 catheters inserted in a retrospective review of 100 cases of severe pre-eclampsia or eclampsia).[64] Central venous catheters can be used if fluid balance is difficult though interpretation of the information provided can be difficult.

Fluid restriction is undertaken to prevent pulmonary and cerebral oedema. The incidence of pulmonary oedema in pre-eclampsia is around 2%.[5] The synergy of left ventricular diastolic dysfunction, reduced colloid oncotic pressure of pregnancy, and increased capillary permeability make this a dangerous complication of pre-eclampsia.[65] The negative inotropic effect of the commonly used agent labetalol as well as injudicious fluid administration with oliguria also increase the risk of pulmonary oedema. Whilst no specific amount of total fluid input per hour can precisely be defined, it is recommended that clear guidance is given to avoid iatrogenic fluid overload. A regimen in current clinical use is 1mL/kg/h of fluids in total, up to a maximum of 80 mL/h. These can be given by the oral or intravenous route. Given that fluid restriction must take into account oral intake, intravenous crystalloid, magnesium sulphate, and labetalol infusions, careful fluid balance monitoring is vital. Ongoing fluid losses such as haemorrhage should be replaced appropriately. If oxytocin is to be continued post delivery it should be administered in small crystalloid volumes by syringe driver (e.g. 50 units in 50 mL 0.9% saline over 5 hours, i.e. therapeutic dose delivered of 10 units/hour). To facilitate fluid restriction, magnesium sulphate and labetalol should equally be given in a low-volume infusion (e.g. in a 50 mL syringe).

Oliguria is a common feature of pre-eclampsia in the peripartum and early postpartum period. However, this will usually resolve spontaneously with a marked diuresis 24–48 hours after delivery. Glomerular capillary endotheliosis is a classical histological appearance in association with pre-eclampsia. However, acute kidney injury is rare, with an incidence of less than 1/10,000 pregnancies. In pre-eclampsia, circulating volume may be reduced despite increased total body water so hourly monitoring of urine output is necessary, particularly with severe pre-eclampsia.

Postnatally, fluid restriction should be maintained. Urine output should be monitored and 4-hour blocks of urine output considered. If urine output is more than 80 ml in a 4-hour block, this should be considered acceptable. If two consecutive 4-hour blocks have less than 80 mL urine output, a fluid bolus should be considered. However, if the woman is already in positive balance by more than 750 mL then furosemide 20 mg intravenously may be given. If the woman is in less than 750 mL positive balance then crystalloid boluses of up to 250 mL should be given. This will resolve most cases of oliguria. If there is still no improvement in urine output then it would then be appropriate to seek the advice of a renal specialist, especially if there is also a raised serum creatinine. A central venous catheter may be useful here in guiding fluid management, though interpretation of the results can be difficult.

In the presence of pulmonary oedema, hypertension can be treated with a glyceryl-trinitrate infusion (5 mcg/min titrated up to response—maximum 100 mcg/min) as recommended by the European guidelines.[66] Such treatment should only be undertaken in the presence of invasive blood pressure monitoring in the ITU. Sodium nitroprusside is reserved only for resistant cases under expert supervision. The risk of cyanide toxicity, particularly for the fetus, makes sodium nitroprusside a short-term option only.

Massive haemorrhage, particularly placental abruption, which occurs more commonly in pre-eclampsia can, however, precipitate acute renal injury due to hypovolaemia. Whilst this may be prevented with timely replacement of blood loss, there is a risk of renal problems even when blood loss is replaced. There is also the challenge of blood replacement leading to fluid overload and pulmonary oedema. In these cases, accurate measuring of blood loss with suction jar measurements and swabs weighting is mandatory. Treatment includes strict attention to electrolyte balance, particularly potassium and fluid balance. Rarely, if renal function does not return to normal or deteriorates, advice from renal physicians may be warranted, especially an assessment of whether dialysis is indicated, though this is rarely required in women who do not have pre-existing renal disease,

Mode of delivery

As previously discussed, the ultimate cure for pre-eclampsia is delivery of the placenta. Intuitively, expediting delivery can therefore seem the most logical solution in treating poorly controlled pre-eclampsia with severe hypertension. However, stabilizing the mother should be a priority over delivery as failure to do this will increase maternal complications (e.g. stroke). Control of the blood pressure to target values of below 140–150 mmHg systolic and 80–100 mmHg diastolic, should be undertaken before the decision to deliver the fetus is made. For this reason the majority of caesarean deliveries for pre-eclampsia are category 2 according to the NICE classification with 'maternal or fetal compromise which is not immediately life-threatening'.[67] In the advent of eclampsia, in particular with fulminant pulmonary oedema or treatment-resistant seizures, it may occasionally be necessary to precipitate the delivery of the fetus before satisfactory blood pressure control can be gained.

Once the decision to deliver has been determined, the mode of delivery should be chosen. This should take into account the woman's wishes and the clinical circumstances. These include:

- hypertensive control
- symptoms
- complications such as HELLP syndrome
- eclampsia
- timing of magnesium sulphate administration
- fetal condition and likely outcome
- unit resource and staffing availability, both maternity and neonatal staff
- the prospects for a reasonably timely vaginal birth

The fetus will be monitored throughout labour regardless of gestation, due to the potentially reduced placental function associated with pre-eclampsia and due to the increased risk of complications, which may affect the fetus such as placental abruption.

There is no evidence supporting the limitation of the second stage of labour in women who have mild or moderate hypertension, but operative delivery is advised for those women with severe hypertension who have not responded to initial treatment in order to expedite delivery. Note that ergometrine should be avoided in the management of the third stage in hypertensive women due to its propensity to aggravate hypertension.

Anaesthetic considerations

In the anaesthetic management of hypertensive diseases of pregnancy, the overarching goals are to ensure adequate tissue perfusion and oxygenation of parturient and fetus whilst treating hypertension to minimize maternal stroke risk. Providing effective analgesia in labour and optimal surgical conditions for caesarean delivery are integral to achieving these goals. There are a number of excellent reviews on this subject.[68,69]

Labour analgesia

Epidurals are the analgesia of choice for labour in the pre-eclamptic patient. The reduction in pain afforded by an epidural prevents catecholamine surges and thus reduces the risk to the mother of stroke or cardiac events. There are advantages to the fetus and Jouppila et al. have shown that placental blood flow is increased in labour by epidural analgesia.[70] This is postulated to occur via decreased uterine vascular resistance which is secondary to the epidural-induced sympathectomy. Further, there is a lower threshold for obstetric interventions with pre-eclamptics and a working epidural can quickly facilitate these. It should be noted that oedema may be present over the lumbar spines and sacrum making insertion of neuraxial anaesthesia challenging.

In the United Kingdom, many obstetric units provide neuraxial anaesthesia to pre-clamptics with platelets down to 75 × 10^9/L based on the observed hypercoagulability seen in severe pre-eclamptics on thromboelastography.[71,111] A postal survey of obstetric anaesthetists from 1996 had already documented that 62% of responding anaesthetists would place epidural catheters in otherwise healthy patients with platelets counts as low as 80 × 10^9/L.[72] Some units advocate the use of platelet transfusion prior to regional anaesthesia if the platelet count is between 50 and 70 × 10^9/L.[72] Platelet transfusion for levels below 50 × 10^9/L prior to delivery may not only be indicated to perform neuraxial anaesthesia but may also be warranted prior to caesarean delivery to reduce the risk of postpartum haemorrhage. Some units would consider neuraxial anaesthesia at lower levels of platelet count especially if they are able to undertake platelet function testing. A careful risk:benefit analysis is required given the concerns of general anaesthesia (GA) in this group of women, due to the risk of surges in blood pressure or failed intubation with laryngeal oedema. Before the removal of epidural catheters in pre-eclamptics, a platelet count is warranted if the count has been low prior to insertion of the epidural or if there has been intervening haemorrhage.

Neuraxial anaesthesia for operative delivery in the pre-eclamptic woman

In the absence of a contraindication to neuraxial anaesthesia, epidural and spinal anaesthesia are currently the anaesthetics of choice for caesarean delivery in pre-eclampsia. Contraindications to neuraxial anaesthesia are no different than in patients without pre-eclampsia/eclampsia, namely untreated coagulopathy including disseminated intravascular coagulation, seizure, pulmonary oedema requiring invasive ventilation, and lack of informed consent. Risk and benefit analysis for cases of eclampsia must be taken on a case-by-case basis by senior anaesthetists and obstetricians.

There have been retrospective and prospective studies with evidence to support the safe use of neuraxial anaesthesia[73–75] in severe pre-eclampsia. A number of studies have compared spinal and epidural anaesthesia in pre-eclamptics[76,77] and found that with spinal anaesthesia, blood pressure drops much less in pre-eclampsia than in healthy partunients.[78] In the context of neuraxial anaesthesia-induced sympathectomy with hypotension, because of an increased sensitivity to vasopressors, ephedrine in small dose increments (3–6 mg) or phenylephrine (50 mcg) may be used. Anaesthetists should have a low threshold for inserting arterial lines as continuous blood pressure measurement will guide vasopressor use.

It is reassuring to know that no significant difference has been found in neonatal outcomes to date when comparing spinal and epidural anaesthesia in pre-eclampsia,[78] although this study by Aya et al.[78] was powered to find haemodynamic differences rather than differences in neonatal outcomes. Other advantages of spinal anaesthesia over epidural are that the former is usually quicker and less traumatic to perform and this may be pertinent when the platelet count is low. Further, some studies have shown that epidurals for caesarean delivery are not as effective as in normotensive patients and require higher conversion rates to spinals or GA.[77,79]

The current evidence thus supports the view that a single-shot spinal anaesthetic is recommended in the pre-eclamptic patient. Similar doses of intrathecal local anaesthetic should be used unless the fetus is premature, when a larger spinal dose is needed. Alternatively, a combined subarachnoid and epidural injection has been found to be a suitable technique. Low-dose subarachnoid bupivacaine (maximum 7.5 mg) with sufentanil in the sitting position followed by an epidural catheter insertion for titrating supplemental anaesthesia was studied prospectively in 30 severely pre-eclamptic parturients.[80]

General anaesthesia in the pre-eclamptic

GA versus neuraxial anaesthesia has been the subject of a 2012 Cochrane review in which there were no differences found in terms of major maternal and neonatal outcomes.[81] The Cochrane review, however, was only able to retain data from 1793 women, of whom none died. There are two potential challenges for the obstetric anaesthetist managing the pre-eclamptic patient requiring a GA. Firstly, there is the risk of dramatic hypertension and cerebral haemorrhage upon direct laryngoscopy at induction and secondly there is the risk of the failed intubation in patients who are well known to have oedematous larynxes.[82] Neuraxial anaesthesia avoids both these potential complications.

However, GA is the recommended anaesthetic technique when patient oxygenation is at risk because of uncontrolled seizures (treatment-resistant eclampsia), or pulmonary oedema requiring invasive ventilation, or if severe coagulopathy is present. In the context of severe thrombocytopenia, the patient declining neuraxial anaesthesia or having disseminated intravascular coagulation, GA is unavoidable. On top of usual considerations for GA for obstetrics (see Chapter 22), considerations must be given to the conduct of a rapid sequence induction and intubation in the presence of hypertension. The use of the ramped position for pre-oxygenation should negate the risk of passive regurgitation and limit the rise in blood pressure seen at direct laryngoscopy by facilitating venous pooling in the lower limbs.

With the aim to secure the airway with a cuffed endotracheal tube, but without hypertensive response to direct laryngoscopy, two broad options are available, namely avoidance of direct laryngoscopy and obtunding the response to laryngeal manipulation with pharmacological options.

The choice of antihypertensives prior to laryngoscopy should be based on the anaesthetist's experience. Drug options include the use of intravenous alfentanil (10–20 mcg/kg 1 minute prior to induction), or remifentanil.[83] A remifentanil dose–response study of 75 parturients with severe pre-eclampsia found that the ED_{50} of remifentanil as a bolus dose for attenuating a hypertensive response 90 seconds before induction was 0.59 mcg/kg.[84] A meta-analysis of remifentanil prior to induction, either as a 1 mcg/kg bolus or a 0.5 mcg/kg bolus followed by an infusion, found that remifentanil was effective in attenuating hypertensive response to laryngoscopy and that fetal base excess was statistically higher, although the clinical significance of the latter is unclear as Apgar values were similar.[85] The choice of opioid will be guided by the opioid onset time, the urgency of the caesarean delivery, and the fetal effects. Discussions about the merits of indirect laryngoscopy (e.g. AirTraq® and Glidescope®), optical stylets (e.g. Levitan FPS and Shikani Optical Stylet), and fibreoptic intubations to avoid hypertension are beyond the scope of this text, but may be increasingly relevant as new equipment is developed and studied.[86,87] Details of this equipment can be found in Chapter 26 on the difficult or failed obstetric airway.

The problem of failed intubation amongst pre-eclamptics is well known and steps must be taken to avoid a 'can't intubate, can't ventilate' scenario. Senior anaesthetists should be present at induction if at all possible and the difficult airway trolley (see Chapter 26 for an example of such a trolley) must be to hand including small endotracheal tubes (down to 5.5 mm). Induction and maintenance of GA, and use of intraoperative analgesia, is similar to that of healthy parturients. The use of magnesium sulphate infusion in pre-eclampsia does not seem to affect the reversal of non-depolarizing neuromuscular blockers in clinical practice, despite the theoretical risks to do so.

Extubation after GA in a pre-eclamptic patient is another potential challenge as there may be more mucosal swelling of the trachea in response to the presence of the endotracheal tube. There is nothing more frightening for an obstetric anaesthetist than to have a pre-eclamptic develop stridor on extubation. To avoid this and after positioning the patient in the sitting position, the cuff of the endotracheal tube should be deflated and if a leak is present, extubation can be performed but if there is no leak, signifying significant mucosal swelling of the trachea, it is better to re-inflate the cuff, re-administer GA, and transfer the patient to intensive care. Diuresis postpartum will result in a reduction of oedema including that of the mucosa and extubation should be subsequently uneventful.

Uterotonics in pre-eclampsia

Oxytocin can cause haemodynamic changes in parturients, namely hypotension, so its dose is usually limited to 5 IU by slow intravenous injection post delivery.[88] Ergometrine is contraindicated in hypertension in pregnancy or with pre-eclampsia[89] because of its hypertensive effect and the consequent risk of cerebral haemorrhage.

Postoperative care

Apart from the usual standards of postoperative care and postanaesthetic care,[90] Level 2 critical care (HDU care) is required particularly in the presence of invasive monitoring and oliguria.

Regular analgesia should be prescribed as paracetamol 1 g 6-hourly *per os* or *per rectum* only to avoid intravenous fluid bolus. Care should be taken to avoid non-steroidal anti-inflammatory drugs (NSAIDs). In the presence of hypertension or pre-existing renal impairment, which pre-eclamptic patients have by definition, NSAIDs can lead to renal failure, papillary necrosis, or interstitial fibrosis.[91] Tramadol may be useful in this setting, particularly in breastfeeding mothers. If the patient has had a caesarean delivery under GA and no neuraxial opiate has been given, patient-controlled analgesia with opioid is necessary. Transversus abdominis plane (TAP) blocks have been shown to reduce morphine requirements postoperatively.[92] TAP blocks should probably be avoided in the presence of abdominal wall oedema or eclampsia owing to the risk of local anaesthetic toxicity.

Postoperative care includes continuation of magnesium sulphate infusion for 24 hours after the delivery or the last seizure in cases of eclampsia. Pre-eclampsia is a risk factor for thromboembolic disease so thromboembolic stockings should be in place and LMWH prophylaxis prescribed as soon as the platelets count is above 80×10^9/L.

Complications and specific treatment

Coagulopathy

Disseminated intravascular coagulation requires close coordination of care with involvement of the haematologists and blood transfusion specialists. Blood products including packed red calls, clotting factors (both cryoprecipitate and fresh frozen plasma), and platelets may all be required (see Chapter 35 and Chapter 48). Supportive haematological care benefits from point-of-care testing and some centres are developing thromboelastography-guided treatment plans.[93]

Renal failure

Acute kidney injury should be treated with supportive treatment in the first instance. Cessation of all nephrotoxic drugs (e.g. NSAIDs and ACE inhibitors) should be undertaken. Strict management of the fluid balance with 250 mL crystalloid boluses in case of oliguria is currently recommended. There is no evidence for the use of dopamine in pre-eclampsia according to a Cochrane review.[94] Indications for renal replacement therapy are as per the usual clinical criteria: refractory hyperkalaemia, severe acidosis, refractory pulmonary oedema, or symptomatic uraemia.

Pulmonary oedema and cardiac failure

Peripartum cardiac failure is a complication in around 3% of parturients with severe pre-eclampsia. It may be a direct complication of pre-eclampsia along with inappropriate fluid management. However an important differential to exclude is peripartum cardiomyopathy (see Chapter 41). Heart failure secondary to pre-eclampsia is characterized by left diastolic dysfunction and is managed with non-invasive respiratory support, fluid restriction, diuretics, antihypertensives, and careful fluid balance especially in cases of haemorrhage and/or pulmonary oedema. More severe cases will require Level 3 critical care with invasive ventilation, intravenous furosemide, intravenous morphine, and as discussed earlier all drug infusions should be in high-concentration/low-volume syringe drivers to minimize fluid intake. But typically, pre-eclampsia-induced cardiac failure resolves in the 24–48 hours after delivery, unlike peripartum cardiomyopathy. Transthoracic echocardiography can be used to differentiate between pathologies and aid appropriate management. Findings usually seen in pre-eclampsia-induced heart failure include left diastolic dysfunction, preserved ejection fraction, and left ventricular hypertrophy with a normal sized ventricle. In peripartum cardiomyopathy, there is more systolic dysfunction, reduced ejection fraction, minimal left ventricular hypertrophy, and a dilated ventricle.[95]

Eclampsia

The 2009–2012 maternal mortality report[2] did not state whether any maternal deaths occurred from eclampsia per se. However, the overall incidence of eclampsia seems to be reducing. In 1992, the estimated incidence of eclampsia was 4.9/10,000 in the United Kingdom. In Yorkshire between 1999 and 2003, it was 3.89/10,000[5] and by the time of the UKOSS survey in 2005/2006, it was 2.75/10,000 cases.[1] Whilst this reduction in the level of eclampsia is consistent with the reduction achieved by using magnesium sulphate in severe pre-eclampsia, much of the reduction had happened before the widespread use of magnesium sulphate for prophylaxis. Therefore some of the reduction must be due to better management of pre-eclampsia in general.

Eclampsia is one of the well-known complications of pre-eclampsia. However, other neurological complications can occur including cerebral haemorrhage/stroke due to uncontrolled hypertension or seizures, encephalopathy, and amaurosis fugax. Loss of autoregulation and perfusion pressures due to pre-eclampsia can account for some of these complications. Thromboembolic disease may contribute to further morbidity as counterintuitively, pre-eclampsia is associated with a hypercoagulable state.

Women with a single typical eclamptic seizure in the first 24–48 hours after birth probably do not need neuroimaging. However, any focal neurological sign should be investigated in the context of hypertension in pregnancy but the syndrome of pre-eclampsia itself, AFLP, and treatment with magnesium sulphate may all serve to generate non-specific neurological symptoms such as confusion, memory loss, inattention, drowsiness, visual disturbance, and tremor. It can thus be difficult to differentiate these signs and symptoms from a focal neurological insult. Careful assessment must be made in consultation with obstetricians, anaesthetists, neurologists, and radiologists whether neurological imaging is required, how it would affect immediate management, and whether the woman is stable enough to move to the computed tomography (CT) or magnetic resonance imaging scanner. Usually the former is sufficient to rule out major neurological change. However, the decision for the final mode of investigation should rest with the neurology and radiological team. Women who have a seizure more than 48 hours after birth, even when there are no focal neurological signs, probably should have neuroimaging to exclude the risk of a cerebral event, especially cerebral venous thrombosis.

Attention to thromboprophylaxis must always thus be taken during antenatal admission due to moderate or severe disease and in the postnatal period if there is no concern about postpartum haemorrhage, low platelets, and the removal of epidural catheters.

Magnesium sulphate

Women who have had an eclamptic fit should be put in the recovery position or wedged if antenatal. The airway should be secured and high-flow oxygen given by a Hudson mask. They should receive intravenous magnesium sulphate. A 4 g intravenous bolus should be given over 15–20 minutes with a further intravenous infusion over 24 hours of 1 g per hour.[96] Diazemuls,[97] phenytoin,[98] or lytic cocktail[99] (chlorpromazine, promethazine, and pethidine) are no longer recommended. These latter treatments, while stopping seizure activity, increase morbidity and mortality by complicating communication, obtunding the airway and masking symptoms of ongoing disease. Prior to the publication of the Eclampsia Trial Collaborative in 1995[96] there was much debate about the appropriate treatment of eclampsia. The trial established that women allocated magnesium sulphate had a 52% lower risk of recurrent convulsions (95% CI 37–64% reduction) than those allocated diazepam and a 67% lower risk of recurrent convulsions (95% CI 47–79% reduction) than women randomized to phenytoin. Women allocated magnesium sulphate were also less likely to be ventilated, develop pneumonia, or require critical care admission than those treated with phenytoin. The babies of women who had been allocated magnesium sulphate before delivery were less likely to require intubation at delivery or require admission to a specialist neonatal unit than the babies born to women treated with phenytoin.

Recurrent seizures should be treated with a 2–4 g bolus of magnesium sulphate given over 5 minutes.[96] In eclampsia, magnesium sulphate infusion should continue for 24 hours after the last seizure. Oral magnesium is not used in the management of pre-eclampsia or eclampsia—this route is reserved for use as a laxative only.

Women on magnesium sulphate should have additional observations to monitor the signs of magnesium toxicity. Regular neurological observations, including orientation and signs of confusion should be noted along with deep tendon reflexes. Pulse oximetry and respiratory rate should also be measured. Since magnesium is renally excreted, urine output should also be monitored. Usually it is not required to measure magnesium levels. But if the patient is confused, has absent reflexes, or urine output of below 0.5 mL/kg (of lean body mass) per hour then magnesium levels should be sent. The infusion should be stopped until the magnesium levels are available. Should magnesium toxicity be diagnosed, that is, levels greater than 5 mmol/L, the standard treatment for magnesium overdose is 10 mL of intravenous calcium gluconate 10%.

Consideration should also be given to commencing the same magnesium regimen in women with severe pre-eclampsia if birth is planned within 24 hours. Again, these women should be treated in a critical care setting. In 2002, the Magpie[100] trial followed up the success of the Eclampsia Collaborative trial group and examined the use of magnesium sulphate in women with pre-eclampsia. Almost 10,000 women in 33 countries were randomized and received allocated treatment. Women allocated magnesium sulphate had a 58% lower risk of eclampsia (95% CI 40–71) than those allocated placebo (40, 0.8%, vs 96, 1.9%) which equated to approximately 11 fewer women with eclampsia per 1000. In the magnesium sulphate arm, 24% of women complained of side effect symptoms compared to 5% of women recruited to the placebo arm. Maternal mortality was also lower among women allocated magnesium sulphate, though the confidence interval crosses unity, so it was not statistically significant, the trend is towards reduction in mortality (RR 0.55; 95% CI 0.26–1.14). For women randomized and receiving treatment before delivery, there was no clear difference in the risk of the baby dying (576 (12.7%) vs 558 (12.4%) RR 1.02; 99% CI 0.92–1.14).

The indications for magnesium are severe pre-eclampsia or mild or moderate hypertension and proteinuria with one or more of the following:

- symptoms of severe headache
- problems with vision, such as blurring or flashing before the eyes
- severe pain just below the ribs or vomiting
- papilloedema
- signs of clonus (≥3 beats)
- liver tenderness
- HELLP syndrome
- platelet count falling to below 100×10^9/L
- abnormal liver enzyme tests (ALT or AST rising to above 70 IU/L)

Anaesthetic management following eclampsia

Delivery of the fetus becomes a priority after an eclamptic fit. However, stabilization of the mother should not be superseded by hasty delivery. Blood pressure control must be achieved as described previously and blood tests taken in anticipation of imminent delivery and possible neuraxial anaesthesia. Delaying delivery also allows time for recovery of maternal cerebral function so that explanation and informed consent can be done. This will also facilitate cooperation for neuraxial anaesthesia or pre-oxygenation prior to GA.

Randomized control trials are not feasible for a study of anaesthesia for delivery after eclampsia—case reports, expert opinion, and the rare retrospective review can give insight into appropriate management. One such review presented 66 'stable' eclamptic parturients who had caesarean deliveries.[101] Of these patients, two had intrathecal anaesthesia while 37 had epidural and the remaining had a GA. We must bear in mind that these 66 patients had a Glasgow Coma Scale score of 14 or 15 and are a 12.4% subset of the eclamptic patients seen in one South African centre over a 4.5-year period.

HELLP syndrome

HELLP syndrome is a serious complication of pregnancy related to pre-eclampsia. It is characterized by *h*aemolysis, *e*levated *l*iver enzymes and a *l*ow *p*latelet count, thus generating the accepted acronym.[102]

United Kingdom obstetric surveillance system definition

Diagnosis is based upon laboratory investigations including FBC, liver function tests, and blood film. Box 36.4 lists the diagnostic signs of HELLP.

Incidence estimates vary from 0.5 to 7.6/1000 deliveries and between 8% and 24% of cases with severe pre-eclampsia/eclampsia.[103,104] Although there have been reports that women with HELLP syndrome are more likely to be older, of white ethnicity, and multiparous,[105–107] and the majority, although not all, have signs of pre-eclampsia,[108] there is no current strong evidence to confirm or refute these risk factors.

UKOSS has completed a study of HELLP syndrome. A total of 210 women met the case definition from an estimated 799,003 pregnancies; 129 had evidence of haemolysis giving an incidence of 1.6/10,000

Box 36.4 Signs of HELLP syndrome

- *Elevated liver enzymes*: defined as serum aspartate aminotransferase (AST) ≥70 units/L *or* gamma-glutamyl transferase (γ-GT) ≥70 units/L *or* alanine aminotransferase (ALT) ≥70 units/L
- *And low platelets*: defined as platelet count < 100 × 10^9/L
- *And either haemolysis*: defined by abnormal peripheral blood smear *or serum lactate dehydrogenase* (LDH) levels ≥ 600 units/L or total bilirubin ≥ 20.5 μmol/L
- *Or hypertension*, defined as a systolic blood pressure ≥ 140 mmHg or a diastolic blood pressure ≥ 90 mmHg *or* proteinuria, defined as 1 + (0.3 g/L) or more on dipstick testing, a protein:creatinine ratio of 30 mg/mmol or more on a random sample, or a urine protein excretion of 300 mg or more per 24 hours

maternities (95% CI 1.3–1.9) but in 79 cases there was no haemolysis, meaning they had ELLP, or no information about haemolysis. This gives an incidence of 1.0/10,000 maternities (95% CI 0.8–1.3).[109]

Previously HELLP was considered to be a discreet entity from pre-eclampsia. However, the overlap in some of the symptoms including the manifestation of hypertension at some point in the disease course in most women and the similarity in some of the biochemical changes along with shared placental histology and molecular biomarkers has led to an acceptance that HELLP lies within the same spectrum of disease as pre-eclampsia.

Presentation

Women may present with oedema, headache, visual disturbance, and epigastric pain in a similar way to pre-eclampsia with additional symptoms of nausea, vomiting, and general malaise. However, they may also be asymptomatic.

To date, there is no robust evidence or data which can be used to formulate risk factors for the development of the HELLP syndrome. Therefore, in the pregnant population, the principal screening methods and measures are currently the same as those for pre-eclampsia.

Management

Treatment overlaps with that of pre-eclampsia should hypertension develop. However, additional monitoring of liver function and symptoms is mandated as rare complications such as liver ischaemia, intrahepatic or subcapsular haemorrhage, and haematoma can occur. All of these complications pose a significant risk of mortality, though conservative management may be appropriate in the stable patient. Hepatological or hepatic surgical support input is required in unstable patients.

Debate exists regarding the optimal management of women with HELLP prior to 34 weeks of gestation, when the maternal and fetal status remains stable. Though this is rare, there is no clear evidence that active management (i.e. plan prompt delivery) or a 'watch and wait' policy of maternal and fetal monitoring with delivery upon signs of worsening HELLP results in best outcomes while minimizing harm. The earlier point that robust, accurately predictive risk factors to guide management have not been elucidated by the current evidence base complicates this.

There is no evidence that corticosteroids effectively manage HELLP syndrome, therefore, do not use dexamethasone or betamethasone for the treatment of HELLP syndrome (unless this is for the benefit of fetal lung maturation).

Thus the clinical management of HELLP syndrome is much the same as for other variants of severe pre-eclampsia. The maternal condition should be optimized, with haematological support (Chapter 48), then birth should be planned. It may be possible to defer for 48 hours for the benefit of antenatal corticosteroids for the fetus but that would require very close maternal monitoring for any signs of deterioration, particularly of renal function. After birth, the recovery of women with HELLP is often much slower than in women with more common pre-eclampsia. They will commonly need 5–6 days of HDU-type care to await the improvement of liver, renal, and haematological function. However, they rarely need significant amounts of treatment for hypertension.

Acute fatty liver of pregnancy

Background and epidemiology

AFLP is a rare but dangerous disorder which may present in combination with pre-eclampsia, is difficult to differentiate from HELLP, and is largely a diagnosis of exclusion. It is said to be more common in primigravidae and in pregnancies carrying a male fetus[110] and twins.[111] AFLP virtually always occurs in the latter part of the third trimester with an average gestational age of 37.5 weeks[112] and may only become clinically apparent after delivery.[113] The UKOSS survey of AFLP in 2005–2006[111] estimated the incidence at 5.0/100,000 pregnancies (95% CI 3.8–6.5/100,000). Case fatality was 1.8%—just one case. However, 60% of women needed critical care.

Definition and diagnosis

Given the non-specific clinical and biochemical changes associated with AFLP, there is a necessity and a difficulty in differentiating non-pregnancy-related liver disease from AFLP. Many women will report persistent nausea and vomiting and these symptoms, while non-specific and unhelpful in pregnancy, may predate any biochemical change. Half of affected women might have hypertension, proteinuria, and oedema, alone or in combination. Accordingly, the Swansea criteria[114] have been developed and are widely accepted as the best international definition and set of diagnostic measures.[115] They are listed in Box 36.5.

The systemic complications of AFLP are due to fulminant hepatic failure and may include encephalopathy, acute kidney injury, infection, pancreatitis, haemorrhage, coagulopathy, and hypoglycaemia. Symptoms may vary and may not progress beyond nausea, vomiting, and epigastric pain but can rapidly deteriorate to encephalopathic symptoms such as restlessness, confusion, disorientation through to asterixis, seizures, psychosis, and ultimately coma. Other, non-hepatic complications are possible, including respiratory failure, sometimes requiring assisted ventilation,[116] gastrointestinal bleeding from gastric ulceration, and Mallory–Weiss tears as a consequence of excessive nausea and vomiting. Hepatorenal

Box 36.5 Features of acute fatty liver of pregnancy

A patient must have six or more of the signs or symptoms, in the absence of other explanations, to be deemed to have the syndrome:

- Vomiting, abdominal pain
- Polydipsia/polyuria
- Encephalopathy
- Elevated bilirubin > 14 μmol/L
- Hypoglycaemia < 4 mmol/L
- Elevated urate > 340 μmol/L
- Leucocytosis > 11 × 10 ^{9}/L
- Ascites or bright liver on ultrasound
- Elevated transaminases
- Elevated ammonia > 47 μmol/L
- Renal impairment creatinine > 150 μmol/L
- Coagulopathy (PT >14 seconds or APTT > 34 seconds), or microvesicular steatosis on liver biopsy

syndrome may eventually develop and cause kidney injury failure due to oliguria and acute tubular necrosis.

Investigation

If AFLP is suspected, investigations should include a FBC, clotting profile, renal and liver function tests, and urate and a cross-match would be prudent.

Imaging

Ultrasound and CT scans of the liver can be used for diagnosis, but the specificity and sensitivity of these tests are limited, may be insufficient to make a firm diagnosis and the likelihood of false negative results is high.[113] Imaging may show hepatic steatosis but, unfortunately, findings are inconsistent as the fat deposits are microvesicular and the liver can appear normal. Ultrasound imaging is a helpful, but not definitive, test as approximately 20% of the general population will demonstrate a hepatic echogenic appearance suggestive of fatty changes to the liver.

Liver biopsy is the gold standard diagnostic test but, given the potential for coagulopathy, biopsy should only be used where the diagnosis is unclear and where delivery will not be delayed. The characteristic findings on biopsy are of microvesicular fatty infiltration, fibrin deposition, and haemorrhage.

Management

Care of patients with AFLP is centred on supportive care and should include careful monitoring for evidence of progressive hepatic failure, hypoglycaemia, and coagulopathy. This usually requires admission to areas that can provide high dependency levels of care. Some hospitals have dedicated high dependency facilities within delivery suites, but this is not universal. The local service setup and a multidisciplinary team approach will determine the most appropriate area for patient management. As treatment and disease progress, the situation may need review. The likelihood is that these women will suffer at least one organ failure, thus level two care should be considered as these women will be best cared for in a critical care setting. The required multidisciplinary team effort will involve the obstetricians and midwives initially, the anaesthetic team throughout, and the input, advice, and review by intensivists and physicians with gastroenterological or hepatological expertise.

A plan of care should include:

- ventilatory support if required
- attention to fluid balance
- fluid restriction to 80 mL/h
- regular monitoring of liver function tests, coagulopathy, haemoglobin, platelets and glucose, and renal function
- antihypertensive medication as required
- vitamin K
- intravenous vitamins $B_{1,2,3,6}$ and vitamin C
- delivery.

Spontaneous resolution usually follows delivery; however, liver damage can be sufficient to require liver transplant. Maternal deaths are caused by sepsis, haemorrhage, aspiration, renal failure, pancreatitis, and gastrointestinal bleeding. Although maternal mortality rates in the past approached 75%, an average mortality rate of 7% has been cited. Early diagnosis, prompt therapy, adequate supportive care, and a multidisciplinary approach are the key to a good outcome.

Differentiating between HELLP and acute fatty liver of pregnancy

In both conditions women may or may not have significant hypertension. They may well have proteinuria. They will have abnormal liver function and commonly disordered renal function. However, in AFLP the liver disorder will be the primary dysfunction. The bilirubin level is likely to be higher and disordered coagulation will be more prominent. Platelets may still be reduced but the urate, if measured, will be significantly higher.

Hypoglycaemia is more common with AFLP. If the plasma ammonia can be measured it will be significantly higher with AFLP. The primary management is not different between the two conditions—stabilization of the mother and then delivery of the baby. However, the likelihood of deterioration of liver function with encephalopathy means that specialist hepatology involvement is more likely to be needed with AFLP.

Chapter 48 has a useful table to help in the differential diagnosis of HELLP, AFLP, and the rarer idiopathic thrombocytopenic purpura and haemolytic uraemic syndrome where presentation may be similar.

Breastfeeding and anti-hypertensives

NICE Clinical Guideline 107 provides a comprehensive overall summary of antihypertensives suitable for use in pregnancy and the postnatal period.[30]

Women who are breastfeeding or expressing milk after birth should not be given diuretics for the treatment of hypertension. Suitable drugs are listed in Box 36.6.

Box 36.6 Antihypertensives suitable for the breastfeeding mother as no known or documented evidence of adverse effects upon infants

- Atenolol
- Captopril
- Enalapril
- Labetalol
- Metoprolol
- Nifedipine

National Institute for Health and Clinical Excellence (2011) CG 107 Hypertension in pregnancy: the management of hypertensive disorders during pregnancy. Manchester: NICE. Available from www.nice.org.uk/CG107 Reproduced with permission. Information accurate at time of press. For up-to-date information, please visit www.nice.org.uk

There remains insufficient evidence to support the safe use of other antihypertensives such as angiotensin receptor blocking agents, amlodipine, and ACE inhibitors (other than enalapril and captopril) in the postnatal period.

Gestational hypertension: postnatal follow-up and longer-term care

Women with GH should receive close monitoring of their blood pressure postpartum, with daily monitoring for 2 days and a further check between day 3 and day 5 as they are at risk of significant hypertension in the early postpartum period. Between 29% and 57% of women with hypertension will have normal blood pressure 3 days after delivery, rising to 50–80% by day 7.[117] Women with GH should continue antihypertensive medication, though this should be reduced if their hypertension falls below 130/80 mmHg. If antihypertensive treatment is modified postpartum, either as a change of dose or medication, additional monitoring should be in place as clinically indicated. Women who had mild antenatal hypertension may become more hypertensive postpartum and treatment is recommended if this increases to 149/99 mmHg or above.

Traditionally, women have continued to take the medication prescribed antenatally, except in the case of methyldopa, which should be changed to an alternative as soon as possible postpartum. This is in direct opposition to a Medicines and Healthcare products Regulatory Agency directive that methyldopa is the only recommended antihypertensive in the postnatal period,[118] due to its minimal excretion in breast milk. However, this directive does not take into account the significant increases in postnatal depression associated with methyldopa. Increasingly, obstetricians are acknowledging that more modern antihypertensives offer better blood pressure control, fewer side effects, are largely considered safe in breastfeeding, and complement recommendations on adult hypertension. Typically women will be changed from medications such as labetalol to slow-release formulations of nifedipine or ACE inhibitors which are safe postnatally, even for the breastfed infant.

A careful plan for postnatal care should be routine for women with GH who return home, with provision for home visits, medical review if warranted, a specified frequency of blood pressure monitoring, along with indications for stopping treatment and seeking medical review, should the degree of hypertension or clinical situation change while under community follow-up.

Women with GH who remain on antihypertensive medication postnatally should be reviewed 2 weeks after delivery in primary care. All women with GH require medical follow-up at 6–8 weeks after delivery.[30] There should be a check of the blood pressure and of the urine for protein. This will normally form part of the GP review common in most areas in the United Kingdom. If the blood pressure has not returned to normal, specialist review of the woman's blood pressure should be sought including potential discussion with cardiologists. In these situations, it is likely that a degree of chronic hypertension or subclinical causative pathology existed prior to pregnancy and this was not discovered until the first antenatal appointment, or the physiological stress of the pregnancy has revealed an underlying predisposition.[21]

Pre-eclampsia: postnatal investigation, monitoring, and treatment

The cure for pre-eclampsia is delivery, as it probably removes the source of abnormal inflammatory cytokines released by the placenta. However, it may take several days or even weeks for maternal physiology to return to normal parameters for the healthy postnatal population. The proportion of eclampsia in the United Kingdom is higher among women who have delivered, possibly due to the mistaken perception that they are no longer at risk. Similarly, a small but significant number of women die due to complications, which are a direct result of pre-eclampsia and associated hypertension, including stroke, liver failure, and hepatic rupture. With this in mind, when reviewing women with pre-eclampsia postnatally, all practitioners should continue to ask about symptoms, specifically headache and epigastric pain/discomfort.

All women who have had pre-eclampsia should be closely monitored in the days following delivery, while they are an inpatient, with blood pressure monitoring performed at least four times per day. Women who have not received antihypertensive medication to treat their pre-eclampsia can expect monitoring on at least one occasion between day 3 and day 5. If this latest reading is elevated, blood pressure should continue to be monitored on alternate days until normal. If this persists at 1 week, medical review is indicated.[43]

Occasionally, women who have not required treatment antenatally will have postnatal hypertension above 150/100 mmHg, in which case antihypertensive medication is indicated to avoid complications. Women who have delivered, but required antihypertensive medication, should have their blood pressure monitored four times daily while an inpatient, and then every other day for up to 2 weeks, until they are normotensive and have stopped medication. If neither of these has occurred, medical review is indicated.[30]

Women who have required antenatal treatment should remain on treatment until their blood pressure falls below 140/90 mmHg and begin to titrate down antihypertensive treatment if their blood pressure falls below 130/80 mmHg. Again, after delivery, women who have been taking methyldopa should be switched to an alternate antihypertensive medication as soon as possible after delivery to avoid an unnecessary increased risk of postnatal depression.

As a general rule, clinicians caring for women in the puerperium whose blood pressure is 140/90 on several occasions, should consider commencing, or increasing antihypertensive medication. If women have a blood pressure reading of 150/100 mmHg, commencing or increasing treatment is recommended. Readings of 160/100 mmHg or above should prompt immediate referral to an obstetric unit and/or senior review. HDU and/or invasive monitoring should be considered.[117]

Women who had pre-eclampsia but are no longer symptomatic, whose blood pressure is below 149/99 mmHg (treated or untreated) and whose blood results are improving, may be transferred from the inpatient to the community setting with an appropriate plan for care. This should include information to the women regarding symptoms to watch out for, a defined team who will review the women in the community, and a plan of who should provide medical review if required. Reviews at 2 and 6–8 weeks should also be organized at this point as medically indicated. All women should receive a medical review at 6–8 weeks; those still on medication should be seen 2 weeks postnatally. If they still require medication at 6–8 weeks, specialist referral is warranted to investigate further causes of hypertension.[11,119,120] Similarly, these women will need specialist advice regarding the increased risk of pre-eclampsia in future pregnancies.[30]

All women with moderate or severe pre-eclampsia, especially those being stepped down from critical care need a postnatal check of biochemical and haematological indices of disease at 48–72 hours. If these are normal, further tests are not necessary; however, if they are improving but remain abnormal, these will need repeating at the 6–8-week postnatal review, unless clinically indicated in the interim.

All women with pre-eclampsia should have their urine checked using a reagent strip for proteinuria at 6–8 weeks. If proteinuria persists, a further test should be undertaken 4 weeks later and specialist renal review requested if this remains positive.

Counselling of long-term risks and lifelong maternal health

It is important that women who have suffered pre-eclampsia in this pregnancy are informed of future risks to their health, both in future pregnancy and in later life.[30]

Women who have suffered an episode of GH or pre-eclampsia have an increased risk of developing cardiovascular disease, compared to the general female population, in later life. Given that there are familial and therefore genetic tendencies towards developing high blood pressure in pregnancy, this may represent a pre-existing propensity to developing cardiovascular disease in later life, compared to the background population. There is some evidence to suggest that pre-eclampsia may actually cause underlying vascular damage on a cellular level in some women and thus, increase their risk of developing pre-eclampsia.[121]

Later life complications include:[21,121]

- hypertension
- ischaemic heart disease
- cerebrovascular accident
- venous thromboembolism
- end-stage renal disease (increased but low absolute risk in women with no proteinuria at 8 week postnatal review).[122]

Thrombophilia screening is not recommended in postnatal women by NICE solely on the basis of an episode of pre-eclampsia.[30] There is some suggestion that some thrombophilic conditions predispose women to pre-eclampsia (including hyperhomocysteinaemia, prothrombin heterozygosity, anticardiolipin antibody positivity, factor V Leiden heterozygosity, and methylene tetrahydrofolate reductase (MTHFR) homozygosity), while others do not (factor V Leiden homozygosity, antithrombin III deficiency, protein C deficiency, protein S deficiency, lupus anticoagulant positive, and acquired activated protein C resistance), though the evidence for this is of mixed quality.[30] If this has been associated with a history of recurrent miscarriage, prematurity, or small-for-gestational-age fetus, then thrombophilia screening may be warranted.

Antenatal and intrapartum venous thromboembolism prophylaxis should be risk assessed as normal, as per guidance from the Royal College of Obstetricians and Gynaecologists.[123]

Future pregnancy

The risk of GH in a future pregnancy ranges from about 1 in 8 (13%) pregnancies to about 1 in 2 (53%) pregnancies, while the risk of pre-eclampsia in a future pregnancy rises to approximately 1 in 6 (16%) pregnancies.[124–127] If their recent episode of pre-eclampsia was severe, or complicated by HELLP syndrome, or led to a pre-term birth prior to 34 weeks, this risk rises to 1 in 4 (25%) of pre-eclampsia recurrence in a future pregnancy. If a pre-term birth occurred before 28 weeks, the risk rises to 55%.[128] There is no evidence to suggest that an interpregnancy interval of 10 years increases the risk of pre-eclampsia.

Conclusion

The hypertensive disorders of pregnancy cover a wide range of conditions, most of which are relatively mild with a low risk of complications for mother and baby. However, they are still an important cause of maternal and fetal mortality. They can present in a number of ways and require multidisciplinary care to achieve an optimum outcome. The more serious complications of eclampsia, hepatic, renal, and haematological abnormalities will commonly involve the care of the anaesthetic and critical care team and will present challenges to the provision of anaesthesia. A full understanding of the nature of the condition, its various presentations, complications, and ability to affect all organ symptoms will be important for obstetric anaesthetists. Anaesthetic care focuses on providing effective analgesia, safe surgical anaesthesia, and individually tailored supportive critical care to parturients with hypertensive diseases of pregnancy in a context of potentially fatal cardiovascular, pulmonary, cerebral, and haematological pathology.

References

1. Knight M, UKOSS. Eclampsia in the United Kingdom 2005. *BJOG* 2007; 114(9):1072–8.
2. Knight M, Kenyon S, Brocklehurst P, *et al. Saving Lives, Improving Mothers' Care – Lessons Learned to Inform Future Maternity Care from the UK and Ireland Confidential Enquiries into Maternal Deaths*

and Morbidity 2009–12. Oxford: National Perinatal Epidemiology Unit, University of Oxford; 2014.

3. Schutte JM, Schuitemaker NW, Van RJ, *et al.* Substandard care in maternal mortality due to hypertensive disease in pregnancy in the Netherlands. *BJOG* 2008; 115(6):732–6.
4. Tuffnell DJ, Jankowicz D, Lindow SW, *et al.* Outcomes of severe pre-eclampsia/eclampsia in Yorkshire 1999/2003. *BJOG* 2005; 112(7):875–80.
5. Confidential Enquiry into Maternal and Child Health (CEMACH). *Perinatal Mortality 2007.* London: CEMACH; 2009
6. Roberts CL, Bell JC, Ford JB, *et al.* The accuracy of reporting of the hypertensive disorders of pregnancy in population health data. *Hypertens Pregnancy* 2008; 27(3):285–97.
7. National Collaborating Centre for Chronic Conditions. *Hypertension. Management of Adults in Primary Care: Pharmacological Update.* London, Royal College of Physicians; 2006.
8. National Institute for Health and Clinical Excellence. *Obesity: The Prevention, Identification, Assessment and Management of Overweight and Obesity in Adults and Children.* Clinical Guidance 43. London: NICE; 2006.
9. Meads CA, Cnossen JS, Meher S, *et al.* Methods of prediction and prevention of pre-eclampsia: systematic reviews of accuracy and effectiveness literature with economic modelling. *Health Technol Assess* 2008; 12(6):iii–iv, 1–270.
10. Action on Pre-eclampsia. PRECOG: *The Pre-eclampsia Community Guideline.* London: Action on Pre-eclampsia; 2004.
11. Report on the National Blood Pressure Education Program Working Group on High Blood Pressure in Pregnancy. *Am J Obstet Gynaecol* 2000; 183:S1–22.
12. Hernandez-Diaz S, Toh S, Cnattingius S. Risk of pre-eclampsia in first and subsequent pregnancies: prospective cohort study. *BMJ* 2009; 338:b2255.
13. Altman D, Carroli G, Duley L, *et al.* Do women with pre-eclampsia and their babies benefit from magnesium sulphate? The Magpie Trial: a randomised placebo controlled trial. *Lancet* 2002; 359:1877–90.
14. National Collaborating Centre for Women's and Children's Health. *Antenatal Care: Routine Care for the Healthy Pregnant Woman.* London: RCOG Press; 2008.
15. Davey DA, MacGillivray I. The classification and definition of the hypertensive disorders of pregnancy. *Am J Obstet Gynecol* 1988; 158(4):892–8.
16. Brown MA, Lindheimer MD, de Swiet M, *et al.* The classification and diagnosis of the hypertensive disorders of pregnancy: statement from the International Society for the Study of Hypertension in Pregnancy (ISSHP). *Hypertens Pregnancy* 2001; 20(1):IX–XIV.
17. Roberts CL, Bell JC, Ford JB, *et al.* The accuracy of reporting of the hypertensive disorders of pregnancy in population health data. *Hypertens Pregnancy* 2008; 27(3):285–97.
18. World Health Organization. *Trends In Maternal Mortality: 1990 to 2008. Estimates developed by WHO, UNICEF, UNFPA and The World Bank.* Geneva: World Health Organization; 2010. http://whqlibdoc.who.int/publications/2010/9789241500265_eng.pdf
19. Slattery MM, Geary M, Morrison JJ. Obstetric antecedents for preterm delivery. *J Perinat Med* 2008; 36(4):306–9.
20. Rasmussen S, Irgens LM. The effects of smoking and hypertensive disorders on fetal growth. *BMC Pregnancy Childbirth* 2006; 6:16.
21. Bellamy L, Casas JP, Hingorani AD, *et al.* Pre-eclampsia and risk of cardiovascular disease and cancer in later life: systematic review and meta-analysis. *BMJ* 2007; 335(7627):974.
22. Maynard SE, Min JY, Merchan J, *et al.* Excess placental soluble fms-like tyrosine kinase 1 (sFlt1) may contribute to endothelial dysfunction, hypertension, and proteinuria in preeclampsia. *J Clin Invest* 2003; 111:649–58.
23. Andraweera PH, Dekker GA, Roberts CT. The vascular endothelial growth factor family in adverse pregnancy outcomes. *Hum Reprod Update* 2012; 18(4):436–57.
24. Nevo O, Soleymanlou N, Wu Y, *et al.* Increased expression of sFlt-1. *Am J Physiol* 2006; 291:R1085–R1093.
25. Venkatesha S, Toporsian M, Lam C, *et al.* Soluble endoglin contributes to the pathogenesis of pre-eclampsia. *N Engl J Med* 2006; 12:642–9.
26. Levine RJ, Lam C, Qian C, *et al.* Soluble endoglin and other circulating anti-angiogenic factors in pre-eclampsia. *N Engl J Med* 2006; 355:992–1005.
27. Cudmore M, Ahmed S Al-Ani B, *et al* which consequently down-regulates heme oxygenase-1 release *Circulation* 2007; 115:1789–97.
28. *Pravastatin for Prevention of Preeclampsia. NCT01717586.* ClinicalTrials.gov [Online] https://clinicaltrials.gov/ct2/show/NCT01717586
29. *Early Prevention of Pre-eclampsia Study (EPAPP). NCT01547390.* ClinicalTrials.gov [Online] https://clinicaltrials.gov/ct2/show/NCT01547390
30. National Institute for Health and Clinical Excellence. *Hypertension in Pregnancy: The Management of Hypertensive Disorders During Pregnancy.* Clinical Guideline 107. London: NICE; 2010 (reviewed 2014).
31. Duckitt K, Harrington D. Risk factors for pre-eclampsia at antenatal booking: systematic review of case controlled studies. *BMJ* 2005; 330:576–80.
32. Duley L, Henderson-Smart DJ, Meher S, *et al.* Antiplatelet agents for preventing pre-eclampsia and its complications. *Cochrane Database Syst Rev* 2007; 2:CD004659.
33. *Regional Anaesthesia in patients with Abnormalities in Coagulation.* A guidance document produced by a Joint Working Party of the: Association of Anaesthetists of Great Britain & Ireland (AAGBI), Obstetric Anaesthetists' Association (OAA),Regional Anaesthesia UK (RA-UK). 2011. http://www.aagbi.org/sites/default/files/RAPAC%20for%20consultation.pdf
34. Meher S, Duley L. Nitric oxide for preventing pre-eclampsia and its complications. *Cochrane Database Syst Rev* 2007; 2:CD006490.
35. Meher S, Duley L. Progesterone for preventing pre-eclampsia and its complications. *Cochrane Database Syst Rev* 2006; 4:CD006175.
36. Churchill D, Beevers GD, Meher S, *et al.* Diuretics for preventing pre-eclampsia. *Cochrane Database Syst Rev* 2007; 1:CD004451.
37. Makrides M, Duley L, Olsen SF. Marine oil, and other prostaglandin precursor, supplementation for pregnancy uncomplicated by pre-eclampsia or intrauterine growth restriction. *Cochrane Database Syst Rev* 2006; 3:CD003402.
38. Meher S, Duley L. Garlic for preventing pre-eclampsia and its complications. *Cochrane Database Syst Rev* 2006; 3:CD006065.
39. Rumbold A, Duley L, Crowther CA, *et al.* Antioxidants for preventing pre-eclampsia. *Cochrane Database Syst Rev* 2008; 1:CD004227.
40. Spinnato JA, Freire S, Pinto E, *et al.* Antioxidant therapy to prevent preeclampsia: a randomized controlled trial. *Obstet Gynecol* 2007; 110(6):1311–18.
41. *High Dose Folic Acid Supplementation Throughout Pregnancy for Preeclampsia Prevention (FACT).* ClinicalTrials.gov NCT01355159. [Online] https://clinicaltrials.gov/ct2/show/NCT01355159
42. Li W, Tang L, Wu T, *et al.* Chinese herbal medicines for treating pre-eclampsia. *Cochrane Database Syst Rev* 2006; 2:CD005126.
43. Atallah AN, Hofmeyr GJ, Duley L. Calcium supplementation during pregnancy for preventing hypertensive disorders and related problems. *Cochrane Database Syst Rev* 2006; 1:CD001059.
44. O'Brien E, Petrie J, Litteler W, *et al*, An outline of the revised British Hypertension Society protocol for the evaluation of blood pressure measuring devices. *J Hypertens* 1993; 11:677–9.
45. O'Brien E, Asmar R, Beilin L, *et al.* European Society of Hypertension recommendations for conventional ambulatory and home blood pressure measurement. *J Hypertens* 2003; 21:821–48.
46. Brown MA, Buddle ML, Farrel T, *et al.* Randomised trial of management of hypertensive pregnancies by Korotkoff phase IV or V. *Lancet* 1998; 352:777–81.

47. Shennan A, Gupta M, Halligan A, *et al.* Lack of reproducibility in pregnancy of Korotkoff phase IV as measured by mercury sphygmomanometer. *Lancet* 1996; 347:139–42.
48. National Institute of Health and Clinical Excellence. *Antenatal Care.* Clinical Guideline 62. London: NICE; 2008
49. Waugh JJ, Clark TJ, Divakaran TG, *et al.* Accuracy of urinalysis dipstick techniques in predicting significant proteinuria in pregnancy. *Obstet Gynaecol* 2004; 103:769–77.
50. Côté AM, Brown MA, Lam E, *et al.* Diagnostic accuracy of urinary spot protein:creatinine ratio in hypertensive pregnant women: systematic review. *BJOG* 2005; 11:412–7.
51. Sibai BM, Mercer BM, Schiff E, *et al.* Aggressive versus expectant management of severe preeclampsia at 28 to 32 weeks' gestation: a randomized controlled trial. *Am J Obstet Gynecol* 1994; 171(3):818–22.
52. Dyer RA, Piercy JL, Reed AR. The role of the anaesthetist in the management of the pre-eclamptic patient. *Curr Opin Anaesthesiol* 2007, 20:168–74.
53. Pickles CJ, Broughton PF, Symonds EM. A randomised placebo controlled trial of labetalol in the treatment of mild to moderate pregnancy induced hypertension. *Br J Obstet Gynaecol* 1992; 99(12):964–8.
54. Cruickshank DJ, Robertson AA, Campbell DM, *et al.* Maternal obstetric outcome measures in a randomised controlled study of labetalol in the treatment of hypertension in pregnancy. *Hypertens Pregnancy* 1991; 10(3):333–44.
55. Cruickshank DJ, Robertson AA, Campbell DM, *et al.* Does labetalol influence the development of proteinuria in pregnancy hypertension? A randomised controlled study. *Eur J Obstet Gynecol Reprod Biol* 1992; 45(1):47–51.
56. Rubin PC, Butters L, Clark DM, *et al.* Placebo-controlled trial of atenolol in treatment of pregnancy-associated hypertension. *Lancet* 1983; 1(8322):431–4.
57. El-Qarmalawi AM, Morsy AH, al-Fadly A, *et al.* Labetalol vs. methyldopa in the treatment of pregnancy-induced hypertension. *Int J Gynecol Obstet* 1995; 49(2):125–30.
58. Sibai BM, Mercer BM, Schiff E, *et al.* Aggressive versus expectant management of severe preeclampsia at 28 to 32 weeks' gestation: a randomized controlled trial. *Am J Obstet Gynecol* 1994; 171(3):818–22.
59. Odendaal HJ, Pattinson RC, Bam R, *et al.* Aggressive or expectant management for patients with severe preeclampsia between 28–34 weeks' gestation: a randomized controlled trial. *Obstet Gynecol* 1990; 76(6):1070–5.
60. GRIT Study Group. A randomised trial of timed delivery for the compromised preterm fetus: short term outcomes and Bayesian interpretation. *BJOG* 2003; 110(1):27–32.
61. Roberts D, Dalziel S, Shaw BNJ. Antenatal corticosteroids for accelerating fetal lung maturation for women at risk of preterm birth. *Cochrane Database Syst Rev* 2007; 2:CD004454.
62. Koopmans CM, Bijlenga D, Groen H, *et al.* Induction of labour versus expectant monitoring for gestational hypertension or mild pre-eclampsia after 36 weeks' gestation (HYPITAT): a multicentre, open-label randomised controlled trial. *Lancet* 2009; 374(9694):979–88.
63. Assessment of changes in coagulation in parturients with preeclampsia using thromboelastography. *Anesthesiology* 1999; 90:385–90.
64. Gilbert WM, Towner DR, Field NT, *et al.* The safety and utility of pulmonary artery catheterization in severe preeclampsia and eclampsia. *Am J Obstet Gynecol* 2000; 182:1397–403.
65. Engelhardt T, MacLennan FM. Fluid management in pre-eclampsia. *Int J Obstet Anesth* 1999; 8(4):253–9.
66. European Society of Cardiology Guidelines on the management of cardiovascular diseases during pregnancy: the Task Force on the Management of Cardiovascular Diseases during Pregnancy of the European Society of Cardiology (ESC). *Eur Heart J* 2011; 32:3147–97.
67. National Institute for Clinical Excellence. *Caesarean Section.* Clinical Guideline 132. London: NICE; 2011 (reviewed 2014).
68. Dennis AT. Management of pre-eclampsia: issues for anaesthetists. *Anaesthesia* 2012; 67:1009–20.
69. Dyer RA, Piercy JL, Reed AR. The role of the anaesthetist in the management of the pre-eclamptic patient. *Curr Opin Anaesthesiol* 2007; 20:168–74.
70. Jouppila P, Jouppila R, Hollmen A, *et al.* Lumbar epidural analgesia to improve intervillous blood flow during labor in severe preeclampsia. *Obstet Gynecol* 1982; 59:158–61.
71. Obstetric Anaesthetists' Association. *Clinical Guidelines.* [Online] http://www.oaa-anaes.ac.uk/ui/content/content.aspx?id=188
72. Beilin Y, Bodian CA, Haddad EM, *et al.* Practice patterns of anesthesiologists regarding situations in obstetric anesthesia where clinical management is controversial. *Anesth Analg* 1996; 83:735–41.
73. Wallace DH, Leveno KJ, Cunningham FG, *et al.* Randomized comparison of general and regional anesthesia for cesarean delivery in pregnancies complicated by severe preeclampsia. *Obstet Gynecol* 1995; 86:193–9.
74. Santos AC, Birnbach DJ. Spinal anesthesia for cesarean delivery in severely preeclamptic women: don't throw out the baby with the bathwater! *Anesth Analg* 2005; 101:859–61.
75. Moslemi F, Rasooli S. Comparison of spinal versus general anesthesia for cesarean delivery in patients with severe preeclampsia. *J Med Sci* 2007; 7(6):1044–8.
76. Hood DD, Curry R. Spinal versus epidural anesthesia for cesarean section in severely pre-eclamptic patients: a retrospective review. *Anesthesiology* 1999; 90:1276–82.
77. Visalyaputra S, Rodanant O, Somboonviboon W, *et al.* Spinal versus epidural anesthesia for cesarean section in severe preeclampsia: a prospective randomized, multicenter study. *Anesth Analg* 2005; 101:862–8.
78. Aya AGM, Mangin R, Vialles N, *et al.* Patients with severe preeclampsia experience less hypotension during spinal anesthesia for elective cesarean delivery than healthy parturients: a prospective cohort comparison. *Anesth Analg* 2003; 97:867–72.
79. Sharwood-Smtih G, Clark VA, Watson E. Regional anesthesia for caesarean section in severe pre-eclampsia: Spinal anaesthesia is the preferred choice. *Int J Obstet Anesth* 1999; 8 (2):85–9.
80. Berends N, Teunkens A, Vandermeersch E, *et al.* A randomized trial comparing low-dose combined spinal-epidural anesthesia and conventional epidural anesthesia for cesarean section in severe preeclampsia. *Acta Anaesthesiol Belg* 2005; 56 (2):155–62.
81. Afolabi BB, Lesi FEA. Regional versus general anaesthesia for caesarean section. *Cochrane Database Syst Rev* 2012; 10:CD004350.
82. Brock-Utne JG, Downing JW, Seedat F. Laryngeal oedema associated with pre-eclamptic toxaemia. *Anaesthesia* 1977; 32:556–8.
83. Allen RW, James MF, Uys PC. Attenuation of the pressor response to tracheal intubation in hypertensive proteinuric pregnant patients by lignocaine, alfentanil and magnesium sulphate. *Br J Anaesth* 1991; 66(2):216–23.
84. Yoo KY, Kang DH, Jeong H, *et al.* A dose-response study of remifentanil for attenuation of the hypertensive response to laryngoscopy and tracheal intubation in severely preeclamptic women undergoing caesarean delivery under general anaesthesia. *Int J Obstet Anesth* 2013; 22(1):10–18.
85. Heesen M, Klöhr S, Hofmann T, *et al.* Maternal and foetal effects of remifentanil for general anaesthesia in parturients undergoing caesarean section: a systematic review and meta-analysis. *Acta Anaesthesiol Scand* 2013; 57(1):29–36.
86. Liem EB, Bjoraker DJ, Gravenstein D. New options for airway management: intubating fibreoptic stylets. *Br J Anaesth* 2003; 91(3):408–18.
87. Kimura A, Yamakage M, Chen X, *et al.* Use of the fibreoptic stylet scope (Styletscope) reduces the hemodynamic response to intubation in normotensive and hypertensive patients. *Can J Anaesth* 2001; 48(9):919–23.

88. Langesæter E, Rosseland LA, Stubhaug A. Haemodynamic effects of oxytocin in women with severe pre-eclampsia. *Int J Obstet Anesth* 2011; 20:26–9.
89. Joint Formulary Committee. *British National Formulary* (65th ed). London: BMJ Publishing Group Ltd and Royal Pharmaceutical Society; 2013.
90. Association of Anaesthetists of Great Britain and Ireland. *Immediate Post-Anaesthesia Recovery 2013. Anaesthesia* 2013; 68:288–97.
91. Joint Formulary Committee. *British National Formulary* (66th ed). London: BMJ Group and Pharmaceutical Press; 2013.
92. Abdallah FW, Halpern SH, Margarido CB. Transversus abdominis plane block for postoperative analgesia after Caesarean delivery performed under spinal anaesthesia? A systematic review and meta-analysis. *Br J Anaesth* 2012; 109(5):679–87.
93. Hill JS, Devenie G, Powell M. Point-of-care testing of coagulation and fibrinolytic status during postpartum haemorrhage: developing a thrombelastography-guided transfusion algorithm. *Anaesth Intensive Care* 2012 Nov; 40(6):1007–15.
94. Steyn DW, Steyn P. Low-dose dopamine for women with severe pre-eclampsia. *Cochrane Database Syst Rev* 2007; 1:CD003515.
95. Dennis AT, Castro JM. Echocardiographic differences between pre-eclampsia and peripartum cardiomyopathy. *Int J Obstet Anesth* 2014; 23:260–6.
96. The Eclampsia Trial Collaborative Group. *Lancet* 1995; 345:1455–63.
97. Duley L, Henderson-Smart D, Walker GJ, *et al.* Magnesium sulphate versus diazepam for eclampsia. *Cochrane Database Syst Rev* 2010; 12:CD000127.
98. Duley L, Henderson-Smart D, Chou D. Magnesium sulphate versus phenytoin for eclampsia. *Cochrane Database Syst Rev* 2010; 10:CD000128.
99. Duley L, Gulmezoglu AM, Chou D. Magnesium sulphate versus lytic cocktail for eclampsia. *Cochrane Database Syst Rev* 2010; 9:CD002960.
100. The Magpie Trial Collaborative Group. Do women with pre-eclampsia, and their babies, benefit from magnesium sulphate? The Magpie Trial: a randomised placebo-controlled trial. *Lancet* 2002; 359:1877–90.
101. Moodley J, Jjuuko G, Rout C. Epidural compared with general anaesthesia for caesarean delivery in conscious women with eclampsia. *BJOG* 2001; 108(4):378–82.
102. Weinstein L. Syndrome of hemolysis, elevated liver enzymes, and low platelet count: a severe consequence of hypertension in pregnancy. *Am J Obstet Gynecol* 1982; 142(2):159–67.
103. Waterstone M, Bewley S, Wolfe C. Incidence and predictors of severe obstetric morbidity: case-control study. *BMJ* 2001; 322(7294):1089–93.
104. Martin JN, Rinehart BK, May WL, *et al.* The spectrum of severe preeclampsia: comparative analysis by HELLP (hemolysis, elevated liver enzyme levels, and low platelet count) syndrome classification. *An J Obstet Gynecol* 1999; 180(6 Pt 1):1373–84.
105. Sibai BM, Taslimi MM, el-Nazer A, *et al.*, Maternal-perinatal outcome associated with the syndrome of hemolysis, elevated liver enzymes, and low platelets in severe preeclampsia-eclampsia. *An J Obstet Gynecol* 1986; 155(3):501–9.
106. Sibai BM. The HELLP syndrome (hemolysis, elevated liver enzymes, and low platelets): much ado about nothing? *An J Obstet Gynecol* 1990; 162(2):311–16.
107. Audibert F, Friedman SA, Frangieh AY, *et al.*, Clinical utility of strict diagnostic criteria for the HELLP (hemolysis, elevated liver enzymes, and low platelets) syndrome. *An J Obstet Gynecol* 1996; 175(2):460–4.
108. Sibai BM. Diagnosis, controversies, and management of the syndrome of hemolysis, elevated liver enzymes, and low platelet count. *Obstet Gynecol* 2004; 103(5 Pt 1):981–91.
109. Fitzpatrick KE, Hinshaw K, Kurinczuk JJ, *et al.* Risk factors, management, and outcomes of hemolysis, elevated liver enzymes, and low platelets syndrome and elevated liver enzymes, low platelets syndrome. *Obstet Gynecol* 2014; 123(3):618–27.
110. Fesenmeier MF, Coppage KH, Lambers DS, *et al.* Acute fatty liver of pregnancy in 3 tertiary care centres. *Am J Obstet Gynaecol* 2005; 192:1416–19.
111. Knight M, Nelson-Piercy C, Kurinczuk JJ, *et al.* A prospective national study of acute fatty liver of pregnancy in the UK, *Gut* 2008; 57:951–6.
112. Castro MA, Goodwin TM, Shaw KJ, *et al.* Disseminated intravascular coagulation and antithrombin III depression in acute fatty liver of pregnancy. *Am J Obstet Gynecol* 1996; 174:211–16.
113. Bacq Y. Liver diseases unique to pregnancy: a 2010 update. *Clin Res Hepatol Gastroenterol* 2011; 35:182–93.
114. Ch'ng CC, Morgan M, Hainsworth I, *et al.* Prospective study of liver dysfunction in pregnancy in South Wales. *Gut* 2002; 51:876–80.
115. Joshi D, James A, Quaglia A, *et al.* Liver disease in pregnancy. *Lancet* 2010; 375:594–605.
116. Castro MA, Fassett MJ, Reynolds TB, *et al.* Reversible peripartum liver failure: a new perspective on the diagnosis, treatment, and cause of acute fatty liver of pregnancy, based on 28 consecutive cases. *Am J Obstet Gynecol* 1999; 181:389–95.
117. Bramham K, Nelson-Piercy C, Brown MJ, *et al.* Postpartum management of hypertension. *BMJ* 2013; 346:30–4.
118. Medicines and Healthcare products Regulatory Agency. ACE inhibitors and angiotensin II receptor antagonists: recommendations on use during breastfeeding. *Drug Safe Update* 2009; 2(10)3–4. www.mhra.gov.uk/publications/safetyguidance/drugsafetyupdate/con046451
119. National Institute for Health and Clinical Excellence. *Clinical Management of Primary Hypertension in Adults.* Clinical Guideline 127. London: NICE; 2011. www.nice.org.uk/CG127
120. Berks D, Steegers EA, Molas M, *et al.* Resolution of hypertension and proteinuria after preeclampsia. *Obstet Gynecol* 2009; 114:1307–14.
121. McDonald SD, Malinowski A, Zhou Q, *et al.* Cardiovascular sequelae of preeclampsia/eclampsia: a systematic review and meta- analyses. *Am Heart J* 2008; 156(5):918–30.
122. Vikse BE, Irgens LM, Leivestad T, *et al.* Preeclampsia and the risk of end-stage renal disease. *N Engl J Med* 2008; 359(8):800–9.
123. Royal College of Obstetricians and Gynaecologists. *Reducing the Risk of Thrombosis and Embolism during Pregnancy and the Puerperium.* Green-top Guideline No. 37s. London: RCOG Press; 2013.
124. Hjartardottir S, Leifsson BG, Geirsson RT, *et al.* Recurrence of hypertensive disorder in second pregnancy. *Am J Obstet Gynecol* 2006; 194(4):916–20.
125. Zhang J, Troendle JF, Levine RJ. Risks of hypertensive disorders in the second pregnancy. *Paediatr Perinal Epidemiol* 2001; 15(3):226–31.
126. Basso O, Christensen K, Olsen J. Higher risk of pre-eclampsia after change of partner. An effect of longer interpregnancy intervals? *Epidemiology* 2001; 12(6):624–9.
127. Trogstad L, Skrondal A, Stoltenberg C, *et al.* Recurrence risk of preeclampsia in twin and singleton pregnancies. *Am J Med Genet A* 2004; 126A(1):41–5.
128. Sibai BM, Mercer B, Sarinoglu C. Severe preeclampsia in the second trimester: recurrence risk and long-term prognosis. *Am J Obstet Gynecol* 1991; 165(5 Pt 1):1408–12.

CHAPTER 37

Thromboembolic disorders in pregnancy

Salma Ballal and Ian A. Greer

Introduction

Thromboembolism in pregnancy remains a major cause of direct maternal mortality in the Western world. It was the leading cause of death in the United Kingdom from 1985 and after dropping to third place with sepsis taking pole position in 2006–2008, thromboembolism has once more re-emerged as the most common cause of direct maternal death in the United Kingdom and Ireland in the latest 2009–2012 national maternal mortality report by MBRRACE-UK[1] (Table 37.1).

Deaths previously from thromboembolism were associated with failures in (1) obtaining objective diagnoses and investigating chest symptoms in at-risk women (often because of unfounded concerns such as radiation exposure for the fetus), (2) lack of provision of adequate thromboprophylaxis, (3) inadequate risk assessment, and (4) failure to ensure multidisciplinary care.[1]

The physiological changes of pregnancy, considered to be hormonally driven, are associated with alterations in the coagulation and fibrinolytic systems. There is an increase in procoagulant factors, such as factors VII, VIII, X, and von Willebrand factor, and a substantial rise in fibrinogen. The endogenous anticoagulant activity and fibrinolysis are suppressed, such as through reduced protein S and increased placentally derived plasminogen activator 2 inhibitor respectively. These changes lead to a physiological hypercoagulable state in pregnancy, which physiologically may prepare the body for the haemostatic challenge of delivery, but will also increase the risk of thrombosis during pregnancy. It is important to emphasize that thrombosis is usually a 'multi-hit' disorder and a single risk factor such as the procoagulant effects of pregnancy is rarely sufficient to cause a clinical event, rather events are more likely when multiple risk factors are present at the same time.

Thromboembolic events in pregnancy are spread across the three trimesters with over 50% of events occurring in the first 20 weeks of pregnancy.[2] However, the puerperium is the time of greatest risk with a relative risk of around 20-fold compared to the non-pregnant population. This is likely to reflect trauma to the pelvic vessels in the course of delivery causing endothelial damage. When this is added to the hypercoagulable changes of pregnancy, and venous stasis, which is also a feature of normal pregnancy, the three components of Virchow's triad, which underlies venous thrombosis will coexist, so increasing the risk. Indeed, in relation to postpartum events, around 80% occur in the first 3 weeks after delivery.[3]

Importantly, when compared to the non-pregnant population where distal deep vein thrombosis (DVT) is most common, most events in pregnancy are iliofemoral and left sided. This is thought to occur due to the compression of the left iliac vein by the right iliac artery which leads to decreased blood flow on the left side.

The relative risk of antenatal venous thromboembolism (VTE) is about fivefold higher than in non-pregnant women of the same age and this is increased further postpartum, but the absolute risk is low, with an overall incidence of VTE in pregnancy and the puerperium of 1–2/1000.[4–6]

Risk factors for thrombosis in pregnancy

Pregnancy is itself a risk factor for thrombosis but it is important, given the multi-hit nature of the problem, for clinicians to be aware of additional risk factors (Table 37.2) that will increase that risk further.[3,10,12] A clear example of this is the dramatic increase in risk when immobility is combined with a body mass index (BMI) of 25 kg/m^2 or higher (Figure 37.1). The two most significant single risk factors in pregnancy for thromboembolism are history of previous VTE and thrombophilia.

Previous venous thromboembolism

In pregnant women with a history of VTE, the risk of recurrence is increased three- to fourfold (relative risk 3.5; 95% confidence interval (CI) 1.6–7.8).[7] Recurrent events account for 15–25% of all thromboembolic events in pregnancy.

A previous single VTE can be provoked (e.g. combined contraceptive pill, pregnancy, trauma, immobility, surgery, and thrombophilia) or unprovoked, where no additional risk factor is apparent. Some of these women will require antenatal prophylaxis but all should receive postpartum prophylaxis, as this is the period of greatest risk.[8,9] Women with a history of an unprovoked or idiopathic, known thrombophilia or oestrogen-related VTE should be treated as a high-risk group and thromboprophylaxis should be recommended antenatally and for 6 weeks postpartum. A history of a VTE provoked by a risk factor that is no longer present in a woman with no other risk factors requires close observation antenatally with thromboprophylaxis commenced after delivery and continued for 6 weeks postpartum.[9]

For women on pharmacological thromboprophylaxis in pregnancy, the rate of recurrence has been reported to range from 0% to 2.4%.[10,11] However, the rate of recurrent VTE in women who

Table 37.1 Maternal mortality rates by cause, per 100,000 maternities, 2006–2012

Cause of death	2006–08			2009–11			2010–12		
	n	Rate	95% CI	n	Rate	95% CI	n	Rate	95% CI
All Direct and Indirect deaths†	261	11.39	10.09–12.86	253	10.63	9.36–12.03	243	10.12	8.89–11.47
Direct deaths									
Genital tract sepsis*	26	1.13	0.77–1.67	15	0.63	0.35–1.04	12	0.50	0.26–0.87
Pre-eclampsia and eclampsia	19	0.83	0.53–1.30	10	0.42	0.20–0.77	9	0.38	0.18–0.71
Thrombosis and thromboembolism	18	0.79	0.49–1.25	30	1.26	0.85–1.80	26	1.08	0.71–1.59
Amniotic fluid embolism	13	0.57	0.33–0.98	7	0.29	0.12–0.61	8	0.33	0.14–0.66
Early pregnancy deaths	11	0.48	0.27–0.87	4	0.17	0.05–0.43	8	0.33	0.14–0.66
Haemorrhage	9	0.39	0.20–0.75	14	0.59	0.32–0.99	11	0.46	0.23–0.82
Anaesthesia	7	0.31	0.15–0.64	3	0.12	0.03–0.37	4	0.17	0.05–0.43
Other Direct‡	4	0.17	0.07–0.47	‡	‡	‡	‡	‡	‡
All Direct	107	4.67	3.86–5.64	83	3.49	2.78–4.32	78	3.25	2.57–4.05
Indirect									
Cardiac disease	53	2.31	1.77–3.0.	51	2.14	1.60–2.82	54	2.25	1.69–2.93
Other indirect causes	49	2.14	1.62–2.83	72	3.03	2.37–3.81	61	2.54	1.94–3.26
Indirect neurological conditions	36	1.57	1.13–2.18	30	1.26	0.85–1.80	31	1.29	0.88–1.83
Psychiartic causes	13	0.57	0.33–0.98	13	0.55	0.29–0.93	16	0.67	0.38–1.08
Indirect neurological conditions	3	0.13	0.04–0.41	4	0.17	0.05–0.45	3	0.13	0.0.–0.37
All Indirect	154	6.72	5.74–7.87	170	7.15	6.11–8.30	165	6.87	5.86–8.00
Coincidental	50	2.18	1.65–2.88	23	0.98	0.61–1.45	26	1.08	0.71–1.59
Late deaths	33†	†	†	325	13.66	12.22–15.33	313	13.03	11.63–14.56

*Genital tract sepsis deaths only including early pregnancy deaths as the result of genital tract sepsis. Other deaths from infectious causes are classified under other indirect causes.

‡Acute fatty liver and genital tract trauma: included with pre-eclampsia and eclampsia and haemorrhage respectively from 2009 onwards.

†Figures on late deaths for 2006–08 include only cases reported to CMACE and not all deaths. therefore rates are not calculated. Cases from 2009–12 identified through direct report and linked national birth and death data and include late direct. late indirect and late coincidental deaths. These deaths will be described fully in the 2015 report.

Sources: CMACE. MBRRACE-UK. Office for National Statistics. National Records Scotland. Northern Ireland Statistics and Research Agency.

Reproduced from Knight M, Kenyon S, Brocklehurst P, *et al. Saving Lives, Improving Mothers' Care – Lessons Learned to Inform Future Maternity Care from the UK and Ireland Confidential Enquiries into Maternal Deaths and Morbidity 2009–12.* Oxford: National Perinatal Epidemiology Unit, University of Oxford; 2014.

did not receive prophylactic anticoagulation has been reported to range from 2.4% to 12.2%.[12,13]

Thrombophilia

Thrombophilia is also an important risk factor[10] and can be divided into heritable and acquired. Heritable thrombophilia is a positive finding in 20–50% of women who experience VTE during pregnancy and the postpartum period.[14,15] Although thrombophilia is a risk factor for VTE, performing a thrombophilia screen before commencing anticoagulant therapy is not routinely recommended as it will not influence the immediate management of acute VTE. Furthermore, although the results of genetic texts for heritable thrombophilia will be unaltered, such as for factor V Leiden, other investigations such as protein S are markedly altered by pregnancy, or the presence of thrombus (e.g. antithrombin) making such investigations less reliable, often confusing rather than clarifying the situation.

Women with multiple previous VTE, or a previous VTE and a problem such as antiphospholipid syndrome, are considered to be at a high risk of recurrence and may require higher doses of low-molecular-weight heparin (LMWH) in pregnancy. They are likely to be on long-term anticoagulation with warfarin prior to conception. An intermediate or treatment dose of LMWH is required throughout pregnancy and should be continued postpartum for a minimum of 6 weeks or until converted back to long-term warfarin.[9]

Diagnosis of thromboembolism in pregnancy

The clinical diagnosis of DVT and pulmonary thromboembolism (PTE) is unreliable in pregnancy. Indeed, following objective testing only a minority of those with clinically suspected VTE will have the diagnosis confirmed.[12,16] Nonetheless, given the

Table 37.2 Risk factors and their odds ratios for risk of venous thromboembolism in pregnancy[3,10–12]

Risk factor	Adjusted odds ratios	95% CIs
Previous VTE	24.8	17.1–36
Immobility:	7.7	3.2–19
If combined with BMI ≥ 25	62	
BMI > 30	5.3	2.1–13.5
Smoking	2.7	1.5–4.9
Weight gain > 21 kg (vs 7–21 kg)	1.6	1.1–2.6
Parity > 1	1.5	1.1–1.9
Age > 35 years	1.3	1.0–1.7
Pre-eclampsia	3.1	1.8–5.3
Preeclampsia with fetal growth restriction	5.8	2.1–16
Assisted reproductive techniques	4.3	2.0–9.4
Twin pregnancy	2.6	1.1–6.2
Antepartum haemorrhage	2.3	1.8–2.8
Postpartum haemorrhage	4.1	2.3–7.3
Caesarean section	3.6	3.0–4.3
Medical conditions, e.g. systemic lupus erythematosus, heart disease, anaemia, active infection, varicose veins	2.0–8.7	
Blood transfusion	7.6	6.2–9.4

Data from various sources (see references).

life-threatening nature of this condition, anticoagulant therapy should be commenced if there is a delay in obtaining objective testing unless there are strong contraindications to its use. The condition should be suspected during pregnancy where symptoms and signs are consistent with a possible VTE, such as dyspnoea, chest pain, haemoptysis, unilateral leg pain and swelling (especially on the left side), lower abdominal pain, low-grade pyrexia (a feature of thrombosis), and collapse.

Clinical probability assessment in pregnancy still has a role in pregnancy despite differing from the non-pregnant assessment. The LEFt rule reported on 194 suspected DVT cases in pregnancy looked at symptoms in the left leg (L), calf circumference difference of at least 2 cm (E for (o)edema), and first-trimester presentation (Ft) are the components of the LEFt rule. It was found that 0/89 with no component had DVT compared with 7/105 with one or more components.[17] Righini et al. assessed 157 pregnant women with suspected DVT; the diagnosis was confirmed in 11.7% of women with one or more LEFt component versus 0% in women with no components. Therefore the LEFt rule may be useful in excluding the diagnosis but meanwhile objective testing remains important.[18]

Diagnosis of deep venous thrombosis in pregnancy

Compression ultrasonography

Compression ultrasonography (CUS) of the entire proximal venous system is considered the optimal first-line diagnostic test for DVT in pregnancy.[19,20] If the initial ultrasound shows an abnormality in the popliteal or femoral veins, the diagnosis of proximal DVT is confirmed and therapeutic anticoagulation should be employed. As the majority of gestational DVTs are iliofemoral these are usually easily visualized confirming the diagnosis. Where the initial CUS is negative and where the clinician has ongoing suspicion of DVT then repeat ultrasound examinations on days 3 and 7 should be considered. Treatment should be stopped pending the repeat test. An apparently normal ultrasound examination in a patient with significant symptoms and signs or risk factors for VTE does not completely exclude a calf DVT.[19] Results from the recently published EDVIGE study found that following a single CUS for suspected DVT in pregnancy only 10.5% had the diagnosis confirmed. Of 177 women who had a negative CUS and who did not receive anticoagulation, only 1.1% (95% CI 0.3–4.0%) had a VTE on 3 months of follow-up.[21] In women reporting swelling of the entire leg with or without back, buttock, or flank pain, an iliac vein thrombosis should be suspected. Serial CUS of the proximal venous system is not helpful in the diagnosis of iliac vein thrombosis and pulsed Doppler of the iliac vein, magnetic resonance imaging (MRI), venography, or conventional contrast venography should be considered.[19,20]

D-Dimer

D-dimer, a specific fibrin degradation product, has been extensively used in the exclusion of DVT in the non-pregnant population, but its use in pregnancy requires further studies and evaluation. Some authorities employ D-dimer measurements in pregnancy following the initial negative ultrasound scan, and where there is an elevated D-dimer a repeat ultrasound is performed. However, D-dimer levels increase in normal pregnancy as gestation advances. D-dimer levels will be outside the normal range at term and postpartum in most normal pregnancies. D-dimer levels also increase with complications such as pre-eclampsia, and abruption, which are themselves associated with an increase in risk for VTE.[8,19,20] Further, false-negative D-dimer results have been reported with VTE in pregnancy.[22] In view of these issues and because D-dimer assays have not been evaluated in prospective management studies, it is the authors' practice to proceed direct to CUS in women with suspected DVT, and repeat this as required rather than rely on D-dimer measurements.

Venography

Venography is the gold standard test for the diagnosis and exclusion of DVT outside of pregnancy.[23,24] In pregnancy, concerns about *in utero* fetal exposure to ionizing radiation and potential teratogenicity and oncogenicity during testing have limited the use of venography and the number of studies involved. When venography is used with abdominal shielding the risk from radiation to the fetus is very low, and the fear of fetal irradiation is often overstated[25] (Table 37.3). For the majority of cases CUS is sufficient, particularly as over 70% of DVTs are iliofemoral in pregnancy. If difficulty is encountered in imaging possible pelvic thrombus then MRI venography can be safely used in pregnancy.

Computed tomography scan venography

Computed tomography venography may be useful in detecting pelvic vein thrombosis but it is associated with significant radiation exposure to the fetus, and in practice is rarely required to make a diagnosis.[26]

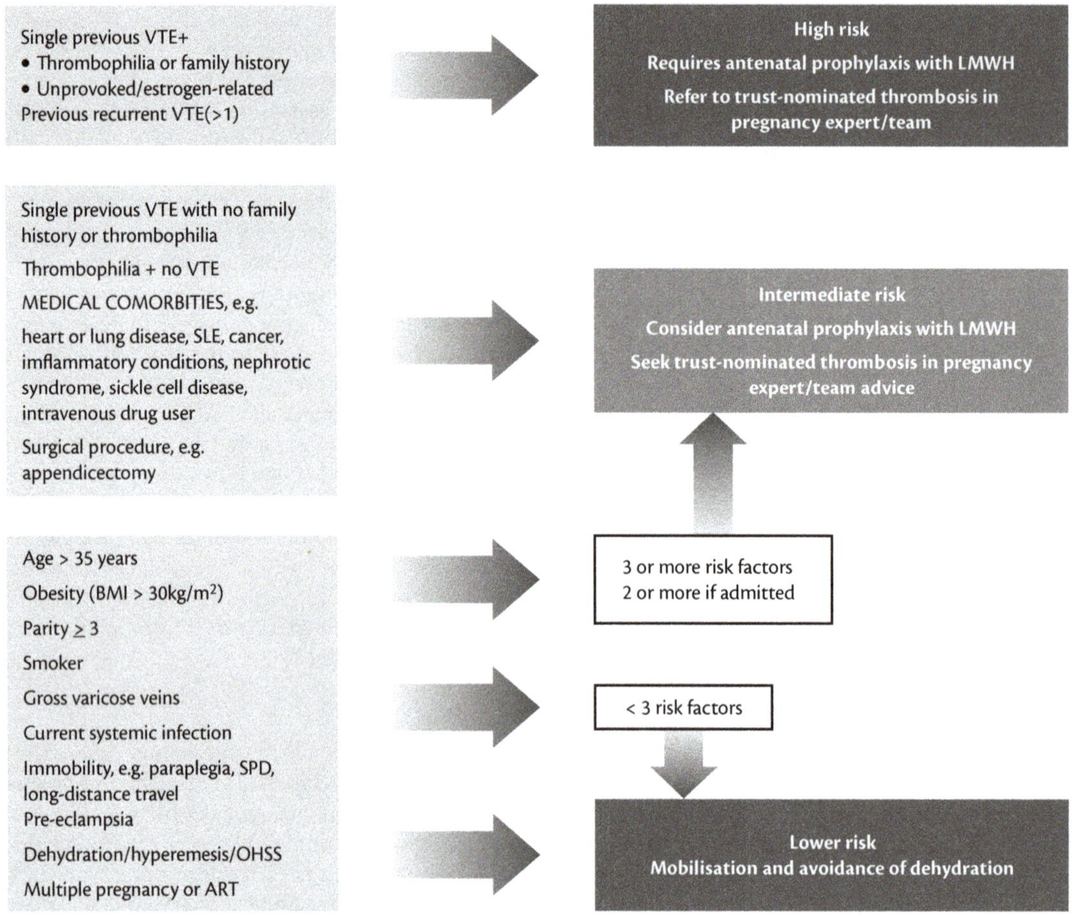

Figure 37.1 Obstetric thromboprophylaxis risk assessment.

Reproduced from Royal College of Obstetricians and Gynaecologists, *Reducing the risk of thrombosis and embolism during pregnancy and the puerperium.* Green-top Guideline No. 37a. London: RCOG; 2015, with the permission of the Royal College of Obstetricians and Gynaecologists.

Diagnosis of pulmonary thromboembolism

Firstly it is useful to note that the CUS is valuable in assessing women with suspected PTE in pregnancy, because the treatment of DVT and PTE is the same. Therefore specific chest imaging may be avoided with a positive diagnosis of DVT. However, it is also important to consider the role of specific thoracic imaging modalities and the electrocardiogram (ECG).

Chest X-ray

In a pregnant woman with a suspected PTE who is haemodynamically stable, a chest X-ray (CXR) is valuable. It may identify other pulmonary disease such as pneumonia, lobar collapse, or pneumothorax. Pregnant women in general have low rates of pre-existing pulmonary disease and in over 50% of cases the CXR will be normal. Non-specific features of PTE on CXR include atelectasis, effusion, focal opacities, regional oligaemia, and pulmonary oedema. The radiation dose to the fetus from a CXR performed at any stage of pregnancy is negligible and a CXR should not be withheld from a pregnant woman with a potentially fatal condition.

Electrocardiogram

The ECG is a non-specific investigation for the diagnosis of pulmonary embolus in pregnancy. In normal pregnancy the electrical axis of the heart changes, which can make the ECG lack specificity. The ECG may also be normal, however in massive pulmonary embolus features of acute right heart strain such as right bundle branch block, right axis deviation and peaked P-waves may be present. The classical S_1, Q_3, T_3 is infrequently seen. It is, however, valuable in relation to alternative cardiac diagnoses.

Computed tomography pulmonary angiography and ventilation perfusion lung scan

The main techniques for objective diagnosis of PTE are ventilation/perfusion (V/Q) lung scan or computed tomography pulmonary angiography (CTPA). Local availability and guidelines may be the determining factor for which diagnostic technique is employed in pregnancy. In the non-pregnant population, the British Thoracic Society recommends CTPA as first-line investigation for non-massive PTE due to better sensitivity and specificity than V/Q lung scanning,[27] and also the possibility to identify other potential pathology contributing to the patients symptoms (e.g. aortic dissection). Furthermore, older non-pregnant patients with chest symptoms will often have co-morbid chest pathology so limiting the value of V/Q scans, but this is not usually the case in most young pregnant women.

When weighing up the risks and benefits of these techniques it is important to consider not only the diagnostic accuracy, but also the issue of radiation exposure in the context of diagnosis of PTE.

Table 37.3 Estimated fetal radiation exposure with venous thromboembolism investigation

Radiologic procedure	Radiation mGy
Bilateral venography without abdominal shield	0.628
Unilateral venography without abdominal shield	0.314
Limited venography	< 0.05
Pulmonary angiography (femoral route)	0.221–0.374
Pulmonary angiography (brachial route)	< 0.05
Ventilation lung scan:	
^{133}Xenon	0.004–0.019
^{99m}Tc-DTPA	0.007–0.035
^{99m}Tc-SC	0.001–0.005
Perfusion lung scan using ^{99m}Tc-MAA:	
3 mCi	0.018
1–2 mCi	0.006–0.012
Chest radiograph	< 0.001

DTPA: diethylenetriamine penta-acidic acid, SC: sulphur colloid; Tc: technetium.

NB 1 Gy = 100 Rad. Threshold for fetal abnormality induced in *in utero* exposure is 100–200 mGy.

Reproduced with permission from Ginsberg JS, Hirsh J, Rainbow AJ, *et al.*, Risks to the fetus of radiological procedures used in the diagnosis of maternal/venous thromboembolic disease, *Thrombosis and Haemostasis*, Volume 61, pp. 189–96, Copyright © 1989 John Wiley & Sons.

Concerns over radiation exposure for the fetus are often cited as reasons to avoid radiation-based investigation in pregnancy. However, the commonly employed investigations are not associated with high levels of fetal exposure (Table 37.3). In addition, it is important to take into account the clinical context—a potentially fatal disorder for the mother, and the fetus if the event is antenatal. CTPA is associated with less radiation exposure to the fetus than V/Q lung scanning in all trimesters of pregnancy. It has been estimated that the risk of fatal cancer to the age of 15 years is <1/1,000,000 after *in utero* exposure to CTPA and 1/280,000 following a perfusion scan.[19] Perhaps of more concern is that CTPA, while associated with a lower dose of radiation for the fetus than a V/Q scan, exposes the mother to a relatively high radiation dose of as much as 20 mGy to the thorax and in particular exposure of breast tissue is a concern, as calculations suggest a significant increase in lifetime risk of breast cancer.

Therefore, where available, V/Q scans are generally preferred in pregnancy because of the lower radiation dose to the mother, and the low incidence of co-morbid pulmonary problems that often reduce the value of such scans in the non-pregnant patient.[19] Further, during pregnancy, and especially if the CXR is normal, the ventilation component can often be omitted thereby minimizing the radiation dose for the fetus. Thus the authors generally prefer V/Q lung scanning over CTPA for the first-line investigation of PTE in pregnancy because of its high negative predictive value, low incidence of co-morbid pulmonary pathology, and lower radiation dose to the mother.

Pulmonary angiography

Pulmonary angiography carries the highest radiation exposure (at least 0.5 mSv to fetus, and 5 –30 mSv to mother)[19] and should be used mainly in severe cases prior to embolectomy.

Management of venous thromboembolism in pregnancy

Initial assessment

In the initial assessment of the patient before commencing therapeutic anticoagulation for VTE, a full blood count, coagulation screen, urea, electrolytes, and liver function tests should be checked to exclude renal or hepatic dysfunction, which are relevant for anticoagulant therapy. As noted earlier, thrombophilia screening is not usually performed as many components of the thrombophilia screen are altered by both pregnancy (e.g. lower protein S) and the presence of thrombus (lower antithrombin), and because the results will not alter the acute management of VTE.

Anticoagulants in pregnancy

Vitamin K antagonists

Warfarin is an oral anticoagulant that interferes with hepatic synthesis of vitamin K-dependent clotting factors, which leads to depletion of prothrombin, and factors VII, IX, and X with resultant anticoagulation. Warfarin crosses the placenta and is associated with an increased risk of fetal complications, specifically congenital malformations and an increased risk of pregnancy loss with first-trimester exposure. While congenital abnormalities are reported in up to 5%[8,28–32] of cases with first-trimester warfarin exposure, only a small number (<1%) develop the specific warfarin embryopathy (midfacial hypoplasia, limb hypoplasia, and stippled epiphyses).[33,34] There is some evidence to suggest that if the woman is taking a dose greater than 5 mg/day this is associated with a higher risk of congenital abnormalities.[32,35,36] In the third trimester, there is a significant risk of maternal and fetal bleeding if taken after 36 weeks, as the fetus is also anticoagulated. This is of particular concern at delivery. Warfarin can, however, be used in the postpartum period if required as there is no significant excretion in breast milk.

Low-molecular-weight heparin

Heparins remain the agents of choice for treatment and prophylaxis of VTE in pregnancy.[19,20] LMWHs have now largely replaced unfractionated heparin (UFH) for the immediate management of VTE in pregnancy. LMWH acts by inactivating thrombin and factor Xa without depleting circulating levels of clotting factors. It does not cross the placenta and is not present in breast milk in appreciable amounts, and in any event is orally inactive, so there is no risk of anticoagulation in the fetus or the newborn. There are now substantial data from randomized controlled trials in non-pregnant patients confirming that LMWH is more effective than vitamin K antagonists in preventing recurrent VTE and post-thrombotic syndrome without increasing the risk of serious bleeding events.[8,37] Furthermore, LMWH is more effective, has a lower risk of bleeding, and is associated with lower mortality than UFH in the initial treatment of DVT in non-pregnant patients.[8,19,38] Indeed, a meta-analysis of randomized controlled trials has shown equivalent efficacy of LMWH to UFH in the initial treatment of PTE.[8,38] While data on efficacy of LMWH in pregnancy are extrapolated from the non-pregnant, direct data on safety are available for pregnancy. A systematic review of LMWH in pregnancy has confirmed its safety and also describes efficacy consistent with the extrapolation from the non-pregnant in the management of acute VTE,[11] supported by further data from a large retrospective review of over 1000 pregnancies exposed to a

LMWH.[39] Heparin-induced thrombocytopenia (HIT) resulting in thrombosis, an immune-mediated reaction, is extremely rare with LMWHs and therefore in women only exposed to LMWH, platelet monitoring is unnecessary. Some patients may develop skin reaction similar to UFH with LMWH in the form of pruritic skin eruption or local irritation at the injection site. The incidence of this has been reported to range from 1.8% to 29%,[8] but in systematic reviews has been of the order of 2%.[11]

Compared with UFH, LMWH is associated with a substantially lower risk of HIT, haemorrhage, and osteoporosis.[11,14,40]

Although useful in monitoring UFH (see 'Unfractionated Heparin'), the activated partial thromboplastin time (aPTT) is not meaningfully changed in patients on LMWH and cannot be used to assess response to therapy. Monitoring anti-Xa levels for women on LMWH is no longer recommended[20] and is difficult to justify in pregnancy due to the satisfactory results with weight-based dosing and also because anti-Xa monitoring does not reliably predict either recurrent thrombosis or bleeding risk, at least in part because of variability in the assay.[8,20,41] There may be a case for monitoring levels at extremes of body weight (<50 kg and >90 kg), where compliance is in doubt, and in women with other complicating factors including renal disease, severe thrombophilia, and recurrent VTE (if LMWH therapy requires monitoring, the aim is to achieve peak anti-Xa activity, 3 hours post injection of 0.5–1.2 units/mL for women with VTE). Routine platelet count monitoring to identify HIT is not required in obstetric patients who have received only LMWH. However, if the obstetric patient is receiving LMWH after first receiving UFH, or if she has received UFH in the past, making HIT more likely, the platelet count should be monitored every other day from day 4 to day 14, or until LMWH is stopped, whichever occurs first.[42]

Unfractionated heparin

UFH, as with LMWH, does not cross the placenta. It was used in the past for treatment and prophylaxis of VTE in pregnancy, but in contemporary practice it has been widely replaced by LMWH due to the evidence discussed earlier. Therefore, in current practice, UFH use has been limited to specific circumstances, such as women considered to be at high risk of haemorrhage who require thromboprophylaxis or treatment prior to delivery. Prophylactic UFH is administered subcutaneously in divided doses. If UFH is required in therapeutic doses it is administered either by an intravenous continuous infusion or subcutaneous injection twice a day. The aPTT is used to monitor UFH with the dose adjusted accordingly to maintain the aPTT in the therapeutic range. The effect of UFH can be limited by stopping the intravenous infusion and also by protamine sulphate, which cannot be so readily achieved with subcutaneous LMWH.

Any exposure to UFH is associated with an increased risk of HIT, which occurs in 3% of non-pregnant patients receiving UFH.[43] Long-term use of UFH has been associated with increased risk of osteoporosis and fractures.[44] Up to 30% reduction in bone density and approximately 2–3% vertebral fractures with long-term use has been reported.[45,46] Adverse skin reactions to UFH include bruising, urticarial rashes, vasculitis which can lead to skin necrosis, and well-circumscribed, erythematous lesions (because of a delayed type 4 hypersensitivity reaction).[8]

Danaparoid

This heparinoid crosses the placenta in negligible quantities. Therefore there is no demonstrable fetal toxicity with maternal danaparoid use.[8] It has an anti-IIa and anti-Xa effects with a long anti-Xa half-life of about 24 hours. Danaparoid can be administered intravenously or subcutaneously. It is usually used in pregnant women who develop HIT or a skin reaction from heparin and require ongoing anticoagulant therapy. However, the quality of evidence available to support its safety is scarce and advice should be sought from experts in haemostasis and thrombosis.

Fondaparinux

There are limited data on this anticoagulant as its use in pregnancy is relatively new. Fondaparinux is a pentasaccharide that acts, like heparins, by inhibiting factor Xa through enhancing the effect of antithrombin. In an *ex vivo* model, no placental passage of fondaparinux was demonstrated[47] but anti-Xa activity of about 10% of that in maternal plasma was found in the umbilical cord plasma in newborn infants of five mothers being treated with 2.5 mg during pregnancy.[48] It is recommended that the use of fondaparinux be restricted to those with severe adverse reactions to heparin such as HIT or who cannot receive danaparoid.[8]

Oral anti-Xa and thrombin inhibitors

There are no significant data supporting the use of new oral direct thrombin inhibitors such as dabigatran, or the new anti-Xa inhibitors such as rivaroxaban, or apixaban in pregnancy. As they are orally active they are likely to cross the placenta with resultant fetal anticoagulation and risk of bleeding. These agents should be avoided in pregnancy at the present time[9] due to lack of safety data and also because a highly effective and safe alternative exists with LMWH although not as an oral preparation.

Parenteral direct thrombin inhibitor

There are insufficient data to evaluate the safety of recombinant hirudin, and no published reports on the use of bivalirudin in pregnancy.[8]

Thrombolysis during pregnancy

Thrombolysis reduces clot burden by breaking down fibrin. Thrombolytic agents include streptokinase, urokinase, recombinant tissue plasminogen activator, and anisoylated plasminogen streptokinase activator complex. These markedly enhance the conversion of plasminogen to plasmin, with resultant degradation of fibrin to fibrin degradation products. There is growing evidence on the use of thrombolytic agents in pregnancy.[8,49,50] Streptokinase, and probably other thrombolytic agents, do not cross the placenta.[51–54] No maternal deaths associated with thrombolytic therapy have been reported, and the maternal bleeding complication rate is approximately 6%, which is consistent with that in non-pregnant patients receiving thrombolytic therapy. Most bleeding events occur around catheter and puncture sites, and in pregnant women, from the genital tract. Currently, given the limited data on the safety and efficiency of thrombolysis in pregnancy, the use of these agents should be reserved for life-threatening maternal thromboembolism.[8]

Treatment of acute venous thromboembolism

In pregnancy, it is recommended that the initial treatment of acute VTE is by a twice-daily dosage regimen of LMWH.[19] This is because of the recognized pregnancy-related alterations in the pharmacokinetics of LMWH, which is cleared by the kidney. However, there are growing data, mostly with tinzaparin, that once-daily dosing may be satisfactory (tinzaparin, 175 units/kg) and may be appropriate in the initial acute treatment of VTE in pregnancy.[39,55] As there is greater experience with twice-daily dosing and the possibility of reduced anticoagulant activity towards the end of the 24-hour period due to increased renal clearance, the authors prefer a twice-daily dose in the initial treatment of acute VTE with enoxaparin (1 mg/kg twice daily) or dalteparin (100 units/kg twice daily) until the situation is stable, then converting if required to a once-daily regimen of (1.5 mg/kg enoxaparin or dalteparin 10,000–18,000 units once daily depending on body weight). There are other techniques that are also of value in the management of acute DVT in pregnancy. Leg elevation should be employed and graduated elastic compression stockings should be fitted to reduce oedema.

The prophylactic and treatment dose of LMWHs as recommended by the Royal College of Obstetrician and Gynaecologists is described in Table 37.4.

Treatment of DVT by thrombolysis can reduce post-thrombotic syndrome, but at the expense of increased bleeding.[37] In the non-pregnant patient, the current American College of Chest Physicians recommendation is to prefer anticoagulation over systemic thrombolysis, reserving consideration of the latter only to patients with all of the following criteria: iliofemoral DVT, symptoms for less than 14 days, good functional status, life expectancy of 1 year or longer, and low risk of bleeding.[37] Catheter-directed thrombolysis is considered the preferable approach. Because of the uncertainty regarding the balance of risks and concerns relating to major bleeding, in pregnancy anticoagulant therapy alone appears preferable to systemic thrombolysis unless there is massive occlusive iliofemoral DVT threatening leg viability through venous gangrene.

Graduated elastic compression stockings

The woman should be encouraged to mobilize whilst wearing compression stockings, as in non-pregnant patients[37] this has been shown to reduce pain and swelling. Studies in non-pregnant patients have shown that early mobilization, with compression therapy, does not increase the likelihood of developing PTE.[56,57] This approach may also help prevent the development of post-thrombotic syndrome as there are some trial data from outside pregnancy to suggest that compression stockings started within 2 weeks of DVT and continued for 2 years reduce the likelihood of post-thrombotic syndrome by around 50% but does not impact on the frequency of recurrent VTE.[37] Although there are no data demonstrating an impact from compression stockings on clinical outcomes in gestational DVT, the effect of these stockings on the venous system in postpartum women has been studied, where they are associated with reduced diameter of the common femoral vein along with increased blood flow velocity.[58]

Life-threatening pulmonary thromboembolism

A massive PTE is a serious, life-threatening obstetric and medical emergency that may be defined as a pulmonary embolus associated with haemodynamic compromise (systolic blood pressure <90 mmHg or a drop in systolic blood pressure of ≥40 mmHg from baseline for a period > 15 minutes), not otherwise explained by hypovolaemia, sepsis, or new arrhythmia. The collapsed, shocked pregnant woman requires rapid assessment by a multidisciplinary resuscitation team of experienced clinicians including senior obstetricians, anaesthetists, physicians, and radiologists. This situation needs a quick but thorough assessment and decision for treatment usually are made on an individual basis taking into account the available resources and expertise. The options include intravenous UFH, thrombolytic therapy, catheter-assisted thrombus removal, or surgical embolectomy. In the initial response, oxygen should be administered and circulatory support provided with intravenous fluids and inotropic agents as required. Intravenous UFH is the traditional method of heparin administration in acute VTE and remains the preferred treatment in massive PTE because of its rapid effect and extensive experience of its use in this situation. The aim is to prolong the a PTT by 1.5–2 times control. As anticoagulant therapy will not reduce the obstruction of the pulmonary circulation, there is a strong case for considering systemic thrombolytic therapy. An infusion of UFH can be given following thrombolytic therapy. If the patient is not suitable for thrombolysis or moribund, cardiothoracic surgeons should be consulted urgently with a view to emergency thoracotomy.

Inferior vena cava filters

It is the authors' experience that inferior vena cava (IVC) filters are rarely necessary. In general, these should be restricted to women with proven VTE and who have continuing PTE despite

Table 37.4 Prophylaxis and treatment dose of LMWHs in pregnancy

Weight (kg)	Enoxaparin	Dalteparin	Tinzaparin
<50	20 mg daily	2500 units daily	3500 units daily
50–90	40 mg daily	5000 units daily	4500 units daily
91–130	60 mg daily[a]	7500 units daily[a]	7000 units daily[a]
131–170	80 mg daily[a]	10,000 units daily[a]	9000 units daily[a]
>170	0.6 mg/kg/day[a]	75 units/kg/day[a]	75 units/kg/day[a]
High prophylactic (intermediate) dose for women weighing 50–90 kg	40 mg 12-hourly	5000 units 12-hourly	4500 units 12-hourly
Treatment dose	1 mg/kg/12 hourly antenatal; 1.5 mg/kg/daily postnatal	100 units/kg/12-hourly or 200 units/kg/daily postnatal	175 units/kg/daily (antenatal and postnatal)

[a]May be given in two divided doses.

Data from the Royal College of Obstetrician and Gynaecologists.

adequate anticoagulation or where anticoagulation cannot be used. Temporary IVC filters can be considered in the perinatal period for large iliac DVT, but their value is uncertain. Each case requires individual assessment as there are hazards from filter placement including filter migration (occurring in >20%), filter fracture (around 5%), and IVC perforation (up to 5%), and lifelong anticoagulation may be required.

In the non-pregnant patient, filters reduce PTE, but increase DVT, and have no change in overall frequency of VTE.[8,19,37] It is important to note that temporary filters are sometimes not retrieved and so remain *in situ* in a proportion of patients.

Where a woman enters pregnancy with a filter *in situ*, her anticoagulation must be reviewed. Pregnancy substantially increases the risk of thrombosis, therefore in women with a filter in place who become pregnant, anticoagulation should be continued or restarted (with LMWH) as soon as pregnancy is diagnosed. Outside pregnancy, increasingly patients with filters in place do not remain on life-long anticoagulation, such as where the risk factor for thrombosis resolves. This is because of the risk of bleeding on long-term warfarin relative to the risk of thrombosis. With regard to anticoagulation of such women in pregnancy it is important to remember that LMWH does not carry the same risk of serious bleeding problems as long-term coumarin therapy. If she enters pregnancy on coumarin therapy then this should be switched to intermediate or treatment dose LMWH by 6 weeks' gestation to avoid the risk of warfarin embryopathy.

Duration and intensity of maintenance treatment of venous thromboembolism

Women with antenatal VTE can be managed with subcutaneous LMWH for the remainder of the pregnancy. It is uncertain whether dose adjustment is required in pregnancy in relation to pregnancy-associated weight gain. It is the authors' practice to continue with the initial dose regimen throughout pregnancy for the majority of cases despite the pregnancy-associated weight gain (since LMWH does not cross the placenta and therefore the weight of the fetoplacental unit is not relevant).[8,19] It is not yet established whether the initial dose of LMWH can be reduced to an intermediate dose (75% of treatment dose) after an initial period of several weeks of therapeutic anticoagulation. However, this practice has been successfully employed outside pregnancy in patients with contraindications to coumarin therapy and in patients with underlying malignancy.[8] Although there have been no studies directly comparing these two types of dosing strategies in pregnant women, this type of modified dosing regimen may be useful in pregnant women at increased risk of bleeding or osteoporosis. For pregnant women with acute VTE, it is recommended that anticoagulants should be continued for at least 6 weeks postpartum and for a minimum total duration of therapy of 3 months.[8,19]

Delivery in women on anticoagulant treatment for venous thromboembolism

For women on therapeutic anticoagulation, a planned delivery, either through induction of labour or elective caesarean delivery, may allow optimal timing of events and minimizes the risk of the woman from an unplanned delivery on full anticoagulation. Each case requires individual management depending on the thrombotic and bleeding risks.

The dose of LMWH should be reduced to a once-daily thromboprophylactic dose on the day prior to induction of labour or caesarean delivery. When a woman presents in labour on therapeutic LMWH, neuraxial anaesthetic techniques should usually be avoided for at least 24 hours after the last dose of LMWH due to the risk of neuraxial haematomas. In patients receiving prophylactic doses of LMWH, epidural anaesthetic techniques should usually be avoided for at least 12 hours after the last dose. A problem that frequently causes concern is where the thrombotic event occurs close to term with a consequently high risk of spontaneous labour. Consideration should be given to the use of UFH (since it can be relatively easily reversed using protamine sulphate and has a short duration of action) in this circumstance. If spontaneous labour occurs in women receiving therapeutic doses of subcutaneous UFH, assessment of the anticoagulant effect by the aPTT is required. Subcutaneous UFH should be discontinued 12 hours and intravenous UFH stopped 6 hours before induction of labour.

There is an increased risk of wound haematoma following caesarean delivery with both UFH and LMWH of around 2%.[9] For this reason, wound drains should be considered at caesarean delivery, and the skin incision should ideally be closed with staples or interrupted sutures to allow easy drainage of any haematoma.

A further thromboprophylactic dose of LMWH (enoxaparin 40 mg; dalteparin 5000 IU; tinzaparin 75 IU/kg) should be given by 3 hours postoperatively or more than 4 hours after a spinal anaesthetic or removal of the epidural catheter, if appropriate. The treatment dose should be recommenced around 12 hours after delivery.

Postnatal anticoagulation

Heparin and warfarin are not excreted in breast milk and are satisfactory for use postpartum and when breastfeeding. In the authors' experience, most women prefer to use LMWH (which can be used with once-daily dosing postpartum) because they have become accustomed to its administration, and they appreciate the convenience of not having to attend clinics for monitoring of coumarin therapy when caring for a new baby. Before discontinuing treatment the ongoing risk of thrombosis should be assessed including a review of personal and family history of VTE. Thrombophilia screening should be discussed and arranged if required. Recently it has been reported that low-dose aspirin (LDA) can prevent recurrence of VTE in non-pregnant patients following completion of 6–18 months of anticoagulant therapy, with a low risk of bleeding.[58] These data do not suggest that LDA can replace therapeutic anticoagulation for VTE, but do suggest that where prolonged therapy is considered of benefit following completion of a full course of therapeutic anticoagulation, that LDA may be valuable. Nor do these data suggest that LDA can replace LMWH in pregnancy for women with a previous VTE. In view of the risk of VTE and its importance for maternal mortality and morbidity, LMWH, where there is now a substantial evidence base of efficacy and safety, remains the leading therapeutic option for secondary prevention of VTE in pregnancy.

Conclusion

Although VTE remains a challenge in obstetric practice, an awareness of risk factors and use of thromboprophylaxis, along with objective diagnosis of possible events with prompt treatment, usually with LMWH, can reduce the burden of disease.

References

1. Knight M, Kenyon S, Brocklehurst P, *et al. Saving Lives, Improving Mothers' Care - Lessons Learned to Inform Future Maternity Care from the UK and Ireland Confidential Enquiries into Maternal Deaths and Morbidity 2009-12.* Oxford: National Perinatal Epidemiology Unit, University of Oxford; 2014.
2. Gherman RB, Goodwin TM, Leung T, *et al.* Incidence, clinical characteristics, and timing of objectively diagnosed venous thromboembolism during pregnancy. *Obstet Gynecol* 1999; 94:730–4.
3. Jacobsen AF, Skjeldestad FE, Sandset PM. Incidence and risk patters of venous thromboembolism in pregnancy and puerperium: a register-based case–control study. *Am J Obstet Gynecol* 2008; 198:233–4.
4. Macklon NS, Greer IA. Venous thromboembolic disease in obstetrics and gynaecology: the Scottish experience. *Scott Med J* 1996; 41:83–6.
5. Andersen BS, Steffensen FH, Sorensen HT, *et al.* The cumulative incidence of venous thromboembolism during pregnancy and puerperium—an 11 year Danish population-based study of 63,300 pregnancies. *Acta Obstet Gynecol Scand* 1998; 77:170–3.
6. Pomp ER, Lenselink AM, Rosendaal FR, *et al.* Pregnancy, the postpartum period and prothrombotic defects: risk of venous thrombosis in the MEGA study. *J Thromb Haemost* 2008; 6:632–7.
7. Pabinger I, Grafenhofer H, Kyrle PA, *et al.* Temporary increase in the risk for recurrence during pregnancy in women with a history of venous thromboembolism. *Blood* 2002; 100(3):1060–2.
8. Bates SM, Greer IA, Middeldorp S, *et al.* VTE, thrombophilia, antithrombotic therapy, and pregnancy: Antithrombotic Therapy and Prevention of Thrombosis, 9th ed: American College of Chest Physicians Evidence-Based Clinical Practice Guidelines. *Chest* 2012; 141(2 Suppl):e691S–e736S.
9. Nelson-Piercy C, MacCallum P, Mackillop L. *Reducing the Risk of Venous Thromboembolism during Pregnancy and the Puerperium.* Green-top Guideline No. 37a. London: Royal College of Obstetricians and Gynaecologists; 2015.
10. Brill-Edwards P, Ginsberg JS, Gent M, *et al.* Safety of withholding heparin in pregnant women with a history of venous thromboembolism. Recurrence of clot in this pregnancy study group. *N Engl J Med* 2000; 343(20):1439–44.
11. Greer IA, Nelson-Piercy C. Low-molecular-weight heparins for thromboprophylaxis and treatment of venous thromboembolism in pregnancy: a systematic review of safety and efficacy. *Blood* 2005; 106(2):401–7.
12. Hull RD, Raskob GF, Carter CJ. Serial IPG in pregnancy patients with clinically suspected DVT. Clinical validity of negative findings. *Ann Intern Med* 1990; 112:663–7.
13. Chan WS, Ray JG, Murray S, *et al.* Suspected pulmonary embolism in pregnancy: clinical presentation, results of lung scanning, and subsequent maternal and pediatric outcomes. *Arch Intern Med* 2002; 162:1170–5.
14. McColl MD, Walker ID, Greer IA. The role of inherited thrombophilia in venous thromboembolism associated with pregnancy. *BJOG* 1999; 75:387–8.
15. Gerhardt A, Scharf RE, Zotz RB. Effect of hemostatic risk factors on the individual probability of thrombosis during pregnancy and the puerperium. *Thromb Haemost* 2003; 90:77–85.
16. Pabinger I, Grafenhofer H, Kyrle PA, *et al.* Temporary increase in the risk for recurrence during pregnancy in women with a history of venous thromboembolism. *Blood* 2002; 100(3):1060–2.
17. Chan WS, Lee A, Spencer FA, *et al.* Predicting deep venous thrombosis in pregnancy: out in "LEFt" field? *Ann Intern Med* 2009; 151(2):85–92.
18. Righini M, Jobic C, Boehlen F, *et al.* Predicting deep venous thrombosis in pregnancy: external validation of the "left" clinical prediction rule. *Haematologica* 2013; 98(4):545–8.
19. Thomson AJ, Greer IA. *Thromboembolic Disease in Pregnancy and the Puerperium: Acute Management.* Green-top Guideline No. 37b. London: Royal College of Obstetricians and Gynaecologists; London; 2015.
20. Bates SM, Jaeschke R, Stevens SM, *et al.* Diagnosis of DVT. *Chest* 2012; 141(2 Suppl):e351S–e418S.
21. Le Gal G, Kercret G, Ben Yahmed K, *et al.* Diagnostic value of single complete compression ultrasonography in pregnant and postpartum women with suspected deep vein thrombosis: prospective study. *BMJ* 2012; 344:e2635
22. To MS, Hunt BJ, Nelson-Piercy C. A negative D-dimer does not exclude venous thromboembolism (VTE) in pregnancy. *J Obstet Gynaecol* 2008; 28(2):222–3
23. Rabinov K, Paulen S. Roentgen diagnosis of venous thrombosis in the leg. *Arch Surg* 1972; 104:134–44.
24. Hull R, Hirsh J, Sackett DL, *et al.* Clinical validity of a negative venogram in patients with clinically suspected venous thrombosis. *Circulation* 1981; 64(3):622–5.
25. Wall BF, Bury RF, Murray M, *et al. Diagnostic Medical Exposures Advice on Exposure to Ionising Radiation During Pregnancy.* London: National Radiological Protection Board, College of Radiographers and Royal College of Radiologists; 2009.
26. Rademaker J, Griesshaber V, Hidajat N, *et al.* Combined CT pulmonary angiography and venography for diagnosis of pulmonary embolism and deep vein thrombosis: radiation dose. *J Thorac Imaging* 2001; 16(4):297–9.
27. Ryu JH, Swensen SJ, Olson EJ, *et al.* Diagnosis of pulmonary embolism with use of computed tomographic angiography. *Mayo Clin Proc* 2001; 76:59–65.
28. Holzgreve W, Carey JC, Hall BD. Warfarin-induced fetal abnormalities. *Lancet* 1976; 2:914–15.
29. Born D, Martinez EE, Almeida PA, *et al.* Pregnancy in patients with prosthetic heart valves: the effects of anticoagulation on mother, fetus, and neonate. *Am Heart J* 1992; 124:413–17.
30. Sareli P, England MJ, Berk MR, *et al.* Maternal and fetal sequelae of anticoagulation during pregnancy in patients with mechanical heart valve prosthesis. *Am J Cardiol* 1989; 63:1462–5.
31. Schaefer C, Hannemann D, Meister R, *et al.* Vitamin K antagonists and pregnancy outcome. A multicentre prospective study. *Thromb Haemost* 2006; 95:949–57.
32. Vitale N, De Feo M, De Santo LS, Dose-dependent fetal complications of warfarin in pregnant women with mechanical heart valves. *J Am Coll Cardiol* 1999; 33:1637–41.
33. Wesseling J, van Driel D, Heymans HAS, *et al.* Coumarins during pregnancy: long term effects on growth and development in school age children. *Thromb Haemost* 2001; 85:609–13.
34. Pauli RM, Haun J. Intrauterine effects of coumarin derivatives *Dev Brain Dysfunct* 1993; 6:229–47.
35. Cotrufo M, De Feo M, De Santo LS, *et al.* Risk of warfarin during pregnancy with mechanical valve prostheses. *Obstet Gynecol* 2002; 99:35–40.
36. Sbarouni E, Oakley CM. Outcome of pregnancy in women with valve prostheses. *Br Heart J* 1994; 71:196–201.
37. Kearon C, Akl EA, Comerota AJ, *et al.* Antithrombotic therapy for VTE disease: antithrombotic therapy and prevention of thrombosis, 9th ed: American College of Chest Physicians evidence-based clinical practice guidelines. *Chest* 2012; 141(2 Suppl):e419S–e494S.
38. Quinlan DJ, McQuillan A, Eikelboom JW. Low-molecular-weight heparin compared with intravenous unfractionated heparin for treatment of pulmonary embolism: a meta-analysis of randomized, controlled trials. *Ann Intern Med* 2004; 140:175–83.
39. Nelson-Piercy C, Powrie R, Borg JV, *et al.* Tinzaparin use in pregnancy: an international, retrospective study of the safety and efficacy profile. *Eur J Obstet Gynecol* 2011; 159:293–9.
40. James AH, Tapson VF, Goldhaber SZ. Thrombosis during pregnancy and the postpartum period. *Am J Obstet Gynecol* 2005; 193:216–19.
41. Greer I, Hunt BJ. Low molecular weight heparin in pregnancy: current issues. *Br J Haematol* 2005; 128:593–601.

42. Warkentin TE, Greinacher A. Heparin-induced thrombocytopenia: recognition, treatment, and prevention: the Seventh ACCP Conference on Antithrombotic and Thrombolytic Therapy. *Chest* 2004; 126(3 suppl):311S–337S.
43. Warkentin TE, Levine MN, Hirsh J, *et al.* Heparin-induced thrombocytopenia in patients treated with low-molecular weight heparin or unfractionated heparin. *N Engl J Med* 1995; 332(20):1330–5.
44. Nelson-Piercy C. Hazards of heparin: allergy, heparin-induced thrombocytopenia and osteoporosis. In Greer IA (ed) *Baillière's Clinical Obstetrics and Gynaecology: Thromboembolic Disease in Obstetrics and Gynaecology.* London: Baillière Tindall; 1997:489–509.
45. Douketis JD, Ginsberg JS, Burrows RF, *et al.* The effects of long-term heparin therapy during pregnancy on bone density. A prospective matched cohort study. *Thromb Haemost* 1996; 75(2):254–7.
46. Dahlman TC. Osteoporotic fractures and the recurrence of thromboembolism during pregnancy and the puerperium in 184 women undergoing thromboprophylaxis with heparin. *Am J Obstet Gynecol* 1993; 168(4):1265–70.
47. Lagrange F, Vergnes C, Brun JL, *et al.* Absence of placental transfer of pentasaccharide (Fondaparinux, Arixtra) in the dually perfused human cotyledon in vitro. *Thromb Haemost* 2002; 7(5):831–5.
48. Dempfle CE. Minor transplacental passage of fondaparinux in vivo. *N Engl J Med.* 2004; 350(18):1914–15.
49. Holden EL, Ranu H, Sheth A, *et al.* Thrombolysis for massive pulmonary embolism in pregnancy—a report of three cases and follow up over a two year period. *Thromb Res* 2011; 127(1):58–9.
50. Ahearn GS, Hadjiliadis D, Govert JA, *et al.* Massive pulmonary embolism during pregnancy successfully treated with recombinant tissue plasminogen activator: a case report and review of treatment options. *Arch Intern Med* 2002; 162(11):1221–7.
51. Pfeifer GW. Distribution and placental transfer of 131-I streptokinase. *Australas Ann Med* 1970; 19 Suppl 1:17–18.
52. Leonhardt G, Gaul C, Nietsch HH, *et al.* Thrombolytic therapy in pregnancy. *J Thromb Thrombolysis* 2006; 1(3):271–6.
53. Ahearn GS, Hadjiliadis D, Govert JA, *et al.* Massive pulmonary embolism during pregnancy successfully treated with recombinant tissue plasminogen activator: a case report and review of treatment options. *Arch Intern Med* 2002; 162(11):1221–7.
54. te Raa GD, Ribbert LSM, Snijder RJ, *et al.* Treatment options in massive pulmonary embolism during pregnancy; a case-report and review of literature. *Thromb Res* 2009; 124(1):1–5.
55. Smith MP, Norris LA, Steer PJ, *et al.* Tinzaparin sodium for thrombosis treatment and prevention during pregnancy. *Am J Obstet Gynecol* 2004; 190:495–501.
56. Blättler W, Partsch H. Leg compression and ambulation is better than bed rest for the treatment of acute deep vein thrombosis. *Int Angiol* 2003; 22:393–400.
57. Brandjes DP, Buller HR, Heijboer H, *et al.* Randomised trial of effect of compression stockings in patients with symptomatic proximal-vein thrombosis. *Lancet* 1997; 349:759–62.
58. Jamieson R, Calderwood C, Greer IA. The effect of graduated compression stockings on blood velocity in the deep venous system of the lower limb in the postnatal period. *BJOG* 2007; 114:1292–4.

CHAPTER 38

Amniotic fluid embolism (anaphylactoid syndrome of pregnancy)

John A. Anderson, Pierre-Antoine Laloë, and Derek J. Tuffnell

Background

The definition of amniotic fluid embolism (AFE) has evolved since first being recognized as a cause of maternal death. Amniotic fluid and fetal debris in the maternal pulmonary circulation was initially described in 1926 by a Brazilian pathologist, RJ Meyer.[1] However, this Portuguese language publication received little attention. In 1941,[2] Steiner and Lushbaugh identified fetal squames and lanugo hair in the lungs of eight women who had collapsed and died shortly after giving birth. The term 'amniotic fluid embolism' was subsequently coined and born with it, the concept that women died from the physical emboli of fetoplacental material released into the maternal circulation by unspecified means. As a result, historical diagnosis has been pathological with the observation of fetal squames and hair in the maternal circulation postmortem. Attempts to histologically diagnose this condition in survivors have previously been attempted by aspirating maternal blood from pulmonary catheters in an effort to find histological evidence of fetal material, without much success.

More recently, the presence of amniotic fluid and fetoplacental material in the circulation of healthy pregnant women has been proven to occur regularly without resulting harm. Thus, the mere presence of amniotic fluid in the circulation as a cause of morbidity or mortality has been challenged. Focus has turned to an associated immunological cascade, which is now accepted to be the principal cause of the catastrophic pathophysiological sequelae and clinical features of AFE. Subsequently an alternative and more accurately descriptive name for AFE has been put forward by Clark et al.,[3] 'anaphylactoid syndrome of pregnancy'.

Definition

The diagnosis of AFE is clinical and must be considered as part of the differential diagnosis and resuscitation of any acutely unwell or collapsed woman who is pregnant, peripartum, puerperal, or who has undergone any recent invasive uterine procedure. Symptoms or signs may be non-specific and include dyspnoea, reduced oxygen saturation, or coagulopathy. The UK Obstetric Surveillance System (UKOSS) uses defined criteria to determine if a patient had AFE (Box 38.1).[4]

Maternal collapse has many differential diagnoses (see later) and AFE should be considered. If, after investigation for other causes of sudden maternal collapse, no obvious cause is found, a diagnosis of AFE becomes likely. In the event of death, pathological findings of fetal material in the maternal circulation will confirm the diagnosis.

Incidence

The incidence of AFE has not significantly changed over the last 5 years and is equal to approximately 2.0/100,000 in the United Kingdom.[4] Despite being very rare, there is some variation in the Western world with estimated incidences of 7.7/100,00 in the United States,[3] 3.3/100,000 in Australia,[5,6] and 6/100,000 in Canada[7], though it is worth noting that collection methodologies for these data vary between nations and uncertainties surrounding diagnosis complicate inclusion criteria. In the United Kingdom, mortality rates remain stable between triennia.[8]

Mortality and morbidity

AFE is the seventh most common cause of all maternal deaths.[8] In the United Kingdom, it has accounted for over 90 deaths since 1985 and in the United States and Australia, it was responsible for between 7.5% and 27% of direct maternal deaths.[5,9] In the United Kingdom, it has fallen from the second to the fourth leading cause of direct death, accounting for 0.57 deaths per 100,000 maternities.[10]

In the developing world, maternal mortality rates are much higher overall, eclipsing the impact of this rare disease. However the importance of AFE in maternal mortality in the developed world demonstrates that improvements such as better antenatal and intrapartum care, which have improved maternal mortality rates in the 40 years until the 1990s, had little or no impact on AFE. Historically case mortality rates were reported as being in excess of 85%;[11] however, they are now within the range of 16.5–61% in the United Kingdom, Australia, and the United States [4,6,9] This is possibly as a result of advances in supportive critical care and clinical diagnosis of milder cases.[12] Perhaps more importantly, as underlined by Margarson, the high reported mortality

Box 38.1 UKOSS case definition

Summary

- *Either*: a clinical diagnosis of AFE (acute hypotension or cardiac arrest, acute hypoxia, or coagulopathy in the absence of any other potential explanation for the symptoms and signs observed)
- *Or*: a pathological diagnosis (presence of fetal squames or hair in the lungs).

Adapted with permission from D. Tuffnell, M. Knight, F. Plaat., Amniotic fluid embolism – an update, *Anaesthesia*, volume 66, issue 1, pp. 3–6 Copyright © 2011 John Wiley & Sons.

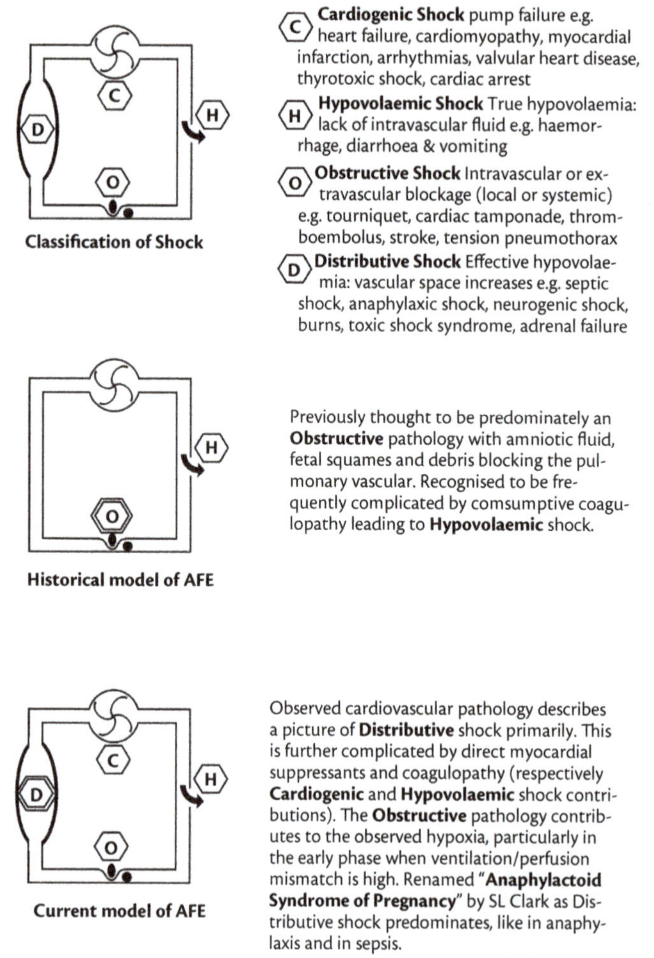

Figure 38.1 Classification of shock with historical and current AFE models.

of the 1979 review was from published cases, which should not be confused with the overall AFE mortality rate.[13] However, given the lack of change in the actual number of deaths, this improved survival may be due to a greater readiness to make a clinical diagnosis rather than a genuine reduction in case survival.

AFE carries significant risk for the fetus. Earlier evidence demonstrated that approximately half of the babies born to women who die of AFE will die, and up to 20% of babies born to women who survive AFE will die. Of the surviving infants, up to a third may suffer hypoxic ischaemic encephalopathy (HIE), a proportion of whom will go on to develop cerebral palsy.[14] The most recent information demonstrates that AFE carries with it a perinatal mortality rate of 135 per 1000 cases.[4]

Pathophysiology

Historical theory underpinning AFE postulated multiple physical emboli of fetoplacental material leading directly to cardiorespiratory collapse (Figure 38.1). Multiple animal studies and biochemical research have failed to substantiate this theory, due to methodological considerations and conflicting results,[15] thus supporting the idea that the main mechanism of action in AFE is secondary to abnormal activation of multiple inflammatory markers and clotting cascades, unique to humans. Furthermore, the physical mechanisms have been hypothesized to include abnormal contractions, cervical tears, or the involvement of placental abruption. However, none have been proven. Indeed, the presence of amniotic fluid and fetal material in the uterine arteries of women undergoing routine obstetric procedures such as a caesarean delivery, who did not display signs of AFE, suggests further yet undiscovered mechanisms.

The observation of rapid circulatory collapse, fluid shift out of the intravascular space, and the invariable onset of consumptive coagulopathy and consequent cardiac and pulmonary complications are hallmarks of AFE. The underlying mechanism of this is thought to be an immune-mediated response to amniotic fluid or trophoblastic cellular components. A host of *in vitro* experiments have produced evidence of coagulant and humoral responses. Mediators such as prostaglandins, serotonin, proteolytic enzymes, leukotrienes, tryptase, and histamine have all been implicated.[12]

Coagulation

Amniotic fluid has been shown to activate complement in certain situations and also causes cells exposed to it to externalize procoagulants such as phosphatidylserine and tissue factor. Fetal surfactant, present in amniotic fluid in increasing levels towards term, has a similar structure to thromboplastin and possesses some thromboplastic action. Cysteine protease, found in amniotic fluid and the amniochorion, can activate factor-X *in vitro*. Platelets will also irreversibly aggregate in amniotic fluid[16] and release platelet factor III. Amniotic fluid itself contains activated factors II, VII, and X. Stimuli to the clotting cascade at multiple points may well trigger the disseminated intravascular coagulation (DIC) and subsequent coagulopathy seen in AFE. Furthermore, amniotic fluid is known to contain high concentrations of anticoagulants such as thrombomodulin, annexin V, and tissue factor pathway inhibitor-2. Correlation between the ability of amniotic fluid to shorten plasma re-calcification time and amniotic fluid surfactant concentrations have been demonstrated.[16] It has also been observed that some patients entered into various AFE registers or case series did not have coagulopathy, while thought to have AFE. This may underline either the difficulty of final diagnosis, or variation in the disease, which would substantiate inconsistent findings in animal studies. One possible confounding explanation for this is that patients in whom coagulopathy was not observed tended to die, despite resuscitation measures, in the early phase of the disease. DIC may not have had time to develop. However, when caring for women who clinically are suspected to have suffered AFE, it must be assumed that a consumptive coagulopathy is very likely to occur and can occur very early in the course of the disease.

Humoral

Other biochemically active substances found in high levels in amniotic fluid include endothelin, a potent vasoconstrictor which will also reduce myocardial contractility, perhaps explaining the reduction in cardiac function seen in AFE cases and animal models. A variety of inflammatory markers such as cytokines, leukotrienes, and prostaglandins have also been implicated. Although performed in 30 pregnant goats, Hankins et al. conducted a carefully matched study with five study groups, including one group who had injectates of 5 μm filtered and boiled amniotic fluid.[17] The allantoic fluid group served as control group and showed that the volume of the injectate (2.5 mL/kg) was not a confounding factor, adding to the argument that humoral mediators are central to the pathology of AFE, much like in sepsis and other forms of distributive shock.

The presence of these substances in amniotic fluid and their production by the fetoplacental unit may be protective against episodes of fetomaternal haemorrhage and may play a crucial role in continuation of pregnancy. Animal studies include the observation that transgenic mice with low tissue factor concentrations have a 42% incidence of spontaneous mid-gestational miscarriage.

Haemodynamic

Consequent to the humoral factors described in the previous section, the initial haemodynamic insult is probably due to pulmonary vasospasm, pulmonary hypertension, and right ventricular dysfunction resulting in profound hypoxia. In a reported case who underwent transoesophageal echocardiography in the hyper-acute setting (performed just after the return of spontaneous circulation near the end of an emergency caesarean section), acute right ventricular failure with prominent septal bulging from right to left was seen.[18] Physical embolization of the pulmonary microvasculature by fetoplacental material would have contributed to this clinical picture. This may be transient but may lead to a primary lung injury and acute respiratory distress syndrome (ARDS). Animal model work supports this as an early rise in pulmonary vascular resistance and extravascular lung water are seen in goats who had meconium-stained amniotic fluid injectates.[17] Early studies suggested that pulmonary hypertension was the prominent feature of the condition, thus requiring treatment with pulmonary vasodilators. Subsequent studies, which included invasive monitoring during the acute phases of the disease, demonstrated an initial period of pulmonary hypertension, which was less than previously thought and then left ventricular failure due to impaired left ventricular function. The initial right ventricular failure followed by left ventricular failure led Clark to suggest that AFE, pending survival of the initial phase, is a bi-phasic disease.[3] As the subsequent reduction in left-sided pre-load causes left ventricular failure and systemic hypotension, this aggravates the cardiogenic shock by reducing myocardial perfusion.[19] Figure 38.2 displays the biphasic response in terms of postulated contributions from the four causes of shock.

Reduced maternal cardiac output and hypoxia will lead to reduced oxygen availability to the fetus. Also, normal physiological uterine contractions will temporarily cut off uterine blood flow during labour. However, this is resumed during uterine relaxation. The concurrent release of catecholamines into the maternal circulation during the acute phase of AFE is thought to induce a tetanic pattern of contraction. Both of these factors may result in fetal distress.

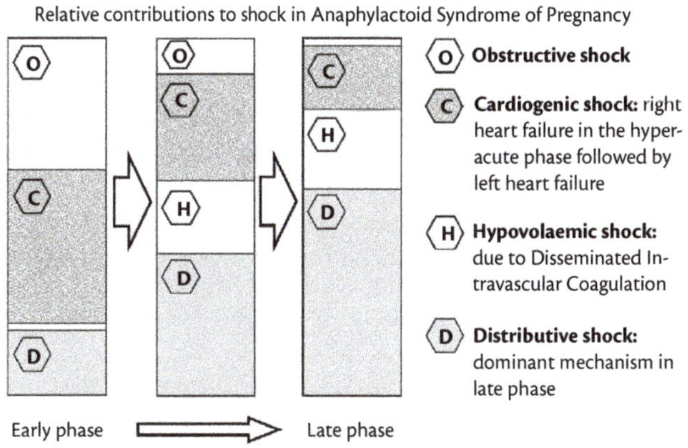

Figure 38.2 Postulated contributions of types of shock seen in AFE with biphasic response.[3,17,19]
Data from various sources (see references).

Sequelae

AFE carries serious consequences for both mother and fetus, including the following:

- Maternal: pulmonary oedema, ARDS, DIC, pulmonary embolus, haemorrhage, left cardiac failure, cardiac arrhythmias, cerebrovascular events, cardiorespiratory arrest, and death
- Fetal: fetal distress, HIE, learning difficulties, cerebral palsy, and intrauterine and neonatal death.

Risk factors

The most recent, comprehensive review of cases within the United Kingdom was performed utilizing data collected by UKOSS, using the specific diagnostic criteria outlined previously. Box 38.2 lists the risk factors that were identified.

There was no association with other risks which were previously felt to predispose women to AFE.[3] These include ethnicity (however, black or ethnic minority women are more likely to die from AFE; this may reflect their overall poor outcomes in relation to all causes of maternal mortality), assisted vaginal delivery,

Box 38.2 Risk factors for AFE

- Maternal age over 35 years old
- Induction of labour (relative risk (RR) 3.86, 95% confidence interval (CI) 2.06–7.31)
- Multiple pregnancy
- Caesarean delivery (RR 12.5, 95% CI 6.25–25.8).

Data from UK Obstetric Surveillance System.

placenta praevia, placental abruption, eclampsia, fetal distress, and hyperstimulation

Some observational studies have suggested that mothers carrying a male fetus are at higher risk of AFE. This could corroborate similar postulates that rhesus or ABO incompatibilities may be a factor in the development of AFE.[20]

One of the concerns about cell salvage in the obstetric setting has been the possibility that it could lead to AFE. That has not been the case either in the literature or clinical practice. Cell salvage should therefore not be seen as a risk factor for AFE (see Chapter 35).

Presentation

Cases of AFE have been reported prior to labour, during and after normal labour, after instrumental delivery, and after caesarean delivery. Less commonly, AFE can occur during uterine evacuation and amniocentesis.

Maternal signs and symptoms may include dyspnoea, loss of consciousness, cough, wheeze, headache, chest pain, cyanosis, hypoxia, hypotension, cardiac arrhythmia, cardiopulmonary arrest, seizure and signs of heart failure, and/or pulmonary oedema (Box 38.3). Less specific symptoms may include premonitory feelings, restlessness, agitation, numbness, tingling and seizures. In many women, one of these presentations will quickly evolve into maternal collapse. As such, AFE should be at the forefront of any differential diagnosis when presented with this obstetric emergency. Fetal monitoring, if running, is likely to show fetal compromise.

Immediate treatment

A working diagnosis of AFE should be considered in any women displaying any of the symptoms just described in the 'Presentation' section during labour and postpartum, or after any surgical evacuation of the uterus which cannot be explained by an alternative diagnosis. Clark and others have best summarized this as an ABCD approach to the collapsed pregnant with Airway, Breathing, Circulation, and Delivery being the key elements.[15,21] The patient must be wedged as a priority if still pregnant as aortocaval compression will worsen the cardiovascular collapse.

Box 38.3 Consider AFE in the presence of:

- Acute fetal compromise
- Cardiac arrest
- Cardiac dysrhythmias
- Coagulopathy
- Hypotension
- Maternal haemorrhage (with evidence of early coagulopathy or cardiorespiratory compromise)
- Premonitory symptoms, e.g. restlessness, numbness, agitation, and tingling
- Seizure
- Shortness of breath.

Call for help

Any maternal collapse requires the immediate expertise of senior obstetricians, midwives, anaesthetists at the bedside, and the support of critical care and haematology departments. Get help immediately.

Ensure airway patency

In the event of collapse, gravid women's airways are at particular risk of airway compromise and of subsequent complications such as Mendelson's syndrome owing to delayed gastric emptying. Concerns regarding the airway changes of pregnancy are reviewed in Chapter 26. Cardiopulmonary resuscitation (CPR), should it be warranted, raises intra-abdominal pressure thus increasing the risk. Practitioners must maintain airway patency. Consider immediate intubation especially if the patient is still pregnant, requires CPR, or is at risk of cardiorespiratory collapse (e.g. profound hypoxia).

Maintain oxygenation

In spontaneously breathing patients, apply high-flow oxygen (>12 L/min) via a non-rebreathing mask with a reservoir bag. As the gravid uterus displaces abdominal viscera, pulmonary functional reserve capacity typically decreases by 20% in pregnancy.[22] A progesterone-mediated physiological rise in respiratory rate throughout pregnancy, means that patients already have an increased minute alveolar volume despite typical 4 cm diaphragmatic displacement.[23] In the presence of respiratory distress, pregnant patients therefore have reduced compensatory mechanisms. The management of hypoxia must therefore be acutely and aggressively managed in proportion with the clinical picture. Symptoms (dyspnoea, collapse), signs (tachypnoea, cyanosis), and monitoring (pulse oximetry, arterial blood gas) should guide care. Invasive positive pressure ventilation via a cuffed endotracheal tube is required in cases of severe respiratory distress, or imminent or actual cardiorespiratory arrest. Consider the use of positive end-expiratory pressure, particularly in the presence of cardiogenic and non-cardiogenic pulmonary oedema.

Cardiovascular support

Women with AFE are prone to sudden circulatory collapse secondary to acute right heart failure, left heart failure, cardiac arrhythmias, pulmonary embolism, and sudden fluid shifts associated with massive haemorrhage and/or disseminated intravascular coagulation. CPR must be started immediately in case of cardiac arrest.

Despite there being no robust evidence of benefit to the arrested mother, delivery should be expedited as a necessary adjunct to maximize the effectiveness of CPR. An accepted threshold within UK practice is that if CPR is proving unsuccessful after 3 minutes, action to deliver the fetus should be taken.[21] Perimortem caesarean delivery of a viable fetus is a time-critical intervention with reported fetal outcomes varying from 67% intact survival to 0% survival if the fetus is delivered respectively within 5, or beyond 35, minutes of maternal arrest.[3] However, this kind of intervention should be performed to aide maternal treatment, regardless of fetal condition, including fetuses which have already died *in utero*.

Continuous monitoring and aggressive management form the basis of personalized cardiovascular support of patients with AFE.

If still pre-delivery, a left lateral tilt remains indicated. Monitoring should include a continuous electrocardiogram (ECG) and invasive blood pressure in a suitable critical care environment, with urgent bloods taken for full blood count, coagulation, urea and electrolytes, and crossmatching. Cardiac output monitors and transoesophageal echocardiography may provide valuable information in the management of AFE-induced shock. Supportive care should be individualized and may include two large-bore intravenous cannulae, replacing intravascular fluid loss with crystalloid, colloid and blood products. Identified arrhythmias should be treated, with particular consideration of the possibility of abnormal electrolytes. Vasopressor, chronotropic, and/or inotropic support will be guided by cardiac output monitoring. The use of cardiopulmonary bypass, extracorporeal membrane oxygenation, and intra-aortic balloon pump devices have all been reported in the management of AFE-induced cardiovascular collapse.[24]

Delivery of the fetus

If CPR is being performed, its success will be impaired by the gravid uterus making chest compression difficult and reducing cardiac venous return despite left lateral tilt. There is good evidence that pregnant women are more vulnerable to hypoxic brain injury in the event of circulatory collapse.[21] High-quality CPR is therefore paramount in preventing such injures should the women survive. To this end, if CPR has not been successful after 3 minutes, plans for immediate delivery should be made, with the aim of delivering by 5 minutes. CPR should not be interrupted wherever possible.

The fetus is also at risk, but this is of secondary concern to maternal well-being. The fetus is at risk of significant mortality or morbidity. The known UK case series cohort is small but suggests that survival is 50/50 if born to a dead mother, rising to over 70% if born to a live women.[15]

If instrumental delivery is not possible, an emergency caesarean delivery should be performed. Considerations of sterility and precise anatomical dissection are secondary, to expediting delivery, and an obstetrician will only need a scalpel. A modified Joel–Cohen or similar technique could be used, or whatever the clinician feels most comfortable with. To this end, a disposable scalpel should be on the resuscitation trolley in every clinical area that pregnant women can present.

Delivery of the fetus, though necessary, is likely to compound the problems presented by DIC. Haemorrhage is likely to ensue. The full armamentarium of postpartum haemorrhage treatments should be employed (see Chapter 35).

A significant proportion of women will need a hysterectomy (20%) and early recourse to hysterectomy is reasonable. The other systemic effects of AFE mean that early cessation of any haemorrhage is a priority to optimize maternal outcome.

Intermediate treatment

Correct hypoperfusion

Consider cardiac output monitoring, especially in the presence of pulmonary oedema, haemodynamic instability, or end-organ hypoperfusion. Liaise with obstetricians, intensivists, other anaesthetists, and cardiologists for ongoing support. These professionals are vital in planning continuing care should the woman survive the initial insult.

Correct coagulopathy

Early transfusion of blood and blood products is often required in managing AFE. Liaise early with senior haematologists to prepare for and treat DIC with fresh frozen plasma, cryoprecipitate, platelets, and red blood cells. The aim of management should be to re-establish and maintain normal coagulation profiles. Point-of-care testing such as thromboelastography will help individualize care (see Chapter 48).

In the UKOSS survey of AFE, seven women with confirmed AFE were successfully treated with plasma exchange transfusion. It is believed that removal of cytokines, cellular debris, and coagulation by-products may moderate and shorten the impact of the humoral response. Any acidosis, hypocalcaemia, and hypothermia should also be corrected. Due to the small numbers of women involved we do not have definitive evidence of additional survival or reduced morbidity.

Uterine tone

In instances of concurrent postpartum haemorrhage, whether this is in the presence of DIC or not, consideration must be given to the use of uterotonic agents in order to limit blood loss and maintain a circulating volume. Surgical options, including emergency hysterectomies, have been used when required.

Further investigation

Obtain a chest X-ray. In many cases of AFE, the appearances of the chest X-ray of women show a shadowing consistent with ARDS, however this seems to improve within a short space of time.[14]

Retrospective diagnosis

Classically, AFE was diagnosed by the presence of fetal squames found in maternal circulation postmortem; however, with AFE survival rates increasing, diagnosis is increasingly clinical. A maternal collapse can be caused by a number of differential diagnoses (see Box 38.4).[24–26]

In the immediate milieu surrounding the management of a maternal collapse due to any of the situations in Box 38.4, treatment will overlap regardless of diagnosis, and uncertainty should not delay treatment. After immediate resuscitation, diagnosis regains importance, some causes may require reversal through particular treatment. Diagnosis of AFE is principally one of exclusion. Thus an ECG should be performed (if not already done), and a repeat arterial blood gas, full blood count, and clotting profile are required along with liver function tests and serum electrolytes. An echocardiogram should be considered to exclude myocardial problems. Similarly a ventilation perfusion scan or computed tomography pulmonary angiogram will diagnose or exclude abnormalities such as a pulmonary embolism.

Zinc coproporphyrin and tryptase levels are not used in the diagnoses of AFE as conflicting results in their use to aid diagnosis have been published.

Ongoing management

If not already involved, senior intensive care input is invaluable. After an episode of maternal collapse and successful resuscitation, transfer to intensive care is inevitable and the only treatment available for AFE is supportive. Failure to provide such care reduces survival. In such an environment women can be closely

Box 38.4 Differential diagnosis of the collapsed gravid patient

Obstetric causes

- Placental abruption
- Uterine rupture
- Pre-eclampsia/HELLP syndrome
- Peripartum cardiomyopathy
- Uterine atony
- Eclampsia
- Amniotic fluid embolus
- Postpartum haemorrhage

Anaesthetic causes

- High intrathecal anaesthesia
- Local anaesthetic systemic toxicity
- Aspiration
- Local anaesthetic toxicity.

Other causes

- Transfusion reaction
- Pulmonary embolism
- Air embolism
- Anaphylaxis
- Septic shock
- Acute myocardial infarction.

Data from Gist RS, Stafford IP, Leibowitz AB, Beilin Y, Amniotic fluid embolism, *Anesthesia & Analgesia*, volume 108, issue 5, pp. 1599–602, copyright © 2009 Wolters Kluwer and Davies S, Amniotic fluid embolus: a review of literature. *Canadian Journal of Anesthesia*, volume 48, pp. 88–98, copyright © 2001 Springer.

monitored, using invasive techniques if necessary, and receive one-to-one nursing care, with the option of treatments for complications such as diuretics, inotropes, and steroids. The timing of movement to an intensive care unit should be discussed with the specialists involved and is likely to follow initial resuscitation. Some units may have the facilities and expertise to provide level one intensive care on the labour ward, but outreach support from intensivists is paramount.

Following initial fluid resuscitation inotropic support should be considered in the event of declining cardiac function.[10] Pulmonary artery monitoring will sometimes be necessary. Once the blood pressure has improved, fluid restriction may act to prevent iatrogenic overload. On the basis that AFE resembles an anaphylactoid process, use of adrenaline and hydrocortisone has been suggested. There is no supportive literature on this point.

Documentation

Good documentation should be clear, concise, and contemporaneous where possible. High-dependency maternity charts improve care by prompting carers for important observations on a regular basis and collating results allowing trends and changes to be identified. Contemporaneous reporting of AFE and maternal collapse is also important, not only for the internal hospital risk reporting but for national data collection. Critical information will include possible precipitant factors, complications, resuscitation timing, and neonatal outcomes.

Nationally, if AFE is suspected or maternal collapse occurs, the case should be reported to UKOSS. This can be done online at http://www.npeu.ox.ac.uk/ukoss. If the woman does not survive, her death should be reported to the confidential enquiry (MBRRACE) which can be found at http://www.npeu.ox.ac.uk/mbrrace-uk.

Conclusion

Despite being first recognized nearly 90 years ago, AFE remains an acute obstetric emergency which carries a high morbidity and mortality. The mainstay of treatment continues to be supportive care of all affected organ systems. The use of prompt supportive treatment, invasive monitoring, and individually tailored care of respiratory, cardiovascular, and haematological complications maximizes each woman's chance of survival and provides an increasing knowledge base about AFE. Multiprofessional expertise must be sought immediately when managing acutely unwell pregnant patients. Owing to thankfully low disease incidence, ongoing surveillance and reporting of all AFE cases to national registrars, such as UKOSS in the United Kingdom, remains a research priority for the benefit of families worldwide.

References

1. Meyer JR. Embolia pulmonar amnio caseosa. *Bra Med* 1926; 2:301–3.
2. Steiner PE, Lushbaugh CC. Maternal pulmonary embolism by amniotic fluid as a cause of obstetric shock and unexpected deaths in obstetrics. *JAMA* 1941; 117:1245–54, 1341–5.
3. Clark SL, Hankins GS, Dudley DA, *et al.* Amniotic fluid embolism: analysis of the national registry. *Am J Obstet Gynaecol* 1995; 172:1158–67.
4. Knight M, Tuffnell D, Brocklehurst P, *et al.* Incidence and risk factors for amniotic fluid embolism. *Obstet Gynecol* 2010; 115:910–17.
5. Sullivan EA, Hall B, King JF. *Maternal deaths in Australia 2003–2005.* Maternal Deaths Series No. 3. Cat. No. PER 42. Sydney: AIHW National Perinatal Statistics Unit; 2007. http://www.aihw.gov.au/WorkArea/DownloadAsset.aspx?id=10737421514
6. Roberts C, Algert C, Knight M, *et al.* Amniotic fluid embolism in an Australian population-based cohort. *Br J Obstet Gynaecol* 2010; 117:1417–21.
7. Kramer MS, Rouleau J, Baskett TF, *et al.* Amniotic-fluid embolism and medical induction of labour: a retrospective, population-based cohort study. *Lancet* 2006; 368:1444–8.
8. Centre for Maternal and Child Enquiries (CMACE). Saving Mothers' Lives: Reviewing Maternal Deaths to make Motherhood Safer—2006–2008. The Eighth Report on Confidential Enquiries into Maternal Deaths in the United Kingdom. *Br J Obstet Gynaecol* 2011; 118 Suppl 1):1–208.
9. Berg CJ, Callaghan WM, Syverson C, *et al.* Pregnancy-related mortality in the United States, 1998 to 2005. *Obstet Gynecol* 2010; 116(6):1302–9.
10. Clark SL. Amniotic fluid embolism. *Crit Care Clin* 1991; 7:877–82.
11. Morgan M. Amniotic fluid embolism. *Anaesthesia* 1979; 34:20–32.
12. Conde-Agudelo A, Romero R. Amniotic fluid embolism: an evidence-based review. *Am J Obstet Gynecol* 2009; 201:445.e1–13.

13. Margarson MP. Delayed amniotic fluid embolism following caesarean section under spinal anaesthesia. *Anaesthesia* 1995; 50(9):804–6.
14. Tuffnell DJ. United Kingdom amniotic fluid embolism register. *Br J Obstet Gynaecol* 2005; 112:1625–9.
15. Dildy GA, Clark SL. Anaphylactoid syndrome of pregnancy (amniotic fluid embolus). In Dildy GA, Belfort MA, Saade GR, *et al.* (eds) *Critical Care Obstetrics* (4th ed). Oxford: Blackwell Science; 2008:466–74.
16. Leighton BL, Wall MH, Lockhart EM, *et al.* Use of recombinant factor VIIa in patients with amniotic fluid embolism: a systematic review of case reports. *Anesthesiology* 2011; 115(6):1201–8.
17. Hankins GD, Snyder RR, Clark SL, *et al.* Acute hemodynamic and respiratory effects of amniotic fluid embolism in the pregnant goat model. *Am J Obstet Gynecol* 1993; 168(4):1113–29.
18. Shechtman M, Ziser A, Markovits R, *et al.* Amniotic fluid embolism: early findings of transesophageal echocardiography. *Anesth Analg* 1999; 89(6):1456–8.
19. Moore J, Baldisseri MR. Amniotic fluid embolism. *Crit Care Med* 2005; 33(10 Suppl):S279–85.
20. Powrie RO, MF Greene MF, Camann W (eds). *de Swiet's Medical Disorders in Obstetric Practice* (5th ed). Hoboken, NJ: Wiley-Blackwell; 2010.
21. Royal College of Obstetricians and Gynaecologists. *Maternal Collapse in Pregnancy and the Puerperium*. Green-top Guideline No. 56. London: RCOG; 2011.
22. Reitman E, Flood P. Anaesthetic considerations for non-obstetric surgery during pregnancy. *Br J Anaesth* 2011; 107 Suppl 1:i72–8.
23. Heidemann BH, McClure JH. Changes in maternal physiology during pregnancy. *CEACCP CEPD Reviews* 2003; 3:65–8.
24. Gist RS, Stafford IP, Leibowitz AB, *et al.* Amniotic fluid embolism. *Anesth Analg* 2009; 108(5):1599–602.
25. Davies S. Amniotic fluid embolus: a review of literature. *Can J Anaesth* 2001; 48:88–98.
26. Tuffnell D, Knight M, Plaat F. Amniotic fluid embolism—an update. *Anaesthesia* 2011; 66(1):3–6.

PART 9

Systemic disease in pregnancy

CHAPTER 39

The obese parturient

Fiona C. Denison and Alistair Milne

The global phenomenon of obesity

Obesity is defined by the World Health Organization (WHO) as a body mass index (BMI) greater than 30 kg/m^2 (Table 39.1).[1] Although obesity has been prevalent throughout human history, the rising prevalence of obesity in developed and more recently in developing countries[2] is a relatively recent phenomenon. The exponential rise in obesity across the world ('globesity') has prompted the WHO to describe it as one of the most important global health problems today, estimating that by 2020, two-thirds of the global burden of disease will be due to non-communicable diseases associated with diet.[1,3]

The aetiology of obesity is complex and multifactorial with increasing urbanization,[4] social deprivation,[5,6] greater use of sugar-sweetened drinks and edible oils, a reduction in physical activity, increase in sedentary lifestyle, and developmental exposure to endocrine disruptors[7] being some of the factors implicated in causing the current global epidemic.

Amongst developed countries, recent estimates for the prevalence of obesity amongst adults are 26% in England,[8] 24% in Canada,[9] and 36% in the United States.[10] In developing countries, the prevalence of obesity is also rising with more women than men being obese.[2,11] In 2008, overweight and obesity were estimated to affect 1.6 billion adults worldwide. Although more recent data suggest a slowing or levelling out of obesity prevalence in some countries (including the United States),[10] the prevalence continues to rise rapidly in other countries. By 2030, it is therefore estimated that 1.12 billion adults will be obese and a further 2.16 billion will be overweight.

The incidence of maternal obesity lags behind that of the general population, primarily due to the relationship between obesity and impaired fertility and age at peak prevalence of obesity. Despite this, maternal obesity is now the commonest pre-existing morbidity in pregnant women in the United Kingdom with an estimated one in five pregnant women being obese.[12,13] In the United States, given that one in three women are obese,[10] the prevalence of obesity in pregnancy is even higher.

Obesity is associated with increased risk of maternal and offspring morbidity and mortality antenatally, intrapartum, and postnatally (Table 39.2).[14–17,156–162] Although it has been suggested that limiting maternal weight gain during pregnancy may reduce the excess maternal and offspring risk associated with maternal obesity (Table 39.3),[18] this is debated and there is currently insufficient evidence to recommend any particular intervention or weight gain targets.[19]

Women with pre-gravid obesity also have higher rates of coronary artery disease, non-alcoholic fatty liver, diabetes mellitus, hypertension, gallbladder disease, and depression. The offspring of obese mothers are at greater risk of long-term health problems including early-onset obesity and hypertension.[20]

From a practical perspective, maternal obesity poses significant technical challenges including availability of appropriate equipment and practical issues such as moving and handling. All anaesthetists and obstetricians, from those with a special interest in high-risk obstetric anaesthesia and obstetrics, to those covering the delivery suite out of hours, will therefore inevitably encounter maternal obesity.[21] It is therefore essential that all clinicians have the knowledge and expertise to manage the anaesthetic implications of maternal obesity and its obstetric complications during pregnancy and labour.

Physiological changes of obesity

The respiratory system

Obesity has several significant effects on lung function. The most marked of these is the change in functional residual capacity (FRC) which decreases in an exponential manner with increasing BMI.[22] This is due to a mass effect of adipose tissue on the chest wall, abdomen, around the viscera, and diaphragm. In the obese, this decreased FRC encroaches on the closing volume which leads to the closure of small airways during normal breathing and is associated with ventilation/perfusion mismatch, leading to reduced oxygen saturation.[23] Figure 39.1 shows the effect of obesity on lung volumes. The decrease in FRC also means that obese patients are breathing in the less compliant part of the pressure volume curve. Increased effort is required to overcome the respiratory system elasticity at these reduced lung volumes.[24] Residual volume usually shows little change, therefore expiratory reserve volume is significantly decreased. Total lung capacity shows a small decrease with increasing BMI.[25]

Compliance of the respiratory system also decreases, partly due to a decrease in chest wall compliance. This is again due to adipose tissue loading on the chest wall, abdomen, and diaphragm.[26] A decrease in lung compliance may also be the result of an increased pulmonary blood volume,[25] along with the reduction in FRC.

Forced expiratory volume in 1 second (FEV_1) is often reduced in morbid obesity, but the FEV_1/forced vital capacity ratio is often normal, thereby showing a mild restrictive defect.[26] However Lazarus et al. found an obstructive pattern that worsened with increasing BMI.[27] These factors result in an increased work of breathing in a population who have ventilation/perfusion mismatch causing reduced oxygen saturations. The obese patient is also well recognized to have increased oxygen consumption.[28]

Table 39.1 Classification of body mass index according to World Health Organization criteria

Classification	Body mass index (kg/m²)
Underweight	<18.5
Normal weight	18.6–24.9
Overweight	25.0–29.9
Obesity I	30.0–34.9
Obesity II	35.0–39.9
Obesity III	≥40.0

Reprinted from *Obesity: Preventing and managing the global epidemic.* Report of a WHO Consultation (WHO Technical Report Series 894), WHO, p. i–xii, Copyright (2000).

Obesity can lead to obesity hypoventilation syndrome and is also associated with sleep apnoea. These two conditions share many physiological and pathological features. Abnormal ventilatory drive, hypoventilation, and hypoxia lead to pulmonary vasoconstriction, which can in turn result in pulmonary hypertension.[26] This can exacerbate the cardiovascular pathology of obesity discussed in the following section.

The cardiovascular system

Obese patients have an increased blood volume and cardiac output in response to the increased metabolic requirements of excess fat. Cardiac output increases by 50 mL/min for every extra 100 g of fat.[29] This can lead to left ventricular dilatation, hypertrophy, and diastolic dysfunction. Systolic dysfunction may also occur due to fat deposition in the myocardial fibres. Left ventricular afterload is also raised due to increased peripheral resistance.[30] Pulmonary hypertension related to obesity hypoventilation syndrome can lead to the right ventricle being affected in a similar way. The above changes can lead to heart failure, and are collectively the changes of obesity cardiomyopathy.[31,32] Obese subjects have double the risk of heart failure of those with a normal BMI.[33] The increase in cardiac workload that leads to obesity cardiomyopathy is exacerbated by the increase in plasma volume and cardiac output that occurs in pregnancy, further reducing cardiovascular reserve.

Table 39.2 Risks of obesity in pregnancy

Problem	Level of increased risk
Miscarriage[156,157]	1–3-fold
Fetal abnormality (spina bifida, heart defect, omphalocele)[158]	2–4-fold
Iatrogenic preterm birth[159,160]	1.5–2-fold
Gestational diabetes[14,16]	4-fold
Venous thromboembolism[161]	3–4-fold
Pre-eclampsia[57]	2-fold
Induction of labour[14,16]	2-fold
Caesarean section1[4,16]	2-fold
Postpartum haemorrhage[16]	1–2-fold
Infection (wound, urinary tract, genital tract)[16]	2-fold
Stillbirth[162]	1–5-fold
Maternal death[107]	Increased

Data from various sources (see references).

Table 39.3 Institute of Medicine recommendations for weight gain during pregnancy, by pre-pregnancy BMI

Pre-pregnancy BMI	BMI (kg/m²)	Total weight gain range (lbs)/(kg)[a]
Underweight	<18.5	28–40/12.5–18
Normal weight	18.6–24.9	25–35/11.5–16
Overweight	25.0–29.9	15–25/7–11.5
Obese (includes all classes)	≥30.0	11–20/5–9

[a]Weight gain during pregnancy.

Reprinted with permission from *Weight Gain During Pregnancy: Reexamining the Guidelines*, K.M. Rasmussen and A.L. Yaktine (Editors), 2009, by the National Academy of Sciences, Courtesy of the National Academies Press, Washington, D.C.

Obesity is also a risk factor for hypertension[34] and coronary heart disease.[35] A significant number of asymptomatic obese patients have ischaemic changes on their electrocardiogram. Echocardiography may be used as an assessment of myocardial function in these patients,[36,37] but quality of scans is often poor due to the increased layers of adipose on the chest wall. Gestational hypertension and pre-eclampsia are also more common in the obese.[38]

Obese women are more susceptible to supine hypotensive syndrome in late pregnancy and require to be carefully positioned. Tsueda et al.[39] described obesity supine death syndrome in the super morbidly obese non-pregnant patient, where death on lying supine probably occurs due to a combination of aortocaval compression causing a sudden reduction in venous return, coupled with hypoxaemia, resulting in cardiac arrest.

The gastrointestinal system

Obese patients have an increase in residual gastric contents[40] and hiatus hernia is common. Coupled with the hormonal changes of pregnancy that lead to an increased risk of gastro-oesophageal reflux, it is probable that the obese are at higher risk of pulmonary aspiration of gastric contents.

The endocrine system

An increased BMI is the strongest risk factor for developing type 2 diabetes mellitus,[41] and gestational diabetes mellitus (GDM) is more common in the obese.[42]

Pharmacology

Pharmacokinetics

Despite the current prevalence and increasing rate of obesity, pharmacokinetic data in obesity is available for a very limited number of drugs.

The obese do not simply have an increased amount of fat. They also have an increase in lean body weight which can be as much as 40% of their excess weight.[43] This means that drug doses based on

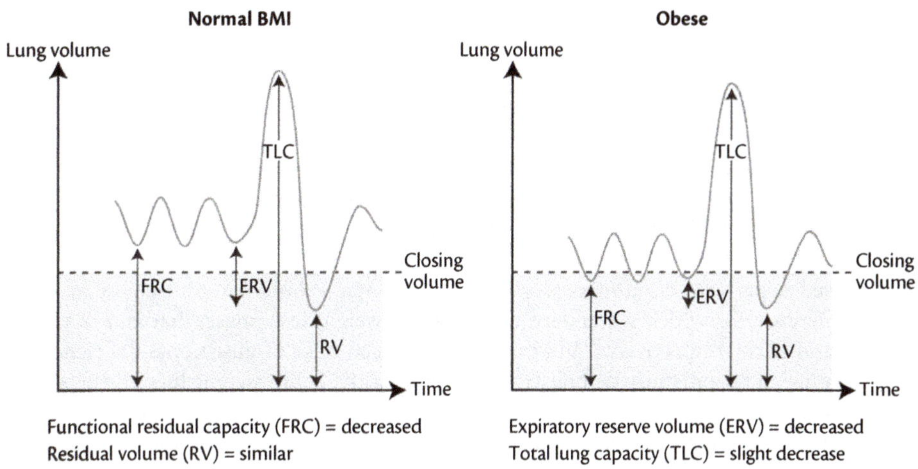

Figure 39.1 The effect of obesity on lung volumes. A decreased functional residual capacity (FRC) encroaching on closing volume is largely at the expense of a decreased expiratory reserve volume (ERV).

their ideal body weight may result in under-dosing. Calculation of lean body weight is not routine in clinical practice, although equations exist to allow its estimation.[44] Due to its relationship with cardiac output, lean body weight is important in the early distribution kinetics of drugs.[45] Therefore a morbidly obese patient with an increased lean body weight and cardiac output will require an increase in initial dosing of some drugs.

The volume of distribution (Vd) is a determinant of drug loading-dose selection.[46] The Vd of a drug can be significantly altered in obesity, dependent on its hydrophilic or lipophilic nature. Hydrophilic drugs do not widely distribute into fat, and their Vd is therefore more dependent on ideal body weight. Total body weight has much more of an influence on lipophilic drugs that distribute extensively into fat.[47] This, however, is a generalization that does not hold true for all drugs, nor even all drugs of a similar group. Information should always be sought for a specific drug, if it is available. Wurtz et al.[48] discuss calculating ideal body weight and then using a 'dosing weight correction factor'—a fraction of the difference between actual and ideal body weights—to achieve a weight on which to base antimicrobial dosing. This correction factor differs dependent on the lipophilic or hydrophilic nature of the antibiotic in question. With no correction factor employed in the morbidly and super morbidly obese, therapeutic tissue levels of antibiotics are often not achieved.[49]

Plasma protein binding is another determinant of Vd. Drug binding to albumin does not appear to be affected by obesity. However, data as to whether drug binding to α_1-acid glycoprotein is affected has been contradictory.[46]

Selection of a maintenance dose regimen is primarily determined by drug clearance. Varying hepatic and renal changes have been postulated to result in changes to drug clearance in the obese. Some have shown changes in clearance suggesting an increase in cytochrome P450 activity, others an increase in phase II conjugation pathways such as glucuronidation and sulphation.[46] Glomerular filtration has been shown to increase in some studies, yet decrease in others.[50] Again, data on the effects of obesity on drug clearance is very limited, although clearance does increase proportionately with increasing lean body weight.[51] Changes in clearance may be the result of obesity itself, or a result of disease processes associated with obesity.

Pharmacodynamics

Morbid obesity can alter the pharmacodynamic profile of some drugs. For example, the morbidly obese patient with sleep apnoea can be very sensitive to the side effects of opiates, resulting in increased episodes of hypoxia. This effectively narrows the therapeutic window of the drug.

Further information on specific drugs can be found in the general anaesthesia section of this chapter.

Obesity and pregnancy

Maternal obesity is associated with increased risk of short- and long-term morbidity and mortality for both mother and offspring. Some of this excess morbidity is due to significant pre-existing morbidities such as essential hypertension and GDM.[52,53] However, much of the disease burden is due to increased risk of complications, such as pre-eclampsia, developing *de novo* during pregnancy due to maternal obesity. These complications in isolation have implications for obstetric and anaesthetic management.

Pre-existing morbidity

Obesity is associated with higher risk for pre-existing medical complications including chronic hypertension, type 2 diabetes, non-alcoholic fatty liver disease, and asthma.[15] For chronic hypertension, the incidence is 12-fold higher in a study of 117 severely obese women compared to normal weight control by term (24% vs 2%, respectively).[54] Pre-existing medical complications increase the risk of developing pregnancy-specific morbidities such as pre-eclampsia during pregnancy. Due to greater utilization of healthcare resources, pre-existing and *de novo* onset of disease have substantial resource implications for healthcare providers.[55]

De novo morbidity during pregnancy

Maternal obesity increases the risk of hypertensive disorders of pregnancy. In nulliparous women, the risk of gestational hypertension is estimated to be 2.5 times greater for obese and 3.2 times greater with severe obesity.[56] For pre-eclampsia, the risk doubles for each 5–7 kg/m^2 increase in weight over normal[57] being 1.6 times and 3.3 times higher in obese and severely obese women, respectively.[56] In women with pre-existing essential hypertension, the risk of developing pre-eclampsia is up to 25%.[58]

Pre-eclampsia causes significant maternal morbidity and is the most common indication for medically indicated pre-term delivery by caesarean delivery. Diagnosis of pre-eclampsia depends on an accurate measurement of blood pressure, which can be challenging in obese women. To measure blood pressure correctly, it is essential that an appropriately sized cuff be used with the cuff bladder encircling at least 80% of the arm. In obese women, this can be difficult due to increased upper arm circumference. The maximum upper arm circumference for which a standard and large cuff can be used is 28 cm and 48 cm, respectively.[59] In women with a BMI greater than 30 kg/m^2, a recent study demonstrated that 44% needed a large cuff with this rising to 100% in women with a BMI greater than 40 kg/m^2.[60] Even for some women, a large cuff may still be too small. Although the thigh cuff can be used up to a maximum arm circumference of 52 cm, it is not available in all settings and the brachial artery is often obscured after bladder inflation due to the width of the cuff. Given that there is a direct relationship between upper arm circumference and maternal BMI during pregnancy,[61] the diagnosis of pre-eclampsia and other hypertensive disorders and their subsequent anaesthetic management will be affected if the correct cuff size is not used. The Pre-eclampsia Community Guidelines (PRECOG) guidelines therefore advise a different size of cuff depending on arm circumference (Table 39.2).[62] The diagnosis of hypertensive disorders of pregnancy is often further complicated in obese women due to the presence of co-morbidities such as pre-existing hypertension, renal compromise, non-alcoholic fatty liver, and diabetes which can mask diagnostic signs. This diagnostic uncertainty can prove challenging to the anaesthetist particularly when delivery by caesarean section is required.

GDM is also much more common in obese women. Although as a single risk factor, obesity has a low predictive value, the unadjusted odds ratio (OR) for developing GDM for overweight, moderately obese, and severely obese were estimated as being 1.97 (95% confidence interval (CI) 1.77–2.19), 3.01 (95% CI 2.34–3.87), and 5.55 (95% CI 4.27–7.21), respectively.[63] Although the evidence base is lacking, recent UK national guidelines[64,65] recommend that women with GDM should be delivered by term and that induction of labour should be considered if spontaneous labour does not occur. GDM is an independent risk factor for caesarean delivery and many obese women with GDM will therefore require anaesthetic input intrapartum.[66]

Maternal obesity is also associated with increased risks of 'minor complications' of pregnancy with higher BMI during the first trimester (BMI ≥ 30 kg/m^2 compared with BMI < 25 kg/m^2) including symphysis pubis dysfunction (OR 3.97; 95% CI 2.19–7.18), heartburn (OR 2.65; 95% CI 1.42–4.94), and chest infection (OR 8.71; 95% 2.20–34.44) and with drugs used to treat these complications including Gaviscon® (OR 3.52; 95% CI 1.78–6.96). Although for an individual woman the burden of disease may be relatively low, at a population level, the burden is substantial due to these conditions being relatively common.

Pregnancy after bariatric surgery: obstetric implications

Bariatric surgery is recognized as the most effective treatment for weight loss in morbidly obese patients.[67] For many women it may be the only way to attain healthy BMI, achieve better regulated hormones, and improve fertility. Pregnancies conceived following bariatric surgery have a reduced risk of GDM, pregnancy-induced hypertension, and pre-eclampsia.[68] However, these benefits need to be balanced by the increased risk of preterm and small-for-gestational-age births[69] and nutritional deficiencies[70] in women. Women with a history of bariatric surgery should therefore be regarded as a high-risk group during pregnancy regardless of their BMI.[69]

Women should be advised to avoid pregnancy during the acute weight loss phase, that is, 1–2 years postoperatively due to increased risks of nutritional deficiencies.[71] Whether conception during the acute weight loss phase is associated with increased risk of adverse pregnancy outcomes is less certain. Although earlier studies suggested an increased risk of premature birth and spontaneous miscarriage in pregnancies conceived within 2 years of a gastric bypass, more recent studies have failed to demonstrate an excess in maternal and perinatal complications.

The three most common bariatric surgical procedures are laparoscopic adjustable gastric banding, laparoscopic sleeve gastrectomy and laparoscopic Roux-en-Y bypass. Laparoscopic adjustable gastric banding is a restrictive procedure that comprises of a silicone band that encircles the proximal stomach, creating a pouch at the top of the stomach. This is connected by a fine-bore tube to a subcutaneously placed port, attached to the abdominal muscle. The band's inner surface has the ability to be inflated thus exerting pressure on the stomach and restricting the passage of food from the proximal stomach to the larger part of the stomach. The band inflation or decompression is carried out by injecting or withdrawing saline solution through the port using a syringe and Huber needle.

Laparoscopic sleeve gastrectomy is a restrictive procedure which involves surgical stapling along the longitudinal reservoir of the stomach following the line of the lesser curve from the cardiac sphincter to the pylorus. This provides a stomach sleeve of approximately 150 mL capacity. The fundus and greater curve of the stomach are then surgically removed.

The laparoscopic Roux-en-Y bypass is both a restrictive and malabsorptive procedure. It involves fashioning a small gastric pouch of 20–50 mL capacity; the remainder of the stomach is detached and left *in situ*. Approximately 150 cm of the small intestine is surgically bypassed so that food from the gastric pouch empties into the jejunum. The small pouch restricts the amount of food the patient is able to consume and the intestinal bypass of the duodenum provides the malabsorptive effect.

Both restrictive and malabsorptive bariatric surgery are associated with nutritional deficiencies due to a combination of malabsorption, food intolerances, and poor dietary intake. Maternal weight and nutritional status should therefore be assessed at the beginning of pregnancy for women who have had bariatric surgery and identified deficiencies should be treated and monitored.[72] Complications of bariatric surgery such as bowel obstruction, anastomotic leak, and band erosion can be difficult to diagnose because they may present with nausea, vomiting, and abdominal pain which are common features of pregnancy. Early and continuous engagement of bariatric surgeons is therefore recommended throughout pregnancy. Even after bariatric surgery, many patients remain obese and are therefore at increased risk of developing GDM during pregnancy. Patients with malabsorptive procedures will experience dumping following ingestion of the normal glucose used for the oral glucose tolerance test. This is caused by hyperinsulinaemia and hypoglycaemia and manifests clinically as nausea, vomiting, bloating, and diarrhoea. Alternative tests such as a fasting blood glucose or a 2-hour postprandial blood sugar between 24 and 28 weeks may need to be used to diagnose GDM.

Pregnancy after bariatric surgery: anaesthetic implications

Restrictive and malabsorptive gastric procedures, coupled with the anatomical distortion of the stomach in pregnancy, may put parturients at even higher risk of delayed gastric emptying. They should be treated as having a full stomach at all times. The nutritional deficiencies that occur after bariatric surgery can result in anaemia due to iron and vitamin B_{12} deficiency and electrolyte disturbance. Reduction in fat-soluble vitamin absorption can lead to vitamin K deficiency and therefore potentially coagulopathy.[73] Recommendation that pregnancy should be delayed for at least 12–18 months post bariatric surgery may not avoid many of these issues. Iron, vitamin B_{12}, and vitamin K deficiencies are often present several years after surgery.[74] Non-steroidal anti-inflammatory drugs should be avoided due to the increased risk of marginal ulceration in post-bariatric surgery patients.[75] Whilst bariatric surgery may result in a significant loss of excess weight, many patients will still be morbidly obese. Therefore all the problems related to obesity remain.

Anaesthetic management of the obese parturient

Assessment of the obese parturient: the anaesthetic clinic

All women with a BMI over 40 kg/m^2 should be seen prior to labour and delivery by an anaesthetist.[76] Early assessment allows for review of current management of any co-morbidities, further investigations to be carried out, and involvement of other specialties as appropriate in a timely manner. Reduced exercise tolerance may signal a decreased cardiorespiratory reserve and the need for further investigations to aid assessment. Symptoms of sleep apnoea should be investigated as the use of continuous positive airway pressure can reduce hypoxaemic episodes and prevent right ventricular failure.

Airway assessment can identify the potentially difficult airway. The increased incidence of failed intubation in the obstetric population is well recognized—approximately 1:250 compared to 1:2000 in the general population.[77] The risk of difficult intubation in the morbidly obese parturient has been reported to be as high as one in three.[78] Whilst difficult intubation in the non-pregnant obese patient is also high (15.5% by Juvin et al.[79] with BMI > 35 kg/m^2), it is worth noting that a low incidence of significant problems has been reported when there is involvement of senior experienced personnel.[80] Neck circumference is more predictive of difficult intubation than BMI in the morbidly obese.[81]

Assessment of ease of venous access is also useful. Peripheral cannulation can be aided by the use of ultrasound where veins are neither visible nor palpable, but in those with extremely difficult access a central venous line may be required.

Examination of the patient's back will give an early indication as to the ease with which neuraxial analgesia or anaesthesia may be established. In those without a palpable midline or spinous processes, ultrasound (Figure 39.2) may be a useful tool to aid neuraxial analgesia or anaesthesia.

Early assessment of the morbidly obese pregnant patient in the clinic environment also allows explanation of available options. Challenges faced in terms of neuraxial analgesia, and neuraxial and general anaesthesia can be discussed. This will help with managing the mother's expectations, and allow anaesthetic involvement at an early stage of labour should she wish it. An anaesthetic plan should be discussed and documented.[76]

Preparation for the morbidly obese parturient involves many considerations, including equipment. Firstly, a clinic area equipped with patient transport chairs, chairs, and examination couches suitable for morbidly obese patients must be available. Beds must be large and robust enough for the patient. Some delivery suite beds will have a weight limit of around 180 kg, which is also the approximate limit for standard operating tables. Bed hydraulic adjustments must be able to operate effectively. Bariatric operating tables have an upper weight limit of around 450 kg and have appropriate side adjusters to alter the table width. Consideration will need to be given to the method of tilting the patient safely to minimize aortocaval compression. This may involve the use of additional side supports attached to the operating table, or straps to hold the patient in place. Patient hoists and hover mattresses will be necessary for patient movement. Bed mattresses must be specifically designed to minimize the risk to pressure areas. Calf compression stockings and inflatable compression boots must be of appropriate sizes.

Blood pressure cuff should exceed the circumference of the arm by 20% in order to read accurately. However, the extremely conical shaped upper arm that some morbidly obese patients have may still make upper arm non-invasive blood pressure recording impossible. A forearm blood pressure cuff could be used, but their accuracy is not as reliable. Singer et al. found that the differences between forearm and upper arm systolic and diastolic blood pressures were within 20 mmHg in 86% and 94% of patients, respectively in non-obstetric, non-obese subjects.[82] Forearm blood pressures are higher. This would be a useful temporizing measure in an emergency situation, but an arterial line would be preferable, especially in a group where arterial blood gases may be beneficial and venous access poor for peripartum blood samples.

Long spinal epidural needles and combined spinal–epidural (CSE) kits will need to be available. The distance between skin and epidural space increases in a linear fashion with increasing BMI.[83,84] However, Hamza et al.[85] found that—despite this correlation—very few parturients had an epidural space deeper than 8 cm.

Equipment should be available to help achieve optimal patient positioning for intubation. Several commercially available wedge-shaped pillows exist for this purpose (see Figure 39.3). If using these wedges, elevating blocks may require to be secured onto arm boards to bring the board level up to that of the patient's shoulders on the wedge. An ultrasound machine may be helpful to attain peripheral or central intravenous access, or to assist with surface skin marking prior to neuraxial anaesthesia. Equipment may be necessary to suspend or lift the fat pannus to aid surgical access.

Staffing levels will also need to be considered. Extra staff will be required to care for the morbidly obese parturient. Moving

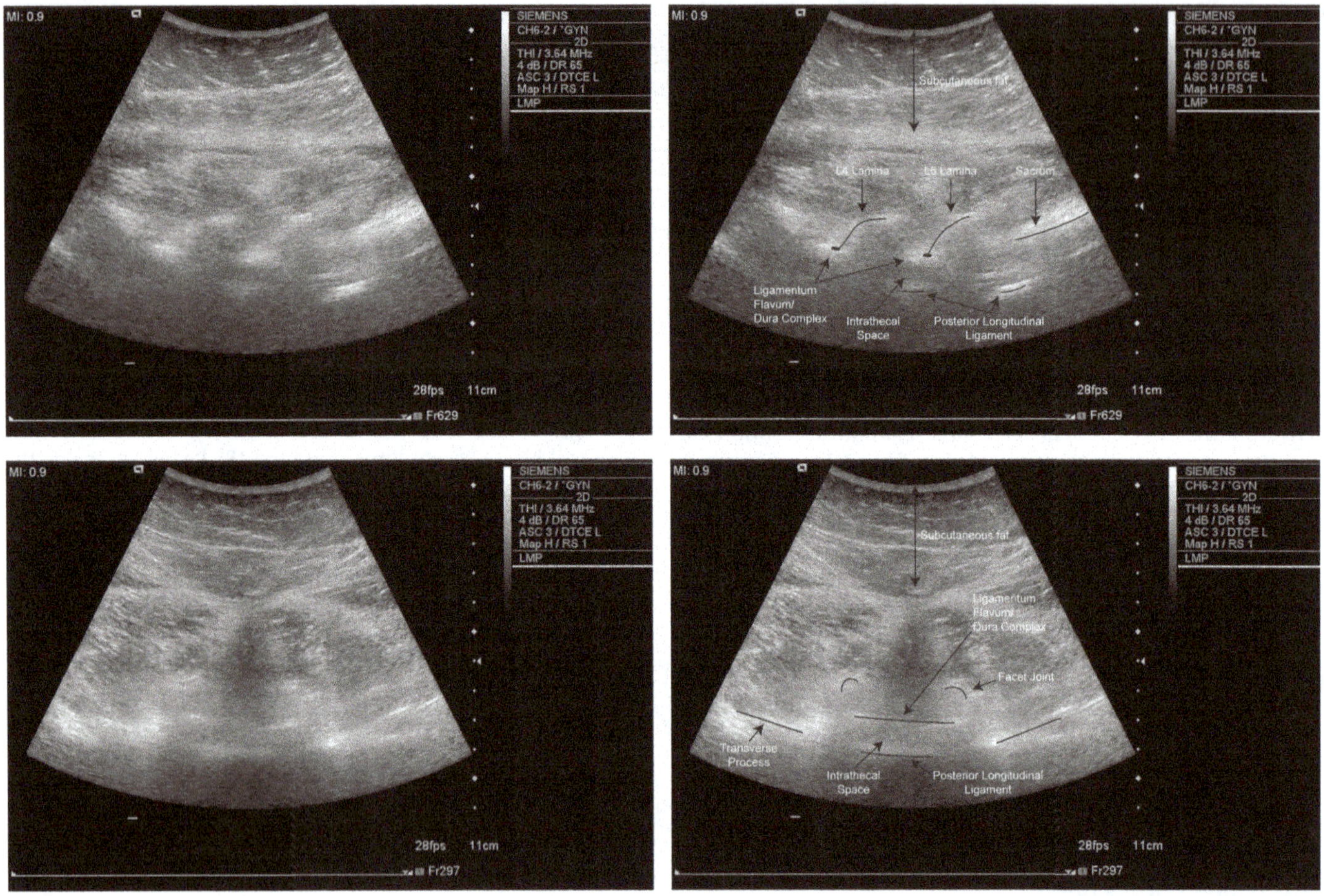

Figure 39.2 Epidural ultrasound images in a patient with BMI > 40 kg/m^2. Top left: paramedian view. Bottom left: transverse view. Right: images repeated with landmarks identified. Note the much poorer quality images obtained in the obese patient compared with those often published from non-obese subjects, due to the layer of subcutaneous fat.

patients may require extra personnel, and those operating hoists need to be familiar with them. Theatre, anaesthetic, and obstetric staffing numbers will all likely need to be increased to assist with the increased technical complexity of morbidly obese patients.

Anaesthetic management in labour

Entonox® and opioids are readily available forms of pain relief in most delivery suites. Both of these have been shown to increase the incidence of hypoxaemia in the morbidly obese[86] and often provide suboptimal analgesia.[87,88]

Epidural analgesia is not only more effective, it also allows conversion to anaesthesia for instrumental or caesarean delivery in a patient population where establishing neuraxial anaesthesia *de novo* could take considerable time and general anaesthesia carries significantly increased risks.

Placement of an epidural catheter can be very challenging and time-consuming in the morbidly obese with more attempts required to site the epidural than in a patient of normal body habitus. Once in place, there is a higher failure rate and an increased likelihood of requiring resited.[54,89] The lack of bony landmarks and increased skin to epidural space distance no doubt contribute to this. Identification of the midline is difficult and any small errors in needle direction will only be magnified by the increased distance traversed by the needle to reach the epidural space. Taking the patient to theatre where the lighting is optimal, the theatre bed rigid, and skilled help is available can all make the insertion easier. Sitting the patient with her pannus between her knees, heels together, and with the table slightly tilted backward to promote her bending forward may also facilitate opening up the lumbar interspaces. Placing the morbidly obese patient on her side for neuraxial block placement is not helpful as the skin folds fall over the midline.

The use of ultrasound imaging to aid epidural insertion can be of great benefit. Ultrasound is used to identify the midline, desired interspace, depth of the epidural space, and needle direction required. Skin surface markings are made to identify needle insertion points and standard techniques then used to insert the epidural. Studies have shown the use of ultrasound to reduce the number of needle punctures and the number of different levels attempted to insert an epidural.[90] They have also shown a decrease in pain scores and an increase in patient satisfaction.[91,92] Vallejo et al. found that ultrasound use prior to epidural insertion for labour analgesia significantly reduced the number of initial attempts taken by first-year trainees and the number of replacements required thereafter.[93] Figure 39.2 shows ultrasound images from a parturient with a BMI greater than 40 kg/m^2. A curved probe is best suited for the obese subject. Real-time insertion is difficult due to the needle and ultrasound beam being parallel rather than perpendicular to each other, so the needle is not easily visualized. Technology is now available that will indicate the needle position on the real-time ultrasound image even when the tip is not visible. This uses multiple position sensors embedded in the probe and needle. Other technologies use a magnetic field and the ferromagnetic properties of the needle to delineate its position on the ultrasound image.

Once successfully inserted, epidurals in the morbidly obese require careful management. Skin to epidural space distance can be altered by a change in patient position.[85] Moving from a sitting, flexed position for insertion to an upright position can result in an indrawing of the catheter at the skin. Carefully sitting the patient upright prior to fixation of the catheter will mean that movement of the catheter occurs inward at the skin rather than the catheter being pulled back out of the epidural space if the change in position is made after fixation. There is increased mobility of the skin over the lumbar spine due to the intervening fat pad. This, coupled with the increased depth from skin to epidural space, means that any movement on the bed could result in the catheter being pulled back out of the space.[94,95] Leaving an increased length of catheter within the epidural space would seem to be a sensible idea. The higher failure rate of epidurals in the morbidly obese dictates that careful attention must be paid to these women and the functioning of their epidurals throughout labour especially as the obstetric intervention rate in obese women is high and the epidural may be needed for anaesthesia.

Remifentanil patient-controlled analgesia (PCA) is a method used for labour analgesia that has become more prevalent in recent years. Epidural analgesia results in lower pain scores than remifentanil PCA.[96,97] However, some studies have shown remifentanil PCA to be similar to epidural analgesia in terms of patient satisfaction.[98] Its use in the morbidly obese must be undertaken with extreme caution. Remifentanil is a potent respiratory depressant. Virtually all studies report patient desaturation with its use,[99] and it has been associated with several incidents of respiratory[100,101] and cardiorespiratory arrest.[102,103] Van de Velde[104] noted that if all studies reporting respiratory side effects are combined, 32% of patients using remifentanil experience some degree of respiratory depression. There is currently no significant data available regarding remifentanil PCA use in the morbidly obese. Its unlicensed use in a subgroup of patients who already have an increased risk of respiratory complications and a narrowed therapeutic window when using opiates should only be undertaken after considerable thought and discussion. If a dosing regimen based on body weight is used, it is imperative that this is based on lean body weight and not total body weight. Due to the pharmacokinetics of the drug, dosing based on total body weight could result in significant overdosing in the morbidly obese. The strict implementation of written local monitoring standards is essential. A recent report highlighted compliance of these in one unit to be 70%, falling to 10% after withdrawal of supervision by their acute pain team.[105] Meticulous attention should therefore be paid to ensure that monitoring—including the continuous presence of an appropriately trained midwife—is instigated appropriately and continues throughout PCA use.

Caesarean delivery

Obstetric issues

There are many factors to consider in the morbidly obese parturient undergoing caesarean delivery. This is a patient population which is at increased risk of morbidity and mortality, both from a global obstetric[11] and anaesthesia-specific perspective, particularly when under general anaesthesia.[106] The 2007 Confidential Enquiries into Maternal and Child Health (CEMACH) report highlighted these increased risks, especially of difficult intubation and aspiration.[107] Wound asepsis is very important as maternal obesity is an independent risk factor for wound infection and subsequent complications including panniculus necrosis.[108] The limited available data suggest that use of prophylactic antibiotic before caesarean delivery,[109] maintaining normothermia intraoperatively and closure of the subcutaneous space if it is greater than 2 cm,[110] may help reduce the incidence of postoperative wound complications. Specific surgical equipment including longer retractors, malleable copper retractors or circular self-retaining rigid or flexible retractors may be required to facilitate access to the pelvis in an obese woman.

Neuraxial anaesthesia for caesarean delivery

An established and effective labouring epidural can be used to provide anaesthesia for delivery. Care should be taken as standard doses of local anaesthetic may produce a higher block in the obese[111] as both the intrathecal and epidural space are reduced with the deposition of adipose tissue. If an epidural is not already *in situ*, then a CSE should be considered. Firstly, the epidural needle can act as a longer introducer needle for the spinal needle compared to the introducers that accompany the normal length spinal needles. With the increased depth required in the obese, the flexible spinal needles often bend but will be unable to do this within an epidural needle. Secondly, a single-shot spinal (SSS) in the morbidly obese is often less predictable. It can result in a higher block[112,113] although other studies have found no correlation between BMI and anaesthetic block height.[114,115] Further, the rapid onset of the sympathetic block due to spinal anaesthesia in the obese can result in catastrophic hypotension when combined with the aortocaval compression caused by fetus and fat pannus and too high a block resulting in intercostal muscle blockade along with the decreased FRC of the obese parturient can lead to hypoxaemia. Therefore using a smaller than normal spinal dose in the first instance can provide a block to appropriate height with less hypotension and the epidural component can be used if that block height was not achieved. Another advantage of the CSE is that augmentation or prolongation of the block is obviously also possible with an epidural catheter *in situ* if operative time is prolonged as is common in the morbidly obese.

However, a SSS with a normal dose is preferred by some operators in the obese parturient. But meticulous care must be taken with positioning and the judicious use of vasopressors to prevent high block and hypotension respectively. The rationale for a SSS is that if the epidural catheter cannot be passed in the CSE technique then one must rely only on the smaller spinal dose with the potential that this will wear off if surgery is prolonged and a general anaesthetic becomes necessary. The two-space technique has been advocated to allow placement of the epidural catheter followed by a SSS in a lower space but in modern practice this is almost obsolete and one could argue that one was fortunate to site the spinal, much less the epidural in the two-space technique in the morbidly obese. The decision of which neuraxial technique to use depends on individual expertise and familiarity with either technique.

Appropriate patient positioning on the operating table is vital. Some super morbidly obese patients will be unable to lie horizontally, even with a left lateral tilt. Indeed, Tsueda et al.[39] described two cases of 'obesity supine death syndrome' in super morbidly obese patients who had cardiovascular collapse when lying supine. A parturient who cannot lie supine, or who cannot lie supine when their fat pannus is manipulated, will not tolerate a caesarean delivery under neuraxial anaesthesia. The ability of the super morbidly obese parturient to tolerate this should be tested towards the end of pregnancy to allow updated and informed anaesthetic and obstetric plans to be made.

The operating table itself should, as discussed earlier, be suitable for the patient's weight, have robust side extenders available, and have side supports and straps for securing the patient when tilted.

The patient should also be positioned on the table in the ideal position for intubation, as the need for conversion to general anaesthesia may arise. This will often be a ramped position (discussed later). This position can obviously lead to significant effects on the spread of spinal anaesthesia when using hyperbaric bupivacaine and so this must be considered when establishing a block. Positioning for surgical access may involve methods for elevating the fat pannus if a Pfannenstiel incision is planned. This can involve moving and taping the pannus in a cephalad direction. Some women will not tolerate this, however, due to cardiorespiratory compromise. A method of suspending the pannus vertically will be required in these cases.

Blood pressure monitoring may require an arterial line. This should be inserted prior to neuraxial anaesthesia to allow for careful monitoring during onset of the block and when positioning the patient supine.

Obese patients have a higher incidence of postpartum haemorrhage which is mainly due to uterine atony and increased technical challenges of operating on the obese parturient. Intraoperative blood loss may be significant, so consideration should be given to the use of Syntocinon® infusion and cell salvage.

General anaesthesia for caesarean delivery

The risks of general anaesthesia in the morbidly obese parturient are significant. Antacid prophylaxis should be used to decrease the risk of pneumonitis from gastric acid aspiration in this population who are known to have increased residual gastric contents. Sodium citrate has been shown to significantly increase gastric pH when given shortly before induction.[116] A recent meta-analysis of ranitidine versus proton pump inhibitors showed ranitidine to be more effective in reducing the volume of gastric acid secretions and increasing gastric pH.[117] A combination of antacids plus H_2 antagonists has been shown to significantly reduce the risk of gastric pH of less than 2.5 compared with antacids alone,[118] therefore many will choose to use this combination.

The immediate increased risks of difficult and failed intubation in the pregnant and obese populations are well recognized, as mentioned earlier. Each patient undergoing general anaesthesia should have an intubation plan made. This may be a rapid sequence induction (RSI) ideally involving senior, experienced personnel with close attention paid to the factors discussed below, or it may be an awake fibreoptic intubation if the risks of an RSI are felt to be too great.

If planning a RSI, close attention should be paid to factors that can delay the time to onset of critical hypoxia at induction of general anaesthesia. FRC, metabolic rate, and alveolar oxygen concentration are the factors which have the greatest effect on this time. The morbidly obese parturient has a significantly reduced FRC. They also have a significantly increased metabolic rate. Oxygen consumption is approximately 250 mL/min in the normal BMI patient at rest. This increases to approximately 330 mL/min in the term parturient.[119] In the morbidly obese at rest, an oxygen consumption of up to 453 mL/min has been reported.[28] Figures for the morbidly obese parturient at term are not readily available, but would be assumed to be significantly elevated. Increasing oxygen consumption from 250 to 400 mL/min reduces the time to 50% oxygen saturations by around 40%.[120] Jense et al. investigated the time to 90% saturations after the onset of closed airway apnoea in preoxygenated patients with normal BMI versus the morbidly obese. These times were 364 seconds in the normal BMI group versus 163 seconds in the morbidly obese group.[121] Alveolar oxygen concentration can be optimized prior to induction by careful preoxygenation with 100% oxygen. Using 90% oxygen has been shown to halve the time to critical hypoxia compared to using 100%, with an open airway during apnoea.[120] Attention to maintaining a patent airway with 100% oxygen during the apnoeic phase of RSI will also significantly increase the time to critical hypoxia. This is due to the fact that during the apnoeic phase the rate of oxygen extraction from the alveoli is tenfold that of carbon dioxide reaching the alveoli. This quickly creates a reduction of intrathoracic pressure if the airway is obstructed which rapidly reduces the partial pressure of oxygen remaining in the lungs still further. An open airway allows bulk movement of oxygen to the lungs and prevents this reduction of intrathoracic pressure. Studies using a physiology simulator have shown the time to 50% saturations as 66 minutes with open airway apnoea and 100% oxygen compared to 8 minutes with a closed airway.[122]

Preoxygenation in a 45° head-up position has also been shown to significantly increase the time to desaturation in the obese non-pregnant population.[123] However, Baraka et al.[124] found no difference with the head-up position in the pregnant population. When severe hypoxia does develop, the oxygen saturation decreases extremely rapidly at a rate of approximately 30% per minute.[120]

Appropriate positioning prior to induction of anaesthesia is vital, both to optimize position for laryngoscopy and to aid respiratory function. Figure 39.3A shows poor positioning for induction of general anaesthesia. Figure 39.3B shows a better, ramped position. This position, with horizontal alignment of the sternum and external auditory meatus is an optimized position for laryngoscopy.[125] The ramping also helps improve respiratory function by moving the weight off the chest wall and diaphragm, increasing the FRC. This may result in an increased time to hypoxia at induction.

Many drugs used in the management of the morbidly obese parturient undergoing general anaesthesia have altered pharmacokinetics as discussed earlier.

- Thiopental—induction doses should be adjusted for lean body weight. Peak plasma concentrations are reduced in the obese due to their increased cardiac output.[126] Thiopental is highly lipid-soluble, which results in an increased volume of distribution in the obese. Clearance is also significantly increased.
- Suxamethonium—dosing should be based on total body weight. The morbidly obese have an increase in both extracellular fluid volume and pseudocholinesterase activity, both of which determine the duration of action of the drug.[127]
- Non-depolarizing neuromuscular blockers—dosing should be based on ideal body weight. Both vecuronium[128] and rocuronium[129] duration of action is significantly increased in the obese when dosing is based on total body weight. Most studies also show the same for atracurium,[130] although Weinstein et al. showed no difference in the recovery times of obese surgical patients.[128] However, it would seem sensible to also base atracurium dosing on ideal body weight.
- Volatile anaesthetic agents—the lipid solubility of isoflurane is greater than that of sevoflurane which is again greater than desflurane. However, the clinical effects that these differences produce in the morbidly obese are the relevant factors. Torri et al.[131] found the difference between the wash out curves of isoflurane and sevoflurane only statistically significant in the first 60 seconds after discontinuation of the agents. This was after surgical procedures significantly over an hour in length. Some studies have shown no difference in time to follow commands and extubation when comparing sevoflurane with desflurane in the morbidly obese, if anaesthetic concentration is carefully titrated.[132] Others have shown a significantly more rapid time to obeying commands and extubation using desflurane—and higher oxygen saturation on arrival to the post-anaesthetic care unit.[133] Emergence and both early and intermediate recovery—for at least 2 hours postoperatively—have been reported as more rapid with desflurane than isoflurane in morbidly obese patients.[134]
- Remifentanil—dosing should be based on lean body weight. Pharmacokinetics are not significantly different in the obese. Dosing based on total body weight results in significantly increased blood levels of the drug in obese patients.[135]
- Opiates—fentanyl dosing should be based on lean body weight.[45] Dosing of longer-acting opiates such as morphine and diamorphine must be carefully titrated due to the risk of respiratory depression and upper airway obstruction in the morbidly obese. Respiratory physiological changes in this group of patients along with the increased occurrence of sleep apnoea make opioid-induced hypoxia much more likely to occur.[136,137]

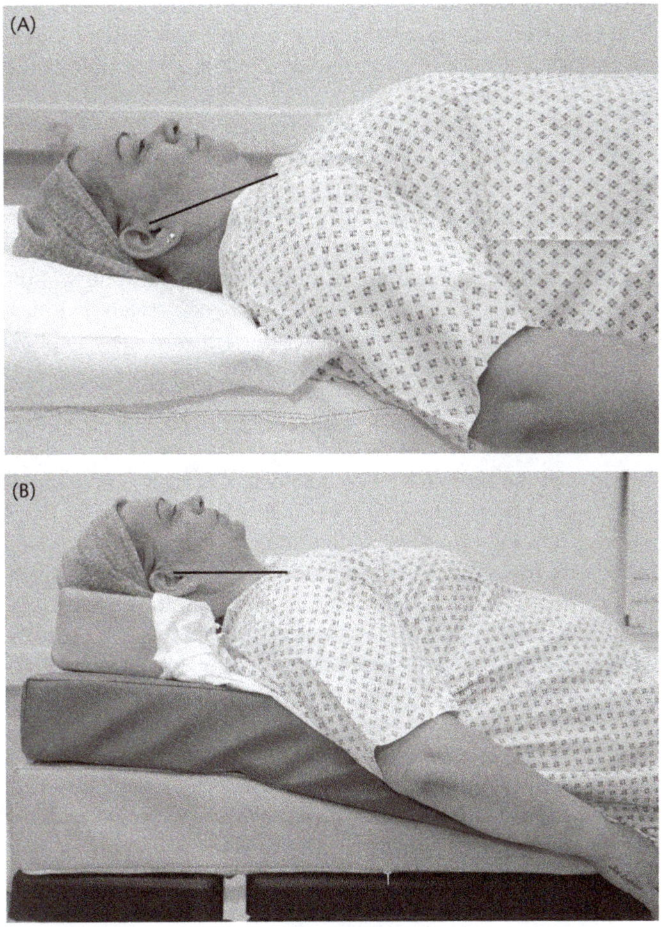

Figure 39.3 Optimal positioning for tracheal intubation. (A) A single pillow provides a poor position. (B) Horizontal alignment of the sternum and external auditory meatus provides an optimized position for laryngoscopy. This is achieved with the use of wedges.

The incidence of respiratory complications has been reported to be significantly higher at tracheal extubation than at intubation.[138] One-third of events reported to the 4th National Audit Project into major complications of airway management in the United Kingdom occurred during emergence or recovery.[139] The most common of these events was airway obstruction. The morbidly obese are in a higher risk category for problems occurring at extubation. They are more sensitive to the side effects of opiates and at an increased risk of airway obstruction. Decreased FRC and increased metabolic rate will lead to more rapid desaturation should a problem occur and there is an increased risk of difficult intubation should reintubation be required. As such, all patients should have an extubation plan made. The Difficult Airway Society published guidelines for the management of tracheal extubation in 2012.[140] These highlight the need to optimize patient and other factors—such as location and assistance—prior to extubation. The threshold for delaying extubation if any factors are not optimized should be low, as extubation is an elective procedure

Postoperative analgesia

This would ideally result in manageable pain levels with minimal side effects—such as drowsiness and respiratory depression—and would allow the patient to breathe deeply to minimize atelectasis and mobilize early to minimize risks of deep venous thrombosis.

If a CSE technique has been used intraoperatively, consideration should be given to running an epidural infusion in the early postoperative period. This not only provides optimal analgesia and minimize opiate-related side effects, it will also provide a method of re-establishing anaesthesia should this be necessary in the early postoperative period when the morbidly obese are at a higher risk of complications such as postpartum haemorrhage.[141] Multimodal analgesia with non-opiate analgesics should be used if appropriate. This will have a morphine-sparing effect.[142,143]

If intrathecal or epidural opiates are used, appropriate regular postoperative monitoring of adequacy of ventilation, oxygenation, and level of consciousness should be in place.[144] Morbid obesity is a risk factor for respiratory depression from neuraxial opiates. In one study of 856 patients, all of the eight patients who suffered respiratory depression were markedly obese.[145] If available, neuraxial diamorphine has been reported as having an improved side effect profile compared with morphine in terms of pruritis and drowsiness.[146] Intravenous morphine is associated with higher pain scores than neuraxial morphine after caesarean delivery,[147] and is well known to cause respiratory depression and sleep-disordered breathing[137] However, morphine PCA after gastric bypass surgery in the morbidly obese has been reported as safe and effective.[148]

Several different local anaesthetic blocks have been used in an attempt to provide improved analgesia and reduce opiate requirements postoperatively, such as ilioinguinal–iliohypogastric nerve blockade and transversus abdominis plane (TAP) blocks. Bilateral ilioinguinal nerve blockade after caesarean delivery has been shown to reduce opiate requirement in the first 24 hours postoperatively,[149,150] but other studies have shown no significant difference between this technique and wound infiltration.[151] TAP blocks are a more recent technique shown by meta-analysis to reduce postoperative morphine consumption in analgesic regimens that exclude neuraxial morphine.[152] In the morbidly obese patient, the landmark technique—identifying the triangle of Petit—would prove difficult. The ultrasound approach, while also more difficult in the morbidly obese, may be better suited which allows accurate placement of local anaesthetic into the correct tissue plane.

A multimodal postoperative analgesic approach with the aim to minimize intravenous opiates would seem sensible, although vigilant, appropriate monitoring is probably the most vital ingredient in avoiding postoperative respiratory complications in the morbidly obese.

Postoperative care

There should be a low threshold for the morbidly obese to be cared for in a high dependency or intensive care area postoperatively, with continuous monitoring. This is especially so after general anaesthesia when the risk of postoperative respiratory failure is elevated.[81] Any morbidly obese patient with sleep apnoea or a history suggestive of this should be cared for in a high dependency unit postoperatively. A high level of medical and nursing care is required with close attention to detail in order to minimize increased risks in the morbidly obese from many postpartum complications such as haemorrhage, deep venous thrombosis, and wound infection.[89,108,153]

Obesity is a significant risk factor for venous thromboembolism and warrants particular consideration. All women should have an assessment of risk factors for venous thromboembolism in the antenatal period. This assessment should be repeated at any hospital admission or on development of any new risk factors. Detailed guidelines from the Royal College of Obstetricians and Gynaecologists describe this risk assessment.[154] A BMI greater than 30 kg/m^2 is one of a range of risk factors. All women with a BMI of over 40 kg/m^2 should be offered 7 days of low-molecular-weight

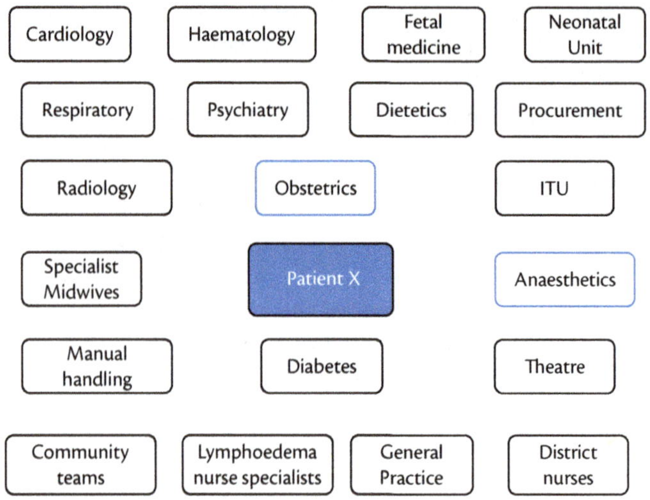

Figure 39.4 The multidisciplinary team involved in the care of one super morbidly obese patient in our institution.

heparin (LMWH) post delivery, even after a normal delivery and in the absence of other risk factors.[154] Dosing of LMWH is calculated on patient weight.

Many of the equipment and staffing needs mentioned earlier are equally as relevant in postpartum patient care, such as appropriate mattresses to minimize pressure area risk, patient hoists, appropriately sized calf compression stockings, inflatable boots, and blood pressure cuffs.

The postpartum period provides women with a unique opportunity to lose weight to reduce the risk of adverse pregnancy outcome in a subsequent pregnancy and also improve maternal health. To facilitate this and to enable pregnancy spacing, it is therefore important that obese women are given appropriate contraceptive advice postpartum. Although the overall quality of the evidence is low, a 2013 Cochrane review demonstrated that most studies do not demonstrate an association between maternal BMI and effectiveness of hormonal contraceptives.[155]

Conclusion

The care of the morbidly obese parturient is truly a multidisciplinary affair which must be coordinated by a named consultant obstetrician. Figure 39.4 lists the different specialities involved in the care of just one super morbidly obese patient in our institution. This care involves a high level of communication and great attention to detail in all aspects of patient management. Continuity of care from the anaesthetic team, from prenatal assessment through to postnatal care, will aid optimum patient management. It can aid peer group discussion through a lead anaesthetist to gain consensus opinion on patient care. This will not only help to provide optimum patient care, but will also help to manage patient expectation, especially in the super morbidly obese patient where differing opinions may exist in terms of their management.

References

1. Anonymous. Obesity: preventing and managing the global epidemic. Report of a WHO consultation. *World Health Organ Tech Rep Ser* 2000; 894:i–xii, 1–253.

2. Popkin BM, Adair LS, Ng SW. Global nutrition transition and the pandemic of obesity in developing countries. *Nutr Rev* 2012; 70(1):3–21.
3. Allison DB, Fontaine KR, Manson JE, *et al.* Annual deaths attributable to obesity in the United States. *JAMA* 1999; 282(16):1530–8.
4. Swinburn BA, Sacks G, Hall KD, *et al.* The global obesity pandemic: shaped by global drivers and local environments. *Lancet* 2011; 378(9793):804–14.
5. Braveman P. A health disparities perspective on obesity research. *Prev Chronic Dis* 2009; 6(3):A91.
6. Dinsa GD, Goryakin Y, Fumagalli E, *et al.* Obesity and socioeconomic status in developing countries: a systematic review. *Obes Rev* 2012; 13(11):1067–79.
7. Newbold RR, Padilla-Banks E, Snyder RJ, *et al.* Developmental exposure to endocrine disruptors and the obesity epidemic. *Reprod Toxicol* 2007; 23(3):290–6.
8. Health and Social Care Information Centre. *Health Survey for England: 2010 Trend Tables.* London: Health and Social Care Information Centre; 2012.
9. Public Health Agency of Canada, Canadian Institute for Health Information. *Obesity in Canada: A Joint Report from the Public Health Agency of Canada and the Canadian Institute for Health Information.* Ottawa, ON: Public Health Agency of Canada, Canadian Institute for Health Information; 2012.
10. Flegal KM, Carroll MD, Kit BK, *et al.* Prevalence of obesity and trends in the distribution of body mass index among US adults, 1999–2010. *JAMA* 2012; 307(5):491–7.
11. Dixit A, Girling JC. Obesity and pregnancy. *J Obstet Gynaecol* 2008; 28(1):14–23.
12. Heslehurst N, Ells LJ, Simpson H, *et al.* Trends in maternal obesity incidence rates, demographic predictors, and health inequalities in 36,821 women over a 15-year period. *BJOG* 2007; 114(2):187–94.
13. Heslehurst N, Rankin J, Wilkinson JR, *et al.* A nationally representative study of maternal obesity in England, UK: trends in incidence and demographic inequalities in 619 323 births, 1989–2007. *Int J Obes (Lond)* 2009; 34(3):420–8.
14. Denison FC, Norrie G, Graham B, *et al.* Increased maternal BMI is associated with an increased risk of minor complications during pregnancy with consequent cost implications. *BJOG* 2009; 116(11):1467–72.
15. Denison FC, Price J, Graham C, *et al.* Maternal obesity, length of gestation, risk of postdates pregnancy and spontaneous onset of labour at term. *BJOG* 2008; 115(6):720–5.
16. Sebire NJ, Jolly M, Harris JP, *et al.* Maternal obesity and pregnancy outcome: a study of 287,213 pregnancies in London. *Int J Obes Relat Metab Disord* 2001; 25(8):1175–82.
17. Tennant PW, Rankin J, Bell R. Maternal body mass index and the risk of fetal and infant death: a cohort study from the North of England. *Hum Reprod* 2011; 26(6):1501–11.
18. Rasmussen KM, Yaktine AL (eds). *Weight Gain During Pregnancy: Reexamining the Guidelines.* Washington, DC: National Academies Press; 2009.
19. Poston L, Chappell LC. How should women be advised on weight management in pregnancy? *BMJ* 2012; 344:e2774.
20. Drake AJ, Reynolds RM. Impact of maternal obesity on offspring obesity and cardiometabolic disease risk. *Reproduction* 2010; 140(3):387–98.
21. Alexander CI, Liston WA. Operating on the obese woman—a review. *BJOG* 2006; 113(10):1167–72.
22. Pelosi P, Croci M, Ravagnan I, *et al.* The effects of body mass on lung volumes, respiratory mechanics, and gas exchange during general anesthesia. *Anesth Analg* 1998; 87(3):654–60.
23. Adams JP, Murphy PG. Obesity in anaesthesia and intensive care. *Br J Anaesth* 2000; 85(1):91–108.
24. Lin CK, Lin CC. Work of breathing and respiratory drive in obesity. *Respirology* 2012; 17(3):402–11.
25. Salome CM, King GG, Berend N. Physiology of obesity and effects on lung function. *J Appl Physiol* 2010; 108(1):206–11.
26. Parameswaran K, Todd DC, Soth S. Altered respiratory physiology in obesity. *Can Respir J* 2006; 13(4):203–10.
27. Lazarus R, Sparrow D, Weiss ST. Effects of obesity and fat distribution on ventilatory function: the normative aging study. *Chest* 1997; 111(4):891–8.
28. Zavala DC, Printen KJ. Basal and exercise tests on morbidly obese patients before and after gastric bypass. *Surgery* 1984; 95(2):221–9.
29. Veille JC, Hanson R. Obesity, pregnancy, and left ventricular functioning during the third trimester. *Am J Obstet Gynecol* 1994; 171(4):980–3.
30. Vasan RS. Cardiac function and obesity. *Heart* 2003; 89(10):1127–9.
31. Alpert MA. Obesity cardiomyopathy: pathophysiology and evolution of the clinical syndrome. *Am J Med Sci* 2001; 321(4):225–36.
32. Alpert MA, Hashimi MW. Obesity and the heart. *Am J Med Sci* 1993; 306(2):117–23.
33. Kenchaiah S, Evans JC, Levy D, *et al.* Obesity and the risk of heart failure. *N Engl J Med* 2002; 347(5):305–13.
34. Peluso L, Vanek VW. Efficacy of gastric bypass in the treatment of obesity-related comorbidities. *Nutr Clin Pract* 2007; 22(1):22–8.
35. Eckel RH. Obesity and heart disease: a statement for healthcare professionals from the Nutrition Committee, American Heart Association. *Circulation* 1997; 96(9):3248–50.
36. Lean ME. Obesity and cardiovascular disease: the waisted years. *Br J Cardiol* 1999; 6:269–73.
37. Saravanakumar K, Rao SG, Cooper GM. The challenges of obesity and obstetric anaesthesia. *Curr Opin Obstet Gynecol* 2006; 18(6):631–5.
38. Weiss JL, Malone FD, Emig D, *et al.* Obesity, obstetric complications and cesarean delivery rate—a population-based screening study. *Am J Obstet Gynecol* 2004; 190(4):1091–7.
39. Tsueda K, Debrand M, Zeok SS, *et al.* Obesity supine death syndrome: reports of two morbidly obese patients. *Anesth Analg* 1979; 58(4):345–7.
40. Lotia S, Bellamy MC. Anaesthesia and morbid obesity. *CEACCP* 2008; 8(5):151–6.
41. Rios MS. Relationship between obesity and the increased risk of major complications in non-insulin-dependent diabetes mellitus. *Eur J Clin Invest* 1998; 28:14–8.
42. Chu SY, Callaghan WM, Kim SY, *et al.* Maternal obesity and risk of gestational diabetes mellitus. *Diabetes Care* 2007; 30(8):2070–6.
43. Forbes GB, Welle SL. Lean body mass in obesity. *Int J Obes* 1983; 7(2):99–107.
44. Janmahasatian S, Duffull SB, Ash S, *et al.* Quantification of lean bodyweight. *Clin Pharmacokinet* 2005; 44(10):1051–65.
45. Ingrande J, Lemmens HJ. Dose adjustment of anaesthetics in the morbidly obese. *Br J Anaesth* 2010; 105 Suppl 1:i16–23.
46. Hanley MJ, Abernethy DR, Greenblatt DJ. Effect of obesity on the pharmacokinetics of drugs in humans. *Clin Pharmacokinet* 2010; 49(2):71–87.
47. Abernethy DR, Greenblatt DJ. Pharmacokinetics of drugs in obesity. *Clin Pharmacokinet* 1982; 7(2):108–24.
48. Wurtz R, Itokazu G, Rodvold K. Antimicrobial dosing in obese patients. *Clin Infect Dis* 1997; 25(1):112–18.
49. Edmiston CE, Krepel C, Kelly H, *et al.* Perioperative antibiotic prophylaxis in the gastric bypass patient: do we achieve therapeutic levels? *Surgery* 2004; 136(4):738–47.
50. Blouin RA, Warren GW Pharmacokinetic considerations in obesity. *J Pharm Sci* 1999; 88(1):1–7.
51. Salazar DE, Corcoran GB. Predicting creatinine clearance and renal drug clearance in obese patients from estimated fat-free body mass. *Am J Med* 1988; 84(6):1053–60.
52. Catalano PM. Management of obesity in pregnancy. *Obstet Gynecol* 2007; 109(2 Pt 1):419–33.
53. Kaaja RJ, Greer IA. Manifestations of chronic disease during pregnancy. *JAMA* 2005; 294(21):2751–7.
54. Hood DD, Dewan DM. Anesthetic and obstetric outcome in morbidly obese parturients. *Anesthesiology* 1993; 79(6):1210–18.

55. Chu SY, Bachman DJ, Callaghan WM, *et al.* Association between obesity during pregnancy and increased use of health care. *N Engl J Med* 2008; 358(14):1444–53.
56. Sibai BM, Ewell M, Levine RJ, *et al.* Risk factors associated with preeclampsia in healthy nulliparous women. The Calcium for Preeclampsia Prevention (CPEP) Study Group. *Am J Obstet Gynecol* 1997; 177(5):1003–10.
57. O'Brien TE, Ray JG, Chan WS. Maternal body mass index and the risk of preeclampsia: a systematic overview. *Epidemiology* 2003; 14(3):368–74.
58. Sibai BM, Lindheimer M, Hauth J, *et al.* Risk factors for preeclampsia, abruptio placentae, and adverse neonatal outcomes among women with chronic hypertension. National Institute of Child Health and Human Development Network of Maternal-Fetal Medicine Units. *N Engl J Med* 1998; 339(10):667–71.
59. Pickering TG, Hall JE, Appel LJ, *et al.* Recommendations for blood pressure measurement in humans and experimental animals: Part 1: blood pressure measurement in humans: a statement for professionals from the Subcommittee of Professional and Public Education of the American Heart Association Council on High Blood Pressure Research. *Hypertension* 2005; 45(1):142–61.
60. Hogan JL, Maguire P, Farah N, *et al.* Body mass index and blood pressure measurement during pregnancy. *Hypertens Pregnancy* 2011; 30(4):396–400.
61. Cooley SM, Maguire P, Farah N, *et al.* The relationship between body mass index and mid-arm circumference in a pregnant population. *J Obstet Gynaecol* 2011; 31(7):594–6.
62. Action on Pre-eclampsia. *PRECOG: The Pre-eclampsia Community Guideline.* London: Action on Pre-eclampsia; 2004.
63. Torloni MR, Betrán AP, Horta BL, *et al.* Prepregnancy BMI and the risk of gestational diabetes: a systematic review of the literature with meta-analysis. *Obes Rev* 2009; 10(2):194–203.
64. Scottish Intercollegiate Guidelines Network. *Management of Diabetes: A National Clinical Guideline.* SIGN Publication No. 116. Edinburgh: SIGN; 2010.
65. National Institute of Health and Care Excellence. *Diabetes in Pregnancy: Management from Preconception to the Postnatal Period.* NICE Guideline NG3. London: NICE; 2015.
66. Gillespie P, Cullinan J, O'Neill C, *et al.* Modeling the independent effects of gestational diabetes mellitus on maternity care and costs. *Diabetes Care* 2012; 36(5):1111–16.
67. Buchwald H, Avidor Y, Braunwald E, *et al.* Bariatric surgery: a systematic review and meta-analysis. *JAMA* 2004; 292(14):1724–37.
68. Magdaleno R Jr, Pereira BG, Chaim EA, *et al.* Pregnancy after bariatric surgery: a current view of maternal, obstetrical and perinatal challenges. *Arch Gynecol Obstet* 2012; 285(3):559–66.
69. Roos N, Neovius M, Cnattingius S, *et al.* Perinatal outcomes after bariatric surgery: nationwide population based matched cohort study. *BMJ* 2013; 347:f6460.
70. Uzoma A, Keriakos R. Pregnancy management following bariatric surgery. *J Obstet Gynaecol* 2013; 33(2):109–14.
71. Karmon A, Sheiner E. Timing of gestation after bariatric surgery: should women delay pregnancy for at least 1 postoperative year? *Am J Perinatol* 2008; 25(6):331–3.
72. Poitou Bernert C, Ciangura C, Coupaye M, *et al.* Nutritional deficiency after gastric bypass: diagnosis, prevention and treatment. *Diabetes Metab* 2007; 33(1):13–24.
73. Davies DJ, Baxter JM, Baxter JN. Nutritional deficiencies after bariatric surgery. *Obes Surg* 2007; 17(9):1150–8.
74. Kalfarentzos F, Kechagias I, Soulikia K, *et al.* Weight loss following vertical banded gastroplasty: intermediate results of a prospective study. *Obes Surg* 2001; 11(3):265–70.
75. Sapala JA, Wood MH, Sapala MA, *et al.* Marginal ulcer after gastric bypass: a prospective 3-year study of 173 patients. *Obes Surg* 1998; 8(5):505–16.
76. Modder J, Fitzsimmons KJ. *Management of Women with Obesity in Pregnancy: CMACE/RCOG Joint Guideline.* London: CMACE/RCOG; 2010.
77. Barnardo PD, Jenkins JG. Failed tracheal intubation in obstetrics: a 6-year review in a UK region. *Anaesthesia* 2000; 55(7):690–4.
78. D'Angelo, R, Dewan DD. Obesity. In Chestnut DH (ed) *Obstetric Anesthesia: Principles and Practice.* St. Louis, MO: Elsevier Mosby; 2004:893–903.
79. Juvin, P, Lavaut E, Dupont H, *et al.* Difficult tracheal intubation is more common in obese than in lean patients. *Anesth Analg* 2003; 97(2):595–600.
80. Bellamy M, Struys M. Obesity and the airway. In *Anaesthesia for the Overweight and Obese Patient.* Oxford: Oxford University Press; 2007:75–82.
81. Vallejo MC. Anesthetic management of the morbidly obese parturient. *Curr Opin Anaesthesiol* 2007; 20(3):175–80.
82. Singer AJ, Kahn SR, Thode HC Jr, *et al.* Comparison of forearm and upper arm blood pressures. *Prehosp Emerg Care* 1999; 3(2):123–6.
83. Clinkscales P, Greenfield ML, Vanarase M, *et al.* An observational study of the relationship between lumbar epidural space depth and body mass index in Michigan parturients. *Int J Obstet Anesth* 2007; 16(4):323–7.
84. Ravi KK, Kaul TK, Kathuria S, *et al.* Distance from skin to epidural space: correlation with body mass index (BMI). *J Anaesthesiol Clin Pharmacol* 2011; 27(1):39–42.
85. Hamza J, Smida M, Benhamou D, *et al.* Parturient's posture during epidural puncture affects the distance from skin to epidural space. *J Clin Anesth* 1995; 7(1):1–4.
86. Arfeen Z, Armstrong PJ, Whitfield A. The effects of Entonox and epidural analgesia on arterial oxygen saturation of women in labour. *Anaesthesia* 1994; 49(1):32–4.
87. Elbourne D, Wiseman RA. Types of intra-muscular opioids for maternal pain relief in labour. *Cochrane Database Syst Rev* 2000; 2:CD001237.
88. Howell CJ. Epidural versus nonepidural analgesia for pain relief in labour. *Cochrane Database Syst Rev* 2000; 2:CD000331.
89. Perlow JH, Morgan MA. Massive maternal obesity and perioperative cesarean morbidity. *Am J Obstet Gynecol* 1994; 170(2):560–5.
90. Grau T, Leipold RW, Conradi R, *et al.* Efficacy of ultrasound imaging in obstetric epidural anesthesia. *J Clin Anesth*, 2002; 14(3):169–75.
91. Howell CJ. Epidural versus non-epidural analgesia for pain relief in labour. *Cochrane Database Syst Rev* 2000; 2:CD000331.
92. Grau T, Leipold RW, Conradi R, *et al.* Ultrasound control for presumed difficult epidural puncture. *Acta Anaesthesiol Scand* 2001; 45(6):766–71.
93. Vallejo MC, Phelps AL, Singh S, *et al.* Ultrasound decreases the failed labor epidural rate in resident trainees. *Int J Obstet Anesth* 2010; 19(4):373–8.
94. Wasson, C. Failed epidural in an obese patient—blame it on Pythagoras! *Anaesthesia* 2001; 56(6):605–6.
95. Faheem M, Sarwar N. Sliding of the skin over subcutaneous tissue is another important factor in epidural catheter migration. *Can J Anaesth* 2002; 49(6):634.
96. Volmanen P, Sarvela J, Akural EI, *et al.* Intravenous remifentanil vs. epidural levobupivacaine with fentanyl for pain relief in early labour: a randomised, controlled, double-blinded study. *Acta Anaesthesiol Scand* 2008; 52(2):249–55.
97. Schnabel A, Hahn N, Broscheit J, *et al.* Remifentanil for labour analgesia: a meta-analysis of randomised controlled trials. *Eur J Anaesthesiol* 2012; 29(4):177–85.
98. Muchatuta NA, Kinsella SM. Remifentanil for labour analgesia: time to draw breath? *Anaesthesia* 2013; 68(3):231–5.
99. Hinova A, Fernando R. Systemic remifentanil for labor analgesia. *Anesth Analg* 2009; 109(6):1925–9.
100. Pruefer C, Bewlay A. Respiratory arrest with remifentanil patient-controlled analgesia—another case. *Anaesthesia* 2012; 67(9):1044–5.
101. Bonner JC, McClymont W. Respiratory arrest in an obstetric patient using remifentanil patient-controlled analgesia. *Anaesthesia* 2012; 67(5):538–40.

102. Marr R, Hyams J, Bythell V. Cardiac arrest in an obstetric patient using remifentanil patient-controlled analgesia. *Anaesthesia* 2013; 68(3):283–7.
103. Kinney MA, Rose CH, Traynor KD, *et al.* Emergency bedside cesarean delivery: lessons learned in teamwork and patient safety. *BMC Res Notes* 2012; 5:412.
104. Van de Velde M. Controversy. Remifentanil patient-controlled analgesia should be routinely available for use in labour. *Int J Obstet Anesth* 2008; 17(4):339–42.
105. Buehner U, Broadbent JR, Chesterfield B. Remifentanil patient-controlled analgesia for labour: a complete audit cycle. *Anaesth Intensive Care* 2011; 39(4):666–70.
106. Hawkins JL. Anesthesia-related maternal mortality. *Clin Obstet Gynecol* 2003; 46(3):679–87.
107. Lewis G. *The Confidential Enquiry into Maternal and Child Health (CEMACH), Saving Mothers' Lives: Reviewing Maternal Deaths to Make Motherhood Safer—2003–2005. The Seventh Report on Confidential Enquiries into Maternal Deaths in the United Kingdom.* London: CEMACH; 2007.
108. Chiswick C, Cooper ES, Norman JE, *et al.* Fat necrosis of the abdominal pannus following caesarean section in patients with morbid obesity. *Eur J Obstet Gynecol Reprod Biol* 2012; 160(1):118–19.
109. Smaill FM, Gyte GM. Antibiotic prophylaxis versus no prophylaxis for preventing infection after cesarean section. *Cochrane Database Syst Rev* 2010; 1:CD007482.
110. Chelmow D, Rodriguez EJ, Sabatini MM. Suture closure of subcutaneous fat and wound disruption after cesarean delivery: a meta-analysis. *Obstet Gynecol* 2004; 103(5 Pt 1):974–80.
111. Hodgkinson R, Husain FJ. Obesity and the cephalad spread of analgesia following epidural administration of bupivacaine for Cesarean section. *Anesth Analg* 1980; 59(2):89–92.
112. McCulloch WJ, Littlewood DG. Influence of obesity on spinal analgesia with isobaric 0.5% bupivacaine. *Br J Anaesth* 1986; 58(6):610–4.
113. Taivainen T, Tuominen M, Rosenberg PH. Influence of obesity on the spread of spinal analgesia after injection of plain 0.5% bupivacaine at the L3-4 or L4-5 interspace. *Br J Anaesth* 1990; 64(5):542–6.
114. Norris MC. Height, weight, and the spread of subarachnoid hyperbaric bupivacaine in the term parturient. *Anesth Analg* 1988; 67(6):555–8.
115. Norris MC. Patient variables and the subarachnoid spread of hyperbaric bupivacaine in the term parturient. *Anesthesiology* 1990; 72(3):478–82.
116. Dewan DM, Floyd HM, Thistlewood JM, *et al.* Sodium citrate pretreatment in elective cesarean section patients. *Anesth Analg* 1985; 64(1):34–7.
117. Clark K, Lam LT, Gibson S, *et al.* The effect of ranitidine versus proton pump inhibitors on gastric secretions: a meta-analysis of randomised control trials. *Anaesthesia* 2009; 64(6):652–7.
118. Paranjothy S, Griffiths JD, Broughton HK, *et al.* Interventions at caesarean section for reducing the risk of aspiration pneumonitis. *Int J Obstet Anesth* 2011; 20(2):142–8.
119. Pernoll ML, Metcalfe J, Schlenker TL, *et al.* Oxygen consumption at rest and during exercise in pregnancy. *Respir Physiol* 1975; 25(3):285–93.
120. Sirian R, Wills J. Physiology of apnoea and the benefits of preoxygenation *CEACCP* 2009; 9(4):105–8.
121. Jense HG, Dubin SA, Silverstein PI, *et al.* Effect of obesity on safe duration of apnea in anesthetized humans. *Anesth Analg* 1991; 72(1):89–93.
122. Hardman JG, Wills JS, Aitkenhead AR. Factors determining the onset and course of hypoxemia during apnea: an investigation using physiological modelling. *Anesth Analg* 2000; 90(3):619–24.
123. Altermatt FR, Muñoz HR, Delfino AE, *et al.* Pre-oxygenation in the obese patient: effects of position on tolerance to apnoea. *Br J Anaesth* 2005; 95(5):706–9.
124. Baraka AS, Hanna MT, Jabbour SI, *et al.* Preoxygenation of pregnant and nonpregnant women in the head-up versus supine position. *Anesth Analg* 1992; 75(5):757–9.
125. El-Orbany M, Woehlck H, Salem MR. Head and neck position for direct laryngoscopy. *Anesth Analg* 2011; 113(1):103–9.
126. Wada DR, Björkman S, Ebling WF, *et al.* Computer simulation of the effects of alterations in blood flows and body composition on thiopental pharmacokinetics in humans. *Anesthesiology* 1997; 87(4):884–99.
127. Bentley JB, Borel JD, Vaughan RW, *et al.* Weight, pseudocholinesterase activity, and succinylcholine requirement. *Anesthesiology* 1982; 57(1):48–9.
128. Weinstein JA, Matteo RS, Ornstein E, *et al.* Pharmacodynamics of vecuronium and atracurium in the obese surgical patient. *Anesth Analg* 1988; 67(12):1149–53.
129. Leykin Y, Pellis T, Lucca M, *et al.* The pharmacodynamic effects of rocuronium when dosed according to real body weight or ideal body weight in morbidly obese patients. *Anesth Analg* 2004; 99(4):1086–9.
130. Kirkegaard-Nielsen H, Helbo-Hansen HS, Lindholm P, *et al.* Anthropometric variables as predictors for duration of action of atracurium-induced neuromuscular block. *Anesth Analg* 1996; 83(5):1076–80.
131. Torri G, Casati A, Comotti L, *et al.* Wash-in and wash-out curves of sevoflurane and isoflurane in morbidly obese patients. *Minerva Anestesiol* 2002; 68(6):523–7.
132. Arain SR, Barth CD, Shankar H, *et al.* Choice of volatile anesthetic for the morbidly obese patient: sevoflurane or desflurane. *J Clin Anesth* 2005; 17(6):413–19.
133. Strum EM, Szenohradszki J, Kaufman WA, *et al.* Emergence and recovery characteristics of desflurane versus sevoflurane in morbidly obese adult surgical patients: a prospective, randomized study. *Anesth Analg* 2004; 99(6):1848–53.
134. Juvin P, Vadam C, Malek L, *et al.* Postoperative recovery after desflurane, propofol, or isoflurane anesthesia among morbidly obese patients: a prospective, randomized study. *Anesth Analg* 2000; 91(3):714–19.
135. Egan TD, Huizinga B, Gupta SK, *et al.* Remifentanil pharmacokinetics in obese versus lean patients. *Anesthesiology* 1998; 89(3):562–73.
136. Benumof JL. Obesity, sleep apnea, the airway and anesthesia. *Curr Opin Anaesthesiol* 2004; 17(1):21–30.
137. Yue HJ, Guilleminault C. Opioid medication and sleep-disordered breathing. *Med Clin North Am* 2010; 94(3):435–46.
138. Asai T, Koga K, Vaughan RS. Respiratory complications associated with tracheal intubation and extubation. *Br J Anaesth* 1998; 80(6):767–75.
139. Cook TM, MacDougall-Davis SR. Complications and failure of airway management. *Br J Anaesth* 2012; 109 Suppl 1:i68–i85.
140. Popat M, Mitchell V, Dravid R, *et al.* Difficult Airway Society Guidelines for the management of tracheal extubation. *Anaesthesia* 2012; 67(3):318–40.
141. Lennox C, Marr J. *Scottish Confidential Audit of Severe Maternal Morbidity; Reducing Avoidable Harm.* Edinburgh: Healthcare Improvement Scotland; 2012.
142. Hodsman NB, Burns J, Blyth A, *et al.* The morphine sparing effects of diclofenac sodium following abdominal surgery. *Anaesthesia* 1987; 42(9):1005–8.
143. Montgomery JE, Sutherland CJ, Kestin IG, *et al.* Morphine consumption in patients receiving rectal paracetamol and diclofenac alone and in combination. *Br J Anaesth* 1996; 77(4):445–7.
144. Carvalho B. Respiratory depression after neuraxial opioids in the obstetric setting. *Anesth Analg* 2008; 107(3):956–61.
145. Abouleish E, Rawal N, Rashad MN. The addition of 0.2 mg subarachnoid morphine to hyperbaric bupivacaine for cesarean delivery: a prospective study of 856 cases. *Reg Anesth* 1991; 16(3):137–40.

146. Husaini SW, Russell IF. Intrathecal diamorphine compared with morphine for postoperative analgesia after caesarean section under spinal anaesthesia. *Br J Anaesth* 1998; 81(2):135–9.
147. Lim Y, Jha S, Sia AT, *et al.* Morphine for post-caesarean section analgesia: intrathecal, epidural or intravenous? *Singapore Med J* 2005; 46(8):392–6.
148. Choi YK, Brolin RE, Wagner BK, *et al.* Efficacy and safety of patient-controlled analgesia for morbidly obese patients following gastric bypass surgery. *Obes Surg* 2000; 10(2):154–9.
149. Bell EA, Jones BP, Olufolabi AJ, *et al.* Iliohypogastric-ilioinguinal peripheral nerve block for post-Cesarean delivery analgesia decreases morphine use but not opioid-related side effects. *Can J Anaesth* 2002; 49(7):694–700.
150. Bunting P, McConachie I. Ilioinguinal nerve blockade for analgesia after caesarean section. *Br J Anaesth* 1988; 61(6):773–5.
151. Ganta R, Samra SK, Maddineni VR, *et al.* Comparison of the effectiveness of bilateral ilioinguinal nerve block and wound infiltration for postoperative analgesia after caesarean section. *Br J Anaesth* 1994; 72(2):229–30.
152. Abdallah FW, Halpern SH, Margarido CB. Transversus abdominis plane block for postoperative analgesia after Caesarean delivery performed under spinal anaesthesia? A systematic review and meta-analysis. *Br J Anaesth* 2012; 109(5):679–87.
153. Robinson HE, O'Connell CM, Joseph KS, *et al.* Maternal outcomes in pregnancies complicated by obesity. *Obstet Gynecol* 2005; 106(6):1357–64.
154. Royal College of Obstetricians and Gynaecologists. *Reducing the Risk of Thrombosis and Embolism During Pregnancy and the Puerperium*. Green-top Guideline 37a. London: RCOG; 2009.
155. Lopez LM, Grimes DA, Chen-Mok M, *et al.* Hormonal contraceptives for contraception in overweight or obese women. *Cochrane Database Syst Rev* 2013; 4:CD008452.
156. Lashen H, Fear K, Sturdee DW. Obesity is associated with increased risk of first trimester and recurrent miscarriage: matched case-control study. *Hum Reprod* 2004; 19(7):1644–6.
157. Boots C, Stephenson MD. Does obesity increase the risk of miscarriage in spontaneous conception: a systematic review. *Semin Reprod Med* 2011; 29(6):507–13.
158. Watkins ML, Rasmussen SA, Honein MA, *et al.* Maternal obesity and risk for birth defects. *Pediatrics* 2003; 111(5 Part 2):1152–8.
159. McDonald SD, Han Z, Mulla S, *et al.* Overweight and obesity in mothers and risk of preterm birth and low birth weight infants: systematic review and meta-analyses. *BMJ* 341:c3428.
160. Khatibi A, Brantsaeter AL, Sengpiel V, *et al.* Prepregnancy maternal body mass index and preterm delivery. *Am J Obstet Gynecol* 2012; 207(3):212.e1–7.
161. Jacobsen AF, Skjeldestad FE, Sandset PM. Ante- and postnatal risk factors of venous thrombosis: a hospital-based case-control study. *J Thromb Haemost* 2008; 6(6):905–12.
162. Chu SY, Kim SY, Lau J, *et al.* Maternal obesity and risk of stillbirth: a metaanalysis. *Am J Obstet Gynecol* 2007; 197(3):223–8.

CHAPTER 40

Moderate to complex congenital heart disease

Daryl P. Dob, Elspeth E. Pickering, and Michael A. Gatzoulis

Introduction

Children born with congenital heart disease no longer face the prospect of early death and a poor quality of life. In fact, most neonates with moderate to complex congenital heart disease have a survival rate to adulthood of over 80%.

The ratio of adults to children with congenital heart disease is increasing, due to better surgical repairs, and longer survival with a better quality of life. In the Western world, there are more adults than children alive with congenital heart disease. This remarkable medical effort has allowed young women with congenital heart disease to mature to an age where they wish to have babies of their own.

Early generations of women, palliated with the Mustard or Senning intra-atrial switch repairs, have shown it is possible to face the cardiovascular challenges of pregnancy and survive. Consequently, more women with congenital heart disease are taking on possibly the greatest cardiovascular challenge of a woman's life—pregnancy and childbirth.

In Europe, maternal death occurred in 0.5% of mothers with congenital heart disease compared with 0.007% in the normal population.[1] As the number of women with congenital heart disease is predicted to grow by 25% in the next decade[2] and more women with congenital heart disease become pregnant, a better understanding of moderate to complex heart disease, different surgical repair procedures, and residual anomalies is paramount. We will examine the management of parturients with transposition complexes (both classical and congenitally corrected), tetralogy of Fallot, the Fontan circulation, Eisenmenger's syndrome, and congenital aortic stenosis, taking into consideration the effect of pregnancy, labour, delivery, and anaesthesia on each circulation.

History

The development of neonatal and paediatric cardiac surgery and cardiology represents one of the greatest medical advances of the last century. This achievement began in the 1930s when the first closure of a patent ductus arteriosus (PDA) was carried out by Robert Gross in Boston. In 1944, Alfred Blalock and Helen Taussig began to palliate babies with their shunt from the aorta to the pulmonary artery which increased pulmonary blood flow.

In 1953, John Gibbon performed the first surgery using a heart–lung bypass machine or pump oxygenator as it was originally known. Quickly after this, repair of Fallot's tetralogy became possible in 1954, and for the first time palliation of transposition of the great arteries was performed in the 1960s by Mustard in Canada and Senning in Sweden. The Jatene arterial switch was performed in 1976 in Brazil and popularized by Professor Sir Magdi Yacoub throughout the 1970s and 1980s in London, United Kingdom.

This was followed by palliation of even more complex congenital heart disease. For the first time babies with univentricular circulations could be palliated with an atriopulmonary or cavopulmonary connection and grow up with the Fontan circulation, a revolutionary idea to separate oxygenated and deoxygenated blood and increase systemic arterial saturations, accepting the loss of the hypoplastic right ventricle.

With more babies growing to adulthood, the understanding of moderate to complex congenital heart disease, the surgical repairs to treat it, and the residual defects left after surgery are paramount to allow safe passage through pregnancy and delivery.

The role of prepregnancy counselling and the high-risk anaesthetic clinic

In line with the top ten recommendations of the 2006–2008 Confidential Enquiries into Maternal and Child Health report published in 2011,[3] pre-conception counselling is essential. Issues such as risks of mortality and morbidity may be understandably difficult to approach, but need and can be handled sensitively. Accurate documentation is important.

The following factors should be specifically considered: a poor functional class before pregnancy (New York Heart Association (NYHA) functional class higher than II), cyanosis, impaired systemic ventricular function (ejection fraction $< 40\%$), left heart obstruction (mitral valve area $< 2\ cm^2$, aortic valve area $< 1.5\ cm^2$, or left ventricular outflow tract peak blood pressure gradient > 30 mmHg before pregnancy), or a preconception history of adverse cardiac events such as symptomatic arrhythmia, stroke, transient ischaemic attack, and pulmonary oedema. The expected cardiac event rate with none, one, or more than one of these factors is 5%, 27%, and 75% respectively.[4–6]

Multidisciplinary working is essential to ensure a safe outcome for mothers and babies. A regular clinic which allows the mother with congenital heart disease to see her obstetrician, cardiologist, midwife, anaesthetist, intensivist, and neonatologist is paramount.

Normal cardiac configuration

In order to understand the circulations and physiology of moderate to complex congenital heart disease it is important to have a logical understanding of the connections in the normal heart. To do this we have divided the normal circulation into seven features.[7,8]

Figure 40.1 shows a schematic drawing of the normal circulation and the features are described as follows:

1. Venoatrial concordance, that is, all (right and left) veins (systemic and pulmonary) are connected to the corresponding atria normally.
2. No atrial septal defect (ASD).
3. Atrioventricular concordance, that is, the atria are normally connected to the corresponding ventricles (right atrium to right ventricle, etc.).
4. No valvular abnormalities between the atria and the ventricles.
5. No ventricular septal defect (VSD).
6. Ventriculoarterial concordance, that is, the ventricles are connected normally to the corresponding great arteries.
7. No semilunar valvular abnormalities and no connections between the great vessels such as PDA.

Knowledge of these features allows a logical means of communication about different surgical repairs and their residual effects on each circulation.

Physiological changes of pregnancy in the normal cardiovascular system

Systemic vascular resistance is reduced due to peripheral vasodilatation mediated by progesterone, oestrogen, and prostacyclin, as well as low-pressure arteriovenous connections in the placenta. In the normal circulation, central venous and pulmonary artery pressures are unchanged during pregnancy, although central venous pressure is increased during labour and may remain elevated for a few hours postpartum. Blood volume also increases throughout pregnancy and is 45–50% greater than prepregnancy values by term. This represents an increase in both red cell volume and plasma volume. The increase in plasma volume is relatively greater, resulting in physiological anaemia. Cardiac output increases steadily until 20 weeks of gestation when it is maintained at 40–50% above normal until term. This is due to an increase in both stroke volume and heart rate. In labour, cardiac output may increase by a further 25–50% with an additional increase of 15–30% during contractions. It remains elevated for a few hours after delivery. Aortocaval compression by the gravid uterus can lead to reduced venous return, cardiac output, and uterine blood flow. Autotransfusion of blood from the placenta also occurs during the third stage of labour.

Functional residual capacity steadily decreases as pregnancy continues. This, in combination with the increasing oxygen demands of the growing fetus, means arterial oxygen desaturation occurs faster than in the non-pregnant state.[9]

Transposition of the great arteries

Transposition of the great arteries is the commonest cyanotic congenital heart disease seen in neonates.[10] In the presence of an intact ventricular septum, cyanosis is seen on the first day or so of life, when the ductus arteriosus usually closes.

Pathophysiology

In transposition of the great arteries there is ventriculoarterial discordance. This is a feature 6 type abnormality in the classification of cardiac configuration previously described. Figures 40.2

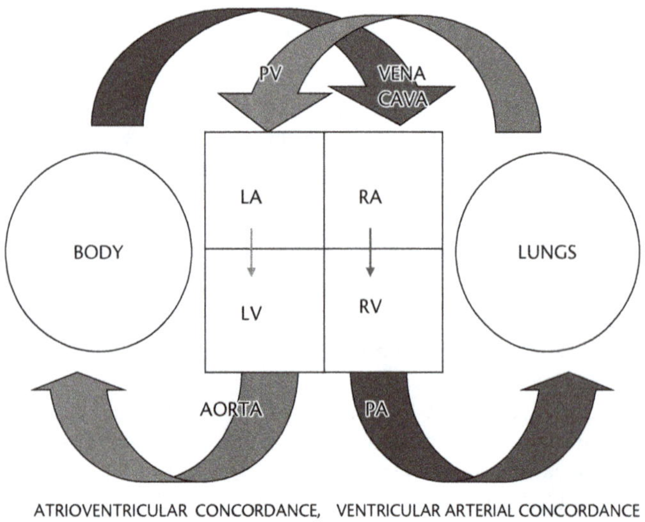

Figure 40.1 (See colour figure section). The normal configuration.
Reprinted from *International Journal of Obstetric Anesthesia*, Volume 19, edition 3, D.P. Dob, M.A. Naguib, M.A. Gatzoulis, A functional understanding of moderate to complex congenital heart disease and the impact of pregnancy. Part I: The transposition complexes, pp. 298–305, Copyright (2010), with permission from Elsevier.

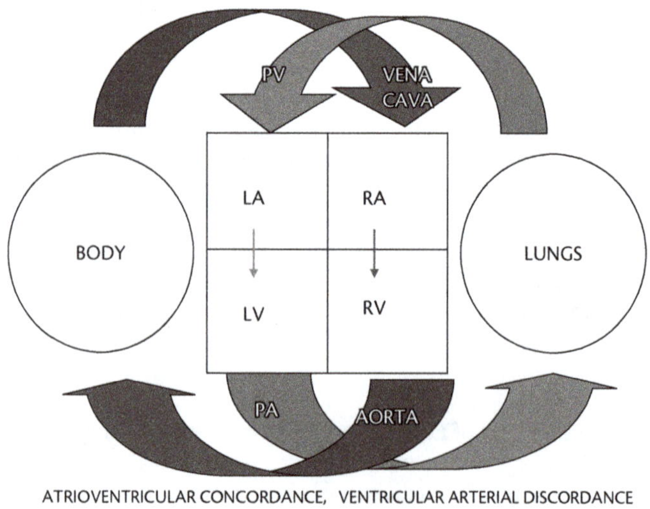

Figure 40.2 (See colour figure section). Classic transposition of the great arteries.
Reprinted from *International Journal of Obstetric Anesthesia*, Volume 19, edition 3, D.P. Dob, M.A. Naguib, M.A. Gatzoulis, A functional understanding of moderate to complex congenital heart disease and the impact of pregnancy. Part I: The transposition complexes, pp. 298–305, Copyright (2010), with permission from Elsevier.

and 40.3 demonstrate the lesion. The aorta and pulmonary artery are incorrectly connected to the left and right ventricles respectively. There is still normal atrioventricular concordance (feature 3). The aorta is connected to the right ventricle and the pulmonary artery to the left ventricle. If there is no connection between pulmonary and systemic circulations this pattern is incompatible with life as the pulmonary circulation receives all the oxygenated blood and the systemic circulation none, that is, there are two completely separate circuits and the patient is severely cyanosed.

Neonates usually survive because mixing between the two circulations allows oxygenated blood to pass through to the systemic circulation. Blood mixes in the heart via a VSD (in >50% of cases), an ASD, or outside the heart via the ductus arteriosus. The ductus arteriosus allows oxygenated blood from the aorta to cross to the pulmonary arteries.

For patients with a large VSD or PDA, high flow through the pulmonary circulation eventually leads to pulmonary hypertension and reversal of flow (Eisenmenger's syndrome—see later). These patients then have differential cyanosis, in which oxygenated blood from the left ventricle entering the pulmonary artery crosses the PDA because of pulmonary hypertension, supplying the lower body with more oxygenated blood than the ascending aorta, leaving them with a blue upper body and head and a pink lower body.

Management

Rashkind atrial balloon septostomy

Early management in cyanotic babies includes prostaglandin E_1 to maintain the patency of the ductus arteriosus and a Rashkind atrial balloon septostomy. This procedure creates a sizeable ASD to improve oxygenation until surgery can be performed.[11] It is performed by passing a catheter through the foramen ovale, blowing a balloon up then pulling the catheter back through, creating the defect. A Blalock–Hanlon surgical atrial septectomy is effectively the same as the Rashkind procedure but carried out as an open operation for infants presenting later when the septum is too thick for balloon septostomy.[12]

Atrial switch (senning or mustard) procedure

From the 1960s to the 1980s repairs concentrated on switching blood flow at atrial level, because arterial switch operations were technically too difficult. Atrial switching was achieved with an atrial baffle, so that deoxygenated blood could be channelled through to the left ventricle and round to the pulmonary circulation, while oxygenated blood could be channelled into the right ventricle (systemic ventricle) to go around the systemic circulation. The inferior vena cava and the superior vena cava are transected and connected to a trouser shaped baffle which conducts the venous blood across to the mouth of the mitral valve. This allows the deoxygenated blood to be pumped around the pulmonary circulation by the subpulmonary (morphological left) ventricle. Oxygenated blood from the lungs returns via the four pulmonary veins into the left atrium. From here it is channelled across to the mouth of the tricuspid valve and into the right ventricle. This allows oxygenated blood to be pumped through the aorta around the systemic circulation, by the subaortic (morphological right) ventricle. These are known as Senning and Mustard repairs and represent physiological rather than anatomical repair. The Senning procedure, in which an atrial baffle was fashioned from autologous tissue, was first described in 1959.[13] This was followed by the Mustard procedure in 1964 where the baffle used was made of synthetic material[14] (Figure 40.4). The 30-year survival rate after atrial switch repair (Mustard or Senning) is 80%.[15]

During surgery for insertion of the atrial baffle, the sinus node may be damaged or compressed, leading to arrhythmia.[16] Pregnancy carries a 20% risk of arrhythmia especially supraventricular tachycardia. This is usually related to the presence of atrial scar tissue, in addition to the physiological changes of pregnancy.[17]

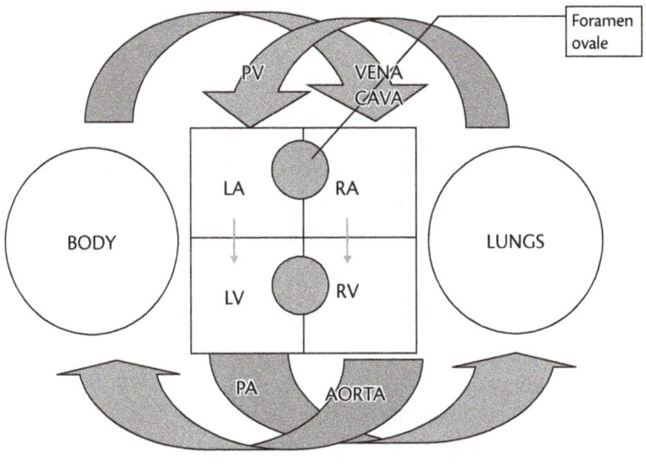

Figure 40.3 (See colour figure section). Classic transposition of the great arteries with a large shunt.

Reprinted from *International Journal of Obstetric Anesthesia*, Volume 19, edition 3, D.P. Dob, M.A. Naguib, M.A. Gatzoulis, A functional understanding of moderate to complex congenital heart disease and the impact of pregnancy. Part I: The transposition complexes, pp. 298–305, Copyright (2010), with permission from Elsevier.

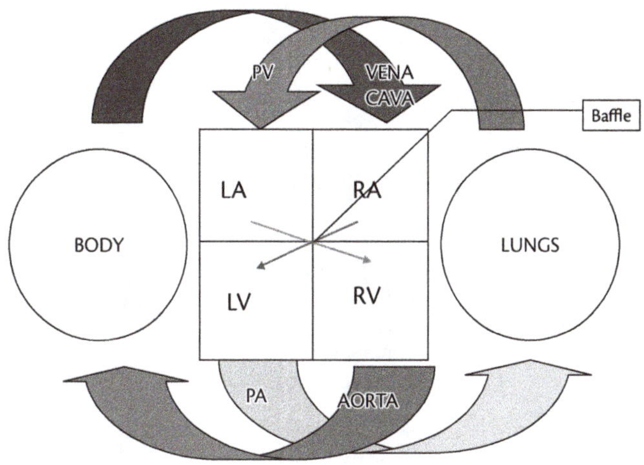

Figure 40.4 (See colour figure section). Intra-atrial baffle (Mustard or Senning atrial switch), represented by the red and blue crossed arrows.

Reprinted from *International Journal of Obstetric Anesthesia*, Volume 19, edition 3, D.P. Dob, M.A. Naguib, M.A. Gatzoulis, A functional understanding of moderate to complex congenital heart disease and the impact of pregnancy. Part I: The transposition complexes, pp. 298–305, Copyright (2010), with permission from Elsevier.

Tachycardia is often more haemodynamically compromising, because of the systemic right ventricle. The presence of artificial tissue, atrial scarring, and complex anatomy makes treatment of arrhythmias by radiofrequency ablation and pacemaker insertion challenging.[18–20]

Baffle obstruction is an infrequent late complication. Obstruction of the superior vena cava is more common than that of the inferior vena cava. Jugular engorgement with facial oedema (superior vena caval syndrome) is usually a late sign indicating obstruction of both superior and inferior venae cavae.[21] Baffle obstruction can be managed by percutaneous balloon dilatation, stent insertion, or occasionally surgical refashioning of the baffle.[22]

Pulmonary hypertension occurs in 7% of patients with Mustard or Senning repairs. Predisposing factors include operation at more than 2 years of age, shunts prior to repair, raised pulmonary pressures, and pulmonary venous baffle obstruction.[23] Some patients with transposition of the great arteries have a degree of pulmonary hypertension at presentation because the left ventricle pumps blood into the pulmonary circulation generating a high pressure, particularly in patients with a large VSD. The most common cause of pulmonary hypertension after baffle procedure is pulmonary venous obstruction secondary to pericardial baffle constriction. The incidence has been reduced since the use of polytetrafluoroethylene baffles.[24]

Women with Mustard or Senning atrial switch repairs for transposition of the great arteries used to represent the majority of patients with moderate to complex congenital heart disease attending high-risk obstetric clinics. This has changed as more women present following an arterial switch operation performed in the 1980s, as this became the operation of choice for transposition of the great arteries. [25] (See 'Arterial Switch (Jatene) Procedure'.)

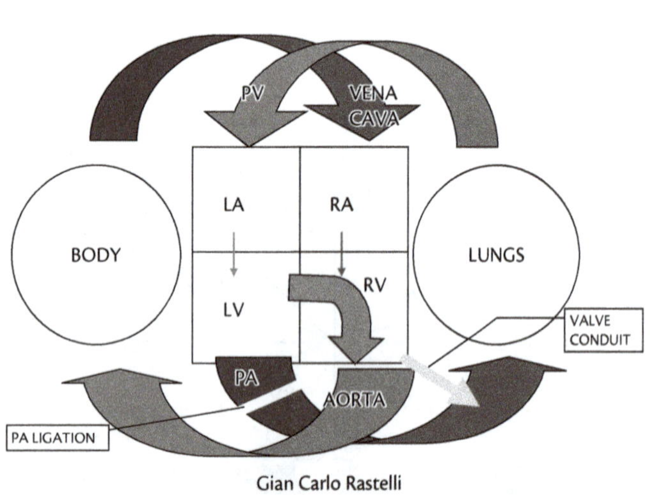

Figure 40.5 (See colour figure section). Rastelli procedure. The large red arrow represents the Dacron tunnel from the left ventricle to the aorta. The blue arrow represents the valved conduit from the right ventricle to the pulmonary artery. The pulmonary trunk is transected and sewn up.

Rastelli procedure

This operation is performed in patients with transposition of the great arteries, VSD, and pulmonary stenosis. Oxygenated blood is directed through the VSD to the aorta using a tunnel made of Dacron® (Figure 40.5). After inserting a large ventricular septal patch, the pulmonary valve is over-sewn and the right ventricle connected to the pulmonary artery via a valved conduit.[26] The Rastelli procedure is a low-risk operation, but later conduit replacement operations are required for most patients. This can be done with low risk.[27] The perceived advantage of this repair is that the systemic ventricle is the left ventricle. In one series, early deaths were related to conduit compression and sepsis, while late deaths were related to residual VSD and infections.[28] The Réparation à l'Etage Ventriculaire (REV; literally repair of the ventricular floor)[29] can be used to dissect off the aorta and pulmonary trunk and change them round without using a valved conduit from the right ventricle. This has the advantage of not having to operate again to replace the conduit. The modified Nikaidoh operation can also be used to dissect off the main arteries in bulk along with the morphologically correct valves and the coronary arteries. These repairs are currently producing good survival and reoperation free numbers but longer follow-up is required.[30]

Arterial switch (Jatene) procedure

The arterial switch procedure (Figure 40.6) was first attempted by Mustard and Senning in the 1950s but was unsuccessful due to early technical problems with cardiopulmonary bypass in small babies. The first successful cases were described in 1976 by Jatene in Brazil and by the 1980s the arterial switch procedure became the operation of choice for transposition of the great arteries.[31] It leaves the patient with a repair that is closer to the normal anatomy, in that the aorta and pulmonary artery are connected to the correct ventricles. The advantages are that the left ventricle now becomes the systemic pumping chamber, and the mitral valve becomes the systemic atrioventricular valve.

The operation is technically demanding as the coronary arteries must be dissected off the pulmonary trunk and re-implanted on to the neo-aorta, without being stretched or kinked.

Coronary events may occur in 7% of patients. They are the main cause of early morbidity and mortality in the postoperative period. They are often related to abnormal coronary anatomy. Kinking, torsion, or extrinsic compression by biological glue are some of the causes of early coronary events and require immediate surgical revision. Late coronary events are uncommon and they are mostly due to progressive intimal thickening due to abnormal coronary blood flow or stretching of the coronary arteries with normal growth.[32] Coronary function must be assessed regularly following surgery, aiming for early diagnosis.[33] This prevents sudden cardiac death due to coronary obstruction.

Ideally the arterial switch operation should be performed before the left ventricle becomes adjusted to the lower pulmonary pressures and thus potentially unable to support the systemic circulation. Left ventricular function may deteriorate gradually after arterial switch operation in patients with transposition of the great arteries with an intact ventricular septum,[34] functional impairment can be observed as early as 2 weeks of life.[35] Pulmonary artery banding is used before surgery to prepare the left ventricle to take over as the systemic ventricle. Unfortunately this is not always successful and left ventricular failure may still

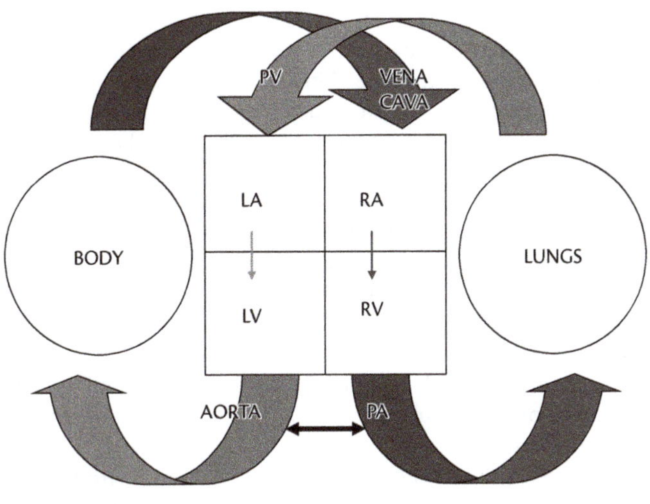

Figure 40.6 (See colour figure section). Arterial switch (Jatene) procedure. Aorta and pulmonary artery switched to the correct ventricle (represented by the black arrow). The coronary arteries are transected with a 'button' of pulmonary artery wall and re-implanted into the neo-aorta, which was the old pulmonary artery.
Reprinted from *International Journal of Obstetric Anesthesia*, Volume 19, edition 3, D.P. Dob, M.A. Naguib, M.A. Gatzoulis, A functional understanding of moderate to complex congenital heart disease and the impact of pregnancy. Part I: The transposition complexes, pp. 298–305, Copyright (2010), with permission from Elsevier.

develop.[36–38] Right ventricular outflow obstruction is the most common late complication of arterial switch procedures. The obstruction can occur at the level of the right ventricle in the form of infundibular stenosis or more commonly in the supravalvular area at the level of the pulmonary artery.[39–41] The mechanism is not clear, but the pulmonary artery may be stretched with growth. In 10% of cases it can be severe enough to require intervention.

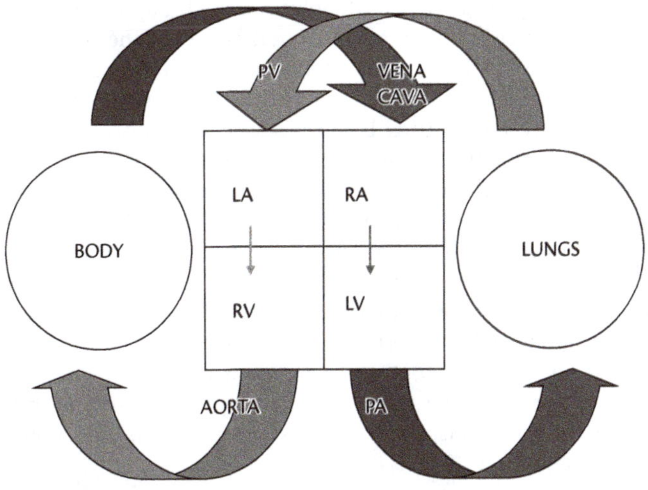

Figure 40.7 (See colour figure section). Congenitally corrected transposition of the great arteries showing double discordance.
Reprinted from *International Journal of Obstetric Anesthesia*, Volume 19, edition 3, D.P. Dob, M.A. Naguib, M.A. Gatzoulis, A functional understanding of moderate to complex congenital heart disease and the impact of pregnancy. Part I: The transposition complexes, pp. 298–305, Copyright (2010), with permission from Elsevier.

Survival rate after the Jatene arterial switch operation can be as high as 96% after 23 years and freedom from reoperation as high as 81.9%.[42] Factors associated with increased mortality include complex transposition of the great arteries, associated cardiac lesions, major intensive care unit events, and re-operation.[43] Patients with arterial switch procedures are now entering early adulthood and increasing numbers are attending high-risk obstetric clinics.[25]

Congenitally corrected transposition of the great arteries

This is an uncommon condition with an incidence of about 1% of all forms of congenital heart diseases.[44] These patients have two abnormalities that nearly correct each other in terms of physiology. They have ventriculoarterial discordance (feature 6, as in patients with classic transposition of the great arteries) but they also have atrioventricular discordance (feature 3), which means they have a natural intra-atrial switch leaving them with an essentially normal circulation in terms of oxygenation (Figure 40.7). However, they have a systemic right ventricle with all the concerns previously discussed. Associated lesions are also common and have an impact on outcome, namely VSD, Ebstein's anomaly of the tricuspid valve (which is the systemic atrioventricular valve), subpulmonary stenosis, and acquired complete heart block.

Since oxygenation is normal at birth, congenitally corrected transposition of the great arteries may present later in life than classic transposition, usually with cardiac failure.[45,46] The median age of death is 40 years, with a 10-year survival of 64–83% from the time of diagnosis, depending on associated anomalies. The main cause of death is heart failure due to the systemic right ventricle.[47–49]

Medical management of congenitally corrected transposition should be aimed at treating complications such as heart failure and arrhythmias. Permanent pacing for complete heart block may be required and biventricular pacing may have an advantage in selected patients.

Surgical treatment such as valvuloplasty or valve replacement for pulmonary stenosis with VSD closure may be required. Pulmonary artery banding increases left ventricular pressure and shifts the interventricular septum to the right. This reduces tricuspid regurgitation and right ventricular dysfunction.

A double-switch procedure (Figure 40.8), in which an arterial switch procedure is combined with an atrial switch procedure, may be used for selected patients, on occasion in preparation for pregnancy. In the atrial switch procedure, the intra-atrial baffle directs oxygenated blood from the left atrium across to the left ventricle, and deoxygenated blood to flow across from the right atrium to the right ventricle. Then the aorta and pulmonary arteries are switched so that the aorta is now connected to the left ventricle and pumps oxygenated blood around the systemic circulation. The right ventricle is connected to the pulmonary artery and pumps deoxygenated blood round to the lungs.[50–52]

The parturient with transposition complexes

Pregnancy

Although the arterial switch procedure is now the gold standard for treatment of transposition of the great vessels, atrial correction was performed regularly until the 1980s and many such patients present to antenatal clinics. They can present with a multitude of

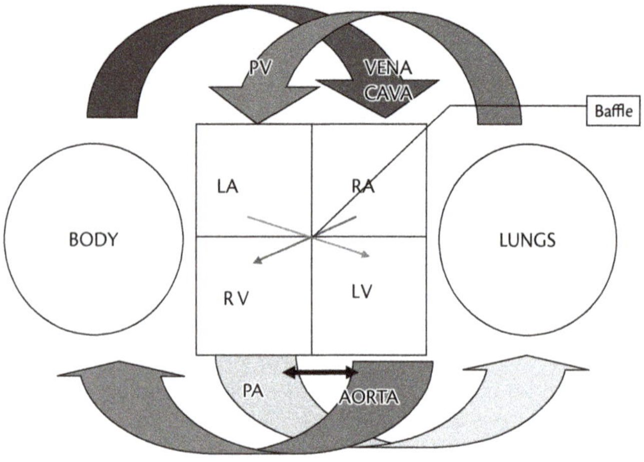

Figure 40.8 (See colour figure section). Double-switch procedure—an intra-atrial switch is combined with an arterial switch to give a near normal circulation to repair congenitally corrected transposition of the great arteries.
Reprinted from *International Journal of Obstetric Anesthesia*, Volume 19, edition 3, D.P. Dob, M.A. Naguib, M.A. Gatzoulis, A functional understanding of moderate to complex congenital heart disease and the impact of pregnancy. Part I: The transposition complexes, pp. 298–305, Copyright (2010), with permission from Elsevier.

problems during pregnancy.[47,53] The most common and potentially life-threatening is right (systemic) ventricular failure or dysfunction. This can be secondary to the pregnancy-induced increase in cardiac output, heart rate, and plasma volume.[53] Strain on the systemic morphological tricuspid valve leads to annular dilatation and subsequent regurgitation, so worsening ventricular failure. Labour puts further strain on the weaker right ventricle. This particular complication can occur any time during pregnancy and delivery.[54]

Patients with more than moderate to severe systemic right ventricular dysfunction should be discouraged from becoming pregnant (and given appropriate contraception) as there is a risk to themselves and a risk of incomplete cardiovascular remodelling even after successful pregnancy, which ultimately compromises their prognosis. It is sometimes necessary to make therapeutic improvements such as baffle reconstruction, before contemplating the demands of pregnancy.

Once pregnant, the woman must be watched carefully for systemic ventricular failure as cardiac output increases with gestation. She will need frequent review by her cardiologist and obstetrician. Cardiac output rises to a peak at around 20 weeks and must then be sustained for the rest of the pregnancy. This is often the time when systemic ventricular failure and pulmonary oedema occur. They can be managed medically. Occasionally, in very severe cases surgical intervention, such as baffle reconstruction, is necessary.

If the woman can sustain the increased ventricular workload, it is a good sign that her circulation is robust. However, if there are signs of decompensation, such as arrhythmias, pulmonary oedema or even simply fatigue, then admission to hospital for bed rest is essential. Delivery should be considered if the gestational age allows.

Mothers with transposition complexes can present with haemodynamically significant arrhythmias, which need to be dealt with promptly. Both DC cardioversion and adenosine are safe and should be offered in any patient with haemodynamic compromise. Beta blockers may convey some protection in arrhythmia control and prevention of recurrence. Patients with a history of arrhythmia should be counselled for catheter-based ablative procedures, which in the right environment and for well selected patients may prevent arrhythmia recurrence during pregnancy.

As gestation progresses, functional residual capacity decreases and respiratory function worsens. This is greatly improved after delivery, so the needs of the mother must be weighed against the needs of a premature fetus. Consultation with the neonatologists is very helpful. Risks to the fetus are associated with poor maternal functional class before pregnancy or maternal cyanosis, left heart obstruction as outlined, maternal age less than 20 or over 35 years, maternal smoking, and treatment with anticoagulants.[55,56]

For patients with congenitally corrected transposition of the great arteries, potential problems in pregnancy include dysfunction of the systemic right ventricle with low cardiac output, increased systemic atrioventricular valve regurgitation with heart failure, atrial arrhythmias, and atrioventricular block. Occasionally, surgery to repair the circulation such as the double-switch operation, may have to be performed prior to conception. The rate of fetal loss is increased.

Labour and delivery in patients with transposition of the great arteries

In the transposition complexes there is a trend towards vaginal delivery and instrumental second stage. If pregnancy is well tolerated and systemic ventricular function is unimpaired, then it is possible to wait for spontaneous labour. A low-dose neuraxial technique can be used for labour analgesia to reduce pain and cardiovascular stress. A traditional epidural or a combined spinal–epidural (CSE) technique that maintains haemodynamic stability[57] are both appropriate. In the CSE technique, 1 mL of plain 0.25% bupivacaine with fentanyl 25 mcg is injected intrathecally and epidural 10–15 mL boluses of 0.1% bupivacaine with fentanyl 2 mcg/mL may be given half-hourly at the request of the patient.[58–60] If systemic ventricular function is good, and the woman appears well in labour, then it is sensible to use non-invasive monitoring: blood pressure, electrocardiography, and pulse oximetry. If systemic ventricular function deteriorates then intra-arterial continuous blood pressure monitoring is useful. It is important to remember that if a Blalock–Taussig shunt has been performed, pulsations in the radial artery may not be present on the operated side. Central venous pressure monitoring is rarely needed unless progress is poor. Pulmonary artery catheterization (PAC) to ascertain pulmonary capillary wedge pressure is not used as a routine, because of technical difficulties in getting through the heart to the pulmonary artery, particularly in an atrial switch (Mustard or Senning) repair and the induction of arrhythmias as the PAC is floated.

In past decades, general anaesthesia was regarded as the mainstay for caesarean delivery in moderate to complex heart disease. It is now rarely used for delivery in mothers with transposition complexes. The presence of a full stomach with delayed gastric emptying in labour necessitates tracheal intubation, which leads to a stress response.[61] It is possible to modify traditional general anaesthesia induction techniques, for example, using high doses of short-acting opioids such as fentanyl, alfentanil, or remifentanil to allow smoother induction. This may help to avoid ventricular depression and hypotension in congenital heart disease but the baby may suffer respiratory depression after birth and need naloxone to counteract residual opiates in the circulation. General anaesthesia tends not to be used for caesarean delivery in women with transposition complexes.

The increased haemodynamic stability associated with low-dose sequential CSE[62,63] or incremental spinal anaesthesia,[64] or *de novo* epidural anaesthesia, has made neuraxial anaesthesia acceptable for caesarean delivery in women with moderate to complex congenital heart disease. Following intrathecal hyperbaric bupivacaine 5 mg with diamorphine 300 mcg, block height is assessed and carefully increased with 5 mL epidural boluses of plain 0.5% bupivacaine/levobupivacaine or ropivacaine 7.5 mg/mL with or without epinephrine 5 mcg/mL, so as to increase block height to a level necessary for surgery. Unfortunately, post-dural puncture headache after intrathecal catheter placement for continuous spinal anaesthesia may be troublesome in obstetric patients.[65]

The blood pressure can be maintained with vasopressors and inotropes. Phenylephrine 25–50 mcg, metaraminol 0.5–1 mg, or epinephrine 5 mcg are useful and can be given in repeated doses. Epinephrine is particularly useful for severe hypotension, as it not only provides vasoconstriction, but positive inotropy and chronotropy. Intra-arterial continuous blood pressure monitoring is a useful guide to vasopressor therapy, but not always necessary for robust circulations. Central venous pressure monitoring may also be useful, but not always necessary. Women with transposition complexes tend to suffer systemic ventricular failure, and small doses of furosemide (5–10 mg) may be given at the time of delivery, to help mobilize and eliminate the extra plasma volume built up during pregnancy. Using these techniques it is possible to deliver babies safely by caesarean delivery and for the mother to be awake to enjoy the experience.

Tetralogy of fallot

Pathology

First described in 1888 by the French physician Etienne-Louis Arthur Fallot,[66,67] tetralogy of Fallot is a common cyanotic congenital heart disease with an incidence of 10% of all reported congenital heart diseases.[68] It is characterized by four components (Figure 40.9):

1. Large VSD.
2. Right ventricular outflow tract obstruction: the severity may vary but it is almost universally at subvalvular level. It is often associated with an abnormality in the pulmonary valve itself. This obstruction causes a right-to-left shunt, a reduction in blood flow to the pulmonary artery, and subsequent cyanosis.
3. Overriding aorta: the aorta receives blood from both the right and left ventricles through the VSD.
4. Right ventricular hypertrophy: progressive right ventricular outflow tract obstruction results in right ventricular hypertrophy which adds to the obstruction and worsens the condition.

Prognosis for patients who do not undergo surgical repair is poor; the most common causes of death are pulmonary haemorrhage, brain abscess, and thromboembolic complications.[69] In 1945, the first surgical treatment for tetralogy of Fallot was performed by Alfred Blalock.[70] This was followed by the first intracardiac repair in 1954, and 1 year later, the first repair using a pump oxygenator by Kirklin.[71] Palliation of tetralogy of Fallot with systemic to pulmonary shunts such as the Blalock–Taussig shunt has been the accepted standard for symptomatic neonates and infants.[72] The Blalock shunt procedure involves fashioning a conduit from the subclavian to the pulmonary artery to increase blood flow to the lungs and bypass pulmonary stenosis. Indications for palliative treatment include cyanotic spells or persistent profound arterial desaturation, very young age, or unfavourable pulmonary arterial anatomy.[73,74]

Surgical repair

Primary repair of tetralogy of Fallot is routinely performed in stable patients aged 6 months or older with suitable pulmonary artery anatomy. Optimal timing for repair remains somewhat controversial, varying between 6 months and 2 years, although currently many surgeons are considering primary neonatal repair.[75,76] Repair involves relieving the right ventricular outflow obstruction and closure of the VSD.

Several complications may follow surgical repair. Up to 80% of patients develop a degree of pulmonary regurgitation.[77] This is made worse by factors that elevate pulmonary artery pressure. Although well tolerated in early life, pulmonary regurgitation may lead to right ventricular dilatation and failure, reduced exercise capacity, arrhythmia, and sudden cardiac death in the long term. The pulmonary valve may eventually need replacement.[78,79]

Aortic valve regurgitation may also occur and is mainly caused by dilatation of the aortic root secondary to increased aortic blood flow before surgical repair. Intrinsic abnormalities of the aortic wall also predispose to aortic root dilatation and secondary aortic regurgitation.[80,81] Other postulated causes are lack of support due to a septal defect and retraction of the surgical patch.[82]

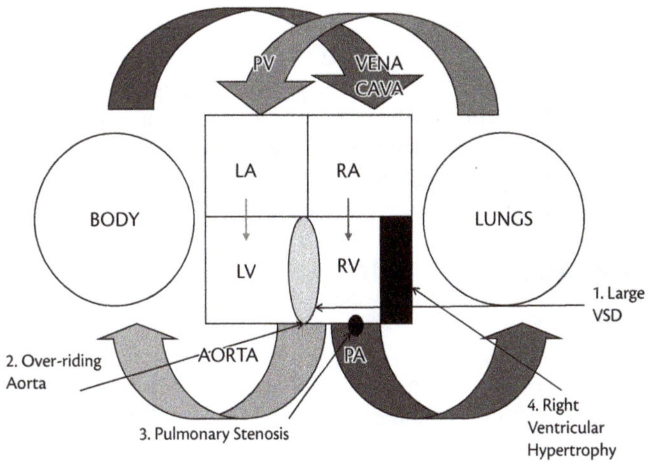

Figure 40.9 (See colour figure section). Fallot's tetralogy. The purple colour represents mixed oxygenated and de-oxygenated blood.

Reprinted from *International Journal of Obstetric Anesthesia*, Volume 19, edition 3, M.A. Naguib, D.P. Dob, M.A. Gatzoulis, A functional understanding of moderate to complex congenital heart disease and the impact of pregnancy. Part II: Tetralogy of Fallot, Eisenmenger's syndrome and the Fontan operation, pp. 306–312, Copyright (2010), with permission from Elsevier.

Further problems after repair include residual or recurrent right ventricular outflow obstruction, right ventricular dilatation, and residual VSD. Atrial and ventricular arrhythmias can also occur. Ventricular arrhythmias are the most common cause of sudden late cardiac death after repair of tetralogy of Fallot.[83]

Pregnancy

Before the introduction of surgical repair, few patients with tetralogy of Fallot reached childbearing age and thus successful pregnancy was uncommon. The haemodynamic burden of pregnancy combined with residual cardiovascular lesions after repair result in a 7% reported incidence of complications. The most important is progressive dilatation of the right ventricle and ventricular failure, in some patients. The circulation should be reviewed with particular reference to severe right ventricular outflow tract obstruction, severe pulmonary regurgitation, and pre-existing right ventricular dysfunction.[84] Other complications include atrial and ventricular arrhythmias, thromboembolism, progressive aortic root dilatation, and endocarditis.[85] There is a 6% incidence of fetal congenital anomaly, including heart disease and pyloric stenosis. Intrauterine growth restriction and spontaneous fetal loss due to low maternal cardiac output may also occur.[86] Early admission to hospital for rest and control of associated complications should be discussed and a plan for delivery agreed and documented. Close follow-up, repeat echocardiography, and treatment of associated complications such as heart failure, arrhythmias, or deterioration of NYHA class is paramount. Preterm delivery should be considered if clinical right ventricular failure and decompensation occur.

Labour and delivery

Vaginal delivery with epidural analgesia is becoming more common, with forceps or ventouse extraction to shorten the second stage. Low-dose epidural or CSE analgesia for labour works well and can avoid haemodynamic instability.[60] If caesarean delivery is planned, low-dose combined spinal with incremental epidural anaesthesia,[62] or incremental *de novo* epidural or incremental spinal catheter anaesthesia[64] are both suitable. If the regional technique fails or there is a life-threatening emergency, general anaesthesia may be necessary. Invasive blood pressure monitoring is useful, but central venous pressure monitoring should be considered carefully, as the information gained can be difficult to interpret and is not always needed. Prophylaxis against thromboembolism and bacterial endocarditis should be considered and postpartum high-dependency care is advised.

Eisenmenger's syndrome

Pathology

Victor Eisenmenger, an Austrian physician, first described this syndrome in 1897, but it was Paul Wood who named it after him and gave us our current understanding of the condition in 1958.[87] It is important as 5–10% of patients with congenital heart disease develop some degree of pulmonary arterial hypertension, which in turn affects functional class and survival prospects.[88]

In patients with intracardiac shunting (ASD or VSD), blood usually flows from left to right, as the pressure on the left side is approximately four times higher. When this shunting is prolonged, exposure of the pulmonary vasculature to systemic arterial pressure leads to progressive changes in the microvasculature causing increased pulmonary vascular resistance. A wide variety of mediators is released, resulting in vasoconstriction and vascular remodelling. The pressure in the pulmonary circulation rises and eventually equals, or, in certain circumstances, exceeds systemic pressures.[89] Figure 40.10 demonstrates that when the pressure on the right side of the heart has increased to equal systemic pressure, a significant amount of blood flows across the VSD from right to left. This dilutes well-oxygenated blood arriving from the lungs with deoxygenated blood, which has completely bypassed the lungs. In pulmonary hypertensive crisis, the pressure on the right side of the heart rises even higher, resulting in more deoxygenated blood entering the systemic circulation, worsening cyanosis (Figure 40.10).

When the shunt reverses from right to left, usually in teenage years or early adulthood, chronic cyanosis and secondary erythrocytosis develop. Some patients with Eisenmenger's syndrome have minimal cyanosis at rest but desaturate profoundly with exercise. General symptoms are usually non-specific and may include breathlessness, fatigue, chest pain, and syncope.[90]

Cerebrovascular accidents result from low oxygen delivery to the tissues, paradoxical embolism, or cerebral abscess. Haemoptysis is also common and may be caused by pulmonary infarction or rupture of a pulmonary vessel, although this is not usually a terminal event. There is also a risk of hepatic and renal impairment and bacterial endocarditis. Arrhythmias are common and may lead to sudden cardiac death. Although exercise limitation and exertional dyspnoea may remain stable for years, poor exercise capacity identifies patients at risk of dying and in need of hospitalization. Congestive cardiac failure is a late ominous sign.[91,92]

Management of Eisenmenger's syndrome

Eisenmenger's syndrome affects many systems and effective management spans a wide variety of treatments.[93–95] Ventricular failure

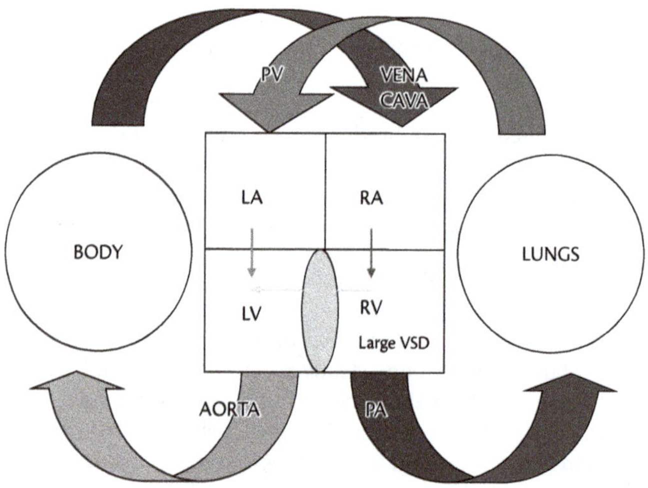

Figure 40.10 (See colour figure section). Eisenmenger's circulation. The purple colour represents mixed oxygenated and de-oxygenated blood.

and associated arrhythmia must be treated promptly. Cyanosis leads to secondary erythrocytosis and blood viscosity increases.[96] As blood viscosity increases, flow and potentially oxygen transport may decrease, leading to symptoms of the 'hyperviscosity syndrome' (headache, loss of concentration, muscle weakness, and fatigue). There is increased risk of cerebrovascular accident[97] and myocardial ischaemia associated with hyperviscosity syndrome. It used to be routinely treated with venesection. However, repeated venesection although useful for primary erythrocytosis, has been shown to result in chronic iron deficiency, microcytosis, and increased whole-blood viscosity in congenital heart disease and so actually increases the risk of cerebrovascular accidents.[98]

Symptoms of iron deficiency are similar to those of hyperviscosity syndrome. In fact, the majority of patients with Eisenmenger's syndrome and chronic secondary erythrocytosis do not exhibit symptoms of overt hyperviscosity and do not require phlebotomies.[99] Iron deficiency should be treated with oral iron supplementation because anaemia limits exercise tolerance and increases the risk of stroke.[100,101] Large intrapulmonary thrombi, occurring in up to a quarter of patients with Eisenmenger's syndrome, may require anticoagulation. Conversely coagulation disorders may occur and must be corrected.

Over the last decade, there has been much interest in pulmonary vasodilators often referred to as pulmonary arterial hypertension-specific therapies. Prostacyclin, produced by vascular endothelium, is a short-acting vasodilator and an inhibitor of platelet aggregation. Prostacyclin analogues, such as epoprostenol, have been shown to improve functional residual capacity and oxygen saturation, and to reduce pulmonary vascular resistance providing both haemodynamic and symptomatic improvement. [102] Patients treated with epoprostenol for up to 3 years live longer than those receiving standard therapy.[103] Endothelins are powerful vasoconstrictors produced by vascular endothelium; competitive antagonists of endothelin-1, such as bosentan, are effective vasodilators. Sildenafil, a selective phosphodiesterase-5 inhibitor, results in increased nitric oxide levels and pulmonary vasodilatation.[104] Both these classes of drug have been used in the management of pulmonary hypertension in Eisenmenger's syndrome, and they are joined by ambrisentan and tadalafil.[105] In the acute situation, inhalation of nitric oxide itself may reduce total pulmonary vascular resistance in 30% of patients.

Heart and lung transplantation or lung transplantation with repair of the defect is the only surgical treatment.[106] However, it is a remote option only in highly selected patients, and there are currently major problems with shortage of donor organs. Currently, the results of the pulmonary arterial hypertension-specific therapies mentioned above have improved oxygenation and quality of life so much that the decision to offer heart transplantation to patients with Eisenmenger's syndrome is now even more challenging. Nevertheless, short-term survival for patients undergoing single or bilateral lung transplant is 70–80% at 1 year while long-term results are less favourable with only 50% surviving 4 years. Heart and lung transplant recipients have a 1-year survival of 60–80% and a 10-year survival less than 30%.[107,108] Life expectancy without transplantation in Eisenmenger's syndrome may be up to 20 years.[109]

Pregnancy

Although maternal morbidity has decreased significantly over the past decade compared with previous decades, it still remains extremely high.[110] This change is due to the availability of pulmonary artery hypertension specific therapies mentioned previously. In the case of patients with pulmonary artery hypertension due to congenital heart disease, the mortality rate in a large British study was 28%[111] (from 36% in a previous study[112]), with the majority of deaths occurring within the first month after delivery due to right heart failure. In patients with pulmonary artery hypertension secondary to congenital heart disease, the systemic vasodilation induced by pregnancy together with the increase in cardiac output may enhance right-to-left shunting, exacerbating pre-existing hypoxia and leading to further pulmonary vasoconstriction. Additional stress occurring during labour and delivery, when hypercarbia and acidosis may lead to an acute increase in pulmonary hypertension, can also lead to refractory right heart failure, the main cause of postnatal death in women with pulmonary arterial hypertension due to congenital heart disease.

The spontaneous abortion rate is up to 40% and surviving infants suffer from intrauterine growth restriction.

Pregnancy prevention or early termination is the preferred measure for improving long-term survival. Combined oral contraceptives carry an increased risk of thrombosis while progesterone only contraceptives have a high failure rate. Laparoscopic sterilization carries the risk of general anaesthesia. Intrauterine coil and subdermal devices offer good safety and efficacy profiles and compare favourably with sterilization. Sterilization of the male partner may be an alternative.[113,114]

Labour and delivery

For the patient who opts to continue pregnancy, coordination of a multidisciplinary team consisting of obstetrician, midwife, cardiologist, anaesthetist, intensive care physician, neonatologist, and social worker is essential. Antenatal counselling is very important and should be carried out in a multidisciplinary forum. Accurate records are necessary, because discussions, particularly those involving mortality, are often forgotten in the aftermath of subsequent events. Early detection and treatment of pregnancy-induced complications is important. The most common is ventricular failure.[115] Patients are usually admitted to the hospital early in the third trimester for bed rest and supplemental oxygen. The use of anticoagulation is controversial, but should be considered on an individual basis.

The pulmonary vasodilators mentioned earlier may be used, with the exception of endothelin antagonists, which are contraindicated in pregnancy because of concerns about teratogenicity. Inhaled nitric oxide may be useful, particularly during the peripartum period.

To allow a planned delivery, most patients with Eisenmenger's syndrome are delivered by elective caesarean delivery, frequently between 30 and 34 weeks, when the infant is viable and before major maternal decompensation ensues. *De novo* incremental epidural, low-dose sequential CSE,[62,116] or incremental spinal anaesthesia[64] are useful, as both allow slow titration of block height with minimal effects on the peripheral circulation, sometimes without the need for vasoconstrictors. Care must be taken not to reduce the systemic vascular resistance too much with the neuraxial technique such that the shunt from right to left worsens. Fluid balance must be meticulous to prevent excessive fluid overload or hypovolaemia both of which will affect shunting. If general anaesthesia is used, transoesophageal echocardiography and invasive monitoring are easier to perform. High-dose opioids may be used to obtund the stress response to tracheal intubation.

Prophylaxis against deep venous thrombosis and infective endocarditis are imperative.[117] All mothers with Eisenmenger's syndrome should be cared for in a high dependency or intensive care unit for at least 48 hours, and close monitoring for 7–10 days is recommended

Fontan procedure

Pathology

First described in 1971 by Francis Fontan for the treatment of tricuspid atresia,[118] the Fontan procedure is now used in the treatment of most congenital heart defects which feature a single functional ventricle, a configuration that cannot be refashioned into a biventricular circulation.[119] Figure 40.11 shows the circulation of a patient with tricuspid atresia and a functional single ventricle.

The Fontan procedure separates pulmonary and systemic circulations, therefore normalizing the oxygen content of systemic blood. It involves either a direct connection between the systemic venous return and the pulmonary artery (the total cavopulmonary connection (TCPC)) or via the right atrium (atriopulmonary connection or classic Fontan circulation), bypassing the right ventricle.[120] This has the advantage that deoxygenated blood is oxygenated in the lungs and does not mix with deoxygenated systemic venous return in the single ventricle. Because the right ventricle is hypoplastic and, after the Fontan procedure, disconnected from the lungs, pulmonary flow must come from the remaining kinetic energy of the systemic circulation driven by the single ventricle. Therefore high venous pressures are usually required. The two circulations are separated and systemic oxygen saturation is high, while the single ventricle (left and hypoplastic right together) promotes flow only through the aorta (Figure 40.12).

Early versions of the Fontan procedure involved connecting the right atrium directly to the pulmonary artery with a valved conduit. This was called the atriopulmonary Fontan or classic Fontan procedure. Unfortunately, with time these versions resulted in sluggish, turbulent, and diminished blood flow through the lungs. Furthermore the relatively underdeveloped pulmonary vasculature was not ready to accept the venous blood flow, and back pressure on the venous system inevitably built up. This caused multiple complications such as right atrial dilatation, pleural effusions, ascites, liver venous engorgement, cirrhosis, and protein-losing enteropathy.

Marc de Leval developed the concept of the modern TCPC.[121] This is now completed in stages to avoid overburdening the developing pulmonary circulation.

After palliation such as a modified Blalock–Taussig [122] shunt to increase pulmonary blood flow, the first stage is to perform a bi-directional Glenn shunt operation.[123] This involves transecting the superior vena cava from the right atrium and connecting it to the right pulmonary artery. In this operation the venous blood from the upper body, head, and neck, flows passively through the lungs via the right and left pulmonary arteries (bi-directional), becoming oxygenated and returning to the left atrium. The inferior vena cava is still connected to the right atrium and so deoxygenated blood from the lower body still mixes in the single ventricle with the oxygenated blood from the lungs. The blood pumped out has an overall oxygen saturation of about 85–90%. This is an improvement on the previous oxygen saturation of about 80%, and allows the pulmonary blood vessels to accommodate a higher blood flow than before. The final stage of the procedure is to complete the TCPC. This involves transecting

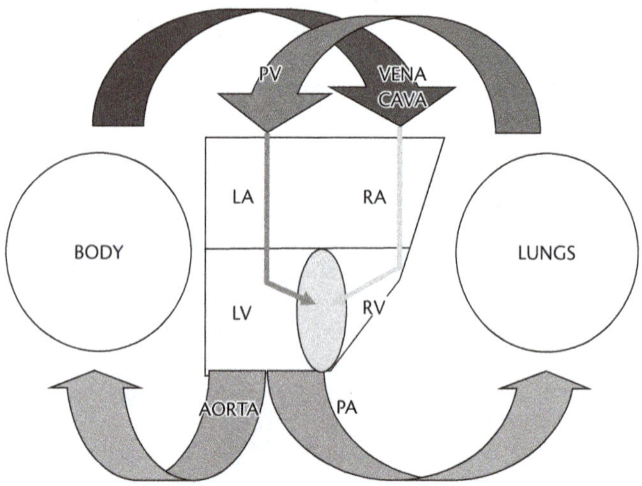

Figure 40.11 (See colour figure section). Univentricular circulation suitable for the Fontan operation. The purple colour represents mixed oxygenated and de-oxygenated blood.

Reprinted from *International Journal of Obstetric Anesthesia*, Volume 19, edition 3, M.A. Naguib, D.P. Dob, M.A. Gatzoulis, A functional understanding of moderate to complex congenital heart disease and the impact of pregnancy. Part II: Tetralogy of Fallot, Eisenmenger's syndrome and the Fontan operation, pp. 306–312, Copyright (2010), with permission from Elsevier.

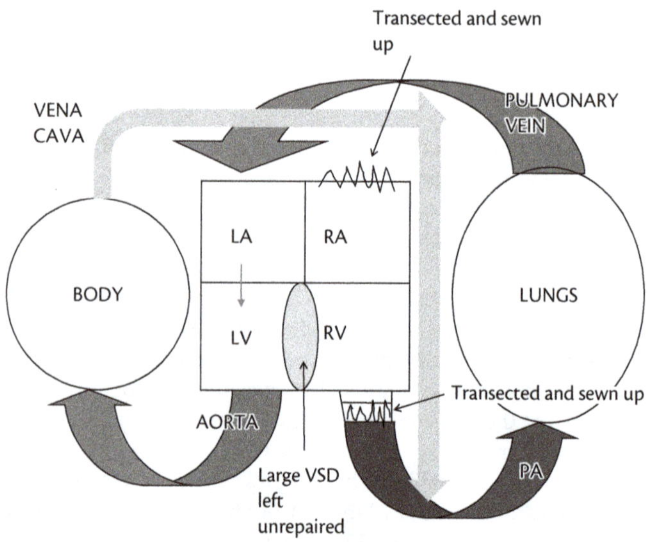

Figure 40.12 (See colour figure section). Total cavopulmonary connection (TCPC), the modern Fontan circulation.

LA = left atrium, LV = left ventricle, RA = right atrium, ASD = atrial septal defect, RV = right ventricle, VSD = ventricular septal defect, PA = pulmonary artery, PV = pulmonary veins. Reprinted from *International Journal of Obstetric Anesthesia*, Volume 19, edition 3, M.A. Naguib, D.P. Dob, M.A. Gatzoulis, A functional understanding of moderate to complex congenital heart disease and the impact of pregnancy. Part II: Tetralogy of Fallot, Eisenmenger's syndrome and the Fontan operation, pp. 306–312, Copyright (2010), with permission from Elsevier.

the inferior vena cava, and connecting it to the pulmonary artery. This means that oxygenated and deoxygenated blood are completely separated, and arterial oxygen saturations reach 94–100%. The completely oxygenated blood is pumped out of the aorta by the single ventricle. It delivers oxygen to the body and then returns via the superior and inferior venae cavae directly to the pulmonary artery through the lungs, using the remaining kinetic energy of the single ventricle pump.

To overcome the problems of turbulent flow, the inferior vena cava is transected and connected to a conduit or 'tunnel' which takes blood through to the pulmonary artery, without eddying through the atrium. This allows smooth laminar blood flow.

In the early period after this operation, the problem of high venous back pressure can still occur. It is possible to make a small hole or 'fenestration' in the tunnel. If pulmonary venous pressure rises, then deoxygenated blood can vent out of the tunnel into the right atrium. This stops the venous pressure rising too high, at the expense of deoxygenated blood shunting through to the single ventricle. Although this slightly reduces systemic arterial saturation, it is worth it to allow the pulmonary vasculature time to recover from bypass surgery. At a later age it is possible to close the fenestration, usually with a catheter technique. In more recent times, the tunnel has been placed outside the right atrium forming an extracardiac conduit, with a small fenestration connected to the atrium.

In children with slightly better developed right ventricular morphology, the 'one-and-a-half ventricle' approach can be used. In this operation, the pulmonary trunk is not transected and the right ventricle is sealed up and allowed to pump blood from the inferior vena cava through the lungs, while the superior vena cava deoxygenated blood goes directly to the lungs through the bi-directional Glenn shunt. Long-term results are good and these patients may avoid the cyanosis and other venous back-pressure problems seen with the TCPC, because the small right ventricle provides some useful kinetic energy for the pulmonary blood flow.[124] Figure 40.13 shows a TCPC which is the modern version of the older atriopulmonary connection or classic Fontan procedure. The superior vena cava is transected and the top part connected to the right pulmonary artery. Subsequently, the inferior vena cava is connected to the underside of the pulmonary artery confluence either with an intra-atrial baffle or more recently with an extracardiac conduit. The proximal pulmonary artery is then transected and sewn up. All the systemic venous blood is thus directed to the lungs and all the oxygenated blood from the lungs travels through the pulmonary veins to the left atrium and into the single ventricle, then to the aorta (as there is no connection of the ventricle with the transected pulmonary artery). This oxygenated blood supplies the systemic circulation and is returned via the venae cavae to repeat the cycle.

The great advantage of the Fontan procedure that the oxygenated and deoxygenated blood are completely separated comes at a price; there is sluggish blood flow through the lungs, driven only by the remaining kinetic energy of the single ventricle pumping blood round the entire circuit. Venous return and pulmonary flow are particularly vulnerable to any extrinsic compression of the veins, for example, by positive pressure pulmonary ventilation, aortocaval compression, or pneumoperitoneum for laparoscopy.[125]

Survival following the Fontan operation is 85–98% at 1 month, 97% at 1 year, 94% at 5 years, and 90% at 10 years.[126–129]

Complications of a fontan circulation

Complications after the Fontan procedure are common and relate to increased venous pressure congestion and low cardiac output.[130,131] Exercise tolerance is reduced mainly due to impaired

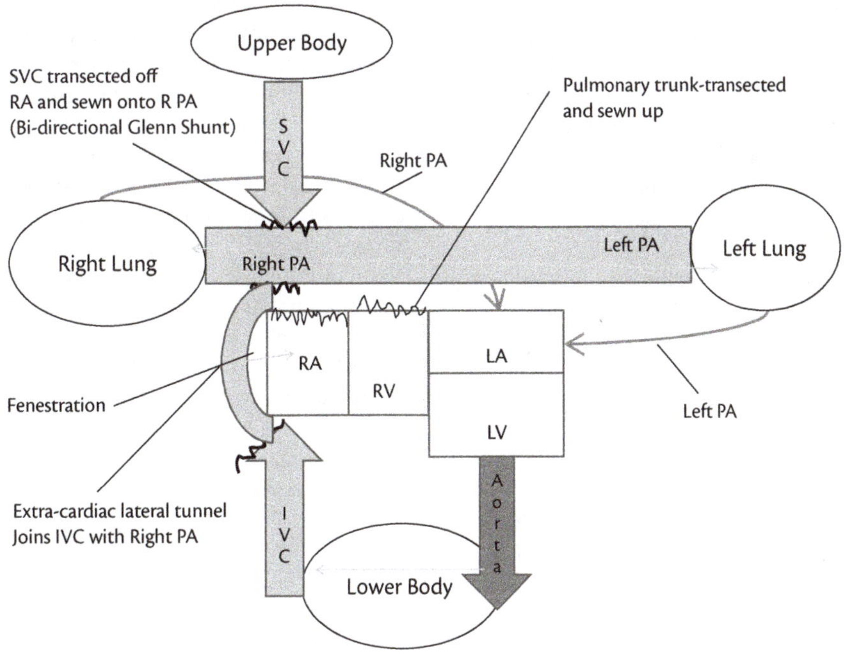

Figure 40.13 (See colour figure section). Total cavopulmonary connection (TCPC) in detail with extracardiac lateral tunnel and fenestration (the modern Fontan). The superior vena cava is transected and connected to the right pulmonary artery. This is known as a bi-directional Glenn shunt and is usually the first part of the palliation. Subsequently, the inferior vena cava is transected and connected to the underside of the pulmonary artery confluence with an extracardiac conduit. The proximal pulmonary trunk is then transected and sewn up.

ventricular function and difficulty in increasing preload. The common ventricle can become dilated, hypertrophic, and hypocontractile. This is caused by the congenital malformation itself, previous surgery, or the very abnormal working conditions at the various stages of palliation before and after a Fontan operation. Low to moderate exercise training may improve cardiopulmonary fitness and should be preceded by exercise testing with electrocardiography.[132] Unfortunately atrial arrhythmias occur in up to 45% of patients and are due to incorporation of the atrial wall in the repair, causing atrial dilatation and hypertrophy. The sinoatrial node, its arterial supply, or its innervations may also be injured at the time of Fontan surgery.

Protein-losing enteropathy secondary to increased venous pressure is a serious complication of Fontan surgery occurring in 3–13% of late survivors. Protein loss results in hypoalbuminaemia and clinical features of oedema, pleural effusion, ascites, immunodeficiency, and hypocalcaemia.[133,134] Treatment includes a low-salt, high-calorie, high-protein diet with medium-chain triglyceride supplements, diuretics, steroids, heparin, protein infusions, and octreotide (synthetic somatostatin).

Thromboembolic complications have a major impact on long-term prognosis. There is also evidence to suggest an increased risk of intracardiac thrombus formation in patients with the Fontan circulation, which is associated with an increased risk of systemic thromboembolism, not necessarily eradicated by warfarin or aspirin therapy.[135]

Pregnancy

Modified Fontan procedures have improved the long-term survival of patients with single-ventricle physiology, who are now reaching childbearing age. The combination of chronic hypoxaemia before palliation and chronic venous congestion afterwards may influence ovarian function resulting in menstrual cycle disorders and infertility.[136] For those who do become pregnant the most common obstetric complications are preterm rupture of membranes, and premature delivery between 26 and 33 weeks. There is a significant risk of neonatal death and postpartum haemorrhage. Arrhythmias, most commonly supraventricular, complicate at least 26% of pregnancies mostly in those with atriopulmonary connection (the older type of Fontan operation.)[137]

Labour and delivery

It is important to avoid dehydration, which may reduce central venous pressure and blood flow through the cavopulmonary connection to the lungs. Avoidance of aortocaval compression by the gravid uterus and thromboprophylaxis are equally important. Since negative intrathoracic pressure helps draw venous return around the pulmonary circulation, it is important to avoid positive pressure ventilation, which will decrease pulmonary blood flow and thus cardiac output. The use of low-dose epidural analgesia or sequential low-dose CSE anaesthesia is preferred to general anaesthesia.

Any form of pneumoperitoneum for laparoscopic procedures will decrease venous return and should be avoided.

Left ventricular outflow tract disorders

Obstructive lesions of the left ventricular outflow tract can occur at three different levels. The aortic stenosis may be subvalvular, valvular, or supravalvular aortic stenosis. Subvalvular and valvular aortic stenosis are more commonly found in males than females. In fact, valvular congenital bicuspid aortic stenosis is four times less common in women than men.

Many women with aortic stenosis will have had a repair during childhood. This is commonly done by the Ross procedure.[138] The stenotic aortic valve is removed and replaced by the native pulmonary valve, with the allograft valve taking the place of the pulmonary valve. This puts the allograft under less pressure.[139,140]

Pregnancy is usually well tolerated in women with isolated mild to moderate aortic obstruction and good left ventricular function. However, women with severe aortic stenosis may be at risk from 20 weeks of gestation onwards as cardiac output has increased by as much as 50%, and this increase must be sustained for a further 18–20 weeks if possible. Women who are pregnant with severe aortic stenosis are at risk of angina, left ventricular failure, and pulmonary oedema as well as sudden death.

It is possible that these symptoms occur for the first time in pregnancy, and management of severe congenital aortic stenosis will depend on the individual mother's needs and her gestation. In pregnancy, because of increased cardiac output, transvalvular pressure gradients measured by echocardiography are not as useful as valve area measurements. Mild aortic stenosis has a valve area of more than 1.5 cm^2, moderate 0.8–1.5 cm^2, and severe aortic stenosis a valve area of less than 0.7 cm^2. Severe aortic stenosis gives a transvalvular pressure gradient of more than 50 mmHg in the non-pregnant state and more than 80 mmHg in pregnancy. If the gradient falls without treatment this may indicate left ventricular failure and prompt immediate action.[60]

Medical treatment is aimed at reducing heart rate to allow better ventricular ejection and coronary filling. Beta blockers may be used in conjunction with bed rest and oxygen therapy to allow the fetus to grow.

If the mother's condition deteriorates and the fetus is not mature enough for delivery, aortic valve balloon dilatation can be considered. It does, however, carry the risk of severe aortic regurgitation, embolism, and cardiac tamponade. Nevertheless, in severe aortic stenosis it may be used as a bridging device to prolong the pregnancy and mature the fetus to a stage where it can be delivered and a definitive aortic valve replacement performed.[141]

Cardiopulmonary bypass during pregnancy carries a high risk of death to both mother (15%) and fetus (19–33%), so definitive aortic valve replacement during pregnancy should only be undertaken in the most exceptional circumstances. Heparinization for cardiopulmonary bypass also carries the risk of placental bleeding.

If, however, the fetus is viable, it can be delivered by caesarean delivery and then aortic valve replacement carried out under cardiopulmonary bypass after delivery, usually with the same general anaesthetic.

Beating heart aortic valve replacement and catheter aortic valve replacement are alternative strategies for these mothers.

Conclusion

Women with moderate to severe congenital heart disease are now presenting to maternity services with increasing frequency; they pose additional risks to themselves and their offspring during pregnancy and the peripartum period. Better awareness of underlying anatomy, physiology, and common complications together with a multidisciplinary approach including expertise in obstetric anaesthesia can improve the chances of safe delivery for both mother and baby and allow this growing patient population to reach their full life potential.[142]

Acknowledgements

We would like to acknowledge the clinical contributions of our colleagues at Chelsea and Westminster Hospital and the Royal Brompton Hospital, London, particularly Dr M.A. Naguib in Rotorua, New Zealand, and the teamwork which makes it possible to look after this challenging, but rewarding, population of patients.

References

1. Roos-Hesselink JW, Ruys TP, Stein JI, *et al.* Outcome of pregnancy in patients with structural or ischaemic heart disease: results of a registry of the European Society of Cardiology. *Eur Heart J* 2013; 34(9):657–65.
2. Department of Health. *Report of the Paediatric and Congenital Cardiac Services Review Group.* London: Department of Health; December 2003. http://webarchive.nationalarchives.gov.uk/20130107105354/http://www.dh.gov.uk/prod_consum_dh/groups/dh_digitalassets/@dh/@en/documents/digitalasset/dh_4070818.pdf
3. Cantwell R, Clutton-Brock T, Cooper G, *et al.* Saving Mothers' Lives: Reviewing maternal deaths to make motherhood safer: 2006–2008. The Eighth Report of the Confidential Enquiries into Maternal Deaths in the United Kingdom. *BJOG* 2011; 118 Suppl 1:1-203.
4. Siu SC, Colman JM. Heart disease and pregnancy. *Heart* 2001; 85(6):710–15.
5. Drenthen W, Boersma E, Balci A, *et al.* Predictors of pregnancy complications in women with congenital heart disease. *Eur Heart J* 2010; 31(17):2124–32.
6. Lui GK, Silversides CK, Khairy P, *et al.* Heart rate response during exercise and pregnancy outcome in women with congenital heart disease. *Circulation* 2011; 123(3):242–8.
7. Dob DP, Naguib MA, Gatzoulis MA. A functional understanding of moderate to complex congenital heart disease and the impact of pregnancy. Part I: The transposition complexes. *Int J Obstet Anaesth* 2010; 19(3):298–306.
8. Naguib MA, Dob DP, Gatzoulis MA. A functional understanding of moderate to complex congenital heart disease and the impact on pregnancy. Part II: Tetralogy of Fallot, Eisenmenger's syndrome and the Fontan operation. *Int J Obstet Anaesth* 2010; 19(3):306–12.
9. Carlin A, Alfirevic Z. Physiological changes of pregnancy and monitoring. *Best Pract Res Clin Obstet Gynaecol* 2008; 22(5):801–23.
10. Levin DL, Paul MH, Muster AJ, *et al.* D-transposition of the great vessels in the neonate. A clinical diagnosis. *Arch Inter Med* 1977; 137(10):1421–5.
11. Rashkind WJ, Miller WW. Creation of ASD without thoracotomy: a palliative approach to complete transposition of the great vessels. *JAMA* 1966; 196(11):991–2.
12. Blalock A, Hanlon CR. Surgical treatment of complete transposition of the aorta and pulmonary artery. *Surg Gynecol Obstet* 1950; 90(1):1–15.
13. Senning A. Surgical correction of transposition of the great vessels. *Surgery* 1959; 45(6):966–80.
14. Mustard WT. Successful two stage correction of transposition of the great vessels. *Surgery* 1964; 55:469–72.
15. Moons P, Gewilling M, Sluymans T, *et al.* Long term outcome up to 30 years after Mustard or Senning operation: a nationwide multicentre study in Belgium. *Heart* 2004; 90(3):307–13.
16. Dos L, Teruel L, Ferreira IJ, *et al.* Late outcome of Senning and Mustard procedures for correction of transposition of the great arteries. *Heart* 2005; 91(5):652–6.
17. Drenthen W, Pieper PG, Ploeg M, *et al.* Risk of complications during pregnancy after Senning or Mustard repair of complete transposition of the great arteries. *Eur Heart J* 2005; 26(23):2588–95.
18. Schwerzerman M, Salehian O, Harris L, *et al.* Ventricular arrhythmias and sudden death in adults after Mustard operation for transposition of great arteries. *Eur Heart J* 2009; 30(15):1873–9.
19. Human-Sorduna I, Sabine E. Ablation of atrial tachycardias post Mustard or Senning surgeries for d-transposition of the great arteries. *Prog Paediatr Cardiol* 2012; 34(1); 75–8.
20. Koyak Z, de Groot J, Mulder BJ. Interventional and surgical treatment of cardiac arrhythmias in adults with congenital heart disease. *Expert Rev Cardiovasc Ther* 2010; 8(12):1753–66.
21. Patel S, Shah D, Chintala K, *et al.* Atrial Baffle problems following the mustard operation in children and young adults with dextro-transposition of the great arteries: the need for improved clinical detection in the current Era. *Congenit Heart Dis* 2011; 6(5):466–74.
22. Warnes CA. Congenital heart disease for the adult cardiologist. Transposition of the great arteries. *Circulation* 2006; 114(24):2699–709.
23. Chan E, Alejos J. Pulmonary hypertension in patients after repair of transposition of the great arteries. *Congenit Heart Dis* 2010; 5(2):161–4.
24. Champsaur GL, Sokol D, Truslar GA, *et al.* Repair of transposition of the great arteries in 123 paediatric patients: early and long term results. *Circulation* 1973; 47(5):1032–41.
25. Tobler D, Fernandes SM, Wald RM, *et al.* Pregnancy outcomes in women with transposition of the great arteries and arterial switch operation. *Am J Cardiol* 2010; 106(3):417–20.
26. Rastelli GC, McGoon DC, Wallace RB. Anatomic correction of transposition of the great arteries with ventricular septal defect and subpulmonary stenosis. *J Thorac Cardiovasc Surg* 1969; 58(4): 545–52.
27. Brown JW, Ruzmetov M, Huynh D, *et al.* Rastelli operation for transposition of the great arteries with ventricular septal defect and pulmonary stenosis. *Ann Thorac Surg* 2011; 91(1):188–93.
28. Moulton AL, De Lavel MR, Macartney FJ, *et al.* Rastelli procedure for transposition of the great arteries, VSD and left ventricular outflow obstruction, early and late results in 41 patients. *Br Heart J* 1981; 45(1):20–8.
29. Lecompte Y, Neveux JY, Leca F, *et al.* Reconstruction of the pulmonary outflow tract without prosthetic conduit. *J Thorac Cardiovasc Surg* 1982; 84(5):727–33.
30. Hu SS, Liu ZG, Li SJ, *et al.* Strategy for biventricular outflow tract reconstruction: Rastelli, REV, or Nikaidoh procedure? *J Thorac Cardiovasc Surg* 2008; 135(2):331–8.
31. Jatene AD, Fontes VF, Paulista PP, *et al.* Anatomic correction of transposition of the great vessels. *J Thorac Cardiovasc Surg* 1976; 72(3):364–70.
32. Legendre A, Losay J, Touchot-Koné A, *et al.* Coronary events after arterial switch operation for transposition of the great arteries. *Circulation* 2003; 108 Suppl 1:186–90.
33. Raisky O, Bergoend E, Agnoletti G, *et al.* Late coronary artery lesions after neonatal arterial surgical correction: results of surgical coronary revascularisation. *Eur J Cardiothoracic Surg* 2007:31(5): 894–8.
34. Pettersen E, Fredriksen PM, Urheim S, *et al.* Ventricular function in patients with transposition of the great arteries operated with arterial switch. *Am J Cardiol* 2009; 104(4):583–9.
35. Hui L, Chau AKT, Leung MP, *et al.* Assessment of left ventricular function long term after arterial switch operation for transposition of the great arteries by dobutamine stress echo. *Heart* 2005; 91(1):68–72.
36. Grotenhuis HB, Ottenkamp J, Fontein D, *et al.* Aortic elasticity and left ventricular function after arterial switch operation: MR-imaging initial experience. *Radiology* 2008; 249(3):801–9.

37. Chen RH, Wong SJ, Wong WH, *et al.* Left ventricular contractile reserve after arterial switch operation for complete transposition of the great arteries: an exercise echocardiographic study. *Eur Heart J Cardiovasc Imaging* 2013; 14(5):480–6.
38. Lacour-Gayet F, Piot D, Zoghbi J, *et al.* Surgical management and indications of left ventricular retraining in arterial switch operation for transposition of the great arteries with an intact ventricular septum. *Eur J Cardiothorac Surg* 2001; 20(4):824–9.
39. Swartz MF, Sena A, Atallah-Yunes N, *et al.* Decreased incidence of supravalvar pulmonary stenosis after arterial switch operation. *Circulation* 2012; 126(11, Suppl 1):118–22.
40. Delmo Walter EM, Miera O, Nasseri B, *et al.* Onset of pulmonary stenosis after arterial switch operation for transposition of great arteries with intact ventricular septum. HSR Proceedings in Intensive Care and Cardiovascular *Anesthesia* 2011; 3(3):177–87.
41. Santoro G, Di Carlo D, Formigari R, *et al.* Late onset pulmonary valvular stenosis after arterial switch operation for transposition of the great arteries. *Heart* 1998; 79(3):311–12.
42. Lim HG, Kim WH, Lee JR, *et al.* Long-term results of the arterial switch operation for ventriculo-arterial discordance. *Eur J Cardiothorac Surg* 2013; 43(2):325–34.
43. Losay J, Touchot A, Serraf A, *et al.* Late outcome after arterial switch operation for transposition of the great arteries. *J Am Coll Cardiol* 2001; 81(12 Suppl 1):121–6.
44. Cordone M, Wolfson A, Wolfson M, *et al.* Anesthetic management of labor in a patient with congenitally corrected transposition of the great arteries. *IJOA* 2008; 17(1):57–60.
45. Beauchesne LM, Warnes CA, Connolly HM, *et al.* Outcome of unoperated patients who present with congenitally corrected transposition of the great arteries. *J Am Coll Cardiol* 2002; 40(2):285–90.
46. Shinbane JS, Shriki J, Hindoyan A, *et al.* Unoperated congenitally corrected transposition of the great arteries, nonrestrictive ventricular septal defect, and pulmonary stenosis in middle adulthood do multiple wrongs make a right? *World J Pediatr Congenit Heart Surg* 2012; 3(1):123–9.
47. Gelson E, Curry R, Gatzoulis M A, *et al.* Pregnancy in women with a systemic right ventricle after surgically and congenitally corrected transposition of the great arteries. *Eur J Obstet Gynaecol Reprod Biol* 2011; 155(2):146–9.
48. Arendt KW, Connolly HM, Warnes CA, *et al.* Anesthetic management of parturients with congenitally corrected transposition of the great arteries: 3 cases and a review of the literature. *Anesth Analg* 2008; 107(6):1973–7.
49. Connolly HM, Grogan M, Warnes CA. Pregnancy among women with congenitally corrected transposition of the great arteries. *J Am Coll Cardiol* 1999; 33(6):1692–5.
50. Ly M, Belli E, Leobon B, *et al.* Results of the double switch operation for congenitally corrected transposition of the great arteries. *Eur J Cardiothorac Surg* 2009; 35(5):879–83.
51. Hiramatsu T, Matsumura G, Konuma T, *et al.* Long-term prognosis of double-switch operation for congenitally corrected transposition of the great arteries. *Eur J Cardiothoracic Surg* 2012; 42(6):1004–8.
52. Therrien J, Barnes I, Somerville J. Outcome of pregnancy in patients with congenitally corrected transposition of the great arteries. *Am J Cardiol* 1999; 84: 820–4.
53. Guedes A, Mercier LA, Leudc L, *et al.* Impact of pregnancy on systemic right ventricle after Mustard operation for transposition of the great arteries. *J Am Coll Cardiol* 2004; 44(2):433–7.
54. Jain VD, Moghbeli N, Webb G, *et al.* Pregnancy in women with congenital heart disease: the impact of a systemic right ventricle. *Congenit Heart Dis* 2011; 6(2):147–56.
55. Uebing A, Steer PJ, Yentis SM, *et al.* Pregnancy and congenital heart disease. *BMJ* 2006; 332(7538):401–6.
56. Hidano G, Uezono S, Terui K. A retrospective survey of adverse maternal and neonatal outcomes for parturients with congenital heart disease. *Int J Obstet Anaesth* 2011; 20(3):229–35.
57. Collis RE, Baxendall ML, Srikantharajah ID, *et al.* Combined spinal epidural analgesia with the ability to walk throughout labour. *Lancet* 1993; 341(8847):767–8.
58. Dob DP, Yentis SM. UK registry of high-risk obstetric anaesthesia: report on cardiorespiratory disease. *Int J Obstet Anesth* 2001; 10(4):267–72.
59. Lewis NL, Dob DP, Yentis SM. UK registry of high-risk obstetric anaesthesia: arrhythmias, cardiomyopathy, aortic stenosis, transposition of the great arteries and Marfan's syndrome. *Int J Obstet Anesth* 2003; 12(1):28–34.
60. Suntharalingam G, Dob D, Yentis SM. Obstetric epidural analgesia in aortic stenosis: a low dose technique for labour and instrumental delivery. *Int J Obstet Anesth* 2001; 10(2):129–34.
61. Douglas J. General anaesthesia for obstetrics: a deadly or a winning combination. *Can J Anesth* 2004; 51(1 Suppl):R17–20.
62. Chan TML, Dob DP. The anaesthetic management of a parturient with polymorphic catecholamine sensitive ventricular tachycardia. *Int J Obstet Anesth* 2002; 11(2):122–4.
63. Hamlyn EL, Douglas CA, Plaat F, *et al.* Low dose sequential combined spinal epidural: an anaesthetic technique for caesarean delivery in patients with significant cardiac disease. *Int J Obstet Anesth* 2005; 14(4):355–61.
64. Cole PJ, Cross MH, Dresner M. Incremental spinal anaesthesia for elective caesarean delivery in a patient with Eisenmenger's syndrome. *Br J Anaesth* 2001; 86(5):723–6.
65. Dresner M, Pinder A. Anaesthesia for caesarean delivery in women with complex congenital heart disease: 34 cases using the Braun Spinocath® spinal catheter. *Int J Obstet Anesth* 2009; 18(2):131–6.
66. Fallot E. Contribution a l'anatomie pathologique de la maladie bleue (cyanose cardiaque). *Marseille Med* 1888; 25:77ff.
67. Evans WN. "Tetralogy of Fallot" and Etienné-Louis Arthur Fallot. *Ped Cardiol* 2008; 29(3):637–40.
68. Bashore TM. Congenital heart disease for the adult cardiologist. *Circulation* 2007; 115(14):1933–47.
69. Yang MC, Chiu SN, Wang JK, *et al.* Natural and unnatural history of tetralogy of Fallot repaired during adolescence and adulthood. *Heart Vessels* 2012; 27(1):65–70.
70. Blalock A, Taussig HB. The surgical treatment of malformation of the heart in which there is pulmonary stenosis or pulmonary atresia. *JAMA* 1945; 128(3):189–202.
71. Kirklin JW, DuShane JW, Patrick RT, *et al.* Intracardiac surgery with the aid of a mechanical pump-oxygenator system (Gibbon type): report of 8 cases. *Proc Staff Meet Mayo Clin* 1955; 30(10):201–6.
72. Kanter KR, Kogon BE, Kirshbom PM, *et al.* Symptomatic neonatal tetralogy of Fallot: Repair or shunt? *Ann Thorac Surg* 2010; 89(3):858–63.
73. Al Habib HF, Jacobs JP, Mavroudis C, *et al.* Contemporary patterns of management of tetralogy of Fallot: data from the Society of Thoracic Surgeons Database. *Ann Thorac Surg* 2010; 90(3):813–20.
74. Van Arsdell GS, Maharaj GS, Tom J, *et al.* What is the optimal age for repair of tetralogy of Fallot? *Circulation* 2000; 102:123–9.
75. Apitz C, Webb GD, Redington AN. Tetralogy of Fallot. *Lancet* 2009; 374(9699):1462–71.
76. Tamesburger MI, Lechner E, Mair R, *et al.* Early primary repair of tetralogy of Fallot in neonates and infants less than four months of age. *Ann Thorac Surg* 2008; 86(6):1928–35.
77. Ho KW, Tan R, Wong KY, *et al.* Late complications following tetralogy of Fallot repair: the need for long term follow up. *Ann Acad Med Singapore* 2007; 36(11):947–53.
78. wan der Wall EE, Mulder BJ. Pulmonary valve replacement in patients with tetralogy of Fallot and pulmonary regurgitation: early surgery similar to optimal timing of surgery? *Eur Heart J* 2005; 26(24):2614–5.
79. Harrild DM, Berul CI, Cecchin F, *et al.* Pulmonary valve replacement in tetralogy of Fallot. *Circulation* 2009; 119(3):445–51.

80. François K, Zaqout M, Bové T, *et al.* The fate of the aortic root after early repair of tetralogy of Fallot. *Eur J Cardiothorac Surg* 2010; 37(6):1254–8.
81. Niwa K, Siu SC, Webb GD, *et al.* Progressive aortic root dilatation in adults late after repair of tetralogy of Fallot. *Circulation* 2002; 106(11):1374–8.
82. Ruiz O. Congenital heart disease in adults: Sequelae and complications of cardiac defects repaired at an early age. *Rev Esp Cardiol* 2003; 56(1):73–88.
83. Diller GP, Kempny A, Liodakis E, *et al.* Left ventricular longitudinal function predicts life-threatening ventricular arrhythmia and death in adults with repaired tetralogy of Fallot. *Circulation* 2012; 125(20):2440–6.
84. Balci A, Drenthen W, Mulder BJ, *et al.* Pregnancy in women with corrected tetralogy of Fallot: occurrence and predictors of adverse events. *Am Heart J* 2011; 161(2):307–13.
85. Pijuan Domènech A, Gatzoulis MA. Pregnancy and heart disease. *Rev Esp Cardiol* 2006; 59(9):971–84.
86. Veldman GR, Connolly HM, Grogan M, *et al.* Outcome of pregnancy in women with tetralogy of Fallot. *J Am Coll Cardiol* 2004; 44(1):74–80.
87. Wood P. The Eisenmenger syndrome or pulmonary hypertension with reversed central shunt. *Br Med J* 1958; 2(5099):755–62.
88. Lowe BS, Therrien J, Ionescu-Ittu R, *et al.* Diagnosis of pulmonary hypertension in the congenital heart disease population. *J Am Coll Cardiol* 2011; 58(5):538–46
89. Beghetti M, Galiè N. Eisenmenger syndrome: a clinical perspective in a new therapeutic era of pulmonary arterial hypertension. *J Am Coll Cardiol* 2009; 53(9):733–40.
90. Diller GP, Gatzoulis MA. Congenital heart disease for the adult cardiologist. Pulmonary vascular disease in adults with congenital heart disease. *Circulation* 2007; 115(8):1039–50.
91. Diller GP, Alonso-Gonzalez R, Kempny A, *et al.* B-type natriuretic peptide concentrations in contemporary Eisenmenger syndrome patients: predictive value and response to disease targeting therapy. *Heart* 2012; 98(9):736–42.
92. Diller GP, Dimopoulos K, Okonko DO, *et al.* Exercise intolerance in adult congenital heart disease: comparative severity, correlates and prognostic implications. *Circulation* 2005; 112:828–35.
93. Diller GP, Alonso-Gonzalez R, Dimopoulos K, *et al.* Disease targeting therapies in patients with Eisenmenger syndrome: response to treatment and long-term efficiency. *Int J Cardiol.* 2013; 167(3):840–7.
94 Daliento L, Somerville J, Presbitero P *et al.* Eisenmenger syndrome. Factors relating to deterioration and death. *Eur Heart J* 1998; 19:1845–55.
95. Spence MS, Balaratnam MS, Gatzoulis MA. Clinical update: cyanotic adult congenital heart disease. *Lancet* 2007; 370(9598):1530–2.
96. Broberg CS, Bax BE, Okonko DO, *et al.* Blood viscosity and its relationship to iron deficiency, symptoms and exercise capacity in adults with cyanotic congenital heart disease. *J Am Coll Cardiol* 2006; 48(2):356–65.
97. Hoffmann A, Chockalingam P, Balint OH, *et al.* Cerebrovascular accidents in adult patients with congenital heart disease. *Heart* 2010; 96(15):1223–6.
98. Ammash N, Warnes CA. Cerebrovascular events in adult patients with cyanotic congenital heart disease. *J Am Coll Cardiol* 1996; 28(3):768–72.
99. Galie N, Manes A, Palazzini M, *et al.* Management of pulmonary arterial hypertension associated with congenital systemic-to-pulmonary shunts and Eisenmenger syndrome. *Drugs* 2008; 68(8):1049–66.
100. Tay EL, Peset A, Papaphylactou M, *et al* Replacement therapy for iron deficiency improves exercise capacity and quality of life in patients with cyanotic congenital heart disease and/or the Eisenmenger syndrome. *Int J Cardiol* 2011; 151(3):307–12.
101. Perloff JK, Rosove MH, Child JS, *et al.* Adults with cyanotic congenital heart disease: haematologic management. *Ann Int Med* 1988; 109(5):406–13.
102. Geohas C, McLaughlin VV. Successful management of pregnancy in a patient with Eisenmenger syndrome with Epoprostenol. *Chest* 2003; 124(3):1170–3.
103. Barst RJ, Rubin LJ, Long WA, *et al.* A comparison of intravenous epoprostenol (prostacyclin) with conventional therapy for primary pulmonary hypertension. *New Engl J Med* 1996; 334(5):296–301.
104. Mikhail GW, Prasad SK, Li W, *et al.* Clinical and haemodynamic effects of sildenafil in pulmonary hypertension. *Eur Heart J* 2004; 25(5):431–6.
105. Humbert M, Simmoneau G, Rubin LJ. A decade of achievement in pulmonary hypertension. *Eur Respir Rev* 2011; 20(122):215–7.
106. Hayes D, Galantowicz M, Hoffman TM. Combined heart–lung transplantation: a perspective on the past and the future. *Pediatr Cardiol* 2013; 34(2):207–12.
107. Goerler H, Simon A, Gohrbandt B, *et al.* Heart–lung and lung transplant in grown up congenital heart disease, long term single centre study. *Eur J Cardiothorac Surg* 2007; 32(6):926–31.
108. Karamlou T, Hirsch J, Welke K, *et al.* A United Network for Organ Sharing analysis of heart transplantation in adults with congenital heart disease: outcomes and factors associated with mortality and retransplantation. *J Thorac Cardiovasc Surg* 2010; 140(1):161–8.
109. Gatzoulis MA. The management of Eisenmenger syndrome in the modern treatment era: a case report. *Eur Respir Rev* 2011; 20(122):293–6.
110. Maxwell BG, El Sayed YY, Riley ET, *et al.* Peripartum outcomes and anaesthetic management of parturients with moderate to complex congenital heart disease or pulmonary hypertension. *Anaesthesia* 2013; 68(1):52–9.
111. Bédard E, Dimopoulos K, Gatzoulis MA. Has there been any progress made on pregnancy outcomes among women with pulmonary hypertension? *Eur Heart J* 2009; 30(3):256–65.
112. Bonnin M, Mercier FJ, Sitbon O, *et al.* Severe pulmonary hypertension during pregnancy: mode of delivery and anesthetic management of 15 consecutive cases. *Anesthesiology* 2005; 102(6):1133–7.
113. Report of British Cardiac Society working party. Grown up congenital heart disease (GCHD): current needs and provisions of service for adolescents and adults with congenital heart disease in the UK. *Heart* 2002; 88:11–14.
114. Moons P, Engelfreit P, Kaemmerer H, *et al.* Delivery of care for adult patients with congenital heart disease in Europe: results from the Euro Heart Survey. *Eur Heart J* 2006; 27(11):1324–30.
115. Midwall J, Jaffin H, Herman MV, *et al.* Shunt flow and pulmonary hemodynamics during labour and delivery in the Eisenmenger syndrome. *Am J Cardiol* 1978; 42(2):299–303.
116. Parneix M, Faonou L, Morau E, *et al.* Low-dose combined spinal-epidural anaesthesia for caesarean delivery in a patient with Eisenmenger's syndrome. *Int J Obstet Anesth* 2009; 18:81–4.
117. Dob DP, Yentis SM. UK registry of high-risk obstetric anaesthesia: report on cardiorespiratory disease. *Int J Obstet Anesth* 2001; 10(4):267–72.
118. Fontan F, Baudet E. Surgical repair of tricuspid atresia. *Thorax* 1971; 26(3):240–8.
119. AboulHosn JA, Shavelle DM, Castellon Y *et al.* Fontan operation and the single ventricle. *Congenit Heart Dis* 2007; 2(1):2–11.
120. Reul GJ, Gregoric ID. Recent modifications of the Fontan procedure for complex congenital heart disease. *Texas Heart Inst J* 1992; 19:223–42.
121. de Leval MR, Kilner P, Gewillig M, *et al.* Total cavopulmonary connection: a logical alternative to atriopulmonary connection for complex Fontan operations. Experimental studies and early clinical experience. *J Thorac Cardiovasc Surg* 1988; 96(5):682–95.
122. Ahmad U, Fatimi SH, Naqvi I, *et al.* Modified Blalock–Taussig shunt: immediate and short-term follow-up results in neonates. *Heart Lung Circ* 2008; 13(1):54–8.
123. Tanoue Y, Kado H, Boku N, *et al.* Three hundred and thirty-three experiences with the bidirectional Glenn procedure in a single institute. *Interact Cardiovasc Thorac Surg* 2007; 6(1):97–101.

124. Lee YO, Kim YJ, Lee JR, *et al.* Long term results of one-and-a-half ventricle repair. *Eur J Cardiothorac Surg* 2011; 39(5):711–15.
125. Koichi Y, Casta A, Uezono S. Anesthetic management of noncardiac surgery for patients with single ventricle physiology. *J Anesth* 2011; 25(2):247–56.
126. Driscoll DJ. Long-term results of the Fontan operation. *Pediatr Cardiol* 2007; 28(6):438–42.
127. Gentles TL, Mayor JE Jr, Gauvreau K, *et al.* Fontan operation in 500 consecutive patients: factors influencing early and late outcome. *J Thorac Cardiovasc Surg* 1997; 114(3):376–91.
128. Khairy P, Fernandes SM, Mayer Jr JE, *et al.* Long-term survival, modes of death, and predictors of mortality in patients with Fontan surgery. *Circulation* 2008; 117(1):85–92.
129. Tweddell JS, Nersesian M, Mussatto KA, *et al.* Fontan palliation in the modern era: factors impacting mortality and morbidity. *Ann Thorac Surg* 2009; 88(4):1291–9.
130. Gewillig M. The Fontan circulation. *Heart* 2005; 91(6):839–46.
131. Gersony WM. Fontan operation after 3 decades: what we have learned. *Circulation* 2008; 117(1):13–5.
132. Takken T, Hulzebos HJ, Blank AC, *et al.* Exercise prescription for patients with Fontan circulation: current evidence and future directions. *Nether Heart J* 2007; 15(4):142–7.
133. Thorne SA, Hooper J, Kemp M, *et al.* Gastrointestinal protein loss in late survivors of Fontan surgery and other congenital heart disease. *Eur Heart J* 1998; 19(3):514–20.
134. Silvilairat S, Cabalka AK, Cetta F, *et al.* Protein losing enteropathy after the Fontan operation: associations and predictors of clinical outcome. *Congenit Heart Dis* 2008; 3(4):262–8.
135. Walker HA, Gatzoulis MA. Prophylactic anticoagulation following Fontan operation. *Heart* 2005; 91(7):854–6.
136. Cannobbio MM, Mair DD, Rapkin AJ, *et al.* Menstrual patterns in females after the Fontan repair. *Am J Cardiol* 1990; 66(2):238–40.
137. Drenthen W, Pieper PG, Roos-Hesselink JW, *et al.* Pregnancy and delivery in women after Fontan palliation. *Heart* 2006; 92(9):1290–4.
138. Ross D. Homograft replacement of the aortic valve. *Lancet* 1962; 7524; 487.
139. Yacoub M, Klieverik L, Melina G, *et al.* An evaluation of the Ross operation in adults. *J Heart Valve Dis* 2006; 15(4): 531–9.
140 Chambers J, Somerville J, Stone S, *et al.* Pulmonary autograft procedure for aortic valve disease: long-term results of the pioneer series. *Circulation* 1997; 96(7):2206–14
141. Thorne SA. Mitral and aortic stenosis. In Steer PJ, Gatzoulis MA, Baker P (eds) *Heart Disease and Pregnancy*. London: RCOG Press; 2006:183–9.
142. Gatzoulis MA, Swan L, Therrien J, *et al.* *Adult Congenital Heart Disease: A Practical Guide*. Oxford: BMJ Books, Blackwell Publishing; 2005.

CHAPTER 41

Acquired heart disease

Linzi Peacock and Rachel Hignett

Introduction

In the United Kingdom, recent maternal mortality reports highlight cardiac disease as the leading cause of maternal death.[1,2] (see Table 37.1 in Chapter 37). Similarly, the Centers for Disease Control and Prevention (CDC) report cardiovascular diseases as the commonest cause of maternal death for 2006–2009 in the United States.[3] The European Registry on Pregnancy and Heart Disease (ERPHD) has recently published mortality rates of 1%, over 100 times the background rate of death, for women with structural heart disease (congenital, ischaemic, cardiomyopathy, and valvular).[4] Morbidity is also increased in women with cardiovascular disease which causes 3.3% of severe maternal morbidity.[5]

Heart disease affects approximately 1% of pregnant women in the United Kingdom.[6] Although congenital heart disease (CHD) accounts for 75–82% of heart disease in pregnancy in the Western world, numbers of women dying from CHD form the minority.[1,2] The majority of cardiac deaths are due to acquired heart disease (AHD) which is increasing due to factors such as obesity, older maternal age, hypertensive disease, and diabetes mellitus becoming more prevalent in the female reproductive population.[7] Table 41.1 shows the rise in cardiac deaths over the triennia in the United Kingdom from 1994 to 2008. Women with CHD are usually diagnosed prior to pregnancy enabling them to have counselling and optimization of treatment before conception. In contrast, many women with AHD present for the first time during pregnancy.

In the 'Saving Mothers Lives' report 2006–2008,[2] 53 women died of heart disease which was associated with or worsened by pregnancy. Of these 53 deaths, 50 were in women with acquired cardiac disease. A further eight deaths which occurred in women with cardiac disease were classified as *late* deaths. The leading causes of cardiac death were sudden adult death syndrome (SADS), myocardial infarction (MI), mostly as a consequence of ischaemic heart disease (IHD), dissection of the thoracic aorta, and cardiomyopathy (Table 41.1). Worldwide, the ERPHD demonstrated the highest rates of maternal mortality in patients with cardiomyopathy.[4] In 'Saving Mothers Lives' 2006–2008, there were no deaths attributable to rheumatic heart disease (RHD). This is in stark contrast to resource-limited countries which have a significant disease burden in pregnancy due to RHD.

In addition to maternal and neonatal morbidity and mortality, there are many other factors which need to be taken into consideration in a woman known to have cardiac disease either prior to or during pregnancy. Pregnancy may accelerate disease progression in the mother, and may alter her life expectancy after pregnancy. The baby may be at risk of being born with cardiac defects. Drug regimens will need to be monitored and adjusted to avoid teratogenicity, and to accommodate the physiological changes encountered in pregnancy. Finally, invasive therapeutic and investigative procedures may need to be undertaken antenatally.

Early identification of heart disease in pregnancy will enable prompt referral to a specialist multidisciplinary team consisting of cardiologists with expertise in cardiac disease in pregnancy, obstetricians, and obstetric anaesthetists. This team will stratify risk, and will plan antenatal, intrapartum, and postnatal care accordingly.

This chapter will focus on the general principles of management of women with AHD in pregnancy, and will look in detail at IHD, arrhythmias, cardiac transplantation, aortic pathology, cardiomyopathies, valvular heart disease, and infective endocarditis (IE).

General principles

Risk assessment

All patients with known cardiac disease should have pre-pregnancy counselling undertaken by a cardiologist with an interest in pregnancy or by an obstetric physician. This advice should commence in adolescence for those with CHD and at the time of diagnosis for women with acquired cardiac disease.

The 2006–2008 triennial report[2] states that *all* women who died from MI and IHD had identifiable risk factors for IHD, and 60% of all the cardiac deaths occurred in women who were classified as overweight or obese. This has led to the recommendation that women with risk factors for IHD (i.e. diabetes, hypertension, obesity, a family history of IHD, and > 35 years old) should receive pre-pregnancy counselling.[8] Women should also be assessed for risk factors for IHD at booking of antenatal care. These recommendations were made in the 2003–2005 Confidential Enquiries report and were re-iterated in the 2006–2008 Confidential Enquiries report as lessons have not yet been learnt.[2,8]

The European Society of Cardiology (ESC) has produced comprehensive guidelines for the management of women with cardiac disease in pregnancy.[9] These guidelines include the modified World Health Organization (WHO) classification of maternal cardiovascular risk (Table 41.2). This classification is applicable to women with both CHD and AHD. It is based on the New York Heart Association (NYHA) classification (Box 41.1) of diagnosis and disease severity. In 2013, the ERPHD demonstrated a strong correlation between WHO risk classification and cardiac,

Table 41.1 Causes of maternal death from heart disease in the United Kingdom from 1994 to 2008

Type and cause of death	1994–96	1997–99	2000–02	2003–05	2006–08
Acquired					
Aortic dissection	7	5	7	9	7
Myocardial infarction (MI)	6	5	8	12	6
Ischaemic heart disease (no MI)	0	0	0	4	5
Sudden adult death syndrome (SADS)	0	0	4	3	10
Peripartum cardiomyopathy	4	7	4	0[a]	9[b]
Other cardiomyopathy	2	3	4	1	4
Myocarditis or myocardial fibrosis	3	2	3	5	4
Mitral stenosis or valve disease	0	0	3	3	0
Thrombosed aortic or tricuspid valve	1	0	0	0	2
Infective endocarditis	0	2	1	2	2
Right or left ventricular hypertrophy or hypertensive heart disease	1	2	2	2	1
Congenital					
Pulmonary hypertension (PHT)	7	7	4	3	2
Congenital heart disease (not PHT or thrombosed aortic valve)	3	2	2	3	1
Other	5	0	2	0	0
Total	39	35	44	48[c]	53

[a]Twelve late deaths reported in 2003–2005.

[b]Two late deaths reported in 2006–2008.

[c]Includes one woman for whom information or cause was not available.

Reproduced from Confidential Enquiry on Maternal and Child Health, Saving mothers iives: reviewing maternal deaths to make motherhood safer 2006–2008, *BJOG: An International Journal of Obstetrics and Gynaecology*, 118, pp. 1–203, Copyright 2011, with permission from Centre for Maternal and Child Enquiries (CMACE), BJOG, and Wiley.

obstetric, and fetal outcome in its series of 1321 consecutive pregnancies from mainly developed nations.[4] The ESC recommends that all women with cardiac disease are risk assessed against the modified WHO criteria (Table 41.2 and Table 41.3).

Box 41.1 New York Heart Association Classification of Heart Disease

- NYHA class I No limitation to physical activity
- NYHA class II Slight limitation to physical activity
- NYHA class III Marked limitation to physical activity
- NYHA class IV Symptoms at rest

Reprinted from *The Journal of Heart and Lung Transplantation*, 28, 6, Stevenson LW, Pagani FD, Young JB, Jessup M, Miller L, Kormos RL, Naftel DC, Ulisney K, Desvigne-Nickens P, Kirklin JK, INTERMACS profiles of advanced heart failure: the current picture, pp. 535–541, Copyright (2009) with permission from Elsevier.

Women will have their antenatal care planned based on this assessment of risk (Table 41.3). Women with class 1 disease are usually treated as low-risk peripartum. It is recommended that women with class 2 disease should be referred to a multidisciplinary team consisting of cardiologists, obstetricians, and obstetric anaesthetists and should be seen each trimester. Class 3 and 4 disease require much closer surveillance, with assessment and management by the multidisciplinary team every 2–4 weeks.

The Royal College of Obstetricians and Gynaecologists (RCOG)[10] recommend that a formalized multidisciplinary care plan is agreed at 32–34 weeks of gestation (Figure 41.1). This should include consideration of mode of delivery, plan for optimal pain relief in labour, mechanisms to avoid and treat atonic postpartum haemorrhage (including safe drug regimens), postpartum care, thromboprophylaxis, and personnel named to oversee labour and delivery.

Physiological changes in pregnancy

Major cardiovascular system (CVS) physiological changes begin to occur from the earliest stages of pregnancy.[11]

- Cardiac output (CO) increases by 30–50% by the end of the second trimester to accommodate the rapidly growing fetoplacental unit. This is achieved by an increase in stroke volume (SV), and to a lesser extent due to some increase in heart rate (HR) later in pregnancy.
- Blood volume will also increase significantly by 50–70% by the end of the second trimester. Red cell mass increases by up to 40%: as the increase in plasma volume is proportionately greater, red cell concentration is diluted which commonly results in physiological anaemia.
- Systemic vascular resistance (SVR) and blood pressure (BP) fall, due to maturation of placental development and circulating vasodilators, to a nadir between the 20th and 32nd week. SVR and BP rise again to early pregnancy levels at term.
- Inferior vena caval compression by the gravid uterus causes a positional reduction in CO from the middle of pregnancy.
- Pregnancy is a hypercoagulable state.
- Drug metabolism may be altered in pregnancy which may require alteration of dose or drug regimen.

Most healthy women are able to adapt easily to these physiological changes, but women with significant heart disease may develop

Table 41.2 Modified WHO classification of maternal cardiovascular risk: application

WHO classification of maternal cardiovascular risk
WHO I
◆ Uncomplicated, small or mild • pulmonary stenosis • patent ductus arteriosus • mitral valve prolapse
◆ Successfully repaired simple lesions (atrial or ventricular septal defect, patent ductus arteriosus, anomalous pulmonary venous drainage)
◆ Atrial or ventricular ectopic beats, isolated
WHO II conditions (if otherwise well and uncomplicated)
◆ Unoperated atrial or ventricular septal defect
◆ Repaired tetralogy of Fallot
◆ Most arrhythmias
WHO II–III (depending on individual)
◆ Mild left ventricular impairment
◆ Hypertrophic cardiomyopathy
◆ Native or tissue valvular heart disease not considered WHO I or IV
◆ Marfan syndrome without aortic dilatation ◆ Aorta < 45 mm in aortic disease associated with bicuspid aortic valve
◆ Repaired coarctation
WHO III
◆ Mechanical valve
◆ Systemic right ventricle
◆ Fontan circulation
◆ Cyanotic heart disease (unrepaired)
◆ Other complex congenital heart disease
◆ Aortic dilatation 40–45 mm in Marfan syndrome ◆ Aortic dilatation 45–50 mm in aortic disease associated with bicuspid aortic valve
WHO IV (pregnancy contraindicated)
◆ Pulmonary arterial hypertension of any cause
◆ Severe systemic ventricular dysfunction (LVEF < 30%, NYHA III–IV)
◆ Previous peripartum cardiomyopathy with any residual impairment of left ventricular function
◆ Severe mitral stenosis, severe symptomatic aortic stenosis
◆ Marfan syndrome with aorta dilated > 45 mm ◆ Aortic dilatation > 50 mm in aortic disease associated with bicuspid aortic valve
◆ Native severe coarctation

Table 41.3 Modified WHO classification of maternal cardiovascular risk: principles

Risk class	Risk of pregnancy by medical condition
I	No detectable increased risk of maternal mortality and no/mild increase in morbidity
II	Small increased risk of maternal mortality or moderate increase in morbidity
III	Significantly increased risk of maternal mortality or severe morbidity. Expert counselling required. If pregnancy is decided upon, intensive specialist cardiac and obstetric monitoring needed throughout pregnancy, childbirth and the puerperium.
IV	Extremely high risk of maternal mortality or severe morbidity; pregnancy contraindicated. If pregnancy occurs termination should be discussed. If pregnancy continues, are as for class III.

new symptoms or worsening of pre-existing symptoms as they struggle to adapt cardiovascularly. Further dramatic physiological changes occur in labour and during delivery which may cause or worsen cardiac decompensation.[11] CO increases by 10% in labour due to autotransfusion of up to 500 mL blood with each contraction, and catecholamine release due to pain. Further increases in CO are seen in the second stage: in addition to autotransfusion and catecholamine release, pushing by the mother contributes to a further increase in CO. CO peaks by up to 80% immediately after delivery due to autotransfusion and sudden relief of aortocaval compression. CO falls to pre-labour levels 1 hour after delivery. Cardiovascular physiology does not return fully to prepregnancy levels until 3–6 months postpartum.

Cardiovascular investigations in pregnancy

Electrocardiogram

Twelve-lead electrocardiograms (ECG) are usually normal, but may differ from the non-pregnant ECG due to the effect of the gravid uterus on heart position:

- Up to 15° left axis deviation
- Non-specific ST-segment and T-wave changes
- Relative tachycardia
- Left ventricular (LV) hypertrophy
- Q wave and inverted T wave in lead III
- Attenuated Q wave in AVF
- Supraventricular and ventricular ectopic beats.

Exercise testing

Exercise testing provides an objective measurement of functional capacity as well as assisting in the diagnosis of IHD and exercise-induced arrhythmias. Unlike some more invasive tests, there is no radiation exposure, but there is an increased false-positive rate in non-pregnant women.[11] Exercise testing is recommended prior to pregnancy in women with known heart

Cardiac diagnosis	....	Please circle agreed plan
If admitted to LW, please inform	Consultant obstetrician on call **Yes / No**	If advice is needed, please contact one of the following consultants via switchboard:
	Obstetric SpR on call **senior / junior**	
	Consultant anaesthetist on call **Yes / No**	
	Anaesthetic SpR on call **senior / junior**	
	Special midwifery team **Yes / No**	
Mode of delivery	Elective LSCS / trial of vaginal delivery	
Elective LSCS	Prophylactic compression suture	Inform consultant on call if admitted in labour before scheduled date
(see anaesthetic sheet for anaesthetic details)	Syntocinon 2 units over 10–20 minutes	
	Syntocinon low-dose infusion (8–12 mU/minute – see over for details)	
	Anaesthetic echnique.................	Epid/Spin/CSE/GA
	Maternal monitoring.................	ECG/SaO2/non-invasive BP/arterial line BP/CVP
Vaginal delivery	TED stockings in labour/HDU chart	Medications to be continued:
1st stage Mx	Prophylactic antibiotics:	
(see anaesthetic sheet for anaesthetic details)	If operative delivery / in all situations	....
	Epidural for analgesia.................	◆ As soon as in established labour
		◆ If and when requested
	Maternal monitoring.................	ECG/SaO2/non-invasive BP/arterial line BP/ CVP
	Continuous EFM is recommended for all women with cardiac disease	
Vaginal delivery 2nd stage Mx	Normal second stage	Assist if not delivered in .... minutes
	Short second stage.....................	
	Elective assisted delivery only	
Vaginal delivery 3rd stage Mx	Normal active Mx (oxytocin 5 i.u. IM and CCT, or 2 i.u. IV over 10 minutes) or	DO NOT GIVE ergometrine
	Syntocinon infusion 8–12 mU/minutes ...... (for details, see overleaf)	Continue .... hours
Postdelivery	High-dependency unit **Yes / No** For .... hours	
	LMW heparin **Yes / No** Dose.....................Duration.........................	
	List medications to be given...	
	and continued for.........................days/weeks	
	Recommended post-natal stay ......days	
	Cardiac review **Yes / No** weeks...........	
	Contraceptive plans discussed **Yes / No**	

Please inform the consultant obstetrician on call if there is departure from planned management or if unexpected clinical situations develop in women with cardiac disease.

Figure 41.1 Clinical management plan for delivery.
Reproduced with kind permission from Ms Gubby Aiyida, FRCOG, Chelsea and Westminster Hospital, London.

Examples of clinical situations	Consider the following:
Spontaneous labour and recent thromboprophylaxis use (e.g. LMWH/warfarin)	Inform anaesthetist asap
	D/W consultant anaesthetist on call
An epidural can be given more than 12 hours after prophylactic dose or more than 24 hours after therapeutic dose, or earlier at the discretion of the anaesthetist	For additional advice, contact .... via switchboard, or obstetricians listed overleaf
Need for syntocinon augmentation in labour	Use double-strength syntocinon but halve rate to reduce total volume of fluids given (this decision needs to be taken at consultant level)
Syntocinon as prophylaxis against postpartum haemorrhage	Low-dose infusion (12 mU/minute): use either 5 i.u. in 50 ml at 7 ml per hour or 10 i.u. in 500 ml at 36 ml per hour Continue for 4 hours (longer if concerns)
Postpartum haemorrhage	Inform anaesthetic and obstetric consultants on call
	For uterotonic, misoprostol 600 micrograms rectally is preferred, but monitor for hyperpyrexia
	Avoid hemabate or high-dose syntocinon
	Consider use of compression suture
	Consider use of intrauterine balloon (antibiotic cover is recommended)
	Strict input/output charts to be maintained
	Consider central access or arterial monitoring
Preterm labour	Atosiban (tractocile) is the first-line Mx Do not use ritodrine or salbutamol
Pacemaker	Do not use unipolar diathermy Beware pacemaker in unusual places (e.g. abdominal wall) when performing caesarean section
	De-activate implantable defibrillators

Please seek advice from a consultant if there are concerns or if clarification is required on clinical management.

The RCOG is grateful to Ms Gubby Ayida FRCOG (Chelsea and Westminster Hospital) for permission to use this clinical management plan.

Figure 41.1 Continued

disease as it can aid risk assessment.[9] The ESC Task Force recommends performing submaximal tests to reach 80% of the predicted maximal HR in asymptomatic pregnant patients with suspected coronary vessel disease.

Echocardiography

Due to the hyperdynamic circulation in pregnancy, echocardiograms should be interpreted by cardiologists with expertise in caring for women with cardiac disease in pregnancy. Confusion may arise, for example, where cardiac impairment is not appreciated due to an apparently normal ventricular cardiac function (which should be hyperdynamic). Stenotic valve lesion severity may also be misinterpreted: increased velocity due to higher CO in pregnancy will increase peak gradients across valves.

Cardiac interventions in pregnancy

Interventions maybe required in pregnancy for diagnosis and treatment of disease. Cardiac catheterization for diagnosis of coronary artery disease is safest if performed in the second trimester. By this time, organogenesis is complete and the fetal thyroid is inactive. Fetal irradiation can be minimized by shielding the abdomen, by using the brachial artery or radial artery approach and by limiting duration of fluoroscopy.[12]

Cardiac surgery is very rarely performed during pregnancy, and is a last resort after other modes of management have failed. Cardiac surgery during pregnancy carries mortality rates of 6%. This is comparable to non-pregnant women undergoing similar procedures.[13,14] Fetal mortality is very considerable with rates of 20–30%,[14–16] and survivors have significant late neurological morbidity in childhood principally as a result of preterm delivery.[9,12] Maternal risk is higher if surgery is emergent, if the mother has significant co-morbidities, and if surgery is for aortic dissection and pulmonary embolectomy (compared with a lower risk for valvular surgery). Surgery at delivery and postnatally is known to substantially increase maternal risk.[17]

The optimum timing of cardiac surgery for the fetus is in the second trimester.[9] If surgery is planned after 28 weeks the fetus is usually delivered by caesarean delivery (CD) immediately prior to cardiac surgery. Between 24 and 28 weeks of gestation, cases are risk assessed on an individual basis. Risk to the baby may be reduced by giving steroids prior to surgery for fetal lung maturation, monitoring of uterine contractions and fetal HR if possible, use of prophylactic tocolytics, and employment of high-flow, high-pressure, pulsatile, normothermic cardiopulmonary bypass.[17]

Aims of intrapartum care

After monitoring and optimization of disease in pregnancy, the multidisciplinary team should formalize a plan for mode of delivery.

Fundamentals of intrapartum care in women with cardiac disease include:

1. Minimization of cardiorespiratory stress. In general, a vaginal delivery with incremental epidural analgesia and assisted second stage (i.e. delivery by low cavity forceps or ventouse) will be advised. Assisted second stage will reduce the cardiorespiratory stress in the mother associated with pushing. Effective incremental epidural analgesia will minimize catecholamine release due to the pain of labour. Planned CD is usually reserved for those with obstetric indications or very severe disease. These include severe aortic stenosis, severe pulmonary hypertension, intractable heart failure, acute or chronic aortic dissection, and a significantly dilated aortic root where the physiological stress of a vaginal birth would be very high risk. Advantages of a vaginal delivery compared with CD include a reduction in blood loss, reduced risk of infection, reduction in pulmonary complications, lower risk of venous thromboembolic complications, and reduced stress response.
2. Avoidance of aortocaval compression.
3. Optimization of fluid balance.
4. Use of invasive monitoring in those with significant disease. Invasive arterial BP monitoring prior to epidural insertion, neuraxial anaesthesia (NA) or general anaesthesia (GA) will enable rapid detection of cardiovascular instability in those women with WHO class 2 to 4 disease.
5. Provision of aspiration prophylaxis.

Anaesthesia for caesarean delivery

Underlying disease and disease severity, preference of the anaesthetist, and choice of the mother will influence mode of anaesthesia, and use of invasive monitoring.

Over recent years, NA has been increasingly advocated for use in women with cardiac disease.[18] Compared with GA, NA is associated with less blood loss, avoids the CVS response to intubation, and avoids the cardiac depressant and vasodilating effects of GA agents. In a study published in 2003[19] of 125 voluntary reports of women with heart disease in pregnancy, 38% of emergency CD and 62% of elective CD were performed using NA. In addition to the usual considerations of use of NA in pregnancy, it is particularly desirable to use a technique which allows for titration of anaesthesia and therefore optimization and stability of haemodynamics in women with heart disease. The most familiar options are:

- Slow epidural top-up
- Combined spinal–epidural (CSE) with a low-dose spinal component for haemodynamic stability[20]
- Continuous spinal anaesthesia technique[21] via a spinal catheter is used in some centres, but this is an unfamiliar technique to most anaesthetists and has been associated with a high incidence of postdural puncture headache.

Whichever NA technique is used care should be taken to:

- Induce anaesthesia slowly to minimize haemodynamic instability
- Control hypotension due to vasodilatation. Phenylephrine is useful in stenotic valve lesions as tachycardia is avoided; ephedrine is useful in regurgitant lesions where a relative tachycardia is beneficial
- Carefully control fluid balance.

Where GA is the preferred technique, CVS stability can be achieved by using a 'cardiac' type GA:

- Hypertensive response to intubation should be obtunded, for example, by the use of 1–2 mg of intravenous alfentanil, or 0.5 mcg/kg intravenous remifentanil.
- Induction agent carefully titrated.
- Avoidance of tachycardia (which will increase myocardial work) and large swings in BP.
- Transoesophageal echocardiography (TOE), if available, is very useful in giving accurate information about ventricular filling and ventricular function. However, this requires the patient to be anaesthetized.
- Analgesia should be optimized to reduce circulating catecholamines. Epidural analgesia may be advantageous in reducing cardiac preload and afterload. Alternatively intravenous opiates and transversus abdominis plane (TAP) blocks may be used.

Invasive monitoring is beneficial in moderate- or high-risk cases: most commonly invasive arterial blood pressure (IABP) monitoring. Central venous pressure (CVP) monitoring may also be required, for example, where inotropic support is anticipated. There are some caveats for the use of CVP monitoring in pregnant women both with and without cardiac disease:

- CVP measurement may be an unreliable guide as to the fluid status of the patient especially in women with pregnancy-induced hypertension.
- Central venous catheter (CVC) tip may not lie in the desired position in the superior vena cava due to anatomical abnormalities or variations.
- Right-sided heart pressures may not accurately reflect left-sided pressures depending on the underlying disease.
- CVC tip may precipitate dangerous arrhythmias.

Drugs used in the management of atonic postpartum haemorrhage

Standard drugs used in the management of atonic postpartum haemorrhage have profound CVS effects:

- Syntocinon® causes a sudden fall in SVR and causes a compensatory tachycardia and increase in CO. In women with significant heart disease, 2–5 IU should be given by infusion over 15–30 minutes to minimize these CVS effects.

- Ergometrine: smooth muscle contraction causes vasoconstriction and hypertension. Contraindicated in women with significant heart disease.
- Carboprost: causes smooth muscle contraction leading to pulmonary hypertension, bronchospasm, shunting, hypoxaemia, hypertension, and pulmonary oedema. Generally contraindicated in women with significant heart disease.
- Misoprostol: may cause pyrexia and shivering. Can be used in heart disease but some concern if pyrexia and shivering occur because of increased O_2 consumption.

Where drug therapies are limited due to significant heart disease, early recourse to surgical interventions such as B-Lynch uterine compression sutures, Bakri/Rusch uterine tamponade balloons should be used. (See Chapter 35 for more details of these techniques.)

Postnatal care

Women with moderate- or high-risk disease should be cared for on a high dependency unit (HDU) for 24–48 hours after delivery. HDU care will enable more frequent observation of vital signs, use of invasive monitoring, and optimization of analgesia. The majority of deaths in women with cardiac disease occur postnatally due to lapses in the intensity of monitoring, fluid shifts which may precipitate cardiac failure, and poor analgesia which results in catecholamine surges.

Ischaemic heart disease

Epidemiology

IHD is rare in women of childbearing age.[22] The incidence of acute MI in pregnancy has been estimated at 1.3–6.7/100,000 births in population-based studies[23–25] although a recent UK Obstetric Surveillance System (UKOSS) study reported a lower incidence of only 0.7 cases/100,000 maternities.[26]

MI is a rare event in pregnancy with devastating consequences for both mother and baby. Maternal mortality due to MI has fallen from 37% in the 1980s but rates remain high at 5–11%.[23,24,28] Mortality is twice as high in women diagnosed with an acute MI during the peripartum period compared to the antepartum or postpartum periods.[28] During the 1990s, fetal mortality was reported as 21–34%:[27,29] again more recent data records a fall to 9%[28] with most deaths occurring in association with maternal death.

In the 2006–2008 Confidential Enquiries report,[2] six women died from acute MI and five deaths were attributed to chronic IHD where no acute MI was recorded. Death in these cases was presumed to be the consequence of arrhythmia or heart failure.

Acute coronary syndrome (ACS) is often a new diagnosis in pregnancy. The recurrence of ACS in pregnancy is unknown. In the European Registry only one patient out of 20 who had previously had an MI suffered a new ACS event whilst pregnant,[3] whilst five new cases occurred in previously well women.

The majority of MIs occur in the latter half of pregnancy or in the puerperium.[26]

Risk factors

Pregnancy increases the risk of acute MI by three to four times.[23,24] The physiological changes of pregnancy with increases in blood volume, stroke volume, and HR, increase myocardial oxygen demand, whilst the physiological anaemia and reduction in diastolic BP reduce myocardial oxygen supply.[30] Thus pregnancy can result in worsening of known IHD but may also reveal disease in previously well women.

The risk factors for MI in pregnancy are similar to those in the general population:

- Hypertension.
- Obesity.
- Diabetes mellitus.
- Family history of MI.
- Advanced maternal age significantly increases the risk of MI. In the UKOSS report, the mean age of women suffering MI was 37 years compared to the mean age in the control group of 29 years.[26] This study found that for every year increase in maternal age the odds of MI increased by 30% whilst James et al.[24] found the risk of MI was 30 times higher in women over 40 compared to those under 20. This is of particular concern as maternal age is rising in developed countries due to the tendency of mothers to delay the age at which they start to have children,[31] and the use of *in vitro* fertilization. UKOSS is currently conducting a study of pregnancy at advanced maternal age. This study is looking at mothers aged 48 years and older to establish the characteristics, management, and outcomes, and to estimate the risk of adverse events attributable to advanced maternal age.
- Smoking has been shown to increase the risk of MI in pregnancy eightfold[24] which is in contrast to non-pregnant female smokers in whom this risk is increased twofold.[32] It may be that the hypercoagulable state of pregnancy and the increase in vascular reactivity[29] compound the risk of acute MI in women who smoke.
- Thrombophilia.
- Several obstetric complications are associated with an increased risk of MI. Endothelial dysfunction is involved in both the pathogenesis of pre-eclampsia and cardiovascular disease. Haemorrhage is associated with a hypercoagulable response[33] which may increase the risk of coronary artery thrombosis.[24] The association of haemorrhage with increased risk of MI may also be due to the use of ergot alkaloids, such as ergometrine, to treat uterine atony. These drugs are well known to cause coronary vasospasm and have been implicated in cases of acute MI.[34] Postpartum infection, mulitparity, and blood transfusion are also associated with an increased risk of MI.[24,28]

Pathophysiology

The underlying pathology for MI in pregnancy differs from that in the general population where atherosclerotic disease with subsequent plaque rupture and thrombus formation predominates.

Information regarding coronary anatomy has been collated in several reviews of MI in pregnancy. These have shown that atherosclerotic disease ± thrombus accounted for only 40–50% of cases of pregnancy-related MI.[26,28,29] Coronary dissection, which is rarely seen outside pregnancy, accounted for 16–27%, coronary thrombus without atherosclerosis accounted for 6–21%, and normal coronary arteries were documented in up to 29%.[26,28,29] Anterior wall MIs occurred more commonly than inferior or lateral.[24,26]

Coronary dissection is the primary cause of MI in the peripartum period. Spontaneous coronary dissection in pregnancy is thought to result from hormonal and haemodynamic changes.[35] Excess progesterone results in biochemical and structural changes in the vessel wall that persists for up to 3 months postpartum.[36] These changes combined with the elevated shear forces from the increased blood volume and CO of pregnancy result in a greater susceptibility to dissection.

Coronary thrombosis without evidence of atherosclerosis may occur as a consequence of the hypercoagulable state of pregnancy, whilst coronary vasospasm may be responsible for the MIs that have been observed in patients with normal vessels.

Diagnosis

The diagnosis of acute MI or ACS in pregnancy or the puerperium is the same as the non-pregnant state and consists of a history of chest pain associated with ECG changes and cardiac enzyme rise. Troponin levels may be higher in women with pre-eclampsia but they do not reach the threshold for diagnosis of ACS out with pregnancy.[11] In the UKOSS study,[26] all the women presented with typical symptoms of MI except for two who developed ECG changes whilst undergoing CD. However, there is concern that pregnant women may present with atypical symptoms such as abdominal or epigastric pain, vomiting, and dizziness, and symptoms may be attributed to pregnancy per se resulting in a failure to consider ACS.[2]

The differential diagnoses of ACS in pregnancy are acute pulmonary embolism, aortic dissection and pre-eclampsia. Echocardiography (Echo) may be a useful diagnostic tool to differentiate between these diagnoses. Coronary angiography is both diagnostic and allows treatment simultaneously.

Management

Pregnancy

- There are no guidelines advising women who have suffered an ACS on how long to defer pregnancy. In general, 1 year is felt to be an appropriate length of time as this allows full recovery, cardiac remodelling,[11] 12 months of dual antiplatelet therapy for those with drug-eluting stents, and full preconception stress testing. The ESC advocates that pregnancy can be considered in the absence of ongoing cardiac ischaemia and LV dysfunction.[9]
- For women who suffer ST elevation MI (STEMI) during pregnancy due to coronary thrombosis, primary percutaneous coronary intervention (PCI) is preferred to thrombolytic therapy as the initial mode of treatment provided that therapy is started promptly. Although thrombolysis using tissue plasminogen activator (which does not cross the placenta) has been used successfully,[37] subplacental haemorrhage can occur. Haemorrhage may be catastrophic particularly if thrombolysis is used in the first few weeks postnatally.[38] STEMI due to coronary dissection can also be treated by PCI whilst thrombolysis may aggravate it. All reports of stenting during STEMI in pregnancy have been with bare metal stents.[9] The safety of drug-eluting stents is unknown in pregnancy and requires prolonged use of dual antiplatelet treatment. There are case reports of the use of clopidogrel in pregnancy.[39,40] However, its safety is uncertain. The ESC advises that it should only be used when absolutely necessary and for as short a duration as possible.
- For patients with non-STEMI with intermediate- and high-risk features (i.e. raised cardiac biomarkers and ST segment changes) PCI should be considered, whilst those who are more stable can be managed medically.[9]
- Beta blockers, nitrates, calcium channel antagonists, and low-dose salicylates (e.g. aspirin 75 mg) can be used safely in pregnancy but angiotensin-converting enzyme (ACE) inhibitors, angiotensin II receptor blockers (ARBs), and statins are contraindicated. There is no safety data on glycoprotein IIb/IIIa inhibitors in pregnancy and as such they are not recommended.

Labour

- The mode of delivery is determined by obstetric considerations and the clinical status of the mother. Vaginal delivery with assisted second stage and slow incremental epidural analgesia is the preferred mode. Despite these recommendations, CD occurred in 60% of women with IHD/MI in the European Registry which was the highest rate for all the cardiac conditions studied.[4]
- Slow incremental epidural analgesia attenuates the progressive rise in CO that occurs during labour, and allows for haemodynamic stability by slow initiation of pain relief. Addition of epinephrine to local anaesthetic mixtures should be avoided.
- Cardiac medication such as aspirin and beta blockers should be continued throughout labour.
- The third stage should be managed actively with an infusion of Syntocinon® (e.g. 2–5 IU of Syntocinon® infused over 15–30 minutes).
- A woman with known IHD should receive supplemental oxygen and have continuous ECG, pulse oximetry, BP, and cardiotocography monitoring throughout labour.
- Invasive BP monitoring should be instituted in women with LV dysfunction.
- Postnatal care should be undertaken in the HDU.
- Haemodynamic goals are:
  - reduction of cardiac workload and myocardial oxygen demand
  - avoidance of tachycardia
  - SVR should only be allowed to fall slowly and modestly to prevent reflex tachycardia and to maintain coronary perfusion
  - avoidance of aortocaval compression.

Caesarean delivery

- For operative delivery, slow-onset NA with either incremental epidural or low-dose spinal component CSE allow for haemodynamic stability.[41] A standard single-shot spinal is relatively contraindicated as this produces a rapid sympathetic block with resultant hypotension and tachycardia.
- GA should be reserved for those women with a contraindication to neuraxial block such as the use of dual antiplatelet agents, or for women who are unable to lie flat due to congestive cardiac failure. Rapid sequence induction should be modified with opioids or beta blockers to obtund the pressor response to laryngoscopy and use of invasive BP monitoring is advised.
- Good postoperative analgesia is necessary to reduce pain-induced catecholamine surges. This should be provided with intrathecal or epidural opiates if NA has been used, or a combination of patient-controlled opioid analgesia and TAP blocks if the patient has undergone GA.
- Postoperatively, women should be monitored on a HDU for 24–28 hours and should receive cardiology input.
- Women who are not breastfeeding can start statins and ACE inhibitors postnatally as required.

Arrhythmias

Arrhythmias during pregnancy are common and may manifest for the first time or recur more frequently. Premature atrial and ventricular beats occur in up to 59% of pregnant women investigated for palpitations,[42] whilst sinus tachycardia is observed in 39% of healthy women during the third trimester.[43] Although sustained tachyarrhythmias are rare (2–3/1000),[44] symptomatic exacerbation of paroxysmal supraventricular tachycardia (SVT) is common and occurs in 22–44% of women during pregnancy.[45]

The majority of arrhythmias are benign and occur in women who are otherwise healthy and have a structurally normal heart. In these circumstances, advice on managing symptomatic episodes and reassurance is sufficient. However, arrhythmias may have serious implications. Silversides et al. observed that arrhythmia recurrence during pregnancy resulted in a significant increase in the risk of adverse fetal events, in particular prematurity,[45] and arrhythmias are a predictor of an adverse cardiac event during pregnancy in women with structural heart disease.[46] Whilst no deaths have been documented from a primary arrhythmia in the United Kingdom, 20% of the cardiac deaths (ten deaths) in the 2006–2008 Confidential Enquiries[2] report were attributed to sudden adult/arrhythmic death syndrome (SADS) where a primary arrhythmia was presumed to be the cause of cardiac arrest.

Pathophysiology

There are a number of cardiovascular adaptations that occur during pregnancy that are thought to result in the increased incidence of arrhythmias in pregnancy (Box 41.2). Pregnancy may also affect the trigger for arrhythmias as most tachycardic episodes are initiated by ectopic beats. These occur more commonly in pregnancy and may contribute to the increased frequency of arrhythmias.[47]

Box 41.2 Pathophysiological mechanisms responsible for arrhythmias during pregnancy

- Elevated heart rate: modifies the effective refractory period and the velocity of conduction
- Reduced potassium levels
- Increased sympathetic tone
- Increased intravascular volume results in mechanical stretch of atria and ventricles which can unveil an arrhythmogenic focus
- Direct effect of hormones on cardiac excitability
- Increased number of myocardial alpha adrenoceptors due to oestrogen

Diagnosis

The most common symptom reported is palpitations. Shortness of breath and chest pain may occur with relatively minor arrhythmias in late pregnancy. Syncope and presyncope may reflect underlying cardiac disease, but may also be attributed to a fall in BP due to peripheral vasodilatation particularly in the second trimester.[48] Patient enquiry should focus on any family history of arrhythmias or sudden death as these may be an indicator of hereditary cardiac disease.

It is important to attempt to diagnose the type of arrhythmia as this will determine appropriate treatment as well as providing prognostic information. Investigations should aim to establish whether any underlying cardiac disease exists, or whether there are underlying systemic disorders such as thyroid disease, pulmonary embolism, or sepsis.

Resting ECG is often unremarkable but may reveal a delta wave due to pre-excitation in Wolff–Parkinson–White (WPW) syndrome. Holter monitors, event recorders, or implantable loop recorders in conjunction with an accurate patient diary may all be used in pregnancy. Echo should be performed to diagnose structural and functional heart disease. Exercise ECG may be performed with care taken to avoid exceeding the woman's normal exercise capacity whilst tilt-table testing is avoided beyond 24 weeks of pregnancy due to supine hypotension from inferior vena cava (IVC) compression. Electrophysiological studies are usually delayed until after delivery.[11]

General principles of treatment

Antiarrhythmic drugs are required in a minority of cases where there have been severe symptoms or significant haemodynamic compromise. Digoxin can be used for ventricular rate control but does not prevent recurrence. Beta blockers, class I antiarrhythmics, and sotalol should be used with caution with right ventricular (RV) or LV impairment and amiodarone is only used if all other drugs have failed.[9]

DC cardioversion may be used for women who are haemodynamically compromised by sustained tachyarrhythmia. DC cardioversion can be used safely in all stages of pregnancy as the amount of current reaching the fetus is small.[44]

Arrhythmias associated with structural and congenital heart disease

Supraventricular and ventricular arrhythmias requiring treatment develop in up to 15% (mean 5%) of patients with CHD during pregnancy.[49] In the European Registry, supraventricular arrhythmias occurred most commonly in patients with valvular heart disease, whilst ventricular arrhythmias were most common in patients with cardiomyopathy.[4] Where a patient has repaired CHD the prevalence of arrhythmias increases with age and is the result of surgical scarring, the underlying lesion, and ageing. Patients who have undergone atrial surgery or who have RV impairment are particularly vulnerable to atrial flutter.

Supraventricular tachycardia

The majority of episodes of paroxysmal SVT (PSVT) occur during the third trimester of pregnancy, labour, delivery, or postpartum.[48] Atrioventricular (AV) node re-entry tachycardia and AV re-entry tachycardia involving an accessory pathway can be treated with vagal manoeuvres, or intravenous adenosine. Adenosine is the first-line drug for terminating PSVT with doses of 6–12 mg successfully terminating 89% of episodes[50] although up to 24 mg has been used. Metoprolol is an alternative. Intravenous verapamil may cause fetal distress secondary to maternal hypotension.

Prophylactic treatment is only required when symptoms have been intolerable or haemodynamic compromise has occurred. Digoxin and metoprolol are first-line agents followed by sotalol, flecainide, and propafenone.[9] AV nodal blocking agents are contraindicated in patients with WPW as this can result in uncontrolled conduction down the accessory pathway resulting in maternal compromise.

Catheter ablation should only be considered during pregnancy for drug refractory or poorly tolerated arrhythmias. Women with a preceding history of SVT should be considered for catheter ablation prior to pregnancy. If this does not occur then the decision to stop or continue prophylactic medication should be made on an individualized basis following careful consideration of the risks versus the benefits.

Atrial flutter/Atrial fibrillation

Atrial fibrillation (AF) and atrial flutter (AFl) are rare in pregnancy unless there is structural heart disease, hyperthyroidism, or electrolyte disturbance. Serious haemodynamic compromise to the mother and fetus may occur, particularly in women with valvular heart disease. Management is as the same as for non-pregnant patients with cases involving haemodynamic compromise being treated with DC cardioversion. Amiodarone is avoided due to fetal toxicity. It is preferable to attempt either electrical or chemical cardioversion in patients acutely as this avoids the need for anticoagulation. Flecainide may be used to cardiovert women with structurally normal hearts, whilst alternatives include beta blockers such as atenolol and sotalol, verapamil and procainamide. Digoxin may be used for rate control. Where AF/AFl is present for more than 48 hours, anticoagulation should be considered.

Ventricular tachycardia

Ventricular tachycardia (VT) is rare in pregnancy. In healthy women, the most common cause of VT in pregnancy is due to idiopathic RV outflow tract tachycardia. It originates from the RV outflow tract just below the pulmonary valve and may cause ectopic beats, bigeminy or short runs of non-sustained VT. VT occurring in women with structural heart disease or ventricular dysfunction is associated with an increased risk of sudden cardiac death.[51] VT results in hypotension with subsequent reduced coronary perfusion and ischaemia resulting in VF. New onset of VT in the last month of pregnancy or in the early postpartum period should alert clinicians to the possibility of peripartum cardiomyopathy.

Irrespective of the underlying cause for VT, DC cardioversion should be performed in all women who are haemodynamically compromised. In those who are stable, lidocaine, procainamide, sotalol, and amiodarone may be considered. In patients with stable polymorphic VT, electrolytes should be corrected including magnesium and any precipitating drugs should be stopped. Temporary overdrive pacing may be required. Amiodarone, verapamil, and cardioselective beta blockers may be used for prophylaxis. Automatic implantable cardiac defibrillators (AICDS) have been used successfully in pregnancy[52] and should be considered where drug treatment for VT fails and for women surviving a cardiac arrest. Catheter ablation may be used when drug therapy fails.

In women with a family history of sudden death arrhythmogenic disorders, long QT syndrome (LQTS) should be considered. This occurs in both autosomal dominant and recessive forms. The risk of cardiac events is significantly increased in the postpartum period in such women but not during pregnancy and delivery.[53] LQTS may also be acquired as a result of certain drugs, electrolyte imbalance and metabolic conditions. If untreated the annual mortality is 1–2%. It is associated with an increased risk of polymorphic VT (torsades de pointes) which unless self-terminating may degenerate to ventricular fibrillation (VF). Beta blockers and occasionally cardiac pacing are used as prophylaxis. If the QT interval is greater than 550 ms or a patient survives a cardiac arrest then an implantable defibrillator should be inserted.

Many drugs used in theatres and anaesthetics are capable of either prolonging the QT interval directly, or predispose or exacerbate QT prolongation secondary to haemodynamic changes. In particular hypertension, bradycardia, tachycardia, hypoxaemia and electrolyte disturbances should be avoided in patients at risk.

- Terbutaline and ritodrine which are used to arrest preterm labour or for tachyphylaxis should be avoided.
- Oxytocin as a bolus of 10 units intravenously prolonged the QTc at 1 minute in normal women with a return to normal at 3 minutes.[54] Thus oxytocin should be administered as an infusion of 5 units over 20 minutes in women with LQTS for the prevention of postpartum haemorrhage.
- Antibiotics: macrolides should be avoided, and the quinolone group and antifungals fluconazole and ketoconazole may have variable effects on QTc.
- Antiemetics: ondansetron, granisetron, and droperidol should be avoided. Cyclizine can be used safely.[55]
- Volatile agents: all volatile agents prolong the QTc.[56] However, volatile agents have been used successfully in patients with LQTS receiving beta blockers.[55] In general, reference books tend to advocate the use of isoflurane over sevoflurane although there are very few studies comparing the safety amongst volatile anaesthetics. Propofol does not have any effect on the

QT interval thus total intravenous anaesthesia may be used although this may not be feasible in an emergency situation.

- Phenylephrine has been used successfully in LQTS patients with hypotension secondary to neuraxial blockade. Ephedrine should be avoided due to sympathomimetic effects.
- Some anaesthetists recommend omission of epinephrine from the epidural solution. This is not a universally accepted practice.[55]
- An up-to-date list of drugs to be avoided or used with caution in patients with LQTS can be found at http://www.crediblemeds.org

Bradyarrhythmias

Bradyarrhythmias are rare in pregnancy and usually have a favourable outcome in the absence of underlying heart disease. Sinus bradycardia may occur secondary to supine hypotension or the Valsalva manoeuvre. First-degree AV block can occur without underlying heart disease. Second-degree AV block is more commonly associated with drugs or structural heart disease and may result following repair of tetralogy of Fallot or a ventricular septal defect. Women with isolated congenital complete heart block usually have a favourable outcome and rarely require insertion of a permanent pacemaker. Permanent pacemaker insertion is reserved for symptomatic women with complete heart block and ideally should be performed after the first trimester with shielding of the uterus to minimize irradiation of the fetus.

Sudden Adult/Arrhythmic Death Syndrome

SADS is defined as sudden unexpected cardiac death (i.e. presumed fatal arrhythmia) where all other causes of sudden collapse are excluded including a drug screen for stimulants. SADS is a pathological diagnosis and includes those unexplained cases with a morphologically normal heart by both gross and histological examination.[2] The incidence of SADS appears to be rising with ten deaths recorded in the 2006–2008 Confidential Enquiries report. Six of the ten women had booking BMIs ranging from 30 to 45 kg/m^2 and obesity has been suggested as a potential risk factor. Cardiac hypertrophy is associated with obesity in the absence of hypertension, and both obesity and cardiac hypertrophy are risk factors for arrhythmia and sudden cardiac death.

Management of pregnant women with arrhythmias

Pregnancy

- Women with a history of arrhythmias should have preconception review by a cardiologist to discuss the risks of pregnancy.
- The use of antiarrhythmic drugs should be reviewed to optimize dose and to select drugs which are safe to take in pregnancy.
- Anticoagulant medication may need to be altered as warfarin is contraindicated in the first trimester.
- Catheter ablation should be considered prior to pregnancy in women with a history of SVT.
- Women with pacemakers tolerate pregnancy well and the presence of an AICD is not a contraindication to pregnancy nor does pregnancy increase the risk of major AICD complications or frequency of discharge.[52]

Labour

- The mode of delivery is determined by obstetric considerations. Vaginal delivery is preferred and the decision on whether to allow maternal expulsive efforts during the second stage should be decided on a case-by-case basis. Expulsive efforts can cause reflex bradycardia but can also increase circulating catecholamine levels and thus trigger an arrhythmia.
- Women with a history of arrhythmias should have continuous ECG monitoring as well as pulse oximetry and regular BP measurements during labour.
- Neuraxial analgesia is recommended for women who are symptomatic or have haemodynamic compromise due to arrhythmia. Slow incremental epidural analgesia preserves maternal haemodynamic stability and minimizes the increase in circulating catecholamines.
- Phenylephrine is the vasopressor of choice for those with tachyarrhythmias whilst ephedrine should be used for women with bradycardia.

Caesarean delivery

- Low-dose spinal component CSE or *de novo* slow incremental epidural may be preferred for CD as single-shot spinal results in rapid reduction in SVR with resultant reflex tachycardia.
- Syntocinon® should be given by slow intravenous infusion to avoid tachycardia.
- Following delivery women should continue to be monitored in a high dependency setting for a minimum period of 24 hours.

Cardiac transplantation

The number of cardiac transplants performed in children and women of childbearing age is increasing.[57] Survival rates at 1 year and 5 years are 84% and 85% respectively (conditional on 1-year survival).[57] The commonest reason for heart transplantation in these groups is viral cardiomyopathy although the number of people being transplanted for CHD is increasing. Combined heart–lung transplants occur more frequently than solitary heart transplants. The majority of recipients have the underlying aetiology of CHD, idiopathic pulmonary artery hypertension, and cystic fibrosis.[58] Many women who have undergone cardiac transplantation regain normal functional status and may desire children. In general, pregnancy is well tolerated in cardiac transplant recipients provided the functional status of the patient pre-pregnancy is good.[59] The incidence of graft rejection during pregnancy and the postpartum period is unaltered and despite the use of immunosuppressant drugs the incidence of birth defects is similar to the general population.[58] The most frequent maternal complications are thought to be secondary to immunosuppressive therapy and include hypertension, pre-eclampsia, and infection.[60] Episodes of acute allograft rejection are usually mild and do not require treatment.[59] Fetal complications include preterm delivery and low birth weight.[60,61]

Pathophysiological changes of pregnancy after cardiac transplantation

The transplanted heart lacks autonomic and somatic innervation. As a result the baseline HR is 100–120 beats per minute. Drugs acting via the vagus nerve such as atropine have no effect whilst indirectly acting vasopressors may have unpredictable effects. Phenylephrine is the vasopressor of choice. Directly acting sympathomimetics such as isoprenaline reliably produce inotropy and chronotropy. The denervated heart responds to the increased cardiovascular demands of pregnancy by atypical adaptive mechanisms. An increase in stroke volume occurs in response to higher CVP and intravascular volume, and a delayed increase in HR and contractility occur in response to circulating catecholamines from the adrenal medulla. The denervated heart is therefore more susceptible to hypovolaemia.

Multivessel coronary artery occlusion develops in 30% of cardiac transplant recipients at 3 years and 50% at 5 years.[62] Due to the lack of innervation episodes of myocardial ischaemia are silent and paroxysmal dyspnoea may be the only symptom.

Management

Pregnancy

- All cardiac transplant patients should have a recent Echo and cardiac catheterization report as these provide assessment of ventricular function, the extent of atherosclerosis and permits endomyocardial biopsy to assess rejection.
- Exercise tolerance during pregnancy should be recorded at every visit as this may be the only indication of cardiac ischaemia.
- Regular monitoring of blood concentrations of immunosuppressants is required as the increase in blood volume may necessitate an alteration to their dose.
- Patients should have regular BP assessment due to the risk of hypertension and pre-eclampsia.

Labour

- The mode of delivery is determined by obstetric indications with vaginal delivery being preferred.
- All staff need to take particular care with asepsis for all procedures including examinations due to the increased risk of sepsis secondary to immunosuppression.
- Cardiac transplant patients generally tolerate the haemodynamic changes of labour and delivery well.[63] Although central venous and pulmonary artery pressure monitoring may be useful for assessing intravascular volume and gauging fluid therapy, the risks from introducing infection may outweigh any perceived benefit.[64] Intravascular volume should be maintained with intravenous hydration and avoidance of IVC compression.
- Patients should have continuous ECG, pulse oximetry, and regular BP monitoring throughout labour.
- Additional steroid cover may be required for patients receiving higher doses.
- Epidural anaesthesia is advocated during labour and delivery to minimize the hyperdynamic cardiovascular responses that may occur.[65] Camann et al.[65] had recommended the avoidance of epinephrine containing local anaesthetics due to concerns of increasing the HR further. However, this has been used without any untoward effect.[64]

Caesarean delivery

- Epidural or low-dose spinal component CSE is preferred over single-shot spinal for operative delivery as this allows a slower onset of block, and therefore more haemodynamic stability.
- Antibiotic prophylaxis should be given for all operative deliveries
- Phenylephrine is recommended for treating hypotension.
- Patients should be monitored for 24–48 hours post delivery in a high dependency area.

Aortic disease and aortic dissection

Due to hormonal changes in pregnancy and up to 6 months postpartum, aortic dissection may occur both in women with and without underlying vascular disease. Approximately one-half of aortic dissections in women below 40 years of age are pregnancy related.[66] Aortic dissection can occur at any time during pregnancy and the puerperium but more than half of dissections occur during the third trimester. Aortic dissection is a devastating condition: the mortality rate associated with pregnancy is 25%.[67]

Risk factors

- Acute or chronic hypertension. This is usually, but not always present when aortic dissection occurs
- Collagen vascular diseases:
  - Marfan syndrome (MFS)
  - Ehlers–Danlos (ED) syndrome type IV
- Bicuspid aortic valve
- Previous repair of aortic coarctation.

Marfan syndrome

Medical literature traditionally quotes the risk of aortic dissection in women with MFS as 1% in pregnancy even in the absence of dilatation of the aortic root.[9] This is mainly based on case reports and retrospective studies. A recent prospective study of 199 pregnancies in 69 women with MFS did not document any aortic dissections even in the 14 women who started pregnancy with an aortic root diameter between 45 and 51 mm.[68] This study also evaluated the aortic root diameter with echocardiography regularly during 55 pregnancies in 35 women. Aortic root diameters are known to increase by up to 1 mm in normal women in pregnancy. In women with MFS, slightly more aortic root dilatation was seen which did not entirely return to baseline postnatally.[68] Pregnancy may therefore have long-term implications for women with MFS.[68] Women who have aortic root diameters greater than 40 mm prior to pregnancy, or who are seen to have progressively increasing aortic root diameters during pregnancy, are thought to be at significantly increased risk of aortic dissection and need careful monitoring during pregnancy.[9] In women who have already undergone aortic root replacement, aortic dissection may still occur in the native aorta.

Mitral valve prolapse and regurgitation may progress in pregnancy with signs and symptoms of heart failure and arrhythmias.[9]

Ehlers–Danlos syndrome Type IV

ED syndrome Type IV carries a very high risk of morbidity and mortality in pregnancy compared to the other nine ED subtypes. Type IV is transmitted as an autosomal dominant syndrome. In the general population, type IV EDS is very rare with an incidence of 1/50,000–1/100,000.[69]

Morbidity and mortality in pregnancy may occur due to:

- Spontaneous rupture and dissection of large vessels, including the aorta, even in the absence of vessel dilatation
- Uterine rupture
- Vascular fragility puts women at risk of postpartum haemorrhage.

Bicuspid aortic valve

Congenital bicuspid aortic valve occurs in the general population with a rate of 1–2%. A high proportion of patients with bicuspid aortic valves will have some degree of aortic root dilatation whether or not there is dysfunction of the valve.[70] However, the risk of aortic dissection is less compared with women who have MFS: women with bicuspid valves are considered WHO class IV when aortic dilatation is greater than 50 mm.[9] Aortic dilatation may occur in the distal aorta which makes conventional imaging with echocardiography less reliable.

Pathophysiology of aortic dissection

Progesterone causes changes in vascular collagen. Dissections occur if tears in vascular intima and adventitia propagate and create a false lumen. In the aorta, dissection may extend proximally and or distally. Signs and symptoms of aortic dissection are due to ischaemia and infarction of end organs (such as limb ischaemia, cerebrovascular accident (CVA), renal hypoperfusion) as dissection interrupts arterial supply. Vessel rupture may occur into the pericardium, abdomen, thoracic cavity and mediastinum. If dissection occurs proximally through the aortic arch, interruption of blood supply to organs supplied by the aortic arch will occur causing CVA, myocardial ischaemia and infarction, aortic regurgitation, pericardial tamponade, upper limb ischaemia, bronchial compression and recurrent laryngeal nerve palsy.

Classification of aortic dissection

Aortic dissection may be classified as Stanford type A (i.e. involving the ascending aorta with or without involvement of the descending aorta: DeBakey types I and II) and Stanford type B (i.e. involving the descending aorta distal to the origin of the left subclavian artery only: DeBakey type III) (Figure 41.2). Most dissections occurring in pregnancy are type A (78.9%).[71]

Presentation

A typical presentation of acute aortic dissection is a woman presenting with severe chest pain radiating through to the back. 'Saving Mothers' Lives' urges medical staff to thoroughly investigate women who need strong opiates for analgesia for chest pain.[2] Other symptoms depend on the location and extent of the dissection and presence of aortic rupture, but may include:

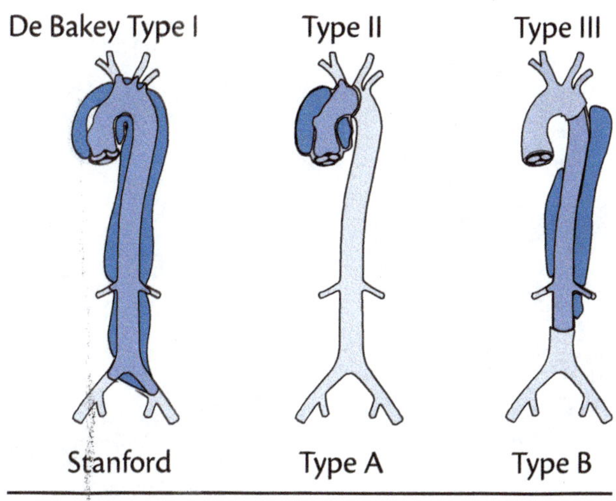

De Bakey

Type I Originates in the ascending aorta, propagates at least to the aortic arch and often beyond it distally.

Type II Originates in and as confined to the ascending aorta.

Type III Originates in the descending aorta and extends distally down the aorta or, rarely retrograde into the aortic arch and ascending aorta.

Stanford

Type A All dissections involving the ascending aorta, regardless of the site of orgin.

Type B All dissections not involving the ascending aorta.

Tsai T T et al. *Circulation*. 2005;AA2:3802-38A3

Figure 41.2 The most common classification systems of thoracic aortic dissection: Stanford and DeBakey.

Reproduced with permission from Christoph A. Nienaber, Kim A. Eagle, Aortic Dissection: New Frontiers in Diagnosis and Management: Part I: From Etiology to Diagnostic Strategies, *Circulation*, Volume 108, Issue 5, pp. 628–635, Copyright © 2003 Wolters Kluwer Health, Inc. Data from Daily PO *et al.*, 'Management of acute aortic dissections', *The Annals of Thoracic Surgery*, 1970, 10, 3, pp. 237–247; and DeBakey ME *et al.*, 'Surgical management of dissecting aneurysms of the aorta', *Journal of Thoracic Cardiovascular Surgery*, 1965, 49, pp. 130–149.

- Differential BP measurements in the arms and legs
- Ischaemic limbs
- CVA
- Dyspnoea
- Myocardial ischaemia and infarction
- Signs of acute aortic regurgitation
- Signs of pericardial tamponade
- Lower abdominal pain.

Investigations

The gold standard for diagnosis is computed tomography (CT) or magnetic resonance (MR) angiogram[72] (Figure 41.3). These imaging modalities will reveal the location and extent of dissection. Abnormalities on chest X-ray (CXR), ECG, and Echo may point to the diagnosis before confirmation by CT or MR. CXR may reveal a widened mediastinum, signs of heart failure due to acute aortic incompetence, pericardial and pleural effusions, or may appear normal. ECG may reveal ST segment elevation due

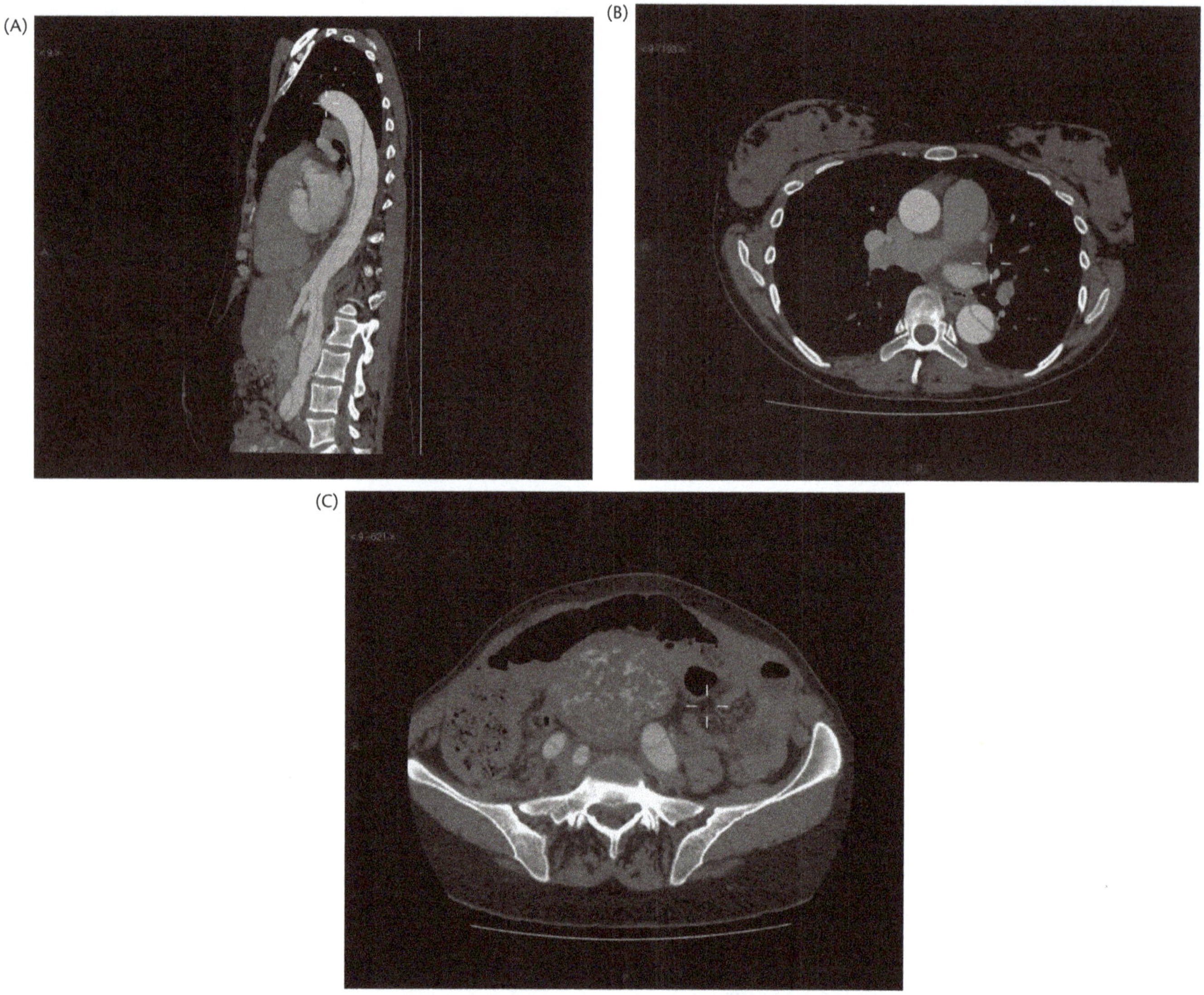

Figure 41.3 Computed tomography angiogram (CTA) of thoracic dissecting aneurysm. (A) Sagittal CTA showing dissection flap extending down from thoracic to abdominal aorta. (B) Axial image from CTA thorax. (C) Axial CTA image showing flap extending into both common iliac arteries with top of postpartum uterus.
Thanks to Dr. Hamish Ireland for the CTA Images of the aortic dissection.

to acute myocardial ischaemia and infarction. Echocardiography may reveal a widened aortic root and dissection flap if dissection has occurred in the proximal aorta, pericardial effusion, and aortic regurgitation. TOE will enable imaging of the descending aorta.[72]

Management of women with aortic disease in pregnancy

Women who have very significant aortic dilatation (>45 mm in MFS, >50 mm associated with bicuspid aortic valves) prior to pregnancy are advised to avoid conception until surgical repair has been carried out.[9] Women with underlying aortic pathology, require frequent assessment of aortic diameter with echocardiography and good control of BP throughout pregnancy. The ESC guidelines[9] recommend that women with MFS are treated with beta blockers in pregnancy: this has been shown to limit aortic dilatation and reduce the risk of dissection. Celiprolol is specifically recommended in women with ED type IV.

Over 60% of patients with MFS may have dural ectasia: up to 90% may be asymptomatic. Patients with EDS may also be at risk of dural ectasia.[73] If this is moderate or severe, narrowing of the epidural space may make the risk of dural puncture unacceptably high. In addition dural ectasia may make the spinal dose difficult to estimate as CSF volume may be increased.[74] MRI evaluation of the lumbar spine should be considered to assist diagnosis.

Intrapartum management aims to limit cardiovascular stress by controlling maximal BP and rapid swings in BP. The ESC taskforce recommends controlled vaginal delivery with incremental epidural analgesia and assisted second stage for women with MFS and aortic diameters between 40 and 45 mm.[9]

If women with MFS have an aortic diameter greater than 45 mm, elective CD is recommended due to the high risk of aortic dissection.

An early elective CD should be planned for all women with ED type IV.

Both during labour and delivery, invasive BP monitoring enables accurate control of BP.

Management of women with aortic dissection in pregnancy

Women who suffer aortic dissection in pregnancy require immediate aggressive control of BP to limit further dissection. Acute type A aortic dissections require surgical correction. Definitive surgical management of the dissection will be undertaken with or without CD depending on gestation.[62] Where aortic rupture and organ malperfusion have not occurred, type B dissections are usually treated conservatively.[71]

Cardiomyopathy

Cardiomyopathy (CMP) is encountered rarely in pregnancy.[9] CMP may be inherited (hypertrophic cardiomyopathy (HCM), some types of dilated cardiomyopathy (DCM), arrhythmogenic RV cardiomyopathy, LV non-compaction cardiomyopathy, and some restrictive cardiomyopathies) or acquired. CMPs may be of toxic, infiltrative, ischaemic, and idiopathic aetiology. The symptoms of CMP overlap with normal symptoms of pregnancy, especially in the later stages of pregnancy, which can make diagnosis difficult.

The commonest forms of CMP encountered in pregnancy in the United Kingdom are peripartum cardiomyopathy (PPCM), DCM, and HCM. Both PPCM and DCM are acquired LV cardiomyopathies.

Peripartum cardiomyopathy and dilated cardiomyopathy

PPCM and DCM may manifest in similar ways in pregnancy, but DCM may be pre-existing or may present early in pregnancy when CVS physiological changes cause cardiac decompensation. In contrast, PPCM presents at the end of pregnancy or within 5 months after delivery. The Heart Failure Association of the European Society of Cardiology Working Group on PPCM (2010) have suggested an alternative definition of PPCM to include idiopathic heart failure occurring due to LV systolic dysfunction which presents towards the end of pregnancy or in the months following pregnancy.[75] Seventy-eight per cent of PPCM cases occur 4 months postnatally, compared with 9% in the last month of pregnancy.[75] LV dilatation is not necessarily present in PPCM in contrast to DCM.

Incidence and aetiology

The limited data available regarding the incidence of PPCM suggests that the incidence varies widely in different populations ranging between 1/300 (Haiti) and 1/4000 (United States) pregnancies.[75] Whilst the aetiology of PPCM is unknown, possible causes include:

- Viral infection
- Inflammation
- Autoimmune
- Haemodynamic stress of pregnancy
- Prolactin (excessive production)[76]
- Genetic predisposition.[76]

In contrast to PPCM where aetiology is speculative, the cause of DCM may be identified in up to 50% of cases as:

- Infections (e.g. viral)
- Connective tissue diseases
- Haematological (e.g. sickle cell anaemia)
- Endocrine (e.g. thyroid disorders)
- Drugs (e.g. alcohol)
- Nutritional deficiencies
- Kawasaki
- Ischaemic
- Arrhythmogenic RV CMP
- Muscular dystrophy
- Metabolic (e.g. haemochromatosis).

Box 41.3 Risk factors for peripartum cardiomyopathy

- Older or very young maternal age
- Black ethnicity
- Multiple gestations
- Increasing parity
- Obesity
- Family history
- Smoking
- Diabetes mellitus
- Prolonged use of beta agonists
- Hypertension

Risk factors

The risk factors for PPCM are listed in Box 41.3.

Diagnosis

Presentation of PPCM and DCM in pregnancy may be insidious, or may be due to an acute decompensation causing florid cardiac failure. This may be difficult to differentiate from the normal symptoms of pregnancy. However, progressive exertional dyspnoea, paroxysmal nocturnal dyspnoea (PND), orthopnoea, recumbent cough, tachypnoea, and auscultatory chest signs are rarely features of a normal pregnancy.[77]

A typical presentation might include the following signs and symptoms:

- Fatigue, lassitude
- Progressive exertional dyspnoea, orthopnoea, PND
- Cough
- Wheeze (which may confuse the diagnosis with asthma), bilateral basal crepitations
- Tachypnoea
- Hypoxaemia
- Peripheral oedema
- Chest pain
- Palpitations, tachycardia, arrhythmias
- Raised JVP
- Gallop rhythm

- Hepatomegaly
- Embolic phenomenon due to pulmonary emboli or due to emboli secondary to mural thrombus.

Investigations

- CXR: typically will reveal cardiomegaly and pulmonary oedema. Pulmonary effusions may be seen.
- ECG: likely to show tachycardia. May reveal dysrhythmias. ST segment, T-wave changes, Q waves, and ventricular ectopic beats are common. Left bundle branch block is present in up to 50% of cases.[78]
- Echo will demonstrate reduced LV systolic function with an ejection fraction (EF) less than 45%, usually with global cardiac dilatation. Mitral regurgitation is often seen.[78] Echo will also detect intracardiac thrombus.

Management

This will depend on the stage of pregnancy. Immediate management is focussed on stabilization of the mother's cardiac function and is the treatment of heart failure:[9,79]

Pregnancy

- Oxygen therapy to optimize oxygen saturation. Non-invasive ventilation may be required.
- Diuretics such as 20–40 mg furosemide intravenously for treatment of pulmonary congestion (which may reduce placental blood flow).
- Nitrates, nifedipine, hydralazine (to reduce afterload) where systolic BP is adequate.
- Anticoagulation in prophylactic or treatment doses (if very poor EF less than 35%, if cardiac thrombus is present or the patient is in persistent AF).
- Antiarrhythmics for AF or atrial flutter (digoxin) or careful rate control with cardioselective beta blockers in women whose CO is preserved.
- ACE inhibitors and ARBs are used postnatally (ACE inhibitors and ARBs are teratogenic early in pregnancy, and may cause fetal hypotension and reduced fetal renal blood flow later in pregnancy).
- More intensive therapies may be needed: inotropic support, counter-pulsation intra-aortic balloon device, ventricular assist devices, and sometimes cardiac transplantation.
- Bromocriptine, which blocks prolactin release, is a potential novel therapy which has reported some success in case reports and one randomized pilot study for postnatal treatment.[80]

Labour

- Depending on response to treatment, mode of delivery will be planned by the multidisciplinary team. Delivery will relieve the physiological burden of pregnancy on the mother's CVS. If the mother's cardiac failure can be stabilized, vaginal delivery with assisted second stage and early incremental epidural pain relief will usually be planned.[5]
- Invasive arterial BP monitoring would be useful prior to epidural insertion.

Caesarean delivery

- CD would be needed for women with obstetric indications, who are fully anticoagulated or in whom stabilization of heart failure cannot be achieved.[9]
- For women who are not fully anticoagulated, anaesthesia for CD may be provided by a low-dose spinal component CSE, or a slow incremental epidural. Both techniques are titratable and preserve myocardial contractility and reduce afterload. Invasive arterial BP monitoring should be used before commencement of anaesthesia.
- GA will be needed for women who are unable to lie flat.

Prognosis for PPCM

In data from the United States, Turkey, and Haiti, between 23% and 41% of women regain normal LV systolic function.[75] This is more likely if EF at diagnosis is higher. Mortality rates for PPCM are not known in Europe, but worldwide, mortality rates of between 10% and 16% at 6 months after diagnosis have been reported.[75] It is strongly advised that women undergo preconception counselling prior to subsequent pregnancies. Limited studies suggest that there are very significant risks in future pregnancies even if LV function has returned to normal.[9,75,28] Subsequent pregnancy is not advised if LV EF was less than 25% at diagnosis, or where LV EF has not normalized.[5,22] Where LV function has normalized, risks include a 26% chance of developing cardiac failure, and 9% risk of persistent fall in LV EF of more than 20%. In women whose LV function has not normalized, there is a 50% chance of worsening cardiac failure, 42% chance of persistent fall in LVEF greater than 20%, and a 25% risk of maternal death.[11]

Hypertrophic cardiomyopathy

Incidence and aetiology

Ninety per cent of HCM is familial and is inherited in an autosomal dominant pattern.[81] The prevalence of HCM is 1/500.[82] HCM consists of asymmetrical hypertrophy of the LV and interventricular septum which causes diastolic LV dysfunction, atrial and ventricular arrhythmias and left ventricular outflow tract obstruction (LVOTO). Systolic LV dysfunction may also occur and mitral regurgitation may be present with LVOTO. When LVOTO occurs the cardiomyopathy may be termed 'hypertrophic obstructive cardiomyopathy'.

Presentation

Many patients with HCM are asymptomatic, but symptoms may include chest pain, dyspnoea, arrhythmias (atrial and ventricular), presyncope and syncope (due to LVOTO), heart failure, and sudden death which may present at any age.

Management

Pregnancy

- HCM is usually well tolerated in pregnancy: the risk of pregnancy correlates well with NYHA class before conception,[9,81] degree of LVOTO, and presence of arrhythmias.
- For women deemed to be very high risk before embarking on pregnancy, surgery may be an option to reduce LVOTO.
- Beta blockers should be continued in women who take them prior to pregnancy. Beta blockers may be started in pregnancy for symptoms or where LVOTO is significant or if interventricular septal thickness is greater than 15 mm.[9]

- Some women with HCM may have implantable cardiac defibrillators for prevention of ventricular arrhythmias and sudden death. Rates of cardiac events in HCM are similar in pregnant and non-pregnant patients: pregnancy does not appear to alter disease progression.[81]

Labour

- In low-risk cases, a vaginal birth may be considered.
- Tachycardias (which will reduce LV diastolic filling, thereby reducing LV preload and increasing LVOTO), and sudden decreases in preload (e.g. due to Valsalva during expulsive efforts and significant blood loss) and afterload should be avoided.
- The degree of LVOTO needs to be considered before using neuraxial analgesia and anaesthesia as these may be relatively contraindicated.
- A pure alpha agonist such as phenylephrine is the vasopressor of choice as tachycardia and increased contractility are to be avoided.[81]
- Fluid balance needs to be carefully maintained.
- Assisted delivery should be considered for women with significant LVOTO to avoid reduction in venous return and CO due to the Valsalva manoeuvre.[83]
- Syntocinon® for active management of the third stage should be given slowly over 15–30 minutes by infusion.

Caesarean delivery

- CD is indicated for women with obstetric indications, decompensated heart failure, and symptomatic LVOTO.[81]
- LVOTO, if severe, would favour GA as sudden falls in SVR and BP can be avoided.[83]
- GA would be required for women who cannot lie flat due to decompensated heart failure.
- Syntocinon® for active management of the third stage should be given slowly over 15–30 minutes by infusion.

Valvular heart disease

Most valvular heart disease in pregnancy in resource-rich countries is due to CHD. This is in contrast to resource-limited countries where the majority of valvular heart disease is acquired due to RHD.[9] The UK triennial Confidential Enquiries into Maternal Deaths have stressed the importance of evaluating non-UK born residents from resource-limited backgrounds early in pregnancy for signs of valvular heart disease.[8]

In general, right-sided lesions are better tolerated than left-sided lesions, and due to the physiological changes which occur in pregnancy, regurgitant lesions are better tolerated than stenotic lesions for the following reasons:

- Rapidly increasing CO leads to higher peak gradients across stenotic valves which causes higher upstream pressures in the heart.
- The relative tachycardia in pregnancy increases oxygen demand to the myocardium.
- A fixed stenotic lesion will limit the heart's ability to increase CO.
- The lowered SVR and increase in HR in pregnancy are beneficial for regurgitant lesions and conversely detrimental to stenotic lesions.

Aortic stenosis

Aortic stenosis (AS) may present for the first time during pregnancy. Usually mild to moderate AS is well tolerated in pregnancy. In contrast, severe AS poses a high risk with heart failure occurring in 10% and arrhythmias in 3–25%.[9] Death is rare in developed countries.

Aetiology

In resource-rich countries, AS is most frequently congenital due to a bicuspid aortic valve. In contrast, in resource-limited countries, AS is usually due to RHD. More than 50% of women who have a bicuspid valve will have associated abnormality and dilatation of the aorta whether the bicuspid valve causes haemodynamic compromise or not:[70] women with bicuspid valves should have careful monitoring of aortic diameter during pregnancy. Anatomically, AS may be supravalvular, valvular, or subvalvular.

Presentation

Women may present for the first time during pregnancy as the stenosed aortic valve struggles to cope with the increasing CO, HR, and reduction in SVR in pregnancy. A woman with AS may present with:

- Dyspnoea
- Angina
- Presyncope or syncope
- Signs and symptoms of cardiac failure
- Sudden death may occur.

Typical signs of AS are:

- Slow rising pulse
- Narrow pulse pressure
- Heaving apex beat
- Ejection systolic murmur heard loudest at the upper right sternal edge with carotid radiation.

Investigations

- ECG: may reveal LVH, left axis deviation, lateral ST segment depression in severe disease.
- CXR: may show signs of cardiac failure.
- Echo: will diagnose valve lesion, and severity, associated pathology such as dilated aortic root and enables assessment of cardiac function. Due to the increase in CO in pregnancy, pressure gradients across the valve will increase which may be misleading. For this reason, valve area is used to categorize severity where a normal valve area is 2.6–3.5 cm^2. Mild AS is greater than 1.5 cm^2, moderate AS 1.0–1.5 cm^2, and severe AS less than 1.0 cm^2.[84]

Management

Pregnancy

- Tachycardia should be avoided: beta blockers may be very useful to slow HR enabling increased LV filling, increased coronary perfusion and limiting oxygen demand. Diuretics are required for heart failure. For symptomatic and severe disease medical treatment will include bed rest and oxygen therapy aiming to prolong gestation.

- Surgical management for severe disease not responding to medical therapy is either by means of percutaneous valvuloplasty or more rarely aortic valve replacement.

Labour

- Assisted vaginal delivery with slow early incremental epidural analgesia is the preferred option. Good epidural analgesia will limit the work of labour minimizing tachycardia and surges in CO.
- Careful monitoring should be undertaken with continuous ECG, SaO_2, and non-invasive BP.
- Invasive monitoring with IABP ± CVP is useful for moderate and severe disease.
- Care after delivery should be either intensive therapy or high dependency.
- Haemodynamic goals are:
  - avoidance of aortocaval compression
  - maintenance of sinus rhythm. Tachycardia should be avoided. Bradycardia should also be avoided to prevent falls in CO
  - optimization of LV filling by keeping the woman well filled
  - avoidance of sudden falls in SVR.

Caesarean delivery

- CD is planned for women who have severe disease and especially those who are symptomatic in the third trimester, or for those with obstetric indications.
- Traditionally GA has been used for severe AS,[19] but there are increasing numbers of case reports which have safely used neuraxial techniques either with low-dose CSE or slow incremental epidural.[85]
- Invasive monitoring is essential for moderate or severe disease. IABP is very useful ± CVP. If the patient undergoes GA, TOE is useful if available.
- For GA, CVS response to induction should be obtunded with either alfentanil or remifentanil.
- Syntocinon® bolus during the third stage should be avoided. An infusion of 2–5 units over 20–30 minutes will limit CVS changes. Ergometrine and carboprost are contraindicated.
- As with vaginal deliveries, women with significant AS after CD should be cared for in a level 2 or 3 area.
- Haemodynamic goals are as listed earlier under 'Labour'.

Mitral stenosis

Significant valve stenosis may lead to left atrial dilatation with risk of AF, pulmonary hypertension, and RV hypertrophy and dilatation. Women who are most at risk include:

- Moderate or severe MS. Risk of death of up to 3%.[9] Women with severe disease are WHO class IV. Pre-pregnancy counselling should advise against pregnancy.
- Women who decompensate during pregnancy either due to poor tolerance of physiological burden or development of AF.
- Pulmonary hypertension with peak systolic pressure greater than 50 mmHg.

Aetiology

In both the developed and the developing world, mitral stenosis (MS) is usually due to RHD.

Presentation

Women may present for the first time during pregnancy especially during the second and third trimesters as CO peaks and SVR falls to a nadir. Symptoms and signs are those of left- and-right sided heart failure including:

- Fatigue, lethargy
- Dyspnoea, PND, orthopnoea
- Cough
- AF
- Systemic embolism (from AF and or dilated LA)
- Chest pain
- Haemoptysis (with pulmonary hypertension)
- Pleural effusions, peripheral oedema, hepatomegaly, ascites
- Symptoms of compression by LA: hoarse voice (recurrent laryngeal nerve compression), dysphagia (oesophageal compression)
- Typically a mid-diastolic rumbling murmur is heard on auscultation.

Investigations

- ECG: may show bifid p waves due to LA enlargement. AF may be present
- CXR: may reveal enlarged LA, cardiac failure, prominent pulmonary arteries
- Echo: valve area is used to assess severity in pregnancy where an area of 4–6 cm^2 is normal, less than 1.5 cm^2 indicates moderate disease, and an area of 1.0 cm^2 or less indicates severe disease. Degree of gradient across the valve, and pulmonary hypertension are used as prognostic indicators.

Management

Pregnancy

- Prevention of tachyarrhythmia and aggressive treatment of AF using beta blockers. Digoxin may be used as a second-line drug treatment or DC cardioversion if drug treatment fails.
- Diuretics will treat fluid overload due to heart failure.
- Low-molecular-weight heparin (LMWH) is required for AF or LA dilatation.
- Bed rest and O_2 therapy may enable a woman to reach a more desirable gestation.
- Surgical intervention for poorly controlled severe disease may be life-saving. Percutaneous balloon valvuloplasty may be offered if the valve looks amenable, that is, absence of significant valve regurgitation and a pliable valve. Mitral valve replacement is rarely performed in pregnancy.

Labour

- Assisted vaginal delivery with early slow incremental epidural is usually advised for women with mild disease or women with more severe disease who are NYHA 1 or 2 and without pulmonary hypertension. Otherwise planned CD is advised.[9]
- Monitor continuously in labour with ECG, SaO_2, non-invasive BP.
- Invasive BP ± CVP are useful for moderate or severe disease.
- After delivery, care should take place in a level 2 or 3 area.
- Haemodynamic goals:
  - avoid aortocaval compression.
  - incremental epidural analgesia will reduce the work of labour by limiting increases in CO and HR due to pain and Valsalva. Epidural analgesia is useful in the immediate postpartum period to reduce preload.
  - prevention of fluid overload. A dose of diuretic should be considered at the time of delivery to offset the effect of autotransfusion. Venous return should be maintained by avoiding aortocaval compression. Excessive fluids should be avoided.
  - maintain sinus rhythm and avoid tachycardia. AF should be treated promptly.
  - avoid rapid reductions in SVR. If vasoconstriction is required, phenylephrine is rapidly titratable, and does not cause tachycardia.
  - avoid factors likely to increase pulmonary arterial pressure: give O_2, avoid acidosis, hypercarbia, and pain.

Caesarean delivery

- CD is planned for women who have severe disease, that is, those who are NYHA class 3 or 4, and for those with pulmonary hypertension, or for women with obstetric indication.
- Invasive monitoring is essential for moderate or severe disease. IABP is very useful ± CVP.
- If NA is used, low-dose spinal component CSE or slow incremental epidural provide slow-onset titratable anaesthesia.
- If the patient undergoes GA, TOE is useful if available.
- For GA, cardiovascular response to induction should be obtunded with either alfentanil or remifentanil.
- Syntocinon® bolus during the third stage should be avoided. An infusion of 2–5 units over 20–30 minutes will limit cardiovascular changes. Ergometrine and carboprost are contraindicated.
- As with vaginal deliveries, women with significant MS after CD should be cared for in a level 2 or 3 area.
- Haemodynamic goals are as listed earlier under 'Labour'.

Aortic and mitral regurgitation

Both aortic and mitral regurgitation (AR and MR) are usually well-tolerated in pregnancy unless regurgitation is severe or of sudden onset. The reduction in SVR and tachycardia in pregnancy favour regurgitant lesions.

Aetiology

- AR and MR may be both congenital and acquired.
- AR may be due to bicuspid valves, dilated aortic root (e.g. MFS), IE, aortic dissection, and RHD.
- MR may be due to mitral valve prolapse, RHD, after valvuloplasty, IE, and functional due to LV dilatation.

Presentation

Both conditions may present with dyspnoea, and signs and symptoms of heart failure. AR may present with angina due to reduction in coronary blood flow. MR may present with palpitations due to AF in association with dilatation of the LA.

Typical signs of AR are:

- collapsing pulse
- wide pulse pressure
- high-pitched early diastolic murmur at upper left sternal edge especially in expiration with woman sitting forward.

A typical sign of MR is:

- pan-systolic murmur radiating to apex.

Investigations

- Both conditions should be investigated with ECG, CXR, and Echo.
- ECG: may show LVH for both valve lesions. Ischaemia may be seen in AR, and AF in MR.
- CXR: both conditions may lead to cardiomegaly and signs of cardiac failure. In MR, a dilated LA may be seen.
- ECHO: Doppler will enable quantification of severity of valve regurgitation.

Management

Pregnancy

- Regular monitoring of cardiac function should be undertaken.
- Medical management is the mainstay of treatment in pregnancy:
  - heart failure is treated with diuretics
  - hydralazine and nitrates may be necessary to reduce afterload.

Labour

- Assisted vaginal delivery with incremental epidural analgesia is planned for women with significant disease. Good epidural analgesia will limit increases in SVR due to pain and Valsalva manoeuvre.
- Haemodynamic goals:
  - Relative tachycardia and lowered SVR are the physiological goals to reduce valve regurgitation
  - Aortocaval compression should be avoided
  - SR should be maintained.

Operative delivery

- If GA is needed, cardiac depression should be minimized.

Prosthetic heart valves

Women with prosthetic heart valves should be referred for cardiology assessment early in pregnancy. In general, women with well-functioning tissue valves do well in pregnancy. In contrast, the risk of mortality with mechanical valves is 1–4%.[86] This risk of valve thrombosis is low for tissue valves and generally women are not anticoagulated. The risk of valve thrombosis is much higher with mechanical valves and lifelong anticoagulation is required. The risk of valve thrombosis is higher again in pregnancy due to hypercoagulability.[87]

Anticoagulation poses risks to both the mother and baby:

- Risk of bleeding from the placental bed
- Fetal loss (one-third with warfarin. Dose dependent)
- Embryopathy in 5–6% fetuses with warfarin between 6 and 12 weeks gestation. Dose dependent
- Fetal bleeding in second and third trimester.[9]

Unlike warfarin, heparin does not cross over the placenta to the fetus: therefore there are no fetal risks. However, the risk of mechanical valve thrombosis is 25% with unfractionated heparin compared with warfarin. Most women will therefore be maintained on LMWH anticoagulation during pregnancy, with monitoring of peak anti-factor Xa levels and also trough levels, as guided by expert haematology advice, in high-risk women. Unfractionated heparin is reserved for situations where rapid reversal of anticoagulation is needed. Consensus guidelines do not exist for optimal anticoagulation regimes in pregnancy. Each patient should therefore be referred for specialist advice early in pregnancy and an individual plan for optimal anticoagulation made on a case-by-case basis.[88] Multidisciplinary planning for labour and delivery will be required. Unless there are obstetric indications for CD, vaginal delivery will usually be the preferred option. To limit the risks of maternal haemorrhage at delivery, and haematomas associated with neuraxial block, induction of labour is often planned to enable step-down or rapid reversal of anticoagulation. UKOSS are currently investigating the outcomes of pregnancy in women with mechanical heart valves.

Infective endocarditis

In contrast to resource-limited countries where RHD is common, resource-rich countries have a very low incidence of IE in pregnancy: 1/100,000 pregnancies.[9] The main at-risk group in resource-rich countries are intravenous drug misusers where IE may occur on normal heart valves. IE may be associated with diseased or prosthetic heart valves, septal defects, shunts, baffles, and AVMs. The risk for these groups rises to 0.5%.[9] The main causative organism in pregnancy is *Streptococcus*. Mortality rates are very high in pregnancy with up to 33% of mothers dying.[9] The major complications are due to heart failure precipitated by acute valvular regurgitation, and embolic disease.

IE is diagnosed in the same way as in non-pregnant patients, and is treated with long-term antibiotics. Surgical treatment is reserved for patients whose medical treatment has failed.

Routine antibiotic prophylaxis for the prevention of IE, for women with valve disorders or other predisposing heart lesions, is not required for women undergoing obstetric procedures. These include urinary catheterization, amniocentesis, chorionic villus sampling, normal vaginal delivery, instrumental vaginal delivery, and CD.[89]

Conclusion

Heart disease is a leading cause of maternal death throughout the world. In many resource-rich countries it is the most common overall cause of maternal mortality: the vast majority of these deaths are due to AHD. AHD is also a significant cause of severe maternal and fetal morbidity. As risk factors for AHD become more prevalent in women of reproductive age, mortality and severe morbidity may increase. However, the majority of pregnant women even with the most severe types of AHD achieve safe deliveries. Assessment, treatment, and detailed peripartum plans agreed by a multidisciplinary team, consisting of cardiologists, obstetricians, and obstetric anaesthetists, are fundamental to a safe approach to pregnancy in women with AHD. Most women will undergo a vaginal delivery: in this instance an early incremental epidural will reduce the cardiorespiratory work of labour. Where operative delivery is undertaken, slow-onset NA is becoming a more accepted approach even in severe cardiac disease.

In stark contrast to patterns of cardiac disease in the Western world, RHD is still highly prevalent in developing countries. Without the same available resources, many more women are dying in pregnancy as a result of their cardiac disease compared with women in developed countries.

Acknowledgement

Thanks to Dr Hamish Ireland for the CT angiography images of the aortic dissection.

References

1. Knight M, Kenyon S, Brocklehurst P, *et al. Saving Lives, Improving Mothers' Care. Lessons Learned to Inform Future Maternity Care from the UK and Ireland Confidential Enquiries into Maternal Deaths and Morbidity 2009–12.* Oxford: National Perinatal Epidemiology Unit, University of Oxford; 2014.
2. Cantwell R, Clutton-Brock T, Cooper G, Dawson A, Drife J, Garrod D, *et al.* Saving Mothers' Lives: Reviewing maternal deaths to make motherhood safer: 2006--2008. The Eighth Report of the Confidential Enquiries into Maternal Deaths in the United Kingdom. *BJOG : an international journal of obstetrics and gynaecology.* 2011; 118 Suppl 1: 1–203.
3. Centers for Disease Control and Prevention. *Pregnancy Mortality Surveillance System.* [Online] http://www.cdc.gov/reproductive-health/maternalinfanthealth/pmss.html#1
4. Roos-Hesselink JW, Ruys TP, Stein JI, *et al.* Outcome of pregnancy in patients with structural or ischaemic heart disease: results of a registry of the European Society of Cardiology. *Eur Heart J* 2013; 34(9):657–65.
5. Huisman CM, Zwart JJ, Roos-Hesselink JW, *et al.* Incidence and predictors of maternal cardiovascular mortality and severe morbidity in the Netherlands: a prospective cohort study. *PLoS One* 2013; 8(2):e56494.
6. Steer PJ. Pregnancy and contraception. In Gatzoulis M, Swan L, Therrien J (eds) *Adult Congenital Heart Disease A Practical Guide.* London: Blackwell; 2005:16–36.
7. Gelson, E, Gatzoulis MA, Steer P, *et al.* Heart disease – why is maternal mortality increasing? *BJOG* 2009; 116(5):609–11.
8. Lewis G (ed). *The Confidential Enquiry into Maternal and Child Health (CEMACH). Saving Mothers' Lives: Reviewing Maternal Deaths to make Motherhood Safer 2003–05. The Seventh Report on*

Confidential Enquiries into Maternal Deaths in the United Kingdom. London: CEMACH; 2007.

9. Regitz-Zagrosek V, Lundquist CB, Borghi C, *et al.* ESC guidelines on the management of cardiovascular diseases during pregnancy. *Eur Heart J* 2011; 32(24):3147–97.
10. Royal College of Obstetricians and Gynaecologists. *Cardiac Disease and Pregnancy*. Good Practice No. 13. London: RCOG; 2011.
11. Adamson DL, Dhanjal MK, Nelson-Piercy C. Physiological changes in pregnancy. In *Heart Disease in Pregnancy*. Oxford: Oxford University Press; 2011:2–11.
12. Pieper PJ, Hoendermis ES, Drijver YN. Cardiac surgery and percutaneous intervention in pregnant women with heart disease. *Neth Heart J* 2012; 20:125–8.
13. Barth WH. Cardiac surgery in pregnancy. *Clin Obstet Gynae* 2009; 52:630–46.
14. John AS, Gurley F, Schaff HV, *et al.* Cardiopulmonary bypass during pregnancy. *Ann Thorac Surg* 2011; 91:1191–6.
15. Chambers CE, Clark SL. Cardiac surgery during pregnancy. *Clin Obstet Gynaecol* 1994; 37:316–23.
16. Parry AJ, Westaby S. Cardiopulmonary bypass during pregnancy. *Ann Thorac Surg* 1996; 61:1865–9.
17. Jafferani, A, Malik A, Khawaja RDA, *et al.* Surgical management of valvular heart diseases in pregnancy. *Eur J Obstet Gynecol Reprod Biol* 2011; 159(1):91–4.
18. Langesaeter E, Dragsund M, Rosseland LA. Regional anaesthesia for a Caesarean section in women with cardiac disease: a prospective study. *Acta Anaesthesiol Scand* 2010; 54(1):46–54.
19. Lewis NL, Dob DP, Yentis SM. UK registry of high-risk obstetric anaesthesia: arrhythmias, cardiomyopathy, aortic stenosis, transposition of the great arteries and Marfan's syndrome. *Int J Obstet Anesth* 2003; 12(1):28–34.
20. Hamlyn EL, Douglass CA, Plaat F, *et al.* Low-dose sequential combined spinal-epidural: an anaesthetic technique for caesarean section in patients with significant cardiac disease. *Int J Obstet Anesth* 2005; 14(4):355–61.
21. Dresner M, Pinder A. Anaesthesia for caesarean section in women with complex cardiac disease: 34 cases using the Braun Spinocath® spinal catheter. *Int J Obstet Anesth* 2009; 18(2):131–6.
22. Centers for Disease Control and Prevention. Prevalence of coronary heart disease. *MMWR* 2011; 60(40):1377–81. http://www.cdc.gov/mmwr/preview/mmwrhtml/mm6040a1.htm
23. Ladner HE, Danielsen B, Gilbert WM. Acute myocardial infarction in pregnancy and the puerperium: a population-based study. *Obstet Gynecol* 2005; 105(3):480–4.
24. James AH, Jamison MG, Biswas MS, *et al.* Acute myocardial infarction in pregnancy: a United States population-based study. *Circulation* 2006; 113(12):1564–71.
25. Wen SW, Huang L, Liston R, *et al.* Severe maternal morbidity in Canada, 1991-2001. *CMA J* 2005; 173(7):759–64.
26. Bush N, Nelson-Piercy C, Spark P, *et al.* Myocardial infarction in pregnancy and postpartum in the UK. *Eur J Prevent Cardiol* 2013; 20(1):12–20.
27. Hankins GD, Wendel GD Jr, Leveno KJ, *et al.* Myocardial infarction during pregnancy: a review. *Obstet Gynecol* 1985; 65(1):139–46.
28. Roth A, Elkayam U. Acute myocardial infarction associated with pregnancy. *J Am Coll Cardiol* 2008; 52(3):171–80.
29. Roth A, Elkayam U. Acute myocardial infarction associated with pregnancy. *Ann Intern Med* 1996; 125(9):751–62.
30. Kealey AJ. Coronary artery disease and myocardial infarction in pregnancy: a review of epidemiology, diagnosis, and medical and surgical management. *Can J Cardiol* 2010; 26(6):e185–e189.
31. Jacobsson B, Ladfors L, Milsom I. Advanced maternal age and adverse perinatal outcome. *Obstet Gynecol* 2004; 104(4):727–33.
32. Prescott E, Hippe M, Schnohr P, *et al.* Smoking and risk of myocardial infarction in women and men: longitudinal population study. *BMJ* 1998; 316(7137):1043.
33. Blair SD, Janvrin SB, McCollum CN, *et al.* Effect of early blood transfusion on gastrointestinal haemorrhage. *Br J Surg* 1986; 73(10):783–5.
34. Sutaria N, O'Toole L, Northridge, D. Postpartum acute MI following routine ergometrine administration treated successfully by primary PTCA. *Heart* 2000; 83(1):97–8.
35. Appleby CE, Barolet A, Ing D, *et al.* Contemporary management of pregnancy-related coronary artery dissection: a single-centre experience and literature review. *Exp Clin Cardiol* 2009; 14(1):e8–e16.
36. Koul AK, Hollander G, Moskovits N, *et al.* Coronary artery dissection during pregnancy and the postpartum period: two case reports and review of literature. *Catheter Cardiovasc Interv* 2001; 52(1): 88–94.
37. Schumacher B, Belfort MA, Card RJ. Successful treatment of acute myocardial infarction during pregnancy with tissue plasminogen activator. *Am J Obstet Gynecol* 1997; 176(3):716–19.
38. Leonhardt G, Gaul C, Nietsch HH, *et al.* Thrombolytic therapy in pregnancy. *J Thromb Thrombolysis* 2006; 21(3):271–6.
39. De Santis M, De Luca C, Mappa I *et al.* Clopidogrel treatment during pregnancy: a case report and a review of the literature. *Intern Med* 2011; 50:1769–73.
40. Klinzing P, Markert UR, Liesaus K, *et al.* Case report: successful pregnancy and delivery after myocardial infarction and essential thrombocythemia treated with clopidogrel. *Clin Exp Obstet Gynecol* 2001; 28:215–16.
41. Smith RL, Young SJ, Greer IA. The parturient with coronary heart disease. *IJOA* 2008; 17:46–52.
42. Shotan A, Ostrzega E, Mehra A. Incidence of arrhythmias in normal pregnancy and relation to palpitations, dizziness and syncope. *Am J Cardiol* 1997; 79:1061–4.
43. Carson MP, Powrie RO, Rosene-Montella K. The effect of obesity and position on the heart rate in pregnancy. *J Matern Fetal Neonatal Med* 2002; 11:40–5.
44. Blomstrom-Lundqvist C, Scheinman MM, Aliot EM, Alpert JS, *et al.* ACC/AHA/ESC guidelines for the management of patients with supraventricular arrhythmias-executive summary. *Eur Heart J* 2003; 24:1857–97.
45. Silversides CK, Harris L, Haberer K, *et al.* Recurrence rates of arrhythmias during pregnancy in women with previous tachyarrhythmia and impact on fetal and neonatal outcomes. *Am J Cardiol* 2006; 97:1206–12.
46. Siu SC, Smer M, Harrison DA, *et al.* Risk and predictors for pregnancy related complications in women with heart disease. *Circulation* 1997; 96:2789–94.
47. Adamson DL, Nelson-Piercy C. Managing palpitations and arrhythmias during pregnancy. *Heart* 2007; 93:1630–6.
48. Li JM, Nguyen C, Joglar JA, *et al.* Frequency and outcome of arrhythmias complicating admission during pregnancy: experience from a high volume and ethnically diverse obstetric service. *Clin Cardiol* 2008; 31:538–41.
49. Drenthen W, Pieper PG, Roos-Hesselink JW, *et al.* Outcome of pregnancy in women with congenital heart disease: a literature review. *J Am Coll Cardiol* 2007; 49:2303–11.
50. Elkayam U, Goodwin TM. Adenosine therapy for SVT during pregnancy. *Am J Cardiol* 1995; 75:521–3.
51. Bauce B, Daliento L, Frigo G, *et al.* Pregnancy in women with arrhythmogenic right ventricular cardiomyopathy/dysplasia. *Eur J Obstet Gynecol Reprod Biol* 2006; 127:186–9.
52. Natale A, Davidson T, Geiger MJ, *et al.* Implantable cardioverter-defibrillators and pregnancy: a safe combination? *Circulation* 1997; 96:2808–12.
53. Rashba EJ, Zareba W, Moss AJ, *et al.* Influence of pregnancy on the risk for cardiac events in patients with hereditary long QT syndrome. *Circulation* 1998; 97:451–6.
54. Charbit B, Funck-Brentano C, Samain E, *et al.* QT interval prolongation after oxytocin bolus during surgical induced abortion. *Clin Pharmacol Ther* 2004; 76:359–64.

55. Kies SJ, Pabelick CM, Hurley HA, *et al.* Anaesthesia for patients with congenital long QT syndrome. *Anesthesiology* 2005; 102:204–10.
56. Nagele P, Swatilika P, Brown F, *et al.* Postoperative QT interval prolongation in patients undergoing non-cardiac surgery under general anaesthesia. *Anesthesiology* 2012; 117(2):321–8.
57. Lund LH, Edwards LB, Kucheryavaya AY, *et al.* The Registry of the International Society for Heart and Lung Transplantation: Thirtieth Official Adult Heart Transplant Report – 2013. *J Heart Lung Transplant* 2013; 32:951–64.
58. Yusen RD, Christie JD, Edwards LB, *et al.* The Registry of the International Society for Heart and Lung Transplantation: Thirtieth Adult Lung and Heart-Lung Transplant Report-2013; focus theme: age. *J Heart Lung Transplant* 2013; 32:965–78.
59. Coscia LA, Cosntantinescu S, Moritz MJ, *et al.* Report from the National Transplantation Pregnancy Registry (NTPR): outcomes of pregnancy after transplantation. *Clin Transpl* 2010; 2010:65–85.
60. Scott JR, Wagoner LE, Olsen SL, *et al.* Pregnancy in heart transplant recipients: Management and outcome. *Obstet Gynecol* 1988; 82:324–7.
61. Miniero R, Tardivo I, Centofanti P, *et al.* Pregnancy in heart transplant recipients. *J Heart Lung Transplant* 2004; 23:898–901.
62. Uretsky BF, Murali S, Reddy PS, *et al.* Development of coronary disease in cardiac transplant patients receiving immunosuppressive therapy with cyclosporine and prednisolone. *Circulation* 1987; 76:827–34.
63. Ray P, Murphy GJ, Shutt LE. Recognition and management of maternal cardiac disease in pregnancy. *Br J Anaesth* 2004; 93:428–39.
64. Kim KM, Sukhnai R, Slogoff S, *et al.* Central hemodynamic changes associated with pregnancy in a long-term cardiac transplant recipient. *Am J Obstet Gynecol* 1996; 174:1651–3.
65. Camann WR, Goldman GA, Johnson MD, *et al.* Caesarean delivery in a patient with a transplanted heart. *Anaesthesiology* 1989; 71:618–20.
66. Hirst AE Jr, Varner JJ Jr, Kime SW Jr. Dissecting aneurysm of the aorta: a review of 505 cases. *Medicine* 1958; 37(3):217.
67. Lipscomb KJ, Clayton Smith J, Clarke B, *et al.* Outcome of pregnancy in women with Marfan's syndrome. *BJOG* 1997; 104(2):201–6.
68. Donnelly RT, Pinto NM, Kocolas I, *et al.* The immediate and long-term impact of pregnancy on aortic growth rate and mortality in women with Marfan syndrome. *J Am Coll Cardiol* 2012; 60(3):224–9.
69. Palmquist M, Pappas JG, Petrikovsky B, *et al.* Successful pregnancy outcome in Ehlers–Danlos syndrome, vascular type. *J Matern Fetal Neonatal Med* 2009; 22(10):924–7.
70. Hahn RT, Roman MJ, Mogtadek AH, *et al.* Association of aortic dilation with regurgitant, stenotic and functionally normal bicuspid aortic valves. *J Am Coll Cardiol* 1992; 19(2):283–8.
71. Immer FF, Bansi AG, Immer-Bansi AS, *et al.* Aortic dissection in pregnancy: analysis of risk factors and outcome. *Ann Thorac Surg* 2003; 76(1):309–14.
72. Thrumurthy SG, Karthikesalingam A, Patterson BO, *et al.* The diagnosis and management of aortic dissection. *BMJ* 2011; 344:d8290.
73. Pyeritz RE, Fishman EK, Bernhardt BA, *et al.* Dural ectasia is a common feature of the Marfan syndrome. *Am J Hum Genet* 1988; 43(5):726.
74. McNeilly G, Nicholl A, Broadway J, *et al.* Dural ectasia in Marfan's syndrome: magnetic resonance imaging appearances and anaesthetic experience of three deliveries. *Int J Obstet Anesth* 2013; 22(4):337–9.
75. Sliwa K, Hilfiker-Kleiner D, Petrie MC, *et al.* Current state of knowledge on aetiology, diagnosis, management, and therapy of peripartum cardiomyopathy: a position statement from the Heart Failure Association of the European Society of Cardiology Working Group on peripartum cardiomyopathy. *Eur J Heart Fail* 2010; 12(8):767–78.
76. Fett JD, McTiernan CF. Towards a unifying hypothesis for the pathogenesis of peripartum cardiomyopathy. *Int J Cardiol* 2011; 153(1):1–3.
77. Howlett JG, McKelvie RS, Costigan J, *et al.* The 2010 Canadian Cardiovascular Society guidelines for the diagnosis and management of heart failure update: heart failure in ethnic minority populations, heart failure and pregnancy, disease management, and quality improvement/assurance programs. *Can J Cardiol* 2010; 26(4):185–202.
78. Blauwet LA, Cooper LT. Diagnosis and management of peripartum cardiomyopathy. *Heart* 2011; 97(23):1970–81.
79. McMurray JJ, Adamopoulos S, Anker SD, *et al.* ESC guidelines for the diagnosis and treatment of acute and chronic heart failure 2012. The Task Force for the Diagnosis and Treatment of Acute and Chronic Heart Failure 2012 of the European Society of Cardiology. Developed in collaboration with the Heart Failure Association (HFA) of the ESC. *Eur Heart J* 2012; 33(14):1787–847.
80. Sliwa K, Blauwet L, Tibazarwa K, *et al.* Evaluation of bromocriptine in the treatment of acute severe peripartum cardiomyopathy a proof-of-concept pilot study. *Circulation* 2010; 121(13):1465–73.
81. Krul SP, van Der Smagt JJ, van den Berg MP, *et al.* Systematic review of pregnancy in women with inherited cardiomyopathies. *Eur J Heart Fail* 2011; 13(6):584–94.
82. Pieper PG, Walker F. Pregnancy in women with hypertrophic cardiomyopathy. *Neth Heart J* 2013; 21(1):14–18.
83. Stergiopoulos K, Shiang E, Bench T. Pregnancy in patients with pre-existing cardiomyopathies. *J Am Coll Cardiol* 2011; 58(4):337–50.
84. Wolff GA, Weitzel NS. Management of acquired cardiac disease in the obstetric patient. *Semin Cardiothorac Vasc Anesth* 2011; 15(3):85–97.
85. Ioscovich AM, Goldszmidt E, Fadeev AV, *et al.* Peripartum anesthetic management of patients with aortic valve stenosis: a retrospective study and literature review. *IJOA* 2009; 18(4):379–86.
86. Chan WS, Anand S, Ginsberg JS. Anticoagulation of pregnant women with mechanical heart valves: a systematic review of the literature. *Arch Intern Med* 2000; 160(2):191.
87. Bowater SE, Thorne SA. Management of pregnancy in women with acquired and congenital heart disease. *Postgrad Med J* 2010; 86:100–5.
88. Bates SM, Greer IA, Middeldorp S, *et al.* VTE, thrombophilia, antithrombotic therapy, and pregnancy: Antithrombotic Therapy and Prevention of Thrombosis, 9th ed: American College of Chest Physicians Evidence-Based Clinical Practice Guidelines. *Chest* 2012; 141(2 Suppl):e691S–736S.
89. National Institute of Health and Clinical Excellence. *Prophylaxis Against Infective Endocarditis*. Clinical Guideline No. 68. London: NICE; 2008.

CHAPTER 42

Respiratory disease

Wendy H. L. Teoh

Cystic fibrosis

Epidemiology and prevalence

Cystic fibrosis (CF) is a fatal autosomal recessive genetic disease involving chloride channels, affecting 1/2500–3200 live Caucasian births. CF was first distinguished from coeliac disease in 1938 when the autopsy studies of malnourished infants revealed 'cystic fibrosis of the pancreas'. Previously regarded as a uniformly fatal childhood disease, it has transitioned to a chronic, progressive disease of adults.[1] Since genetic identification in 1989 and improvements in diagnosis and therapeutic advances, CF sufferers have attained significant gains in quality of life, pregnancy, and longevity. The median survival age of patients with CF is now 38 years and increasing.[2] Declines in newborn CF incidence from 1975 to 2009 have been reported consecutive to the availability of prenatal diagnosis in France[3] and Australia.[3,4]

Genetics

The cause of CF is a mutation in a single gene on chromosome 7, that encodes the cystic fibrosis transmembrane conductance regulator (CFTR).[5,6] CFTR functions as an adenosine triphosphate- and cyclic adenosine monophosphate (cAMP)-dependent chloride channel that is found at the apical border of epithelial cells lining most exocrine glands. Clinical CF is associated with mutations in the *CFTR* gene (of which the most common mutation among Caucasians, DeltaF508, was identified in 1989[7]) where epithelial cells are unable to alter chloride permeability in response to changes in cAMP, decreasing the water content of various secretions, and resulting in increased viscosity and luminal obstruction. Organs that express CFTR in their epithelial cells are affected, notably the airways (including sinuses and lungs), gastrointestinal tract (including pancreas and biliary system), the sweat glands, and the genitourinary system.

Clinical manifestations

Pulmonary disease is responsible for more than 90% of the morbidity and mortality in patients with CF[8] stemming from the inability to clear thickened and inspissated mucus from the airways. Chronic airway obstruction with decreased forced expiratory volume in 1 second (FEV_1) and peak expiratory flow (PEF), and increased residual volume is seen. Colonization with *Pseudomonas aeruginosa, Staphylococcus aureus, Haemophilus influenza, Stenotrophomonas maltophilia*, and other Gram-negative organisms commonly occurs. *Burkholderia cepacia* and *Aspergillus fumigatus* are associated with high morbidity and mortality. Recurrent bacterial infections result in dilation of the conducting airways and bronchiectasis.[9] With disease progression, there is destruction of parenchyma and loss of pulmonary arterial vascular cross-sectional area. Ventilation/perfusion inequality results in chronic hypoxaemia, an increase in pulmonary vascular resistance (PVR), pulmonary hypertension, and cor pulmonale. Spontaneous pneumothorax is prevalent in older patients and those with more severe pulmonary impairment (FEV_1 of <40% predicted).[10]

Non-respiratory manifestations of CF include exocrine pancreatic deficiency, malabsorption, failure to thrive, fat-soluble vitamin deficiencies, recurrent pancreatitis, CF-related diabetes mellitus, hepatobiliary cirrhosis and portal hypertension, intestinal obstruction, increased gastroesophageal reflux, infertility, obstructive azoospermia, and salt-losing syndromes.

Diagnosis

Diagnosis is based on sweat chloride measurements greater than 60 mEq/L plus the following characteristic clinical symptoms: presence of chronic obstructive lung disease (cough, chronic purulent sputum production, exertional dyspnoea) or a family history of CF. Chronic pansinusitis is universal. Malabsorption responsive to pancreatic enzyme treatment is evidence of exocrine insufficiency associated with CF. Obstructive azoospermia confirmed by testicular biopsy is also strong evidence of CF. Other laboratory findings include *CFTR* genotype with two known CF mutations, and nasal potential difference testing to detect CFTR dysfunction.[2]

Impact of pregnancy on cystic fibrosis

With improvement in clinical care and longer survival of patients with CF, pregnancy has become commonplace. Deterioration of pulmonary function occurs as CF patients may be unable to meet the required increases in pregnancy-associated minute ventilation and oxygen uptake. Blood volume and cardiac output increments precipitate right heart strain, congestive heart failure, and pulmonary hypertension in those with moderate-to-severe pulmonary disease.

Of 20 pregnancies from 18 women with CF during the period 1995–2009, all women delivered live births apart from one therapeutic abortion. Three mothers either died or required lung transplantation after pregnancy (range 2.5–8.0 years).[11] Factors associated with poor outcome in pregnant CF patients are weight gain less than 4.5 kg, forced vital capacity (FVC) less than 50% predicted, pulmonary colonization with *B. cepacia*, frequent pulmonary infections, diabetes mellitus, malnutrition, and pancreatic insufficiency.[12,13]

Despite these negative effects, pregnancy can be managed without a persisting decrement in lung function beyond what may be expected in non-pregnant CF.[14] Successful pregnancy outcome has even been reported in a CF patient following heart, lung, and renal transplant.[15]

With the increasingly positive outcomes for people with CF, it is likely that more couples will chose to pursue pregnancy, cognisant of the risks and longer-term issues for mother, child, and family. Successful outcomes for mother and child can be achieved with appropriate multidisciplinary care. The process begins prior to conception and requires frequent monitoring of the mother's respiratory status, level of glycaemic control and obstetric well-being. Overall long-term survival appears unaffected[16] but intensive health monitoring, more frequent use of intravenous (IV) antibiotics, and hospitalization[17] is evident in pregnant CF patients (due to respiratory exacerbations, diabetic treatment, supplementary nutrition, etc.).[18] A multidisciplinary team of providers is optimal to address the variety of issues that arise in such a pregnancy.

Impact of cystic fibrosis on pregnancy

The incidence of intrauterine growth retardation, low birth weight infants, and preterm labour and delivery is increased for women with CF, especially those with the worst pulmonary, nutritional, and pancreatic function.[19,20] FEV_1 less than 60% predicted and body mass index (BMI) less than 20 kg/m^2 were significant predictors of fetal complications.[11] A recent review of 523 pregnancies in 401 women showed 83.1% of 516 pregnancies resulted in live births, of which 24% delivered preterm; miscarriage occurred in 6.3% and therapeutic abortion in 10% of pregnancies.[21]

Medical management

Comprehensive care at adult subspecialty centres decreases hospitalization, and improves morbidity and mortality. Respiratory management includes chest physiotherapy with postural drainage: breathing exercises, high-frequency chest compression with an inflatable vest, and airway oscillation with a flutter valve are less time-consuming and do not require trained personnel. Adrenergic agonists (e.g. salbutamol) can be used for bronchial hyper-reactivity; bronchodilator therapy is considered if patients have an increase of 10% or more in FEV_1 in response to an inhaled bronchodilator. Chronic suppressive antibiotic therapy with aerosolized tobramycin[22] and oral azithromycin[23] decreases exacerbations of CF. The abnormal viscosity of airway secretions is due primarily to neutrophils and their degradation products. DNA released from neutrophils forms long fibrils that increase viscosity. Recombinant human deoxyribonuclease 1 (dornase alfa (Pulmozyme®)) cleaves this DNA, and increases sputum clearance, reduces air trapping,[24] improves FEV_1, and decreases pulmonary exacerbation rate.[25] Inhaled aztreonam lysine is also beneficial for chronic airway *Pseudomonas aeruginosa*.[26,27] Hypertonic saline acutely increases mucociliary clearance and has emerged as a safe and inexpensive adjunct therapy.[28] CF patients have a significant inflammatory component with asthma or asthma-like symptoms and benefit from oral or inhaled glucocorticoids. Continuous supplemental oxygen is the only medical therapy effective in treating pulmonary hypertension and improving right ventricle performance.[29] After lung transplantation, 1- and 5-year survival rates of 89% and 71% respectively have been reported, with the presence of diabetes not associated with a worse outcome.[30] Antithymocyte globulin induction therapy confers a significant survival benefit in CF patients undergoing lung transplantation and reduces rejection.[31] Nasal polyps, hypertrophy, and hyperplasia of nasal/sinus mucosa may benefit from use of decongestants or topical glucocorticoids, saline irrigation, and surgical drainage of sinonasal passages.

Obstetric management

The primary issue is whether pregnancy is advisable, dependent on pregravid CF maternal health. CF is the first genetic disorder for which universal screening of preconceptional or prenatal patients became a component of standard prenatal care. Carrier screening facilitates risk assessment for prospective parents to have an affected offspring, although there remains a small residual risk for carrying a mutation even with a negative screening result.[32] There has been a modest reduction in the live-birth prevalence of CF since the introduction of newborn screening.[33]

Anaesthetic management

CF sufferers have usually established long-term relationships with their respiratory physicians or CF specialists, are familiar with their disease, and have knowledge of healthcare systems. These strengths should be harnessed by the obstetric anaesthetist, and management decisions made in tandem with the CF parturient's multidisciplinary care team throughout the delivery and perioperative period. Neuraxial anaesthetic techniques are promoted to avoid airway instrumentation and exacerbating risk of pulmonary complications.

Preoperative assessment and optimization

A thorough pulmonary evaluation is indicated. The interview should elicit the history of CF, disease progression, presence of cough, quality and quantity of mucus production, frequency of respiratory infections and airway reactivity, wheezing and response to bronchodilators, and functional exercise capacity. It is perfectly acceptable to order a chest radiograph, and a recent one is crucial to diagnose pneumothorax, pneumonic processes, or bullous disease. Lung hyperinflation is evidenced by diaphragm flattening, prominence of the retrosternal space, and kyphoscoliosis in late disease. Bronchovascular markings, initially present in upper lobes, progress to the lower lobes later in the disease process. Peribronchial cuffing and parallel-lined 'tram tracks' will be seen with bronchiectasis and cyst formation. Chest computed tomography may be helpful to delineate the extent of bronchiectasis, but does not correlate with exercise tolerance, and may appear worse than the patient's actual physical capabilities.[34] Baseline arterial blood gas analysis should be performed looking for CO_2 retention. Pulmonary function testing typically shows an obstructive pattern: increased ratio of residual volume to total lung capacity and decreased forced expiratory flow at 25–75% of lung volume. Greater reductions in FEV_1 and FEV_1/FVC ratio epitomize disease progression. Late findings of increased PVR, right ventricular hypertrophy, and cor pulmonale indicate advanced and decompensated CF, with great mortality. The perioperative management of patients with CF also encompasses a pancreatic and hepatobiliary evaluation. Coagulopathy resulting from vitamin K deficiency or general malnutrition should be excluded with prothrombin time and partial thromboplastin time. Aspiration prophylaxis is imperative due to increased incidence of gastroesophageal reflux disease (GORD) in CF patients. Glucose intolerance is rife and may require escalating insulin therapy.

Issues affecting labour and vaginal delivery

Labour pain relief from neuraxial anaesthesia should aim to provide adequate analgesia, prevent maternal hyperventilation to limit the increased work of breathing, avoid high thoracic motor blockade that will impair the CF parturient's cough reflex and ability to expectorate thick secretions, and include avoidance of respiratory depression (e.g. parenteral opioids). Intrathecal opioids have been used successfully[35] but should be monitored closely for respiratory depression. Continuous lumbar epidural analgesia (avoiding a high block) with dilute bupivacaine solutions is ideal.[36–38] Continuous pulse oximetry monitoring and supplemental oxygen therapy are advisable due to the high incidence of hypoxaemia in CF patients.

Issues regarding caesarean delivery

Neuraxial anaesthesia techniques (e.g. single-shot spinal, combined spinal–epidural (CSE), or epidural top-up) are ideal in minimizing postoperative pulmonary complications, with the same treatment goals as outlined above for labour and vaginal delivery. However, if general anaesthesia cannot be avoided, the increased risk of aspiration (from GORD) and bronchospasm need to be factored into the anaesthetic plan. The goal would be to have a parturient with minimal respiratory depression and full recovery of airway reflexes at the end of surgery and anaesthesia. Nasopharyngeal airways should be avoided due to sinonasal disease including sinus polyps. A rapid sequence induction should be preceded by non-particulate antacids and H_2 antagonists. CF is an obstructive process, and prolonged expiratory times may be necessary, as well as humidification of inspired gases and minimization of peak airway pressures to reduce the risk of barotrauma and pneumothorax. Nitrous oxide should be used with caution because of the increased risk of pneumothorax formation with positive pressure ventilation, as well as the likely presence of multiple blebs. Volatile anaesthetic agents produce bronchodilation and may be preferable in CF patients to total IV anaesthesia techniques. Adjunctive pain medications should be administered for post-caesarean delivery (CD) analgesia (e.g. non-steroidal anti-inflammatory drugs, IV paracetamol to reduce opioid-related respiratory depression). Bilateral transversus abdominis plane blocks are useful in reducing morphine consumption following CD under general anaesthesia.[39] Before extubation, consider lung recruitment manoeuvres to avoid atelectasis and endotracheal suction to mobilize secretions. The patient should be extubated fully awake, and high dependency care for 24 hours to monitor respiratory function is necessary. Immediate postoperative chest physiotherapy may be beneficial to some patients.

Asthma

Definition

Asthma is derived from the Greek word *aazein* meaning 'to pant' and was first used in 450 BC by Hippocrates to describe a condition characterized by spasms of breathlessness. The present Global Initiative for Asthma (GINA) definition of asthma covers a triad of airway pathology (chronic airway inflammation), disordered airway function (reversible airway obstruction and airway hyper-responsiveness), and typical symptomatology.[40]

Epidemiology and prevalence

Asthma is the most common respiratory disorder to complicate pregnancy. The burden of asthma in pregnancy is increasing worldwide,[41] with European estimates of at least 4% of women having asthma, and at least 8% of women in antenatal clinics in the United Kingdom having asthma.[42] From 1976 to 2001,the prevalence of asthma in the United States has risen from 3% to 8.8%[43] and is 12% in Australia.[44]

Genetics

Genes and environmental exposures interact to influence the risk of asthma susceptibility and severity; implicated genes indicate pathways for therapeutic intervention and provide insight into mechanisms of asthma severity progression.[45] Two large meta-analyses of asthma susceptibility identified four chromosomal regions that were consistently associated with development of asthma in ethnically different individuals: loci in the *ORMDL3* gene region of 17q21, interleukin (IL)-1 receptor-like 1 isoform 1 (*IL-1RL*/*IL-18R*) on chromosome 2q, thymic stromal lymphopoietin (*TSLP*) on 5q22, and *IL-33* on chromosome 9p24.[46,47] Genetic variants in the major histocompatibility complex gene region (human leucocyte antigen region) on chromosome 6p21 indicated asthma susceptibility in Asian populations.[48] Pharmacogenetic genome-wide screens also identified two correlated genetic variants in the glucocorticoid-induced transcript 1 (*GLCCI1*) gene that related to decreased response to inhaled glucocorticoids.[49]

Pathophysiology

The underlying mechanisms involve (a) airway smooth muscle (ASM)-related bronchial hyper-responsiveness, (b) airway inflammation, and (c) remodelling changes in airway epithelium. This occurs against a backdrop of various genetic, environmental, biochemical, and immunological host characteristics affecting asthma phenotype and severity.

Changes in ASM contractile properties or impaired function of relaxant receptors play an important role in the development of bronchial hyper-responsiveness. G-protein coupled receptor (GPCR)-associated calcium responses in ASM can be modulated by a variety of inflammatory stimuli like tumour necrosis factor gamma, IL-13 (a T-helper type 2 (Th2) mediator in allergic asthma), or IL-1b.[50] Vagal and sympathetic factors directly modulate airway tone. Asthmatic ASM is infiltrated by both mast cells (mast cell myositis) and T lymphocytes but apparently not eosinophils. Mast cell migration is further induced by the production of various chemotactic mediators secreted by the ASM itself, which is closely related to the ASM inflammatory microenvironment.[50] This complex relationship between ASM cells and inflammatory cells is postulated to be a possible way for ASM to organize inflammation.

Placental growth factor (PlGF) and its receptor vascular endothelial growth factor receptor 1 (VEGFR1) play an important role in pathological conditions related to angiogenesis, vascular leakage, and inflammation. PlGF and its receptor VEGFR1 were found to be up-regulated in allergic asthma, playing a proinflammatory role by inducing tissue oedema, increasing tissue neutrophilia and the production of IL-17.[51]

Asthmatic bronchial remodelling is characterized by various structural changes, including abnormal epithelium, subepithelial membrane thickening, alteration of the extracellular matrix deposition, neoangiogenesis, mucus gland hypertrophy, and increased ASM mass.[52] Inflammatory oedema and mucous plugging exacerbate airflow limitation and progressively impair the response to bronchodilator therapy. Recent evidence suggests that the increased ASM mass is the key feature of bronchial remodelling in asthma because of its association with a more severe asthma phenotype, and correlates with a decrease in lung function.[50] The airway remodelling, thickening, and aberrant communication between the injured airway epithelium and the pulmonary mesenchyme contributes to disease chronicity and refractoriness to corticosteroids.[53] Genome-wide association studies of asthma provide strong evidence of the biological importance of pathways that communicate epithelial damage to the adaptive immune system, ultimately leading to airway inflammation. Moreover, cytokines derived from epithelial cells such as TSLP and IL-33 are thought to promote the TH2 response through activation of receptors such as IL-1RL1 on cell types such as mast cells, TH2 cells, and regulatory T cells.[45]

Diagnosis

Many patients with asthma during pregnancy will already be known asthmatics. A new diagnosis of asthma is usually suspected on the basis of characteristic symptoms (wheezing, chest tightness, cough, shortness of breath), temporal relationships (fluctuating intensity, worse at night) and triggers (e.g. allergens, exercise, and infections). Chest auscultation may reveal wheezing (but its absence does not exclude it) and a prolonged expiration phase.

The most common differential diagnosis is dyspnoea of pregnancy, which can occur in early pregnancy in approximately 70% of women. This breathlessness is differentiated from asthma by its lack of association with cough, wheezing, or airway obstruction. Other differential diagnoses include GORD, allergic rhinitis with chronic cough from postnasal drip, bronchitis, pneumonia, pulmonary oedema, and pulmonary embolism.[54]

Spirometry reliably demonstrates airflow obstruction, and is the diagnostic tool of choice.[55] The diagnosis of asthma is confirmed by a reduced FEV_1 with greater than 12% improvement after inhalation of a short-acting bronchodilator like salbutamol, or by an increase of greater than 10% of predicted FEV_1 post salbutamol.[55,56] The peak expiratory flow rate (PEFR) is another commonly used pulmonary function parameter. Peak flow meters are designed for monitoring asthma control and should not be used as diagnostic tools in the office because of significant variability in their reference values for predicted peak expiratory flow measurements. Current National Asthma Education and Prevention Program (NAEPP) guidelines suggest classifying degree of asthma severity in patients not on controller medication and degree of asthma control in patients on controller medication. Assessing severity or control involves determining the frequency of daytime symptoms, night-time symptoms, activity limitation, frequency of rescue therapy, and FEV_1.[57]

In patients with normal pulmonary function, methacholine testing is often performed to confirm bronchial hyper-reactivity. However, methacholine testing is not recommended in pregnancy due to lack of available safety data. If reversibility of airway obstruction cannot be elicited after bronchodilator therapy, yet has a clinical picture consistent with asthma, the parturient should be empirically treated for presumed asthma until methacholine testing can be performed postpartum.[58] Skin testing for allergens is recommended for most non-pregnant patients with persistent asthma[55] to help identify potential triggers such as mites, animal dander, mould, and cockroachs, for which specific environmental control instructions can be given; however, it is not recommended in pregnancy as it is associated with systemic reactions and anaphylaxis. As an alternative, pregnant patients with persistent asthma may undergo blood testing for immunoglobulin E antibodies to specific allergens.[58]

Effects of pregnancy on asthma

The rule of thirds

Most women with asthma experience a change in their disease control while pregnant. One-third of women will improve, one-third will worsen, the remainder will remain unchanged. These changes are unpredictable from woman to woman and from pregnancy to pregnancy,[59,60] necessitating careful regular review of asthma during pregnancy. While exacerbations may occur at any time during gestation, they appear to be more common in the late second trimester. This 'one-third hypothesis' of worsening asthma stemmed from a large prospective study of 330 parturients in the 1980s whose symptoms of wheeze and sleep and activity limitation due to asthma were significantly increased between 29 and 36 weeks' gestation.[61] Exacerbations of asthma during labour and delivery can be predicted by severity: Women with mild asthma had an exacerbation rate of 12.6% and hospitalization rate of 2.3%; those with moderate asthma had an exacerbation rate of 25.7% and hospitalization rate of 6.8%; and severe asthmatics had exacerbation of 51.9% and hospitalization rate of 26.9%.[62]

Risk factors for asthma exacerbations during pregnancy

Atopy, sinusitis, and gastroesophageal reflux may also worsen in pregnancy, exacerbating asthma. Other risk factors for asthmatic exacerbations include inadequate prenatal care, obesity, and inhaled corticosteroids nonadherence.[63,64] The use of medication have profound effects on the course of asthma. One study found that asthma severity during pregnancy is similar to severity in the year before pregnancy, provided patients continue to use their prescribed medication. If women discontinue medication, even mild asthma becomes significantly more severe.[65] Respiratory tract viral infection is another culprit.[64] Pregnant women and those with asthma are certainly two groups with significantly increased susceptibility to infection with influenza strains, including seasonal and H1N1 influenza[66,67] due to a reduced production of interferon gamma and IL-10 from peripheral blood mononuclear cells and attenuation of antiviral and regulatory immunity,[68] which can be significantly improved by vaccination.[69] During the H1N1 pandemic in the United States, 7% of hospitalized patients were pregnant and 22% of these women had asthma. In total, 9% of all admissions to intensive care units (ICUs) and 16% of all deaths were among pregnant women, indicating that both the prevalence of illness and its severity is increased with pregnancy.[66,70–74]

Assessment of asthma severity

Different benchmarks have been used to assess asthma severity, be it clinical symptoms or pharmacological therapeutic requirements, therefore leading to variations in reported studies. Women with severe exacerbations in pregnancy have significantly lower asthma-specific quality of life, which may be a more sensitive measure of limitations due to asthma than symptoms alone.[75] Teeter[76] found that asthma symptoms correlated poorly with objective measures of airway obstruction FEV_1 and PEF, as post-treatment improvement in those parameters were not seen despite a subjective improvement in asthma symptoms. This reinforces the recommendation to measure airway obstruction objectively when assessing adult patients with chronic asthma.

Juniper and colleagues[77] described an overall improvement in methacholine airway responsiveness (dose change required to lower FEV_1 by 20%) in 16 parturients in the second trimester compared with preconception or postpartum values, with an associated improvement in clinical asthma severity as indicated by a reduction in minimum medication requirements. However, this did not result from better asthmatic control, as both symptoms and spirometry remained unchanged during pregnancy. They found no relationship with serum progesterone or oestriol concentrations, suggesting that other non-hormonal factors may also contribute to the improvement during pregnancy.[78]

Mechanisms for changes in asthma during pregnancy

Hormonal involvement, altered immune function, and fetal-sex have been proposed as mechanisms in pregnancy-related changes in asthma.

Hormonal factors

Physiological factors that may improve asthma during pregnancy include higher levels of circulating cortisol, increased production of bronchodilating prostaglandins, and increased progesterone with advancing gestation that contributes to increased minute ventilation and cAMP-induced relaxation of ASM. Factors that may worsen asthma during pregnancy are decreased sensitivity to beta-adrenergic agonists, increased production of bronchoconstricting prostaglandins, and reduced sensitivity to circulating cortisol due to binding of steroid hormones (e.g. progesterone) to cortisol receptors. Juniper's work showed that increasing levels of progesterone in pregnancy does not play a central role in attenuating airway hyper-responsiveness in asthmatics.[77] Data has emerged that progesterone may actually worsen asthma by aggravating eosinophilic airway inflammation by enhancing systemic IL-5 production, and increasing bronchial hyperreactivity.[79] Thus, effects of pregnancy on asthma appear to involve factors *other* than direct hormonal effects on ASM.

Non-hormonal factors

Alterations in the maternal immune system during pregnancy such as a suppression of cell-mediated immunity may contribute to changes in asthma. Pregnancy-induced increases in regulatory T-cell prevalence was found to be absent in asthmatic pregnancies that interfere with physiological intrauterine growth.[80] In a study of 208 pregnant women, asthmatic atopic women with pets in the home during pregnancy were found to have lower percentages of regulatory T cells than atopic women who did not have pets.[81] Others have also found that lymphocyte activation of CD4 and CD8 T cells and the number of natural killer T cells were found to be blunted in pregnancy.[82] As lymphocyte activation characterizes bronchial asthma, these pregnancy-associated immunological alterations may explain why some mothers experience an improvement in their asthma.

Heat shock protein (Hsp)-70 is a novel marker of the immunotolerance of pregnancy. It is decreased in the circulation of healthy pregnant women compared with non-pregnant adults[83] but asthmatic women exhibit higher levels of Hsp70 than their non-asthmatic counterparts.[84] The role of this marker in the chronic inflammation of asthma and impact on perinatal outcomes has not been fully elucidated yet.

IL-4 and gamma-interferon producing T-lymphocyte subsets were found to be significantly increased in pregnant women with asthma, compared with healthy pregnant women and non-pregnant asthmatic women, but was not related to whether women perceived their asthma to have improved or worsened during pregnancy.[85] Bronchial epithelial cells have demonstrated increased production of IL-8 and soluble intercellular adhesion molecule 1 in the presence of plasma from pregnant women with asthma, and results were suggestive of an increased chemotactic capacity[86] which may be a mechanism contributing to worsening asthma in some pregnant women.

Progression of maternal asthma symptoms in pregnancy were thought to be influenced by the sex of the fetus,[87–89] with female fetus having a higher incidence of hospitalization for asthma during pregnancy.[90] However, other reports do not support this association.[91,92] The largest study in this area of more than 10,000 asthmatic pregnancies in Quebec found no differences between women pregnant with male and female fetuses with regard to the occurrence of severe exacerbations, or the use of inhaled corticosteroids or short-acting beta agonist.[92]

Effects of asthma on the parturient and fetus

A large meta-analysis of 40 publications between 1975 and March 2009 involving 1,637,180 subjects confirmed the link between maternal asthma and increased risk of adverse perinatal outcomes. Maternal asthma was associated with an increased risk of low birthweight (relative risk (RR) 1.46; 95% confidence interval (CI) 1.22–1.75), small for gestational age (SGA) (RR 1.22; 95% CI 1.14–1.31), preterm delivery (RR 1.41; 95% CI 1.22–1.61), and pre-eclampsia (RR 1.54; 95% CI 1.32–1.81). Encouragingly, the relative risk of preterm delivery and preterm labour were reduced to non-significant levels by active asthma management.[93] The increased perinatal risks in pregnant asthmatic women have been postulated to be due to (a) hypoxia and other physiological sequelae of poorly controlled asthma, (b) medications used to treat asthma, and (c) pathogenic or demographic factors (e.g. race, ethnicity, smoking, and obesity) associated with asthma but not actually caused by the disease or its treatment, such as abnormal placental function.[94] Other publications confirm that mothers with asthma during pregnancy are also more likely to have CDs, diabetes mellitus,[95] fertility treatments,[58] membrane-related disorders and antepartum hemorrhage,[95,96] pulmonary embolism and maternal ICU admissions,[95] and SGA, low birth weight, or preterm birth infants than non-asthmatic women.[97] A large Canadian cohort of 41,637 pregnancies found an increased risk of congenital malformations (especially the nervous system (excluding spina bifida), respiratory, and digestive systems) in patients with maternal asthma compared to non-asthmatics, postulated to be due to fetal oxygen impairment from the disease itself, although the authors stated that further research would be needed to disentangle the relative effect of asthma and medications used to treat this disease.[98] Lower maternal FEV_1 has also been shown to be associated with increased gestational hypertension and prematurity in asthmatic pregnancies.[99] Racial disparity also exists. Asthma during pregnancy was found to be a risk factor for low birth weight outcomes in black non-Hispanics but not white non-Hispanic women. Higher BMI and increased alcohol, tobacco, and illicit drug use were found in the black non-Hispanics. [100] Pregnant asthmatics with disease of mild-to-moderate severity can have excellent maternal and fetal outcomes. Conversely, mothers with severe or suboptimally controlled asthma during pregnancy have an increased maternal and fetal risk[101,102] including increased perinatal mortality.[103]

New evidence suggests that circulating antioxidant profiles of pregnant women with asthma may impact fetal growth. Antioxidants are important during pregnancy due to their protective role against a state of high oxidative stress as gestation progresses. McLernon et al.[104] characterized the circulating profile of tocopherols and carotenoids in pregnant women with asthma to determine whether asthma severity and dietary intake were associated with an altered antioxidant profile, to account for the increased incidence of intrauterine growth restriction in pregnant asthmatics. They found that pregnant women with moderate/severe asthma had increased plasma concentrations of total carotenoids, lutein, and alpha-tocopherol late in gestation compared to those women with mild asthma and healthy pregnant controls. Moderate/severe asthmatics had higher erythrocyte alpha-tocopherol quinone levels early in gestation relative to the controls but this marker of oxidative stress decreased as gestation progressed. Tocopherols and carotenoids were positively associated with birth weight centile. These findings suggest that the maternal system adjusts antioxidant pathways in response to the presence of a high oxidative load induced by asthma during pregnancy in an attempt to ensure continued fetal growth in an adverse environment.[104]

Medical management

The genetic predisposition to asthma and bronchial hyperactivity persists throughout life, and the adage that children outgrow their asthma is refuted.[105] The ultimate goal of asthma therapy during pregnancy is to maintain adequate fetal oxygenation by prevention of maternal hypoxic episodes. Other goals include minimization or eradication of asthmatic exacerbations, daytime or nocturnal maternal symptoms, limitations of activities, maintenance of normal or near normal pulmonary function, minimal use of short-acting bronchodilators, and minimal or no adverse effects from medications.

A team approach is advised for the management of the asthmatic parturient, involving the obstetrician, anaesthetist, and respiratory physician. Consultation with an asthma specialist is indicated for evaluation of the role of allergy and irritants, complete pulmonary function studies, or evaluation of the medication plan if there are difficulties in achieving the goals of therapy, especially if the asthma is severe.

The effective management of asthma during pregnancy relies on four integral components: objective measures for assessment and monitoring, patient education, avoidance or control of asthma triggers, and stepwise titration of asthma pharmacotherapy. Asthma medications should be continued during pregnancy and while breastfeeding.[106]

Objective measures for assessment and monitoring

FEV_1 after a maximal inspiration is the single best measure of pulmonary function. A mean FEV_1 less than 80% predicted has been found to be significantly associated with increased preterm delivery between 32 and 37 weeks, and birth weight less than 2500 g.[99] However, measurement of FEV_1 requires a spirometer. The PEFR correlates well with the FEV_1, and can be reliably measured with inexpensive, disposable, portable peak flow meters by the parturient herself. This self-monitoring of PEFR can provide valuable insight to the course of asthma throughout the day, assess circadian variation in pulmonary function, and detect early signs of deterioration so that timely therapy can be instituted. Parturients with persistent asthma should be evaluated at least monthly and those with moderate-to-severe asthma should have daily home PEFR monitoring.[57] The typical PEFR in pregnancy should be 380–550 L/min. The pregnant woman should establish her 'personal best' PEFR, then calculate her individualized PEFR zones: green zone greater than 80% of personal best, yellow zone 50–80% of personal best, and red zone less than 50% of personal best PEFR as suggested by the American Lung Association.[106]

Management of asthma in pregnancy can also be guided by measurement of fraction of exhaled nitric oxide (FENO).[107] A recent double-blind, randomized controlled trial involving 220 parturients who had their treatment adjusted at monthly visits by an algorithm using clinical symptoms (control group) or FENO concentrations (active intervention group) to uptitrate (FENO > 29 ppb) or downtitrate (FENO <16 ppb) their inhaled corticosteroid dose, found that asthma exacerbations during pregnancy and neonatal hospitalizations could be significantly reduced with a validated FENO-based treatment algorithm.[107]

Patient education and smoking cessation

Proper asthma management should ideally be started in the preconception period. Patients should be made aware that controlling asthma during pregnancy is especially important for the well-being of their fetus. Vital patient education should include a basic understanding of the medical management of asthma, adherence to controller medication, and early treatment of exacerbations. She should be instructed on the proper PEFR technique (performed standing, after maximal inspiration, and note the reading on the peak flow meter), monitoring of PEFRs, the correct use of inhalers, and strongly encouraged to quit smoking. Smoking is a well-recognized contributor to poor perinatal outcomes, and remains the most modifiable risk factor of asthma, so pregnant woman should avoid active and passive smoking. In pregnant women with asthma, current and former smokers had higher rates of severe exacerbation,[108] and greater number of symptomatic days and nights of sleep disturbance were found among active smokers than in non-smokers with asthma.[109] A recent meta-analysis found a 20% increase in wheeze and asthma in children exposed to passive smoking, therefore preventing parental smoking is crucial to the prevention of asthma.[110]

Avoidance or control of asthma triggers

75-80% of patients with asthma have positive skin tests to common allergens like animal dander, house dust mites, cockroach antigens, pollens, and moulds. Avoiding or controlling triggers can reduce asthma symptoms, airway hyper-responsiveness, and need for medication.[57] Other non-immunological triggers include tobacco smoke, air pollutants, food additives such as sulphites, and certain drugs including aspirin and beta blockers. Exercise-induced asthma can be mitigated by inhalation of salbutamol 10–30 minutes before starting.

Pharmacological therapy

Medications used for asthma control in the non-pregnant population are generally the same in pregnancy with a few exceptions. They are divided into two groups: the long-term controllers that prevent asthma manifestations (inhaled corticosteroids (ICS), long-acting beta-2-agonists (LABAs), leukotriene-receptor antagonists (LRTAs), cromoglicate, and theophylline) and rescue therapy such as salbutamol that provides quick relief of symptoms. Current pharmacological therapy emphasizes treatment of airway inflammation to decrease airway hyper-responsiveness and prevent asthma symptoms. The 'step-care' therapeutic approach uses the least amount of drug intervention necessary to control a patient's severity of asthma, and increases the number and frequency of medications with increasing asthma severity[106] (Table 42.1).

Bronchodilators: inhaled short-acting beta-2 agonists (SABAs) salbutamol, levalbuterol, and pirbuterol are currently recommended for all levels of asthma during pregnancy as quick relievers. Rapid onset of action by smooth muscle relaxation occurs within 5 minutes, peaking within 1 hour and lasts 4–6 hours. Side effects of tremor, tachycardia, and palpitations occur but are not common at standard doses. SABAs do not block the development of airway hyper-responsiveness. Increased frequency of SABA use would indicate the need for additional anti-inflammatory therapy. In 2004, the NAEPP released an updated expert panel report on the management of asthma in pregnant women.[57] Safety concerns of asthma medications in pregnancy were addressed, and a significant amount of reassuring data on the safety of SABAs were found, particularly salbutamol. A prospective cohort study found no significant differences in perinatal mortality, congenital malformations, preterm delivery, and low birth weight in asthmatic women who used SABAs compared with women who did not use treatment for asthma during pregnancy.[111,112] In non-pregnant patients, a possible association between LABAs and increased risk of severe and fatal asthmatic exacerbations was observed. Limited data exist on the use of LABAs like salmeterol and formoterol during pregnancy. An epidemiological study reported no adverse outcomes among 65 women who used salmeterol while pregnant, out of a cohort exceeding 15,000 patients in the United Kingdom.[113] Recent information suggest there is no such increased risk when LABAs are used in conjunction with inhaled corticosteroids[114], as in pregnancy. Current guidelines recommend salmeterol as the preferred LABA used in pregnancy, as it has been available for longer in the United States.[57] A recent study investigated the association between exposure to SABAs and LABAs in the first trimester of pregnancy and the risk of congenital malformations in 13,117 asthmatics[115]. It confirmed evidence of SABA safety during pregnancy, but found significant increased risks of major congenital malformations observed with LABA use. The authors cautioned that more research was required to assess whether the increased risk of malformations among LABA users was due to the medication, bias by asthma severity, or chance alone.[115]

Table 42.1 Step therapy medical management of asthma during pregnancy

Step asthma severity and medications
Mild intermittent
1. No daily medications, salbutamol as needed
Mild persistent
2. Low-dose inhaled corticosteroid (alternative: Cromoglicate, LTRA, or theophylline
Moderate persistent
3. Medium-dose inhaled corticosteroid (alternative: low-dose inhaled corticosteroid and LABA, LTRA, or theophylline)
4. Medium-dose inhaled corticosteroid and LABA (alternative: medium-dose inhaled corticosteroid plus LTRA, or theophylline
Severe persistent
5. High-dose inhaled corticosteroid and LABA
6. High-dose inhaled corticosteroid and LABA and oral prednisone

LABA indicates long-acting β agonist; LTRA, leukotriene-receptor antagonist.

Reproduced from Dombrowski MP, Schatz M, Asthma in pregnancy, *Clinical Obstetrics and Gynecology*, Volume 53, Issue 2, pp.301-10, Copyright © 2010 Wolters Kluwer Health, Inc.

Theophylline is an alternative treatment for mild persistent asthma and an alternative add-on treatment for the step 3 or 4 management of moderate persistent asthma during pregnancy (see Table 42.1). Theophylline is only indicated for chronic therapy and is not effective for the treatment of acute maternal exacerbations. Theophylline's long duration of action (10–12 hours with sustained-release preparations) makes it especially useful for nocturnal asthma. Inhaled corticosteroids are preferred over theophylline because they lead to a greater improvement in FEV_1, have fewer side effects, and do not require serum monitoring. Serum theophylline concentrations should be maintained at 5–12 mcg/mL during pregnancy.[57] Theophylline can have significant interactions with other drugs, which can cause decreased clearance with resultant toxicity, for example, 70% increase in theophylline serum levels with cimetidine and 35% with erythromycin.

LRTAs (e.g. zafirlukast (Accolate®), montelukast (Singulair®), and modifier zileuton that inhibits the leukotriene pathway) are all pregnancy category B drugs. Their use originated from the observation that leukotrienes are released into the airways by immune cells, contributing to the inflammatory process. They are not useful for acute treatment of bronchospasm. Leukotriene modifiers are less effective as single agents than inhaled corticosteroids and less effective than LABA as add-on therapy.[57] Zileuton use has been associated with hepatic injury, and LRTA use with Churg–Strauss vasculitis, especially when steroid dosage is decreased. Human data are limited for their use in pregnancy. Investigators found that LRTA use in 96 pregnancies was not associated with a specific pattern of major structural anomalies but cautioned interpretation of the results due to the limited sample size.[116] A recent systematic review found that congenital malformations had been reported with LRTA exposure during pregnancy, but those women also had exposure to other medications, including oral corticosteroids.[117]

Corticosteroids: ICS (e.g. beclometasone, budesonide, fluticasone, and triamcinolone) are the preferred controller therapy for all levels of persistent asthma during pregnancy, of which budesonide is the safest. However, if a woman is well-controlled by a different ICS before pregnancy (e.g. beclometasone dipropionate and fluticasone), it would be reasonable to continue that medication during pregnancy. No clinically important adrenal suppression has been found with their administration in low to moderate doses. LABAs are the preferred add-on therapy to medium to high-dose ICS.[64] Their beneficial effect on airway mechanics can take 4–6 hours in acute bronchospasm. Maternal glucose levels should be monitored during pregnancy. Adrenal suppression, infection, delayed healing, hyperglycaemia, and fluid retention are common complications of prolonged therapy.

Cromoglicate sodium and *nedocromil sodium* are mast cell stabilizers but of limited benefit, requiring several weeks for action, and have been replaced by ICS and leukotriene modifiers. Limited studies suggest cromolglicate's safety during pregnancy,[116] and greater clinical experience with its use for longer, hence its preferred use over nedocromil.

Anti-immunoglobulin E therapy, specifically *omalizumab*, is reserved for patients with moderate-to-severe persistent asthma who do not respond to standard treatment. It is costly and has no role in the acute management of bronchospasm.

Overall safety of asthmatic medications

Women with asthma tend to significantly decrease their asthma medication use from 5 to13 weeks of pregnancy due to concerns about safety of medications for the fetus.[118] Prospective population or birth cohort studies have shown that acute asthma medications, SABAs, and controller medications (ICS, cromones, theophylline, leukotriene inhibitors) have no or minimal effects on fetal growth, and perinatal complications are reduced when maternal asthma is adequately controlled.[119] The NAEPP has found that the potential risks associated with asthma medications are lower than the risks associated with uncontrolled asthma, and it is imperative that women continue to use their asthma medications in pregnancy.[57]

A direct causal relationship is difficult to establish. When National Birth Defects Prevention Study data for 2853 infants with one or more selected birth defects (diaphragmatic hernia, oesophageal atresia, small intestinal atresia, anorectal atresia, neural tube defects, omphalocele, or limb deficiencies) were analysed, no statistically significant associations were observed for maternal periconceptional asthma medication use and most defects studied. However, positive associations were observed for anorectal atresia, oesophageal atresia, and omphalocele. These may be chance findings or may be a result of maternal asthma severity and related hypoxia rather than medication use.[120] Munsie et al. observed a statistically significant association between maternal bronchodilator use and the risk of orofacial clefts. They too concluded uncertainty on whether the increased odds ratios they found were due to the bronchodilators, the severity of asthma, or both, or to chance alone. Further studies to disentangle the role of asthma or asthma medications would help clarify these findings.[121] In a large retrospective insurance claims cohort study comprising approximately 12 million covered lives and more than 277,000 pregnancies linked to a live-birth outcome, Nelsen et al. did not find any cases similar to the six postmarketing surveillance events of limb-reduction defects among the 1535 infants born to mothers taking montelukast. Other anomalies, confirmed by medical chart review with blinded adjudication, were reported at rates that were similar in the montelukast, ICS, and general population cohorts. The conclusion from this study, together with findings from other pregnancy databases, was that there was no epidemiological evidence to support a causal relationship between montelukast and limb-reduction or other birth defects.[122]

Obstetric management

Women with poorly controlled asthma are at increased risk of pregnancy complications, and would benefit from increased fetal surveillance: monthly ultrasounds for growth, and antepartum testing beginning at 32 weeks. Pregnant asthmatics should continue their medication regimen as prescribed throughout labour and delivery. If systemic corticosteroids have been used in the previous 4 weeks, the American College of Obstetricians and Gynaecologists (ACOG) guidelines recommend administering stress-dose corticosteroids (hydrocortisone 100 mg every 8–12 hours during labour and for 24 hours postpartum)[56] although there is little information about the benefit of corticosteroid replacement during labour. A recent study found maternal asthma was associated with less fetal movements per hour, but computerized cardiotocography did not demonstrate an association between the abnormal parameters of fetal heart rate and maternal asthma. The authors suggested further studies on the counting of fetal movements in pregnant women with asthma.[123]

The obstetric management of an asthmatic parturient may further differ from that of non-asthmatics at induction of labour, management of postpartum haemorrhage and treatment of hypertension. For labour induction, prostaglandin E_2 has a known risk of bronchospasm, and should be avoided. Misoprostol (a synthetic prostaglandin E_1 analogue) can be used in pregnant asthmatics for cervical ripening, and the management of spontaneous or induced abortions, but respiratory status should still be monitored for bronchospasm.[56] For management of postpartum haemorrhage, ergot alkaloids (ergometrine, ergonovine, and methylergonovine) and 15-methyl prostaglandin $F_{2\alpha}$ (carboprost, Hemabate®) should be used cautiously in asthmatics, as they have been associated with episodes of acute bronchospasm.[124,125] Oxytocin does not significantly affect airway tone and is the preferred uterotonic agent in asthmatics. Some hypertensive women are treated with beta-adrenergic receptor antagonists. In asthmatic women, these provoke bronchospasm, and should be avoided. There are no reports of bronchospasm associated with calcium channel blockers, hydralazine, and sodium nitroprusside, making them suitable alternatives. If tocolysis is needed, magnesium sulphate and terbutaline have bronchodilator effects and can be used safely; in contrast, indomethacin might induce bronchospasm in aspirin-sensitive patients.[56]

Anaesthetic management

Preoperative assessment and optimization

Ideally the severe asthmatic (a patient with prior admissions to the high dependency/intensive therapy unit (HDU/ITU) with asthma or is on oral steroids) should be seen at the high-risk anaesthetic clinic. However, not infrequently, the time frame for anaesthetic preoperative intervention is too short, with problematic cases presenting on the delivery suite. Additionally, the practitioner can be misled by the variable nature of the disease and symptoms may be completely absent before labour or delivery, with no less a potential for intraoperative bronchospasm. The anaesthetist should assess the severity of the disease, and whether an acute attack is occurring. A thorough history should elicit symptoms of wheezing, dyspnoea, and cough; the frequency and severity of acute asthma exacerbations, its course during pregnancy, past hospitalizations, history of intubation and mechanical ventilation; prior oral steroid use; and known environmental asthma triggers. Physical examination is focused on the pulmonary system. Chest auscultation may reveal wheezing ± a prolonged expiratory phase. A 'silent' chest devoid of wheezing can occur if air movement is markedly reduced. Tachypnoea, use of accessory muscles of respiration, and pulsus paradoxus of 20 mmHg or greater point to an acute asthmatic exacerbation. A simple screening test for prolonged exhalation is the forced expiratory time (FET), which can be assessed by listening over the trachea while the patient exhales forcibly and fully. An FET longer than 6 seconds correlates with a substantially lowered FEV_1/FVC ratio and should initiate further investigation. Laboratory investigations in pregnant women with stable asthma have little yield in adding to management. A chest radiograph may reveal hyperinflation and flattening of the diaphragm, and helps diagnose exacerbating conditions like pneumonia, pneumothorax, and heart failure. Arterial blood gas analysis may show hypoxaemia and respiratory alkalosis during acute attacks, with hypercarbia secondary to fatigue. Blood eosinophil counts often parallel the degree of airway inflammation. If the patient is being evaluated in a pre-anaesthesia clinic with facilities for referral to respiratory physicians, then spirometry may be useful; however, PEFR measurements are perhaps a more useful bedside test. Chest physiotherapy, antibiotics, and bronchodilator therapy during the perioperative period can often improve reversible components of asthma. Ideally, the patients should be wheeze-free and have a PEF of more than 80% predicted or at the level of their personal best value before labour and CD.

Issues affecting labour and vaginal delivery

The goal of adequate labour pain relief does not differ for pregnant asthmatics in labour. It is even more important to reduce maternal stress and hyperventilation in asthmatics describing exercise or stress-induced triggers. Maternal paralysis of respiratory muscles, maternal sedation, and neonatal depression should be minimized in seeking out the optimal labour analgesia technique. In contemporary obstetric anaesthetic practice, this is often achieved by a CSE or an epidural infusion employing dilute local anaesthetic solutions with a modest dose of opioids (delivered as a continuous infusion, patient-controlled epidural analgesia (PCEA), computer-integrated-PCEA, or programmed intermittent boluses).[126] The advantage of lumbar epidurals include continuous pain relief and reduction in the stimulus to hyperventilate in pregnant asthmatics. High thoracic motor blocks should be avoided to avoid respiratory insufficiency. The epidural catheter also allows extension of the sensory block for CD should the need arise, thereby avoiding the risk of general anaesthesia and endotracheal intubation in asthmatic parturients.

Other possible labour analgesic regimens include systemic opioids (e.g. fentanyl patient-controlled analgesia (PCA) and remifentanil PCA) but maternal respiratory depression, sedation, and neonatal depression remain real issues[127] that would disadvantage the pregnant asthmatic. Alternative neuraxial anaesthesia techniques of paracervical block and pudendal nerve block performed mostly by obstetricians, and the lumbar sympathetic block are rarely utilized these days in modern obstetric anaesthetic practice.

Issues regarding caesarean delivery

Neuraxial anaesthesia techniques are preferred for CD in stable asthmatic parturients as it obviates airway instrumentation, and minimizes risk of bronchospasm. General anaesthesia for CD traditionally mandates a rapid sequence induction and endotracheal intubation which markedly increases airway resistance due to several pathophysiological mechanisms, for example, depression of the cough reflex, impairment of mucociliary function, reduction in palatopharyngeal musculature tone, depression of diaphragmatic function, and increased airway wall fluid.

A standard dose of spinal anaesthetic is appropriate in stable asthmatics, but high thoracic blocks that might impair accessory muscles of respiration required in a brittle asthmatic are undesirable. Thoracic adrenergic nerve blockade due to spinal anaesthesia might trigger asthmatic attacks by influencing the cholinergic ganglia of the lung and/or pulmonary blood flow, as was postulated to be the cause of bronchospasm triggered by a spinal anaesthetic in two women with T2 sensory levels.[128] Severe bronchospasm has also occurred during epidural anaesthesia for CD, postulated to be related to sympathetic nervous blockade allowing unopposed parasympathetically mediated bronchoconstriction.[129] Notwithstanding, many asthmatic patients have a subjective sensation of inability to breathe even with an appropriate level of neuraxial block as their intercostals are non-functioning and they need reassurance. Showing them their pulse oximetry often allays their fears.

When general anaesthesia cannot be avoided, rapid sequence induction and endotracheal intubation is indicated. Bronchospasm can be provoked by laryngoscopy, tracheal intubation, airway suctioning, cold inspired gases, and tracheal extubation. Airway tone is increased by vagal stimulation caused by endoscopy, peritoneal, or visceral stretch. Propofol or ketamine are the preferred IV induction agents in asthmatics.[130] Propofol is superior to thiopental and etomidate in constraining increases in airway resistance.[131] Propofol formulations containing metabisulphite induce higher airway resistance than that preserved with calcium edetate in heavy smokers undergoing anaesthesia,[132] and should be taken into consideration in asthmatics as well. Ketamine is a sympathomimetic agent which induces bronchodilation and inhibits neural reflexes, and should be administered with antisialogogue and benzodiazepine (post delivery of baby) due to its propensity to increase secretions and cause dysphoria. IV lidocaine can prevent bronchospasm by attenuating sensory responses to airway instrumentation or irritation.[133,134] Warm, humidified gases should be provided at all times. Anaesthetic maintenance with a volatile agent such as isoflurane or sevoflurane confers protective bronchodilation. However, there is evidence that desflurane provokes bronchoconstriction in smokers.[135] Histamine-releasing neuromuscular blocking drugs like atracurium should be avoided.[136] Rocuronium would be preferred in this setting. An adequately long expiratory time should be given during mechanical ventilation to avoid the build-up of intrinsic or auto-PEEP. This can be facilitated by using higher inspiratory flow rates or smaller tidal volumes than usual.[137] Patients should be kept adequately hydrated as usual, but fluid overload/pulmonary congestion should be avoided as it can precipitate 'cardiac asthma'. Intraoperative bronchospasm can be managed by administering beta-2 agonists by aerosol or increasing concentration of volatile agents, the latter risks increasing blood loss due to haemorrhage from increased uterine relaxation. IV adrenaline or ketamine may be required to break the spasm, and hydrocortisone should be administered. Intraoperative analgesia with fentanyl is associated with less histamine release than morphine[138,139] and should be considered in brittle asthmatics, who would also benefit from PCA fentanyl over PCA morphine for postoperative analgesia, and a transversus abdominus plane block.[39] Upon tracheal extubation, bronchodilator therapy, incentive spirometry, deep breathing exercises, and early mobilization are beneficial. HDU care postoperatively could be considered. Severe asthmatics might benefit from a spell in ITU postoperatively if a general anaesthetic has been necessary.

Mask induction of general anaesthesia with sevoflurane in a parturient in status asthmaticus has been described.[140] The combination of non-invasive mechanical ventilation with neuraxial anaesthesia may be of value in selected parturients with acute or chronic respiratory insufficiency requiring surgery.[141] In cases of life-threatening status asthmaticus refractory to standard medical and ventilatory therapies in the third trimester, CD should be considered as a final effort to increase tidal volumes and improve maternal gas exchange. In one such case, significant maternal respiratory acidosis and difficulty with ventilation necessitated CD at 33 weeks of gestation in the medical ICU.[142] Cardiopulmonary resuscitative efforts are difficult in near-term parturients, and a promptly performed CD might have saved an infant and mother who suffered recurrent cardiopulmonary arrest due to status asthmaticus.[143]

Pneumonias

Epidemiology and prevalence

The reported incidence of antepartum pneumonia was 6/1000 deliveries (pre-1970s) that then declined in the 1970s and 1980s to 0.4/1000, with studies published in 1990–2003 reporting an increase to 2.72/1000 deliveries.[144] The latter reflects women with chronic illnesses now being able to conceive, prevalence of human immunodeficiency virus (HIV) infection, and rising illicit drug use in pregnant women. Rates tend to be higher in large urban hospitals than in community settings due to different risk populations, and also because the available data generally come from those hospitalized.

The odds of being admitted with pneumonia in the postpartum period are more than twice as high for patients who underwent CDs compared with vaginal deliveries,[145] purportedly due to more abdominal discomfort and splinting after CD. Pre-existing comorbidities in these women (asthma, obesity, diabetes, advanced maternal age) which may have necessitated the CD in the first place, may predispose them to infections.

Pathophysiology

These alterations in pregnancy lead to an increased incidence and risk of complications from pneumonia:

- *Maternal physiological changes* predispose pregnant women to a more severe pneumonia course. The diaphragm is elevated up to 4 cm, a decrease in functional residual capacity, increase in oxygen consumption and increase in lung water makes a parturient less tolerant to even brief hypoxic episodes.[146] These alterations also decrease the ability of the pregnant woman to clear respiratory secretions and potentially aggravate airway obstruction associated with pulmonary infections.
- *Maternal immunological changes* in the second and third trimester are thought to occur generally to protect the fetus from rejection by the mother. Substances produced by the trophoblast block maternal recognition of major fetal histocompatibility antigens, resulting in a reduced lymphokine response to alloantigens. Other alterations in maternal cellular immunity include a reduced lymphocyte proliferative response, diminished cell-mediated cytotoxicity, decreased natural killer cell activity and reduced number of circulating helper T cells.[147,148] Hormonal changes during pregnancy (increased progesterone, human gonadotropin, alphafetoprotein, and cortisol) may also inhibit cell-mediated immune function.[147] These changes can predispose to infection with certain virus, fungi, and tuberculosis. Catanzaro showed the *in vitro* growth of *Coccidioides immitis* was enhanced by increased 17-oestradiols leading to increased pulmonary mycosis in pregnant women.[149]
- *Comorbidities:* maternal risk factors associated with increased incidence of pneumonia development during pregnancy include a history of underlying pulmonary disease (e.g. asthma, CF, and recent viral respiratory infection), smoking, anaemia (haemoglobin level < 10g/dL),[150] illicit drug use, HIV infection, other immunosuppressive illness, and therapy.
- *Labour and delivery* increases risk of aspiration pneumonia (although this is modifiable with antacids and H_2 antagonists).

Aetiology

The bacterial, viral, and fungal pathogens causing pneumonia in pregnancy are similar to those in non-pregnant adults. The commonest is *Streptococcus pneumoniae*, which is identified in 15–20% of community-acquired pneumonia cases in pregnancy, followed by *Hemophilus influenzae*.[151] Atypical pathogens include *Legionella* species, *Mycoplasma pneumoniae*, and *Chlamydia pneumoniae*; whereas influenza A and varicella are common viral agents in pregnancy. *Pseudomonas aeruginosa* is common in parturients with bronchiectasis and CF. In a patient suffering from acquired immunodeficiency syndrome (AIDS), *Pneumocystis jirovecii* is the most frequent pathogen.

Clinical manifestations

A detailed history and high index of suspicion is needed in pregnant women presenting with cough and shortness of breath, as initial clinical symptoms of mild pneumonia may be subtle and mimic many other pathologies of pregnancy. Cough, fever, chills, rigors, pleuritic chest pain, sputum production, and dyspnoea usually present later in the clinical course. Non-respiratory symptoms include nausea, headache, myalgias, and fever. Chest auscultation may reveal decreased or bronchial breath sounds or occasional wheezing. Dullness to percussion may be elicited if consolidation is present. The new American Thoracic Society/Infectious Diseases Society of America (ATS/IDSA) guidelines have criteria for characterizing severe community-acquired pneumonia, but these are not specific to pregnant women: presence of at least one major criterion (e.g. mechanical ventilation requirement or septic shock requiring vasopressors) or the presence of three minor criteria (respiratory rate of at least 30 breaths per minute, PaO_2/FiO_2 ratio ≤250 mmHg, multilobar infiltrates, confusion or disorientation, blood urea nitrogen ≥ 20 mg/dL, white blood cell count < 400/mm^3, platelet count < 100,000/mm^3, hypotension requiring aggressive fluid resuscitation, and hypothermia). The guideline also suggested that criteria such as hypoglycaemia, hyponatraemia, asplenia (as in sickle cell disease), and unexplained acidosis be considered in deciding the need for ICU admission.[152]

Diagnosis

Pregnancy should not prevent the use of standard radiographic techniques[153] and *chest radiographs* should be obtained to confirm the diagnosis. The most common site of pneumonia was the left lower lobe (53.4%), followed by the right lower lobe (26.3%) and right middle lobe (8.3%); 9.8% were complicated with pleural effusion.[154] The differential diagnosis of pneumonia in pregnancy includes pulmonary embolism, infectious aetiologies with systemic inflammatory findings, pulmonary oedema consequent to tocolytic therapy, severe pre-eclampsia, and cardiomyopathy. With the increasing availability of portable ultrasound machines in perioperative anaesthesia settings to aid central venous catheter insertions, peripheral nerve blockade, and ultrasound-guided neuraxial blocks, the use of ultrasonography has become increasingly prevalent. *Lung ultrasonography* (LUS) has been described in the bedside detection of pneumonia.[155] It enables diagnosis and treatment of interstitial syndrome, lung consolidation, atelectasis, pleural effusion, and differentiation of the causes of acute breathlessness.[155] The use of LUS is ideal in parturients due to the lack of ionizing radiation and its non-invasiveness, allowing repeated scans to not only diagnose but guide and monitor therapy.[156] All admitted patients should have an assessment of gas exchange (arterial blood gas or oximetry), routine blood chemistry, and blood counts. Sputum culture, Gram stain, and blood cultures are recommended in severe pneumonia, as are *Legionella* and pneumococcal urinary antigen.

Management

Patients should be admitted for evaluation, empirical initiation of antimicrobial therapy, fetal evaluation, and maintenance of normal maternal respiratory function. For patients with mild symptoms, the ATS recommends an advanced generation macrolide. For more severe disease, a macrolide and beta-lactam antibiotic should be initiated.[152] Doxycycline, recommended as a second-line antibiotic therapy, should be avoided in pregnancy as administration of tetracycline in the second and third trimesters of pregnancy has been associated with staining and banding of teeth and depression of bone growth, especially the fetal fibula, and fulminant maternal hepatitis. Patients at-risk of hospital-acquired pneumonia or aspiration pneumonia should receive an aminoglycoside for the coverage of *Pseudomonas* and enteric Gram-negative organisms.[152,157] IV aciclovir is indicated for varicella pneumonia. Trimethoprim/sulfamethoxazole is effective in prevention and treatment of pneumocystis pneumonia in immunocompromised individuals. Supplemental oxygen should be administered in patients with an increased alveolar–arterial gradient as reduction in maternal functional residual capacity predisposes them to overt respiratory distress, and oxygen delivery to the fetus will decrease when maternal oxygen saturation is less than 90%. The criteria for intubation in pregnancy are the same as in the non-pregnant state: inadequate oxygenation, inadequate ventilation, systemic sepsis, need for invasive haemodynamic monitoring, or persistent metabolic acidosis. The pneumococcal vaccine is recommended for pregnant women with underlying illnesses (e.g. immunocompromised states, asplenia, sickle cell disease, diabetes, or chronic cardiopulmonary diseases) to reduce the incidence of community-acquired pneumonia in these high-risk populations.

Maternal and perinatal outcomes

In two nationwide population-based datasets,[158] 1462 women with pneumonia during pregnancy were found to have a significantly higher risk of low birth weight, preterm birth, SGA, low Apgar score infants, CD, and pre-eclampsia/eclampsia compared to 7310 unaffected women. Pneumonia was also significantly associated with placental abruption and intrauterine growth restriction but no significant differences were noted between the groups regarding labour induction, second stage non-progressive labour, and post-partum haemorrhage.[154]

H1N1 influenza

The H1N1 virus is the subtype of influenza A virus that was the most common cause of 'swine flu' in 2009. It is an orthomyxovirus that contains the glycoproteins haemagglutinin and neuraminidase, and thus is described as H1N1, H1N2, etc. depending on the type of H or N antigens it expresses. Haemagglutinin causes red blood cells to clump together and binds the virus to the infected cell. Neuraminidase is a glycoside hydrolase enzyme which helps to move the virus particles through the infected cell and assist in budding from the host cells.

Epidemiology and prevalence

Influenza A H1N1 drew worldwide attention when identification of this new viral strain in humans was found to be a 'quadruple reassortant' virus containing gene segments from human, avian, and two swine lineages.[159] It spread rapidly after the first outbreak in Mexico and the United States, and was declared a global pandemic by the WHO in June 2009. The rate of admission for pandemic H1N1 influenza virus infection in pregnant women during the first month of the outbreak was higher than it was in the general population (0.32/100,000 pregnant women vs 0.076/100,000 population at risk).[73] When population-based data from the Emerging Infections Program in ten US states were examined, pregnant women represented 23.5% and 31.0% of all reproductive-aged women (15–44 years) hospitalized for seasonal (2005/2006 through 2008/2009) and 2009 H1N1 pandemic influenza A (pH1N1) virus infection respectively.[160] Worldwide, pregnancy was found to be a major risk factor for increased mortality and morbidity. The US Centers for Disease Control and Prevention (CDC) reported a 13% mortality in pregnant women in the first 2 months of the outbreak.[73] In a Brazilian series, the rate of maternal and perinatal mortality was 9.7%.[161]

Pathophysiology

Little is known about the biological reasons for pregnant women being at high risk for influenza virus infection, but it is postulated to be due to the altered innate immunity and physiological changes of pregnancy. It was suggested that pregnant women had a greater likelihood of developing a Th2 response to H1N1 influenza which may be responsible for the systemic inflammatory response syndrome that causes pulmonary oedema and death.[162] When peripheral blood mononuclear cells (PBMCs) were isolated from 26 healthy non-pregnant women and 28 healthy pregnant women and cultured with the 2009 pandemic influenza A (pH1N1) virus, PBMCs from pregnant women produced significantly less interferon alpha and interferon lambda.[69] Messenger RNA expression of protein kinase R (PKR) and toll-like receptors 3, 7, and 9 measured from cell lysates were also significantly reduced in PBMCs from pregnant women. This response improved with vaccination.[69] These novel findings help in understanding the increased susceptibility and disease severity to influenza virus infection during pregnancy and the importance of influenza vaccination.

Clinical manifestations

Presenting features of the largest published cohort (N = 211) of H1N1-infected pregnant women presenting to a single tertiary referral centre over 4 months, were cough (90.5%), fever (62.6%), rhinorrhoea (62.1%), sore throat (58.8%), breathlessness (13.3%), headache (18.0%), and myalgia (32.2%).[163] Diarrhoea and vomiting were also a feature of the 2009 outbreak. Other parturients may have varying degrees of dyspnoea and tachypnoea, pneumonia, and increasing hypoxia requiring intubation and mechanical ventilation in the ICU. Severe H1N1 pneumonia, acute respiratory distress syndrome, multiorgan failure, and maternal deaths have all been reported.[73,164]

Maternal age and the time interval between onset of symptoms and hospital admission were not found to be risk factors for hospitalized pregnant women developing respiratory and multiple organ failure. The significant risk factor associated with critical illness was gestational age, with an odds ratio of 1.034 (95% CI 0.968–1.106) during the first trimester, 9.667 (95% CI 0.750–124.59) during the second trimester, and 87 (95% CI 6.750–1121.39) during the third trimester.[165] H1N1-infected pregnant women who went on to require mechanical ventilation tended to have more advanced gestational age, lower early oxygenation index, wider early-stage pneumonic lesions, and adverse pregnancy outcomes compared to those patients that did not require mechanical ventilation.[166]

Diagnosis

Detection of influenza-specific RNA by real-time reverse-transcriptase *polymerase chain reaction* (rRT-PCR) is the recommended test for confirmation of novel influenza A H1N1 cases.[167] The H1N1 virus will test positive for influenza A and negative for H1 and H3. Samples can be obtained with a nasopharyngeal swab, nasal aspirate, or a combined nasopharyngeal and oropharyngeal swab. Duration of viral shedding is unknown but infected persons are assumed to be shedding virus and potentially infectious from the day prior to onset of symptoms up to resolution of fever. *Viral culture* does not yield timely results to guide clinical management, but serological tests on paired acute (within 1 week of illness onset) and convalescent (collected 2–3 weeks later) sera can help establish a retrospective diagnosis for epidemiological and research studies. Commercially available *rapid influenza diagnostic test kits* (RIDTs) can provide results within 30 minutes or less, but were initially varied in their sensitivities from 10% to 70% in detecting H1N1 compared to RT-PCR. Therefore a negative RIDT did not rule out H1N1 infection.[168,169] Newer assays have higher sensitivity and specificity for A(H1N1) virus of 76–95%.[170,171]

Management

Oseltamivir (trade name Tamiflu®) and *zanamivir* (Relenza®) are two antivirals (neuraminidase inhibitors) currently recommended for H1N1 infection.[73] Early treatment (<2 days from diagnosis)[163,172,173] with oseltamivir prevents serious complications associated with H1N1 infection in pregnant women and does not affect perinatal outcome. The existing information on the safety of oseltamivir and zanamivir, the most used antivirals is limited but reassuring.[174] There is a significant association between late treatment with oseltamivir and increased hospitalization[173] and increased systemic complications in pregnancy.[161]

Anaesthetic technique for CD will depend on disease severity. Spinal or epidural anaesthesia for CD in mild H1N1 cases are acceptable. Most parturients in respiratory distress or failure would already be intubated and CD performed under general anaesthesia with postoperative ITU care.[175]

Pregnant women who come in close contact with a suspected or confirmed H1N1 infected person also need preventive antiviral therapy. Use of personal protective equipment (e.g. surgical masks) and *isolation precautions* to mitigate spread differ from country to country depending on whether the disease is in the containment or mitigation phase[176] and existing national resources.[177] Containment strategies include the triage of febrile patients at frontline healthcare settings, admission and isolation of confirmed cases, mandatory Quarantine Orders (QO) for close contacts, and temperature screening at border entry points. After sustained community transmission becomes established, containment shifts to mitigation. Hospitals only need to admit H1N1-2009 cases based on clinical indications, not for isolation. Mild cases are managed in the community. Contact tracing and QOs are tapered off, and border temperature screening ended.

Maternal and perinatal outcomes

Pregnant women with mild clinical illness secondary to H1N1 virus are not at a greater risk of adverse pregnancy outcomes. However, severely infected women were more likely to deliver SGA babies and CD may be required.[178] There is a causal relationship between early exposure and fetal demise, as the H1N1 virus can be identified in maternal and fetal tissue confirming transplacental passage.[179] Not all patients require hospitalization, or result in preterm delivery when vigilance in assessment, early presentation, diagnosis and prompt treatment is initiated.[163,172,180] Indeed, complete recovery from H1N1 with no mortality was seen in all 235 infected parturients in one series.[172]

Myocarditis has also been reported, where two pregnant Caucasian women (aged 29 and 30 years) presented with respiratory manifestations of H1N1 influenza virus infection in their third trimester and developed evidence of myocarditis (one woman developed acute respiratory distress syndrome, nearly requiring extracorporeal membrane oxygenation, and subsequently developed persistent cardiomyopathy; the other recovered without any long-term consequence).[181] While it was not possible to ascertain retrospectively if myocarditis was caused by either infection with H1N1 virus or as a result of pregnancy (in the absence of endomyocardial biopsies), the significant association with myocardial involvement in both women demonstrates the increased risk of exposure to H1N1 influenza virus in pregnant women.

Efficacy of H1N1 vaccination

With the emergence of the pH1N1 influenza, the US CDC recommended that pregnant women be one of five initial target groups to receive the 2009 monovalent H1N1 vaccine, regardless of prior infection with this influenza strain. Performance of haemagglutination inhibition assays (HAIs) for pH1N1 and maternal and umbilical venous cord blood sampling at delivery revealed that pH1N1 vaccination conferred a similar HAI antibody response as compared to pH1N1 infection during pregnancy, both in quantity and quality. Illness or vaccination during pregnancy therefore confers passive immunity to the newborn.[182]

Safety of H1N1 vaccination

Vaccination is imperative for parturients as unvaccinated women fare worse. A perinatal database of 55,570 mothers in Ontario, Canada reported that 23,340 (42.0%) mothers who had received H1N1 vaccination during the 2009–2010 H1N1 pandemic had improved fetal and neonatal outcomes (fewer SGA infants, preterm delivery, and fetal death) compared to unvaccinated women.[183] In the United States, for the 2009–2012 combined influenza seasons, a prospective cohort of 841 pregnant women who received the H1N1 monovalent or trivalent influenza (pH1N1) vaccine were not found to have increased relative risks for major birth defects, spontaneous abortion, or SGA infants when compared to 191 unexposed women.[184] These conclusions were also echoed by a Swiss medical birth registry[185] and a large French observational cohort study of 12,120 people in their French prescription database that compared 1645 women who were administered A/H1N1 vaccine during pregnancy to 3290 non-vaccinated women and found no increased risk of adverse pregnancy outcomes (all-cause pregnancy loss, preterm delivery, SGA, and neonatal pathology) in vaccinated pregnant women. The rate of SGA was also lower in the vaccinated group than in the non-vaccinated group.[186] Data from four regional centres in the United States collected as part of the Slone Epidemiology Center's Birth Defects Study found no meaningful evidence of increased risk for specific congenital malformations following pH1N1 influenza vaccinations in the 2009–2010 and 2010–2011 seasons.[187] Similarly, in a large Danish cohort, exposure to the adjuvanted influenza A(H1N1) pdm09 vaccine during pregnancy was not associated with a significantly increased risk of major birth defects, preterm birth, or fetal growth restriction.[188,189]

Rare side effects of vaccination

A rare occurrence of Guillain-Barre syndrome was reported after immunization to influenza during the last trimester of pregnancy.[190]

Conclusion

Respiratory illness in pregnant women is not uncommon. A multidisciplinary approach to care of these women is essential and anaesthetists play a vital role in diagnosis and management of these patients. Asthma is very common and usually does not cause a problem during pregnancy or delivery. CF on the other hand can pose a challenge and patients with CF may deteriorate such that severe maternal morbidity and mortality can ensue. The pneumonias and H1N1 disease can affect previously healthy women but appropriate therapy instituted in a timely fashion will usually result in effective treatment. Vaccination against H1N1 is recommended for pregnant women.

References

1. Salvatore D, Buzzetti R, Baldo E, *et al.* An overview of international literature from cystic fibrosis registries. Part 3. Disease incidence, genotype/phenotype correlation, microbiology, pregnancy, clinical complications, lung transplantation, and miscellanea. *J Cyst Fibros* 2011; 10:71–85.
2. Boyle MP. Adult cystic fibrosis. *JAMA* 2007; 298:1787–93.
3. Scotet V, Dugueperoux I, Saliou P, *et al.* Evidence for decline in the incidence of cystic fibrosis: a 35-year observational study in Brittany, France. *Orphanet J Rare* Dis 2012; 7:14.
4. Massie RJ, Curnow L, Glazner J, *et al.* Lessons learned from 20 years of newborn screening for cystic fibrosis. *Med J Aust* 2012; 196:67–70.
5. Riordan JR, Rommens JM, Kerem B, *et al.* Identification of the cystic fibrosis gene: cloning and characterization of complementary DNA. *Science* 1989; 245:1066–73.
6. Rommens JM, Iannuzzi MC, Kerem B, *et al.* Identification of the cystic fibrosis gene: chromosome walking and jumping. *Science* 1989; 245:1059–65.
7. Chandrasekharan S, Heaney C, James T, *et al.* Impact of gene patents and licensing practices on access to genetic testing for cystic fibrosis. *Genet Med* 2010; 12:S194–211.
8. Huffmyer JL, Littlewood KE, Nemergut EC. Perioperative management of the adult with cystic fibrosis. *Anesth Analg* 2009; 109:1949–61.
9. Gibson RL, Burns JL, Ramsey BW. Pathophysiology and management of pulmonary infections in cystic fibrosis. *Am J Respir Crit Care Med* 2003; 168:918–51.
10. Flume PA, Strange C, Ye X, *et al.* Pneumothorax in cystic fibrosis. *Chest* 2005; 128:720–8.
11. Lau EM, Barnes DJ, Moriarty C, *et al.* Pregnancy outcomes in the current era of cystic fibrosis care: a 15-year experience. *Aust N Z J Obstet Gynaecol* 2011; 51:220–4.
12. Gilljam M, Antoniou M, Shin J, *et al.* Pregnancy in cystic fibrosis. Fetal and maternal outcome. *Chest* 2000; 118:85–91.
13. Muammar M, Marshall P, Wyatt H, *et al.* Caesarean section in a patient with cystic fibrosis. *Int J Obstet Anesth* 2005; 14:70–3.
14. Lau EM, Moriarty C, Ogle R, *et al.* Pregnancy and cystic fibrosis. *Paediatr Respir Rev* 2010; 11:90–4.
15. Dhonnchu TN, Regan C, Egan JJ. Successful pregnancy outcome in a patient following heart, lung and renal transplant. *Transpl Int* 2012; 25:e43–4.
16. Goss CH, Rubenfeld GD, Otto K, *et al.* The effect of pregnancy on survival in women with cystic fibrosis. *Chest* 2003; 124:1460–8.
17. McArdle JR. Pregnancy in cystic fibrosis. *Clin Chest Med* 2011; 32:111–20, ix.
18. Cheng EY, Goss CH, McKone EF, *et al.* Aggressive prenatal care results in successful fetal outcomes in CF women. *J Cyst Fibros* 2006; 5:85–91.
19. McMullen AH, Pasta DJ, Frederick PD, *et al.* Impact of pregnancy on women with cystic fibrosis. *Chest* 2006; 129:706–11.
20. Odegaard I, Stray-Pedersen B, Hallberg K, *et al.* Maternal and fetal morbidity in pregnancies of Norwegian and Swedish women with cystic fibrosis. *Acta Obstet Gynecol Scand* 2002; 81:698–705.
21. Ciavattini A, Ciattaglia F, Cecchi S, *et al.* Two successful pregnancies in a woman affected by cystic fibrosis: case report and review of the literature. *J Matern Fetal Neonatal Med* 2012; 25:113–15.
22. Ramsey BW, Pepe MS, Quan JM, *et al.* Intermittent administration of inhaled tobramycin in patients with cystic fibrosis. Cystic Fibrosis Inhaled Tobramycin Study Group. *N Engl J Med* 1999; 340:23–30.
23. McArdle JR, Talwalkar JS. Macrolides in cystic fibrosis. *Clin Chest Med* 2007; 28:347–60.
24. Robinson TE, Goris ML, Zhu HJ, *et al.* Dornase alfa reduces air trapping in children with mild cystic fibrosis lung disease: a quantitative analysis. *Chest* 2005; 128:2327–35.
25. Fuchs HJ, Borowitz DS, Christiansen DH, *et al.* Effect of aerosolized recombinant human DNase on exacerbations of respiratory symptoms and on pulmonary function in patients with cystic fibrosis. The Pulmozyme Study Group. *N Engl J Med* 1994; 331:637–42.
26. Retsch-Bogart GZ, Quittner AL, Gibson RL, *et al.* Efficacy and safety of inhaled aztreonam lysine for airway pseudomonas in cystic fibrosis. *Chest* 2009; 135:1223–32.

27. McCoy KS, Quittner AL, Oermann CM, *et al.* Inhaled aztreonam lysine for chronic airway Pseudomonas aeruginosa in cystic fibrosis. *Am J Respir Crit Care Med* 2008; 178:921–8.
28. Reeves EP, Molloy K, Pohl K, *et al.* Hypertonic saline in treatment of pulmonary disease in cystic fibrosis. *ScientificWorldJournal* 2012; 2012:465230.
29. Bright-Thomas RJ, Webb AK. The heart in cystic fibrosis. *J R Soc Med* 2002; 95 Suppl 41:2–10.
30. Hofer M, Schmid C, Benden C, *et al.* Diabetes mellitus and survival in cystic fibrosis patients after lung transplantation. *J Cyst Fibros* 2011; 11:131–6.
31. Jaksch P, Wiedemann D, Augustin V, *et al.* Antithymocyte globulin induction therapy improves survival in lung transplantation for cystic fibrosis. *Transpl Int* 2012; 26:34–41.
32. Dungan JS. Carrier screening for cystic fibrosis. *Obstet Gynecol Clin North Am* 2010; 37:47–59.
33. Massie J, Curnow L, Gaffney L, *et al.* Declining prevalence of cystic fibrosis since the introduction of newborn screening. *Arch Dis Child* 2010; 95:531–3.
34. Edwards EA, Narang I, Li A, *et al.* HRCT lung abnormalities are not a surrogate for exercise limitation in bronchiectasis. *Eur Respir J* 2004; 24:538–44.
35. Hyde NH, Harrison DM. Intrathecal morphine in a parturient with cystic fibrosis. *Anesth Analg* 1986; 65:1357–8.
36. Deshpande S. Epidural analgesia for vaginal delivery in a patient with cystic fibrosis following double lung transplantation. *Int J Obstet Anesth* 1998; 7:42–5.
37. Duggal KN, Douglas MJ, Bright S. Anaesthesia for the parturient with cystic fibrosis. *Int J Obstet Anesth* 1994; 3:122–3.
38. Howell PR, Kent N, Douglas MJ. Anaesthesia for the parturient with cystic fibrosis. *Int J Obstet Anesth* 1993; 2:152–8.
39. Tan TT, Teoh WH, Woo DC, *et al.* A randomised trial of the analgesic efficacy of ultrasound-guided transversus abdominis plane block after caesarean delivery under general anaesthesia. *Eur J Anaesthesiol* 2012; 29:88–94.
40. Olaguibel JM, Quirce S, Julia B, *et al.* Measurement of asthma control according to Global Initiative for Asthma guidelines: a comparison with the Asthma Control Questionnaire. *Respir Res* 2012; 13:50.
41. Baiz N, Annesi-Maesano I. Is the asthma epidemic still ascending? *Clin Chest Med* 2012; 33:419–29.
42. Clark JM, Hulme E, Devendrakumar V, *et al.* Effect of maternal asthma on birthweight and neonatal outcome in a British inner-city population. *Paediatr Perinat Epidemiol* 2007; 21:154–62.
43. Kwon HL, Triche EW, Belanger K, *et al.* The epidemiology of asthma during pregnancy: prevalence, diagnosis, and symptoms. *Immunol Allergy Clin North Am* 2006; 26:29–62.
44. Clifton VL, Engel P, Smith R, *et al.* Maternal and neonatal outcomes of pregnancies complicated by asthma in an Australian population. *Aust N Z J Obstet Gynaecol* 2009; 49:619–26.
45. Slager RE, Hawkins GA, Li X, *et al.* Genetics of asthma susceptibility and severity. *Clin Chest Med* 2012; 33:431–43.
46. Moffatt MF, Gut IG, Demenais F, *et al.* A large-scale, consortium-based genomewide association study of asthma. *N Engl J Med* 2010; 363:1211–21.
47. Torgerson DG, Ampleford EJ, Chiu GY, *et al.* Meta-analysis of genome-wide association studies of asthma in ethnically diverse North American populations. *Nat Genet* 2011; 43:887–92.
48. Hirota T, Takahashi A, Kubo M, *et al.* Genome-wide association study identifies three new susceptibility loci for adult asthma in the Japanese population. *Nat Genet* 2011; 43:893–6.
49. Tantisira KG, Lasky-Su J, Harada M, *et al.* Genomewide association between GLCCI1 and response to glucocorticoid therapy in asthma. *N Engl J Med* 2011; 365:1173–83.
50. Black JL, Panettieri RA Jr, Banerjee A, *et al.* Airway smooth muscle in asthma: just a target for bronchodilation? *Clin Chest Med* 2012; 33:543–58.
51. Bobic S, Seys S, De Vooght V, *et al.* Placental growth factor contributes to bronchial neutrophilic inflammation and edema in allergic asthma. *Am J Respir Cell Mol Biol* 2012; 46:781–9.
52. Bara I, Ozier A, Tunon de Lara JM, *et al.* Pathophysiology of bronchial smooth muscle remodelling in asthma. *Eur Respir J* 2010; 36:1174–84.
53. Holgate ST, Polosa R. The mechanisms, diagnosis, and management of severe asthma in adults. *Lancet* 2006; 368:780–93.
54. Orzechowski KM, Miller RC. Common respiratory issues in ambulatory obstetrics. *Clin Obstet Gynecol* 2012; 55:798–809.
55. Hardy-Fairbanks AJ, Baker ER. Asthma in pregnancy: pathophysiology, diagnosis and management. *Obstet Gynecol Clin North Am* 2010; 37:159–72.
56. Dombrowski MP, Schatz M. ACOG practice bulletin: clinical management guidelines for obstetrician-gynecologists number 90, February 2008: asthma in pregnancy. *Obstet Gynecol* 2008; 111:457–64.
57. NAEPP. NAEPP expert panel report. Managing asthma during pregnancy: recommendations for pharmacologic treatment-2004 update. *J Allergy Clin Immunol* 2005; 115:34–46.
58. Sheiner E, Mazor M, Levy A, *et al.* Pregnancy outcome of asthmatic patients: a population-based study. *J Matern Fetal Neonatal Med* 2005; 18:237–40.
59. Schatz M. Interrelationships between asthma and pregnancy: a literature review. *J Allergy Clin Immunol* 1999; 103:S330–6.
60. Kircher S, Schatz M, Long L. Variables affecting asthma course during pregnancy. *Ann Allergy Asthma Immunol* 2002; 89:463–6.
61. Schatz M, Harden K, Forsythe A, *et al.* The course of asthma during pregnancy, post partum, and with successive pregnancies: a prospective analysis. *J Allergy Clin Immunol* 1988; 81:509–17.
62. Schatz M, Dombrowski MP, Wise R, *et al.* Asthma morbidity during pregnancy can be predicted by severity classification. *J Allergy Clin Immunol* 2003; 112:283–8.
63. Murphy VE, Gibson PG. Asthma in pregnancy. *Clin Chest Med* 2011; 32:93–110, ix.
64. Vatti RR, Teuber SS. Asthma and pregnancy. *Clin Rev Allergy Immunol* 2012; 43:45–56.
65. Belanger K, Hellenbrand ME, Holford TR, *et al.* Effect of pregnancy on maternal asthma symptoms and medication use. *Obstet Gynecol* 2010; 115:559–67.
66. Jain S, Kamimoto L, Bramley AM, *et al.* Hospitalized patients with 2009 H1N1 influenza in the United States, April-June 2009. *N Engl J Med* 2009; 361:1935–44.
67. Scriven J, McEwen R, Mistry S, *et al.* Swine flu: a Birmingham experience. *Clin Med* 2009; 9:534–8.
68. Vanders RL, Gibson PG, Wark PA, *et al.* Alterations in inflammatory, antiviral and regulatory cytokine responses in peripheral blood mononuclear cells from pregnant women with asthma. *Respirology* 2013; 18(5):827–33.
69. Forbes RL, Wark PA, Murphy VE, *et al.* Pregnant women have attenuated innate interferon responses to 2009 pandemic influenza A virus subtype H1N1. *J Infect Dis* 2012; 206:646–53.
70. CDC. 2009 pandemic influenza A (H1N1) in pregnant women requiring intensive care—New York City, 2009. *MMWR Morb Mortal Wkly Rep* 2010; 59:321–6.
71. CDC. Maternal and infant outcomes among severely ill pregnant and postpartum women with 2009 pandemic influenza A (H1N1)—United States, April 2009-August 2010. *MMWR Morb Mortal Wkly Rep* 2011; 60:1193–6.
72. Creanga AA, Johnson TF, Graitcer SB, *et al.* Severity of 2009 pandemic influenza A (H1N1) virus infection in pregnant women. *Obstet Gynecol* 2011; 115:717–26.
73. Jamieson DJ, Honein MA, Rasmussen SA, *et al.* H1N1 2009 influenza virus infection during pregnancy in the USA. *Lancet* 2009; 374:451–8.
74. Louie JK, Acosta M, Jamieson DJ, *et al.* Severe 2009 H1N1 influenza in pregnant and postpartum women in California. *N Engl J Med* 2010; 362:27–35.

75. Schatz M, Dombrowski MP, Wise R, *et al.* The relationship of asthma-specific quality of life during pregnancy to subsequent asthma and perinatal morbidity. J Asthma 2010; 47:46–50.
76. Teeter JG, Bleecker ER. Relationship between airway obstruction and respiratory symptoms in adult asthmatics. *Chest* 1998; 113:272–7.
77. Juniper EF, Daniel EE, Roberts RS, *et al.* Improvement in airway responsiveness and asthma severity during pregnancy. A prospective study. *Am Rev Respir Dis* 1989; 140:924–31.
78. Juniper EF, Daniel EE, Roberts RS, *et al.* Effect of pregnancy on airway responsiveness and asthma severity. Relationship to serum progesterone. *Am Rev Respir Dis* 1991; 143:S78.
79. Hellings PW, Vandekerckhove P, Claeys R, *et al.* Progesterone increases airway eosinophilia and hyper-responsiveness in a murine model of allergic asthma. *Clin Exp Allergy* 2003; 33:1457–63.
80. Bohacs A, Cseh A, Stenczer B, *et al.* Effector and regulatory lymphocytes in asthmatic pregnant women. *Am J Reprod Immunol* 2010; 64:393–401.
81. Wegienka G, Havstad S, Bobbitt KR, *et al.* Within-woman change in regulatory T cells from pregnancy to the postpartum period. *J Reprod Immunol* 2011; 88:58–65.
82. Bohacs A, Pallinger E, Tamasi L, *et al.* Surface markers of lymphocyte activation in pregnant asthmatics. *Inflamm Res* 2010; 59:63–70.
83. Molvarec A, Tamasi L, Losonczy G, *et al.* Circulating heat shock protein 70 (HSPA1A) in normal and pathological pregnancies. *Cell Stress Chaperones* 2010; 15:237–47.
84. Tamasi L, Bohacs A, Tamasi V, *et al.* Increased circulating heat shock protein 70 levels in pregnant asthmatics. *Cell Stress Chaperones* 2010; 15:295–300.
85. Tamasi L, Bohacs A, Pallinger E, *et al.* Increased interferon-gamma- and interleukin-4-synthesizing subsets of circulating T lymphocytes in pregnant asthmatics. *Clin Exp Allergy* 2005; 35:1197–203.
86. Osei-Kumah A, Wark PA, Smith R, *et al.* Asthma during pregnancy alters immune cell profile and airway epithelial chemokine release. *Inflamm Res* 2010; 59:349–58.
87. Beecroft N, Cochrane GM, Milburn HJ. Effect of sex of fetus on asthma during pregnancy: blind prospective study. *BMJ* 1998; 317:856–7.
88. Dodds L, Armson BA, Alexander S. Use of asthma drugs is less among women pregnant with boys rather than girls. *BMJ* 1999; 318:1011.
89. Kwon HL, Belanger K, Holford TR, *et al.* Effect of fetal sex on airway lability in pregnant women with asthma. *Am J Epidemiol* 2006; 163:217–21.
90. Bakhireva LN, Schatz M, Jones KL, *et al.* Fetal sex and maternal asthma control in pregnancy. *J Asthma* 2008; 45:403–7.
91. Baibergenova A, Thabane L, Akhtar-Danesh N, *et al.* Is fetal gender associated with emergency department visits for asthma during pregnancy? *J Asthma* 2006; 43:293–9.
92. Firoozi F, Ducharme FM, Lemiere C, *et al.* Effect of fetal gender on maternal asthma exacerbations in pregnant asthmatic women. *Respir Med* 2009; 103:144–51.
93. Murphy VE, Namazy JA, Powell H, *et al.* A meta-analysis of adverse perinatal outcomes in women with asthma. *BJOG* 2011; 118:1314–23.
94. Namazy JA, Schatz M. Asthma and pregnancy. *J Allergy Clin Immunol* 2011; 128:1384–5 e2.
95. Mendola P, Laughon SK, Mannisto TI, *et al.* Obstetric complications among US women with asthma. *Am J Obstet Gynecol* 2013; 208:127. e1–8
96. Enriquez R, Griffin MR, Carroll KN, *et al.* Effect of maternal asthma and asthma control on pregnancy and perinatal outcomes. *J Allergy Clin Immunol* 2007; 120:625–30.
97. Firoozi F, Lemiere C, Beauchesne MF, *et al.* Impact of maternal asthma on perinatal outcomes: a two-stage sampling cohort study. *Eur J Epidemiol* 2012; 27:205–14.
98. Blais L, Kettani FZ, Elftouh N, *et al.* Effect of maternal asthma on the risk of specific congenital malformations: a population-based cohort study. *Birth Defects Res A Clin Mol Teratol* 2010; 88:216–22.
99. Schatz M, Dombrowski MP, Wise R, *et al.* Spirometry is related to perinatal outcomes in pregnant women with asthma. *Am J Obstet Gynecol* 2006; 194:120–6.
100. Aly H, Nada A, Ahmad T, *et al.* Maternal asthma, race and low birth weight deliveries. *Early Hum Dev* 2011; 87:457–60.
101. Firoozi F, Lemiere C, Ducharme FM, *et al.* Effect of maternal moderate to severe asthma on perinatal outcomes. *Respir Med* 2010; 104:1278–87.
102. Blais L, Forget A. Asthma exacerbations during the first trimester of pregnancy and the risk of congenital malformations among asthmatic women. *J Allergy Clin Immunol* 2008; 121:1379–84.
103. Kallen B, Otterblad Olausson P. Use of anti-asthmatic drugs during pregnancy. 2. Infant characteristics excluding congenital malformations. *Eur J Clin Pharmacol* 2007; 63:375–81.
104. McLernon PC, Wood LG, Murphy VE, *et al.* Circulating antioxidant profile of pregnant women with asthma. *Clin Nutr* 2011; 31:99–107.
105. Gershwin ME, Albertson TE. The practical understanding and treatment of asthma. *Clin Rev Allergy Immunol* 2012; 43:1–2.
106. Dombrowski MP, Schatz M. Asthma in pregnancy. *Clin Obstet Gynecol* 2010; 53:301–10.
107. Powell H, Murphy VE, Taylor DR, *et al.* Management of asthma in pregnancy guided by measurement of fraction of exhaled nitric oxide: a double-blind, randomised controlled trial. *Lancet* 2011; 378:983–90.
108. Murphy VE, Clifton VL, Gibson PG. The effect of cigarette smoking on asthma control during exacerbations in pregnant women. *Thorax* 2010; 65:739–44.
109. Newman RB, Momirova V, Dombrowski MP, *et al.* The effect of active and passive household cigarette smoke exposure on pregnant women with asthma. *Chest* 2010; 137:601–8.
110. Burke H, Leonardi-Bee J, Hashim A, *et al.* Prenatal and passive smoke exposure and incidence of asthma and wheeze: systematic review and meta-analysis. *Pediatrics* 2012; 129:735–44.
111. Schatz M, Zeiger RS, Harden KM, *et al.* The safety of inhaled beta-agonist bronchodilators during pregnancy. *J Allergy Clin Immunol* 1988; 82:686–95.
112. Schatz M, Dombrowski MP, Wise R, *et al.* The relationship of asthma medication use to perinatal outcomes. *J Allergy Clin Immunol* 2004; 113:1040–5.
113. Mann RD, Kubota K, Pearce G, *et al.* Salmeterol: a study by prescription-event monitoring in a UK cohort of 15,407 patients. *J Clin Epidemiol* 1996; 49:247–50.
114. Nelson HS, Carr W, Nathan R, *et al.* Update on the safety of long-acting beta-agonists in combination with inhaled corticosteroids for the treatment of asthma. *Ann Allergy Asthma Immunol* 2009; 102:11–15.
115. Eltonsy S, Forget A, Blais L. Beta2-agonists use during pregnancy and the risk of congenital malformations. *Birth Defects Res A Clin Mol Teratol* 2011; 91:937–47.
116. Bakhireva LN, Jones KL, Schatz M, *et al.* Safety of leukotriene receptor antagonists in pregnancy. *J Allergy Clin Immunol* 2007; 119:618–25.
117. Lim A, Stewart K, Konig K, *et al.* Systematic review of the safety of regular preventive asthma medications during pregnancy. *Ann Pharmacother* 2011; 45:931–45.
118. Enriquez R, Wu P, Griffin MR, *et al.* Cessation of asthma medication in early pregnancy. *Am J Obstet Gynecol* 2006; 195:149–53.
119. Rocklin RE. Asthma, asthma medications and their effects on maternal/fetal outcomes during pregnancy. *Reprod Toxicol* 2011; 32:189–97.
120. Lin S, Munsie JP, Herdt-Losavio ML, *et al.* Maternal asthma medication use and the risk of selected birth defects. *Pediatrics* 2012; 129:e317–24.
121. Munsie JW, Lin S, Browne ML, *et al.* Maternal bronchodilator use and the risk of orofacial clefts. *Hum Reprod* 2011; 26:3147–54.
122. Nelsen LM, Shields KE, Cunningham ML, *et al.* Congenital malformations among infants born to women receiving montelukast,

inhaled corticosteroids, and other asthma medications. *J Allergy Clin Immunol* 2012; 129:251–4.e1–6.

123. Nemer DS, Nomura RM, Ortigosa C, *et al.* Computerized cardiotocography in pregnancies complicated by maternal asthma. *J Matern Fetal Neonatal Med* 2011; 25:1077–9.
124. Johnston D, Hughes D. Bronchospasm following ergometrine in a non-asthmatic patient. *Int J Obstet Anesth* 2013; 22:261–2.
125. Louie S, Krzanowski JJ Jr, Bukantz SC, *et al.* Effects of ergometrine on airway smooth muscle contractile responses. *Clin Allergy* 1985; 15:173–8.
126. Loubert C, Hinova A, Fernando R. Update on modern neuraxial analgesia in labour: a review of the literature of the last 5 years. *Anaesthesia* 2011; 66:191–212.
127. Tveit TO, Halvorsen A, Seiler S, *et al.* Efficacy and side effects of intravenous remifentanil patient-controlled analgesia used in a stepwise approach for labour: an observational study. *Int J Obstet Anesth* 2013; 22:19–25.
128. Kawabata KM. [Two cases of asthmatic attack caused by spinal anesthesia]. *Masui* 1996; 45:102–6.
129. Wang CY, Ong GS. Severe bronchospasm during epidural anaesthesia. *Anaesthesia* 1993; 48:514–15.
130. Brown RH, Wagner EM. Mechanisms of bronchoprotection by anesthetic induction agents: propofol versus ketamine. *Anesthesiology* 1999; 90:822–8.
131. Eames WO, Rooke GA, Wu RS, *et al.* Comparison of the effects of etomidate, propofol, and thiopental on respiratory resistance after tracheal intubation. *Anesthesiology* 1996; 84:1307–11.
132. Rieschke P, LaFleur BJ, Janicki PK. Effects of EDTA- and sulfite-containing formulations of propofol on respiratory system resistance after tracheal intubation in smokers. *Anesthesiology* 2003; 98:323–8.
133. Chang HY, Togias A, Brown RH. The effects of systemic lidocaine on airway tone and pulmonary function in asthmatic subjects. *Anesth Analg* 2007; 104:1109–15.
134. Maslow AD, Regan MM, Israel E, *et al.* Inhaled albuterol, but not intravenous lidocaine, protects against intubation-induced bronchoconstriction in asthma. *Anesthesiology* 2000; 93:1198–204.
135. Goff MJ, Arain SR, Ficke DJ, *et al.* Absence of bronchodilation during desflurane anesthesia: a comparison to sevoflurane and thiopental. *Anesthesiology* 2000; 93:404–8.
136. Caldwell JE, Lau M, Fisher DM. Atracurium versus vecuronium in asthmatic patients. A blinded, randomized comparison of adverse events. *Anesthesiology* 1995; 83:986–91.
137. Woods BD, Sladen RN. Perioperative considerations for the patient with asthma and bronchospasm. *Br J Anaesth* 2009; 103 Suppl 1:i57–65.
138. Rosow CE, Moss J, Philbin DM, *et al.* Histamine release during morphine and fentanyl anesthesia. *Anesthesiology* 1982; 56:93–6.
139. Flacke JW, Flacke WE, Bloor BC, *et al.* Histamine release by four narcotics: a double-blind study in humans. *Anesth Analg* 1987; 66:723–30.
140. Que JC, Lusaya VO. Sevoflurane induction for emergency cesarean section in a parturient in status asthmaticus. *Anesthesiology* 1999; 90:1475–6.
141. Erdogan G, Okyay DZ, Yurtlu S, *et al.* Non-invasive mechanical ventilation with spinal anesthesia for cesarean delivery. *Int J Obstet Anesth* 2010; 19:438–40.
142. Lo JO, Boltax J, Metz TD. Cesarean delivery for life-threatening status asthmaticus. *Obstet Gynecol* 2013; 121:422–4.
143. Lurie S, Mamet Y. Caesarean delivery during maternal cardiopulmonary resuscitation for status asthmaticus. *Emerg Med J* 2003; 20:296–7
144. Brito V, Niederman MS. Pneumonia complicating pregnancy. *Clin Chest Med* 2011; 32:121–32, ix.
145. Belfort MA, Clark SL, Saade GR, *et al.* Hospital readmission after delivery: evidence for an increased incidence of nonurogenital infection in the immediate postpartum period. *Am J Obstet Gynecol* 2010; 35:e1–7.
146. Khan S, Niederman MS: Pneumonia in the pregnant patient. In Rosene-Montela K, Bourjeily G (eds) *Pulmonary Problems in Pregnancy*. New York: Humana Press; 2009:177–96.
147. Lederman MM. Cell-mediated immunity and pregnancy. *Chest* 1984; 86:6S-9S.
148. Rodrigues J, Niederman MS. Pneumonia complicating pregnancy. *Clin Chest Med* 1992; 13:679–91.
149. Catanzaro A. Pulmonary mycosis in pregnant women. *Chest* 1984; 86:14S–9S.
150. Benedetti TJ, Valle R, Ledger WJ. Antepartum pneumonia in pregnancy. *Am J Obstet Gynecol* 1982; 144:413–17.
151. Sheffield JS, Cunningham FG. Community-acquired pneumonia in pregnancy. *Obstet Gynecol* 2009; 114:915–22.
152. Mandell LA, Wunderink RG, Anzueto A, *et al.* Infectious Diseases Society of America/American Thoracic Society consensus guidelines on the management of community-acquired pneumonia in adults. *Clin Infect Dis* 2007; 44 Suppl 2:S27–72.
153. ACOG. Guidelines for diagnostic imaging during pregnancy. American College of Obstetricians and Gynecologists Committee Opinion No. 299. *Obstet Gynecol* 2004; 104:647–51.
154. Romanyuk V, Raichel L, Sergienko R, *et al.* Pneumonia during pregnancy: radiological characteristics, predisposing factors and pregnancy outcomes. *J Matern Fetal Neonatal Med* 2011; 24:113–17.
155. Kristensen MS, Teoh WH, Graumann O, *et al.* Ultrasonography for clinical decision-making and intervention in airway management: from the mouth to the lungs and pleurae. *Insights Imaging* 2014; 5(2):253–79.
156. Teoh WH, Kristensen MS. Utility of ultrasound in airway management. *Trends Anaesth Crit Care* 2014; 4(4):84–90.
157. Torres A. The new American Thoracic Society/Infectious Disease Society of North America guidelines for the management of hospital-acquired, ventilator-associated and healthcare-associated pneumonia: a current view and new complementary information. *Curr Opin Crit Care* 2006; 12:444–5.
158. Chen YH, Keller J, Wang IT, *et al.* Pneumonia and pregnancy outcomes: a nationwide population-based study. *Am J Obstet Gynecol* 2012; 207:288 e1–7.
159. Smith GJ, Vijaykrishna D, Bahl J, *et al.* Origins and evolutionary genomics of the 2009 swine-origin H1N1 influenza A epidemic. *Nature* 2009; 459:1122–5.
160. Creanga AA, Kamimoto L, Newsome K, *et al.* Seasonal and 2009 pandemic influenza A (H1N1) virus infection during pregnancy: a population-based study of hospitalized cases. *Am J Obstet Gynecol* 2011; 204:S38–45.
161. Figueiro-Filho EA, Oliveira ML, Pompilio MA, *et al.* Obstetric, clinical, and perinatal implications of H1N1 viral infection during pregnancy. *Int J Gynaecol Obstet* 2012; 116:214–18.
162. McAlister VC. H1N1-related SIRS? *CMAJ* 2009; 181:616–17.
163. Lim ML, Chong CY, Tee WS, *et al.* Influenza A/H1N1 (2009) infection in pregnancy—an Asian perspective. *BJOG* 2010; 117:551–6.
164. Bowkalow S, Brauer M, Gross W, *et al.* Severe H1N1-infection during pregnancy. *Arch Gynecol Obstet* 2011; 284:1133–5.
165. Liu J, Li Q, Cui H, *et al.* Severe and critical cases of H1N1 influenza in pregnancy: a Chinese perspective. *J Postgrad Med* 2011; 57:298–301.
166. Chang C, Gao HL, Yao WZ, *et al.* Early clinical characteristics and pregnancy outcomes of patients with influenza A (H1N1) infection requiring mechanical ventilation during pregnancy. *J Obstet Gynaecol* 2013; 33:561–5.
167. Shu B, Wu KH, Emery S, *et al.* Design and performance of the CDC real-time reverse transcriptase PCR swine flu panel for detection of 2009 A (H1N1) pandemic influenza virus. *J Clin Microbiol* 2011; 49:2614–19.
168. Hurt AC, Baas C, Deng YM, *et al.* Performance of influenza rapid point-of-care tests in the detection of swine lineage A(H1N1) influenza viruses. *Influenza Other Respir Viruses* 2009; 3:171–6.

169. Faix DJ, Sherman SS, Waterman SH. Rapid-test sensitivity for novel swine-origin influenza A (H1N1) virus in humans. *N Engl J Med* 2009; 361:728–9.
170. Pierro A, Gaibani P, Rossini G, *et al.* Clinical application of a molecular method based on real time RT-PCR for detection of influenza A(H1N1)v virus. *New Microbiol* 2013; 36:405–8.
171. Barbas MG, Gallego SV, Castro GM, *et al.* Performance of a commercial assay for the diagnosis of influenza A (H1N1) infection in comparison to the Centers for Disease Control and Prevention protocol of real time RT-PCR. *Rev Argent Microbiol* 2012; 44:26–9.
172. Lim ML, Lim WY, Tee NW, *et al.* Obstetric outcomes of influenza A H1N1 (2009) infection in pregnancy—experience of a Singapore tertiary hospital. *Ann Acad Med Singapore* 2010; 39:295–304.
173. Hansen C, Desai S, Bredfeldt C, *et al.* A large, population-based study of 2009 pandemic Influenza A virus subtype H1N1 infection diagnosis during pregnancy and outcomes for mothers and neonates. *J Infect Dis* 2012; 206:1260–8.
174. Bozzo P, Djokanovic N, Koren G. H1N1 influenza in pregnancy: risks, vaccines, and antivirals. *J Obstet Gynaecol Can* 2009; 31:1172–5.
175. Shanker N, Aneja S, Jayalalitha MV, *et al.* Perioperative management of a parturient for cesarean section with confirmed H1N1 influenza. *J Obstet Anaesth Crit Care* 2013; 3:104–7.
176. Tay J, Ng YF, Cutter JL, *et al.* Influenza A (H1N1-2009) pandemic in Singapore—public health control measures implemented and lessons learnt. *Ann Acad Med Singapore* 2010; 39:313–412.
177. Mukherjee P, Lim PL, Chow A, *et al.* Epidemiology of travel-associated pandemic (H1N1) 2009 infection in 116 patients, Singapore. *Emerg Infect Dis* 2010; 16:21–6.
178. Brown CM: Severe influenza A virus (H1N1) infection in pregnancy. *Obstet Gynecol* 2010; 115:412–14.
179. Lieberman RW, Bagdasarian N, Thomas D, *et al.* Seasonal influenza A (H1N1) infection in early pregnancy and second trimester fetal demise. *Emerg Infect Dis* 2011; 17:107–9.
180. Malinowski AK, McGeer A, Robertson J, *et al.* H1N1 in pregnancy: a tertiary care centre experience. *J Obstet Gynaecol Can* 2011; 33:698–704.
181. Chan K, Meek D, Chakravorty I. Unusual association of ST-T abnormalities, myocarditis and cardiomyopathy with H1N1 influenza in pregnancy: two case reports and review of the literature. *J Med Case Rep* 2011; 5:314.
182. Fisher BM, Van Bockern J, Hart J, *et al.* Pandemic influenza A H1N1 2009 infection versus vaccination: a cohort study comparing immune responses in pregnancy. *PLoS One* 2012; 7:e33048.
183. Fell DB, Sprague AE, Liu N, *et al.* H1N1 influenza vaccination during pregnancy and fetal and neonatal outcomes. *Am J Public Health* 2012; 102:e33–40.
184. Chambers CD, Johnson D, Xu R, *et al.* Risks and safety of pandemic h1n1 influenza vaccine in pregnancy: birth defects, spontaneous abortion, preterm delivery, and small for gestational age infants. *Vaccine* 2013; 31:5026–32.
185. Kallen B, Olausson PO. Vaccination against H1N1 influenza with Pandemrix® during pregnancy and delivery outcome: a Swedish register study. *BJOG* 2012; 119:1583–90.
186. Beau AB, Hurault-Delarue C, Vidal S, *et al.* Pandemic A/H1N1 influenza vaccination during pregnancy: a comparative study using the EFEMERIS database. *Vaccine* 2014; 32(11):1254–8.
187. Louik C, Ahrens K, Kerr S, *et al.* Risks and safety of pandemic H1N1 influenza vaccine in pregnancy: exposure prevalence, preterm delivery, and specific birth defects. *Vaccine* 2013; 31:5033–40.
188. Pasternak B, Svanstrom H, Molgaard-Nielsen D, *et al.* Risk of adverse fetal outcomes following administration of a pandemic influenza A(H1N1) vaccine during pregnancy. *JAMA* 2012; 308:165–74.
189. Ludvigsson JF, Zugna D, Cnattingius S, *et al.* Influenza H1N1 vaccination and adverse pregnancy outcome. *Eur J Epidemiol* 2013; 28:579–88.
190. Campanharo FF, Santana EF, Sarmento SG, *et al.* Guillain-Barre syndrome after H1N1 shot in pregnancy: maternal and fetal care in the third trimester-case report. *Case Rep Obstet Gynecol* 2012; 2012:323625.

CHAPTER 43

Liver disorders

Chris Verslype, David Cassiman, and Johan Verhaeghe

Introduction

Nearly 5% of pregnancies are complicated by liver disorders and this may result in considerable harm to mother and child. Early diagnosis and treatment of liver disease is challenging, given the wide spectrum of liver diseases that may be related or unrelated (either pre-existing or coincidental) to pregnancy. Before discussing liver disorders in detail, we focus on how to diagnose and assess liver disease in pregnant women. Special attention is also devoted to the management of clinically significant portal hypertension and to the guidelines regarding pregnancy in patients who have undergone liver transplantation.

Diagnosis and assessment of liver disease in pregnant women

Clinical assessment of patients with suspected liver disease during pregnancy

The assessment of pregnant patients with liver disorders is challenging due to the physiological changes of pregnancy that can be mistaken for liver dysfunction. Cardiovascular changes (fall in systemic vascular resistance and blood pressure, rise in cardiac output) seen in normal pregnancy are similar to the hyperdynamic circulatory state in the context of advanced liver disease. Increased splanchnic blood flow and compression of the inferior vena cava in the supine position by the uterus may induce transient portal hypertension.[1,2] The hyperoestrogenic state of pregnancy induces palmar erythema and spider naevi—considered as typical signs of chronic liver disease—that resolve by the seventh postpartum week in the majority of women.[3] During pregnancy, microscopic liver architecture appears normal and liver blood flow remains constant.[4]

Cholestasis, portal hypertension, and liver failure represent three major clinical entities that should be recognized early because of the prognostic implications for mother and child. *Cholestatic liver disease* should be suspected in a patient with pruritus and/or jaundice. The presence of ascites or enlarged portosystemic collateral veins (abdominal wall, gastrointestinal tract, and retroperitoneal space) or a history of gastrointestinal bleeding may point to *clinically significant portal hypertension*. Hepatic encephalopathy, which may range from mild confusion to deep coma, often preceded or accompanied by jaundice, and clotting failure is indicative of *liver failure*. In some patients, a combination of these clinical entities may exist.

Of note, significant liver disease may present without symptoms or signs. In these patients, a history of risk factors for liver disease (e.g. alcohol or drug intake, familial history of liver failure, tattoos, or blood transfusions prior to the introduction of tests for hepatitis C (1989)) may influence the choice of additional biochemical and/or imaging tests, which will be discussed below.

Biochemical tests to detect liver disease and assess liver function during pregnancy

Biochemical tests are commonly used to screen and confirm the presence of liver disease, to estimate severity, prognosis, and to evaluate therapy. The 'liver function tests' (LFTs) include aminotransferases, alkaline phosphatase (AP), gamma-glutamyltransferase (GGT) and serum bilirubin. Strictly speaking, these tests do not assess liver function but a rise in their serum levels or activity may point to the presence of liver cell necrosis, impairment of bile flow (cholestasis), and hyperbilirubinaemia. The prothrombin time (after vitamin K administration) and, to a lesser extent, serum albumin are more indicative of hepatic synthetic capacity.

The aminotransferases (aspartate transaminase (AST) and alanine transaminase (ALT)) catalyse the reversible transformation of α-ketoacids into amino acids. Their serum level activity reflects the amount of liver cell injury and death on a day-by-day basis. The aminotransferases (predominantly AST) are not only found in hepatocytes but also in other tissues (muscles, kidney, brain, pancreas, lung, and red blood cells).

The liver contains 400 units of ALT/g protein (mainly cytoplasmic) and 500 units of AST/g protein (>80% contained in mitochondria and endoplasmic reticulum). Damage to 1 g of liver tissue results in a significant increase in the serum ALT and AST activity.[5,6] Serum aminotransferase levels can rise to over ten times the upper limit of normal (ULN) in hepatic hypoxia, acute viral hepatitis, toxin-induced necrosis, and acute bile duct obstruction. In chronic hepatitis, the levels are generally less than five times the ULN. The sensitivity and specificity of ALT for the detection of liver disease is around 83%.[5,6] The diagnostic sensitivity of AST is significantly lower (70%) and less specific. Serial assessment of transaminases can be used to monitor progress in an individual patient but correlation is poor between absolute values and the extent of necrosis. Serum ALT activity, but not AST, is slightly higher during the second trimester of pregnancy compared with non-pregnant women, but remains below the ULN.[7] Increased AST and ALT levels noted during labour may be secondary to uterine muscle contractions.[8,9] In conclusion, serum AST and ALT activities remain normal during pregnancy prior to labour, and increased values should lead to further investigation.

AP is found in the biliary pole of hepatocytes, bile duct epithelia, osteoblasts, kidney, lung, intestine, and placenta. Levels of AP rise in cholestasis and to a lesser extent with hepatocyte injury. Serum AP levels increase significantly in late pregnancy due to placental and bone production. This limits the utility of AP as a test to diagnose cholestasis of pregnancy. Hepatic and non-hepatic causes of AP elevation can be differentiated by determination of AP isoenzymes or more easily by testing for GGT, which rises in liver but not in bone disease. GGT is found in hepatocytes, cholangiocytes, kidney, pancreas, epididymis, heart, lung, intestine, bone marrow, salivary glands, thymus, spleen, and brain, and therefore is not very specific for liver disease. Elevated values of GGT are caused by damage to cellular membranes, cellular regeneration, or by enhanced synthesis as a result of induction of the biotransformation enzyme system.[6] Known inducers are bile acids (cholestasis), prolonged regular abuse of alcohol, and especially antiepileptic drugs (phenytoin, carbamazepine). A decline in GGT can be observed during oestrogen administration or during the second and third trimester of pregnancy.[7] Fasting total bile acid concentrations are unaltered in normal pregnancy, and are therefore a specific test for the diagnosis of cholestasis. Conjugated bilirubin can be elevated in cholestatic and hepatocellular disease and is associated with a rise in the above-mentioned serum enzymes. An isolated rise in serum bilirubin (without enzyme elevation) may be familial (Gilbert's phenomenon) or due to haemolysis. Conjugated bilirubin concentrations are significantly lower during the second and third trimesters compared to non-pregnant women. This can be partially explained by haemodilution because albumin is the bilirubin transporting protein.[7]

The hepatocyte is the principal site of synthesis of coagulation proteins. The prothrombin time (after vitamin K administration) represents a good indicator of liver synthetic function, due to the short half-life of factor VII (100–300 minutes). Estimation of individual clotting factors is rarely necessary, although the level of factor V (not vitamin K dependent) is related to outcome in acute liver failure. Serum albumin levels[10] provide some indication of hepatic synthetic capacity. However, serum albumin levels may be normal with acute liver failure because the half-life of albumin is about 22 days. Low levels can be caused by increased loss through the kidneys or gastrointestinal tract, increased catabolism and altered vascular permeability. Because of haemodilution, serum albumin levels are significantly lower during all trimesters of pregnancy compared with non-pregnant women.[7] Alterations in the concentration of serum albumin must therefore be interpreted with caution.

Liver function scoring systems

Several scoring systems have been developed to assess and classify liver function (Table 43.1). The Child–Pugh score reflects the severity of chronic liver disease according to the degree of ascites, the prothrombin time, the plasma concentrations of bilirubin and albumin, and the stage of encephalopathy. A total score of 5–6 signifies a well-compensated state (grade A), 7–9 is grade B, and 10–15 is grade C (decompensated disease). These grades correlate with 1- and 2-year patient survival.

More recently, the Model of End Stage Liver Disease (MELD) has been introduced in clinical practice to predict prognosis in patients with cirrhosis and to guide listing for liver transplantation. This score uses the prothrombin time, serum bilirubin, and creatinine as input values.[11] Patients having a MELD score <9 face a 2% 3-month mortality, whereas patients having a MELD score of 40 or higher have a mortality rate of 70% within 3 months.

Table 43.1 Assessment of liver function

(A) Child–Pugh classification

Factor	Units	1 point	2 points	3 points
Serum bilirubin	μmol/L	<34	34–51	>51
	mg/dL	<2.0	2.0–3.0	>3.0
Serum albumin	g/L	>35	30–35	<30
	g/dL	>3.5	3.0–3.5	<3.0
Prothrombin time	Seconds prolonged	0–4	4–6	>6
	INR	<1.7	1.7–2.3	>2.3
Ascites		None	Moderate	Severe
Hepatic encephalopathy		None	Mild	severe

The score is calculated by adding the scores of the five factors:
Child–Pugh A: 5–6; B: 7–9; C: > 9.

(B) Model of End-stage Liver Disease (MELD)

$$\text{Formula} = \begin{bmatrix} \left(0.957 \times \log_e \text{Creat mg / dL}\right) + 0.378 \times \\ \left(\log_e \text{Br mg / dL}\right) + \left(1.120 \times \log_e \text{INR}\right) + 0.643 \end{bmatrix} \times 10$$

MELD calculator available through http://www.esot.org/elita/meldcalculator.aspx

Reproduced with permission from Pugh RNH *et al.*, Transection of the oesophagus for bleeding oesophageal varices, *British Journal of Surgery*, Volume 60, pp. 646–649, Copyright © 1973 John Wiley and Sons and from Wiesner RH *et al.*, MELD and PELD: Application of survival models to liver allocation, *Liver Transplantation*, Volume 7, pp. 567–580, Copyright © John Wiley and Sons.

Imaging of the liver during pregnancy

Real-time ultrasonography represents the most widely used imaging modality in clinical hepatology and is used to evaluate biliary tract obstruction, to identify splenomegaly and collateral vessels in portal hypertension, and to examine tumour vascularity. It is also valuable in diagnostic assessment of portal or hepatic vein thrombosis. More recently, liver elastography is used by many hepatologists to evaluate liver stiffness. This non-invasive technique uses both ultrasound (US) (5 MHz) and low-frequency (50 Hz) elastic waves, whose propagation velocity is directly related to elasticity.[12] There is no published experience in pregnancy and unfortunately, pregnancy has been a contraindication in clinical studies.

Magnetic resonance imaging (MRI) is a popular modality in pregnancy because of the lack of ionizing radiation. The classical T1- and T2-weighted images of MRI can be distinguished by considering the signal intensity of water: water has a low signal intensity ('black') on T1-weighted images while it has a high signal intensity ('white') on T2-weighted images. No contrast injection is needed for blood vessel or bile duct visualization. Image quality has improved to such a degree that MRI-cholangiography has replaced diagnostic ERCP.[13] Contrast agents (such as gadolinium) can be used to differentiate among focal liver lesions, but should be avoided during pregnancy because of transplacental transfer and unknown fetal effects.[14] More recently, diffusion-weighted imaging has been introduced allowing characterization of liver lesions, without contrast administration.[15]

Liver disorders during pregnancy

In this section we will review the most frequent liver diseases that can be encountered during pregnancy. Liver disease in pregnancy is generally separated into disorders that are unique to pregnancy and those that coincide with pregnancy. We recommend a systematic approach that focuses on the major differential diagnostic characteristics of pregnancy-related liver diseases (Table 43.2) and a limited set of tests for pregnancy-unrelated liver diseases (Box 43.1).

Pregnancy-related liver diseases

Hyperemesis gravidarum

Hyperemesis gravidarum occurs in 0.3–2% of pregnancies and is characterized by intractable vomiting in the first half of pregnancy resulting in dehydration, electrolyte imbalance, weight loss, and ketosis.[16–18] Thiamine deficiency may lead to a superimposed Wernicke's encephalopathy. The aetiology is poorly understood and likely involves a combination of hormonal, genetic, and immunological factors. Serum ALT and AST are usually mildly elevated, but levels up to 20 times the ULN have been reported. Jaundice is uncommon and there is no risk of liver failure. Liver biopsy is not indicated but when performed shows focal necrosis, steatosis, or bile-plugs. Therapy involves frequent small low-fat meals, intravenous fluids, thiamine and folate supplementation, and antiemetic medication. Liver test abnormalities usually return to normal levels within a few days of volume expansion and the cessation of vomiting. Persistently elevated transaminases are indicative of an alternative diagnosis such as acute viral hepatitis. Other pregnancy-related conditions such as acute fatty liver of pregnancy (AFLP) and the haemolysis, elevated liver enzymes, and low platelets (HELLP) syndrome typically present in the third trimester of pregnancy and are as such easily distinguished from hyperemesis gravidarum.

Intrahepatic cholestasis of pregnancy

Intrahepatic cholestasis of pregnancy (ICP) is characterized by generalized pruritus (particularly affecting soles and palms and worse at night) and high fasting serum bile acid levels (>10 µmol/L) in the late second or third trimester.[17,18] Mild jaundice (serum bilirubin < 5 mg/dL) is present in 10–25% of women and appears 1–4 weeks after the start of pruritus.[16,17] Aminotransferase levels may be normal to mildly elevated with levels 10–20 times the ULN in rare cases. There is no evolution to liver failure. Diagnosis is made based on these clinical and biochemical findings. Liver ultrasound shows no dilated bile ducts. A liver biopsy may show signs of cholestasis and inflammatory changes, but is not required for the diagnosis. The incidence of ICP varies among different geographic areas and populations: from less than 0.5% in the United States and Australia, to 10-16% in Chile and Scandinavia. The condition is associated with a relatively high rate of fetal morbidity, due to premature birth and meconium-stained amniotic fluid and intrauterine fetal death (0.4–1.6%) from fetal anoxia.[16] The risk of adverse fetal outcome appears to increase with increasing bile acid levels, especially once a level of greater than 40 µmol/L is reached.[19]

Prognosis for the mother is good, despite the pruritus and an increased risk for postpartum haemorrhage (because of cholestasis-induced vitamin K malabsorption). The rapid and complete recovery following delivery (within 2 weeks) is a typical feature. Risk factors include multiparity, advancing maternal age, and multiple gestation and recurrence rates are high. Women with

Table 43.2 Major differential diagnostic characteristics of pregnancy-related liver diseases in the second half of pregnancy

	Intrahepatic cholestasis of pregnancy	Acute fatty liver of pregnancy	HELLP syndrome
Trimester	(2)–3	3	(2)–3
Symptoms	Pruritus	Malaise—fatigue—vomiting	Abdominal pain
Jaundice (bilirubin)	<5 mg/dL	Variable, >5 mg/day severe cases	Rare, and if present <5 mg/dL
Liver failure	No	Yes	No
Hypoglycaemia	No	Yes	No
Mental status	Normal	HE (NH_3↑)	Headache, seizures,
Cause ↑ PT	Low vitamin K	Liver dysfunction	DIC
Thrombocytopenia	No	No	Per definition
↑ Transaminases	Variable, 2–20 × ULN	Variable, up to 10 × ULN	Per definition, up to 10 × ULN
Haemolysis	No	No	Per definition
Arterial hypertension	No	25–50%	85%
Imaging	Normal	Fatty changes	Hepatic infarction, haematoma
Liver histology	Cholestasis, limited inflammation	Microvesicular steatosis (zone 3)	Patchy necrosis, sinusoidal thrombi and haemorrhage

DIC, disseminated intravascular coagulation; HE, hepatic encephalopathy; HELLP, haemolysis-elevated liver enzymes-low platelets; PT, prothrombin time; ULN, upper limit of normal.

Adapted with permission from Hay JE., Liver disease in pregnancy, *Hepatology*, Volume 47, pp. 1067–76, Copyright © 2008 John Wiley & Sons. Adapted from *The Lancet*, Volume 375, issue 9714, Deepak Joshi, Andra James, Alberto Quaglia, Rachel H Westbrook, Michael A Heneghan, Liver disease in pregnancy, pp. 594–605, Copyright (2010), with permission from Elsevier.

Box 43.1 Non-invasive evaluation of patients with clinical or biochemical suspicion of liver disease

1. **Clinical history (medication!) and physical examination**
2. **Liver disease**

- Hepatobiliary imaging: liver ultrasound (or if in doubt MRI)
- Liver synthetic and excretory function: prothrombin time, albumin, bilirubin
- Specific tests:
  a. Viral hepatitis A*, B, C, D, E* and CMV*, HSV*, EBV*
  b. Autoimmune disease: antinuclear antibody, antimitochondrial antibody, smooth muscle cell antibody; liver-kidney microsomal antibodies; immunoglobulins
  c. α-1-antitrypsin deficiency: protein electrophoresis (genetic testing)
  d. Wilson's disease: serum ceruloplasmin, urinary copper excretion

3. **Excluding non-hepatic causes of elevated aminotransferases**

- Thyroid disorders: TSH
- Coeliac disease: tissue transglutaminase antibodies
- Muscle pathology: creatine kinase

*Only relevant to test in case of markedly elevated AST and ALT levels (>10 × ULN).

a history of ICP have more gallstone-related disease (pancreatitis, cholecystitis) and cholestasis due to oral contraceptive use.

The pathogenesis of the disease is only partially understood. Hormonal changes in oestrogen and progesterone metabolites, together with genetically determined mutations in bile transporter proteins, such as multidrug resistance glycoprotein 3 (MDR3) and bile salt export pump (BSEP) play a role.[20] The link between high bile salt concentrations and fetal morbidity is possibly related to induction of myometrial contractions and placental vasoconstriction.[17]

Intrahepatic cholestasis of pregnancy is associated with an approximately 1% risk of fetal death that occurs at a median gestational age of 38 weeks.[16] Delivery at 37–38 weeks is therefore commonly performed to minimize perinatal morbidity and mortality.[21] Fetal monitoring is recommended despite the inability to prevent cases of sudden fetal death. Ursodeoxycholic acid (UDCA) is considered the drug of choice for the treatment of ICP. In a double-blind, placebo-controlled study, 130 Swedish women with ICP were randomized to UDCA (1 g/day, 3 weeks) or dexamethasone (12 mg/day, 1 week). The patients that were treated with UDCA had significant improvement of pruritus and biochemical parameters of cholestasis.[22] There was no difference in fetal complications, but this may be due to the small group of patients (N = 34) with bile salt levels greater than 40 μmol/L. A management proposal for women with ICP, as followed in the University Hospitals Leuven (Belgium), is given in Figure 43.1.

'Haemolysis, elevated liver enzymes, low platelets' (HELLP syndrome)

HELLP syndrome occurs in 0.5–0.9% of pregnancies and in about 70% of the cases before delivery with a peak frequency between the 27th and 37th gestational weeks (see Chapter 36 and Chapter 48 for more detailed information).[23] It is considered the hepatic manifestation of preeclampsia. However, in 20% of cases there are no signs of (pre-)eclampsia, and HELLP is more often seen in older Caucasian multiparous women.[24] HELLP is thought to result from an acute rejection of the fetal allograft and the clinical picture is a reflection of a microangiopathic haemolytic anaemia with platelet consumption and fibrin degradation. The liver damage resembles a sinusoidal obstruction syndrome (previously called veno-occlusive disease) with reduction of liver blood flow,[25] and liver ischaemia.

By definition, the transaminases are variably elevated (up to ten times ULN), platelets drop in severe cases below 50,000/μL and there are signs of haemolysis (abnormalities in blood smear with contracted or fragmented red blood cells, anaemia, rise in serum lactate dehydrogenase (LDH), low haptoglobin, increased reticulocytes, and moderately elevated indirect bilirubin (<5 mg/dL)).[23] Two classifications for HELLP syndrome have been put forward. The Tennessee System classification is based on the following parameters: AST greater than 70 IU/L, LDH greater than 600 IU/L and platelets less than 100,000/μl. Accordingly, there are two forms: complete (all elements present) and partial HELLP syndrome (one or two elements present).[24] The Mississippi classification relies on the nadir of platelet counts: class I (<50,000/μL), class II (50,000–100,000/μL), and class III (100,000–150,000/μL).[26]

The combination of upper abdominal pain, 'malaise', nausea, and vomiting in the third trimester or postpartum (up to 8 days), should alert the physician. Approximately 80% of patients demonstrate signs of (pre-)eclampsia (hypertension and proteinuria). Liver imaging may show intrahepatic haemorrhage, subcapsular haematoma, or haemoperitoneum due to hepatic rupture (occurring in 1–2% of patients with HELLP).[27] Other serious maternal complications include placental abruption, disseminated intravascular coagulation (DIC), renal failure, and pulmonary oedema with variable maternal and especially fetal mortality ranging from 8% to 80%.[28,29] Interestingly, in women with postpartum HELLP syndrome, the risk of renal failure and pulmonary oedema is significantly increased compared to those with an antenatal onset.[30]

Most neonates born from a woman with HELLP have a normal long-term development. Prematurity at delivery is the main problem rather than HELLP in itself.[23]

The management of the patient with HELLP is similar to that applied for severe pre-eclampsia (control of hypertension, fetal monitoring, and seizure prophylaxis) and urgent delivery is needed. Severe maternal complications are more frequent when the induction of pregnancy is delayed. At a gestational age between 24–34 weeks and a stable maternal condition, corticosteroids are advocated to accelerate fetal pulmonary maturity. A randomized, double-blind, placebo-controlled study of high-dose dexamethasone included 132 women with the HELLP syndrome (60 patients with HELLP occurring in pregnancy and 72 after delivery).[31] Dexamethasone treatment did not reduce maternal complications (such as acute kidney injury, pulmonary oedema, and oliguria). There was no statistically significant difference between dexamethasone-treated and placebo-treated patients with respect to the time that was required to achieve a platelet count of greater than 100,000/mm^3. The rates of platelets and fresh frozen plasma transfusions were not significantly

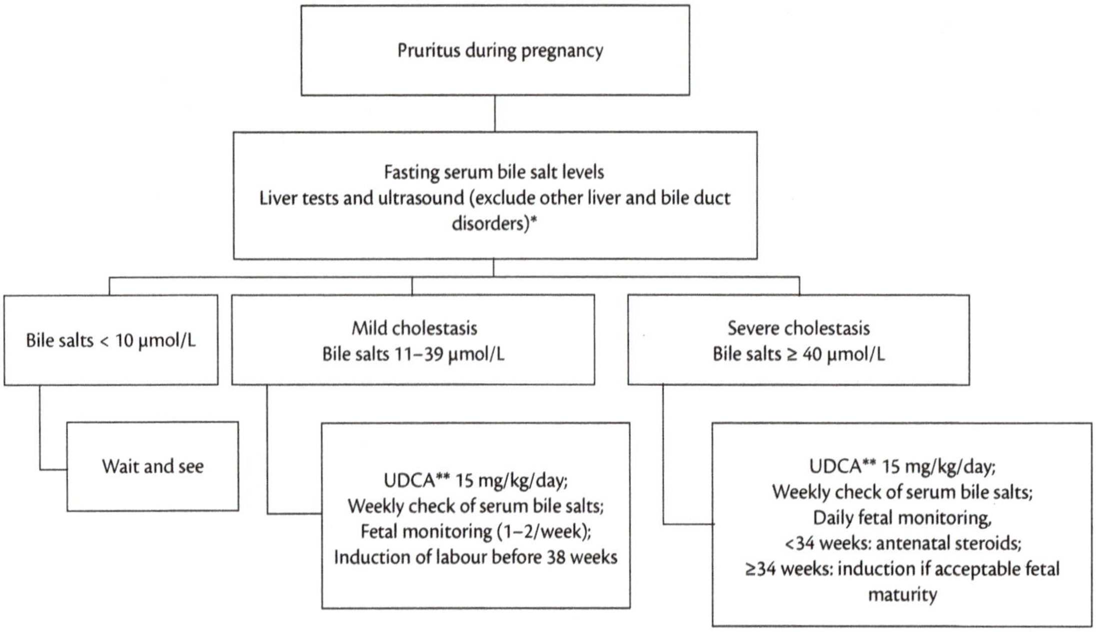

Figure 43.1 Management algorithm for women with intrahepatic cholestasis of pregnancy, used at the University Hospital Leuven, Belgium.
*See Box 43.1; **UCDA: ursodeoxycholic acid.

reduced, nor was the time of recovery of laboratory test shortened, or the duration of hospital stay.[31]

The rupture of a subcapsular liver haematoma represents a surgical emergency (packing with gauze is preferable to lobectomy). Other options include arterial ligation, selective arterial embolization, or even liver transplantation.[23]

Acute fatty liver of pregnancy

AFLP affects approximately 5/100,000 pregnancies and is associated with a 1–2% maternal and 10% perinatal mortality rate in the Western world.[32] Mothers with twin pregnancies are at greater risk. AFLP is caused by a defect in mitochondrial beta-oxidation and in up to 20% of cases a deficiency of the long-chain 3-hydroxyacyl-coenzyme A-dehydrogenase (L-CHAD syndrome) can be identified in the fetus which is usually male. The transfer of non-oxidated long-chain fatty acids from the fetus is most likely the cause of toxic liver damage of the mother. The characteristic microscopic alteration is microvesicular steatosis.[33] Patients usually present in the third trimester and may exhibit acute liver failure with hepatic encephalopathy, jaundice, marked elevation of transaminases, prolonged prothrombin time, and hypoglycaemia. The differential diagnosis includes acute viral hepatitis and HELLP syndrome (Table 43.2). The liver may have a bright appearance on ultrasound imaging, but this is not conclusive as nearly 20% of the general population has a fatty liver nowadays (see below). Management of AFLP involves intensive supportive care and prompt delivery. The clinical condition may deteriorate further within the first 48 hours following delivery and liver transplantation may be indicated in the absence of liver regeneration.[16] According to a retrospective evaluation of 54 admissions with pregnancy-related liver disease, the classical King's College criteria of acute liver failure were not effective in predicting outcome. Instead, a serum lactate of at least 2.8 mg/dL and the presence of encephalopathy had sensitivity of 90% and a specificity of 86% to predict liver transplantation or death.[34]

Following delivery, a rapid reversal of the clinical condition is expected, with no long-term sequelae. The risk of recurrence in future pregnancies is difficult to predict and genetic counselling of the newborn and parents should be offered.

Liver diseases unrelated to pregnancy

Several viruses may induce hepatitis. The natural history of the disease is dependent upon the host's immune response to the virus. Most cases of acute hepatitis are characterized by malaise, nausea, anorexia, and vomiting. Jaundice and marked elevation of transaminases may develop. The occurrence of hepatic encephalopathy and prolongation of prothrombin time are indicative of acute liver failure. Several viruses (e.g. hepatitis A (HAV) and E (HEV), herpes simplex, cytomegalovirus, and Epstein–Barr viruses) that usually cause an acute self-limited hepatitis may occasionally result in acute liver failure.

Infections with hepatitis B, C, or D (HBV, HCV or HDV) may run a chronic course and the viral genome can be detected in the serum more than 6 months after infection. Most of these patients are asymptomatic, and are only diagnosed after detection of liver tests abnormalities. A longstanding infection can induce cirrhosis, which includes marked fibrosis, nodular regeneration, vascular shunt formation, and clinically significant portal hypertension. In addition to viruses, the pregnant women may develop autoimmune, drug-induced (including toxins) or metabolic liver disease.

Hepatitis A

HAV is transmitted via the faecal–oral route and complicates 1/1000 pregnancies. Diagnosis is made by detection of anti-HAV immunoglobulin M. The clinical presentation and disease course are similar to non-pregnant patients. Acute hepatitis A in the third trimester of pregnancy is associated with preterm labour in approximately 60% of patients.[18,35] In case of acute liver failure, liver transplantation may be indicated. Perinatal HAV transmission is uncommon and most cases remain subclinical. A safe and effective vaccine against HAV is available. After birth, children of mothers with hepatitis A in the last trimester should receive the vaccine and some experts also recommend administration of immunoglobulin.

Hepatitis B and delta

HBV is highly infectious and transmitted parenterally by percutaneous or mucosal exposure, sexually, and from mother to infant. The clinical presentation and course of the disease are similar to non-pregnant infected individuals. Diagnosis of HBV infection is made by detection of hepatitis B surface antigen (HbsAg) in the serum. It is difficult to determine, in the absence of previous serology, if a patient acquired a new infection or has a flare of chronic hepatitis B. Although intrauterine infection has been reported, the intrapartum period is the time of greatest risk. Women with a high HBV viral load or those positive for the hepatitis B e antigen have an 80–90% chance of transmitting the virus to their infant.[17,18] Perinatal infection commonly progresses to chronic infection in the offspring, which is associated with an increased risk of cirrhosis and liver cancer. Because of the risk of vertical transmission, HbsAg status should be assessed early in pregnancy and unimmunized high-risk patients should be vaccinated, even during pregnancy. Administration of HBV human immune globulin and the HBV vaccine within 12 hours of birth to all neonates born to HbsAg positive women reduces the vertical transmission rate by 85–95%.[36] The use of antiviral drugs such as lamivudine or tenofovir during the third trimester in women with a high viral load appears to be safe during pregnancy and may further reduce the risk of vertical transmission.[16,36,37] There is no consensus concerning the cut-off of high viral load in this setting, but the risk of transmission seems very high if more than 10^8 copies/mL are present. The vertical transmission rate does not appear to be affected by mode of delivery or breastfeeding.

Hepatitis delta is dependent upon the presence of HBV for replication. The diagnosis of HDV is established by serological testing. Vertical transmission is possible but preventable by using the measures to prevent HBV infection.

Hepatitis C

HCV is transmitted through the parenteral route and is nowadays mainly a disease of intravenous drug users and men who have sex with men. Following a mostly asymptomatic acute infection, more than 80% of patients will develop chronic hepatitis and are at risk for developing cirrhosis or primary liver cancer over the following two to three decades. The incidence of chronic HCV infection in pregnant women is similar to that of the general population and ranges from less than 1% to 2.4%.[16,37] Screening for HCV exposure is performed by screening for HCV antibodies. Diagnosis of HCV infection is confirmed by the detection of HCV-RNA in the serum. The antibodies that are detectable are not protective and no effective vaccine is available. Transaminase activity levels may fall in the second half of pregnancy with a concurrent rise in serum HCV-RNA levels, but this is not clinically significant. Women with chronic HCV infection usually experience an uneventful pregnancy except when advanced fibrosis and portal hypertension are present.

Unlike HBV infection, vertical transmission of HCV is generally below 10%. Factors that increase this risk include co-infection with HIV, high viral load (>10^6 copies/mL) and membrane rupture greater than 6 hours.[16] Risk of transmission is unaffected by mode of delivery or breastfeeding. The presence of serum HCV-RNA at 6 months of age is indicative of congenital HCV infection. Vertically acquired neonatal HCV infection usually manifests as mild liver disease though spontaneous clearance later on is possible. Antiviral therapy is generally postponed until young adulthood. Current antiviral therapy for HCV includes interferon and ribavirin, which are contraindicated during pregnancy (Table 43.3). There are no new data yet on the newer direct acting antiviral agents.

Hepatitis E

HEV is endemic to large areas of Africa, Asia, and Central America and shares the same faecal–oral transmission route as HAV. Sporadic cases are increasingly diagnosed in developed countries. Pregnant women are especially susceptible to this viral infection and HEV infection during the last two trimesters of pregnancy is associated with a 60% risk of fulminant hepatic failure, resulting in high maternal (41–54%) and fetal (69%) mortality rates.[18,38] Delivery does not affect maternal outcome and there is no therapy to prevent transmission. HEV vaccines are under development.

Herpes simplex virus hepatitis

Pregnancy increases susceptibility to herpes simplex virus (HSV) hepatitis, which is otherwise rarely seen in adults. Maternal and neonatal mortality rates may be as high as 40%. Mucocutaneous lesions are not always present. High transaminase values and coagulopathy in the absence of jaundice ('anicteric' hepatitis) should raise suspicion of HSV hepatitis, for which intravenous therapy with aciclovir is effective.[39]

Autoimmune hepatitis

Autoimmune hepatitis (AIH) has a prevalence of 0.1–1.2 cases/100,000 in the Caucasian population. The clinical manifestations of this condition vary widely and include asymptomatic patients, those with acute fulminant hepatitis and those with chronic hepatitis and cirrhosis. Although AIH is typically associated with infertility, a patient with well-controlled disease and even cirrhosis can become pregnant. AIH is classically treated with corticosteroids as induction therapy and azathioprine in maintenance. More recently, budesonide was shown to control the disease with less systemic side effects than dexamethasone. Autoimmune hepatitis tends to run a highly variable course in pregnancy. Postpartum flares are common (in at least 30% of patients), which is similar to other autoimmune conditions. The risk of fetal loss, preterm birth, and fetal growth restriction appears to be increased in women with AIH. However, successful pregnancy outcome is anticipated in women with well-controlled disease.[40–42] Treatment commonly consists of corticosteroids and/or azathioprine. Corticosteroids are considered safe during pregnancy. Azathioprine (US Food and Drug Administration (FDA) pregnancy category D) may be associated with fetal growth restriction and preterm birth, but teratogenic effects have not been documented.[43] In a recent series of 53 women with 81 pregnancies, flares in AIH were more likely in patients who were not on therapy or who had a disease flare in the year prior to conception.[44]

In patients with cholestatic autoimmune liver diseases, such as primary sclerosing cholangitis (PSC) or primary biliary cirrhosis, limited data are available concerning pregnancy outcome.[45] In patients with PSC, concomitant inflammatory bowel disease may pose specific problems that are out of the scope of this review. For

Table 43.3 Indication and safety of drugs for liver disease during pregnancy

Medication	FDA category	Indication	Remarks	Breastfeeding
Prednisone	C	Autoimmune hepatitis, post-liver transplantation	Safe	No, except low dose
Azathioprine	D		Safe	No
Ciclosporin	C		Safe	No
Tacrolimus	C		Safe	No
Mycophenolate mofetil	D		Not recommended, limited data	
Everolimus				
Ursodeoxycholic acid	B	Intrahepatic cholestasis of pregnancy (ICP)	Indicated for ICP and safe	Yes
Lamivudine	C	HBV	Safe	No
Entecavir	C	HBV	Not recommended	No
Tenofovir	B	HBV	Safe	No
Interferon	C	HBV, HCV	Not recommended, high dose may induce abortion	No
Ribavirin	X	HCV	Contraindicated, fetal toxicity	Unknown
Penicillamine	D	Wilson's disease	Embryopathy, but need to continue therapy	No
Zinc	C		Safe	Yes
Beta blockade	C/D Depending on agent	Oesophageal varices	Risk of fetal bradycardia and intrauterine growth retardation, but necessary to prevent variceal bleeding	Yes
Terlipressin	X	Variceal bleeding	Contraindicated, uterine ischaemia	No data

Adapted with permission from Hay JE., Liver disease in pregnancy, *Hepatology*, Volume 47, pp. 1067–76, Copyright © 2008 John Wiley & Sons.

both diseases, UDCA is a standard treatment and is safe during pregnancy.

Non-alcoholic fatty liver disease

Non-alcoholic fatty liver disease (NAFLD) is becoming the most frequent liver disease in the Western world, with a prevalence of at least 20% in unselected populations.[46,47] NAFLD is a spectrum of liver disease, ranging from steatosis to steatohepatitis, with advanced fibrosis and eventually cirrhosis. NAFLD is the hepatic manifestation of the metabolic syndrome that includes obesity, arterial hypertension, hyperlipidaemia, and type 2 diabetes mellitus. The influx of free fatty acids together with insulin resistance on a susceptible genetic background is a possible mechanism, but the pathogenesis remains poorly understood.[48] Patients may remain asymptomatic for decades. The diagnosis is made by the combination of abnormal liver tests (typically with the ALT:AST ratio > 2:1), the suggestion of liver steatosis on imaging, and (rarely) a liver biopsy. The histological findings are similar to alcoholic liver disease, and therefore the differential diagnosis can only be made in patients who abstain from alcohol. Therapy includes control of the components of the metabolic syndrome and lifestyle changes. Despite the supposed high prevalence of NAFLD in the general population, there are virtually no data in the literature concerning NAFLD and pregnancy.[49] Despite the lack of data, an increased risk of pre-eclampsia is expected in women with NAFLD due to the associated comorbidities such as obesity and hypertension.

Hepatic vein thrombosis (Budd–Chiari syndrome)

Pregnancy, along with other hypercoagulable states (i.e. myeloproliferative disorders and inherited thrombophilia), are risk factors for the rare condition of hepatic vein thrombosis.[50] The clinical picture is dependent upon the number of veins involved. Prognosis is poor in patients with painful hepatomegaly, jaundice, and marked ascites. Therapy consists of low molecular weight heparin and the timely placement of a transjugular portosystemic shunt to decompress the liver. Liver transplantation may be indicated in case of overt liver failure.

Treatment in pregnancy involves anticoagulation (low molecular weight heparins in the therapeutic dose as given outside pregnancy), though thrombosis may occur despite therapy. Maternal outcome is generally favourable but an increased rate of miscarriage and preterm delivery has been reported.[51]

Wilson's disease

Wilson's disease is a rare autosomal recessive disorder of copper metabolism characterized by deposition of excess copper in the liver, brain, and kidney. Patients may present with jaundice, elevated transaminases, and haemolytic anaemia, which may be mistaken for HELLP syndrome.

Pregnant patients should continue anticopper therapy throughout pregnancy to prevent disease flare and acute liver failure. The dose of penicillamine, an FDA category D medication, should be decreased by 25–50% in pregnancy.[52] The authors demonstrated an excellent outcome of 12 pregnancies in patients with Wilson's disease who received D-penicillamine.[53] Zinc appears to be a safe and effective alternative.[54]

Drug-induced liver disease, including alcohol

The liver is susceptible to damage by drugs and toxins as it has an important role in metabolizing xenobiotics. The degree of drug-induced liver injury (DILI) can vary from mild transient elevation of liver tests to severe injury and acute failure. Hepatotoxicity is a result of multiple factors and is difficult to predict. Few drugs that cause DILI have a predictable, dose-dependent toxic mechanism of action, the most widely recognized being acetaminophen/paracetamol. When acetaminophen/paracetamol overdose is excluded, most cases of DILI are due to rare, unpredictable reactions to commonly used drugs.[55] The drug itself or its metabolite may be inherently hepatotoxic. The level of exposure, environmental factors, and genetic factors play a role in hepatotoxicity. During pregnancy, the liver remains vulnerable to these toxic drug reactions. Catastrophic cases of DILI have been reported in pregnancy, even with drugs that were presumed 'safe' in pregnancy.[56]

Ethanol ingestion in pregnancy may be associated with dangerous consequences for mother and child. In non-pregnant women, the intake of more than 2 units a day and especially binge drinking, is associated with many health risks, including but not limited to liver disease. The histologic liver changes caused by alcohol are similar to those seen with NAFLD. In contrast with NAFLD, patients with acute alcoholic hepatitis (without cirrhosis) may present with the clinical picture of acute liver failure (marked jaundice, prolonged prothrombin time, encephalopathy, portal hypertension, and moderately elevated serum transaminases), with a high risk of death (up to 50%). The pathogenesis of liver disease relates to ethanol metabolism with generation of acetaldehyde that is highly toxic because of the formation of protein and DNA adducts that promote glutathione depletion, lipid peroxidation, and mitochondrial damage.[57]

Alcohol ingestion may have several negative effects on pregnancy. The age-adjusted relative risk of second-trimester spontaneous abortions (15–27 weeks) was 1.03 (non-significant), 1.98 ($P < 0.01$), and 3.53 ($P < 0.01$) for women taking less than 1, 1–2, and more than 3 units daily, compared with non-drinkers.[58] Alcohol exposure in pregnancy may lead to fetal alcohol spectrum disorder that includes craniofacial, cardiac, growth, and behavioural abnormalities. Fetal injury may occur with alcohol exposure at any time in pregnancy, though the risk of birth defects is highest with first trimester consumption. Abstinence from alcohol is recommended during pregnancy because a safe level of consumption has not been determined.[59]

Clinically significant portal hypertension during pregnancy

Portal hypertension may arise in the context of liver disease (most often cirrhosis due to various causes discussed earlier) or in non-cirrhotic cases (most often due to portal vein thrombosis). Fertility is unaffected in women with non-cirrhotic portal hypertension. Cirrhosis is associated with a high incidence of amenorrhea, making pregnancy less likely to occur.[60] The spontaneous abortion rate can be as high as 40% of pregnancies in women with cirrhosis.

Clinically significant portal hypertension is defined by the presence of oesophagogastric varices and/or ascites that correlate with an invasively measured hepatic venous pressure gradient of greater than 10 mmHg. The increased blood volume that occurs during pregnancy may worsen portal hypertension and increase the risk of variceal bleeding, which develops in 20–25% of patients.[16] Pregnancy outcome in women with cirrhosis and portal hypertension is variable. Fetal and maternal mortality rates up to 50% were reported in older studies. In a 2011 retrospective series of 62 pregnancies in 29 women with cirrhosis, maternal complications (ascites, encephalopathy, or variceal haemorrhage) occurred in 10% of patients and one mother died.[34] The reduction in complications in recent studies is likely due to the implementation of evidence-based treatments, such as the use of non-selective beta blockers propranolol and/or endoscopic band ligation of the varices. Mortality rates are higher in cirrhotic (10–50%) than non-cirrhotic patients (<10%).[61]

The existing prognostic models of cirrhosis severity are useful in determining outcomes in pregnant women with cirrhosis. Higher MELD and Child–Pugh scores (discussed in 'Liver Function Scoring Systems') are associated with poorer outcomes for mother and newborn. In the study of Westbrook,[34] a MELD score at the time of conception of 10 or higher predicted, with 83% sensitivity and 83% specificity, which patients were likely to have significant, liver-related complications. No patient who had a MELD score of 6 or below at the time of conception developed significant hepatological complications. Women with a MELD score of 10 or more should be advised against pregnancy.

Every patient with suspicion of cirrhotic or non-cirrhotic portal hypertension (history of liver disease and upper gastrointestinal bleeding, imaging suggestive of cirrhosis, and low platelets) who considers pregnancy should undergo upper endoscopy to identify varices. During pregnancy, the best timing of gastroscopy would be the second trimester. Primary prophylaxis with a non-selective beta blocker may be indicated. In case of intolerance to beta blockers or if gastrointestinal bleeding does occur during pregnancy, urgent endoscopic ligation of the varices is indicated.[62] The administration of vasoactive drugs like terlipressin is contraindicated because of uterine ischaemia and ischaemia of fetal digits (see Table 43.3).

In patients with known varices on a stable regimen of beta blockers before pregnancy, the role of repeated endoscopy during pregnancy is unknown. Interruption of beta blockers may be associated with rebound portal hypertension, so continuation of beta blockers during pregnancy (including labour) is mandatory.

Patients with portal hypertension may have significant varicose veins on the abdominal wall and in the epidural space.[63] Visualization of these collaterals by MRI may minimize the risk of neuraxial anaesthesia or caesarean delivery (Figure 43.2). An additional reason to perform an MRI in pregnant patients with portal hypertension is to look for splenic artery aneurysms. These vascular abnormalities are prone to rupture during the third trimester resulting in high fetal and maternal mortality rates.[64] Preconceptional screening and treatment (coiling) of splenic aneurysms in patients with known portal hypertension is recommended.[65]

Operative vaginal delivery following passive fetal descent is suggested to avoid Valsalva and minimize the risk of variceal bleeding.

Special situations

Pregnancy in women after liver transplantation

Nearly 90% of women of child-bearing age return to a fertile state by 7 months after liver transplantation. Women are generally

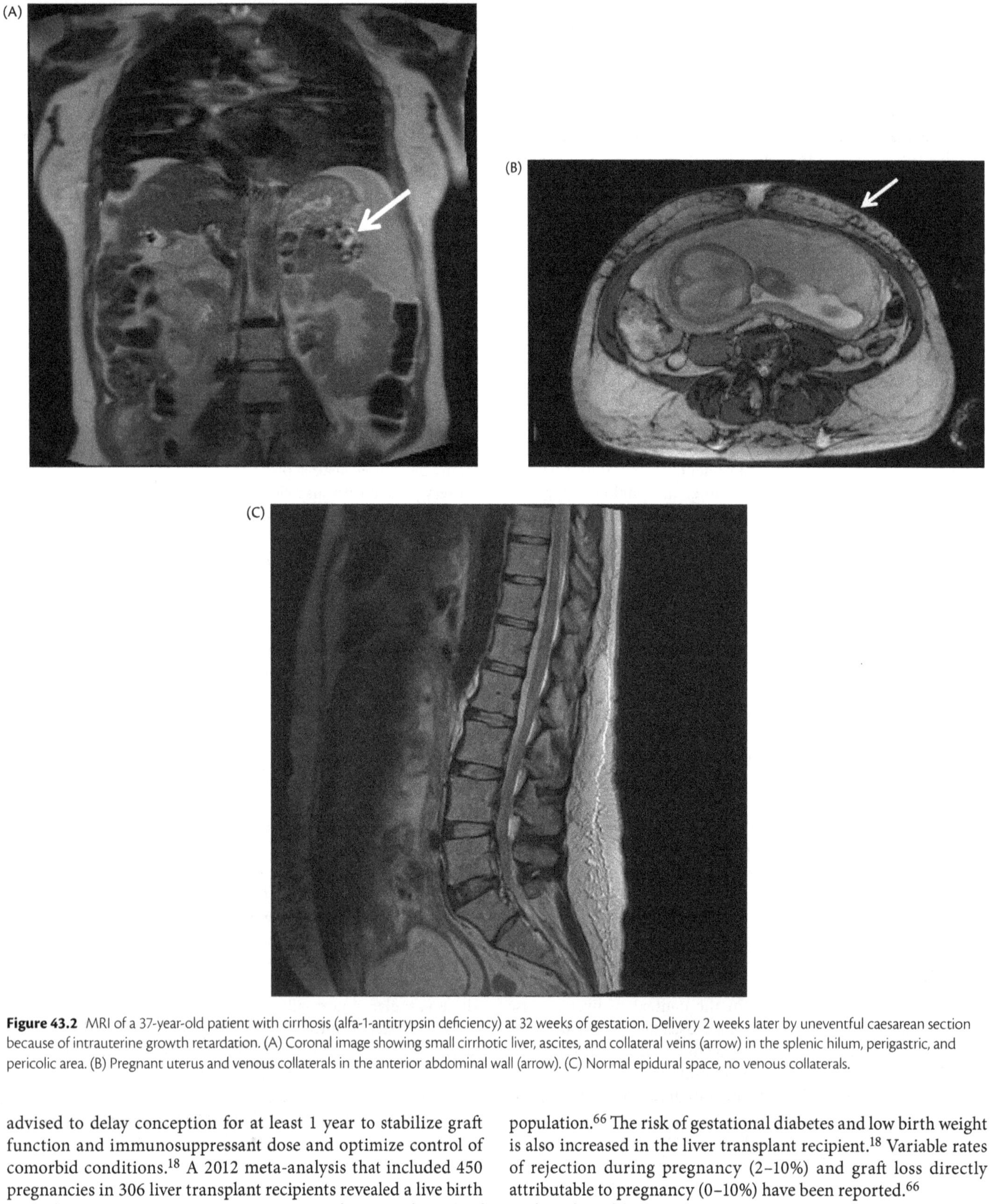

Figure 43.2 MRI of a 37-year-old patient with cirrhosis (alfa-1-antitrypsin deficiency) at 32 weeks of gestation. Delivery 2 weeks later by uneventful caesarean section because of intrauterine growth retardation. (A) Coronal image showing small cirrhotic liver, ascites, and collateral veins (arrow) in the splenic hilum, perigastric, and pericolic area. (B) Pregnant uterus and venous collaterals in the anterior abdominal wall (arrow). (C) Normal epidural space, no venous collaterals.

advised to delay conception for at least 1 year to stabilize graft function and immunosuppressant dose and optimize control of comorbid conditions.[18] A 2012 meta-analysis that included 450 pregnancies in 306 liver transplant recipients revealed a live birth rate of nearly 77% and a miscarriage rate of 15.6%. The risk of pre-eclampsia (21.9%), preterm delivery (39.4%), and caesarean delivery (44.6%) were increased compared to the general US population.[66] The risk of gestational diabetes and low birth weight is also increased in the liver transplant recipient.[18] Variable rates of rejection during pregnancy (2–10%) and graft loss directly attributable to pregnancy (0–10%) have been reported.[66]

The safety of the immunosuppressive drugs is given in Table 43.3. Most data are available for corticosteroids, azathioprine, ciclosporin, and tacrolimus-based regimens. Mycophenolate mofetil and everolimus should be avoided in pregnancy. Breastfeeding is contraindicated in women taking immunosuppressant drugs.

Hepatocellular adenomas and bleeding risk

Hepatocellular adenomas (HCAs) are a rare but important problem. Some HCAs have a tendency for malignant transformation, but during pregnancy life-threatening bleeding is the major concern. The lesion typically develops in women and most often in long-term oral contraceptive users. The yearly incidence has been estimated in (older) case–control studies to be less than 5/100,000 long-term (>5 years) oral contraceptive users.

HCAs arise in a normal liver while a similar lesion in a cirrhotic liver is called a regenerative or dysplastic nodule.[67] Studies that correlate lesional genotype with phenotype form the basis of a new histological/molecular classification of hepatocellular adenomas. Based on molecular criteria (hepatocyte nuclear factor-1α and β-catenin mutations) and histological criteria (the presence/absence of inflammation, cytological and architectural atypia, steatosis, sinusoidal congestion, and mild ductular reaction), subgroups of hepatocellular adenoma can be defined with variable risks of bleeding and malignant transformation.

The occurrence of haemorrhage seems to cluster with the inflammatory HCA.[68] There are two types of haemorrhage: internal bleeding usually admixed with necrotic changes (this type is mostly observed in adenomas > 4 cm) and spontaneous rupture that causes subcapsular haematoma and possible haemoperitoneum. The diameter of bleeding adenomas in the literature varies between 6.5 and 19 cm. These tumours are prone to bleed in the third trimester, but one-third rupture in the postpartum period. Mortality rates of 44% and 38% respectively for mother and fetus have been described, when rupture occurred during pregnancy.[69] Other benign lesions, such as focal nodular hyperplasia or haemangiomas have no bleeding risk.

Preconceptional detection of an HCA by ultrasound, contrast-enhanced CT, and especially MRI allow for a specific diagnosis. Resection of an HCA before pregnancy is necessary with large (≥4–5 cm) tumours or when there are factors that suggest malignant transformation such as rapid growth, change in radiological characteristics or elevated serum alpha-fetoprotein. HCAs that are discovered during pregnancy should be followed by ultrasound at monthly intervals and should be treated according to the criteria above after multidisciplinary discussion.

Conclusion

The management of liver disease during pregnancy requires a multidisciplinary collaboration between obstetrician, hepatologist, anaesthetist, and neonatologist in order to optimize outcome for mother and child. Interpretation of abnormal liver tests in pregnancy may be difficult, given the normal physiological changes that occur in this condition. The timely recognition of cholestasis, clinically significant portal hypertension, and liver failure is essential to minimize fetal and maternal morbidity and mortality. The differentiation of diseases related or unrelated to pregnancy is important and determines management.

References

1. Scott DB, Kerr MG. Inferior vena caval pressure in late pregnancy. *J Obstet Gynaecol Br Commonw* 1963; 70:1044–9.
2. Britton RC. Pregnancy and esophageal varices. *Am J Surg* 1982; 143:421–5.
3. Bean WB, Cogswell R, Dexter M, *et al.* Vascular changes of the skin in pregnancy: vascular spiders and palmar erythema. *Surg Gynecol Obstet* 1949; 88:739–52.
4. Perez V, Gorodisch S, Casavilla F, *et al.* Ultrastructure of human liver at the end of normal pregnancy. *Am J Obstet Gynecol* 1971; 110:428–31.
5. Pratt DS, Kaplan MM. Evaluation of abnormal liver-enzyme results in asymptomatic patients. *N Engl J Med* 2000; 342:1266–71.
6. Kuntz E. Laboratory diagnostics. In Kuntz E, Kuntz HD (eds) *Hepatology, Principles and Practice.* Heidelberg: Springer–Verlag; 2001:78–112.
7. Bacq Y, Zarka O, Bréchot JF, *et al.* Liver function tests in normal pregnancy: a prospective study of 103 pregnant women and 103 matched controls. *Hepatology* 1996: 23:1030–4.
8. Meade BW, Rosalki SB. Serum enzyme activity in normal pregnancy and the newborn. *J Obstet Gynaecol* 1963; 70:693–700.
9. David AL, Kotecha M, Girling JC. Factors influencing postnatal liver function tests. *BJOG* 2000; 107:1421–6.
10. Rothschild MA, Oratz M, Schreiber SS. Serum albumin. *Hepatology* 1988; 8:385–401.
11. Wiesner R, Edwards E, Freeman R, *et al.* Model for end-stage liver disease (MELD) and allocation of donor livers. *Gastroenterology* 2003; 124:91–6.
12. Sandrin L, Fourquet B, Hasquenoph JM, *et al.* Transient elastography: a new noninvasive method for assessment of hepatic fibrosis. *Ultrasound Med Biol* 2003; 29:1705–13.
13. Van Hoe L, Vanbeckevoort D, Van Steenbergen W. *Atlas of Cross-Sectional and Projective MR Cholangio-Pancreatography.* Berlin-Heidelberg: Springer-Verlag; 1999.
14. Shellock FG, Kanal E. Safety of magnetic resonance imaging contrast agents. *J Magn Reson Imaging* 1999; 10:477–84.
15. Vandecaveye V, De Keyzer F, Verslype C, *et al.* Diffusion-weighted MRI provides additional value to conventional dynamic contrast-enhanced MRI for detection of hepatocellular carcinoma. *Eur Radiol* 2009; 19:2456–66.
16. Hay JE. Liver disease in pregnancy. *Hepatology* 2008; 47:1067–76.
17. Lee N, Brady C. Liver disease in pregnancy. *World J Gastroenterol* 2009; 15:897–906.
18. Joshi D, James A, Quaglia A, *et al.* Liver disease in pregnancy. *Lancet* 2010; 375:594–605
19. Glantz A, Marschall HU, Mattsson LA. Intrahepatic cholestasis of pregnancy: relationships between bile acid levels and fetal complication rates. *Hepatology* 2004; 40:467–74.
20. Wasmuth HE, Glantz A, Keppeler H, *et al.* Intrahepatic cholestasis of pregnancy: the severe form is associated with common variants of the hepatobiliary phospholipid transporter ABCB4 gene. *Gut* 2007; 56:265–70.
21. Mays JK. The active management of intrahepatic cholestasis of pregnancy. *Curr Opin Obstet Gynecol* 2010; 22:100–3.
22. Glantz A, Marschall HU, Lammert F, *et al.* Intrahepatic cholestasis of pregnancy: a randomized controlled trial comparing dexamethasone and ursodeoxycholic acid. *Hepatology* 2005; 42:1399–405.
23. Haram K, Svendsen E, Abildgaard U. The HELLP syndrome: clinical issues and management. A review. *BMC Pregnancy Childbirth* 2009; 9:8.
24. Sibai BM, Ramadan MK, Usta I, *et al.* Maternal morbidity and mortality in 442 pregnancies with hemolysis, elevated liver enzymes, and low platelets (HELLP syndrome). *Am J Obstet Gynecol* 1993; 169:1000–6.
25. Kawabata I, Nakai A, Takeshita T. Prediction of HELLP syndrome with assessment of maternal dual hepatic blood supply by using Doppler ultrasound. *Arch Gynecol Obstet* 2006; 274:303–9.
26. Martin JN Jr, Rose CH, Briery CM. Understanding and managing HELLP syndrome: the integral role of aggressive glucocorticoids for mother and child. *Am J Obstet Gynecol* 2006; 195:914–34.

27. Wicke C, Pereira PL, Neeser E, *et al.* Subcapsular liver hematoma in HELLP syndrome: evaluation of diagnostic and therapeutic options—a unicenter study. *Am J Obstet Gynecol* 2004; 190:106–12.
28. Barton JR, Sibai BM. Diagnosis and management of hemolysis, elevated liver enzymes, and low platelets syndrome. *Clin Perinatol* 2004; 31:807–33.
29. Mihu D, Costin N, Mihu CM, *et al.* HELLP syndrome—a multisystemic disorder. *J Gastrointestin Liver Dis* 2007; 16:419–24.
30. Sibai BM, Ramadan MK. Acute renal failure in pregnancies complicated by hemolysis, elevated liver enzymes, and low platelets. *Am J Obstet Gynecol* 1993; 168:1682–7.
31. Fonseca JE, Mendez F, Catano C, *et al.* Dexamethasone treatment does not improve the outcome of women with HELLP syndrome: a double-blind, placebo-controlled, randomized clinical trial. *Am J Obstet Gynecol* 2005; 193:1591–8.
32. Knight M, Nelson-Piercy C, Kurinczuk JJ, *et al.* A prospective national study of acute fatty liver of pregnancy in the UK. *Gut* 2008; 57:951–6.
33. Rolfes DB, Ishaj KG. Liver disease in pregnancy. *Histopathology* 1986; 10:555–70.
34. Westbrook RH, Yeoman AD, O'Grady JG, *et al.* Model for end-stage liver disease score predicts outcome in cirrhotic patients during pregnancy. *Clin Gastroenterol Hepatol* 2011; 9:694–9.
35. Elinav E, Ben-Dov IZ, Shapira Y, *et al.* Acute hepatitis A infection in pregnancy is associated with high rates of gestational complications and preterm labor. *Gastroenterology* 2006; 130:1129–34.
36. Lee C, Gong Y, Brok J, *et al.* Effect of hepatitis B immunisation in newborn infants of mothers positive for hepatitis B surface antigen: systematic review and meta-analysis. *BMJ* 2006; 332:328–36.
37. Sookoian S. Liver disease during pregnancy: acute viral hepatitis. *Ann Hepatol* 2006; 5:231–6.
38. Banait VS, Sandur V, Parikh F, *et al.* Outcome of acute liver failure due to acute hepatitis E in pregnant women. *Indian J Gastroenterol* 2007; 26:6–10.
39. Kang AH, Graves CR. Herpes simplex hepatitis in pregnancy: a case report and review of the literature. *Obstet Gynecol Surv* 1999; 54:463–8.
40. Heneghan MA, Norris SM, O'Grady JG, *et al.* Management and outcome of pregnancy in autoimmune hepatitis. *Gut* 2001; 48:97–102.
41. Buchel E, Van Steenbergen W, Nevens F, *et al.* Improvement of autoimmune hepatitis during pregnancy followed by flareup after delivery. *Am J Gastroenterol* 2002; 97:3160–5.
42. Terrabuio DR, Abrantes-Lemos CP, Carrilho FJ, *et al.* Follow-up of pregnant women with autoimmune hepatitis: the disease behavior along with maternal and fetal outcomes. *J Clin Gastroenterol* 2009; 43:350–6.
43. Akbari M, Shah S, Velayos FS, *et al.* Systematic review and meta-analysis on the effects of thiopurines on birth outcomes from female and male patients with inflammatory bowel disease. *Inflamm Bowel Dis* 2013; 19(1):15–22.
44. Westbrook RH, Yeoman AD, Kriese S, *et al.* Outcomes of pregnancy in women with autoimmune hepatitis. *J Autoimmun* 2012; 38:J239–44.
45. Heathcote E. Management of primary biliary cirrhosis. *Hepatology* 2000; 31:105–13.
46. Browning JD, Szczepaniak LS, Dobbins R, *et al.* Prevalence of hepatic steatosis in an urban population in the United States: impact of ethnicity. *Hepatology* 2004; 40:1387–95.
47. Bedogni G, Miglioli L, Masutti F, *et al.* Prevalence of and risk factors for nonalcoholic fatty liver disease: the Dionysos nutrition and liver study. *Hepatology* 2005; 42:44–52.
48. Cohen JC, Horton JD, Hobbs HH. Human fatty liver disease: old questions and new insights. *Science* 2011; 24; 332:1519–23.
49. Page L, Girling J. A novel cause for abnormal liver function tests in pregnancy and the puerperium: non-alcoholic fatty liver disease. *BJOG* 2011; 118:1532–5.
50. Rautou PE, Plessier A, Bernuau J, *et al.* Pregnancy: a risk factor for Budd-Chiari syndrome? *Gut* 2009; 58:606–8.
51. Rautou PE, Angermayr B, Garcia-Pagan JC, *et al.* Pregnancy in women with known and treated Budd-Chiari syndrome: maternal and fetal outcomes. *J Hepatol* 2009; 51:47–54.
52. Roberts EA, Schilsky ML. A practice guideline on Wilson disease. *Hepatology.* 2003; 37:1475–92.
53. Lowette KF, Desmet K, Witters P, *et al.* Wilson's disease: long-term follow-up of a cohort of 24 patients treated with D-penicillamine. *Eur J Gastroenterol Hepatol* 2010; 22:564–71.
54. Brewer GJ, Johnson VD, Dick RD, *et al.* Treatment of Wilson's disease with zinc. XVII: treatment during pregnancy. *Hepatology* 2000; 31:364–70.
55. Björnsson E. Drug-induced liver injury: Hy's rule revisited. *Clin Pharmacol Ther* 2006; 79:521–8.
56. Sequeira E, Wanyonyi S, Dodia R. Severe propylthiouracil-induced hepatotoxicity in pregnancy managed successfully by liver transplantation: a case report. *J Med Case Rep* 2011; 5:461.
57. Joenje H. Metabolism: alcohol, DNA and disease. *Nature* 2011; 475:45–6.
58. Anokute CC. Epidemiology of spontaneous abortions: the effect of alcohol consumption and cigarette smoking. *Natl Med Assoc* 1996; 78:771–5.
59. de Sanctis L, Memo L, Pichini S, *et al.* Fetal alcohol syndrome: new perspectives for an ancient and underestimated problem. *J Matern Fetal Neonatal Med* 2011; 24 Suppl 1:34–7.
60. Cundy TF, O'Grady JG, Williams R. Recovery of menstruation and pregnancy after liver transplantation. *Gut* 1990; 31:337–8.
61. Kochhar R, Kumar S, Goel RC, *et al.* Pregnancy and its outcome in patients with noncirrhotic portal hypertension. *Dig Dis Sci* 1999; 44:1356–61.
62. Starkel P, Horsmans Y, Geubel A. Endoscopic band ligation: a safe technique to control bleeding esophageal varices in pregnancy. *Gastrointest Endosc* 1998; 48:212–14.
63. Hirabayashi Y, Shimizu R, Fukuda H, *et al.* Effects of the pregnant uterus on the extradural venous plexus in the supine and lateral positions, as determined by magnetic resonance imaging. *Br J Anaesth* 1997; 78:317–19.
64. Barrett JM, Caldwell BH. Association of portal hypertension and ruptured splenic artery aneurysm in pregnancy. *Obstet Gynecol* 1981; 57:255–7.
65. Sunagozaka H, Tsuji H, Mizukoshi E, *et al.* The development and clinical features of splenic aneurysm associated with liver cirrhosis. *Liver Int* 2006; 26:291–7.
66. Deshpande NA, James NT, Kucirka LM, *et al.* Pregnancy outcomes of liver transplant recipients: a systematic review and meta-analysis. *Liver Transpl* 2012; 18:621–9.
67. Verslype C, Libbrecht L. The multidisciplinary management of gastrointestinal cancer. The diagnostic and therapeutic approach for primary solid liver tumours in adults. *Best Pract Res Clin Gastroenterol* 2007; 21:983–96.
68. Cobey FC, Salem RR. A review of liver masses in pregnancy and a proposed algorithm for their diagnosis and management. *Am J Surg* 2004; 187:181–91.
69. Zucman-Rossi J, Jeannot E, Nhieu JT, *et al.* Genotype-phenotype correlation in hepatocellular adenoma: new classification and relationship with HCC. *Hepatology* 2006; 43:515–24.

CHAPTER 44

Kidney disease

Kate Wiles, Kate Bramham and Catherine Nelson-Piercy

Renal physiology in pregnancy

Critical renal physiological adaptations occur early in pregnancy, including increased erythropoietin production and vitamin D hydroxylation[1] which appear to be fundamental to successful maternal and fetal outcomes.

Glomerular filtration

Glomerular filtration rate (GFR) increases from the first day of menstruation and rises by approximately 10–20% until day 21 before returning to baseline levels.[2] Relaxin is a circulating peptide hormone released by the corpus luteum which increases in the luteal phase of the menstrual cycle, correlating with this transient rise in GFR.[3] Following conception, relaxin appears to be an important mediator of pregnancy-associated change in renal physiology. When the ovum is fertilized, the corpus luteum is maintained and relaxin production increases dramatically, stimulated by human chorionic gonadotropin (hCG).[4] At the same time, effective renal plasma flow increases by 80% over the next 16 weeks with a rise in glomerular filtration of 50%.

Relaxin has been shown to be essential for mediating increased renal blood flow in pregnant and non-pregnant rats.[5] Women with *in vitro* fertilization and embryo transfer, with undetectable relaxin levels, have a blunted gestational increase in GFR.[6] In addition, administration of intravenous recombinant human relaxin to non-pregnant volunteers leads to a 47% increase in renal blood flow. However, this increased blood flow does not lead to a parallel increase in glomerular filtration, suggesting that there are also additional unknown mechanisms mediating pregnancy-associated changes in GFR.

An increase in GFR is noted in both renal transplants and women with single kidneys.[7,8] Furthermore, healthy pregnant women given amino acid infusions have a further increase in GFR suggesting that the kidneys have a remarkable capacity for increased filtration on top of pregnancy-associated change.[9] Outside of pregnancy, hyperfiltration has been shown to be a precursor to progressive renal damage.[10] However, despite a sustained period of increased GFR in pregnancy there are no renal consequences. The preservation of renal function in normal pregnancy is proposed to be due to a lack of increase in transglomerular hydrostatic pressure demonstrated by single-nephron GFR studies in rat models.[11]

Increased renal blood flow results in up to a 70% rise in renal volume, and an approximately 1 cm increase in kidney length.[12] Hydronephrosis is a common finding in pregnancy due to progesterone mediated dilatation of the whole renal tract, and compression of the ureters by the enlarging uterus or iliac vessels. The right renal pelvicalyceal system dilates by a maximum of 0.5 mm each week from 6 to 32 weeks, reaching a maximal diameter of about 20 mm which is maintained until term. The left pelvicalyceal system reaches a maximal diameter of 8 mm at 20 weeks' gestation.[13]

Proteinuria

Proteinuria increases in normal pregnancy and it is widely accepted that the upper limit of normal is 300 mg/24 h.[14] Women with pre-existing proteinuria usually have an approximate doubling of protein excretion in normal pregnancy. This increase in proteinuria is due to increased renal blood flow and alterations in the selectivity and charge of the glomerular basement membrane.[15] Albumin accounts for approximately 30% of urine protein excretion. Albuminuria increases two- to threefold during pregnancy and may not return to normal until 12 weeks postpartum.[16] There are also increases in urinary excretion of low-molecular-weight proteins, glucose, amino acids, calcium, and uric acid suggesting physiological compromise of proximal tubular reabsorption during pregnancy.

Acute kidney injury in pregnancy

Epidemiology

Acute kidney injury (AKI) is characterized by a rapid reduction in kidney function resulting in a failure to maintain fluid, electrolyte, and acid–base homoeostasis. AKI is a common clinical problem. Data from the United Kingdom estimate the incidence of AKI to be 486–630/million population/year[17] and between 5% and 20% of critically ill patients experience an episode of AKI during the course of their illness.[18]

The incidence of AKI in pregnancy varies depending upon the socioeconomic conditions of the population studied. The incidence of AKI in developed countries is estimated to be 1/15,000–20,000 pregnancies.[19] However, in developing nations, obstetric AKI remains a serious problem, complicating up to 1/2000 pregnancies[20] and resulting in as many as 25% of referrals to dialysis centres.[21] Improved prenatal care and the liberalization of abortion laws with consequent reduction in septic abortion are significant factors in explaining this variance.[6]

The presence of AKI is associated with an increased mortality regardless of the underlying aetiology.[22] The estimated maternal mortality from pregnancy-related AKI, although rare in the developed world, is up to 20% in developing countries.[23] Despite its decreasing incidence, AKI remains a serious complication in pregnancy.

Table 44.1 RIFLE classification scheme for acute kidney injury

RIFLE category	Creatinine (Cr), glomerular filtration rate (GFR)	Urine output
Risk	Cr ≥ 1.5 × baseline or decrease in GFR ≥ 25%	<0.5 mL/kg/h for ≥6 hours
Injury	Cr ≥ 2 × baseline or decrease in GFR ≥ 50%	<0.5 mL/kg/h for ≥12 hours
Failure	Cr ≥ 3 × baseline or Cr ≥ 354 µM with a rise of at least 44 µM or decrease in GFR ≥ 75%	<0.3 mL/kg/h for ≥24 hours or anuria ≥ 12 hours
Loss	Loss of kidney function for >4 weeks	
End-Stage	Loss of kidney function for >3 months	

Reproduced from Bellomo R, Ronco C, Kellum JA *et al*., Acute renal failure–definition, outcome measures, animal models, fluid therapy and information technology needs: the Second International Consensus Conference of the Acute Dialysis Quality Initiative (ADQI) Group, *Critical Care*, volume 8, issue 4, R204–12. http://ccforum.com/content/8/4/R204.

Definitions of acute kidney injury: difficulties in pregnancy

In the past, studies of AKI were limited by the way AKI was defined and classified. Collaborative groups therefore worked to produce consensus definitions of AKI based on changes in serum creatinine and urine output (see Table 44.1 and Table 44.2).

However, the physiology of pregnancy includes an increase in renal blood flow and an associated 50% increase in GFR. In addition, there is an expansion in plasma volume causing haemodilution. Consequently, such consensus definitions of AKI are not valid in the pregnant woman.

In the United Kingdom, laboratories calculate an estimated GFR (eGFR) on all samples sent for creatinine measurement using the Modification of Diet in Renal Disease (MDRD) equation. When assessing for kidney injury it needs to be remembered that not only does this formula require plasma creatinine levels to be in steady state thereby precluding accurate assessment of acute changes in renal function, it also underestimates a gestational GFR calculated by inulin clearance by more than 40 mL/min.[26]

Clinicians are therefore limited to the interpretation of creatinine as a surrogate marker for renal function. Even then, the physiological changes of pregnancy mean that serum creatinine falls by an average of 35 µmol/L (0.4 mg/dL) in pregnancy.[27] Although a 'normal' laboratory value for creatinine can therefore still mask kidney injury in the pregnant patient, a creatinine of higher than 90 µmol/L is indicative of renal impairment in pregnancy.[28] In the context of the limitations of biochemical parameters to assess for AKI, the value of urine output criteria should be remembered, although oliguria is very common intra- and postpartum especially in the context of pre-eclampsia (see 'Pre-Eclampsia' section).

Table 44.2 Acute Kidney Injury Network (AKIN) staging system for acute kidney injury

AKIN stage	Serum creatinine (Cr)	Urine output
1	Cr ≥ 1.5–1.9 × baseline or Cr increase by ≥26.2 µM	<0.5 mL/kg/h for ≥6 hours
2	Cr ≥ 2–2.9 × baseline	<0.5 mL/kg/h for ≥12 hours
3	Cr ≥ 3 × baseline or Cr ≥ 354 µM with a rise of at least 44 µM or initiation of renal replacement therapy	<0.3 mL/kg/h for ≥24 hours or anuria ≥ 12 hours

Reproduced from Mehta RL, Kellum JA, Shah SV *et al.* Acute Kidney Injury Network. Acute Kidney Injury Network: report of an initiative to improve outcomes in acute kidney injury, *Critical Care*, volume 11, issue 2, R31. http://www.ccforum.com/content/11/2/R31.

Aetiology of acute kidney injury

AKI is a common medical problem affecting 5% of hospital in-patients and 30% of critically ill patients.[25] It is less common in the pregnant population ranging from 1/2000 to 1/20,000 pregnancies depending on the socioeconomic status of the population.[29] As in the non-pregnant patient, the aetiology of AKI can be considered as 'pre-renal' due to pathology of renal perfusion, 'renal' with intrinsic renal damage, or 'post-renal' caused by interruption to the normal outflow of the kidney. The pregnancy-related causes of AKI are listed in Table 44.3.

Acute kidney injury in pregnancy: general principles

Supportive measures in the management of AKI apply to the pregnant population as in the non-pregnant population. Renal perfusion needs to be maintained. Fluid requirements need to be assessed in the context of a careful clinical examination of the pregnant patient remembering the physiological reduction in both blood pressure and oncotic pressure that occur in pregnancy. Doses of antibiotics, anticoagulants, insulin, and opiates may need to be adjusted when there is a decrease in GFR. Erythropoietin requirements can increase with AKI. Nephrotoxic drugs including aminoglycosides, postpartum non-steroidal anti-inflammatory drugs (NSAIDs), and radiocontrast agents should be avoided. Treatment of hyperkalaemia with ion-exchange resin, insulin, and glucose

Table 44.3 Causes of acute kidney injury in pregnancy

Pre renal	Renal	Post renal
Vomiting/hyperemesis	Pre-eclampsia	Gravid uterus
Postpartum haemorrhage	HELLP	Papillary necrosis
Placental abruption	AFLP	Urinary retention
Sepsis	TTP and HUS	Damaged ureters
Heart failure	Acute tubular necrosis	
	Interstitial nephritis	
	Glomerulonephritis	

AFLP, acute fatty liver of pregnancy; HELLP, haemolysis, elevated liver enzymes, and low platelet count; HUS, haemolytic uraemic syndrome; TTP, thrombotic thrombocytopenic purpura.

Adapted from Alsuwaida AO., Challenges in diagnosis and treatment of acute kidney injury during pregnancy. *Nepro-Urology Monthly*, volume 4, issue 1, pp. 340–344. Adapted from: *Handbook of Obstetric Medicine. 4th Edition.* Nelson-Piercy C, can, and should, be given if required in pregnancy. Maternal and fetal indications for renal replacement therapy are considered below (see 'Dialysis' section).

Acute kidney injury in pregnancy: specific conditions

Pre-Eclampsia

Pre-eclampsia is a pregnancy-specific disorder characterized by new-onset hypertension and proteinuria after 20 weeks' gestation. Hypertension is defined as a blood pressure above 140/90 mmHg. Proteinuria is an excretion of greater than 300 mg/24 h. A 24-hour urine collection is considered the gold standard for quantification of proteinuria but a spot urinary protein:creatinine ratio greater than 50 mg/mmol may also be used for diagnosis.[27] Pre-eclampsia is a multisystem disorder which can affect any maternal organ including the kidney. Pre-eclampsia is the most common cause of AKI in pregnancy. In addition, as pre-eclampsia affects approximately 5% of pregnancies it is also the commonest glomerular disease in the world.[32]

The primary locus for kidney injury in pre-eclampsia is the glomerular endothelium. This substantiates the epidemiology of pre-eclampsia whereby diseases that are associated with endothelial dysfunction such as diabetes and antiphospholipid syndrome carry an increased risk for the development of pre-eclampsia. Endothelial cell swelling leads to capillary occlusion and endotheliosis (a swelling of the glomerulus, the degree of which correlates with disease severity).[33] Electron microscopy confirms the loss of renal fenestrae. Antiangiogenic factors are hypothesized to play a role in the interruption of normal endothelial health leading to a diffuse endotheliosis that is pathognomonic for pre-eclamptic renal injury. Impaired hydraulic permeability of glomerular capillary wall leads to a reduced plasma flow and a fall in GFR.[34] In pre-eclampsia, GFR and renal plasma flow decrease by 24–40% compared with normal pregnancy of the same gestation.[35,36] Of note, milder glomerular endotheliosis is seen in up to 50% of pregnancies complicated by hypertension without coexisting proteinuria suggesting that pregnancy-induced hypertension is part of the spectrum of pre-eclamptic renal disease.[33]

Although oedema is not a criterion for the diagnosis of pre-eclampsia it remains a common presenting symptom. The oedema in pre-eclampsia is not due to vascular underfilling driving the renin axis and causing renal sodium retention. It is better comparable to the 'overflow' state of acute nephritic syndromes in which GFR decreases disproportionately to renal plasma flow and glomerular–tubular imbalance is hypothesized to cause salt retention.[37] Decreased GFR, increased capillary permeability, and hypoalbuminaemia may all contribute to the oedematous clinical state.

The treatment of pre-eclampsia aims to maintain blood pressure at less than 140/90 mmHg to reduce the risk of hypertension in the mother whilst maintaining adequate uteroplacental perfusion. Treatment is mandatory for a blood pressure greater than 160/110 mmHg due to the risk of both maternal cerebral haemorrhage and placental abruption. Common agents used in the treatment of hypertension are outlined in Table 44.4.

Fluid management is important in pre-eclampsia. Aggressive hydration in women with pre-eclampsia is associated with increased maternal mortality and it is advised that women are 'kept dry' to avoid these risks.[39] Oliguria is common in pre-eclampsia and does not imply volume depletion.[40] There is no evidence of benefit of fluid expansion in pre-eclampsia[41] and a fluid challenge with either crystalloid or colloid does not ensure improved utero-placental perfusion.[42] Equally, from an anaesthetic perspective it should be remembered that women with pre-eclampsia firstly, are vasoconstricted and not at increased risk of hypotension either during or after regional anaesthesia and secondly, that there is no evidence that a bolus of crystalloid as a preload prevents hypotension.[39,43]

There is a natural diuresis at 36–48 hours postpartum. Judicious fluid management is needed until this occurs. A fluid restriction of 80 mL/h is suggested.[39,44] Before the postpartum diuresis, oliguria is common and does not require further management. It is suggested that a urine output greater than 40 mL in 4 hours is sufficient in the immediate postpartum period[39] but there is no evidence that maintenance of a specific urine output prevents the rare development of overt renal failure. Urine output is, however, used to guide magnesium treatment in severe pre-eclampsia and eclampsia. The kidney is the key player in magnesium homeostasis and a fall in GFR increases the potential for developing hypermagnesaemia. When urine output falls to less than 20 mL/h, dose adjustment of magnesium sulphate is required. However in the event of eclampsia, the usual loading bolus dose of 4 g should be given.

The reversible glomerular endothelial pathology in pre-eclampsia that temporarily compromises renal function may be complicated both by hypovolaemia and overzealous fluid restriction. Permanent renal damage in pre-eclampsia is unusual suggesting that restriction of fluid in pre-eclampsia is either not clinically significant or that permanent clinical sequelae are rare.[44] Renal function is, however, vulnerable in patients with pre-eclampsia and a nephrotoxic hit from NSAIDs should be avoided with alternative postpartum analgesia prescribed.

The glomerular swelling and renal endothelial changes in pre-eclampsia usually resolve by 8 weeks postpartum coinciding with the clinical regression of hypertension and proteinuria.[37] However, research has demonstrated a longer regression trajectory in those with higher blood pressures and greater quantities of gestational proteinuria. It has been found that 14% of women have persistent proteinuria at 3 months, falling to 2% at 2 years postpartum with an estimate of 16% longer to remission for every 1 g/day increase in proteinuria during pregnancy.[45] However, it is advised that patients who continue to demonstrate proteinuria at 6–8 week postpartum are reviewed again at 3 months postpartum and a referral to a nephrologist is considered to exclude underlying renal disease.

Pre-eclampsia is known to increase the risk of vascular disease in later life including chronic hypertension, ischaemic heart disease, cerebrovascular disease, and venous thromboembolism.[46] For this reason, women who have developed pre-eclampsia are advised to undergo annual assessment of their vascular risk, appropriate modification of lifestyle factors, and treatment when risk thresholds are reached. In addition, pre-eclampsia is an independent risk factor for both renal biopsy and subsequent end-stage renal disease (ESRD). Women with pre-eclampsia whose babies weigh less than 1.5 kg have a 17-fold increase risk of proceeding to renal biopsy.[47] In addition, although the absolute risk of ESRD is low, pre-eclampsia increases that risk by 3–15 times depending on the number of pregnancies in which pre-eclampsia develops.

Table 44.4 Common pharmacological agent used to treat hypertension in pregnancy and the postpartum period

Agent	Dose	Side effects	Comments
Antenatal			
Methyldopa	250 mg bd–1 g tds	Lethargy Depression	Documented safety profile 7-year follow-up of offspring
Labetalol	200 mg bd–500 mg tds or intravenous infusion		Avoid in asthma
Nifedipine slow release	10 mg–40 mg bd	Headache Flushing Swollen lower limbs	Tocolytic Synergistic interaction with magnesium sulphate
Hydralazine	Intravenous infusion or 25 mg bd–75 mg tds	Headache Flushing Tachycardia	
Amlodipine	5–10 mg od	Swollen lower limbs	
Doxazosin	1 mg od–8 mg bd		
Angiotensin-converting enzyme inhibitors Angiotensin receptor blockers	CONTRAINDICATED	Congenital cardiac and CNS anomalies Fetopathy Oligohydramnios Fetal growth restriction Neonatal renal failure	
Postnatal			
Enalapril	5–20 mg bd		Safe in breastfeeding
Nifedipine slow release	10–40 mg bd		Safe in breastfeeding
Amlodipine	5–10 mg od		Safe in breastfeeding
Atenolol	25–50 mg od		Safe in breastfeeding

Data from *Hypertension in pregnancy: The management of hypertensive disorders in pregnancy*, National Institute for Health and Clinical Excellence, 2011.

These data include correction for pre-existing renal disease, rheumatic disease, essential hypertension, and diabetes mellitus.[48]

Haemolysis, elevated liver enzymes, and low platelets (HELLP syndrome)

Severe pre-eclampsia is complicated by a consumptive coagulopathy and microangiopathy in 10–20% of cases.[33] HELLP syndrome is the constellation of haemolysis, elevated liver enzymes, and low platelets and is an important variant of severe pre-eclampsia. AKI may complicate any pre-eclampsia but the incidence of renal failure is much higher in HELLP syndrome. HELLP affects 10–20% of patients with severe pre-eclampsia and the largest study estimates that AKI complicates 3% of HELLP.[49] Abruption, disseminated intravascular coagulation, sepsis, haemorrhage, and intrauterine death all increase the risk of AKI in HELLP. A rise in serum creatinine in association with HELLP worsens prognosis.[50]

Although AKI in HELLP can be severe enough to require renal replacement therapy, it is observed that most patients will recover renal function. In addition, successful cadaveric renal transplantation from patients with HELLP and renal involvement are described.[51] This potential for renal recovery means that there are limited biopsy data on the nature of the renal insult in HELLP. Limited case reports describe the glomerulosis of pre-eclampsia with additional thrombotic microangiopathy. It is therefore hypothesized that the endothelial pathology which triggers kidney injury in pre-eclampsia, can extend to produce a thrombotic microangiopathy in HELLP. The resulting renal tissue ischaemia is more severe, producing both tubular and cortical necrosis.[52,53]

The management of HELLP is supportive and mirrors that of pre-eclampsia. A double-blind randomized controlled trial showed that the use of steroids did not alter hospital stay, recovery of laboratory parameters, or complication rates.[54] Although the renal pathology is that of a thrombotic microangiopathy, there are no prospective trial data to either support or refute the use of plasmapheresis.

Thrombotic microangiopathy

Thrombotic thrombocytopenic purpura

Thrombotic thrombocytopenic purpura (TTP) is characterized by thrombocytopenia, microangiopathic haemolytic anaemia, and organ dysfunction which can include AKI. Pregnancy-associated TTP usually occurs in the second or third trimesters or in the postpartum period.[55] The average gestational age at diagnosis is 26 weeks. Pregnancy is both a trigger factor for new disease and for disease flare in those with a history of TTP. (See Chapter 48 for more haematological details of TTP.)

The pathogenesis of TTP is characterized by the deposition of platelet-rich thrombi in the microcirculation of multiple organs, including the kidneys. Von Willebrand factor (vWF) plays a haemostatic role by inducing the formation of platelet plugs. In TTP, von Willebrand proteins do not undergo their normal rapid breakdown due to either a quantitative or functional deficiency of the vWF cleaving protein, ADAMTS13. This leads to platelet aggregation, red cell fragmentation, and the clinical picture of TTP. Pregnancy is a procoagulant state with increased levels of factor VIIa, factor VIII, vWF, and fibrinogen as well as increased amounts of fibrin degradation products. This suggests that mild intravascular coagulation is a phenomenon of normal pregnancy.[53] In addition, levels of ADAMTS13 decrease in normal pregnancy during the second and third trimesters. A severe deficiency of ADAMTS13 has been recorded in pregnancy-associated TTP with 20% of patients having levels of less than 5%.[56]

TTP can be difficult to diagnose in pregnancy as thrombocytopenia, haemolysis, renal dysfunction, and neurological symptoms exist in both TTP and HELLP. Twenty per cent of woman with pregnancy-associated TTP are diagnosed with coexisting pre-eclampsia/HELLP.[53] Clotting abnormalities are, however, more common (20%) in HELLP and so elevated antithrombin and fibrinogen levels may increase the clinical suspicion of TTP.[53] ADAMTS13 levels may not be diagnostically helpful as a reduced level has been described in HELLP without evidence of concurrent TTP.[57] Levels below 5% are diagnostic of TTP. The presence of antibodies against ADAMTS13 suggest the more common acquired form as opposed to congenital TTP.

Renal disease in TTP is due to thrombotic microangiopathy within the kidney and is common in pregnancy-associated TTP; 30–80% of pregnant women with TTP will demonstrate renal dysfunction which is a higher rate than in TTP outside of pregnancy.[53] Treatment is with fresh frozen plasma infusion and/or plasma exchange which will replace the deficiency of normal anticoagulant factors and/or neutralize circulating antibodies against them. Plasma exchange has improved maternal mortality from over 50% to less than 10%.[55] Fetal outcome, however, remains poor with a perinatal mortality rate of 30–80% attributed to microangiopathy of the placental arterioles.[58] Reports of long-term renal outcome are variable. The literature describes renal recovery as 'typical' in some cohorts.[53] In patients with a known history of TTP who subsequently become pregnant, serial monitoring of ADAMTS13 levels is advised where a quantitative deficiency is measurable, with prophylactic plasma exchange instituted to prevent disease flare.

Haemolytic uraemic syndrome

Haemolytic uraemic syndrome (HUS) and TTP are clinically similar disorders, traditionally segregated on the basis of clinical presentation. Those with microangiopathic haemolytic anaemia causing neurological deficit were traditionally classified as TTP, whereas microangiopathy without neurological symptoms but predominant renal impairment was labelled HUS. The same patient might have been labelled as HUS by a nephrologist and TTP by a haematologist.[59] The term TTP/HUS was therefore coined to avoided uncertainty of diagnosis.

However, a more detailed understanding of the molecular basis of both TTP and HUS has facilitated clinical distinction once more. An acquired or constitutional deficiency of ADAMTS13 is associated with the clinical picture of TTP, whereas mutations to proteins involved in the complement pathway are described in HUS. Patients with microangiopathy in association with complement dysregulation have significant renal disease and 76% progress to ESRD.[60]

In the same way that pregnancy can trigger the onset and/or relapse of ADAMTS13-deficient TTP, it can also initiate complement dysregulation-associated HUS. Interestingly, complement dysfunction is also described in HELLP[61] which, as discussed, can be difficult to distinguish from isolated microangiopathy (see 'Thrombotic thrombocytopenic purpura' section).

Pregnancy-associated HUS accounts for up 21% of non-diarrhoea-associated HUS in women of whom 86% have a detectable complement gene mutation.[60] In contrast to TTP, most cases (>75%) of pregnancy-associated HUS occur in the postpartum period. It is theorized that placental expression of complement regulatory proteins is protective in pregnancy and when this control is lost at delivery HUS can present.[60]

As for TTP, treatment of HUS includes plasma infusion and exchange. In addition, eculizumab is now licensed for the treatment of non-diarrhoea-associated HUS. Eculizumab inhibits activation of the alternative complement pathway in HUS via anti-C5 blocking antibody. Small prospective studies show an improvement in GFR including dialysis-requiring patients becoming independent of renal replacement for the duration of treatment.[62] Data on eculizumab are limited in pregnancy but use at a lower dose for paroxysmal nocturnal haemoglobinuria is reported.[63,64]

Pre-pregnancy counselling of women with known complement dysregulation is difficult as there is incomplete penetrance at a molecular level and pregnancy may, or may not, be a sufficient trigger for clinical disease. A 20% risk of pregnancy-associated disease is quoted.[60]

Acute fatty liver of pregnancy

Acute fatty liver of pregnancy (AFLP) is a rare obstetric emergency, which has the potential to progress to fulminant liver failure. This disorder has been linked to genetic mutations in maternal and fetal mitochondrial fatty acid oxidation genes leading to an excessive hepatotoxic fatty acid load and impaired liver function.

AKI is a common complication occurring in 20–100% of patients.[53] The underlying renal pathology is variable and includes acute tubular necrosis and the endotheliosis of coexisting pre-eclampsia. Tubular free fatty acid deposition has also been seen which links directly with current theories of liver pathogenesis.[65]

Treatment requires early diagnosis, supportive care, and prompt delivery. Maternal and perinatal mortality is between 10–20% but in most women there is complete liver and renal recovery after delivery.[66]

Systemic lupus erythematosus

Systemic lupus erythematosus (SLE) is primarily a disease of young women. It therefore has the potential to present for the first time in pregnancy with AKI. The diagnostic difficulty and management of lupus in pregnancy plus the indications for renal biopsy in pregnancy are considered below in the sections on lupus nephritis and renal biopsy in pregnancy.

Urinary tract infection

Physiological changes to the urinary tract increase the risk of bacterial colonization. These include increased bladder volume, decreased detrusor muscle tone, progesterone-driven ureteric dilatation, and glycosuria. The incidence of urinary tract infection (UTI) in pregnancy is approximately 2%[67] with a 0.07% incidence of pyelonephritis.[68] However, pyelonephritis carries a high (23%) risk of recurrence in the same pregnancy.[69]

Any infection of the urinary tract is associated with increased risk of adverse outcomes for both mother and child. Pyelonephritis represents the most serious type of infection which if untreated leads to pyonephrosis, abscess formation, septicaemia, and organ failure. Antepartum pyelonephritis is associated with adverse perinatal outcomes and is an independent risk factor for preterm delivery.[68]

Screening and effective treatment of asymptomatic bacteriuria and cystitis will reduce the risk of pyelonephritis. Treatment of asymptomatic bacteriuria should be directed by urine culture and continued for a minimum of 7 days.[70] Cystitis and pyelonephritis should be treated empirically with broad-spectrum agents until culture and sensitivity results are available. A 10-day course of antimicrobial therapy is advocated for symptomatic infection with up to 21 days recommended for pyelonephritis.[71] It is important to exclude renal tract anomaly with persistent, recurrent, or clinically significant infection. Recurrent infection carries the same risks as primary infection and low-dose antibiotic prophylaxis may be required for the remainder of the pregnancy.[72]

Women with vesicoureteric reflux have a higher incidence of UTI in pregnancy but this is not associated with excess maternal or fetal morbidity provided there is no renal scarring. It is the existence of renal scarring, rather than the presence or absence of reflux, which increases the risk of hypertension and pre-eclampsia in pregnancy [73] (see 'Reflux Nephropathy' section).

Obstructive nephropathy

AKI secondary to an obstructive nephropathy is rare although patients with a single kidney, multiple pregnancy, or polyhydramnios have an increased risk.[74] Bladder neuropathy in those with transplant-treated diabetic renal disease or neurological disorders (e.g. spina bifida) needs to be remembered.

Evaluation of renal tract obstruction is made difficult in pregnancy as the pelvicalyceal system and ureter dilate from as early as 6–10 weeks' gestation, particularly on the right. Certain radiological features are, however, useful in the distinction between physiological and pathological renal obstruction in pregnancy. Firstly, a dilated ureter distal to the pelvic brim suggests a cause other than pregnancy for the dilatation. Secondly, resistance indices (Doppler sonography of arcuate or interlobar renal arteries) are normal in physiological hydronephrosis and an increased index, particularly where there is an inter-renal difference, is suggestive of an alternative pathology. Finally, an absence of ureteric jets can suggest obstruction, but the pregnant patient should be examined both supine and in the contralateral decubitus position in order to negate the effect of the gravid uterus before conclusions can be made.[75]

Chronic kidney disease

Prevalence

Chronic kidney disease (CKD) is estimated to affect 3% of women of childbearing age.[76] A 2012 population cohort study in the United States demonstrated a significant increase in chronic hypertension due to renal disease from 1995 to 2008.[77] Both increasing age and body mass index are associated with CKD.[78] Therefore, the trend of women delaying pregnancy and increasing obesity in women of childbearing age are likely to result in a greater number of pregnancies complicated by CKD. Table 44.5 and Table 44.6 offer practical guidance in the prepregnancy and antenatal management of women with CKD.

In 1975, a review of renal disease in pregnancy reported that 'Children of women with renal disease used to be born dangerously or not at all—not at all if their doctors had their way'.[79] Dramatic improvements in pregnancy outcomes have occurred over recent decades, such that the majority of women with CKD have successful pregnancies. However, a meta-analysis of studies, including 2682 women with CKD, confirmed a high incidence of both maternal and neonatal adverse outcomes.[80]

Influence of pregnancy on renal disease

Despite the increasing demands of pregnancy on renal function, pregnancy has no detrimental effect on renal function for the majority of women with CKD. However, in some individuals pregnancy may precipitate a rapid decline in renal function, which may result in ESRD. The complexities of life as a new mother combined with the practical and psychological issues of commencing dialysis needs to be considered and explained carefully to women at risk.

There are few studies exploring the incidence of pregnancy-associated decline in renal function. Renal outcomes from 908 pregnancies which reached 24 weeks' gestation reported in the literature between 1985 and 2007, are shown in Table 44.7.

An earlier study of 89 pregnancies in 62 women with initial serum creatinine greater than 125 μmol/L reported 20% of women experiencing a decline in renal function during pregnancy and 23% having a decline in renal function postpartum.[81] A prepregnancy GFR of less than 40 mL/min/1.73 m^2 and proteinuria greater than 1 g/24 hours were risk factors for a 50% decline in renal function and requirement for renal replacement therapy.[82]

Temporary deterioration in renal function in women with CKD is common and frequently this can be difficult to distinguish from the normal physiological rise in creatinine towards the end of pregnancy. A study of 105 pregnancies in renal transplant recipients reported that 38% of women had a greater than 20% rise in creatinine during their pregnancy.[83] Causes for AKI should be explored, before pregnancy-associated decline in renal function is assumed.

Influence of renal disease on pregnancy

Hypertension in pregnancy

Women with CKD and associated prepregnancy hypertension may have an initial fall in blood pressure due to the physiological changes during pregnancy, and may be able to discontinue antihypertensive treatment. However, many women have an increase in blood pressure towards term. Normotensive women with CKD are also more likely to develop gestational hypertension than healthy controls.[80]

Pre-eclampsia is more common in women with CKD, and the likelihood of occurrence is related to both severity of underlying renal disease,[1] and the aetiology of renal disease. Women with lupus nephritis, reflux nephropathy, and renal transplants are more susceptible to pre-eclampsia than women with other causes of renal impairment with the same level of renal function.[84] Presence and severity of pre-existing hypertension and proteinuria have also been identified as risk factors for the development of pre-eclampsia in women with CKD.[85]

Table 44.5 Prepregnancy counselling strategy for women with renal disease

Gynaecological and obstetric history	Review current menstrual cycle, previous pregnancies, current contraceptive use Discuss effects of age, weight, and renal function on fertility Consider investigations for infertility if necessary
Pregnancy and renal outcomes	Discuss effects of renal disease on pregnancy, e.g. pre-eclampsia Discuss effects of pregnancy on renal disease Discuss implications of loss of renal function if relevant, e.g. symptoms of chronic kidney disease, lifestyle of renal replacement therapy Inform of necessity of hospital-based antenatal care Advise that vaginal delivery is achievable and desired, but that caesarean delivery may be required
Medication	Start folic acid 5 mg daily Advise to start aspirin 75 mg daily at conception Review medication and switch to non-teratogenic alternatives Discuss drug safety in pregnancy and breastfeeding Optimize haemoglobin and iron stores Treat vitamin D deficiency
Disease activity and/or stability	Advise not to conceive if disease flare or episode of transplant rejection within 6 months Consider delaying conception if renal function rapidly deteriorating Consider renal biopsy if underlying disease unknown
Disease-specific issues	Discuss inheritance and screening for adult polycystic kidney disease and reflux nephropathy Inform of risk of neonatal lupus if anti-Ro/La positive Discuss importance of glycaemic control in type 1 and type 2 diabetes prior to conception and during pregnancy
Other medical history	Assess for other concurrent medical disorders which may impact on pregnancy outcome, e.g. pulmonary hypertension, cardiac disease, respiratory disease
Advice for when conceives	Do not stop all medications other than those discussed If problems taking medication due to nausea or vomiting to seek medical advice Give contact details in order to inform relevant health professionals when conceives to allow early pregnancy assessment and viability scan

The diagnosis of pre-eclampsia that is superimposed on pre-existing hypertension may be difficult. Research definitions of superimposed pre-eclampsia specify that additional features are required in order to confirm the diagnosis including clinical symptoms or changes in other parameters such as liver function tests or platelet count.[86] In practice, additional features may be absent but women with CKD may have a rapid rise in blood pressure or dramatic increase in proteinuria, coupled with non-specific clinical features such as oedema or headache. Frequently women with suspected superimposed pre-eclampsia may require inpatient admission for maternal and fetal assessment. A decision to deliver is made by a multidisciplinary team evaluating the risk of deterioration of renal disease in the mother versus the complications of preterm delivery.

There is limited evidence for the role of novel markers for the diagnosis of pre-eclampsia in women with CKD. However, soluble FMS-like tyrosine kinase-1 and placental growth factor ratios have been found to be significantly higher in women with pre-eclampsia compared to women with CKD[87] suggesting they may be useful discriminators.

Uterine artery Doppler has not been formally evaluated in women with CKD although one study of women with CKD due to lupus nephritis has calculated a mid-trimester negative predictive value of only 47%.[88] Despite this, most clinicians would measure uterine artery Doppler indices in women with CKD and plan ongoing fetal assessment according to estimated risk. There is some evidence that normal flow velocity waveforms distinguish women with CKD from those with pre-eclampsia, but the role of Doppler for diagnosing superimposed pre-eclampsia is unclear.[89]

Aspirin has been shown to be of benefit in reducing the risk of pre-eclampsia by 17%.[90] The absolute risk reduction is greater in higher-risk populations including women with CKD.

Fetal loss

The majority of women with CKD have successful pregnancies. Data on rates of early fetal loss and termination of pregnancy for medical reasons are limited due to under-reporting, but both early and late miscarriage are more common in women with CKD, particularly in those with severe renal impairment.[1]

Preterm delivery and fetal growth restriction

Preterm delivery is more common in women with CKD than the general population.[80] The majority of preterm deliveries are iatrogenic, predominantly for maternal reasons including progression of hypertension, proteinuria, or renal dysfunction.[91] Women should be counselled carefully about the short- and long-term consequence of a preterm delivery prior to conception, particularly those with severe renal impairment, as the challenges of managing deteriorating maternal health, and the emotional

Table 44.6 Antenatal and postnatal care of women with chronic kidney disease

Antenatal care	Target blood pressure < 140/90 mmHg
	Monitor serum creatinine and proteinuria
	Thromboprophylaxis if albumin < 20 g/dL or proteinuria > 2 g/24 h or protein:creatinine ratio > 200 mg/mmol
	Low-molecular-weight heparin if serum creatinine < 200 μmol/L
	Unfractionated heparin if serum creatinine > 200 μmol/L
	Regular urine culture, and start antibiotic prophylaxis after one infection
	Aim to keep haemoglobin 10–11 g/dL—use oral or intravenous iron and erythropoietin as necessary
	Monitor tacrolimus or ciclosporin levels every 4 weeks—aim for non-pregnant therapeutic range
	Treat vitamin D deficiency—cholecalciferol and/or 1-alpha-calcidol depending on level of renal impairment
	Consider haemodialysis if urea > 20 mmol/L, or problems with hyperkalaemia or acidosis
	Uterine artery Dopplers at 20–22 weeks' gestation, and repeat if notching at 24 weeks
	Serial growth scans in women with CKD stage 3–5 or CKD 1–5 with hypertension
Postnatal care	Review blood pressure and fluid balance—target blood pressure <140/90 mmHg
	Reduce tacrolimus or ciclosporin to prepregnancy dose and monitor levels
	Continue thromboprophylaxis for 6 weeks postpartum
	Stop aspirin if not required for long-term cardiovascular disease prophylaxis
	Assess for proteinuria at 6 weeks and revise target blood pressure accordingly:
	<130/80 mg/mmol if protein creatinine ratio > 150 mg/mmol
	<140/90 mg/mmol if protein creatinine ratio < 150 mg/mmol
	Discuss future contraception

demands of having a very preterm infant in intensive care may be underestimated.[92] The rate of preterm delivery is higher in women with more severe renal impairment and reaches more than 90% in women with serum creatinine greater than 180 μmol/L.[1]

Fetal growth restriction is estimated to be up to five times more common in women with CKD,[93] with risks increasing with severity of renal disease.[1,80] Serial growth scans are recommended from 24 weeks' gestation in women with a reduced GFR, hypertension, or significant proteinuria.

Chronic kidney disease: specific conditions

Transplantation

Women with renal transplants frequently have successful pregnancies;[83] however, their pregnancies are associated with more complications than women with matched levels of kidney function.[84] This is likely to reflect irreversible endothelial damage from previous ESRD. Pre-eclampsia is increased sixfold and low-dose aspirin should be offered to all these women after conception to try and reduce this. A prospective study of 105 pregnancies in renal transplant recipients in the United Kingdom demonstrated a higher risk of pregnancy complications compared to healthy controls with 20% of women requiring high dependency care at some point during their pregnancy.[83] An additional finding of this study was that 45% of women with a second or subsequent graft had poor pregnancy outcomes possibly reflecting the vascular damage of reaching ESRD on two or more occasions.

Transplant recipients are seen frequently by medical professionals and are a population who should be able to plan pregnancies and receive appropriate prepregnancy counselling. A 2013 study in the United Kingdom of pregnancies in renal transplant recipients found that only 64% were taking folic acid at conception, suggesting that a third of women had unplanned pregnancies.[83]

The timing of conception following renal transplantation is controversial. The first year post transplantation is associated with most episodes of acute rejection, and therefore it is felt that pregnancy should be avoided during this time. A transplant-to-pregnancy interval of 12–24 months is suggested by the European Best Practice Guidelines for renal transplantation.[94] The American Society of Transplantation Guidelines recommended that pregnancy may be considered after 1 year in women who are at low risk of complications[95] on the basis of favourable outcomes.[96,97] However, a meta-analysis of 50 studies of pregnancy following renal transplantation did not identify an association between time from transplant and pregnancy outcome.[98]

Remarkably, physiological changes seen in native kidneys are also reported in renal transplants.[8] An increase in GFR is expected in women with a preserved GFR prepregnancy. Hydronephrosis may be identified and positional scanning is recommended to

Table 44.7 Pregnancy and renal outcomes

	Effects on pregnancy outcome				Loss of >25% renal function		
Mean prepregnancy creatinine (μmol/L)	**Fetal growth restriction**	**Preterm delivery**	**Pre-eclampsia**	**Perinatal deaths**	**During pregnancy**	**Persists postpartum**	**ESRF after 1 year**
<125	25%	30%	22%	1%	2%	0%	0%
125–180	40%	60%	40%	5%	40%	20%	2%
>180	65%	>90%	60%	10%	70%	50%	35%
On dialysis	>90%	>90%	75%	50%	N/A	N/A	N/A

ESRF, end stage renal failure; N/A, not applicable.

Reproduced from *The BMJ*, Chronic kidney disease in pregnancy, David Williams, John Davison, volume 336, p. 211, Copyright 2008 with permission from BMJ Publishing Group Ltd.

assess whether or not this is pregnancy associated. Causes for a decline in transplant renal function are listed in Table 44.8.

Most studies report no significant effects of pregnancy on graft function,[96,99–102] although a single study of 48 pregnancies reported a 20% decline in function at 6 months postpartum.[103] Women at risk of pregnancy-associated accelerated decline in function are those with impaired GFR, hypertension, and one or more previous transplants.[104] There is no evidence of increased rates of acute rejection in the postpartum period with the restoration of cellular immunity.

Kidney–pancreas transplantation

There are now several successful pregnancies reported in women with simultaneous kidney–pancreas transplants (SPK). Unfortunately these pregnancies appear to be more complicated than those of women with single-organ transplants. The intraperitoneal position of the graft makes obstructive nephropathy more common.[105] The United States National Transplant Pregnancy Register records high rate of fetal loss (29%), hypertension (66%), infection (48%), pre-eclampsia (34%), preterm delivery (77%), and low birthweight (62%).[106] Graft loss of one or both organs postpartum is reported to be up to 19% in one series of 43 women.[106] Prepregnancy creatinine does not appear to be a predictor of graft loss.[107] There is no evidence for an adjustment in immunosuppressive regimens other than switching to non-teratogenic medication prior to pregnancy and maintaining calcineurin inhibitor levels in the desired non-pregnant range for that individual.

Table 44.8 Causes of rise in serum creatinine in pregnant transplant recipients

Cause	Features
Normal physiological return to prepregnancy levels in third trimester	No concerning features identified
Urinary tract infection	Positive MSU, clinical features may be absent due to denervated kidney
Pre-eclampsia	Worsening pre-existing or new onset hypertension, worsening pre-existing or new onset proteinuria, possibly abnormal liver function tests, low platelets
Obstruction	Improved renal function after bed rest with patient lying on opposite side to transplanted kidney. Hydronephrosis on ultrasound with no other cause found. Exclude urinary retention.
Calcineurin inhibitor (tacrolimus/ciclosporin) toxicity	High trough drug levels
Hypovolaemia	Hyperemesis, antepartum haemorrhage, sepsis
Viral infections	Polyoma virus (decoy cells in urine), cytomegalovirus (CMV PCR)
Acute rejection	Diagnosis confirmed on renal biopsy. Consider pulsed steroids, or intravenous immunoglobulin Avoid monoclonal antibodies or antithymocyte globulin[95]

MSU, midstream specimen of urine; PCR, polymerase chain reaction.

Pre-existing complications of diabetes need to be considered, including the risk of deterioration in diabetic retinopathy associated with pregnancy and chronic urinary retention due to bladder neuropathy.[105]

Dialysis

Women on dialysis (stage 5 CKD) are frequently amenorrhoeic due to suppression of the hypothalamic–pituitary–gonadal axis associated with severe renal impairment.[108] This coupled with a reduced libido makes conception on dialysis uncommon. Rates of pregnancy in women of child-bearing age on dialysis are as low as 1–1.5%.[109] Fetal loss is probably under-reported but up to 25% miscarry in the first trimester.[109]

With the advent of improved dialysis regimens and treatment of erythropoietin deficient anaemia, pregnancy on dialysis is becoming more frequent,[110] and contraception should be discussed with women of child-bearing age. The majority of women with stage 5 CKD are hypertensive and oestrogen-containing contraception should be avoided, but progesterone preparations can be considered. Pregnancy may be difficult to identify early in women with oligo- or amenorrhoea and increased erythropoietin requirements may be the only clinical feature.

Live birth rates have dramatically increased over recent decades for women on dialysis. Recent series have reported 100% successful pregnancy outcomes[111,112] compared with 23% in 1980.[113] These improvements are likely to be a consequence of advances in neonatal care, and the introduction of intensive dialysis regimens as soon as conception is confirmed, with some women receiving up to 48 hours/week of nocturnal haemodialysis. A small study has suggested that women receiving greater than 20 hours of dialysis per week have better pregnancy outcomes when established on dialysis with a viable pregnancy in the second trimester.[114]

A systematic review of 222 pregnancy outcomes of women on renal replacement therapy found a mean delivery gestation of 32 ± 6.7 weeks, mean birth weight of 1810 ± 1193 g, and high rates of neonatal (11.9%) and perinatal deaths (17.9%).[115] Women who conceive on dialysis compared with women who start dialysis during pregnancy tend to have worse pregnancy outcomes. Years of dialysis prior to conception is also a negative confounder.[115]

Urea is fetotoxic and it is recommended that dialysis should be commenced when maternal urea levels are 15–20 mmol/L.[110] Polyhydramnios is a consequence of placental transfer of raised maternal urea, but has been shown to be associated with better pregnancy outcomes, possibly reflecting adequacy of function of the fetoplacental unit.[116] Ideally fluid shifts during dialysis should be minimized in order to maintain placental perfusion, and this should be achieved by restricting ultrafiltration during dialysis to 1–1.5 L per session.[110] This needs to be titrated to the woman's fluid intake and hours of dialysis. Volume status should be assessed regularly during pregnancy to allow for dry weight increases due to fetal and placental growth. Increased dialysis frequency allows a relaxation of potassium and phosphate restriction, and dialysate may need to be supplemented with potassium and phosphate in order to maintain serum levels.[110] Water-soluble vitamins should be prescribed including folic acid 5 mg daily.

Anaemia in women with CKD should be treated promptly and aggressively. Those already requiring intravenous iron and/or subcutaneous erythropoietin usually need up to a 50% increase in dose.[117] Women on haemodialysis with higher third-trimester haematocrits have been shown to have better pregnancy outcomes.[116] There have been no reports of teratogenicity in women taking recombinant human erythropoietin and there does not appear to be significant placental transfer.[118,119] Whilst there have been no reports of thrombosis associated with recombinant erythropoietin use, this is a possibility due to the hypercoagulable state during pregnancy and it is advisable to reduce or temporarily withhold treatment in women with haemoglobin levels higher than 11 g/dL. Anticoagulation doses should be increased in pregnant women on dialysis due to hypercoagulability.[120]

Lupus nephritis

Women with lupus nephritis have more complex pregnancies than those matched for renal function,[84] and even those with treated renal disease and preserved renal function have worse pregnancy outcomes than women with SLE without renal involvement.[88] Risk factors for pregnancy complications include black ethnicity, low complement at conception, pre-existing hypertension, positive antiphospholipid antibodies, and severity of renal impairment.[121] Fetal loss is higher particularly in those with hypertension, proteinuria and antiphospholipid antibodies. It is recommended that women conceive after their disease is quiescent for 6 months as active disease at conception is also associated with worse pregnancy outcomes.[122] Class of lupus nephritis does not appear to be a risk factor for complications.[121]

Disease flare during pregnancy has been variably reported including both renal and extrarenal disease. A meta-analysis of 37 studies published between 1984 and 2009, including 1842 women with lupus nephritis with varying baseline renal function and 2751 pregnancies, showed lupus flare rates of 26% with 16% renal disease.[121] Diagnosis of new or a flare of pre-existing lupus nephritis during pregnancy can be challenging as many features are present in normal pregnancy or with the onset of pre-eclampsia. Table 44.9 shows common and distinguishing features between the conditions.

A renal biopsy may be required to confirm the diagnosis of lupus nephritis flare. Indications and risks of biopsy in pregnancy are discussed later (see 'Renal Biopsy in Pregnancy' section). Treatment for active lupus nephritis during pregnancy includes methylprednisolone. Cyclophosphamide and mycophenolate mofetil are contraindicated in the first trimester due to teratogenicity, but can be considered in the second or third trimesters, although pregnancy outcomes reported are variable[123] and fetal bone marrow toxicity is possible. Rituximab may be given but if used later in pregnancy has been shown to be associated with absent B cells in infants for up to 6 months, and the long-term effects are unknown.[124]

All women with SLE should be assessed for the presence of anti-Ro or anti-La antibodies. Offspring of women with anti-Ro/anti-La antibodies are at risk of congenital heart block due to the placental transfer of the antibody resulting in fibrosis of the fetal cardiac conducting system. Fetal cardiac scans should be performed at 18–25 weeks' gestation and assessment of the fetal heart rate during obstetric examination is mandatory. The risk of congenital heart block is 2%, but if a previous child has been affected the risk increases to 15–20%, and if two children have been affected the risk may be as high as 50%.[125] Treatment options are limited although hydroxychloroquine may confer some benefit.[126] High-dose steroids, plasma exchange, and intravenous immunoglobulin have not shown any significant beneficial effect.[125,127] Fetal mortality is up to 30% and a neonatologist should be present at the delivery of an affected infant.

Table 44.9 Features of systemic lupus erythematosus (SLE) compared to problems in normal pregnancy and pre-eclampsia

Features	SLE	Pregnancy
General	Fatigue and malaise	Fatigue
Hair	Loss	Loss or gain
Skin	Malar rash	Melasma/chloasma Facial flushing
Joint pain and swelling	Inflammatory synovitis	Mechanical arthralgia Bland knee effusion
Anaemia	Haemolytic anaemia Anaemia of chronic disease	Haemodilution
Thrombocytopenia	Immune thrombocytopenia	Pre-eclampsia HELLP syndrome
Deranged liver function tests	Lupus hepatitis (usually transaminases)	Pre-eclampsia HELLP syndrome Obstetric cholestasis
Erythrocyte sedimentation rate	Elevated	Elevated
Features	**Lupus nephritis**	**Pre-eclampsia**
Haematuria/red cell casts	Present	Absent
Anti-DNA antibodies	Raised	Normal
Complement C3 and C4	Low	Normal or raised
Liver function tests	Normal	Normal or raised
Hypertension	Present	Present and rising
Proteinuria	Present	Present
Oedema	Present	Present
Low platelets	Present	Present
Rising creatinine	Present	Present

Approximately 5% of infants of women with anti-Ro/anti-La antibodies may develop neonatal cutaneous lupus.[128] This is a benign condition which resolves spontaneously after 6 months, when maternal antibody levels fall. It does not usually require any specific treatment.

Immunoglobulin A nephropathy

Women with immunoglobulin A (IgA) nephropathy tend to have successful pregnancies and there is no evidence that disease progression is affected by pregnancy, other than in women with more severe disease. Women with prepregnancy creatinine higher than 120 μmol/L, eGFR less than 50 mL/min/1.73m^2, heavy proteinuria, or severe histological lesions on renal biopsy are most likely to have pregnancies complicated by pre-eclampsia, fetal growth restriction, preterm labour, and a pregnancy-associated decline in renal function.[129,130] A multicentre case–control study has shown that pregnancy does not affect long-term renal function in women with IgA nephropathy with prepregnancy creatinine less than 110 μmol/L over a median follow-up period of 10 years.[131]

Polycystic kidney disease

Adult polycystic kidney disease (APKD) in women of childbearing age is usually associated with normal or mild renal impairment. Hypertension and renal impairment are associated with worse pregnancy outcomes.[132] Cyst growth has not been found to progress with pregnancy and uterine expansion is not compromised by the presence of enlarged kidneys. Urinary tract and cyst infection are more common in pregnancy, and should be treated promptly and aggressively.[132]

Genetic defects for APKD have been identified and whilst prenatal screening is possible many women choose not to have genetic testing. Cysts are not usually present until an individual is in their teens or early twenties and therefore the absence of cysts in the fetus or baby does not provide any reassurance about inheritance.

Reflux nephropathy

Reflux nephropathy is a common cause of renal impairment in women of childbearing age and may be associated with worse renal and pregnancy outcomes. High rates of superimposed pre-eclampsia (up to 75%), recurrent UTIs (28–65%), decline in renal function (13%), and ureteral obstruction requiring drainage (5%) are reported.[133] Reflux nephropathy is diagnosed after the identification of cortical scarring, usually in an individual with a history of childhood urinary tract infections. Antenatal care should include vigilance for UTIs and prophylaxis after infection. Offspring should be screened for the presence of reflux, as inheritance can be autosomal dominant.

Diabetic nephropathy

Women with diabetic nephropathy have complicated pregnancies. Women with prepregnancy microalbuminuria may develop macroalbuminuria when pregnant, although one study has suggested that urinary albumin excretion in women with type 1 diabetes is unchanged in early pregnancy.[134] Proteinuria, including microalbuminuria, at conception has been shown to be associated with worse pregnancy outcomes in women with type I diabetes.[134] In a review of nine studies of pregnancies in women with diabetic nephropathy, proteinuria increased from 1–3 g/24 h at baseline to 4–8 g/24 h in the third trimester[135] but proteinuria usually returns to baseline levels after delivery, even in women with nephrotic range excretion.[136] Associated problems with nephrotic range proteinuria include severe oedema that may require judicious use of diuretics, and increased thrombotic risk that should be managed with thromboprophylaxis. Although women with diabetes are at risk for macrosomia, the presence of renal impairment appears to outweigh the effects of hyperglycaemia and nearly 50% of infants of mothers with diabetic nephropathy are small for gestational age.[134]

Glycaemic control and blood pressure treatment have been shown to be associated with better pregnancy outcomes.[137] A small study of intensive angiotensin-converting enzyme inhibition for 6 months preconception together with improved glycaemic management in women with diabetic nephropathy, showed a reduction in proteinuria that was maintained during and after pregnancy, compared to women with no treatment.[138] Angiotensin-converting enzyme inhibitors and/or angiotensin II receptor blockers should probably be continued until conception if possible in women with significant proteinuria prepregnancy.

Chronic kidney disease: drugs in pregnancy

Preconception counselling should include a review of a woman's medication. All women with CKD who are considering conception within 3 months should start folic acid 5 mg daily. Aspirin should be continued or commenced with confirmation of pregnancy. Statins and bisphosphonates should be discontinued. Specific considerations of commonly used drugs in women with CKD are outlined in Table 44.10.

Renal biopsy in pregnancy

The indications to perform a renal biopsy in pregnancy include rapidly deteriorating renal function and severe nephrotic syndrome. A biopsy should only be performed if the findings are likely to change management and renal biopsy should not be used to diagnose pre-eclampsia. After 28 weeks, delivery should be considered with biopsy performed postpartum. Complexities of performing a renal biopsy in a pregnant woman include difficulties in positioning due to the gravid uterus. In addition, vasopressin to reduce biopsy-associated bleeding is not usually given due to the increased thrombotic risk of pregnancy. A recent systematic review including 243 renal biopsies performed during pregnancy suggested that the risks of major or minor bleeding, haematoma, or loin pain were 7% when performed antenatally compared with 1% postpartum.[139]

Mode of delivery and anaesthesia

The mode of delivery depends on many factors including the progression of renal disease, the development of pregnancy-related complications (e.g. pre-eclampsia), and the well-being of the fetus.

Unless renal function is severely impaired and hypertension is present, non-invasive monitoring should suffice for both labour and caesarean delivery. If arteriovenous fistulae are present, care should be taken to avoid that arm for blood pressure cuffs or arterial lines.

There is hyperacidity in renal patients and these patients will require a histamine H_2-receptor antagonist, for example, ranitidine, during labour. Women with renal disease attempting vaginal birth can be offered an early epidural providing there are no contraindications to neuraxial anaesthesia. Patients with CKD may be anticoagulated due to their thrombotic risk in the context of antenatal proteinuria or for vascular indications, but labour and delivery can usually be timed to allow neuraxial anaesthesia, for example, 4 hours since the last dose of unfractionated heparin or 12 hours post prophylactic low-molecular-weight heparin. The patient must also be euvolaemic following dialysis or else hypotension may follow neuraxial blockade. An early epidural would not only provide analgesia but eliminate the catecholamine surges with pain which increase the risk of hypertension, particularly if pre-eclampsia is also present. Further, there will be a lower threshold for operative delivery in a patient with CKD, and an epidural can be topped-up to facilitate this. Ropivacaine is the local anaesthetic of choice for epidural top-up as its pharmacokinetics are not affected by renal failure.[140]

Table 44.10 Commonly used drugs in chronic kidney disease

Drug	Trans-placental passage	Teratogenicity	Fetal/neonatal effects	Safe in pregnancy	Safe in breastfeeding	FDA classification
Angiotensin-converting enzyme inhibitor (ACEI), angiotensin receptor blocker (ARB)	✓	✓	Cardiovascular, central nervous system defects in 1st trimester and oligohydramnios, intrauterine growth restriction, and neonatal anuria in 2nd and 3rd trimesters	× Stop at conception	✓ Enalapril is recommended treatment of hypertension during breastfeeding by NICE × Other ACEI/ARB breastfeeding safety unknown	D
Prednisolone	Limited	Possible increase in oral clefts	Rare—except at large doses. (cataract, adrenal insufficiency and infection)	✓	✓ (Breastfeeding is not encouraged if > 60 mg prednisolone daily)	C
Hydroxychloroquine	✓	×	×	✓	✓	C
Azathioprine	✓	×	Sporadic congenital abnormalities, transient immune alterations in neonates	✓	✓	D
Mycophenolate mofetil	✓	✓		× Stop 3/12 preconception	×	D
Tacrolimus	✓	×	Hyperkalaemia and renal impairment	✓ Usually increased doses required to achieve prepregnancy target levels	✓	C
Cyclophosphamide	✓ Animal data	✓	Chromosomal abnormalities and cytopenia	✓ (Only after the 1st trimester in life-threatening maternal disease.)	×	D
Ciclosporin	✓	×	Transient immune alterations	✓ Usually increased doses required to achieve prepregnancy target levels	Probably possible	D
Intravenous immunoglobulin	✓	×	None reported	✓	✓	C
Recombinant erythropoietin	×	×		✓ Increased doses usually required Possible risk of hypertension	No reports, but neonates frequently treated with erythropoietin safely Protein likely to be broken down in infants' gastrointestinal tract	C

Reproduced with permission from Bramham K, Lightstone L., Pre-pregnancy counseling for women with chronic kidney disease, *Journal of Nephrology*, Volume 25, Issue 4, pp. 450–459, Copyright © 2012 courtesy of the Italian Society of Nephrology-SIN.

The rate of caesarean delivery is high in women with CKD even in those with a preserved GFR.[91] Neuraxial anaesthesia is the technique of choice and either topped-up epidurals, single-shot spinals, or combined spinal–epidurals can be used. Provided the patient has a normal volume status before surgery, hypotension associated with neuraxial block is best treated with phenylephrine rather than fluid to avoid overloading and possible pulmonary oedema.

General anaesthesia should be avoided if at all possible. But if this is the only possible option, measures should be taken to obtund the hypertensive response to laryngoscopy, using a short-acting opiate like remifentanil or alfentanil. The conventional rapid sequence induction with suxamethonium may result in a rise of potassium and should not be given if the starting potassium is over 5.5 mEq/L. Atracurium is the non-depolarizing relaxant of choice due to its Hoffman degradation which is independent of renal function. Renal blood flow is maintained with desflurane and isoflurane but reduced with sevoflurane.[141] Morphine can accumulate in renal patients as can fentanyl.[142]

Patients with significant renal dysfunction should have their postpartum care in the high dependency unit. Thromboprophylaxis post caesarean delivery is important in women with heavy proteinuria and should be continued for 6 weeks postpartum.[143]

A reduced dose of low-molecular-weight heparin should be considered in women with impaired renal function (serum creatinine > 200 umol/l), or alternatively, a switch to twice-daily unfractionated heparin. Women with CKD should not be prescribed non-steroidal analgesia due to the risk of deterioration in renal function and exacerbation of hypertension.

Conclusion

AKI can develop during pregnancy but may be masked by a normal serum creatinine due to a physiological increase in glomerular filtration. The prevalence of pre-eclampsia makes it the most common cause of AKI in pregnancy and the most common glomerular disease worldwide. Other pregnancy-related diseases can also result in AKI and non-pregnant aetiologies should not be missed. The management of AKI in pregnancy is supportive and aims to maintain renal perfusion and avoid nephrotoxicity whilst treating the underlying cause.

Women with pre-existing CKD are likely to have successful pregnancies, but require heightened antenatal surveillance. Monitoring of haemoglobin, renal function, vitamin D, albumin, proteinuria, and bacteriuria throughout pregnancy is recommended. Prepregnancy counselling is important to optimize maternal health and medication, inform women of possible pregnancy outcomes, and in a minority, to explain the potential risk of accelerated progression of renal impairment.

References

1. Williams D, Davison J. Chronic kidney disease in pregnancy. *BMJ* 2008; 336:211–15.
2. Davison JM, Noble MC. Serial changes in 24 hour creatinine clearance during normal menstrual cycles and the first trimester of pregnancy. *Br J Obstet Gynaecol* 1981; 88(1):10–17.
3. Stewart DR, Celniker AC, Taylor CA, *et al.* Relaxin in the peri-implantation period. *J Clin Endocrinol Metab* 1990; 70(6):1771–3.
4. Sherwood OD. Relaxin. In Knobil ENJ (ed) *The Physiology of Pregnancy*. New York: Raven Press; 1994:861–1009.
5. Debrah DO, Conrad KP, Danielson LA, *et al.* Effects of relaxin on systemic arterial hemodynamics and mechanical properties in conscious rats: sex dependency and dose response. *J Appl Physiol* 2005; 98(3):1013–20.
6. Smith MC, Murdoch AP, Danielson LA, *et al.* Relaxin has a role in establishing a renal response in pregnancy. *Fertil Steril* 2006; 86(1):253–5.
7. Davison JM. Changes in renal function in early pregnancy in women with one kidney. *Yale J Biol Med* 1978; 51(3):347–9.
8. Davison JM. The effect of pregnancy on kidney function in renal allograft recipients. *Kidney Int* 1985; 27(1):74–9.
9. Sturgiss SN, Wilkinson R, Davison JM. Renal reserve during human pregnancy. *Am J Physiol* 1996; 271(1 Pt 2):F16–20.
10. Anderson S, Brenner BM. The role of intraglomerular pressure in the initiation and progression of renal disease. *J Hypertens* 1986; 4(5):S236–8.
11. Baylis C. The mechanism of the increase in glomerular filtration rate in the twelve-day pregnant rat. *J Physiol* 1980; 305:405–14.
12. Linheimer MD DJ. Renal disorders. In Barron WM, Linheimer MD (eds) *Medical Disorders During Pregnancy*. London: Mosby; 1990:42–72.
13. Faundes A, Bricola-Filho M, Pinto e Silva JL. Dilatation of the urinary tract during pregnancy: proposal of a curve of maximal caliceal diameter by gestational age. *Am J Obstet Gynecol* 1998; 178(5):1082–6.
14. Airoldi J, Weinstein L. Clinical significance of proteinuria in pregnancy. *Obstet Gynecol Surv* 2007; 62(2):117–24.
15. Roberts M, Lindheimer MD, Davison JM. Altered glomerular permselectivity to neutral dextrans and heteroporous membrane modeling in human pregnancy. *Am J Physiol* 1996; 270(2 Pt 2):F338–43.
16. Taylor AA, Davison JM. Albumin excretion in normal pregnancy. *Am J Obstet Gynecol* 1997; 177(6):1559–60.
17. Hegarty J, Middleton R, Krebs M, *et al.* Severe acute renal failure. Place of care, incidence and outcomes. *QJM* 2005; 98:661–6.
18. Metnitz PGH, Krenn CG, Steltzer H, *et al.* Effect of acute renal failure requiring renal replacement therapy on outcome in critically ill patients. *Crit Care Med* 2002; 30:2051–8.
19. Stratta P, Besso L, Canavese C, *et al.* Is pregnancy-related acute renal failure a disappearing clinical entity? *Ren Fail* 1996; 18(4):5.
20. Alsuwaida AO. Challenges in the diagnosis and treatment of acute kidney injury during pregnancy. *Nephro-Urol Mon* 2012; 4(1):340–4.
21. Goplani KR, Shah PR, Gera DN, *et al.* Pregnancy-related acute renal failure: a single center experience. *Indian J Nephrol* 2008; 18(1):17–21.
22. Murugan R, Kellum JA. Acute kidney injury: what's the prognosis? *Nat Rev Nephrol* 2011; 7(4):209–17.
23. Prakash J, Niwas SS, Parekh A, *et al.* Acute kidney injury in late pregnancy in developing countries. *Clin Stud* 2010; 32:309–13.
24. Bellomo R, Ronco C, Kellum JA, *et al.* Acute renal failure—definition, outcome measures, animal models, fluid therapy and information technology needs: the Second International Consensus Conference of the Acute Dialysis Quality Initiative (ADQI) Group. *Crit Care* 2004; 8(4):R204–12.
25. Mehta RL, Kellum JA, Shah SV, *et al.* Acute Kidney Injury Network. Acute Kidney Injury Network: report of an initiative to improve outcomes in acute kidney injury. *Crit Care* 2007; 11(2):R31.
26. Smith MC, Moran P, Ward MK, *et al.* Assessment of glomerular filtration rate during pregnancy using the MDRD formula. *Br J Obstet Gynaecol* 2008; 115:109–12.
27. Fischer MJ. Chronic kidney disease and pregnancy maternal and fetal outcomes. *Adv Chronic Kidney Dis* 2007; 14:132–45.
28. Girling JC. Reevaluation of plasma creatinine concentration in normal pregnancy. *J Obstet Gynecol* 2000; 20:128–31.
29. Ventura JE, Villa M, Mizraji R, *et al.* Acute renal failure in pregnancy. *Ren Fail* 1997; 19(2):217–20.
30. Alsuwaida AO. Challenges in diagnosis and treatment of acute kidney injury during pregnancy. *Nepro-Urol Mont* 2012; 4(1):340–4.
31. Nelson-Piercy C. *Handbook of Obstetric Medicine* (4th ed). London: Informa Healthcare, 2010.
32. Stillman IE, Karumanchi SA. The glomerular injury of pre-eclampsia. *J Am Soc Nephrol* 2007; 18:2281–4.
33. Nochy BP, Hinglais N, Freund M, *et al.* Renal lesions in the hypertensive syndromes of pregnancy: immunomorphological and ultrastructural studies in 114 cases. *Clin Nephrol* 1980; 19:754–60.
34. Dragun D, Haase M. Acute kidney failure during pregnancy and post-partum. In Jorres A, Ronco C, Kellum JA (eds) *Management of Acute Kidney Problems*. Berlin: Springer-Verlag; 2010:445–58.
35. Moran P, Baylis PH, Lindheimer MD, *et al.* Glomerular ultrafiltration in normal and pre-eclamptic pregnancy. *J Am Soc Nephrol* 2003; 14:648–52.
36. Lafayette RA. The kidney in pre-eclampsia. *Kidney Int* 2005; 67:1194–203.
37. Karumanchi SA, Maynard SE, Stillman IE, *et al.* Preeclampsia: a renal perspective. *Kidney Int* 2005; 67:2101–13.
38. National Clinical Guideline Centre London, Royal College of Obstetricians and Gynaecologists. *Hypertension in Pregnancy: The Management of Hypertensive Disorders in Pregnancy.* London: National Institute for Health and Clinical Excellence; 2011.
39. Von Dadelszen P, Menzies J, Gilgoff S, *et al.* Evidence-based management for pre-eclampsia. *Front Biosci* 2007; 12:2876–89.
40. Lee W, Gonik B, Cotton DB. Urinary diagnostic indices in pre-eclampsia-associated oliguria: correlation with invasive hemodynamic monitoring. *Am J Obstet Gynecol* 1987; 156:100–3.

41. Duley L, Williams J, Henderson-Smart DJ. Plasma volume expansion for treatment of women with pre-eclampsia. *Cochrane Database Syste Rev* 2000; 2:CD000065.
42. Sehgal NN, Hitt JR. Plasma volume expansion in the treatment of pre-eclampsia. *Am J Obstet Gynecol* 1980; 138:165–8.
43. Aya AG, Mangin R, Vialles N, *et al.* Patients with severe preeclampsia experience less hypotension during spinal anesthesia for elective cesarean delivery than healthy parturients: a prospective cohort comparison. *Anesth Analg* 2003; 97(3):867–72.
44. Engelhardt T, MacLennan FM. Fluid management in pre-eclampsia. *International Journal of Obstetric Anesthesia* 1999; 8:253–9.
45. Berks D, Steegers EA, Molas M, *et al.* Resolution of hypertension and proteinuria after pre-eclampsia. *Obstet Gynecol* 2009; 114(6):1307–14.
46. Bellamy L, Casas J-P, Hingorani AD, *et al.* Pre-eclampsia and risk of cardiovascular disease and cancer in later life: systematic review and meta-analysis. *BMJ* 2007; 335:974.
47. Vikse BE, Irgens LM, Bostad L, *et al.* Adverse perinatal outcome and later kidney biopsy in the mother. *J Am Soc Nephrol* 2006; 17(3):837–45.
48. Vikse BE, Irgens LM, Leivestad T, *et al.* Pre-eclampsia and the risk of end-stage renal disease. *N Engl J Med* 2008; 359:800–9.
49. Martin JN, Blake PG, Perry KG, *et al.* The natural history of HELLP syndrome: patterns of disease progression and recession. *Am J Obstet Gynecol* 1991; 164:1500–9.
50. Guidelines and Audit Committee of the Royal College of Obstetricians and Gynaecologists. *The Management of Severe Pre-Eclampsia/Eclampsia*. Green-top Guideline No. 10(A). London: RCOG Press; 2006.
51. Flynn MF, Power RE, Murphy DM, *et al.* Successful transplantation of kidneys from a donor with HELLP syndrome-related death. *Transpl Int* 2001; 14:108–10.
52. Abraham KA, Kennelly M, Dorman AM, *et al.* Pathogenesis of acute renal failure associated with HELLP syndrome: a case report and review of the literature. *Eur J Obstet Gynecol Reprod Biol* 2003; 108:99–102.
53. Ganesan C, Maynard SE. Acute kidney injury in pregnancy: the thrombotic microangiopathies. *J Nephrol* 2011; 24:554–63.
54. Fonseca JE, Mendez F, Catano C, *et al.* Dexamethasone treatment does not improve the outcome of women with HELLP syndrome: a double-blind, placebo-controlled, randomized clinical trial. *Am J Obstet Gynecol* 2005; 193:1591–8.
55. Martin JN, Bailey AP, Rehberg JF, *et al.* Thrombotic thrombocytopenic purpura in 1666 pregnancies: 1995–2006. *Am J Obstet Gynecol* 2008; 199:98–104.
56. Vasely SK, George JN, Lammle B, *et al.* ADAMTS13 activity in thrombotic thrombocytopenic purpura-hemolytic uraemic syndrome: relation to presenting features and clinical outcomes in a cohort of 142 patients. *Blood* 2003; 102:60–8.
57. Lattuada A, Rossi E, Calzarossa C, *et al.* Mild to moderate reduction of a von Willebrand factor cleaving protease (ADAMTS-13) in pregnant women with HELLP microangiopathic syndrome. *Haematologica* 2003; 88:1029–34.
58. Gammill HS, Jeyabalan A. Acute renal failure in pregnancy. *Crit Care Med* 2005; 33(s10):S372–S384.
59. Furlan M, Lammle B. Haemolytic-uraemic syndrome and thrombotic thrombocytopenic purpura—new insights into underlying biochemical mechanisms. *Nephrol Dial Transplant* 2000; 15:1112–14.
60. Fakhouri F, Roumenina L, Provot F, *et al.* Pregnancy-associated hemolytic uremic syndrome revisited in the era of complement gene mutations. *J Am Soc Nephrol* 2010; 21(5):859–67.
61. Fakhouri F, Jablonski M, Lepercq J. Factor H, membrane cofactor protein, and factor I mutations in patients with hemolysis, elevated liver enzymes, and low platelet count syndrome. *Blood* 2008; 112:4542–5.
62. European Medicines Agency. *Solaris: Summary of Product Characteristics* [Online] http://www.ema.europa.eu/docs/en_GB/document_library/EPAR_-_Product_Information/human/000791/WC500054208.pdf
63. Kelly R, Arnold L, Richards S, *et al.* The management of pregnancy in paroxysmal nocturnal haemoglobinuria on long-term eculizumab. *Br J Haematol* 2012; 149(3):446–50.
64. Marasca R, Coluccio V, Santachiara R, *et al.* Correspondence: Pregnancy in PNH: another eculizumab baby. *Br J Haematol* 2010; 150(6):707–8.
65. Slater DN, Hague WM. Renal morphological changes in idiopathic acute fatty liver of pregnancy. *Histopathology* 1984; 8(4):567–81.
66. Machado S, Figueiredo N, Borges A, *et al.* Acute kidney injury in pregnancy: a clinical challenge. *J Nephrol* 2012; 25:19–30.
67. Mazor-Dray E, Levy A, Schlaeffer F, *et al.* Maternal urinary tract infection: is it independently associated with adverse pregnancy outcome? *J Matern Fetal Neonatal Med* 2009; 22(2):124–8.
68. Evelina Farkash E, Weintraub A, Sergienko R. Acute antepartum pyelonephritis in pregnancy: a critical analysis of risk factors and outcomes. *Eur J Obstet Gynecol Reprod Biol* 2012; 162(1):24–7.
69. Gilstrap LC, Cunningham FG, Whalley PJ. Acute pyelonephritis in pregnancy: an anterospective study. *Obstet Gynecol* 1981; 57:409–13.
70. Smaill F. Antibiotics for aymptomatic bacteriuria in pregnancy. *Cochrane Database Syst Rev* 2000; 2:CD00049.
71. McCormick T, Ashe RG, Kearney PM. Urinary tract infection in pregnancy. *Obstetrician Gynaecologist* 2008; 10(3):156–62.
72. Romero R, Oyarzun E, Mazor M, *et al.* Meta-analysis of the relationship between asymptomatic bacteruria and preterm delivery/low birth weight. *Obstet Gynecol* 1989; 73:576–82.
73. Hollowell JG. Outcome of pregnancy in women with a history of vesico-ureteric reflux. *BJU Int* 2008; 102(7):780–4.
74. Madhumita J, Mitch WE. Rapidly reversible acute renal failure from ureteral obstruction in pregnancy. *Am J Kidney Dis* 1996; 28(3):457–60.
75. Webb JAW. Ultrasonography and Doppler studies in the diagnosis of renal obstruction. *BJU Int* 2000; 86(S1):25–32.
76. Coresh J, Selvin E, Stevens LA, *et al.* Prevalence of chronic kidney disease in the United States. *JAMA* 2007; 298(17):2038–47.
77. Bateman BT, Bansil P, Hernandez-Diaz S, *et al.* Prevalence, trends, and outcomes of chronic hypertension: a nationwide sample of delivery admissions. *Am J Obstet Gynecol* 2012; 206(2):134.e1–34.
78. Floege J, Johnson R, Feehally J (eds). *Comprehensive Clinical Nephrology* (4th ed.) Oxford: Mosby Elsevier; 2010.
79. Anonymous. Pregnancy and renal disease. *Lancet* 1975; 2(7939):801–2.
80. Nevis IF, Reitsma A, Dominic A, *et al.* Pregnancy outcomes in women with chronic kidney disease: a systematic review. *Clin J Am Soc Nephrol* 2011; 6(11):2587–98.
81. Jones DC, Hayslett JP. Outcome of pregnancy in women with moderate or severe renal insufficiency. *N Engl J Med* 1996; 335(4):226–32.
82. Imbasciati E, Gregorini G, Cabiddu G, *et al.* Pregnancy in CKD stages 3 to 5: fetal and maternal outcomes. *Am J Kidney Dis* 2007; 49(6):753–62.
83. Bramham K, Nelson-Piercy C, Gao H, *et al.* Pregnancy in renal transplant recipients: a UK national cohort study. *Clin J Am Soc Nephrol* 2013; 2013; 8(2):290–8.
84. Stratta P, Canavese C, Quaglia M. Pregnancy in patients with kidney disease. *J Nephrol* 2006; 19(2):135–43.
85. Bramham K, Lightstone L. Pre-pregnancy counseling for women with chronic kidney disease. *J Nephrol* 2012; 25(4):450–9.
86. Brown MA, Lindheimer MD, de Swiet M, *et al.* The classification and diagnosis of the hypertensive disorders of pregnancy: statement from the International Society for the Study of Hypertension in Pregnancy (ISSHP). *Hypertens Pregnancy* 2001; 20(1):IX–XIV.
87. Rolfo A, Attini R, Nuzzo AM, *et al.* Chronic kidney disease may be differentially diagnosed from preeclampsia by serum biomarkers. *Kidney Int* 2013; 83(1):177–81.
88. Bramham K, Hunt BJ, Bewley S, *et al.* Pregnancy outcomes in systemic lupus erythematosus with and without previous nephritis. *J Rheumatol* 2011; 38(9):1906–13.
89. Piccoli GB, Gaglioti P, Attini R, *et al.* Pre-eclampsia or chronic kidney disease? The flow hypothesis. *Nephrol Dial Transplant* 2013; 28:1199–206.

90. Duley L, Henderson-Smart DJ, Meher S, *et al.* Antiplatelet agents for preventing pre-eclampsia and its complications. *Cochrane Database Syst Rev* 2007; 2:CD004659.
91. Piccoli GB, Attini R, Vasario E, *et al.* Pregnancy and chronic kidney disease: a challenge in all CKD stages. *Clin J Am Soc Nephrol* 2010; 5(5):844–55.
92. Davison JM, Nelson-Piercy C, Kehoe S, *et al.* Consensus views arising from the 54th study group: renal disease in pregnancy. In Davison JM, Nelson-Piercy C, Kehoe S, *et al.* (eds) *Renal Disease in Pregnancy.* London: RCOG Press 2008:249–51.
93. Holley JL, Bernardini J, Quadri KH, *et al.* Pregnancy outcomes in a prospective matched control study of pregnancy and renal disease. *Clin Nephrol* 1996; 45(2):77–82.
94. EBPG Expert Group on Renal Transplantation. European Best Practice Guidelines for renal transplantation. Long term management of the transplant patient Section IV: pregnancy in renal transplant patients. *Nephrol Dial Transplant* 2002; 17(Suppl 4):50–5.
95. McKay DB, Josephson MA, Armenti VT, *et al.* Reproduction and transplantation: report on the AST Consensus Conference on Reproductive Issues and Transplantation. *Am J Transplant* 2005; 5(7):1592–9.
96. Fischer T, Neumayer HH, Fischer R, *et al.* Effect of pregnancy on long-term kidney function in renal transplant recipients treated with cyclosporine and with azathioprine. *Am J Transplant* 2005; 5(11):2732–9.
97. Kim HW, Seok HJ, Kim TH, *et al.* The experience of pregnancy after renal transplantation: pregnancies even within postoperative 1 year may be tolerable. *Transplantation* 2008; 85(10):1412–19.
98. Deshpande NA, James NT, Kucirka LM, *et al.* Pregnancy outcomes in kidney transplant recipients: a systematic review and meta-analysis. *Am J Transplant* 2011; 11(11):2388–404.
99. Crowe AV, Rustom R, Gradden C, *et al.* Pregnancy does not adversely affect renal transplant function. *QJM* 1999; 92(11):631–5.
100. Gutierrez MJ, Acebedo-Ribo M, Garcia-Donaire JA, *et al.* Pregnancy in renal transplant recipients. *Transplant Proc* 2005; 37(9):3721–2.
101. Keitel E, Bruno RM, Duarte M, *et al.* Pregnancy outcome after renal transplantation. *Transplant Proc* 2004; 36(4):870–1.
102. Stratta P, Canavese C, Giacchino F, *et al.* Pregnancy in kidney transplantation: satisfactory outcomes and harsh realities. *J Nephrol* 2003; 16(6):792–806.
103. Thompson BC, Kingdon EJ, Tuck SM, *et al.* Pregnancy in renal transplant recipients: the Royal Free Hospital experience. *QJM* 2003; 96(11):837–44.
104. Sibanda N, Briggs JD, Davison JM, *et al.* Pregnancy after organ transplantation: a report from the UK Transplant pregnancy registry. *Transplantation* 2007; 83(10):1301–7.
105. Bramham K, Lightstone L, Taylor J, *et al.* Pregnancy in pancreas-kidney transplant recipients; report of 3 cases and review of the literature. *Obstetric Medicine* 2010; 3:73–7.
106. Gilbert-Hayn L SN, McGrory CH. Pregnancy outcomes in female pancreas-kidney (PK) transplant recipients. *Am J Transplant* 2007; 7(S2):250.
107. Wilson GA, Coscia LA, McGrory CH, *et al.* National transplantation pregnancy registry: postpregnancy graft loss among female pancreas-kidney recipients. *Transplant Proc* 2001; 33(1–2):1667–9.
108. Hou S. Pregnancy in women with chronic renal disease. *N Engl J Med* 1985; 312(13):836–9.
109. Okundaye I, Abrinko P, Hou S. Registry of pregnancy in dialysis patients. *Am J Kidney Dis* 1998; 31(5):766–73.
110. Hladunewich M, Hercz AE, Keunen J, *et al.* Pregnancy in end stage renal disease. *Semin Dial* 2011; 24(6):634–9.
111. Barua M, Hladunewich M, Keunen J, *et al.* Successful pregnancies on nocturnal home hemodialysis. *Clin J Am Soc Nephrol* 2008; 3(2):392–6.
112. Haase M, Morgera S, Bamberg C, *et al.* A systematic approach to managing pregnant dialysis patients—the importance of an intensified haemodiafiltration protocol. *Nephrol Dial Transplant* 2005; 20(11):2537–42.
113. Registration Committee of the European Dialysis and Transplant Association. Successful pregnancies in women treated by dialysis and kidney transplantation. *Br J Obstet Gynaecol* 1980; 87(10):839–45.
114. Hou S. Modification of dialysis regimens for pregnancy. *Int J Artif Organs* 2002; 25(9):823–6.
115. Yang LY, Thia EWH, Tan LK. Obstetric outcomes in women with end-stage renal disease on chronic dialysis: a review. *Obstet Med* 2010; 3:48–53.
116. Luders C, Castro MC, Titan SM, *et al.* Obstetric outcome in pregnant women on long-term dialysis: a case series. *Am J Kidney Dis* 2010; 56(1):77–85.
117. Holley JL, Reddy SS. Pregnancy in dialysis patients: a review of outcomes, complications, and management. *Semin Dial* 2003; 16(5):384–8.
118. Yankowitz J, Piraino B, Laifer S, *et al.* Erythropoietin in pregnancies complicated by severe anemia of renal failure. *Obstet Gynecol* 1992; 80(3 Pt 2):485–8.
119. Hou S, Orlowski J, Pahl M, *et al.* Pregnancy in women with end-stage renal disease: treatment of anemia and premature labor. *Am J Kidney Dis* 1993; 21(1):16–22.
120. Hou S. Pregnancy in women requiring dialysis for renal failure. *Am J Kidney Dis* 1987; 9(4):368–73.
121. Smyth A, Oliveira GH, Lahr BD, *et al.* A systematic review and meta-analysis of pregnancy outcomes in patients with systemic lupus erythematosus and lupus nephritis. *Clin J Am Soc Nephrol* 2010; 5(11):2060–8.
122. Wagner S, Craici I, Reed D, *et al.* Maternal and foetal outcomes in pregnant patients with active lupus nephritis. *Lupus* 2009; 18(4):342–7.
123. Clowse ME, Magder L, Petri M. Cyclophosphamide for lupus during pregnancy. *Lupus* 2005; 14(8):593–7.
124. Chakravarty EF, Murray ER, Kelman A, *et al.* Pregnancy outcomes after maternal exposure to rituximab. *Blood* 2011; 117(5):1499–506.
125. Friedman DM, Rupel A, Buyon JP. Epidemiology, etiology, detection, and treatment of autoantibody-associated congenital heart block in neonatal lupus. *Curr Rheumatol Rep* 2007; 9(2):101–8.
126. Izmirly PM, Costedoat-Chalumeau N, Pisoni CN, *et al.* Maternal use of hydroxychloroquine is associated with a reduced risk of recurrent anti-SSA/Ro-antibody-associated cardiac manifestations of neonatal lupus. *Circulation* 2012; 126(1):76–82.
127. Pisoni CN, Brucato A, Ruffatti A, et al. Failure of intravenous immunoglobulin to prevent congenital heart block: Findings of a multicenter, prospective, observational study. *Arthritis Rheum* 2010; 62(4):1147–52.
128. Cimaz R, Spence DL, Hornberger L, *et al.* Incidence and spectrum of neonatal lupus erythematosus: a prospective study of infants born to mothers with anti-Ro autoantibodies. *J Pediatr* 2003; 142(6):678–83.
129. Jungers P, Forget D, Houillier P, *et al.* Pregnancy in IgA nephropathy, reflux nephropathy, and focal glomerular sclerosis. *Am J Kidney Dis* 1987; 9(4):334–8.
130. Abe S. (1991). Pregnancy in IgA nephropathy. *Kidney Int* 40(6):1098–102.
131. Limardo M, Imbasciati E, Ravani P, *et al.* Pregnancy and progression of IgA nephropathy: results of an Italian multicenter study. *Am J Kidney Dis* 2010; 56(3):506–12.
132. Chapman AB, Johnson AM, Gabow PA. Pregnancy outcome and its relationship to progression of renal failure in autosomal dominant polycystic kidney disease. *J Am Soc Nephrol* 1994; 5(5):1178–85.
133. Jungers P, Houillier P, Chauveau D, *et al.* Pregnancy in women with reflux nephropathy. *Kidney Int* 1996; 50(2):593–9.
134. Ekbom P, Damm P, Feldt-Rasmussen B, *et al.* Pregnancy outcome in type 1 diabetic women with microalbuminuria. *Diabetes Care* 2001; 24(10):1739–44.

135. Star J, Carpenter MW. The effect of pregnancy on the natural history of diabetic retinopathy and nephropathy. *Clin Perinatol* 1998; 25(4):887–916.
136. Gordon M, Landon MB, Samuels P, *et al.* Perinatal outcome and long-term follow-up associated with modern management of diabetic nephropathy. *Obstet Gynecol* 1996; 87(3):401–9.
137. Reece EA, Leguizamon G, Homko C. Pregnancy performance and outcomes associated with diabetic nephropathy. *Am J Perinatol* 1998; 15(7):413–21.
138. Hod M, van Dijk DJ, Karp M, *et al.* Diabetic nephropathy and pregnancy: the effect of ACE inhibitors prior to pregnancy on fetomaternal outcome. *Nephrol Dial Transplant* 1995; 10(12):2328–33.
139. Piccoli G, Daidola G, Attini R, *et al.* Kidney biopsy in pregnancy: evidence for counselling? A systematic narrative review. *BJOG* 2013; 120(4):412–27.
140. Pere PJ, Ekstrand A, Salonen M, *et al.* Pharmacokinetics of ropivacaine in patients with chronic renal failure. *Br J Anaesth* 2011; 106:512–21.
141. Beilin Y, Reid RW. Renal disease. In Chestnut DH, Polley LS, Tsen LC, *et al.* (eds) *Chestnut's Obstetric Anesthesia: Principles and Practice* (4th ed). Philadelphia, PA: Mosby Elsevier; 2009:1095–108.
142. Koehntop DE, Rodman JH. Fentanyl pharmacokinetics in patients undergoing renal transplantation. *Pharmacotherapy* 1997; 17:746–52.
143. Williams D. Pregnancy with pre-existing kidney disease. In Floege J, Johnson R, Feehally J (eds) *Comprehensive Clinical Nephrology* (4th ed). Oxford: Mosby Elsevier, 2010:495–504.

CHAPTER 45

Neurological disease

James Griffiths and Kate Drummond

Introduction

Neurological disease is an important cause of maternal morbidity and mortality,[1] and presents a significant challenge to the obstetric anaesthetist. The eighth Confidential Enquiries into Maternal Deaths (CEMD) reported 36 women who died from neurological causes. These women died from such conditions as subarachnoid haemorrhage, intracerebral haemorrhage, thrombosis, and epilepsy. Overall, the rate of maternal mortality related to neurological disease (1.57/100,000 maternities) has remained little changed over the past several decades, despite significant improvements in overall maternal morbidity and mortality. Eleven of the 36 deaths in the reported triennium had major elements of substandard care 'where different treatment might have altered the outcome'.[2] It is critical that any anaesthetist involved in the care of pregnant women is aware of the implications of neurological disease for the safe provision of both neuroanaesthesia and obstetric anaesthesia, sometimes in combination.[3,4]

This chapter will predominantly focus on the provision of obstetric anaesthesia and analgesia for the parturient with neurological disease. However, there are some important principles and considerations when undertaking neurosurgical procedures in pregnant women and these will also be outlined briefly.[3,5,6]

Anaesthetists may be asked to care for the parturient with neurological disease in several clinical settings. Firstly, women may present at any stage of pregnancy requiring urgent surgical intervention for neurosurgical disease, such as space-occupying lesions or subarachnoid haemorrhage. Secondly, women with pre-existing neurological disease may present requesting analgesia for labour and delivery or anaesthesia for caesarean delivery. Also, anaesthetists are often requested to assist in the evaluation and management of women who present whilst pregnant or immediately postpartum with a new onset of neurological symptoms, such as headache or peripheral numbness.[7] It is important that the anaesthetist is aware that pregnant women may present with neurological symptoms associated with obstetric disease, such as pre-eclampsia, those indirectly related to or exacerbated by pregnancy, such as cerebral venous thrombosis or subarachnoid haemorrhage, and also those conditions related to anaesthesia, such as postdural puncture headache and neuropraxia following obstetric neuraxial blockade.[8,9]

Although a pregnant woman is, in general, no more likely to suffer from a serious neurological or neurosurgical condition than a non-pregnant woman, the physiological and anatomical changes associated with pregnancy and the concern for both maternal and fetal welfare, which may be conflicting, add to the complexity of management. This is hampered by the lack of class I or II evidence for these complex decisions in the majority of instances. Case reports and case series provide some important guidance but the majority of management is based on general principles. Care of the pregnant woman with a neurological condition thus requires a coordinated approach involving a multidisciplinary team, including neurosurgeon, neurologist, obstetrician, anaesthetist, midwife, neonatologist, and potentially, interventional radiologist. Surgery is generally avoided in pregnancy, occurring in less than 2% of parturient women,[10] with neurosurgical procedures being rare. However, recent studies suggest the safety of planned neurosurgical procedures during pregnancy when warranted, and undue delay may result in neurological deterioration with poor outcomes for mother and child.[5,6,11,12] Care is likely to be optimal in a tertiary setting, particularly if neurosurgical, obstetric, and neonatal management can occur on the same site.

Care for the fetus involves consideration of the timing of delivery (which may be before, after, or coincidental with a neurosurgical procedure), fetal monitoring, and maternal positioning during procedures to minimize the impact on placental perfusion. Fetal welfare may be compromised by any derangement of maternal physiology, including hypotension, hypoxaemia, and hypocarbia, and by many drugs commonly used in neurological disorders and neuroanaesthesia. Intraoperative fetal monitoring is only of benefit if sufficiently experienced staff are available to interpret the data, and clinical facilities are available to expedite delivery should this be indicated. Careful planning with specialist radiologists should be undertaken to optimize the diagnostic utility of neuroimaging, with due consideration to the use of contrast and radiation shielding to optimize fetal outcomes.[13]

General considerations

Many of the principles of anaesthesia for neurosurgery in the pregnant women are identical to those when undertaking any non-obstetric procedure.[14] These include planning for a potentially difficult airway, appropriate aspiration prophylaxis and airway protection, maternal positioning to avoid aortocaval compression and optimize placental perfusion, fetal monitoring, suppression of preterm labour, and the risk of postpartum haemorrhage if caesarean delivery is combined with a non-obstetric procedure.

The great majority of procedures will be undertaken under general anaesthesia, although spinal surgery under epidural anaesthesia has been reported.[15] There is no evidence that any specific anaesthetic technique is contraindicated in pregnancy. Early studies suggested prolonged occupational exposure to nitrous oxide may be associated with increased risk of fetal loss; however, more recent studies have refuted this.[16–20] When propofol is used for maintenance of anaesthesia during caesarean delivery, it has been shown to result in reduced neurobehavioural performance in the neonate.[21] It is unlikely this would be clinically significant in a neurosurgical setting. Potent opioids (such as remifentanil and alfentanil) are useful to ablate the haemodynamic responses to laryngoscopy and intubation, but, however, may result in neonatal chest wall rigidity and respiratory depression.[22,23] Intra-arterial monitoring of blood pressure should be used for all but the most minor procedure in a pregnant patient with neurosurgical disease.

Positioning

Depending on the nature of the procedure, neurosurgery may be undertaken in a variety of positions including supine, lateral, prone, and sitting. Great care must be undertaken when positioning pregnant patients for surgery. The prone position may add to difficulties with fetal heart rate monitoring, emergency caesarean delivery, and potentially increases epidural venous bleeding.[3] It has been proposed that surgery in the prone position should be avoided altogether in pregnancy.[24]

Raised intracranial pressure

Strategies for maintaining stable intracranial pressure are critical in any intracranial surgical procedure. A number of common approaches need to be modified in the pregnant patient. The physiological increase in ventilation in later pregnancy results in a respiratory alkalosis, with arterial carbon dioxide tension (P_ACO_2) falling to around 4–4.2 kPa. Excessive hyperventilation has been associated with worsening of neurosurgical outcomes due to cerebral ischaemia from intense vasoconstriction, but also may result in uterine artery vasoconstriction and decreased placental blood flow.[3] Animal studies have demonstrated that the administration of mannitol may result in a number of adverse fetal effects including hyperosmolarity, hypernatraemia, and reduced lung fluid production.[25,26] However, published cases report the use of small doses of mannitol (0.25–0.5 mg/kg) and it appears to be safe.[3,14]

Oxytocics

There is limited data available regarding the use of oxytocics in the setting of neurological and neurosurgical disease. Syntocinon® causes a brief but significant decrease in systemic blood pressure with a corresponding increase in heart rate and cardiac output.[27] Ergometrine causes significant systemic hypertension which may be associated with a corresponding increase in intracranial pressure, and should be used with caution in patients with raised intracranial pressure. There is limited data to support the use of prostaglandins such as E_1 and $F_{2\alpha}$ in a neurosurgical/obstetric setting, although it has been proposed.[28]

Steroids

Glucocorticoids are frequently used in neurosurgical disease (such as to reduce oedema surrounding brain tumours) but also in neurological disease (e.g. to treat acute exacerbations of multiple sclerosis (MS)). Single doses or short courses of dexamethasone or methylprednisolone have not been shown to be harmful to the fetus, and will actually contribute to fetal lung maturity.[29]

Epilepsy

Aetiology

Epilepsy is a common neurological disorder in pregnancy, with an incidence in the order of 0.3–0.7%.[30] The condition is characterized by repeated paroxysmal seizures in the absence of another cause (such as drug withdrawal or hypoglycaemia). A variety of types of seizures and patterns of epilepsy have been classified, based on the clinical description of the seizure event.[31] Clinically observed seizures are triggered as a result of excessive neuronal firing, which can either be localized or generalized. Seizures from a localized source reflect the abnormal activity related neuroanatomically to that site. Seizures are considered simple or complex, depending on whether consciousness is affected, and focal (partial) or generalized depending on whether a localized area or the entire cerebral cortex is involved.

Obstetric considerations

Epilepsy remains a major cause of morbidity and mortality in pregnancy, with 14 deaths reported in the 2006–2008 CEMD report published in 2011.[2] The hypoxia and respiratory acidosis associated with maternal seizures may also increase the risk of fetal loss. In a case series of 154 pregnancies in women with epilepsy, only 31% were seizure free throughout pregnancy. Seizure frequency increased in 32%, decreased in 14%, and remained unchanged in 23% of cases.[32]

Women with epilepsy require carefully coordinated care between their neurologist and obstetrician, preferably commencing prior to conception. In most patients, effective seizure prophylaxis must continue through pregnancy, as the adverse effects of seizures during pregnancy outweigh the risk to the fetus of antiepileptic medication. However, choice of agent remains controversial.[33] There is evidence that the risk of fetal abnormalities increases with the use of multiple agents, so in general, the aim should be monotherapy, at the lowest possible effective dose.[33] Many antiepileptic drugs (AEDs) are known to increase the risk of fetal abnormalities.[34] Older AEDs, including phenytoin, valproate, carbamazepine, and barbiturates, are all known to cause abnormalities in humans, whereas data is lacking for newer agents (such as lamotrigine, gabapentin, and levetiracetam).[35] It appears that valproate is the least acceptable agent for use in pregnancy. Common abnormalities for all AEDs include neural tube defects, orofacial abnormalities, alimentary tract atresia, diaphragmatic hernia, and congenital heart disease.[35]

Low maternal plasma levels of folate have been shown to be associated with major fetal malformations particularly neural tube defects.[36] Folate supplementation appears to decrease this risk and all pregnant women should take low-dose (0.4 mg/day) supplemental folate. Animal studies have shown that carbamazepine and valproate both act to decrease maternal folate plasma concentrations and high-dose supplementation (4 mg/day) may be of benefit.[37]

In addition to folate supplementation, consideration should be given to prescribing vitamin K supplementation to women taking AEDs in late pregnancy. AEDs (particularly phenytoin and carbamazepine) cross the placenta and induce hepatic microenzymes, resulting in degradation of neonatal vitamin K. There are published data to both support and refute the possibility that this increases the risk of neonatal haemorrhage.[38,39] Whilst neonatal vitamin K should be administered routinely, many practitioners recommend the additional administration of maternal vitamin K as a cheap and low-risk intervention.[40]

There are many reasons why seizure frequency may increase during pregnancy, including non-compliance with medication, altered metabolism of drugs, fluid and electrolyte retention, hyperventilation leading to respiratory alkalosis, stress, sleep deprivation, and hormonal changes. If available, drug levels should be monitored during pregnancy and dosage adjusted accordingly especially phenytoin, carbamazepine, and lamotrigine. Consideration should be given to parenteral administration of AED if gastric absorption in labour is uncertain. Many antiepileptic drugs are unavailable parenterally, so an alternative agent may be needed in labour (such as phenytoin or levetiracetam).

While most pregnancies proceed uneventfully, it is possible that pregnant women with epilepsy taking AEDs may be at increased risk of a number of obstetric complications, including pre-eclampsia, preterm labour, and peripartum bleeding.

In addition to the risk of major malformations, associated with AEDs, women with epilepsy appear to be at higher risk of low birth weight babies (<2500g). Infants of epileptic mothers also may be at higher risk of developmental delay.

Anaesthetic implications

A patient presenting with a seizure during pregnancy is a medical emergency. Whilst standard resuscitation measures are instituted, a broad differential diagnosis must be considered (Box 45.1), even in a known epileptic.[32] If eclampsia is likely, then seizures should be treated with magnesium sulphate and delivery should be expedited once the patient is stabilized. Magnesium sulphate is, however, not appropriate treatment for epileptic seizures, which should be treated with a benzodiazepine. In the setting of emergency caesarean delivery, general anaesthesia is indicated if the airway is compromised by the postictal conscious state.

Many AEDs have the potential to cause important but complex pharmacokinetic interactions with a wide variety of other classes of medication.[41] Some (including carbamazepine, phenytoin, and phenobarbitone) can induce hepatic microenzymes of the cytochrome P450 subtype, leading to the accelerated metabolism—and hence lower plasma levels—of many other medications. Medications which may be affected include antibacterials, immunosuppressants, and cardiovascular medications such as amiodarone and beta blockers.[42] Conversely, other AEDs, such as valproate, can inhibit enzyme activity leading to delayed metabolism and hence higher plasma levels of other drugs. Benzodiazepines, valproate, and phenytoin are highly protein bound and may compete for protein binding sites, increasing the free concentrations of other drugs.

Box 45.1 Differential diagnosis of seizures in pregnancy

- (Pre-) Eclampsia
- Epilepsy
- Local anaesthetic toxicity
- Amniotic fluid embolism
- Cerebral venous thrombosis
- Space-occupying lesion (e.g. tumour, haemorrhage)
- Drug withdrawal (e.g. alcohol)
- Electrolyte abnormality (e.g. hyponatraemia, hypoglycaemia)
- Pseudo-seizure

Many anaesthetic agents have the potential to either increase or decrease the seizure threshold.[41] Benzodiazepines and barbiturates are all anticonvulsant. Opioids, particularly pethidine (meperidine), may cause seizures, as may etomidate. Somewhat confusingly, propofol has been associated with excitatory activity including seizures and seizure-like phenomena; however, it also has a role in status epilepticus.[43] Neuraxial analgesia and anaesthesia is safe, although high doses of local anaesthetic may also reduce the seizure threshold and thus, these agents should be titrated judiciously.

Cerebrovascular disease

Introduction

Cerebrovascular disorders are the neurological diseases most commonly seen during pregnancy and include cerebral aneurysm, arteriovenous malformation (AVM), cavernous haemangioma, intracerebral haematoma, ischaemic stroke, and cerebral venous sinus thrombosis (CVT), as well as a number of newly defined cerebral vasoconstriction entities, including reversible cerebral vasoconstriction syndrome (RCVS), and posterior reversible encephalopathy syndrome (PRES).[7] Overall, these lesions are uncommon in pregnancy, but the risk is increased compared to the general population[44] and there is some evidence that the rate is increasing.[45] The reported rates for ischaemic stroke are 4–11/100,000 live births, for intracerebral haematoma 3.7–9/100,000 live births, and for subarachnoid haemorrhage 2.4–11/100,000 live births.[44–51] The risk may be increased in Asian patients.[52] Despite their rarity, cerebrovascular disorders account for more than 10% of all non-obstetric maternal deaths.[47,53–55] Anaesthetic considerations are twofold; firstly there is the patient presenting with an acute event, such as a subarachnoid haemorrhage or intracerebral haemorrhage from an aneurysm or AVM, who needs treatment during pregnancy and the second is management of delivery in the patient with a known lesion at risk for rupture. The natural history of many of these lesions in pregnancy is unknown due to their rarity. Guidelines that exist for management of the non-pregnant patient[56,57] may not apply due to the physiological changes associated with pregnancy, which may change the risk profile of the lesion, and the paucity of pregnant patients included in most large trials. Most studies are case series or case reports.[11,58–60] However, from these limited reports it would appear that neurosurgical treatment of these lesions, as dictated by standard neurosurgical care, may result in good maternal and fetal outcomes, with minimal additional morbidity and mortality associated with the surgical procedure.

It should be remembered that the differential diagnosis between these uncommon lesions and the much more common pre-eclampsia and eclampsia (which occur in up to 8% of pregnancies)[61] can be difficult. Acute neurological symptoms in pregnancy are more likely to be due to these latter conditions, but there is a significant overlap, and symptoms such as hypertension and proteinuria can also be present in neurological disorders such as aneurysmal subarachnoid haemorrhage.[62] Pre-eclampsia can result in ischaemic stroke, intracerebral hypertensive haematoma, subarachnoid haemorrhage, and CVT.[7] Severe vasoconstriction can also occur in pre-eclampsia, resulting in cerebral infarction or haemorrhage, and is associated with RCVS and PRES.[63]

Pre-eclampsia and eclampsia are the cause of up to 50% of strokes in pregnancy.[47,48,64]

The clinical presentation of these lesions is with the sudden onset of a severe headache (thunderclap headache), often described as 'the worst headache of my life', which is the result of haemorrhage into the subarachnoid space from a ruptured aneurysm or AVM, CVT, or severe hypertension in pre-eclampsia. Cerebral vasospasm, arterial dissection or pituitary apoplexy can result in a similar headache.[65] Intracerebral bleeding may present with a more gradual onset headache with evolving neurological deficit and decreased level of consciousness and ischaemic stroke with the sudden onset of a neurological deficit. Each of these presentations requires immediate expert review[66] and thorough investigation, initially with computed tomography (CT) scan, but if negative, with lumbar puncture and, if necessary, advanced imaging such as magnetic resonance imaging (MRI) or angiography. The risk of a missed serious diagnosis far outweighs the negligible risk of a brain CT scan with lead shielding of the fetus.[67–69]

The association of pregnancy with intracranial haemorrhage, particularly from an aneurysm or AVM, has been suggested to be due to hormonal and physiological effects on the cerebral blood vessels, but often with scanty evidence. These effects include vascular wall weakening due to hyperplasia of arterial smooth muscle and loss of normal elastic fibre alignment.[70] Pregnancy-induced hypertension, increased plasma volume, and increased cardiac output are also thought to play a role.[47,62,71] However, the literature is inconclusive as to whether the incidence of bleeding is actually higher in pregnancy and depends on the methodology and population used to determine incidence.[46,53,54,58,62,64,72,73]

Many of the cerebrovascular disorders discussed above are important causes of neurological presentations in pregnancy, but are unlikely to require neuroanaesthesia for surgical intervention or to have serious implications for mode of delivery. These include arterial dissection,[74–76] CVT,[77,78] RCVS,[63,79] and PRES.[80–82] Thus, they will not be considered further and the reader is directed to the relevant reviews cited. Those most relevant to obstetric anaesthesia are cerebral aneurysm, AVM, cavernous haemangioma, and ischaemic stroke and these are discussed in further detail.

Cerebral aneurysms and arteriovenous malformation

Ruptured aneurysms and AVM

Spontaneous subarachnoid haemorrhage occurs in 0.01–0.05% of pregnancies and is due to ruptured aneurysm in 77% of cases and ruptured AVM in 23%, with a reported maternal mortality varying widely between 10% and 83%, but probably closest to 10–20% with aggressive modern multimodality management. The fetal mortality is 17–26%.[47,53,55] The incidence of rupture rises with advancing trimester, being 6% in the first trimester and 55% in the third for cerebral aneurysms.[6,83] Once ruptured, the risk of recurrent haemorrhage from an untreated aneurysm or AVM is 25–50%, with an associated maternal mortality of 50–70%. For AVM, the calculated 26% rebleeding rate in the same pregnancy is higher than the 6–7.3% re-bleed rate in the first year in the general population.[73,84,85] Due to this risk of devastating recurrent haemorrhage, aggressive management is particularly warranted. Thus, standard neurosurgical management of ruptured lesions is advocated, with immediate securing of the ruptured aneurysm or resection or other treatment of the AVM. Standard medical management of symptomatic vasospasm, which complicates approximately one-third of aneurysmal subarachnoid haemorrhages, should also be as for non-pregnant patients. The mainstay of this treatment, 'triple H therapy', that is, intravenous fluid with or without pressors to achieve 'hypertension, hypervolaemia, and haemodilution' may not need to be as aggressively pursued due to the hypervolaemia of pregnancy. Nimodipine, a calcium channel antagonist, is widely used for vasospasm prophylaxis and treatment in both aneurysmal subarachnoid haemorrhage and pre-eclampsia and eclampsia, but is of unproven safety for the fetus and may cause maternal and fetal hypotension.[6,62,86]

Management of ruptured lesions along reported neurosurgical principles, results in the most favourable maternal and fetal outcomes and is almost universally recommended.[11,53,58–60,71,73,85,87] In pregnant patients with a pre-viable fetus, neurosurgical or endovascular treatment of the lesion should occur during pregnancy with later delivery. For a viable fetus, delivery by caesarean delivery under general anaesthesia followed immediately by definitive treatment is recommended.

Aneurysm rupture usually results in subarachnoid haemorrhage (Figure 45.1A), with thunderclap headache, vomiting, photophobia, focal neurological signs, and decreased level of consciousness. However, AVM may present with either haemorrhage or seizures. Rupture is more commonly into the cerebral parenchyma, rather than the subarachnoid space, with more gradual headache and focal neurological deficit. Initial imaging is with CT scan, as described above, but definitive imaging of the lesion requires either CT angiography or digital subtraction angiography (Figure 45.1B).[13] In general, imaging involving ionizing radiation is avoided in pregnancy, however, the gravity of an aneurysm or AVM diagnosis warrants their judicious use. Most reports would suggest minimal or no risk to the fetus with properly planned imaging[68,69,88] and consideration of the risks of hypothyroidism in the neonate after administration of iodinated contrast agents.[89–92] MRI is also useful to determine the position and characteristics of an AVM. MRI is safe in pregnancy and is further discussed in the section on intracranial tumours.[90,93–96]

The choice of treatment modality, either surgical or endovascular (Figure 45.1C), of ruptured aneurysms in the pregnant patient is controversial. In the non-pregnant population, the International Subarachnoid Aneurysm Trial (ISAT) study[56] reported improved outcomes with coiling over clipping and has resulted in an exponential increase in endovascular coiling of aneurysms if technically feasible. However, in the pregnant patient, concerns for ionizing radiation with a prolonged neuro-interventional procedure, iodinated contrast load, the risk of only partial obliteration of the aneurysm, and the possible need for short- and long-term anticoagulation are pertinent.[6] The literature would suggest that clipping, with definitive occlusion of the aneurysm, continues to be favoured by neurosurgeons for pregnant patients.[54] However, safe and successful endovascular coil embolization has been described in pregnancy with phantom calculations of radiation dose to the fetus being within acceptable limits.[88,97] For AVM, treatment options include surgery, endovascular obliteration, and stereotactic radiosurgery, or combinations thereof. Treatment decisions are complex, particularly in pregnancy, and largely based on incomplete and retrospective data, with no level 1 evidence.[98] Thus, decisions should be made in the context of a multidisciplinary discussion including the cerebrovascular team,

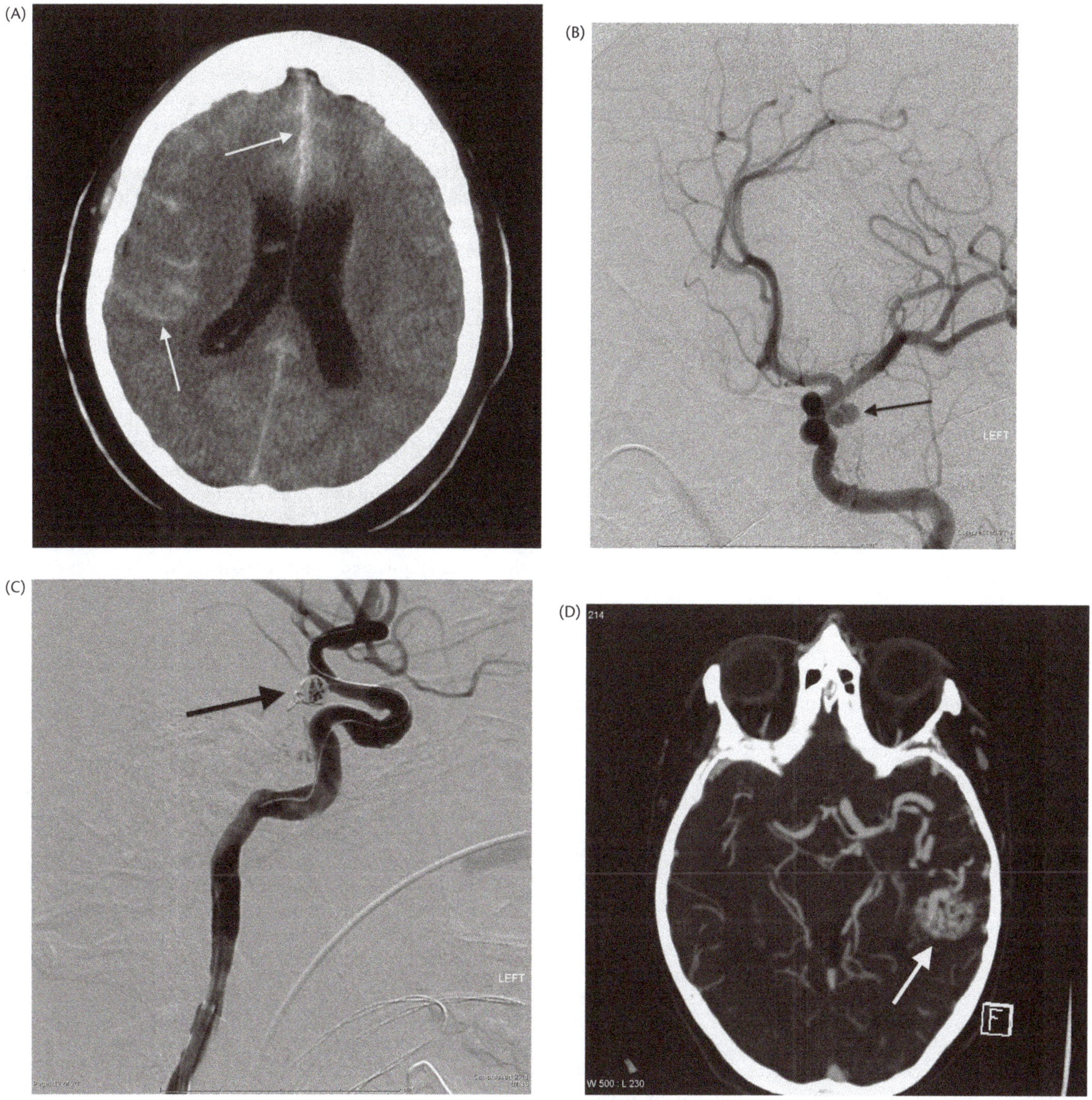

Figure 45.1 (A) Axial CT scan brain showing subarachnoid haemorrhage with hyperdense blood in the interhemispheric region and cortical sulci (arrows). (B) Oblique projection of a left internal carotid angiogram showing a posterior communicating artery aneurysm (arrow). (C) Left internal carotid angiogram during endovascular coiling of the posterior communicating artery aneurysm in (B) showing the loosely packed coil mass (arrow). (D) Axial CT angiogram showing a left temporal arteriovenous malformation.

obstetrician, neonatologist, and anaesthetist. Facilities offering both neurosurgical and obstetric care are optimal.[99]

During routine surgery for clipping of a cerebral aneurysm, induced hypotension is commonly used to facilitate clipping of the aneurysm; however, this should be avoided in pregnancy due to the risk of uterine hypoperfusion, as uterine blood flow is not autoregulated. Similarly, vigorous osmotic diuresis should be avoided to avoid hypotension and fetal hyperosmolarity, although small doses of mannitol (0.5–1 g/kg) can probably be used safely.[62]

As for all neurosurgical procedures, hypertension during induction of anaesthesia, endotracheal intubation, or application of skull clamp pins should be avoided.

Unruptured aneurysms and AVM

The risk of rupture of an unruptured aneurysm during pregnancy and delivery is unknown and it has been suggested that pregnancy and labour confers increased risk,[46,53,58] although not all authors agree.[72] A recent, large, 20-year population-based study suggested the risk of rupture during pregnancy to be 1.4% and during delivery to be 0.05%, which is similar to that of the general population. Interestingly, the caesarean delivery rate amongst patients with a known unruptured aneurysm was over 70%, almost triple that of the general population, and the authors suggested that this may be unwarranted based on their estimates.[54] Neurosurgical or endovascular management of an unruptured aneurysm diagnosed in or before pregnancy should be along standard neurosurgical practice, with no evidence to suggest benefit of treatment during or before pregnancy of an aneurysm that would otherwise be observed based on guidelines from large international trials.[57] Enlarging, symptomatic, or high-risk aneurysms can be considered for treatment, with decisions regarding the timing and mode of therapy being made by a multidisciplinary team considering the characteristics of the aneurysm and the risk to maternal and fetal welfare.[54]

For AVM (Figure 45.1D), the risk of rupture is probably higher in the pregnant patient compared to that in the non-pregnant female population, although, as for aneurysms, the data is conflicting. The risk of a primary haemorrhage from an unruptured AVM in a pregnant patient is reported to be between 3.5% and 9.3%.[58,59,73,85,100–102] An increased haemorrhage rate is attributed to, as for cerebral aneurysms, pregnancy-related hormonal and physiological effects on the vessel wall, plasma volume, blood pressure, and cardiac output, and is highest in the second trimester.[53,85,100] Thus, treatment of the unruptured AVM, if feasible, is often recommended prior to conception. If discovered during pregnancy, a caesarean delivery under general anaesthesia is usually recommended, although, as for cerebral aneurysms, there is scant evidence on which to base this recommendation.[73,84,103]

Overall, the most appropriate mode of delivery for women with treated, untreated or partially treated aneurysms and AVM is unknown, although commonly caesarean delivery under general anaesthetic is recommended unless the aneurysm or AVM has been definitively treated with clipping or complete excision. Only 2% of aneurysms actually rupture during labour, with 90% of ruptures occurring during pregnancy and 8% postpartum[53,54] but if the rupture rate is corrected for the time spent in each of the stages of pregnancy, labour and the postpartum period carry the highest risk.[44,47,50,62,71] However, the literature is inconclusive, and there is no evidence to suggest improved outcomes or a reduced rupture rate with caesarean delivery over closely supervised vaginal delivery, particularly under epidural anaesthesia.[53,58,60,85] Broadly, the mode of delivery of ruptured aneurysms and AVM should be based on neurosurgical considerations and the management of unruptured or definitively treated lesions should be based on obstetric considerations. Generally, the use of epidural anaesthesia and an assisted second stage of labour to avoid hypertension and the Valsalva manoeuver are advised, unless the lesion is confidently obliterated.[6,105] Less certain methods of treatment with respect to completeness of exclusion from the circulation, such as partial endovascular coiling or embolization should be considered with caution. It has been suggested that spinal anaesthesia, and also inadvertent dural puncture during epidural anaesthesia, should be avoided in unruptured or incompletely obliterated aneurysms and AVM, due to the risk of rupture with cerebrospinal fluid (CSF) drainage and reduction in the lesion transmural pressure.[106]

Cavernous haemangioma

Cavernous haemangiomas ('cavernomas') are common vascular malformations consisting of sinusoidal venous channels within the cerebral parenchyma. They are present in 0.4% of the population and are frequently asymptomatic.[107] Symptomatic presentation is with seizure or bleeding with intracerebral haematoma, although catastrophic haemorrhage is uncommon unless located in the brainstem or other eloquent area. Similar to other vascular malformations, an increased propensity to bleed during pregnancy is reported or assumed.[50,53,108] However, two large recent studies would suggest no increased risk from pregnancy and found no contraindication to normal vaginal delivery.[109,110]

Ischaemic stroke

Ischaemic stroke is uncommon in pregnant and postpartum women but the incidence is three times higher than in the age-matched non-pregnant female population.[44,46,47] This increased incidence is likely to be related to the hypercoagulability of pregnancy and the risk is increased by hypertension (including pre-eclampsia), dehydration, anaemia, electrolyte and acid–base disturbance, haemorrhage, transfusion, infection, and caesarean delivery.[111] There is some evidence that women with pre-eclampsia undergoing caesarean delivery under general anaesthesia may have more than double the incidence of stroke compared to women receiving neuraxial anaesthesia[112].

Most strokes occur in the days before or after delivery and the mortality can approach 13%.[44,46] Management is as for ischaemic stroke in the non-pregnant population, including the use of intravenous or intra-arterial tissue plasminogen activator, although the safety profile in pregnancy is not yet clear.[113,114] Increasingly, ischaemic strokes are managed using chemical thrombolysis or mechanical thrombectomy or embolectomy in the interventional neuroradiology suite, with similar concerns to those outlined for endovascular coil embolization of cerebral aneurysms. These interventions are generally performed under general anaesthesia. Considerations are of raised intracranial pressure due to the mass effect of the stroke, similar to that for an intracranial tumour, and meticulous blood pressure control to avoid hypertensive bleeding into the ischaemic brain or hypotension with uterine hypoperfusion.

Multiple sclerosis

Introduction

MS is a chronic immune-mediated disease resulting in demyelinated plaques within the central nervous system. The disease is more common in women than men, and commonly presents in women of reproductive age.[115] Estimates of the prevalence vary widely but typically range between 66 and 168/100,000.[116] There is evidence that the incidence of the disease may be increasing in some parts of the world, particularly in females.[102,117]

Pathology

MS is thought to be fundamentally an organ-specific autoimmune disease. The initial pathology is thought to be inflammation, demyelination, and axonal degeneration secondary to autoreactive lymphocytes. This is followed, in more chronic stages, by microglial activation and chronic neurodegeneration.[118]

Aetiology

Whilst the disease is primarily autoimmune in nature, a wide variety of genetic, environmental, and immunological factors have been implicated in the aetiology. Current theories suggest that susceptible individuals are more likely to develop the disease if they are exposed to certain environmental triggers, such as smoking. Susceptible individuals include those with a family history, certain ethnic groups, and particular human leucocyte antigen subtypes. Epidemiological studies in Australia and Canada suggest an association with exposure to ultraviolet light (and/or vitamin D levels). Previous infection with a viral illness such as Epstein–Barr virus may also be implicated,[119,120] and this raises the controversy as to whether previous viral immunization may be associated with MS.[119]

Clinical course

MS is characterized by episodic relapses and remissions of discrete neurological deficits. There may be complete recovery between episodes ('relapsing remitting MS') or a gradual progression of underlying disability ('chronic progressive MS'). Many patients over time with relapsing remitting MS will gradually develop chronic progressive symptoms. Relapses tend to evolve over several days. Common presentations include optic neuritis (with decreased vision and pain in one eye), limb ataxia, limb weakness and paraesthesia, bladder dysfunction, and progressive symptoms of respiratory weakness and fatigue.

Diagnosis is based on a characteristic clinical course and the presence of diagnostic lesions on T2-weighted and fluid-attenuated inversion recovery (FLAIR) MRI images of the brain, optic nerve, or spinal cord.[121] There may also be characteristic abnormalities in CSF or changes in visual or somatosensory evoked potentials.

Treatment of MS aims to accelerate resolution of symptomatic episodes, prevent recurrent episodes, and slow the progression of the disease. Treatment of acute episodes may include high-dose methylprednisolone or plasma exchange transfusion. Interferon and glatiramer are both used to prevent recurrence of attacks.[122] Interferon slows progression of the disease by immune modulation, reducing T cell proliferation and tumour necrosis factor alpha production. Side effects include flu-like symptoms, liver enzyme elevation, and leucopenia. Glatiramer is structurally similar to myelin and hence may act as an alternative target for T-helper cells in the inflammatory pathway. Glatiramer may reduce relapse by as much as 29%.[123] Other features of progressive disease such as spasticity and depression may be treated with baclofen and standard antidepressants. Patients may develop bladder spasticity requiring anticholinergics or intermittent catheterization. Depression and epilepsy are both more common in patients with MS,[119] and may be treated with routine medications.

Obstetric considerations

A meta-analysis of several large studies demonstrated a reduction in the likelihood of relapse during pregnancy (particularly during the third trimester), but then an increase in the 3 months postpartum.[124–126] This postpartum increase may be due to fatigue, intercurrent infection, or the removal of antepartum immunosuppression. Consideration between patient and neurologist should be given to the choice of disease modifying therapy during pregnancy. There is limited data to support the safety of either interferon or glatiramer in pregnant women.[127] Some patients with severe progressive disease may be treated with immunosuppressant medication, such as cyclophosphamide or methotrexate. These medications are associated with congenital malformations and should be avoided in pregnancy.[128]

There is no evidence that mode of delivery, breastfeeding, or the use of epidural labour analgesia influence the rate of relapse. There is no evidence that pregnancy has any impact on the long-term progression of the disease.[129,130] However, it is important for these women to have careful specialist follow-up as minor postpartum symptoms such as bladder dysfunction and paraesthesia may be misinterpreted as MS relapse.

There is inconclusive evidence to suggest that women with MS may be at some increased risk of a variety of obstetric complications. Several large studies have suggested women with MS had an increased risk of giving birth to babies of low birth weight, and a higher rate of requiring induction of labour and operative interventions for delivery.[131,163]

Anaesthetic issues

Neuraxial anaesthesia

It has previously been proposed that areas of demyelinated neurons within the spinal cord may be damaged by the direct application of concentrated local anaesthetic, such as during spinal anaesthesia. There was concern that this may either result in direct toxicity, or increase the risk of MS relapse. This concern led initially to a reluctance to perform neuraxial anaesthesia at all, and later, a preference to perform epidural rather than spinal anaesthesia, in order to reduce the concentration of local anaesthetic directly reaching the spinal cord.[132] In fact, there is little evidence to support these contentions, and neuraxial anaesthesia (both spinal and epidural) appears safe.[133] Recent surveys suggest that most anaesthetists are now happy to proceed with neuraxial anaesthesia in the setting of MS.[134] Patients with autonomic dysfunction may be at increased risk of hypotension following neuraxial anaesthesia.

General anaesthesia

Many of the potential issues associated with administering general anaesthesia in the setting of MS are more likely to be relevant in severe advanced disease, which is unlikely to be seen in an obstetric setting. A brief overview is provided, and more detail is available elsewhere.[120]

A thorough preoperative assessment is critical for planning intraoperative and postoperative management. A careful documentation of the current neurological state is valuable if there are concerns later about postoperative relapse. An assessment of bulbar symptoms and respiratory weakness is important as this can increase the risk of aspiration and atelectasis postoperatively. Demyelinating lesions in the thoracic cord can lead to autonomic dysfunction, leading to intraoperative haemodynamic instability, particularly hypotension that can be resistant to treatment. This may also be relevant in the setting of neuraxial anaesthesia. Consideration should be given to the patient's current medications, and their potential relevance to anaesthesia. Recent high-dose steroid use may require perioperative supplementation to avoid adrenal insufficiency. Use of baclofen may increase sensitivity to non-depolarizing neuromuscular blocking drugs.

Patients with advanced MS and an element of limb spasticity are potentially at risk of exaggerated hyperkalaemia in response to suxamethonium. It is possible that high-dose rocuronium may be more appropriate in this setting; however, there are several reasons why patients with MS may have unpredictable responses to non-depolarizing muscle relaxants. Denervation may result in upregulation of postsynaptic acetylcholine receptors and increased resistance to non-depolarizing neuromuscular blocking drugs. Conversely, pre-existing weakness and reduced muscle mass may result in increased sensitivity. As previously stated, baclofen treatment for limb spasticity may also contribute to sensitivity to non-depolarizing neuromuscular blocking drugs.

Hyperthermia has been implicated in recurrence of MS. Temperature should be monitored and excessive warming should be avoided.

Brain tumours

Incidence and presentation

Central nervous tumours are uncommon neoplasms, with an annual incidence of 5.1–7 cases/100,000 population, but only 1.8–3.2 cases/100,000 women between the ages of 20 and 39.[135] The incidence is not increased in pregnant women compared to the non-pregnant female population,[136,137] but an increased growth rate during pregnancy may occur in some tumour types. Studies in various Western countries estimate that this translates to peripartum diagnosis of malignant brain tumour of 3.6–32/100,000 live births.[136,138] These studies excluded common benign tumours such as meningiomas and pituitary adenomas. The relative frequencies of common brain tumour types in the normal population are shown in Table 45.1; however, these vary between reports and populations. In particular, meningiomas are three times more common in women than men. Brain metastases are often not included when tumour incidence is considered, but with the increasingly aggressive treatment of common cancers such as breast, lung, renal, and bowel cancer and melanoma, these are most commonly seen and treated. In practice, the tumours most likely to present as a clinical dilemma in pregnancy are low- and high-grade gliomas (Figure 45.2A), meningiomas (Figure 45.2B, C), acoustic neuromas, pituitary tumours, and the multiple lesions associated with the phacomatoses (neurofibromatosis (NF)-1, NF-2, and von Hippel–Lindau disease) (Figure 45.2D). One large population-based study of pregnant women with brain tumours found an increased risk of maternal mortality, preterm labour, and intrauterine growth retardation associated with malignant brain tumours and of preterm labour associated with benign brain tumours. Both were associated with an increase in caesarean delivery rates,[139] and similar outcomes have been reported in smaller studies.[140,141] Although uncommon, brain tumours can precipitate catastrophic neurological deterioration with devastating fetal and maternal outcomes.[138]

Table 45.1 Relative frequencies of common brain tumours in the general population

Histological type		Percentage
Glioma	High-grade (malignant) glioma	25
	Low-grade glioma	20
Meningioma		25
Acoustic neuroma		8
Pituitary tumour		8

Brain tumours generally present in one of three ways: symptoms of raised intracranial pressure, seizures, or focal neurological deficit related to the location of the tumour. Other presentations, such as with catastrophic haemorrhage, are uncommon. Dramatic presentation with a seizure, which occurs in 30–50% of patients,[142] presents no diagnostic challenge unless eclampsia is suspected—seizures occurring in late pregnancy are more likely to be due to eclampsia.[143] The clinical features of raised intracranial pressure, including headache, nausea, vomiting, and lethargy are frequent in normal pregnancy, making diagnosis more difficult. New, constant, progressive, or morning headache, nausea or vomiting occurring in, or persisting into, the second or third trimester, drowsiness, confusion, or new neurological deficit should always be investigated. Headaches that are worse with bending, lying down, coughing, and other manoeuvers that increase intracranial pressure are particularly suspicious.

A small percentage of brain tumours grow significantly during pregnancy, although the exact incidence of this is difficult to assess, and some reports show no relationship of tumour growth to pregnancy.[144] Tumour growth usually presents in the second and third trimesters.[145] For malignant tumours growth would be expected over the time period of a normal pregnancy, but there have also been reports of unusual growth of benign tumours during pregnancy. This has classically been attributed to hormonal effects on cell proliferation, which is probably true for pituitary tumours. The normal pituitary gland increases in size during pregnancy[146] and pituitary adenomas may undergo significant enlargement due to hormonal stimulatory effects. This is particularly the case for prolactin-secreting macroadenomas (>1 cm in diameter), 24% of which may appreciably enlarge during pregnancy.[147] More than 80% of meningiomas also express receptors for progesterone or oestrogen;[67] however, their significance is unclear as many meningiomas do not grow during pregnancy, the receptors are equally present in meningiomas in children and men, and treatment directed against these receptors has been fruitless. Additionally, the increased mass effect with neurological deficit occurring in pregnancy may improve after delivery, which should not occur if the effect is due to enhanced cell proliferation. Therefore, it has also been suggested that the hypervolaemic state of pregnancy may exacerbate the mass effect of the tumour. One study of meningiomas requiring resection for mass effect during pregnancy showed no particular change in proliferation rate but features of hypervascularity, intracellular and stromal oedema, and haemorrhage when compared to meningiomas in non-pregnant women.[145] This may also occur in other benign tumours, such as acoustic neuromas,[148] and low-grade gliomas, and the risk of deterioration due to mass effect continues into the immediate postpartum period.[149] Immunological tolerance has also been suggested as an aetiological factor in brain tumour growth in pregnancy.

Diagnosis and investigation

In a patient suspected to harbour a brain tumour, imaging should not be delayed due to pregnancy. If possible, a CT scan should be avoided to limit exposure to ionizing radiation; however, if MRI is not readily available and clinical presentation warrants urgent imaging, then CT scan should be performed with lead shielding of the fetus, which results in a negligible radiation exposure.[68,69] MRI does not involve ionizing radiation, is not known to have harmful effects on humans[90,94] and is frequently used safely for imaging of the fetus.[96] Thus, it is the preferred maternal brain imaging modality in pregnancy, and indeed in the non-pregnant patient suspected to suffer from a brain tumour as it provides more detailed and sensitive brain tumour imaging than CT scan. Intravenous contrast agents improve the diagnostic yield of cranial imaging and have not been specifically shown to have mutagenic or teratogenic effects[89] but are generally avoided in pregnancy based on the general principle of drug avoidance. Iodinated contrast used for CT scan may cause anaphylaxis and is nephrotoxic and has been reported to cause hypothyroidism in the fetus.[90–92] Gadolinium-based contrast used for MRI is less likely to cause allergic reactions and is not nephrotoxic and has no known adverse effects for the fetus.[92] Nonetheless, a non-contrast MRI scan is usually sufficient for diagnosis of the majority of lesions and can be performed in the first instance. Consultation with the radiologist to ensure maximal benefit from limited imaging is essential.[13]

Anaesthetic and obstetric considerations

The management of a brain tumour is complex in the non-pregnant patient, requiring the expertise of a multidisciplinary team including neurosurgeons, radiation oncologists, medical oncologists, and epilepsy specialists. The complexity of management in the pregnant patient is amplified and the team expands to include obstetricians, neonatologists, and anaesthetists. Decisions relating to both maternal and fetal welfare need to be balanced, with many routine therapies such as radiotherapy or chemotherapy used with caution, or contraindicated. A detailed outline of brain tumour management in pregnancy is not warranted here, but is found elsewhere.[149,150] Anaesthetic considerations are twofold; the first is the pregnant patient with a non-viable fetus who requires urgent surgery to remove a brain tumour, usually for mass effect or suspected malignancy. The second is delivery of the child in a patient with a brain tumour, which may be followed by immediate surgical resection.

In the patient with raised intracranial pressure, steroids can be used to reduce cerebral oedema, which is usually a component of the mass effect, and may delay surgery. These are generally considered safe in pregnancy and have the additional advantage of promoting fetal lung maturity but the benefit needs to be weighed against the possibility of growth retardation and adrenal insufficiency in the fetus. Increased maternal cortisol secretion in the second trimester may be somewhat protective against brain tumour associated oedema.[151] Management of seizures is considered in the epilepsy section. Many AEDs are teratogens or of unknown risk,[68] therefore choice of agent is limited. However, the risk of uncontrolled seizures outweighs the potential side effects of many medications. Prophylactic AEDs would commonly be used for the patient with a brain tumour but no seizures, at least perioperatively, but should be avoided in pregnancy. Surgery can be avoided for pituitary tumours in some cases using medications with an acceptable safety profile including bromocriptine and other dopamine analogues for prolactin-secreting tumours.[152]

In pregnant patients who are known to have a brain tumour, frequent clinical review is necessary to monitor signs of raised intracranial pressure and neurological deficit as appropriate to the location of the lesion. Thus, catastrophic deterioration can be avoided and semi-elective, rather than emergency, surgery can be undertaken. This would include a careful history, examination of the fundi for papilloedema, neurological examination, and imaging as indicated. For pituitary tumours, regular visual field examination is necessary.

Surgery during pregnancy is usually required when the mass effect of the tumour threatens life or function. Up to 48% of hospital admissions of pregnant patients with malignant brain tumours will result in a neurosurgical procedure, and 19% of those for benign tumours.[139] The histological type of tumours detected during pregnancy, such as after a seizure, can be accurately predicted with advanced imaging, therefore tissue diagnosis and treatment of many tumours can be safely delayed until after delivery.[11,143] However, a large tumour, or that in a critical location, can be safely removed during pregnancy if necessary, without an increase in adverse outcomes.[5,11,139] Thus, delay of an indicated procedure is not warranted and most studies suggest that delayed surgery after neurological deterioration results in worse outcomes.[5,12] Small tumours, such as pituitary microadenomas or meningiomas that have not grown during pregnancy (Figure 45.2B), are unlikely to result in significantly raised intracranial pressure and normal vaginal delivery can be planned.

There are a number of considerations for the pregnant patient who is to undergo surgery for removal of a brain tumour. The prone or supine position may not be possible, therefore the sitting, semi-lateral, or lateral position is often preferred to avoid aortocaval or fetal compression.[153] Fluid shifts and haemodynamic changes that are tolerated by the normal pregnant patient may exacerbate cerebral oedema, hypotension may result in inadequate cerebral perfusion pressure, and hypertension may result in intracranial haemorrhage and worsening of cerebral oedema, thus hypotension, hypertension, hypotonic fluids, and fluid overload should be avoided. Intubation should occur without hypertension or raised intracranial pressure. Emergence and extubation should avoid haemodynamic instability, coughing, and the Valsalva manoeuver.

If delivery prior to surgery or other therapy for a brain tumour with significant mass effect is planned, the mode of delivery will need to be considered. The decision should involve the neurosurgical, obstetric, and anaesthetic teams. Intracranial pressure may rise to over 70 cmH_2O with the Valsalva manoeuvre in labour,[154] normal being less than 20 cmH_2O. Thus, in the patient with even mildly elevated intracranial pressure due to an intracranial mass, the risk of cerebral herniation is high and vaginal delivery may be contraindicated. Inhaled nitrous oxide and systemic narcotics may result in drowsiness and hypoventilation and are contraindicated. Epidural anaesthesia is potentially contraindicated due to the risk of inadvertent dural puncture, increasing the risk of herniation,[155] and of raised intracranial pressure with bolus injection into the epidural space.[156] Therefore, caesarean delivery under general anaesthesia is most commonly recommended,[11,27] particularly if surgery is to immediately follow delivery. However, others have advocated careful epidural anaesthesia with caesarean delivery or instrumental vaginal delivery to avoid pushing with a pain-free second-stage labour.[157] Neuraxial anaesthesia has the advantage of allowing neurological assessment during delivery.

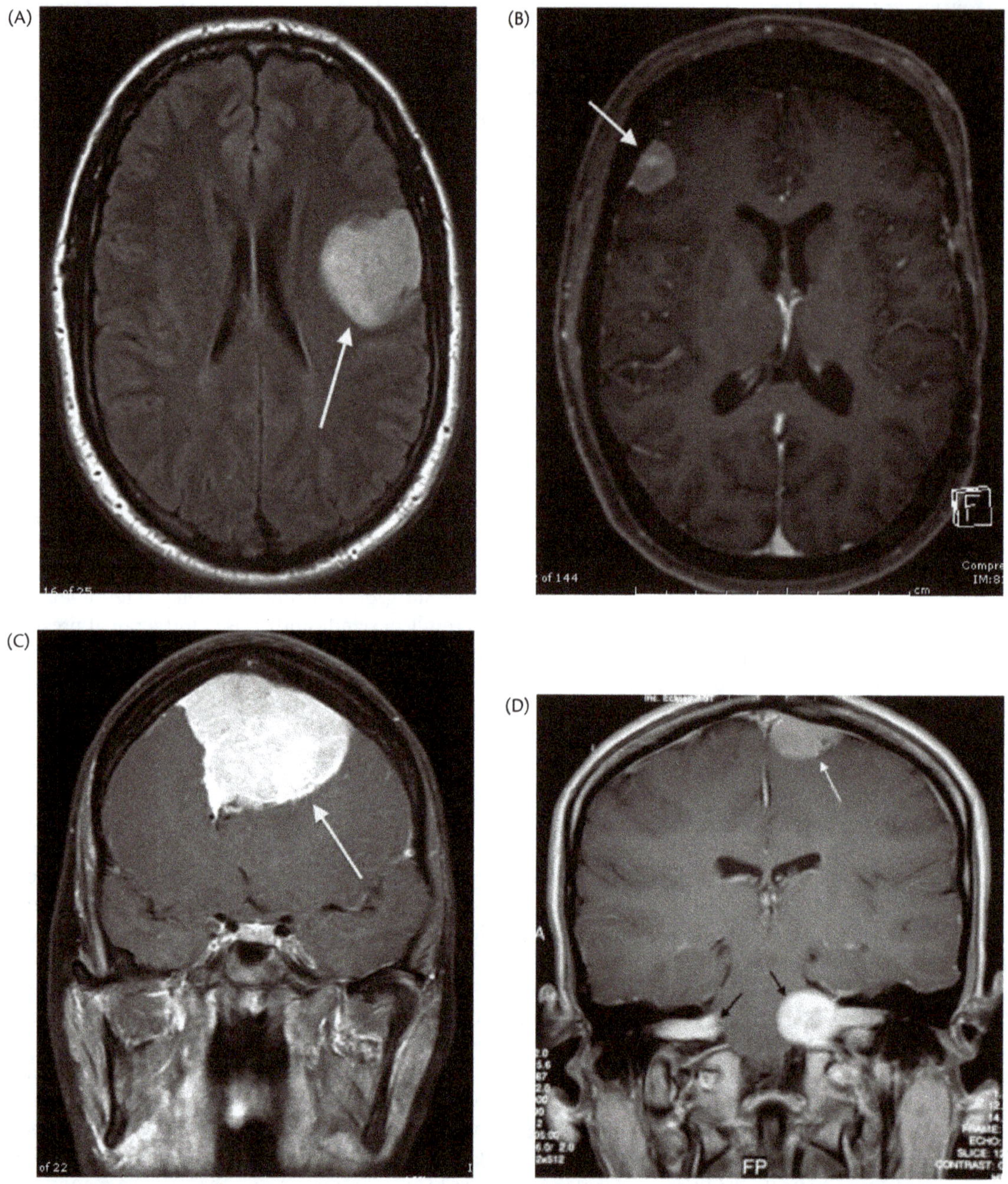

Figure 45.2 (A) Axial fluid-attenuated inversion recovery (FLAIR) brain MRI showing a left parietal low grade glioma. This tumour was diagnosed during pregnancy when the patient suffered sensory seizures. In retrospect she had suffered similar episode during a previous pregnancy that she had ignored. (B) Axial T1-weighted contrast-enhanced brain MRI showing a small right frontal meningioma (arrow). Small benign tumours can be observed during pregnancy with a low risk of significant enlargement. This tumour did not grow during pregnancy and the patient had a normal vaginal delivery. (C) Coronal T1-weighted contrast-enhanced brain MRI showing a large frontal falcine meningioma with significant mass effect. This tumour was not diagnosed during pregnancy and the patient had a normal vaginal delivery before suffering seizures in the postpartum period. (D) Coronal T1-weighted contrast-enhanced brain MRI showing typical lesions of neurofibromatosis-2 including bilateral acoustic neuromas (black arrows) with brainstem compression on the left, and a small convexity meningioma (white arrows). Decisions regarding pregnancy and delivery in the patients with an autosomal dominant inherited disorder and multiple intracranial and spinal lesions of varying size and severity are complex and should be made in a multidisciplinary setting.

Hydrocephalus, idiopathic intracranial hypertension, and cerebrospinal fluid shunts

Hydrocephalus

Hydrocephalus is a condition in which there is an abnormal accumulation of CSF in the cerebral ventricles. It may be obstructive (non-communicating) hydrocephalus, where there is a mechanical obstruction to CSF flow within the ventricular system, or communicating hydrocephalus, where there is an abnormality of CSF absorption from the ventricles into the venous system. In obstructive hydrocephalus, the enlarged ventricles act as an intracranial mass, with the resulting risk of tonsillar herniation.

In communicating hydrocephalus, the raised pressure is distributed evenly throughout the neuraxis, with no risk of herniation. There are many causes of hydrocephalus, both congenital and acquired, particularly after intracranial infection, haemorrhage, or tumour.

The mainstay of treatment of hydrocephalus is insertion of a CSF shunt. This is a CSF diversion system that comprises three parts. The first is a catheter in the CSF space, usually the lateral ventricles, but less commonly in the lumbar theca. The second is a valve system to regulate the pressure or flow of CSF, of which there are many types, and the third is a drainage catheter that diverts CSF into a body cavity, most commonly the peritoneal cavity, but the pleural cavity or right atrium are also utilized. Thus, the most common types of CSF shunt are ventriculoperitoneal and lumboperitoneal; however, ventriculopleural and ventriculoatrial shunts are also used for various indications, including an unsuitable peritoneal cavity due to adhesions, infection, or peritoneal dialysis. Increasingly, endoscopic third ventriculostomy is used to treat hydrocephalus in suitable patients. An opening is made in the floor of the third ventricle to allow ventricular outflow into the basal cisterns, but is dependent on normal CSF absorption capacity.[158]

Women with a shunt report increased headache and abdominal pain, and have an increased incidence of shunt complications, during pregnancy. In one study, 76% of patients had a shunt complication during pregnancy, including 59% with worsening symptoms of raised intracranial pressure. Symptoms generally resolve after delivery. The risk of shunt obstruction is probably increased, with a reported 23% of patients requiring surgical shunt revision during pregnancy.[159,160] Patients with hydrocephalus who have not required a shunt prior to pregnancy may decompensate during pregnancy and require shunt insertion.[160] Differential diagnosis from the headache of pre-eclampsia, CVT, and other causes of headache due to raised intracranial pressure in pregnancy may be difficult.

The reasons for worsening of hydrocephalus and shunt malfunction in pregnancy include physiological changes such as increased plasma volume and increased intra-abdominal pressure. Anatomical changes associated with the enlarging uterus may also be relevant.[161,162] Premature uterine contractions have been attributed to irritation from a shunt peritoneal catheter.[5]

Idiopathic intracranial hypertension

Idiopathic intracranial hypertension (IIH), previously known as pseudotumour cerebri or benign intracranial hypertension, is raised intracranial pressure with normal CSF composition and in the absence of hydrocephalus, a mass lesion, or impaired consciousness. It is likely a disorder of CSF absorption, being associated with cerebral venous sinus outflow obstruction.[164] It is common in obese women of child-bearing age and the chief symptoms are severe headache and visual loss due to chronic papilloedema. If medical treatment of the headache or visual failure is inadequate, a lumboperitoneal, or less commonly, ventriculoperitoneal shunt may be inserted.[162]

The symptoms of IIH worsen with pregnancy and exogenous oestrogens. The onset of the disease may also occur during pregnancy, particularly the first and second trimesters, although the incidence is probably not increased in pregnancy.[165,166] Generally, maternal and fetal outcomes are good and visual outcomes are similar to non-pregnant patients.[165–168] If there is severe papilloedema, caesarean delivery to minimize raise intracranial pressure during delivery can be considered to avoid irreversible visual loss, but generally vaginal delivery is appropriate. Neuraxial anaesthesia is not contraindicated if the patient does not have a lumboperitoneal shunt. Lumbar puncture is often used therapeutically and does not result in herniation due to the even distribution of pressure throughout the neuraxis.[167,177]

Anaesthetic concerns

Parturients with raised intracranial pressure present a major challenge to the obstetric anaesthetist. Dural puncture in the setting of obstructive hydrocephalus may allow a rapid decrease in CSF pressure, potentially leading to tonsillar herniation or intracranial haemorrhage. Intracranial subdural haematoma and subarachnoid haemorrhage have been described following epidural and spinal anaesthesia.[170,171] As mentioned previously, intracranial pressure increases significantly during labour contractions, particularly during the second stage.[172] A planned assisted instrumented delivery will reduce the increase in intracranial pressure associated with pushing and the Valsalva manoeuver. This is advisable even for those patients with IIH or communicating hydrocephalus, who are not at risk of herniation, or those with obstructive hydrocephalus and a functioning ventriculoperitoneal shunt or ventriculostomy.[174]

Patients with a functioning ventriculoperitoneal shunt or communicating hydrocephalus can safely receive neuraxial analgesia or anaesthesia and a vaginal delivery is not contraindicated.[174,176] It would seem reasonable to administer prophylactic antibiotics to shunt patients, although this is not universally recommended.[176] Patients with a lumboperitoneal shunt for IIH should not receive neuraxial blockade. Firstly, there is the potential for unpredictable spread of local anaesthetic, and secondly, the risk of damaging the catheter itself with the spinal or epidural needle.[177] There have, however, been reports of successful epidural anaesthesia in patients with lumboperitoneal shunts.[41]

Overall, treatment of hydrocephalus, IIH and shunt malfunction in pregnancy using standard neurosurgical guidelines and in consultation with the obstetric and anaesthetic team is associated with good maternal and fetal outcomes. [5,11,165,166,174,176]

Spina bifida

Introduction

Spina bifida is one of a spectrum of congenital disorders relating to failure of closure of the neural tube. Subtypes of spina bifida describe the anatomical extent of the abnormality. The mildest form of the disease is known as spina bifida occulta, implying that there is no external defect visible, although there is frequently a patch of hair or dimpling of the skin overlying the abnormality. In the more severe forms, collectively known as spina bifida cystica, the neuraxis is exposed along the dorsal aspect of the body to a variable degree by defects in the formation of covering structures.[178] The incidence is falling due to maternal folate supplementation and a rise in prenatal diagnosis with termination of significantly affected pregnancies.[179] The current incidence is in the order of 0.1–0.3% of the population, although it is much higher in the offspring of sufferers, and may be as high as 3–4%.[180,181]

Obstetric considerations

Survivors of spina bifida who reach reproductive age frequently suffer kyphoscoliosis, abnormal pelvic shape, and neuropathic bladder, and may have undergone multiple corrective procedures for musculoskeletal, neurological, or urological abnormalities.[182] Recurrent urinary tract infections and latex allergy are common.[181] Whilst normal vaginal delivery of women with spina bifida has been reported, the combination of abnormal pelvic shape and lower body muscular weakness means instrumental and operative delivery is frequently required. Great care needs to be taken at caesarean delivery to avoid ureteric trauma in the setting of previous urological procedures.[181]

Anaesthetic considerations

Neuraxial anaesthesia may be challenging (or impossible) in the parturient with spina bifida for several reasons, and many anaesthetists would consider spina bifida to be a contraindication for neuraxial techniques. Firstly, the procedure may be technically difficult to perform due to abnormal anatomy such as kyphoscoliosis or scarring from previous corrective surgery. Secondly, local anaesthetic spread is unpredictable due to abnormalities in CSF flow and the abnormal structure and integrity of the epidural space. This may lead to a variety of problems, including inadequate caudal spread of local anaesthetic beyond the level of the defect, excessive cephalad spread of anaesthetic, possibly related to decreased epidural space volume and increased dural permeability, or unilateral block.[178] Thirdly and most significantly, abnormal anatomy may increase the risk of trauma to the spinal cord, spinal nerves, or dura. A significant proportion of patients with spina bifida have a 'tethered' spinal cord, where the spinal cord ends below the normal level due to a shortened filum terminale, or other spinal dysraphism (a congenital abnormality of the spine). The incidence of tethered spinal cord may be as high as 60%.[1,183] Hydrocephalus and CSF shunts are also common in these patients. Thus, close liaison with the treating neurosurgeon to define the anatomical abnormalities and the potential for complications is essential. It is wise to have imaging available before embarking on the route of a neuraxial anaesthetic technique.

Arnold–Chiari malformation and syringomyelia

The Arnold–Chiari malformations are a spectrum of disorders of varying severity resulting from the descent of hindbrain structures through the foramen magnum.[184] They may be associated with obstruction to CSF flow and hydrocephalus, syringomyelia, and spina bifida.[185] Syringomyelia is the formation of a longitudinal cystic cavity within the spinal cord.[186] Arnold–Chiari malformations are divided into four subtypes, associated with greater degrees of hindbrain displacement and worsening clinical severity. In type 1, the mildest form, only the cerebellar tonsils extend beyond the foramen magnum (Figure 45.3). This malformation is often asymptomatic and diagnosed incidentally, but may become symptomatic in adolescence and young adulthood.[185] Type 2 is more severe, with displacement of the cerebellar vermis, brainstem, and fourth ventricle, and is more likely to be associated with hydrocephalus and a lumbar myelomeningocoele and diagnosed in the pre-natal period or at birth. Types 3 and 4 are rare, and describe more severe descent of hindbrain structures. The most common clinical manifestations include headache (particularly 'cough' headache), neck and upper limb pain, ataxia, and nystagmus, which may worsen with the Valsalva manoeuver. Surgical correction most commonly involves suboccipital craniectomy and upper cervical laminectomy, which provides bony and dural decompression of the structures crowded within the foramen magnum and upper cervical canal. Treatment is only required in symptomatic patients or those developing syringomyelia. Insertion of a CSF shunt is commonly necessary to treat hydrocephalus.[185]

The uneventful use of both neuraxial analgesia and anaesthesia has been described in parturients with Arnold–Chiari type 1 malformation[184,186–189] and syringomyelia.[190,191] However, there are also reports of exacerbation of neurological symptoms postpartum (specifically headache and nystagmus) following the use of neuraxial anaesthesia.[192,193] Some authors propose that dural puncture should be avoided, due to abnormalities in CSF circulation and the potential for a differential pressure gradient to develop between the brain and spinal cord, particularly during straining.[194–196] Chantigian and colleagues reported on 50 years' experience at the Mayo Clinic, during which only 12 women with known Arnold–Chiari malformations delivered a total of 30 babies. A variety of techniques were used including general, epidural, and spinal anaesthesia. None of the patients undergoing neuraxial anaesthesia experienced exacerbation of their neurological symptoms (although one required an epidural blood patch for a postdural puncture headache).[189] In patients with asymptomatic or adequately treated Arnold–Chiari malformations, delivery based on obstetric considerations would seem reasonable, with additional caution for symptomatic, untreated patients.

Spinal trauma, paraplegia, and quadriplegia

Incidence

It is estimated that in the United States approximately 52,000 women are affected by spinal injury and approximately 2400 new spinal injuries are reported each year.[197] Causes include motor vehicle accidents, gunshot wounds, horse-riding accidents, and diving accidents.[198] Lesions below T1 result in paraplegia whereas lesions above T1 result in quadriplegia. There may be complete loss of neurological control (motor, sensory, and autonomic) below the lesion or varying degrees of incomplete loss. There may be associated bony deformity.

Obstetric considerations

Fertility is not generally affected in women with spinal cord injury (SCI).[198] Complications of SCI relevant to obstetrics include iron deficiency anaemia, folate deficiency, urinary tract infection, and decubitus ulcers. Asymptomatic bacteriuria and urinary tract infection are extremely common in women with SCI, and routine urinary culture at each antenatal visit is recommended.[199] Antibiotic prophylaxis should be considered. Thromboprophylaxis may be warranted, but is not universally recommended.[198]

Ability to detect labour pain depends on the level of the injury. Women with injuries above T10 may experience painless labour and delivery. Preterm labour appears to be no more common than in the general population; however, consideration should be given to how these women will diagnose the onset of labour, in order to avoid unattended delivery from undetected contractions. Possible options include home uterine activity monitoring, teaching women to palpate their own uterine contractions, and recognition of sympathetic nervous system activity such as leg or abdominal wall spasms or increased lower limb spasticity. Some authors recommend frequent assessment of cervical dilatation after 28 weeks and inpatient management of women with cervical dilatation.[200,201]

Published case series suggest that whilst vaginal delivery is possible in women with SCI, the likelihood of instrumental or operative delivery is increased, especially in women with higher cord lesions.

Anaesthetic considerations

Women with high thoracic or cervical SCI should have an assessment of respiratory function either prior to conception or early in pregnancy.[202] Baseline spirometry should be performed with subsequent serial assessment of vital capacity, due to the increased respiratory requirements in late pregnancy. Careful attention to pulmonary care is important, and non-invasive ventilatory support may be required in labour.[202] Hypo- or hyperthermia may occur as a result of impaired thermoregulation.

Autonomic dysreflexia is very common in labour, and may be seen in 75% of women with higher SCI (above T6).[199] Precipitants may include cervical dilatation, bladder or bowel distention, vaginal examination, urinary catheterization, and temperature change in the lower limbs (e.g. placing the legs into cold or hot water).[202] The syndrome results from sympathetic hyperactivity below the level of the lesion. Symptoms include severe hypertension (may be confused with pre-eclampsia), bradycardia, tachycardia, or other arrhythmias. Uterine vasoconstriction may result in fetal distress. Reported complications of autonomic dysreflexia include intracerebral haemorrhage and myocardial infarction. Invasive monitoring of blood pressure should be considered.[198]

Epidural analgesia should be used early in labour to prevent these complications, even if the patient is insensate to labour pain.[198] If epidural analgesia has not yet been administered, or is contraindicated, other agents such as labetalol and nifedipine can be used. Sodium nitroprusside may be required. The use of magnesium sulphate has also been described.[203] Epidural anaesthesia has also been successfully used for caesarean delivery in a quadriplegic patient.[204]

Acute spinal cord injury during pregnancy

Acute SCI has been reported during pregnancy via mechanisms such as motor vehicle accident, gunshot wounds, or traumatic falls.[198] Management is complex, and requires input from a specialized multidisciplinary team with experience in both high-risk obstetrics and spinal trauma. Care must be taken with immobilization of the entire spine to prevent worsening of injury. Pelvic tilt must be achieved in pregnant women beyond 24 weeks' gestation, where aortocaval compression may contribute to hypotension.

Acute SCI may also be associated with haemodynamic instability. Neurogenic shock is a syndrome of hypotension, bradycardia, and hypothermia resulting from loss of sympathetic tone below the level of the lesion (and resulting unopposed parasympathetic tone). Adequate volume resuscitation and pressor support should be instituted. Bradycardia resulting from neurogenic shock may complicate assessment of volume status. In addition to this, the gravid uterus may make examination of the abdomen more difficult. There should be a high index of suspicion for internal bleeding. Deep venous thrombosis is very common following acute SCI, and routine thromboprophylaxis should be considered.[198]

Peripheral neuropathy

This section will briefly consider several conditions associated with peripheral neuropathy in the obstetric population, including Guillain–Barré syndrome (GBS) and poliomyelitis. In clinical practice, obstetric anaesthetists will far more commonly be asked to assess patients presenting with new peripheral neurological symptoms, especially postpartum. A thorough knowledge of the aetiology, pathology, and relevant anatomy of the peripheral nervous system are important for developing a framework for adequately assessing these patients.

Guillain–Barré syndrome

GBS is an acute post-infectious inflammatory polyneuropathy. It typically develops within a few weeks of an infectious illness such as an upper respiratory tract infection or gastroenteritis, and presents with a syndrome of ascending motor weakness and numbness, with loss of deep tendon reflexes.[118] *Campylobacter jejuni* has been implicated as a common causative pathogen.[205] Symptoms may develop over 1–2 weeks, reaching peak severity after 4 weeks, but in severe cases may deteriorate over a few hours. Patients with severe disease may develop respiratory weakness requiring mechanical ventilation (up to 30% of patients) and autonomic dysfunction (up to 70% of patients). Symptoms of autonomic dysfunction may include tachycardia, urinary retention, and hypo- or hypertension. Other supportive care includes physiotherapy, thromboprophylaxis, and antibiotics, which may be required as nosocomial infection such as pneumonia and urinary tract infection are common. Disease-modifying treatment may include plasma exchange transfusion or intravenous gammaglobulin.[206]

GBS does not appear to occur with increased frequency in pregnancy.[205] The successful use of plasma exchange transfusion and intravenous gammaglobulin are both well established.[205] Uncomplicated GBS does not appear to influence the rates of assisted or operative delivery, which should be undertaken on obstetric grounds.[207] The occurrence of GBS in the neonate of a parturient with GBS has been described in a single case report.[165]

Whilst it has been proposed that the use of neuraxial analgesia and anaesthesia may have the potential to exacerbate the severity of GBS,[161] this has largely been discredited.[205] Parturients may, however, be sensitive to the effects of local anaesthetic medications, requiring reduced doses to achieve adequate anaesthesia. Also, patients may be at risk of exaggerated haemodynamic instability during establishment of neuraxial anaesthesia. Careful titration of epidural anaesthesia has been recommended in favour of single-shot spinal anaesthesia.[207]

Suxamethonium should be used with caution due to the potential for exaggerated release of potassium due to postsynaptic receptor proliferation. Succinylcholine-induced cardiac arrest has been reported in a patient recovering from GBS.[167] However, patients can also be highly sensitive to non-depolarizing muscle relaxants,[207] which should be titrated in small doses, with appropriate monitoring. Facilities for postoperative ventilation should be available.

Autonomic instability may also be prominent during general anaesthesia and should be treated aggressively.

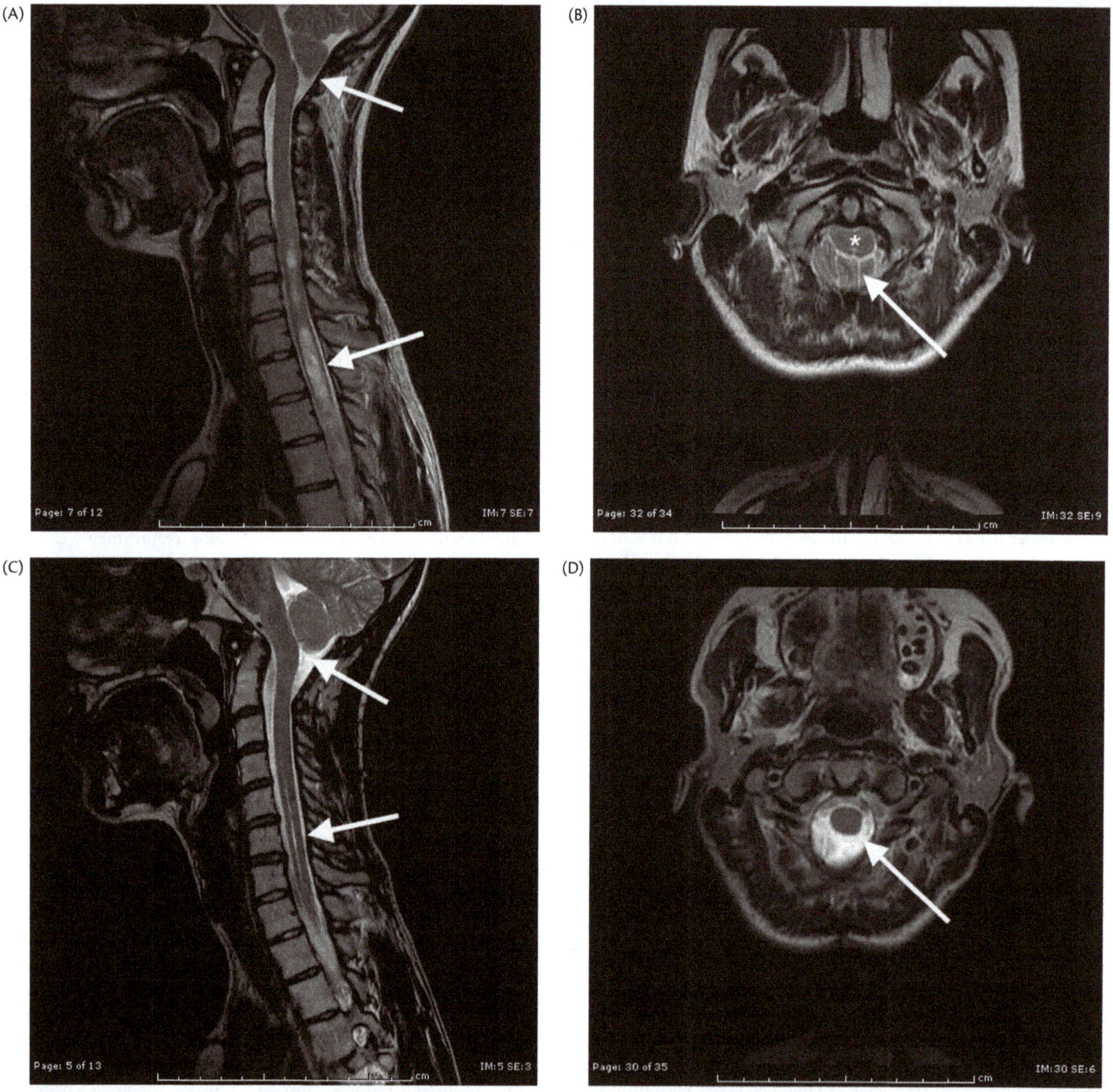

Figure 45.3 (A) Sagittal T2-weighted MRI of the craniocervical junction showing a Chiari 1 malformation with displacement of the cerebellar tonsils into the foramen magnum (upper arrow) and an extensive cervical syrinx (lower arrow). (B) Axial T2-weighted MRI at the level of C1/2 showing the medulla/spinal cord (asterisk) compressed by the cerebellar tonsils (same patient as Figure 45.3A). (C) Sagittal T2-weighted MRI of the patient in Figure 45.3A,B after surgical posterior fossa decompression with a capacious foramen magnum region (upper arrow) and resolution of the cervical syrinx (lower arrow). (D) Axial T2-weighted MRI of the patient in Figure 45.3 A,B showing the decompressed medulla/spinal cord.

Charcot–Marie–Tooth disease (hereditary motor sensory neuropathy)

Charcot–Marie–Tooth disease is a rare inherited defect in myelin structure and function, also known as hereditary motor sensory neuropathy. It has an incidence of approximately 36/100,000. It results in a progressive distal limb weakness and muscle atrophy, leading to gait disturbance and deformity.[118] Parturients with Charcot–Marie–Tooth disease appear to have higher rates of malpresentation, higher rates of operative delivery, and an increased incidence of postpartum haemorrhage.[166] Symptoms of the disease may be temporarily or permanently worsened by pregnancy.[169] Neuraxial analgesia and anaesthesia are not contraindicated in these patients, although it may be challenging if there is kyphoscoliosis.[208]

Polio (and post-polio syndrome)

Infective poliomyelitis ('polio') is a highly infectious viral illness predominantly affecting children under the age of 5. The enterovirus replicates in the gut and is spread rapidly by faecal–oral contamination. Most sufferers only experience a mild influenza-like illness. However, one in 200 sufferers develops an acute flaccid paralysis as a result of spread to the motor neurones in the anterior horn of the spinal cord. Five to ten per cent of these patients die from respiratory failure. It is not known why such a small proportion of sufferers develop paralysis, although risk factors are known to include pregnancy, previous tonsillectomy, strenuous physical activity, and minor trauma such as intramuscular injections.[158] Survivors of spinal paralysis may have lifelong sequelae, including deformity and physical disability such as limb contractures, kyphoscoliosis, and chest wall deformity, which may contribute to respiratory insufficiency.

Around 40% of patients who survive paralytic polio will go on to develop additional worsening symptoms 15–40 years following the illness. This worsening of symptoms is known as post-polio syndrome (PPS). These symptoms include muscle weakness, chronic pain, fatigue, and impaired activities of daily living.[209] The number of worldwide cases of polio has dropped by 99% due to highly successful vaccination programmes, from an estimated 350,000 cases in 1998 to 650 reported cases in 2011.[173] Polio is now endemic in only three countries—Pakistan, Afghanistan, and Nigeria.

There is a paucity of data in the recent literature examining obstetric outcomes in female survivors of polio. One study searched the Medical Birth Register of Norway and reported on 2495 births between 1967 and 1998. The authors found that women with a past history of polio were significantly more likely to develop pre-eclampsia (3.4% vs 2.8%), urinary tract infection (3.5% vs 2.4%), and antepartum haemorrhage (3.8% vs 2.4%).[175] Labours were more likely to become obstructed (6.1% vs 2.0%) and caesarean delivery was more common (13.2% vs 8.3%). Infants of mothers with polio were significantly smaller (3383 vs 3483 g) and had a higher risk of perinatal death (2.1% vs 1.1%).

The patient with post-polio sequelae may present a number of significant challenges to the anaesthetist, in the performance of either neuraxial anaesthesia or general anaesthesia. Issues of general anaesthesia include concern over using both depolarizing and non-depolarizing muscle relaxants, sensitivity to analgesic and sedative medication, and the risk of postoperative respiratory depression and aspiration.[133]

Issues requiring preoperative assessment include the degree of respiratory compromise, which may be due to anatomical deformity, particularly kyphoscoliosis, but also due to obstructive or central sleep apnoea. Patients may also have bulbar dysfunction, increasing the risk of aspiration.[210] Other issues include management of chronic pain, which is a common feature of PPS, and cold intolerance. As with many other conditions associated with denervation of peripheral muscle, the use of suxamethonium carries the risk of exaggerated release of potassium and cardiac arrest. However, the safe use of suxamethonium has been described for caesarean delivery in the post-polio patient.[211] Patients may also be sensitive to normal doses of non-depolarizing muscle relaxants.[212]

Whilst neuraxial anaesthesia represents an attractive option, there are still several areas of concern. These include the potential for neuraxial anaesthesia to temporarily affect accessory muscles required for respiration, potential to exacerbate the underlying disease process, and also the difficulty in adequately assessing for complications of neuraxial anaesthesia in the setting of pre-existing neurological pathology. Achieving successful neuraxial anaesthesia may also be technically challenging in the patient with abnormal neuraxial anatomy.[133] The use of ultrasound-guidance has been proposed as a technique for improving success rate in patients with complex kyphoscoliosis.[172]

There is no convincing evidence in the literature that neuraxial anaesthesia worsens neurological disability in patients with post-polio sequelae or PPS [133]. However, it has been proposed that spinal neurons in these patients may be both damaged and reduced in number, and therefore these patients may be at risk of direct local anaesthetic neurotoxicity.

Bell's palsy

Bell's palsy is the paralysis of the facial nerve resulting in asymmetrical facial expression and unilateral weakness of eye closure. Bell's palsy is idiopathic and a wide variety of immunological and viral mechanisms have been considered.[213] The condition is two- to fourfold more common during pregnancy.[118] Treatment options are identical during pregnancy and in the non-pregnant population, and consist of supportive care, particularly to avoid trauma to the non-closing eye, and early treatment with oral glucocorticoids, for which there is limited evidence of benefit. Oral glucocorticoids are not recommended in the first trimester in pregnancy due to a risk of increased cleft palate.[214] The prognosis of Bell's palsy depends on the severity of the paralysis. Incomplete lesions are more likely to resolve than complete lesions. Whilst overall, 85% of patients will regain normal or near normal function, this may be significantly less in pregnancy.[4,215] Possible explanations for this are that pregnant patients may be less likely to receive treatment, or may be more likely to develop complete lesions.

Carpal tunnel syndrome

Carpal tunnel syndrome is an extremely common condition resulting from compression of the median nerve as it passes under the flexor retinaculum at the wrist. This results in pain, paraesthesia and/or numbness of the thumb, index and middle fingers, as well as the radial half of the ring finger, which may wake the patient from sleep. The condition is thought to be more common in pregnancy as a result of fluid retention and peripheral oedema.[118] Symptoms commonly occur in the third trimester and may last for several weeks or months postpartum. The condition has a good prognosis for resolution after delivery and should rarely be treated surgically during pregnancy, unless there is the threat of permanent neurological disability.

Postpartum peripheral neuropathy

The process of labour and delivery, either vaginally or at caesarean delivery, can potentially damage peripheral nerves by excessive compression or traction. Several case series have been published suggesting that the incidence of postpartum compression neuropathy is in the order of 0.5% of pregnancies.[216–218] Risk factors include nulliparity and a prolonged second stage of labour. Neuraxial anaesthesia may contribute either directly or indirectly to peripheral neuropathy. Indirectly, it may allow women to push for longer periods without changing position, unaware of impending nerve injury.[216] The incidence of neuropraxia directly related to obstetric analgesia (spinal or epidural) is probably in the order of 1–2/10,000 parturients.[217,220,221] Although rare, the consequences of neuraxial abscess or haematoma can be devastating. Careful consideration should be given to this possibility and urgent radiological imaging (preferably MRI) and neurosurgical opinion should be sought in a patient with motor or sensory dysfunction after delivery.[8,222] Further details of the presentation, investigation, and treatment of neuraxial abscesses and haematomas are to be found in Chapter 28.

The most commonly affected peripheral nerve is the lateral femoral cutaneous nerve of the thigh, which can be stretched by retraction during caesarean delivery, or compressed beneath the inguinal ligament, especially with prolonged hip flexion. This results in the condition known as 'meralgia paraesthetica'. Associated risk factors include obesity, exaggerated lumbar lordosis, and an anatomical variant where the lateral femoral cutaneous nerve bisects the inguinal ligament. Other commonly injured peripheral nerves include the femoral nerve, the lumbar component of the sacral nerve (compressed as the fetal head enters the pelvis, especially during mid-cavity forceps deliveries), and the common peroneal nerve (compressed against the head of the fibula in the lithotomy position).

Assessment of new neurological symptoms in the postpartum period requires a careful history and thorough examination, including detailed documentation of the findings. In patients who have received neuraxial anaesthesia, consideration should always be given to the potential diagnosis of a neuraxial space-occupying collection (such as abscess or haematoma). If this possibility exists, then urgent imaging (preferably MRI) and early neurosurgical intervention is required to optimize neurological recovery. Otherwise, assessment should focus on the likely causative peripheral nerves. The lateral femoral cutaneous nerve is sensory only, and causes pain and noxious paraesthesia and numbness over the anterolateral part of the thigh, without motor deficit. Femoral nerve injury results in quadriceps weakness and numbness or paraesthesia over the lower anterior thigh. Peroneal nerve compression at the fibular head may result in foot drop and numbness over the lateral lower leg and dorsum of the foot. Compression of the obturator nerve is less common, but results in numbness and paraesthesia of the medial thigh and weakness of hip adduction.

The natural history of postpartum neuropraxia is one of gradual improvement to normal (or near-normal) function. In most patients, complete recovery occurs over 2–3 months, although in some this may take up to 2 years.[218]

Myasthenia gravis

Aetiology and presentation

Myasthenia gravis (MG) is an autoimmune disease resulting in fatigable weakness of skeletal muscle. The disorder is caused by T-cell dysfunction which results in the production of antibodies against the nicotinic acetylcholine receptor on the neuromuscular end-plate of skeletal muscle.[223] The disease commonly affects young women (male:female ratio 1:3), frequently in the third or fourth decade of life. The incidence is approximately 1/10,000[224] and may present for the first time in pregnancy.[225] Patients present with symptoms of skeletal muscle weakness, which worsens after a period of activity. MG may be isolated to ocular muscles (presenting with diplopia or ptosis), or more generalized, affecting a variable combination of ocular, bulbar, peripheral, and respiratory muscles. Weakness may fluctuate throughout the day, but tends to be worse in the evening. Approximately 10–15% of patients with MG have an underlying thymoma.

Treatment

Treatment priorities are similar to non-pregnant patients and should include exclusion of coexisting autoimmune disease (such as thyroid disease), evaluation of respiratory muscle dysfunction, and aggressive treatment of infections (such as endometritis and mastitis), which may precipitate MG exacerbation. Acute worsening of MG, particularly of respiratory function, is known as *myasthenic crisis*, and may require intubation and mechanical ventilation. Increased dosage of cholinesterase inhibitors is indicated and immunoglobulin or plasmapheresis may be required in this setting. Excessive treatment with cholinesterase inhibitors may also lead to a clinical syndrome of weakness, known as *cholinergic crisis*. The two crises may be difficult to distinguish, although cholinergic crisis may be accompanied by excessive sweating, salivation, and bradycardia. A single dose of edrophonium can also be given—symptoms will improve in the setting of myasthenic crisis and worsen or remain unchanged in cholinergic crisis.[226]

Obstetric considerations

The disease has a variable progression in pregnancy.[227,228] In a published case series, symptoms improved during pregnancy in 39% of patients, worsened in 19%, and remained unchanged in 42%.[229] If exacerbation occurs it is likely to be in the first trimester or in the immediate postpartum period.

Acetylcholinesterase inhibitors (such as pyridostigmine) are the first-line treatment for MG, and may require dose adjustment in pregnancy. They should be given parenterally during labour, due to variable gastric absorption. Other treatments may include glucocorticoids, and immunosuppressive therapy such as ciclosporin and azathioprine. Ciclosporin and azathioprine have been associated with spontaneous abortion, preterm labour, and low birth weight infants.[223] They should also be avoided in breastfeeding.

Magnesium sulphate must be avoided as it may precipitate myasthenic crisis. Hypertension should be treated with methyldopa or hydralazine. Beta blockers and calcium channel blockers should also be avoided if possible. If seizure prophylaxis is required in the setting of pre-eclampisa, levetiracetam or valproate should be used. Phenytoin may also exacerbate skeletal muscle weakness.

Uterine smooth muscle is not affected by MG and therefore the first stage of labour usually progresses uneventfully. However, the second stage of labour may be slowed by the weakening of skeletal muscle, and an assisted instrumental or operative delivery may be required. Stress and excessive exertion may also precipitate respiratory weakness and myasthenic crisis and should be avoided. Epidural analgesia should be strongly considered in this setting.

All infants born to mothers with MG should be observed in a special care nursery. Up to 10–20% of infants may develop neonatal MG as a result of passive transfer of maternal antibodies.[227]

Anaesthetic considerations

MG presents a number of challenges for the anaesthetist mainly due to the risk of respiratory weakness, and the difficulty of managing neuromuscular blockade if required.[226] Patients are also at risk of perioperative myasthenic (or cholinergic) crisis. Because patients with MG have a reduced number of normally functioning acetylcholine receptors, they may display abnormal responses to both depolarizing and non-depolarizing neuromuscular blocking agents. If the patient is treated with cholinesterase inhibitors, these medications also inhibit plasma cholinesterase, and therefore may result in a prolonged effect of suxamethonium. However, if untreated, due to the reduced number of normally functioning receptors, they may be relatively resistant to suxamethonium, but for the same reason, highly sensitive to non-depolarizing neuromuscular blockers. Neostigmine may be ineffective at reversing neuromuscular blockade as the cholinesterase may be already maximally inhibited. If rapid sequence induction is required, muscle relaxation with rocuronium followed by reversal with sugammadex may provide an attractive alternative to reversal with cholinesterase inhibitors.[225,230]

Neuraxial anaesthesia is both safe and recommended both for labour analgesia and caesarean delivery.[225,226] The potential for respiratory weakness resulting from a high block should be considered, and a carefully titrated epidural may be more prudent than single-shot spinal anaesthesia. Alternatively a combined spinal–epidural may be suitable with a small dose of spinal and then a titrated epidural dose to bring the block up. Acute respiratory muscle weakness requiring intubation and mechanical ventilation has been described following single-shot spinal anaesthesia for caesarean delivery.[225]

Conclusion

Although most neurological conditions are relatively rare, many can occur in women of child-bearing age. A number of important issues may need to be considered during the pregnancy, particularly with regard to planning for labour and delivery. Some patients may need to modify ongoing treatments (e.g. antiepileptic medications) due to potential adverse effects for the fetus. Patients with peripheral muscle weakness (such as MG and MS) may be at risk of respiratory failure in the later stages of pregnancy. Many neurological conditions also have important implications for the safe conduct of neuraxial anaesthesia and analgesia, such as spina bifida, hydrocephalus, and raised intracranial pressure. Parturients with neurological disease will benefit from coordinated care by a multidisciplinary team including an obstetrician, neurologist, neurosurgeon, and anaesthetist.

References

1. May AE, Fombon FN, Francis S. UK registry of high-risk obstetric anaesthesia: report on neurological disease. *Int J Obstet Anesth* 2008; 17:31–6.
2. Wilkinson H. Saving mothers' lives. Reviewing maternal deaths to make motherhood safer: 2006–2008. *BJOG* 2011; 118:1402–3.
3. Wang LP, Paech MJ. Neuroanesthesia for the pregnant woman. *Anesth Analg* 2008; 107:193–200.
4. Shehata HA, Okosun H. Neurological disorders in pregnancy. *Curr Opin Obstet Gynecol* 2004; 16:117–22.
5. Nossek E, Ekstein M, Rimon E, *et al.* Neurosurgery and pregnancy. *Acta Neurochir* 2011; 153:1727–35.
6. Ng J, Kitchen N. Neurosurgery and pregnancy. *J Neurol Neurosurg Psychiatry* 2008; 79:745–52.
7. Edlow JA, Caplan LR, O'Brien K, *et al.* Diagnosis of acute neurological emergencies in pregnant and post-partum women. *Lancet Neurol* 2013; 12:175–85.
8. Russell R. Neurological complications in obstetric regional anaesthesia. *Anaesth Intensive Care Med* 2007; 11:323–5.
9. Wong CA. Neurologic deficits and labor analgesia. *Reg Anesth Pain Med* 2004; 29:341–51.
10. Kuczkowski KM. Nonobstetric surgery in the parturient: anesthetic considerations. *J Clin Anesth* 2006; 18:5–7.
11. Cohen-Gadol AA, Friedman JA, Friedman JD, *et al.* Neurosurgical management of intracranial lesions in the pregnant patient: a 36-year institutional experience and review of the literature. *J Neurosurg* 2009; 111:1150–7.
12. Isla A, Alvarez F, Gonzalez A, *et al.* Brain tumor and pregnancy. *Obstet Gynecol* 1997; 89:19–23.
13. Mortimer AM, Bradley MD, Likeman M, *et al.* Cranial neuroimaging in pregnancy and the post-partum period. *Clin Radiol* 2013; 68(5):500–8.
14. Reitman E, Flood P. Anaesthetic considerations for non-obstetric surgery during pregnancy. *Br J Anaesth* 2011; 107 Suppl 1: i72–8.
15. Brown MD, Levi AD. Surgery for lumbar disc herniation during pregnancy. *Spine* 2001; 26:440–3.
16. Cohen EN, Gift HC, Brown BW, *et al.* Occupational disease in dentistry and chronic exposure to trace anesthetic gases. *J Am Dent Assoc* 1980; 101:21–31.
17. Hemminki K, Kyyronen P, Lindbohm ML. Spontaneous abortions and malformations in the offspring of nurses exposed to anaesthetic gases, cytostatic drugs, and other potential hazards in hospitals, based on registered information of outcome. *J Epidemiol Community Health* 1985; 39:141–7.
18. Jones HE, Balster RL. Inhalant abuse in pregnancy. *Obstet Gynecol Clin North Am*1998; 25:153–67.
19. Rowland AS, Baird DD, Shore DL, *et al.* Nitrous oxide and spontaneous abortion in female dental assistants. *Am J Epidemiol* 1995; 141:531–8.
20. Rowland AS, Baird DD, Weinberg CR, *et al.* Reduced fertility among women employed as dental assistants exposed to high levels of nitrous oxide. *N Engl J Med* 1992; 327:993–7.
21. Van de Velde M, Teunkens A, Kuypers M, *et al.* General anaesthesia with target controlled infusion of propofol for planned caesarean section: maternal and neonatal effects of a remifentanil-based technique. *Int J Obstet Anesth* 2004; 13:153–8.
22. Carvalho B, Mirikitani EJ, Lyell D, *et al.* Neonatal chest wall rigidity following the use of remifentanil for cesarean delivery in a patient with autoimmune hepatitis and thrombocytopenia. *Int J Obstet Anesth* 2004; 13:53–6.
23. Draisci G, Valente A, Suppa E, *et al.* Remifentanil for cesarean section under general anesthesia: effects on maternal stress hormone secretion and neonatal well-being: a randomized trial. *Int J Obstet Anesth* 2008; 17:130–6.
24. Al-areibi A, Coveney L, Singh S, *et al.* Case report: anesthetic management for sequential Cesarean delivery and laminectomy. *Can J Anaesth* 2007; 54:471–4.
25. Ross MG, Leake RD, Ervin MG, *et al.* Fetal lung fluid response to maternal hyperosmolality. *Pediatr Pulmonol* 1986; 2:40–3.
26. Lumbers ER, Stevens AD. Changes in fetal renal function in response to infusions of a hyperosmotic solution of mannitol to the ewe. *J Physiol* 1983; 343:439–46.
27. Chang L, Looi-Lyons L, Bartosik L, *et al.* Anesthesia for cesarean section in two patients with brain tumours. *Can J Anaesth* 1999; 46:61–5.
28. Korula G, Farling P. Anesthetic management for a combined Cesarean section and posterior fossa craniectomy. *J Neurosurg Anesth* 1998; 10:30–3.
29. Roberts D, Dalziel S. Antenatal corticosteroids for accelerating fetal lung maturation for women at risk of preterm birth. *Cochrane Database Syst Rev* 2006; 3:CD004454.

30. Borthen I, Gilhus NE. Pregnancy complications in patients with epilepsy. *Curr Opin Obstet Gynecol* 2012; 24:78–83.
31. Proposal for revised classification of epilepsies and epileptic syndromes. Commission on Classification and Terminology of the International League Against Epilepsy. *Epilepsia* 1989; 30:389–99.
32. Bardy AH. Incidence of seizures during pregnancy, labor and puerperium in epileptic women: a prospective study. *Acta Neurol Scand* 1987; 75:356–60.
33. Adab N, Tudur SC, Vinten J, *et al.* Common antiepileptic drugs in pregnancy in women with epilepsy. *Cochrane Database Syst Rev* 2004; 3:CD004848.
34. Borthen I, Eide MG, Veiby G, *et al.* Complications during pregnancy in women with epilepsy: population-based cohort study. *BJOG* 2009; 116:1736–42.
35. Tomson T, Battino D. Teratogenic effects of antiepileptic drugs. *Lancet Neurol* 2012; 11:803–13.
36. Hernandez-Diaz S, Werler MM, Walker AM, *et al.* Folic acid antagonists during pregnancy and the risk of birth defects. *N Engl J Med* 2000; 343:1608–14.
37. Prevention of neural tube defects: results of the Medical Research Council Vitamin Study. MRC Vitamin Study Research Group. *Lancet* 1991; 338:131–7.
38. Kaaja E, Kaaja R, Matila R, *et al.* Enzyme-inducing antiepileptic drugs in pregnancy and the risk of bleeding in the neonate. *Neurology* 2002; 58:549–53.
39. Cornelissen M, Steegers-Theunissen R, Kollee L, *et al.* Supplementation of vitamin K in pregnant women receiving anticonvulsant therapy prevents neonatal vitamin K deficiency. *Am J Obstet Gynecol* 1993; 168:884–8.
40. Schachter SC. Management of epilepsy and pregnancy. In Basow DS (ed) *UpToDate*. Waltham, MA; 2013. http://www.uptodate.com/contents/management-of-epilepsy-and-pregnancy
41. Bedard JM, Richardson MG, Wissler RN. Epidural anesthesia in a parturient with a lumboperitoneal shunt. Anesthesiology 1999;90(2):621–3.
42. Perks A, Cheema S, Mohanraj R. Anaesthesia and epilepsy. *Br J Anaesth* 2012; 108:562–71.
43. San-juan D, Chiappa KH, Cole AJ. Propofol and the electroencephalogram. *Clin Neurophysiol* 2010; 121:998–1006.
44. James AH, Bushnell CD, Jamison MG, *et al.* Incidence and risk factors for stroke in pregnancy and the puerperium. *Obstet Gynecol* 2005; 106:509–16.
45. Kuklina EV, Tong X, Bansil P, *et al.* Trends in pregnancy hospitalizations that included a stroke in the United States from 1994 to 2007: reasons for concern? *Stroke* 2011; 42:2564–70.
46. Salonen Ros H, Lichtenstein P, Bellocco R, *et al.* Increased risks of circulatory diseases in late pregnancy and puerperium. *Epidemiology* 2001; 12:456–60.
47. Kittner SJ, Stern BJ, Feeser BR, *et al.* Pregnancy and the risk of stroke. *N Engl J Med* 1996; 335:768–74.
48. Jaigobin C, Silver FL. Stroke and pregnancy. *Stroke* 2000; 31:2948–51.
49. Lanska DJ, Kryscio RJ. Stroke and intracranial venous thrombosis during pregnancy and puerperium. *Neurology* 1998; 51:1622–8.
50. Sharshar T, Lamy C, Mas JL. Incidence and causes of strokes associated with pregnancy and puerperium. A study in public hospitals of Ile de France. Stroke in Pregnancy Study Group. *Stroke* 1995; 26:930–6.
51. Lanska DJ, Kryscio RJ. Risk factors for peripartum and postpartum stroke and intracranial venous thrombosis. *Stroke* 2000; 31:1274–82.
52. Liu XJ, Wang S, Zhao YL, *et al.* A single-center study of hemorrhagic stroke caused by cerebrovascular disease during pregnancy and puerperium in China. *Int J Gynaecol Obstet* 2011; 113:82–3.
53. Dias MS, Sekhar LN. Intracranial hemorrhage from aneurysms and arteriovenous malformations during pregnancy and the puerperium. *Neurosurgery* 1990; 27:855–65.
54. Kim YW, Neal D, Hoh BL. Cerebral aneurysms in pregnancy and delivery: pregnancy and delivery do not increase the risk of aneurysm rupture. *Neurosurgery* 2013; 72:143–9.
55. Wong MC, Giuliani MJ, Haley EC, Jr. Cerebrovascular disease and stroke in women. *Cardiology* 1990; 77 Suppl 2:80–90.
56. Molyneux AJ, Kerr RS, Yu LM, *et al.* International subarachnoid aneurysm trial (ISAT) of neurosurgical clipping versus endovascular coiling in 2143 patients with ruptured intracranial aneurysms: a randomised comparison of effects on survival, dependency, seizures, rebleeding, subgroups, and aneurysm occlusion. *Lancet* 2005; 366:809–17.
57. Unruptured intracranial aneurysms—risk of rupture and risks of surgical intervention. International Study of Unruptured Intracranial Aneurysms Investigators. *N Engl J Med* 1998; 339:1725–33.
58. Horton JC, Chambers WA, Lyons SL, *et al.* Pregnancy and the risk of hemorrhage from cerebral arteriovenous malformations. *Neurosurgery* 1990; 27:867–71.
59. Sadasivan B, Malik GM, Lee C, *et al.* Vascular malformations and pregnancy. *Surg Neurol* 1990; 33:305–13.
60. Minielly R, Yuzpe AA, Drake CG. Subarachnoid hemorrhage secondary to ruptured cerebral aneurysm in pregnancy. *Obstet Gynecol* 1979; 53:64–70.
61. Duley L, Meher S, Abalos E. Management of pre-eclampsia. *BMJ* 2006; 332:463–8.
62. Selo-Ojeme DO, Marshman LA, Ikomi A, *et al.* Aneurysmal subarachnoid haemorrhage in pregnancy. *Eur J Obstet Gynecol Reprod Biol* 2004; 116:131–43.
63. Ducros A. Reversible cerebral vasoconstriction syndrome. *Lancet Neurol* 2012; 11:906–17.
64. Bateman BT, Olbrecht VA, Berman MF, *et al.* Peripartum subarachnoid hemorrhage: nationwide data and institutional experience. *Anesthesiology* 2012; 116:324–33.
65. Schwedt TJ, Matharu MS, Dodick DW. Thunderclap headache. *Lancet Neurol* 2006; 5:621–31.
66. Dahl J, Myhr KM, Daltveit AK*et al.* Planned vaginal births in women with multiple sclerosis: delivery and birth outcome. *Acta Neurol Scand Supplementum* 2006; 183:51–4.
67. Hsu DW, Efird JT, Hedley-Whyte ET. Progesterone and estrogen receptors in meningiomas: prognostic considerations. *J Neurosurg* 1997; 86:113–20.
68. Klein JP, Hsu L. Neuroimaging during pregnancy. *Semin Neurol* 2011; 31:361–73.
69. Osei EK, Faulkner K. Fetal doses from radiological examinations. *Br J Radiol* 1999; 72:773–80.
70. Manalo-Estrella P, Barker AE. Histopathologic findings in human aortic media associated with pregnancy. *Arch Pathol* 1967; 83:336–41.
71. Stoodley MA, Macdonald RL, Weir BK. Pregnancy and intracranial aneurysms. *Neurosurg Clin N Am* 1998; 9:549–56.
72. Tiel Groenestege AT, Rinkel GJ, van der Bom JG, *et al.* The risk of aneurysmal subarachnoid hemorrhage during pregnancy, delivery, and the puerperium in the Utrecht population: case-crossover study and standardized incidence ratio estimation. *Stroke* 2009; 40:1148–51.
73. Gross BA, Du R. Hemorrhage from arteriovenous malformations during pregnancy. *Neurosurgery* 2012; 71:349–55.
74. Arnold M, Camus-Jacqmin M, Stapf C, *et al.* Postpartum cervicocephalic artery dissection. *Stroke* 2008; 39:2377–9.
75. Borelli P, Baldacci F, Nuti A, *et al.* Postpartum headache due to spontaneous cervical artery dissection. *Headache* 2011; 51:809–13.
76. McKinney JS, Messe SR, Pukenas BA, *et al.* Intracranial vertebrobasilar artery dissection associated with postpartum angiopathy. *Stroke Res Treat* 2010; 2010:pii: 320627.
77. Cantu C, Barinagarrementeria F. Cerebral venous thrombosis associated with pregnancy and puerperium. Review of 67 cases. *Stroke* 1993; 24:1880–4.
78. Srinivasan K. Cerebral venous and arterial thrombosis in pregnancy and puerperium. A study of 135 patients. *Angiology* 1983; 34:731–46.
79. Sattar A, Manousakis G, Jensen MB. Systematic review of reversible cerebral vasoconstriction syndrome. *Expert Rev Cardiovasc Ther* 2010; 8:1417–21.

80. Fugate JE, Claassen DO, Cloft HJ, *et al.* Posterior reversible encephalopathy syndrome: associated clinical and radiologic findings. *Mayo Clinic Proc Mayo Clinic* 2010; 85:427–32.
81. Li Y, Gor D, Walicki D, *et al.* Spectrum and potential pathogenesis of reversible posterior leukoencephalopathy syndrome. *J Stroke Cerebrovasc Dis* 2012; 21:873–82.
82. Roth C, Ferbert A. Posterior reversible encephalopathy syndrome: is there a difference between pregnant and non-pregnant patients? *Eur Neurol* 2009; 62:142–8.
83. Hunt HB, Schifrin BS, Suzuki K. Ruptured berry aneurysms and pregnancy. *Obstet Gynecol* 1974; 43:827–37.
84. Ogilvy CS, Stieg PE, Awad I, *et al.* Recommendations for the management of intracranial arteriovenous malformations: a statement for healthcare professionals from a special writing group of the Stroke Council, American Stroke Association. *Circulation* 2001; 103:2644–57.
85. Robinson JL, Hall CS, Sedzimir CB. Arteriovenous malformations, aneurysms, and pregnancy. *J Neurosurg* 1974; 41:63–70.
86. Khan M, Wasay M. Haemorrhagic strokes in pregnancy and puerperium. *Int J Stroke* 2012; 8(4):265–72.
87. Trivedi RA, Kirkpatrick PJ. Arteriovenous malformations of the cerebral circulation that rupture in pregnancy. *J Obstet Gyanecol* 2003; 23:484–9.
88. Marshman LA, Rai MS, Aspoas AR. Comment to "Endovascular treatment of ruptured intracranial aneurysms during pregnancy: report of three cases". *Arch Gynecol Obstet* 2005; 272:93.
89. Nelson JA, Livingston GK, Moon RG. Mutagenic evaluation of radiographic contrast media. *Invest Radiol* 1982; 17:183–5.
90. Patel SJ, Reede DL, Katz DS, *et al.* Imaging the pregnant patient for nonobstetric conditions: algorithms and radiation dose considerations. *Radiographics* 2007; 27:1705–22.
91. Rodesch F, Camus M, Ermans AM, *et al.* Adverse effect of amniofetography on fetal thyroid function. *Am J Obstet Gynecol* 1976; 126:723–6.
92. Webb JA, Thomsen HS, Morcos SK, *et al.* The use of iodinated and gadolinium contrast media during pregnancy and lactation. *Eur Radiol* 2005; 15:1234–40.
93. Delgado Almandoz JE, Schaefer PW, *et al.* Diagnostic accuracy and yield of multidetector CT angiography in the evaluation of spontaneous intraparenchymal cerebral hemorrhage. *AJNR Am J Neuroradiol* 2009; 30:1213–21.
94. Edelman RR, Warach S. Magnetic resonance imaging (1). *N Engl J Med* 1993; 328:708–16.
95. Gross BA, Frerichs KU, Du R. Sensitivity of CT angiography, T2-weighted MRI, and magnetic resonance angiography in detecting cerebral arteriovenous malformations and associated aneurysms. *J Clin Neurosci* 2012; 19:1093–5.
96. Levine D, Barnes PD, Madsen JR, *et al.* Central nervous system abnormalities assessed with prenatal magnetic resonance imaging. *Obstet Gynecol* 1999; 94:1011–19.
97. Meyers PM, Halbach VV, Malek AM, *et al.* Endovascular treatment of cerebral artery aneurysms during pregnancy: report of three cases. *AJNR Am J Neuroradiol* 2000; 21:1306–11.
98. van Beijnum J, van der Worp HB, Buis DR, *et al.* Treatment of brain arteriovenous malformations: a systematic review and meta-analysis. *JAMA* 2011; 306:2011–19.
99. Agarwal N, Guerra JC, Gala N, *et al.* Current treatment options for cerebral arteriovenous malformations in pregnancy: a review of the literature. *World Neurosurg* 2014;81(1):83–90.
100. Forster DM, Kunkler IH, Hartland P. Risk of cerebral bleeding from arteriovenous malformations in pregnancy: the Sheffield experience. *Stereotact Funct Neurosurg* 1993; 61 Suppl 1:20–2.
101. Hernesniemi JA, Dashti R, Juvela S, *et al.* Natural history of brain arteriovenous malformations: a long-term follow-up study of risk of hemorrhage in 238 patients. *Neurosurgery* 2008; 63:823–9.
102. Koch-Henriksen N, Sorensen PS. The changing demographic pattern of multiple sclerosis epidemiology. *Lancet Neurol* 2010; 9:520–32.
103. Sharma SK, Herrera ER, Sidawi JE, *et al.* The pregnant patient with an intracranial arteriovenous malformation. Cesarean or vaginal delivery using regional or general anesthesia? *Reg Anesth* 1995; 20:455–8.
104. Trojano M, Pellegrini F, Paolicelli D, *et al.* Real-life impact of early interferon beta therapy in relapsing multiple sclerosis. *Ann Neurol* 2009; 66:513–20.
105. Viscomi CM, Wilson J, Bernstein I. Anesthetic management of a parturient with an incompletely resected cerebral arteriovenous malformation. *Reg Anesth* 1997; 22:192–7.
106. Eggert SM, Eggers KA. Subarachnoid haemorrhage following spinal anaesthesia in an obstetric patient. *Br J Anaesth* 2001; 86:442–4.
107. Vernooij MW, Ikram MA, Tanghe HL, *et al.* Incidental findings on brain MRI in the general population. *N Engl J Med* 2007; 357:1821–8.
108. Aiba T, Tanaka R, Koike T, *et al.* Natural history of intracranial cavernous malformations. *J Neurosurg* 1995; 83:56–9.
109. Kalani MY, Zabramski JM. Risk for symptomatic hemorrhage of cerebral cavernous malformations during pregnancy. *J Neurosurg* 2013; 118:50–5.
110. Witiw CD, Abou-Hamden A, Kulkarni AV, *et al.* Cerebral cavernous malformations and pregnancy: hemorrhage risk and influence on obstetrical management. *Neurosurgery* 2012; 71:626–30.
111. Tate J, Bushnell C. Pregnancy and stroke risk in women. *Womens Health* 2011; 7:363–74.
112. Huang CJ, Fan YC, Tsai PS. Differential impacts of modes of anaesthesia on the risk of stroke among preeclamptic women who undergo Caesarean delivery: a population-based study. *Br J Anaesth* 2010; 105:818–26.
113. Johnson DM, Kramer DC, Cohen E, *et al.* Thrombolytic therapy for acute stroke in late pregnancy with intra-arterial recombinant tissue plasminogen activator. *Stroke* 2005; 36: e53–5.
114. Murugappan A, Coplin WM, Al-Sadat AN, *et al.* Thrombolytic therapy of acute ischemic stroke during pregnancy. *Neurology* 2006; 66:768–70.
115. Alonso A, Hernan MA. Temporal trends in the incidence of multiple sclerosis: a systematic review. *Neurology* 2008; 71:129–35.
116. Pugliatti M, Sotgiu S, Rosati G. The worldwide prevalence of multiple sclerosis. *Clin Neurol Neurosurg* 2002; 104:182–91.
117. Simpson S Jr, Pittas F, van der Mei I, *et al.* Trends in the epidemiology of multiple sclerosis in Greater Hobart, Tasmania: 1951 to 2009. *J Neurol Neurosurg Psychiatry* 2011; 82:180–7.
118. Lee MJ, Hickenbottom S. Neurologic disorders complicating pregnancy. In Basow DS (ed) *UpToDate.* Waltham, MA; 2013. http://www.uptodate.com/contents/neurologic-disorders-complicating-pregnancy
119. Olek MJ. Epidemiology and clinical features of multiple sclerosis in adults. In Basow DS (ed) *UpToDate.* Waltham, MA; 2013. http://www.uptodate.com/contents/pathogenesis-and-epidemiology-of-multiple-sclerosis
120. Dorotta IR, Schubert A. Multiple sclerosis and anesthetic implications. *Curr Opin Anaesth* 2002; 15:365–70.
121. Polman CH, Reingold SC, Banwell B, *et al.* Diagnostic criteria for multiple sclerosis: 2010 revisions to the McDonald criteria. *Ann Neurol* 2011; 69:292–302.
122. Comi G, Filippi M, Barkhof F, *et al.* Effect of early interferon treatment on conversion to definite multiple sclerosis: a randomised study. *Lancet* 2001; 357:1576–82.
123. Johnson KP, Brooks BR, Cohen JA, *et al.* Copolymer 1 reduces relapse rate and improves disability in relapsing-remitting multiple sclerosis: results of a phase III multicenter, double-blind, placebo-controlled trial. 1995. *Neurology* 2001; 57:S16–24.
124. Finkelsztejn A, Brooks JB, Paschoal FM Jr, *et al.* What can we really tell women with multiple sclerosis regarding pregnancy? A systematic review and meta-analysis of the literature. *BJOG* 2011; 118:790–7.
125. Vukusic S, Hutchinson M, Hours M, *et al.* Pregnancy and multiple sclerosis (the PRIMS study): clinical predictors of post-partum relapse. *Brain* 2004; 127:1353–60.

126. Confavreux C, Hutchinson M, Hours MM, *et al.* Rate of pregnancy-related relapse in multiple sclerosis. Pregnancy in Multiple Sclerosis Group. *N Engl J Med* 1998; 339:285–91.
127. Waubant E, Sadovnick AD. Interferon beta babies. *Neurology* 2005; 65:788–9.
128. Weinreb HJ. Demyelinating and neoplastic diseases in pregnancy. *Neurol Clin* 1994; 12:509–26.
129. Stenager E, Stenager EN, Jensen K. Effect of pregnancy on the prognosis for multiple sclerosis. A 5-year follow up investigation. *Acta Neurol Scand* 1994; 90:305–8.
130. Verdru P, Theys P, D'Hooghe MB, *et al.* Pregnancy and multiple sclerosis: the influence on long term disability. *Clin Neurol Neurosurg* 1994; 96:38–41.
131. Kelly VM, Nelson LM, Chakravarty EF. Obstetric outcomes in women with multiple sclerosis and epilepsy. *Neurology* 2009; 73:1831–6.
132. Jones RM, Healy TE. Anaesthesia and demyelinating disease. *Anaesthesia* 1980; 35:879–84.
133. Lirk P, Birmingham B, Hogan Q. Regional anesthesia in patients with preexisting neuropathy. *Int Anesthesiol Clin* 2011; 49:144–65.
134. Drake E, Drake M, Bird J, Russell R. Obstetric regional blocks for women with multiple sclerosis: a survey of UK experience. *Int J Obstet Anesth* 2006; 15:115–23.
135. Centers for Disease Control. *National Program of Cancer Registries.* [Online] http://www.cdc.gov/cancer/npcr/
136. Haas JF, Janisch W, Staneczek W. Newly diagnosed primary intracranial neoplasms in pregnant women: a population-based assessment. *J Neurol Neurosurg Psychiatry* 1986; 49:874–80.
137. Roelvink NC, Kamphorst W, van Alphen HA, *et al.* Pregnancy-related primary brain and spinal tumors. *Arch Neurol* 1987; 44:209–15.
138. Tewari KS, Cappuccini F, Asrat T, *et al.* Obstetric emergencies precipitated by malignant brain tumors. *Am J Obstet Gynecol* 2000; 182:1215–21.
139. Terry AR, Barker FG, 2nd, Leffert L, *et al.* Outcomes of hospitalization in pregnant women with CNS neoplasms: a population-based study. *Neuro Oncol* 2012; 14:768–76.
140. Dugoff L, Sujansky E. Neurofibromatosis type 1 and pregnancy. *Am J Med Genet* 1996; 66:7–10.
141. Johnson N, Sermer M, Lausman A, *et al.* Obstetric outcomes of women with intracranial neoplasms. *Int J Gynaecol Obstet* 2009; 105:56–9.
142. van Breemen MS, Wilms EB, Vecht CJ. Epilepsy in patients with brain tumours: epidemiology, mechanisms, and management. *Lancet Neurol* 2007; 6:421–30.
143. DeAngelis LM. Central nervous system neoplasms in pregnancy. *Adv Neurol* 1994; 64:139–52.
144. Ye DY, Bakhtian KD, Asthagiri AR, *et al.* Effect of pregnancy on hemangioblastoma development and progression in von Hippel-Lindau disease. *J Neurosurg* 2012; 117:818–24.
145. Lusis EA, Scheithauer BW, Yachnis AT, *et al.* Meningiomas in pregnancy: a clinicopathologic study of 17 cases. *Neurosurgery* 2012; 71:951–61.
146. Dinc H, Esen F, Demirci A, *et al.* Pituitary dimensions and volume measurements in pregnancy and post partum. MR assessment. *Acta Radiol* 1998; 39:64–9.
147. Molitch ME. Pituitary tumors and pregnancy. *Growth Horm IGF Res* 2003; 13 Suppl A: S38–44.
148. Kachhara R, Devi CG, Nair S, *et al.* Acoustic neurinomas during pregnancy: report of two cases and review of literature. *Acta Neurochir* 2001; 143:587–91.
149. Stevenson CB, Thompson RC. The clinical management of intracranial neoplasms in pregnancy. *Clin Obstet Gynecol* 2005; 48:24–37.
150. Bonfield CM, Engh JA. Pregnancy and brain tumors. *Neurol Clin* 2012; 30:937–46.
151. Trainer PJ. Corticosteroids and pregnancy. *Semin Reprod Med* 2002; 20:375–80.
152. Imran SA, Ur E, Clarke DB. Managing prolactin-secreting adenomas during pregnancy. *Can Fam Physician* 2007; 53:653–8.
153. Giannini A, Bricchi M. Posterior fossa surgery in the sitting position in a pregnant patient with cerebellopontine angle meningioma. *Br J Anaesth* 1999; 82:941–4.
154. Marx GF, Zemaitis MT, Orkin LR. Cerebrospinal fluid pressures during labor and obstetrical anesthesia. *Anesthesiology* 1961; 22:348–54.
155. Su TM, Lan CM, Yang LC, *et al.* Brain tumor presenting with fatal herniation following delivery under epidural anesthesia. *Anesthesiology* 2002; 96:508–9.
156. Hilt H, Gramm HJ, Link J. Changes in intracranial pressure associated with extradural anaesthesia. *Br J Anaesth* 1986; 58:676–80.
157. Finfer SR. Management of labour and delivery in patients with intracranial neoplasms. *Br J Anaesth* 1991; 67:784–7.
158. Kelly PJ. Stereotactic third ventriculostomy in patients with nontumoral adolescent/adult onset aqueductal stenosis and symptomatic hydrocephalus. Journal of neurosurgery 1991;75(6):865–73.
159. Liakos AM, Bradley NK, Magram G, *et al.* Hydrocephalus and the reproductive health of women: the medical implications of maternal shunt dependency in 70 women and 138 pregnancies. *Neurol Res* 2000; 22:69–88.
160. Wisoff JH, Kratzert KJ, Handwerker SM, *et al.* Pregnancy in patients with cerebrospinal fluid shunts: report of a series and review of the literature. *Neurosurgery* 1991; 29:827–31.
161. Kleinman G, Sutherling W, Martinez M, Tabsh K. Malfunction of ventriculoperitoneal shunts during pregnancy. Obstetrics and gynecology 1983;61(6):753–4.
162. Tang RA, Dorotheo EU, Schiffman JS, *et al.* Medical and surgical management of idiopathic intracranial hypertension in pregnancy. *Curr Neurol Neurosci Rep* 2004; 4:398–409.
163. Dahl J, Myhr KM, Daltveit AK, *et al.* Pregnancy, delivery, and birth outcome in women with multiple sclerosis. *Neurology* 2005; 65:1961–3.
164. Friedman DI, Jacobson DM. Diagnostic criteria for idiopathic intracranial hypertension. *Neurology* 2002; 59:1492–5.
165. Digre KB, Varner MW, Corbett JJ. Pseudotumor cerebri and pregnancy. Neurology 1984;34(6):721–9.
166. Huna-Baron R, Kupersmith MJ. Idiopathic intracranial hypertension in pregnancy. Journal of neurology 2002;249(8):1078–81.
167. Bagga R, Jain V, Das CP, Gupta KR, Gopalan S, Malhotra S. Choice of therapy and mode of delivery in idiopathic intracranial hypertension during pregnancy. MedGenMed : Medscape general medicine 2005;7(4):42.
168. Koontz WL, Herbert WN, Cefalo RC. Pseudotumor cerebri in pregnancy. *Obstet Gynecol* 1983; 62:324–7.
169. Sax TW, Rosenbaum RB. Neuromuscular disorders in pregnancy. *Muscle Nerve* 2006; 34:559–71.
170. Vos PE, de Boer WA, Wurzer JA, *et al.* Subdural hematoma after lumbar puncture: two case reports and review of the literature. *Clin Neurol Neurosurg* 1991; 93:127–32.
171. Yildirim GB, Colakoglu S, Atakan TY, *et al.* Intracranial subdural hematoma after spinal anesthesia. *Int J Obstet Anesth* 2005; 14:159–62.
172. Hopkins EL, Hendricks CH, Cibils LA. Cerebrospinal fluid pressure in labor. American journal of obstetrics and gynecology 1965;93(7):907–16
173. The Global Polio Eradication Initiative. Website. [Online] http://www.polioeradication.org
174. Littleford JA, Brockhurst NJ, Bernstein EP, *et al.* Obstetrical anesthesia for a parturient with a ventriculoperitoneal shunt and third ventriculostomy. *Can J Anaesth* 1999; 46:1057–63.
175. Veiby G, Daltveit AK, Gilhus NE. Pregnancy, delivery and perinatal outcome in female survivors of polio. *J Neurol Sci* 2007; 258:27–32.
176. Landwehr JB, Jr, Isada NB, Pryde PG, *et al.* Maternal neurosurgical shunts and pregnancy outcome. *Obstet Gynecol* 1994; 83:134–7.
177. Abouleish E, Ali V, Tang RA. Benign intracranial hypertension and anesthesia for cesarean section. *Anesthesiology* 1985; 63:705–7.
178. Tidmarsh MD, May AE. Epidural anaesthesia and neural tube defects. *Int J Obstet Anesth* 1998; 7:111–14.

179. Pitkin RM. Folate and neural tube defects. *Am J Clin Nutr* 2007; 85:285S–8S.
180. Rietberg CC, Lindhout D. Adult patients with spina bifida cystica: genetic counselling, pregnancy and delivery. *Eur J Obstet Gynecol Reprod Biol* 1993; 52:63–70.
181. Richmond D, Zaharievski I, Bond A. Management of pregnancy in mothers with spina bifida. *Eur J Obstet Gynecol Reprod Biol* 1987; 25:341–5.
182. Kuczkowski KM. Labor analgesia for pregnant women with spina bifida: what does an obstetrician need to know? *Arch Gynecol Obstet* 2007; 275:53–6.
183. Azimullah PC, Smit LM, Rietveld-Knol E, *et al.* Malformations of the spinal cord in 53 patients with spina bifida studied by magnetic resonance imaging. *Childs Nerv Syst* 1991; 7:63–6.
184. Semple DA, McClure JH. Arnold-chiari malformation in pregnancy. *Anaesthesia* 1996; 51:580–2.
185. Paul KS, Lye RH, Strang FA, *et al.* Arnold-Chiari malformation. Review of 71 cases. *J Neurosurg* 1983; 58:183–7.
186. Newhouse BJ, Kuczkowski KM. Uneventful epidural labor analgesia and vaginal delivery in a parturient with Arnold-Chiari malformation type I and sickle cell disease. *Arch Gynecol Obstet* 2007; 275:311–13.
187. Landau R, Giraud R, Delrue V, *et al.* Spinal anesthesia for cesarean delivery in a woman with a surgically corrected type I Arnold Chiari malformation. *Anesth Analg* 2003; 97:253–5.
188. Kuczkowski KM. Spinal anesthesia for Cesarean delivery in a parturient with Arnold-Chiari type I malformation. *Can J Anaesth* 2004; 51:639.
189. Chantigian RC, Koehn MA, Ramin KD, *et al.* Chiari I malformation in parturients. *J Clin Anesth* 2002; 14:201–5.
190. Nel MR, Robson V, Robinson PN. Extradural anaesthesia for caesarean section in a patient with syringomyelia and Chiari type I anomaly. *Br J Anaesth* 1998; 80:512–15.
191. Roelofse JA, Shipton EA, Nell AC. Anaesthesia for caesarean section in a patient with syringomyelia. A case report. *S Afr Med J* 1984; 65:736–7.
192. Hullander RM, Bogard TD, Leivers D, *et al.* Chiari I malformation presenting as recurrent spinal headache. *Anesth Analg* 1992; 75:1025–6.
193. Barton JJ, Sharpe JA. Oscillopsia and horizontal nystagmus with accelerating slow phases following lumbar puncture in the Arnold-Chiari malformation. *Ann Neurol* 1993; 33:418–21.
194. Penney DJ, Smallman JM. Arnold-Chiari malformation and pregnancy. *Int J Obstet Anesth* 2001; 10:139–41.
195. Sicuranza GB, Steinberg P, Figueroa R. Arnold-Chiari malformation in a pregnant woman. *Obstet Gynecol* 2003; 102:1191–4.
196. Nielsen JL, Bejjani GK, Vallejo MC. Cesarean delivery in a parturient with syringomyelia and worsening neurological symptoms. *J Clin Anesth* 2011; 23:653–6.
197. Sterling L, Keunen J, Wigdor E, *et al.* Pregnancy outcomes in women with spinal cord lesions. *J Obstet Gynaecol Can* 2013; 35:39–43.
198. Pereira L. Obstetric management of the patient with spinal cord injury. *Obstet Gynecol Surv* 2003; 58:678–87.
199. Westgren N, Hultling C, Levi R, *et al.* Pregnancy and delivery in women with a traumatic spinal cord injury in Sweden, 1980–1991. *Obstet Gynecol* 1993; 81:926–30.
200. Wanner MB, Rageth CJ, Zach GA. Pregnancy and autonomic hyperreflexia in patients with spinal cord lesions. *Paraplegia* 1987; 25:482–90.
201. Greenspoon JS, Paul RH. Paraplegia and quadriplegia: special considerations during pregnancy and labor and delivery. *Am J Obstet Gynecol* 1986; 155:738–41.
202. ACOG committee opinion. Obstetric management of patients with spinal cord injuries. Number 275, September 2002. Committee on Obstetric Practice. American College of Obstetrics and Gynecology. *Int J Gynaecol Obstet* 2002; 79:189–91.
203. Maehama T, Izena H, Kanazawa K. Management of autonomic hyperreflexia with magnesium sulfate during labor in a woman with spinal cord injury. *Am J Obstet Gynecol* 2000; 183:492–3.
204. Burns R, Clark VA. Epidural anaesthesia for caesarean section in a patient with quadriplegia and autonomic hyperreflexia. *Int J Obstet Anesth* 2004; 13:120–3.
205. Chan LY, Tsui MH, Leung TN. Guillain-Barre syndrome in pregnancy. *Acta Obstet Gynecol Scand* 2004; 83:319–25.
206. Hughes RA, Cornblath DR. Guillain-Barre syndrome. *Lancet* 2005; 366:1653–66.
207. Brooks H, Christian AS, May AE. Pregnancy, anaesthesia and Guillain Barre syndrome. *Anaesthesia* 2000; 55:894–8.
208. Greenwood JJ, Scott WE. Charcot-Marie-Tooth disease: peripartum management of two contrasting clinical cases. *Int J Obstet Anesth* 2007; 16:149–54.
209. Howard RS. Poliomyelitis and the postpolio syndrome. *BMJ* 2005; 330:1314–18.
210. Lambert DA, Giannouli E, Schmidt BJ. Postpolio syndrome and anesthesia. *Anesthesiology* 2005; 103:638–44.
211. Wernet A, Bougeois B, Merckx P, *et al.* Successful use of succinylcholine for cesarean delivery in a patient with postpolio syndrome. *Anesthesiology* 2007; 107:680–1.
212. Gyermek L. Increased potency of nondepolarizing relaxants after poliomyelitis. *J Clin Pharmacol* 1990; 30:170–3.
213. Ronthal M. Bells palsy: pathogenesis, clinical features and diagnosis in adults. In Basow DS (ed) *UpToDate*. Waltham, MA; 2013. http://www.uptodate.com/contents/bells-palsy-pathogenesis-clinical-features-and-diagnosis-in-adults
214. Vrabec JT, Isaacson B, Van Hook JW. Bell's palsy and pregnancy. *Otolaryngol Head Neck Surg* 2007; 137:858–61.
215. Gillman GS, Schaitkin BM, May M, *et al.* Bell's palsy in pregnancy: a study of recovery outcomes. *Otolaryngol Head Neck Surg* 2002; 126:26–30.
216. Wong CA, Scavone BM, Dugan S, *et al.* Incidence of postpartum lumbosacral spine and lower extremity nerve injuries. *Obstet Gynecol* 2003; 101:279–88.
217. Dar AQ, Robinson AP, Lyons G. Postpartum neurological symptoms following regional blockade: a prospective study with case controls. *Int J Obstet Anesth* 2002; 11:85–90.
218. Loo CC, Dahlgren G, Irestedt L. Neurological complications in obstetric regional anaesthesia. *Int J Obstet Anesth* 2000; 9:99–124.
219. Birnbach DJ, Bader A, Ostheimer GW. Anesthesia and multiple sclerosis. *JAMA* 1988; 260:2838.
220. Holdcroft A, Gibberd FB, Hargrove RL, *et al.* Neurological complications associated with pregnancy. *Br J Anaesth* 1995; 75:522–6.
221. Paech MJ, Godkin R, Webster S. Complications of obstetric epidural analgesia and anaesthesia: a prospective analysis of 10,995 cases. *Int J Obstet Anesth* 1998; 7:5–11.
222. Moen V, Irestedt L. Neurological complications following central neuraxial blockades in obstetrics. *Curr Opin Anaesth* 2008; 21:275–80.
223. Bird SJ, Stafford IP, Dildy GA. Management of myasthenia gravis in pregnancy. In Basow DS (ed) *UpToDate*. Waltham, MA; 2013. http://www.uptodate.com/contents/management-of-myasthenia-gravis-in-pregnancy
224. Hoff JM, Daltveit AK, Gilhus NE. Myasthenia gravis: consequences for pregnancy, delivery, and the newborn. *Neurology* 2003; 61:1362–6.
225. Almeida C, Coutinho E, Moreira D, *et al.* Myasthenia gravis and pregnancy: anaesthetic management—a series of cases. *Eur J Anaesth* 2010; 27:985–90.
226. Blichfeldt-Lauridsen L, Hansen BD. Anesthesia and myasthenia gravis. *Acta Anaesthesiol Scand* 2012; 56:17–22.
227. Plauche WC. Myasthenia gravis in mothers and their newborns. *Clin Obstet Gynecol* 1991; 34:82–99.
228. Stafford IP, Dildy GA. Myasthenia gravis and pregnancy. *Clin Obstet Gynecol* 2005; 48:48–56.
229. Batocchi AP, Majolini L, Evoli A, *et al.* Course and treatment of myasthenia gravis during pregnancy. *Neurology* 1999; 52:447–52.
230. Garcia V, Diemunsch P, Boet S. Use of rocuronium and sugammadex for caesarean delivery in a patient with myasthenia gravis. *Int J Obstet Anesth* 2012; 21:286–7.

CHAPTER 46

Musculoskeletal disorders

James P. R. Brown and M. Joanne Douglas

Introduction

Musculoskeletal diseases present challenges for obstetricians and anaesthetists. The physiological changes of pregnancy and labour may exacerbate existing symptoms and stress cardiorespiratory reserve; this may also result in the first presentation of previously undiagnosed musculoskeletal disorders.

Many musculoskeletal conditions are rare. Anaesthetic management is based mainly on case reports that are subject to reporting and publication bias and may represent worst-case scenarios. Musculoskeletal diseases have a spectrum of phenotypic expression, associations, and functional consequences. Anaesthetic management needs to be tailored to the individual parturient and should, where possible, be planned in advance by the multidisciplinary team with the mother.

Malignant hyperthermia

Malignant hyperthermia (MH) is a pharmacogenetic disease of muscle with an autosomal dominant (AD) inheritance.[1] Mutations for MH have been found in genes encoding the ryanodine (RYR1) and dihydropyridine (DHPR) receptors, but not all mutations have been identified.[2,3]

The volatile anaesthetic agents may trigger a MH episode, either alone or in combination with suxamethonium. There is debate as to whether suxamethonium alone can trigger MH.[4] In MH susceptible (MHS) individuals, volatile agents can lead to prolonged excitation–contraction coupling (ECC) due to excessive release of calcium from the sarcoplasmic reticulum.[5,6] This ECC results in muscle rigidity and a hypermetabolic syndrome that presents as an increase in carbon dioxide, lactate, and eventually temperature with a decrease in bicarbonate, pH, and oxygen. If untreated, rhabdomyolysis will occur with myoglobinaemia, myoglobinuria, hyperkalaemia and an increase in creatine kinase (CK).[1] MH may not be triggered with every anaesthetic exposure;[1] rarely it occurs in the absence of triggering agents.[7]

Following suxamethonium, masseter muscle rigidity can be the first sign[1] and may prevent endotracheal intubation. When suxamethonium is not used, an increase in end-tidal carbon dioxide, unrelated to ventilation, may be the initial presentation. Spontaneously breathing patients will become tachypnoeic. Sympathetic stimulation leads to tachycardia, arrhythmias, and hypotension. Generalized muscle rigidity, rhabdomyolysis, and hyperthermia may occur if the episode is not treated early.

Treatment of MH consists of calling for help, stopping volatile agents, administering 100% oxygen (provides additional oxygen, purges anaesthetic machine), administration of dantrolene, and supportive treatment of acidosis, hyperthermia, and hyperkalaemia.[8]

Dantrolene sodium is the specific treatment for MH[9] and has been used successfully in parturients. Dantrolene crosses the placenta[10] and may be found in breast milk after its use.[11] A report of uterine atony following use[12] may have been related to mannitol in the formulation, rather than dantrolene itself.[13]

Confirmatory evidence of a MH episode is by a positive *in vitro* contracture test,[8] unless the individual has one of the known genetic mutations. If the genetic mutation is known it may be possible to diagnose MHS in a newborn using umbilical cord blood.[14]

Case reports of MH occurring in parturients during anaesthesia for obstetric surgery are rare, possibly because neuraxial anaesthesia (NA) is commonly used. There are multiple reports of anaesthesia for MHS parturients.[15] Ideally, NA will be used for obstetric surgery in MHS parturients, but when contraindicated, general anaesthesia (GA) can be safe, providing trigger agents are avoided and the parturient fully monitored.[16] Some recommend avoidance of triggers in non-MHS parturients who may be carrying a MHS fetus (father MHS). Most medications used in obstetrics are safe in MHS parturients, although the prostaglandins may cause maternal fever; as may prolonged epidural analgesia and sepsis. Fever may lead to erroneous diagnosis of MH in a MHS parturient. Prior to use the anaesthetic machine should be purged of volatile agents.[17] Many anaesthetic agents may be safely used in patients with MH (Box 46.1).

Backache

Pregnancy-related backache

Backache has a background population prevalence of approximately 25%.[18] At term, pregnancy-related backache (PRB) is present in up to 50% of parturients. Proposed aetiologies include weight gain, altered posture and mechanical loading of the spine (especially posterior elements e.g. facet joints), increased lumbar lordosis, and forward tilting of the pelvis with a gravid uterus (Figure 46.1), ligament laxity secondary to oestrogen, and relaxin. PRB is a significant cause of sick leave and can impair activities of daily living.[19]

PRB can be divided into lumbar pain or pelvic girdle pain, which commonly involves the symphysis pubis or the sacroiliac joints and radiates into the thighs. There is no radicular or neurological component to PRB. Pelvic pain is linked to greater levels of dysfunction and increased sick leave compared with lumbar backache.[18]

In one survey, 50% of parturients had backache 12–15 months post delivery. For many, backache at this stage is not a direct

Box 46.1 Anaesthetic drugs that may be used safely in parturients susceptible to malignant hyperthermia

Induction agents

- Propofol
- Thiopentone
- Ketamine
- Benzodiazepines
- Etomidate

Analgesics

- Remifentanil
- Alfentanil
- Fentanyl
- Sufentanil
- Morphine
- Oxycodone
- Pethidine

Muscle relaxants

- Atracurium
- Rocuronium
- Vecuronium

Anaesthetic gases

- Nitrous oxide

Local anaesthetics

- Lidocaine
- Prilocaine
- Bupivacaine
- Ropivacaine
- 2-Chloroprocaine

result of labour and delivery; 21% of those with postpartum backache did not have backache during pregnancy.[20] The most significant predictor of postpartum backache is an antenatal history of backache.[21] Prospective studies suggest labour epidurals may be associated with an increase in acute backache in the first 24 hours postpartum, but do not increase chronic backache.[22–24] Physical fitness is protective against PRB and physiotherapy aimed at strengthening core muscles, providing increased stability to the pelvis and lumbar region, is first-line treatment.

Prolapsed intervertebral disc

Acute disc herniation causing radiculopathy is rare in pregnancy, 1/10,000,[25] although there are case reports of cauda equina syndrome requiring urgent back surgery.[26] Symptoms in parturients with pre-existing disc disease commonly deteriorate during pregnancy. A study investigating parturients who have had previous

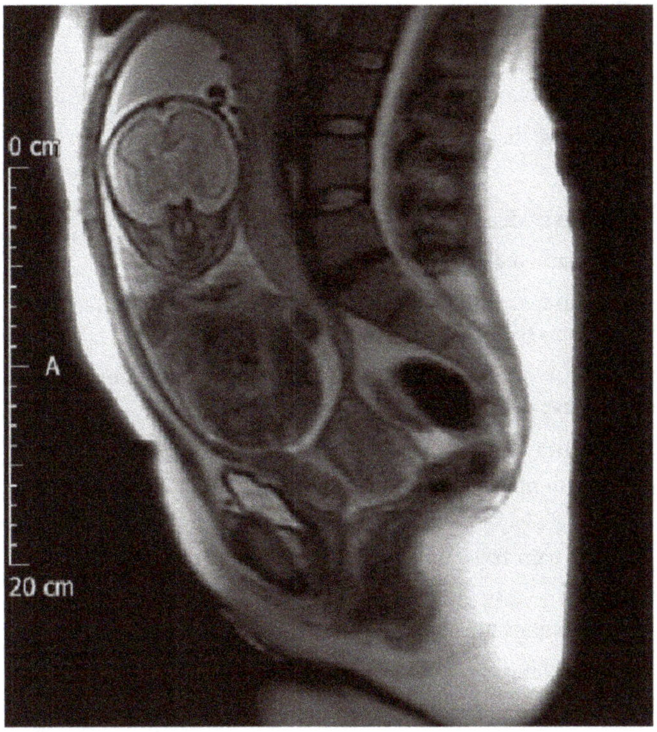

Figure 46.1 Sagittal MRI of lumbar spine, demonstrating increased lumbar lordosis and forward tilting of pelvis at 25 weeks of gestation.

microdiscectomy, demonstrated worsening radiculopathy in 24% of patients; 6% developing a motor deficit.[25]

Stable pre-existing neurology from a prolapsed intervertebral disc is not necessarily an absolute contraindication to NA (epidurals are commonly used in treatment). A pragmatic approach can be taken, clinically evaluating existing neurological deficit, discussing the risks and benefits of epidural versus alternative labour analgesia, or NA versus GA for operative delivery. These patients need to be actively followed up; including doing a postpartum neurological exam. If the level of disc herniation is known, risk may be reduced by avoiding this level when inserting NA.[26]

Spondylolisthesis

This is a misalignment of the lumbar vertebrae, most commonly an anterior displacement of L5 relative to L4 as a result of degenerative change. Pregnancy does not appear to worsen symptoms associated with pre-existing spondylolisthesis.[27]

Anaesthetic considerations

Antenatal

- Confirm diagnosis/cause of backache:
  - PRB
  - Other cause (e.g. prolapsed disc, spondylolisthesis)
- Prolapsed intervertebral disc:
  - Full neurological assessment of lower limbs
  - Evidence of cauda equina:
    - Magnetic resonance imaging (MRI)
    - Neurosurgical consultation

- Consider physiotherapy referral
- Anaesthetic review:
  - Any previous spinal imaging
  - Review, discuss, and agree anaesthetic plan
  - PRB:
    - No evidence epidurals increase chronic backache
  - Prolapsed disc:
    - Discuss rare possibility of worsening neurological symptoms (exact risk unknown)
    - Risk/benefit of alternative labour analgesia or GA for operative delivery.

Peripartum

- Confirm no acute deterioration or development of new neurological signs or symptoms
- Assess pain-free range of movement of legs prior to NA
- Ensure passive positioning does not exceed pain-free active range of movement:
  - Lithotomy may not be possible
- Ensure symmetrical movement of legs when positioning
- Consider passive second stage if prolapsed disc.

Postpartum

- Neurological exam to rule out deterioration.

Scoliosis

Scoliosis is defined as a lateral curvature of the spine of greater than 10°. It is commonly accompanied by vertebral rotation and rib deformity. There is a female to male preponderance of 3.5:1;[28] the majority of cases are idiopathic. Table 46.1 lists other causes with their specific anaesthetic considerations. Changing aetiology (e.g. lower rates of polio and tuberculous osteomyelitis) and modern management with evolving surgical techniques have improved outcomes. Management is guided by severity of scoliosis Figure 46.2. Traditional scoliosis surgery involves fusing the spine posteriorly.[29]

Obstetric considerations

- Generally tolerate pregnancy, labour, and delivery well; complications similar to normal population[35]
- Abnormal pelvic weight-bearing alters anatomy, possible labour dystocia, fetal malpresentation
- Increased labour induction (odds ratio (OR) 1.6)[28]
- Increased caesarean delivery (CD) (OR 1.8):[28]
  - Uterine forward displacement increases fetal malpresentation
- Possible classical uterine incision for surgical access:[36]
  - Risk of uterine rupture/dehiscence with subsequent pregnancies.

Anaesthetic considerations

General anaesthesia

There are 34 cases in the literature describing GA for CD in parturients with idiopathic scoliosis,[36–40] including 13 cases with severe restrictive respiratory disease.[36,37] Most were uncomplicated, but one required prolonged ventilation following CD.[40]

Reduced neck flexion and spinal hump may make positioning for intubation challenging. Difficult intubation[41] and respiratory dysfunction[30] are more likely in patients with scoliosis secondary to another disorder.

Respiratory problems are rare if respiratory volumes are greater than 50% of predicted: mortality and morbidity increase with vital capacities less than 1 L.[42] Several respiratory defects may occur (Box 46.2).

Neuraxial anaesthesia

An early labour epidural reduces the stress response and ensures time to achieve adequate function if operative delivery required. However, NA can be difficult due to:

- Failure to locate epidural or intrathecal space:
  - Rotation of vertebrae makes identification of midline difficult
  - If surgically corrected, anatomy is distorted causing risk of subdural or intrathecal placement[43,44] (> 5% epidurals following surgical correction)
- Unpredictable anaesthetic block:
  - Short stature and decreased volume of cerebrospinal fluid:[45]
    - Risk high block
  - Abnormal intrathecal spread of hyperbaric local anaesthetic:
    - Although the intrathecal space is usually not affected by surgery,[46] abnormal curvature and rotation affect gravitational spread
    - Positioning or mixing iso- and hyperbaric anaesthetic may overcome[47 48]
  - If surgically corrected:
    - Possible adhesions in epidural space or indentation by instrumentation (20% inadequate subarachnoid block despite locating space).[38,49,50]

In 89 labour epidurals reported in parturients with scoliosis, 96% were successful in non-operated compared to 60% in operated.

Methods to improve success:

- Angle of approach (Figure 46.3)[42,58]
- Level of approach:
  - L5/S1 interspace:
    - 20% of fixations extend to L3/4—potentially more problematic[51]
    - Fusion unlikely to involve L5/S1[46]
  - Caudal epidural[52]
- Guided approach—prepuncture ultrasound[53] (see Chapter 54):
  - Assess vertebral rotation (asymmetry of transverse processes), guiding needle direction[54]
  - If surgically corrected:
    - Identify lower extent of fixation; may not correspond to scar[55]
    - Spinal instrumentation: lateral marker of midline[56]

Table 46.1 Aetiology of scoliosis with summary of anaesthetic considerations

	Aetiology	Considerations	
Vertebral anomalies	Congenital defects, e.g. hemivertebrae	Ensure isolated defect rather than part of syndrome	
	Velocardiofacial[30]	Facial dysmorphism, difficult airway Cardiac defects 75% Thymic dysplasia, immune defects	
	VACTERL syndrome[31]	Difficult airway Cardiac defects	
	Spina bifida[32]	Pelvic abnormalities, CD likely Risk inadvertent dural puncture with epidural Tethered cord, risk trauma with spinal Previous spinal surgery common Possible shunt for hydrocephalus	
Osteochondrodystrophies	Achondroplasia	See 'Achondroplasia' and 'Osteogenesis Imperfecta' in main text	
	Osteogenesis imperfecta		
Neurological	UMN	Cerebral palsy	Scoliosis
	LMN	Postpolio syndrome[32]	Respiratory impairment, sensitivity to opioids and anaesthetic agents Bulbar dysfunction, aspiration risk
		Spinal muscular atrophy[32]	Respiratory muscle weakness, sensitivity to NDMR Hyperkalaemia with suxamethonium
	Other	Syringomyelia[33]	Hyperkalaemia with suxamethonium Prolonged neuromuscular block with NDMR Aspiration risk if syringobulbia Deterioration with increased ICP, e.g. pressor response to intubation
		Neurofibromatosis[34]	Spinal cord neuromas; relative contraindication to NA Raised ICP Respiratory impairment Associated phaeochromocytoma
		Friedreich (spinocerebellar) ataxia[34]	Hyperkalaemia with suxamethonium Unpredictable response to NDMR Respiratory muscle weakness Associated cardiomyopathy, arrhythmias, diabetes mellitus Aspiration risk
Muscular	Muscular dystrophy	See 'Muscular Dystrophy' in main text	
Infection	Tuberculosis (Pott disease)	Respiratory impairment	
Connective tissue disease	Marfan syndrome	See Chapter 41	
	Ehlers–Danlos syndrome	See 'Ehler-Danlos syndrome' in main text	

CD, caesarean delivery; ICP, intracranial pressure; LMN, lower motor neuron; NA, neuraxial anaesthesia; NDMR, non-depolarizing muscle relaxants; UMN, upper motor neuron; VACTERL, Vertebral, Anal, Cardiac, Tracheo-oEsophageal fistula, Renal, Limb.

Data from various sources (see references).

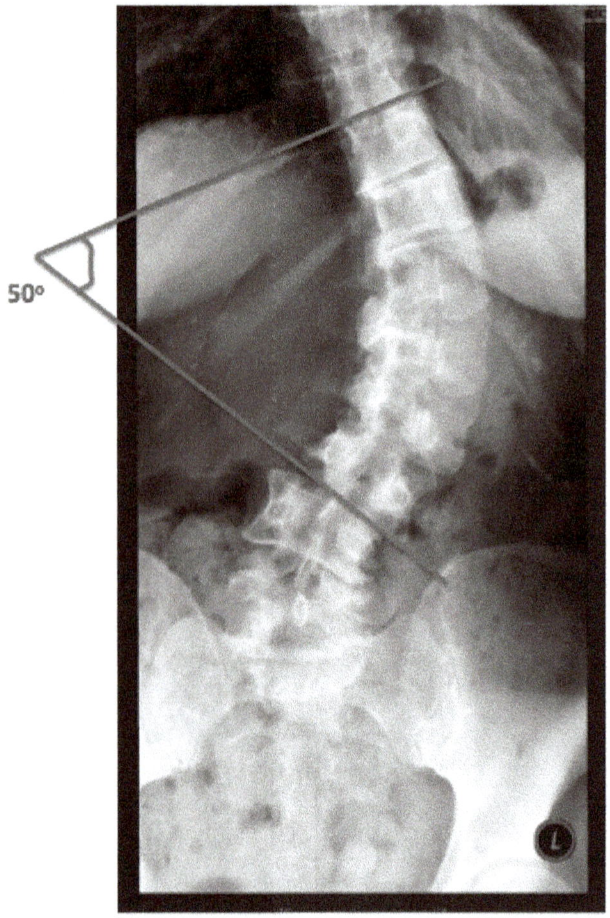

Figure 46.2 Severity of scoliosis can be described by Cobb angle. This X-ray demonstrates a severe thoracolumbar scoliosis (Cobb angle of 50°) with an apex at L2, with marked rotation and convexity to the left.

- Continuous spinal anaesthesia (CSA):[49]
    - Ability to titrate:
    - Reduces cardiovascular and respiratory compromise
    - Control block height
- Dural puncture epidurals:[57]
    - Puncture dura (25 G needle through epidural needle), without injecting intrathecal anaesthetic. Improves quality and adequacy of epidural block in parturients without scoliosis, probably by direct spread of local anaesthetic to subarachnoid space.

Box 46.2 Respiratory defects associated with scoliosis

- Reduced lung volumes
- Reduced compliance
- Restrictive defect
- Hypoxaemia
- Increased pulmonary vascular resistance
- Pulmonary hypertension
- Cor pulmonale

Summary of anaesthetic considerations

Antenatal

- Assess specific co-morbidities (secondary scoliosis (Table 46.1))
- Cardiology:
    - Electrocardiogram (ECG):
        - Right atrial dilatation or ventricular hypertrophy
    - Echocardiography:
        - Right ventricular hypertrophy or pulmonary hypertension
- Respiratory:
    - Pulmonary function tests
- Anaesthetics:
    - Spinal anatomy:
        - Previous radiological imaging
            - Operative report from spinal surgery
        - Ultrasound assessment: lower extent of scoliosis or operative correction
    - Discuss labour and delivery analgesia and anaesthesia:

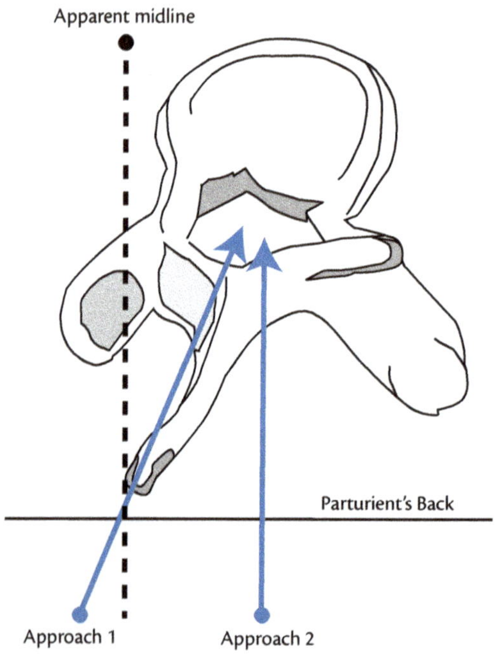

Figure 46.3 Suggested approach to epidural space in parturients with scoliosis. Lumbar vertebra in a parturient with scoliosis, convexity is to the right of apparent midline. The vertebra is rotated, with a wider angle between the transverse and distorted spinous process on the convex (right) side.

Approach 1: aim towards the convexity of the scoliosis, in-line with spinous processes. Advantage: starting in the apparent midline and approaching through familiar tissue planes.

Approach 2: approach via the paramedian route, away from the midline on the side of convexity; advance needle onto lamina, prior to '*walking off*'. Advantages: a familiar perpendicular approach and aiming for larger interlaminar space.

Adapted with permission from Jeffrey Huang, Paramedian Approach for Neuroaxial Anesthesia in Parturients with Scoliosis, *Anesthesia & Analgesia*, Volume 111, Issue 3, pp. 821–22, Copyright © 2010 Wolters Kluwer Health, Inc., and from Gambling D, Douglas M, McKay R, *Obstetric Anesthesia and Uncommon Disorders*, Cambridge University Press, Cambridge, UK, Copyright © 2008.

- Potential technical difficulties with insertion, increased risk of failure and complications with NA (especially following operative repair)
- Explore patient concerns and wishes.

Peripartum

- Establish early labour epidural:
  - Assess effectiveness
  - Actively manage
  - Titrate anaesthetic, use low-dose local anaesthetic with opioid—high blocks may precipitate cardiovascular/respiratory deterioration if no functional reserve
- If GA:
  - Exclude associated MH risks with secondary scoliosis
  - Anticipate difficult intubation and ventilation.

Postpartum

- Severe cardiorespiratory compromise:
  - Invasive arterial monitoring
  - Manage in high dependency unit.

If secondary scoliosis, please see Table 46.1 for additional specific anaesthetic considerations.

Myopathies

A myopathy is a primary disease of muscle. Causes of myopathy are:

- Inherited:
  - Muscular dystrophies
  - Myotonia
  - Congenital:
    - Central core
    - Nemaline
    - Centronuclear
  - Familial periodic paralysis
  - Metabolic:
    - Glycogen storage
    - Lipid metabolism
    - Mitochondrial
    - Myoadenylate deaminase (MADA) deficiency
- Acquired:
  - Inflammatory:
    - Dermatomyositis, polymyositis, inclusion body myositis
  - Endocrine:
    - Thyroid, adrenal
  - Metabolic:
    - Hypokalaemia, hypocalcaemia, hypercalcaemia
  - Drug induced:
    - Glucocorticoid, alcohol
  - Infectious:
    - Human immunodeficiency virus (HIV)
  - Paraneoplastic
  - Critical illness.

Anaesthetic implications

Antenatal

- Multidisciplinary input:
  - Cardiology
    - Electrocardiography, 24-hour tape, echocardiography
    - Implantable pacemaker or defibrillator
    - Reduced exercise tolerance:
      - Skeletal muscle weakness
      - Respiratory insufficiency
      - Cardiomyopathy
  - Respiratory:
    - Restrictive respiratory defect:
      - Pulmonary function tests
    - Associated sleep apnoea:
      - Screening questionnaire (e.g. STOP BANG[59])
      - Sleep studies
    - Presence of pulmonary hypertension:
      - Echocardiography
  - Anaesthetic:
    - Consider and discuss implications of myopathy
    - Agree anaesthetic plan for delivery.

Peripartum

- Assess progression of symptoms with pregnancy
- Increased incidence of assisted delivery or CD:
  - Early senior anaesthetic review
  - Consider early labour epidural
- CD:
  - Titratable NA where possible:
    - Avoid high block; may precipitate respiratory compromise
  - Reduce risk of rhabdomyolysis with GA:
    - Avoid suxamethonium, caution with volatile agents
    - Consider non-depolarizing muscle relaxants (NDMRs) and total intravenous anaesthesia
    - Purge anaesthetic machine
    - Measure serum potassium and CK perioperatively, continue cardiac monitoring into recovery period
    - Dantrolene immediately available
  - Prepare for difficult intubation.

Postpartum

- Anticipate respiratory compromise:
  - Multimodal analgesia for operative delivery:
    - Opioid sparing
    - Consider postoperative epidural analgesia
    - Consider tranversus abdominis plane block
  - High dependency
  - Invasive arterial line, monitoring adequacy of ventilation
  - Respiratory physiotherapy.

Despite different underlying causes, all myopathies have similar anaesthetic considerations (Table 46.2). Specific considerations for different causes of myopathy are discussed in their respective sections below.

Risk of malignant hyperthermia with myopathies

The pathophysiology of rhabdomyolysis in myopathies differs to MH;[60] the two do not appear to be linked. In myopathies, the muscle membrane integrity is unstable and even in the resting state can lead to increased serum potassium and CK release. Depolarizing muscle relaxants and halogenated agents can further stress the membrane causing rhabdomyolysis and hyperkalaemia. The exceptions are myopathies involving the RYR1 receptor, which are associated with MH: central core disease (CCD) and King–Denborough syndrome.[61,62]

Consensus is that suxamethonium should be avoided in all myopathies.[63,64] There is limited evidence to quantify risk of volatile agents; use an alternative technique where possible to avoid MH risk, that is, NA or total intravenous anaesthesia.

Muscular dystrophies

This is a collection of inherited degenerative muscle disorders which, depending on the specific genetic defect, lead to progressive weakness of variable distribution and severity. The progressive nature and age of onset mean that they may first present peripartum. Molecular genetics are refining the traditional clinical classification (Box 46.3)[65] and each has different anaesthetic considerations (Table 46.3).

Table 46.2 Anaesthetic implications of myopathy, in general

System	Manifestation	Implication
Airway	Dysmorphia	Difficult intubation
	Bulbar involvement	Aspiration risk
Respiratory	Muscle weakness	Respiratory failure
	Associated scoliosis	See 'Scoliosis' in main text
Cardiovascular	Cardiomyopathy or conduction defects	Arrhythmias Cardiac failure
Musculoskeletal	Unpredictable rhabdomyolysis with suxamethonium or volatile agents	Hyperkalaemia Myoglobulinuria

Box 46.3 Classification of muscular dystrophies

- X-Linked:*
  - Duchenne
  - Becker
  - Emery–Dreifuss (also AD form, chromosome (Chr) 1)[66]
- Limb-girdle:[66]
  - 6 AD subtypes
  - 9 AR subtypes
- Distal:
  - Late onset (AD), e.g. Welander, Markesbery
  - Early onset (mostly AR), e.g. Miyoshi, Nonaka, Laing (AD)
- Congenital (mostly AR), e.g. Fukuyama, muscle–eye–brain disease, Walker–Warburg, merosin-deficient, merosin positive, integrin deficient
- Other:
  - Fascioscapulohumeral (AD), Chr 4
  - Oculopharyngeal (AD), Chr 14
  - Myotonic dystrophy:
    - Type 1, Chr 19
    - Type 2, Chr 3

*Parturients who are carriers may suffer mild disease.[64]

Data from various sources (see references).

Other myopathies

Congenital myopathies

This heterogeneous group[63,71,80–82] of over 40 different disorders (autosomal recessive (AR), AD, or X-linked[80]) present with neonatal hypotonia and muscle weakness.[64] Cardiac involvement is rare but reported.[63] Nemaline myopathies are associated with dysmorphic features that may cause difficult intubation (e.g. high-arched palate, mandibular abnormalities).[82,83] Central core disease is a result of AD or AR abnormality of RYR1 and is associated with MH.[61,84]

Metabolic myopathies

Metabolic myopathies are inborn errors of metabolism that affect myocyte adenosine triphosphate (ATP) production (Figure 46.4). Metabolic myopathies are caused by inherited enzyme abnormalities: either defects in the conversion of glycogen to pyruvate, fatty acids to acetyl CoA, or in the respiratory chain.

Glycogen storage disorders

There are 11 enzyme disorders of glucose (glucose-6-phosphate) metabolism (type I—XI),[85] leading to abnormal deposition of glycogen. Collectively known as glycogen storage disorders (Table 46.4) they present with exercise intolerance; resting energy production is usually sufficient.

Lipid metabolism disorders

Lipid metabolism disorders (Table 46.5) are a result of failure in processing fatty acids. They present during periods of starvation or physiological stress, as a result of defects in the following:[96]

Table 46.3 Muscular dystrophies and anaesthetic implications

Dystrophy	Characteristics	Implications
Duchenne or Becker[67]	X-linked, 12% carriers have skeletal muscle weakness; 18% cardiac abnormalities, e.g. dilated cardiomyopathy (7%), arrhythmias Phenotypically similar to limb-girdle[66]	Consider screening ECG, Holter monitoring, echocardiography
Limb-girdle[68–70] prevalence 8/million[66]	Pelvis and shoulder, wasting and weakness Restrictive respiratory impairment Cardiomyopathy (some subtypes only)[66] Conduction defects	Risk of deterioration peripartum (>50%)[71] Likely require assisted VD or CD because of pelvic involvement (>50%)[71]
Fascioscapulo-humeral[72,73] prevalence 8/million[66]	Usually presents in childhood >90% affected by age 20 Asymmetrical facial weakness, especially orbicularis oris and oculi. Shoulder girdle weakness Legs affected later (10% wheelchair bound)	Relatively less cardiomyopathy and conduction defects,[74] although described[66,73] Bulbar and respiratory muscles relatively spared[73]
Emery–Dreifuss[75–77]	Childhood onset Tendon contractures of: Achilles, elbow, posterior cervical; predates weakness[66] Humeral and peroneal weakness and wasting Cardiomyopathy (age < 30)[76] Arrhythmias (97%) including conduction blocks, VT, VF, sudden death	Contractures limit neck movement: difficult intubation Risk of intracardiac thromboembolic disease, may require anticoagulation[77] Often need implantable cardiac defibrillator Consider echocardiography
Oculopharyngeal[66,78]	Extraocular muscles Ptosis Weakness neck, proximal arms Dysphagia	No case reports Typical onset after child-bearing age[78] Aspiration risk
Congenital[79] prevalence 25/million[66]	Heterogeneous group Hypotonia, weakness at birth Weakness non-progressive Cardiac involvement unusual May affect intelligence	Respiratory muscle weakness Aspiration risk

CD, caesarean delivery; ECG, electrocardiogram; VD, vaginal delivery; VF, ventricular fibrillation; VT, ventricular tachycardia.

Data from various sources (see references).

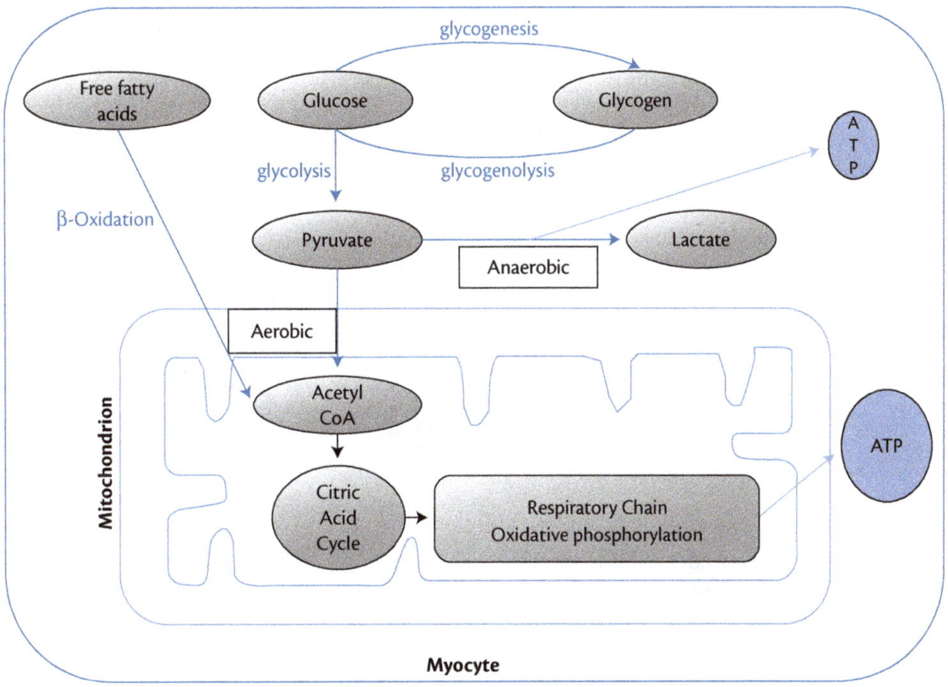

Figure 46.4 Normal myocyte adenosine triphosphate (ATP) production.

Table 46.4 Adult presentations of glycogen storage disorders and anaesthetic implications, all AR

Glycogen storage disease	Features	Implications	Case reports
II Pompe[86] (acid maltase deficiency)	Incidence 1/40,000[86] Glycogen abnormally deposited in all cells Dysphagia Macroglossia Obstructive sleep apnoea Cardiac impairment Progressive muscular weakness Scoliosis	Aspiration Difficult intubation Opioid sensitivity Arrhythmias Cardiac failure Slowly progressive respiratory failure See section 'Scoliosis' in main text	1 parturient 2 pregnancies 1st pre-eclampsia and IUGR, CD at 27 weeks: neonatal death 2nd uncomplicated CD with CSE[86]
III Cori–Forbes[85,87–90] (debranching enzyme deficiency)	Incidence 1/100,000[87] Onset 3rd–4th decade Hepatic, myocardial, erythrocyte, leucocyte, skeletal muscle involvement Risk of hypoglycaemia with starvation Ketosis and lactic acidosis with physiological stress, including pregnancy Risk intrauterine death Associated with hepatic adenomas	**Screen**: echocardiography, liver function tests **Prevent hypoglycaemia**: cornstarch, IV dextrose, nocturnal NG feed **Labour or CD**: Consider invasive arterial pressure monitoring Monitor serum lactate	6 parturients with 9 deliveries 4 CD[85,87,89,90] 1 stillbirth 28 weeks[90] 1 emergency CD for fetal distress at 34 weeks, following maternal hypoglycaemia associated with coma and seizures[89]
IV Anderson (branching enzyme deficiency)	Most commonly an isolated myopathy		No reports
V McArdle (phosphorylase deficiency[91–94])	Exercise intolerance Muscle cramps Myoglobinuria with exercise (50%)[95] Rhabdomyolysis, associated renal impairment (27%)[95] 'Second-wind' effect as muscle switches to alternate substrate[94]	Pregnancy and delivery usually well tolerated	16 parturients with 24 pregnancies[91–94] 2 assisted deliveries 5 CD 2 worsening muscle cramps 1 mild myoglobinuria post delivery
VII Tarui (phospho-fructokinase deficiency) (Also X, XI)	Presentation similar to McArdles[96] Tarui is associated with haemolysis		No reports

I and VI have no associated myopathy.

VIII and IX are X-linked.

AR, autosomal recessive; CD, caesarean delivery; CSE, combined spinal–epidural; IUGR, intrauterine growth restriction; IV, intravenous; ng, nasogastric.

Data from various sources (see references).

- Transport of long chain fatty acids across mitochondrial membrane (e.g. carnitine-palmitoyl-transferase deficiency—types 1 and 2)
- Transport of carnitine into the cell (e.g. carnitine transporter deficiency)
- Enzymes responsible for β-oxidation (e.g. acetyl-CoA dehydrogenase).

Mitochondrial myopathies

This is a heterogeneous group[96,110–115] of over 100 different defects in the respiratory chain.[113] Parturients may not be able to meet the increased energy demands of pregnancy (20% increased oxygen consumption) or labour (63% increase) leading to lactic acidosis.[112]

Depending on severity of the defect it may cause multiorgan dysfunction, especially in organs with higher energy requirements; brain, muscle, and heart, for example, MELAS syndrome (mitochondrial encephalopathy, lactic acidosis, and stroke-like episodes).[112]

Anaesthetic Considerations

- Antenatal:
  - Baseline: renal, liver function, clotting studies, glucose, lactate
- Peripartum:
  - Monitor serum lactate
  - Supplementary oxygen
  - Early labour epidural (25% reduction oxygen consumption)
  - Elective CD avoids increased labour oxygen consumption
  - Prevent hypothermia:
    - Shivering increases oxygen consumption
  - Avoid lactate-containing crystalloid solutions

Table 46.5 Lipid metabolism disorders and anaesthetic implications

	Presentation	Cases	Implications
Carnitine-palmitoyl-transferase (CPT) deficiency Two enzyme complexes CPT 1 on outer and CPT 2 on inner mitochondrial membrane	Commonly presents in childhood with hypoketotic hypoglycaemia, hepatomegaly, seizures and cardiomyopathy Adult presentation: most commonly myopathy after prolonged exercise May be associated with rhabdomyolysis, myoglobinuria[96]	8 parturients, 10 pregnancies: 2 with CPT 1[97,98], 4 with CPT 2[99–101,102] 2 unknown[103,104] 2 first presented in pregnancy[97,98] 6 term VD[97,99,100,102–104], 1 induction 34 weeks **Labour analgesia and VD:** 1 spinal[104] 1 CSE,[102] 2 epidurals,[99,100] All: IV glucose during labour 4: increased CK, 1: hypoglycaemia, 1: myoglobinuria **3 CD:**[98,101,103] 1 spinal, 2 anaesthetic not described 1 abruption, preterm labour 26 weeks,[101] 1 massive haemorrhage, hysterectomy, renal replacement therapy to treat metabolic acidosis[98]	Prevent hypoglycaemia, hypothermia Early labour epidural or elective CD Hydration reduces risk of renal impairment if myoglobinuria Monitor CK Check liver function and clotting (HELLP syndrome from associated fatty liver)[98]
Carnitine transporter deficiency Systemic (hepatic, cardiac) or isolated skeletal disease[105] AR inherited carnitine transporter defect OCTN 1 and 2 genes[106]	50% present as infants with hypoketotic hypoglycaemia, hepatomegaly, hepatic encephalopathy 50% present ages 1–7 with cardiomyopathy ± progressive muscle weakness Can present as sudden death or remain asymptomatic[107]	Serum carnitine decreases with pregnancy, symptoms may progress intrapartum with significant deterioration[105,107–109] 1 uncomplicated CD: OCTN 2 deficiency, anaesthetic technique not described[106]	Treat: carnitine supplementation Screen: liver, cardiac involvement Prevent: hypoglycaemia, hypothermia Early labour epidural or elective CD

AR, autosomal recessive; CD, caesarean delivery; CK, creatine kinase; CSE, combined spinal–epidural; HELLP, Haemolysis, Elevated Liver enzymes, Low Platelets; IV, intravenous; VD, vaginal delivery.

Data from various sources (see references).

- Postpartum:
  - Ensure good postoperative analgesia.

Both local and general anaesthetic agents have been used successfully in mitochondrial myopathies,[113] but theoretically some could adversely affect the respiratory chain (e.g. propofol infusion syndrome).[112]

Myoadenylate deaminase deficiency

Myoadenylate deaminase (MADA)[96,116] is unique to skeletal muscle and catalyses conversion of adenosine monophosphate to inosine monophosphate. A defect in this enzyme is present in up to 2% of the population[96] and affects muscle ATP availability. Although often asymptomatic, MADA may present with exercise intolerance, cramps, progressive weakness, exertional myoglobinuria, and rhabdomyolysis.[116] There is a report of two uncomplicated vaginal deliveries (VDs) in one parturient.[116]

Idiopathic inflammatory myopathies

Polymyositis and dermatomyositis are autoimmune-mediated diseases, characterized by inflammatory muscular infiltrates, proximal muscle weakness, abnormal electromyography, and increased serum CK. They can occur in isolation or in combination with other autoimmune diseases such as rheumatoid arthritis, systemic lupus erythematosus, or systemic sclerosis.[117] Myositis has a bimodal age distribution peaking at 10–25 and 30–60 years, with a prevalence of 2.5–10/100,000.[118] A heliotrope (purple) periorbital, butterfly rash is typical of dermatomyositis, 20% are associated with malignancy.

Obstetric implications

Fetal outcome is related to maternal disease activity and is worst in parturients presenting with myositis for the first time in early pregnancy.[117]

- Outcome is better when in remission (72% healthy)[117]
- Active disease:[117]
  - Fetal loss, 43%[117]
  - Intrauterine growth restriction (IUGR), 33%[117]
  - Premature delivery.

Theoretically proximal muscle weakness may increase assisted or CD rates, but this is not reported in the limited case literature. Uterine muscle is not involved.[64]

Management of acute disease is challenging as many drugs used for treatment are contraindicated in pregnancy. Corticosteroids appear relatively safe and immunoglobulin therapy has been used successfully.[119]

Anaesthetic implications

There is only one report discussing the anaesthetic management of a parturient with myositis.[120] There is no evidence that one anaesthetic technique is superior.

Myotonic dystrophy

Myotonic dystrophy (type 1) is the commonest cause of myotonia (delayed muscular relaxation). The incidence in Europe is 3–5/100,000.[121] Also known as myotonia dystrophica, myotonia atrophica, or Steinert disease, there is an inherited defect of the myosin kinase gene in skeletal, smooth, and cardiac muscle. The condition is caused by an unstable trinucleotide code (CTG) on chromosome 19,[121] the defect is amplified by meiosis; offspring have a greater number of repeated CTG sequences. Because of this, myotonic dystrophy demonstrates anticipation: subsequent generations are affected at an earlier age by more severe disease.

Subtypes of myotonic dystrophy are classified by age of onset: congenital, childhood, adult, or late.[121] Adult onset (classical disease) is most relevant to obstetrics (Box 46.4).

There are 27 reports of anaesthesia for myotonic parturients (Box 46.5).[122–138] Maternal diagnosis is frequently made only after the congenital form is found in offspring.[129,130,133,137] These are high-risk patients. There was a 24% incidence of postpartum haemorrhage (PPH), abnormal placentation, and postoperative respiratory complications, as well as a parturient suffering arrhythmia with cardiogenic shock.[127] Table 46.6 presents methods of mitigating risks.

The disease process is distal to the neuromuscular junction therefore NA and NDMR will not improve myotonia. Treatment of a crisis (generalized myotonia, masseter spasm, chest rigidity, arching of spine) is with quinine, procainamide, or phenytoin.[139] Localized myotonia may be treated with local anaesthetic infiltration, for example, abdominal muscles stimulated with diathermy or uterine myotonia.[122,132]

Anaesthetic considerations are similar for parturients with non-dystrophic myotonias (Table 46.7), although cardiac risks and uterine myotonia are not seen.

Connective tissue disease

Ehlers–Danlos syndrome

Ehlers–Danlos is a group of genetically inherited collagen diseases. Collagen is a product of 19 proteins, coded for on 15 different chromosomes: disease severity, organ involvement, and clinical manifestations depend on the specific genetic defect.[149] Shared characteristics include joint hypermobility, tissue fragility with poor wound healing, and easy bruising and bleeding. There are two classifications based on clinical and genetic findings.

- Berlin classification:
  - Types I—XI
- Villefranche classification:[150]
  - Common subtypes, prevalence:[149]
    - Classical (formerly type I and II), 1/20,000–40,000
    - Hypermobility (formerly type III), 1/10,000–15,000 (*some authorities suggest this is a spectrum of joint hypermobility syndrome*)

Box 46.4 Features of myotonic dystrophy (adult onset)

First diagnosis 20–50 years

- Skeletal muscle:
  - Progressive weakness and wasting:
    - Facial:
      - Ptosis
      - Masseter and temporalis
    - Accessory respiratory muscles, e.g. sternocleidomastoid
    - Distal limbs
  - Myotonia, e.g. inability to relax grip
  - Stiffness improving with repetitive movement:
    - 'Warm-up phenomenon'
  - Raised serum creatine kinase
- Smooth muscle:
  - Dysphagia
  - Uterine myotonia
- Cardiac:
  - Arrhythmias, can be exercise induced
  - Cardiomyopathy
  - Sudden death
- Respiratory:
  - Progressive restrictive defect
  - Aspiration risk
- Cataracts
- Frontal balding
- Endocrine:
  - Gonadal hypotrophy
  - Hypothyroidism
  - Diabetes mellitus
- Low intelligence quotient
- Premature death, aged 48—60

Obstetric implications

Increased risk

- Spontaneous abortion (uterine myotonia)
- Genetic inheritance with anticipation:
  - Neonatal myotonic dystrophy
  - Consider:
    - Preconception counselling
    - Genetic screening of fetus
    - Medical termination
- Weakness and myotonia:[122]
  - Possible first presentation[123]
  - Progressive disease, possible previous uncomplicated delivery[122]

- Polyhydramnios
- Preterm labour

Peripartum

- Labour exacerbates weakness and myotonia
- Risk fetal malpresentation

First stage:

- Slow progress; abnormal uterine contractions, slow cervical dilatation:
    - Likely require oxytocin augmentation
- May be rapid: uterine functional incompetence

Second stage:

- Ineffective uterine contractions
- Maternal muscular weakness and fatigue
- Muscular stiffness may make vaginal delivery (VD) difficult
- Often require assisted delivery

Third stage:

- Retained placenta
- Abnormal placentation, e.g. accreta
- Uterine atony and postpartum haemorrhage (PPH) risk

Anaesthetic implications

Antenatal

- Cardiology:
    - Electrocardiography, 24-hour tape, echocardiography
- Respiratory:
    - Pulmonary function tests
- Endocrine:
    - Thyroid function
    - Diabetic screening
- Obstetric:
    - Assess for abnormal placentation (ultrasound/MRI)
    - Consider neonatal involvement and availability of care required
- Anaesthetic:
    - Consider and discuss implications of myotonia, agree anaesthetic plan for delivery—consider early labour epidural

Peripartum

- Temperature (prevent hypothermia, monitor for MH):
    - Monitor continually
    - Active warming
- Be prepared for PPH
- If requires GA:
    - Avoid suxamethonium—consider rapid sequence intubation with rocuronium
    - Monitor peripheral nerve stimulator
    - Avoid anticholinestereases—consider sugammadex for reversal of rocuronium

Postpartum

- Postoperative respiratory failure:
    - Postoperative analgesia:
        - Multimodal, opioids sparing
            - Consider continuing epidural postoperatively
            - Consider tranversus abdominis plane block
    - High dependency:
        - Consider invasive arterial monitoring
    - Respiratory physiotherapy

Data from various sources (see references).

    - Vascular (formerly type IV), 1/100,000—200,000
- Rare subtypes (<100 cases worldwide). Few reports, but available information suggests these are high risk and to manage as vascular subtype:[150]
    - Kyphoscoliotic
    - Arthrochalasia
    - Dermatosparaxis

Common subtypes are inherited in an AD manner and share similar obstetric and anaesthetic implications. The vascular subtype has additional risks.

Obstetric implications

- PPH 20%
- Poor wound healing, abnormal scar formation (episiotomy or caesarean) 46%
- Uterine (15%) or rectal (11%) prolapse
- 50% neonatal disease.[151]

Anaesthetic implications

- General considerations:
    - Bleeding or easy bruising, no specific associated coagulation defect:
        - Anticipate PPH
    - Friable skin, care with pressure points
    - Deep venous thrombosis risk (4.2%)[151]
    - Chronic joint pain—complex pain management
    - Resistance to local anaesthetic agents[149]
    - Arrhythmias (autonomic dysfunction, conduction defects)
    - Valvular heart disease
- Neuraxial anaesthesia—consider:
    - Reducing risk of epidural haematoma: spinal (smaller needle), epidural (flexible catheter)
    - Combined spinal-epidural (CSE)

Box 46.5 Anaesthetic management for 27 parturients with myotonic dystrophy

- Two VDs:[124,133]
  - Uncomplicated with epidural[124]
  - Forceps delivery[133]
- 25 CD:
  - Five elective[126,130,136,137]
  - Nine emergency[123,125,129,131,132,134,135,138]
  - Rest undisclosed
- Anaesthetic technique:
  - Seven GA[123,132,135,137,138]
  - Three spinal[122,132] (one converted to GA for haemorrhage)[132]
  - Three epidural[129,131,136]
  - Three CSE[126,128,134]
- Complications (N = 25) (some > 1):
  - Four uncomplicated[128,129,131,134]
  - Six haemorrhage[122,123,130,132]
  - Six abnormal placentation[122,123,125,130,132]
  - Three hysterectomy[123,130,132]
  - Four uterine atony[122,123,129,132]
  - Four postoperative pneumonia[123,126,133,137]
  - Two postoperative ventilatory failure requiring reintubation[133,135]
  - One required supplementary oxygen postoperatively[138]
  - One masseter spasm, vigorous shivering following epidural top-up, intravenous fentanyl for inadequate block—no complications[136]
  - One paroxysmal atrial fibrillation, ventricular tachycardia, cardiogenic shock[127]

Data from various sources (see references).

Table 46.6 Type 1 myotonic dystrophy, anaesthetic implications, and methods of mitigating risk

Manifestations	Implications	Mitigate risk
Myotonia precipitated by:		
Cold	Avoid hypothermia	Temperature monitoring Warm fluids Forced air warmer
Depolarizing muscle relaxants	Suxamethonium may cause masseter spasm or respiratory muscle myotonia Difficult intubation and ventilation	Avoid GA if possible Avoid suxamethonium Risk prolonged blockade with NDMR
Anticholinesterases[140]	Avoid reversal	Use sugammadex for rocuronium[141]
Shivering	NA-induced[125]	Risk epidural>spinal
Respiratory muscle weakness and myotonia	Postoperative respiratory failure Poor secretion clearance	Use sedatives with caution Physiotherapy
Obstructive sleep apnoea Abnormal central response to hypoxia, hypercarbia	Sensitivity to opioids, barbiturates[140]	Postoperative monitoring in high dependency Monitor $PaCO_2$
Dysphagia	Aspiration pneumonitis, postoperative respiratory failure	Adequate fasting Antacid prophylaxis
Cardiac involvement	Arrhythmias[127] Cardiac failure[127] Sudden death[140]	Monitor ECG postoperatively
	Arrhythmia risk with sympathetic response to labour/delivery	Reduce stress response: early labour epidural, elective CD
Uterine involvement	Abnormal placentation[130] APH[123]/PPH[122] Increased risk hysterectomy[123,130,132]	Prepare for PPH

APH, antepartum haemorrhage; CD, caesarean delivery; ECG, electrocardiogram; GA, general anaesthesia; NA, neuraxial anaesthesia; NDMR, non-depolarizing muscle relaxants; $PaCO_2$, arterial partial pressure carbon dioxide; PPH, postpartum haemorrhage.

Data from various sources (see references).

    - Possible prolonged surgery, difficult closure (tissue friability, bleeding)
    - Low-dose spinal component improves cardiovascular stability in presence of autonomic dysfunction
  - Stringent testing of sensory block:
    - Possible reduced effectiveness of local anaesthetics[149]
  - Monitor lower limb neurological recovery postpartum:
    - Proactively investigate abnormal or persisting neurology suggesting epidural haematoma, MRI
- General anaesthesia—consider:
  - Consent:
    - Risk dental and airway trauma (periodontal disease, friable tissue upper airway)
  - Careful cricoid pressure:
    - Potentially makes intubation more difficult[142]
  - Use airway adjuncts or awake fibreoptic intubation:
    - Reduce manipulation of hypermobile cervical spine, avoids cord trauma
  - Avoid high airway pressures:
    - Risk of pneumothorax
  - Attention to positioning and padding on operating table:
    - Skin friability

Table 46.7 Other causes of myotonia

Diagnosis	Inheritance	Features of note[142]
Myotonic dystrophy type 2 (proximal myotonic myopathy)	AD ZNF9 Chr 3	Proximal weakness. Milder than type 1 Similar multisystem involvement and anaesthetic implications
Non-dystrophic myotonias		
Myotonia congenita Thomson disease[143,144]	AD CLCN1 mutation Chr 7 Defect chloride channel	Muscular hypertrophy Not progressive or periodic
Myotonia congenita Becker disease[145]	AR CLCN1 mutation	Myotonia predominantly affects lower limbs; weakness upper limbs Progressive, periodic
Paramyotonia congenita[146,147]	AD Sodium channel defect SCN4A Possible spectrum of disease with hyperkalaemic periodic paralysis[148]	Generalized myotonia, presents in childhood Stiffness worsens with exercise
Hyperkalaemic periodic paralysis[148] (adynamia episodica heredita)	AD Sodium channel defect Chr 17 SCN4A	Flaccid paralysis with increased serum potassium, cold or emotional stress Reduce extracellular potassium with diuretics, β-agonists

AD, autosomal dominant; AR, autosomal recessive; Chr, chromosome.

Data from various sources (see references).

Vascular (type IV) Ehlers–Danlos

Parturients with vascular subtype have a defect in type III collagen increasing the risk of vascular (aorta, vena cava) or visceral (bowel or uterine) rupture, with a peripartum mortality of up to 25%.[152] Identify this subgroup through genetic screening.

Preconception counselling is advised including discussing the option of medical termination in unplanned pregnancies. There is debate concerning optimum mode and timing of delivery. Both VD and CD have been described successfully.[152,153]

Reduce maternal risk by:

- Delivering in specialist centre
- Screening for existing major vessel disease (e.g. carotid dopplers, echocardiography, MRI)[154]
- Giving desmopressin (DDAVP)[153]
- Early labour epidural
- Extreme caution with labour induction or augmentation[155]
- Invasive blood pressure monitoring
- GA, obtund pressor response at intubation:
  - Use rapid-onset, short-acting opioids (e.g. remifentanil or alfentanil)
- Monitoring postpartum in high dependency area.

Marfan syndrome

See Chapter 41.

Autoimmune-associated musculoskeletal disease

Autoimmune function is affected by pregnancy:

- Maternal exposure to fetal antigens
- Proinflammatory effect of oestrogen, stimulating tumour necrosis factor alpha (TNF-α) production[119]
- Susceptibility to viral illnesses: possible trigger for autoimmune disease.

Rheumatoid arthritis

Rheumatoid arthritis is a multisystem autoimmune disease, characterized by a distal, symmetrical deforming polyarthropathy. Disease-modifying antirheumatic drugs (DMARDs) reduce disease progression and side effects of long-term or high-dose corticosteroid therapy. Many DMARDs are teratogenic: conception should be planned when disease is stable on a low-risk drug. Biological agents (e.g. anti-TNF-α) are being used to treat severe disease; their effects on pregnancy and fetus are unknown.

Symptoms usually improve in 70–80% of rheumatoid patients by the second trimester.[156] Unfortunately nearly all experience a disease flare in the year following delivery.

Obstetric implications

- Teratogenic risk, especially unplanned pregnancies
- Balance risk from drug therapy and disease activity
- Hip involvement may require CD.

Anaesthetic implications

See Table 46.8 and Table 46.9.

Antenatal

- Assess:
  - Airway:
    - Predictors of difficult intubation—temporomandibular joint involvement
    - Presence of atlantoaxial subluxation
  - Respiratory:
    - Presence of fibrotic lung disease
    - Any functional deterioration with progression of pregnancy—consider lung function tests
  - Cardiovascular:
    - ECG—exclude conduction blocks
    - Echocardiogram—if functional limitation; exclude pericardial effusion
  - Haematology and biochemistry:
    - Anaemia:
      - Multiple causes—ensure haematinics optimised
    - Thrombocytopaenia—associated splenomegaly and platelet sequestration (Felty syndrome)

Table 46.8 Complications of rheumatoid arthritis and anaesthetic implications

System	Manifestation	Implications
Airway	Temporomandibular involvement	Avoid GA when possible Difficult intubation, reduced mouth opening, mandibular protrusion
	Cricoarytenoid involvement	Difficulty passing endotracheal tube Use smaller tube
	Atlantoaxial subluxation	Risk spinal cord injury Consider intubation adjuncts
Respiratory	Interstitial lung disease (fibrosis)	Respiratory impairment May decompensate with pregnancy or anaesthesia
	Pleural effusions	
Cardiac	Nodules in cardiac conduction system	Heart block Ventricular dysfunction May decompensate with pregnancy, delivery, or anaesthesia
	Pericarditis	
	Pericardial effusions	
Musculoskeletal	Hip/lumbar spine involvement	Difficult positioning for VD Consider CD NA difficult
	Skin at risk from long-term steroid therapy and joint deformity	Skin breakdown and neuropraxias at pressure points
Haematological	Anaemia	Reduced reserve if peripartum haemorrhage
	Associated Felty syndrome	Rheumatoid with splenomegaly, thrombocytopaenia Risk: epidural haematoma
Other	Associated Sjögren syndrome (10%)[157]	Risk: corneal abrasion with GA Consider eye lubrication
	Drug therapy	See Table 46.9

CD, caesarean delivery; GA, general anaesthesia; NA, neuraxial anaesthesia; VD, vaginal delivery.

Data from various sources (see references).

- Disease-modifying medication—ensure no associated neutropaenia or abnormal liver function
- Thyroid function—common associated autoimmune disease

- Discuss labour and delivery analgesia and anaesthesia:
  - Discuss anaesthetic options, risks and benefits
  - Explore patient concerns and wishes.

Peripartum

- Assess for any deterioration in cardiorespiratory function with advancing pregnancy
- Careful positioning and pressure point care:
  - Reduced joint mobility
    - Assess range of movement prior to NA, do not exceed

Table 46.9 Drugs for autoimmune disease and fetal concerns

Drug	Fetal and neonatal implications
Corticosteroids	Increased rates of: ◆ Gestational diabetes ◆ Pregnancy induced hypertension ◆ Infection ◆ Premature rupture of membranes ◆ IUGR Risks increase with prednisolone dose > 20 mg
Non-steroidal anti-inflammatory drugs	Considered safe to 32 weeks' gestation[156] Risk premature closure ductus arteriosus Potential increased bleeding in neonates
COX-2 inhibitors	Avoid: affects neonatal cardiac and renal genesis
Hydroxychloroquine	Theoretical risk: oculo- and ototoxicity Appears safe Safe in breastfeeding (2% transferred)[156]
Sulfasalazine	Possible increased teratogenicity Considered safe with folate supplementation[156]
Azathioprine Ciclosporin	Appear safe in pregnancy, but not breastfeeding.[156] Possible IUGR Both can cause leucopenia, thrombocytopaenia.
Methotrexate	Not safe in pregnancy or breastfeeding
Cyclophosphamide	Teratogenic
Leflunomide	Teratogenicity seen in animal studies, no human cases Current recommendations to avoid for 2 years prior to conception (enterohepatic recirculation)[156]
Immunoglobulins (pooled donor IgG)	Safely used to manage various autoimmune conditions in pregnancy Increased thromboembolic risk
Biological agents: anti-TNF-α e.g. infliximab, etanercept or B-cell depletion, e.g. rituximab	Limited clinical experience in pregnancy or breastfeeding Current recommendation to avoid[156]

COX 2, cyclooxygenase 2; IUGR, intrauterine growth restriction; TNF, tumour necrosis factor.

Data from various sources (see references).

    - Increased risk of pressure sores
- If hip involvement, increased likelihood of CD
- May need steroid supplementation
- NA:
  - Technically challenging
- GA:
  - Potential difficult intubation
  - Reduce manipulation and movement of cervical spine
    - Use intubation aids
    - Consider fibreoptic intubation
  - Consider protective eye lubrication (Sjögren syndrome).

Postpartum

- Impaired cardiovascular reserve:
  - Recovery in high dependency area
- Relatively immunosuppressed:
  - Monitor for postoperative infection:
    - Wound
    - Epidural abscess
- Increased thromboembolic risk
- May suffer flare of rheumatoid disease postpartum:
  - Involve rheumatologist in management of immunosuppressive therapy.

Ankylosing spondylitis

Ankylosing spondylitis is a human leucocyte antigen-B27 associated seronegative spondyloarthropathy, characterized by sacroiliac joint arthritis progressing to spinal fusion, 'bamboo spine'. It is typically a slowly progressing disease, therefore few suffer severe symptoms at child-bearing age.[158] The effect of pregnancy on symptoms is variable: 38% improve, 62% worsen.[158]

Obstetric implications

Pelvic or hip (30%)[159] involvement may affect VD. Biological agents (i.e. anti-TNF-α) may increase susceptibility to infection.[160]

Anaesthetic implications

Both GA and NA may be challenging (Table 46.10). There are a few case reports describing different methods of anaesthesia in parturients, all were successful.

- Spinal for emergency CD[161]
- Labour epidural analgesia, fifth attempt[162]
- Labour epidural, easy insertion, topped-up for emergency CD[158]
- Planned CSE (failed to feed epidural catheter)[163]
- Two awake fibreoptic intubations for elective CD[164,165]
- CSA for labour (two failed epidurals, abnormal spread of local anaesthetic).[166]

Although epidurals are possible,[158] one should anticipate difficulty as evidenced by larger studies of anaesthesia for non-obstetric patients.[159] The risk of epidural haematoma[167] and total spinal[168] appears to be greater.

Spinals are probably more reliable than epidurals in patients with ankylosing spondylitis. One retrospective study reported a 77% (10/13) success rate with spinals for lower limb surgery, compared to 0% (0/3) for epidurals.[159]

Considerations

- Labour:
  - Progress may be affected by pelvic or hip disease
  - Epidural analgesia may be difficult or impossible to establish and relatively high risk
  - In emergency, NA and GA may be challenging, placing fetus at risk

Table 46.10 Ankylosing spondylitis and anaesthetic implications

System	Manifestation	Implications
Airway	Temporomandibular dysfunction (10–30%)[160]	Potential difficult intubation. Consider awake fibreoptic
	Reduced cervical spine mobility	Difficult airway equipment immediately available
	Cricoarytenoid involvement	
	Atlantoaxial subluxation (up to 21%)[160]	Potential cervical cord injury with intubation
Respiratory	Restrictive defect	May decompensate with pregnancy or anaesthesia
	Fibrosis (especially apical)	Consider screening pulmonary function tests
Cardiac	Aortic regurgitation (up to 43%)[158]	May decompensate with pregnancy, labour, or anaesthesia.
	Conduction defects	Consider screening ECG, echocardiogram
Neuraxial	Vertebral fractures: 47% have associated sensory or motor neurological disease, e.g. cauda equina syndrome, nerve root compression[160]	Relative contraindication to NA Document existing neurological findings
	Restricted spinal flexion	Difficult NA
	Calcification of ligaments	Paramedian approach may be more successful[169] Increased risk epidural haematoma[160] Careful neurological follow-up postpartum
Other	Peripheral disease	Care with positioning patient, reduced range of movement

ECG, electrocardiogram; NA, neuraxial anaesthesia.

Data from various sources (see references).

- Elective CD:
  - Spinal anaesthesia: approximately 75% success; risk of requiring emergency GA if complication
  - Elective awake fibreoptic intubation allows controlled, safe induction, with minimal cervical manipulation; requires compliant parturient.
- For all cases:
  - Difficult intubation equipment should be immediately available.

Achondroplasia

Achondroplasia is the commonest of over 100 causes of dwarfism with an incidence of approximately 1.5/10,000 live births with an AD inheritance, although 80% are *de novo* mutations.[170] The typical short tubular bones and other features (Table 46.11) are the

Table 46.11 Features of achondroplasia, anaesthetic implications, and methods to mitigate

Features		Implications	Suggestions to mitigate
Cranial abnormalities: Macrocephaly Frontal bossing Mid-face hypoplasia Flattened nose Large mandible Large tongue Short neck[172]		Difficult ventilation (poor seal with mask) Difficult intubation Risk of obstructive sleep apnoea[172] Reduced neck extension	Prepare for difficult airway Choose endotracheal tube on weight rather than age[173] Consider awake fibreoptic[174] ENT surgeon available for urgent tracheostomy Attention to extubation and recovery
Foramen magnum stenosis		Extreme cases, hydrocephalus	Avoid increased ICP Avoid spinal anaesthesia
Atlantoaxial subluxation		Risk cervical cord injury with hyperextension[173]	Care at intubation
Short stature		Dose of NA unpredictable, risk high block	Use titratable NA, e.g. epidural, CSE, or CSA
Pelvis broad and flat with wide iliac wings. Pelvic inlet narrow.[175]	Uterus displaced from pelvis	Head will not engage in pelvis	Cephalopelvic disproportion, likely CD (especially if fetus achondroplastic with macrocephaly)[172]
		Greater encroachment on diaphragm decreasing FRC (exacerbated by short stature)	Elective CD: anaesthetic provided by experienced obstetric anaesthetist Maximal preoxygenation
Marked lumbar lordosis and osteophytes	Displaces uterus further into abdominal cavity	Greater aortocaval compression, supine hypotension	Attention to positioning Alpha agonist for hypotension
		Increased abdominal pressure, risk of regurgitation and aspiration	Ensure antacid prophylaxis, adequate fasting
		Increased epidural vein engorgement, risk of IV cannulation with epidural	Use flexible epidural catheter
		Bony landmarks indistinct Reduced lumbar intervertebral spaces NA difficult	Use prepuncture ultrasound Insert low thoracic, rather than lumbar epidural[176]
Thoracic scoliosis		See 'Scoliosis' in main text	
Pectus carinatum and rib hypoplasia[170]		Risk of respiratory compromise	Use titratable NA May require early delivery
Short pedicles Thickened laminae Spinal stenosis		Difficulty threading epidural catheter[177]	Consider paramedian approach[178]
		Increased risk of dural puncture[179]	
		Appropriate dose NA unknown Risk of high block[173]	Use titratable NA, e.g. epidural,[176] CSE, CSA. Possible lower limb neurological deterioration post NA[26]
		Possible lumbar laminectomy for spinal stenosis[180]	Difficult NA, may be inadequate
Normal size spinal cord in small vertebral canal[181]		CSF may not flow freely	Failure to identify intrathecal space, despite being in it Affects local anaesthetic spread, inadequate block[179]

CD, caesarean delivery; CSA, continuous spinal anaesthetic; CSE, combined spinal–epidural; CSF, cerebrospinal fluid; ENT, ear nose throat; FRC, functional residual capacity; ICP, intracranial pressure; IV, intravenous; NA, neuraxial anaesthesia.

Data from various sources (see references).

result of a mutation in fibroblast growth factor receptor 3, causing failure in endochondral ossification at growth plates.[171]

General versus neuraxial anaesthetic

Some suggest achondroplastic patients should have a GA for CD, due to concerns over the safety of spinal anaesthesia.[175] There are, however, reports of safe administration of intrathecal anaesthesia, although there is debate about appropriate dosing: in three reported cases, 5 mg bupivacaine produced adequate anaesthesia.[171,182,183] Using a titratable technique (epidural, CSE, or CSA) is an alternative.[182]

The spinal cord appears to terminate at a similar level to the normal population, therefore spinal injection below L3 should not result in cord or conus injury.[184]

There are nine reports describing GA for CD in achondroplastic parturients:[41,174,179,185–189] two after failed NA,[174,185] one awake fibreoptic for predicted difficult intubation,[174] one where intubation was not attempted (spontaneous ventilation with face mask),[185] and one intubation was described as difficult.[188] A retrospective study reported 35 cases without complication.[175]

Antenatal

- Confirm diagnosis of achondroplasia; ensure not an alternative cause of dwarfism, for example, syndrome or metabolic disorder
- Consider investigating those with history of associated complications:
  - Obstructive sleep apnoea—polysomnography
  - Spinal stenosis—MRI spine
  - Raised intracranial pressure—MRI head
- Airway:
  - Examine for predictors of difficult airway
  - Cervical spine mobility—symptoms of cervical cord compression
- Spinal anatomy:
  - Examine lumbar spine
  - Ultrasound assessment
- Perform neurological examination of lower limbs:
  - Abnormal, consider MRI spine
- Discuss labour and delivery analgesia and anaesthesia:
  - Discuss anaesthetic options, risks and benefits:
    - Potential technical difficulties with insertion: increased risk of high block
    - Increased risk of dural puncture
  - Potential advantages of controlled setting and elective CD
  - Agree on technique if presents as an emergency:
    - If not enough time to establish epidural, are the risks of single shot spinal acceptable?
  - Explore patient concerns and wishes.

Peripartum

- Increased likelihood of CD
- Non-invasive blood pressure may be difficult because of limb proportions:
  - Consider invasive arterial monitoring
- Care with supine positioning: cardiorespiratory compromise:
  - Relative increased uterine size:
    - Pronounced aortocaval compression
    - Increased respiratory compromise
- If no evidence of lower limb neurology or spinal stenosis, titratable NA technique ideal:
  - Increased risk of difficult or failed insertion
  - Low-thoracic or paramedian approaches may be easier
- Reduce dose of single-shot spinal:
  - Risk of high block
- Anticipate difficult airway:
  - Fibreoptic equipment
  - Ear nose and throat (ENT) surgeon available.

Postpartum

- If obstructive sleep apnoea:
  - Consider high dependency care
  - Multimodal analgesia to reduce opioids requirements—consider epidural for post CD analgesia.

Osteogenesis imperfecta

Osteogenesis imperfecta (OI) is the result of a defect in type I collagen, the main provider of tensile strength in bone, ligaments, sclera, and dentine. OI results in a disease spectrum, characterised by multiple fractures, often from trivial injury. It occurs in approximately 1/25,000 pregnancies[190] and is classified into four subtypes on the basis of clinical presentation and inheritance (Table 46.12).[172,190,191]

Obstetric implications

Pelvic fractures and deformity lead to cephalopelvic disproportion or malpresentation, increasing risk of CD.[172]

Anaesthetic implications

Most anaesthetic techniques have been successfully reported without complication: general,[193–198] epidural,[191,192,199–201] spinal,[190,191] CSE,[202] and local infiltration (Table 46.13).[192]

Table 46.12 Subtypes of osteogenesis imperfect

Type I	Most prevalent
Mild	AD inheritance, with incomplete penetrance
	Normal stature
	Blue sclera (choroid pigment seen through sclera)[192]
	Several fractures a year, starting in childhood, decreasing after puberty[193]
Type II	AR
Severe	Multiple *in utero* fractures, deformity
	Early fetal or neonatal demise
Type III	AD and AR
Severe	Some suffer fractures *in utero*
	Dentinogenesis imperfecta
Type IV	AD
Mild to moderate	Multiple fractures
	Short stature
	Normal sclera
	Multiple fractures, resulting in deformity
	Dentinogenesis imperfecta

AD, autosomal dominant; AR, autosomal recessive.

The classification system for subtypes of OI was originally proposed by DO Sillence: Adapted by permission from BMJ Publishing Group Limited. *Journal of Medical Genetics*, DO Sillence, A Senn, DM Dank, volume 16, issue 2, pp. 101–116, Copyright © 1979.

Table 46.13 Osteogenesis imperfect: anaesthetic implications and methods of mitigating risks

Manifestation	Consequences	Method of reducing risk
Bone fractures with minimal force	Fractures with normal VD (e.g. pubic rami)[192] or assisted VD[172]	Consider elective CD in severe disease Extra padding for positioning[200]
	Brittle teeth, may dislodge (dentinogenesis imperfecta) Mandible fractures with minimal force[197]	Avoid GA where possible Consider intubation aids, awake fibreoptic intubation
	Potential for fracture with high inflation pressures with non-invasive BP cuff[203]	Consider invasive arterial monitoring[199]
	Possible fracture from suxamethonium fasciculations[197]	Avoid GA Use rocuronium for intubation
	Vertebral collapse, scoliosis[191]	See 'Scoliosis' in main text
Joint hypermobility Odontoid peg hypoplasia[191]	Cervical cord damage with neck hyperextension	Care with intubation Consider intubation aids
Blood vessel involvement[191]	Risk: haemorrhage	Prepare for blood loss
Uterine muscle involvement	Risk: rupture, tearing, uterine atony[190,192]	
Platelet function abnormalities (adhesion and aggregation)[191]	Risk: haemorrhage	History/examination looking for platelet function Avoid NSAIDs
	Risk: epidural haematoma	Risk/benefit of NA: Spinal < epidural[204] Use flexible epidural catheter[204]
Endocrine and metabolic abnormalities Thyroid activity increased by 50%[197]	Hyperthermia (non-MH)[196] Increased oxygen utilization	Monitor temperature, $EtCO_2$ with GA (exclude MH) Active cooling[199] Supplemental oxygen Check thyroid function
Hereditary	Risk *in utero* fractures May influence delivery method	Some evidence delivery mode does not affect fetal outcome[172,202]
Otosclerosis and hearing impairment (25–50%)[193]	Challenge with communication	Counsel preoperatively Ensure has hearing aid, as appropriate Alternate communication, e.g. written

BP, blood pressure; CD, caesarean delivery; $EtCO_2$, end-tidal carbon dioxide; GA, general anaesthesia; MH, malignant hyperthermia; NA, neuraxial anaesthesia; NSAIDs, non-steroidal anti-inflammatory drugs; VD, vaginal delivery.

Data from various sources (see references).

Antenatal

- History:
  - Previous fractures:
    - Site, mechanism, and frequency—indication of severity of disease
  - Platelet function:
    - Easy bleeding/bruising
- Physical examination:
  - Presence of blue sclera; suggestive of type I and milder disease
  - Petechiae around pressure points, for example, non-invasive blood pressure
- Investigation:
  - Thyroid function
- Discussion:
  - Discuss benefits of the controlled setting of an elective CD in severe disease
  - Risks/benefits of GA versus NA
  - Explore patient concerns and wishes.

Peripartum

- GA:
  - Prepare for difficult intubation
  - Avoid suxamethonium
- NA:
  - Caution if history of platelet dysfunction
  - Spinal less risk than epidural
- Anticipate and prepare for PPH
- History of platelet dysfunction:
  - Caution with NSAIDs
- Consider:
  - Extra padding for operating table
  - Invasive arterial monitoring
  - Temperature monitoring.

Postpartum

- NA:
  - Postoperative neurological monitoring of lower limbs
    - Exclude epidural haematoma formation.

Conclusion

Women with musculoskeletal disease may have their first presentation around delivery, but as most know their diagnosis antenally they generally have the opportunity to be reviewed in an obstetric anaesthetic high-risk clinic. A multidisciplinary approach is essential, along with detailed examination and appropriate investigations. Formal obstetric delivery and anaesthetic plans should be made, discussed, and documented in this challenging group of patients.

References

1. Larach M, Gronert G, Allen G, *et al.* Clinical presentation, treatment, and complications of malignant hyperthermia in North America from 1987-2006. *Anesth Analg* 2010; 110:498–507.
2. Rosenberg H. Continued progress in understanding the molecular genetics of malignant hyperthermia. *Can J Anesth* 2011; 58:489–93.
3. Dirksen S, Larach M, Rosenberg H, *et al.* Future directions in malignant hyperthermia research and patient care. *Anesth Analg* 2011; 113:1108–19.
4. Hopkins P. Malignant hyperthermia: pharmacology of triggering. *Br J Anaesth* 2011; 107:48–56.
5. Hopkins P. Malignant hyperthermia: advances in clinical management and diagnosis. *Br J Anaesth* 2000; 85:118–28.
6. Rossi A, Dirksen R. Sarcoplasmic reticulum: the dynamic calcium governor of muscle. *Muscle Nerve* 2006; 33:715–31.
7. Lehmann-Horn F, Klingler W, Jurkat-Rott K. Nonanesthetic malignant hyperthermia. *Anesthesiology* 2011; 115:915–17.
8. Glahn K, Ellis F, Halsall P, Müller C, *et al.* Recognizing and managing a malignant hyperthermia crisis: guidelines from the European Malignant Hyperthermia group. *Br J Anaesth* 2010; 105:417–20.
9. Krause T, Gerbershagen M, Fiege M, *et al.* Dantrolene—a review of its pharmacology, therapeutic use and new developments. *Anaesthesia* 2004; 59:364–73.
10. Craft J, Goldberg N, Lim M, *et al.* Cardiovascular effects and placental passage of dantrolene in the maternal-fetal sheep model. *Anesthesiology* 1988; 68:68–72.
11. Fricker R, Hoerauf K, Drewe J, *et al.* Secretion of dantrolene into breast milk after acute therapy of a suspected malignant hyperthermia crisis during cesarean section. *Anesthesiology* 1998; 89:1023–5.
12. Weingarten A, Korsh J, Neuman G, *et al.* Postpartum uterine atony after intravenous dantrolene. *Anesth Analg* 1987; 66:269–70.
13. Shin Y, Kim Y, Collea J, *et al.* Effect of dantrolene sodium on contractility of isolated human uterine muscle. *Int J Obstet Anesth* 1995; 4:197–200.
14. Girard T, Jöhr M, Schaefer C, *et al.* Perinatal diagnosis of malignant hyperthermia susceptibility. *Anesthesiology* 2006; 104:1353–4.
15. Pollock N, Langton E. Management of malignant hyperthermia susceptible parturients. *Anaesth Intensive Care* 1997; 25:398–407.
16. Wappler F. Anesthesia for patients with a history of malignant hyperthermia. *Curr Opin Anaesthesiol* 2010; 23:417–22.
17. Kim T, Nemergut M. Preparation of modern anesthesia workstations for malignant hyperthermia-susceptible patients. *Anesthesiology* 2011; 114:205–12.
18. Sneag DB, Bendo JA. Pregnancy-related low back pain. *Orthopedics* 2007; 30:839–45.
19. Malmqvist S, Kjaermann I, Andersen K, *et al.* Prevalence of low back and pelvic pain during pregnancy in a Norwegian population. *J Manip Physiol Ther* 2012; 35:272–8.
20. Groves P, Breen T, Ransil B, *et al.* The natural history of postpartum back pain and its relationship with epidural anesthesia. *Anesthesiology* 1994; 81:A1167.
21. Breen T, Ransil B, Groves P, *et al.* Factors associated with back pain after childbirth. *Anesthesiology* 1994; 81:29–34.
22. MacArthur A, MacArthur C, Weeks S. Epidural anaesthesia and low back pain after delivery: a prospective cohort study *BMJ* 1995; 311:1336–9.
23. MacArthur A, MacArthur C, Weeks S. Is epidural anesthesia in labor associated with chronic low back pain? A prospective cohort study. *Anesth Analg* 1997; 85:1066–70.
24. Howell C, Kidd C, Roberts W, *et al.* A randomised controlled trial of epidural compared with non-epidural analgesia in labour. *Br J Obstet Gynaecol* 2001; 108:27–33.
25. Berkmann S, Fandino J. Pregnancy and childbirth after microsurgery for lumbar disc herniation. *Acta Neurochir* 2012; 154:329–34.
26. Vercauteren M, Waets P, Pitklnen M, *et al.* Neuraxial techniques in patients with pre-existing back impairment or prior spine interventions: a topical review with special reference to obstetrics. *Acta Anaesth Scand* 2011; 55:910–17.
27. Sanderson P, Fraser R. The influence of pregnancy on the development of degenerative spondylolisthesis. *J Bone Joint Surg* 1996; 78B:951–4.
28. Lebel D, Sergienko R, Wiznitzer A, *et al.* Mode of delivery and other pregnancy outcomes of patients with documented scoliosis. *J Matern Fetal Neonatal Med* 2012; 25:639–41.
29. Maruyama T, Takeshita K. Surgical treatment of scoliosis: a review of techniques currently applied. *Scoliosis* 2008; 3:6.
30. Cohen V, Powell E, Lake C. Failure of neuraxial anaesthesia in a patient with velocardiofascial syndrome. *Int J Obstet Anaesth* 2011; 20:256–9.
31. Luce V, Mercier F, Benhamou D. Anesthetic management for a parturient affected by the VACTERL association. *Anesth Analg* 2004; 98:874.
32. Preston R. Spinal cord disorders. In Gambling D, Douglas M, McKay R (eds) *Obstetric Anesthesia and Uncommon Disorders*. Cambridge: Cambridge University Press; 2008:191–214.
33. Agusti M, Adalia R, Fernandez C, *et al.* Anaesthesia for caesarean section in a patient with syringomyelia and Arnold-Chiari type I malformation. *Int J Obstet Anesth* 2004; 13:114–16.
34. Grange C. Miscellaneous skeletal and connective tissue disorders in pregnancy. In Gambling D, Douglas M, McKay R (eds) *Obstetric Anesthesia and Uncommon Disorders*. Cambridge: Cambridge University Press; 2008:145–65.
35. Orvomaa E, Hiilesmaa V, Poussa M, *et al.* Pregnancy and delivery in patients operated by the Harrington method for idiopathic scoliosis. *Eur Spine J* 1997; 6:304–7.
36. To W, Wong M. Kyphoscoliosis complicating pregnancy. *Int J Gynaecol Obstet* 1996; 55:123–8.
37. Chopra S, Adhikari K, Agarwal N, *et al.* Kyphoscoliosis complicating pregnancy: maternal and neonatal outcome. *Arch Gynecol Obstet* 2011; 284:295–7.
38. Russell R, Comara S. Regional blocks for delivery in women with scoliosis or previous spinal surgery. *Int J Obstet Anesth* 2003; 12:308–10.
39. Taylor S, Wilson R, McLure H, *et al.* Catheter techniques succeed in scoliosis. *Int J Obstet Anesth* 2009; 18:S6.
40. Saxena K, Gupta A. Combined spinal epidural for caesarean section in patients with kyphoscoliosis. *J Anaesthesiol Clin Pharmacol* 2009; 25:501–2.
41. Aedla N, Duncan A. Achondroplasia and pregnancy—a case report. *Br J Obstet Gynaecol* 2012; 119:108.
42. Crosby E. Disorders of the vertebral column. In Gambling D, Douglas M, McKay R (eds) *Obstetric Anesthesia and Uncommon Disorders*. Cambridge: Cambridge University Press; 2008:129–44.

43. Gerancher J, D'Angelo R, Carpenter R. Caudal epidural blood patch for the treatment of postdural puncture headache. *Anesth Analg* 1998; 87:394–5.
44. Howard R, Anderson W. Subdural catheterization and opiate administration in a patient with Harrington rods. *Can J Anaesth* 1990; 37:712.
45. Bansal N, Gupta S. Anaesthetic management of a parturient with severe kyphoscoliosis. *Kathmandu Univ Med J* 2008; 6: 379–82.
46. Kardash K, King B, Datta S. Spinal anaesthesia for caesarean section after Harrington instrumentation. *Can J Anaesth* 1993; 40:667–9.
47. Moran D, Johnson M. Continuous spinal anesthesia with combined hyperbaric and isobaric bupivacaine in a patient with scoliosis. *Anesth Analg* 1990; 70:445–7.
48. Douglas MJ. Unusual regional block. *Can J Anaesth* 1995; 42:362–3.
49. Smith P, Wilson R, Robinson A, *et al.* Regional blockade for delivery in women with scoliosis or previous spinal surgery. *Int J Obstet Anesth* 2003; 12:17–22.
50. Pascoe H, Jennings G, Marx G. Successful spinal anesthesia after inadequate epidural block in a parturient with prior surgical correction for scoliosis. *Reg Anesth* 1993; 18:191–2.
51. Crosby E, Halpern S. Obstetric epidural anaesthesia in patients with Harrington instrumentation. *Can J Anaesth* 1989; 36:693–6.
52. Sudunagunta S, Eckersall S. Continuous caudal analgesia in labour for a patient with Harrington rods. *Int J Obstet Anesth* 1998; 7:128–30
53. Costello J, Balki M. Cesarean delivery under ultrasound-guided spinal anesthesia in a parturient with poliomyelitis and Harrington instrumentation. *Can J Anaesth* 2008; 55:606–11.
54. Cavalho J. Ultrasound-facilitated epidurals and spinals in obstetrics. *Anesthesiology Clinics* 2008; 26:145–58.
55. Daley M, Morningstar B, Rolbin S, *et al.* Epidural anaesthesia for obstetrics after spinal surgery. *Reg Anesth* 1990; 15:280–4.
56. Yeo S, French R. Combined spinal-epidural in the obstetric patient with Harrington rods assisted by ultrasonography. *Br J Anaesth* 1999; 83:670–2.
57. Ko J, Leffert L. Clinical implications of neuraxial anesthesia in the parturient with scoliosis. *Anesth Analg* 2009; 109:1930–4.
58. Huang J. Paramedian approach for neuraxial anesthesia in parturients with scoliosis. *Anesth Analg* 2010; 111:821–2.
59. Farney R, Brandon S, Farney R, *et al.* The STOP-Bang equivalent model and prediction of severity of obstructibve sleep apnea: Relation to polysomnographic measurements of the apnea/hypopnea index. *J Clin Sleep Med* 2011; 7:459–65.
60. Gurnaney H, Brown A, Litman R. Malignant hyperthermia and muscular dystrophies. *Anesth Analg* 2009; 109:1043–8.
61. Quane K, Healy J, Keating K. Mutations in the ryanodine receptor gene in central core disease and malignant hyperthermia. *Nature Genet* 1993; 5:51–5.
62. Dowling J, Lillis S, Amburgey K, *et al.* King-Denborough syndrome with and without mutations in the skeletal muscle ryanodine receptor (RYR1) gene. *Neuromuscul Disord* 2011; 21:420–7.
63. Wang C, Dowling J, Nirth K, *et al.* Consensus statement of standard of care for congenital myopathies. *J Child Neurol* 2012; 27:363–82.
64. Crochetiere C. Myopathies. In Gambling D, Douglas M, McKay R (eds) *Obstetric Anesthesia and Uncommon Disorders.* Cambridge: Cambridge University Press, 2008:101–14.
65. Kissel J, Mendell J. Muscular dystrophy: historical overview and classification in the genetic era. *Semin Neurol* 1999; 19:5–7.
66. Emery E. The muscular dystrophies. *Lancet* 2002; 359:687–95.
67. Grain L, Cortina-Borja M, Forfar C, *et al.* Cardiac abnormalities and skeletal muscle weakness in carriers of Duchennes and Becker muscular dystrophies and contrals. *Neuromusc Disorder* 2001; 11:186–91.
68. Pash M, Balaton J, Eagle C. Anaesthetic management of a parturient with severe muscular dystrophy, lumbar lordosis and a difficult airway. *Can J Anaesth* 1996; 43:959.
69. Allen T, Maguire S. Anaesthetic management of a woman with autosomal recessive limb-girdle muscular dystrophy for emergency caesarean section. *Int J Obstet Anesth* 2007; 16:370–4.
70. Ekblad U, Kanto J. Pregnancy outcome in an extremely small woman with muscular dystrophy and respiratory insufficiency. *Acta Anaesthesiol Scand* 1993; 37:228–30.
71. Rudnik-Schoneborn S, Glauner B, Rohrig D, *et al.* Obstetric aspects in women with fascioscapulohumeral muscular dystrophy, limb-girdle muscular dystrophy and congenital myopathies. *Arch Neurol* 1997; 54:888–94.
72. Franco N, Rocha C, Paula C. Spinal anesthesia for operative delivery in a patient with facioscapulohumeral muscular dystrophy. *Pain Practice* 2009; 9:127.
73. Kissel J. Fascioscapulohumeral dystrophy. *Semin Neurol* 1999; 19:35–43.
74. Dresner D, Ali H. Anaesthetic management of a patient with Facioscapulohumeral muscular dystrophy. *Br J Anaesth* 1989; 63:331–4.
75. Kim O, Elliott D. Elective caesarean section for a woman with Emery-Dreifuss muscular dystrophy. *Anaesth Inten Care* 2010; 38:744–7.
76. Aedla N, Duncan A. Emery-Dreifuss muscular dystrophy—case report and discussion of pregnancy complications. *Br J Obstet Gynaecol* 2012; 119:109.
77. Zacharias A, Wagener M, Warren S, *et al.* Emery-Dreifuss muscular dystrophy. *Semin Neurol* 1999; 19:67–79.
78. Brais B, Rouleau G, Bouchard J, *et al.* Oculopharyngeal muscular dystrophy. *Semin Neurol* 1999; 19:59–66.
79. Nonaka I, Kobayashi O, Osari S. Nondystrophinopathic muscular dystrophies including myotonic dystrophy. *Semin Ped Neurol* 1996; 3:110–21.
80. Goebel H. Cogenital myopathies. *Semin Ped Neurol* 1996; 3:152–61.
81. Wallgren-Pettersson C, Hiilesmaa VK, Paatero H. Pregnancy and delivery in congenital nemaline myopathy. *Acta Obstet Gynecol Scand* 1995; 74:659–61.
82. Stackhouse R, Chelmow D, Dattel BJ. Anesthetic complications in a pregnant patient with nemaline myopathy. *Anesth Analg* 1994; 79:1195–7.
83. Eskandar O, Eckford S. Pregnancy in a patient with nemaline myopathy. *Obstet Gynecol* 2007; 109:501–4.
84. Klingler W, Rueffert H, Lehmann-Horn F, *et al.* Core myopathies and risk of malignant hyperthermia. *Anesth Analg* 2009; 109:1167–73.
85. Bolton S, Clark V, Norman J. Multidisciplinary management of an obstetric patient with glycogen storage disease type 3. *Int J Obstet Anesth* 2012; 21:86–9.
86. Cilliers H, Yeo S, Salmon N. Anaesthetic management of an obstetric patient with Pompe disease. *Int J Obstet Anesth* 2008; 17:170–3.
87. Bhatti S, Parry E. Successful pregnancy in a woman with glycogen storage disease type III. *Aust N Z J Obstet Gynaecol* 2006; 46:168–9.
88. Lee P, Fisher N, Green A, *et al.* Successful pregnancy in a patient with type III glycogen storage disease managed with cornstarch supplements *Br J Obstet Gynaecol* 1999; 106:181–2.
89. Confino E, Pauzner D, Lidor A, *et al.* Pregnancy associated with amylo-1,6-glucosidase deficiency (Forbe's disease). *Br J Obstet Gynaecol* 1984; 91:494–7.
90. Mendoza A, Fisher N, Duckett J, *et al.* Successful pregnancy in a patient with type III glycogen storage disease managed with cornstarch supplements. *Br J Obstet Gynaecol* 1998; 105:677–80.
91. Coleman P. McArdle's disease. Problems of anaesthetic management for caesarean section. *Anaesthesia* 1984; 39:784–7.
92. Cochrane P, Alderman B. Normal pregnancy and successful delivery in myophosphorylase deficiency (McArdle's disease). *J Neurol Neurosurg Psychiatry* 1973; 36:225–7.
93. Samuels T, Coleman P. McArdle's disease and caesarean section. *Anaesthesia* 1988; 43:161–2.

94. Quinlivan R, Buckley J, James M, *et al.* McArdle disease: a clinical review. *J Neurol Neurosurg Psychiatry* 2010; 81:1182–8.
95. Tein I. Metabolic myopathies. *Semin Ped Neurol* 1996; 3:59–98.
96. van Adel B, Tarnopolsky M. Metabolic myopathies: update 2009. *J Clin Neuromuscul Dis* 2009; 10:97–121.
97. Innes A, Seargeant L, Balachandra K, *et al.* Hepatic carnitine palmitoyltransferase I deficiency presenting as maternal illness in pregnancy. *Pediatr Res* 2000; 47:43–5.
98. Ylitalo K, Vanttinen T, Halmesmaki E, *et al.* Serious pregnancy complications in a patient with previously undiagnosed carnitine palmitoyltransferase 1 deficiency. *Am J Obstet Gynecol* 2005; 192:2060–2.
99. Slater P, Grivell R, Cyna A. Labour management of a woman with carnitine palmitoyl transferase type 2 deficiency. *Anaesth Intensive Care* 2009; 37:305–8.
100. Lilker S, Kasodekar S, Goldszmidt E. Anaesthetic management of a parturient with carnitine palmitoyltransferase 2 deficiency. *Can J Anaesth* 2006; 53:482–6.
101. Ramsey P, Biggio J. Carnitine palmitoyltransferase deficiency in pregnancy. *J Matern Fetal Neonatal Med* 2005; 18:357–9.
102. Moundras J, Wattrisse G, Leroy B, *et al.* Labour analgesia in a patient with carnitine palmityl transferase deficiency. *Ann Fr Anesth* 2000; 19:611–6.
103. Dreval D, Bernstein D, Zakut H. Carnitine palmitoyl transferase deficiency in pregnancy—a case report. *Am J Obstet Gynecol* 1994; 170:1390–2.
104. Mardirosoff C, Dumont L, Cobin L, *et al.* Labour analgesia in a patient with carnitine palmityl transferase deficiency and idiopathic thrombocytopenic purpura. *Int J Obstet Anesth* 1997; 7:134–6.
105. Angelini C, Govoni E, Bragaglia M, *et al.* Carnitine deficiency: acute postpartum crisis. *Ann Neurol* 1978; 4:558–61.
106. Donnelly C, Hameed A, Abdenur J, *et al.* Carnitine deficiency in pregnancy. *Obstet Gynecol* 2007; 110:480–2.
107. El-Hattab A, Li F, Shen J, *et al.* Maternal systemic primary carnitine deficiency uncovered by newborn screening: clinical, biochemical, and molecular aspects. *Genet Med* 2010; 12:19–24.
108. Cornelio F, Didonato S, Peluchetti D, *et al.* Fatal cases of lipid storage myopathy with carnirine deficiency. *J Neurol Neurosurg Psychiatry* 1977; 40:170–8.
109. Boudin G, Mikol J, Guillard A. Fatal systemic carnitine deficiency with lipid storage in skeletal muscle, heart, liver and kidney. *J Neurol Sci* 1976; 30:313–25.
110. Rosaeg OP, Morrison S, MacLeod JP. Anaesthetic management of labour and delivery in the parturient with mitochondrial myopathy. *Can J Anaesth* 1996; 43:403–7.
111. Braham D, Bell R. Anaesthetic considerations for caesarean section in a patient with mitochondrial myopathy (complex I and IV deficiency) with respiratory weakness: a case report. *Int J Obstet Anesth* 2010:S30.
112. Maurtua M, Torres A, Ibarra V, *et al.* Anesthetic management of an obstetric patient with MELAS syndrome: case report and literature review. *Int J Obstet Anesth* 2008; 17:370–3.
113. Shipton E, Prosser D. Mitochondrial myopathies and anaesthesia. *Eur J Anaesthesiol* 2004; 21:173–8.
114. Blake L, Shaw R. Mitochondrial myopathy in a primigravid pregnancy. *Br J Obstet Gynaecol* 1999; 106:871–3.
115. Berkowitz K, Monteagudo A, Marks F, *et al.* Mitochondrial myopathy and preeclampsia associated with pregnancy. *Am J Obstet Gynecol* 1990; 162:146–7.
116. Bellver J, Cervera J, Boldo A, *et al.* Myoadenylate deaminase deficiency myopathy in pregnancy. *Arch Gynecol Obstet* 1997; 259:157–9.
117. Silva C, Sultan S, Isenberg D. Pregnancy outcome in adult-onset idiopathic inflammatory myopathy. *Rheumatology* 2003; 42:1168–72.
118. Chopra S, Suri V, Bagga R, *et al.* Autoimmune inflammatory myopathy in pregnancy. *Medscape J Med* 2008; 10:17.
119. Linardaki G, Cherouvim E, Goni G, *et al.* Intravenous immunoglobulin treatment for pregnancy-associated dermatomyositis. *Rheumatol Int* 2011; 31:113–5.
120. Gunusen I, Karaman S, Nemli S, *et al.* Anesthetic management for cesarean delivery in a pregnant woman with polymyositis: a case report and review of literature. *Cases J* 2009; 2:1–4.
121. Turner C, Hilton-Jones D. The myotonic dystrophies: diagnosis and management. *J Neurol Neurosur Ps* 2010; 81:358–67.
122. Cope D, Miller J. Local and spinal anesthesia for cesarean section in a patient with myotonic dystrophy. *Anesth Analg* 1986; 65:687–90.
123. Blumgart CH, Hughes DG, Redfern N. Obstetric anaesthesia in dystrophia myotonica. *Anaesthesia* 1990; 45:26–9.
124. Atlas I, Smolin A. Combined maternal and congenital myotonic dystrophy managed by a multidisciplinary team. *Eur J Obstet Gyn Reprod Biol* 1999; 87:175–8.
125. Camann W, Johnson M. Anesthetic management of a parturient with myotonia dystrophica: a case report. *Reg Anesth* 1990; 15:41–3.
126. Campbell A, Thompson N. Anaesthesia for Caesarean section in a patient with myotonic dystrophy receiving warfarin therapy. *Can J Anaesth* 1995; 45:409–14.
127. Chung HT, Tam AYC, Wong V. Dystrophia myotonica and pregnancy—an instructive case. *Postgrad Med J* 1987; 63:555–7.
128. Driver I, Broadway J. Dystrophia myotonica: combined spinal-epidural anaesthesia for caesarean section. *Int J Obstet Anesth* 1996; 5:275–7.
129. Dufour P, Berard J, Vinatier D, *et al.* Myotonic dystrophy and pregnancy a report of two cases and a review of the literature. *Eur J Obstet Gyn R B* 1997; 72:159–64.
130. Freeman R. Placenta accreta and myotonic dystrophy: two case reports. *Br J Obstet Gynaecol* 1991; 98:594–5.
131. Harris M. Extradural analgesia and dystrophia myotonia. *Anaesthesia* 1984; 39:1032–3.
132. Hook R, Anderson EF, Noto P. Anesthetic management of a parturient with myotonia atrophica. *Anesthesiology* 1975; 43:689–92.
133. Hughes RG, Lyall EGH, Liston WA. Obstetric and neonatal complications of myotonic dystrophy. *J Obstet Gynaecol* 1991; 11:191–4.
134. O'Connor P, Caldicott L, Braithwaite P. Urgent caesarean section in a patient with myotonic dystrophy: a case report and review. *Int J Obstet Anesth* 1996; 5:272–4.
135. Owen PM, Chu C. Emergency caesarean section in a patient with myotonic dystrophy: a case of failed postoperative extubation in a patient with mild disease. *Anaesth Intensive Care* 2011; 39:293–8.
136. Paterson R, Tousignant M, Skene D. Caesarean section for twins in a patient with myotonic dystrophy. *Can J Anaesth* 1985; 32:418–21.
137. Risseeuw JJ, Oudshoorn JH, Van Der Straaten PJC, *et al.* Myotonic dystrophy in pregnancy: A report of two cases within one family. *Eur J Obstet Gyn Reprod Biol* 1997; 73:145–8.
138. Walpole A, Ross A. Acute cord prolapse in an obstetric patient with myotonia dystrophica. *Anaesth Intensive Care* 1992; 20:526–8.
139. Butwick AJ, Riley ET. Successful spinal blockade in a parturient with myotonia congenita. *Int J Obstet Anesth* 2007; 16:292–3.
140. Aldridge L. Anaesthetic problems in myotonic dystrophy. A case report and review of the Aberdeen experience comprising 48 general anaesthetics in a further 16 patients. *Br J Anaesth* 1985; 57:1119–30.
141. Petrovski J. The use of sugammadex to reverse rocuronium in a patient with myotonic dystrophy. *Anaesth Intensive Care* 2011; 39:505–6.
142. Russell S, Hirsch N. Anaesthesia and myotonia. *Br J Anaesth* 1994; 72:210–6.
143. Farrow C, Carling A. Successful spinal blockade in a parturient with myotonia congenita. *Int J Obstet Anesth* 2007; 16:89–90.
144. Basu A, Nishanth P, Ifaturoti O. Pregnancy in women with myotonia congenita. *Int J Gynecol Obstet* 2009; 106:62–3.

145. Butwick A, Riley E. Anesthetic management for cesarean section in a parturient with myotonia congenita. *Anesthesiology* 2005; 102:A110.
146. Howell P, Douglas M. Lupus anticoagulant, paramyotonia congenital and pregnancy. *Can J Anaesth* 1992; 39:992–6.
147. Grace R, Roach V. Caesarean section in a patient with paramyotonia congenita. *Anaesth Intensive Care* 1999; 27:534–7.
148. Mackenzie M, Pickering E, Yentis S. Anaesthetic management of labour and caesarean delivery of a patient with hyperkalaemic periodic paralysis. *Int J Obstet Anaesth* 2006; 15:329–31.
149. Volkov N, Nisenblat V, Ohel G, *et al.* Ehlers-Danlos syndrome: insights on obstetric aspects. *Obstet Gynecol Surv* 2007; 62:51–7.
150. Esaka E, Golde S, Stever M, *et al.* A maternal and perinatal mortality in pregnancy complicated by the kyphoscoliotic form of Ehlers-Danlos syndrome. *Obstet Gynecol* 2009; 113:515–18.
151. Castori M, Morlino S, Dordoni C, *et al.* Gynecologic and obstetric implications of the joint hypermobility syndrome (a.k.a. Ehlers-Danlos syndrome hypermobility type) in 82 Italian patients. *Am J Med Genet A* 2012; 158:2176–82.
152. Erez Y, Ezra Y, Rojansky N. Ehlers-Danlos type IV in pregnancy: a case report and a literature review. *Fetal Diagn Ther* 2008; 23:7–9.
153. Hammond R, Oligbo N. Ehlers Danlos syndrome type IV and pregnancy. *Arch Gynecol Obstet* 2012; 285:51–4.
154. Palmquist M, Pappas J, Petrikovsky B, *et al.* Successful pregnancy outcome in Ehlers-Danlos syndrome, vascular type. *J Matern Fetal Neonatal Med* 2009; 22:924–7.
155. Brighouse D, Guard B. Anaesthesia for caesarean section in a patient with Ehlers-Danlos syndrome type IV. *Br J Anaesth* 1992; 69:517–9.
156. Keeling S, Oswald A. Pregnancy and rheumatic disease: "By the book" or "by the doc". *Clin Rheumatol* 2009; 28:1–9.
157. Grange C. Autoimmune Diseases. In Gambling D, Douglas M, McKay R, editors. *Obstetric Anesthesia and Uncommon Disorders.* Cambridge: Cambridge University Press; 2008:404–22.
158. Bourlier R, Birnbach D. Anesthetic management of the parturient with ankylosing spondylitis. *Int J Obstet Anaesth* 1995; 4:244–7.
159. Schelew B, Vaghadia H. Ankylosing spondylitis and neuraxial anaesthesia—a 10 year review. *Can J Anaesth* 1996; 43:65–8.
160. Woodward L, Kam P. Ankylosing spondylitis: recent developments and anaesthetic implications. *Anaesthesia* 2009; 64:540–8.
161. Sivrikaya G, Hanci A, Dobrucali H, *et al.* Cesarean section under spinal anesthesia in a patient with ankylosing spondylitis-a case report. *Middle East J Anesth* 2010; 20:865–8.
162. Andic V, Kovacevic M, Skok I, *et al.* Epidural analgesia for pregnant with ankylosing spondylitis: Case report. *Region Anesth Pain M* 2012; 37:E255.
163. Sng B, Shah M. Regional anaesthesia for Caesarean section in an ankylosing spondylitic patient with twin pregnancy. *Eur J Anaesth* 2008; 25:767–9.
164. Broomhead C, Davies W, Higgins D. Awake oral fibreoptic intubation for caesarean section. *Int J Obstet Anaesth* 1995; 4:172–4.
165. Hiruta A, Fukuda H, Hiruta M, *et al.* Anesthetic management of caesarean section in a parturient with ankylosing spondylitis complicated with severe cervical myelitis. *Masui* 2002; 51:759–61.
166. Hoffman S, Zaphiratos V, Girard M, *et al.* Failed epidural analgesia in a parturient with advanced ankylosing spondylitis: a novel explanation. *Can J Anaesth* 2012; 59:871–4.
167. Wulf H. Epidural anaesthesia and spinal haematoma. *Can J Anaesth* 1996; 43:1260–71.
168. Batra Y, Sharma A, Rajeev S. Total spinal anaesthesia following epidural test dose in an ankylosing spondylitic patient with anticipated difficult airway undergoing total hip replacement. *Eur J Anaesthesiol Clin Pharmacol* 2006; 23:897–8.
169. Wetzl R. Anaesthesiological aspects of pregnancy in patients with rheumatic diseases. *Lupus* 2004; 13:699–702.
170. Berkowitz I, Raja S, Bender K, *et al.* Dwarfs: pathophysiology and anesthetic implications. *Anesthesiology* 1990; 73:739–59.
171. Mitra S, Dey N, Gomber K. Emergency cesarean section in a patient with achondroplasia: an anesthetic diliemma. *J Anaesthesiol Clin Pharmacol* 2007; 23:315–8.
172. Chetty S, Shaffer B, Norton M. Management of pregnancy in women with genetic disorders, part 1: Disorders of the connective tissue, muscle, vascular, and skeletal systems. *Obstet Gynecol Surv* 2011; 66:699–709.
173. Brimacombe J, Caunt J. Anaesthesia in a gravid achondroplastic dwarf. *Anaesthesia* 1990; 45:132–4.
174. Huang J, Babins N. Anesthesia for cesarean delivery in an achondroplastic dwarf: a case report. *AANA J* 2008; 76:435–6.
175. Allanson J, Hall J. Obstetric and gynecologic problems in women with chondrodystrophies. *Obstet Gynecol* 1986; 67:74–8.
176. Carstoniu J, Yee I, Halpern S. Epidural anaesthesia for Caesarean section in an achondroplastic dwarf. *Can J Anaesth* 1992; 39:708–11.
177. Keller C, Brimacombe J, Lirk P, *et al.* Failed obstetric tracheal intubation and postoperative respiratoy support with the Proseal LMA. *Anesth Analg* 2004; 98:1467–70.
178. Cohen S, Ulla S, Burley E. Epidural anesthesia for cesarean section in an achondroplastic dwarf. *Int J Obstet Anaesth* 2000; 9:293–4.
179. Cohen S. Anesthesia for cesarean section in achondroplastic dwarfs. *Anesthesiology* 1980; 52:264–6.
180. DeRenzo J, Vallejo M, Ramanathan S. Failed regional anesthesia with reduced spinal bupivacaine dosage in a parturient with achondroplasia presenting for urgent cesarean section. *Int J Obstet Anaesth* 2005; 14:175–8.
181. Lutter L, Lonstein J, Winters R, *et al.* Anatomy of the achondroplastic lumbar canal. *Clin Orthop Relat Res* 1977; 126:139–42.
182. Crawford M, Dutton D. Spinal anaesthesia for Caesarean section in an achondroplastic dwarf. *Anaesthesia* 1992; 47:1007.
183. Palomero Rodriguez M, Vargas M, Pelaez E, *et al.* Spinal anaesthesia for emergency Caesarean section in an achondroplastic patient. *Eur J Anaesthesiol* 2007; 24:981–2.
184. Modi H, Sus S, Hong J, *et al.* Magnetic resonance imaging study determining cord level and occupancy at thoracolumbar junction in achondroplasia—a prospective study. *Indian J Orthop* 2011; 45:63–8.
185. Ekwere I, Edomwonyi N, Imarengiaye C. Anaesthetic challenges associated with achondroplasia: a case report. *Afr J Reprod Health* 2010; 14:149–55.
186. Bancroft G, Lauria J. Ketamine induction for cesarean section in a patient with acute intermittent porphyria and achondroplastic dwarfism. *Anesthesiology* 1983; 59:143–4.
187. Cevik B, Colakoglu S. Anesthetic management of achondroplastic dwarf undergoing cesarean section: a case report. *Middle East J Anesth* 2010; 20:907–10.
188. Lattanzi D, Harger J. Achondroplasia and pregnancy. *J Reprod Med* 1982; 27:363–6.
189. McArthur R. Obstetric anaesthesia in an achondroplasic dwarf at a regional hospital. *Anaesth Intensive Care* 1992; 20:376–8.
190. Sharma A, George L, Erskin K. Osteogenesis imperfecta in pregnancy: two case reports and review of literature. *Obstet Gynecol Surv* 2001; 56:563–6.
191. Yeo S, Paech M. Regional anaesthesia for multiple caesarean sections in a parturient with osteogenesis imperfecta. *Int J Obstet Anesth* 1999; 8:284–7.
192. Key T, Horger E. Osteogenesis imperfecta as a complication of pregnancy. *Obstet Gynecol* 1978; 51:67–71.
193. Sauer A, Joyce T. Management of a patient with osteogenesis imperfecta: a case study. *AANA J* 1981; 49:580–1.
194. Roberts J, Soloman C. Management of pregnancy in osteogenesis imperfecta: new perspectives. *Obstet Gynecol* 1975; 45:168–70.
195. Evans H. Severe osteogenesis imperfecta with pregnancy. *Obstet Gynecol* 1966; 28:394–6.

196. Fiegel M. Cesarean delivery and colon resection in a patient with type III osteogenesis imperfecta. *Semin Cardiothorac Vasc Anesth* 2011; 15:98–101.
197. Cho E, Dayan S, Marx G. Anaesthesia in a parturient with osteogenesis imperfecta. *Br J Anaesth* 1992; 68:422–3.
198. Broadway J. Osteogenesis imperfecta: regional anaesthesia not always possible. *Int J Obstet Anesth* 2000; 9:213–14.
199. Cunningham A, Donnelly M, Comerford J. Osteogenesis imperfecta: anesthetic management of a patient for cesarean section: a case report. *Anesthesiology* 1984; 61:91–3.
200. Vogel T, Ratner E, Thomas R Jr, *et al.* Pregnancy complicated by severe osteogenesis imperfecta: a report of two cases. *Anesth Analg* 2002; 94:1315–17.
201. Price J, Reynolds F. Management of pregnancy complicated by severe osteogenesis imperfecta. *J Obstet Gynaecol* 1987; 7:178–80.
202. Murray S, Shamsuddin W, Russell R. Sequential combined spinal-epidural for caesarean delivery in osteogenesis imperfecta. *Int J Obstet Anesth* 2010; 19:127–8.
203. Libman R. Anesthetic considerations for the patient with osteogenesis imperfect. *Clin Orthop Relat R* 1981; 159:123–5.
204. Douglas M. Platelets, the parturient and regional anesthesia. *Int J Obstet Anesth* 2001; 10:113–20.

CHAPTER 47

Endocrine and autoimmune disorders

Mirjana Kendrisic and Borislava Pujic

Diabetes mellitus

Definition

Diabetes mellitus (DM) is defined as a clinical and metabolic disorder of the pancreas and characterized by hyperglycaemia.

Epidemiology

DM is one of the most common chronic diseases worldwide and continues to increase both in numbers and severity. Changing lifestyles of the world population lead to reduced physical activity and increased obesity. According to World Health Organization (WHO) published estimates, the number of people with diabetes in the world is expected to approximately double between 2000 and 2030, based solely upon demographic changes.[1] Prevalence of diabetes in Europe will continue to rise from 8.6% to 10% between 2010 and 2030. Although the highest incidence is registered in developed countries, the largest increase in number of people with diabetes is expected to occur in developing countries.

The main types of DM are type 1 (T1D, insulin-dependent), type 2 (T2D, insulin-independent) and gestational diabetes. All of them may be present during pregnancy. Approximately 87.5% of pregnancies complicated by diabetes are due to gestational diabetes. Prevalence of gestational diabetes in European countries varies from 2.0% to 6.0%. Data from Northern Europe showed less than 4% of gestational diabetes in that region comparing to Southern Europe where more than 6% was estimated. Another 7.5% of pregnant women with diabetes have T1D and the remaining 5% are due to T2D. The prevalence of T1D and T2D continues to rise in pregnant women worldwide.[2]

Type 1 diabetes

T1D (previously known as insulin-dependent diabetes) is a chronic inflammatory disease in which destruction of the beta-cells in the islets of Langerhans results in insulin deficiency and hyperglycaemia. This type of diabetes, also known as juvenile-onset diabetes, accounts for 10–15% of all people with the disease. It can appear at any age, although commonly under the age of 40, so women of childbearing age may be affected. It is important to know that it is now possible to identify people at risk of future disease accurately, by using islet cell autoantibody assays.

Disease can be triggered by environmental factors such as viruses, diet, or chemicals in people who are genetically predisposed. This type of diabetes is divided into three groups, according to aetiology—autoimmune, idiopathic, and mixed (double):

1. Autoimmune DM is associated with appearance of islet autoantibodies.
2. Idiopathic DM has the clinical features of T1D, but the autoimmune component is not detected.
3. Mixed or double DM is a combination of autoimmunity and characteristics of T2D such as obesity, insulin resistance, and dyslipidaemia.

Pathophysiology of T1D

Genetic predisposition for T1D

T1D is considered to be a heterogeneous disease. To date, several loci at different chromosomes have been linked to T1D susceptibility in humans.[3,4] Population studies confirmed that children with a first-degree relative withT1D have higher risk for the development of T1D and this risk increases further if both parents are affected.[5,6] The risk for offspring of a mother with T1D is 1.3–4%, while the risk for offspring of a father with T1D is 6–9%. It has been suggested that pregnancy may protect the infant from T1D. A possible explanation is that autoantibodies transmitted from the mother with T1D may protect the child from the development of autoantibodies and T1D later in life.[7,8] Such protection could be due to fetal and neonatal exposure to antibody-mediated presentation of autoantigen. The exposure provides a state of immune ignorance against autoantigen or a more efficient elimination of autoreactive T-cell clones, especially in offspring without a high-risk human leucocyte antigen (HLA) genotype.[9] The concordance of T1D between monozygotic twins is high (up to 50%), while between dizygotic twins it is only 10%.[10] However, the lack of 100% concordance shows that some environmental factors increase the risk of developing T1D.

Islet autoimmunity

The selective destruction of beta cells of pancreatic islets in T1D is the result of the interaction among beta cells, the immune system, and environmental factors in genetically susceptible individuals. However, the mechanisms which start the changes in this interaction and lead to the development of T1D have not been fully clarified yet. In the beginning of the autoimmune process against beta cells, patients produce several different antigens.[11] After presentation of the antigen by the macrophages to T lymphocytes, cellular and humoral immune responses are induced. The most important mechanism of cellular response is a decrease in number and function of regulatory T cells. Regulatory T cells are essential for many aspects of immune tolerance, including the suppression of autoimmune responses.

Humoral immune response is represented by islet autoantibodies. Islet cell autoantibodies are strongly associated with the development of T1D. The autoimmune process may persist subclinically in the majority of patients. Pancreatic autoantibodies are commonly present years before the diagnosis of T1D. Childhood onset of T1D is associated with the first signs of islet autoimmunity by the age of 2 years.[12] Risk of progressing to T1D is increased by the number of antibody types, so it rises from 60% to 100% in individuals with three to four antibody types. Clinical symptoms do not appear until up to 80% of cells have been destroyed. Therefore, detection of autoantibodies in the pre-diabetes phase has been most useful.[13–15]

Environmental factors

Environmental factors play an important role in the pathogenesis of T1D. The most important factors are infectious, dietary, perinatal, and psychosocial ones. Viral infections, breastfeeding, the early presence or lack of certain foods, birth weight, childhood over-nutrition, and negative stressful events are related to the prevalence of T1D.[16]

Viruses may trigger islet autoimmunity by molecular mimicry with islet antigens. Some viral infections including enteroviruses (especially Coxsackie B virus), rubella, mumps, rotavirus, parvovirus, and cytomegalovirus have long been suggested as potential environmental triggers for the disease.[17]

Cows' milk-based infant formulas and consumption of cows' milk within the first 3 months of life are associated with increased risk of T1D. The gut-associated immune system plays a major role in disease development, probably because of disturbed oral tolerance mechanisms and normal maturation of the gut.[18]

The concept of dietary regulation of autoimmunity cannot be applied only to cows' milk protein, but also to other dietary proteins. Early introduction of gluten-containing foods has been found to be a risk factor for the development of T1D-associated autoimmunity in children with certain genotype of parents with T1D.[19]

Type 2 diabetes

T2D (previously known as non-insulin dependent diabetes) is the most common form of diabetes, affecting 85–90% of all diabetic cases. This type of diabetes, also known as late-onset diabetes, is characterized by insulin resistance and relative insulin deficiency. T2D is increasingly common throughout the world in younger people and children. Lifestyle factors, such as excess weight, inactivity, high blood pressure, and poor diet, are major risk factors.[20]

Genetic Predisposition for T2D

T2D is a heterogeneous disorder caused by a combination of genetic and acquired abnormalities that affect insulin sensitivity and insulin secretion. At least 36 genes are identified to be associated with a risk of T2D. However, only about 10% of the heritability of T2D can be explained. The concordance of T2D between monozygotic twins is high (34–58%), while the rate of impaired glucose tolerance is up to 100%.[21,22] Despite the statistical significance of genetic data, it is not clinically possible to predict the risk of T2D. To date, most of the discovered gene variants have been linked to beta-cell dysfunction. There is no evidence that genetic variations may cause insulin resistance.

Pathogenesis of T2D

The metabolic changes underlying T2D are insulin resistance, beta-cell dysfunction, and impaired hepatic glucose production. Insulin resistance is defined as the inability of exogenous or endogenous insulin to increase glucose uptake and utilization in an individual compared to the normal population. Possible causes underlying the development of insulin resistance include genetic abnormalities of proteins of the insulin action cascade, fetal malnutrition, and increase in visceral adiposity.[23] T2D is characterized by impaired insulin secretion. Some evidence suggests that a decrease in beta-cell mass contributes to this. Progression of the disease is associated with decline in beta-cell function.[24]

Gestational diabetes mellitus

Gestational diabetes mellitus (GDM) is defined as glucose intolerance with an onset or first recognition during pregnancy. Pregnant women with GDM are a heterogeneous group. Some of the patients have unrecognized pre-existing T2D and a minority of them has T1D with first onset during pregnancy. This condition may persist after pregnancy leading to a significant risk of developing permanent diabetes.[25] The risk factors for GDM are found in Box 47.1.

About 40–60% of women with GDM do not have any of these risk factors. According to the recent guidelines from areas with significant prevalence, screening of all pregnant women should be done to diagnose patients at risk for GDM.[26]

Genetic predisposition and pathophysiology of GDM

Genetic susceptibility for GDM has not been proven despite the higher risk of hyperglycaemia during pregnancy in patients from families with either T1D or T2D.[27,28] During normal pregnancy, particularly in the third trimester, there is a physiological increase in insulin resistance. Normally, the mother's beta cells can produce additional insulin to overcome the insulin resistance. Patients with GDM are more insulin resistant than pregnant non-diabetic women because their insulin resistance precedes pregnancy and continues to increase in pregnancy.

Box 47.1 Risk factors for gestational diabetes mellitus

- Family history of T2D
- Maternal age (>35 years)
- Maternal obesity (BMI > 30)
- Ethnicity (African, black Caribbean, South Asian, Hispanic, Middle Eastern origin)
- Polycystic ovarian syndrome
- Past history of GDM or glucose intolerance
- Previous poor obstetric history
- Fetal macrosomia (body weight > 4000 g at term) in previous pregnancy

Data from Working group on gestational diabetes. National guidelines for gestational diabetes. *Duodecim* 2008; 124:1556–1569.

Placental products, such as human placental growth hormone (GH) and tumour necrosis factor alpha (TNF-α), have been suggested to be the mediators of insulin resistance. This effect of placental hormones usually begins 20–24 weeks into the pregnancy. The growing placenta in the third trimester has a greater effect on insulin resistance in patients with GDM. Excessive secretion of proinsulin, is often observed in women with GDM. Persistent insulin resistance leads to beta-cell dysfunction. The precise mechanism still remains unknown because the deficit in beta-cell function is multifactorial and polygenetic.[29]

Preconceptual care of patients with diabetes

T1D and T2D are associated with a greater risk of congenital malformations and poor pregnancy outcome. Women with diabetes who are planning pregnancy should be informed about the importance of strict glycaemic control, diet, and exercise in the preconception period and the level of haemoglobin (HbA1C) should be maintained below 6.1%. If possible, HbA1C values should be targeted towards normal (3.5–5.5%), although this runs the risk of hypoglycaemia. Pregnancy is not recommended for diabetic patients with HbA1C above 8.6%. Women with diabetes who are hyperglycaemic should be tested for ketones in blood and urine.[30] Guidelines advocate blood glucose self-monitoring and prescription of insulin for better glycaemic control. Metformin has been a safe alternative in patients resistant to insulin or in cases of insulin refusal.[31]

Retinal and renal assessment should be performed preconceptually in diabetic patients. Pregnancy is not recommended for women undergoing islet transplantation. There are insufficient data showing potential adverse effects of immunosuppressive drugs (daclizumab and rapamycin) on pregnancy.

Box 47.2 Signs and symptoms of diabetes in pregnancy

Common symptoms

- Excessive thirst
- Increased hunger
- Frequent urination
- Unusual fatigue

Less common signs and symptoms

- Blurred vision
- Dry itchy skin and skin infections
- Impaired healing of cuts or sores
- Tingling or numbness in hands or feet
- Urinary tract infections
- Vaginal infection (usually fungal)
- Psychological symptoms (irritability, lethargy, agitation)

Data from The Expert Committee on the Diagnosis and Classification of Diabetes Mellitus: Report of the Expert Committee on the Diagnosis and Classification of Diabetes Mellitus. *Diabetes Care* 1997; 20:1183–1197.

Clinical presentation of diabetes in pregnancy

Gestational diabetes is usually asymptomatic or the symptoms are mild and not life-threatening to the pregnant woman. Many of the signs of T1D and T2D are similar (Box 47.2).

Type 1 diabetes and pregnancy

Pregnancy is considered to be a diabetogenic state due to increases in cytokines (TNF-α) and hormones such as cortisol, progesterone, oestrogen, prolactin, and human placental lactogen. Activities of these factors and hormones result in elevation of postprandial glucose levels and decreased insulin sensitivity. Pregnancy in women with T1D is associated with an increased risk of poor maternal and fetal outcome. Complications during pregnancy related to a mother with T1D are hypoglycaemia, diabetic ketoacidosis (DKA), retinopathy, and nephropathy.

Hypoglycaemia

Avoidance of hyperglycaemia and tight glycaemic control increase the likelihood of insulin overdose and hypoglycaemia. It is recommended that blood glucose levels are maintained higher than 3.9 mmol/L. Nocturnal hypoglycaemia is a relatively common complication of T1D during the first and third trimester. The most severe complication of hypoglycaemia is hypoglycaemic coma, where urgent management is needed.[32]

Diabetic ketoacidosis (DKA)

DKA is a potentially life-threatening complication in patients with DM. In pregnancy, DKA is usually precipitated by stressful events, such as vomiting, infections of urinary and respiratory tracts, insulin delivery system failure, and poor management of DM. It usually occurs in the later stages of pregnancy.

Relative or absolute lack of circulating insulin and an excess of counter-regulatory hormones (e.g. glucagon) result in DKA. Hyperglycaemia and ketosis develop, leading to polyuria, polydipsia, and dehydration. Although DKA is less frequent in diabetic patients compared to hypoglycaemia, it can result in fatal complications—death (rarely) and fetal demise (reported in up to 35% of cases).

Patients with DKA need aggressive intravenous (IV) isotonic fluid replacement with 15–20 mL/kg/h of normal saline in the first 2 hours.

The average fluid deficit in these patients is around 100 mL/kg and it should be replaced within 24 hours. If possible, 50% of the fluid deficit should be given in the first 12 hours. A fixed rate IV insulin infusion (0.1 unit/kg/h based on estimate of weight) of 50 units human soluble insulin (Actrapid® or Humulin S®) made up to 50 mL with 0.9% sodium chloride solution should be commenced.[33] Total body potassium is decreased, but serum potassium levels are unreliable in DKA. Replacement is commenced if serum potassium is lower than 5 mmol/L. Use of bicarbonate is recommended in DKA at admission only if pH is lower than 6.9. Administration of bicarbonate can increase blood lactate and ketone bodies.[34]

Retinopathy

The progression of diabetic retinopathy in pregnancy is often associated with poor glycaemic control, hypertension, and duration of diabetes for longer than 15 years. Laser photocoagulation is a proven effective treatment and may protect patients against rapid progressive diabetic retinopathy (PDR). Vaginal delivery is debatable in cases of severe PDR. A multidisciplinary approach is needed for a decision with respect to mode of delivery.[35]

Nephropathy

Diabetes nephropathy is not a common complication of pregnancy and renal function remains preserved in patients with a normal serum creatinine level and normoalbuminuria. Hypertension is likely to be an aggravating factor in patients with microalbuminuria (albumin excretion is between 30 and 300 mg/day (20–200 mcg/min)). Therefore, intensive antihypertensive therapy is strongly recommended in combination with low-dose aspirin. In patients with macroalbuminuria (albumin excretion above 300 mg/day (200 mcg/min)), risk of pre-eclampsia and preterm delivery is significantly higher.[36]

Pre-eclampsia

Pregnancies affected by T1D are at increased risk of pre-eclampsia, which might lead to serious complications for both mother and baby. Appropriate metabolic control and antihypertensive therapy are essential for preventing eclampsia.[37]

Impact of T1D on fetal and neonatal outcome

Strict glycaemic control is needed in early pregnancy during organogenesis, because of a higher risk of miscarriage and fetal abnormalities. Diabetic nephropathy is associated with fetal growth restriction. In late pregnancy, poor glycaemic control increases the risk of macrosomia and birth trauma.[38]

Type 2 diabetes and pregnancy

Patients with T2D are older compared with other groups of diabetic patients and usually multiparous. There is a higher incidence of T2D in certain ethnic groups such as people of African, black Caribbean, South Asian, Middle Eastern, or Chinese family origin. Language and cultural barriers may result in poor preconception care. Cessation of oral hypoglycaemic therapy is important before conception due to its possible teratogenic effects.

Risk of perinatal mortality is similar to that of patients with T1D, but significantly higher compared to healthy patients (2.5–6.7% cf 0.7%). The incidence of caesarean and preterm delivery is significantly higher. Risk of congenital malformations, macrosomia, and neonatal hypoglycaemia, hypocalcaemia, and hyperbilirubinaemia is also significant.[39]

Gestational diabetes mellitus and pregnancy

Pregnant women with GDM are mostly overweight and have an increased risk of developing T2D after pregnancy. Children of mothers with GDM are also at higher risk of obesity and T2D later in life.[40]

Blood glucose levels are mostly in the normal range in GDM patients during the first trimester. Therefore, the risk of congenital birth defects is lower compared to patients with T1D. GDM is associated with perinatal complications—macrosomia, stillbirth, shoulder dystocia, and birth injuries. Rates of hypoglycaemia and hyperbilirubinaemia in the babies are higher immediately after delivery.[41]

Diagnosis of GDM

Diabetes screening for gestational diabetes is divided into three phases:

Phase 1: Risk assessment

Risk of developing GDM should be assessed in all pregnant women. If any of the risk factors are present, testing for GDM is strongly recommended. However, if only these women are tested, approximately 40% of GDM patients will remain undiagnosed. It is still debatable whether universal screening is beneficial and cost-effective.

Phase 2: Early detection of GDM in high-risk group

Selective screening for GDM is recommended for women diagnosed with GDM in a previous pregnancy. Recommended screening tests are early self-monitoring of blood glucose and oral glucose tolerance test (OGTT) at 16–18 weeks. The 2-hour 75 g OGTT should be used to test for GDM. If results are within the reference range, a further OGTT should be repeated at the 28th week.

Phase 3: Late detection of GDM

Screening for GDM is recommended for all pregnant women without diagnosed diabetes before pregnancy (except for those at very low risk) at 24–28 gestational weeks using the OGTT test after overnight fasting.[42]

Threshold values for diagnosis of GDM

The significant threshold values for the OGTT which have an impact on pregnancy outcome have not been clarified yet. According to WHO criteria, the threshold for fasting plasma glucose (FPG) should remain at 6.1 mmol/L.

The threshold values on the 2-hour 75 g OGTT for the diagnosis of GDM have been derived from Hyperglycemia and Adverse Pregnancy Outcome (HAPO) study data (Table 47.1). For the diagnosis of GDM, one or more of these values have to equal or exceed the threshold. Using these criteria, the total incidence of GDM in the HAPO study was 17.8%. According to the study, a rise in glucose levels was associated with the greater frequency of adverse pregnancy outcomes.[43]

Diagnosis of overt diabetes

Overt DM during pregnancy is associated with significantly increased risks of adverse perinatal outcomes compared to GDM. Identification of women with overt diabetes should be at the earliest possible opportunity. Targets for blood glucose control should be determined in the same way as for women with pre-existing diabetes. Early testing is recommended at the first prenatal visit, especially in the high-risk population.

Overt diabetes can be confirmed by measurement of FPG, HbA1C, or random plasma glucose. In the absence of a reliable gold standard test for detecting overt diabetes early in pregnancy, the International Association of Diabetes and Pregnancy Study Groups (IADPSG) suggested using standard laboratory

Table 47.1 Threshold values of the oral glucose tolerance test for diagnosis of gestational diabetes mellitus

Glucose concentration threshold		
Glucose measure	**mmol/L**	**mg/dL**
FPG	5.1	92
1 h plasma glucose	10.0	180
2 h plasma glucose	8.5	153

Data from The HAPO study cooperative research group. Metzger BE, Lowe LP, Dyer AR, Trimble ER *et al.* Hyperglycemia and Adverse Pregnancy Outcomes. *N Engl J Med* 2008; 358:1991–2002.

Table 47.2 Standard laboratory methods for diagnosis of overt diabetes

Measure of glycaemia	Threshold for diagnosis of overt diabetes
FPG	≥7.0 mmol/L (126 mg/dL)
HbA1C	≥6.5% (DCCT/UKPDS standardized essay)
Random plasma glucose	≥11.1 mmol/L (200 mg/dL)[a]

DCCT, Diabetes Control and Complications Trial; UKPDS, United Kingdom Prospective Diabetes Study.

[a]If random plasma glucose is used for screening of DM, diagnosis of overt diabetes in pregnancy should be confirmed by FPG or HbA1C.

Data from Metzger BE, Gabbe SG, Persson B, Buchanan TA, Catalano PA, Damm P, *et al.* International association of diabetes and pregnancy study groups recommendations on the diagnosis and classification of hyperglycemia in pregnancy. *Diabetes Care* 2010; 33(3):676–82.

methods for measuring glucose (FPG, random plasma glucose, or HbA1C)[44] (Table 47.2).

Management of diabetes in pregnancy

The aim of diabetes therapy in pregnancy is normoglycaemia. The key to achieving this goal is management of women with diabetes by a specialized multidisciplinary team.

Diet and physical activity

A dietary plan should be individualized for every patient and recommended by a nutritionist. The recommended calorie intake for pregnant woman is 30–35 kcal/kg/day. Obese women with a pregestational body mass index (BMI) greater than 27 have to reduce their caloric intake to 24 kcal/kg/day. Plasma glucose concentration and morning insulin requirements suddenly increase between 5:00 and 9:00 a.m. (dawn phenomenon), even in healthy people. Women with GDM have deficiency in the first phase of insulin secretion. It is necessary to adjust the morning meal and insulin therapy in order to avoid hyperglycaemia and its consequences. During the night, insulin requirements increase and nocturnal hypoglycaemia may be a significant problem in diabetic patients. An evening snack is recommended for pregnant women receiving insulin therapy due to the inability of insulin preparations to maintain normoglycaemia overnight.[45]

Moderate exercise is associated with better glycaemic control and improved maternal and fetal outcome. If there is no medical or obstetric contraindication, physical activity should be maintained until the last weeks of pregnancy.

Insulin therapy

Before the introduction of insulin in everyday practice, women were counselled to avoid pregnancy due to an extremely high risk of fetal mortality (up to 100%) and maternal mortality (30%). Since 1980, insulin therapy and better glycaemic control have led to improved maternal and fetal outcomes.[46]

Insulin is the first-line pharmacotherapy in women with GDM if medical nutritional therapy results in inadequate glucose control. Patients with T1D require lifelong insulin therapy to substitute endogenous secretion, but the insulin regimen needs to be adapted in pregnancy.

Insulin is considered safe for the treatment of diabetes in pregnancy and a large body of research evidence supports its safety and efficacy. It was not initially thought that insulin can be transferred from the maternal to fetal circulation, but it is now confirmed that small amounts of insulin (1–5%) do cross the human placenta. Maternal hyperglycaemia, rather than maternal hyperinsulinaemia, results in fetal hyperinsulinaemia. Fetal hyperglycaemia and consequent hyperinsulinaemia cause macrosomia, the most prevalent complication in offspring of diabetic mothers.[47]

Box 47.3 Basic types of insulin and duration of action

- Rapid-acting insulins: lispro, aspart, and glulisine (2–4 hours)
- Short-acting insulin: regular insulin (4–6 hours)
- Intermediate-acting insulins: neutral protamine Hagedorn (NPH) insulin (14–20 hours)
- Long-acting insulins: glargine and detemir (20–24 hours)

To date, only human neutral protamine Hagedorn (NPH) insulin, regular human insulin, and the rapid-acting insulin analogues lispro and aspart are approved for use in pregnancy. Older types of insulin are considered safe for use during pregnancy. It is less clear if the newer insulin medications are also safe. Box 47.3 contains basic types of insulin and their duration of action.

Combination insulins are:

- Intermediate-acting plus short-acting: NPH insulin/regular insulin.
- Intermediate-acting plus rapid-acting: insulin lispro protamine/insulin lispro.

Human insulin is available in two forms, a short-acting (regular) form and an intermediate-acting (NPH) form (Table 47.3).

Insulin analogues are developed in order to achieve pharmacokinetic properties of endogenous insulin by changing the primary amino acid sequence (Box 47.4 and Tables 47.4 and 47.5).[48–51]

Table 47.3 Characteristics of short-acting and intermediate-acting insulin forms

	Short-acting (regular) form	Intermediate-acting (NPH) form
Multiple-dose regimen insulin (well-controlled patients)	Pre meal (three times daily)	Basal requirements pre breakfast + bedtime (twice daily)
Patients with poor glycaemic control	Continuous subcutaneous insulin infusion	
Advantages	Extensively used during pregnancy	Well studied during pregnancy
Disadvantages	Increases risk of macrosomia Postprandial hyperglycaemia	Nocturnal hypoglycaemia
Onset/peak/ duration of action	30–60 min/1–2 h/4–6 h	1–2 h/5–7 h/14–20 h

Data from International Society for Pediatric and Adolescent Diabetes DKA Guidelines. *Pediatric Diabetes* 2009: 10 (Suppl. 12): 118–133. http://www.bsped.org.uk/professional/guidelines/docs/DKAGuideline.pdf

Box 47.4 Short-acting and long-acting insulin analogues

- Short acting:
  - Insulin lispro
  - Insulin aspart
- Long acting:
  - Insulin glargine
  - Insulin detemir

Data from Angelina L. Trujillo. Insulin Analogs and Pregnancy. *Diabetes Spectrum* 2007; 20(2):94–101.

Oral hypoglycaemic agents

Oral hypoglycaemic agents, such as glibenclamide and metformin, have been approved for use in pregnancy, especially for treatment of GDM. Some of the patients diagnosed with T2D can also be treated with oral therapy. These agents are possible alternatives in patients who refuse insulin therapy.

Metformin

Metformin has become increasingly popular in pregnancy, since published data suggested its safety and efficacy in patients with polycystic ovary syndrome (PCOS). Although it crosses the placenta, teratogenic effects are not found. Metformin has been shown to improve fertility in patients with PCOS and may prevent early pregnancy loss. However, evidence of its effects on maternal outcome is still controversial.[52]

Glibenclamide (Glyburide)

Glibenclamide is an oral sulfonylurea long-acting hypoglycaemic agent. Most women with GDM who are treated with glibenclamide can achieve adequate glycaemic control. Risk of neonatal hypoglycaemia is significantly lower in comparison with patients on insulin therapy. There are no published data about teratogenic effects of glibenclamide.[53]

Table 47.4 Characteristics of short-acting insulin analogues when compared to regular human insulin

	Insulin lispro	Insulin aspart
Chemical structure	Inversion of prolin-lysin into lysin–prolin (positions 28–29)	Aspart instead of prolin at the 28th position
Pharmacokinetic properties	Fast rise and higher pick of insulin concentration	Similar to insulin lispro
	Better glycaemic control Lower risk of postprandial hypoglycaemia	Similar to insulin lispro
Neonatal outcome	No difference in perinatal outcome	In patients with T1D, reduces fetal mortality
Duration of action	2–4 h, onset of action 15–30 min	2–4 h, onset of action 10–20 min

Data from García-Domínguez M, Herranz L, Hillman N, Martín-Vaquero P. *et al.* Use of insulin lispro during pregnancy in women with pregestational diabetes mellitus. *Medicina Clínica*, 2011, volume 137, issue 13, pp. 581–586; and Mathiesen ER. Insulin aspart in diabetic pregnancy: state of the art. *Women's Health*, 2008, volume 4, issue 2, pp. 119–24.

Table 47.5 Characteristics of long-acting insulin analogues when compared to regular human insulin

	Insulin glargine	Insulin detemir
Chemical structure	2 molecules of arginine have been added (B chain) Aspartic acid replaced by glycine (A chain at position 21)	Threonine is removed at B30 Myristic acid is added to lysine at position 29
Pharmacokinetic properties	High affinity for insulin-like growth factor I receptor	Weak affinity for insulin-like growth factor I receptor
Advantages	Glycaemic stability Reduced incidence of nocturnal hypoglycaemia	Reduce fasting glucose levels Reduced HbA1C levels
Neonatal outcome	Risk for macrosomia was not confirmed	Lower incidence of macrosomia
Duration of action	>24 h, onset of action 4–5 h	20 h, onset of action 4–6 h

Data from Pollex EK, Feig DS, Lubetsky A, Yip PM, Koren G. Insulin glargine safety in pregnancy: a transplacental transfer study. *Diabetes Care*, 2010, volume 33, issue 1, pp. 29–33; and McElduff A. Insulin Detemir in Pregnancy: A Small but Significant Step Forward? *Diabetes Care*, 2012, volume 35, issue 10, pp. 1968–69.

Chlorpropamide and tolbutamide

Chlorpropamide and tolbutamide are oral sulfonylurea long-acting hypoglycaemic agents. They are shown to cross the placenta in higher proportion than glibenclamide. Due to their potential teratogenic effects, their use in patients who are planning pregnancy or who are pregnant is not recommended.

Obstetric management of women with diabetes

All women diagnosed with diabetes during pregnancy carry a higher risk for obstetric complications and careful obstetric follow-up is needed from the first antenatal visit. The purpose of this follow-up is to provide good perinatal outcome by:

- antenatal fetal surveillance techniques.
- meticulous selection of the most appropriate timing and route of delivery.

Obstetricians should be aware that severity of the disease and poor metabolic control may worsen fetal well-being. Therefore, multidisciplinary strategies for metabolic optimization should be performed together with diabetologists to reduce consequences of maternal hyperglycaemia on fetal growth.[54]

Fetal surveillance

- Serial monitoring by ultrasound is recommended. In the first trimester, an ultrasound scan should be performed at 7–10 weeks to confirm viability. During the second trimester, an ultrasound between 18 and 20 weeks is recommended to exclude fetal anomalies. During the third trimester, a minimum of two ultrasound scans should be performed for evaluation of fetal growth.
- Monitoring of fetal movements. Self-monitoring of fetal movements should start from the 32nd week of gestation. Reduction in fetal movements over a period of 2 hours should be reported immediately to the obstetrician.

- Non-stress testing (NST) has been suggested from the 32nd week of gestation in high-risk patients and 'near term' in patients with low risk for complications.[55]
- Biophysical profiles and amniotic fluid index are suggested only if they are clinically indicated.

Timing and route of delivery

- In diabetic patients with good metabolic control and fetal surveillance, medically indicated delivery should be performed between 37 and 38^{+6} weeks of pregnancy.[31] Delivery before 37 weeks' gestation is not recommended in the absence of evidence of fetal compromise due to increased risk of fetal lung immaturity.
- Diabetes itself in pregnancy is not an indication for caesarean delivery. However, neonatal complications, such as macrosomia, shoulder dystocia, clavicular fracture, brachial palsy, and unexplained intrauterine fetal death, are significantly higher in diabetic patients. Therefore, patients with an ultrasound confirmation of a macrosomic fetus should be informed of the risks and benefits of vaginal birth.
- Women affected by pre-existing DM need tertiary-level obstetric care due to an extremely high risk of adverse perinatal outcomes.[56]

Anaesthetic management of women with diabetes

Low-risk diabetic patients

Labour and delivery

Most pregnant women with diabetes and good metabolic control may have an induction of labour. Labour epidural analgesia can have a positive effect in these patients, due to its superior pain relief. Epidural analgesia also removes the stress response to the pain of labour and helps to facilitate blood glucose control. Attenuation of the stress response and reduction in maternal hyperventilation may have a beneficial effect on fetal metabolic acidosis.[57] Avoidance of fetal metabolic acidosis is one of the possible factors which can reduce the risk of stillbirth in diabetic mothers.

Pregnant women, who were offered information based on the current available evidence during antenatal care, were more likely to receive labour epidural analgesia than women with no pregnancy risk factors.[58] Furthermore, according to some evidence, epidural analgesia was not found to be an independent risk factor for caesarean delivery, but rather a protective factor.[59] However, there is insufficient evidence from well-designed studies on the influence of epidural analgesia on labour in women with diabetes. Despite being at a high risk for infection, there are no published data on the higher incidence of epidural abscesses in diabetic patients.

Fasting during induction of labour is still a controversial issue independently of DM. During established labour, blood glucose levels should be maintained between 4 and 7 mmol/L. Measurement of capillary blood glucose should be performed hourly. IV fluids and insulin should be administered during labour and adjusted according to the blood sugar—the 'sliding scale', especially in patients with T1D.[31]

Elective caesarean delivery

Diabetic patients with obstetric complications and/or poor metabolic control are candidates for elective caesarean delivery.

Women with complications of diabetes and/or obesity should have an anaesthetic assessment in the antenatal period, or immediately after admission to the delivery suite. During the anaesthetic evaluation, the presence of diabetic complications (nephropathy, diabetic heart disease) and medical comorbidities should be assessed.

If the patient is scheduled for planned caesarean delivery, the operation should be performed early in the morning, to enable better glucose control. Monitoring of blood glucose levels is essential perioperatively. Diabetic patients require a minimum of hourly glucose monitoring and titration of short-acting insulin for successful glycaemic target achievement.

Neuraxial anaesthesia (NA) is the preferred choice. Both spinal and combined spinal–epidural (CSE) anaesthesia are well known for its safety and reliability. Diabetic women are likely to have pre-eclampsia and autonomic neuropathy. Therefore, there has been concern regarding severe hypotension following subarachnoid block.[60] Preloading with crystalloid or colloid has not always been found to be effective. Once the placenta is delivered, insulin requirements decrease dramatically and any insulin infusion is usually stopped. Blood sugars are monitored thereafter and many patients can resume their prepregnancy insulin doses soon after delivery. Caesarean delivery results in moderate to severe postoperative pain. Management of postoperative pain relief in diabetic mothers leads to better glycaemic control and enables breastfeeding.[61]

High-risk diabetic patients

Urgent caesarean delivery

Urgent caesarean delivery is needed in patients with maternal or fetal compromise, which is not immediately life-threatening. The preferred anaesthetic technique is NA (see chapters in Part 6).

Emergency caesarean delivery

Emergency caesarean delivery is needed if an immediate life-threatening condition exists for mother and/or fetus. General anaesthesia (GA) with rapid sequence induction is the usual technique. Obesity and pregnancy each increase the risk of difficult airway. Obesity in diabetic mothers, especially with T2D, is associated with a higher likelihood of unanticipated difficult airway. There may also be difficult airway challenges with T1D due to the 'stiff joint syndrome'—problems with the atlanto-occipital joint resulting in reduced neck extension.

Fetal compromise is more frequent in diabetic mothers due to an increased risk of fetal hypoxia. Fetal hyperglycaemia and hyperinsulinaemia increase oxygen consumption by up to 30%. Patients with pre-existing diabetes are more likely to have placental insufficiency. The placenta has a limited ability to increase oxygen delivery, but insufficiency remains largely subclinical during pregnancy. Pain during labour may decrease the oxygen supply to the fetus. Intermittent hypoxia that occurs with uterine contractions of normal labour leads to fetal asphyxia in the compromised fetus of diabetic mother.

Unstable diabetics will require care in the high dependency unit as close monitoring of their blood sugars and insulin regimen is required.[62]

Acute neonatal complications in offspring of diabetic mothers

Acute neonatal complications are hypoglycaemia, hypocalcaemia, hypomagnesaemia, hyperbilirubinaemia, and respiratory distress.

Neonatal hypoglycaemia is the most common complication in the newborn of diabetic mothers. During pregnancy, prolonged maternal hyperglycaemia leads to fetal hyperglycaemia and consequent fetal hyperinsulinaemia. After delivery, there is a sudden drop in blood glucose levels in the presence of hyperinsulinaemia. This condition usually occurs within 2 hours after delivery and persists up to 72 hours. Hourly blood glucose testing is needed in high-risk infants.

Hypocalcaemia and hypomagnesaemia are caused by low parathyroid levels and the immaturity of neonatal parathyroid gland. Calcium can be easily transferred through the placenta. Hypocalcaemia occurs within 72 hours of birth, if parathyroid hormone response is delayed. Hyperbilirubinaemia is precipitated by expansion of fetal red cell mass. The immature neonatal liver is unable to conjugate and excrete larger amounts of bilirubin, caused by polycythaemia. Common causes of respiratory distress are lack of surfactant before 38 weeks of gestation and meconium aspiration in macrosomic babies. Babies of mothers who have DM are more likely to develop the disease in later life. This is even more likely if the father has T1D.[63]

Breastfeeding

Breastfeeding is recommended in patients with T1D.[64] However, it may be delayed due to neonatal morbidity and poor maternal metabolic control. In women with GDM and T2D, breastfeeding has been found to have numerous advantages for both mother and newborn. Women who breastfeed their babies have a lower risk of breast and ovarian cancer. Breastfed offspring may have lower risks of obesity, cardiovascular disease, hypertension, and T2D later in life.[65,66]

Pituitary gland

The pituitary gland ('master gland') is a small endocrine organ that controls a multitude of important functions in the body. It is located in a sella turcica and is functionally connected to the hypothalamus. It is composed of three lobes—anterior, intermediate, and posterior—which secrete nine hormones (Box 47.5).

Box 47.5 Products of the anterior and the posterior pituitary

Products of the anterior pituitary

- Growth hormone (GH)
- Thyroid-stimulating hormone (TSH)
- Adrenocorticotropic hormone (ACTH)
- Prolactin (PRL) or 'luteotropic' hormone (LTH)
- Luteinizing hormone (LH) or 'lutropin'
- Follicle-stimulating hormone (FSH)
- Melanocyte-stimulating hormones (MSHs)

Products of the posterior pituitary

- Oxytocin
- Antidiuretic hormone (ADH, vasopressin)

Data from Karaca ZF, Unluhizarci K, Kelestimur F. Pregnancy and pituitary disorders. *Eur J Endocrinol* 2010; 162(6):453–475.

Pregnancy and the pituitary

Pituitary volumes during pregnancy are increased from 45% to 120%. The highest volumes were observed during the first 3 days postpartum.[67] It returns to normal size within 6 months postpartum. Anterior pituitary cells (lactotrophs) produce prolactin (PRL). PRL secretion is also stimulated by progesterone. Increased PRL secretion during pregnancy is important for the preparation of breast tissue for lactation.

Normal gestation is associated with increased maternal hypothalamic–pituitary–adrenal axis (HPA) activity. The placenta is the source of elevated corticotropin-releasing hormone (CRH) and appears to be the major stimulus for the HPA axis, especially during the third trimester.[68] Placental GH is detectable by the fifth week of pregnancy and levels increase exponentially and peak at 35–37 weeks.[69]

Hyperpituitarism

Hyperpituitarism is a condition in which the pituitary gland is overactive. The most common causes are pituitary tumours (Box 47.6).

Prolactinomas are the most common cause of persistent hyperprolactinemia.[70] The risk of tumour growth in pregnant patients with macroprolactinomas is higher than that in those with microprolactinomas. Medical treatment with bromocriptine has been recommended, but it should be stopped if pregnancy is confirmed.[71] Prolonged treatment with dopamine agonists is associated with the higher probability of conception.[72]

In healthy individuals, hormonal activity of the pituitary returns to normal 11 months after delivery. The abnormal enlargement of the pituitary gland during pregnancy might shrink spontaneously after delivery and these patients might have a higher risk of postpartum hypopituitarism.[73]

Hypopituitarism

Hypopituitarism is a rare disorder, characterized by deficient or diminished production of pituitary hormones and can be caused by disease in the pituitary or in the hypothalamus. The lack of hormone results in a loss of function of the gland or organ that it controls. Damage to the pituitary gland can be caused by tumour, radiation, surgery, infections, postpartum haemorrhage (Sheehan's syndrome), or other conditions. The symptoms

Box 47.6 Types of pituitary tumours

- By function:
  - Tumours which produce hormones (~35%)
  - Tumours which do not produce hormones (65%)
- By size:
  - Microadenomas (<1 cm)
  - Macroadenomas (>1 cm)

Data from Arafah BM, Nasrallah MP. Pituitary tumors: pathophysiology, clinical manifestations and management. *Endocrine-Related Cancer* 2001; 8:287–305.

depend on which hormone is involved.[74] The pituitary gland can also revert spontaneously to normal after delivery and the patient remains asymptomatic in a subsequent pregnancy. If the disorder has been diagnosed before or during the pregnancy and hormone replacement therapy has also been started, it should be continued. Surgical treatment should be avoided during pregnancy, except if symptoms worsen. After neurosurgery, hormone replacement is needed throughout life.

Diagnosis

This depends on the specific lack of hormones. Magnetic resonance imaging (MRI) without contrast is mandatory. The enlarged pituitary gland can cause visual problems and together with hypertension can mimic pre-eclampsia.

Anaesthetic management

Delivery can be undertaken under epidural, spinal, or CSE. GA has been described in a patient who had her pituitary tumour removed after delivery under NA.[75]

Complications

Ischaemia and necrosis may also occur in the pituitary gland at the end of pregnancy or in the postpartum period. Modest hypertension of 140/70 mmHg in younger patients (during pre-eclampsia/eclampsia) can cause cerebral oedema and haemorrhage and further increases the risk of pituitary necrosis.[76] Haemorrhage in the gland, ischaemia, and necrosis may cause death. Emergency treatment is needed for pituitary necrosis: surgical or medical (bromocriptine, hydrocortisone, thyroid hormone replacement).[77] The severe consequences of missing the diagnosis underline the importance of this potentially lethal endocrine emergency.[78]

Thyroid gland

The thyroid gland is responsible for the synthesis of thyroxine (T_4) and triiodothyronine (T_3). Thyroid-stimulating hormone (TSH) released from the pituitary gland binds the TSH receptor on the thyroid cells and stimulates them. Thyroxine is produced as the precursor of thyroglobulin which is cleaved by enzymes to produce active T_4. The lysosomal enzymes cleave the T_4 from the iodinated thyroglobulin. Activity of thyroid hormone depends on free T_4 and T_3. Thyroid hormones have negative feedback on thyroid-releasing hormone and TSH production. Therefore, TSH is a very sensitive and specific marker of thyroid function.

TSH secretion has a daily circadian rhythm. The highest TSH level is reached during the second part of the night. TSH level is the best screening test for both hyperthyroidism (decreased TSH level) and hypothyroidism (increased TSH level) diagnosis.

Thyroid cells release T_4 and T_3 into the bloodstream. There is 0.03% free T_4 and 0.03% free T_3, which is three- to five-fold more active than T_4. The levels are regulated by iodothyronine transporters.[79] All cells in the body are targets for thyroid hormones and their metabolic effects are summarized in Box 47.7.

Plasma concentration of cholesterol and triglycerides is inversely correlated with thyroid hormone levels. One of the diagnostic signs of hypothyroidism is increased blood cholesterol concentration. Thyroid hormones stimulate gluconeogenesis and glycogenolysis to generate free glucose.

Normal levels of thyroid hormones are essential for the development of the fetal and neonatal brain. In the first trimester and at the end of pregnancy, serum TSH level is sometimes below the normal range outside of pregnancy.[80,81] Serum TSH is a more accurate indication of thyroid status in pregnancy than any of the other markers. In the first trimester, the fetus is totally dependent on maternal hormones. In the second trimester the fetal thyroid gland starts the production of its own hormones, but it is still dependent on the mother.[82] Fetal T_3 remains low until 30 weeks of gestation and increases at term. The increased demand for thyroid hormones (and iodine) is reached by about 20 weeks of gestation and persists until term. Additionally, the placenta contains deiodinases that can convert T_4 to T_3. The WHO recommends increasing iodine intake from the standard 100–150 mcg/day to 200 mcg/day during pregnancy, because lack of iodine results in maternal goitres.[83]

Box 47.7 Metabolic effects of thyroid hormones

- Basal metabolism regulation
- Thermoregulation
- Control of energy production in brain, heart, and muscles
- Protein, fat, vitamin, and carbohydrate metabolism

Data from *Thyroid Disease and Pregnancy 2012*. The American Thyroid Association. http://www.thyroid.org.

Thyroid disease

Thyroid disease is not uncommon in pregnancy. Thyroid dysfunction may be detected for the first time during pregnancy. The most common cause (80–85%) of maternal hyperthyroidism is Graves' disease (1/1500 pregnancies). If untreated, thyroid disorders can have profound effects on both mother and fetus.

Limited amounts of T_3 and T_4 cross the placenta and influence fetal thyroid function. In mild thyroid disorders, there is no implication for the fetus.[84]

Hyperthyroidism

Hyperthyroidism affects 0.1–0.4% of pregnancies. Approximately 0.2% of cases of hyperthyroidism are diagnosed before pregnancy and only 0.05% are diagnosed during pregnancy. Symptoms of hyperthyroidism may be difficult to recognize in pregnancy, because normal pregnancy may mimic them (Box 47.8). The effects of hyperthyroidism on the pregnancy and fetus are shown in Box 47.9.

Box 47.8 Symptoms of hyperthyroidism

- Fatigue
- Tachycardia
- Heat intolerance
- Appetite changes
- Emesis and hyperemesis

Data from *Thyroid Disease and Pregnancy 2012*. The American Thyroid Association. http://www.thyroid.org.

Box 47.9 The effects of hyperthyroidism on pregnancy and fetus

The effects of hyperthyroidism on pregnancy

- Infection
- Miscarriage
- Molar pregnancy
- Pregnancy-induced hypertension
- Congestive heart failure
- Pre-eclampsia
- Preterm delivery

Effects of maternal hyperthyroidism on fetus

- Low weight
- Prematurity
- Neonatal hyperthyroidism
- Stillbirth

Data from *Thyroid Disease and Pregnancy 2012*. The American Thyroid Association. http://www.thyroid.org.

Medical and surgical management

Thyroid hormones should be assessed monthly during the treatment in pregnancy. Hyperthyroidism is diagnosed by high free T_4 and reduced TSH levels. Thyroidectomy is relatively contraindicated in pregnancy. If it is necessary, the optimum time to perform thyroidectomy is in the late second trimester. All antithyroid drugs (Box 47.10) cross the placenta. Propylthiouracil (PTU) may cause hepatotoxicity.[85–87] Beta blockers are recommended only for thyroid crisis. Radioactive iodine is contraindicated in pregnancy. Pregnancy should be postponed until 6 months after radioactive iodine treatment.

Anaesthetic management

Ideally, parturients presenting for labour should be euthyroid. Early epidural analgesia is the method of choice for vaginal delivery in order to avoid pain and potential thyroid crisis. Epidural, spinal, or GA can be used for caesarean delivery. IV administration of hydrocortisone 100 mg may be considered preoperatively to prevent adrenal insufficiency. Prehydration prior to NA is useful to minimize haemodynamic changes. Phenylephrine is recommended for the treatment of hypotension. It should be administered as a 20–40 mcg an IV bolus or by infusion. NA should be performed with caution to minimize maternal anxiety and to avoid maternal and fetal respiratory depression. If GA is needed, careful airway assessment has to be performed preoperatively. An enlarged thyroid gland can affect the airway, making endotracheal intubation difficult. Thiopentone, the induction agent of choice for caesarean delivery under GA, can have an antithyroid effect. Light anaesthesia, atropine, and ketamine are not recommended because they can stimulate the sympathoadrenal axis. Volatile anaesthetic agents of choice for maintenance of anaesthesia are isoflurane and sevoflurane. Muscular weakness may occur and neuromuscular monitoring can be useful.

Box 47.10 Medical management of hyperthyroidism

- Propylthiouracil (PTU): 100–150 mg/8 h increasing up to 250–300 mg/8 h—*first choice*
- Carbimazole: second trimester, nursing period, more potent

Data from Stagnaro-Green A, Abalovich M, Alexander E, *et al.* Guidelines of the American Thyroid Association for the diagnosis and management of thyroid disease during pregnancy and postpartum. *Thyroid* 2011; 21(10):1081; and Rosenfeld H, Ornoy A, Shechtman S, Diav-Citrin O. Pregnancy outcome, thyroid dysfunction and fetal goitre after in utero exposure to propylthiouracil: a controlled cohort study. *Br J Clin Pharmacol* 2009; 68:609.

Complications

Thyroid storm or thyrotoxic crisis can occur during vaginal delivery or induction of GA. Thyrotoxicosis is defined as 'the clinical syndrome of hypermetabolism and hyperactivity that results when the serum concentrations of free T_4 and/or free T_3 are high'. Symptoms are found in Box 47.11. It is associated with high serum hCG levels.[88,89] The most common cause is Graves' disease.

The differential diagnosis of thyroid storm includes malignant hyperpyrexia. Patient should be admitted to the intensive care unit and managed by a multidisciplinary team (anaesthetist, intensivist, endocrinologist, obstetrician, and neonatologist). The treatment of thyroid storm is summarized in Box 47.12.

Postpartum thyroiditis is the most common complication within the first 3 months after delivery, especially in Graves' disease. Therefore close monitoring of thyroid function tests is important during this period.

Hypothyroidism

Hypothyroidism has been defined as the presence of an elevated TSH concentration and is found in 2–3% of apparently healthy, non-pregnant women of childbearing age. It is estimated that 0.3–0.5% of these women have overt hypothyroidism with raised TSH and reduced free T_4, while 2–2.5% have subclinical hypothyroidism where TSH is elevated but free T_4 levels are normal.[90]

Deficiency in thyroid hormones is not compatible with normal health. Hashimoto thyroiditis is the most common cause of hypothyroidism in pregnant women. According to data

Box 47.11 Symptoms of thyroid storm

- Fever > 38°C
- Tachycardia > 130 beats/min
- Confusion
- Diarrhoea
- Jaundice
- Coma

Data from Braverman LE. Utiger RD. Introduction to thyrotoxicosis. In: Braverman LE, editor; Utiger RD, editor. Werner and Ingbar's *The Thyroid: A Fundamental and Clinical Text*. 9th. Lippincott, Williams and Wilkins; Philadelphia 2005; 453–455; and Patil-Sisodia K. Mestman JH. Grave's hyperthyroidism and pregnancy: a clinical update. *Endocr Pract* 2010; 16:118–129.

Box 47.12 Treatment of thyroid storm

- PTU (400–600 mg, followed by 150–300 mg every 6 h)—*first line*
- Potassium iodine IV or Lugol's solution orally—*second line*
- Corticosteroids
- Beta blockers
- Acetaminophen
- Cold fluids, cooling blankets

Data from Braverman LE. Utiger RD. Introduction to thyrotoxicosis. In: Braverman LE, editor; Utiger RD, editor. Werner and Ingbar's *The Thyroid: A Fundamental and Clinical Text.* 9th. Lippincott, Williams and Wilkins; Philadelphia 2005; 453–455; and Patil-Sisodia K. Mestman JH. Grave's hyperthyroidism and pregnancy: a clinical update. *Endocr Pract* 2010; 16:118–129.

from the United States, hypothyroidism affects up to 2.2% of pregnant women. Prevalence is higher in countries with iodine insufficiency.[91] Causes of hypothyroidism are found in Box 47.13.

Almost all patients with Hashimoto disease are positive for antithyroid peroxidase antibody. Of these patients, 50–70% also have positive results for antithyroglobulin antibodies. Over-treatment with antithyroid drugs can cause hypothyroidism, especially in the postpartum period. Overt maternal hypothyroidism is usually associated with infertility. Signs and symptoms of severe hypothyroidism are found in Box 47.14.

Hypothyroidism may also manifest itself with other conditions (Box 47.15).

Subclinical hypothyroidism has been associated with spontaneous abortion, preterm labour, increased risk for severe pre-eclampsia, developmental disease, and can influence children's intellect. Fetal self-sufficiency of thyroid hormones protects the fetus against brain development abnormalities caused by maternal hypothyroidism.[92]

If the mother suffers from autoimmune hypothyroidism, her antibodies could cross the placenta and destroy the fetal thyroid gland. Most children with isolated fetal hypothyroidism are without symptoms at birth, due to the presence of their mother's hormones. It is therefore important to recognize the disease and start with treatment as soon as possible after the birth. If the treatment has not been started on time the result may be permanent damage.[93]

Iodine deficiency is the most common cause of combined maternal and fetal hypothyroidism and endemic iodine deficiency remains a substantial public health problem in many parts of Europe, Asia, Africa, and South America.

Box 47.13 Common causes of hypothyroidism

- Autoimmune disease (Hashimoto thyroiditis)
- Surgical removal of the thyroid gland
- Post irradiation
- Congenital
- Lack of iodine in mother's diet
- Medication
- Inflammation

Data from Allan WC. Haddow JE. Palomaki GE. Williams JR. Mitchell ML. Hermos RJ. Faix JD. Klein RZ. Maternal thyroid deficiency and pregnancy complications: implications for population screening. *J Med Screen* 2000; 7:127–130.

Box 47.14 Symptoms and signs of severe hypothyroidism

- Anaemia
- Muscle pain
- Weakness
- Congestive heart failure
- Miscarriage
- Pre-eclampsia
- Placental abnormalities
- Low-birth-weight infants
- Postpartum haemorrhage

Data from *Thyroid Disease and Pregnancy 2012.* The American Thyroid Association. www.thyroid.org; and Stagnaro-Green A, Abalovich M, Alexander E, *et al.* Guidelines of the American Thyroid Association for the diagnosis and management of thyroid disease during pregnancy and postpartum. *Thyroid* 2011; 21(10):1081.

Obstetric management

The Endocrine Society recommends screening of all pregnant women for serum TSH abnormalities by 9 weeks of gestation or at the first prenatal visit.[94] Women at risk of developing hypothyroidism are those with a goitre, or prior treatment for hyperthyroidism or a positive family history of thyroid disease.

Box 47.15 Clinical manifestations of hypothyroidism

- Decreased intravascular volume
- Hypoglycaemia
- Anaemia
- Hyponatraemia
- Hypothermia
- Platelet dysfunction
- Abnormal coagulation factors
- Postpartum haemorrhage

Data from *Thyroid Disease and Pregnancy 2012.* The American Thyroid Association. www.thyroid.org; and Stagnaro-Green A, Abalovich M, Alexander E, *et al.* Guidelines of the American Thyroid Association for the diagnosis and management of thyroid disease during pregnancy and postpartum. *Thyroid* 2011; 21(10):1081.

Fetal thyroid dysfunction should be screened during pregnancy by ultrasound between the 18th to 22nd week of gestation and repeated every 4–6 weeks.

If hypothyroidism develops during pregnancy, treatment should be started immediately with levothyroxine. If iodine supplementation has been started in the third trimester, it will harm the developing fetus. Ideally, women with hypothyroidism should have their levothyroxine dose optimized prior to becoming pregnant. Women should increase their dose by 25–50% during pregnancy and check thyroid function every 6–8 weeks. After delivery, a woman may return to her usual prepregnancy dose.

Anaesthetic management

Epidural analgesia has been recommended for labour. If caesarean delivery has been indicated, NA with prehydration is the preferred choice. Coagulation should be assessed before initiation of neuraxial analgesia/anaesthesia. Administration of sedatives may cause respiratory depression. Ketamine might be a preferred induction agent for GA.[95] Volatile agents should be avoided because of potential myocardial depression. Opioids have not been recommended for postoperative pain relief in these patients.

Adrenal glands

The adrenal glands are endocrine glands located above the kidneys. The adrenal cortex and the adrenal medulla secrete different hormones. They are responsible for releasing hormones in response to stress (cortisol and catecholamines—epinephrine and norepinephrine), androgens, and aldosterone. These hormones exert their effect on every tissue in the body and under stressful conditions help them to maintain homeostasis.

The adrenal cortex produces glucocorticoids and mineralocorticoids. The release of glucocorticoids is triggered by the hypothalamus and pituitary gland. The hypothalamus produces CRH and it stimulates the pituitary gland to release adrenocorticotropic hormone (ACTH). ACTH than stimulates the adrenal cortex to produce hormones and release them in the bloodstream via a positive feedback system. Corticosteroids are involved into the metabolism of fat, carbohydrates, and proteins and also have an effect on the immune system by suppression of inflammatory reactions. Aldosterone regulates the level of sodium excreted into the urine and blood pressure. Androgen hormones are converted in the body to female hormones (oestrogens) and male hormones (androgens).[96]

The adrenal medulla secretes epinephrine (adrenaline) and norepinephrine (noradrenaline). Epinephrine is responsible for increasing heart rate, facilitates blood flow to the muscles and brain, causes relaxation of smooth muscles, and helps with conversion of glycogen to glucose in the liver. Epinephrine is critical in life-threatening situations as it rapidly prepares the body to spring into action. Norepinephrine has a strong vasoconstrictive effect, and thus increases blood pressure.

Pregnancy and adrenal glands

Pregnancy dramatically affects the HPA axis leading to increased circulating cortisol and ACTH levels during gestation.[97] The hormones reach levels similar to that in Cushing's syndrome (CS).The cause of increased secretion of ACTH may also be placental synthesis and release of CRH and ACTH, pituitary desensitization to cortisol feedback, or enhanced pituitary responses to corticotropin-releasing factors.[98]

Normal pregnancy is characterized by adaptation of the renin–angiotensin system (RAS) to increased demands upon the maternal circulation. Normal pregnant women retain 200–300 mEq of sodium, which results in an increase in extracellular fluid by 4–6 L.[99] Elevations in mineralocorticoid levels are necessary for maintenance of normal sodium balance and volume homeostasis.[100] In normal pregnancy, levels of plasma and urinary aldosterone rise and result in a 10- to 20-fold increase until the 38th week of gestation.

Ability to handle stress in pregnancy is preserved. Cortisol and ACTH levels are subsequently increased during the stress of labour. ACTH secretion is elevated 10-fold during labour and delivery. CRH concentrations fall rapidly after delivery.[101] Vaginal delivery is associated with a higher level of plasma cortisol when compared with caesarean delivery.[102] In the immediate postpartum period (within 2 hours), plasma CRH and ACTH tend to decrease to normal levels, whereas normalization of plasma cortisol levels is more protracted.

Cushing's syndrome

CS occurs in the presence of hypercortisolism. The most common cause is prolonged treatment with corticosteroids. This type of CS is called iatrogenic CS and can be a side effect of corticosteroid treatment of allergies, asthma, autoimmune diseases, and transplanted patients. Less common non-iatrogenic causes include excessive ACTH secretion or adrenal hypersecretion of cortisol independent of ACTH. Hypersecretion of ACTH can be induced by pituitary adenomas. A common cause of adrenal hypersecretion of cortisol is an adrenal cortex tumour.[103] The clinical manifestations of CS are found in Box 47.16.

Diagnosis

If CS is suspected, midnight plasma or salivary cortisol may be a better diagnostic alternative than morning levels. The dexamethasone 1 mg suppression test has limited utility in pregnancy. Ultrasound appears to be less sensitive for detecting small tumours, so MRI is recommended. Pituitary MRI should

Box 47.16 Clinical features of Cushing's syndrome

- Weight gain
- Hypertension
- Bruising
- Hypokalaemia
- Muscle weakness
- Pathological fractures
- Extensive purple abdominal striae
- Hirsutism
- Hyperglycaemia

Data from Lindsay JR, Nieman LK. The Hypothalamic-Pituitary-Adrenal Axis in Pregnancy: Challenges in Disease Detection and Treatment. *Endocr Rev* 2005; 26(6):775–799.

be obtained in all non-pregnant patients with ACTH-dependent CS.[104] MRI has been considered safe for pregnant women after 32 weeks of gestation. Surgical treatment of CS in pregnancy is recommended, except in the late third trimester, while medical treatment is preferable choice. Most patients undergo adrenalectomy, trans-sphenoidal surgery (for pituitary tumours), or receive medical therapy with metyrapone.[105,106]

Obstetric management

This disturbance is seen extremely rarely during pregnancy because it prevents normal follicular development and ovulation. The first case was reported by Hunt and McConahey in 1953 and some sporadic cases were reported later.[107] It is often not detected until 12–26 weeks' gestation. The most common complications of CS in pregnancy are hypertension and diabetes. Maternal death is rare. In a series of 136 pregnancies complicated by CS there were 107 (79%) live births, almost half of which were premature.[97]

Anaesthetic management

These patients are often hypertensive and hypervolaemic. Many of them are receiving long-term antihypertensive drugs. All antihypertensive agents have to be continued until the morning of surgery.[108]

Hyperglycaemia is problematic in these patients. The aim of the treatment is to maintain blood glucose levels within 7–10 mmol/L, using regular subcutaneous insulin.[109] Patients with CS are usually overweight. Obesity is often associated with hypertension, hyperglycaemia, and hypercoagulability. Therefore, prevention of perioperative venous thromboembolism and pulmonary embolism using low-molecular-weight heparin (LMWH) and compression of lower extremities must be provided. Care must be taken during positioning of the patient to prevent bone fractures and skin damage. The airway must be assessed properly because of the risk of difficult intubation caused by the buffalo hump. Arterial blood gases and pulmonary functional tests are useful to predict postoperative respiratory failure.

GA is usually required for laparoscopic adrenalectomy. Due to the risk of possible gastric aspiration, ranitidine 50 mg IV and sodium citrate should be administered orally prior to surgery. Standard and invasive monitoring of the patient is mandatory. Large-bore peripheral vein cannulae must be placed. Central vein cannulation should be considered. Antibiotic prophylaxis is necessary to prevent infection. Patients undergoing adrenalectomy may require intraoperative glucocorticoid replacement, for example, hydrocortisone 100 mg.

In the postoperative period, pulmonary atelectasis can be prevented by effective pain relief (patient-controlled analgesia or epidural) and physiotherapy. Early mobilization is recommended in order to avoid pulmonary embolism. Postoperative glucose, cortisol, and electrolyte levels must be routinely checked. Replacement therapy should be continued postoperatively.

Addison's disease (adrenal insufficiency)

Addison's disease in pregnancy is uncommon. It affects mostly the Caucasian population and its range varies from 39 to 117 per million.[110] Adrenal insufficiency (AI) can be primary, caused by damage of adrenal cortex. Atrophy or insult of the adrenal cortex results in impairment of aldosterone and/or cortisol secretion. Autoimmune adrenalitis and tuberculosis are the most common causes of primary AI. Secondary adrenal insufficiency is most commonly caused by discontinuation of glucocorticoids. Current asthma guidelines support the use of inhaled corticosteroids as opposed to oral steroids for treatment in pregnancy due to less systemic absorption and therefore reduced likelihood of suppression of the adrenals.[111] Less frequently, ACTH deficiency may be caused by pituitary insufficiency or tumours. Pregnancies in women with panhypopituitarism should be considered high risk.[112] The signs and symptoms of Addison's disease are found in Box 47.17.

Diagnosis

Urinary and plasma cortisol and aldosterone levels are low or undetectable in these patients. Severe hyponatraemia and hyperkalaemia are present, as well as unexplained orthostatic hypotension. Adrenal antibodies can be present in some cases. There is no reliable diagnostic test for use in pregnancy. If a diagnosis has been made during pregnancy, it is necessary to confirm it after the first week postpartum. Patients with positive adrenal antibodies have an autoimmune aetiology and do not require imaging.[113] Ultrasound imaging has limited resolution, especially during pregnancy. Therefore, MRI without gadolinium administration is recommended.

Obstetric management

Treatment includes mineralocorticoid and/or corticosteroid replacement therapy in the antenatal period, during labour, and in the postpartum period. An endocrinologist, obstetrician, and experienced surgeon should provide multidisciplinary management. Surgery, if necessary, may be postponed to the postpartum period in selected cases. The second trimester is the optimal time to perform surgery. During the first and the second trimesters, careful monitoring and titration of therapy is required to avoid corticosteroid over-replacement, and in women with coexisting T1D, to prevent recurrent hypoglycaemia. Hydrocortisone is the recommended choice due to its inactivation by the placenta. Replacement dose of hydrocortisone varies between 20 and 25 mg.[114] The total daily dose is usually divided into two doses: two-thirds in the morning and

Box 47.17 Signs and symptoms of adrenal insufficiency

- Excessive fatigue
- Malaise
- Weight loss
- Vomiting
- Biochemical disturbances
- Seizures
- Mental confusion

Data from Lebbe M, Arlt W. What is the best diagnostic and therapeutic management strategy for an Addison patient during pregnancy? *Clin Endocrinol* 2013; 78:497–502.

one-third in the afternoon. Mineralocorticoids are required only in primary Addison's disease at the time of diagnosis. Mineralocorticoid dosages are usually stable throughout pregnancy, but sometimes doses are reduced during the third trimester to avoid the side effects of oedema or exacerbation of hypertension.

Anaesthetic management

Vaginal delivery should be offered to women with Addison's disease. The oral dose of hydrocortisone should be doubled during labour in these patients. Patients undergoing caesarean delivery should be given stress doses of hydrocortisone: 100 mg IV or intramuscularly, before induction of anaesthesia followed by 100 mg IV at 6- to 8-hour intervals after delivery for the first 48 hours.

Adrenal crisis

Adrenal crisis is often associated with hypotension, hypoglycaemia, or coma. Hydrocortisone bolus 100–200 mg IV is required, followed by 50–100 mg IV every 6–8 hours. Infusion of 5% dextrose or saline is also recommended.

Phaeochromocytoma

Most phaeochromocytomas (90%) are adrenal medullary tumours, characterized by excessive production of catecholamines. A phaeochromocytoma can develop at any age and may be life-threatening if unrecognized or untreated. The prevalence of phaeochromocytomas in patients with hypertension is only 0.1–0.6%.[115] Most phaeochromocytomas are benign and unilateral. The signs and symptoms of phaeochromocytoma are found in Box 47.18.

Obstetric management

The reported incidence is less than 0.2/10,000 pregnancies.[116] Untreated phaeochromocytomas carry a risk of mortality for both mother and fetus, as high as 58%.[117] Conversely, early detection and proper treatment during pregnancy decrease the maternal and fetal mortality to less than 5% and 15% respectively.[118] Pregnancy limits diagnostic imaging methods. Tumour activity may be triggered by the enlarging uterus. If hypertension develops in a pregnant woman in the first 20 weeks' gestation, it could be misdiagnosed as gestational hypertension or pre-eclampsia. On the other hand, the presence of unexplained orthostatic hypotension in a pregnant hypertensive patient should arouse immediate suspicion of a phaeochromocytoma.[119,120]

Box 47.18 Symptoms of phaeochromocytoma

- Hypertension
- Sweating
- Pallor
- Palpitations
- Headache
- Tachycardia
- Flushing
- Anxiety
- Weight loss

Data from Lenders JW, Eisenhofer G, Mannelli M, Pacak K. Phaeochromocytoma. *Lancet* 2005; 36:665–675.

Diagnosis

Blood and urine metanephrines testing are diagnostic methods of choice.[121] Sensitivity of plasma-free metanephrines varies between 95% and 100%. Some authors prefer ultrasound imaging. MRI is increasingly being used in diagnosis of phaeochromocytoma with a sensitivity of greater than 90%. Genetic tests could be useful, especially in cases with a positive family history of phaeochromocytoma.[122]

Surgery

The best treatment for most phaeochromocytomas is surgery. Before surgery alpha- and beta blockers have been used to treat high blood pressure.

Alpha blockers (phenoxybenzamine, prazosin, and terazosin) exert their activity by preventing the vasoconstriction caused by norepinephrine and thus reduce blood pressure. Phenoxybenzamine is a non-competitive alpha-1- and alpha-2-adrenoceptor antagonist. The recommended starting dose is 10 mg twice a day. The dose should be increased at 2–3-day intervals by 20 mg up to a final dose of 1 mg/kg per day. Its prolonged action after tumour removal may be predisposing factor of postoperative hypotension.[123] Phenoxybenzamine crosses the placenta and neonates must be monitored for the first few postnatal days, because of possible hypotension and respiratory depression.[124] Doxazosin is an effective alternative to phenoxybenzamine. The recommended initial dose of doxazosin should be gradually increased from 2 mg to 16 mg, up to 32 mg per day.[125]

Beta blockers (atenolol, metoprolol, and propranolol) exert their effects by blocking norepinephrine, preventing arrhythmias and inhibiting the release of renin from kidneys. Beta-adrenergic blockade should be started a few days after appropriate alpha-adrenergic blockade in order to prevent a hypertensive crisis.[126] Both propranolol (40mg three times daily) and atenolol (25–50 mg once daily) are considered suitable for this purpose.

Box 47.19 Drug therapy for management of hypertension during phaeochromocytoma surgery

- Sodium nitroprusside (initially 0.5–1.5 mcg/kg/min, maintenance 3–5 mcg/kg/min)
- Phentolamine boluses of 1–2 mg
- Nitroglycerine

Data from Lenders JW, Eisenhofer G, Mannelli M, Pacak K. Phaeochromocytoma. *Lancet* 2005; 366:665–675; Boutros AR, Bravo EL, Zanettin G, Straffon RA. Perioperative management of 63 patients with phaeochromocytoma. *Cleveland Clinic Journal of Medicine* 1990; 57:613–617; Weingarten TN, Cata JP, O'Hara JF, *et al.* Comparison of two preoperative medical management strategies for laparoscopic redelivery of phaeochromocytoma. *Urology* 2010; 76:508–511.

Box 47.20 Drug therapy for management of tachycardia during phaeochromocytoma surgery

- Beta blockers:
  - Esmolol 500 mcg or 50–200 mcg/kg/min
  - Metoprolol 1–2 mg
  - Atenolol 2.5–10 mg
  - Propranolol 1–10 mg
  - Labetalol 0.25 mg/kg up to 20 mg over a period of 10 min
- Calcium channel blockers: amlodipine, nifedipine, verapamil, or diltiazem
- Magnesium sulphate: bolus 40–60 mg/kg, maintenance 1–2 g/h

Data from Lenders JW, Eisenhofer G, Mannelli M, Pacak K. Phaeochromocytoma. *Lancet* 2005; 366:665–675; Boutros AR, Bravo EL, Zanettin G, Straffon RA. Perioperative management of 63 patients with phaeochromocytoma. *Cleveland Clinic Journal of Medicine* 1990; 57:613–617; Weingarten TN, Cata JP, O'Hara JF, *et al.* Comparison of two preoperative medical management strategies for laparoscopic redelivery of phaeochromocytoma. *Urology* 2010; 76:508–511.

Anaesthetic management

A multidisciplinary team consisting of an anaesthetist, endocrinologist, cardiologist, obstetrician, and surgeon should arrange a management plan to reduce risks in perioperative care. Surgical removal of phaeochromocytoma is usually performed by laparoscopy or laparotomy. If the tumour has been diagnosed during the first 24 weeks of gestation, it should be removed by laparoscopic adrenalectomy, after 10–14 days of medical preparation. The second trimester is the safest period to perform surgery in pregnancy.[127] Hypertension may persist after the surgical treatment in almost 50% of patients. The tumour recurrence rate during follow-up has been estimated to be 14% in adrenal disease and 30% in extra-adrenal disease.[128]

If the tumour is still *in situ*, caesarean delivery with immediate tumour removal is the best option, because catecholamine release and intra-abdominal pressure are higher in vaginal labour. The best anaesthesia option is a combination of GA and epidural. Hypotension should be avoided, if possible.

Box 47.21 Drug therapy for treatment of post-resection hypotension during phaeochromocytoma surgery

- Norepinephrine
- Dopamine
- Phenylephrine

Data from Lenders JW, Eisenhofer G, Mannelli M, Pacak K. Phaeochromocytoma. *Lancet* 2005; 366:665–675; Boutros AR, Bravo EL, Zanettin G, Straffon RA. Perioperative management of 63 patients with phaeochromocytoma. *Cleveland Clinic Journal of Medicine* 1990; 57:613–617; Weingarten TN, Cata JP, O'Hara JF, *et al.* Comparison of two preoperative medical management strategies for laparoscopic redelivery of phaeochromocytoma. *Urology* 2010; 76:508–511.

Box 47.22 Perioperative corticosteroid therapy in patients with phaeochromocytoma

- Prior to surgery: methylprednisolone 40 mg IV
- On the day of surgery: 40 mg (three times a day)
- Postoperative day 1: 20 mg (three times a day)
- Postoperative day 2: 10 mg (three times a day)
- Postoperative day 3: prednisone 5 mg orally + fludrocortisone 0.1 mg in the morning and prednisone 25 mg orally in the evening

Data from Lenders JW, Eisenhofer G, Mannelli M, Pacak K. Phaeochromocytoma. *Lancet* 2005; 366:665–675.

- Phenoxybenzamine should be withdrawn 48 hours prior to surgery. Alpha-adrenergic blockers therapy should be stopped the night before surgery.
- If surgery is performed on both glands, corticosteroid therapy should be started before the surgery.
- Premedication with an anxiolytic (benzodiazepine) is advised, but the neonatologist should be informed.
- Two large-bore IV cannulae, an arterial line for continuous monitoring of blood pressure, and central venous catheter for intravascular volume monitoring should be inserted preoperatively.
- A GA or a GA combined with epidural anaesthesia can be started. Intraoperative epidural analgesia can be achieved with an initial bolus of 10 mL bupivacaine 0.25% in divided doses, followed by a continuous infusion of bupivacaine (0.1%) and opiate (e.g. fentanyl 2 mcg/mL) at a rate of 6–12 mL/h.
- The hypertensive response to laryngoscopy should be avoided during induction of GA (as this may cause intracranial haemorrhage and myocardial failure).
- After the tumour has been removed, blood glucose and blood pressure may fall. Therefore, the infusion of glucose is necessary at the end of surgery. Hypotension should be treated by sympathomimetic adrenergic stimulation or vasoconstrictor drugs.
- These patients should be managed postoperatively in the intensive care unit.

Boxes 47.19, 47.20, and 47.21, summarize drugs which may be useful in controlling blood pressure and tachycardia. Perioperative steroids are necessary and a suggested regimen can be found in Box 47.22.

Autoimmune diseases in pregnancy

Immunological response changes during normal pregnancy by transient immune tolerance of maternal cell-mediated immunity to protect the fetus, a genetically foreign body, from rejection. It was originally thought that the immune response was diminished, but recent data show that the change of ratio and function of leucocytes is the possible mechanism of reduced autoimmunity in pregnancy.

Immunomodulatory T-helper cells and their cytokines are found to be associated with pregnancy outcome. Type 1 CD4+ T cells (Th1) produce inflammatory cytokines including interferon-gamma (IFN-γ), interleukin (IL)-2, and TNF-α. Type 2 CD4+ T cells (Th2) produce IL-4, IL-5, IL-13, IL-10, and IL-6. Th 1 and Th 2 ratio play an important role in immunological maternal responses in early pregnancy.

Th1 cytokine domination and lack of adequate Th2 type response are associated with a greater incidence of miscarriages. Activation of the proinflammatory Th1 profile in late pregnancy may provoke preterm labour. Autoimmune diseases with predominant Th1 response, such as rheumatoid arthritis (RA), may improve during pregnancy. On the other hand, diseases with predominant Th2 response (e.g. systemic lupus erythematosus (SLE)) tend to worsen.[129,130]

Production of maternal alloantibodies to paternally inherited fetal HLA is the expected immune process during pregnancy. Mothers who carry histocompatible fetuses are at higher risk of pregnancy loss, due to lack of alloantibodies. Maternal alloantibodies against the trophoblast and its products may activate complement cascade. Complement activation is important in the pathogenesis of pre-eclampsia.

Successful pregnancy outcome depends on the balance of Th1/Th2-type lymphocytes response. The imbalance in the Th1/Th2 response could provoke an increase in natural killer (NK) cell levels. NK cells produce numerous proinflammatory cytokines (TNF-α, IFN-γ, and IL-10), which can cause recurrent spontaneous abortion.

Rheumatoid arthritis

RA is a chronic autoimmune disorder that mostly affects synovial joints. The immune response is directed against an individual's own tissues, such as tendons, bones, lung, and kidney, resulting in inflammation and destruction. Extra-articular manifestations include vasculitis, subcutaneous nodules, pericarditis, peripheral neuropathy, lung disease, anaemia, and thrombocytosis. Progression of disease results in destruction of articular cartilage, ankylosis of the joints, and organ insufficiency.

The prevalence of RA is about 1% and increases with age. Onset is usually slow, over weeks or even months. Older age and female gender are risk factors both for the development of RA and for a worse outcome. It has been suggested that the largest genetic susceptibility to LA is associated with the *HLA-DRB1* gene.[131] Presence of antibodies against citrullinated peptides (ACPA) and rheumatoid factor (RF) precedes the development of clinical RA in genetically susceptible persons. Rheumatoid inflammation is mediated by activated pro-inflammatory Th1 cells. Immunomodulatory Th2 cells and their cytokines are rarely found.[132]

Influence of pregnancy on RA

Immune tolerance in pregnancy is probably the most important factor of improvement of clinical symptoms and signs of RA. It is estimated that in 70% of patients, improvement of clinical signs or even remission have been found during pregnancy. Disparity in maternal and paternally inherited *HLA-DRB1* and *HLA-DQα* alleles is associated with improvement of the disease. Pregnancy-induced immune response towards an anti-inflammatory Th2 profile has been also suggested to have positive effects on RA symptoms.[133] Evidence suggesting that pregnancy may decrease the risk of RA is still controversial. On the other hand, exacerbation of the disease has been observed postpartum.

Influence of RA on pregnancy outcomes

There are insufficient data of impact of RA on pregnancy outcomes. However, some authors suggest an increase in the rate of premature and small for gestational age infants in women diagnosed with RA.[134]

Treatment of RA in pregnancy

The use of corticosteroids and non-steroidal anti-inflammatory drugs (NSAIDs) is approved in pregnancy, although the latter is stopped in the third trimester due to potential closure of the patent ductus arteriosus. Glucocorticoids modulate the immune response. They are the most potent inhibitors of pro-inflammatory cytokines and promote Th2 response. Cytostatic agents (methotrexate and leflunomide) and biologics (anti-TNF agents, rituximab, and abatacept) are not recommended for use in pregnancy.[135]

Anaesthetic management of RA

NA for caesarean delivery is the preferable choice for RA patients. Some patients may find positioning for spinal or epidural insertion difficult due to limited or painful movement of the spine. Long-term treatment with NSAIDs has not been associated with higher risk of epidural haematoma.[136] If GA is performed, there is higher risk of atlanto- axial subluxation during intubation. In patients with temporomandibular joint involvement, mouth opening is restricted. Neck flexion or extension can also be restricted, making intubation challenging. Further details of anaesthetic management can be found in Chapter 46.

Scleroderma

Systemic sclerosis (SS; systemic scleroderma) is an autoimmune disorder of connective tissue. Endothelial cells along with muscle cells of the small blood vessels (arterioles) in the skin and other organs have been destroyed by programmed cell death (apoptosis). These cells have been replaced by collagen. Further damage of the tissue is caused by inflammatory cell infiltration.

Scleroderma occurs predominantly in women and can be divided into two types—limited cutaneous scleroderma and diffuse cutaneous scleroderma. In limited cutaneous scleroderma, the severity of skin fibrosis is more important than the duration of the disease. Skin manifestations include Raynaud's phenomena, non-pitting oedema, and 'tight' skin. Diffuse cutaneous scleroderma is associated with organ involvement: the kidney, heart, and particularly lung.[137] In the severe disease, there may be renal insufficiency, cardiomyopathy, malignant hypertension, pericarditis, arrhythmia, pulmonary fibrosis, and malabsorption.[138] The aetiology of SS remains unknown but numerous risk factors have been suggested including various environmental agents, genetic influences, viruses, and more recently, microchimerism. Microchimerism is the presence of an increased number of circulating cells transferred from fetus to mother. These fetal cells lie dormant in the mother for many years and then initiate a host-versus-graft reaction.[139]

Pregnancy and scleroderma

There is a relative paucity of literature concerning pregnancy and scleroderma. Women with scleroderma tend to have successful pregnancies. Adverse pregnancy outcomes have been associated with severity of the disease. There is increased frequency of miscarriages, preterm births, and small-for-date babies. Careful antenatal surveillance is needed in these patients. Pregnancy does not seem to affect long-term prognosis of women with scleroderma.[140]

Anaesthetic management

Multidisciplinary evaluation of the patient should be done prior to labour and delivery. Examination and investigation should be directed towards detection of underlying systemic dysfunction. An electrocardiogram (ECG) and an echocardiogram should be performed to assess cardiac function which, if reduced, may preclude NA. The skin over the lumbar area is usually devoid of the fibrous contractures so spinal, CSE anaesthesia, and epidural anaesthesia may be used with caution. Spinal anaesthesia is associated with higher risk of hypotension due to relative hypovolaemia and chronic vasoconstriction. If epidural anaesthesia is used, prolongation of motor and sensory blockade can be expected because of poor blood flow to the neural tissue and reduced local anaesthetic uptake. Patients with SS have been thought to be at a greater risk of difficult airway and/or difficult intubation, due to neck flexion contractures and restricted mouth opening. An awake fibreoptic intubation will be necessary if NA is contraindicated or unsuccessful.[141]

Systemic lupus erythematosus

SLE is an autoimmune disease which may affect different organs and connective tissue in the whole body. It is more common in women of childbearing age. The course of SLE is unpredictable, with periods of remissions and relapses. Prognosis of SLE ranges from relatively benign to rapidly progressive and even fatal disease. The highest rates of prevalence have been reported in Italy, Spain, Martinique, and the United Kingdom, especially in the Afro-Caribbean population.[142]

SLE can involve the nervous system, lungs, kidneys, heart, blood vessels, liver, skin, and joints.[143] Lupus may imitate other diseases making the diagnosis extremely difficult. The signs and symptoms of SLE are summarized in Box 47.23.

These patients also have increased mortality from comorbidities such as infections, DM, atherosclerosis, coronary disease, lipid disorders, and malignancy.[144]

SLE is an illness of unknown aetiology. This autoimmune disease is characterized by the presence of antinuclear antibodies (ANAs) or anti-double-stranded DNA (dsDNA) antibodies. Acute lupus often flares following bacterial infections. Chronic infections may also induce lupus-like symptoms. Invading pathogens stimulate the immune system to proliferation and production of autoantibodies against the cell's nucleus.[145–147] Immune complexes form deposits in the microvasculature, on the basement membranes of skin and kidneys.

All patients with SLE are found to have serum ANAs. However, antibodies to native dsDNA are relatively specific for the diagnosis of SLE.[148,149]

Box 47.23 Symptoms and signs of SLE

- Musculoskeletal:
  - Myalgia
  - Fatigue
  - Fever
  - Arthralgia
- Skin and mucosal:
  - Face rash—butterfly rash
  - Discoid skin lesion
  - Dry eyes
  - Skin and mucosal ulcers
- Lungs:
  - Shortness of breath
  - Chest pain
- Heart:
  - Endocarditis
  - Myocarditis
  - Pericarditis
- Renal:
  - Proteinuria
  - Haematuria
  - Lupus nephritis
- Neurological:
  - Headaches
  - Polyneuropathy
  - Cerebrovascular disease
- Psychiatric:
  - Depression
  - Psychosis
  - Cognitive dysfunction
  - Anxiety disorder
- Haematology:
  - Low white cell count
  - Low platelets
  - Anaemia

Data from *Harrison's Internal Medicine, 17th ed.* Chapter 313. Systemic Lupus Erythematosus. Accessmedicine.com. Retrieved 2011-08-06.

Diagnosis

The American College of Rheumatology (ACR) has recommended criteria for SLE diagnosis, revised in 2012. According to this classification, SLE is diagnosed if the person has had biopsy-proven lupus nephritis with ANAs or anti-dsDNA antibodies or if four of the 11 diagnostic criteria, including at least one clinical and one immunological criterion, have been satisfied.[150] Increased levels of anti-dsDNA and decreased levels of complement (C3, C4, CH50) are specific for lupus flare. Diagnostic tests for SLE in pregnancy are listed in Box 47.24.

Box 47.24 Diagnostic tests for SLE in pregnancy

- Increased anti-dsDNA levels
- Positive direct Coombs' test
- Red blood cells in the urine
- Antiplatelet antibodies in thrombocytopenic pregnant women
- Complement level—not specific in pregnancy due to oestrogen-induced synthesis

Data from Bertsias G, Ioannidis JP, Boletis J, *et al.* EULAR recommendations for the management of systemic lupus erythematosus. Report of a Task Force of the EULAR Standing Committee for International Clinical Studies Including Therapeutics. *Ann Rheum Dis* 2008; 67(2):195–205.

Obstetric management

Pregnant women with SLE should be managed by a multidisciplinary team including a rheumatologist, obstetrician, and, if necessary, a nephrologist, neurologist, haematologist, cardiologist, and respiratory physician. Thrombophilia is often present. It is necessary to check platelets and other coagulation tests. Mild elevations of serum creatinine and blood pressure may be precursors of impending complications during pregnancy and daily proteinuria which exceeds approximately 200 mg is significant.[151] Pregnancy produces an environment of immune suppression in order to prevent fetal rejection, but cellular and humoral function has been modulated rather than suppressed. Diagnosis of SLE in pregnancy is a challenge for obstetricians. Many of these symptoms can be seen in normal pregnancy (e.g. backache, swollen ankles, and arthralgia). Pre-eclampsia and eclampsia can mimic lupus. Expectant mothers with lupus have a greater likelihood of miscarriage, intrauterine growth retardation, preterm birth, and intrauterine death. Lupus tends to worsen during pregnancy. However, maternal death is uncommon in pregnancies complicated by SLE. It can occur if active renal or central nervous system disease has been involved.

Fetal outcome

This depends on placental pathology: ischaemia/hypoxia, decidual vasculopathy, decidual and fetal thrombi, chronic villitis, decreased placental weight and placental infarctions along with deposits of fibrin, immunoglobulin (Ig)-G, IgM, IgA, and C3 in the trophoblastic membrane.[152,153]

Previous history of lupus nephritis is not a contraindication to pregnancy, particularly if conception occurs 6 month after the nephritis. Patients with lupus nephritis with a previous renal transplant can have successful outcomes.[154]

Immunosuppressive medication required to control lupus disease should be continued despite a risk of minor fetal anomalies.[155] Corticosteroids are relatively safe. Prednisolone is the first-line treatment. Although methotrexate has been contraindicated, azathioprine, ciclosporin, and sulfasalazine might be used in combination with immunoglobulin therapy.[156] The presence of ANAs can produce congenital heart block. Thus, some tests should be performed at birth to exclude neonatal lupus (Box 47.25). Sun exposure is best avoided in infants of mothers with SLE.

Box 47.25 Tests for neonates if the mother has SLE

- ECG
- Complete blood count
- Alkaline phosphatase test
- Transaminases

Data from Buyon JP, Clancy RM. Neonatal lupus: review of proposed pathogenesis and clinical data from the US-based Research Registry for Neonatal Lupus. *Autoimmunity* 2003; 36:41–50.

Anaesthetic management

SLE parturients are likely to be on unfractionated heparin or LMWH and anticoagulation should be discontinued prior to delivery. Mode of delivery depends on the condition of the mother and baby. Delivery can be performed by the vaginal or caesarean route. Epidural and spinal analgesia has been considered safe for delivery provided sufficient time has elapsed between the heparin and epidural/spinal insertion (see Chapter 48). GA can be used in emergency situations.[157,158]

Corticosteroid therapy should be withdrawn gradually postpartum together with reintroduction of immunosuppressive therapy. Anticoagulant therapy should be continued for 3 months after the delivery. Breastfeeding is not recommended for these mothers.

Antiphospholipid syndrome

Antiphospholipid syndrome (APS), also known as Hughes syndrome, is an autoimmune, hypercoagulable state, characterized by anticardiolipin antibodies and beta-2 glycoprotein I. APS causes non-traumatic thrombosis or thromboembolism, stroke, unexplained transient ischaemic attacks (including amaurosis fugax), autoimmune thrombocytopaenia, autoimmune haemolytic anaemia, and neurological and behavioural dysfunction. Antiphospholipid (APL) antibodies react against proteins on plasma membranes. Destruction of APL antibodies activates coagulation and produces blood clots in any organ system. APS has been commonly associated with other similar diseases, such as SLE (with which it shares many features).[159] During infectious disease processes (viral, bacterial, spirochetal, or parasitic) the disruption of cellular membranes may stimulate APL antibody production.

Diagnosis

Diagnostic criteria include one clinical and one laboratory positive test (anticardiolipin antibodies, lupus anticoagulant, and/or anti-beta-2-glycoprotein I antibodies).[160,161] Patients with all three positive tests have been at greater risk for clinical events (thrombosis or pregnancy loss), when compared with patients with only one or two positive tests.[162] Activated partial thromboplastin time is prolonged but there is no evidence of coagulopathy.

Obstetric management

Pregnant women with APS should be considered high-risk obstetric patients as they can have many complications (Box 47.26).

The rate of fetal loss due to placental infarction may exceed 90% in untreated patients with APS. Fetal ultrasonography has been

Box 47.26 Effects of APL antibodies on pregnancy

APL antibodies may cause:

- Miscarriage
- Stillbirth
- Preterm delivery
- Severe pre-eclampsia

Data from Cowchock FS, Reece EA, Balaban D, Branch DW, Plouffe L. Repeated fetal losses associated with antiphospholipid antibodies: a collaborative randomized trial comparing prednisone with low-dose heparin treatment. *Am J Obstet Gynecol* 1992; 166(5):1318–23.

recommended monthly starting at 18–20 weeks of pregnancy. It is recommended to assess the presence of fetal growth retardation at 30–32 weeks of gestation. Multiorgan failure (Asherson's syndrome) has been described in pregnancy and during the postpartum period.[163,164]

A low dose of aspirin combined with prophylactic doses of LMWH have been recommended if there have not been thrombotic episodes in the past. Patients with a history of thrombotic episodes should be treated with therapeutic doses of LMWH—it can reduce the rate of fetal loss up to 25%. Splenectomy has been recommended in patients who suffer from the chronic form of idiopathic thrombocytopenic purpura.

Anaesthetic management

The management of a patient with APS is not dissimilar to that of patient with SLE. The presence of lupus anticoagulant antibodies is not a contraindication for RA. Patients receiving anticoagulant therapy with heparins can receive NA provided an appropriate period has elapsed since the last dose of heparin (see Chapter 48).

In patients receiving or recently treated with corticosteroid therapy, supplementation is needed to cover the labour or caesarean delivery. Anticoagulant prophylaxis has to be continued for 6 weeks after the delivery.[165]

Conclusion

Pregnancy itself influences specific endocrine changes caused by development of the fetoplacental unit. The function of this unique endocrine organ stimulates metabolic changes which can mimic endocrine diseases. Endocrine diseases, such as diabetes and thyroid disease, are not uncommon in pregnancy. If endocrine diseases remain untreated, they can have adverse effects on both mother and fetus. Therefore, early recognition and appropriate treatment during pregnancy is essential for good pregnancy outcome.

Immunological response is modulated during normal pregnancy and the course of autoimmune disease might be altered. RA may improve during pregnancy while SLE tends to worsen. Pregnant women with autoimmune disease are considered high risk. The rate of fetal loss is higher in these patients, especially in APS.

Every anaesthetist should have the basic knowledge of pathophysiology, diagnostic tests, and treatment of endocrine and autoimmune diseases. Anaesthetic management of these patients has significant differences when compared with healthy parturients.

References

1. Wild S, Roglic G, Green A, *et al.* Global prevalence of diabetes: estimates for the year 2000 and projections for 2030. *Diabetes Care* 2004; 27:1047–53.
2. Fleming DM, Schellevis FG, Van Casteren V. The prevalence of known diabetes in eight European countries. *Eur J Public Health* 2004; 14:10–14.
3. Lambert AP, Gillespie KM, Thomson G, *et al.* Absolute risk of childhood-onset type 1 diabetes defined by human leukocyte antigen class II genotype: a population-based study in the United Kingdom. *J Clin Endocrinol Metab* 2004; 89:4037–43.
4. Gillespie KM, Gale EA, Bingley PJ. High familial risk and genetic susceptibility in early onset childhood diabetes. *Diabetes* 2002; 51:210–14.
5. Noble JA, Valdes AM, Cook M, *et al.* The role of HLA class II genes in insulin-dependent diabetes mellitus: molecular analysis of 180 Caucasian, multiplex families. *Am J Hum Genet* 1996; 59(5):1134–48.
6. Hyttinen V, Kaprio J, Kinnunen L, *et al.* Genetic liability of type 1 diabetes and the onset age among 22,650 young Finnish twin pairs: a nationwide follow-up study. *Diabetes* 2003; 52:1052–5.
7. Harjutsalo V, Lammi N, Karvonen M, *et al.* Age at onset of type 1 diabetes in parents and recurrence risk in offspring. *Diabetes* 2010; 59(1):210–14.
8. Harjutsalo V, Reunanen A, Tuomilehto J. Differential transmission of type 1 diabetes from diabetic fathers and mothers to their offspring. *Diabetes* 2006; 55:1517–24.
9. Koczwara K, Bonifacio E, Ziegler AG. Transmission of maternal islet antibodies and risk of autoimmune diabetes in offspring of mothers with type 1 diabetes. *Diabetes* 2004; 53(1):1–4.
10. Redondo MJ, Yu L, Hawa M, *et al.* Heterogeneity of type I diabetes: analysis of monozygotic twins in Great Britain and the United States. *Diabetologia* 2001; 44:354–62.
11. Von Herrath M, Sanda S, Herold K. Type 1 diabetes as a relapsing-remitting disease? *Nat Rev Immunol* 2007; 7:988–94.
12. Achenbach P, Bonifacio E, Kocwara K, *et al.* Natural history of type 1 diabetes. *Diabetes* 2005; 54(2):25–30.
13. Pociot F, Norgaard K, Hobolth N, *et al.* A nationwide population-based study of the familial aggregation of type 1 (insulin dependent) diabetes mellitus in Denmark: Danish Study Group of Diabetes in Childhood. *Diabetologia* 1993; 36:870–5.
14. Stanley HM, Norris JM, Barriga K, *et al.* Is presence of islet autoantibodies at birth associated with development of persistent islet autoimmunity? The Diabetes Autoimmunity Study in the Young (DAISY). *Diabetes Care* 2004; 27:497–502.
15. Barker JM, Barriga KJ, Yu L, *et al.* Prediction of autoantibody and progression to type 1 diabetes: Diabetes Autoimmunity Study in the Young (DAISY). *J Clin Endocrinol Metab* 2004; 89:3896–902.
16. Peng H, Hagopian W. Environmental factors in the development of type 1 diabetes. *Rev Endocr Metab Disord* 2006; 7(3):149–62.
17. Coppieteters KT, Boettler T, Von Herrath M. Virus infections in type 1 diabetes. *Cold Spring Harb Perspect Med* 2012; 2(1):a007682.
18. Wasmuth HE, Kolb H. Cow's milk and immune-mediated diabetes. *Proc Nutr Soc* 2000; 59(4):573–9.
19. Ziegler A, Schmid S, Huber D, *et al.* Early infant feeding and risk of developing type 1 diabetes-associated autoantibodies. *JAMA* 2003; 290(13):1721–8.
20. Herder C, Roden M. Genetics of type 2 diabetes: pathophysiologic and clinical relevance. *Eur J Clin Inves* 2011; 41(6):679–92.
21. Newman B, Selby JV, King MC, *et al.* Concordance for type 2 (non-insulin-dependent) diabetes mellitus in male twins. *Diabetologia* 1987; 30(10):763–8.
22. Medici F, Hawa M, Ianari A, *et al.* Concordance rate for type II diabetes mellitus in monozygotic twins: actuarial analysis. *Diabetologia* 1999; 42(2):146–50.
23. Lebovitz HE. Insulin resistance: definition and consequences. *Exp Clin Endocrinol Diabetes* 2001; 109(2):S135–48.

24. The Expert Committee on the Diagnosis and Classification of Diabetes Mellitus: Report of the Expert Committee on the Diagnosis and Classification of Diabetes Mellitus. *Diabetes Care* 1997; 20:1183–97.
25. Hoffman L, Nolan C, Wilson JD, *et al.* Gestational diabetes mellitus—management guidelines. The Australasian Diabetes in Pregnancy Society. *Med J Aust* 1998; 169(2):93–7.
26. Working group on gestational diabetes. National guidelines for gestational diabetes. *Duodecim* 2008; 124:1556–69.
27. Shaat N, Groop L. Genetics of gestational diabetes mellitus. *Curr Med Chem* 2007; 14(5):569–83.
28. Watanabe RM. Inherited destiny? Genetics and gestational diabetes mellitus *Genome Med* 2011; 3:18.
29. Genuth S, Alberti KG, Bennett P, *et al.* Follow-up report on the diagnosis of diabetes mellitus. *Diabetes Care* 2003; 26:3160–7.
30. Mahmud M, Mazza D. Preconception care of women with diabetes: a review of current guideline recommendations. *BMC Women's Health* 2010; 10:5.
31. National Institute of Health and Care Excellence. *Diabetes in Pregnancy: Management from Preconception to the Postnatal Period.* NICE Guidelines NG3. London: NICE; 2015. http://www.nice.org.uk/guidance/ng3
32. terBraak EW, Evers IM, Willem Erkelens D, *et al.* Maternal hypoglycemia during pregnancy in type 1 diabetes: maternal and fetal consequences. *Diabetes Metab Res Rev* 2002; 18(2):96–105.
33. Wolfsdorf J, Craig ME, Daneman D, *et al.* Diabetic ketoacidosis in children and adolescents with diabetes. *Pediatr Diabet* 2009: 10 Suppl 12: 118–33.
34. Savage MW, Dhatariya KK, Kilvert A, *et al.* Joint British Diabetes Societies guideline for the management of diabetic ketoacidosis. *Diabetic Med* 2011; 28(5):508–15.
35. Impe JV. Pregnancy and its effect on the progression of diabetic retinopathy. *MJM* 2005; 8(2):142–8.
36. Nielsen LR, Damm P, Mathiesen ER. Improved pregnancy outcome in type 1 diabetic women with microalbuminuria or diabetic nephropathy: effect of intensified antihypertensive therapy? *Diabetes Care* 2009; 32(1):38–44.
37. Mathiesen ER, Ringholm L, Feldt-Rasmussen B, *et al.* Obstetric nephrology: pregnancy in women with diabetic nephropathy—the role of antihypertensive treatment *CJASN* 2012; 7:2081–8, 2012.
38. Bonifacio E, Pflüger M, Marienfeld S, *et al.* Maternal type 1 diabetes reduces the risk of islet autoantibodies: relationships with birthweight and maternal HbA(1c). *Diabetologia* 2008; 51(7):1245–52.
39. deValk HW, van Nieuwaal NHG, Visser GHA. Pregnancy outcome in type 2 diabetes mellitus: a retrospective analysis from the Netherlands. *Rev Diabet Stud* 2006; 3(3):134–42.
40. Bellamy L, Casas JP, Hingorani AD, *et al.* Type 2 diabetes mellitus after gestational diabetes: a systematic review and meta-analysis. *Lancet* 2009; 373(9677):1773–9.
41. Kaaja R, Rönnemaa T. Gestational diabetes: pathogenesis and consequences to mother and offspring. *Review Diab Stud* 2008; 5(4):194–202.
42. Savona-Ventura C, Chircop M. Significant thresholds for the 75-g oral glucose tolerance test in pregnancy. *J Diabetes Complications* 2008; 22(3):178–80.
43. The HAPO Study Cooperative Research Group, Metzger BE, Lowe LP, *et al.* Hyperglycemia and adverse pregnancy outcomes. *N Engl J Med* 2008; 358:1991–2002.
44. Metzger BE, Gabbe SG, Persson B, *et al.* International association of diabetes and pregnancy study groups recommendations on the diagnosis and classification of hyperglycemia in pregnancy. *Diabetes Care* 2010; 33(3):676–82.
45. Allen KV, Frier BM. Nocturnal hypoglycemia: clinical manifestations and therapeutic strategies toward prevention. *Endocr Pract* 2003; 9(6):530–43.
46. Trujillo AL. Insulin analogs and pregnancy. *Diabetes Spectrum* 2007; 20(2):94–101
47. Inge M, Evers IM, de Valk HW, *et al.* Risk of complications of pregnancy in women with type 1 diabetes: nationwide prospective study in the Netherlands. *BMJ* 2004; 328(7445):915.
48. García-Domínguez M, Herranz L, Hillman N, *et al.* Use of insulin lispro during pregnancy in women with pregestational diabetes mellitus. *Medicina Clínica* 2011; 137(13):581–6.
49. Mathiesen ER. Insulin aspart in diabetic pregnancy: state of the art. *Women's Health* 2008; 4(2):119–24.
50. Pollex EK, Feig DS, Lubetsky A, *et al.* Insulin glargine safety in pregnancy: a transplacental transfer study. *Diabetes Care* 2010; 33(1):29–33.
51. McElduff A. Insulin detemir in pregnancy: a small but significant step forward? *Diabetes Care* 2012; 35(10):1968–9.
52. Morin-Papunen L, Rantala AS, Unkila-Kallio L, *et al.* Metformin improves pregnancy and live-birth rates in women with polycystic ovary syndrome (PCOS): a multicenter, double-blind, placebo-controlled randomized trial *JCEM* 2012; 97:1492–500.
53. Langer O. Oral antidiabetic drugs in pregnancy: the other alternative. *Diabetes Spectrum* 2007; 20(2):101–15.
54. Melcer SJ. Effects of treatment in women with gestational diabetes mellitus: systematic review and meta-analysis *BMJ* 2010; 340:c1395.
55. American College of Obstetricians and Gynecologists Committee on Practice Bulletins—Obstetrics. ACOG Practice Bulletin No. 30: Gestational diabetes. *Obstet Gynecol* 2001; 98(3):525–38.
56. Conway DL. Obstetric management in gestational diabetes. *Diabetes Care* 2007; 30(2):S175–S179.
57. Reynolds F. Labour analgesia and the baby: good news is no news. *IJOA* 2011; 20:38–50.
58. Osterman MJ, Martin JA. Epidural and spinal anesthesia use during labor: 27-state reporting area, 2008. *Natl Vital Stat Rep* 201; 59(5):1–13, 16.
59. O'Hana HP, Levy A, Rozen A, *et al.* The effect of epidural analgesia on labor progress and outcome in nulliparous women. *J Matern Fetal Neonatal Med* 2008; 21(8):517–21.
60. Chaudhary S. Salhotra R. Subarachnoid block for caesarean delivery in severe preeclampsia. *J Anaesthesiol Clin Pharmacol* 2011; 27(2):169–73.
61. Wong JY, Carvalho B, Riley ET. Intrathecal morphine 100 and 200 µg for post-cesarean delivery analgesia: a trade-off between analgesic efficacy and side effects. *IJOA* 2013; 22(1):36–41.
62. Klemetti M, Nuutila M, Tikkanen M, *et al.* Trends in maternal BMI, glycaemic control and perinatal outcome among type 1 diabetic pregnant women in 1989–2008. *Diabetologia* 2012; 55(9):2327–34.
63. Nold JL, Georgieff MK. Infant of diabetic mothers. *Pediatr Clin N Am* 2004; 51:619–37.
64. Stage E, Nørgård H, Damm P, *et al.* Long-term breast-feeding in women with type 1 diabetes. *Diabetes Care* 2006; 29(4):771–4.
65. Owen CG, Martin MM, Whincup PH, *et al.* Does breastfeeding influence risk of type 2 diabetes in later life? A quantitative analysis of published evidence. *Am J Clin Nutr* 2006; 84:1043–54.
66. Gunderson EP. Breastfeeding after gestational diabetes pregnancy: subsequent obesity and type 2 diabetes in women and their offspring. *Diabetes Care* 2007; 30(2):S161–S168.
67. Dinc H, Esen F, Demirci A, *et al.* Pituitary dimensions and volume measurements in pregnancy and post partum. MR assessment. *Acta Radiol* 1998; 39:64–9.
68. Fadalti M, Pezzani I, Cobellis L, *et al.* Placental corticotropin-releasing factor. An update. *Ann N Y Acad Sci* 2000; 900:89–94.
69. Rigg LA, Lein A, Yen SS. Pattern of increase in circulating prolactin levels during human gestation. *AJOG* 1977; 129:454–6.
70. Arafah BM, Nasrallah MP. Pituitary tumors: pathophysiology, clinical manifestations and management. *Endocr Relat Cancer* 2001; 8:287–305.
71. Casanueva FF, Molitch ME, Schlechte JA, *et al.* Guidelines of the Pituitary Society for the diagnosis and management of prolactinomas. *Clin Endocrinol* 2006; 65:265–73.
72. Holmgren U, Bergstrand G, Hagenfeldt K, *et al.* Women with prolactinoma—effect of pregnancy and lactation on serum prolactin and on tumour growth. *Acta Endocrinol* 1986; 111:452–9.
73. Chen HW, Su DH, Chen HW, *et al.* Abnormal enlargement of pituitary gland during pregnancy remitted spontaneously after delivery. *Chang Gung Med J* 2007; 30:81–6.

74. Karaca ZF, Unluhizarci K, Kelestimur F. Pregnancy and pituitary disorders. *Eur J Endocrinol* 2010; 162(6):453–75.
75. Paech MJ. An unusual presentation of a pituitary tumour in the early postpartum period. *Anaesth Intensive Care* 2006; 34(1):79–82.
76. Lachmansingh J, Chaudhuri K, Vogt-Harenkamp C, *et al. Pituitary Apoplexy Mimicking Post-Dural Puncture Headache.* Abstract number: S-60, SOAP 2012. http://soap.org/display_2012_abstract.php?id=S-60
77. Janssen NM, Dreyer K, van der Weiden RMF. Management of pituitary tumour apoplexy with bromocriptine in pregnancy. *JRSM* 2012; 3(6):43.
78. Okafor UV, Onwuekwe IO, Ezegwui HU. Management of pituitary adenoma with mass effect in pregnancy: a case report. *Cases J* 2009; 2:9117.
79. Dietrich JW, Brisseau K, Boehm BO. Absorption, transport and bio-availability of iodothyronines. *Deutsche Medizinische Wochenschrift* 2008; 133(31/21):1644–8.
80. Soldin OP, Tractenberg RE, Hollowell JG, *et al.* Trimester-specific changes in maternal thyroid hormone, thyrotropin, and thyroglobulin concentrations during gestation: trends and associations across trimesters in iodine sufficiency. *Thyroid* 2004; 14:1084–90.
81. Negro R. Significance and management of low TSH in pregnancy. In Lazarus J, Pirags V, Butz S (eds) *The Thyroid and Reproduction.* New York: Georg Thieme Verlag; 2009:84–95.
82. Calvo RM, Jauniaux E, Gulbis B, *et al.* Fetal tissues are exposed to biologically relevant free thyroxine concentrations during early phases of development. *J Clin Endocrinol Metab* 2002; 87(4):1768–77.
83. American Thyroid Association. *New ATA Guidelines for Managing Thyroid Disease in Pregnancy – Hypothyroidism Effects Maternal and Fetal Health.* 2011. [Online] http://www.thyroid.org/new-ata-guidelines-for-managing-thyroid-disease-in-pregnancy-hypothyroidism-effects-maternal-and-fet al-health/
84. Stagnaro-Green A, Abalovich M, Alexander E, *et al.* Guidelines of the American Thyroid Association for the diagnosis and management of thyroid disease during pregnancy and postpartum. *Thyroid* 2011; 21(10):1081–125.
85. Rosenfeld H, Ornoy A, Shechtman S, *et al.* Pregnancy outcome, thyroid dysfunction and fetal goitre after in utero exposure to propylthiouracil: a controlled cohort study. *Br J Clin Pharmacol* 2009; 68:609–17.
86. Bowman P, Vaidya B. Suspected spontaneous reports of birth defects in the UK associated with the use of carbimazole and propylthiouracil in pregnancy. *J Thyroid Res* 2011; 2011:235130.
87. Chen CH, Xirasagar S, Lin CC, *et al.* Risk of adverse perinatal outcomes with antithyroid treatment during pregnancy: a nationwide population-based study. *BJOG* 2011; 118:1365.
88. Braverman LE. Utiger RD. Introduction to thyrotoxicosis. In Braverman LE, Utiger RD (eds) *Werner and Ingbar's The Thyroid: A Fundamental and Clinical Text* (9th ed). Philadelphia, PA: Lippincott, Williams and Wilkins; 2005:453–5.
89. Patil-Sisodia K, Mestman JH. Grave's hyperthyroidism and pregnancy: a clinical update. *Endocr Pract* 2010; 16:118–29.
90. Casey BM, Dashe JS, Wells CE, *et al.* Subclinical hypothyroidism and pregnancy outcomes. *Obstet Gynecol* 2005; 105:239–45.
91. Allan WC, Haddow JE, Palomaki GE, *et al.* Maternal thyroid deficiency and pregnancy complications: implications for population screening. *J Med Screen* 2000; 7:127–30.
92. Zoeller RT. Transplacental thyroxine and fetal brain development. *J Clin Invest* 2003; 111(7):954–7.
93. Lazarus JH, Bestwick JP, Channon S, *et al.* Antenatal thyroid screening and childhood cognitive function. *N Engl J Med* 2012; 366:493–8.
94. Brent GA. The debate over thyroid-function screening in pregnancy. *N Engl J Med* 2012; 366:562–3.
95. Chu F, Fuller AJ. *Manual of Clinical Anesthesiology.* Philadelphia, PA: Lippincott Williams & Wilkins; 2012.
96. Johns Hopkins Medicine. *Health Library: The Adrenal Glands.* http://www.hopkinsmedicine.org/healthlibrary/conditions/adult/endocrinology/adrenal_glands_85,p00399/
97. Lindsay JR, Nieman LK. The hypothalamic-pituitary-adrenal axis in pregnancy: challenges in disease detection and treatment. *Endocr Rev* 2005; 26(6):775–99.
98. Gabbe SG. *Obstetrics: Normal and Problem Pregnancies* (4th ed). New York: Churchill and Livingston; 2002.
99. Mirshahi M, Ayani E, Nicolas C, *et al.* The blockade of mineralocorticoid hormone signaling provokes dramatic teratogenesis in cultured rat embryos. *Int J Toxicol* 2002; 21:191–9.
100. Costa A, De Filippis V, Voglino M, *et al.* Adrenocorticotropic hormone and catecholamines in maternal, umbilical and neonatal plasma in relation to vaginal delivery. *J Endocrinol Invest* 1988; 11:703–9.
101. Mukherjee K, Swyer GI. Plasma cortisol and adrenocorticotrophic hormone in normal men and non-pregnant women, normal pregnant women and women with pre-eclampsia. *J Obstet Gynaecol Br Commonw* 1972; 79:504–12.
102. Oh HC, Koh JM, Kim MS, *et al.* A case of ACTH-producing pheochromocytoma associated with pregnancy. *Endocr J* 2003; 50:739–44.
103. Lubin V, Gautier JF, Antoine JM, *et al.* Cushing's syndrome during pregnancy. *Presse Med* 2002; 31:1706–13.
104. Arnaldi G, Angeli A, Atkinson AB, *et al.* Diagnosis and complications of Cushing's syndrome: a consensus statement. *J Clin Endocrinol Metab* 2003; 88:5593–602.
105. Shaw JA, Pearson DW, Krukowski ZH, *et al.* Cushing's syndrome during pregnancy: curative adrenalectomy at 31 weeks gestation. *Eur J Obstet Gynecol Reprod Biol* 2002; 105:189–91.
106. Hana V, Dokoupilova M, Marek J, *et al.* Recurrent ACTH-independent Cushing's syndrome in multiple pregnancies and its treatment with metyrapone. *Clin Endocrinol* 2001; 54:277–81.
107. Hunt AB, McConahey CW. Pregnancy associated with diseases of the adrenal glands. *Am J Obstet Gynecol* 1953; 66:970–87.
108. Domi R. Cushing's surgery: role of the anesthesiologist. *Indian J Endocrinol Metab* 2011; 15 Suppl 4: S322–S328.
109. Moghissi ES, Korytkowski MT, DiNardo M, *et al.* American Association of Clinical Endocrinologists and American Diabetes Association consensus statement on inpatient glycemic control. *Endocr Pract* 2009; 15:353–69.
110. Lovas K, Husebye ES. High prevalence and increasing incidence of Addison's disease in western Norway. *Clin Endocrinol* 2002; 56:787–91.
111. Chrisoulidou A, Williamson C, De Swiet M. Assessment of adrenocortical function in women taking exogenous glucocorticoids during pregnancy. *J Obstet Gynaecol* 2003; 23:643–4.
112. Overton CE, Davis CJ, West C, *et al.* High risk pregnancies in hypopituitary women. *Hum Reprod* 2002; 17:1464–7.
113. Kelestimur F. The endocrinology of adrenal tuberculosis: the effects of tuberculosis on the hypothalamo-pituitary-adrenal axis and adrenocortical function. *J Endocrinol Invest* 2004; 27:380–6.
114. Lebbe M, Arlt W. What is the best diagnostic and therapeutic management strategy for an Addison patient during pregnancy? *Clin Endocrinol* 2013; 78:497–502
115. Lo CY, Lam KY, Wat MS, *et al.* Adrenal phaeochromocytoma remains a frequently overlooked diagnosis. *Am J Surg* 2000; 179:212–15.
116. Dugas G, Fuller J, Singh S, *et al.* Pheochromocytoma and pregnancy: a case report and review of anesthetic management. *Can J Anaesth* 2004; 51:134–8.
117. Smith CM, Wigent PJ. Pheochromocytoma in pregnancy. Considerations for the advanced practice nurse. *J Perinat Neonatal Nurs* 1998; 12:11–25.
118. Sarathi V, Lila AR, Bandgar TR, *et al.* Phaeochromocytoma and pregnancy: a rare but dangerous combination. *Endocr Pract* 2010; 16:300–9.

119. Manger WM. An overview of pheochromocytoma: history, current concepts, vagaries, and diagnostic challenges. *Ann NY Acad Sci* 2006; 1073:1–20.
120. Desai AS, Chutkow WA, Edelman E, *et al.* Clinical problem-solving. A crisis in late pregnancy. *N Engl J Med* 2009; 361:2271–7.
121. Lenders JW, Eisenhofer G, Mannelli M, *et al.* Phaeochromocytoma. *Lancet* 2005; 366:665–75.
122. Comino-Mendez I, Gracia-Aznarez FJ, Schiavi F, *et al.* Exome sequencing identifies MAX mutations as a cause of hereditary pheochromocytoma. *Nature Genetics* 2011; 43:663–7.
123. Boutros AR, Bravo EL, Zanettin G, *et al.* Perioperative management of 63 patients with phaeochromocytoma. *Cleve Clin J Med* 1990; 57:613–17.
124. Santeiro ML, Stromquist C, Wyble L. Phenoxybenzamine placental transfer during the third trimester. *Ann Pharmacother* 1996; 30:1249–51.
125. Weingarten TN, Cata JP, O'Hara JF, *et al.* Comparison of two preoperative medical management strategies for laparoscopic redelivery of phaeochromocytoma *Urology* 2010; 76:508–11.
126. Sibal L, Jovanovic A, Agarwal SC, *et al.* Phaeochromocytomas presenting as acute crises after beta blockade therapy. *Clin Endocrinol* 2006; 6:186–90.
127. Fernandez-Cruz L, Taura P, Saenz A, *et al.* Laparoscopic approach to phaeochromocytoma: hemodynamic changes and catecholamine secretion. *World J Surg* 1996; 20:762–8.
128. Amar L, Servais A, Gimenez-Roqueplo A, *et al.* Year of diagnosis, features at presentation and risk of recurrence in patients with phaeochromocytoma or secreting paraganglioma. *JCEM* 2005; 90:2110–16.
129. Sykes L, MacIntyre DA, Teoh TG, *et al.* Targeting immune activation in the prevention of preterm labour. *Eur Obstet Gynaecol* 2011; 6(2):100–16.
130. Wilczynski JR. Th1/Th2 cytokines balance—yin and yang of reproductive immunology. *Eur J Obstet Gynecol Reprod Biol* 2005; 122(2):136–43.
131. Buyon JP. The effects of pregnancy on autoimmune diseases. *J Leukoc Biol* 1998; 63(3):281–7.
132. Schulce-Koops H, Kalden JR. The balance of Th1/Th2 cytokines in rheumatoid arthritis. *Best Pract Res Clin Rheumatol* 2001; 15(5):677–91.
133. Golding A, Haque UJ, Giles JT. Rheumatoid arthritis and reproduction. *Rheum Dis Clin N Am* 2007; 33:319–44.
134. Skomsvoll JF, Østensen M, Irgens LM, *et al.* Perinatal outcome in pregnancies of women with connective tissue disease and inflammatory rheumatic disease in Norway. *Scand J Rheumatol* 1999; 28:352–6.
135. Partlett R, Roussou E. The treatment of rheumatoid arthritis during pregnancy. *Rheumatol Int* 2011; 31(4):445–9.
136. Ruppen W, Derry S, McQuay H, *et al.* Incidence of epidural hematoma, infection, and neurologic injury in obstetric patients with epidural analgesia/anesthesia. *Anesthesiology* 2006; 105(2):394–9.
137. Lidar M, Langevitz P. Pregnancy issues in scleroderma. *Autoimmun Rev* 2012; 11(6–7):A515–19.
138. Steen VD, Medsger TA Jr. Severe organ involvement in systemic sclerosis with diffuse scleroderma. *Athritis Rheum* 2000; 43(11):2437–44.
139. Artlett CM. Microchimerism and scleroderma: an update. *Curr Rheumatol Rep* 2003; 5(2):154–9.
140. Miniati I, Guiducci S, Mecacci F, *et al.* Pregnancy in systemic sclerosis. *Rheumatology* 2008; 47(3):16–18.
141. Bailey AR, Wolmarans M, Rhodes S. Spinal anaesthesia for Caesarean delivery in a patient with systemic sclerosis. *Anaesthesia* 1999; 54(4):355–58.
142. Danchenko N, Satia JA, Anthony MS. Epidemiology of systemic lupus erythematosus: a comparison of worldwide disease burden. *Lupus* 2006; 15(5):308–18.
143. Rahman A, Isenberg DA. Systemic lupus erythematosus. *N Engl J Med* 2008; 358:929–39.
144. Bertsias G, Ioannidis JP, Boletis J, *et al.* EULAR recommendations for the management of systemic lupus erythematosus. Report of a Task Force of the EULAR Standing Committee for International Clinical Studies Including Therapeutics. *Ann Rheum Dis* 2008; 67(2):195–205.
145. Martens HA, Nolte IM, van der Steege G, *et al.* An extensive screen of the HLA region reveals an independent association of HLA class I and class II with susceptibility for systemic lupus erythematosus. *Scand J Rheumatol* 2009; 38(4):1–7.
146. Cooper GS, Dooley MA, Treadwell EL, *et al.* Hormonal, environmental, and infectious risk factors for developing systemic lupus erythematosus. *Arthritis Rheum* 1998; 41(10):1714–24.
147. Rahman A, Isenberg DA. Systemic lupus erythematosus. *N Engl J Med* 2008; 358(9):929–39
148. Hanly JG, Urowitz MB, Su L, *et al.* Autoantibodies as biomarkers for the prediction of neuropsychiatric events in systemic lupus erythematosus. *Ann Rheum Dis* 2011; 70(10):1726–32.
149. Bosch X. Systemic lupus erythematosus and the neutrophil. *N Engl J Med* 2011; 365(8):758–60.
150. Petri M, Orbai AM, Alarcón GS, *et al.* Derivation and validation of the Systemic Lupus International Collaborating Clinics classification criteria for systemic lupus erythematosus. *Arthritis Rheum* 2012; 64(8):2677–86.
151. Branch DW. Physiologic adaptations of pregnancy. *Am J Reprod Immunol* 1992; 28:120–2.
152. Magid MS, Kaplan C, Sammaritano LR, *et al.* Placental pathology in systemic lupus erythematosus: a prospective study. *AJOG* 1998; 179:226–34.
153. Ogishima D, Matsumoto T, Nakamura Y, *et al.* Placental pathology in systemic lupus erythematosus with antiphospholipid antibodies. *Pathol Int* 2000; 50:224–9.
154. Moroni G, Ponticelli C. The risk of pregnancy in patients with lupus nephritis. *J Nephrol* 2003; 16:161–7.
155. Buyon JP, Clancy RM. Neonatal lupus: review of proposed pathogenesis and clinical data from the US-based Research Registry for Neonatal Lupus. *Autoimmunity* 2003; 36:41–50.
156. Clowse ME, Magder LS, Witter F, *et al.* The impact of increased lupus activity on obstetric outcomes. *Arthritis Rheum* 2005; 52:514–21.
157. Thakur A, Kiranpreet C, Chhabra B, *et al.* Anaesthetic management of systemic lupus erythematosus with pregnancy: a case report. *J Anaesthesiol Clin Pharmacol* 2002; 18(2):215–17.
158. Iqbal RK, Russell R. Anaesthesia for caesarean delivery in a parturient following a recent cerebrovascular event. *Int J Obstet Anesth* 2009; 18(1):55–9.
159. Wikipedia. *Antiphospholipid Syndrome.* https://en.wikipedia.org/wiki/Antiphospholipid_syndrome
160. Kochenour NK, Branch DW, Rote NS, *et al.* A new postpartum syndrome associated with antiphospholipid antibodies. *Obstet Gynecol* 1987; 69(3 Pt 2):460–8.
161. The American College of Obstetricians and Gynecologists. Antiphospholipid syndrome. *ACOG Pract Bull* 2011; 118:1–8.
162. Miyakis S, Lockshin MD, Atsumi T, *et al.* International consensus statement on an update of the classification criteria for definite antiphospholipid syndrome (APS). *J Thromb Haemost* 2006; 4(2):295–306.
163. Cowchock FS, Reece EA, Balaban D, *et al.* Repeated fetal losses associated with antiphospholipid antibodies: a collaborative randomized trial comparing prednisone with low-dose heparin treatment. *Am J Obstet Gynecol* 1992; 166(5):1318–23.
164. Asherson RA, Khamashta MA, Ordi-Ros J, *et al.* The "primary" antiphospholipid syndrome: major clinical and serological features. *Medicine (Baltimore)* 1989; 68(6):366–74.
165. Sciascia S, Murru V, Sanna G, *et al.* Clinical accuracy for diagnosis of antiphospholipid syndrome in SLE: evaluation of 23 possible combinations of antiphospholipid antibody specificities. *J Thromb Haemost* 2012; 10:2512–18.

CHAPTER 48

Obstetric haematology

Sapna Ladani, Beverley J. Hunt, and Sue Pavord

Introduction

The aim of this chapter is to cover aspects of haematology of pregnancy, delivery, and postpartum that are not addressed in other chapters. Obstetric haematology is a vast and complex area, the importance of which has promoted the development of this as a unique subspecialty.

Thrombosis and bleeding, anaemia, and haemoglobinopathies still account for significant morbidity and mortality in pregnancy, despite improvements in recognition, prevention, and management. The management of postpartum haemorrhage is discussed in Chapter 35, while thrombosis and thromboprophylaxis is covered in Chapter 37. This chapter addresses the management of anaemia, haemoglobinopathies (mainly sickle cell disease), thrombocytopenia, microangiopathies, and the inherited bleeding disorders.

Anaemia

Anaemia affects 1.62 billion people globally, corresponding to 24.8% of the world population.[1] Iron deficiency is the most common cause and even in the developed world an estimated 30–40% of preschool children and pregnant women have iron depletion. Other relatively common causes of anaemia in pregnancy in the United Kingdom include folate deficiency, haemoglobinopathies, and haemolytic anaemia.

Anaemia is defined as haemoglobin (Hb) less than 2 standard deviations below the mean for a healthy matched population. However, there is variation in what are considered normal values for pregnancy. The World Health Organization (WHO) defines anaemia in pregnancy as a Hb concentration of less than 110 g/L. However, in view of the relative plasma expansion being particularly marked in the second trimester, it would seem reasonable to take 105 g/L as the cut-off from 12 weeks, as suggested by the UK guidelines from the British Committee for Standards in Haematology.[2]

Iron deficiency

Iron deficiency is the most common deficiency state in the world. Effective management is needed to prevent adverse maternal and pregnancy outcomes and avoidable blood transfusion. Iron deficiency represents a spectrum ranging from iron depletion to iron deficiency anaemia. In iron depletion, the amount of stored iron (measured by serum ferritin concentration) is reduced and there are insufficient iron stores to mobilize if the body requires additional iron. In iron-deficient erythropoiesis, transport iron (measured by transferrin saturation) is also reduced and the shortage of iron limits red blood cell production and results in increased erythrocyte protoporphyrin concentration. In iron deficiency anaemia, the most severe form of iron deficiency, there is shortage of iron stores, transport iron, and functional iron, resulting in reduced Hb in addition to low serum ferritin, low transferrin saturation, and increased erythrocyte protoporphyrin concentration. Tissue enzyme malfunction occurs even in the early stages of iron-deficient erythropoiesis and adverse effects have been described on maternal morbidity and mortality, fetal and infant development, and pregnancy outcomes.

Iron deficiency and its contribution to morbidity and mortality

Iron deficiency may contribute to maternal morbidity through effects on immune function with increased susceptibility or severity of infections, poor work capacity and performance, and disturbances of postpartum cognition and emotions. Mortality at delivery is potentially increased by the heightened bleeding risk, low reserves, and poorer tolerance of blood loss.

The fetus is relatively protected from the effects of iron deficiency by upregulation of placental iron transport proteins. However, evidence suggests that maternal iron depletion increases the risk of iron deficiency in the first 3 months of life, through a variety of mechanisms.[3] Impaired psychomotor and/or mental development are well described in infants with iron deficiency anaemia and it may be associated with adult-onset diseases[4]. There is some evidence for the association between maternal iron deficiency and preterm delivery, low birth weight, possibly placental abruption, and increased peripartum blood loss. However, further research on the effect of iron deficiency, independent of confounding factors, is necessary to establish a clear causal relationship with pregnancy and fetal outcomes.

Diagnosis of iron deficiency

Clinical symptoms and signs of iron deficiency anaemia in pregnancy are usually non-specific, unless the anaemia is severe. Fatigue is the most common symptom but patients may also complain of weakness, headache, palpitations, dizziness, dyspnoea, and irritability. Rarely pica develops where there is a craving for non-food items such as ice and dirt. Iron deficiency anaemia may also impair temperature regulation and cause pregnant women to feel colder than normal.

Storage iron is depleted before a fall in Hb and as iron is an essential element in all cells, symptoms of iron deficiency may occur even without anaemia; these include fatigue, irritability, poor concentration, and hair loss.

A full blood count (FBC) is taken routinely in pregnancy and may show low Hb, mean cell volume (MCV), mean cell

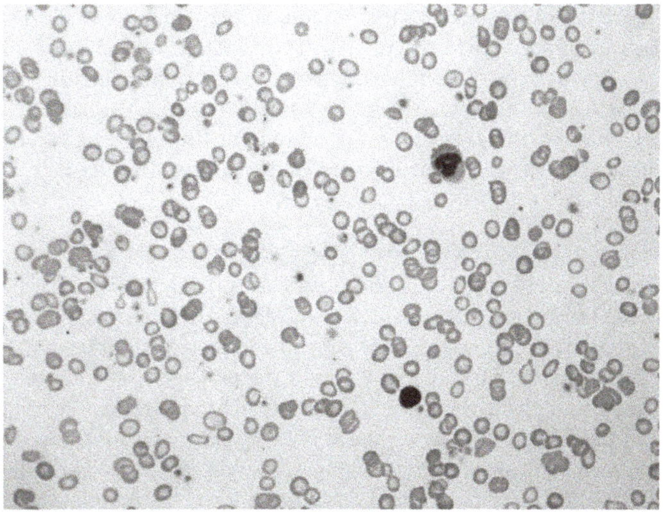

Figure 48.1 A blood film of a patient with iron deficiency anaemia depicting microcytic hypochromic red cells and target cells.

haemoglobin (MCH), and mean cell haemoglobin concentration (MCHC). A blood film may confirm the presence of microcytic hypochromic red cells (Figure 48.1) and characteristic 'pencil cells'. However, microcytic, hypochromic indices may also occur in haemoglobinopathies. In addition, for milder cases of iron deficiency, the MCV may not have fallen below the normal range.

Some analysers will give a percentage of hypochromic red cells present. This is said to be a sensitive marker of functional iron deficiency, but is not available on all analysers, and there is little information on its use in pregnancy.

Other tests either assess iron stores or the adequacy of iron supply to the tissues.

Serum ferritin

Serum ferritin is a stable glycoprotein which accurately reflects iron stores in the absence of inflammatory change. It is the first laboratory test to become abnormal as iron stores decrease and it is not affected by recent iron ingestion. It is generally considered the best test to assess iron deficiency in pregnancy,[5] although it is an acute-phase reactant and levels will rise when there is active infection or inflammation.

During pregnancy, in women with adequate iron stores at conception, the serum ferritin concentration initially rises, followed by a progressive fall by 32 weeks to about 50% of prepregnancy levels. This is due to haemodilution and mobilization of iron. The levels increase again mildly in the third trimester. Even though the ferritin level may be influenced by the plasma dilution later in pregnancy, a concentration below 15 mcg/L indicates iron depletion in all stages of pregnancy. In women of reproductive age, a level less than 15 mcg/L has shown specificity of 98% and sensitivity of 75% for iron deficiency, as defined by no stainable bone marrow iron. There are a variety of levels for treatment, quoted in different studies, but in general, treatment should be considered when serum ferritin levels fall below 30 mcg/L, as this indicates early iron depletion which will worsen unless treated. Van den Broek et al. found that serum ferritin is the best single indicator of storage iron provided a cut-off point of 30mcg/L is used, with sensitivity of 90%, and specificity of 85%.[5] Concurrent measurement of the C-reactive protein (CRP) may be useful in excluding inflammatory disease. The CRP concentration is largely independent of pregnancy and gestational age.

Trial of iron therapy

A trial of iron therapy is simultaneously diagnostic and therapeutic and is both cost- and time-effective. Ferritin should be checked first if the patient is known to have a haemoglobinopathy but otherwise microcytic or normocytic anaemia can be assumed to be caused by iron deficiency until proven otherwise. Assessment of response to iron should be carried out at 2 weeks when a rise in Hb confirms iron deficiency. If haemoglobinopathy status is unknown, it is reasonable to start iron whilst screening is carried out immediately, in accordance with the UK NHS sickle cell and thalassaemia screening programme guidelines. Severe anaemia can affect the results of haemoglobinopathy testing, with a reduction in HbA_2 of up to 0.5%, but there is no justification for delay. If there has been no improvement in Hb by 2 weeks, referral should be made to secondary care to consider other causes of anaemia, such as folate deficiency.

Dietary iron

The amount of iron absorption depends upon the amount of iron in the diet, its bioavailability, and physiological requirements. The main sources of dietary haem iron are haemoglobin and myoglobin from red meats, fish, and poultry. Haem iron is absorbed two to three times more readily than non-haem iron. Meat also contains organic compounds which promote the absorption of iron from other less bioavailable non-haem iron sources. However, approximately 95% of dietary iron intake is from non-haem iron sources. Vitamin C significantly enhances iron absorption from non-haem foods, the size of this effect increasing with the quantity of vitamin C in the meal. Germination and fermentation of cereals and legumes improve the bioavailability of non-haem iron by reducing the content of phytate, a food substance that inhibits iron absorption. Tannins in tea and coffee inhibit iron absorption when consumed with a meal or shortly after.

Oral iron supplements

Education and counselling regarding diet may improve iron intake and enhance absorption but this is insufficient to correct established iron deficiency and medication is required.

Oral iron is an effective, cheap, and safe way to replace iron. Ferrous salts show only marginal differences between one another in efficiency of absorption of iron. Ferric salts are much less well absorbed. The recommended dose of elemental iron for treatment of iron deficiency is 100–200 mg daily. Higher doses should not be given, as absorption is saturated and side effects increased.

Available ferrous salts include ferrous fumarate, ferrous sulphate, and ferrous gluconate. The amount of elemental iron in each salt varies as detailed in Table 48.1. Combined iron and folic acid preparations may also be used but it should be noted that use of these preparations does not obviate the need to take the recommended dose of folic acid for prevention of neural tube defects preconception and during the first 12 weeks of pregnancy.

Oral iron supplementation should be taken on an empty stomach, as absorption is reduced or promoted by the same factors that affect absorption of dietary non-haem iron.

Parenteral iron therapy

Parenteral iron therapy is indicated when there is absolute non-compliance with, or intolerance to, oral iron therapy or proven malabsorption.[6] It circumvents the natural gastrointestinal

Table 48.1 Dose and elemental iron content per tablet of oral iron preparations

Iron salt	Dose per tablet	Elemental iron
Ferrous fumarate	200 mg	65 mg
Ferrous gluconate	300 mg	35 mg
Ferrous sulphate (dried)	200 mg	65 mg
Ferrous sulphate	300 mg	60 mg
Ferrous feredetate (Sytron®)	190 mg/5 mL elixir	27.5 mg/5 mL

Reproduced with permission from *British National Formulary*, Copyright © 2010 Royal Pharmaceutical Society.

regulatory mechanisms to deliver non-protein bound iron to the red cells.

Faster increases in Hb and better replenishment of iron stores in comparison with oral therapy have been demonstrated, particularly for iron sucrose and iron (III) carboxymaltose. A large retrospective study reported fewer postpartum transfusions in the group treated with intravenous (IV) iron.[7] However, there is a paucity of good quality trials that assess clinical outcomes and safety of these preparations.

As free iron may lead to the production of hydroxyl radicals with potential toxicity to tissues, iron deficiency should be confirmed by ferritin levels before use of parenteral preparations. Contraindications include a history of anaphylaxis or reactions to parenteral iron therapy, first trimester of pregnancy, active acute or chronic infection, and chronic liver disease. Facilities and staff trained in management of anaphylaxis should be available.

The IV iron preparations currently available in the United Kingdom and their properties are summarized in Table 48.2. The different preparations have not been compared to each other in pregnancy. Iron sucrose has a higher availability for erythropoiesis than iron dextran and experience suggests a good safety profile in pregnancy.[8] Its use is limited by the total dose that can be administered at any one time, requiring multiple infusions which may limit patient compliance. The newer preparations, iron III carboxymaltose and iron III isomaltoside, aim to overcome this problem, with single dose administration in an hour or less.

Fast-acting intravenous iron preparations

Iron III carboxymaltose (Ferrinject®) is a ferric hydroxide carbohydrate complex, which allows for controlled delivery of iron within the cells of the reticuloendothelial system (primarily bone marrow) and subsequent delivery to the iron binding proteins ferritin and transferrin. It is administered intravenously, as a single dose of 1000 mg over 15 minutes (maximum 15 mg/kg by injection or 20 mg/kg by infusion). Randomized controlled trials have shown non-inferiority[9,10] and superiority[11] to oral ferrous sulphate in the treatment of iron deficiency anaemia in the postpartum period, with rapid and sustained increases in Hb. Animal studies have shown it to be rapidly eliminated from the plasma, giving minimal risk of large amounts of ionic iron in the plasma. By 28 days, in iron-deficient rats most of the iron has been incorporated into new erythrocytes.[12]

Iron III isomaltoside (Monofer®) is an IV preparation with strongly bound iron in spheroid iron-carbohydrate particles, providing slow release of bioavailable iron to iron binding proteins. There is rapid uptake by the reticuloendothelial system and little risk of release of free iron. An erythropoietic response is seen in a few days, with an increased reticulocyte count. Ferritin levels return to the normal range by 3 weeks as iron is incorporated into new erythrocytes. Doses of more than 1000 mg iron can be administered in a single infusion and it has been used safely in pregnancy.

Intramuscular preparations

The only preparation available in the United Kingdom that may be given intramuscularly (IM) is low-molecular-weight iron dextran. However injections tend to be painful and there is significant risk of permanent skin staining. Its use is therefore generally discouraged but if given, the Z-track injection technique should be used to minimize risk of iron leakage into the skin. The advantage of IM iron dextran is that, following a test dose, it can be administered in primary care, although facilities for resuscitation should be available as there is a small risk of systemic reaction.

A recent Cochrane review on treatments for iron deficiency in anaemia[13] highlighted the need for good quality randomized controlled trials in this setting, in particular to assess clinical outcomes and adverse events. Pending further good quality evidence, centres should review their policies and systems for use of parenteral therapy in iron deficiency anaemia in pregnancy.

Management of delivery in anaemic women

With good practice this situation should generally be avoided; however, there are instances when women book late, have recently come from abroad, or have not engaged with antenatal care. In these situations it may be necessary to take active measures to minimize blood loss at delivery. Consideration should be given to delivery in hospital, IV access, and blood availability. Whilst this should be done on an individual basis, a suggested cut off would be Hb less than 100 g/L for delivery in hospital, including hospital-based midwifery-led unit and less than 95 g/L for delivery in an obstetrician-led unit, with an intrapartum care plan discussed and documented.

The third stage of labour should be actively managed to minimize postpartum blood loss.

Indications for and risks of blood transfusion

Concerns about safety, high costs, and availability of donor blood have promoted greater scrutiny of blood transfusion practice. Potential dangers of transfusion are numerous but most commonly arise from clinical and laboratory errors.[14] In addition, the potential for transfusion-induced sensitization to red cell antigens, confer a potential risk of fetal haemolytic disease.

Massive obstetric haemorrhage is widely recognized as an important cause of morbidity and mortality and requires prompt use of blood and components as part of appropriate management. Chapter 35 covers the multidisciplinary approach required, together with the implementation of intraoperative cell salvage as a transfusion sparing strategy. However, outside the setting of massive haemorrhage, audits indicate that a high proportion of blood transfusions administered in the postpartum period may be inappropriate,[15] with under-utilization of iron supplements.

Postpartum anaemia

The WHO defines postnatal anaemia as Hb less than 10 g/dL. FBC should be checked within 48 hours of delivery in all women with

Table 48.2 Summary of intravenous iron preparations available in the United Kingdom

	Cosmofer® iron (III) hydroxide dextran complex	Venofer® iron (III) hydroxide sucrose complex	Ferinject® iron (III) carboxymaltose	Monofer® iron (III) isomaltoside
Dose of elemental iron	50 mg/mL	20 mg/mL	50 mg/mL	100 mg/mL
Test dose required as per manufacturer	Yes, before every IV dose, once before IM treatment	First dose new patients only	No	No
Routes of administration	Slow IV injection IV infusion of total dose IM injection total dose	Slow IV injection IV infusion	Slow IV injection IV infusion	Slow IV injection IV infusion
Able to administer total dose	Yes (up to 20 mg/kg body weight over 4–6 hours)	No	Yes (up to 20 mg/kg body weight maximum of 1000 mg/week over 15 min)	Yes (up to 20 mg/kg body weight over 1 hour)
Half-life	5 hours	20 hours	7–12 hours	5 hours
Dosage	100–200 mg per IV injection up to 3 times a week Total dose infusion up to 20 mg/kg body weight over 4–6 hours) (100 mg IM into alternate buttocks daily in active patients in bed ridden up to 3 times a week)	Total IV single dose no more than 200 mg, can be repeated up to 3 times in 1 week	1000 mg by IV injection up to 15 mg/kg/week Total dose infusion up to 20 mg/kg body weight. Maximum weekly dose of 1000 mg that can be administered over 15 min.	100–200 mg per IV injection up to 3 times a week Total dose infusion up to 20 mg/kg body weight per week. Doses up to 10 mg/kg body weight can be administered over 30 min, doses greater than 10 mg/kg body weight should be administered over 60 min
Adverse drug-related events	5% patients may experience minimal adverse events (dose related) Risk of severe anaphylaxis < 1/10,000 Risk of anaphylactoid symptoms >1/1000 <1/100	0.5–1.5% of patients may experience adverse events Risk of anaphylactoid reaction >1/10,000 <1/1000	3% of patients may experience adverse events Risk of anaphylactoid reaction >1/1000 <1/100	>1% of patients may experience adverse events Risk of anaphylaxis <1/10,000 >1/1000 to <1/100 Anaphylactoid reactions

Reproduced with permission from *British National Formulary*, Copyright © 2010 Royal Pharmaceutical Society.

an estimated blood loss greater than 500 mL and in women with uncorrected anaemia in the antenatal period or symptoms suggestive of postpartum anaemia. Where there is no bleeding, the decision to transfuse should77 be made on an informed individual basis. In fit, healthy, asymptomatic patients there is little evidence of the benefit of blood transfusion, which should be reserved for women with continued bleeding or at risk of further bleeding, imminent cardiac compromise, or significant symptoms requiring urgent correction. Women with Hb levels less than 100 g/L, who are haemodynamically stable, asymptomatic, or mildly symptomatic, should be offered elemental iron 100–200 mg daily for at least 3 months and a repeat FBC and ferritin to ensure Hb and iron stores are replete.

If, after careful consideration, elective transfusion is required, women should be fully counselled about potential risks, including written information, and consent should be obtained.

Folate deficiency

Folate deficiency is an unusual cause of anaemia in pregnancy, largely due to the fortification of foods with folic acid and the wide-scale supplementation of low-dose folic acid in early pregnancy for the prevention of neural tube defects. It is found in a wide variety of food sources including green leafy vegetables, citrus fruits, nuts, bread, and dairy products; however, it is heat labile and often lost in the cooking process.

Body stores last for several months. It is absorbed mainly in the jejunum and will be affected by malabsorptive syndromes such as coeliac disease, although it is most unusual for these to first become manifest in pregnancy.

Secondary folate deficiency can result from increased erythropoiesis, as occurs in haemolytic anaemias and myeloproliferative disorders, and also from anticonvulsant therapy, which induces metabolic enzymes.

Diagnosis of folate deficiency

Mean cell volume (MCV) rises in pregnancy by around 6 fL but an increase to over 100 fL is suggestive of vitamin B_{12} or folate deficiency. Other clues on the blood film are the presence of oval macrocytes, hypersegmented neutrophils (Figure 48.2) and possible mild leucopenia or thrombocytopenia. If iron deficiency coexists the mean cell volume may be normal but the blood film shows dimorphism, with microcytes as well as macrocytes.

Red cell folate gives a more accurate assessment than serum folate but neither has particularly good sensitivity or specificity in pregnancy. Bone marrow examination would reveal the presence of megaloblasts, where there is loss of synchrony between nuclear

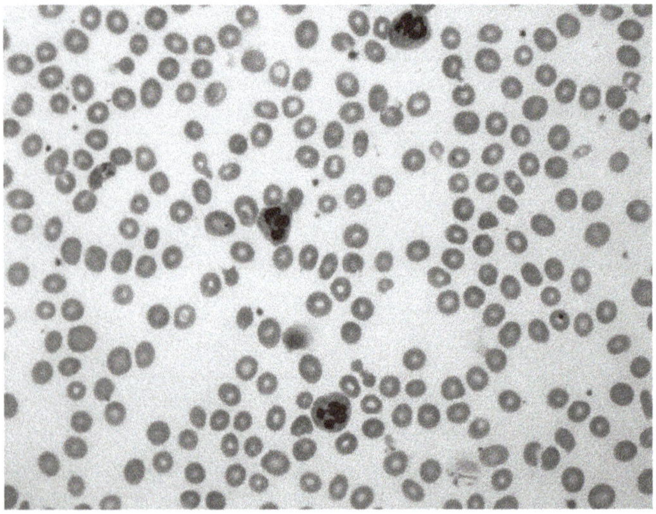

Figure 48.2 A blood film from a patient with folate deficiency showing hypersegmented neutrophils and macrocytes.

Table 48.3 Causes of haemolysis

	Primary
Autoimmune	In association with connective tissue disorders or neoplastic disease
Hereditary	Disorders of Hb synthesis
	Red cell membrane disorders
	Enzymopathies
Mechanical	Mechanical heart valves
	Disseminated intravascular coagulation (DIC)
	Microangiopathic haemolytic anaemia (MAHA)
Drugs	Immune-mediated
	Oxidative stress
Infections	Bacterial enzymes, e.g. *Clostridium perfringens*
Paroxysmal nocturnal haemoglobinuria	Clonal disorder causing increased susceptibility to complement lysis

and cytoplasmic maturation but the investigation is invasive and a trial of supplementation for suspected cases would be preferred. Proven folate deficiency requires treatment with 5 mg folic acid three times per day. The improvement in Hb levels can mask an undiagnosed B_{12} deficiency and this should be excluded first.

Vitamin B_{12} deficiency

Vitamin B_{12} deficiency is extremely rare in pregnancy but is often incorrectly diagnosed due to the physiological fall in serum B_{12} levels as B_{12} binding globulin increases. Genuine vitamin B_{12} deficiency is usually associated with infertility and the most common cause, pernicious anaemia, usually develops after the age of 40 years. Vitamin B_{12} is found in foods of animal origin, such as meat and dairy but even vegans rarely develop B_{12} deficiency due to the synthesis of B_{12} by bacteria in the gut or on legumes. In suspected cases, oral cyanocobalamin can be tried first but if IM hydroxycobalamin is thought necessary, proper investigation should be performed outside of pregnancy to avoid unnecessary lifelong supplements.

Haemolytic anaemia

Haemolysis is defined as shortened red cell survival, the average lifespan of a red cell being 120 days. Mild haemolysis in compensated by an increase in bone marrow erythropoiesis and may not affect the Hb concentration, however anaemia will develop when the degree of shortened red cell survival exceeds the bone marrow's ability to compensate. Causes of haemolysis are listed in Table 48.3.

The most common cause is autoimmune haemolytic anaemia, either idiopathic or in association with underlying autoimmune disease such as systemic lupus erythematosus.

Laboratory markers of haemolysis include elevated lactate dehydrogenase (LDH), increased reticulocytes, fall in haptoglobins, and rise in bilirubin. Autoimmune haemolysis is characterized by a positive direct antiglobulin test (Coombs' test), giving evidence of antibody bound to the surface of erythrocytes.

Where there is intravascular haemolysis, such as in microangiopathic haemolytic anaemia (MAHA), free haemoglobin will be present in the urine and shed in tubal cells, showing as urine haemosiderin.

Management depends on the underlying cause. Autoimmune haemolysis can be treated with immunosuppressants such as steroids and immunoglobulin. Transfusion is sometimes necessary but provision of compatible donor units can be delayed by specialist investigation to identify the specificity of the antibody. Patients with cold haemagglutinin disease may benefit from receiving transfusion via a blood warmer.

Haemoglobinopathies

Introduction

The haemoglobinopathies are common genetic disorders. They may result in significant morbidity and mortality, affecting all age groups and genders. The abnormalities of haemoglobin can either be:

- *structural:* such as in sickle cell disease, where a single nucleotide change in the beta (β)-globin gene leads to the substitution of valine for glutamine at position 6 on the β-globin chain
- *disorders resulting from unbalanced globin chain production:* the thalassaemias, the globin chains produced are structurally normal but reduced in quantity.

It has long been known that morbidity and mortality in children with sickle cell disease is high in the first 5 years of life. The protective effects of high levels of fetal haemoglobin (HbF) in the newborn decline over the first 4–6 months of life, thereafter much of childhood mortality is due to pneumococcal septicaemia and acute splenic sequestration. Successful antibiotic prophylaxis, vaccination, and education programmes have all but eliminated these problems and are perhaps the single most important step in the improved survival of sickle cell disease. In adulthood, morbidity is predominated by end-organ damage from microvascular disease.

In β thalassaemia major, the failure of beta globin chain production results in a severe transfusion dependent anaemia which is manifest as HbF levels reduce in the first few months of life. From this point on, the management of thalassaemia is based upon regular transfusion and iron chelation to reduce the risk of organ damage, particularly cardiac. Care of the patient with thalassaemia requires collaboration between haematologists, endocrinologists, diabetologists, cardiologists, and occasional input from other specialities such as hepatology. With appropriate care and good compliance, life expectancy may be normal. However, early cardiac death is common in those who do not comply with iron chelation.

Sickle cell disease

The sickling disorders are a group of inherited chronic haemolytic anaemias with clinical manifestations occurring as a result of the polymerization of haemoglobin S. The disorders in which sickling occur are:

- homozygous sickle cell disease—HbSS. The most common and generally the most severe.

Compound heterozygous states associated with clinical disease include:

- haemoglobin SC disease
- haemoglobin Sβ thalassaemia
- haemoglobin SD Punjab
- haemoglobin SO Arab
- haemoglobin SLepore Boston.

Carriage of haemoglobin S is not associated with significant disease but its significance in pregnancy is in terms of genetic counselling and the need for partner testing.

Sickle cell disease is characterized by chronic intravascular and extravascular haemolysis; red cell lifespan is shortened from 120 days to 16–20 days. This chronic haemolysis leads to the liberation of free haemoglobin which mops up nitric oxide released from the vascular endothelium. This in turn leads to endothelial activation and vasoconstriction providing ideal conditions for adherence of cellular blood components. The combination of poorly deformable red blood cells, increased viscosity, endothelial activation and vasoconstriction causes ongoing vaso-occlusion in the microvasculature. The process is further exacerbated by leucocytosis, platelet activation, and increased levels of pro-inflammatory cytokines. Vaso-occlusion leads to both the acute complications of sickle cell disease, such as painful crises, as well as chronic organ damage, including cardiac and renal impairment seen in older patients.

Much of the published information on pregnancy in sickle cell disorders relates to homozygous (SS) sickle cell disease. This, and Sbeta^{0}thalassaemia, are in general the most severe forms. Patients with milder sickle conditions such as SC disease and Sβ$^+$thalassaemia can also have complicated pregnancies though the risks are lower. All patients with sickling disorders should be jointly managed by an obstetrician and haematologist with interest and experience in these diseases. Since these pregnancies are high risk, patients will require frequent review by the multidisciplinary team. Twin and multiple birth pregnancies are associated with a higher rate of serious complications. Despite the potential complications, more than one-quarter of these pregnancies occur without problems.

Prior to the 1970s, 30–40% of women with sickle cell disease did not survive pregnancy, but recent decades have seen a marked improvement; currently mortality has been shown to be 1–2% in studies from the United States and Europe. A National Confidential Enquiry into Patient Outcome and Death (NCEPOD) report[16] highlights difficulties with death certification and autopsy in sickle cell disorders. Few pathologists have significant experience and non-specialist sickle clinicians are in a similar position. It is recommended that pathologists with appropriate experience perform such autopsies though there are now national guidelines for autopsy in sickle cell disease. Clinicopathological correlation is crucial, for example, in differentiating sickle chest from pneumonia or whether thrombosis is likely to have been *in situ* or embolic. These women may have complex coexisting medical problems which can make the management of their pregnancy even more challenging.

Perinatal mortality was reported to be as high as 50–80% prior to the 1970s. More recent studies in the United States and Europe have reported a perinatal mortality rate of between 1% and 8%. Since the 1970s, it has been known that women with sickling disorders are more likely to have premature deliveries. This has been reported at an average of between 34.1 to 38.5 weeks' gestation. In a recent Jamaican study, the mean gestational age was found to be 37.0 weeks compared to 38.7 weeks in controls. In African Americans, the mean gestational age was 37 weeks. Infants born to HbSS mothers are twice as likely to be preterm compared to HbSC mothers. Intrauterine growth retardation is a well-documented complication of sickle cell pregnancy. This is probably a consequence of maternal anaemia and impaired placental function resulting from vaso-occlusion in uteroplacental circulation. Histological studies have shown placental infarction with abruptions and villous oedema.

Seventy-seven per cent of infants born to mothers with sickle cell anaemia have a birth weight below the 50th centile, with 21% below the 10th centile. Neonates born to mothers with HbSS disease are significantly smaller than babies born to mothers with HbSC disease.

Patients with sickle cell disease have hyposplenism. Urinary tract infections are increased in normal pregnancies and can lead to pyelonephritis and premature labour. There may be a further increase in risk in sickle pregnancy. Other common sites of infection include chest and bone. Common pathogens include *Pneumococcus, Salmonella, Escherichia coli*, and *Mycoplasma*. Infection is a common precipitant of painful crises.

Pregnancy-induced hypertension and pre-eclampsia complicate one-third of pregnancies in sickle cell disease. There is an association between hypertension with proteinuria and simultaneous sickling complications. The pregnant patient with sickle cell disease should be regarded as at high risk of venous thromboembolism. Pulmonary embolism is difficult to diagnose in this setting but should be considered within the differential of a patient presenting with dyspnoea and chest pain.

General management of sickle cell pregnancy

All couples should receive preconceptual advice. Maternal and fetal risks of pregnancy and availability of prenatal diagnosis should be discussed in the light of partner screening. Crisis prevention measures should be advised, including avoidance of cold, overexertion, and dehydration. Medications should be reviewed, with assessment of risks versus benefits for individual drugs. Folic acid supplements and antibiotic prophylaxis are a necessity. Hydroxycarbamide should be discontinued at least 3 months before conception and the need for an antenatal top-up or exchange transfusion programme should be considered.[17]

Throughout pregnancy, women require continued health education and review of compliance with medications. The clinical condition of the patient, degree of haemolysis, and urine culture should be monitored regularly, along with fetal growth scans.

There should be a low threshold for admission especially if there is limb, bone, abdominal, or chest pain after 28 weeks' gestation, with a 24-hour admission policy and contact numbers if any features of sickle cell crisis develop. All women should have an appropriate plan for use of analgesia in pregnancy, aiming to avoid non-steroidal anti-inflammatory drugs (NSAIDs) after 34 weeks. The obstetric anaesthetist needs to be involved early to discuss management in labour. Transfusion should only occur after discussion with a haematologist.

The majority of severe crises occur in the third trimester often at the time of delivery. Often the complications of sickle cell disease precipitate labour rather than labour precipitating sickling complications. Crises in pregnancy are more common in women with HbSS pregnancies (30–80%) than in women with HbSC (30%). SC disease is generally a milder condition outside pregnancy but patients may present with pain, thrombosis, and other sickle complications in the third trimester.

Labour and early puerperium are risk periods for development of pain. This becomes more likely in the presence of infection, dehydration, or acidosis. Sickle patients have a renal concentrating defect from early childhood and pass large volumes of dilute urine. Attention to hydration status is therefore crucial. Crises in pregnancy often present as abdominal pain which can be difficult to distinguish from obstetric complications.

Those with a sickle cell crisis should be admitted only to an obstetric or haematology ward. In the final trimester, with the high risk of obstetric problems, the obstetric setting is most appropriate, and the patient should be rested and given adequate hydration of 3–4 L of fluid per 24 hours. Strict fluid balance is essential and oxygen if hypoxic. Pain relief should be initiated within 30 minutes, taking account of the previous analgesic history.[18] Regular paracetamol should be given and NSAIDs if the pregnancy is less than 34 weeks. However, subcutaneous opiates are often necessary. Pethidine is not recommended for the treatment of sickle pain, as it can induce seizures. Morphine, diamorphine, or oxycodone is appropriate. Linear analogue scales are used to assess pain control. Patient-controlled analgesia or subcutaneous pumps are occasionally required. Regular assessment of sedation and conscious level is essential if the patient is on strong opiates. Investigations should include a FBC, reticulocyte count, urea and electrolytes, group and screen, pulse oximetry and arterial blood gases if appropriate, a mid-stream specimen of urine, blood cultures and throat swabs, and a chest X-ray. Antibiotics are not routinely required unless there is evidence of infection. Low-grade fever of less than 38°C is common in painful crisis, even in the absence of infection. Low-molecular-weight heparin (LMWH) thromboprophylaxis and compression stockings should be given routinely. Indications for transfusion or exchange transfusion should be discussed with a haematologist. Chest physiotherapy including incentive spirometry will reduce the risk of a subsequent chest syndrome in patients with rib pain. Chest crises in pregnancy require even closer monitoring and the use of a broad-spectrum antibiotic. Transfusion, either exchange or top-up, should be considered in hypoxaemia (SaO_2 < 5% lower than patient's steady-state level), deteriorating clinical status, or progressive multilobe involvement.

Labour and delivery

The aim should be to achieve a vaginal delivery, as there is no benefit from elective caesarean delivery. Induction leads to a higher caesarean delivery rate, with its own complications, plus the implication that future pregnancies will need a trial of scar and be associated with a risk of subsequent operative delivery. The mother needs to be kept warm and well hydrated, with IV fluids commenced at time of admission in labour, at a rate of 1 L 8-hourly, to maintain good urine output. Strict fluid balance should be ensured. A FBC, group and screen should be taken and continuous pulse oximetry used, with continuous cardiotocography monitoring throughout labour.

Epidural analgesia is the pain relief of choice. Therefore careful timing of LMWH should be taken into consideration if labour is induced. The woman should not be allowed to labour for more than 12 hours and prolonged rupture of membranes should be avoided as it increases the risk of infection and dehydration. If operative delivery is necessary, this should be discussed with the haematologist. Neuraxial (rather than general) anaesthesia reduces the likelihood of sickle crisis and postoperative acute chest syndrome. Thromboprophylaxis with LMWH and compression stockings is required postpartum and the neonatologist should be alerted.

Postpartum

Baby and mother need close monitoring, with good hydration. The baby needs to be monitored for signs of respiratory depression if opiates have been used intrapartum.

Prophylactic transfusion

The role of transfusion in sickle cell disease in pregnancy is controversial, although it is generally accepted that transfusion is not required as part of the management of uncomplicated sickle pregnancy. Transfusion should be reserved for high-risk pregnancies. This would include twin pregnancies, women with previous poor obstetric history, chest crises, recurrent pain, and severe anaemia. Cell salvage is contraindicated in women with sickle cell disease as the fragile cells are lysed in the machine.

Summary

Maternal mortality is significantly increased for women with sickle cell disorders and the key to successful outcome lies in the close interaction between obstetric teams, the anaesthetist, and haematologists. Close monitoring and awareness of risks and complications is essential and the majority of pregnancies will have a successful outcome. Where possible, delivery should be allowed to proceed with minimal intervention; there being little evidence that transfusion or operative delivery are of any benefit in the majority of cases.

Thalassaemia and pregnancy

The thalassaemias are almost always autosomal recessive disorders caused by mutations or deletions in the alpha (α)- or β-globin genes, leading to diminished or absent production of one or more globin chains. The other globin chain is produced in relative excess and precipitates within erythroid precursors, causing chronic haemolysis and ineffective erythropoiesis.

α thalassaemia

Four α-globin genes are inherited as a pair from each parent. The severity of the condition depends on the number of α-globin genes deleted.

α-thalassaemia carrier (αα/−−), (α−/α−) or (−α/αα)

Carriers of α thalassaemia are asymptomatic and are usually first detected at antenatal screening. Their haemoglobin is in the normal range or minimally decreased with low MCV and MCH.

Haemoglobin H disease (−−/−α)

Those affected by haemoglobin H disease have three non-functioning α-globin genes. The haemoglobin is commonly in the range 8–9 g/dL with microcytic, hypochromic red cell indices, and splenomegaly. HbH disease is a mild form of thalassaemia intermedia, those affected rarely need transfusion. The anaemia may worsen in pregnancy and with infection.

Haemoglobin Bart's hydrops (−−/−−)

A complete absence of α chains is incompatible with life and results in the unopposed chains forming tetramers called haemoglobin Bart's. This is a common cause of stillbirth in areas with a high frequency of (−−/αα) such as SE Asia and the Eastern Mediterranean. The fetus is stillborn at 34–40 weeks or dies soon after birth. The Hb Bart's binds oxygen poorly, impairing tissue oxygenation. The fetus appears oedematous and jaundiced with massive hepatosplenomegaly and ascites.

β-thalassaemia carrier

Individuals are asymptomatic and diagnosed at antenatal screening or during investigation of microcytic, hypochromic indices. The haemoglobin is rarely less than 100 g/L. HbA_2 is raised. Iron replacement need not be given unless a deficiency state is proven by reduced serum ferritin.

β-thalassaemia intermedia

A range of interacting genetic lesions may lead to a thalassaemic phenotype of varying severity. Some will be asymptomatic whilst others require intermittent transfusion. The haemoglobin is usually 100–120 g/L but can be as low as 50–60 g/L in severe forms. Hepatosplenomegaly may be present.

Management in pregnancy

Carriers of α and β thalassaemia and those with HbH disease or other mild forms of thalassaemia intermedia can be managed as a normal pregnancy. Anaemia may worsen during pregnancy because of the normal physiological changes. Oral iron supplements should be given where there is a reduced ferritin but not for microcytosis and hypochromia alone.

It is important to identify couples at risk of a baby affected by Hb Bart's. This should be picked up by the antenatal screening programme and parents offered counselling, education and prenatal diagnosis. The mother may also develop 'mirror syndrome' a severe pre-eclampsia, and delivery of a hydropic fetus and placenta can cause obstetric problems.

β-thalassaemia major and severe forms of intermedia require careful multidisciplinary management in specialist centres. Cardiac and liver damage from iron overload should be assessed prior to pregnancy and organ function monitored. Transfusion regimens should be carefully reviewed as pregnancy proceeds and physiological haemodilution occurs and iron chelation therapy at delivery should be considered.

Neuraxial anaesthesia can be used for labour and delivery as long as there is no thrombocytopaenia,[19] which may occur if there is splenomegaly. Cell salvage can be used during caesarean delivery.[20]

Normal haemostasis

Haemostasis is the process by which a fibrin platelet plug forms at the site of vascular injury. The reactions responsible for the formation of this haemostatic plug take place on phospholipid cell membranes, particularly endothelial cells, platelets, and monocytes, and are usually due to the expression of tissue factor (TF), which activates the coagulation pathway. In the resting state, the cells in contact with the blood do not support procoagulant reactions, but when activated, the negatively charged phospholipid, normally present on the inside of the cell, becomes exposed on the outside and provides a catalytic site for haemostatic reactions to occur. To further increase the procoagulant surface area, activated or apoptotic cells shed microparticles, pieces of membrane with exposed negatively charged phospholipid.

Laboratory investigations

Laboratory screening tests of coagulation attempt to replicate haemostatic processes *in vitro*. However, this does not necessarily reflect the *in vivo* status and normal results do not exclude a bleeding disorder. Results should therefore be interpreted in conjunction with the bleeding history, particularly the response to haemostatic challenges and drug history. A coagulation screen will usually include the prothrombin time (PT) and activated partial thromboplastin time (aPTT). The thrombin time (TT) and fibrinogen level can also be easily measured.

The easiest way to understand *in vitro* tests of coagulation is to refer to the traditional cascade model of blood coagulation which uses a Y-shaped cascade of protease activation, with two pathways (intrinsic and extrinsic) converging to a final common pathway. Although this has little *in vivo* validity, it is a useful concept for interpreting laboratory tests. Figure 48.3 illustrates a simplified version of the coagulation cascade, and the factors which affect the PT and aPTT.

Prothrombin time

The PT measures the extrinsic pathway. It is calculated by measuring the time taken for a clot to form after the addition of TF, phospholipid, and calcium to platelet-poor plasma.

Activated partial thromboplastin time

The aPTT measures the intrinsic pathway. It is the time taken for a clot to form after addition of calcium to platelet-poor plasma, phospholipids, and a contact activator, such as kaolin, to activate factor XII (FXII).

Thrombin time

The TT involves the addition of thrombin to platelet-poor plasma. It reflects the conversion of fibrinogen to fibrin but is also sensitive to the presence of inhibitors that may be present in the plasma (e.g. heparin).

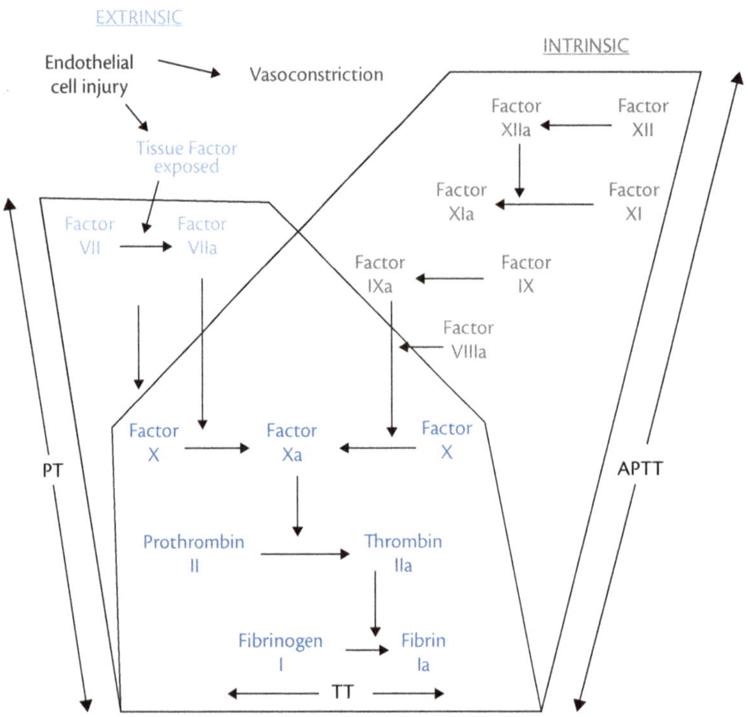

Figure 48.3 A simplified model of the coagulation cascade.

Fibrinogen

There are numerous methods of measuring fibrinogen levels. Most commonly performed is the Clauss assay, which is a functional or qualitative measure of fibrinogen. The immunological method measures the quantity of fibrinogen (fibrinogen antigen) and the comparison between the two can detect dysfibrinogenaemias.

The potential causes of abnormal coagulation tests are summarized in Table 48.4.

Near-patient assessment of coagulation—thromboelastography (TEG®) and Rotational elastometry (ROTEM®)

Thromboelastography® (TEG®) and thromboelastometry (ROTEM®) provide a global assessment of clot formation, stabilization, and dissolution at the bedside. They give a dynamic assessment of coagulation compared to conventional methods, and assess the whole haemostatic process rather than isolated aspects. Near-patient testing allows rapid assessment.

Table 48.4 Potential causes of abnormal coagulation tests

Isolated prolonged PT	Isolated prolonged aPTT	Prolonged PT and aPTT	Prolonged TT	Decreased fibrinogen
Factor VII deficiency	Factor VIII deficiency	Vitamin K deficiency	Congenital and acquired deficiencies in fibrinogen	DIC
Warfarin therapy	Factor IX deficiency	Liver disease	Dysfibrinogenaemia	Liver disease
Vitamin K deficiency	Factor XI deficiency	DIC	Heparin	Massive transfusion
	Factor XII deficiency	Massive transfusion	Direct thrombin inhibitors	Inherited deficiencies including afibrinogenaemia, hypofibrinogenaemia, and dysfibrinogenaemia
	Lupus anticoagulant	Common pathway including factor V, factor X, prothrombin, and fibrinogen deficiencies	Elevated fibrin degradation products	
	Heparin therapy	Warfarin/heparin therapy	Paraproteinaemias	
		Direct thrombin inhibitors		

aPTT, activated partial thromboplastin time; DIC, disseminated intravascular coagulation; PT, prothrombin time; TT, prothrombin time.

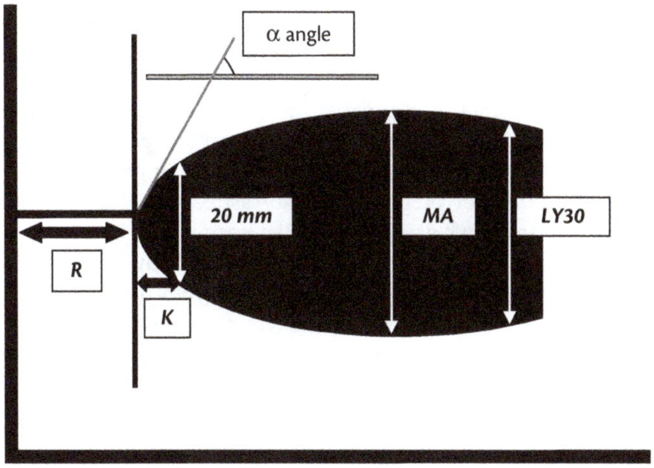

Figure 48.4 A normal TEG® trace.

Reproduced from da Luz LT, Nascimento B, Rizoli S., Thromboelastography (TEG): practical considerations on its clinical use in trauma and resuscitation, *Scandinavian Journal on Trauma, Resuscitation and Emergency Medicine.*, Volume 21: 29. 2013 © 2013 da Luz *et al.* This is an Open Access article distributed under the terms of the Creative Commons Attribution License (http://creativecommons.org/licenses/by/2.0), which permits unrestricted use, distribution, and reproduction in any medium, provided the original work is properly cited.

Classical thromboelastography (TEG®) involves placing a small sample of citrated blood into a cuvette which is gently rotated to imitate sluggish venous blood flow, activating coagulation. The blood is also recalcified to initiate coagulation, and an activator is added to standardize the test. The speed and strength of the clot is then measured, and a trace is formed. Four values which determine clot formation are measured in this test: the R time, the K value, the 'α' angle, and the maximal amplitude (MA). These are illustrated in Figure 48.4.

The R time represents the time from the start of test to the initial detection of the clot. The K time represents the time from the R time to the time taken for the clot to reach 20 mm in size. This represents the speed of coagulation. The 'α' angle is the tangent of the curve made as the K is reached and offers similar information to the K. The MA is a reflection of clot strength, assessing the properties of platelet and fibrin adhesion. The LY30 can also be calculated, which measures the percentage decrease in amplitude 30 minutes post MA, which gives a measure of the degree of haemolysis.

A heparinized cup can also be used with is sensitive to heparin. The use of paired plain and heparinized cups can be used to detect whether residual heparin is present. The generated curves and values can be used to detect and classify coagulopathies, and aid use of blood products, as suggested in Table 48.5. Some commonly seen curves are illustrated in Figure 48.5.[21]

ROTEM® uses similar principles to TEG®, but it is the sensor shaft rather than the cup which rotates. Formation of fibrin strands impedes the rotation of the sensor shaft and a trace is generated.[22]

Inherited bleeding disorders

Women who are sufferers or carriers of a congenital bleeding disorder need to be carefully managed to allow them to cope with the haemostatic challenges of pregnancy, labour, and delivery. Cases should be managed in a multidisciplinary setting by experienced obstetricians, anaesthetists, and haematologists. Individually tailored management plans are needed, taking into account bleeding risks to mother and fetus, as well as obstetric risk factors. Key features in the management of mothers and babies at risk of bleeding disorders are listed in Boxes 48.1 and 48.2.

Table 48.5 Potential causes of abnormal TEG® results

Value	Causes	Suggested therapy
Increased R time	Factor deficiency, anticoagulation, severe hypofibrinogenaemia, severe thrombocytopenia	Fresh frozen plasma (FFP), consider cryoprecipitate if grossly prolonged
Increased K time	Factor deficiency, thrombocytopenia, thrombocytopathy, hypofibrinogenaemia	Do FibTem or functional fibrinogen to determine whether need of FFP and/or cryoprecipitate. Give platelets if count <50 × 10^9/L
Decreased α angle	Hypofibrinogenaemia, thrombocytopenia	Perform a FibTem or functional fibrinogen to determine whether need of FFP and/or cryoprecipitate, Give 1 pool of platelets if platelet count is <50 × 10^9/L
Decreased MA	Thrombocytopenia, thrombocytopathy, hypofibrinogenaemia	Perform a FibTem or functional fibrinogen and platelet count to determine if fibrinogen and/or platelet defect
Increased LY30	Hyperfibrinolysis	Tranexamic acid

The commonest disorders likely to be encountered are haemophilia A and B, and von Willebrand disease (VWD). However the rarer coagulation disorders also need to be considered.

Haemostatic agents

Treatments available for women with inherited bleeding disorders are similar in the obstetric and non-obstetric setting. Most commonly used agents include tranexamic acid, desmopressin,

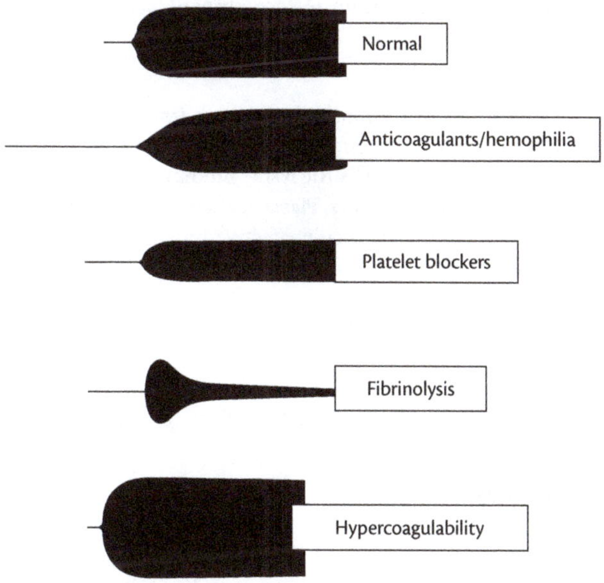

Figure 48.5 Commonly seen TEG® traces.

Reproduced from da Luz LT, Nascimento B, Rizoli S., Thromboelastography (TEG): practical considerations on its clinical use in trauma and resuscitation, *Scandinavian Journal on Trauma, Resuscitation and Emergency Medicine.*, Volume 21: 29. 2013 © 2013 da Luz *et al.* This is an Open Access article distributed under the terms of the Creative Commons Attribution License (http://creativecommons.org/licenses/by/2.0), which permits unrestricted use, distribution, and reproduction in any medium, provided the original work is properly cited.

Box 48.1 Management of mothers with bleeding disorders

- Care should be in a unit by a multidisciplinary team of obstetricians, anaesthetists, and haematologists with expertise in managing patients with bleeding disorders
- Plan of management should be discussed before pregnancy or as early as possible and a detailed labour plan documented during the third trimester
- Avoid IM injections
- Use NSAIDs with caution
- Avoid anticoagulation
- Establish baseline levels of deficiency/abnormality prior to intervention or labour
- Obtain good IV access during labour
- Ensure adequate haemostasis during labour and delivery with the use of appropriate therapy
- Avoid excessive genital or perianal trauma
- Active management of the third stage of labour
- Consider risk of thrombosis, especially postpartum
- Levels of deficient factor should be raised to at least 50 IU/dL before considering neuraxial anaesthesia

plasma-derived clotting factor concentrates, and recombinant factor concentrates.

Plasma-derived and recombinant factor concentrates

If possible, plasma-derived clotting factors should be avoided, as although virucidal methods are used to eliminate the risk of HIV and hepatitis B and C there is a risk of transmission of hepatitis A and parvovirus infection. Fetal parvovirus infection can lead to hydrops fetalis and fetal death.[23] Recombinant factor concentrates are therefore preferred.

Tranexamic acid

Tranexamic acid is an antifibrinolytic which competitively inhibits the activation of plasminogen to plasmin. It is a synthetic form of the amino acid lysine, and blocks the lysine binding sites on plasminogen and plasminogen receptors. Plasmin enzymatically breaks down many molecules and it especially effective in lysing fibrin, fibrinogen, and factor V. Tranexamic acid can be used prophylactically to reduce bleeding. It can also be used to treat bleeding. It is indicated in fibrinolysis which is diagnosed via thromboelastometry where fibrinolysis produces the classic 'tadpole' trace as seen in Figure 48.5. Fibrinolysis cannot be diagnosed by current standard laboratory tests. The dose is 1 g given slowly IV which can be repeated 8-hourly. Limited evidence on the use of tranexamic acid in pregnancy suggests it is safe[24] for pregnancy and breastfeeding. Currently the utility of tranexamic acid in managing postpartum haemorrhage is being assessed in the WOMAN study (Worldwide Maternal Antifibrinolytics Trial) randomizing 15,000 women with postpartum haemorrhage to tranexamic acid versus placebo.

Concurrent use of tranexamic acid with factor XI concentrate should be avoided, due to the potential risk of arterial or venous thrombosis that has been associated with factor XI concentrate.

Box 48.2 Management of delivery for babies at risk of bleeding disorders

- Establish, if relevant, whether prenatal diagnosis has been made
- Avoid invasive monitoring
- Avoid prolonged labour
- Avoid ventouse extraction
- Avoid mid cavity forceps
- Obtain cord blood for baseline levels
- Avoid IM injections until cord results is known
- Give oral vitamin K rather than IM

Desmopressin

Desmopressin (DDAVP®) can be used as prophylaxis or treatment of bleeding in carriers of haemophilia A, some subtypes of VWD, and some platelet function disorders. It has no effect in patients with haemophilia B. Desmopressin acts by stimulating exocytosis of Weibel–Palade bodies in endothelial cells, to release von Willebrand factor (VWF), and in some tissues also factor VIII (FVIII). FVIII levels rise approximately threefold after treatment with desmopressin. It also increases platelet responsiveness. The effect is maximal 30 minutes after IV administration, and 60 minutes after subcutaneous or intranasal treatment. The half-life of released FVIII is 8 hours. Repeated doses can be given, however tachyphylaxis occurs and the second dose can produce a rise of only 30% of the first. Desmopressin also has a fibrinolytic effect as it also stimulates the release of tissue plasminogen activator from the endothelium, so concurrent use of tranexamic acid is common. Lastly it has an antidiuretic activity, so fluid intake should be restricted for 24 hours.

There have been concerns about the safe use of desmopressin in pregnancy because of potential risks of placental insufficiency due to arterial vasoconstriction, and miscarriage or preterm labour due to an oxytocin effect.[23] A recent systematic review looked at 30 studies on the use of desmopressin in 216 pregnancies, in women with inherited bleeding disorders. They found that desmopressin was effective in preventing and reducing bleeding complications associated with pregnancy and delivery. There was one case of a water intoxication seizure, and one case of premature labour reported. There were no other maternal or fetal adverse outcomes.[25] Our practice is to use desmopressin in pregnancy where indicated (Box 48.3), but with careful attention to fluid balance.

General measures

Antenatal management

Antenatal management of women with a bleeding disorder, or at risk of a child with bleeding disorder, should include involvement by

Box 48.3 Indications for DDAVP®

- Low factor VIII levels in carriers for haemophilia
- Type 1 VWD
- Some cases of type 2 VWD where response to DDAVP® is demonstrated
- Platelet function disorders

experienced obstetricians, haematologists, and anaesthetists. There are a number of haemostatic challenges in the antenatal period including miscarriage, termination of pregnancy, cervical cerclage, and prenatal diagnostic tests.[5,23,26,27] It is therefore essential to be aware of the level of the deficient or abnormal factor. The United Kingdom Haemophilia Centre Doctors' Organisation (UKHCDO) recommends measuring relevant coagulation factor levels at booking, and at 28 and 34 weeks' gestation.[28] They should also be checked prior to any intervention, and ideally after treatment to assess response.

Patients with factor XIII deficiency and afibrinogenaemia are at risk of early pregnancy loss and placental abruption[29–31] and often need prophylactic treatment throughout pregnancy. Patients with other inherited bleeding disorders do not usually need prophylaxis throughout pregnancy, but may do so before any interventions, delivery and during episodes of bleeding.

Prenatal diagnosis

Prenatal diagnosis is often considered where the fetus is at risk of severe disease. This is usually performed by chorionic villus sampling at 11–14 weeks' gestation or amniocentesis between 16 and 20 weeks. These procedures may need to be covered with appropriate haemostatic support. Third-trimester amniocentesis is sometimes performed in women who are not considering termination of pregnancy, but wish to know whether the fetus is affected, to aid decisions made for delivery. For X-linked conditions such as haemophilia, it is clearly crucial to know the gender of the baby before planning delivery.

Antenatal haemorrhage

Patients presenting with antenatal haemorrhage need assessment by the obstetric team to establish the cause. Conservative treatment is usually appropriate for most but those with severe bleeding disorders or severe bleeding may need factor replacement. Tranexamic acid is often effective in antenatal haemorrhage.[23]

Labour and delivery

A detailed intrapartum care plan should be formulated by the multidisciplinary team during the third trimester for the management of labour and delivery. The mother's preferences with regards to caesarean delivery should be taken into account. It should include haemostatic measures that need to be taken and preferred mode of delivery. The plan should be made available for all involved, including the mother.

Women with moderate to severe haemophilia will need to be delivered in a unit with the necessary expertise in managing patients with bleeding disorders, and availability of appropriate coagulation assays and clotting factor treatments. Cell salvage is useful in these cases.

It is usually necessary to maintain haemostatic levels during labour and delivery up to those needed for major surgery because of the unpredictable need for emergency caesarean delivery.[31] If factor levels are not available in the acute setting, those obtained during the third trimester should be used. IV access should be obtained for patients with abnormal coagulation assays, and factor replacement is often needed to cover labour and delivery.

The mode of delivery can be controversial, and the decision should be made on a case-by-case basis. The aim is to minimize the risk of neonatal intracranial haemorrhage. A review of 117 deliveries of infants affected by haemophilia in Sweden reported rates of intracranial haemorrhage of 5.9%, 2.3%, and 0% among 17 ventouse deliveries, 87 spontaneous vaginal deliveries, and five emergency caesarean deliveries respectively.[32] There were eight elective caesarean deliveries, with one intracranial haemorrhage in a delivery at 27 weeks, where it was thought that the haemorrhage related to the prematurity of the neonate, rather than the coagulation defect.

The UKHCDO states that normal spontaneous vaginal delivery can be allowed, even for babies at risk of severe haemophilia, with early recourse to caesarean delivery if labour is prolonged or complicated. However, fear of a caesarean delivery becoming necessary in the second stage of labour prompts many to consider surgery electively. Furthermore, the decision to allow spontaneous vaginal delivery will often depend on the resources of the hospital, 24-hour availability of on-call senior obstetricians, anaesthetists and haematologists with experience in patients with haemophilia, and 24-hour laboratory support to allow processing of samples for factor assays. If these are not available, which may be the case in many hospitals, elective caesarean delivery may be a safer course of action.

Interventions such as fetal scalp monitoring, ventouse delivery, mid-cavity forceps, and forceps involving rotation of the head should be avoided in all male babies at risk of haemophilia, to minimize the risk of intracranial or scalp haemorrhage.

Care needs to be taken to avoid excessive maternal genital or perineal trauma to reduce the risk of excessive bleeding during delivery.[31]

Neuraxial anaesthesia

Use of neuraxial anaesthesia in patients with bleeding disorders is a much debated issue. A systematic review in 2009 looked at the use of neuraxial techniques in obstetric and non-obstetric patients with bleeding disorders. A total of 507 procedures were included, 107 in patients with haemophilia, 74 in patients with VWD, and 326 in patients with idiopathic thrombocytopenic purpura (ITP), after review of 30 articles. Haemostatic treatments were not standardized. There was one case of spinal haematoma, which was in an infant with an undiagnosed haemophilia which resulted in paraplegia.[33]

Decisions on neuraxial anaesthesia should be made by the multidisciplinary team, after thorough counselling and consenting of the mother. The UKHCDO states that neuraxial anaesthesia is not contraindicated if the coagulation screen is normal, and the relevant factor level is above 50 IU/dL, either due to the spontaneous rise in pregnancy, or following prophylactic treatment (2006). The procedure needs to be performed by an experienced anaesthetist with meticulous technical skill. However, a non-traumatic insertion of a spinal or epidural cannot be guaranteed. The lowest concentration of local anaesthetic agent should be used to allow adequate analgesia but preserving motor function[32] and regular assessment of neurological function should be carried out to allow early recognition of complications. Suspicion of a spinal epidural haematoma should lead to an urgent MRI and surgical decompression if appropriate. As adverse neurological outcome is directly related to time interval to surgical decompression, early recognition is essential. Removal of epidural catheter is also associated with a risk of spinal epidural haematoma. Coagulation screen and factor assays should therefore be performed before removal of epidural catheter, and appropriate treatment given if abnormal.[31,34]

Postpartum management

Women with inherited bleeding disorders are at significantly increased risk of primary and secondary postpartum haemorrhage especially those with severe disease. Perineal and vaginal haematomas are also more common at a rate of 1–6% versus 0.2% in the normal population.[35,36] Secondary postpartum haemorrhage is more common as coagulation factor levels return back to baseline after a rise in the third trimester.

Steps should be taken to reduce the risk of postpartum haemorrhage. The third stage of labour should be actively managed to reduce the risk of uterine atony. Agents used should be given IV rather than IM.

Normal factor levels should be maintained for 3–5 days after vaginal delivery, and 5–7 days after caesarean delivery. Close follow-up is needed after discharge, to identify and manage secondary postpartum haemorrhage.

Risk of thrombosis will need to be considered, particular in those receiving replacement therapy with FXI concentrate, recombinant activated factor VII and prothrombin complex concentrate. Antithrombotic measures such as hydration, early mobilization and the use of pharmacological thromboprophylaxis and antiembolic stockings should be considered in all.

Management of the newborn

Early diagnosis of inherited bleeding disorders is essential to reduce the risk of complications. A cord sample should be taken for the appropriate factor assay in all neonates at risk. It should be remembered however that for mild and moderate disease, the result may not be representative, as some factors increase with the stress of delivery and some have not reached normal adult values. In these cases, the test may need to be repeated at a later stage. In neonates in whom haemophilia has not been excluded, IM injections including vitamin K should be avoided. The UKHCDO recommends cranial ultrasound for all neonates at risk of a severe or moderate bleeding tendency, prior to discharge,[37] however, for neonates with suspected intracranial haemorrhage, CT or MRI are more sensitive imaging modalities. Intracranial haemorrhage tends to occur at around 4 days of life, so parents should be warned which signs to look for.

Haemophilia A and B

Pathophysiology

Haemophilia A and B are due to a reduction in factor VIII and IX respectively. Factor VIII and IX together with factor X form the tenase complex, an essential component of the coagulation cascade, needed to produce the thrombin burst and ultimately the fibrin platelet plug. Lack of factor VIII or IX produces loose friable fibrin, which is susceptible to fibrinolysis. Fibrinolysis is further enhanced by the lack of the thrombin-activator fibrinolysis inhibitor, normally activated by the thrombin burst. The lack of thrombin burst leads to a failure to consolidate the primary haemostatic plug, causing the characteristic bleeding pattern of haemophilia A and B, which is delayed after trauma but prolonged.[38]

Presentation

Haemophilia A affects approximately 1 in 10000 live births. Haemophilia B is rarer, affecting 1 in 50000 live births. Patients with haemophilia A and B tend to present in a similar fashion and suffer from similar clinical features. Patients are classified as mild, moderate or severe depending on factor levels (Table 48.6). Many infants are diagnosed because of a positive family history, where the mother is known to be a carrier. A cord sample for factor VIII or IX levels will establish a diagnosis. At least one third of cases have no family history and are due to new mutations. These patients may present with bleeding, such as a cephalohaematoma, after the trauma of delivery. They may otherwise present with bruises from minimal trauma, which can be misinterpreted as non-accidental injury, or with joint and muscle bleeds when the child starts walking. Patients with mild to moderate haemophilia may not suffer from spontaneous bleeding and may not present until later in life with bleeding after surgery or dental work.

Table 48.6 Classification of haemophilia

Severity	Factor VIII/IX level	Clinical features
Severe	< 1%	Spontaneous bleeds into muscle, joints, and internal organs
Moderate	1–5%	Bleeding after minor trauma Occasional spontaneous bleeding,
Mild	5–49%	Bleeding after surgery or major trauma Spontaneous bleeding very rare

Data from White GC, Rosendaal F, Aledort LM, *et al.*, Definitions in haemophilia. Recommendation of the scientific subcommittee on factor VIII and factor IX of the scientific and standardization committee of the International Society on Thrombosis and Haemostasis. *Thromb Haemost*, volume 85, p. 560, copyright © 2001 Schattauer GmbH.

Inheritance

The genes for factor VIII and factor IX are both encoded on the long arm of chromosome X and the conditions are inherited in an X-linked fashion. Daughters of men with haemophilia A or B are obligate carriers and are at risk of having an affected child. Their sons have a 50% chance of being a haemophilia sufferer and daughters have a 50% chance of being a carrier. Carrier females have on average 50% of normal levels and have a higher incidence of bleeding than non-carriers. Where lyonization is unbalanced, with skewed X-chromosome inactivation, baseline levels fall lower than 50% and bleeding risk is further increased.

In a similar manner to non-haemophiliac patients, factor VIII levels are expected to rise from 6 weeks' gestation, although Factor IX levels remain constant. FVIII levels start to fall from 48 hours postpartum.

Outcomes

Of 90 pregnancies in 53 carriers of haemophilia A and B, between 1995 and 2005, there were 65 live births, 13 miscarriages and 12 terminations.[39] Neuraxial anaesthesia was performed in 25 pregnancies with no complications. The caesarean delivery rate was 47%. The incidence of primary and secondary postpartum haemorrhage was 19% and 2%, respectively. Two women required blood transfusion and all survived. There were two neonatal cranial bleeding complications associated with prolonged labour or instrumental delivery. Pregnancy and delivery therefore needs to be carefully managed to prevent bleeding in the mother and the child.

Treatments for haemophilia A and B

Treatment options for the prevention or management of bleeds in women who are carriers of haemophilia include factor replacement, desmopressin, and tranexamic acid. These are in addition to other standard measures used to prevent or treat bleeding in obstetric patients. Decisions on treatment need to be made in conjunction with the haemophilia team.

Tranexamic acid

Tranexamic acid is a very useful agent for carriers of haemophilia A or B. It can be used prophylactically to reduce bleeding prior to procedures, where it is often started the day before the procedure and continued for up to 5 days. It can be used to reduce risk of bleeding during delivery and the postpartum period, when it should be started at the onset of labour, with an initial IV dose of 1 g, followed by 1 g tds orally for at least 5 days. It can also be used as adjunctive therapy for treatment of bleeding in haemophilia carriers.

Desmopressin

Desmopressin can be used as prophylaxis or treatment for carriers of haemophilia A, as well as male sufferers of mild to moderate haemophilia A. It has no effect in patients with haemophilia B. Mechanism of action, half-life, side effects and safety is covered earlier in the chapter. It should be remembered that desmopressin also acts as an antidiuretic, and therefore fluid intake should be monitored and may need to be restricted.

Recombinant factor concentrate

Factor concentrate is needed for haemophilia B carriers with low Factor IX levels. It is only required for haemophilia A carriers with low factor VIII levels if there is contraindication to desmopressin, such as hypertensive disorders. Recombinant factor concentrate is used, so risk of transmission of blood borne infection is not a concern. The main complication of factor replacement is inhibitor formation but this is very rare when used in haemophilia A or B carriers. Dosage is based on weight and increment needed (Box 48.4).

Antenatal management

Female carriers of haemophilia normally have factor levels of around 50 IU/dL. This level is usually sufficient to protect the patient from spontaneous bleeding and bleeding associated with surgery. However some carriers have lower Factor VIII or IX levels, due to unbalanced lyonization, and levels as low as 5 IU/dL have been seen in some patients.[39] Levels should be checked at booking and in the third trimester. They should be known before invasive procedures or delivery, and monitored during therapy. Therapeutic levels should be maintained for a suitable time period depending on the procedure. For minor antenatal procedures, usually 1–2 days of treatment is sufficient but for delivery normal values should be maintained for 3–5 days.

FVIII levels tend to increase during pregnancy, whereas FIX levels tend to remain constant. Chi et al. looked at 90 pregnancies of haemophilia carriers. Haemophilia A carriers had a significant rise in FVIII levels, with 92% achieving levels of greater than 50 IU/dL in the third trimester. Factor IX results were less consistent.[39]

Attempts are often made to establish the risk to the fetus so the pregnancy can be managed appropriately. Establishing the sex of the fetus is crucial. This can be done from 7 weeks' gestation by determining evidence of fetal Y chromosome in maternal blood, or by ultrasound scan at 12 weeks. If the fetus is female special precautions are not needed for delivery. For male fetuses, some women may accept prenatal diagnosis, by chorionic villus sampling or amniocentesis. If termination of pregnancy is not being considered, some parents opt for third trimester amniocentesis of male fetuses to aid decisions on management of labour.

A factor VIII or IX level of 50 IU/dL is necessary for procedures including chorionic villus sampling and amniocentesis. If the level is insufficient, treatment will be needed in the form of DDAVP® or factor VIII replacement for haemophilia A carriers, and factor IX replacement for haemophilia B carriers.

Box 48.4 Dosage of recombinant factor VIII/IX

$$\text{Factor VIII dosage (units)} = [\text{weight (kg)} \times \text{increment needed (units dL)}] / 2$$

$$\text{Factor IX dosage (units)} = [\text{weight (kg)} \times \text{increment needed (units dL)}] / 0.8$$

Management of labour and delivery

At the onset of labour a FBC, clotting screen and group and save should be taken. A factor assay should be taken if less than 50 IU/ dL at the last check. The majority of haemophilia A carriers do not need haemostatic support for delivery, as factor VIII levels usually reach the normal range spontaneously. However as factor IX does not rise in pregnancy these patients often need factor replacement.

As stated earlier, when considering the mode of delivery, factors to be taken into account include the maternal and fetal bleeding risks, other maternal complications and local resources such as availability of on-call senior obstetric, haematology and anaesthetic cover with experience in dealing with patients with bleeding disorders. Risk of intracranial haemorrhage is 4% in babies with severe haemophilias and special precautions need to be taken to avoid unnecessary trauma in potentially affected male babies. If vaginal delivery is opted for, use of ventouse extraction, mid cavity forceps and fetal scalp monitoring should be avoided. A prolonged second stage of delivery should also be avoided, with early recourse to caesarean delivery if necessary.

Neuraxial anaesthesia is considered safe providing the clotting screen is normal and factor VIII/IX levels are above 50 IU/Dl.[40] Levels should be checked again before removal of the epidural catheter as they may have fallen rapidly.

Postpartum management

Postpartum patients should be closely monitored as levels are expected to fall. Levels should be maintained at least 50 IU/dL for 3–5 days, although longer if caesarean delivery has been performed.

Aspirin, NSAIDs, IM injections, and pharmacological thromboprophylaxis should be avoided in patients with factor VIII or IX levels less than 50 IU/dL.

Management of the neonate

A cord sample should be taken to assess factor VIII or IX levels, although these may not be representative of the true baseline, as Factor VIII often rises in response to the stress of delivery and Factor IX does not reach true baseline levels until around 6 months of age. IM vitamin K should be withheld until the factor levels are known, or given orally if needed.

Von Willebrand disease

Pathophysiology

VWF is an essential part of the coagulation system. It is produced in the vascular endothelial cells and megakaryocytes in the bone marrow and binds to Factor VIII which inactivates rapidly in the absence of VWF. It is also important in platelet adhesion to wound sites.

VWF is released from the Weibel–Palade storage granules in response to a number of agonists including thrombin, epinephrine, histamine and vasopressin. This can be taken advantage of therapeutically by the use of desmopressin to treat milder forms of VWD. Increased synthesis and secretion of VWF also occurs as part of an acute-phase response to injury, inflammation, infection, malignancy, emotional stress and also pregnancy. This needs to be kept in mind when managing a pregnant woman with VWD.[38]

For normal von Willebrand function, it must be present in normal amounts, have a normal multimeric structure, and an intact binding site for collagen and platelet glycoproteins GPIb and GPIIb/IIIa. VWD is most commonly inherited, with mutations affecting each of these different aspects leading to the six different subclassifications of inherited VWD (Table 48.7).

During pregnancy, there is a rise in VWF antigen (VWF:Ag). In women with type 1 VWD, this is also accompanied by a rise in VWF activity and FVIII:C, usually reaching normal ranges by term.

Clinical features

The severity of bleeding varies from a mild to moderately severe bleeding tendency. Failure of platelets to adhere to injured vessel walls leads to failure of primary haemostasis and bleeding from small blood vessels in the skin and mucous membranes. Patients often present with bruising, epistaxis, menorrhagia and bleeding after surgery and dental extraction. Importantly, these patients are also vulnerable to postpartum bleeding. Patients with type 3 VWD have absent VWF and FVIII:C levels of 1-2%. These patients have a bleeding tendency similar to severe haemophilia A and suffer from haemarthrosis, muscle bleeds and life-threatening bleeding after trauma, as well as small vessel bleeding which is not normally a feature of haemophilia A.

Outcomes

Women are at risk of bleeding early in pregnancy before VWF and FVIII levels have risen. In one case series 33% of pregnancies in mothers with VWD developed vaginal bleeding.[37] Major antenatal haemorrhage is rare, but can occur after miscarriage or termination. Up to 10% of terminations can be accompanied by excessive bleeding requiring transfusion.[37] Women are at risk of postpartum haemorrhage, as VWF and factor VIII levels fall. 16–29% of women with VWD will develop primary postpartum haemorrhage, and 20–29% of women will develop secondary postpartum haemorrhage.[41]

Table 48.7 Subclassification of von Willebrand disease

Subclassification	Pathology	Inheritance	Severity
Type 1	Quantitative reduction in VWF	Autosomal dominant	Mild to moderate
Type 2a	Reduced high-molecular-weight multimers	Autosomal dominant	Mild to moderate
Type 2b	Increased GpIb binding leading to platelet aggregation and consumption	Autosomal recessive	Mild to moderate
Type 2m	Reduced GpIb binding	Autosomal recessive	Mild to moderate
Type 2n	Reduced VIII binding	Autosomal recessive	Mild to moderate
Type 3	Quantitative complete absence of VWF	Autosomal recessive	Severe

GP, glycoprotein; VWF, von Willebrand factor. Adapted from Sadler JE, Budde U, Eikenboom JCJ, *et al.*, Update on the pathophysiology and classification of von Willebrand disease: a report of the Subcommittee on von Willebrand Factor. *Journal of Thrombosis and Haemostasis*, volume 4, pp. 2103–14. copyright © 2006 John Wiley & Sons.

Laboratory investigations

Investigation of VWD initially involves measurement of the FBC, APTT, von Willebrand factor antigen (VWF:Ag), von Willebrand factor ristocetin cofactor activity (VWF:RCo), von Willebrand collagen binding activity (VWF:CBA) and FVIII level (FVIII:C) (Table 48.8).

VWF:Ag is a quantitative measurement of VWF. VWF:CBA and VWF:RCo are functional measures of VWF activity. If an abnormality is found, further investigations including ristocetin-induced platelet aggregation (RIPA) which measures the ability of VWF to bind to platelets, and VWF multimer factor analysis are performed.

Treatments for Von Willebrand disease

Patients with type 1 VWD and mild to moderate bleeding can often be treated with desmopressin, which acts to release VWF from Weibel–Palade storage granules, producing a brisk rise in VWF and FVIII levels, about 30 minutes after an IV infusion.[38] Desmopressin is less likely to be effective in patients with type 2 VWD due to the release of abnormal VWF. It is contraindicated in type 2b VWD as it will exacerbate platelet consumption and cause worsening thrombocytopenia. However it may be of benefit in type 2a, 2m and 2n VWD and a trial should be carried out before pregnancy. Desmopressin will be ineffective in patients with type 3 VWD.

For patients in whom desmopressin is ineffective or contraindicated, VWF concentrate is required. Intermediate and high purity concentrates are available which vary in the amount of VWF concentrate they contain and how well it is preserved, as well as the VWF/FVIII ratio. Following treatment with DDAVP® or VWF concentrate, FVIII:C levels, VWF:Ag, VWF:RCo, and if appropriate a FBC should be taken to assess response. Further levels may be required to assess if further treatment is needed.

Antenatal management

A baseline FVIII:C level, VWF:Ag, VWF:RCo and FBC should be taken at booking, and at 28 and 36 weeks. Risks to the baby of inheriting VWD need to be determined, although prenatal diagnosis is rarely undertaken as patients with VWD are able to maintain a good quality of life with current treatments. However, where babies are at risk of type 3 VWD, mothers may wish to undergo antenatal diagnosis and the procedure may need to be covered with DDAVP® or von Willebrand concentrate to ensure levels of more than 50 IU/dL.

Management of delivery

At the onset of labour a FBC, coagulation screen, FVIII;C level, VWF;Ag and VWF:RCo should be taken. Patients with type 1 VWD usually show a rise in VWF levels to within the normal range, giving no cause for concern at delivery. However the rise in VWF antigen levels leads to no improvement in activity for most patients with type 2 disease and those with type 2b VWD often develop a worsening of thrombocytopenia due to the heightened platelet binding. Patients with type 3 VWD have no increase in VWF.

Table 48.8 Laboratory investigations in von Willebrand disease

Subclassification	FBC	aPTT	VWF:Ag	VWF:RCo	VWF:CBA	FVIII:C	RIPA	Multimers
Type 1	Normal	Normal or prolonged	Low	Low	Low	Normal or low	No reaction	Normal
Type 2a	Normal	Normal or prolonged	Normal or low	Low	Low	Normal or low	No reaction	Decrease in large multimers
Type 2b	Platelet count 75–100	Normal or prolonged	Normal or low	Low	Low	Normal or low	Positive	Decrease in large multimers
Type 2m	Normal	Normal or prolonged	Normal or low	Low	Low	Normal or low	No reaction	Normal
Type 2n	Normal	Normal or prolonged	Normal or low	Normal or Low	Normal or Low	Low	No reaction	Normal
Type 3	Platelet count reduced/ normal/increased	Prolonged	Absent	Absent	Absent	Low	No reaction	Absent

Ag, antigen; aPTT, activated partial thromboplastin time; CBA, collagen binding activity; FBC, full blood count; RCo, ristocetin cofactor activity; RIPA, ristocetin-induced platelet aggregation; VWF, von Willebrand factor. Adapted from Laffan, M., *et al*, The diagnosis of von Willebrand disease: a guideline from the UK Haemophilia Centre Doctors' Organization. *Haemophilia*, Volume 10: issue 3, pp. 199–217. Copyright © 2004 John Wiley & Sons.

For labour, VWF activity levels and FVIII should be raised to 50 IU/dL. This can be achieved by the use of desmopressin, or if unsuitable, VWF concentrate. A delivery plan should have been made antenatally including the treatment agent of choice.

Neuraxial anaesthesia should only be used if FVIII;C level, VWF;Ag are above 50 IU/dL.[40]

The mode of delivery should be based on obstetric indications. Vaginal delivery is generally safe in type 1 and 2 VWD. Where the baby is at risk of type 2 or 3 VWD, a prolonged second stage of labour should be avoided, with early recourse to caesarean delivery. Interventions such as fetal scalp monitoring, ventouse delivery, mid cavity forceps and forceps involving rotation of the head should be avoided to minimize trauma to mother and baby, although the occurrence of intracranial haemorrhage is very low, even in patients with type 3 VWD.[42] The third stage of labour should be managed actively.

Postpartum management of mother

Women with FVIII and VWF:RCo levels less than 50 IU/d Lare more likely to develop postpartum haemorrhage.[44] Levels should be maintained above 50 IU/dL for up to 5 days postpartum. This can be achieved with the use of desmopressin or VWF concentrate. If complications occur and treatment is needed for more than 3 days, VWF concentrate may be required in addition to desmopressin because of the potential of tachyphylaxis.

Management of the neonate

A cord sample should be taken to establish FVIII:C, VWF:Ag and VWF:RCo levels. However, results may not be representative of true baseline levels as they can rise with the stress of delivery. Oral vitamin K should be given rather than IM, unless the cord sample shows normal levels.

Factor XI deficiency

Inheritance of Factor XI deficiency is autosomal. Homozygotes have levels of less than 15–20 IU/dL. Heterozygotes are partially deficient and have levels ranging between 20 and 70 IU/dL. In Ashkenazi Jews heterozygosity is reported to be as high as 8%.[44]

FXI levels and the degree of bleeding tendency do not correlate and patients can be categorized into those with a non-bleeding phenotype and those at risk during haemostatic challenges. Bleeding intensity tends to be associated with the site of injury. Areas with high fibrinolytic activity such as the oral cavity or urogenital tract have a higher risk of bleeding and women are prone to menorrhagia and bleeding after childbirth. A severe bleeding phenotype is unusual and in many of these patients there is coexistence of other bleeding tendencies such as VWD or platelet function disorders.[31]

Factor XI levels do not rise in pregnancy but the incidence of spontaneous miscarriage or antepartum haemorrhage is no higher than for women with normal Factor XI levels. The risk of postpartum haemorrhage (PPH) is increased, although a study of 105 pregnancies in 33 women showed there to be a highly significant difference between women with a 'bleeding' phenotype compared to those considered to be 'non-bleeders', with a relative risk [RR] of 7.2 (CI 1.99–25.9).[45] A study of women with severe factor XI deficiency (factor IX < 17 IU/dL), found that 24% of 132 untreated vaginal deliveries were accompanied by excessive bleeding. 17% of the 12 women undergoing caesarean delivery without prophylaxis had increased bleeding but this did not occur in any of the 6 who received prophylaxis for surgery.[46]

Standard measures as outlined in Boxes 48.1 and 48.2 should be taken throughout pregnancy, during labour and delivery and the postpartum period. Decisions on prophylaxis for delivery should be made on an individual basis based on previous bleeding tendency, factor XI levels, and mode of delivery.

Treatment options include tranexamic acid, FXI concentrate and FFP. The UKCHDO advise that women with FXI levels between 15 and 70 IU/dL and no significant bleeding history can be managed expectantly, without prophylaxis.[40] Women with levels between 15–70 IU/dL and a significant bleeding history or no previous haemostatic challenges can be given a 3-day course of tranexamic acid, with the first dose being given during labour. Patients with severe deficiency (FXI levels < 10–20 IU/dL) are likely to require factor XI concentrate. As this is associated with an increased risk of thrombotic complications, low dose therapy is usually used (around 10 IU/kg) to raise FXI levels to between 30 IU/dL and 70 IU/dL. Concomitant use of tranexamic acid should be avoided and antithrombotic measures should be used, including anti-embolic stockings, good hydration and early mobilization.

Neuraxial anaesthesia should be avoided unless an adequate response to treatment has been documented, with levels in the normal range. Recombinant activated factor VII has been used to prevent bleeding but this is an unlicensed indication and it is associated with increased thrombotic risk. All women with a bleeding phenotype should receive oral tranexamic acid for 2 weeks after delivery.

Rare inherited bleeding disorders

Standard precautions (as in Boxes 48.1 and 48.2) for patients with bleeding disorders are required for women with a rare inherited bleeding disorder (Table 48.9).

Fibrinogen and FXIII are both needed to support a pregnancy. Therefore women with inherited fibrinogen abnormalities and FXIII deficiency are unique in needing prophylactic replacement therapy throughout pregnancy, from the outset.

Some women with dysfibrinogenaemia and hypofibrinogenaemia also have a paradoxical risk of thrombosis. Bleeding and thrombotic risk should be considered in all patients, and prophylaxis with LMWH is considered in some.

Although most rare inherited bleeding disorders are autosomal recessive, the risk of the fetus inheriting the disorder should be considered in consanguineous marriages.

Analgesia for women with bleeding disorders

Normal analgesics used in the obstetric setting can be problematic for patients with bleeding disorders, due either to the side effects of the medication or its route of administration, and careful consideration should be given in choosing the most suitable form.

Aspirin

Aspirin is commonly used in pregnancy, to prevent hypertensive disorders and placental insufficiency. It inhibits platelet aggregation and activation by inactivating the cyclooxygenase (COX) enzyme, responsible for the synthesis of precursors of prostaglandin and thromboxane. Prostaglandins are involved in transmission of pain sensation, inflammation and modulation of the hypothalamic thermostat. Thromboxane is a potent vasoconstrictor and enhances platelet aggregation and activation of new platelets. The inhibitory effect of aspirin is irreversible and thus persists for the lifetime of the platelet, approximately 7–10 days. Thus aspirin is not recommended for patients with bleeding disorders.

Table 48.9 Summary of rare inherited bleeding disorders

	Incidence	Inheritance	Coagulation results	Preferred therapeutic option	Other options
II	1 per 2 million	Autosomal recessive	Prolonged aPTT and PT	Prothrombin complex concentrate	SD plasma
V	1 per 1 million	Autosomal recessive	Prolonged AaPTT and PT, normal TT	SD plasma	Platelets and recombinant activated factor VII
VII	2 per million	Autosomal recessive	Prolonged PT	Recombinant activated factor VII	Virally inactivated factor VII concentrate Prothrombin complex concentrate or SD plasma—only recommended if alternatives not available
X	1 per million	Autosomal recessive	PT and aPTT prolonged	Prothrombin complex concentrate	SD plasma
Combined V and VIII	1 per million	Autosomal recessive	aPPT more prolonged than PT	SD plasma to raise FVII levels, and Recombinant FVIII	FVIII concentrate
XIII	1 per million	Autosomal recessive	Normal aPTT/PT/TT Positive clot solubility test	FXIII concentrate	SD plasma
Fibrinogen	1 per million	Autosomal recessive/ dominant	Afibrinogenaemia—fibrinogen unmeasurable by function (Clauss) method, and immunoreactive assays. Hypofibrinogenaemia—low fibrinogen by functional and immunoreactive method. Dysfibrinogenaemia—fibrinogen measured lower by functional method than immunoreactive assay	Virally inactivated fibrinogen	Cryoprecipitate only in emergencies

aPTT, activated partial thromboplastin time; PT, prothrombin time; SD, solvent detergent; TT, prothrombin time.

Non-steroidal anti-inflammatory drugs

NSAIDs also inhibit the COX enzyme, reducing production of thromboxane and prostaglandins but inhibition is competitively reversible. This the duration of the inhibitory effect is more dependent on the half-life of the drug. NSAIDs such as ibuprofen and diclofenac, ketoprofen and indomethacin have short half-lives of less than 6 hours, whereas naproxen, celecoxib, meloxicam, nabumetone, and piroxicam have half-lives of more than 6 hours and up to 60 hours. Pessaries and suppositories can have just the systemic effect as oral NSAIDs. Gastric ulceration can occur, both due to direct irritation of the gastric mucosa, and also due to reduction of protective prostaglandin.

NSAIDs are generally not recommended in patients with bleeding disorders. However, short-acting forms can be used with caution in women receiving haemostatic treatment.

Intramuscular analgesia

NSAIDs or opiates are often given by the IM route. However in women with bleeding disorders this can be associated with muscle haematoma. IM injections are not recommended in women with factor levels less than 50%, or a platelet count less than 50×10^9/L.

Patient-controlled analgesia

Patient controlled analgesia is a good option for analgesia in this cohort of women, allowing patients to manage their own analgesia. Long-acting opioids will affect the neonate, so short-acting opioids like remifentanil are more appropriate (see Chapter 13).

Neuraxial anaesthesia

Use of neuraxial analgesia needs to be carefully considered. Epidural analgesia is more of a concern than spinal analgesia as the catheter is left *in situ* and the epidural needle is bigger and potentially causes more trauma. Removal of the catheter can be associated with a higher bleeding risk than insertion. Factor VIII or IX levels should be at least 50% for insertion and removal of the catheter and the platelet count should be at least 50×10^9/L and usually 80×10^9/L.

Spinal analgesia is often preferred as a smaller needle can be used and usually no catheter is left in place. Very rarely spinal catheters are used and would be contra-indicated in a patient with a bleeding tendency. Again a factor level of more than 50% is advised.

Thrombocytopenia

Thrombocytopenia occurs in up to 10% of pregnancies, with gestational thrombocytopenia, MAHAs, and immune thrombocytopenias the most common causes. Figure 48.6 demonstrates the incidence of causes of thrombocytopenia. Box 48.5 lists rarer causes of thrombocytopenia.

General considerations

Serious maternal haemorrhage is rare in those with thrombocytopenia. The bleeding risk depends on the cause of the thrombocytopenia, the level of platelet count, rate of fall and if there is an associated coagulopathy. For example, a patient with ITP will have younger more active platelets, and have a lower bleeding risk than a patient with disseminated intravascular coagulation (DIC) or a platelet function disorder.

Patients with a platelet count over 100×10^9/L can be monitored by the midwife or GP. Those with a platelet count less than 100×10^9/L usually need to be assessed in secondary care. Treatment aims to maintain a safe, rather than normal platelet count and is usually only required to cover invasive procedures and delivery.

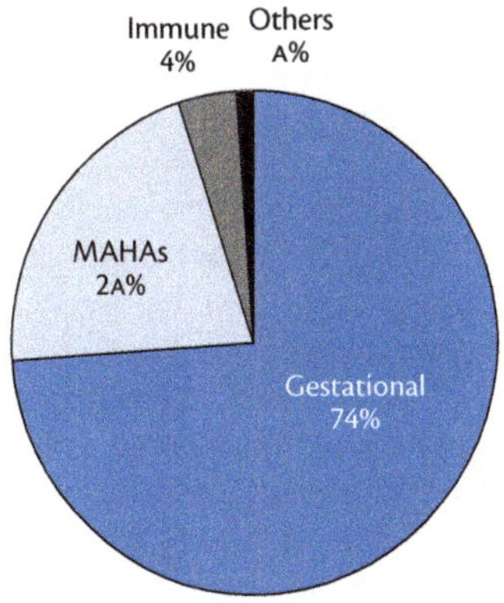

Figure 48.6 Causes of thrombocytopenia in pregnancy.

Anaesthesia

Use of neuraxial anaesthesia is often a source of debate and there is little evidence to support a safe platelet count. A threshold of more than 80×10^9/L is considered safe by most anaesthetists to insert and remove epidural anaesthesia, provided there is no associated coagulopathy, and the patient is not on anticoagulants or antiplatelet agents.[47] Some experienced anaesthetists would consider neuraxial anaesthesia in ITP patients with a platelet count above 50×10^9/L.[48] Patients with a platelet count of $50–80 \times 10^9$/L should be assessed on a case-by-case basis, and a detailed bleeding history should be established to help determine the bleeding risk.

Mode of delivery

Mode of delivery should be based on obstetric factors, as there is no evidence to suggest caesarean delivery is safer than uncomplicated vaginal delivery.[45] If delivery is anticipated to be complicated, an elective caesarean delivery may be a better option.

General considerations for the fetus

Neonatal thrombocytopenia with associated intracranial haemorrhage is the major concern for a baby with a thrombocytopenic mother and the cause of maternal thrombocytopenia needs to be considered. Gestational thrombocytopenia is a benign diagnosis for the fetus. However, maternal ITP can result in transplacental transfer of maternal immunoglobulin G (IgG) autoantibody,

Box 48.5 Rare causes of thrombocytopaenia in pregnancy

- Folate deficiency
- Systemic lupus erythematosus/antiphospholipid syndrome
- Viruses
- Drugs
- Malignancies
- Splenomegaly
- Congenital platelet disorders

leading to thrombocytopenia in the fetus. Thrombocytopenia due to MAHA is not usually associated with thrombocytopenia in the fetus, but can cause placental infarction and high rates of morbidity and mortality.

Standard precautions should be taken for fetuses at risk of thrombocytopenia. This includes avoidance of fetal scalp monitoring, use of ventouse and rotational forceps, and prolonged labour. A cord sample should be taken to assess the platelet count. IM vitamin K should be avoided if the platelet count is less than 50×10^9/L, and can be given orally instead. Infants with a subnormal platelet count should be monitored, as the platelet count may continue to fall, with a nadir at 2–5 days.

Severe thrombocytopenia in infants is rare. Infants with a platelet count less than 20×10^9/L should be tested to exclude fetoneonatal alloimmune thrombocytopenia.

Gestational thrombocytopenia

Gestational thrombocytopenia is the most common cause of thrombocytopenia in pregnancy and complicates 5% of pregnancies. There is approximately a 10% fall in platelet count from baseline, which tends to occur in the second half of pregnancy. The platelet count at term is more than 100×10^9/L in 95% of cases and it is rare for it to fall below 70×10^9/L. Other causes, namely ITP, should be considered if this is the case.

Gestational thrombocytopenia is a diagnosis of exclusion, and it can be difficult to distinguish severe forms of this from ITP. Table 48.10 summarizes the key distinguishing features.

Gestational thrombocytopenia is benign for both mother and baby, and is not associated with haemorrhagic complications. The thrombocytopenia usually resolves within 6 weeks after delivery. Use of neuraxial anaesthesia is considered safe in patients with gestational thrombocytopenia, as the platelet count rarely falls to below 70×10^9/L.

Table 48.10 Differences between gestational and immune thrombocytopaenia

Gestational thrombocytopenia	Immune thrombocytopenic purpura
No specific diagnostic test—diagnosis of exclusion	No specific diagnostic test—diagnosis of exclusion
No associated autoimmune diseases	Associated autoimmune diseases
Normal platelet count prepregnancy	Possible previous history of thrombocytopenia
Platelet count usually $>100 \times 10^9$/L, rarely $< 70 \times 10^9$/L	Median platelet count at delivery 85×10^9/L
Not associated with maternal haemorrhage	Small risk of maternal haemorrhage
Occurs in second half of pregnancy	Can cause thrombocytopenia in the first and second trimester
No improvement with steroids	Improvement with steroids
No fetal haemorrhage	Small risk of fetal haemorrhage
Spontaneous resolution after delivery	Thrombocytopenia can persist after pregnancy
May recur in subsequent pregnancies	May recur in subsequent pregnancies

Immune thrombocytopenic purpura

Although ITP is one of the less frequent causes of thrombocytopenia in pregnancy, it is the most common cause of thrombocytopenia in the first and second trimester. It is due to antibodies against platelet surface glycoproteins, mainly glycoprotein IIb/IIIa and glycoprotein Ib/IX.

Severe bleeding complications are rare in patients with ITP as platelets tend to be younger and more active. Unlike gestational thrombocytopenia, ITP can cause haemorrhagic complications in the fetus as the IgG antibodies can cross the placenta.

Outcomes

Webert et al. looked at 119 pregnancies in mothers with ITP.[49] Although 15.5% of women had a platelet count of lower than 50×10^9/L at the time of delivery, haemorrhagic complications were uncommon and not related to the platelet count. Four women had an estimated blood loss at delivery of more than 1 L and the platelet count in these women ranged from 54×10^9/L to 321×10^9/L. Neuraxial analgesia was used in 42 pregnancies, seven of whom had a platelet count of less than 75×10^9/L. No complications were reported. There was one fetal death related to thrombocytopenia. This was a stillbirth at 27 weeks in a mother with moderately severe ITP who had previously undergone a splenectomy.

Treatments

Decisions on treatments for ITP should be based on the balance of risks of bleeding versus risks of side effects from treatments. The aim is for a safe platelet count for pregnancy, rather than a normal platelet count. Patients with a platelet count more than 20×10^9/L often do not need treatment until 36 weeks, or if delivery is imminent.

Table 48.11 suggests some maternal platelet counts which are generally thought to be acceptable.

Prednisolone is the usual first-line treatment, with 20 mg being a suitable starting dose in pregnancy. A response can be expected within 3–7 days. Patients unresponsive to steroids can be tried on IV immunoglobulin or higher-dose steroids. Other treatment options for ITP have limited use in pregnancy.

Splenectomy is rarely required for treatment of refractory ITP in pregnancy and is best undertaken in the second trimester. It can be performed laparoscopically before 20 weeks, after which the technique becomes difficult. Splenectomy in the first trimester is associated with increased risks of preterm labour.[50] The platelet count often does not need to be raised prior to splenectomy, as it can be expected to rise after the splenic artery is clamped.

Platelet transfusions are ineffective in the treatment of ITP as they are destroyed by the antibody, so are short lived. The only indication for use of platelets in the management of ITP is major

Table 48.11 Acceptable platelet counts for various situations in women with idiopathic thrombocytopenic purpura

Situation	Accepted platelet count
Antenatally	>20 × 109/L
Vaginal delivery	>40 × 109/L
Operational/instrumental delivery	>50 × 109/L
Epidural	>80 × 109/L

haemorrhage or emergency surgery, when bleeding points can be transiently sealed. Concurrent use of IV immunoglobulin can extend the half-life of transfused platelets to some degree.

Antenatal management

Women with a platelet count above 100 × 10^9/L can usually be managed in the community with monthly blood counts by the midwife. Those with a platelet count below 100 × 10^9/L should be referred to a specialized haematology obstetric clinic. In these patients, if the count is relatively stable monitoring can occur every 4 weeks until after 26 weeks, increasing to every fortnight and every week as term approaches.

Treatment for thrombocytopenia is not usually needed unless the platelet count is less than 20 × 10^9/L, a procedure is planned, the patient is bleeding, or delivery is approaching. Potential side effects of treatment need to be considered, such as gestational diabetes, weight gain, or postpartum psychiatric disorders.

Management of labour and delivery

Home delivery is not advised if the platelet count is less than 100 × 10^9/L. Mode of delivery should be based on obstetric factors as there is no evidence that caesarean delivery is safer for the fetus. A blood count should be checked on arrival in labour and neuraxial anaesthesia avoided if the platelet count is too low. Standard precautions mentioned earlier should be taken to reduce the risk of neonatal haemorrhage.

Postpartum management of the mother

Active management of the third stage of labour is recommended, with IV oxytocic drugs. Non-steroidal analgesia should be avoided due to the associated bleeding risk of haemorrhage. Oral tranexamic acid given for 14 days postpartum should be considered.

It needs to be remembered that 25% of mothers with ITP have antiphospholipid antibodies and therefore thromboprophylaxis may well be necessary.

Management of the newborn

Babies born to mothers with ITP are at risk of thrombocytopenia. Reported incident of neonatal thrombocytopenia varies, but between 8% and 30% of infants will have platelet counts less than 50 × 10^9/L, and 1–5% will have a platelet count below 20 × 10^9/L.[51–53]

Table 48.12 Common causes of microangiopathic haemolytic anaemias

Specific to pregnancy	Not specific to pregnancy
Pre-eclampsia	Thrombotic thrombocytopenic purpura
HELLP syndrome	Haemolytic uraemic syndrome
Acute fatty liver of pregnancy	Disseminated intravascular coagulation
	Malignant hypertension
	Burns
	Vasculitides, e.g. Wegener's, systemic lupus erythematosus
	Certain infections, e.g. malaria, babesiosis, bartonellosis, *Clostridium perfringens*

HELLP, haemolysis, elevated liver enzymes, low platelets.

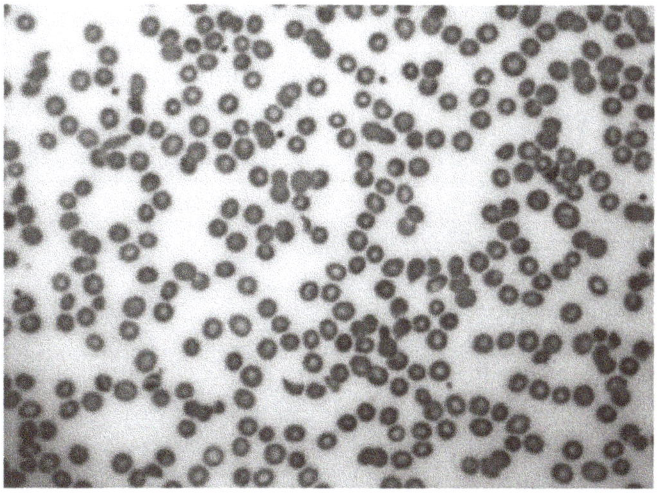

Figure 48.7 A blood film from a patient with MAHA depicting polychromasia and schistocytes.

A cord sample should be taken to assess the platelet count and for those with thrombocytopenia, a repeat count should be considered at 2–5 days when platelets reach their nadir due to splenic development in the neonate.

Microangiopathic haemolytic anaemias

MAHAs are a subgroup of haemolytic anaemias which involve physical destruction of red blood cells in blood vessels. Destruction can occur in the large vessels because of abnormal vasculature or cardiac valves, or more commonly in pregnancy in the small vessels due to deposition of thrombi. Destruction of red cells leads to anaemia and the presence of red cell fragments, known as schistocytes in the blood film (Figure 48.7). Consumption of platelets in deposited thrombi leads to thrombocytopenia

There is overlap in the presenting features of MAHAs, which can cause some diagnostic difficulty. Table 48.13 outlines some of the distinguishing features between the pregnancy-associated MAHAs. Delay in diagnosis, especially of thrombocytopenic purpura, can be life threatening, and often plasma exchange needs to be started immediately, before a diagnosis can be confirmed.

MAHAs secondary to pre-eclampsia

The aetiology of the mechanical damage to red cells during pre-eclampsia is uncertain but is probably due to fracturing of red cells as they pass over microthrombi, reflecting coagulation activation, vasoconstriction, and/or endothelial dysfunction seen in this condition. Up to 50% of women develop thrombocytopenia, secondary to activation of coagulation and formation of microthrombi in the circulation. The severity parallels the pre-eclampsia (Box 48.6).

Management

The FBC and coagulation screen should be monitored in patients with pre-eclampsia. Platelet transfusions should only be given if there is active bleeding, or if delivery is urgent. In this setting and in the presence of a DIC, platelets should be given to maintain a platelet count above 50 ×10^9/L.

Similarly, fresh frozen plasma should be used only if there is active bleeding.

Table 48.13 Distinguishing features between the pregnancy-associated microangiopathic haemolytic anaemias

	Pre-eclampsia	HELLP (haemolysis, elevated liver enzymes, and low platelets)	DIC (disseminated intravascular coagulation)	AFLP (acute fatty liver of pregnancy)	TTP (thrombotic thrombocytopenic purpura)	HUS (haemolytic uraemic syndrome)
Onset of symptoms	Third trimester	Third trimester	Any time	Third trimester	Third trimester	Postpartum
Central nervous system symptoms	+/–	+/–	+/–	+/–	+++	+/–
Renal impairment	+/–	+	+/–	+	++	+++
Fever	–	–	+/–	–	+/–	+/–
Liver impairment	+/–	+++	+/–	+++	+/–	+/–
Hypertension	+++	+/–	–	+	+/–	++
Haemolysis	+	++	+	+/–	+++	++
Thrombocytopenia	+	++	+++	+	+++	++
Prolonged clotting times	+/–	+/–	+++	++	–	–
ADAMTS13 levels	Mildly reduced	Mildly reduced	Mildly reduced	Mildly reduced	Severely deficient (levels < 5%)	Mildly reduced
Resolution post delivery	Rapid	May take 2–3 days	Rapid	Can take weeks	Can take weeks	Can take weeks

Myers B. Thrombocytopenia in pregnancy. *The Obstetrician & Gynaecologist*, volume 11, issue 3, pp. 177–183. copyright © 2009 John Wiley & Sons.

Neuraxial anaesthesia is only recommended if the platelet count is above 80 × 10^9/L and the coagulation screen is normal.

Thrombocytopenia, MAHAs, and coagulopathy associated with pre-eclampsia usually quickly resolve after delivery, but occasionally may worsen or even present postpartum and can continue for up to 14 days after delivery.

HELLP syndrome

HELLP syndrome is characterized by haemolysis, elevated liver enzymes, and low platelets. It occurs in 0.5–0.9% of pregnancies and in 10–20% of cases of severe pre-eclampsia.[54] Seventy per cent of cases occur antenatally, usually in the third trimester, the remainder occur in the 48 hours postpartum (see also Chapter 36).

The pathophysiology of HELLP is thought to be similar to pre-eclampsia, with endothelial damage, possibly more marked in the liver vasculature, with local fibrin deposition and infrequently areas of liver infarction as a consequence. Haemolytic anaemia with the presence of schistocytes on the blood film, and thrombocytopenia are characteristic. Thrombocytopenia reflects the degree of severity and is used in the Mississippi classification of HELLP (Table 48.14). Liver function tests are abnormal and right upper quadrant pain can occur which is the result of obstructed blood flow in the hepatic sinusoids and hepatic necrosis. DIC complicates 80% of severe cases (Box 48.7).[45]

HELLP has a maternal mortality rate of approximately 1%.[55] Perinatal mortality has been reported as between 7% and 34% and is mainly due to prematurity.[56–58]

Box 48.6 Haematological features of severe pre-eclampsia

- Thrombocytopenia
- Anaemia
- Reticulocytosis
- Presence of schistocytes and polychromasia in blood film
- Prolonged aPTT
- Increased fibrin degradation products
- Reduced antithrombin activity

Haematological management

Mode of delivery should be guided by obstetric factors. Clotting screen results are usually normal in HELLP and as this is a prothrombotic condition blood products are rarely needed. Platelets should be avoided unless the patient is bleeding.

Table 48.14 Mississippi classification of HELLP

HELLP class	Mississippi classification
1	Platelets ≤ 50 × 10^9/L AST or ALT ≥ 70 IU/L LDH ≥ 600 IU/L
2	Platelets ≤ 100 × 10^9/L ≥ 50 × 10^9/L AST or ALT ≥ 70 IU/L LDH ≥ 600 IU/L
3	Platelets ≤ 150 × 10^9/L ≥ 100 × 10^9/L AST or ALT ≥ 40 IU/L LDH ≥ 600 IU/L

ALT, alanine transaminase; AST, aspartate aminotransferase; LDH, lactate dehydrogenase.
Adapted from *American Journal of Obstetrics and Gynecology*, volume 195, issue 4, James N. Martin, Carl H. Rose, Christian M. Briery, Understanding and managing HELLP syndrome: The integral role of aggressive glucocorticoids for mother and child pp. 914–934, Copyright (2006), with permission from Elsevier.
Adapted from *American Journal of Obstetrics and Gynecology*, volume 180, issue 6, James N. Martin *et al.*, The spectrum of severe preeclampsia: Comparative analysis by HELLP (hemolysis, elevated liver enzyme levels, and low platelet count) syndrome classification pp. 1373–1384, Copyright (1999), with permission from Elsevier.

Box 48.7 Complications of HELLP

- DIC (15%)
- Placental abruption (15%)
- Acute respiratory distress syndrome
- Hepatorenal syndrome
- Pulmonary oedema (8%)
- Subcapsular hepatic haematoma (1%)
- Hepatic rupture
- Maternal mortality (1%)
- Fetal mortality (7–34%)

Antiphospholipid syndrome is associated with HELLP and patients would benefit from testing for antiphospholipid antibodies after delivery, to guide management of future pregnancies.

Neuraxial anaesthesia is not without risk because of the associated coagulopathy, and should only be performed if the coagulation profile is normal or has been corrected, and the platelet count is above 80×10^9/L.

Thrombotic thrombocytopenic purpura

Thrombotic thrombocytopenic purpura (TTP) is a rare condition with an incidence of less than six cases per million per annum. It has a 90% mortality if it not treated; 50% of deaths occur in the first 24 hours so early recognition is essential.[59] TTP is not unique to pregnancy, but 10–25% of cases can be associated with pregnancy. Presentation can be at any time in pregnancy, but is more common in the third trimester and postpartum. Pregnancy is a risk factor for relapse in women with known TTP especially those with congenital TTP.

TTP is due to a deficiency of the von Willebrand cleaving protein ADAMTS13. This is an enzyme which cleaves large molecules of VWF into smaller units. This deficiency can be due to a congenital deficiency (congenital TTP), or more commonly in adults, due to autoantibodies against ADAMTS13. Immune destruction of ADAMTS13 can be idiopathic/primary, or secondary to one of the conditions listed in Box 48.8. In the absence of ADAMTS13, high-molecular-weight VWF multimers under shear stresses will activate platelets and cause widespread platelet aggregates of clumps, which block vessels.

TTP is typically characterized by a clinical pentad of microangiopathic haemolytic anaemia, thrombocytopenia, renal dysfunction, fever, and neurological impairment, although diagnosis is hopefully

Box 48.8 Conditions associated with TTP not always associated with low ADAMTS13 levels

- HIV
- Drugs including quinine, trimethoprim, and pegylated interferon
- Malignancy, particularly adenocarcinoma
- After bone marrow transplantation
- Pancreatitis
- Autoimmune disease

Table 48.15 Clinical features of TTP

Neurological	Seizures, headaches, drowsiness, confusion, focal neurological signs
Renal	Acute kidney injury, proteinuria, microhaematuria
Cardiac	Ischaemia/infarction
Respiratory	Pulmonary embolism
Haematology	Bruising, haemorrhage, jaundice due to haemolysis
Gastrointestinal	Abdominal pain
Non-specific	Fever, pallor, fatigue, arthralgia, myalgia
Fetal	Miscarriage, intrauterine growth restriction, intrauterine death, pre-eclampsia

made before the full pentad develops and should be considered in the presence of MAHA and thrombocytopenia alone, if there are no other obvious causes. Diagnosis is based on clinical signs and blood film appearances. Other laboratory investigations may be helpful (Box 48.8). A severely low ADAMTS13 of less than 5% is diagnostic of TTP, but this investigation is often not rapidly available. Signs and symptoms are due to widespread multiorgan thrombosis (Table 48.15). Thrombosis in the placenta also has detrimental effects for the fetus, causing intrauterine growth restriction or fetal death.

Management

The diagnosis of TTP is a medical emergency; patients must be prioritized to receive plasma exchange as soon as possible as delays can be life-threatening for the mother. In the last two triennial Confidential Enquiries, TTP accounted for 1% of all maternal deaths due to late diagnosis or delayed treatment resulting in myocardial infarction.[60] Patients presenting with a MAHA and thrombocytopenia which cannot be easily explained by another pregnancy-related MAHA should be assumed to have TTP and treated as such.

Investigations

Investigations listed in Table 48.16 should be performed to aid diagnosis. It is essential that the ADAMTS13 level and antibodies are taken prior to the infusion of plasma products, as this will invalidate the result. A low ADAMTS13 level will confirm the diagnosis of TTP, which is particularly important when the clinical diagnosis is uncertain. The presence of antibodies against ADAMTS13 suggests immune-mediated or acquired TTP, rather than congenital TTP. In addition, a virology sample for HIV and hepatitis B and C should be taken as a baseline prior to infusion of plasma products. A troponin should also be measured to assess for cardiac involvement which is a poor prognostic sign.

Treatment options

Plasma exchange will infuse ADAMTS13, and remove the ADAMTS13 antibody. If there is any delay in plasma exchange, a plasma infusion should be given, ideally solvent detergent plasma if available, otherwise fresh frozen plasma is acceptable. As a new presentation of TTP in this age group is usually immune in nature, immunosuppressants in the form of oral prednisolone or IV methylprednisolone should also be commenced. Although most patients present with thrombocytopenia, platelet transfusions are contraindicated as they will increase the risk of thrombosis. Treatment with plasma exchange and immunosuppressants

Table 48.16 Diagnostic investigations of TTP

Haemoglobin	Reduced—usually 80–100 g/L
Platelet count	Reduced—usually 10–30 × 10^9/L
Reticulocyte count	Increased
Lactate dehydrogenase	Increased
Bilirubin	Increased
Haptoglobin	Reduced
Direct coombs test	Negative
Clotting screen	Usually normal
Urea and electrolytes	Can be abnormal if renal involvement. Acute kidney injury requiring haemodialysis is more indicative of HUS
Blood film	Presence of schistocytes, polychromasia, thrombocytopenia, left shift
ADAMTS13 level	Reduced
ADAMTS13 antibodies	Present in acquired/immune TTP, absent in congenital TTP

should lead to an increase in the platelet count within a few days. Regular plasma exchange should be continued throughout pregnancy, and also in the postpartum period. In the rarer scenario of the mother being found to have congenital rather than immune TTP, they should attend a specialist centre and receive ADAMTS13 supplementation regularly throughout pregnancy and the postpartum period.

Management of delivery

Ideally patients should be stabilized with plasma exchange. Neuraxial anaesthesia should be avoided if the platelet count is below 80 × 10^9/L. It should be remembered, however, that, unlike MAHA associated with pre-eclampsia, TTP is slow to resolve after delivery and treatment needs to be continued.

Supportive care

As TTP is a prothrombotic condition, aspirin and prophylactic LMWH should be commenced once the platelet count is above 50 × 10^9/L. Folic acid is required to support increased erythropoiesis, to compensate for the haemolysis but red cell transfusion is only needed if significant uncontrolled anaemia develops.

Management of patients with a previous history of TTP in pregnancy

Patients with a previous history of TTP are at risk of recurrence during subsequent pregnancies and require preconceptual counselling about potential risks of future pregnancies and the use of the combined oral contraceptive pill. These patients need close monitoring during pregnancy in a joint haematology and obstetric clinic. ADAMTS13 levels can be used to predict likelihood of relapse, and guide prophylactic treatment

Haemolytic uraemic syndrome

Haemolytic uraemic syndrome (HUS) is the clinical trial of a microangiopathic haemolytic anaemia, acute kidney injury, and thrombocytopenia. It is divided into diarrhoea associated due to a toxin produced by *Escherichia coli* and occasionally pneumococci. In atypical HUS, there is no prodrome of diarrhoea and recent research shows the majority relate to a defect in the complement system or occasionally due to antiphospholipid syndrome. The disease most commonly presents in the late postpartum period. It is often associated with a poor outcome with 76% of patients developing end-stage renal failure.[60]

Management of diarrhoea-associated HUS is supportive, plasma exchange has little benefit except in the very old or very young. Atypical HUS is diverse in its response to plasma exchange and some cases do respond to eculizumab. HUS is best managed by experts in this field.

Table 48.17 Common causes of disseminated intravascular coagulation

Pregnancy related	Non-pregnancy related
Placental abruption	Severe sepsis
Amniotic fluid embolism	Trauma and burns
Pre-eclampsia	Malignancy
Acute fatty liver of pregnancy	Acute promyelocytic leukaemia
Septic abortion	Organ destruction, e.g. pancreatitis
	ABO incompatible transfusion reaction
	Liver failure
	Vascular abnormalities
	Massive haemorrhage

Acute fatty liver of pregnancy

Acute fatty liver of pregnancy (AFLP) is a rare complication of late pregnancy, or the postpartum period (see also Chapter 36). Presentation is with nausea, vomiting, right upper quadrant pain, and liver failure. Haematological laboratory findings include a low platelet count, prolonged PT, low fibrinogen, and low antithrombin levels. The associated coagulopathy is due to reduced production of clotting factors by the liver, rather than consumption.

Treatment for AFLP includes fresh frozen plasma, platelets, and cryoprecipitate if the patient is bleeding. Careful attention needs to be paid to fluid balance and use of analgesia and anaesthesia.[61] Early delivery should be considered, as this can correct some of the clinical and laboratory abnormalities.[62]

Disseminated intravascular coagulation

DIC refers to a pathological intravascular activation of coagulation, with severe consumption of coagulation factors and platelets. Deposition of fibrin in small vessels can lead to a MAHA. DIC is a clinicopathological diagnosis, that is, it cannot be made from a set of blood tests but requires a clinical overview to make the diagnosis.

Some of the numerous causes of DIC are listed in Table 48.17. Laboratory features suggestive of DIC are listed in Box 48.9, although not all features are always present.

Thromboelastometry is diagnostic with prolonged clotting time and reduced angle and clot strength. Definitive treatment of

Box 48.9 Laboratory features suggestive of disseminated intravascular coagulation

- Prolonged aPTT
- Prolonged PT
- Thrombocytopenia
- Low fibrinogen
- Increased fibrin degradation products

DIC is to treat the underlying cause. Plasma products and platelet transfusions should be given if there is active bleeding or if delivery is imminent.

Conclusion

Haematological disorders in pregnancy can be varied but often present unique and complex challenges. There is a need for these pregnancies to be carefully managed within the multidisciplinary team to improve maternal and fetal outcomes.

References

1. McLean E, Cogswell M, Egli I, *et al.* Worldwide prevalence of anaemia, WHO Vitamin and Mineral Nutrition Information System 1993–2005. *Public Health Nutr* 2009; 12:444–54.
2. Pavord S, Myers B, Robinson S, *et al.* UK guidelines on the management of iron deficiency in pregnancy. *Br J Haematol* 2012; 156:588–600.
3. Colomer J, Colomer C, Gutierrez D, *et al.* Anaemia during pregnancy as a risk factor for infant iron deficiency: report from the Valencia Infant Anaemia Cohort (VIAC) study. *Paediatr Perinat Epidemiol* 1990; 4:196–204.
4. Insel BJ, Schaefer CA, McKeague IW, *et al.* Maternal iron deficiency and the risk of schizophrenia in offspring. *Arch Gen Psychiatry* 2008; 65:1136–44.
5. Van den Broek, Letsky E, White A, *et al.* Iron status in pregnant women: which measurements are valid? *Br J Haematol* 1998; 103:817–24.
6. Royal College of Obstetricians and Gynaecologists. *Blood Transfusions in Obstetrics*. Green-top Guideline No. 47. London: RCOG; 2007.
7. Broche DE, Gay C, Armand-Branger S, *et al.* Severe anaemia in the immediate post-partum period. Clinical practice and value of intravenous iron. *Eur J Obstet Gynecol Reprod Biol* 2005; 123:21–7.
8. Bayoumeu F, Subiran-Buisset C, Baka NE, *et al.* Iron therapy in iron deficiency anaemia in pregnancy: intravenous route versus oral route. *Eur J Obstet Gynecol Reprod Biol* 2005; 123:15–19.
9. van Wyk DB, Martens MG. Intravenous ferric carboxymaltose compared with oral iron in the treatment of postpartum anaemia: a randomized controlled trial. *Obstet Gynecol* 2007; 110:267–78.
10. Breymann C, Gliga F, Bejenariu C, *et al.* Comparative efficacy and safety of intravenous ferric carboxymaltose in the treatment of postpartum iron deficiency anemia. *Int J Gynecol Obstet* 2007; 101:67–73.
11. Seid MH, Derman RJ, Baker JB, *et al.* Ferric carboxymaltose injection in the treatment of postpartum iron deficiency anemia: a randomized controlled clinical trial. *Am J Obstet Gynecol* 2008; 199:435.e1–7.
12. Funk F, Ryle P, Canclini C, *et al.* The new generation of intravenous iron: chemistry, pharmacology, and toxicology of ferric carboxymaltose. *Arzneimittel-forschung* 2010; 60:345–53.
13. Reveiz L, Gyte GML, Cuervo LG. Treatments for iron-deficiency anaemia in pregnancy. *Cochrane Database Syst Rev* 2007; 2:CD003094.
14. Bolton-Maggs PHB, Cohen H. Serious Hazards of Transfusion (SHOT) haemovigilance and progress is improving transfusion safety. *Br J Haematol* 2013; 163(3):303–14.
15. Parker J, Thompson J, Stanworth S. A retrospective on-year single-centre survey of obstetric red cell transfusions. *Int J Obstet Anesth* 2009; 18(4):309–13.
16. NCEPOD. *A Sickle Crisis?: A Report of the National Confidential Enquiry into Patient Outcome and Death (2008)*. London: NCEPOD; 2008. http://www.ncepod.org.uk/2008report1/Downloads/Sickle_report.pdf
17. Howard RJ, Tuck SM, Pearson TC. Pregnancy in sickle cell disease in the UK: results of a multicentre survey of the effect of prophylactic blood transfusion on maternal and fetal outcome. *Br J Obstet Gynaecol* 1995; 102:947–51.
18. National Institute for Health and Care Excellence. *Sickle Cell Acute Painful Episode: Management of an Acute Painful Sickle Cell Episode in Hospital*. Clinical Guideline CG143. London: NICE; 2012 (reviewed 2014).
19. Butwick A, Findley I, Wonke B. Management of pregnancy in a patient with β thalassaemia major. *Int J Obstet Anaesth* 2005; 14:351–4.
20. Waters JH, Lukauskiene E, Anderson ME. Intraoperative blood salvage during cesarean delivery in a patient with β thalassemia intermedia. *Anesth Analg* 2003; 97:1808–9.
21. da Luz LT, Nascimento B, Rizoli S. Thromboelastography (TEG): practical considerations on its clinical use in trauma and resuscitation. *Scand J Trauma Resusc Emerg Med* 2013; 21:29.
22. Armstrong S, Fernando R, Ashpole R. Assessment of coagulation in the obstetric population using ROTEM® thromboelastometry. *Int J Obstet Anesth* 2011; 20(4):293–8.
23. Huq FY, Kadir RA. Management of pregnancy, labour and delivery in women with inherited bleeding disorders. *Haemophilia* 2011; 17:20–30.
24. Peitsidis P, Kadir RA. Antifibrinolytic therapy with tranexamic acid in pregnancy and postpartum. *Expert Opin Pharmacother* 2011; 12(4):503–11.
25. Trigg D, Peitsidis P, Kadir RA. The use of desmopressin (DDAVP) for treatment and prophylaxis of bleeding disorders in pregnancy—a systematic review. *Haemophila* 2011; 18(1):25–33.
26. Lee CA, Chi C, Pavord SR. The obstetric and gynaecological management of women with inherited bleeding disorders—review with guidelines produced by a taskforce of UK Haemophilia Centre Doctors' Organisation. *Haemophilia* 2006; 12:301–36.
27. Siboni SM, Spreafico M, Calo L. Gynecological and obstetric problems in women with different bleeding disorders. *Haemophilia* 2009; 15:1291–9.
28. Lee CA, Kadir RA, Kouides P. *Inherited Bleeding Disorders in Women*. Chichester: Wiley-Blackwell; 2009.
29. Burrows RF, Ray JG, Burrows E. Bleeding risk and reproductive capacity among patients with factor XIII deficiency: a case presentation and a review of the literature. *Obstet Gynecol Surv* 2000; 55:103–8.
30. Kobayashi T, Kanayama N, Tokunaga N. Prenatal and peripartum management of congenital afibrinogenaemia. *Br J Haematol* 2000; 109:346–66.
31. Kadir RA, Chi C, Bolton Maggs P. Pregnancy and rare bleeding disorders. *Haemophilia* 2009; 15:990–1005.
32. Ljung R, Lindgren AC, Petrini P, *et al.* Normal vaginal delivery is to be recommended for haemophilia carriers gravidae. *Acta Pediatr* 1994; 83:609–11.
33. Choi S, Brull R. Neuraxial techniques in obstetric and non-obstetric patients with common bleeding diatheses. *Anesth Analg* 2009; 109:648–60.
34. Van der Meulen EP, Van Aken H, Vermylen J. Anticoagulants and spinal epidural anesthesia. *Anesth Analog* 1994; 79:1165–77.
35. Greer I, Lyal F, Perera T, *et al.* Increased concentrations of cytokines interleukin-6 and interleukin-1 receptor antagonist in plasma of

women with preeclampsia: a mechanism for endothelial dysfunction. *Obstet Gynecol* 1994; 84(6):903–1089.

36. Kadir RA, Lee CA, Sabin CA, *et al.* Pregnancy in women with von Willebrand's disease or factor XI deficiency. *Br J Obstet Gynaecol* 1998; 105:314–21.
37. Chalmers E, Williams M, Brennand J, *et al.* Guideline on the management of haemophilia in the fetus and neonate. *Br J Haematol* 2011; 154(2):208–15.
38. Hoffbrand A, Catovsky D, Tuddenham E, *et al. Postgraduate Haematology* (6th ed). London: Wiley-Blackwell; 2011.
39. Chi C, Lee CA, Shiltagh N, *et al.* Pregnancy in carriers of haemophilia. *Haemophilia* 2008; 14:56–64.
40. Lee CA, Chi C, Pavord SR. The obstetric and gynaecological management of women with inherited bleeding disorders—review with guidelines produced by a taskforce of UK Haemophilia Centre Doctors' Organisation. *Haemophilia* 2006; 12:301–36.
41. Kouides PA, Phatak PD, Burkart P. Gynaecological and obstetrical morbidity in women with type 1 von Willebrand disease: results of a patient survey. *Haemophilia* 2000; 6:643–8.
42. Wetzstein V, Budde U, Oyen F. Intracranial hemorrhage in a term newborn with severe von Willebrand disease type 3 associated with sinus venous thrombosis. *Haematologica* 2006; 91:60.
43. Pacheco LD, Costantine MM, Saade GR, *et al.* von Willebrand disease and pregnancy: a practical approach for the diagnosis and treatment. *Am J Obstet Gynecol* 2010; 203:194–200.
44. Seligsohn U. Factor XI deficiency. *Thromb Haemost* 1993; 70:68–71.
45. Myers B, Pavord S, Kean L, *et al.* Pregnancy outcome in factor XI deficiency: incidence of miscarriage, antenatal and postnatal haemorrhage in 33 women with factor XI deficiency. *Br J Obstet Gynaecolol* 2007; 114(5):643–6.
46. Salomon O, Steinberg DM, Tamarin I, *et al.* Plasma replacement therapy during labor is not mandatory for women with severe factor XI deficiency. *Blood Coagul Fibrinolysis* 2005; 16:37–41.
47. van Veen JJ, Nokes TJ, Makris M. The risk of spinal haematoma following neuraxial anaesthesia or lumbar puncture in thrombocytopenic individuals. *Br J Haematol* 2010; 148:15–25.
48. Douglas MJ. The use of neuraxial anesthesia in parturients with thrombocytopenia: what is an adequate platelet count? In Halpern SH, Douglas MJ (eds) *Evidence-Based Obstetric Anesthesia*. Oxford: Blackwell Publishing; 2005:165–77.
49. Webert KE, Mittal R, Sigouin C, *et al.* A retrospective 11-year analysis of obstetric patients with idiopathic thrombocytopenic purpura. *Blood* 2003; 102:4306–11.
50. Neunert C, Lim W, Crowther M, *et al.* The American Society of Hematology 2011 evidence-based practice guideline for immune thrombocytopenia. *Blood* 2011; 117(16):4190–207.
51. Neylon AJ, Saunders PW, Howard MR, *et al.* Clinically significant newly presenting autoimmune thrombocytopenic purpura in adults: a prospective study of a population-based cohort of 245 patients. *Br J Haematol* 2003; 122:966–74.
52. Ozkan H, Cetinkaya M, Koksal N, *et al.* Neonatal outcomes of pregnancy complicated by idiopathic thrombocytopenic purpura. *J Perinatol* 2010; 30:38–44.
53. Gasim T. Immune thrombocytopenia in pregnancy: a reappraisal of obstetric management and outcome. *J Reprod Med* 2011; 56:163–8.
54. Kirkpatrick CA. The HELLP syndrome. *Acta Clinica* 2010; 65:91–7.
55. Sibai BM, Ramadan MK, Usta I, *et al.* Maternal morbidity and mortality in 442 pregnancies with haemolysis, elevated liver enzymes, and low platelets (HELLP syndrome). *Am J Obstet and Gynecol* 1993; 169(4):1000–6.
56. Sibai BM. Diagnosis, controversies, and management of the syndrome of hemolysis, elevated liver enzymes, and low platelet count. *Obstet Gynaecol* 2004; 103:981–91.
57. Gul A, Cebeci A, Aslan H, *et al.* Perinatal outcomes in severe preeclampsia-eclampsia with and without HELLP syndrome. *Gynecol Obstet Invest* 2005; 59:113–18.
58. Osmanagaoglu MA, Erdogan I, Zengin U, *et al.* Comparison between HELLP syndrome, chronic hypertension, and superimposed preeclampsia on chronic hypertension without HELLP syndrome. *J Perinat Med* 2004; 32:481–5.
59. Scully M, Yarranton H, Liesner R, *et al.* Neuraxial UK TTP registry: correlation with laboratory ADAMTS 13 analysis and clinical features. *Br J Haematol* 2008; 142:819–26.
60. Cantwell R, Clutton-Brock T, Cooper G, *et al.* Saving Mothers' Lives: Reviewing maternal deaths to make motherhood safer: 2006–2008. The Eighth Report of the Confidential Enquiries into Maternal Deaths in the United Kingdom. *BJOG* 2011; 118 Suppl 1:1–203
61. Fakhouri F, Jablonski M, Lepercq J, *et al.* Factor H, membrane cofactor protein, and factor I mutations in patients with haemolysis, elevated liver enzymes, and low platelet syndrome. *Blood* 2008; 112:4542–5.
62. Gregory TL, Hughes S, Coleman MA, *et al.* Acute fatty liver of pregnancy; three cases and discussion of analgesia and anaesthesia. *Int J Obstet Anesth* 2007; 16:175–9.

CHAPTER 49

Peripartum psychiatric disorders

Roch Cantwell

Epidemiology of mental illness in relation to pregnancy and childbirth

Mental illness is common. Depression has a lifetime prevalence of 4–10% in the general population, with women having a rate 1.5–2.5 times that of men.[1] Bipolar affective disorder and schizophrenia each affects approximately 1% of the population. Pregnancy offers little protection against the continuation or development of mental illness, although risk of suicide[2] and admission to inpatient psychiatric care is reduced at this time.[3] Minor mental illness may be more common in early pregnancy and nearer to delivery. However, the early postpartum period places a woman at greater risk of severe psychiatric disorder and admission to psychiatric care than at any other time in her life. For some women, this risk can be identified, allowing for preventative interventions to be put in place.

Normal emotional changes in early pregnancy

Some 50% of pregnancies are unplanned,[4] and a proportion of those, unwanted. Rates of unplanned pregnancy are even higher among women with severe mental illness. Even in much wanted pregnancies, ambivalence about the pregnancy, health-related anxieties, and fears about inability to cope (especially in first-time mothers) are typical and normal. Increased emotional lability is common in the first trimester, and may be exacerbated by the physical changes typical of early pregnancy. Such emotional changes are largely bound up with the psychological adjustments typical to pregnancy but may be contributed to by hormonal alterations. It is important to be able to distinguish these changes from those more clearly associated with mental illness.

Oates[5] describes certain groups as having particular needs for increased support in relation to childbearing:

- Very young, single, and unsupported mothers, and women who themselves have poor experiences of mothering, may be especially vulnerable. Their own needs may conflict with those of their babies and early planning to provide appropriate support is essential to help develop the woman's ability to care for her baby.
- Older mothers who may have over-idealized expectations of pregnancy and delivery, and have problems adjusting to life changes after the birth.
- Women who have complicated pregnancies, including those with previous pregnancy loss, those who have undergone assisted conception, and those who require an emergency caesarean delivery.

Women also face an increased risk of domestic violence in pregnancy. Fifteen per cent of women report abuse during their pregnancy and 30% of domestic violence begins during pregnancy.[6] It is recommended that women should be seen alone on at least one occasion during their antenatal care, enquiries about violence should be routinely included in the antenatal history, and information provided on legal rights and available supports. In over 50% of cases of domestic abuse, children are also directly abused. All professionals involved in the care of pregnant women should be aware of how to recognize signs of abuse.[7]

Pre-existing mental illness

Bipolar affective disorder

Bipolar disorder is estimated to have a lifetime prevalence of 0.4–1.6%, with peak age of onset for women during reproductive years. Lifetime prevalence is likely to reach 4% when less severe forms of the disorder are included. It is characterized by episodes of elevated (termed mania or hypomania, depending on severity) or depressed mood, and altered behaviour, with relative well-being between periods of illness. Psychotic symptoms (delusions, hallucinations) are typical during episodes, but not essential to the diagnosis. Bipolar disorder is conventionally subdivided into types I and II, depending on the presence or absence of psychotic symptoms or marked behavioural disturbance. Genetic factors play an important role in aetiology, with heritability accounting for approximately 85% of the variance,[8] but episodes of illness may be triggered by stressful life events. Women with bipolar disorder are likely to be on maintenance therapy, which can include lithium, mood-stabilizing antiepileptics, and second-generation antipsychotics. There are teratogenic risks associated with lithium and with the mood-stabilizing antiepileptics, sodium valproate and carbamazepine, but high risk too with regard to relapse of illness on discontinuation. Viguera et al.[9] found that 71% of bipolar women who discontinued prophylactic lithium treatment at onset of pregnancy relapsed at some point during that pregnancy, a two-fold greater risk than for those continuing treatment. Decisions regarding continuation, stopping, or alteration of treatment (for part, or all, of the pregnancy) should be made on an individual basis and with the woman's fully informed involvement. Factors to be taken into account include the previous natural history of the disorder (number, severity, and time interval between episodes of illness), response to previous treatment discontinuations, and time taken to recovery.

Relapse of bipolar disorder in pregnancy (whether with mania, depression, or a mixed presentation) is likely to require use of antipsychotics, antidepressants, mood stabilizers, or sedatives, alone or in combination, depending on the severity and nature of the mood disturbance. Inpatient care is often indicated and, occasionally, electroconvulsive therapy (ECT) may be used. This is discussed more fully later in the chapter.

Pre-existing bipolar disorder is one of the greatest risk factors for postpartum psychosis. Seventy per cent of women with bipolar disorder will experience relapse in the first 6 postnatal months if not taking mood-stabilizing agents.[10] Irrespective of decisions about medication during pregnancy, all women should be offered prophylactic medication (usually lithium or a mood-stabilizing antipsychotic) immediately following delivery. Given that most women with bipolar disorder return to full health between episodes, there is little evidence that they are any less able to care appropriately for their children, except during the acute phase of the illness.

Schizophrenia

Schizophrenia is an enduring mental illness, characterized by *positive symptoms* such as bizarre delusions, hallucinations, and disrupted thinking reflected in speech (thought disorder), and *negative symptoms* such as social withdrawal, blunted affect, and lack of motivation. It affects approximately 1% of the general population, and is slightly more common in men. Fertility is lowered among women with schizophrenia[11] but the move away from institutional care, and increased use of second-generation antipsychotic drugs, which have a lower propensity to elevate prolactin, may contribute to increasing rates of pregnancy in this group. Women who switch from older drugs may not be aware of this and may place themselves inadvertently at risk of unwanted pregnancy. Women with schizophrenia are more likely to have unplanned and unwanted pregnancies and less likely to engage well with routine antenatal care. They have more adverse outcomes of pregnancy including increased risk of pregnancy loss and neonatal death.[12] Some of this increased risk may be due to confounders such as high rates of smoking and poorer physical health.

There is an increased risk of relapse of schizophrenia in the postnatal period, but the pattern of relapse into illness does not show the very early high risk found in bipolar disorder.[13] This may be explained by the likelihood that precipitants to relapse relate more to the psychosocial and emotional demands of increased contact with health and social care professionals, and caring for a developing child. Although not universally poor, the outcome in terms of the mother remaining the primary carer for her child is often unfavourable,[14] leading to great distress for the mother and for those (including health professionals) who support her. Appropriate supports, including social services, should be engaged at an early stage in pregnancy to ensure sufficient help is available to the mother and her family. It is often difficult for women with schizophrenia to cope with frequent contact with health professionals during pregnancy and there is a risk that they will receive suboptimal care due to failure to attend antenatal care.

Most women with schizophrenia will be on maintenance antipsychotic medication. The implications of relapse during pregnancy are severe for both mother and child, and, unless there are strong reasons to the contrary, treatment should continue, with appropriate monitoring, throughout pregnancy. Difficult decisions may have to be made regarding the relative advantages and problems associated with continuing a well-established regimen involving newer antipsychotics or switching to older medication, where the risks associated with pregnancy are better known.

Depressive and anxiety disorders

Depressive disorder is characterized by a triad of symptoms groupings including disturbed mood, negative thinking, and somatic or behavioural change, which may include reduced appetite and energy, disturbed sleep, impaired enjoyment, and difficulty with concentration and memory. Suicidal thoughts, planning, or acts may be present in more severe illness. Given a lifetime prevalence of 4–10%, with rates higher in women than men, many women may have a pre-existing depressive disorder at conception. Studies suggest that 2–10% of women are taking prescribed antidepressant treatment at the time of conception. Women are most likely to discontinue treatment, without consultation, on discovering a pregnancy.[15] This may place them at greater risk of relapse of illness. A past history of depressive illness is one of the strongest risk factors for antenatal depression, which in turn is predictive of postnatal depression. Although depressive symptoms are probably as common in pregnancy as in the postnatal period they often remain undetected.

For anxiety disorders, the course in pregnancy is likely to be related to the severity of illness preconceptually. Physiological changes in respiratory function during pregnancy may lead to an increased propensity to panic and anxiety and panic may worsen in the postnatal period. These disorders may also significantly compromise antenatal care. Women with severe needle phobia are likely to be referred to anaesthetic services to assist in blood taking. The Confidential Enquiry into Maternal Deaths 2006–08 reported one case of refusal to have bloods taken in pregnancy or thromboprophylaxis postnatally in a woman who died of thromboembolism.[16] Such patients require early referral and intervention, using behavioural techniques.

Non-pharmacological treatments include *cognitive therapy* and *behavioural techniques*, such as anxiety management, teaching the patient about the nature and genesis of symptoms, and engaging in relaxation exercises to reverse them. Drug treatments include selective serotonin reuptake inhibitors (SSRIs) and tricyclic antidepressants. Beta blockers should not be used as first-line treatment.[17]

Eating disorders

Core features of eating disorders (anorexia nervosa and bulimia) include distorted body image and a morbid fear of fatness with efforts at weight loss, such as food restriction, excessive exercising, self-induced vomiting, and use of appetite suppressants, laxatives, and diuretics. Bulimic symptoms (binge eating followed by vomiting) are a core feature of bulimia but may also be present in anorexia nervosa. Amenorrhoea is essential to the full anorexic syndrome, but many women have partial syndromes (commonly termed EDNOS (eating disorders not otherwise specified)), which may include presentations where ovulation continues, or returns when weight loss is not so extreme. Eating disorders, including EDNOS, have some of the highest mortality rates of any psychiatric disorder.

Eating disorders (including partial syndromes) affect 5–7% of women of childbearing age.[18] There is some evidence that eating disorder symptoms may improve in pregnancy, but the postnatal period can be associated with a worsening of symptoms, as efforts are made to lose weight gained in pregnancy. With regard to the impact of a pre-existing eating disorder on pregnancy, there is evidence from some studies of intrauterine growth restriction, miscarriage, and preterm delivery.[19,20] Self-induced vomiting may lead to electrolyte imbalance, and severe weight restriction to delayed wound healing after delivery.

The fertility of anorexic women is significantly reduced. Women with bulimia may have menstrual irregularities despite a normal body mass index. During and after pregnancy, women with eating disorders are more likely to experience comorbid depressive disorder. They struggle more with breastfeeding.

Early detection and referral to eating disorders services, where available, is core to management. Guidance on expected weight gain in pregnancy, healthy eating, and bodily changes in pregnancy are of particular importance in this group. Rarely, inpatient refeeding may be required. In the postnatal period, specific enquiry about depressive symptoms and worsening or return of eating disorder should be made.

Substance use disorders

Details of specific substance abuse can be found in Chapter 51. Women with alcohol or drug problems often engage poorly with antenatal care and their impaired physical health, and increased risk of blood-borne virus infection, may place them and their pregnancy at risk. An increasing number of drug-using women contribute to cases reported to the Confidential Enquiries into Maternal Deaths.[21]

As with other maladaptive behaviours, excessive alcohol use tends to decrease during the antenatal period. Physical complications of alcohol misuse, which can threaten or complicate pregnancy, include nutritional deficiencies, liver disease, and pancreatic disease. Withdrawal complications such as delirium tremens and seizures pose particular risk.

Fetal alcohol syndrome, and the more encompassing term, fetal alcohol effects, is characterized by craniofacial abnormalities, growth retardation, and neurodevelopmental abnormalities, including impaired IQ, in the presence of maternal alcohol consumption.[22] The pathway for adverse effects on fetal development is complex but there is evidence that alcohol is a direct teratogen and there appears to be a dose-related response. Animal studies suggest that binge pattern drinking in pregnancy is particularly harmful, but there is no consensus about whether there may be a safe lower limit for consumption in pregnancy.

Other drug use effects vary depending on the properties of the specific drug, although it is important to recognize that patients may frequently use a combination of substances and research in the area is not extensive. Pregnant women who misuse drugs should receive specialist support, with the aim of stabilizing, minimizing, or, where appropriate, stopping their use. Abrupt discontinuation of drug use is not recommended. Although women may be more motivated to stop drug use in pregnancy, there is significant risk of relapse in the postnatal period with potentially serious adverse child welfare consequences. Early involvement of child care social work is an essential component of alcohol and drug misuse management in pregnancy. The children of many of these women are taken into care and some may enter a vicious cycle of repeated pregnancies in an attempt to retain at least one of their children. Contraceptive advice should be a priority postpartum.

Personality disorder

Personality disorders are deeply engrained and enduring patterns of behaviour, resulting in inflexible responses to a broad range of personal and social situations. They are stable and unchanging, usually present from adolescence, and often cause the person, or those around them, to suffer. There are often difficulties in forming and/or sustaining relationships, and this may extend to health professionals involved in the person's care. In one epidemiological study, the prevalence of personality disorder in pregnancy was 6.4%.[23] Of the group of personality disorders, the emotionally unstable type is perhaps the most commonly diagnosed in young women. It is characterized by emotional instability, impulsivity, dysphoric mood, disturbances in self-image, chronic feelings of emptiness, and self-destructive behaviour, including recurrent self-harm, and drug or alcohol misuse. Such difficulties cause high levels of anxiety among health and social care professionals, and may interfere with effective antenatal care. Impaired forward planning and tolerance of distress may increase anxieties regarding child welfare. Effective management is usually provided through good joint working and communication between professionals, and a clear and consistent treatment plan to which the patient agrees. There may be a role for specific psychological and drug therapies.

Newly arising mental disorder

Tocophobia

Tocophobia is a morbid fear of childbirth.[24] Primary tocophobia pre-dates pregnancy and may be associated with previous abusive experiences. Secondary tocophobia arises from previous traumatic delivery. Tocophobia may also present as a symptom of depressive disorder in pregnancy. For some women, the dread of delivery is such that they will proceed to termination despite the pregnancy being wanted. Other women will plan, from the outset, for elective caesarean delivery. Interventions will usually take the form of cognitive therapy and anxiety management techniques, but there is a higher incidence of caesarean delivery even where such approaches are used.

Postpartum psychosis

Psychotic disorders arise after 1 in 500 births. Although the absolute risk for any woman is low, relative to other times in a woman's life, this period carries the highest risk of psychosis and psychiatric hospital admission.[25] The illness has its onset in the early postnatal period, 90% occurring within the first month. Despite the name, a small proportion of cases have onset in late pregnancy. Almost all cases are affective in nature, that is, they present predominantly with mood disturbance in addition to the characteristic symptoms of psychosis—delusions, hallucinations, marked behavioural disturbance, and loss of insight. Non-affective or schizophrenia-like presentations are much less common. Typically, the presentation is one of rapid fluctuations of mood (often with a mixture of manic and depressive symptoms), perplexity, confusion, and markedly altered behaviour. Ideas of self-harm may be driven by delusions of guilt, self-worthlessness, or hopelessness. Thoughts of harm concerning the baby or other children are rare but should always be assessed. Initial symptoms may be non-specific, often including anxiety and labile mood. Failure to recognize such prodromal symptoms, coupled with rapid progression to frank illness over a short period of time, is a recurrent theme in psychiatric deaths reported to the Confidential Enquiry.[21]

Several factors have been identified that significantly increase the risk of psychosis. Of greatest importance is a previous history of postpartum psychosis or bipolar disorder. A first-degree relative with bipolar disorder or previous postpartum psychosis increases this risk further. With one or more of these risks, a woman may have a greater than one in two risk of developing postpartum psychosis. Identification of risk is particularly important, as there is evidence that preventative interventions, when started in the immediate postpartum period, are effective in reducing progression to illness. Interventions include lithium, mood-stabilizing antipsychotic drugs, and measures to protect sleep.

All women with postpartum psychosis should be managed by psychiatric services. Most will require admission to hospital. Where specialist mother and baby facilities are available, her baby will usually accompany her. Treatment consists of a combination of antipsychotic medication, antidepressants, or mood stabilizers depending on the specific presentation. ECT is also an effective and rapid treatment. Supervised support for the patient's care of her infant and help for the family are crucial to good management. Recovery usually takes place over a period of 1–2 months but there is great individual variation. Prognosis for the episode is very good and most women will make a complete recovery, but remain at a one in two risk of future postpartum episodes. There is also a significantly increased risk, perhaps as high as 60%, of non-postpartum recurrence, in which case criteria are likely to be met for bipolar disorder.

The aetiology of postpartum psychosis remains uncertain. The dramatic, early presentation is suggestive of a link with major hormonal changes normally occurring after childbirth. The strong association with bipolar disorder implies a genetic predisposition, and evidence has emerged of a specific familial risk for postpartum episodes in bipolar disorder.[26] It has been suggested that the rapid reduction in oestrogen levels is linked to the development of dopamine receptor hypersensitivity, which in turn may trigger the onset of psychosis in predisposed individuals.[27] Serotonergic neurotransmitter systems have also been implicated in causation. So far, however, there is very limited evidence for the use of hormonal treatments in routine management.

Antenatal and postnatal depression

In contrast to postpartum psychosis, non-psychotic depression often presents later in the postnatal period, with a peak occurrence at around 6 weeks. While there is some evidence of a telescoping in the incidence of depression in the first postnatal weeks, the overall prevalence of 10–15% in the first year is not very different from the prevalence of mild to moderate depression at any other time in a woman's life, including in pregnancy. Similarly, the symptoms of depression in the antenatal and postnatal period do not differ greatly from those at other times, depression usually presenting with a combination of the triad of affective, cognitive, and behavioural symptoms mentioned earlier. Some studies suggest a greater predominance of obsessional symptoms in postnatal depression. For some women, these may take the form of obsessional worries or fears that she may cause harm to her baby. Much less commonly, there may be true infanticidal thoughts. Thoughts of self-harm are not uncommon and should be followed up with sensitive enquiry as to the depth and strength of these feelings.

The majority of depressions occurring at this time are mild and do not require specific psychiatric intervention. Most will be uncovered during routine antenatal and postnatal screening by the midwife, general practitioner (GP), or health visitor. For postnatal depression, the provision of extra support and non-directive counselling by health visitors is usually adequate to bring about resolution. A smaller number of women, approximately 3–5%, will benefit from antidepressant medication, but fewer than half that number will require referral to psychiatric services. Of these, only a small number will be admitted to psychiatric care, though it is important to identify those with the most severe disorders. While previously advocated, there is no evidence that progesterone or synthetic progestagens are effective treatments for postnatal depression.

Unlike postpartum psychosis, where risk factors are largely biological, psychosocial factors play the greatest part in the development of non-psychotic depression. Most important are a past history of depression, psychological problems during pregnancy, poor social support, lack of a confiding relationship, and recent adverse life events.[28] Weaker associations have been found with obstetric complications, history of abuse, lower socioeconomic status, and perception of poor obstetric experience. Unfortunately, these risk factors have poor specificity and so, while allowing for heightened awareness, cannot be used to accurately predict the development of depression in any one individual. Untreated postnatal depression is also closely associated with disturbed mother–baby interaction and with adverse effects on infant cognitive and emotional development.

Psychological aspects of miscarriage, stillbirth, and abortion

Around one in five pregnancies will end in spontaneous loss before 20 weeks. Early loss is often not associated with the same acknowledgement and support attending stillbirth or neonatal death. In the absence of an obvious cause, miscarriage may also lead to a greater sense of self-blame and guilt. Around 40% of women will go through a typical bereavement process, similar to that following stillbirth or neonatal death, with emotional reactions that may include numbness, disbelief, social withdrawal, anger, guilt, sadness and anxiety, leading eventually to acceptance and resolution. Depressive symptoms are present, at a rate two to four times that of the general population in the first 6 months,[29] and anxiety symptoms are similarly elevated. In most cases, symptoms have returned to background levels by 1 year. However, some women may experience an abnormal or prolonged grief reaction, depressive or anxiety disorder.

Interventions to reduce the risk of psychological morbidity are poorly researched. Women consistently say they wish for greater access to psychological support, and there is some evidence for the benefit of psychological interventions. Where benefit has been demonstrated, it has mostly been for interventions targeted at those displaying early difficulties, rather than for general approaches to all women who miscarry. However, an empathic approach, and acknowledgement of the significance of the loss, is important for all women.

Late pregnancy and early neonatal loss is likely to result in a normal grief reaction. Some controversy surrounds the common practice of encouraging parents to spend time with, hold, and dress their dead infants. One study found an increased risk of depression, anxiety, and post-traumatic stress disorder in subsequent pregnancy, where women had time with their infants, and that greater exposure was correlated with more subsequent problems.[30] Best practice is to allow parents to decide for themselves whether they wish contact with their dead infants, without assumption from staff that such exposure is the correct or desired option.[31]

The link between induced abortion and mental health is shrouded in controversy. The most recent, and extensive, review of the literature to date suggests that for women with an unwanted pregnancy, the risk of adverse mental health is the same, whether the outcome is an induced abortion or term delivery.[32] Certain factors, such as a negative attitude to abortion, or pressure from a partner to have an abortion, may increase the risk of adverse mental health outcomes. Overall however, the most reliable predictor of mental health problems post abortion is having a history of mental health problems before the abortion.

Maternal mental illness, child welfare, and infant development

Infanticide is a very rare outcome of maternal mental illness. However, some mental illnesses, such as schizophrenia, may compromise a woman's ability to engage with antenatal care, increasing the risk of adverse outcomes for the pregnancy. Furthermore, persistent anxiety in pregnancy, and untreated postnatal depression, may be linked to impaired social and cognitive development in children as they grow up.[33] Antenatally, this may be mediated through disruption of the fetal hypothalamic–pituitary–adrenal axis. In the postnatal period, maternal depression may alter the quality of interaction between mother and child, leading to poorer social interaction.

The majority of women with mental health problems care for their children without difficulty. Where there are concerns that care may be compromised by severe illness or substance misuse, early involvement of social services is essential, ideally during pregnancy, to allow for a full evaluation of risk and for support, if required, to be coordinated.

Biological management of psychiatric disorder in pregnancy and breastfeeding

The research base for psychotropic medication effects in pregnancy is limited but ever changing. For this reason, it is not possible to give definitive advice. The National Institute of Health and Care Excellence (NICE)[34] and the Scottish Intercollegiate Guidelines Network (SIGN)[35] provide some general principles which should govern prescribing in pregnancy. These are summarized in Box 49.1. NICE and SIGN also recommend that access to psychological therapies, where appropriate, should be promptly available.

Antidepressants

Coincidental antidepressant prescribing at conception is common and SSRI antidepressant use is now more established in pregnancy. There is some evidence of an increased risk of cardiac anomaly, but the absolute risk is likely to be less than 1%. Some studies suggest a greater risk with paroxetine but research to date is imperfect and poorly controlled for potential confounders, such as smoking and alcohol use. There remains uncertainty about whether SSRIs are associated with an increased risk of persistent pulmonary hypertension in the neonate, if given after 20 weeks. A recent meta-analysis suggests an odds ratio of 2.5–2.8, against a baseline risk of 1.9/1000.[36] Again,

Box 49.1 Principles of prescribing in pregnancy

- Involve the woman, and her family where appropriate, in all decisions about treatment, including an individualized assessment of benefit versus risk
- Be aware that not treating mental illness in pregnancy or the postpartum period may in itself be associated with adverse outcomes for the woman, her pregnancy, and her infant
- Establish a clear indication for drug treatment (ie the presence of significant illness in the absence of acceptable or effective alternatives)
- Choose treatments with the lowest known risk
- In choosing medication in pregnancy consider the implications for breast feeding and the benefits of avoiding the need to switch drugs (including the minimization of withdrawal effects)
- Use treatments in the lowest effective dose for the shortest period necessary
- Be aware of potential drug interactions, particularly with non-psychotropics, and aim for monotherapy
- Where there is no clear evidence base that one drug is safer than another, the safest option is not to switch. The only drug with a clear indication for switching on safety grounds is valproate
- Be aware of the potential effects of pregnancy and childbirth on drug pharmacokinetics and pharmacodynamics (eg the need for dose adjustments as pregnancy progresses and specific risks during labour and following birth)
- Be aware that although knowledge of teratogenic effects of psychotropic drugs is increasing, understanding of the long-term neurodevelopmental effects of such medications in pregnancy and breast feeding is extremely limited
- Be aware of the need for close monitoring for change in mental state where a woman decides to cease her usual medication. Stopping medication may lead to relapse of illness
- Where there is known risk, ensure that women are offered appropriate fetal screening and monitoring of the neonate for adverse effects. This may include involvement of neonatal and or paediatric services
- Be aware that premature or ill babies are more at risk of harmful drug effects
- Monitor the infant for specific drug side effects as well as feeding patterns, growth and development
- Caution women against sleeping in bed with the infant, particularly if taking sedative drugs.

Data from National Institute for Health and Clinical Excellence (NICE). *Antenatal and postnatal mental health: clinical management and service guideline*. London: 2007. (NICE publication CG45).

Data from Scottish Intercollegiate Guidelines Network (SIGN). *Management of perinatal mood disorders*. Edinburgh: 2012. (SIGN publication no. 127). [cited 11 Sept 2015].

Available from URL: http://www.sign.ac.uk.

the absolute risk remains low. Similarly, there is limited evidence for growth retardation and premature delivery. Neonatal poor adaptation is increased threefold against background rates. Typical symptoms include irritability, constant crying, shivering, increased tone and tremor, poor feeding and, rarely, seizures. Infants are at increased risk of special care admission and of lower Apgar scores at birth. More recent evidence suggests a possible association between SSRIs and autistic spectrum disorder. Although more research is required, even if increased, the attributable risk remains very low.

Tricyclic antidepressants are likely to have a similar adverse side effect profile in pregnancy. While they have been available for a much greater period of time than the SSRIs and consequently any greater adverse effects might be expected to have emerged, systematic reporting of exposure is less extensive than with the SSRIs and so quality of evidence is poorer. Monoamine oxidase inhibitors may be associated with early teratogenicity and the risk of blood pressure abnormalities, particularly with tyramine-related food interactions, make them unsuitable in pregnancy.

While an evaluation of the risks and benefits of continuing already prescribed antidepressants in pregnancy should be made with the woman, there are also risks of relapse with sudden discontinuation. Women should usually be advised not to abruptly discontinue, but to arrange an early review with their GP. Decisions on new prescribing in pregnancy should take into account the severity of illness, previous treatment response and breastfeeding intentions. Different SSRIs are present in breastfed babies in very varying concentrations.

Antipsychotics

Many antipsychotics raise prolactin levels and reduce fertility. Some are associated with excessive weight gain and impaired glucose tolerance. Because of this, it is recommended that women on antipsychotics be regarded as at increased risk of gestational diabetes and managed accordingly.[37] The evidence of any association with fetal malformation is very limited. Where these drugs are prescribed for the management of severe and enduring mental illness (i.e. schizophrenia and related disorders), the risks of discontinuing will usually outweigh any risks of medication to the developing fetus. In the majority of cases, usual practice would be to continue medication throughout pregnancy. Long-acting depot medication can persist in the neonate for considerable periods and it may be possible to change to an oral preparation during the pregnancy to avoid this risk. Such decisions need to take individual circumstances into account, particularly the significant risk of relapse of illness. There is a theoretical risk of blood dyscrasia in the neonate where clozapine is used in pregnancy but, again, risks for the woman from discontinuation may be very high.

Mood stabilizers

These drugs, most commonly prescribed for prophylaxis of bipolar disorder, include lithium, and the antiepileptics valproate, carbamazepine, and lamotrigine.

Lithium has a narrow therapeutic to toxic ratio and is monitored by regular blood level assay. In early pregnancy, lithium has been associated with an increased risk of cardiac malformation, notably Ebstein's anomaly. The relative risk of Ebstein's anomaly may be increased 10–20-fold, but the absolute risk remains low, at 0.05–0.1%. Overall, risk of cardiac anomaly may have been overestimated in earlier retrospective studies.[38] In later pregnancy, lithium is associated with neonatal complications, including hypotonia, neonatal hypothyroidism, and nephrogenic diabetes insipidus. Lithium crosses the placenta with ease and levels in the neonate are equivalent to those in the mother. There is a close correlation between maternal/neonatal levels, and neonatal complications.[39] Pharmacokinetic changes in pregnancy result in lithium levels lowering, for the same oral dose, from mid trimester. Doses may need to be increased to maintain therapeutic levels, but there is then a risk of toxicity in the mother and neonate after delivery.

Lithium levels should be monitored monthly in pregnancy, and weekly from 36 weeks. It should be discontinued at onset of labour, and some authorities would suggest reducing the dose in late pregnancy, aiming for levels at the lower end of the therapeutic range, particularly where there is a history of rapid delivery or other indicators of early delivery (e.g. twin pregnancy). Other precipitants of toxicity, which may be relevant in pregnancy, include dehydration occurring in hyperemesis or prolonged labour, pre-eclampsia, impaired renal function, and sodium-restricted diets. Drug interactions with diuretics, non-steroidal anti-inflammatory agents, angiotensin-converting enzyme inhibitors, and calcium channel blockers may also cause toxicity.

Sudden lithium discontinuation is associated with greatly increased risk of relapse in bipolar disorder and specialist advice should be sought urgently if a woman presents, on lithium, in early pregnancy.

The antiepileptic mood stabilizers carbamazepine and valproate are associated with a risk of neural tube defects (0.5% for carbamazepine; 1–2% for valproate), including spina bifida. They are also associated with cardiac, gastrointestinal, and facial anomalies, along with a range of other minor malformations. Given that many pregnancies will not be confirmed until after the neural tube closes (day 28), reducing this risk is dependent on preconceptual advice and management. This may include high-dose folate (5 mg/day) from at least 12 weeks prior to conception, although its prescription has not been shown directly to reduce the rate of neural tube defects in women on antiepileptics. For valproate, there is evidence of a dose relationship, with greater risk at doses above 1000 mg/day. Valproate has also been linked to a significant impairment in cognitive function, with 22% of children noted to have exceptionally low verbal IQ, compared with an expected rate of 2% in the general population.[40] Given these concerns, it is recommended that valproate is not prescribed to bipolar women of childbearing potential unless there are no effective alternatives. In such circumstances, women should be on long-acting contraception. Some studies suggest that lamotrigine is associated with increased rate of cleft palate, but findings are conflicting. Lamotrigine is also subject to significantly lowered bioavailability as pregnancy progresses and levels should be monitored in each trimester.

Anxiolytics and hypnotics

Evidence for teratogenicity associated with benzodiazepines is conflicting, with some, but not all, studies suggesting an increased risk of oral cleft. In late pregnancy, there is an increased risk of neonatal sedation or withdrawal. Ideally, doses should be tapered nearing delivery and the infant monitored for withdrawal effects.

Electroconvulsive therapy

Despite a somewhat controversial reputation, ECT is a well-established treatment with a good evidence base for effectiveness in

Box 49.2 Indications for referral to mental health services in pregnancy

- Woman with current illness where there are symptoms of psychosis, severe anxiety, severe depression, suicidality, self-neglect, harm to others, or significant interference with daily functioning. Such illnesses may include psychotic disorders, severe anxiety or depression, obsessive–compulsive disorder, and eating disorders.
- Woman with a history of bipolar disorder or schizophrenia.
- Woman with previous serious postpartum mental illness (postpartum psychosis).
- Women on complex psychotropic medication regimens.
- Referral should be considered for women with illness of moderate severity if developing in late pregnancy or the early postpartum period.
- Referral should be considered for women with current illness of mild or moderate severity where there is a first-degree relative with bipolar disorder or puerperal psychosis. In the absence of current illness, such a family history indicates a raised, but low absolute, risk of early postpartum serious mental illness. Where identified, information should be shared with primary care and any evidence of mood disturbance during pregnancy or in the postpartum period should lead to referral.
- Women with previous periods of inpatient mental health care should be screened by mental health services (either by assessing case records or seeing the woman).
- Maternity services need to ensure that appropriate communication with primary care, and social services where necessary, takes place for women who decline referral to specialized mental health services.

Reproduced from Royal College of Obstetricians and Gynaecologists, *Management of Women with Mental Health Issues during Pregnancy and the Postnatal Period.* Good Practice Paper No. 14. London: RCOG; 2011, with the permission of the Royal College of Obstetricians and Gynaecologists.

severe depressive disorder where, in certain circumstances, it may be the treatment of choice. Less commonly, it is used to manage mania and catatonia. It is also an effective treatment for postpartum psychosis. ECT is most likely to be used where there is a need for rapid recovery because of significant distress, self-neglect, or suicidality, or where there has been a previous good ECT response. There are clear guidelines about the use of ECT, including the use of general anaesthesia and availability of resuscitation and recovery facilities.[41]

The evidence base for the use of ECT in pregnancy is sparse. One case series suggested that the overall risk is low, with 3.2% of fetal or neonatal complications, and 5.3% of maternal complications, attributable to the treatment. The commonest fetal complication was transient cardiac bradyarrhythmia.[42] Modifications to standard ECT administration in pregnancy, particularly in the second and third trimester, include additional fetal monitoring, measures to counteract increased risk of aspiration such as histamine H_2 receptor antagonists, for example, ranitidine, sodium citrate, a rapid sequence induction, cricoid pressure, intubation, antiemetics, avoiding excessive hyperventilation, and positioning of the patient to prevent aortocaval compression.[43]

Managing risk

Guidance for risk management is outlined in NICE[34] and SIGN[35] guidelines on perinatal mental illness.

Prepregnancy

Women who are planning a pregnancy should be asked about a history of significant mental illness. Those at greatest risk of adverse consequences include women with bipolar disorder or schizophrenia (risk of relapse of illness postnatally), and women with schizophrenia, substance misuse, or personality disorder (who may struggle to cope with the challenges of pregnancy and childcare, without appropriate support). Women currently prescribed complex psychotropic regimens should be given advice regarding any known teratogenicity, and specialist review to establish the safest and most effective treatment in advance of pregnancy.

Pregnancy

First contact with maternity services provides an important opportunity to identify women with pre-existing mental illness, or those with a raised risk of postnatal mental illness. All women should be asked about:

- personal history of postpartum psychosis, other psychotic disorders (especially bipolar disorder and schizophrenia), and severe depressive disorder
- family history of bipolar disorder or postpartum psychosis.

Women confirming any of these risk factors should be referred for assessment and management of risk, and should have a detailed plan for their management in late pregnancy and the early postnatal period, which is shared with the woman and all those involved in her care. Services should also respond promptly to any change in mental state reported in late pregnancy or the early postnatal period.

Enquiry should also be made about depressive symptoms at booking and, if there are ongoing concerns, at all subsequent contacts.

Box 49.2 outlines situations where referral to mental health services is indicated during pregnancy.[44]

Conclusion

Pre-existing mental illness presents services with particular challenges during pregnancy, labour, and the postnatal period. Disorders may compromise access to care (such as with schizophrenia or needle phobia), predispose to comorbid physical illness (such as with eating disorders or substance misuse), or result in treatments which require expert management during pregnancy and delivery (such as with lithium or ECT). In addition, the development of early severe postpartum mental illness is, in a substantial proportion of cases, a predictable risk which can be identified and prevented by careful clinical enquiry. All clinicians have a role in the prevention, early detection, referral, and initial management of such disorders.

References

1. Waraich P, Goldner EM, Somers, JM, *et al.* Prevalence and incidence studies of mood disorders: a systematic review of the literature. *Can J Psychiatry* 2004; 49:124–38.
2. Appleby L. Suicide during pregnancy and in the first postnatal year. *BMJ* 1991; 302:137–40.
3. Kendell R, Chalmers J, Platz C. Epidemiology of puerperal psychoses. *Br J Psychiatry* 1987; 150:662–73.
4. Finer LB, Henshaw SK. Disparities in rates of unintended pregnancy in the United States, 1994 and 2001. *Perspect Sex Reprod Health* 2006; 38:90–6.
5. Oates MR. Normal emotional changes in pregnancy and the puerperium. *Baillieres Clin Obstet Gynaecol* 1989; 3:791–804.
6. Lewis G. Chapter 14: Coincidental (fortuitous) deaths. Chapter 16: Domestic vio- lence. In Lewis G, Drife J (eds) *Why Mothers Die 1997–1999. Fifth Report of the Confidential Enquiries into Maternal Deaths.* London: RCOG Press; 2001:225–30, 241–51.
7. Department of Health. *Responding to Domestic Abuse: A Handbook for Professionals.* London: Department of Health; 2005.
8. McGuffin P, Rijsdijk F, Andrew M, *et al.* The heritability of bipolar affective disorder and the genetic relationship to unipolar depression. *Arch Gen Psychiatry* 2003; 60:497–502.
9. Viguera AC, Whitfield T, Baldessarini RJ, *et al.* Risk of recurrence in women with bipolar disorder during pregnancy: prospective study of mood stabilizer discontinuation. *Am J Psychiatry* 2007; 164:1817–24.
10. Viguera AC, Nonacs R, Cohen LS, *et al.* Risk of recurrence of bipolar disorder in pregnant and nonpregnant women after discontinuing lithium maintenance. *Am J Psychiatry* 2000; 157:179–84.
11. Bundy H, Stahl D, MacCabe JH. A systematic review and meta- analysis of the fertility of patients with schizophrenia and their unaffected relatives. *Acta Psychiatr Scand* 2011; 123:98–106.
12. Howard LM. Fertility and pregnancy in women with psychotic disorders. *Eur J Obstet Gynecol Reprod Biol* 2005; 119(1):3–10.
13. Munk-Olsen T, Munk Laursen T, Mendelson T, *et al.* Risks and predictors of readmission for a mental disorder during the postpartum period. *Arch Gen Psychiatry* 2009; 66:189–95.
14. Kumar R, Marks M, Platz C, *et al.* Clinical survey of a psychiatric mother and baby unit: characteristics of 100 consecutive admissions. *J Affect Disord* 1995; 33(1):11–22.
15. Ververs T, Kaasenbrood H, Visser G, *et al.* Prevalence and patterns of antidepressant drug use during pregnancy. *Eur J Clin Pharmacol* 2006; 62:863–70.
16. Centre for Maternal and Child Enquiries (CMACE). Saving Mothers' Lives: reviewing maternal deaths to make motherhood safer: 2006–08. The Eighth Report on Confidential Enquiries into Maternal Deaths in the United Kingdom. *BJOG* 2011; 118(Suppl. 1):1–203.
17. Meidahl Petersen K, Jimenez-Solem E, Andersen JT, *et al.* β-Blocker treatment during pregnancy and adverse pregnancy outcomes: a nationwide population-based cohort study. *BMJ Open* 2012; 2:e001185.
18. Micali N, Treasure J. Biological effects of a maternal ED on pregnancy and foetal development: a review. *Eur Eat Disorders Rev* 2009; 17:448–54.
19. Kouba S, Hallstrom T, Lindholm C, *et al.* Pregnancy and neonatal outcomes in women with eating disorders. *Obstet Gynecol* 2005; 105:255–60.
20. Ward VB, Waller D. Eating disorders in pregnancy. *BMJ* 2008; 336:93–6.
21. Oates MR, Cantwell R. Deaths from Psychiatric Causes. In Centre for Maternal and Child Enquiries (CMACE). Saving Mothers' Lives: reviewing maternal deaths to make motherhood safer: 2006–08. The Eighth Report on Confidential Enquiries into Maternal Deaths in the United Kingdom. *BJOG* 2011; 118(Suppl. 1):132–42.
22. Pruett D, Waterman EH, Caughey AB. Fetal alcohol exposure: consequences, diagnosis and treatment. *Obstet Gynecol Surv* 2013; 68:62–9.
23. Borjesson K, Ruppert S, Bagedahl-Strindlund M. A longitudinal study of psychiatric symptoms in primiparous women: relation to personality disorders and sociodemographic factors. *Arch Womens Ment Health* 2005; 8:232–42.
24. Hofberg K, Brockington IF. Tokophobia: an unreasoning dread of childbirth. *Br J Psychiatry* 2000; 176:83–5.
25. Kendell R, Chalmers J, Platz C. Epidemiology of puerperal psychosis. *Br J Psychiatry* 1987; 150:662–73.
26. Jones I, Craddock N. Familiarity of the puerperal trigger in bipolar disorder: results of a family study. *Am J Psychiatry* 2001; 158:913–17.
27. Wieck A, Kumar R, Hirst AD, *et al.* Increased sensitivity of dopamine receptors and recurrence of affective psychosis after childbirth. *BMJ* 1991; 303:613–16.
28. O'Hara MW, Swain AM. Rates and risk of postnatal depression—a meta-analysis. *Int Rev Psychiatry* 1996; 8:37–54.
29. Neugebauer R, Kline J, Shrout P, *et al.* Major depressive disorder in the six months after miscarriage. *JAMA* 1997; 277:382–8.
30. Hughes P, Turton P, Hopper E, *et al.* Assessment of guidelines for good. practice in psychosocial care of mothers after stillbirth: a cohort study. *Lancet* 2002; 360:114–18.
31. Hughes P, Riches S. Psychological aspects of perinatal loss. *Curr Opin Obstet Gynecol* 2003; 15:107–11.
32. Academy of Medical Royal Colleges. *Induced Abortion and Mental Health: A Systematic Review of the Mental Health Outcomes of Induced Abortion, Including their Prevalence and Associated Factors.* London: Academy of Medical Royal Colleges; 2011.
33. Talge NM, Neal C, Glover V. Antenatal maternal stress and long-term effects on child neurodevelopment: how and why? *J Child Psychol Psychiatry* 2007; 48:245–61.
34. National Institute for Health and Clinical Excellence (NICE). *Antenatal and Postnatal Mental Health: Clinical Management and Service Guideline.* Clinical Guideline CG45. London: NICE; 2007.
35. Scottish Intercollegiate Guidelines Network (SIGN). *Management of Perinatal Mood Disorders.* SIGN Publication No. 127. Edinburgh: SIGN; 2012.
36. Grigoriadis S, VonderPorten EH, Mamisashvili L, *et al.* Prenatal exposure to antidepressants and persistent pulmonary hypertension of the newborn: systemic review and meta-analysis. *BMJ* 2014; 348:f6932.
37. Scottish Intercollegiate Guidelines Network (SIGN). *Management of Schizophrenia.* SIGN Publication No. 131. Edinburgh: SIGN; 2013.
38. Matok I, Pupco A, Koren G. Drug exposure in pregnancy and heart defects. *J Cardiovasc Pharmacol* 2011; 58:20–4.
39. Newport DJ, Viguera AC, Beach AJ, *et al.* Lithium placental passage and obstetrical outcome: implications for clinical management during late pregnancy. *Am J Psychiatry* 2005; 162:2162–70.
40. Adab N, Kini U, Vinten J, *et al.* The longer term outcome of children born to mothers with epilepsy. *J Neurol Neurosurg Psychiatry* 2004; 75:1575–83.
41. Waite J, Easton A (eds). *The ECT Handbook* (3rd ed.) London: Royal College of Psychiatrists; 2013.
42. Anderson EL, Reti IM. ECT in pregnancy: a review of the literature from 1941 to 2007. *Psychosomat Med* 2009; 71:235–42.
43. O'Reardon JP, Cristancho, MA, von Andreae CV, *et al.* Acute and maintenance electroconvulsive therapy for treatment of severe major depression during the second and third trimesters of pregnancy with infant follow-up to 18 months: case report and review of the literature. *J ECT* 2011; 27:e23–e26.
44. Cantwell R, Mahmood TA. *Good Practice No. 14: Management of Women with Mental Health Issues During Pregnancy and the Postnatal Period.* London: Royal College of Obstetricians and Gynaecologists; 2011.

CHAPTER 50

Chronic maternal infections

Kristel Van Calsteren

Introduction

Pregnant women diagnosed with chronic infections are a worldwide problem. In developed countries, the most frequently encountered are hepatitis B and C (see Chapter 43), toxoplasmosis, syphilis, herpes simplex, and *Cytomegalovirus* infections. In developing countries, human immunodeficiency virus (HIV) and malaria are also seen commonly in pregnant women. Maternal infections are associated with various complications in pregnant women, but also with congenital infections with or without structural anomalies and long-term sequelae, fetal growth restriction, preterm delivery, and perinatal mortality.

Moreover, increasing evidence suggests that maternal infection during pregnancy affects the developing immune system of the fetus independently of the vertical transmission of pathogens.[1]

In this chapter, I discuss the pathogen characteristics, ways of transmission, clinical presentation, diagnostic options, treatment, and, if relevant, prophylaxis for the most common infections in pregnant women.

Human immunodeficiency virus

General information

An infection with HIV is a life-long infection that can lead to the acquired immunodeficiency syndrome (AIDS).

The official first registration of the disease occurred in the summer of 1981 when the US Centers for Disease Control and Prevention (CDC) reported on a cluster of *Pneumocystis jirovecii* (previously *carinii*) pneumonia (PCP) in five homosexual men.[2] Soon thereafter, additional gay men developed a previously rare skin cancer called Kaposi's sarcoma (KS).[3,4] However, there is substantial evidence that HIV first crossed the simian–human species barrier much earlier. The identification of a cytopathic retrovirus in 1983 and development of a diagnostic serological test for HIV-1 in 1985 have served as the basis for developing improvements in diagnosis.

HIV is a lentivirus, a slow-replicating retrovirus, that infects vital cells in the human immune system such as helper T cells (specifically CD4+ T cells), macrophages, and dendritic cells.[5] Lentiviruses are transmitted as single-stranded, positive-sense, enveloped RNA viruses. Upon entry into the target cell, the viral RNA genome is converted (reverse transcribed) into double-stranded DNA by a virally encoded reverse transcriptase that is transported along with the viral genome in the virus particle. The resulting viral DNA is then imported into the cell nucleus and integrated into the cellular DNA by a virally encoded integrase and host co-factors. Once integrated, the virus may become latent, allowing the virus and its host cell to avoid detection by the immune system. Alternatively, the virus may be transcribed, producing new RNA genomes and viral proteins that are packaged and released from the cell as new virus particles that begin the replication cycle anew.

Two types of HIV have been identified: HIV-1 and HIV-2. HIV-1 is more virulent, more infective,[6] and is the cause of the majority of HIV infections globally. The lower infectivity of HIV-2 implies that fewer of those exposed to HIV-2 will be infected per exposure. Because of its relatively poor capacity for transmission, HIV-2 is largely confined to West Africa.

HIV infection leads to low levels of CD4+ T cells through a number of mechanisms including apoptosis of uninfected bystander cells, direct viral killing of infected cells, and killing of infected CD4+ T cells by CD8 cytotoxic lymphocytes that recognize infected cells. When CD4+ T cell numbers decline below a critical level, cell-mediated immunity is lost, and the body becomes progressively more susceptible to opportunistic infections (Figure 50.1).

Transmission

Infection with HIV occurs by the transfer of blood, semen, vaginal fluid, pre-ejaculate, or breast milk. Within these bodily fluids, HIV is present as both free virus particles and virus within infected immune cells. If their mothers have HIV, infants can become infected during the pregnancy, during labour and delivery, and, to a lesser degree, through breastfeeding.

Diagnosis

HIV testing is performed by immunoassays (ELISA or combination antibody and antigen immunoassays) and analysed in duplicate. If the result of either duplicate test is reactive, the specimen is reported as repeatedly reactive and undergoes confirmatory testing with Western blot.

When the possibility of an acute HIV infection is considered or the serology is positive, viral load is determined by reverse transcription polymerase chain reaction (RT-PCR) and CD4 cell count is measured.

Testing post exposure is recommended initially and at 6 weeks, 3 months, and 6 months since the time interval between infection and test positivity is 20–45 days for immunoassays, 35–60 days for Western blot, and 5–15 days for viral load.[7]

Many HIV-positive people are unaware that they are infected with the virus. Therefore, it is strongly recommended that all pregnant women undergo serological screening for HIV.

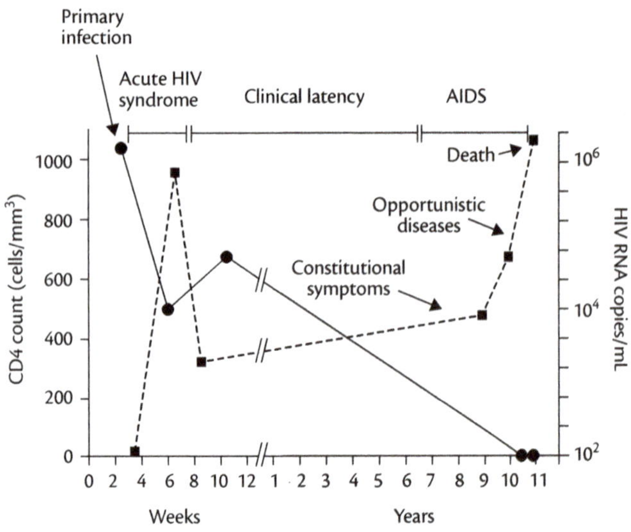

Figure 50.1 HIV infection: CD4 count and viral load throughout disease progression.

Adapted from https://commons.wikimedia.org/wiki/File:Hiv-timecourse_copy.svg. This file is made available under the Creative Commons CC0 1.0 Universal Public Domain Dedication. https://creativecommons.org/publicdomain/zero/1.0/deed.en

Clinical presentation

Ten to 60% of patients with early HIV infection will not experience symptoms. In acute symptomatic HIV infection, a variety of symptoms can be seen: fever, lymphadenopathy, sore throat, rash, myalgia/arthralgia, headache, and diarrhoea. These findings are not specific for acute HIV, but prolonged duration of symptoms and the presence of mucocutaneous ulcers are suggestive of HIV. The usual time from HIV exposure to the development of symptoms is 2–4 weeks.

AIDS is a disease characterized by progressive failure of the immune system allowing life-threatening opportunistic infections and cancers to thrive.

Treatment

At diagnosis, and at regular time intervals, viral load, CD4 T cell count and side effects of medication should be monitored. HIV drug-resistance studies are advised to be performed before starting or modifying antiretroviral regimens in all pregnant women whose HIV RNA levels are above the threshold for resistance testing (above 500–1000 copies/mL).[8] The importance of adherence to prescribed antiretroviral medications should be stressed to reduce the potential for development of resistance.

During pregnancy, all women with HIV are advised to take combination antiretroviral regimens using three HIV drugs. Combination antiretroviral drug regimens will maximally suppress viral replication, which is the most effective strategy for preventing development of resistance and minimizing risk of perinatal transmission.

The 2013 World Health Organization guidelines recommend initiation of a once-daily, fixed-dose combination of tenofovir (300 mg), lamivudine (300 mg) (or emtricitabine (200 mg)), and efavirenz (600 mg) in all HIV-infected pregnant women. Alternative agents are zidovudine to replace tenofovir and nevirapine to replace efavirenz in the three-drug regimen. There are extensive safety and efficacy data on the use of zidovudine and nevirapine in pregnant and breastfeeding women.[9]

Studies suggest that women who start HIV medications earlier in pregnancy are more likely to have a low amount of virus in the blood by the time of delivery. However, some women may prefer to start after the first trimester of pregnancy to avoid unnecessary drug exposure to the embryo. Once started, HIV medications are continued throughout pregnancy.

There are several HIV medications that should not be used in pregnancy. Nevirapine is generally not started in women with a CD4 count higher than 250/mm^3, since it is associated with hepatic toxicity and hypersensitivity reactions. Efavirenz is associated with fetal malformations (neural tube defects), so should not be started during the first few weeks of pregnancy. However, women who become pregnant while taking efavirenz can continue that medication.

Obstetric care

HIV-positive patients are at increased risk for spontaneous abortions and stillbirths, growth restriction, preterm delivery, and perinatal mortality and appear to have a lower risk of pre-eclampsia.[10,11] The latter has been linked to the HIV-1-related immune deficiency and indicates the pivotal role of the immune system in the pathogenesis of pre-eclampsia.[12]

A detailed ultrasound is usually recommended at 18–20 weeks of pregnancy to screen for structural anomalies, especially when antiretroviral drugs were administered in the first trimester of pregnancy. A follow-up ultrasound is often recommended during the third trimester to monitor the fetal growth.

The advised mode of delivery depends on the viral load at that time.[8,9]

Pregnant women with HIV who have been taking HIV medications throughout pregnancy and have an *undetectable HIV viral* load at 34–36 weeks of pregnancy may choose to have a vaginal delivery. The risk of transmission during a vaginal delivery is than very low, and a caesarean delivery has not been shown to decrease this risk any further.

Women with an HIV viral load *between 0 and 1000 copies/mL* who have been taking HIV medications during pregnancy may choose between a vaginal or caesarean delivery. Data are insufficient to evaluate the potential benefit of caesarean delivery used solely for prevention of perinatal transmission in women with HIV RNA levels less than 1000 copies/mL, and given the low rate of transmission in these patients, it is unclear whether scheduled caesarean delivery would confer additional benefit in reducing transmission.

Pregnant women with HIV who have taken HIV medications throughout pregnancy but have a *viral load above 1000 copies/ mL* at 34–36 weeks of pregnancy (or unknown HIV levels and newly diagnosed disease) are advised to have a planned caesarean delivery (at 38 weeks) rather than a vaginal delivery. For these patients it is advised to administer zidovudine intravenously (IV) to reduce the risk of HIV transmission, next to their combination HIV medications which they should continue to take on schedule to provide maximal protection to the mother and infant and to minimize the risk that the mother could develop drug resistance due to a missed dose of medication.[8] Women with newly diagnosed disease or unknown HIV levels at the time of delivery should also have a caesarean delivery and zidovudine IV.

It is not clear whether caesarean delivery after rupture of membranes or onset of labour provides benefit in preventing perinatal transmission. Management of women originally scheduled for caesarean delivery who present with ruptured membranes or in labour must be individualized at the time of presentation based on duration of rupture and/or labour, plasma HIV RNA level, and current antiretroviral drug regimen.[8]

Transmission-increasing procedures, like amniocentesis, artificial rupture of membranes, use of fetal scalp electrodes/scalp pH, operative delivery with forceps/vacuum, and episiotomy, should be avoided unless there are clear obstetric indications.

In case of postpartum haemorrhage resulting from uterine atony, the current antiretroviral drug regimen should be taken into consideration. In women who are receiving a cytochrome P450 (CYP)-3A4 enzyme inhibitor such as a protease inhibitor, methylergometrine should be used only if no alternative treatments are available. If methylergometrine is used, it should be administered in the lowest effective dose for the shortest possible duration. In women who are receiving a CYP3A4 enzyme inducer such as nevirapine, efavirenz, or etravirine, additional uterotonic agents may be needed because of the potential for decreased methylergometrine levels and inadequate treatment effect.

Postpartum care

Decisions about continuing antiretroviral drugs after delivery should take into account current recommendations for antiretroviral therapy, current and nadir CD4 T-lymphocyte counts and trajectory, HIV RNA levels, adherence issues, whether a woman has an HIV-uninfected sexual partner, and patient preference.

Women with HIV who breastfeed can pass HIV to the infant. In one study of over 600 mother–infant pairs from Malawi, the risk of transmitting HIV to the infant through breast milk was 7% for infants who breastfed for 1 year and 10% for infants who breastfed for up to 2 years.

In resource-rich countries, clean water and infant formulas are readily available and are safe alternatives to breastfeeding. Therefore, in resource-rich countries, HIV-positive patients are recommended not to breastfeed their babies, even if the woman is taking HIV medications. While risk of HIV transmission through breast milk can be lowered by HIV medications, HIV can still be transmitted through breast milk. The same advice cannot be given to women in resource-poor countries because safe alternatives to breast milk may not be consistently available.

Newborns of women with HIV should receive post-exposure prophylaxis to prevent transmission from exposure to HIV during delivery/breastfeeding with 6 weeks of zidovudine or nevirapine. Zidovudine or nevirapine should be initiated as close to the time of birth as possible, preferably within 6–12 hours of delivery.

Infants born to HIV-infected women who have not received antepartum antiretroviral drugs should receive prophylaxis with zidovudine given for 6 weeks combined with three doses of nevirapine in the first week of life (at birth, 48 hours later, and 96 hours after the second dose), begun as soon after birth as possible. A longer duration of infant prophylaxis is reasonable in breastfeeding infants in certain circumstances that increase the likelihood of absent or delayed viral suppression in the mother, such as when women do not receive antepartum antiretroviral drugs. The use of antiretrovirals other than zidovudine and nevirapine cannot be recommended in premature infants because of lack of dosing and safety data.[8]

HIV antibody tests are not accurate in infants since HIV antibodies may be transferred from the mother to the baby. This may result in the infant having a positive HIV antibody test. However, this does not mean that the baby necessarily has HIV infection.

For this reason, in infants an HIV PCR test that directly measures the virus itself should be performed to determine whether or not the baby is infected with HIV.

Long-term follow-up of children

Studies of infants who were exposed to zidovudine and who did not become infected with HIV have not shown any increased risk of serious problems with growth, the immune system, brain function, cancers, or other problems for up to 6 years.[13] However, long-term data regarding the safety of HIV medications during pregnancy, particularly combination regimens, are not available.

Prophylaxis

Pregnancy does not appear to worsen HIV or increase the risk of death from HIV. For the baby, patients should understand that the risk of transmission is much lower with an undetectable viral load. Therefore it is important to take HIV medication adequately.[8]

For serodiscordant couples who want to conceive, it is important to recognize that treatment of the infected partner may not be fully protective against sexual transmission of HIV.

For HIV-infected females with HIV-uninfected male partners, the safest conception option is artificial insemination, including the option of self-insemination with a partner's sperm during the periovulatory period.

For HIV-infected men with HIV-uninfected female partners, the use of sperm preparation techniques coupled with either intrauterine insemination or *in vitro* fertilization should be considered if using donor sperm from an HIV-uninfected male is unacceptable.

For serodiscordant couples who want to conceive, initiation of antiretroviral therapy for the HIV-infected partner is recommended. Periconception administration of antiretroviral pre-exposure prophylaxis (PrEP) for HIV-uninfected partners may offer an additional tool to reduce the risk of sexual transmission. The utility of PrEP of the uninfected partner when the infected partner is receiving antiretroviral therapy has yet not been studied.

Partners should be screened and treated for genital tract infections before attempting to conceive.

Perinatal transmission can be reduced by antiretroviral drugs by lowering maternal antepartum viral load and providing infant pre- and post-exposure prophylaxis.

Anaesthetic management

Patients with HIV infection have early HIV virus infection of the central nervous system (CNS). Hence the initial fear of epidural or spinal anaesthesia transferring the virus to the CNS, are unfounded and regional anaesthesia should not be withheld.[14] Also the use of an epidural blood patch whenever indicated seems to be safe.

HIV patients may have mild thrombocytopenia. Hence platelet levels should be tested.

Malaria

General information

Malaria is caused by five species of the protozoan genus *Plasmodium: P. vivax, P. falciparum, P. malariae, P. knowlesi*, and *P. ovale*. The infection is maintained in nature by female mosquitoes of the genus *Anopheles*, in which the parasites' multiplication occurs.

Malaria is an endemic disease in parts of Asia, Africa, Oceania, and Central and South America, where environmental factors including temperature, humidity, and standing water support the breeding of mosquitoes in close contact with humans.

The mosquito feeds on human blood, in which the *Plasmodium* life cycle is completed.

Transmission

When a female *Anopheles* mosquito bites an infected human, male and female gametocytes are ingested into the mosquito stomach. The sexual reproductive cycle produces sporozoites in about 2 weeks' time, which accumulate in the mosquito salivary glands and are infectious for humans. When the mosquito bites again, the sporozoites are infected into the bloodstream. The sporozoites infect liver parenchymal cells during this clinically inapparent pre-erythrocytic or exoerythrocytic phase. After several days merozoites are released into the bloodstream. This form of the parasite is capable of red blood cell invasion and multiplication, a process called schizogony, which lead to red blood cell lysis. When enough parasites are in synchrony, periodic fevers manifest themselves coincident with rupture of red blood cells and release merozoites. The cycle takes 36–72 hours.

Certain haemoglobinopathies and erythrocyte enzyme defects render patients less susceptible to severe complications of malaria. Patients with sickle haemoglobin acquire falciparum malaria as frequently but the clinical disease is attenuated, possibly because the parasite is less able to divide in the abnormal erythrocyte. Certain black populations are less susceptible to *P. vivax* infections because of the absence of Duffy blood group antigen, which acts as an erythrocyte receptor for *P. vivax* merozoites.[15]

Immunity to clinical malaria is acquired gradually as a result of repeated exposure to the infection. In endemic areas, this process takes 5–10 years to develop and immunity is partial, meaning that the parasites are present intermittently in the blood of semi-immune subjects.[16] The development of antibodies and cell-mediated immunity contribute to the pathogenesis of some of the clinical features of chronic malaria such as nephrotic syndrome and tropical splenomegaly. Disruption of the host–parasite balance by malnutrition, pregnancy, or introduction of new strains of parasite, may precipitate recrudescence and clinical manifestations in the semi-immune host.

All types of malaria can be transmitted congenitally, but congenital disease is most often associated with *P. vivax* and *P. falciparum*. In immune mothers, the risk of transplacental transmission of malaria appears to be small (0.1–1.5% had cord blood positive for parasites and clinical disease), when overt attacks occurred during pregnancy the risk was 1–4%.[17] In contrast, in semi-immune or non-immune mothers, transplacental antibody transfer may be deficient, and the incidence of congenital infection appears to be higher (7–10%).[18]

Primiparous women in endemic areas seem to be more susceptible to recrudescent infections than multiparous women.

Diagnosis

Diagnosis is made by Giesma-stained thick and/or thin peripheral blood smears or a rapid diagnostic test. The highest level of parasitaemia will be demonstrable several hours after a rigor and serial thick and thin slides may be needed to demonstrate parasitaemia. It is important to point out that women may have placental parasites that are not circulating in the peripheral blood, and hence, the blood film would be negative. Yet, no reliable peripheral biomarker for the presence of placental malaria has been identified.

Clinical presentation

Patients with acute malaria usually present with rigors and fever (which may or may not be periodic), often associated with headache and myalgia. Non-specific symptoms include malaise, dry cough, abdominal pain, diarrhoea, nausea, anorexia, or vomiting. Physical examination reveals fever, tachycardia, respiratory distress, hepatomegaly, splenomegaly, pallor, and sometimes jaundice.

Fever and related symptoms gradually subside over several weeks in untreated *P. vivax, P. ovale*, and *P. malariae* malaria. Months or years after initial exposure, dormant forms of the parasitic (hypnozoites) may emerge from the liver and cause relapses. With *P. falciparum*, serious complications such as coma, severe haemolytic anaemia, disseminated intravascular coagulation, acute kidney injury, and acute pulmonary oedema may develop rapidly in the non-immune host; however, once eradicated from the blood *P. falciparum* does not relapse.[15]

Compared to non-pregnant women, pregnant women experience more severe disease, severe anaemia (60%), more hypoglycaemia, and more respiratory complications (pulmonary oedema, acute respiratory distress syndrome).[19]

Adverse perinatal outcomes associated with malaria include miscarriage, fetal growth restriction, preterm birth, low birth weight, fetal and maternal anaemia, and congenital infection. Each year, 50 million women living in malaria-endemic areas become pregnant. It is estimated that 10,000 women and 200,000 infants die as a result of malaria infection during pregnancy; severe maternal anaemia, prematurity, and low birth weight contribute to more than half of these deaths.

In endemic areas, it can be difficult to distinguish malaria acquired congenitally from that acquired as a newborn, particularly in infants of asymptomatic mothers. The onset of symptoms is usually at 2–8 weeks of age and includes poor feeding, fever, vomiting, diarrhoea, and irritability. Anaemia, thrombocytopenia, and hyperbilirubinaemia are common. Splenomegaly is more common than hepatomegaly.

Treatment

Acute malaria in the unexposed, pregnant host is a medical emergency requiring immediate treatment.

Patients with malaria during pregnancy should be admitted and started with drug treatment (artesunate, quinine, clindamycin, chloroquine, atovaquone–proguanil) (Table 50.1).[20] Paracetamol (maximum 4 g/day provided the patient is >50 kg) should be started for fever and screening for anaemia should be performed.

These patients should be monitored for hypoglycaemia, pulmonary oedema, acute respiratory distress, and secondary bacterial infection should be screened for if the patient becomes hypotensive. (Exchange) Transfusion might be necessary for anaemia.

Uncomplicated malaria in pregnancy is not a reason for induction of labour.

Table 50.1 Royal College of Obstetricians and Gynaecologists guidelines for treatment and prophylaxis of malaria in pregnancy[20]

Severity	Indication	Drug and dosage
Severe or complicated malaria	Any species	Artesunate IV 2.4 mg/kg at 0, 12, and 24 hours, then daily thereafter. When the patient is well enough to take oral medication she can be switched to oral artesunate 2 mg/kg (or IM artesunate 2.4 mg/kg) once daily, plus clindamycin. If oral artesunate is not available, use a 3-day course of Riamet® or Malarone® or a 7-day course of quinine and clindamycin at 450 mg 3 times a day 7 days
		Alternative: Quinine IV 20 mg/kg loading dose (no loading dose if patient already taking quinine or mefloquine) in 5% dextrose over 4 hours and then 10 mg/kg IV over 4 hours every 8 hours plus clindamycin IV 450 mg every 8 hours (maximum dose quinine 1.4 g). When the patient is well enough to take oral medication she can be switched to oral quinine 600 mg 3 times a day to complete 5–7 days and oral clindamycin 450 mg 3 times a day 7 days (an alternative rapid quinine-loading regimen is 7 mg/kg quinine dihydrochloride IV over 30 minutes using an infusion pump followed by 10 mg/kg over 4 hours) *Note*: quinine dosing should be reduced to 12-hourly dosing if IV therapy extends more than 48 hours or if the patient has renal or hepatic dysfunction. Quinine is associated with severe and recurrent hypoglycaemia in late pregnancy.
Uncomplicated malaria	*P. falciparum*	Oral quinine 600 mg 8-hourly and oral clindamycin 450 mg 8-hourly for 7 days *or* Riamet® 4 tablets/dose for weight > 35 kg, twice daily for 3 days *or* Malarone® 4 standard tablets daily for 3 days
	Vomiting but no signs of severe or complicated malaria	Quinine 10 mg/kg dose IV in 5% dextrose over 4 hours every 8 hours plus IV clindamycin 450 mg every 8 hours. When the patient is well enough to take oral medication she can be switched to oral quinine 600 mg 3 times a day to complete 5–7 days and oral clindamycin can if needed be switched to 450 mg 3 times a day 7 days
Non-falciparum malaria	*P. vivax, P. ovale, P. malariae*	Oral chloroquine (base) 600 mg followed by 300 mg 68 hours later. Then 300 mg on day 2 and again on day 3
	Resistant *P. vivax*	As for uncomplicated malaria *P. falciparum*
	Preventing relapse during pregnancy	Chloroquine oral 300 mg weekly until delivery
	Preventing relapse after delivery	Postpone until 3 months after delivery and G6PD testing
	P. ovale	Oral primaquine 15 mg single daily dose for 14 days
	P. vivax	Oral primaquine 30 mg single daily dose for 14 days
	G6PD (mild) for *P. vivax* or *P. ovale*	Primaquine oral 45–60 mg once a week for 8 weeks

Reproduced from Royal College of Obstetricians and Gynaecologists, *The diagnosis and treatment of malaria in pregnancy*. Green-top Guideline No. 54b. London: RCOG; 2010, with the permission of the Royal College of Obstetricians and Gynaecologists.

Peripartum malaria is an indication for placental histology and placenta, cord, and baby blood films to detect congenital malaria at an early stage.

Prophylaxis

Pregnant travellers should be advised to defer travel until after delivery whenever feasible. For pregnant women who cannot defer travel, mosquito avoidance measures should be used in conjunction with chemoprophylaxis.

Chloroquine or hydroxychloroquine are considered safe to use in all trimesters of pregnancy. Mefloquine is the agent of choice for chloroquine-resistant areas, and evidence suggests it is not associated with an increased risk to the fetus. Although the atovaquone–proguanil drug combination is not currently recommended for use during pregnancy, limited data suggest that it is not harmful to the fetus. Doxycycline and primaquine are not recommended during pregnancy.[21]

Syphilis

General information

Syphilis is a chronic infectious disease caused by the spirochaete, *Treponema pallidum*. It is a sexually transmitted disease that can cause long-term complications and/or death if not treated correctly. Symptoms in adults are divided into four stages: primary, secondary, latent, and late syphilis.

Transmission

Syphilis is transmitted by direct contact with a syphilitic ulcer during anal, vaginal, or oral sex. Ulcers can be found on the penis, vagina, lips, and in the rectum and mouth.

The disease can be found at any stage in a pregnant woman and *T. pallidum* can cross the placenta to infect the fetus, resulting in congenital disease or stillbirth. The risk of congenital syphilis is directly related to the stage of syphilis in the mother and the risk is extremely high for the first 4 years after maternal acquisition of infection when spirochaetaemia is common. Perinatal transmission occurs in 50% of patients with primary or secondary syphilis, with fewer congenital infections among women with early latent (40%), late latent (10%), and tertiary disease (10%).[15]

Diagnosis

Available tests are divided into screening and confirmatory tests.

For screening, a non-treponemal antibody test (Venereal Disease Research Laboratory (VDRL) test and the Rapid Plasma

Reagin (RPR) test) is performed on serum. Positive tests are usually reported as antibody titre and can be used to follow the response to treatment in many patients. These tests are relatively inexpensive, easy to perform, and can also be done on other body fluids, such as cerebrospinal fluid (CSF). Confirmatory tests (treponemal antibody tests) detect antibodies specifically directed at treponemal cellular components (fluorescent treponemal antibody absorption (FTA-ABS), microhaemagglutination assay for antibodies to *T. pallidum* (MHA-TP), and *T. pallidum* particle agglutination assay (TPPA)). These tests are sensitive and specific, but expensive. Furthermore, they remain positive despite treatment and therefore correlate poorly with disease activity.

Lumbar puncture is required for any patient with clinical evidence of neurological involvement and is strongly recommended for patients with coexistent HIV or with latent syphilis for more than 1 year.

In all pregnant women, it is advised to screen for syphilis during the first prenatal medical visit. If the patient is considered to be at high risk this screening should be repeated in the third trimester.

For the diagnosis of congenital syphilis, the VDRL or RPR test should be performed. A thorough physical examination should be performed for evidence of congenital syphilis. Direct visualization of *T. pallidum* by darkfield microscopy or fluorescent antibody staining of infected body fluids (e.g. nasal discharge) or lesions, placenta, or umbilical cord can be performed.

PCR has been used on neonatal blood and CSF for diagnosis of congenital syphilis, but these tests are not widely available.[22]

Maternal clinical presentation

Primary syphilis presents as a papule, which is typically painless, at the site of inoculation (genital or extragenital).[23] This soon ulcerates to produce the classic chancre(s) of primary syphilis. The chancre is a 1–2 cm painless ulcer with an indurated margin, which is associated with regional lymphadenopathy. Chancres heal spontaneously within 3–6 weeks, even in the absence of treatment. The primary stage of syphilis is often missed in women because the lesion is on vaginal or cervical mucosa.

Secondary syphilis is a disseminated systemic process that begins 6 weeks to 6 months after the appearance of the chancre in approximately 25% of untreated patients. This stage of disease is characterized by a generalized maculopapular skin rash involving the palms and soles and mucous membranes, but usually sparing the face. The rash is usually not itchy. Other symptoms that can accompany the skin rash include generalized lymphadenopathy, fever, pharyngitis, weight loss, patchy hair loss, headaches, muscle aches, and fatigue, as well as genital condylomata lata. Although spirochaetes can be found in the CSF of around 40–50% of patients with early syphilis, neurological manifestations are rare. The rash of secondary syphilis typically resolves spontaneously within 2–6 weeks. Secondary syphilis is commonly the stage when women present to a healthcare provider.

Latent disease is usually subclinical, although clinical relapses, particularly of lesions of secondary syphilis, may occur. If syphilis is not treated, it can remain present for years without any signs or symptoms.

Tertiary syphilis occurs in approximately one-third of untreated patients, but is now rarely seen since most patients are treated either deliberately or inadvertently when receiving penicillin for other indications. Tertiary syphilis can occur 10–30 years after the infection begun, or 5–20 years after the disease has become latent. This stage is characterized by slowly progressive signs and symptoms. Clinical manifestations include gumma formation (15%), cardiovascular disease (10%) (aortic aneurysm), and neurosyphilis (6.5%) (general paresis, numbness, blindness, dementia, tabes dorsalis).

Congenital syphilis

The clinical spectrum of congenital infection includes perinatal death, preterm delivery, low birth weight, non-immune hydrops, early congenital syphilis, and late congenital syphilis.

Two-thirds of live-born neonates with congenital syphilis are asymptomatic at birth. Clinical manifestations in untreated infants usually appear by 3 months of age, most often by 5 weeks.[24]

Characteristic findings for early congenital syphilis include a maculopapular rash, hepatosplenomegaly and jaundice, fever, neurosyphilis, pneumonitis, rhinitis or 'snuffles', lymphadenopathy, chorioretinitis, anaemia, thrombocytopaenia, and osteochondritis which may lead to pseudoparalysis. Also condylomata lata and nephrotic syndrome have been described. Chancres do not occur.[25]

If untreated, late congenital syphilis will develop. Manifestations of late congenital syphilis are facial features (frontal bossing, saddle nose, short maxilla, protuberant mandible), oropharyngeal anomalies (Hutchinson's teeth, mulberry molars, perforation of hard palate), ophthalmologic damage (interstitial keratitis, chorioretinitis, secondary glaucoma, corneal scarring, optic atrophy), sensorineural deafness, gummas, skeletal anomalies (saber shins: anterior bowing of the tibia, Higoumenakis sign: enlargement of the sternoclavicular portion of the clavicle, Clutton joints: painless arthritis) and lesions of the CNS (intellectual disability, arrested hydrocephalus, seizures, juvenile general paresis).[25]

Late congenital syphilis develops in approximately 40% of infants born to women with untreated syphilis during pregnancy. Some manifestations of late congenital syphilis can be prevented by treatment of the mother during pregnancy or treatment of the infant within the first 3 months of life. However, other manifestations (e.g. keratitis and saber shins) may occur or progress despite appropriate therapy.

Treatment

Benzathine penicillin G cures maternal infection and prevents congenital infection in 98% of cases.[26] Alternative therapy with other non-penicillin regimens is not recommended for pregnant patients because of treatment failures in preventing congenital infection, especially with erythromycin (Table 50.2).[27] Tetracycline is not recommended because of discolouration of fetal teeth and bones, but may represent a reasonable choice if no other alternatives are available. Ceftriaxone is also effective in adults for the treatment of early syphilis, but there is no information about its efficacy in preventing congenital syphilis.

If non-penicillin alternative regimens are used during the pregnancy, the neonate should be very carefully evaluated for active disease and treated with a single dose of benzathine penicillin G (50,000 units/kg IM).

Patients with a history of penicillin allergy should receive skin testing for the presence of anaphylactic antibodies to both the major determinant antigen, penicilloyl polylysine, and to the minor determinant antigens, benzylpenicillin G and benzyl penicilloic acid. About 90% of patients giving a history of

Table 50.2 Guidelines for treatment of syphilis

Stage of disease	Recommended treatment
Early syphilis (primary, secondary or latent syphilis of <1 year duration)	Benzathine penicillin G 2.4 million units IM in a single dose *Alternatives:* Tetracycline 500 mg orally 4 times daily for 2 weeks Erythromycin 500 mg orally 4 times daily for 2 weeks Ceftriaxone 1 g IM daily for 10 days
Late latent syphilis (>1 year duration and cardiovascular syphilis)	Benzathine penicillin G 2.4 million units IM weekly for 3 consecutive weeks *Alternative:* Tetracycline 500 mg orally 4 times daily for 4 weeks
Neurosyphilis	Aqueous crystalline penicillin G, 3–4 million units IV every 4 h for 10–14 days, followed by benzathine penicillin G 2.4 million units IM weekly for 3 consecutive weeks *Alternative:* Aqueous procaine penicillin G 2.4 million units IM daily and probenecid 500 mg orally 4 times daily, both for 10 to 14 days

Reproduced with permission from James D, Steer P, Weiner C, *et al.* (eds) *High Risk Pregnancy: Management Options*. Second Edition. Philadelphia, USA, W.B Saunders Copyright © 2003. Data from Workowski KA, Berman S. Sexually transmitted diseases treatment guidelines, 2010. *MMWR Recomm Rep* 2010;59: 1–110.

penicillin allergy do not in fact have a true immunoglobulin (Ig)-E-mediated anaphylactic reaction and can be treated with penicillin. Patients who do have an IgE-mediated allergic reaction should be offered penicillin desensitization, as proposed by Wendel et al.[28]

Occasionally, pregnant patients with early syphilis may experience a Jarisch–Herxheimer reaction after therapy. This reaction generally consists of fever 2–12 hours after initiation of therapy for active syphilis. However, cardiovascular collapse, seizures, and death also have been reported. The Jarisch–Herxheimer reaction is thought to be produced by the release of endotoxin-like compounds during penicillin-mediated lysis of *T. pallidum*. Since fever may initiate preterm labour, hospitalization should be considered for these patients.

Follow-up

After treatment, quantitative RPR or VDRL titres should be followed closely until negative (or stable at a low titre of generally less than 1:4 for late latent syphilis). In general, the quantitative titre should decline fourfold by the third or fourth month after therapy for primary and secondary syphilis. Patients should be evaluated for neurosyphilis and retreated for persistently high titres after 3 months, or for a fourfold increase in titre.[29]

Toxoplasmosis

General information

Toxoplasmosis is caused by the protozoan *Toxoplasma gondii*. It is an obligate intracellular parasite that exists in three forms: the oocyst, which is shed only in cat faeces; the tachyzoite, a rapidly dividing form observed in the acute phase of infection; and the bradyzoite, a slow-growing form observed within tissue cysts.

Cats play an important role in the spread of toxoplasmosis. Eating infected rodents, birds, or other small animals infects them. The parasite is then passed in the cat's faeces in oocyst form. During a primary infection, a cat can shed millions of oocysts daily for a period of 1–3 weeks. These oocysts become infective 1–5 days later and may remain infectious for over a year, especially in warm, humid environments. Cats typically develop immunity after a primary infection; therefore, recurrent infection with passage of oocysts is unlikely. Other animals (including pigs, chickens, lambs, and goats) and humans become infected by contact with contaminated soil or water or eating soil-contaminated fruit or vegetables, resulting in meat containing tissue cysts.

Once a person is infected, the parasite lies dormant in neural and muscle tissue and will never be eliminated.[30]

Transmission

There are three principal routes of transmission of *Toxoplasma*:

1. *Foodborne transmission*. This is the main source of human infection in developed, temperate climate countries. People become infected by ingestion of bradyzoites contained in undercooked meat, by eating undercooked contaminated meat or by handling it and not washing hands thoroughly, or by eating food that was contaminated by knives, cutting boards, or other foods that had contact with raw contaminated meat.
2. *Animal-to-human (zoonotic) transmission*. Hereby, people become infected by ingestion of oocysts from contact with contaminated soil or water or eating soil-contaminated fruit or vegetables.
3. *Mother-to-child (congenital) transmission*. A woman who is infected with *Toxoplasma* during pregnancy can pass the infection to her unborn child. Transmission to the fetus occurs predominantly in women who acquire their primary infection during gestation. In rare cases, congenital transmission has occurred in chronically infected women whose infection was reactivated because of their immunocompromised state (e.g. from AIDS or treatment with corticosteroids for their underlying disease). The incidence of maternal infection during pregnancy ranges from 1 to 8/1000 susceptible pregnancies, with the highest reported rates in France.[31]

   The risk of fetal infection increases with advancing gestational age at the time of maternal infection. Meta-analysis of all available cohorts estimated the risk of transmission to be 15% when the mother seroconverted at 13 weeks, 44% at 26 weeks, and 71% at 36 weeks.[32]
4. *Rare instances of transmission*. Rarely, people become infected by receiving infected blood via transfusion or by receiving an organ transplant from a *Toxoplasma*-positive donor. Laboratory workers who handle infected blood can also acquire infection through accidental inoculation.

Diagnosis

Diagnosis is usually achieved by serology. The presence of IgG antibodies shows that a person has been infected. To try to estimate the time of infection, IgM is measured and an avidity test is performed. An IgG avidity test measures how tightly the antibody binds to the antigen. Over time this value increases, so a low avidity means that the infection was recent, a high avidity suggests that the infection was more than 3–4 months ago.

Interpreting serology results of toxoplasmosis is often confusing. A positive IgM is not indicative for an acute infection since the IgM response lasts a median of 10–13 months. Depending on the type of test used, there is substantial variation in duration between individuals, and about one-quarter of infected women have a persistent IgM response lasting years. Although high IgG avidity is a hallmark of latent infection, low avidity is not diagnostic of acute infection; low IgG avidity can persist for years in some women.[33,34] For women whose first prenatal test at 13 weeks of gestation was IgM and IgG positive, the probability that their infection occurred after conception is 1–3%, depending on the test used.

The most accurate diagnosis of a maternal infection is based on seroconversion from negative to positive toxoplasma-specific IgM or IgG. Serial testing can be offered in susceptible asymptomatic pregnant women. Monthly or 3-monthly retesting schedules operate in parts of Europe, while in the United States and Canada, universal screening for toxoplasmosis in pregnancy is not performed.

Apart from serology, diagnosis can be made by direct observation of the parasite in stained tissue sections, CSF, or other biopsy material. These techniques are used less frequently because of the difficulty of obtaining these specimens. Parasites can also be isolated from blood or other body fluids (e.g. CSF) but this process can be difficult and requires considerable time.

Ocular disease is diagnosed based on the appearance of the lesions in the eye, symptoms, course of disease, and often serological testing.

Diagnosis of congenital infections can be achieved by detecting *T. gondii* DNA in amniotic fluid using molecular methods such as PCR; however, accuracy varies among laboratories and techniques and sensitivity is lower in early (<18 weeks of gestation) than in late pregnancy.

Clinical presentation

Most pregnant women with acute acquired infection do not experience obvious symptoms or signs. A minority may experience mild flu-like symptoms (e.g. malaise, low-grade fever, lymphadenopathy, and muscle aches) that last for several weeks. Up to 1% of infected individuals will present with visual changes due to toxoplasmic chorioretinitis as a result of recently acquired infection or reactivation of a chronic infection.[35]

In the fetus and neonate, toxoplasmosis infection presents with chorioretinitis, microcephaly or ventriculomegaly/hydrocephaly, intracerebral calcifications, and mental retardation or other evidence of parenchymal brain damage, hepatosplenomegaly, myocarditis, pericardial and pleural effusion (TORCH syndrome). The later in pregnancy, the less severe the fetal damage of a toxoplasmosis infection will be. The risk of developing clinical signs of infection in the offspring is 60%, 25%, and 10% in the first, second, and third trimesters, respectively.[36]

Of all infected fetuses, 70% are born without obvious lesions, 10% suffer only ocular manifestations, and the remaining 20% have the classic TORCH syndrome.[30]

Treatment

Most healthy persons recover from toxoplasmosis without treatment. In pregnancy, antibiotic treatment will be started to protect and treat the fetus.

In the case of a primary maternal infection before 18 weeks of gestation, spiramycin (3 g/day to the mother) should be started since it reduces the risk of transmission to the fetus by about 60%.[37] The longer the interval between maternal seroconversion and the start of spiramycin, the greater the likelihood of fetal damage. Spiramycin therapy, even over a long period, appears to have no significant maternal or fetal toxicity. Since spiramycin does not readily cross the placenta, it is not reliable for treatment of infection in the fetus.

Therefore, if fetal infection is confirmed by positive PCR of amniotic fluid (at/after 18 weeks) or structural anomalies on prenatal ultrasound, it is recommended to switch treatment to pyrimethamine, sulfadiazine, and folic acid. Because of the high transmission rates observed after 18 weeks of gestation, treatment with pyrimethamine, sulfadiazine, and folic acid is also used for patients who have acquired the infection after 18 weeks of gestation. Pyrimethamine is not used earlier because it is potentially teratogenic.

If ultrasound examination reveals congenital anomalies indicating congenital fetopathy, the option of termination of pregnancy should be discussed with the parents.

Cytomegalovirus

General information

Cytomegalovirus (CMV) is a DNA virus and member of the herpes family of viruses. The rate of seroconversion (primary infection) during pregnancy ranges from 1% to 7%.[38] Like other herpesviruses, CMV establishes latency after the host is initially infected. Non-primary infection, also sometimes called recurrent or secondary infection, may be due to reactivation of latent virus or reinfection with a new strain.

Transmission

Person-to-person transmission usually occurs by contact with infected nasopharyngeal secretions, urine, saliva, semen, cervical and vaginal secretions, breast milk, tissue, or blood, including transfusion of blood and bone marrow and transplacental transfer. The risk of seroconversion is highest in households with young children in daycare centres.[39]

Transmission of CMV from the mother to the fetus or newborn can occur in several ways. Most commonly, CMV infects the placenta (placental cytotrophoblasts are permissive to CMV replication) and is then transmitted to the embryo/fetus, where the virus is replicated in multiple tissues, including renal tubular epithelium.[40] Ascending infection from the maternal genital tract is thought to be rare antepartum, but possible.[41] Intrapartum and postnatal transmission can occur via ingestion/aspiration of cervicovaginal secretions during delivery or via breastfeeding. Rates of cervical CMV excretion vary depending upon various factors, including age, socioeconomic status, and geography of the populations studied.[42]

Perinatal transmission of CMV occurs in 5–8% when the infection occurred within 3 months before conception, in 10–20% when a periconceptional infection occurred, in 30% when the infection occurred in the first trimester, and 40–60% when infection occurred in the second to third trimester of pregnancy.[43] Although perinatal transmission may increase as gestation advances, sequelae in offspring appear to be less severe the later in gestation transmission occurs.

Diagnosis

Diagnosis is made by viral culture from urine, nasopharynx, or blood, or by serology.

Seroconversion of CMV-specific IgG is diagnostic for a new acute infection. The presence of CMV IgM is not helpful for timing the onset of the infection because it usually remains present until 4–8 months after the primary infection, but can persist at low titre for years or increase periodically in women with reactivation or reinfection with a different strain. Therefore determination of the avidity of IgG is used to determine the acuity of the infection, and thus the risk of *in utero* transmission. High avidity (>65%) suggests that the primary infection occurred more than 6 months in the past; low avidity (<30%) suggests a recent primary infection in the last 3 months.[44,45]

Reactivation or reinfection can be suspected when there is a fourfold rise in IgG and presence of IgM titres and patients with positive IgG on former blood analysis.

When CMV infection is diagnosed periconceptionally or in the first trimester of pregnancy, that is, patients at risk for serious abnormalities, an amniocentesis is offered to determine whether or not the fetus is infected based on a PCR analysis for CMV DNA of amniotic fluid. Critical to obtain an adequate sensitivity is to perform the amniocentesis after 21 weeks of gestation and with a time interval of at least 6 weeks between the maternal infection and the amniocentesis.[46,47]

For maternal infections late in gestation, PCR for CMV is performed on a urine sample of the newborn.

Clinical presentation

The most common manifestation of CMV infection is the lack of any demonstrable disease (90%).

Primo-infection in the *immunocompetent* (pregnant) adult may develop a mild febrile illness, atypical lymphocytosis, some malaise (rhinitis, pharyngitis, myalgia, arthralgia, headache, fatigue), mild lymphadenopathy, but generally has a benign course. Rarely, serious complications of the acute infection occur including interstitial pneumonitis, hepatitis, the Guillain–Barré syndrome, meningoencephalitis, myocarditis, thrombocytopenia, and haemolytic anaemia.

The virus may be excreted for weeks, months, or years after a primary infection and can be cultured from urine. A latency period eventually occurs, but reactivation and reinfection are common. Reinfection with a different strain of CMV or reactivation of virus in women with pre-existing antibody generally does not cause clinical illness.

CMV infection in the *immunosuppressed patient* (immunosuppressive drugs, organ transplant, AIDS patients) can be serious. Most commonly is a mononucleosis-like syndrome. The next most frequent manifestation is interstitial pneumonia, which may progress rapidly from asymptomatic to fatal, often in association with pneumocystis infection in AIDS patients. Also frequent are myocarditis, hepatitis, gastrointestinal disease with ulceration leading to haemorrhage and perforation, and meningoencephalitis.[30]

Congenital CMV infection occurs in 5–60% of the maternal primo-infections. The rate of maternofetal transmission increases linearly with the gestational age at infection, while the sequelae in the infected newborn decrease with the gestational age at infection. Twenty to 25% of infected fetuses develop sequelae and 10–15% will be symptomatic at birth or diagnosed prenatally on ultrasound (Table 50.3). These newborns have a mortality rate of about 5%, and 50–60% of survivors will develop severe long-term neurological morbidity (progressive hearing/visual loss and cognitive impairment). Although fetal infection can be detected, there is no way to accurately predict whether or not the fetus will develop significant sequelae. Serial ultrasound examinations every 2–4 weeks can be useful to detect development of sonographic abnormalities. Persistent changes, such as ventriculomegaly, periventricular calcifications, growth restriction, microcephaly, and hydrops, suggest the presence of severe disease and high risk of long-term neurodevelopment impairment. For these patients the option of termination of the pregnancy should be discussed. Magnetic resonance imaging (MRI) may provide additional information about anomalies, particularly neurological abnormalities.[48] However, normal ultrasound and MRI imaging does not exclude the possibility of hearing loss.[49]

Five to 15% of infected fetuses are asymptomatic at birth, but will develop neurodevelopmental damage (learning disabilities, hearing loss) within the first 3 years of life.[50] Non-primary infection results in symptomatic disease at birth in 0.2–2% of cases; perinatal death is rare.[51]

Treatment

Treatment of the acute symptomatic CMV infection in immunocompetent patients consists of supportive care for symptomatic relief.

In immunocompromised patients and neonates, antiretroviral drugs such as ganciclovir, foscarnet, and cidofovir reduce

Table 50.3 Ultrasonographic and clinical signs of congenital CMV infection

Ultrasonographic markers	Clinical symptoms
Periventricular echogenicity	Small for gestational age
Periventricular (pseudo)cysts	Microcephaly
Periventricular calcifications	Chorioretinitis
Cerebral ventriculomegaly	Hepatosplenomegaly
Microcephaly	Thrombocytopenia
Polymicrogyria	Petechiae
Large cisterna magna	Sensorineural hearing loss
Cerebellar hypoplasia	Pneumonitis
Branching linear echogenic areas in the thalami corresponding to arteries in the basal ganglia and thalamus	Visual impairment
Intraventricular adhesions	
Hyperechogenic fetal bowel	
Hepatosplenomegaly	
Fetal growth restriction	
Ascites and/or pleural effusion	
Hydrops	
Placental enlargement	

Data from various sources (see references).

mortality and morbidity. However, antiretroviral drugs have not been shown to decrease perinatal transmission.

Pre-existing maternal antibodies to CMV is the most important protective factor against congenital CMV infection.[53] Studies using passive immunization with specific anti-CMV immunoglobulin reveal promising results, but are still investigational.[54]

Better than the available treatment is prevention by practising good personal hygiene thorough pregnancy and use of CMV-negative blood products when transfusing seronegative pregnant women and newborns. The demonstrated benefits of breastfeeding outweigh the minimal risk of acquiring CMV from an infected breastfeeding mother. There is progress in the development of a specific CMV vaccine; however, it will take several more years until it will be available for use in humans.

Herpes simples virus

General information

The herpes simplex viruses (HSV) are DNA viruses of the herpes family. HSV-1 has been considered to cause orolabial herpes and HSV-2 genital herpes infection; however, there is an important overlap. Up to one-third of the genital herpes infections are caused by HSV-1.

Transmission

Primary orolabial herpes is mainly a disease of childhood, children acquiring the infection from family members through close contact. Genital herpes may occur after sexual contact either genital–genital or orogenital, with an infectious person. The incubation period is less than a week and persons transmitting the virus may be asymptomatic themselves.[55]

Transmission of HSV to the fetus or neonate occurs mostly during labour and delivery as a result of direct contact with virus shed from infected sites (vulva, vagina, cervix, perineal area). The concentration and duration of viral shedding are higher with primary versus non-primary disease and in HSV-2 versus HSV-1 infection. On the other hand, viral shedding can also occur when maternal symptoms and lesions are absent. Rarely *in utero* infection occurs as a result of transplacental or ascending transmembranous infection.[56,57]

Diagnosis

HSV infection can be diagnosed by viral culture, PCR, direct fluorescent antibody testing, and type-specific serological tests. PCR is more sensitive than culture and is becoming the preferred test for diagnostic testing in symptomatic patients and for detecting viral shedding. Serological testing for HSV is of little clinical use since a large proportion of pregnant women are positive. Only a seroconversion and the presence of HSV-specific IgM confirm the diagnosis.[58]

Clinical presentation

Although 90–95% of *primary oral infections* are asymptomatic, a few may consist of a rather florid vesiculoulcerative outbreak in the oropharynx and lips about a week after exposure. Adenopathy and viraemia, along with fever and malaise, may persist for a week or two, with viral shedding for up to 6 weeks. Thereafter, antibody production limits the virus such that it remains dormant, occasionally flaring up as localized blisters on the lips in times of stress, sunburn, or febrile systemic illness. During recurrent disease, viral shedding lasts up to a week.[59]

Primary genital HSV infection can be severe with painful genital ulcers, pruritus, dysuria, tender inguinal lymphadenopathy, and systemic symptoms of fever, malaise, myalgia, and headache. Disseminated infection, mostly in immunosuppressed patients, can lead to death from HSV encephalitis and hepatitis.[60] Lower motor neuron and autonomic dysfunction may lead to bladder atony and urinary retention. Viral shedding occurs for nearly 3 weeks in severe cases. Local disease may reoccur weeks or months later, especially if the offending virus is HSV-2, which recurs more often than HSV-1 does, especially in the genital area.[61] In patients who develop lesions, prodromal symptoms, such as pruritus, burning, or pain, may occur before the lesions are visible. The genital lesions may be non-tender or atypical in appearance (e.g. fissure, vulvar irritation). The duration of lesions and viral shedding during recurrent infection are shorter than that seen during the primary episode.

Disseminated HSV infection to the fetus can lead to abortion, prematurity, and fetal/neonatal infection.

Systemic illness and fever may stimulate preterm contractions. The fetus acquiring HSV, especially if the mother suffers an acute, primary infection,[62] may sustain severe neonatal morbidity including chorioretinitis, meningitis, encephalitis, mental retardation, seizures, and death. Primary infection early in pregnancy, perhaps due to a viral endometritis ascending from cervical infection, may end in spontaneous abortion.

Treatment

Recurrent infections are mild and little symptomatic intervention is necessary. Many practitioners recommend topical aciclovir for pregnant patients on the grounds that it is not significantly absorbed. It is unclear whether it is helpful.

Pregnant women with a significant primary HSV infection or a genital non-primary infection should be treated, regardless of the timing in pregnancy. Aciclovir is administered orally (200 mg five times a day for 7–10 days) or IV (5 mg/kg every 8 hours for the same period).

Active lesions at the time of labour is considered to be an indication for caesarean delivery, although the risk is less with recurrent disease. If there are no active lesions and no prodromal symptoms at the time of labour, vaginal delivery is allowed. Women with preterm premature rupture of the membranes and active lesions are considered individually taking into account gestational age and other relevant factors. It should not, however, be assumed the fetus is infected just because of prolonged rupture of membranes.

In women with symptomatic infection during pregnancy, the American College of Obstetricians and Gynecologists recommends suppressive therapy with aciclovir (400 mg orally three times daily) at 36 weeks of gestation through delivery rather than no therapy. Suppressive therapy reduces the risk of clinical recurrence of HSV and asymptomatic viral shedding at delivery, and thus the need for caesarean delivery. However, the clinical impact on neonatal HSV is unknown.[63]

Conclusion

The impact of the maternal infections discussed in this chapter are both for the mother and the fetus potential life-threatening events which may lead to chronic complications, sometimes lasting throughout life.

This stresses the importance of adequate patient information. The way of transmission of the most common infections—and so the way of prevention—should be discussed preconceptionally. Furthermore, systematic screening for the most important infections should be offered at the first pregnancy consultation. In case an infection is diagnosed, the appropriate treatment and a multidisciplinary follow-up are required to reduce the risk of congenital infections and long-term sequelae.

References

1. Dauby N, Goetghebuer T, Kollmann TR, *et al.* Uninfected but not unaffected: chronic maternal infections during pregnancy, fetal immunity, and susceptibility to postnatal infections. *Lancet Infect Dis* 2012; 12:330–40.
2. Centers for Disease Control (CDC). Pneumocystis pneumonia—Los Angeles. *MMWR Morb Mortal Wkly Rep* 1981; 30:250–2.
3. Friedman-Kien AE. Disseminated Kaposi's sarcoma syndrome in young homosexual men. *J Am Acad Dermatol* 1981; 5:468–71.
4. Hymes KB, Cheung T, Greene JB, *et al.* Kaposi's sarcoma in homosexual men - a report of eight cases. *Lancet* 1981; 2:598–600.
5. Cunningham AL, Donaghy H, Harman AN, *et al.* Manipulation of dendritic cell function by viruses. *Curr Opin Microbiol* 2010; 13:524–9.
6. Gilbert PB, McKeague IW, Eisen G, *et al.* Comparison of HIV-1 and HIV-2 infectivity from a prospective cohort study in Senegal. *Stat Med* 2003; 22:573–93.
7. Tolle MA, Schwarzwald HL. Postexposure prophylaxis against human immunodeficiency virus. *Am Fam Physician* 2010; 82:161–6.
8. AIDS*info*. *Clinical Guidelines Portal.* [Online] http://www.aidsinfo.nih.gov/Guidelines
9. World Health Organization. *Consolidated Guidelines on the Use of Antiretroviral Drugs for Treating and Preventing HIV Infection.* 2013. [Online] http://apps.who.int/iris/bitstream/10665/85321/1/9789241505727_eng.pdf?ua=1
10. Haeri S, Shauer M, Dale M, *et al.* Obstetric and newborn infant outcomes in human immunodeficiency virus-infected women who receive highly active antiretroviral therapy. *Am J Obstet Gynecol* 2009; 201:315.
11. Brocklehurst P, French R. The association between maternal HIV infection and perinatal outcome: a systematic review of the literature and meta-analysis. *Br J Obstet Gynaecol* 1998; 105:836–48.
12. Wimalasundera RC, Larbalestier N, Smith JH, *et al.* Pre-eclampsia, antiretroviral therapy, and immune reconstitution. *Lancet* 2002; 360:1152–4.
13. Culnane M, Fowler M, Lee SS, *et al.* Lack of long-term effects of in utero exposure to zidovudine among uninfected children born to HIV-infected women. Pediatric AIDS Clinical Trials Group Protocol 219/076 Teams. *JAMA* 1999; 281:151–7.
14. Gershon RY, Manning-Williams D. Anesthesia and the HIV infected parturient: a retrospective study. *Int J Obstet Anesth* 1997; 6:76–81.
15. Sampson J, Gravett M. Other infectious conditions in pregnancy. In James D, Steer P, Weiner C, *et al.* (eds) *High Risk Pregnancy: Management Options* (2nd ed). Philadelphia, PA: WB Saunders; 2003:568–9.
16. Playfair JH. Immunity to malaria. *Br Med Bull* 1982; 38:153–9.
17. Bergstrom S, Fernandes A, Schwalbach J, *et al.* Materno-fetal transmission of pregnancy malaria: an immunoparasitological study on 202 parturients in Maputo. *Gynecol Obstet Invest* 1993; 35:103–7.
18. Hulbert TV. Congenital malaria in the United States: report of a case and review. *Clin Infect Dis* 1992; 14:922–6.
19. Whitty CJ, Edmonds S, Mutabingwa TK. Malaria in pregnancy. *BJOG* 2005; 112:1189–95.
20. Royal College of Obstetricians and Gynaecologists. *Malaria in Pregnancy, Diagnosis and Treatment.* Green-top Guideline No. 54B. London: RCOG; 2010. https://www.rcog.org.uk/en/guidelines-research-services/guidelines/gtg54b/
21. Irvine MH, Einarson A, Bozzo P. Prophylactic use of antimalarials during pregnancy. *Can Fam Physician* 2011; 57:1279–81.
22. Michelow IC, Wendel GD, Jr., Norgard MV, *et al.* Central nervous system infection in congenital syphilis. *N Engl J Med* 2002; 346:1792–8.
23. Norwitz E. Syphilis in pregnancy. In *UpToDate*, 2014. [Online] http://www.uptodate.com/contents/syphilis-in-pregnancy
24. Woods CR. Syphilis in children: congenital and acquired. *Semin Pediatr Infect Dis* 2005; 16:245–57.
25. Dobson S. Congenital syphilis: clinical features and diagnosis. In *UpToDate*, 2014. [Online] http://www.uptodate.com/contents/congenital-syphilis-clinical-features-and-diagnosis
26. Thompson SE, III. Treatment of syphilis in pregnancy. *J Am Vener Dis Assoc* 1976; 3:158–67.
27. Workowski KA, Berman S. Sexually transmitted diseases treatment guidelines, 2010. *MMWR Recomm Rep* 2010; 59:1–110.
28. Wendel GD Jr, Stark BJ, Jamison RB, *et al.* Penicillin allergy and desensitization in serious infections during pregnancy. *N Engl J Med* 1985; 312:1229–32.
29. James D, Steer P, Weiner C, *et al.* (eds). *High Risk Pregnancy: Management Options* (2nd ed). Philadelphia, PA: WB Saunders; 2003.
30. Yankowitz J, Pastorek G. Maternal and fetal viral infections. In James D, Steer P, Weiner C, *et al.* (eds) *High Risk Pregnancy: Management Options* (2nd ed). Philadelphia, PA: WB Saunders; 2003:525–58.
31. Gilbert RE, Peckham CS. Congenital toxoplasmosis in the United Kingdom: to screen or not to screen? *J Med Screen* 2002; 9:135–41.
32. Thiebaut R, Leproust S, Chene G, *et al.* Effectiveness of prenatal treatment for congenital toxoplasmosis: a meta-analysis of individual patients' data. *Lancet* 2007; 369:115–22.
33. Gras L, Gilbert RE, Wallon M, *et al.* Duration of the IgM response in women acquiring Toxoplasma gondii during pregnancy: implications for clinical practice and cross-sectional incidence studies. *Epidemiol Infect* 2004; 132:541–8.
34. Lefevre-Pettazzoni M, Le CS, Wallon M, *et al.* Delayed maturation of immunoglobulin G avidity: implication for the diagnosis of toxoplasmosis in pregnant women. *Eur J Clin Microbiol Infect Dis* 2006; 25:687–93.
35. Burnett AJ, Shortt SG, Isaac-Renton J, *et al.* Multiple cases of acquired toxoplasmosis retinitis presenting in an outbreak. *Ophthalmology* 1998; 105:1032–7.
36. Montoya JG, Remington JS. Management of Toxoplasma gondii infection during pregnancy. *Clin Infect Dis* 2008; 47:554–66.
37. Hohlfeld P, Daffos F, Thulliez P, *et al.* Fetal toxoplasmosis: outcome of pregnancy and infant follow-up after in utero treatment. *J Pediatr* 1989; 115:765–9.
38. Lamy ME, Mulongo KN, Gadisseux JF, *et al.* Prenatal diagnosis of fetal cytomegalovirus infection. *Am J Obstet Gynecol* 1992; 166:91–4.
39. Hyde TB, Schmid DS, Cannon MJ. Cytomegalovirus seroconversion rates and risk factors: implications for congenital CMV. *Rev Med Virol* 2010; 20:311–26.
40. Fisher S, Genbacev O, Maidji E, *et al.* Human cytomegalovirus infection of placental cytotrophoblasts in vitro and in utero: implications for transmission and pathogenesis. *J Virol* 2000; 74:6808–20.
41. Raynor BD. Cytomegalovirus infection in pregnancy. *Semin Perinatol* 1993; 17:394–402.
42. Reynolds DW, Stagno S, Hosty TS, *et al.* Maternal cytomegalovirus excretion and perinatal infection. *N Engl J Med* 1973; 289:1–5.
43. Picone O, Vauloup-Fellous C, Cordier AG, *et al.* A series of 238 cytomegalovirus primary infections during pregnancy: description and outcome. *Prenat Diagn* 2013; 33:751–8.
44. Ghaemmaghami F, Hasanzadeh M. Good fetal outcome of pregnancies with gynecologic cancer conditions: cases and literature review. *Int J Gynecol Cancer* 2006; 16 Suppl 1:225–30.

45. Bodeus M, Van Ranst M, Bernard P, *et al.* Anticytomegalovirus IgG avidity in pregnancy: a 2-year prospective study. *Fetal Diagn Ther* 2002; 17:362–6.
46. Azam AZ, Vial Y, Fawer CL, *et al.* Prenatal diagnosis of congenital cytomegalovirus infection. *Obstet Gynecol* 2001; 97:443–8.
47. Liesnard C, Donner C, Brancart F, *et al.* Prenatal diagnosis of congenital cytomegalovirus infection: prospective study of 237 pregnancies at risk. *Obstet Gynecol* 2000; 95:881–8.
48. Lipitz S, Hoffmann C, Feldman B, *et al.* Value of prenatal ultrasound and magnetic resonance imaging in assessment of congenital primary cytomegalovirus infection. *Ultrasound Obstet Gynecol* 2010; 36:709–17.
49. Farkas N, Hoffmann C, Ben-Sira L, *et al.* Does normal fetal brain ultrasound predict normal neurodevelopmental outcome in congenital cytomegalovirus infection? *Prenat Diagn* 2011; 31:360–6.
50. Fowler KB, McCollister FP, Dahle AJ, *et al.* Progressive and fluctuating sensorineural hearing loss in children with asymptomatic congenital cytomegalovirus infection. *J Pediatr* 1997; 130:624–30.
51. Ornoy A, Diav-Citrin O. Fetal effects of primary and secondary cytomegalovirus infection in pregnancy. *Reprod Toxicol* 2006; 21:399–409.
52. Malinger G, Lev D, Zahalka N, *et al.* Fetal cytomegalovirus infection of the brain: the spectrum of sonographic findings. *AJNR Am J Neuroradiol* 2003; 24:28–32.
53. Fowler KB, Stagno S, Pass RF. Maternal immunity and prevention of congenital cytomegalovirus infection. *JAMA* 2003; 289:1008–11.
54. Visentin S, Manara R, Milanese L, *et al.* Early primary cytomegalovirus infection in pregnancy: maternal hyperimmunoglobulin therapy improves outcomes among infants at 1 year of age. *Clin Infect Dis* 2012; 55:497–503.
55. Rooney JF, Felser JM, Ostrove JM, *et al.* Acquisition of genital herpes from an asymptomatic sexual partner. *N Engl J Med* 1986; 314:1561–4.
56. Wald A, Zeh J, Selke S, *et al.* Reactivation of genital herpes simplex virus type 2 infection in asymptomatic seropositive persons. *N Engl J Med* 2000; 342:844–50.
57. Brown ZA, Wald A, Morrow RA, *et al.* Effect of serologic status and cesarean delivery on transmission rates of herpes simplex virus from mother to infant. *JAMA* 2003; 289:203–9.
58. Boggess KA, Watts DH, Hobson AC, *et al.* Herpes simplex virus type 2 detection by culture and polymerase chain reaction and relationship to genital symptoms and cervical antibody status during the third trimester of pregnancy. *Am J Obstet Gynecol* 1997; 176:443–51.
59. Baker DA, Amstey MS. Herpes simplex virus: biology, epidemiology, and clinical infection. *Semin Perinatol* 1983; 7:1–8.
60. Whitley RJ, Soong SJ, Linneman C Jr, *et al.* Herpes simplex encephalitis. Clinical assessment. *JAMA* 1982; 247:317–20.
61. Lafferty WE, Coombs RW, Benedetti J, *et al.* Recurrences after oral and genital herpes simplex virus infection. Influence of site of infection and viral type. *N Engl J Med* 1987; 316:1444–9.
62. Brown ZA, Vontver LA, Benedetti J, *et al.* Effects on infants of a first episode of genital herpes during pregnancy. *N Engl J Med* 1987; 317:1246–51.
63. Hollier LM, Wendel GD. Third trimester antiviral prophylaxis for preventing maternal genital herpes simplex virus (HSV) recurrences and neonatal infection. *Cochrane Database Syst Rev* 2008; 1:CD004946.

CHAPTER 51

Substance abuse

Ross Junkin and Elizabeth M. McGrady

Introduction

Substance abuse can be simply defined as a pattern of harmful use of any substance for mood-altering purposes that deviates from medically or socially accepted use. If prolonged, it can lead to physical or psychological dependence. This dependency is characterized by:

- intermittent or continuous impaired control over substance self-administration (despite awareness of adverse effects)
- preoccupation with substance acquisition
- distortions of mental capacity, most notably denial.

Various attendant terms have also been defined in the *Diagnostic and Statistical Manual of Mental Disorders*, fourth edition (DSM-IV)[1], see Table 51.1. Illegal drugs are not the only substances that can be abused. Alcohol, prescription medication, solvents, caffeine, and tobacco can all be implicated. The line between use and abuse can sometimes be difficult to determine especially when the patient may not even recognize a problem or indeed admit to it.

Social implications of substance abuse in pregnancy

Substance abuse in pregnancy is a cause of morbidity and mortality with 13 deaths directly related to substance abuse highlighted in the 2006–2008 Confidential Enquiry into Maternal Deaths in the United Kingdom.[2] It is easy to focus on the medical complications of substance abuse in pregnancy but there are also wide-ranging general health, social, and psychological problems which are as important, if not more so. The main characteristics of substance-abusing women who died either from medical or psychiatric complications of their abuse were that they were most often young, single, unemployed, and socially deprived. It is difficult to regard substance abuse in isolation without some consideration of the socioeconomic environment and social background with which substance abuse is associated.

Antenatal care is often inadequate in women who misuse drugs because of late presentation. Reasons for this include a chaotic lifestyle and a reluctance to have involvement with social services. Women who misuse substances are often excluded from mainstream society and, on becoming pregnant, feel guilty about their drug misuse and the potential effects this could have on their unborn baby. These women are vulnerable in many ways and agencies must ensure that they are not excluded from antenatal care.[3] The prevalence of antepartum drug abuse is higher in unbooked parturients and has been reported in up to 70% in some centres in the United States.[4,5] One UK study demonstrated increased rates of emergency caesarean deliveries and reduced rates of elective caesarean deliveries in drug-abusing parturients.[6] This may reflect lack of antenatal preparation among the other increased risks in pregnant women who misuse substances.

Extent of the problem

Accurate prevalence statistics regarding drug abuse rates of illicit substances are difficult to ascertain when measuring those engaged in a largely covert or socially unacceptable activity, which may be further heightened by the pregnant state. Health professionals do not always ask specifically about drug abuse and when they do, pregnant women often fail to disclose it. Epidemiological data from the general non-obstetric population are available. Data collected by the Centers for Disease Control and Prevention (CDC) in the United States are displayed in Table 51.2.[7]

The trends suggest that substance abuse is most prevalent among young adults with variation between ethnic groups. Although there is often a male sex preponderance, the problem will also transfer into the obstetric population of young women of child-bearing age. Table 51.3 collates data reported by the European Monitoring Center for Drugs and Drug Addiction (EMCDDA) from population surveys specific to young women who report recent drug use (within the 30 days prior to survey completion).[8]

Direct techniques tend to underestimate the extent of drug use and the incidence of substance misuse in the United Kingdom varies widely by geographical location. Three per cent of under-35s are said to have a drug problem in the United Kingdom, with Data from the UK National Treatment Agency for Substance Misuse (NTASM) estimating overall rates of 8.93/1000 in the general population using heroin and/or crack cocaine with the highest rates in people aged 25–34.[9] Twenty-five years ago, there were relatively few problem drug users in the United Kingdom. Since then, the numbers have increased dramatically. No part of the country has been spared, although inner city areas and especially London, Glasgow, Liverpool, and Manchester have traditionally been considered hotspots. For example, the number of known heroin addicts and the number of heroin confiscations by police increased 10-fold and 15-fold respectively between 1980 and the late 1990s.

In England and Wales, estimates from the 2010/2011 British Crime Survey, which relies upon anonymous questionnaire self-reporting, show that around one in three adults aged 16–59 (36.3%) had used illicit drugs in their lifetime (almost 12 million people) and 8.8% (2.9 million) had used illicit drugs in the last year.[10] The national surveys have consistently shown the highest drug prevalence among young adults (20.4% of 16–24-year-olds in 2010/11) and especially in males (Figure 51.1).

Table 51.1 Definitions of substance-related disorders

Substance use disorder	Definition
Tolerance	Increasing doses of the substance used over time is required to achieve a consistent or desired effect. Equally, persisting with the same dose will result in a lessening effect
Substance abuse	A pattern of substance use which leads to harm, as manifested by ≥1 of the following, occurring within 1 year: ◆ Repeated substance use impacting on ability to fulfil work, school, or home/family commitments ◆ Repeated substance use in situations in which it is dangerous, e.g. driving, work environments ◆ Repeated substance-related legal problems ◆ Repeated social or interpersonal problems caused or exacerbated by the effects of the substance
Substance dependence	A pattern of substance use which leads to harm. Evidence of physiological dependence and the substance use taking a prominent position in the user's life. Manifested by ≥ 3 of the following, occurring within 1 year: ◆ Tolerance ◆ Withdrawal ◆ Increasing dose and duration ◆ Persistent desire or unsuccessful efforts to cut down or control substance use ◆ Prominent substance seeking and associated behaviours requiring significant time and effort acquiring the substance or recovering from it ◆ Social harm—impact on work and career or recreational pastimes reduced because of substance use ◆ Knowing the harmful effects but continuing to use the substance

Data from the *Diagnostic and Statistical Manual of Mental Disorders*, Fourth Edition, 2000, American Psychiatric Association.

Class A drugs represent those deemed most dangerous and carry the harshest criminal punishment as outlined in the United Kingdom Misuse of Drugs Act 1971.[11] The long-term trends in the use of different drugs in England and Wales show variation in the levels of Class A drug use since 1996 (Figure 51.2). Of note, cocaine use appears to have been increasing recently to a peak in 2008/2009.

In Scotland, the most recently available official statistics from the information services division (ISD)[12] uses the 2013 European Standard Population (ESP2013) to calculate the European Age-Sex Standardised Rates (EASRs) regarding hospital admissions directly related to drug misuse. It is based on nationally available information routinely drawn from hospital administrative systems across the country and relate to all patients, both obstetric and non-obstetric. The publication reveals an overall general substance-misuse-related hospital admission rate of 107/100,000 population in Scotland in 2012/2013. In the period 2008/2009 to 2012/2013, the general hospital discharges with a diagnosis of drug misuse increased among older age groups (35 years and over) and decreased among younger age groups. Despite these reductions, the highest rates of drug misuse persisted in the young adults of potentially child-bearing age (Figure 51.3).

The relative proportions of male (around two-thirds) to female (around one-third) have remained roughly the same for 5 years and are consistent with findings from the rest of the United Kingdom.

In 2012/2013, the majority of drug-related general hospital discharges were associated with opioids (67%), followed by multiple/other drugs (14%; includes hallucinogens, volatile solvents, multiple drug use, and use of other psychoactive substances), cannabinoids (11%), and cocaine (6%).

Data subsets specifically concerning pregnancy show that the rate of drug misuse reported per 1000 maternities in Scotland has increased recently to a peak of 19.7/1000 (see Table 51.4[13]). Opiates were the most frequently recorded substance of abuse with 8–9/1000 maternities consistently across the records. The drug using parturients were more likely to come from more deprived areas with 42% residing in the most deprived areas. The rates of preterm and lower birth weight babies were also increased compared with non-drug using parturients.

Maternal use of illicit and prescription drugs is additionally associated with considerable neonatal morbidity. Lifestyle factors, such as illicit substance exposure, have been implicated in restricting fetal growth and causing the onset of preterm birth.[14] Low birth weight and preterm birth are associated with short- and long-term morbidities. One North American study retrospectively examined 669,451 births over an 8-year period (2000–2008) identifying 9024 neonates with prenatal drug exposure. In this cohort, both illicit and prescription maternal drug use was associated with increased risk of prematurity, lower mean birth weight, longer birth hospitalization, feeding problems, and respiratory conditions.[15]

The UK Home Office report entitled 'Hidden Harm' estimates that there are between 200,000 and 300,000 children living in England and Wales where one or both parents have serious drug problems.[16] This represents about 2–3% of children under 16. Only 37% of fathers and 64% of mothers were still living with their children. The more serious the drug problem, the less likely it was for the parent still to be living with the child. Most children not living with their natural parents were living with other relatives and about 5% of all children were in care. In Scotland, the estimated situation is worse still, with between 41,000 and 59,000 children with a problem drug-using parent. This represents about 4–6% of all children under 16 years.

Obstetric anaesthetists may become involved in the care of substance-abusing parturients in controlled settings antenatally when planning labour and delivery or in the emergency setting

Table 51.2 Use of illicit drugs in the past month among persons aged 12 and over by age, sex, race, and ethnic origin in the United States

Age, sex, race, and Hispanic origin	Any illicit drug[1]			Marijuana			Non-medical use of any psychotherapeutic drug[2]		
	2002	2009	2010	2002	2009	2010	2002	2009	2010
	Percent of population								
12 years and over	8.3	8.7	8.9	6.2	6.6	6.9	2.7	2.8	2.7
Age									
12–13 years	4.2	3.6	4.0	1.4	0.8	0.9	1.7	1.6	2.0
14–16 years	11.2	9.0	9.3	7.6	6.3	6.5	4.0	3,3	3,0
16–17 years	19.8	16.7	16.6	15.7	14.0	14.3	6.3	4.3	3.9
18–25 years	20.2	21.2	21.5	17.3	18.1	18.5	5.5	6.3	5.9
26–34 years	10.5	12.3	13.8	7.7	9.6	10.5	3.7	3.8	4.4
35 years and over	4.6	4.9	4.9	3.1	3.4	3.4	1.6	1.7	1.7
Sex									
Male	10.3	10.8	11.2	8.1	8.6	9.1	2.8	3.1	3.0
Female	6.4	6.6	6.8	4.4	4.8	4.7	2.6	2.4	2.5
Age and sex									
12–17 years	11.6	10.0	10.1	8.2	7.3	7.4	4.0	3.1	3.0
Male	12,3	10.6	10.4	9.1	8.3	8.3	3.6	2.8	2.3
Female	10.9	9.4	9.8	7.2	6.3	6.4	4.4	3.5	3.7
Hispanic origin and race[3]									
Not Hispanic or Latino:									
White only	8.5	8.8	9.1	6.5	6.8	7.0	2.8	3.0	3.0
Black or African American only	9.7	9.6	10.7	7.4	7.8	8.6	2.0	2.0	2.0
American Indian or Alaska Native only	10.1	18.3	12.1	6.7	10.6	10.0	3.2	6.2	4.6
Native Hawaiian or Other Pacific Islander only	7.9	*	5.4	4.4	4.3	2.9	3.8	*	2.4
Asian only	3.5	3.7	3.5	1.8	2.4	2.6	0.7	1.4	1.0
2 or more races	11.4	14.3	12.5	9.0	12.2	10.2	3.5	3.4	3.1
Hispanic or Latino	7.2	7.9	8.1	4.3	6.6	5.8	2.9	2.4	2.5

*Estimates are considered unreliable. Data not shown if the relative standard error is greater than 17.5% of the log transformation of the proportion, the minimum effective sample size is less than 68, the minimum nominal sample size is less than 100, or the prevalence is close to 0% or 100%.

[1]Any illicit drug includes marijuana/hashish, cocaine (including crack), heroin, hallucinogens, inhalants, or any prescription-type psychotherapeutic drug used non-medically.

[2]Non-medical use of prescription-type psychotherapeutic drugs includes the nonmedical use of pain relievers, tranquilizers, stimulants, or sedatives and does not include over-the-counter drugs.

[3]Persons of Hispanic origin may be of any race. Data on race and Hispanic origin were collected using the 1997 Revisions to the Standards for the Classification of Federal Data on Race and Ethnicity. Single-race categories shown include persons who reported only one racial group. The category 2 or more races includes persons who reported more than one racial group.

Reproduced from National Center for Health Statistics. *Health, United States, 2012: With Special Feature on Emergency Care.* Hyattsville, MD. 2013.

where substance abuse may be known or indeed covert. Drug abuse is often associated with poor nutrition, poor hygiene, generalized immunosuppression, difficult intravenous access, and altered drug metabolism. Substance abuse therefore poses specific challenges for the obstetric anaesthetist with regard to the delivery of anaesthesia and the management of pain around the peripartum period. Identification of the substance-abusing parturient is difficult when the denial of such abuse is common[17] and clinical signs of illicit drug use can lead to serious obstetric complications and even mimic other diseases such as pre-eclampsia.[18] Local knowledge of obstetric services' catchment areas, specific regional illicit drug prevalence, and popular modes of drug administration will be helpful in recognition of the drug-abusing parturient and the associated co-morbidities.

Substance abuse is thus a major problem facing our society and in particular the young adult population. About half of substance-using women may continue substance use during pregnancy[19] and so form an important subgroup that warrants specific care and attention.

Table 51.3 Population survey data displaying recent (within 30 days) drug use in young women in countries across Europe

Country	Year	Age range of women	Cannabis (%)	Cocaine (%)	Amphetamines (%)	Ecstasy (%)	LSD (%)
Belgium	2008	15–34	3.6	:	:	:	:
Bulgaria	2008	15–34	2.4	0.9	0.9	0.5	0.0
Czech Republic	2011	15–34	4.5	0.0	0.0	0.0	0.0
Denmark	2010	16–34	3.1	0.1	0.2	0.1	0.0
Germany	2009	18–34	3.5	0.2	0.6	0.1	0.0
Estonia	2008	15–34	2.7	0.3	0.0	0.3	0.0
Ireland	2010–11	15–34	1.6	0.4	0.1	0.1	0.0
Greece	2004	15–34	0.9	0.1	0.0	0.0	0.0
Spain	2011	15–34	7.0	0.7	0.3	0.4	:
France	2010	15–34	5.5	:	:	:	:
Italy	2012	18–34	2.4	0.2	0.0	0.0	0.0
Cyprus	2009	15–34	1.5	0.4	0.1	0.1	0.1
Latvia	2011	15–34	1.7	0.1	0.1	0.0	0.0
Lithuania	2008	15–34	1.6	0.0	:	0.4	0.2
Luxembourg	:	:	:	:	:	:	:
Hungary	2007	18-34	1.4	0.0	0.0	0.2	0.0
Malta	2001	18–34	:	:	:	:	:
Netherlands	2009	15–34	:	:	:	:	:
Austria	2008	15–34	2.2	0.5	0.2	0.5	0.0
Poland	2010	15–34	5.1	0.8	0.9	0.3	0.0
Portugal	2007	15–34	1.0	0.2	0.1	0.2	0.0
Romania	2010	15–34	0.2	0.0	0.0	0.0	0.0
Slovenia	2007	15–34	:	:	:	:	:
Slovakia	2010	15–34	0.9	0.0	0.0	0.1	0.0
Finland	2010	15–34	1.2	0.0	0.2	0.2	0.0
Sweden	2008	15–34	0.4	0.3	0.2	0.0	:
Sweden	2011	16-34	1.5	:	:	:	:
United Kingdom	2006	16–34	5.6	1.7	0.6	1.1	0.0
Croatia	2012	15-34	3.7	0.3	0.2	0.1	0.1
Turkey	2011	15-34	:	:	:	0.1	:
Norway	2009	15–34	1.5	0.3	0.6	0.0	0.0

Data from European Monitoring Centre for Drugs and Drug Addiction (EMCDDA). *Problem amphetamine and metamphetamine use in Europe. Selected Issue 2010.* http://www.emcdda.europa.eu. Unavailability of data is indicated explicitly with a colon in the corresponding cell ":"

Tolerance and addiction to drugs in pregnancy creates potential problems for the parturient, her fetus, and the wide range of healthcare professionals involved in her care. Extra vigilance is required in the care of these patients as they are a high risk both to themselves, the fetus, and to healthcare workers.

Screening, assessment, and treatment

Motivation to change unhealthy or harmful behaviours is increased during pregnancy and it is an ideal time to intervene with women who have substance abuse problems.[20] The cessation of substance abuse in pregnancy is a potentially reversible cause of adverse birth outcomes. All pregnant women regardless of socioeconomic status should be screened for past/current alcohol, smoking, and illicit drug use. This should be in a private setting with a non-judgemental tone.

Previous healthcare professionals' attitudes towards pregnant patients who use substances, particularly alcohol and/or illicit drugs, were largely negative and few routinely screened their patients for substance abuse.[21–23] More recently, increased awareness of the importance of this issue among healthcare

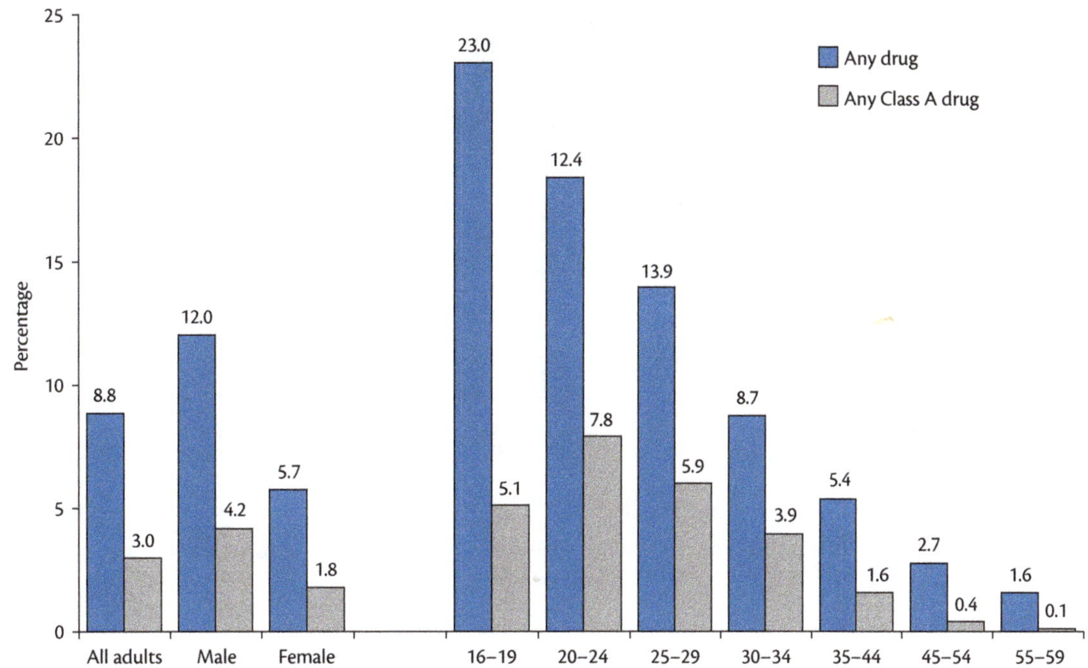

Figure 51.1 Proportions of 16–59-year-olds in England and Wales self-reporting use of any drug by age group and sex in the 2010/2011 British Crime Survey.
Smith K and Flatley J. *Drug Misuse Declared: Findings from the 2010/11 British Crime Survey*, England and Wales. http://www.statistics.gov.uk

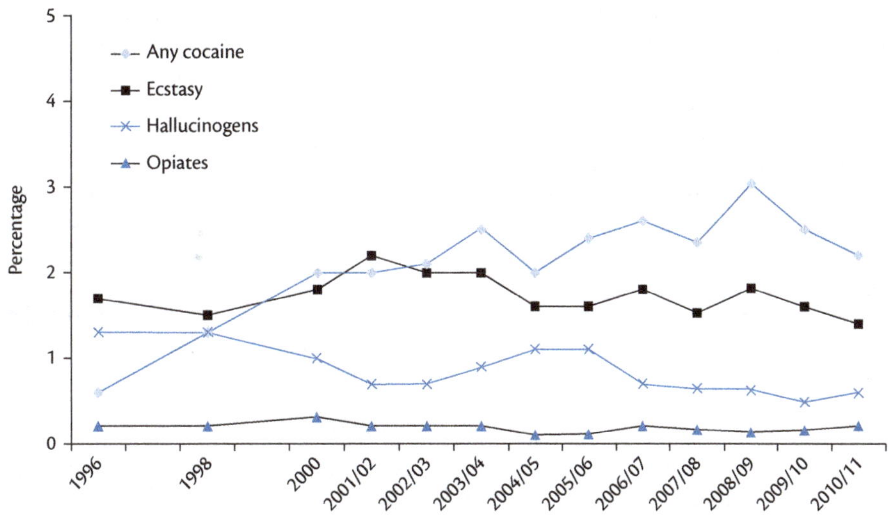

Figure 51.2 Trends in individual class A drug use in England and Wales in 16–59-year-olds.
Smith K and Flatley J. *Drug Misuse Declared: Findings from the 2010/11 British Crime Survey*, England and Wales. http://www.statistics.gov.uk

providers has led to actively asking about tobacco, alcohol, and illicit drugs.[24,25]

Identification of substance abuse most often depends on a history given voluntarily by the patient. Questions about alcohol, smoking, and illicit substances should be routine at the initial prenatal visit. Previous as well as present drug use should be explored including questioning regarding frequency, patterns, quantity, and route of administration. Serum or urine drug screening, hepatitis B and C, and HIV testing may be considered after informed consent from the patient. The CAGE questionnaire[26] or the TACE Screening Tool are often used to assess alcohol use (see Box 51.1).

Polysubstance abuse is common, with single agents rarely used in isolation. Pregnant women who use illicit drugs may be more likely to use a combination of drugs rather than a single drug.[27] Random anonymous testing of all patients now raises several legal and ethical issues including the right to privacy and admissibility of test results.[28] Despite this, anonymous screening of both newborns and mothers has previously been conducted and may be more accurate than reliance on self-reporting rates. A large multisite study based in the eastern United States tested meconium specimens of 8527 newborns for illicit drugs and on average found positive results for cocaine/opiate exposure in 10.7%. The mothers had denied drug

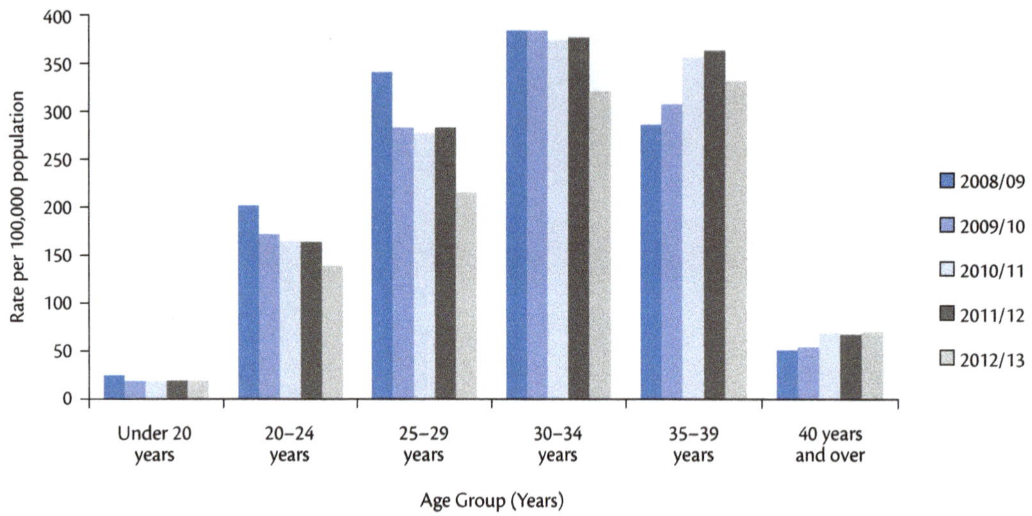

Figure 51.3 Scottish Information Services Division (ISD) data depicting rate per 100,000 population of general acute inpatient and day-case hospital admissions related to drug misuse.
ISD Scotland.

use in 38% of these cases.[29] Geographical variations were demonstrated across different sites with inner city populations again highlighted as having higher prevalence. Prospective screening of newborns in a high-risk urban population in the United States revealed that 44% of babies tested positive for opiates, cocaine, or cannabis.[30] Screening anonymized urine samples of pregnant women in inner city clinics in the United Kingdom has revealed rates of 10.7%[31] to 16%[32]. Substances tested for included cannabinoids, opiates, amphetamines, cocaine, and benzodiazepines.

Rapid urine dipstick testing for multiple illicit drugs can be easily achieved at the bedside and various kits are available.[33] Urine sampling demonstrates high rates of false-negatives, however. Except for chronic marijuana use, most substances or their metabolites are only measurable in urine for less than 72 hours and alcohol for less than 12 hours. It is therefore easy to miss substance abuse on testing unless frequent sampling is carried out. A single negative result may not necessarily be reassuring. Hair analysis of mother or newborn can be used to test for cocaine and opiates. The benefit of hair analysis is the retrospective window of detection that is able to show the trend of a habit over time and identify what drugs were used, serving as a 'diary' of usage. It improves on identification of drug use by random testing, making evasion of detection very difficult if not impossible.[34]

Table 51.4 Year-on-year rates per 1000 Scottish maternities where drug misuse has been recorded

Year of dataset	Rate of drug misuse per 1000 maternities
2006/7–2008/9	9.9
2007/8–2009/10	11.9
2008/9–2010/11	15.8
2009/10–2011/12	18.9
2010/11–2012/13	19.7

Data from ISD Scotland: Scottish Morbidity Records (SMR02).

The most accurate screening method is analysis of meconium, but this is not undertaken routinely in the United Kingdom. Drug metabolites accumulate in meconium by direct deposition from bile or by ingestion of metabolites in the amniotic fluid (or both). Meconium is not usually excreted antenatally and accumulates throughout gestation, thus its composition reflects not only recent drug use but a prolonged antenatal period. It can only be sampled post delivery, is retrospective, and may in effect

Box 51.1 TACE Screening Tool to assess possibility of alcoholism

A total score of 2 or greater indicates potential risk for the purposes of Pregnancy Outreach Program identification of prenatal risk:

Tolerance

1. How many drinks does it take to make you feel high?
   0. Less than or equal to 2 drinks
   1. More than 2 drinks

Annoyance

2. Have people annoyed you by criticizing your drinking?
   0. No
   1. Yes

Cut down

3. Have you felt you ought to cut down on your drinking?
   0. No
   1. Yes

Eye opener

4. Have you ever had a drink first thing in the morning to steady your nerves or to get rid of a hangover?
   0. No
   1. Yes

Reprinted from *American Journal of Obstetrics and Gynecology*, Volume 160, issue 4, American Journal of Obstetrics and Gynecology, The T-ACE questions: Practical prenatal detection of risk-drinking, pp. 863–870, Copyright (1989), with permission from Elsevier.

Table 51.5 Summary of anaesthetic implications of substance abuse in pregnancy

Smoking	*Acute* ◆ Transient hypoxia ◆ Increased blood carbon monoxide levels ◆ Increased airway reactivity *Chronic* ◆ Cardiorespiratory comorbidities with longstanding use including ischaemic heart disease and obstructive airway disease ◆ Chronic respiratory disease compromised by increasingly gravid uterus
Caffeine	*Acute* ◆ Sympathomimetic ◆ Administration has been used as a symptomatic treatment of postdural puncture headache *Withdrawal* ◆ Acute withdrawal in the peripartum period is a common cause of headache and should be considered in postdural puncture headache differential diagnosis
Alcohol	*Acute* ◆ Intoxicated potentially uncooperative patient ◆ Reduced anaesthetic induction agent requirements ◆ Delayed gastric emptying and increased risk of gastric content aspiration ◆ Hypoglycaemia *Chronic* ◆ Multiple comorbidities to which women are more susceptible ◆ Anaemia ◆ Dilatational cardiomyopathy—decompensated by pregnancy ◆ Biochemical derangements potentially confused with abnormalities found in HELLP syndrome ◆ Platelet/coagulation abnormalities may contraindicate neuraxial anaesthesia ◆ Altered drug metabolism (enzyme induction and liver failure) ◆ Poor nutrition and Wernicke's encephalopathy *Withdrawal (starting 48 hours post dose)* ◆ Withdrawal seizures potentially confused with eclampsia ◆ Delirium tremens
Marijuana	Considered a 'gateway drug'—enquire regarding other drug use *Acute* ◆ Intoxicated potentially uncooperative patient ◆ Myocardial depression and tachycardia ◆ Often smoked with tobacco and therefore associated with its harmful effects
Solvents	*Acute* ◆ Intoxicated potentially uncooperative patient ◆ Cardiac arrhythmias ◆ Bronchospasm *Chronic* ◆ Peripheral neuropathy ◆ Autonomic neuropathy
Opioids	*Acute* ◆ Intoxicated sedate patient with respiratory depression *Chronic* ◆ Drug tolerance ◆ Difficult acute pain management—pain often underestimated and undertreated, hyperalgesia ◆ Emphasis on multimodal analgesic regimen ◆ Difficult venous cannulation and risk of blood borne virus transmission if intravenous user ◆ Notoriously poor nutrition, dentition and self-neglect with chronic infections both localized and systemic *Withdrawal (starts 36–72 hours post dose)* ◆ Sweating, pyrexia, abdominal symptoms, tachycardia and hypertension ◆ Continue established maintenance opiate therapy (delay if delivery imminent)

(continued)

Table 51.5 (continued)

Cocaine and amphetamine	*Acute* ◆ Intoxicated potentially uncooperative patient, prominent euphoria, and/or hallucinations ◆ Sympathomimetic ◆ Myocardial ischaemia and arrhythmias ◆ Hypertension and seizures can mimic pre-eclampsia/eclampsia (however, laboratory studies often normal and clinical picture improves before delivery) ◆ Excessive uterine activity causes preterm labour, vaginal bleeding, abruption, and uterine rupture ◆ Obtund exaggerated hypertensive response to laryngoscopy ◆ Consider labetalol for treatment of toxicity ◆ Increased anaesthetic drug requirement *Chronic* ◆ Decreased anaesthetic drug requirement

only represent a missed opportunity for antenatal drug counselling and support.

Antenatal substance abuse management

Substance abuse management may involve behavioural therapy, support groups (e.g. Alcoholics Anonymous and Narcotics Anonymous), nutritional therapy (e.g. replacement of thiamine which is often deficient in alcohol abusers due to malabsorption), close monitoring for complications (e.g. placental abruption), and inpatient or outpatient pharmacotherapy (e.g. methadone to prevent withdrawal symptoms that may affect the fetus).

Drug-specific issues

Substance abuse in pregnancy may be obvious, openly admitted, or occult. It is also subject to geographical variations in the availability of the substance in question and its locally preferred route of administration. The ranges of substances which are abused are diverse chemically, pharmacologically, and physiologically with each bringing with it its own unique subset of challenges. The anaesthetic implications are summarized in Table 51.5.

Smoking

Smoking-related morbidity and mortality affects millions of individuals throughout the world. It is well established that smoking is harmful to general health but it is a socially tolerated form of substance abuse. Since 1998 to present, when *Smoking Kills: A White Paper on tobacco*[35] was published, cigarette smoking prevalence among adults in the United Kingdom has gradually declined from 28% to 21%. Estimates from the 2011 report regarding self-reporting of tobacco smoking among English women in the age range 16–44 years has fallen to a rate of 20–22%.[36] United States CDC data[7] also reveals similar reduction trends in smoking rates over time although they lag behind that seen in the United Kingdom with higher rates overall (see Table 51.6).

Overall there is evidence of a gradual decline in smoking rates over study periods stretching back over the last two decades in the general population. Regarding the obstetric population, Scottish ISD data for maternal smoking rates at booking over the last decade are depicted in Figure 51.4, and similarly demonstrate a small overall decline.[37]

Smoking in pregnancy is decreasing in high-income countries[38] and increasing in low- to middle-income countries.[39] It is strongly associated with poverty, low educational attainment, poor social support, low socioeconomic status, and psychological illness.[40] Figure 51.5 depicts Scottish smoking rates at first booking and their association with degree of maternal deprivation.[41] Depressed women are up to four times more likely to smoke during pregnancy than non-depressed women.[42]

Tobacco smoking remains a preventable factor associated with complications in pregnancy. Educational programmes are well established in pointing out the risks to maternal health and fetal well-being but despite this it has proved very difficult to introduce preventative strategies as nicotine is highly addictive and only a minority will stop smoking when they become pregnant. Smoking in pregnancy has been studied extensively. Mothers should be counselled to reduce and/or stop smoking altogether in early pregnancy; however, approximately 80% of mothers who smoke prior to pregnancy continue to do so when pregnant[43] and of those that do manage to quit around half will resume smoking by 2 weeks postpartum.[44] A meta-analysis of randomized controlled trials where smoking cessation was the primary aim of the intervention included 72 trials and over 25,000 patients. Interventions ranged from maternal counselling, information on fetal well-being, provision of nicotine replacement therapy, and social support. Overall only six women in every 100 stopped smoking.[45]

Smoking: pathophysiology

There are over 4800 substances isolated from cigarette smoke of which nicotine and carbon monoxide are well known. Others include nitrogen oxides, volatile aldehydes, alkenes, and the toxin hydrogen cyanide.

Cigarette smoking causes transient mild hypoxia, cough, mucous hypersecretion, and airflow obstruction progressing to chronic obstructive pulmonary disease in the long term. Morbidity and mortality from smoking is largely related to the effects on cardiovascular disease although increased risk of thromboembolic events and cancer, particularly of the lung, are also prevalent. Passive smokers also have an increased incidence of adverse events.

Smoking: impact on the mother

It appears that actively smoking mothers have reduced incidences of pregnancy-associated hypertension and pre-eclampsia.[46]

Table 51.6 United States Centers for Disease Control and Prevention (CDC) data showing smoking rates among persons age 12 and over by age, sex, race and ethnic origin

Age, sex, race, and Hispanic origin	Any tobacco[1]			Cigarettes			Cigars		
	2002	2009	2010	2002	2009	2010	2002	2009	2010
	Percent of population								
12 years and over	30.4	27.7	27.4	26.0	23.3	23.0	5.4	5.3	5.2
Age									
12–13 years	3.8	2.3	2.4	3.2	1.4	1.8	0.7	0.7	0.5
14–15 years	13.4	9.8	9.5	11.2	7.5	7.4	3.8	3.1	2.0
16–17 years	29.0	21.6	19.6	24.9	16.9	15.4	9.3	7.7	6.2
18–25 years	45.3	41.6	40.8	40.8	35.8	34.2	11.0	11.4	11.2
26–34 years	38.2	39.6	38.5	32.7	34.0	33.6	6.6	7.4	6.8
35 years and over	27.9	24.5	24.6	23.4	20.4	20.4	4.1	3.7	3.8
Sex									
Male	37.0	33.5	33.7	28.7	25.3	25.4	9.4	8.7	8.5
Female	24.3	22.2	21.5	23.4	21.4	20.7	1.7	2.0	2.0
Age and sex									
12–17 years	15.2	11.6	10.7	13.0	8.9	8.3	4.5	4.0	3.2
Male	16.0	13.6	12.2	12.3	9.2	8.6	6.2	5.2	4.3
Female	14.4	9.5	9.1	13.6	8.6	8.1	2.7	2.7	2.1
Hispanic origin and race[2]									
Not Hispanic or Latino:									
White only	32.0	29.6	29.5	26.9	24.5	24.3	5.5	5.2	5.2
Black or African American only	28.8	26.5	27.3	25.3	22.8	22.6	6.8	7.2	7.4
American Indian or Alaska Native only	44.3	41.8	35.8	37.1	33.0	31.1	5.2	6.9	5.6
Native Hawaiian or Other Pacific Islander only	28.8	*	*	*	15.4	*	4.1	*	*
Asian only	18.6	11.0	12.5	17.7	10.9	10.9	1.1	1.5	2.0
2 or more races	38.1	36.6	32.0	35.0	30.7	27.7	5.5	7.7	5.0
Hispanic or Latino	25.2	23.2	21.9	23.0	21.2	20.1	5.0	4.7	4.4

*Estimates are considered unreliable. Data not shown if the relative standard error is greater than 17.5% of the log transformation of the proportion, the minimum effective sample size is less than 68, the minimum nominal sample size is less than 100, or the prevalence is close to 0% or 100%.

[1]Any tobacco product includes cigarettes, smokeless tobacco (i.e. chewing tobacco or snuff), cigars, or pipe tobacco.

[2]Persons of Hispanic origin may be of any race. Data on race and Hispanic origin were collected using the 1997 Revisions to the Standards for the Classification of Federal Data on Race and Ethnicity. Single-race categories shown include persons who reported only one racial group. The category 2 or more races includes persons who reported more than one racial group.

Reproduced from National Center for Health Statistics. *Health, United States, 2012: With Special Feature on Emergency Care.* Hyattsville, MD. 2013.

However, if a smoker does develop pre-eclampsia, she is considerably more likely to develop the more severe early-onset form[47]. Additionally, it is likely that any beneficial reduction in the overall pre-eclampsia rate is superseded by the many other harmful effects of smoking. Encouragingly, if a woman stops smoking during her pregnancy, the deleterious outcomes all decrease.[44] This is an important observation for those caring for pregnant women and supports active promotion of smoking cessation.

Women who smoke are more likely to have preterm rupture of membranes and preterm delivery. The mechanism is not fully understood but is possibly related to a smoking-induced increased sensitivity of the myometrium to oxytocin.[48] Risk of placental abruption and placenta praevia are also increased.[49]

Chronic obstructive pulmonary disease may well be present in women of child-bearing age if they have been heavy smokers from an early age.[50] Chronically impaired respiratory function is further compromised by the gravid uterus due to reduction in functional residual capacity and can be demonstrated by reduced measured performance in pulmonary function tests.

Smoking: impact on the fetus

Carbon monoxide has a much higher affinity for haemoglobin than oxygen resulting in decreased oxygen delivery to the fetus. Nicotine decreases placental blood flow due to vasoconstriction and contributes to development of fetal hypoxia.[51] Smoking during pregnancy increases the risk of miscarriage, preterm labour,

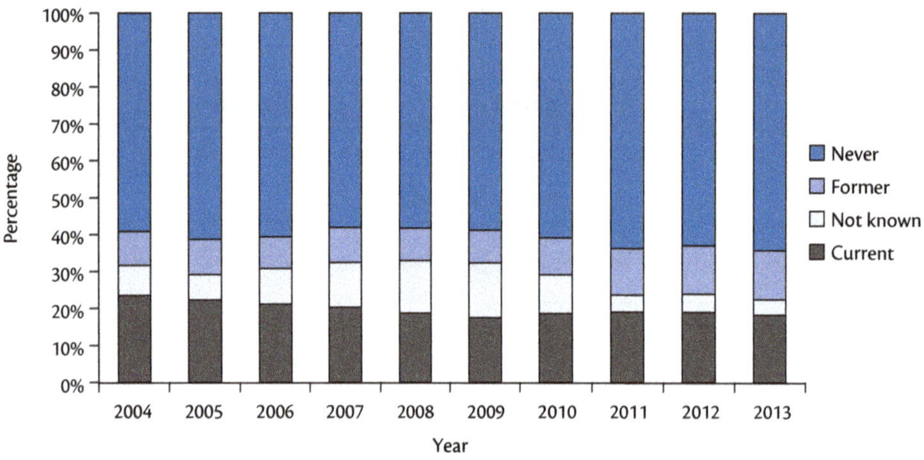

Figure 51.4 A decade of trends in smoking rates (%) in Scottish mothers at booking.
ISD Scotland.

low birth weight, stillbirth, and newborn death. The number of low birth weight neonates increase in proportion to the number of cigarettes smoked[52] and is also influenced by passive smoking.[53] Maternal third-trimester cigarette consumption is the strongest predictor of low birth weight with an estimated 27 g reduction in birth weight with each additional cigarette per day.[54] These reductions in fetal weight may have lifelong consequences with evidence pointing to significant paediatric and adulthood morbidity associated with the reduced birth weight.[55]

Maternal smoking is associated with modestly increased risk of congenital heart defects in the newborn (relative risk 1.11), especially septal defects (relative risk 1.44).[56] Passive smoking also increases the risk of congenital malformations and stillbirth.[57]

Smoking: implications for anaesthesia

Smoking is a risk factor for intraoperative pulmonary complications and a wide range of postoperative pulmonary, cardiovascular, and wound-related complications.[58] If general anaesthesia is required, adequate anaesthesia should be administered for intubation to minimize the risk of provoking bronchospasm.

Neuraxial anaesthesia is well established as the technique of choice in obstetric anaesthesia and has additional advantages for patients who smoke avoiding instrumentation of an airway which may display increased reactivity and postoperative respiratory morbidity.

Long-term smoking-related comorbidities including underlying ischaemic heart disease, chronic obstructive pulmonary disease, and hypertension should be considered and labour analgesia/anaesthesia administered following consideration of these risks on an individual patient basis.

Smokers are usually asked to abstain for at least 24–48 hours before anaesthesia for elective caesarean delivery is administered. Clearly labour is often not predictable in its onset although women should be told not to smoke when imminent labour is suspected or once contractions have started.

Caffeine

Caffeine is a central nervous system (CNS) stimulant and is the most widely consumed drug in the world since it is present in coffee, tea, many carbonated drinks, and some medications. Additional unrecognized caffeine consumption can occur in certain energy drinks and fortified foods.

Caffeine: pathophysiology

Caffeine is a methyl xanthine of which the main action is competitive antagonism of the inhibitory neurotransmitter adenosine.

Caffeine: impact on the mother

Excess caffeine intake can produce a syndrome similar to that of anxiety neurosis including:

- irritability
- nervousness
- excitement
- muscular twitching and tremor
- insomnia
- headache
- myocardial stimulation—tachycardia, inotropy, increased ectopic beats

The most consistent symptom of caffeine withdrawal is headache and typically occurs within 24 hours of abstinence.[59] Indeed, medical-grade caffeine is commonly combined with other simple analgesics for treatment of migraine.[60]

Caffeine: impact on the fetus

Caffeine has not been shown to be teratogenic[61] and does not appear to influence birth weight or length of gestation.[62,63] The effect of caffeine intake during pregnancy has been studied for the past 30 years with inconsistent results. Even though the evidence is limited, it is, however, recommended that very high intakes of caffeine in pregnancy should be avoided due to potential increased risk of stillbirth.[64]

Caffeine can be tested for in the serum and urine of neonates with neonatal caffeine withdrawal presenting with excessive levels of feeding difficulties, vomiting, crying, irritability, and poor sleep. The prevalence of fetal caffeine withdrawal is difficult to estimate due to the non-specific nature of the symptoms.

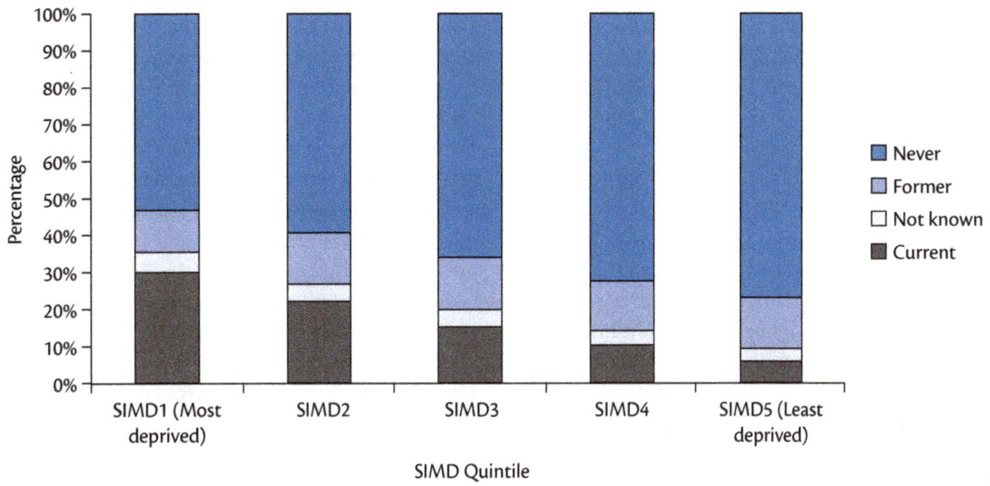

Figure 51.5 Scottish Information Services Division (ISD) data from 2010 showing maternal smoking rates at first booking and its association with degree of deprivation (SIMD= Scottish Index of Multiple Deprivation).
ISD Scotland.

Caffeine administration (either oral or intravenous) is a therapeutic option used in management of the apnoea of prematurity in neonates.[65]

Caffeine: implications for anaesthesia

Caffeine withdrawal has been associated with postoperative headache.[66] Caffeine withdrawal may form part of the differential diagnosis of postpartum headache in mothers who have received neuraxial anaesthesia. Patients may abruptly cease consumption of caffeine which can be either enforced (fasting prior to theatre, nausea, prolonged labour) or voluntary (concerns about breastfeeding etc.). This can often be identified with thorough history taking and be easily rectified by caffeine consumption and alternate diagnoses explored if non-resolution of symptoms. Caffeine administration was also a recognized treatment for headache caused by dural puncture, having been shown to both decrease persistence of headache and need for other therapeutic interventions[67] but its evidence base is poor.[68]

Alcohol

Alcohol use is common and causes problems as a result of both acute intoxication and the health effects of chronic consumption. Most women who drink alcohol before pregnancy tend to reduce or abstain when they become pregnant. Studies have demonstrated pre-pregnancy rates of alcohol consumption (average one drink per day) falling from 44% to 4.6% during pregnancy.[69] Psychological and educational interventions might increase abstinence from alcohol and reduce alcohol consumption among pregnant women.[70] Alcohol addiction can be more subtle and difficult to detect in the pregnant patient than the other illicit drugs.[71]

Alcohol: pathophysiology

Alcohol ingestion causes acute intoxication and liver damage with chronic usage. The spectrum of liver damage ranges with worsening prognosis from normal liver to fatty liver, steatohepatitis and fibrosis or cirrhosis. The severity of disease does not always correlate with the amount of alcohol intake, and environmental and genetic factors likely play a crucial role in alcoholic liver disease development.[72,73] Women appear to be more susceptible to cirrhosis for any given level of alcohol intake developing liver disease after the ingestion of less than half the amount of the equivalent male alcohol intake.[74]

Excessive alcohol intake has many adverse effects on all body systems:

- Haematological—complications result from both direct bone marrow toxicity and indirect associations such as nutritional deficiencies. Results include macrocytic anaemia, poor immunity and impaired platelet production/function
- Cardiac—arrhythmias, dilatational cardiomyopathy, hypertension
- Pancreatitis—chronic and acute
- Brain—mood/behaviour change, Wernicke's encephalopathy, Korsakoff's psychosis, seizures, and cerebral atrophy
- Osteoporosis
- Cancer—associated as a risk factor for various cancers including oropharyngeal, oesophageal, liver, and breast.

Alcohol: impact on the mother

Acute alcohol intoxication causes ataxia, confusion, stupor, and eventually coma. Risks from aspiration of gastric contents are increased as alcohol ingestion increases gastric volume and acidity whilst reducing the ability to protect the airway. Other acute presentations of alcohol abuse include hypoglycaemia, acute or chronic hepatic failure, and Wernicke's encephalopathy. Wernicke's encephalopathy often results from inadequate intake or absorption of vitamin B_1 and is characterized by the classic triad of:

- confusion
- ophthalmoplegia (paralysis of one or more extraocular muscles)
- ataxia.

Alcohol withdrawal may result from physiological dependency and produce blackouts, tremor, hallucinations, delirium, seizures, and cardiac failure. Acute withdrawal occurs around 48 hours after cessation but can occur up to 10 days after.[75]

Chronic alcohol consumption may result in malnutrition, liver disease, altered drug metabolism, coagulopathy, pancreatitis, oesophageal varices, and cardiomyopathy.[76]

Alcohol: impact on the fetus

Alcohol readily crosses the placenta and is the most widely recognized teratogen (chemical causing malformation) among abused substances in pregnancy. The fetal alcohol syndrome (FAS) describes a group of features caused by *in utero* alcohol exposure and may be as infrequent as 4% among heavy daily users.[77] FAS is one of the most severe effects of alcohol use during pregnancy and remains the leading cause of mental retardation in the United States.[78,79] It is a syndrome of mental and physical defects with characteristic features described in Box 51.2.

Acute alcohol intoxication in the mother causes fetal distress. Moderate chronic alcohol use increases the risk of small for gestational age babies (three or more drinks per week)[80] and is associated with increased risk of stillbirth (five or more drinks per week).[81] Use of alcohol in pregnancy also adversely effects exposed children later in life causing poor coordination, behavioural problems such as hyperactivity, learning, and developmental problems.[82,83]

Regardless of gestational period, alcohol causes adverse fetal effects and abstinence appears the safest approach in pregnancy.[84]

Alcohol: implications for anaesthesia

Alcohol-abusing pregnant patients may present to obstetric services acutely intoxicated, acutely withdrawing, or suffering other ill effects of chronic alcohol abuse.

Neuraxial anaesthesia can be safely performed in alcohol-abusing parturients. Contraindications, however, include coagulopathy, platelet dysfunction, and infection. Direct alcohol toxicity and nutritional deficiencies have been implicated in the development of peripheral neuropathy.[85] Alcoholic neuropathy is characterized by spontaneous burning pain, hyperalgesia, and allodynia. Examination and documentation of any pre-existing lower limb peripheral neuropathy should be performed prior to consideration of neuraxial anaesthetic techniques.

Chronic alcohol abuse may result in bleeding tendency. Direct alcohol toxicity can produce thrombocytopenia and alcoholic liver disease may produce a prolonged prothrombin time. Monitoring of prothrombin time and albumin levels are good markers of synthetic liver function, although only really encountered in end-stage disease. Laboratory clotting studies should be checked to ensure acceptable platelet counts and coagulation. Full blood count may reveal anaemia of chronic disease or macrocytic anaemia. Liver transaminases (aspartate transaminase (AST) and alanine transaminase (ALT)) are raised in alcohol abuse. Biochemical and haematological findings of alcoholic liver disease can be confused with those encountered on the spectrum of HELLP syndrome (*H*aemolysis, *E*levated *L*iver enzymes and *L*ow *P*latelet count). A high index of suspicion should prompt reassessment of the patient's alcohol history and clinical examination.

When general anaesthesia is required, acutely intoxicated patients are already partially anaesthetized and will require dose reductions in some anaesthetic agents. Chronic alcohol abuse per se does not alter the requirement, pharmacokinetics, and pharmacodynamics of thiopentone.[86] Chronic alcohol excess induces tolerance to other general anaesthetic agents. Induction dose requirements of propofol have been studied in alcoholic patients and have found to be increased, albeit in the non-obstetric population.[87] Acute intoxication may cause vomiting, hypoglycaemia, and delayed gastric emptying. Risk of aspiration of stomach contents is increased and appropriate airway management should assume a full stomach. Antacid pharmacoprophylaxis should be administered.

Alcoholic cardiomyopathy is characterized by a dilated hypokinetic heart with reduced ejection fraction. The increased cardiac output of pregnancy, together with increased fluid retention and hypoalbuminaemia may present as peripartum congestive cardiac failure. Pregnancy in the cardiomyopathy patient is high risk.[88]

Patients at risk of alcohol withdrawal should be identified on admission to hospital. They may abscond from medical care in order to continue drinking if withdrawal is imminent. Symptoms can be suppressed by benzodiazepine administration in accordance with local policies or resumption of alcohol consumption. Intravenous B vitamin supplementation may be required. Delirium tremens is a potentially life-threatening condition. Alcohol withdrawal should be considered in the differential diagnosis of seizures in the pregnant patient and could potentially mimic eclampsia. Reduced serum potassium and magnesium predispose to alcohol-related seizures.

Marijuana

Marijuana is a naturally occurring preparation of the plant *Cannabis sativa* and has been smoked for its hallucinogenic properties and used both as a recreational psychoactive and medicinal drug. It contains many chemicals classified as cannabinoids but by far the most important and potent agent found is tetrahydrocannabinol (THC). Marijuana has been the most frequently used of

Box 51.2 Characteristic features of fetal alcohol syndrome

- Growth deficiency, both pre- and postnatally
- Central nervous system disturbances that affect intellect and behaviour
- Decreased muscle tone and poor coordination
- Abnormal facial characteristics:
  - Low-set unparallel ears
  - Short, flat philtrum
  - Elongated midface
  - Small upper jaw
  - Small head
  - Small eyes with large epicanthic folds
  - Short upturned nose
- Malformation of major organs, especially heart (VSD and ASD) and skeletal deformities.

the illicit drugs in pregnancy,[89] with varying rates of 9.5–27%[90] of parturient usage described in the United States.

Marijuana is obtained in a variety of preparations such as dried leaves, resins, and oils. It goes by many street names including pot, weed, and herb. Hash, a concentrated form of the drug, is short for hashish. It is most frequently consumed by inhalation through smoking (rolled in paper with tobacco and termed a 'joint') or vaporization (through various dedicated pipes). It may also be consumed orally in any form and its use has been described in cookery and teas.

Marijuana: pathophysiology

High fat-solubility of cannabinoids leads to rapid accumulation in adipose tissue from which they are slowly released into the brain with elimination half-lives up to 7 days. The high lipid-solubility results in their persistence in the body for long periods of time. As a result they can be detected in the body for weeks or longer.

Cannabinoids undergo hepatic metabolism to numerous metabolites all of which have psychoactive properties. They seem to exert their effects by agonist action at cannabinoid receptors in the brain and peripherally. THC indirectly increases dopamine release to produce its psychotropic effects.

Most users take marijuana for its mood altering effects—feelings of 'high' or 'stoned', but the US National Institute on Drug Abuse describes the main psychological effects as quite variable and including euphoria, calmness, anxiety, or paranoia. Aside from a subjective change in perception and, most notably mood, the most common short-term physical and neurological effects include:

- myocardial depression, low blood pressure, increased heart rate
- increased respiratory rate
- red eyes
- dry mouth
- increased appetite and consumption of food
- slowed reaction time.

These effects are reduced after about 3–4 hours.

Marijuana: impact on the mother

Although marijuana usage in pregnancy appears common, the effects are unclear, perhaps due to the close association and combination abuse with alcohol, tobacco, and other drugs.[91] It is seen as a gateway drug which may lead to harder drug abuse.

Studies suggest that medicinal cannabis use may in fact be beneficial for treatment of pregnancy-related nausea and vomiting.[92]

Marijuana: impact on the fetus

Prenatal marijuana use is not associated with increased rates of birth defects, spontaneous abortion, or stillbirth.[93] Most investigators have concluded that marijuana is not an established human teratogen and does not produce structural defects or that insufficient data exists. Evidence regarding adverse neurobehavioural effects is inconclusive but associations with sleep disturbance, hyperactivity, inattention, poorer visual problem-solving skills, and delinquency in children have been suggested [94]. Heavy prenatal marijuana use (≥ 1 cigarette/day) is associated with decreased intelligence scores in children at age 6 years.[95] An association between childhood cancers, most notably leukaemia, has been reported.[96]

Marijuana remains in the baby's fat cells for 7–30 days and can be detected on drug screening.

Marijuana: implications for anaesthesia

Acute cannabis intoxication may augment the sedative and hypnotic effects of anaesthetic agents when co-administered and require relative dose reductions. Similarly chronic marijuana usage can lead to cross-tolerance with alcohol, barbiturates, opioids, benzodiazepines, and phenothiazines.[97] The cardiovascular effects of myocardial depression and tachycardia may be enhanced by the vasoactive side effects of anaesthetic agents and emergency drugs.

Smoking cannabis also leads to effects on the lungs and airways very similar to that of tobacco smoking. Marijuana smoking may lead to oropharyngitis and airway oedema and thorough airway examination should take place.

A careful drug history should be taken, enquiring for use of other more harmful drugs, and general reduction of use should be encouraged.

Solvents/inhalant abuse

Recreational inhalation of solvents causes intoxication, euphoria, and addiction. National surveys in the United States report that nearly 20% of young people have experimented with inhalants at least once.[98] Solvents are a range of chemicals which include almost any household cleaning agent or propellant:

- Aliphatic hydrocarbons (butane): lighter fuels, spray paint, paint thinner, hairspray, deodorants
- Alkyl halides: paint stripper, solvent
- Aromatic hydrocarbons (benzene, toluene): glue, spray paint, nail polish remover.

The method of delivery is inhalation of a solvent from its container ('sniffing'), a soaked rag ('huffing'), or a bag ('bagging'). Rebreathing from a closed bag causes hypercapnia and hypoxia which intensifies the effect of the inhalant.[99] Solvent-abusing patients may be identified by the characteristic odour from their breath or clothes, evidence of solvent residue, or presence of drug-taking paraphernalia. No specific laboratory tests confirm solvent inhalation.

Solvents/inhalant abuse: pathophysiology

These compounds are rapidly absorbed and excreted through the lungs. They are very lipid-soluble and rapidly reach the CNS producing the desirable acute effects. Chronic exposure can lead to permanent CNS damage such as toluene leucoencephalopathy characterized by dementia, ataxia, corticospinal tract damage, brainstem signs, and cranial neuropathies.[100] Chronic inhalant abuse can also cause changes in autonomic cardiac function, ventricular fibrillation, and myocardial infarction.[101,102] Renal and hepatic damage have also been described.

Solvents/inhalant abuse: impact on the mother

Acute respiratory distress, increased airway resistance, pulmonary hypertension, adult respiratory distress syndrome, and liver toxicity have all been reported in pregnant women exposed to solvents.[103] Arrhythmias, hypotension, bronchospasm, seizures, and chronic neurological symptoms are all implicated.

Solvents/inhalant abuse: impact on the fetus

Evidence suggests that the risk for pregnancy problems, as well as developmental delays and neurobehavioral difficulties, is higher for the children of women who have been exposed to high concentrations of organic solvents during pregnancy than for those who have not.[104] There are more than 100 cases reported in the literature of children born to solvent-abusing mothers. Many of these children were small at birth and some have craniofacial abnormalities not unlike that seen in children with FAS. In the few studies reporting the findings of follow-up in these children, some evidence has been obtained for retardation in growth, development and for residual deficits in cognitive, speech, and motor skills.[105]

Solvents/inhalant abuse: implications for anaesthesia

There are no reversal agents for inhalant intoxication and treatment of complications is generally supportive. Like other illicit drugs, the obstetric anaesthetist could be faced with the challenges of dealing with an acutely intoxicated patient. The chronic background neuropathy association with solvent abuse should necessitate accurate documentation of neurological examination prior to neuraxial anaesthesia.

Opioids/heroin

Opioids are strong analgesic drugs with associated recreational properties amenable to abuse. Frequent and regular administration is associated with physical dependence and physical tolerance. Medical-grade opioids are available in a variety of formulations and are typically used to treat severe pain or opiate withdrawal symptoms. Opioid analgesic drugs may be divided into:

- Naturally occurring alkaloids (e.g. morphine and codeine)
- Semisynthetic drugs (e.g. diamorphine and dihydrocodeine)
- Synthetic drugs (e.g. pethidine, fentanyl, and alfentanil).

Each drug has slightly different effects on the body but in general is similar to morphine. They may be abused both legally when prescribed by a medical practitioner and illegally when obtained without prescription. Non-medically processed illicit opioids are also available as street drugs.

Heroin is the name attributed to diamorphine when it is discussed in its illegal (street) form and is also colloquially known by a huge variety of names including H, dope, smack, brown, and tar among many others. Illegally obtained heroin is often supplied in freebase form which has a duller appearance than the bright white powder of diamorphine, has a lower boiling point, and is amenable to smoking. It can also be dissolved in water when mixed with an acid (usually citric acid or lemon juice) and heated to provide a mixture suitable for intravenous injection. Oral use of heroin as a means of recreation is less common due to the lack of a 'rush' associated with the rapid rise in blood concentration. Additionally, combining heroin with other illicit drugs is common practice and there are also locally accepted terminologies to describe these (e.g. snowball—heroin and cocaine, speedball—heroin and amphetamine).

Opioids/heroin: pathophysiology

Opioids mimic the action of the endogenous opioid peptides and are agonists binding to mu-, delta-, and kappa-opioid receptors throughout the CNS. Excessive use leads to receptor down-regulation and tolerance. Heroin readily crosses the placenta.

Classic effects include:

- analgesia
- sedation/euphoria/dysphoria
- respiratory depression
- nausea and vomiting
- constipation
- histamine release causing hypotension, bradycardia, bronchospasm and rash
- meiosis (pinpoint pupils).

Methadone is a long-acting opiate agonist that reduces heroin craving, drug-seeking, and other high-risk behaviours.

Opioids/heroin: impact on the mother

It is difficult to separate out the ill effects of heroin from the coexisting effects of additional agents, multiple diseases, and lifestyle factors among heavy opioid users. Heroin may be contaminated with other substances during preparation (lactose, glucose, mannitol, starch, quinine, amphetamines, strychnine, procaine, or lidocaine among many others). Serious infections can occur due to both biological contamination of heroin batches with bacteria, viruses, or fungi and transmission of blood-borne viruses between individuals sharing needles. Serious recent outbreaks of unusual infections with high mortality rates as a by-product of contaminated heroin use in the United Kingdom have been described. These include anthrax,[106] botulism,[107,108] tetanus,[109] and *Clostridium novyi*[110] infections. Injecting users sharing needles have well-established blood-borne virus transmission, most commonly hepatitis C, but also hepatitis B and HIV.

Opioid withdrawal is characterized by sweating, lacrimation, pyrexia, nausea, vomiting, diarrhoea, abdominal pain, tachycardia, and hypertension. These symptoms peak at 36–72 hours after the last dose. Aims of treatment should be provision of analgesia, prevention of opioid withdrawal, and management of abnormal drug-taking behaviour. Opioid abuse is linked to irregular menstrual cycles and together with chaotic lifestyles, women may not even realize that they are pregnant contributing to lack of antenatal care. The early signs of pregnancy can even be misinterpreted as opioid withdrawal symptoms. Unintended pregnancy is common in these women with 86% of pregnant opioid-abusing women reporting that their pregnancy was unintended in one study.[111] Methadone maintenance has become the 'gold standard' for the management of pregnant heroin users and UK guidelines support its use.[112]

The treatment of opioid dependence with methadone or buprenorphine decreases opioid and other drug abuse, reduces criminal activity, and improves individual functioning and decreases HIV transmission rates.[113] The purpose of substitution therapy is to replace illicit opioid use by the medically controlled oral use of a synthetic opioid. Unfortunately, these medically controlled agents can also be subject to a phenomenon known as pharmaceutical leakage and they themselves appear on the illicit market for abuse.[114] Methadone maintenance is used in the treatment of opioid dependence in pregnancy. Methadone maintenance given during pregnancy reduces maternal illicit opiate use and fetal exposure, enhances compliance with obstetrical care and is associated with improved outcomes like heavier birth weight.[115]

Buprenorphine is a partial agonist–partial antagonist synthetic opioid with around 72 hours; action that has also been used to treat opioid dependence in pregnancy both in Europe and the United States.[116] Buprenorphine's effectiveness during pregnancy as maintenance therapy has not been proven although neonatal withdrawal may be shorter and less severe with buprenorphine than with methadone.[117] Subutex (buprenorphine combined with naloxone to reduce side effects) may also be taken for mild to moderate withdrawal.

Opiates/heroin: impact on the fetus

Heroin rapidly crosses the placenta entering fetal tissues within 1 hour of administration. This can affect the fetus directly (opioid effects). Birth weight is reduced in the offspring of heroin (mean reduction 489 g) and methadone (279 g) users,[118] possibly as a result of malnutrition and frequent infections. Intrauterine growth retardation and intrauterine fetal distress are established consequences.[119] Postnatal growth deficiency, microcephaly, neurobehavioural problems, increase in neonatal mortality, and a 74-fold increase in sudden infant death syndrome have been described.[120] There are no direct teratogenic effects on the fetus but direct harm is caused to the fetus by the associations of high-risk maternal opioid use. These include severe malnutrition, lack of obstetric care, inhabiting a risky environment, and sequelae of medical complications such as infectious diseases, endocarditis, abscesses, and sexually transmitted disease.[121]

Fluctuating opioid concentrations in the maternal blood may lead to cyclical fetal overdose and withdrawal. Maternal drug withdrawal is thus equally experienced by the fetus both *in utero* and post delivery. Around 48–94% of fetuses exposed to *in utero* opioids develop clinical signs of withdrawal following delivery, termed neonatal abstinence syndrome (NAS).[122] There is some correlation between dose and severity of withdrawal[123].

Apart from NAS, many of these health risks to the fetus can be avoided in principle by opioid substitution treatment[124,125] and lifestyle changes. Methadone replacement substantially minimizes the peak and trough in maternal serum opioid levels that typically occur with repeated use of short-acting opioids (i.e. heroin) reducing harm to the fetus of repeated maternal intoxication and withdrawal.[126]

Methadone treatment may well stabilize the maternal lifestyle but one study in Glasgow of 450 drug-dependent mothers prescribed substitute methadone found that 45.5% of infants needed pharmacological treatment for NAS.[127] Neonatal intensive care unit admission was required in 48.8% of infants born to methadone users. The reasons for admission included prematurity (15.8%), respiratory distress (12.6%), and a range of social reasons (13%). Infants born to drug-misusing mothers constituted 2.9% of hospital births, but occupied almost a fifth of neonatal cot days. A prolonged postnatal stay is recommended to help healthcare professionals observe for signs of NAS, conduct social work assessment, and arrange for parenting and community support for the mothers prior to discharge. Additionally, researchers showed that encouraging breastfeeding in mothers, who are established on the lowest dose of methadone to remain stable, helps to protect against the risk of developing NAS.

Opiates/heroin: implications for anaesthesia

Polydrug use is common in opioid-abusing patients and history and examination should reflect this. Heavy users are at risk of acute withdrawal when admitted to hospital and may abscond from medical care in order to continue drug-seeking behaviour. There may be obvious signs of recent needle marks or local skin infection which may require explanation if history taking seems unreliable. It will be difficult to judge appropriate pain management and dosing when illicit opioid drugs have complicated analgesic requirement.

Pregnant patients may present acutely with signs of acute opioid overdose including respiratory depression. Opioid-related hypoxia will be both more rapid and more severe in advanced pregnancy due to the alterations in cardiorespiratory physiology. Patients who present for obstetric reasons acutely under the influence of opioids may require a reduction in the dose of anaesthetic drugs. Similarly patients who are severely malnourished may have unexpectedly low body weights and caution should be noted when calculating appropriate local anaesthetic and non-opioid analgesic safe dosages.

Treatment of acute pain in women with opioid abuse disorders can be very challenging. The pain of many opioid-agonist-maintained patients is often underestimated and undertreated[128] with behavioural and social responses worsening the pain experience. There are common misconceptions when treating the non-opiate naive patient experiencing acute pain (see Box 51.3).

Hyperalgesia is observed in patients with heroin use and this is not altered by maintenance methadone or buprenorphine. Tolerance is one factor that explains why these patients derive little pain relief from long-term maintenance opioids. Pain is subjective, making assessment of its severity objectively difficult. Medical staff experience concern about being manipulated by drug-seeking patients but this can only be reduced by careful clinical assessment. A multimodal analgesic regimen[129] including regular short-acting opioid medications, non-opioid simple analgesics,[130] and neuraxial anaesthesia/analgesia where appropriate will be required in addition to maintenance opioid therapy to achieve adequate acute pain control.[131] It can be difficult to predict response to opioid analgesics in an opioid abusing patient but frequent regular dosing with frequent review seems logical to ascertain a dose–effect relationship in an individual.

In a labouring patient or elective delivery, methadone therapy should be timed wherever possible to avoid peak drug concentration occurring around delivery time of the fetus. Maintenance

Box 51.3 Common misconceptions in the non-opioid naïve patient experiencing acute pain

1. Maintenance medication (e.g. methadone) provides pain relief
2. Opioids prescribed for acute pain will cause a relapse
3. Opioids prescribed for acute pain, in addition to maintenance doses, may cause respiratory depression
4. Acute pain may be assumed to acquire prescribed opioid medication.

Data from Alford D, Compton P and Samet J. Acute pain management for patients receiving maintenance methadone or buprenorphine therapy. *Ann Intern Med* 2006; 144:127–134.

opioid medication is usually inadequate for labour pain management. Neuraxial anaesthesia can provide adequate pain relief in women receiving methadone or buprenorphine for both labour and delivery and is the technique of choice. The dose of opioid in the epidural or spinal should be similar to that in opioid-naïve patients. Patient-controlled analgesia can be used as a mode of opioid administration but settings may need to include a background infusion and a higher bolus dose. The aim is to eventually discharge patients on no more opioid than was used before admission.

The partial agonist (buprenorphine or subutex) maintenance dosing can complicate pain management during labour and delivery. The slow dissociation and low intrinsic activity at the mu receptor[132] result in a favourable safety profile, but also complicate pain management by preventing acute pain medications adequately reaching their target receptors. Another option for consideration is to discontinue partial agonists in advance of delivery and substitute with regular full agonist opioid analgesics, titrating to effect to avoid withdrawal and then to later achieve adequate analgesia as required. Otherwise, higher doses than typical may be required to competitively displace buprenorphine from mu opioid receptors.[111]

Chronic opioid users may be relatively immunosuppressed due to alteration of cell-mediated immune pathways, poor nutrition, and pregnancy. They may also be more likely to be exposed to infectious pathogens through self-administration of contaminated drug, heavy smoking, and breaching of the skin with contaminated needles. Systemic infection may be present due to local cellulitis, endocarditis, and abscesses related to injection sites. Neuraxial anaesthesia may be contraindicated in a systemically septic patient. Chronic opioid-abusing patients have notoriously poor dentition and this should also be examined as part of a thorough airway assessment.

Blood sampling and peripheral venous cannulation (PVC) may be extremely technically difficult in the chronic intravenous drug-abusing patient. This is compounded by the prevalence of blood-borne viruses present in this patient group which increases the infection risk via needlestick injury to healthcare professionals. This represents a significant concern to healthcare professionals performing exposure-prone procedures and universal precautions must apply to all staff in the delivery suite and obstetric theatre. Obstetric patients can have life-threatening emergencies which can be unpredictable and fast paced with time-critical responses needed to prevent morbidity.[133] Emergency resuscitation and/or delivery of the fetus could be delayed when faced with difficult or impossible PVC. Intravenous access traditionally and ultimately falls to the labour ward anaesthetist in the most difficult of patients.

Antenatal anaesthetic assessment may reveal that some patients have required multiple previous central venous catheters on separate occasions during previous medical treatments. Long-term intravenous drug abusing patients are often expert self-phlebotomists and evidence of multiple skin popping (failed venous injection or intentional subcutaneous injection of drug) may herald lack of venous access. These patients should be regarded as high risk of difficult intravenous access when they later present for management of labour and delivery (see Box 51.4).

Management plans regarding vascular access prior to labour should be discussed and equipment such as ultrasound and central venous access catheters be made available. Ultrasound has been recommended for safe placement of central venous access[134] and more recently has gained recognition for its use in siting peripheral venous cannulae.[135] Individual risk assessment should reflect the need for vascular access with particular consideration given to risk factors for sudden massive haemorrhage and/or potential requirements for large volume resuscitation. Pre-existing large-bore vascular access should be optimal in these circumstances permitting appropriate flow rates.

When antenatal assessment is not met, similar assessment of patients at risk of difficult venous access should occur in early labour and vascular access secured appropriately. Difficulty may arise when an intravenous drug abusing patient with difficult access presents with a life-threatening obstetric emergency. If PVC attempts fail, and access must be expedited, intraosseous (IO) access is one alternative to central line insertion which may provide significant time savings,[136] has been used successfully in a previous obstetric emergency[137] and has been recommended in national guidelines.[138,139] A recent national survey of UK obstetric anaesthetists revealed that 81% of respondents would consider the use of IO access in a life-threatening obstetric emergency after failed PVC attempts.[140] The technique of IO needle insertion appears easy to learn among delivery suite staff with a high first-pass success rate demonstrable following simulation training.[141] In our institution, inhalational induction of general anaesthesia in a mother with very difficult venous access has been used rarely to facilitate an emergency caesarean delivery because of immediate threat to life of mother or fetus (category 1 caesarean delivery according to the Lucas et al. classification[142]). A laryngeal mask airway was inserted, and a central line sited once the baby was delivered. Individual risk assessment to all parties including mother, baby, and healthcare professionals in emergency settings should take place.

Once vascular lines are in place it should be remembered that they can be used for 'main-lining' and therefore patients should not be allowed off the ward with them *in situ* and they should be removed as soon as they are no longer medically needed.

Cocaine

Cocaine (benzoylmethylecgonine, $C_{17}H_{21}N_{O4}$) is an alkaloid derived from the plant *Erythroxylon coca*. It is legally available as a topical local anaesthetic but its illegal/recreational use as a CNS stimulant far exceeds the medicinal use. It is illegal for non-medicinal use in almost every country.

Route of administration includes snorting, smoking, ingestion, and injection. It is presented in the following forms:

- Coke—pure cocaine which is a white powder generally snorted through the nasal mucosa.
- Crack—the alkalinized form or free base, known as 'crack' has increased bioavailability, is more dangerous, and is highly

Box 51.4 Risk factors for difficult intravenous access in intravenous drug abusers

- Needle marks in the dominant arm or groins
- Evidence of skin/muscle popping
- Central vein cannulation in previous hospital admission
- Lack of antenatal blood sampling results

addictive.[143] It is produced by mixing cocaine crystal or powder with water and baking soda (sodium bicarbonate, $NaHCO_3$). The mixture is boiled until the water evaporates leaving brown and white rocks which are very hard/brittle. The origin of the name 'crack' comes from the crackling sound that is produced when the cocaine and its impurities (i.e. water and sodium bicarbonate) are heated past the point of vaporization. Crack cocaine is widely smoked throughout the world,[144] usually through special glass pipes or from foil, although it can also be injected when reconstituted with water.

Cocaine: pathophysiology

Cocaine is absorbed rapidly into the bloodstream producing a 'high' in approximately 6–8 minutes and lasts around 30 minutes to an hour, with variations depending on route of intake. Cocaine is a potent nervous system stimulant, readily crossing the blood–brain barrier and acting as a serotonin–norepinephrine–dopamine reuptake inhibitor, also known as a triple reuptake inhibitor (TRI). It is a sympathomimetic, causing an exaggerated response to these chemical messengers. Through this mechanism, prolonged adrenergic stimulation is produced with the following physical manifestations:

- increased motor activity
- tremors
- convulsion
- tachycardia
- generalized vasoconstriction
- hypertension
- hyperpyrexia.

With excessive dosage, tremors, seizures, and increased body temperature are observed.[145]

Mood-altering effects of cocaine produce euphoria by promotion of dopamine's activity in the limbic system. Feelings of high energy, alertness, increased competence, and general well-being are experienced. Anxiety, paranoia, and restlessness are also frequent. Sudden withdrawal of the drug results in fatigue, mental depression, and psychological craving.

Cocaine: impact on the mother

In common with other illicit drug use in pregnancy, denial of use is a likely response to direct questioning. Heavy use may be associated with exhaustion, dehydration, and poor nutrition. Since it is often smoked, it can affect others due to passive smoking which has implications for other family members nearby including the newborn and other children.

Binge cycles are a particular problem and reflect the chaotic lifestyle. Bingeing is associated with preterm birth and an increased incidence of acute complications.[146] Use of cocaine in pregnancy can result in systemic and focal vasoconstriction and abnormal uterine contractions due to increased sensitivity to catecholamines. Cocaine also indirectly increases uterine contractility by promoting endometrial prostaglandin production. Overdoses cause hyperthermia, a marked elevation of blood pressure and seizures which can be life-threatening.

Maternal complications of cocaine ingestion include increased likelihood of placenta-associated syndromes such as placental abruption[147] and infarction.[148] Uterine rupture has been described in association with cocaine abuse in both women who have had previous caesarean delivery (scar rupture)[149] and even in a primigravid unscarred uterus.[150] Preterm labour, hepatic rupture,[151] rhabdomyolysis,[152] cerebral haemorrhage,[153] cardiac arrhythmias, and death[154] are all recognized. Cocaine-induced cardiovascular complications do not seem to be dose dependent, and even small recreational doses can lead to significant morbidity and mortality in an otherwise healthy parturient. The cardiovascular toxicity of cocaine is significantly increased in pregnancy.[155] Increased myocardial oxygen demand together with coronary vasoconstriction and enhanced platelet aggregation can lead to myocardial ischaemia and chest pain. This is most likely to occur within 1 hour after ingestion when blood levels of cocaine are at their highest.[156]

Acute cocaine intoxication in the third trimester can mimic pre-eclampsia and eclampsia. A case series of 11 pregnant women has been described in a report from the United States where patients presented with hypertension, blurred vision, abdominal pain, or seizures in the third trimester, but with a positive urine test for cocaine.[157] All women had a diastolic above 90 mmHg but which returned to the normal range within 45–90 minutes after admission. In these patients all laboratory investigations (liver and renal function tests) for pre-eclampsia were negative and the clinical syndrome improved as the drug wore off. A similar case of acute cocaine intoxication mimicking pre-eclampsia has also been described in the postpartum period.[158] Hypertension, proteinuria, and oedema can all occur with acute cocaine intake. In these cases, the diagnosis was aided by rapid result bedside urine toxicology testing. Normal laboratory testing may be a key differential.

Persistent cocaine abuse is associated with more chronic problems such as small-for-gestational-age infants, systemic infections, anaemia, and low maternal body weight.[142]

Cocaine and other illicit drugs should also be considered in the differential diagnosis of commonly encountered postpartum headache.[159]

Cocaine: impact on the fetus

Cocaine is rapidly transferred across the placenta by simple diffusion.[160] There is no convincing evidence of teratogenic effects although this is difficult to isolate from other attributable factors in 'at-risk' mothers.[161] Infant outcomes in early studies consistently associated prenatal cocaine use with decreased birth weight, prematurity, and decreased fetal growth.[162] These finding have been reinforced by a more recent meta-analysis including 31 studies and accumulating data from nearly 40,000 patients.[163] Links to delayed cognitive development[164] and behavioural problems[165] later in childhood are also present.

Fetal cocaine withdrawal occurs around day 3 of life, with many discharged home before symptoms. Cocaine can be detected in fetal meconium.[166]

Cocaine: implications for anaesthesia

Cocaine abuse is often denied by the pregnant patient and associated risk factors may include cigarette smoking, late booking, and premature labour.[167] A high index of suspicion is required. Cocaine effects should be considered when mothers present with new-onset cardiac arrhythmias or signs of myocardial ischaemia and no previous cardiac history or risk factors. Management of cocaine-induced arrhythmias are usually similar to that in the non-pregnant women but with added consideration of fetal effects and safety profiles.[168]

Excessive uterine activity may result in fetal compromise or abruption and requirements for emergency resuscitation and delivery. Delivery suite anaesthetists should be aware of the increased risks of complications associated with cocaine abuse. High prevalence of obstetric emergencies in cocaine-abusing mothers results in the occasional necessity to expedite delivery of a cocaine-intoxicated patient. Mode of anaesthesia for delivery should be individualized to the specific set of problems presented by a cocaine-abusing parturient.

When neuraxial anaesthesia is selected, combative behaviour, altered pain perception, cocaine-induced thrombocytopenia, and ephedrine-resistant hypotension may be encountered. Phenylephrine should be used for hypotension associated with neuraxial anaesthesia. Neuraxial anaesthesia is still recommended as per non-cocaine abusing mothers but individual consideration should be given to the cardiovascular effects of cocaine use. Changes in opioid receptor densities and alteration in endorphins may result in perception of breakthrough pain despite adequate spinal and epidural blocks.[169,170] Chronic cocaine abuse leads to increased need for opiate analgesia in treatment of acute pain.

If general anaesthesia is required, consideration should be given to obtund the hypertensive response to laryngoscopy which may be exaggerated and anaesthetic volatile agents may worsen incidence of cardiac arrhythmias. Cardiac arrhythmias, hypertension, and myocardial ischaemia may be encountered under general anaesthesia.[171] Myocardial infarction and chest pain are caused by cocaine-induced vasospasm together with increased myocardial oxygen demand. Chest pain should be treated with oxygen, nitrates, benzodiazepines, and consideration of angioplasty.

Beta blockade to obtund cardiovascular responses in cocaine-abusing parturients may be relatively contraindicated due to the resultant unopposed alpha-adrenergic stimulation which can worsen hypertension. Hydralazine has been used but the decrease in systemic vascular resistance may cause reflex tachycardia[172] which is undesirable in cocaine intoxication. Labetalol is a combined alpha and beta blocker which has been widely used in pre-eclampsia treatment and has also been recommended for treatment of cocaine toxicity.[173,174]

Amphetamines

Amphetamine is one compound within its own class of drugs. They are addictive stimulants. Derivatives range from 3,4-methylenedioxy-*N*-methylamphetamine (MDMA) known as ecstasy, to the *N*-methylated form methamphetamine known as 'crystal meth' and to medical decongestants such as ephedrine. Another common street name is 'speed' but there are many others. Population surveys across Europe suggest widespread use in the general population (Figure 51.5),[175] with the Czech Republic highest at 3.2%. Amphetamine use across Europe is generally stable, with most countries reporting broadly constant levels since the 1990s.

In the United States, it has been estimated that 5% of all pregnant women have used methamphetamines[176] and hospitalizations due to amphetamine abuse in pregnancy are increasing.[177] In the United Kingdom, amphetamines are regarded as Class B drugs.[11]

Physical effects reflect its action as a stimulant and include:

- hyperactivity
- pupil dilatation
- hypertension
- tachycardia and palpitations
- headache
- tachypnoea
- fever
- sweating
- conjunctival injection
- tremor
- convulsions.

Users also experience prominent psychological effects which can include euphoria, increased alertness, concentration, energy, confidence, and self-esteem. However, these effects occur on a spectrum also including anxiety, aggression, grandiose behaviour, paranoia, and psychosis. Tolerance to the drug is developed rapidly.

Withdrawal symptoms produce fatigue, mental depression, and somnolence. Amphetamine overdose is fairly common, which is probably due to abusers' ever-increasing need for more and more of the drug (tolerance). Unintentional overdose is a sign of increasing tolerance.

Amphetamine is administered orally, by smoking, by snorting, and by injection. Oral administration in tablet or powder form is the commonest method of recreational use.[178] In some areas amphetamine is also available in a paste which can be mixed with water and drunk. Oral ingestion effects appear within 15–60 minutes and peak at 2–3 hours.[179] Amphetamine can be smoked by heating to vaporization in glass pipes or aluminium foil. Snorting involves inhaling drug in fine powder form into the nose where it is rapidly absorbed through mucus membranes producing effects within minutes but with a shorter duration. If not already in powder form the drug may first be prepared by crushing. Injection is the most dangerous method of administering amphetamine and is prepared by dissolving in water and drawing up through a cigarette filter. This route produces the highest bioavailability and the sensation of an immediate 'rush' but with faster offset of effects. Regional variations among illicit users are seen in choice of route of administration.[180] Polydrug use is common among amphetamine users.[181] Potentiation of both effects and side effects can result from combining amphetamine with other drugs.

Amphetamines: pathophysiology

Amphetamines enhance neurotransmitters in the brain including dopamine, serotonin, and norepinephrine, increasing their concentrations in synaptic clefts. Ecstasy (MDMA) is a derivative of methamphetamine. It causes accumulation of serotonin and dopamine at the synapses and has additional hallucinogenic properties.

Amphetamine and its derivatives, methamphetamine and MDMA, are slowly metabolized and easily distributed to the CNS.

Amphetamines: impact on the mother

Stimulant effects of amphetamine resemble and appear to have significant crossover with those seen in cocaine abuse.

Although the medical literature on the adverse maternal and infant outcomes of cocaine abuse during pregnancy is substantial, less research has been done on amphetamine abuse during pregnancy; however, the reported effects are similar.[188] When cocaine and amphetamine abusing groups are compared with each other, obstetric diagnoses associated with infant morbidity such as premature delivery and poor fetal growth are more common in the cocaine-abusing women, whereas vasoconstrictive effects such as cardiovascular disorders and hypertension complicating pregnancy are more common in the amphetamine-abusing mothers.[175] Amphetamine injection increases the risk of emergencies such as placental abruption.[182]

Patient cooperation and safe positioning for neuraxial anaesthesia may complicate attempts at neuraxial analgesia/anaesthesia in a patient experiencing acute hallucinogenic effects of MDMA. Adverse cardiovascular events have been reported in amphetamine-dependent parturients undergoing operative delivery under both neuraxial and general anaesthesia.

MDMA intoxication has been associated with hyperthermia (> 39° C), disseminated intravascular coagulation, and severe dehydration. Excessive antidiuretic hormone (ADH) release may cause hyponatraemia leading to coma and death. Serum electrolytes should be measured and care taken with fluid administration

Amphetamines: impact on the fetus

Amphetamine abuse during pregnancy has potential fetal side effects as the drugs are fat-soluble and can easily cross the placental barrier.[183] It has been postulated that amphetamines will decrease uterine blood flow and increase uterine vascular resistance in a dose-related manner. Its use in pregnancy is associated with increased risk of adverse pregnancy outcomes such as increased neonatal mortality and worsened Apgar scores at 1 minute and 5 minutes.[184] The problems of amphetamine exposure in pregnancy include intrauterine growth restriction,[185] preterm labour,[186] and low birth weight.[187] One study found a 3.5-fold increased risk of fetal growth restriction among babies of women using methamphetamine in pregnancy.[188] Long-term effects include reduction in childhood growth, intellectual performance,[189] and behavioural problems.[190]

Methamphetamine exposure was also associated with neonatal withdrawal symptoms of agitation, vomiting, and tachypnoea.[191] This withdrawal syndrome is relatively mild and only requires medical intervention in approximately 4% of cases.[192]

Preterm birth rates in amphetamine abusing mothers have been quoted around 26–28.6%.[193,194] As per previous studies, the exact causes are multifactorial and it is difficult to extrapolate whether it is a direct effect of amphetamine itself or associated factors in the substance abusing parturient such as anaemia, poor nutrition, and social factors. Fetal and infant deaths have also been reported in relation to amphetamine abuse.[195]

Amphetamines: implications for anaesthesia

Amphetamine intoxication presenting with seizures, proteinuria, and/or hypertension may be mistaken for pre-eclampsia/eclampsia and is similar to cocaine intoxication in this respect. Psychedelic effects, psychosis, and hallucinations may cause difficulty with cooperation required for siting neuraxial blockade. Caution should be demonstrated with sympathomimetic

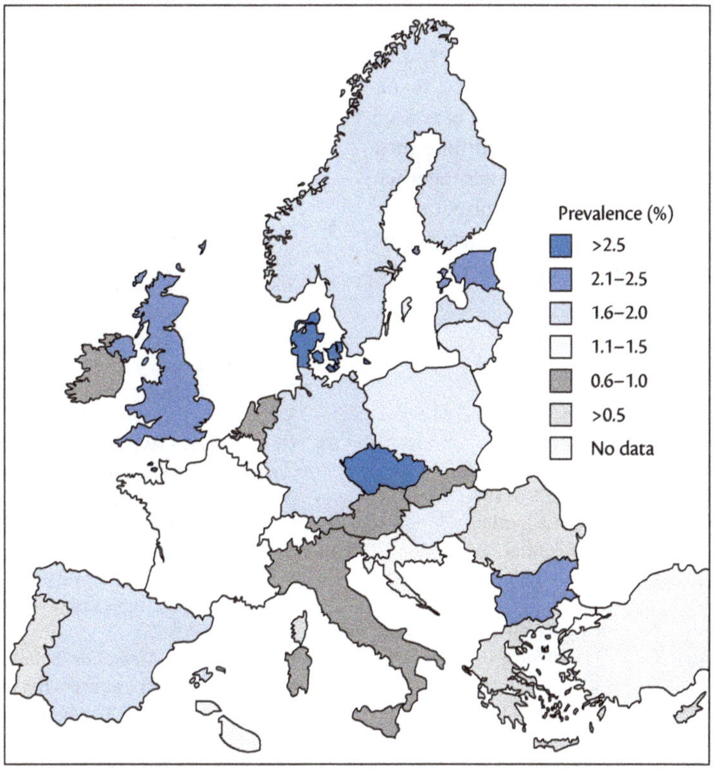

Figure 51.6 Report of population surveys suggesting prevalence of amphetamine use among young adults (15–34 years) in Europe.

European Monitoring Centre for Drugs and Drug Addiction (EMCDDA). *Problem amphetamine and methamphetamine use in Europe. Selected Issue 2010.* © European Monitoring Centre for Drugs and Drug Addiction, 2010.

drugs due to exaggeration of hypertension, arrhythmias, and myocardial ischaemia. Acute amphetamine intoxication tends to increase minimum alveolar concentrations of anaesthetic agents, while chronic usage tends to decrease anaesthetic dose requirements. Electrolytes should be monitored together with careful fluid balance as seizure-induced hyponatraemia has been associated with extreme thirst and ingestion of large volumes of water.

One study has shown that 35% of amphetamine-abusing mothers are anaemic on screening, compared to nearly 8% in the non-substance abusing group.[196] The increased risk of this complication may well result from poor nutrition and lack of antenatal iron supplementation in a patient group demonstrated to have higher incidences of lack of obstetric care. Screening for anaemia should be undertaken.

Conclusion

Substance abuse in pregnancy is a significant problem faced by the obstetric anaesthetist which adds a layer of complexity to the management of labour and delivery. It is difficult to quantify the true extent of the problem given the often socially unacceptable, illegal, and covert nature of this activity although it appears significant, particularly in inner city regions.

Substance abuse may be obvious, openly admitted, or occult. It is also subject to geographical variations in the availability of the substance in question and its locally preferred route of administration. The ranges of substances which are abused are diverse chemically, pharmacologically, and physiologically with each bringing with it its own unique subset of challenges.

Substance-abusing mothers tend to default on antenatal care, present with obstetric and non-obstetric emergencies directly related to drug abuse, mimic other obstetric disease states, and have a tendency towards preterm labour. Neonates tend to be premature, small for gestational age, at risk of stillbirth, at risk of withdrawal, and have behavioural problems which continue into childhood and adult life. Local knowledge and experience together with a high index of suspicion among obstetric care providers is invaluable in supporting substance-abusing mothers throughout their pregnancy to obtain the most favourable outcomes for both mother and baby.

References

1. American Psychiatric Association. *Diagnostic and Statistical Manual of Mental Disorders* (4th ed, Text revision). Arlington, VA: American Psychiatric Publishing Inc; 2000.
2. Centre for Maternal and Child Enquiries (CMACE). Saving Mothers' Lives: reviewing maternal deaths to make motherhood safer: 2006–08. The Eight Report on Confidential Enquiries into Maternal Deaths in the Unites Kingdom. 2011. *BJOG* 118 Suppl. 1:1–203.
3. Moran P, Madgula RM, Gilvarry E, *et al.* Substance misuse during pregnancy: its effects and treatment. *Fetal Matern Med Rev* 2009; 20(1):1–16.
4. Birnbach DJ, Stein DJ, Grunebaum A, *et al.* Cocaine screening of parturients without prenatal care: an evaluation of a rapid screening assay. *Anesth Analg* 1997; 84:76–9.
5. American College of Obstetricians and Gynaecologists. Routine Human Immunodeficiency Virus Screening. *Commitee Opinion* 596, May 2014.
6. Robertson JL, McGrady E, Young S. Drug-using parturients in a tertiary referral centre. *Eur J Anaesthesiol* 2011; 28:166.
7. National Center for Health Statistics. *Health, United States, 2012: With Special Feature on Emergency Care.* Hyattsville, MD: National Center for Health Statistics; 2013.
8. European Monitoring Center for Drugs and Drug Addiction (EMCDDA). *Statistical Bulletin 2013.* [Online] http://www.emcdda.europa.eu/stats13
9. National Treatment Agency for Substance Misuse. *National and Regional Estimates of the Prevalence of Opiate and/or Crack Cocaine Use 2009–10: A Summary of the Key Findings.* 2011. [Online] http://www.nta.nhs.uk
10. Smith K, Flatley J. *Drug Misuse Declared: 2010/11 British Crime Survey, England and Wales.* [Online] http://www.statistics.gov.uk
11. Advisory Council on the Misuse of Drugs, UK. *Misuse of Drugs Act 1971, Chapter 38.* [Online] http://www.legislation.gov.uk
12. Information Services Division (ISD) Scotland. *Drug-Related Hospital Statistics Scotland 2013.* 25 February 2014. [Online] http://www.isdscotland.org
13. Information Services Division (ISD) Scotland. *Derived from Scottish Morbidity records (SMR02) Drug Misuse in Pregnancy: Births in Scottish Hospitals—Year Ending 31st March 2013.* [Online] http://www.isdscotland.org/Health-Topics/Maternity-and-Births/Publications/data-tables.asp
14. Cunningham FG, Haugh JC, Wenstrom KC, *et al.* (eds) *William's Obstetrics* (22nd ed). New York: McGraw-Hill; 2008.
15. Creanga AA, Sabel JC, Ko JY, *et al.* Maternal drug use and its effect on neonates: a population-based study in Washington State. *Obstet Gynecol* 2012; 119(5):924–33.
16. Advisory Council on the Misuse of Drugs. *Hidden Harm: Responding to the Needs of Children and Problem Drug Users.* London: Home Office; 2004. http://www.homeoffice.gov.uk/publications
17. Knisely JS, Spear ER, Green DJ, *et al.* Substance abuse patterns in pregnant women. *NIDA Res Monogr* 1991; 108:280–1.
18. Towers CV, Pircon RA, Nageotte MP, *et al.* Cocaine intoxication presenting as pre-eclampsia and eclampsia. *Obstet Gynecol* 1993; 81:545–7.
19. Chasnoff IJ, McGourty RF, Bailey GF, *et al.* The 4P's Plus screen for substance abuse in pregnancy: clinical application and outcomes. *J Perinatol* 2005; 25(6):368–74.
20. Working Group on Problematic Substance Use in Pregnancy. Substance use in pregnancy. *J Obstet Gynaecol Can* 2011; 33(4):367–84.
21. Moran S, Thorndike AN, Armstrong K, *et al.* Physicians' missed opportunities to address tobacco use during prenatal care. *Nicotine Tob Res* 2003; 5: 363–8.
22. Chappel JN, Schnoll SH. Physician attitudes. Effect on the treatment of chemically dependent patients. *JAMA* 1977; 237:2318–19.
23. Fisher JC, Keeley KA, Mason RL, *et al.* Physicians and alcoholics. Factors affecting attitudes of family-practice residents toward alcoholics. *J Stud Alcohol* 1975; 36:626–33.
24. Hartmann KE, Wechter ME, Payne P, *et al.* Best practice smoking cessation intervention and resource needs of prenatal care providers. *Obstet Gynecol* 2007; 110:765–70.
25. Jordan TR, Dake JA, Price JH. Best practices for smoking cessation in pregnancy: do obstetrician/gynecologists use them in practice? *J Womens Health* 2006; 15:400–41.
26. Ewing JA. Detecting alcoholism: the CAGE questionnaire. *JAMA* 1984; 252:1905–7.
27. Benderskey M, Alessandri S, Gilbert P, *et al.* Characteristics of pregnant substance abusers in two cities in the northeast. *Am J Drug Alcohol Abuse* 1996; 22:349–62.
28. Foley E. Drug screening and criminal prosecution of pregnant women. *J Obstet Gynecol Neonatal Nurs* 2002; 31:133–7.
29. Lester BM, ElSohly M, Wright LL, *et al.* The Maternal Lifestyle Study: drug use by mecoium toxicology and maternal self-report. *Pediatrics* 2001; 107(2):309–17.

30. Ostrea EM, Brady M, Gause S, *et al.* Drug screening of newborns by meconium analysis: a large-scale, prospective, epidemiologic study. *Pediatrics* 1992; 89:107–13.
31. Sanaullah F, Gillian M, Lavin T. Screening of substance misuse during early pregnancy in Blyth: an anonymous unlinked study. *J Obstet Gynaecol* 2006; 26:187–90.
32. Sherwood RA, Keating J, Kavvadia V, *et al.* Substance misuse in early pregnancy and relationship to fetal outcome. *Eur J Pediatr* 1999; 158:488–92.
33. Birnbach DJ. Identification of polysubstance abuse in the parturient. *Br J Anaesth* 2001; 87(3):488–90.
34. Tsanaclis L, Wicks JFC. Patients in drug use in the United Kingdom as revealed through analysis of hair in a large population sample. *Forensic Sci Int* 2007; 170:121–8.
35. Department of Health. *Smoking Kills: A White Paper on Tobacco.* London: Department of Health; 1998.
36. Health and Social Care Information Centre. *Health Survey for England 2011.* 2012. [Online] http://www.ic.nhs.uk/pubs/hse11report
37. Information Services Division (ISD) Scotland. *Births in Scottish Hospitals—Year Ending 31st March 2013.* 26th August 2014. [Online] http://www.isdscotland.org
38. Cnattingius S. The epidemiology of smoking during pregnancy: smoking prevalence, maternal characteristics, and pregnancy outcomes. *Nicotine Tob Res* 2004; 6(S2):S125–S140.
39. Richmond R. You've come a long way baby: women and the tobacco epidemic. *Addiction* 2003; 98:553–7.
40. US Department of Health and Human Services. *The Health Consequences of Smoking. 2004 Surgeon General's Report.* Washington, DC: US Department of Health and Human Services; 2004.
41. Information Services Division (ISD) Scotland. *Births in Scottish Hospitals—Year Ending 31st March 2013.* 26th August 2014. [Online] http://www.isdscotland.org
42. Blalock JA, Fouladi RT, Wetter DW, *et al.* Depression in pregnant women seeking smoking cessation treatment. *Addict Behav* 2005; 30(6):1195–208.
43. Prager K, Malin H, Spiegler D, *et al.* Smoking and drinking behaviour before and during pregnancy of married mothers of live-born infants and stillborn infants. *Publ Health Rep* 1984; 99:117–27.
44. Suplee PD. The importance of providing smoking relapse counselling during the postpartum hospitalization. *J Obstet Gynecol Neonatal Nurs* 2005; 34(6):703–12.
45. Lumley J, Chamberlain C, Dowswell T, *et al.* Interventions for promoting smoking cessation during pregnancy. *Cochrane Database Sys Rev* 2009; 3:CD001055.
46. Conde-Agudelo A, Althabe F, Belizan JM, *et al.* Cigarette smoking during pregnancy and risk of preeclampsia: a systematic review. *Am J Obstet Gynecol* 1999; 181:1026–35.
47. Broughton-Pipkin F. Smoking in moderate/severe pre-eclampsia worsens pregnancy outcome, but smoking cessation limits the damage. *Hypertension* 2008; 51(4, part 2) Suppl:1042–6.
48. Tsuyoshi Nakamoto T, Yasuda K, Yasuhara M, *et al.* Cigarette smoke extract enhances oxytocin-induced rhythmic contractions of rat and human preterm myometrium. *Reproduction* 2006; 132:343–53.
49. Naeye RL. Abruptio placentae and placenta previa: frequency, perinatal mortality, and cigarette smoking. *Obstet Gynecol* 1980; 55:701–4.
50. Corradino ML, Raju L. Pregnancy and chronic obstructive pulmonary disease. *Chest* 1981; 80:759–61.
51. Economides D, Braithwaite J. Smoking, pregnancy and the fetus. *J R Soc Health* 1994; 114:198–201.
52. Luciano A, Bolognani M, Biondani P, *et al.* The influence of maternal passive and light active smoking on intrauterine growth and body composition of the newborn. *Eur J Clin Nutr* 1998; 52:760–3.
53. Van der Veen F, Fox H. The effects of cigarette smoking on the human placenta: a light and electron microscopic study. *Placenta* 1982; 3:243–56.
54. Bernstein IM, Mongeon JA, Badger GJ, *et al.* Maternal smoking and its association with birth weight. *Obstet Gynaecol* 2005; 106 (5, Part 1):986–91.
55. Barker DJ, Gluckman PD, Godfrey KM, *et al.* Fetal nutrition and cardiovascular diseases in adult life. *Lancet* 1993; 341:938–41.
56. Lee LJ, Lupo PJ. Maternal smoking during pregnancy and the risk of congenital heart defects in offspring: a systematic review and metaanalysis. *Pediatr Cardiol* 2013; 34(2):398–407.
57. Leonardi-Bee J, Britton J, Venn A. Secondhand smoke and adverse fetal outcomes in nonsmoking pregnant women: a meta-analysis. *Pediatrics* 2011; 127(4):734–41.
58. Egan TD, Wong KC. Perioperative smoking cessation and anaesthesia. *J Clin Anaesth* 1992; 4:63–72.
59. Shapiro RE. Caffeine and headaches. *Curr Pain Headache Rep* 2008; 12(4):311–15.
60. Matchar DB, Young WB, Rosenberg JH, *et al.* *Evidence-Based Guidelines for Migraine Headache in the Primary Care Setting: Pharmacological Management of Acute Attacks.* St. Paul, MN: American Academy of Neurology; 2001. http://www.aan.com
61. Christian MS, Brent RL. Teratogen update: evaluation of the reproductive and developmental risks of caffeine. *Teratology* 2001; 61(1):51–78.
62. Bech BH, Obel C, Henriksen TB, *et al.* Effect of reducing caffeine intake on birth weight and length of gestation: randomised controlled trial. *BMJ* 2007; 334(7590):409.
63. Maslova E, Bhattacharya S, Lin SW, *et al.* Caffeine consumption during pregnancy and risk of preterm birth: a meta-analysis. *Am J Clin Nutr* 2010; 92(5):1120–32.
64. Wisborg K, Kesmodel U, Bech BH, *et al.* Maternal consumption of coffee during pregnancy and stillbirth and infant death in first year of life: a prospective study. *BMJ* 2003; 326(7386):420.
65. Schmidt B, Roberts RS, Davis P, *et al.* Caffeine therapy for apnea of prematurity. *N Engl J Med* 2006; 354(20):2112–21.
66. Fennelly M, Galletly DC, Purdie GI. Is caffeine withdrawal the mechanism of postoperative headache? *Anesth Analg* 1991; 72:449–53.
67. BasurtoOna X, Martínez García L, Solà I, *et al.* Drug therapy for treating post-dural puncture headache. *Cochrane Database Syst Rev* 2011; 8:CD007887.
68. Camann WR, Murray RS, Mushlin PS, *et al.* Effects of oral caffeine on postdural puncture headache. A double-blind, placebo-controlled trial. *Anesth Anal* 1990; 70:181–4.
69. Day N, Jasperse D, Richardson G, *et al.* Prenatal exposure to alcohol. Effect on infant growth and morphological characteristics. *Pediatrics* 1989; 84:536.
70. Stade BC, Bailey C, Dzendoletas D, *et al.* Psychological and/or educational interventions for reducing alcohol consumption in pregnant women and women planning pregnancy. *Cochrane Database Syst Rev* 2009; 2:CD004228.
71. Andres RL. Effects of therapeutic, diagnostic, and environmental agents and exposure to social and illicit drugs. In Creasy RK, Resnik R (eds) *Maternal-Fetal Medicine* (5th ed). Philadelphia, PA: Saunders; 2003:281–314.
72. Stewart S, Jones D, Day CP. Alcoholic liver disease: new insights into mechanisms and preventative strategies. *Trends Mol Med* 2001; 7:408–13.
73. Rouault TA. Hepatic iron overload in alcoholic liver disease: why does it occur and what is its role in pathogenesis? *Alcohol* 2003; 30:103–6.
74. Gramenzi A, Caputo F, Biselli M, *et al.* Review article: alcoholic liver disease—pathophysiological aspects and risk factors. *Aliment Pharmacol Ther* 2006; 24:1151–61.
75. Beattie MC, Longabaugh R, Elliott G, *et al.* Effect of the social environment on alcohol involvement and subjective well-being prior to alcoholism treatment. *J Stud Alcohol* 1993; 54:283–96.
76. Newman LM. The chemically dependent parturient. *Sem Anesth* 1992; 11:66–75.
77. Abel EL. An update on the incidence of FAS: FAS is not an equal opportunity birth defect. *Neurotoxicol Teratol* 1995; 17:437–43.

78. Abel EL, Hannigan JH. Maternal risk factors in fetal alcohol syndrome: provocative and permissive influences. *Neurotoxicol Teratol* 1995; 17:445–62.
79. National Institute on Alcohol Abuse and Alcoholism. *Alcohol Alert: Fetal Alcohol Exposure and the Brain.* Bethesda, MD: National Institute on Alcohol Abuse and Alcoholism; 2000.
80. Chiaffarino F, Parazzini F, Chatenoud L, *et al.* Alcohol drinking and risk of small for gestational age birth. *Sur J Clin Nutr* 2006; 60(9):1062–6.
81. Kesmodel U, Wisborg K, Olsen SF, *et al.* Moderate alcohol intake during prenancy and the risk of stillbirth and death in the first year of life. *Am J Epidemiol* 2002; 155(4):305–12.
82. Konovalov HV, Kovetsky NS, Bobryshev YV, *et al.* Disorders of brain development in the progeny of mothers who used alcohol during pregnancy. *Early Hum Dev* 1997; 48:153–66.
83. Sokol RJ, Delaney-Black V, Nordstrom B. Fetal alcohol spectrum disorder. *J Am Med Assoc* 2003; 290:2996–9.
84. Council on Scientific Affairs, American Medical Association. Fetal effects of maternal alcohol abuse. *JAMA* 1983; 249: 2517–21.
85. Chopra K, Tiwari V. Alcoholic neuropathy: possible mechanisms and future treatment possibilities. *Br J Clin Pharmacol* 2012; 73(3): 348–62.
86. Swerdlow BN, Holley FO, Maitre PI, *et al.* Chronic alcohol intake does not change thiopental anesthetic requirement, pharmacokinetics, or pharmacodynamics. *Anesthesiology* 1990; 72:455–61.
87. Fassoulaki A, Farinotti R, Servin F, *et al.* Chronic alcoholism increases the induction dose of propofol in humans. *Anesth Analg* 1993; 77(3):553–6.
88. Morton A. Pregnancy outcome in a mother with alcoholic cardiomyopathy. *Aust N Z J Obstet Gynaecol* 2005; 45:328–30.
89. National Institute on Drug Abuse. *National Pregnancy and Health Survey: Drug Use Among Women Delivering Live Births.* Rockville, MD: National Clearing House for Drug and Alcohol Information; 1992.
90. Bell GL, Lau K. Perinatal and neonatal issues of substance abuse. *Pediatr Clin North Am* 1995; 42:261–81.
91. Zuckerman B, Frank DA, Hingson R, *et al.* Effects of maternal marijuana and cocaine use on fetal growth. *N Engl J Med* 1989; 320:762–8.
92. Westfall RE, Janssen PA, Lucas P, *et al.* Survey of medicinal cannabis use among childbearing women: patterns of its use in pregnancy and retroactive self-assessment of its efficacy against "morning sickness". *Comp Ther Clin Pract* 2006; 12:27–33.
93. Kline J, Hutzler M, Levin B, *et al.* Marijuana and spontaneous abortion of known karyotype. *Paediatr Perinat Epidemiol* 1991; 320:5.
94. Kozer E, Koren G. Effects of prenatal exposure to marijuana. *Can Fam Physician* 2001; 47:263–4.
95. Goldschmidt L, Richardson GA, Willford J, *et al.* Prenatal marijuana exposure and intelligence test performance at age 6. *J Am Acad Child Adolesc Psychiatry* 2008; 47(3):254–63.
96. Robison LL, Buckley JD, Daigle AE, *et al.* Maternal drug use and risk of childhood nonlymphoblastic leukaemia among offspring. An epidemiological investigation implicating marijuana (a report from the children's Cancer Study Group). *Cancer* 1989; 63:1904–11.
97. Pertwee RG. Tolerance to and dependence on psychotropic cannabinoids. In Pratt JA (ed) *The Biological Basis of Drug Tolerance and Dependence.* New York: Academic Press; 1991:232–63.
98. Department of Health and Human Services HHS News. *Monitoring the Future Survey Release. Smoking Among Teenagers Decreases Sharply and Increase in Ecstasy Use Slows.* [Online] http://archives.drugabuse.gov/newsroom/01/NR12-19.html
99. Meadows R, Verghese A. Medical complications of glue sniffing. *South Med J* 1996; 89:455–62.
100. Filley CM, Halliday W, Kleinschmidt-DeMasters BK. The effects of toluene on the cemtral nervous system. *J Neuropathol Exp Neurol* 2004; 63:1–12.
101. Murata K, Araki S, Yokoyama K, *et al.* Changes in autonomic function as determined by ECG P-R interval variability in sandal, shoe and leather workers exposed to n-hexane, xylene and toluene. *Neurotoxicology* 1994; 15:867–75.
102. Cunningham SR, Dalzell GWN, McGirr P, *et al.* Myocardial infarction and primary ventricular fibrillation after glue sniffing. *Br Med J* 1987; 294:739–40.
103. Reyes de la Rocha S, Brown MA, *et al.* Pulmonary function abnormalities in intentional spray paint inhalation. *Chest* 1987; 92:100–10.
104. Hannigan JH, Bowen SE. Reproductive toxicology and teratology of abused toluene. *Syst Biol Reprod Med* 2010; 56(2):184–200.
105. Jones HE, Balster RL. Inhalant abuse in pregnancy. *Obstet Gynecol Clin North Am* 1998; 25(1):153–67.
106. Booth MG, Hood J, Brooks TJ, *et al.* Anthrax infection in drug users. *Lancet* 2010; 375:1345–6.
107. Brett MB, Hallas G, Mpamugo O. Wound botulism in the UK and Ireland. *J Med Microbiol* 2004; 53:555–61.
108. Morrison GA, Lang C, Huda S. Botulism in a pregnant intravenous drug abuser. *Anaesthesia* 2006; 61:57–60.
109. Beeching NJ, Crowcroft NS. Tetanus in injecting drug users. *BMJ* 2005; 330:208–9.
110. Brett MM, Hood J, Brazier JS, *et al.* Soft tissue infections caused by spore-forming bacteria in injecting drug users in the United Kingdom. *Epidemiol Infect* 2005; 133(4):575–82.
111. Heil SH, Jones HE, Arria A, *et al.* Unintended pregnancy in opioid abusing women. *J Subst Abuse Treat* 2011; 40:199–202.
112. Department of Health (England), The Scottish Government, Welsh Assembly Government, *et al. Drug Misuse and Dependence: UK Guidelines on Clinical Management.* 2007. [Online] http://ww.smmgp.org.uk
113. Alford D, Compton P, Samet J. Acute pain management for patients receiving maintenance methadone or buprenorphine therapy. *Ann Intern Med* 2006; 144:127–34.
114. Lovell, A. Addiction markets. The case of high-dose buprenorphine in France. In Petryna A, Lakoff A, Kleinman A (eds) *Global Pharmaseuticals. Ethics, Markets, Practices.* Durham, NC: Duke University Press; 2006.
115. Fajemirokun-Odudeyi O, Sinha C, Tutty S, *et al.* Pregnancy outcome in women who use opiates. *Eur J Obstet Gynecol Reprod Biol* 2006; 126(2):170–5.
116. Jones H, Johnson RE, Jasinski DR, *et al.* Buprenorphine versus methadone in the treatment of pregnant opioid dependent patients: effects on the neonatal abstinence syndrome. *Drug Alcohol Depend* 2005; 79:1–10.
117. Jones HE, Kaltenbach K, Heil SH, *et al.* Neonatal abstinence syndrome after methadone or buprenorphine exposure. *N Engl J Med* 2010; 363:2320–31.
118. Hulse GK, Milne E, English DR, *et al.* The relationship between maternal use of heroin and methadone and infant birth weight. *Addiction* 1997; 92:1571.
119. Naeye RL, Blanc W, LeBlanc W, *et al.* Fetal complications of maternal heroin addiction: abnormal growth, infections and episodes of stress. *J Pediatr* 1973; 83:1055–61.
120. Minozzi S, Amato L, Vecchi S, *et al.* Maintenance agonist treatments for opiate dependent pregnant women. *Cochrane Database Syst Rev* 2008; 2:CD006318.
121. Winklbaur B, Kopf N, Ebner N, *et al.* Treating pregnant women dependent on opioids is not the same as treating pregnancy and opioid dependence: a knowledge synthesis for better treatment for women and neonates. *Addiction* 2008; 103:1429–40.
122. Osborn DA, Jeffery HE, Cole MJ. Sedatives for opiate withdrawal in newborn infants. *Cochrane Database Syst Rev* 2010; 10:CD002053.
123. Doberczak TM, Kandall SR, Wilets I. Neonatal opiate abstinence syndrome in term and preterm infants. *J Pediatr* 1991; 118:933–7.
124. Jones HE, Martin PR, Heil SH, *et al.* Treatment of opioid-dependent pregnant women: clinical and research issues. *J Subst Abuse Treat* 2008; 35:245–59.

125. Kahila H, Saisto T, Kivitie-Kallio S, *et al.* A prospective study on buprenorphine use during pregnancy: effects on maternal and neonatal outcome. *Acta Obstet Gynecol* 2007; 86:185–90.
126. Kaltenbach K, Berghella V, Finnegan L. Opioid dependence during pregnancy: effects and management. *Obstet Gynecol Clin North Am* 1998; 25:139–51.
127. Dryden C, Young D, Hepburn M, *et al.* Maternal methadone use in pregnancy: factors associated with the development of neonatal abstinence syndrome and implications for healthcare resources. *BJOG* 200; 9; 116(5):665–71.
128. Mehta V, Langford RM. Acute pain management for opioid dependent patients. *Anesthesia* 2006; 61:269–76.
129. Kehlet H, Dahl JB. The value of "multimodal" or "balanced analgesia" in postoperative pain treatment. *Anesth Analg* 1993; 77:1048–56.
130. Jones HE, O'Grady K, Dahne J, *et al.* Management of acute postpartum pain in patients maintained on methadone or buprenorphine during pregnancy. *Am J Drug Alcohol Abuse* 2009; 35:151–6.
131. White JM. Pleasure into pain: the consequences of long-term opioid use. *Addict Behav* 2004; 29:1311–24.
132. Cowan, A. Update of the general pharmacology of buprenorphine. In Lewis J, Cowan A (eds) *Buprenorphine: Combating Drug Abuse with a Unique Opioid.* New York: Wiley; 1995:31–47.
133. Guise JM. Anticipating and responding to obstetric emergencies. *Best Pract Res Clin Obstet Gynaecol* 2001; 21:625–38.
134. National Institute for Clinical Excellence. *Guidance on the Use of Ultrasound Locating Devices for Placing Central Venous Catheters.* Technology Appraisal Guidance No 49. London: NICE; 2002.
135. Gress SC, Murthi SB, Sisley AC, *et al.* Ultrasound-guided peripheral intravenous access in the intensive care unit. *J Crit Care* 2010; 25(3):514–9.
136. Paxton JH, Knuth TE, Klausner A. Proximal humerus intraosseous infusion: a preferred emergency venous access. *J Trauma Injury Infect Crit Care* 2009; 67(3):606–11.
137. Chatterjee DJ, Bukunola B, Samuels TL, *et al.* Resuscitation in massive obstetric haemorrhage using an intraosseous needle. *Anaesthesia* 2011; 66:306–10.
138. European Resuscitation Council. European resuscitation guidelines. *Resuscitation* 2005 6751:51–2.
139. AAGBI. Blood transfusion and the anaesthetist: management of massive haemorrhage. *Anaesthesia* 2010; 65:1153–61.
140. Junkin R, Selfridge J, Litchfield K. Intraosseous vascular access in obstetric emergencies: an OAA approved national survey. *Int J Obstet Anaesth* 2013; 22:S31.
141. Junkin R, Litchfield K. Intraosseous vascular access skill acquisition in labour ward staff: results of a training programme. *Int J Obstet Anaesth* 2013; 22:S31.
142. Lucas DN, Yentis SM, Kinsella SM, *et al.* Urgency of caesarean section: a new classification. *J R Soc Med* 2000; 93:346–50.
143. Kuczkowski KM. Labour analgesia for the drug abusing parturient: is there cause for concern? *Obstet Gynecol Surv* 2003; 58:599–608.
144. Hatsukami DK, Fischman MW: Crack cocaine and cocaine hydrochloride. Are the differences myth or reality? *JAMA* 1996; 276:1580–8.
145. World Health Organization. *Neuroscience of Psychoactive Substance Use and Dependence.* Geneva: World Health Organization; 2004. http://www.who.int/substance_abuse/publications/en/Neuroscience_E.pdf
146. Burkett G, Yasin SY, Palow D, *et al.* Patterns of cocaine binging: effect on pregnancy. *Am J Obstet Gynaecol* 1994; 171(2):372–8.
147. Dombrowski MP, Wolfe HM, Welch RA, *et al.* Cocaine abuse is associated with abruptio placentae and decreased birth weight, but not shorter labor. *Obstet Gynecol* 1991; 77:130–41.
148. Mbah AK, Alio AP, Fombo DW, *et al.* Association between cocaine abuse in pregnancy and placenta-associated syndromes using propensity score matching approach. *Early Hum Dev* 2012; 88(6):333–7.
149. Hsu CD, Chen S, Feng TI, *et al.* Rupture of uterine scar with extensive maternal bladder laceration after cocaine abuse. *Am J Obstet Gynecol* 1992; 167(1):129–30.
150. Gonsoulin W, Borge D, Moise KJ Jr. Rupture of unscarred uterus in primigravid woman in association with cocaine abuse. *Am J Obstet Gynecol* 1990; 163(2):526–7.
151. Moen MD, Caliendo MJ, Marshall W, *et al.* Hepatic rupture in pregnancy associated with cocaine use. *Obstet Gynecol* 1993; 82:687–9.
152. Lampley EC, Williams S, Myers SA. Cocaine-associated rhabdomyolysis causing renal failure in pregnancy. *Obstet Gynecol* 1996; 87(5 Pt 2):804–6.
153. Mercado A, Johnson G Jr, Calver D, *et al.* Cocaine, pregnancy, and postpartum intracerebral haemorrhage. *Obstet Gynecol* 1989; 73(3 Pt 2):467–8.
154. Burkett G, Bandstra ES, Cohen J, *et al.* Cocaine-related maternal death. *Am J Obstet Gynecol* 1990; 163(1 Pt 1):40–1.
155. Plessinger MA, Woods JR Jr. Maternal, placental, and fetal pathophysiology of cocaine exposure during pregnancy. *Clin Obstet Gynecol* 1993; 36:267–78.
156. Lange RA, Hillis LD. Cardiovascular complications of cocaine use. *N Engl J Med* 2001; 345:351–8.
157. Towers CV, Pircon RA, Nageotte MP, *et al.* Cocaine intoxication presenting as pre-eclampsia and eclampsia. *Obstet Gybecol* 1993; 81(4):545–7.
158. Maagdenberg T, Savci S, Iffy L. Cocaine intoxication mimicking preeclampsia postpartum. *Int J Gynecol Obstet* 2006; 92:73–4.
159. Klein AM, Loder E. Postpartum headache. *Int J Obstet Anaesth* 2010; 19:422–30.
160. Krishna RB, Levitz M, Dancis J. Transfer of cocaine by the perfused human placenta: the effect of binding to serum proteins. *Am J Obstet Gynecol* 1993; 169:1418–23.
161. Frank DA, Augustyn M, Knight WG, *et al.* Growth, development and behavior in early childhood following prenatal cocaine exposure: a systematic review. *JAMA* 2001; 285(12):1613–25.
162. Slutsker L. Risks associated with cocaine use during pregnancy. *Obstet Gynecol* 1992; 79 (5 Pt 1):778–89.
163. Gouin K, Murphy K, Shah PS, *et al.* Effects of cocaine use during pregnancy on low birth weight and preterm birth: a systematic review and meta-analysis. *Am J Obstet Gynecol* 2011; 204(4):340.e1–12.
164. Singer LT, Arendt R, Minnes S, *et al.* Cognitive and motor outcomes of cocaine-exposed infants. *JAMA* 2002; 287(15):1952–60.
165. Bada HS, Das A, Bauer CR, *et al.* Impact of prenatal cocaine exposure on child behavior problems through school age. *Pediatrics* 2007; 119(2):e348–59.
166. Oyler J, Darwin WD, Preston KL, *et al.* Cocaine disposition in the meconium from newborns of cocaine-abusing mothers and urine of adult drug users. *J Analyt Toxicol* 1996; 20:453–62.
167. Ebrahim SH, Gfroerer J. Pregnancy-related substance use in the United States during 1996–1998. *Obstet Gynecol* 2003; 101:374–9.
168. Gowda RM, Khan IA, Mehta NJ, *et al.* Cardiac arrhythmias in pregnancy: clinical and therapeutic considerations. *Int J Cardiol* 2003; 88:129–33.
169. Kreek MJ. Cocaine, dopamine and the endogenous opioid system. *J Addict Dis* 1996; 15:73–96.
170. Kuczkowski KM, Birnbach DJ, van Zundert A. Drug abuse in the parturient. *Semin Anesth Periop Med Pain* 2000; 19:216–24.
171. Kuczkowski KM. Caesarean section in a cocaine-intoxicated parturient: regional vs. general anesthesia? *Anaesthesia* 2003; 58:1042–3.
172. Vertommen JD, Hughes SC, Rosen MA, *et al.* Hydralazine does not restore uterine blood flow during cocaine-induced hypertension in the pregnant ewe. *Anesthesiology* 1992; 76:580–7.
173. Lange RA, Hillis LD. Cardiovascular complications of cocaine use. *N Engl J Med* 2001; 345:351–8.
174. Gay GR, Loper KA. The use of labetalol in the management of cocaine crisis. *Ann Emerg Med* 1988; 17:282–3.
175. European Monitoring Centre for Drugs and Drug Addiction (EMCDDA). *Problem Amphetamine and Methamphetamine Use*

in Europe. Selected Issue 2010. 2010. [Online] http://www.emcdda.europa.eu/publications/selected-issues/problem-amphetamine

176. Arria AM, Derauf C, Lagasse LL, *et al.* Methamphetamine and other substance use during pregnancy: preliminary estimates from the Infant Development, Environment, and Lifestyle (IDEAL) study. *Matern Child Health J* 2006; 10:293–302.
177. Cox S, Posner SF, Kourtis AP, *et al.* Hospitalizations with amphetamine abuse among pregnant women. *Obstet Gynecol* 2008; 111(2 Pt 1):341–7.
178. Uitermark J, Cohen P. Amphetamine users in Amsterdam: patterns of use and modes of self-regulation. *Addict Res Theory* 2006; 14 (2):159–88.
179. Angrist B, Corwin J, Bartlik B, *et al.* Early pharmacokinetics and clinical effects of oral D-amphetamine in normal subjects. *Biol Psychiatry* 1987; 22 (11):1357–68.
180. Peters A, Davies T, Richardson A. Increasing popularity of injection as the route of administration of amphetamine in Edinburgh. *Drug Alcohol Depend* 1997; 48(3):227–34.
181. Darke S, Hall W. Levels and correlates of polydrug use among heroin users and regular amphetamine users. *Drug Alcohol Depend* 1995; 39(3):231–5.
182. Wagner CL, Katikaneni LD, Cox TH, *et al.* The impact of prenatal drug exposure on the neonate. *Obstet Gynecol Clinic North Am* 1998; 25:169–94.
183. Ramamoorthy JD, Ramamoorthy S, Leibach FH, *et al.* Human placental monoamine transporters as targets for amphetamines. *Am J Obstet Gynecol* 1995; 173:1782–7.
184. Good MM. Methamphetamine use during pregnancy: maternal and neonatal implications. *Obstet Gynecol* 2010; 116 (2 Pt 1):330–4.
185. McFarlane J, Parker B, Soeken K. Physical abuse, smoking, and substance use during pregnancy: prevalence, interrelationships, and effects on birth weight. *J Obstet Gynecol Neonatal Nurs* 1996 25:313–20.
186. Gillogley KM, Evans AT, Hansen RL, *et al.* The perinatal impact of cocaine, amphetamine, and opiate use detected by universal intrapartum screening. *Am J Obstet Gynecol* 1990; 163:1535–42.
187. Ladhani NN, Shah PS, Murphy KE. Prenatal ampheatamine exposure and birth outcomes: a systematic review and metaanalysis. *Am J Obstet Gynecol* 2001; 205(3):219.e1–7.
188. Smith LM, LaGasse LL, Derauf C, *et al.* The infant development, environment, and lifestyle study: effects of prenatal metamphetamine exposure, polydrug exposure and poverty on intrauterine growth. *Pediatrics* 2006; 118:1149–56.
189. Cernerud L, Eriksson M, Jonsson B, *et al.* Amphetamine addiction during pregnancy: 14-year follow-up of growth and school performance. *Acta Paediatr* 1996; 85:204–8.
190. Billing L, Eriksson M, Jonsson B, *et al.* The influence of environmental factors on behavioural problems in 8-year-old children exposed to amphetamine during fetal life. *Child Abuse Negl* 1994; 18:3–9.
191. Chomchai C, Na Manorom N, Watanarungsan P, *et al.* Methamphetamine abuse during pregnancy and its health impact on neonates born at Siriraj Hospital, Bangkok, Thailand. *Southeast Asian J Trop Med Public Health* 2007; 35(1):228–31.
192. Winslow BT, Voorhees KI, Pehl KA. Methamphetamine abuse. *Am Fam Physician* 2007; 76 (8):1169–74.
193. Ludlow JP, Evans SF, Hulse G. Obstetric and perinatal outcomes in pregnancies associated with illicit substance abuse. *Aust N Z J Obstet Gynaecol* 2004; 44: 302–6.
194. Furara SA, Carrick P, Armstrong D, *et al.* The outcome of pregnancy associated with amphetamine use. *J Obstet Gynaecol* 1999; 19:377–80.
195. Stewart JL, Mecker JE. Fetal and infant deaths associated with maternal methamphetamine abuse. *J Anal Toxicol* 1997; 21:515–17.
196. Phupong V, Darojn D. Amphetamine abuse in pregnancy: the impact on obstetric outcome. *Arch Gynecol Obstet* 2007; 276:167–70.

PART 10

Recent advances in obstetric anaesthesia

CHAPTER 52

Genetics

Ruth Landau and Clemens Ortner

Introduction

Since the completion of the Human Genome Project over a decade ago, the medical community has been somewhat disillusioned after the promise that pharmacogenomics would transform their practice and result in personalized medicine.[1–4] Undeniably, recommendations based on pharmacogenetic testing to ensure effective and safe analgesia and anaesthesia are still awaited. The National Institutes of Health's Pharmacogenetics Research Network developed a Pharmacogenomics Knowledge Base (PharmGKB)[5] with the goal 'to collect, encode, and disseminate knowledge about the impact of human genetic variations on drug response, curate primary genotype and phenotype data, annotate gene variants and gene–drug–disease relationships via literature review, and summarize important pharmacogenetic genes and drug pathways'. In line with their goals, the Clinical Pharmacogenetics Implementation Consortium (CPIC)[6] was launched in 2011 to establish clinical recommendations for dosing based on genetic testing providing information on genotype–test interpretations and on the scientific evidence supporting the evidence of these tests. Since its inception, genetic/drug dosing guidelines have been established for eight different drugs, out of which only codeine prescription according to cytochrome P450 (CYP)-2D6 genotype[7] may be relevant to the practice of anaesthetists, pain doctors, paediatricians, obstetricians, or perinatologists.

This chapter describes a selection of association studies that have examined the contribution of genetics to (1) preterm labour and the progression of labour, (2) labour analgesia, (3) haemodynamics and vasopressor response during spinal anaesthesia for caesarean delivery, and (4) post-caesarean pain and analgesic response to opioids. Numerous genes influence the overall experience of labour and delivery, but we will focus on the most well-studied genes in the clinical context of obstetric anaesthesia and perinatology: the μ-opioid receptor gene (*OPRM1*), the catechol-*O*-methyltransferase gene (*COMT*), the β_2 adrenergic receptor gene (*ADRB2*), the oxytocin receptor gene (*OXTR*), the ATP-binding cassette, subfamily B, member 1 (*ABCB1*) gene, and the genetics of CYP2D6 metabolism (Table 52.1).

Preterm labour and the progression of labour

The influence of these genetic variants on preterm delivery, preterm labour, as well as the progress of labour has been the focus of several clinical studies in the last decade. The preterm birth phenotype is defined as having five components (maternal conditions that are present before presentation for delivery, fetal conditions that are present before presentation for delivery, placental pathological conditions, signs of the initiation of parturition, and the pathway to delivery),[8] therefore the exact contribution and the weight carried by each genetic variants is probably not very high and remains to be determined.

The beta-2 (β_2)-adrenergic receptor gene (*ADRB2*) and in particular two common polymorphisms found in strong linkage disequilibrium, p.16Arg/Gly and p.27Gln/Glu, have been extensively evaluated in a number of anaesthesia-related studies with relevant clinical effects described in the context of airway responsiveness[9] and cardiac perioperative outcomes.[10] All in all, these two single nucleotide polymorphisms (SNPs) have been studied over the last decade in only a handful of reports evaluating uterine quiescence and the progression of labour.

Homozygosity for Arg16 of *ADRB2* was first shown to confer protection from preterm delivery in a small association study in a North American cohort [11], followed by other studies suggesting that the Glu27 variant of *ADRB2* increases the risk for preterm delivery.[12,13] Thereafter, the response to hexoprenaline, a β_2-agonist administered for tocolysis in a cohort of Swiss women diagnosed with idiopathic preterm labour between 24 and 34 weeks gestation, was found to be more effective in the presence of Arg16 homozygosity,[14] demonstrating a pharmacogenetic effect. This improved response to tocolysis had a significant impact on neonatal outcomes, with higher birth weights and fewer neonatal admissions to the intensive care unit for respiratory or other complications due to prematurity in babies born to mothers with that genotype.

In a larger trial evaluating the impact of *ADRB2* genotype/haplotype on preterm labour, a subanalysis confirmed the hypothesis that Arg16 homozygosity of *ADRB2* is associated with a slower rate of labour progress in successful term and late-preterm labour when compared to women with all other genotypes.[15] In this North American cohort, women Arg16Arg–Gln27Gln (double homozygous) progressed at the slowest rate of active labour ('slow haplotype'), and women Gly16Gly–Glu27Glu (double homozygous) progressed with the fastest cervical rate ('fast haplotype').

Using the previously validated non-linear mixed effects modelling (NONMEM) to predict the pain and labour progress of the first stage of labour in nulliparous women, another smaller study from the same North American group, to evaluate the effect of *ADRB2* and *OPRM1* genotypes on the progress of labour and labour pain demonstrated that women homozygous for the variant Gln27 allele had a slower transition into the active phase labour, resulting in prolonged labour compared to women with the other genotypes.[16] Genotype was strongly correlated with

Table 52.1 Selected genes, genetic variants, and associated phenotype of interest to obstetric anaesthesia and perinatology

Gene	Variant	Phenotype	Anaesthetic and obstetric outcome	Reference
OPRM1	p.118A/G	Pain perception and response to opioids	Labour analgesia (G118 associated with decreased median effective dose of spinal fentanyl and epidural sufentanil)	40–43
			Post-caesarean analgesia (A118 associated with decreased IV PCA morphine use)	41,47,54
			Neonatal exposure to opioid (NAS) (neonatal G118 associated with shorter hospital stay and less medication)	69
COMT	p.472G/A (Val158Met)	Pain perception and response to opioids	Labour analgesia (Met158 associated with poor response to IV fentanyl)	43
			Neonatal exposure to opioid (NAS) (neonatal Val158 associated with shorter hospital stay and less medication)	69
		Uterine activity	Labour progress (rs4633 associated with slow labour progress)	17
ADRB2	Arg16Gly–Gln27Glu	Uterine activity	Preterm labour and delivery (Arg16 associated with protection from preterm delivery; Glu27 associated with increased risk for preterm delivery)	11-13
			Tocolysis efficacy (β_2-agonist) (Arg16 associated with better response to β_2-agonist tocolysis)	14
			Labour progress (Arg16–Gln27 associated with slow labour progress)	15-17
		Response to ephedrine	Spinal hypotension during caesarean (Gly16–Glu27 associated with increased response to ephedrine)	64–66
			Neonatal acidosis (neonatal Arg16 associated with protection from ephedrine-induced neonatal acidosis)	64
OXTR	rs53576 A/G	Uterine activity	Labour progress (G allele at rs53576 associated with slower progress of labour)	17
ABCB1	p.1236C/T p.2677T/A p.3435C/T	Pain perception and response to opioids	Chronic post-caesarean pain (T allele of C3435T associated with increased trend for chronic post-caesarean pain)	61
			Neonatal exposure to opioid (NAS) (no impact of neonatal *ABCB1* genotype on hospital stay)	69
CYP2D6	PM/IM/EM/UM	Drug metabolism	Neonatal exposure to codeine (Maternal CYP2D UM associated with neonatal death due to morphine overdose)	7,75,78–80,83,86

NAS, neonatal abstinence syndrome; PCA, patient-controlled analgesia.
Data from various sources (see references).

ethnicity (none of the Asian women included in the study were Glu27 homozygous), and labour was indeed found to be slower among Asians. The study was underpowered to detect an effect of *OPRM1* genotype on labour pain, but identified that cold sensitivity was the pain modality that may predict the intensity of labour pain.

Using the same model to evaluate the progression of labour, eight SNPs in three different genes, *ADRB2, COMT*, and *OXTR* were examined in a cohort of 233 Saudi Arabian nulliparous women.[17] Three different SNPs of *COMT* were evaluated, and one of them (region sequence rs4633) along with one SNP of *OXTR* (region sequence rs53576) were associated with increased duration of the latent phase of first stage of labour, resulting in longer labours (in the order of 5 hours for *COMT* and 2 hours for *OXTR*). These findings contrast with results from other studies that found no effect of *OXTR* SNPs on the duration of first-stage labour[16] or risk of dystocia.[18] In addition, *ADRB2* genotype/haplotype was not associated with labour progress once demographic factors were accounted for. Data combining all the genetic variants (joined allelic combination) for each woman in the cohort was not reported, so one cannot infer the overall importance of a genetic contribution to the progress of labour.

Taken together, all studies evaluating obstetrical outcomes based on *ADRB2* genotype reported that women carrying Arg16 and/or Gln27 are conferred protection from preterm delivery and have a more 'quiescent' uterus, resulting at the time of labour and delivery in a slower progression and prolonged labour duration. Overall though, factors influencing the progress of labour are multiple, including ethnicity and maternal weight, and genetic variability, out of which *ADRB2* is only one of many candidate genes, is unlikely to contribute in a major manner.

A variety of genomic studies have examined the influence of genetic variants and validation of biomarkers to identify women at risk for preterm labour and delivery is ongoing.[19,20] On the other extreme of the clinical spectrum, a genome-wide scan study in Sweden has identified at least six loci that appear to contribute to the risk of women requiring a caesarean delivery for dystocia,[18] and further prospective studies will need to validate these findings.

Labour analgesia

Clearly, the pain of childbirth is the most severe pain most women will endure in their lifetimes.[21] Nonetheless, despite undeniable advances in our understanding of the physiology of labour pain that have resulted in the ability to provide safe and effective labour analgesia to the majority of women in the developed world, evaluating and measuring labour pain and the response to analgesia remains a remarkable challenge.[22] Therefore, it is no surprise when one realizes that a standard tool such as a numeric pain score, used in all clinical pain studies, does not capture very well the essence of labour pain. Other challenges that are specific to obstetric pain relate to the dynamic nature of labour and labour progress and the consequent changes in nociception that occur over time; pain of first-stage labour is conducted by thin afferent, *visceral* sympathetic fibres, entering the spinal cord at thoracic and lumbar roots (T10–L1) while second-stage labour pain is conducted via thicker *somatic* nerve fibres entering the spinal cord at sacral roots S2–4. The dynamic component of labour pain has been integrated in a recent mathematical modelling technique that attempts to integrate multiple parameters to predict the intensity of pain over the course of labour.[23] Nonetheless, one of the major hurdles in labour pain studies relies on the subjective, individual ability of women to quantify their pain during labour.

We have made numerous assumptions in our attempts to evaluate labour pain and women's response to labour analgesia. We have assumed that asking women to score their pain on a 0–10 scale would result in a meaningful and relevant response, that if women experienced severe pain they would request an epidural, that if women requested an epidural earlier in the process of labour they were surely hurting more than women requesting an epidural at a later stage in labour, that if women required more analgesic medication they may have a poorer response to analgesia, and finally that if women had not requested any medication, they either had better coping skills or hurt less. We have also assumed that we could accurately measure pain scores, average these scores for each woman enrolled in a study, that we could compare these averaged scores between women and infer into which category (more pain, less pain) women belong. Last, analysing and interpreting findings from such studies is a gruelling and perplexing task for the obstetric anaesthetist invested in evaluating labour pain and analgesia. Ultimately, obstetrical factors greatly influence the amount of medication and analgesia women will want to take and agree to receive, based on the belief that the ability to effectively push and deliver the baby may come at the expense of some discomfort and pain. Therefore, any study that has considered overall analgesic consumption during labour and delivery, whether by means of systemic opioids or neuraxial analgesia, as a surrogate to measure pain during childbirth is likely to be meaningless and misconstruing the complexity of the labour pain experience. Labour pain and analgesic requirements in the peripartum period may well be the most intricate pain phenotype to evaluate and surely requires multidimensional tools not yet widely utilized to evaluate obstetrical or acute postoperative pain as clinical models of acute pain. This may in part explain why genetic association studies that have attempted to predict the consumption of opioids in any clinical setting have been disappointing;[24] genotyping is probably useless if the phenotype cannot be well defined and measured.[25]

Among the myriad of candidate genes that have been considered important in opioid response, *OPRM1* is probably the most studied [26]. A common polymorphism of *OPRM1* is a single nucleotide substitution at position 118, with an adenine substitution by a guanine (p.118A/G) reported to occur with an allelic frequency of 10–30% among Caucasians,[27] a higher prevalence among Asians,[28] and a lower one in African Americans.[29] Despite numerous studies in the last two decades to identify the mechanism by which the altered receptor influences opioid analgesia, several hypothesis remain unconfirmed. *In vitro* studies have suggested that p.118A/G of *OPRM1* affects receptor binding characteristics[30,31] or messenger RNA expression levels;[32] however, under some experimental conditions no effect on function[33] or expression levels[34] was confirmed. In a recent humanized mouse model exploring signal transduction pathways that mediate opioid pharmacology, sensory neurons expressing G118 homozygosity displayed reduced morphine (but not fentanyl) potency and efficacy compared with the A118 homozygous version of the gene, suggesting an effect at the level of the sensory neurons.[35]

In a study evaluating the response to different experimental modalities in healthy individuals, there was no significant effect of *OPRM1* genotype on pain sensitivity in the entire sample, but when examining each ethnic group separately (Caucasians, Hispanics, and African Americans), a lower pain sensitivity was found among Caucasians carrying the G118 allele, while there was a trend in the opposite direction among Hispanics and no measurable effect among African Americans (the G allele is under-represented in this ethnicity); of note, there were no Asian women in that study.[36] Also, since the G118 variant allele is extremely common among Asians, studies comparing pain sensitivity between Caucasians and Asians will be of interest. It remains to be determined whether haplotype structure, gene–gene interactions, or DNA methylation[37] rather than the A118G genotype itself are key to explain these inter-ethnic differences in pain sensitivity; nonetheless this ethnicity-dependent genetic association may contribute to some of the discrepancies reported in clinical studies as underlined in the paragraphs that follow.

In a large cohort of Swedish women, labour pain-related behaviours, characterized by the cervical rate upon arrival in the labour room and the use of any type of analgesia (nitrous oxide, epidural, systemic opioids, and acupuncture) were not found to be associated with a particular genotype of *OPRM1*.[38] In other words, women did not seem to have different thresholds for labour pain or epidural request based on p.118A/G genotype, but the response to labour analgesia once provided was not evaluated. Of note though, the overall epidural rate was relatively low (30%) and the epidurals were placed at a relatively advanced stage in labour (at approximately 6 cm of cervical dilatation); therefore the lack of difference in epidural use is more likely to reflect a local clinical practice than a lack of genetic contribution. The same authors also reported that a previously described pain-protective haplotype related with three SNPs of the guanosine triphosphate cyclohydrolase gene (*GCH1*) did not appear to drastically alter labour pain-related behaviours.[39]

The first clinical study evaluating any genetic influence on labour pain and searching for a pharmacogenetic effect in response to labour analgesia is most likely the one conducted in a Swiss cohort of nulliparous women requesting neuraxial analgesia early in labour evaluating p.118A/G of *OPRM1*. Using the up-down sequential allocation model to identify differences in analgesic requirement according to A118G genotype, women carrying the less common G118 variant allele required substantially *lower* doses of spinal fentanyl, with a 1.5-fold difference compared to A118 homozygous women (Figure 52.1).[40] This finding was replicated with a different pharmacological study design using random-dose allocation, with a twofold difference between genetic groups.[40] Of note, cervical dilatation at the time of analgesia request was significantly *less* in A118 homozygous women than that in women carrying one or two variant alleles (A118G heterozygotes or G118 homozygotes). The finding of lower analgesic requirements at a more advanced stage in labour at the time of the analgesic request suggests that women carrying the G118 variant allele have a *higher* pain tolerance, which allows them to wait longer before requesting analgesia. This is of interest because women received the combined spinal–epidural analgesic when they requested pain relief, in other words at the time they experienced painful contractions. Since it has previously been demonstrated that epidural analgesic requirements increase with progress of labour and cervical dilatation, the expectation would be that women carrying the G118 allele should have greater analgesic requirements due to the greater cervical dilatation at which they requested analgesia; the finding that these women required *less* fentanyl may actually underestimate the true effect of genotype. Since provision of optimal labour analgesia remains an ongoing challenge for obstetric anaesthetists with minimal motor impairment and opioid-related side effects such as pruritus and fetal bradycardia (which appear to be dose dependent), this significant difference in median effective dose (ED_{50}) according to genotype may be relevant from a clinical standpoint. Therefore, one may presume that genotyping may well help improve the delivery of neuraxial labour analgesia because a 1.5–2-fold difference in spinal fentanyl dose is not trivial. Meanwhile, another clinical study in a North American cohort determined that the duration of spinal fentanyl analgesia is not influenced by p.118A/G.[41] Taken

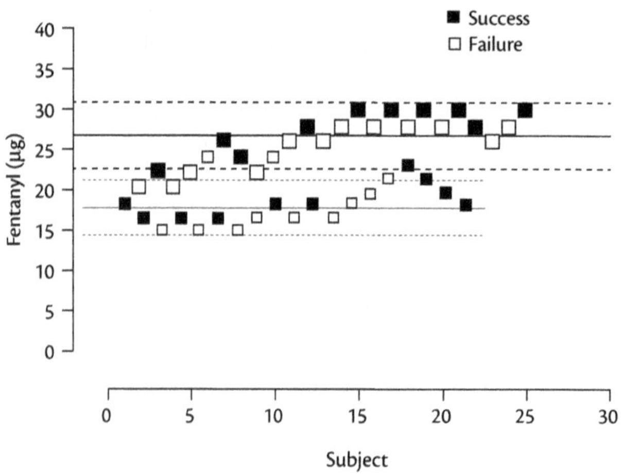

Figure 52.1 Influence of p.118A/G of *OPRM1* on spinal fentanyl dose for labour analgesia. Median effective dose (ED_{50}) of spinal fentanyl according to p.118A/G genotype of *OPRM1* was evaluated using the up-down sequential allocation method. Data show effective (success) and ineffective (failure) analgesic outcome according to genotype; A118 homozygotes are represented within the upper dotted bars, women heterozygous (118A/G) or 118G homozygotes are represented within the lower dotted bars, with solid bars representing ED_{50} and dotted bars representing 95% confidence intervals. ED_{50} of spinal fentanyl was 26.8 mcg (95% CI 22.7–30.9) in women A118 homozygotes (per-protocol analysis, n = 25) versus 17.7 mcg (95% CI 13.4–21.9; P < 0.001) for women heterozygous (118A/G) or 118G homozygotes (per-protocol analysis, n = 19). ED_{50} ratio (A:G) for genotype is 1.51 (95% CI 1.18–2.01), P = 0.009.

Adapted with permission from Landau R, Kern C, Columb MO, Smiley RM, Blouin JL., Genetic variability of the µ-opioid receptor influences intrathecal fentanyl analgesia requirements in laboring women, *Pain*, Volume 139, pp. 5–14, Copyright © 2008 Wolters Kluwer Health, Inc.

together, these studies suggest that this common polymorphism of *OPRM1* influences spinal fentanyl potency without affecting the duration of analgesic action.

Using the same methodology, another recent study in Caucasian women demonstrated a similar pharmacogenetic association of p.118A/G with opioid potency during labour analgesia, although with a more modest clinical effect. In nulliparous women receiving early epidural analgesia, a lower dose requirement (ED_{50}) for epidural sufentanil was found among those carrying the G allele.[42]

The benefits of intravenous (IV) fentanyl for labour analgesia have not been well studied, but fentanyl is offered to women trying to delay or avoid altogether receiving neuraxial analgesia. The rationale for studying the influence of p.118A/G in this clinical context would be to examine the hypothesis that the analgesic response to IV versus spinal fentanyl, under similar clinical conditions (i.e. labour pain) may be influenced differently by this genetic variant. A recent study attempted to explore this question, and determine whether the response to IV fentanyl, and subsequently spinal fentanyl if women went on to request a combined spinal–epidural analgesic would be different according to *OPRM1* genotype alone or in combination with p.472G/A (158Val/Met) of the *COMT* gene.[43] In this North American cohort, most women were Caucasian, and IV analgesic success was found to be relatively low (only 20% of women reported a pain score of <10/100 at 15 minutes after dosing). The average decrease in pain scores 15 minutes after a unique dose of IV fentanyl was only modestly influenced by *OPRM1* genotype, but was found to be lowest among Met/Met158 women compared with women carrying Val/Met or Val/Val of *COMT*; that genotype with the poorer analgesic response was carried by 31% of women. Genotypes of p.118A/G of *OPRM1* in combination with p.472G/A (158Val/Met) of *COMT* seemed to have an impact on the analgesic outcome; IV fentanyl was least effective in women with the A/A–Met/Met combination of *OPRM1* and *COMT*, which was carried by 18% of women in this cohort. The study was ultimately insufficiently powered to explore the hypothesis that spinal and systemic opioid dynamics are different and determine whether enhanced analgesia in response to spinal fentanyl in the presence of the variant *OPRM1* G118 allele may not exist in response to IV fentanyl. Nonetheless, such findings may have useful clinical implications, such as not offering IV fentanyl in labour to women who will most likely not benefit from it.

Overall, findings in labouring women are in disagreement with most if not all other studies examining p.118A/G and opioid analgesia,[24] whether one evaluates postoperative IV fentanyl consumption,[44–46] spinal morphine for post-caesarean pain,[41,47] IV morphine for postoperative pain,[48,49] or oral morphine for chronic cancer pain.[50–52] Potential explanations other than ethnicity for such discrepant results are that labour pain is different from that experienced in other clinical settings (experimental, postoperative or chronic pain), or that the response to systemic rather than spinal fentanyl, is affected differently by *OPRM1* genotype. One could speculate that human spinal cord receptor function and signal transduction is selectively more altered by the G118 variant than supraspinal receptors. Another potential explanation and factor to bear in mind is the different nature of the nociceptive stimulus in labour versus other painful syndromes. Indeed, similar disparate results in human genetic studies of pain sensitivity have been shown to occur with other polymorphisms commonly assessed in pain studies.[53]

Post-caesarean delivery pain and response to postoperative analgesia

The effect of p.118A/G of *OPRM1* on post-caesarean analgesia after spinal and IV *morphine* was evaluated in three studies.[41,47,54] In a North American cohort, the amount of post-caesarean rescue analgesia after a spinal solution of 150 mcg morphine and 15 mcg of fentanyl according to genotype was examined and there was no difference in the duration of spinal morphine analgesia or need for analgesic supplementation over 72 hours in women carrying the G118 allele.[41] The total median morphine equivalent dose was 68 mg (interquartile range; 37–97) in women A118 homozygotes (n = 78) and 75 mg (interquartile range; 37–90) in women carrying at least one G118 variant allele (n = 22 118A/G heterozygotes and n = 3 G118 homozygotes). The time for first opioid rescue analgesia was 22 hours (interquartile range; 12–24) in women A118 homozygotes, and 22 hours (interquartile range; 15–24) in women carrying at least one G118 variant allele. The incidence of nausea was similar between groups; however, pruritus was less frequent in carriers of the G118 variant allele during the first 24 hours.

Sia et al. from Singapore reported that in women undergoing caesarean deliveries under spinal anaesthesia with a morphine spinal dose of 100 mcg, carriers of the G118 variant allele exhibited *increased* 24-hour postoperative consumption of morphine via IV patient-controlled analgesia (PCA).[47,54] In both studies, women were given upon arrival in the post-anaesthesia care unit (PACU) a morphine IV PCA pump (1 mg bolus) and no other analgesics were prescribed. In a first publication reporting on 588 Chinese Singaporean women, 24 hours postoperative morphine IV PCA consumption was lowest in women A118 homozygotes (n = 288) with a mean dose of 5.9 mg (95% confidence interval (CI) 5.1–6.8) versus 8.0 (95% CI 6.9–91) in women 118A/G heterozygotes (n = 234) and 9.4 mg (95% CI 7.3–11.5) in women G118 homozygotes (n = 82) (P = 0.0017).[47] Distribution of morphine use over time (doses were recorded in 4-hour time intervals) demonstrated that most of morphine use occurred in the PACU during the first 4 hours after spinal anaesthesia. It is possible that this early IV morphine use reflects lack of analgesia upon arrival in the PACU; indeed onset of analgesia procured by spinal morphine is known to be slow and has been shown to occur up to 45 minutes after its administration.[55] Consequently, initial differences in IV morphine use may be due to differences in pain perception rather than impaired spinal morphine analgesia in women carrying the G118 variant allele, while differences of morphine use at 24 hours reflect either differences in spinal morphine duration and/or efficacy or more likely differences in IV morphine efficacy. The overall incidence of nausea was low; nonetheless incidence of nausea was higher in women A118 homozygotes versus the other two groups (9.6% vs 5.6% and 1.2% for women 118A/G heterozygotes and G118 homozygotes, respectively; P = 0.02). Since pain scores were lower in women A118 homozygotes, it was concluded that nausea was unlikely to have discouraged women from using the IV PCA morphine button.

In a second publication by the same authors, 994 women from the three main ethnic groups in Singapore were evaluated (n = 617 Chinese, n = 241 Malays, and n = 136 Indians).[54] The overall genotype distribution in the women was 39% A118 homozygotes, 44% 118A/G heterozygotes, and 17% G118 homozygotes, with significant differences between ethnic groups (G118 homozygosity more prevalent among Malays and Indians). The average amount of self-administered morphine was 8.9 mg ± 9.6 over 24 hours. The authors report a large inter-individual range with 65 women not using any, 129 using only one dose, while another 122 administered two doses. The highest amount recorded was 62 mg followed by 55 mg; the remainder of women (n = 676) used between 3 and 40 mg. Total IV morphine use over the first 24 hours was significantly higher in women G118 homozygotes, and incidence of nausea was again lower in women with this genotype. In a multiple regression analysis, the most important factor contributing to morphine usage was maximum pain score, followed by ethnicity and p.118A/G. After correction for *OPRM1* genotype, ethnicity was still a significant contributing factor, with Indian women reporting higher pain scores and using higher doses of IV morphine.

This apparent discrepancy between the North American study reporting no effect of p.118A/G of *OPRM1* on spinal morphine analgesia and the Singaporean findings of a pharmacogenetic effect of this polymorphism, may be explained by differences in study design and primary outcomes. In Sia et al.'s studies evaluating Asian women, the spinal solution did not include fentanyl therefore it is possible that onset of spinal analgesia occurred after women arrived in the PACU. Since women were given IV PCA morphine as the initial rescue analgesic (rather than ibuprofen as in Wong et al.'s study), such study design was more likely to evaluate the effect of p.118A/G of *OPRM1* on IV morphine analgesia rather than the analgesic effect of spinal morphine, at least for the early morphine doses. Another obvious explanation may be that *OPRM1* genotype interacts differently with opioid analgesia in different ethnic groups, as may be suggested by the recent finding of an ethnicity-dependent genetic association for p.118A/G of *OPRM1* recently described in healthy volunteers evaluated with an experimental model of pain.[36]

Finally, the risk for developing chronic pain after childbirth and in particular after caesarean delivery, a topic of interest and subject of several recent publications,[56–60] has been associated with SNPs of the *ABCB1* gene in an Asian cohort of women evaluated in Singapore.[61] Such findings need to be validated with studies evaluating prospectively chronic pain, with pain outcomes that include neuropathic pain descriptors, across multiple ethnicities.

Haemodynamics and vasopressor use during caesarean delivery

The response to vasopressor agents (α- and β-adrenergic agonists) to prevent and/or treat hypotension during spinal anaesthesia for elective caesarean delivery has been extensively studied.[62] Ephedrine is a sympathomimetic amine, the principal mechanism of its action relies on its direct and indirect actions on the adrenergic receptor system (both an α- and β-adrenergic agonist). For decades, ephedrine has been considered the safest and probably the sole acceptable agent in pregnant women, based on a seminal study in the pregnant ewe that suggested deleterious effects of pure α-adrenergic agonists on uteroplacental blood flow.[63] Ephedrine has been widely used in a variety of regimens (different bolus doses, infusions, and in combination with phenylephrine) although no definitive consensus has ever been achieved as to which of these modes of administration provides the most reliable and effective response.

To date, only three studies have evaluated the effect of *ADRB2* genotype/haplotype on maternal haemodynamics and vasopressor requirement during caesarean delivery under spinal anaesthesia.[64–66] In a North American cohort of healthy pregnant women (N = 170), the incidence and severity of maternal hypotension after spinal anaesthesia for caesarean delivery and the response to treatment was clearly affected by *ADRB2* genotype/haplotype.[66] Women Gly16 homozygous and carrying one or two Glu at position 27 (Gln27Glu heterozygous or homozygous for the Glu27 variant allele) were found to require significantly *less* vasopressors (ephedrine) for treatment of hypotension during spinal anaesthesia. The two haplotypes that seemed to 'protect' women from requiring higher doses of ephedrine are relatively common in Caucasians, and in this study 20% of the women carried either one of these haplotypes.

In a small Brazilian cohort (N = 50), homozygosity for Arg16 was suggested to confer protection from hypotension and ephedrine requirements were lower in women with that genotype.[65] Finally in a cohort of Asian women, as expected, the haplotype distribution for p.16Arg/Gly and p.27Gln/Glu was found to be substantially different from that described in Caucasian individuals; the two haplotypes found to be associated with lower ephedrine requirements in the North American study mentioned above[66] were under-represented among Asian women and *ADRB2* genotype/haplotype was not found to influence ephedrine dosage in that study evaluating Asian women.[64]

Further studies would be required to confirm this genetic and pharmacogenetic effect of *ADRB2* genotype/haplotype on maternal hypotension and ephedrine requirement; however, current clinical practice warrants prevention of hypotension with phenylephrine, either given as a bolus or by means of a continuous infusion, therefore this question will most likely remain unanswered. Nonetheless, this possible pharmacogenetic effect may explain in part why two decades of multiple studies trying to define one single optimal strategy (fluid loading, ephedrine, or phenylephrine) to prevent or treat hypotension during spinal anaesthesia for caesarean delivery have failed to identify that one regimen that would 'fit all'.

Fetal and neonatal effects of maternal medication

Neonatal acidosis after maternal ephedrine

The direct effects of ephedrine on the fetus have been revisited.[67] Evidence that ephedrine crosses the placenta to a greater extent and undergoes less early metabolism and redistribution than phenylephrine (a direct α-adrenergic agonist) causing direct fetal metabolic acidosis has made ephedrine less desirable as a first-line treatment.[68] The proposed mechanism is that direct fetal β-adrenergic stimulation increases anaerobic glycolysis and causes a hypermetabolic state. The hypothesis that neonatal *ADRB2* genotype may directly influence the degree of neonatal acidaemia in response to ephedrine given to the mother prior to delivery has been explored. The most clinically relevant and intriguing finding of a study conducted in Asian women was that umbilical artery (UA) pH was overall higher and UA lactate was lower in neonates that were Arg16 homozygous as compared to neonates with the two other genotypes of *ADRB2*.[64] Furthermore, among babies born to mothers receiving ephedrine, ephedrine dose was associated with neonatal acidaemia (decreased UA pH) only in neonates carrying a Gly16 allele, but not in neonates who were Arg16 homozygous. Since there was no significant difference in ephedrine concentration as determined by maternal and umbilical cord assays among genetic groups, any difference in metabolic markers are unlikely to have resulted from differential transplacental transfer of drug or a pharmacokinetic effect. Arg16 homozygous neonates seem to be protected from the risk of developing acidaemia when exposed to ephedrine, irrespective of the dose given to the mother. These findings provide interesting insight on fetal acidosis and metabolic responses in neonates born to mothers who have received β-agonists (ephedrine and/or other β-stimulants prescribed for tocolysis or bronchodilation) prior to delivery.

Neonatal abstinence syndrome after maternal opioids

In a recent prospective cohort study conducted in the Unites States, 86 mother–infant pairs were studied to evaluate the association between p.118A/G of *OPRM1*, p.472G/A (158Val/Met) of *COMT* genes, and three SNPs of the *ABCB1* gene and the risk for neonatal abstinence syndrome (NAS) in neonates exposed *in utero* to methadone or buprenorphine.[69] Neonates carrying the variant G118 allele of *OPRM1* had a shorter length of hospital stay and were less likely to require medication compared to neonates A118 homozygotes. Neonates carrying one or two alleles of the Val158 variant were also protected from a longer hospital stay and the need for medication. There was no effect of any *ABCB1* SNPs and neonatal outcome. The study was truly underpowered to evaluate the joined allelic combination for both SNPs.

This is the first study to evaluate the influence of fetal/neonatal genotype on neonatal outcomes after fetal exposure to opioids, and while epigenetic studies will be of interest as well, these findings do provide some insight into the mechanisms underlying NAS.

Neonatal death after maternal codeine

Codeine was initially prescribed because of the belief that this weak opioid would not result in adverse outcomes. For that reason, codeine has been considered a safe alternative to other opioids for outpatient pain management, and is still available in some countries as an over-the-counter medication, either alone or in combination with paracetamol (acetaminophen). Current use of codeine includes paediatric patients,[70] and treatment of postoperative pain, although large-scale evidence on efficacy is sparse and has been challenged by a meta-analysis.[71] Codeine is a pro-drug, and requires O-demethylation catalysed by CYP2D6 to be converted into morphine and become analgesic; this metabolic pathway accounts for 10% of codeine clearance. The conversion of codeine into norcodeine by CYP3A4 and into codeine-6-glucuronide by glucuronidation represents approximately 80% of codeine clearance. Morphine is further metabolized into morphine-6-glucuronide (M6G) and morphine-3-glucuronide; both morphine and M6G display opioid activity. Individuals with an UM phenotype carry the risk for respiratory depression with codeine, particularly if CYP3A4 activity is inhibited by concomitant use of antibiotics or in the context of kidney dysfunction.[72]

In a recent pilot study, the relationship between CYP2D6 genotype, post-caesarean pain scores, codeine consumption, and side effects were evaluated.[73] The two extremes in CYP2D6 genotype seemed to predict pain response and or adverse effects. Several reports of fatalities after codeine prescription in paediatric cases have been published in recent years.[74] The most striking report is that of the death of a breastfed 13-day-old neonate following a morphine overdose because his mother was taking codeine after childbirth.[75] Toxic blood levels of morphine or its active metabolite M6G may arise in mothers and neonates that are CYP2D6 ultra-rapid or extensive metabolizers. The mother was categorized as a CYP2D6 ultra-rapid metabolizer and her breast milk had a morphine concentration of 87 ng/mL—the typical range being 1.9–20.5 ng/mL at doses of 60 mg codeine every 6 hours. The infant was categorized as a CYP2D6 extensive metabolizer (extensively metabolizing the pro-drug codeine to morphine) and postmortem toxicology tests using gas-chromatography mass spectrometry revealed blood concentrations of morphine at 70 ng/mL. A daily codeine dose of 60 mg for postpartum pain normally results in maximum morphine plasma concentrations of 2.2 ng/mL in breastfed neonates[76] and neonates prescribed morphine for analgesia display serum morphine concentrations in the range of 10–12ng/mL.[77] Codeine and morphine clearance in breastfeeding mothers and their relation to *CYP2D6* genotypes have been extensively evaluated and commented on.[78–86] Since 2007, the US Food and Drug Administration (FDA) requires manufacturers of prescription codeine products to state in the 'Precautions' section of the drug label the risks of prescribing codeine to breastfeeding mothers.[87] An FDA-approved genetic test (AmpliChip CYP450, Roche Diagnostics, Palo Alto, CA, USA) is commercially available to test genetic variants of *CYP2D6*.[88] Overall, the level of evidence linking gene variation (*CYP2D6*) to phenotype (increased biotransformation of

Table 52.2 Codeine therapy recommendations based on CYP2D6 phenotype

Phenotype	Implications for codeine metabolism	Recommendations for codeine therapy	Classification of recommendation for codeine therapy
Ultra-rapid metabolizer (CYP2D5 activity score >2)	Increased morphine formation Higher risk of morphine toxicity	Avoid codeine use (potential for toxicity) Consider alternative such as morphine or non-opioid Consider avoiding tramadol	Strong
Extensive metabolizer (CYP2D6 activity score = 1–2)	Normal morphine formation	15–60 mg every 4 h as needed for pain (label recommendation)	Strong
Intermediate metabolizer (CYP2D6 activity score = 0.5)	Reduced morphine formation	Start at 15–60 mg every 4 h as needed for pain If no response, consider alternative analgesics Monitor tramadol use for response	Moderate
Poor metabolizer (CYP2D6 activity score = 0)	Greatly reduced morphine formation Insufficient pain relief	Avoid codeine use (lack of efficacy) Consider alternative such as morphine or a non-opioid Consider avoiding tramadol	Strong

Reproduced with permission from Crews KR, Gaedigk A, Dunnenberger HM, *et al.*, Clinical Pharmacogenetics Implementation Consortium (CPIC) guidelines for codeine therapy in the context of cytochrome P450 2D6 (CYP2D6) genotype, *Clinical Pharmacology & Therapeutics*, Volume 91, Issue 2, pp. 321–326, Copyright © 2012 John Wiley & Sons.

codeine into morphine) is significant; however, there is no randomized clinical trial assessing the benefits of genetic testing prior to codeine therapy at large. In addition, while insufficient morphine formation from codeine resulting in failure of analgesia can currently be well predicted, extremely high morphine formation still requires the effort of combining genotyping with phenotyping.[89] Finally, the CIPC published guidelines in 2012 based on a focused review and interpretation of the literature by experts in the field (Table 52.2).[7] Because of a wide inter-ethnic genotype distribution not only for CYP2D6 but also of most SNPs assessed in this chapter (Table 52.3), it is important to identify the cohorts in which pharmacogenetic effects and genetic association have been reported, and avoid generalizing findings from one study to different ethnicities.

Conclusion

Overall, whether in the perioperative period or in a more chronic setting, defining relevant clinical outcomes in pain and analgesia studies—or, in other words, identifying meaningful differences in pain perception and opioid response—remains the problem to solve; [25] this has proven to be even more complex in the context of obstetric pain.[22,90] Phenotyping is key in all association studies and designing clinical studies to assess the genetic contribution to pain is challenging. In addition, interpreting results, particularly when multiple genes are evaluated, requires large sample sizes and appropriate statistical analysis to avoid misconstrued findings.[91,92] Last but not least, the genetic contribution to labour pain or even that of pharmacogenetics to explain differences in analgesic response is probably not simple and straightforward,[90] and we are at the beginning of our explorations. On the positive side, these pharmacogenetic studies have enlightened us and have taught us that one should no longer design clinical studies with the sole goal to find 'the one dose for one drug that will fit all' because genetic variants do influence drug response in ways that have clinical implications. Unfortunately, firm recommendations to tailor opioid regimens based on patients' individual genetic profile are not available and are unlikely to become available in the near future other than for the prescription of codeine.[93]

The concept of mathematical modelling of labour progress is certainly promising, and may in the future allow identification of some of the genetic contributions that are important for the progression of labour and the risk for dystocia and will perhaps one day predict labour outcome and labour pain perception. Large prospective studies, well designed, and interpreted with the necessary caution are needed to thoroughly investigate this fascinating topic; meanwhile genome-wide association studies or exome sequencing to examine well-known and yet undiscovered genetic variants resulting in women being outliers for the various phenotypes during labour will be of interest.

Acknowledgements

The author declares receiving funding for research projects that are not related with the topic of this review, from the Millennium Research Institute (Millennium Laboratories).

Ruth Landau is the recipient of Swiss National Foundation Research grant (SNF #3200B0-114129) that funded in part the *OPRM1* genetic research conducted in Switzerland.

Table 52.3 Genotype frequency of selected SNPs studied in the context of obstetric outcomes, labour analgesia and post-caesarean pain

Gene	Nucleotide	Polymorphism	Genotype frequency by ethnicity		
			Caucasian	African American	Asian
OPRM1	c.118A/G	rs1799971—p.40Asn/Asp	AA 65–70%[27]	AA = 100%[94]	AA = 35%[47]
			AG 25–30%	AG = 0	AG = 45%
			GG 0–5%	GG = 0	GG = 20%
COMT	c.472G/A	rs4680—p.158Val/Met	GG = 22%[43]	GG = 52%[95]	GG = 62%[96]
			GA = 47%	GA = 44%	GA = 32%
			AA = 31%	AA = 4%	AA = 5%
CYP2D6		80 SNPs affecting enzymatic activity	UM = 5–10%[97]	UM = 40[97]	UM = 2–5%[97]
		CYP2D6*1—normal	EM = 65–80%	EM = 50%	EM = 90%
		CYP2D6*2—increased	IM = 10–15%	IM = 9%	IM = 5%
		CYP2D6*3, -*4, -*5—none	PM = 5–10%	PM = 1%	PM = 2–5%
		CYP2D6*9, -*10, -*17—decreased			
ABCB1	c.3435C/T	rs1046542—synonymous p.1145Ile	CC = 24%[98]	CC = 68%[98]	CC = 31%[61]
			CT = 48%	CT = 31%	CT = 51%
			TT = 28%	TT = 1%	TT = 18%

ABCB1, ATP binding cassette sub-family B member 1 gene; *COMT*, catechol-O-methyltransferase gene; *CYP2D6*, cytochrome P450 2D6; EM, extensive metabolizer; IM, intermediate metabolizer; *OPRM1*, μ-opioid receptor gene; PM, poor metabolizer; rs, RefSNP; SNP, single nucleotide polymorphism; UM, ultra-rapid metabolizer.

Data from various sources (see references).

References

1. Mogil JS. Are we getting anywhere in human pain genetics? *Pain* 2009; 146:231–2.
2. Candiotti K. Anesthesia and pharmacogenomics: not ready for prime time. *Anesth Analg* 2009; 109:1377–8.
3. Donahue BS, Balser JR. Perioperative genomics. Venturing into uncharted seas. *Anesthesiology* 2003; 99:7–8.
4. Schwinn DA, Booth JV. Genetics infuses new life into human physiology: implications of the human genome project for anesthesiology and perioperative medicine. *Anesthesiology* 2002; 96:261–3.
5. PharmGKB. Website. [Online] http://www.pharmgkb.org/
6. Relling MV, Klein TE. CPIC: Clinical Pharmacogenetics Implementation Consortium of the Pharmacogenomics Research Network. *Clin Pharmacol Ther* 2011; 89(3):464–7.
7. Crews KR, Gaedigk A, Dunnenberger HM, *et al.* Clinical Pharmacogenetics Implementation Consortium (CPIC) guidelines for codeine therapy in the context of cytochrome P450 2D6 (CYP2D6) genotype. *Clin Pharmacol Ther* 2012; 91:321–6.
8. Villar J, Papageorghiou AT, Knight HE, *et al.* The preterm birth syndrome: a prototype phenotypic classification. *Am J Obstet Gynecol* 2012; 206:119–23.
9. Carroll CL, Sala KA, Zucker AR, *et al.* β_2-adrenergic receptor haplotype linked to intubation and mechanical ventilation in children with asthma. *J Asthma* 2012; 49:563–8.
10. Nagele P, Liggett SB. Genetic variation, β-blockers, and perioperative myocardial infarction. *Anesthesiology* 2011; 115:1316–27.
11. Landau R, Xie HG, Dishy V, *et al.* β_2-Adrenergic receptor genotype and preterm delivery. *Am J Obstet Gynecol* 2002; 187:1294–8.
12. Doh K, Sziller I, Vardhana S, *et al.* β_2-adrenergic receptor gene polymorphisms and pregnancy outcome. *J Perinat Med* 2004; 32:413–17.
13. Ozkur M, Dogulu F, Ozkur A, *et al.* Association of the Gln27Glu polymorphism of the β_2-adrenergic receptor with preterm labor. *Int J Gynaecol Obstet* 2002; 77:209–15.
14. Landau R, Morales MA, Antonarakis SE, *et al.* Arg16 homozygosity of the β_2-adrenergic receptor improves the outcome after beta2-agonist tocolysis for preterm labor. *Clin Pharmacol Ther* 2005; 78:656–63.
15. Miller RS, Smiley RM, Daniel D, *et al.* β_2-adrenoceptor genotype and progress in term and late preterm active labor. *Am J Obstet Gynecol* 2011; 205:137.e1–7.
16. Reitman E, Conell-Price J, Evansmith J, *et al.* β_2-adrenergic receptor genotype and other variables that contribute to labor pain and progress. *Anesthesiology* 2011; 114:927–39.
17. Terkawi AS, Jackson WM, Thiet MP, *et al.* Oxytocin and catechol-O-methyltransferase receptor genotype predict the length of the first stage of labor. *Am J Obstet Gynecol* 2012; 207:184.e1–8.
18. Algovik M, Kivinen K, Peterson H, *et al.* Genetic evidence of multiple loci in dystocia—difficult labour. *BMC Med Genet* 2010; 11:105.
19. Esplin MS, Merrell K, Goldenberg R, *et al.* Proteomic identification of serum peptides predicting subsequent spontaneous preterm birth. *Am J Obstet Gynecol* 2011; 204:391.e1–8.
20. Gracie S, Pennell C, Ekman-Ordeberg G, *et al.* An integrated systems biology approach to the study of preterm birth using "-omic" technology—a guideline for research. BMC Pregnancy *Childbirth* 2011; 11:71.
21. Melzack R. The myth of painless childbirth (the John J. Bonica lecture). *Pain* 1984; 19:321–37.
22. Carvalho B, Cohen SE. Measuring the labor pain experience: delivery still far off. *Int J Obstet Anesth* 2013; 22:6–9.
23. Conell-Price J, Evans JB, Hong D, *et al.* The development and validation of a dynamic model to account for the progress of labor in the assessment of pain. *Anesth Analg* 2008; 106:1509–15.
24. Walter C, Lotsch J. Meta-analysis of the relevance of the OPRM1 118A>G genetic variant for pain treatment. *Pain* 2009; 146:270–5.
25. Landau R, Schwinn D. Genotyping without phenotyping: does it really matter? *Anesth Analg* 2013; 116:8–10.
26. Mura E, Govoni S, Racchi M, *et al.* Consequences of the 118A>G polymorphism in the OPRM1 gene: translation from bench to bedside? *J Pain Res* 2013; 6:331–53.
27. Landau R, Cahana A, Smiley RM, *et al.* Genetic variability of μ-opioid receptor in an obstetric population. *Anesthesiology* 2004; 100:1030–3.
28. Tan EC, Tan CH, Karupathivan U, *et al.* μ-opioid receptor gene polymorphisms and heroin dependence in Asian populations. *Neuroreport* 2003; 14:569–72.
29. Crowley JJ, Oslin DW, Patkar AA, *et al.* A genetic association study of the μ-opioid receptor and severe opioid dependence. *Psychiatr Genet* 2003; 13:169–73.
30. Kroslak T, Laforge KS, Gianotti RJ, *et al.* The single nucleotide polymorphism A118G alters functional properties of the human mu opioid receptor. *J Neurochem* 2007; 103:77–87.
31. Bond C, LaForge KS, Tian M, *et al.* Single-nucleotide polymorphism in the human μ-opioid receptor gene alters β-endorphin binding and activity: possible implications for opiate addiction. *Proc Natl Acad Sci U S A* 1998; 95:9608–13.
32. Zhang Y, Wang D, Johnson AD, *et al.* Allelic expression imbalance of human opioid receptor (OPRM1) caused by variant A118G. *J Biol Chem* 2005; 280:32618–24.
33. Beyer A, Koch T, Schroder H, *et al.* Effect of the A118G polymorphism on binding affinity, potency and agonist-mediated endocytosis, desensitization, and resensitization of the human μ-opioid receptor. *J Neurochem* 2004; 89:553–60.
34. Oertel BG, Kettner M, Scholich K, *et al.* A common human μ-opioid receptor genetic variant diminishes the receptor signaling efficacy in brain regions processing the sensory information of pain. *J Biol Chem* 2009; 284:6530–5.
35. Mahmoud S, Thorsell A, Sommer WH, *et al.* Pharmacological consequence of the A118G μ opioid receptor polymorphism on morphine- and fentanyl-mediated modulation of Ca2 channels in humanized mouse sensory neurons. *Anesthesiology* 2011; 115:1054–62.
36. Hastie BA, Riley JL, 3rd, Kaplan L, *et al.* Ethnicity interacts with the OPRM1 gene in experimental pain sensitivity. *Pain* 2012; 153:1610–9.
37. Nielsen DA, Hamon S, Yuferov V, *et al.* Ethnic diversity of DNA methylation in the OPRM1 promoter region in lymphocytes of heroin addicts. *Hum Genet* 2010; 127:639–49.
38. Pettersson FD, Gronbladh A, Nyberg F, *et al.* The A118G single-nucleotide polymorphism of human μ-opioid receptor gene and use of labor analgesia. *Reprod Sci* 2012; 19:962–7.
39. Dabo F, Gronbladh A, Nyberg F, *et al.* Different SNP combinations in the GCH1 gene and use of labor analgesia. *Mol Pain* 2010; 6:41.
40. Landau R, Kern C, Columb MO, *et al.* Genetic variability of the μ-opioid receptor influences intrathecal fentanyl analgesia requirements in laboring women. *Pain* 2008; 139:5–14.
41. Wong CA, McCarthy RJ, Blouin J, *et al.* Observational study of the effect of μ-opioid receptor genetic polymorphism on intrathecal opioid labor analgesia and post-cesarean delivery analgesia. *Int J Obstet Anesth* 2010; 19:246–53.
42. Camorcia M, Capogna G, Stirparo S, *et al.* Effect of μ-opioid receptor A118G polymorphism on the ED50 of epidural sufentanil for labor analgesia. *Int J Obstet Anesth* 2012; 21:40–4.
43. Landau R, Liu SK, Blouin JL, *et al.* The effect of OPRM1 and COMT genotypes on the analgesic response to intravenous fentanyl labor analgesia. *Anesth Analg* 2013; 116:386–91.
44. Fukuda K, Hayashida M, Ide S, *et al.* Association between OPRM1 gene polymorphisms and fentanyl sensitivity in patients undergoing painful cosmetic surgery. *Pain* 2009; 147:194–201.

45. Wu WD, Wang Y, Fang YM, *et al.* Polymorphism of the μ-opioid receptor gene (OPRM1 118A>G) affects fentanyl-induced analgesia during anesthesia and recovery. *Mol Diagn Ther* 2009; 13:331–7.
46. Zhang W, Chang YZ, Kan QC, *et al.* Association of human μ-opioid receptor gene polymorphism A118G with fentanyl analgesia consumption in Chinese gynaecological patients. *Anaesthesia* 2010; 65(2):130–5.
47. Sia AT, Lim Y, Lim EC, *et al.* A118G single nucleotide polymorphism of human μ-opioid receptor gene influences pain perception and patient-controlled intravenous morphine consumption after intrathecal morphine for postcesarean analgesia. *Anesthesiology* 2008; 109:520–6.
48. Chou WY, Wang CH, Liu PH, *et al.* Human opioid receptor A118G polymorphism affects intravenous patient-controlled analgesia morphine consumption after total abdominal hysterectomy. *Anesthesiology* 2006; 105:334–7.
49. Coulbault L, Beaussier M, Verstuyft C, *et al.* Environmental and genetic factors associated with morphine response in the postoperative period. *Clin Pharmacol Ther* 2006; 79:316–24.
50. Klepstad P, Fladvad T, Skorpen F, *et al.* Influence from genetic variability on opioid use for cancer pain: a European genetic association study of 2294 cancer pain patients. *Pain* 2011; 152:1139–45.
51. Klepstad P, Rakvag TT, Kaasa S, *et al.* The 118 A > G polymorphism in the human μ-opioid receptor gene may increase morphine requirements in patients with pain caused by malignant disease. *Acta Anaesthesiol Scand* 2004; 48:1232–9.
52. Reyes-Gibby CC, Shete S, Rakvag T, *et al.* Exploring joint effects of genes and the clinical efficacy of morphine for cancer pain: OPRM1 and COMT gene. *Pain* 2007; 130:25–30.
53. Diatchenko L, Nackley AG, Slade GD, *et al.* Catechol-O-methyltransferase gene polymorphisms are associated with multiple pain-evoking stimuli. *Pain* 2006; 125:216–24.
54. Tan EC, Lim EC, Teo YY, *et al.* Ethnicity and OPRM variant independently predict pain perception and patient-controlled analgesia usage for post-operative pain. *Mol Pain* 2009; 5:32.
55. Baraka A, Noueihid R, Hajj S. Intrathecal injection of morphine for obstetric analgesia. *Anesthesiology* 1981; 54:136–40.
56. Eisenach JC, Pan P, Smiley RM, *et al.* Resolution of pain after childbirth. *Anesthesiology* 2013; 118:143–51.
57. Flood P, Wong CA. Chronic pain secondary to childbirth: does it exist? *Anesthesiology* 2013; 118:16–18.
58. Gutierrez S, Liu B, Hayashida K, *et al.* Reversal of peripheral nerve injury-induced hypersensitivity in the postpartum period: role of spinal oxytocin. *Anesthesiology* 2013; 118:152–9.
59. Landau R, Bollag L, Ortner C. Chronic pain after childbirth. *Int J Obstet Anesth* 2013; 22:133–45.
60. Lavand'homme P. Chronic pain after childbirth. *Curr Opin Anaesthesiol* 2013; 26:273–7.
61. Sia AT, Sng BL, Lim EC, *et al.* The influence of ATP-binding cassette sub-family B member -1 (ABCB1) genetic polymorphisms on acute and chronic pain after intrathecal morphine for caesarean section: a prospective cohort study. *Int J Obstet Anesth* 2010; 19:254–60.
62. Ngan Kee WD, Khaw KS. Vasopressors in obstetrics: what should we be using? *Curr Opin Anaesthesiol* 2006; 19:238–43.
63. Ralston DH, Shnider SM, DeLorimier AA. Effects of equipotent ephedrine, metaraminol, mephentermine, and methoxamine on uterine blood flow in the pregnant ewe. *Anesthesiology* 1974; 40:354–70.
64. Landau R, Liu SK, Blouin JL, *et al.* The effect of maternal and fetal β_2-adrenoceptor and nitric oxide synthase genotype on vasopressor requirement and fetal acid-base status during spinal anesthesia for cesarean delivery. *Anesth Analg* 2011; 112:1432–7.
65. Magalhaes E, Gomes MD, Barra GB, *et al.* Evaluation of the influence of the codon 16 polymorphism of the β_2-adrenergic receptor gene on the incidence of arterial hypotension and ephedrine use in pregnant patients submitted to subarachnoid anesthesia. *Rev Bras Anestesiol* 2010; 60:228–36.
66. Smiley RM, Blouin JL, Negron M, *et al.* beta2-adrenoceptor genotype affects vasopressor requirements during spinal anesthesia for cesarean delivery. *Anesthesiology* 2006; 104:644–50.
67. Cooper DW, Carpenter M, Mowbray P, *et al.* Fetal and maternal effects of phenylephrine and ephedrine during spinal anesthesia for cesarean delivery. *Anesthesiology* 2002; 97:1582–90.
68. Ngan Kee WD, Khaw KS, Tan PE, *et al.* Placental transfer and fetal metabolic effects of phenylephrine and ephedrine during spinal anesthesia for cesarean delivery. *Anesthesiology* 2009; 111:506–12.
69. Wachman EM, Hayes MJ, Brown MS, *et al.* Association of OPRM1 and COMT single-nucleotide polymorphisms with hospital length of stay and treatment of neonatal abstinence syndrome. *JAMA* 2013; 309:1821–7.
70. Lee PJ, Delaney P, Keogh J, *et al.* Catecholamine-o-methyltransferase polymorphisms are associated with postoperative pain intensity. *Clin J Pain* 2011; 27:93–101.
71. Derry S, Moore RA, McQuay HJ. Single dose oral codeine, as a single agent, for acute postoperative pain in adults. *Cochrane Database Syst Rev* 2010; 4:CD008099.
72. Gasche Y, Daali Y, Fathi M, *et al.* Codeine intoxication associated with ultrarapid CYP2D6 metabolism. *N Engl J Med* 2004; 351:2827–31.
73. VanderVaart S, Berger H, Sistonen J, *et al.* CYP2D6 polymorphisms and codeine analgesia in postpartum pain management: a pilot study. *Ther Drug Monit* 2011; 33:425–32.
74. Voelker R. Children's deaths linked with postsurgical codeine. *JAMA* 2012; 308:963.
75. Koren G, Cairns J, Chitayat D, *et al.* Pharmacogenetics of morphine poisoning in a breastfed neonate of a codeine-prescribed mother. *Lancet* 2006; 368:704.
76. Meny RG, Naumburg EG, Alger LS, *et al.* Codeine and the breastfed neonate. *J Hum Lact* 1993; 9:237–40.
77. Madadi P, Koren G, Cairns J, *et al.* Safety of codeine during breastfeeding: fatal morphine poisoning in the breastfed neonate of a mother prescribed codeine. *Can Fam Physician* 2007; 53:33–5.
78. Sistonen J, Madadi P, Ross CJ, *et al.* Prediction of codeine toxicity in infants and their mothers using a novel combination of maternal genetic markers. *Clin Pharmacol Ther* 2012; 91:692–9.
79. Madadi P, Joly Y, Avard D, *et al.* The communication of pharmacogenetic research results: participants weigh in on their informational needs in a pilot study. *J Popul Ther Clin Pharmacol* 2011; 18:e152–5.
80. Madadi P, Ciszkowski C, Gaedigk A, *et al.* Genetic transmission of cytochrome P450 2D6 (CYP2D6) ultrarapid metabolism: implications for breastfeeding women taking codeine. *Curr Drug Saf* 2011; 6:36–9.
81. Kurtz M, Black Golde P, *et al.* Ethical considerations in CYP2D6 genotype testing for codeine-prescribed breastfeeding mothers. *Clin Pharmacol Ther* 2010; 88:760–2.
82. Willmann S, Edginton AN, Coboeken K, *et al.* Risk to the breast-fed neonate from codeine treatment to the mother: a quantitative mechanistic modeling study. *Clin Pharmacol Ther* 2009; 86:634–43.
83. Madadi P, Koren G. Pharmacogenetic insights into codeine analgesia: implications to pediatric codeine use. *Pharmacogenomics* 2008; 9:1267–84.
84. Ferner RE. Did the drug cause death? Codeine and breastfeeding. *Lancet* 2008; 372:606–8.
85. Bateman DN, Eddleston M, Sandilands E. Codeine and breastfeeding. *Lancet* 2008; 372:625–6.
86. Madadi P, Koren G, Cairns J, *et al.* Safety of codeine during breastfeeding: fatal morphine poisoning in the breastfed neonate of a mother prescribed codeine. *Can Fam Physician* 2007; 53:33–5.
87. Lotsch J, Fluhr K, Neddermayer T, *et al.* The consequence of concomitantly present functional genetic variants for the identification of functional genotype-phenotype associations in pain. *Clin Pharmacol Ther* 2009; 85:25–30.
88. de Leon J, Susce MT, Murray-Carmichael E. The AmpliChip CYP450 genotyping test: integrating a new clinical tool. *Mol Diagn Ther* 2006; 10:135–51.

89. Lotsch J, Rohrbacher M, Schmidt H, *et al.* Can extremely low or high morphine formation from codeine be predicted prior to therapy initiation? *Pain* 2009; 144:119–24.
90. Wong CA. The promise of pharmacogenetics in labor analgesia ... tantalizing, but not there yet. *Int J Obstet Anesth* 2012; 21:105–8.
91. Landau R, Ortner C, Carvalho B. Challenges in interpreting joined allelic combinations of OPRM1 and COMT genes. *Anesth Analg* 2011; 113:432.
92. Lotsch J. Basic genetic statistics are necessary in studies of functional associations in anesthesiology. *Anesthesiology* 2007; 107:168–9.
93. Vuilleumier PH, Stamer UM, Landau R. Pharmacogenomic considerations in opioid analgesia. *Pharmgenomics Pers Med* 2012; 5:73–87.
94. Ginosar Y, Birnbach DJ, Shirov TT, *et al.* Duration of analgesia and pruritus following intrathecal fentanyl for labour analgesia: no significant effect of A118G μ-opioid receptor polymorphism, but a marked effect of ethnically distinct hospital populations. *Br J Anaesth* 2013; 111(3):433–44.
95. Al-Hendy A, Salama SA. Catechol-O-methyltransferase polymorphism is associated with increased uterine leiomyoma risk in different ethnic groups. *J Soc Gynecol Investig* 2006; 13:136–44.
96. Liang S, Liu X, Fan P, *et al.* Association between Val158Met functional polymorphism in the COMT gene and risk of preeclampsia in a Chinese population. *Arch Med Res* 2012; 43:154–8.
97. Sistonen J, Sajantila A, Lao O, *et al.* CYP2D6 worldwide genetic variation shows high frequency of altered activity variants and no continental structure. *Pharmacogenet Genomics* 2007; 17:93–101.
98. Ameyaw MM, Regateiro F, Li T, *et al.* MDR1 pharmacogenetics: frequency of the C3435T mutation in exon 26 is significantly influenced by ethnicity. *Pharmacogenetics* 2001; 11:217–21.

CHAPTER 53

Simulation

Mark Wigginton, Miguel Garcia, Timothy J. Draycott, and Neil A. Muchatuta

An introduction to simulation

Simulation enables healthcare professionals to acquire knowledge, attitudes and skills in an environment that is safe both for them and for patients. It is 'a technique to replace or amplify real-patient experiences with guided experiences, artificially contrived, that evokes or replicates substantial aspects of the real world in a fully interactive manner'.[1]

Primum non nocere: 'Above all, do no harm'. This cornerstone principle of medical practice is undone when patients are exposed to avoidable error.[2] In 1999, the Institute of Medicine in the United States produced the landmark report *To Err is Human* which revealed that up to 98,000 deaths a year occurred as a consequence of medical error.[3] Medical simulation aims to reduce errors by improving individual and team performance, and offering the opportunity to improve systems. In obstetric anaesthesia, simulation has been used widely from routine task training to multidisciplinary teamwork training for high risk, rarely occurring events.[4]

History of simulation

It is a common misconception that simulation training in anaesthesia, obstetrics, and medicine is a late twentieth-century concept that has been refined and improved to produce the high-fidelity mannequins in use today. On the contrary, the history of simulation has a long and complex story, to the extent that much of its earliest use has been irrevocably lost to time. When reviewing the history of simulation for which records still remain, it is useful to make a distinction between purely anatomical models and those interactive simulation models that allow an element of feedback to the trainee.

Anatomical models

Anatomical stone sculptures exist from approximately 24,000 years BC but it is difficult to separate the educational value of early models from their likely artistic, religious, or entertainment objectives.[5] The ancient Egyptian and Mayan civilizations produced partially dissected human models in a variety of media displaying good knowledge of anatomy but their use was most likely to be spiritual in nature.[5] Similarly, *memento mori* are carved dissected or skeletal figures, popular throughout the eighteenth and nineteenth centuries, intended primarily as a reminder of the transient and fragile nature of life.[5]

The first anatomical models used specifically for medical training purposes were probably from the Chinese Song dynasty. Wang Wei-Ye (987–1067), the imperial physician, was responsible for standardizing the teaching of acupuncture. He commissioned two life-sized bronze figures with organs; it is believed that the figures were then covered in wax. Students would have to identify acupuncture points from the surface anatomy, and were rewarded if the needle passed through a hole in the bronze structure and emerged with a drip of fluid from the mannequin.[5]

The European development of anatomical models was stimulated by the publication of *De Humani Corporis Fabrica Libri Septum* by Andrea Vesalio in 1543.[6,7] The artistry of wax and bronze models produced after this time compares favourably with models of today. A detailed understanding of anatomy was considered essential training for renaissance artists. Therefore, throughout the seventeenth and eighteenth centuries, European medical students were instructed using *écorché* ('flayed man' models) in addition to cadaveric dissection.[7] By the end of the seventeenth century, the use of polychromatic wax in decaying figures created by Gaetano Giulio Zumbo were said to be so realistic as to 'evoke a sense of overwhelming stench'.[5]

The practice of casting anatomical detail in a variety of media has continued. In some cases, pathological details were cast directly from patients. Wealthy medical schools across the world have built up large collections; some are still used for teaching purposes, whilst others have been consigned to antiquity.

Interactive models

To practise a specific task, or to evaluate the consequences of one's actions using simulated physiology, is clearly an entirely different concept to pure anatomical teaching. What we might now refer to as task trainers or physiological simulators are intended for this purpose. These creations frequently appear far simpler in outward appearance than anatomical models but the ingenuity of internal design or their suitability for a specific training need is what gives them value.

Obstetric simulation has a particularly rich history in the development and widespread use of task trainers. The eighteenth and nineteenth centuries were a prolific era with the introduction of the first simulators to address an identified training need, and also the first recognized regional simulation programme. In 1739, the first British maternity hospital opened with a promise that the students would be taught using an obstetric simulator whereby 'all the inconveniences which might otherwise happen to women from pupils practising too early on real objects will be entirely prevented: for by this method and contrivance each pupil will become in a great measure proficient in his business before he attempts a real delivery'.[5]

Mid-eighteenth-century surgeon Giovanni Antonio Galli was concerned that surgical trainees had theoretical knowledge but limited practical experience and that the midwives assisting with births may also have very limited practical experience. He developed a birthing simulator consisting of a glass uterus in a pelvis with a flexible fetus. This was designed specifically to address a training need and was also used for assessment as students were made to deliver the fetus blindfolded.[5]

No history of simulation could be considered complete without mentioning Angélique Marguerite Le Boursier du Coudray. Tasked by Louis XV to stem the decline in the population of rural France, she developed and ran two-month courses comprised of 40 sessions with an accompanying course manual. For practical training she developed life-sized mannequins with removable uterus, interchangeable nulliparous and multiparous os which could simulate dilatation by means of a silk drawstring, and sponges which released red or clear fluid to simulate blood or amniotic fluid. From 1760, Madame du Coudray toured the country for two decades with her 'machines' and, to facilitate repeated training, left courses running in various places with regional supervisors.[8]

By 1831, we have evidence of sophisticated obstetric simulators in use which are in many ways comparable to some of today's high-fidelity models. Dr Ozenne presented to the French Royal Academy of Medicine a whole-body simulator that had a uterus with radial and longitudinal fibres able to contract. The strength and rate of contractions could be controlled manually. It also had an amniotic sac and an artificial fetus with fontanelles.[5]

By the latter half of the nineteenth century, obstetric simulation had made its way into American medical schools. However, by the start of the twentieth century, damning reports were published on the state of simulation equipment around the country. The *Medical Education in the United States and Canada* report, published in 1909, referring to Southwestern University Medical College, Texas, remarked 'in a corner of one [lecture theatre] is an abused manikin'.[9] This comprehensive report was critical of large sections of the North American medical school system, and served as a damning indictment of medical education as a whole. These attitudes towards medical education were reflected in a neglect of simulation as a teaching modality. An era sometimes referred to as 'the dark age of simulation' began. For much of the twentieth century medical advances were made by practice on real patients. Mistakes and adverse outcomes may have been commonplace but it is difficult to be critical when materials and facilities were made scarce by the ravages of two worldwide conflicts.

During the second half of the twentieth century, there was recognition that significant improvements in safety achieved by the airline industry came as a result of highly technical and realistic simulation training.[10] Medicine again looked to simulation in order to emulate these safety improvements. Resusci-Anne is a mannequin developed by Laerdal, a toy manufacturer, in the 1960s.[11] It has been widely used to teach cardiopulmonary resuscitation (CPR) since then and probably represents the early stages of a simulation resurgence that has subsequently gathered pace and momentum. The 1960s also saw the development of the first computer-controlled patient simulator; although Sim One, as it was called, may have been ahead of its time and never became commercially available.[12]

Since then simulation centres, point-of-care simulation, multidisciplinary team training, and physiological remote-controlled mannequins have become commonplace terms in the burgeoning simulation field. Up-to-date educational theory is now incorporated into courses and instructors are tutored on effective methods of instructing. There is a small but growing evidence base for the usefulness of simulation in reducing adverse events and improving outcome, as well as evidence of its limitations.[13–16] To refer to the latest simulation technology as high-fidelity leaves little scope for superlatives to describe future innovations in a rapidly evolving field. Medicine, art, engineering, and computer technology have come together, working in synergy to produce experiences as close as possible to the real thing. Nevertheless, the human body is potentially the most complex and heterogeneous machine known. To simulate it fully will take many more years of development, and could well prove impossible.

Simulation technology for obstetric anaesthesia

Simulators provide the physical interface between the simulation and its user. Whilst simulators are commonly thought of as a piece of expensive high-technology equipment, tools for simulation form a wide spectrum. At one end are increasingly complex, computer-driven mannequins that can replicate maternal anatomy, physiology, and pathology; at the other are verbal techniques, such as role-play and narrative discussions.[17]

Simulators can be categorized in a number of ways, such as by the way the user interacts with them, by the skill they are used to examine, and by the participants involved.[18–21] Gaba described a spectrum that is based on the technology employed:[17]

- Verbal (role play)
- Standardized patients (actors)
- Part-task trainer (physical or virtual reality)
- Computer patient (screen based)
- Electronic patient (mannequin based)

There have always been examples that cross between these categories, and the march of modern technology is blurring the boundaries still further. Each technique has its own particular advantages, and their relative strengths and weaknesses will help the operator decide which best to employ.

Role play

Verbal role play forms the basis of much of the teaching that occurs in labour wards and obstetric theatres on a daily basis, such as getting a trainee to work through an invented problem or discussing 'what ifs'. By projecting a mental scenario for the learner to temporarily inhabit, the trainer can achieve many of the benefits of a full-scale simulation without relying upon a physical simulator or props.

Standardized patients

Standardized patients, or patient actors, are people who have been coached to portray a specific patient. They appear in medical education literature from the early 1960s[22] and are most commonly used to teach communication skills, although they can also used to teach clinical skills.[23] One of the recent drivers for their use in medical training is an increasing focus on the patient's perspective of the medical care they receive.[24]

Using a patient actor can be at least as effective as using a high-fidelity mannequin. In one study of eclampsia training, groups trained with a patient actor and those trained with a high-end simulator both improved their performance to a similar degree.[25] The same investigators looked at the simulated management of postpartum haemorrhage, where training using patient actors and mannequins were compared.[26] Again the teams improved similarly in terms of clinical outcomes, but the perception of safety and communication were significantly improved in the group trained using a patient actor.

Standardized patients enable a degree of fidelity that is not currently possible with mannequin technology. They can be used to simulate a wide variety of physical findings, although there can be limitations in their use in terms of performing invasive or embarrassing procedures. More recently, patient actors have been combined with part-task trainers to enhance fidelity and patient interaction whilst performing medical interventions, thus creating a convincing learning environment.[27,28] An obstetric part-task trainer has recently been developed which has been specifically designed for use with patient actors (Figure 53.1). It can be used to replicate a variety of obstetric conditions such as postpartum haemorrhage, and further blurs the boundary between patient actors, part-task trainers, and mannequins.

The efficacy and cost-effectiveness of standardized patients, especially when combined with part-task trainers, is an important consideration during times of budgetary constraint. This is particularly true in the developing world, where access to expensive technology is impractical, but effective training is particularly crucial.[29]

Part-task/skills trainers

Part-task trainers are simulators that recreate only a portion of the process or system being examined. They are traditionally used to practice psychomotor skills, but have also been successfully employed to improve higher-level skills such as teamwork and clinical judgement. They have been used to allow the participant to focus upon a particular facet of a scenario, thereby building simple tasks into a complex skill.[30] Part-task trainers are available in a range of levels of complexity; an example of the lowest level could include using the palm of the hand to simulate structures in the palate encountered whilst inserting a laryngeal mask airway,[31] whilst highly complex examples include some virtual reality devices. They can be used for a number of applications relevant to obstetric anaesthetists:

Epidural trainers

Epidural insertion is a core obstetric anaesthetic skill, and many trainees learn or refine their skills whilst on the delivery suite. A simulated spine has the potential to allow novices to safely practise epidural insertion without putting patients at risk. A number of homemade and commercially available devices have been described,[32–34] although few studies have evaluated them against alternatives means of training. One study compared the use of a homemade device with a high-fidelity mannequin to train junior anaesthetists in epidural insertion, and then went on to observe them carrying out epidurals on patients.[35] They were able to show that the homemade version was as good for training as the high-end device.

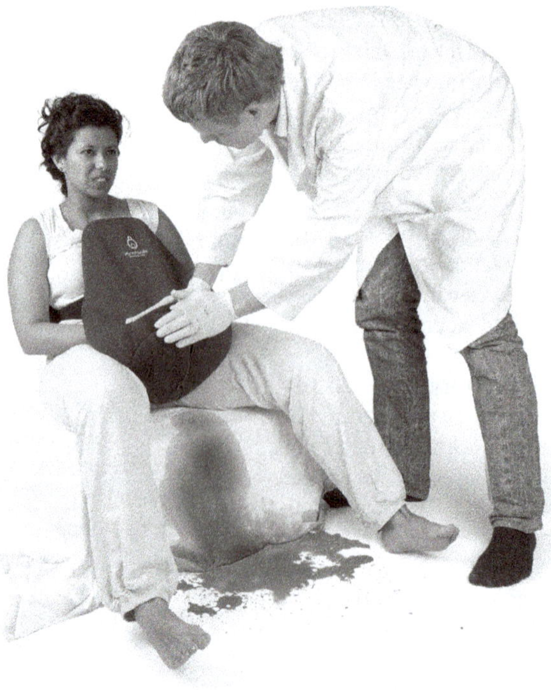

Figure 53.1 Example of an obstetric part-task trainer that can be combined with a patient actor to enhance simulation fidelity.
Reproduced with permission by Laerdal.

Although no study has yet established whether there is an advantage to training with an epidural trainer over traditional patient-based training methods, one study of junior physicians training for lumbar puncture showed improved skills after training with a similar device.[36]

Estimating maternal haemorrhage

Maternal haemorrhage remains an important cause of maternal death in the United Kingdom,[37] and is a leading cause of preventable maternal death worldwide.[38] The successful management of obstetric haemorrhage relies upon an accurate estimation of blood loss. Studies have shown that clinicians underestimate blood loss using visual inspection by as much as 33–50%.[39] Simulation has been used both to demonstrate this discrepancy, and to train staff in how to better recognize the degree of haemorrhage. Bose et al.[40] used simulated stations (Figure 53.2) to replicate the blood lost at the time of delivery; all groups underestimated, with their assessments becoming less accurate with worsening degrees of haemorrhage. Toledo et al.[41,42] demonstrated that simulation stations, both live and web-based, could improve the estimation of blood loss to a clinically insignificant degree of error. However these improvements decayed by 9 months, suggesting that training of this nature needs to be regularly repeated.[43]

Airway trainers

A decline in the use of general anaesthesia for caesarean delivery,[44,45] and the increased risk of failed intubation in the obstetric population,[46,47] means that maintaining competent airway skills in this setting is especially vital. Simulators have been used

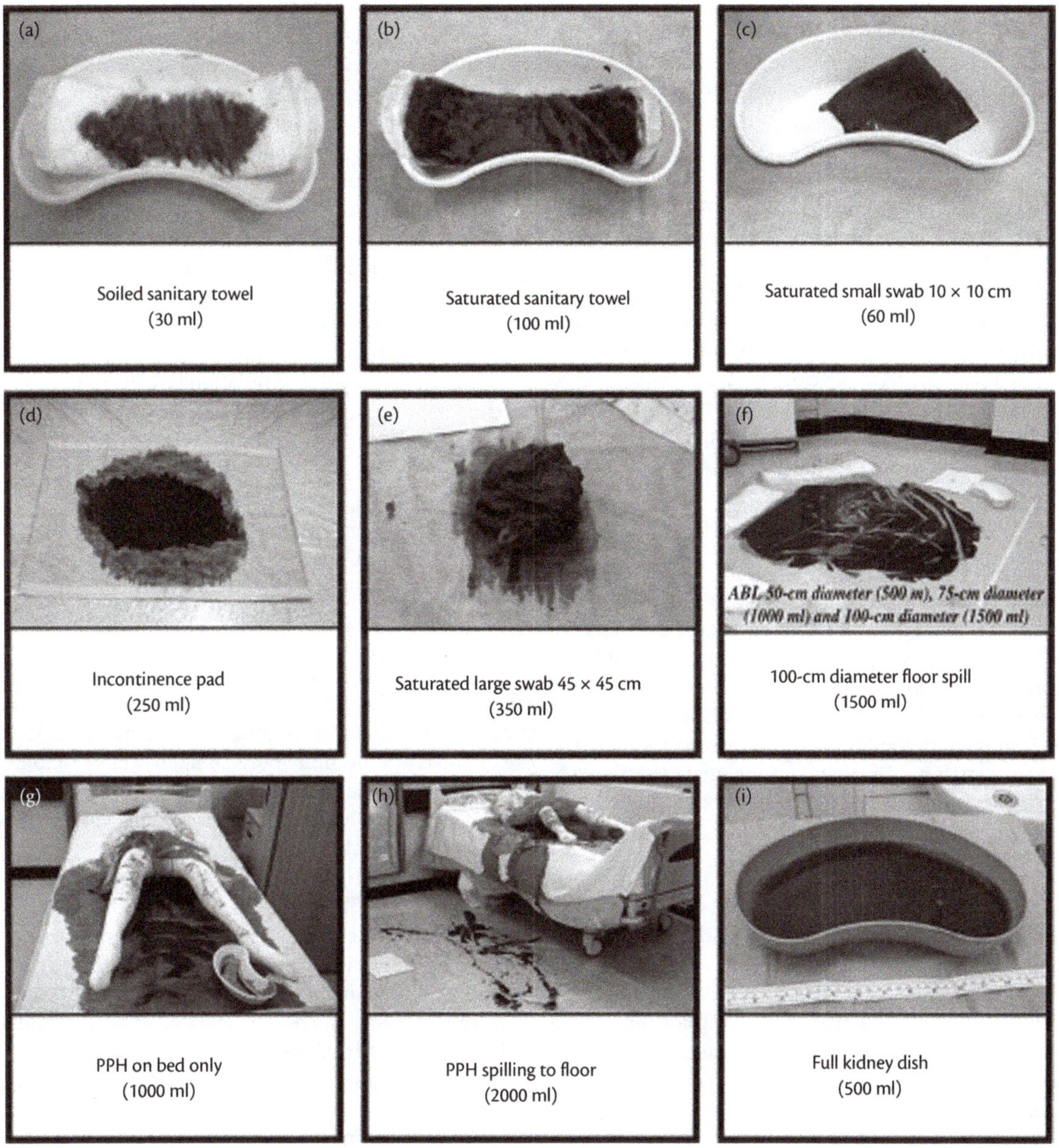

Figure 53.2 Simulation tools used to replicate varying degrees of obstetric blood loss.

to assess and train all aspects of airway management relevant to obstetrics, including to teach the correct application of cricoid pressure.[48]

Goodwin and French [49] used a part-task simulator to assess trainees' management of failed intubation during caesarean delivery. The initial results were mediocre, but improved significantly following training using the simulator. Similarly, using simulators to train for cricothyroidotomy in the event of 'can't intubate can't ventilate' scenarios improved anaesthetists' management of this life-threatening crisis,[50,51] including with real patients.[51] Investigators have found that a single simulation session improved skills for at least 1 year in one study,[50] although this degree of persistence of learning has not been replicated universally.

There are numerous airway trainers available, with complexities ranging from a disposable plastic coffee cup[52] to high-fidelity devices designed to replicate all aspects of airway anatomy. Truly accurate replication of airway anatomy may not be achievable even with the most expensive devices;[53] however, current evidence suggests that it is the quality of the training, rather than the technology employed, that allows effective learning to take place.[54,55]

Cardiopulmonary resuscitation in pregnancy

Studies that have looked at CPR in pregnancy have demonstrated that even experienced clinicians have inconsistent knowledge,[56,57] and that the performance of CPR in simulated scenarios is often poor.[58] However, there is evidence emerging that simulation can be successful in improving the management of simulated maternal cardiac arrest,[59] and possibly in the management of cardiac arrest in real patients.[60] As a result there are calls to further improve resuscitation in pregnancy by developing a simulation-based life support course especially designed for obstetrics.[61] MOET (Managing Obstetric Emergencies and Trauma) is one such course, and has been credited with improving knowledge of managing obstetric emergencies and contributing to an increased use of perimortem caesarean delivery at maternal cardiac arrest.[60]

Ultrasound for epidural insertion

The use of ultrasound is becoming ubiquitous in anaesthesia, and the National Institute for Health and Care Excellence (NICE) in the United Kingdom has suggested that it might be helpful in achieving correct placement of epidural catheters for labour.[62] Evidence suggests that 'phantoms', part-trainers for the acquisition of skills in ultrasound-guided techniques, can facilitate the training of anaesthetists in ultrasound for regional anaesthesia.[63] Further research is needed to see whether the phantoms for epidural insertions that have recently been developed can be successfully used in obstetric anaesthesia.

Virtual reality devices

Virtual reality simulators, in which screens or specialized headsets replicate a physical environment, have been used successfully to train surgical trainees and interventional radiologists for real operations and procedures.[14] Their earliest application within anaesthesia came in the form of vascular access trainers,[21] and they are now used to train for airway management, resuscitation, and spinal anaesthesia.[64–66] One of the pitfalls of virtual reality simulations has been providing convincing haptic (touch) feedback, which is becoming a key area of research and development.[67] Whilst still a relatively nascent form of technology it holds much promise, and further research will help determine its place amongst other available simulation modalities.

Screen-based simulators

Screen-based technology has been used as a simulation tool in a number of ways, ranging from interactive tutorials to whole-body simulators.[21] Numerous websites provide access to simulation programmes, and simulation applications ('apps') for smartphones and tablet computers are now becoming well established. The use of electronically supported learning ('e-learning'), which often includes elements of simulation, has also become widespread within medicine.

The use of screen-based technology seems to provide more effective learning than traditional didactic teaching when preparing for the successful management of medical emergencies.[68–70] It has also been used successfully as a bridging tool for learners before exposing them to a higher-fidelity environment.[68] Indeed the technology has the potential to be at least as effective as highly complex simulation mannequins when training for certain key anaesthetic emergencies.[71]

The widespread use of smartphones and tablets has increased the accessibility and portability of simulation technology significantly, with many apps that support simulation being free or readily affordable. They can also be effective, with studies showing that they can help improve resuscitation skills over traditional teaching methods.[72,73] Some apps allow a smartphone or tablet to replicate a patient monitor, thereby allowing users to create a high-fidelity environment using a low-fidelity mannequin.[74] Such accessible, portable, and affordable technology has the potential to transform the way that simulation is delivered, although its familiarity should not prevent application-based tools being assessed and researched as vigorously as any other simulation modality.

Mannequin-based simulators

The use of patient mannequins has a long history in obstetrics, as the life-sized mannequins used by Madame du Coudray to teach the art of childbirth to doctors in the eighteenth century French court attest. The use of highly technological mannequins to deliver simulation for anaesthesia has grown rapidly from Sim One, a one-off computerized patient mannequin designed and constructed in the 1960s,[12] to the plethora available from various manufacturers today. As mannequin technology has expanded and become more complex, the taxonomy to describe them has become equally complicated.[21] Terms such as high- and low-fidelity are often described, but are variably used, and are often relative to the technology of the era.

All mannequins share the same basic hardware: a life-sized patient model. Those designed for use in anaesthesia typically have a realistic head, an airway that can accept airway devices and adjuncts, and lungs that can be ventilated. More complex models may also allow cannulation of peripheral, central, and arterial vessels; airways that can be manipulated to simulate airway obstruction and failed intubation; chests that permit decompression of pneumothoraces; and many more features. Modern mannequins for obstetrics may combine a full-body anaesthetic simulator with a female pregnancy simulator (Figure 53.3), further enhancing the realism as well as making multidisciplinary interaction more practicable.

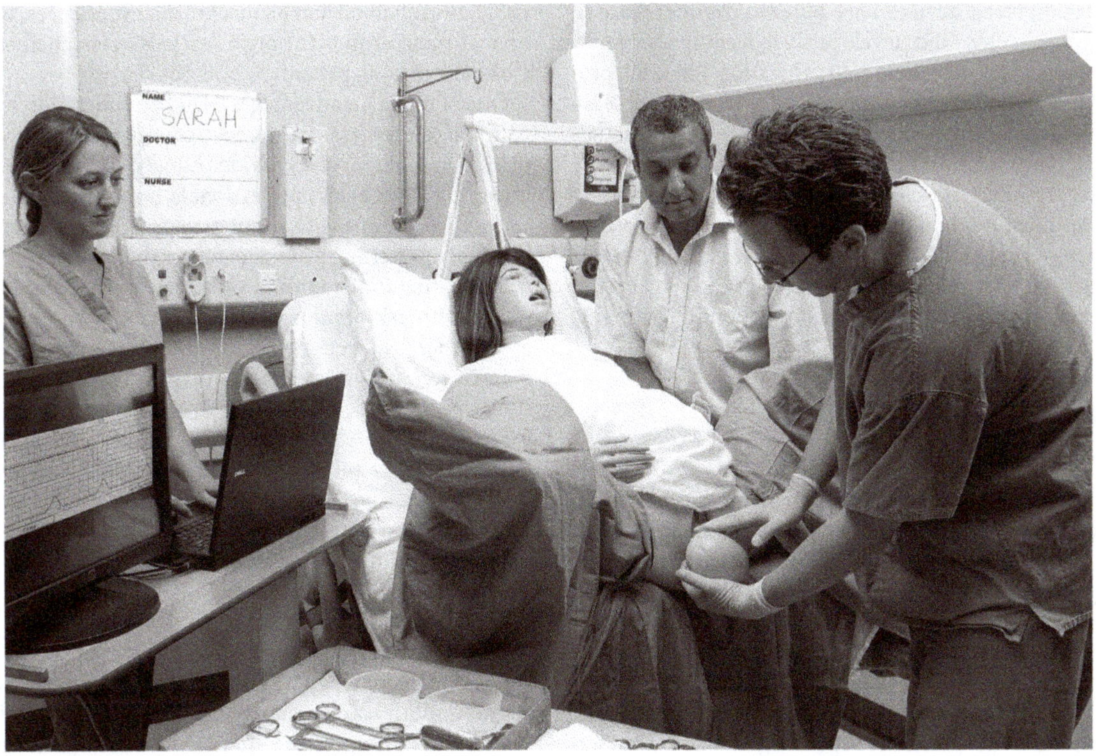

Figure 53.3 Example of a high-fidelity obstetric and anaesthetic mannequin.
Reproduced with permission by Laerdal.

The software that drives the simulation can also vary in complexity. Many mannequins have no intrinsic software; they rely on the use of display screens, verbal cues, pre-prepared graphics, or other simulating devices to present their physiology.

For mannequins that do have software, the physiological parameters are usually computerized.[21] These can be script-controlled, where the changes occur according to a predetermined script or plan, and can be altered in response to the interventions of the participant. This allows the user to retain a degree of control of the simulation and its intended objectives. Alternatively they can be model controlled, where a mathematical model determines the mannequin's physiology and its response to interventions. This can result in a more accurate physiological response, but is sometimes unpredictable and therefore having a manual override available may be helpful.

Fidelity

Fidelity is the degree to which a real environment is simulated.[75] This can be applied in a number of domains, of which the simulation tools themselves form only one part (Figure 53.4). Therefore simulation technology on its own cannot be the key to successful simulation. Equal thought needs to be given to the environment in which the simulation occurs, and the preparation of the participants and those running it.

The ideal level of fidelity for effective simulation is unclear,[76] and most evidence would suggest that increasing the fidelity of the simulator itself does not improve the intended outcomes.[18,35,54,55,77] Concentrating on the complexity of the simulator may be the wrong priority: ultimately, it is the learning requirements that drive the choice of simulation tool. The key to effective simulation is in successfully marrying these.

Conclusion

As technology advances, the options available for simulation are increasing exponentially. Life-sized patient mannequins are able to replicate human anatomy and physiology with ever increasing levels of accuracy and sophistication. Innovative uses for patient actors, part-task trainers, and combinations of both continue to be found. However, it is within screen-based technology that the next explosion of developments is likely to emerge. Smartphones

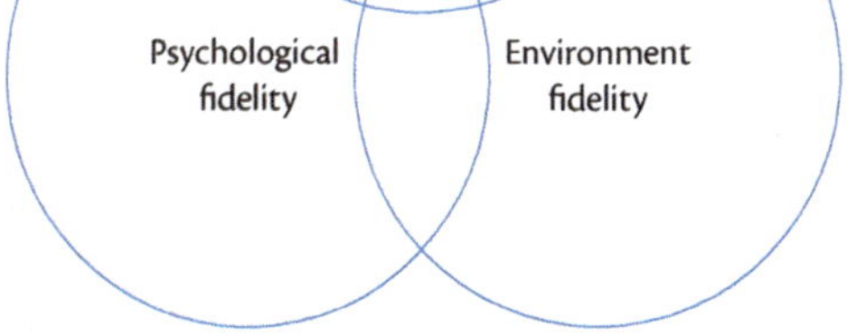

Figure 53.4 The domains of fidelity within simulation.
Adapted by permission from BMJ Publishing Group Limited. *BMJ Quality and Safety*, The use of simulation for training teamwork skills in health care: how low can you go?, JM Beaubien, DP Bake, volume 13, suppl 1, pp. i51–i56, copyright © 2004.

and portable computing devices have become commonplace in healthcare environments, and developers are feeding the frenzy for novel ways to incorporate them into simulation. Since the programming software that creates applications is relatively accessible, this places the future of simulation technology into the hands of people who run simulation.

This is a responsibility as well as an opportunity. The choice of simulation tool must be determined by the learning objectives, and evidence needs to be sought as to how this technology should best be applied. Further research needs to focus on how best to apply the myriad tools available within simulation to improving patient outcomes.

Simulation delivery methods

Simulation centres

Simulation can take place in specifically purpose-built facilities or in any other space refurbished or adjusted to accommodate a simulation facility. Simulation centres are expensive to build and develop. They can usually accommodate many different types of simulation training such as part-task training, full-scale mannequins, and computer-based simulation. In addition, more advanced simulation training for laparoscopic procedures, robotic surgery, or using virtual reality devices may also be available. They sometimes focus on different specialties depending on clinical leadership, local interests, and politics.[78] The Swiss Centre for Medical Simulation at the University Hospital in Basel, Switzerland was amongst the first simulation centres to be established in Europe in 1994.[79] Since then simulator centres have become commonplace, and are available in most major cities in the United Kingdom.

Simulation centres can vary from single rooms placed within a hospital to an entire building with rooms that accommodate different methods of simulation delivery. Rooms designed for full-scale simulation are often flexible allowing them to be converted into different areas such as theatres, emergency resuscitation rooms, or ward bays. This flexibility allows setting up multiple scenarios when performing simulation. Rooms are usually equipped with functioning oxygen and suction equipment. The simulation room may have video and audio links to a control room, which is typically fitted with a one-way mirror (smoked glass) so that the operator or simulation technician can visualize the entire room. Whilst the scenario is being run, the operator can manage the mannequin's physiology, control its voice, and allow the simulation to respond appropriately to the participant's actions. Video and sound equipment are often used to capture images in order to give feedback to participants. Multiple video camera recordings can be synchronized with monitor readings to make the debriefing process more efficient.[80]

Simulation *in situ*

In situ simulation is arguably as old as the medical profession where apprentices would be observed interrogating patients, following the instructions of their masters. In modern medical educational terms, *in situ* simulation is simulation that is physically integrated into the normal clinical environment. *In situ* simulation has enabled the transfer of simulation into hospitals; this allows the potential benefits of training using the environment, equipment, and clinical teams that might be encountered when dealing with real patients. *In situ* training has the potential to enhance individual and team learning experiences, with the additional benefit of allowing organizations to test their safety systems without exposing patients to potential harm.

One of the main advantages of *in situ* simulation over the use of a simulation centre is its low cost. Compared with traditional simulation, it often involves a wider range of participants, potentially including allied health professionals, porters, clerks, and administrators. In contrast with simulation centres, the primary audience is usually practising providers rather than trainees.[81]

Simulating in the normal working environment has the potential to unmask organizational factors that contribute to latent errors, thereby promoting a culture where safety is paramount.[82] It has been shown to be an effective tool to improve organizational performance in trauma as shown by Steinmann and colleagues, with a 76% improvement in task completion and 16% improvement in resuscitation times.[83] It has also shown benefits in obstetrics: Riley and colleagues showed a reduction in perinatal mortality in hospitals trained with *in situ* simulation alongside teamwork training, when compared to hospitals who trained with the teamwork training alone.[84]

In the United Kingdom, the SaFE study (Simulation and Fire drill Evaluation) compared training for obstetric emergencies using high-technology training at simulation centres with *in situ* training. Both teams improved their performance after training. However, training in the simulation centre conferred no additional benefit. Following the SaFE study, the investigators continued to do their obstetric team training *in situ*. Their continued use of in-house simulation has been credited with a reduction in brachial plexus injuries in neonates born following deliveries with shoulder dystocia.[85] Since instituting the training, they have also found a reduction in babies born with low Apgar scores and a decreased incidence of hypoxic-ischaemic encephalopathy.[86–88] This is a powerful demonstration of the potential for successful *in situ* simulation training to translate to improved patient outcomes.

Simulation as a teaching tool

Teaching professionals can be difficult, and using simulation as a teaching tool for professionals is a potentially complex issue. Unlike schoolchildren, adult learners attending a simulation course often do so because they want to learn and improve their skills. They are invariably highly motivated. The common mistake made when teaching professionals is to assume that a lack of learning is due to a lack of motivation and therefore a little inspiration (i.e. simulation) will solve the problem. In fact, perhaps more than any other modality of teaching, simulation must have a secure footing in educational theory. Candidates are placed in potentially stressful situations; they may be tested beyond their current level of expertise in the company of their peers. This combination of circumstances can be potentially damaging. Professionals are used to being successful; consequently they can have great difficulty learning from their own errors. Reactions to errors made in stressful situations include anxiety, embarrassment, and 'defensive reasoning'.[89] Defensive reasoning describes the action of justifying errors by looking at them as the inevitable result of external circumstances or the actions of others. The term was coined by Chris Argyris, an acclaimed educational thinker. Much of his educational theory is relevant to simulation, as are other educational theories too numerous to cover fully here. However it is possible to illustrate with examples some of the educational theory relevant to teaching with simulation.

Behaviourism describes perhaps the most basic of learning strategies; the classic example being Pavlov's conditioning experiments in which the association of the sound of a bell with food eventually lead to the physiological response in dogs of salivation at only the sound of the bell.[90] Operant conditioning introduces the concept of reward and punishment. If an operator performs a task repeatedly and receives reward for doing so then they are conditioned to perform that task again in the same way. This way of learning can often be seen when using task trainers.

Obviously, this is an oversimplification. Cognitive learning, where conceptual knowledge and experience from other areas influence the learning process, also plays a role. Nevertheless, it has been demonstrated that even novice practitioners, who would be expected to have a limited internal cognitive structure upon which to base the learning, will increase their skill at performance on a task trainer with repeated attempts. Crucially though, this does not necessarily translate to increased skill at performance of the task on real patients. Clearly real patients are much more heterogeneous than the average part-task trainer.

One might expect that the higher fidelity the trainer is, the more likely it would be to increase performance on real patients. This is not necessarily the case; Freidman and colleagues[35] took 24 anaesthetic trainees and randomized them into two groups. One group received epidural training with a high-fidelity, anatomically correct, commercially produced simulator that was coupled with a virtual reality display of the needle progression. The other group practised their loss-of-resistance technique by inserting needles into a banana. Blinded expert examiners, utilizing a validated manual skills checklist and global ratings scale, found no difference in subsequent performance of epidural insertion in actual patients between the two groups.

Simulation is often used to increase a participant's knowledge or to train them for a particular skill. It can also be used to train teams of clinicians in crisis resource management (CRM) or 'human factors' training. This type of training has gained popularity due to the realization that decision-making, interpersonal behaviour, and team management can have just as significant an effect on outcome as an individual's knowledge of the algorithms involved.[91]

Different teaching modalities tend to suit different learning environments, candidate selection, and scenario set-up. For example, whilst running knowledge-based teaching scenarios, candidates that will be involved in the scenario at a later stage can benefit from being wallflowers in the room. Conversely, for CRM or human factors training, part of the educational objective is often to examine the flow of information through different members of the team. Obviously this will not happen in a realistic manner if a candidate has been in the room watching the scenario unfold. However, regardless of the simulation modality, the mechanism of learning probably adheres to a similar structure.

In 1984, David Kolb published his experiential learning styles model.[92] It suggests that the learning process cycles through four separate stages and also that people have different learning styles (see Figure 53.5). Kolb proposed that in order to learn it was not sufficient to have the experience, but that reflecting on that experience is a necessity. Learners can engage in the learning process at any part of the cycle. The part of the cycle in which they are likely to engage, and the scale of this engagement, may relate to the type of learner. The Kolb cycle has been elaborated, augmented, and criticized since its inception. The stages may be less distinct than the cycle suggests and learners probably have many styles of learning rather than a clear predilection for one.[93] However, by mapping the stages of simulation to the Kolb cycle, it should be possible to engage all types of learners and complete the learning cycle.

As important as addressing people's learning styles and the learning cycle, is creating an environment in which learning is possible. Maslow's hierarchy of needs (Figure 53.6) is a well-established psychological theory, which asserts that for self-actualization to take place an individual must first have physiological well-being, feel safe, be satisfied in interpersonal relationships and have a sense of self-esteem.[94] It can be argued that many of our most vivid memories are from emotionally charged experiences where in fact we feel unsafe.[95] Indeed many clinicians might attest that much of the 'traditional' practice of medical teaching seemed to be based on seniors undermining their student's sense of self-esteem. Teaching by humiliation is thankfully dying out but, if set up incorrectly, simulation can be equally humiliating.

The aim of increased fidelity is to achieve a situation as close as possible to the real thing. Suspension of disbelief is a term used in the literary, film, and television industries. For example, if a viewer is not able to suspend disbelief and look upon something as 'real' then they will never truly engage with a film. Conversely, if they can view the action as real, then not only will the filmmaker be able to truly immerse them in the story, but may also elicit actual physiological and emotional responses along the way. The same is true for simulation. During high-fidelity simulation, candidates can become anxious and stressed, relieved when things go well, and frustrated even saddened when things go badly. The key is to be able to moderate these feelings to such an extent that learning can take place.

To help understand this there are a number of emotional models: Russell's circumplex model of affect is an accessible and useful example (Figure 53.7).[96] Studies have demonstrated that stimuli that create either an arousal or valence response can lead to increased memory retention.[95] Valence in this respect refers to a scale of positive or negative feeling. For example, feeling happy has a positive valance response, whereas feeling excited would have both positive valance and arousal. High arousal states can be as damaging to effective learning as those in the low end of the spectrum, such as sleepiness or boredom. If candidates become overstimulated by a perceived excess of information, their attention and focus can become narrowed to the extent that they miss the relevant teaching points of the scenario. So the aim is to create realism in simulation that stimulates both arousal and a positive emotional response; to design simulation that will be challenging, but not to the extent that anxiety interferes with the educational objectives.

An interesting case study in this regard is the Managing Emergencies in Paediatric Anaesthesia (MEPA) course that is in widespread use in the United Kingdom and now taught in several centres around the world. The scenarios for MEPA are based on real events and, as occurred in real life, if a certain cue is missed in a scenario, the stress level will build as the simulated patient progressively deteriorates. This can be frustrating, even distressing, for the candidate for whom the scenario is going badly. From the previous discussion it might be assumed that this situation

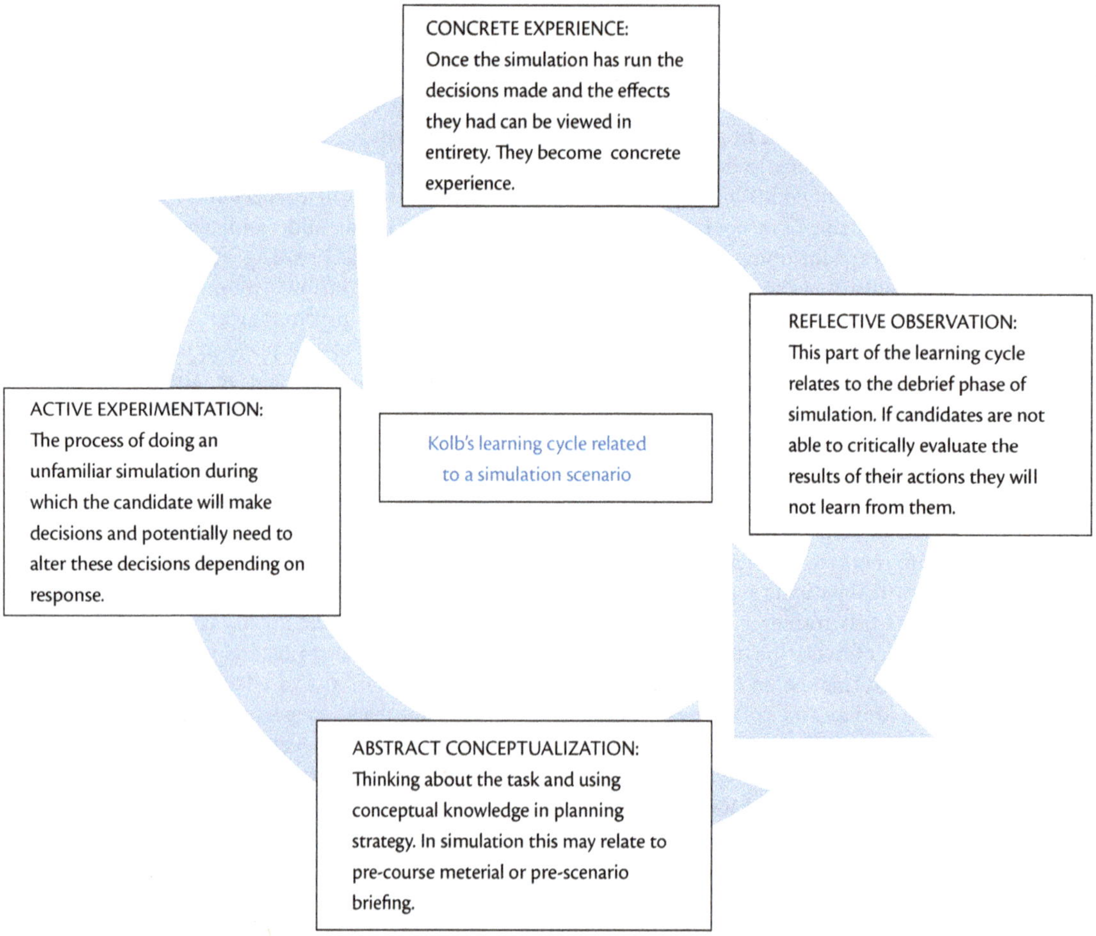
CONCRETE EXPERIENCE:
Once the simulation has run the decisions made and the effects they had can be viewed in entirety. They become concrete experience.
REFLECTIVE OBSERVATION:
This part of the learning cycle relates to the debrief phase of simulation. If candidates are not able to critically evaluate the results of their actions they will not learn from them.
Kolb's learning cycle related to a simulation scenario
ACTIVE EXPERIMENTATION:
The process of doing an unfamiliar simulation during which the candidate will make decisions and potentially need to alter these decisions depending on response.
ABSTRACT CONCEPTUALIZATION:
Thinking about the task and using conceptual knowledge in planning strategy. In simulation this may relate to pre-course meterial or pre-scenario briefing.

Figure 53.5 Kolb's cycle of learning.
Kolb, David A., *Experiential Learning: Experience as a Source of Learning & Development*, 1st, ©1984. Printed and Electronically reproduced by permission of Pearson Education, Inc., New York, New York.

is less than ideal on a simulation course. However, the learning objectives of the scenario are to teach the cues for that particular adverse event, to localize the cause of the problem using a systematic method, and to warn of the dangers of task fixation in

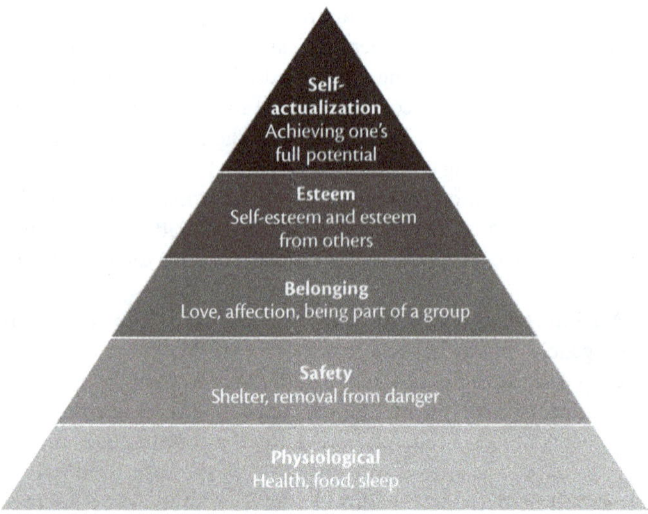

Figure 53.6 Maslow's hierarchy of needs.
Maslow A, A theory of human motivation, *Psychological Review*, Volume 50, Issue 4, pp. 370–96, Copyright © 1943 American Psychological Association. Reprinted with permission.

high-stress situations. Therefore, despite the poor outcome, the arousal and emotion has helped encode and consolidate the learning point. Nevertheless in the eyes of the candidate that outcome may be seen as a failure. As previously stated, professionals and high achievers can have great difficulty learning from failure. How then is it possible to address inevitable failures of judgement and action that will arise during simulation scenarios? This is achieved through debriefing.

The debrief is one of the most crucial aspects of simulation,[76,97] and as Kolb suggested, it is an integral part of the learning process. There are some basic practical points to be borne in mind when considering how to debrief effectively. From a time allocation perspective, an effective and thorough debrief should run for approximately the same duration as the scenario itself. Ideally it should take place away from the area of simulation so that candidates are not constantly distracted by the equipment and faculty setting up for the next group. From the instructor's perspective, the aim of the debrief is firstly to understand the candidates' perceptions of their own actions and then to understand their reasons for acting as they did, before facilitating a group understanding of how things can be done differently to achieve a different result.

This process is more complex than it sounds. Often when someone is asked their reasons for doing something, they will often respond with an 'espoused' theory.[98] That is, they respond with

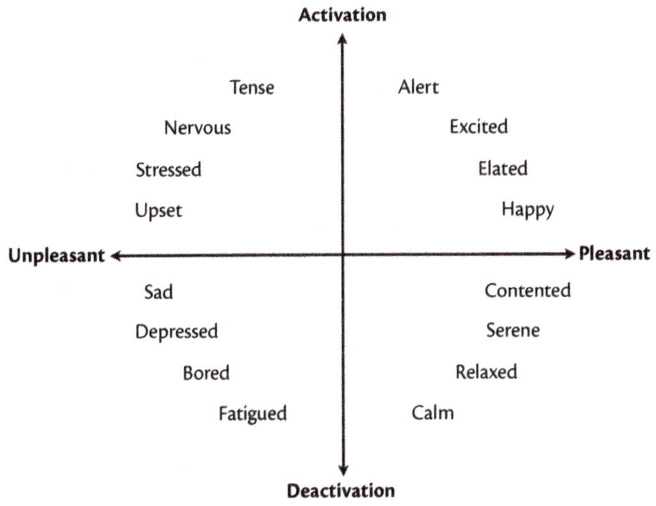

Figure 53.7 Russell's circumplex model of affect.

the theory that they think is the correct answer to the question rather than the 'theory-in-use', which is their underlying personal reason for their actions. For example, if an anaesthetic trainee is asked, 'Why did you use an ultrasound machine to identify vessels for central venous cannulation?' they may respond 'Using ultrasound for this purpose is associated with a reduced risk of inadvertent arterial cannulation'. Which is correct; but it is an espoused theory. The real reason may be that it is the only method they know for identifying the vessel location. To identify the theory-in-use is critical in order to understand the motivation of the candidates. Without an appreciation of a candidate's motivation, a debrief will be didactic and may never serve to change actions in real life.

In 2006, Jenny Rudolph et al. published a debriefing strategy they termed 'debriefing with good judgment'.[99] In essence, the instructor is advised to establish a genuine stance of curiosity in order to elicit the knowledge, assumptions, and feelings that drive the trainee's actions. Following this disclosure the instructor is then able to reframe those feelings and generalize them, which opens up the discussion making it relevant for the entire group, before examining ways of addressing the misapprehensions and if necessary altering behaviour.

Video debriefing has a particular role to play in CRM or human factors training scenarios. Candidates' perception of what happens in high-stress scenarios can differ significantly from that of the impartial observer. Video footage can illustrate this, sometimes quite spectacularly. For this, specialist equipment and a smooth information technology interface is required. Often there is insufficient time when debriefing to scroll through minutes of footage to find a particular incident. Despite the challenges, video debriefing has its enthusiasts.

Simulation as a teaching tool is the topic of various 'Train the Trainers' courses. Teaching theory, mannequin/equipment set-up and use, and lecture and debriefing skills are all covered to varying degrees. Such courses signal that the incorporation of educational theory into simulation design should now be considered a necessity for instructors.

Simulation as an assessment tool

Assessing healthcare providers

Assessments for healthcare providers are generally divided into summative and formative. Formative assessment is a self-reflective process that highlights an individual's strengths and weaknesses, and in simulation typically involves direct observation followed by feedback. Summative assessment is a formal assessment of learning with a specific end point and includes exams, accreditation, and revalidation.[100] Fitness to practice based on simulation assessment is a developing field but to date it is not supported by the current state of simulation knowledge and simulation should not be used with this purpose outside of research.[101]

The current literature of simulation-based assessments describes two main types of scoring, those for explicit process (i.e. based on marking each aspect of a performance) and those for implicit process (marking the process as a whole). Checklists are commonly used to assess explicit processes. Checklists denote the key actions that candidates should successfully accomplish in order to optimally manage the patient. These actions are predetermined by an experienced practitioner and are usually supported by recognized guidelines. Checklists have several limitations. Any single action might have the same weight in the final score, which may not take into account that certain actions are more important than others. Secondly, there is not usually a sequential order in which to achieve the different actions, and thus appropriate prioritization may not be rewarded. Finally, checklist scoring can prompt the candidate into quick-fire action in order to score as highly as possible.

Implicit process scoring is designed to grade the entire scenario in a holistic way, taking in to consideration many factors including non-technical skills. One of the advantages of this type of scoring is the freedom to make observations of overall performance and it is more appropriate for multidimensional complex scenarios.[102]

Studies comparing these two scoring modalities in simulation have found that they are equivalent in their ability to rank the ability of participants in simulation.[103] The main advantages of checklists are their simplicity to mark and their reproducibility. In practice, a combination of assessing implicit and explicit processes is used through a checklist of key actions, and global rating of non-technical skills in the different domains. This seems to be the strategy mostly used to assess participants in simulation.[104]

The use of assessment using simulation is developing rapidly. It is important that the assessment of a participant is reliable and reflects their capability in real clinical practice. Good candidates can be put off by simulation and perform below their abilities; some who are less able may actually do well in the simulation environment, especially as widespread use of simulation means candidates can be 'primed' from past experience during the same or similar scenarios. Before any summative assessment is put in place, rigorous quality assurance needs to be performed to ensure that its outcomes are valid.

Assessing healthcare systems

Simulation-based assessment of healthcare systems is probably best done through *in situ* simulation. This can unmask latent errors within systems, and allow assessment of the interactions between different areas of the hospital such as laboratories and other support services in real time and place.[81]

More than half of the obstetric units in England and Wales conduct *in situ* simulation on a regular basis.[105] There is evidence that drill training improves readiness and reaction times during emergencies, and its frequent use can also improve the availability of equipment and drugs at the point of care.[101]

Setting up a simulation programme

The construction of an effective and enduring simulation programme is rarely a simple and stress-free task. Frequently enthusiasm and good intentions are squandered, along with significant amounts of work, on programmes that either peter out soon after conception or indeed never get past the design stage. Unfortunately there is little empirical evidence to serve as a roadmap to a successful programme. However, testimony from experienced individuals involved in simulation around the world serves to outline the common pitfalls and obstacles encountered when putting a simulation programme together.

Firstly, be realistic with your aims. In a centre with no infrastructure, constructing a unique, self-funding, international programme of simulation may take decades or may even not be possible. On the other hand, a local programme, tailored to address specific issues within your unit could be achievable in a reasonable time frame. If targeted correctly, it could become invaluable and serve as a stepping-stone to future simulation development.

Avoid simulation for simulation's sake. Some individuals are simulation enthusiasts; some are not. Simulation is not the answer to all training needs. It is worthwhile remembering that a poorly constructed simulation can serve to worsen outcome. Expensive high-fidelity simulators are not always the best simulators to teach a specific task. Nevertheless, any type of simulation often necessitates a considerable investment in man-hours if nothing else.

Achieving and maintaining that man-hour investment can make the difference between a short-lived venture and a sustainable training tool, so the importance of involving and encouraging individuals who express enthusiasm for simulation cannot be overstated. If your institution has enthusiastic teachers and trainers, or if there is a local simulation centre, their involvement in the project can be invaluable. Conversely the inception of a simulation programme is not the time to convert sceptics to your cause; their cynicism is only likely to increase as the inevitable faults of a naïve programme are uncovered.

Once these initial considerations have taken place it is time to commit to a repetitive cycle of course or scenario development (Figure 53.8). Each individual stage helps to ensure a robust final product.

Needs assessment

Your needs assessment might examine data from audit, critical incident reporting, feedback survey, or staff perceptions of inefficiency. There are many different models of systematic needs assessment; however, the key with regards to simulation is to be able to target resources with the aim of beneficially affecting outcome.

Scenario/course design

The educational objectives will be determined by the needs assessment. The scenario/course design must draw on the educational theory in order to achieve these objectives. When constructing scenarios it is useful to use a scenario proforma. Not only does this aid in the construction of the scenario but it also enables

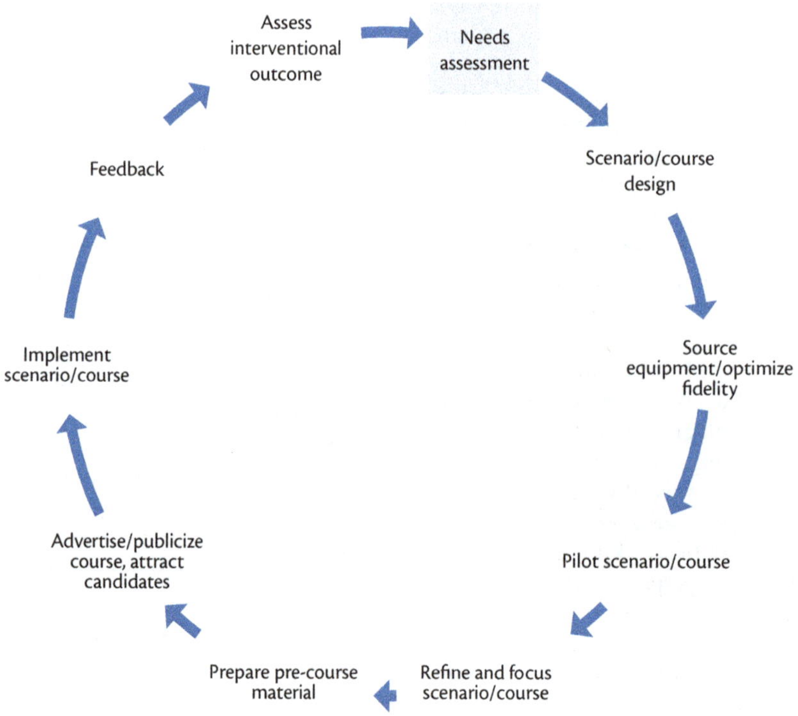

Figure 53.8 The stages required to successfully set up a simulation programme.
Reproduced with permission from Dr. Peter Weinstock.

immediate quantification of the diversity of faculty and equipment required to run the scenario.

Source equipment/optimize fidelity

Equipment may be available from local simulation or education centre. You may be able to borrow from other departments. You may also need to be creative to achieve the desired level of fidelity. Some caveats need to be remembered when sourcing equipment. If ward stock is used it must be documented and replaced so as not to leave clinical areas short of equipment. Similarly, particularly when using point-of-care simulation, a robust system must be in place to ensure simulation equipment is not confused with ward stock after the course has run, with potentially catastrophic consequences.

Attention must be paid to sources of danger in simulation as in real life. Sharps and drugs must be safely disposed of, defibrillators and other electrical devices must be managed appropriately. Also the use of cadaveric products should be carefully considered; cultural and religious objections should be borne in mind.

Pilot the scenario/course

Test runs are important to iron out unanticipated glitches in the running of the course. These teething problems would otherwise have the ability to seriously detract from the course's educational value.

Refine and focus the scenario/course

Following the pilot stage there may be areas that require redesign or elements that clearly need addressing. These should be implemented prior to launching the course.

Prepare pre-course material

The type and scope of pre-course material will depend on various factors including the educational objectives of the course, time constraints for delivering the course, whether the scenarios are to form part of an assessment, and the ratios of human factors to skills and/or knowledge training involved in the course. Resuscitation courses now employ a large degree of online learning and formative assessment to be completed prior to attendance on their courses. This strategy has the advantage of allowing candidates to learn in their own time but crucially aims to ensure that candidates reach a baseline level of knowledge prior to participation. This sort of approach can be important for courses designed primarily to test knowledge and its application. Courses designed to test systems or involve a greater degree of human factors training might benefit from less detailed pre-course material.

Advertise/publicize the course

Intrapartum update simulations have been shown to improve outcomes[106] but to achieve this they are run at least yearly and have 100% participation. If you wish to attract candidates from outside of your unit you will need to publicize your course. In order for that publicity to be successful your own needs assessment will have to be in line with the needs of the potential candidate.

Implement the scenario/course

The faculty for early versions of the course is likely to comprise primarily of the development team. As the course evolves, it becomes increasingly important to develop flexible and motivated faculty members to help with the running and further development of the course. This faculty may be previous candidates on the course or staff with an interest in simulation and training. Either way, encouraging the involvement of new faculty will allow the course to be sustainable. Numerous 'Train the Trainers' courses are available to ensure that faculty is appropriately trained for the various simulation modalities that may be needed, and to ensure that they can deliver the sessions and the feedback in a standardized way.

Feedback

Feedback from candidates and faculty is important to ascertain which parts of the course/scenarios are working and which need to be changed. This is also an appropriate stage to review which bits of simulation equipment require servicing or replacement.

Assess the interventional outcome

There is precious little data on the ability of simulation training to change patient outcome. You should aim to demonstrate that the simulation course fulfils the original needs assessment. To facilitate this process establishing an audit trail alongside the training programme would be appropriate.

The process is cyclical. As the needs of training evolve, so does the course. As the course evolves, so does the course material and the faculty.

The key elements of successful simulation

Whilst 'success' in simulation may be described in many ways, the intended outcome of most medical simulation is to improve patient outcomes. The other key component is a consistent demonstration of improved learning.

Educational outcomes

Issenberg, McGaghie, and their colleagues have examined the outcomes of simulation-based medical education from 1969 onwards, through a systematic review of the published literature.[76,97] They have identified key features and best practices that are found in papers that given rise to effective learning. Those from their latest work, which covers 2003–2009, are summarized in Table 53.1.[107]

Patient outcomes

Given that improving patients' outcomes is the primary aim of most medical simulation, it may seem surprising that there is a paucity of data to support the translation of simulation training into better clinical results.[14] Much of the published evidence demonstrates that simulation training improves performance in future simulations. Does this mean that clinical performance will also improve? And why are there so few data?

Part of the difficulty is that simulation is often geared to prepare for rare emergencies. Rare and unpredictable emergencies are challenging to monitor and capture, their outcomes are often hard to neatly encapsulate, and to ascribe a causal relationship between the clinical outcome and the training can be tenuous. Randomized controlled studies, the highest level of evidence, are difficult to perform in this setting and would likely require multicentre collaboration. Much of the evidence we do have comes from retrospective studies, and even here the discovery of improved patient outcomes has sometimes been fortuitous. However, there

Table 53.1 Features and best practice for effective learning through simulation

Feature	Relevance
Feedback given	The most valuable component for learning
Deliberate practice (expert-level learning)	Continuously challenges learners
Integrated into the whole curriculum	Complements other education
Outcomes measured	Required for valid research
Simulation fidelity appropriate	Technology should be matched to the learning objectives
Skill acquisition and maintenance	Repetition is needed to ensure the learning lasts
Mastery of learning	Accomplish *all* educational objectives
Transferable to clinical practice	Achieves a deeper level of learning[107]
Team training	In addition to clinical tasks
High-stakes testing	Simulation for summative assessment must be reliable
Instructor training	Ability to facilitate is not innate
Set in the learner's educational and professional context	Should be relevant to the leaner's needs

Reproduced with permission from McGaghie WC, Issenberg SB, Petrusa ER, Scalese RJ, A critical review of simulation-based medical education research: 2003–2009, *Medical Education*, Volume 44, Issue 1, pp. 50–63, Copyright © 2010 John Wiley and Sons.

are a number of studies where simulation training has been shown to improve patient outcomes (Table 53.2).

With regard to obstetrics, eight key components are shared by all the hospitals in which obstetric training has yielded improved patient outcomes. These are summarized in Box 53.1.

It is challenging to identify the elements of training programmes that give rise to the best outcomes. This is especially true in simulation, where 'success' can be difficult to quantify, and the clinical denominator is often relatively low. No one can be certain precisely what is required in the ideal simulation recipe, nor in what quantities, nor how much 'cooking' is required, and how often. Using the above components is a good start, but more data needs to be collected about which training leads to improved outcomes in the real world.

Gaba has rightly argued that 'no industry in which human lives depend on the skilled performance of responsible operators has waited for unequivocal proof of the benefits of simulation before embracing it. In my opinion, neither should anesthesiology'.[111] However, unless more irrefutable evidence of real-world benefit is collected, there is a limit to how long we can continue to argue for the investments of manpower, time, and money that good quality simulation requires. Simulation in obstetrics and obstetric anaesthesia probably does save lives; those working in the specialty instinctively believe it, but there is also a need to produce high quality data in order to prove it.

Box 53.1 The components shared by hospitals with obstetric simulation programmes that have led to improved patient outcomes

- Institution-level incentives to training
- Relevant, *in situ* training
- Non-threatening assessment
- 100% penetration: train the entire workforce
- Train in multiprofessional teams
- Clinical training and teamwork training combined
- Realistic tools (high fidelity rather than high technology)
- Self-directed infrastructural change: local solutions to national problems.

Data from Siassakos D *et al.*, The active components of effective training in obstetric emergencies, *BJOG: An International Journal of Obstetrics and Gynaecology*, Volume 116, Issue 8, pp. 1028–1032, Copyright © 2009 Jon Wiley & Sons

Table 53.2 Examples of studies that have shown improved patient outcomes following simulation training

Clinical improvement	Type of training
Improved Apgar scores in infants[15]	*In situ* multidisciplinary team training
Reduction in brachial plexus injury after shoulder dystocia[16]	*In situ* multidisciplinary team training
Reduction in hypoxic-ischaemic encephalopathy in infants[15]	*In situ* multidisciplinary team training
Safer insertion of central venous catheters[108]	Part-task training with screen-based teaching
Reduced catheter-related bloodstream infections from central venous catheters[109]	Part-task training with screen-based teaching
Reduction in complications during eye surgery[110]	Part-task training and structured curriculum

Data from various sources (see references).

References

1. Rosen MA, Hunt EA, Pronovost PJ, *et al.* In situ simulation in continuing education for the health care professions: a systematic review. *J Contin Educ Health Prof* 2012; 32(4):243–54.
2. Smith CM. Origin and uses of primum non nocere—above all, do no harm! *J Clin Pharmacol* 2005; 45(4):371–7.
3. Kohn LT, Corrigan JM, Donaldson MS (eds). *To Err Is Human: Building a Safer Health System.* Washington, DC: The National Academies Press; 2000.
4. Cass GK, Crofts JF, Draycott TJ. The use of simulation to teach clinical skills in obstetrics. *Semin Perinatol* 2011; 35(2):68–73.
5. Owen H. Early use of simulation in medical education. *Simul Healthc* 2012; 7(2):102–16.
6. Porter R. *Blood and Guts: A Short History of Medicine.* New York: W. W. Norton; 2004.
7. Russell KF. Ivory anatomical manikins. *Med Hist* 1972; 16(2):131–42.
8. Gelbart NR. *The King's Midwife: A History and Mystery of Madame Du Coudray.* Berkeley and Los Angeles, CA: University of California Press; 1999.

9. Flexner A, Pritchett HS, Carnegie Foundation for the Advancement of Teaching. *Medical Education in the United States and Canada: A Report to the Carnegie Foundation for the Advancement of Teaching*. New York: Carnegie Foundation for the Advancement of Teaching; 1910.
10. Howard SK, Gaba DM, Fish KJ, *et al.* Anesthesia crisis resource management training: teaching anesthesiologists to handle critical incidents. *Aviat Space Environ Med* 1992; 63(9):763–70.
11. Cooper JB, Taqueti VR. A brief history of the development of mannequin simulators for clinical education and training. *Qual Saf Health Care* 2004; 13 Suppl 1:i11–8.
12. Denson JS, Abrahamson S. A computer-controlled patient simulator. *JAMA* 1969; 208(3):504–8.
13. McGaghie WC, Issenberg SB, Cohen ER, *et al.* Does simulation-based medical education with deliberate practice yield better results than traditional clinical education? A meta-analytic comparative review of the evidence. *Acad Med* 2011; 86(6):706–11.
14. McGaghie WC, Draycott TJ, Dunn WF, *et al.* Evaluating the impact of simulation on translational patient outcomes. *Simul Healthc* 2011; 6 Suppl:S42–7.
15. Draycott T, Sibanda T, Owen L, *et al.* Does training in obstetric emergencies improve neonatal outcome? *BJOG* 2006; 113(2):177–82.
16. Draycott TJ, Crofts JF, Ash JP, *et al.* Improving neonatal outcome through practical shoulder dystocia training. *Obstet Gynecol* 2008; 112(1):14–20.
17. Gaba DM. The future vision of simulation in health care. *Qual Safe Health Care* 2004; 13(Suppl 1):i2–i10.
18. Beaubien JM, Baker DP. The use of simulation for training teamwork skills in health care: how low can you go? *Qual Safe Health Care* 2004; 13 Suppl 1:i51–6.
19. Meller G. A typology of simulators for medical education. *J Digit Imaging* 1997; 10(3 Suppl 1):194–6.
20. Alinier G. A typology of educationally focused medical simulation tools. *Med Teach* 2007; 29(8):e243–50.
21. Cumin D, Merry AF. Simulators for use in anaesthesia. *Anaesthesia* 2007; 62(2):151–62.
22. Barrows HS, Abrahamson S. The programmed patient: a technique for appraising student performance in clinical neurology. *J Med Educ* 1964; 39:802–5.
23. May W, Park JH, Lee JP. A ten-year review of the literature on the use of standardized patients in teaching and learning: 1996–2005. *Med Teach* 2009; 31(6):487–92.
24. Nestel D, Tabak D, Tierney T, *et al.* Key challenges in simulated patient programs: an international comparative case study. *BMC Med Educ* 2011; 11:69.
25. Ellis D, Crofts JF, Hunt LP, *et al.* Hospital, simulation center, and teamwork training for eclampsia management: a randomized controlled trial. *Obstet Gynecol* 2008; 111(3):723–31.
26. Crofts JF, Bartlett C, Ellis D, *et al.* Patient-actor perception of care: a comparison of obstetric emergency training using manikins and patient-actors. *Qual Saf Health Care* 2008; 17(1):20–4.
27. Kneebone R, Kidd J, Nestel D, *et al.* An innovative model for teaching and learning clinical procedures. *Med Educ* 2002; 36(7):628–34.
28. Kneebone RL, Kidd J, Nestel D, *et al.* Blurring the boundaries: scenario-based simulation in a clinical setting. *Med Educ* 2005; 39(6):580–7.
29. Sibanda T, Crofts JF, Barnfield S, *et al.* PROMPT education and development: saving mothers' and babies' lives in resource poor settings. *BJOG* 2009; 116(6):868–9.
30. Johnson KB, Syroid ND, Drews FA, *et al.* Part Task and variable priority training in first-year anesthesia resident education: a combined didactic and simulation-based approach to improve management of adverse airway and respiratory events. *Anesthesiology* 2008; 108(5):831–40.
31. Sivanandan I, Morris E, Soar J. The Palm-LM (laryngeal airway) simulator. *Anaesthesia* 2003; 58(8):825–6.
32. Meek T. An epidural training simulator. *Int J Obstet Anesth* 1998; 7(4):282.
33. Daykin AP, Bacon RJ. An epidural injection simulator. *Anaesthesia* 1990; 45(3):235–6.
34. Uppal V, Kearns RJ, McGrady EM. Evaluation of M43B Lumbar puncture simulator-II as a training tool for identification of the epidural space and lumbar puncture. *Anaesthesia* 2011; 66(6):493–6.
35. Friedman Z, Siddiqui N, Katznelson R, *et al.* Clinical impact of epidural anesthesia simulation on short- and long-term learning curve: High- versus low-fidelity model training. *Reg Anaesth Pain Med* 2009; 34(3):229–32.
36. Barsuk JH, Cohen ER, Caprio T, *et al.* Simulation-based education with mastery learning improves residents' lumbar puncture skills. *Neurology* 2012; 79(2):132–7.
37. Cantwell R, Clutton-Brock T, Cooper G, *et al.* Saving Mothers' Lives: reviewing maternal deaths to make motherhood safer: 2006–2008. The Eighth Report of the Confidential Enquiries into Maternal Deaths in the United Kingdom. *BJOG* 2011; 118 Suppl 1:1–203.
38. Mathai M, Gulmezoglu AM, Hill S. Saving women's lives: evidence-based recommendations for the prevention of postpartum haemorrhage. *Bull World Health Organ* 2007; 85(4):322–3.
39. Patel A, Goudar SS, Geller SE, *et al.* Drape estimation vs. visual assessment for estimating postpartum hemorrhage. *Int J Obstet Anaesth* 2006; 93(3):220–4.
40. Bose P, Regan F, Paterson-Brown S. Improving the accuracy of estimated blood loss at obstetric haemorrhage using clinical reconstructions. *BJOG* 2006; 113(8):919–24.
41. Toledo P, McCarthy RJ, Hewlett BJ, *et al.* The accuracy of blood loss estimation after simulated vaginal delivery. *Anesth Analg* 2007 Dec; 105(6):1736–40.
42. Toledo P, McCarthy RJ, Burke CA, *et al.* The effect of live and web-based education on the accuracy of blood-loss estimation in simulated obstetric scenarios. *Am J Obstet Gynecol* 2010; 202(4):400.e1–5.
43. Toledo P, Eosakul ST, Goetz K, *et al.* Decay in blood loss estimation skills after web-based didactic training. *Simul Healthc* 2012; 7(1):18–21.
44. Johnson RV, Lyons GR, Wilson RC, *et al.* Training in obstetric general anaesthesia: a vanishing art? *Anaesthesia* 2000; 55(2):179–83.
45. Lipman S, Carvalho B, Brock-Utne J. The demise of general anesthesia in obstetrics revisited: prescription for a cure. *Int J Obstet Anesth* 2005; 14(1):2–4.
46. Hawthorne L, Wilson R, Lyons G, *et al.* Failed intubation revisited: 17-yr experience in a teaching maternity unit. *Br J Anaesth* 1996; 76(5):680–4.
47. Quinn AC, Milne D, Columb M, *et al.* Failed tracheal intubation in obstetric anaesthesia: 2 yr national case-control study in the UK. *Br J Anaesth* 2013; 110(1):74–80.
48. Owen H, Follows V, Reynolds KJ, *et al.* Learning to apply effective cricoid pressure using a part task trainer. *Anaesthesia* 2002; 57(11):1098–101.
49. Goodwin MW, French GW. Simulation as a training and assessment tool in the management of failed intubation in obstetrics. *Int J Obstet Anesth* 2001; 10(4):273–7.
50. Boet S, Borges BC, Naik VN, *et al.* Complex procedural skills are retained for a minimum of 1 yr after a single high-fidelity simulation training session. *Br J Anaesth* 2011; 107(4):533–9.
51. Kuduvalli PM, Jervis A, Tighe SQ, *et al.* Unanticipated difficult airway management in anaesthetised patients: a prospective study of the effect of mannequin training on management strategies and skill retention. *Anaesthesia* 2008; 63(4):364–9.
52. de Menezes Lyra R. Glottis simulator. *Anesth Analg* 1999; 88(6):1422–3.
53. Schebesta K, Hupfl M, Rossler B, *et al.* Degrees of reality: airway anatomy of high-fidelity human patient simulators and airway trainers. *Anesthesiology* 2012; 116(6):1204–9.

54. Chandra DB, Savoldelli GL, Joo HS, *et al.* Fiberoptic oral intubation: the effect of model fidelity on training for transfer to patient care. *Anesthesiology* 2008; 109(6):1007–13.
55. Friedman Z, You-Ten KE, Bould MD, *et al.* Teaching lifesaving procedures: the impact of model fidelity on acquisition and transfer of cricothyrotomy skills to performance on cadavers. *Anesth Analg* 2008; 107(5):1663–9.
56. Cohen SE, Andes LC, Carvalho B. Assessment of knowledge regarding cardiopulmonary resuscitation of pregnant women. *Int J Obstet Anesth* 2008; 17(1):20–5.
57. Einav S, Matot I, Berkenstadt H, *et al.* A survey of labour ward clinicians' knowledge of maternal cardiac arrest and resuscitation. *Int J Obstet Anesth* 2008; 17(3):238–42.
58. Lipman SS, Daniels KI, Carvalho B, *et al.* Deficits in the provision of cardiopulmonary resuscitation during simulated obstetric crises. *Am J Obstet Gynecol* 2010; 203(2):179.e1–5.
59. Fisher N, Eisen LA, Bayya JV, *et al.* Improved performance of maternal-fetal medicine staff after maternal cardiac arrest simulation-based training. *Am J Obstet Gynecol* 2011; 205(3):239.e1–5.
60. Dijkman A, Huisman CM, Smit M, *et al.* Cardiac arrest in pregnancy: increasing use of perimortem caesarean section due to emergency skills training? *BJOG* 2010; 117(3):282–7.
61. Lipman SS, Daniels KI, Arafeh J, *et al.* The case for OBLS: a simulation-based obstetric life support program. *Semin Perinatol* 2011; 35(2):74–9.
62. National Institute of Health and Clinical Excellence. *Ultrasound-Guided Catheterisation of the Epidural Space.* London: NICE; 2008. http://www.nice.org.uk/guidance/ipg249
63. Hocking G, Hebard S, Mitchell CH. A review of the benefits and pitfalls of phantoms in ultrasound-guided regional anesthesia. *Reg Anaesth Pain Med* 2011; 36(2):162–70.
64. Kulcsar Z, O'Mahony E, Lovquist E, *et al.* Preliminary evaluation of a virtual reality-based simulator for learning spinal anesthesia. *J Clin Anesth* 2013; 25(2):98–105.
65. Semeraro F, Frisoli A, Bergamasco M, *et al.* Virtual reality enhanced mannequin (VREM) that is well received by resuscitation experts. *Resuscitation* 2009; 80(4):489–92.
66. Goldmann K, Steinfeldt T. Acquisition of basic fiberoptic intubation skills with a virtual reality airway simulator. *J Clin Anesth* 2006; 18(3):173–8.
67. Ullrich S, Kuhlen T. Haptic palpation for medical simulation in virtual environments. *IEEE Trans Vis Comput Graph* 2012; 18(4):617–25.
68. Schwid HA, Rooke GA, Michalowski P, *et al.* Screen-based anesthesia simulation with debriefing improves performance in a mannequin-based anesthesia simulator. *Teach Learn Med* 2001; 13(2):92–6.
69. Ohrn MA, van Oostrom JH, van Meurs WL. A comparison of traditional textbook and interactive computer learning of neuromuscular block. *Anesth Analg* 1997; 84(3):657–61.
70. Bonnetain E, Boucheix JM, Hamet M, *et al.* Benefits of computer screen-based simulation in learning cardiac arrest procedures. *Med Educ* 2010; 44(7):716–22.
71. Nyssen AS, Larbuisson R, Janssens M, *et al.* A comparison of the training value of two types of anesthesia simulators: computer screen-based and mannequin-based simulators. *Anesth Analg* 2002; 94(6):1560–5.
72. Semeraro F, Taggi F, Tammaro G, *et al.* iCPR: a new application of high-quality cardiopulmonary resuscitation training. *Resuscitation* 2011; 82(4):436–41.
73. Low D, Clark N, Soar J, *et al.* A randomised control trial to determine if use of the iResus(c) application on a smart phone improves the performance of an advanced life support provider in a simulated medical emergency. *Anaesthesia* 2011; 66(4):255–62.
74. Castle Andersen ApS. *SimMon.* [Online] https://itunes.apple.com/gb/app/simmon/id364731597?mt=8
75. Schwid HA. Anesthesia simulators—technology and applications. *Isr Med Assoc J* 2000; 2(12):949–53.
76. McGaghie WC, Issenberg SB, Petrusa ER, *et al.* A critical review of simulation-based medical education research: 2003–2009. *Med Educ* 2010; 44(1):50–63.
77. Crabtree NA, Chandra DB, Weiss ID, *et al.* Fibreoptic airway training: correlation of simulator performance and clinical skill. *Can J Anaesth*2008; 55(2):100–4.
78. Seropian M, Lavey R. Design considerations for healthcare simulation facilities. *Simul Healthc* 2010; 5(6):338–45.
79. Gardner R, Raemer DB. Simulation in obstetrics and gynecology. *Obstet Gynecol Clin North Am* 2008; 35(1):97–127, ix.
80. Murray DJ. Current trends in simulation training in anesthesia: a review. *Minerva Anestesiol* 2011; 77(5):528–33.
81. Walker ST, Sevdalis N, McKay A, *et al.* Unannounced in situ simulations: integrating training and clinical practice. *BMJ Qual Saf* 2013; 22(6):453–8.
82. Aggarwal R, Mytton OT, Derbrew M, *et al.* Training and simulation for patient safety. *Qual Saf Health Care* 2010; 19 Suppl 2:i34–43.
83. Steinemann S, Berg B, Skinner A, *et al.* In situ, multidisciplinary, simulation-based teamwork training improves early trauma care. *J Surg Educ* 2011; 68(6):472–7.
84. Riley W, Davis S, Miller K, *et al.* Didactic and simulation nontechnical skills team training to improve perinatal patient outcomes in a community hospital. *Jt Comm J Qual Patient Saf* 2011; 37(8):357–64.
85. Siassakos D, Fox R, Crofts JF, *et al.* The management of a simulated emergency: better teamwork, better performance. *Resuscitation* 2011; 82(2):203–6.
86. Crofts JF, Winter C, Sowter MC. Practical simulation training for maternity care—where we are and where next. *BJOG* 2011; 118 Suppl 3:11–16.
87. Crofts JF, Fox R, Ellis D, *et al.* Observations from 450 shoulder dystocia simulations: lessons for skills training. *Obstet Gynecol* 2008; 112(4):906–12.
88. Crofts JF, Bartlett C, Ellis D, *et al.* Training for shoulder dystocia: a trial of simulation using low-fidelity and high-fidelity mannequins. *Obstet Gynecol* 2006; 108(6):1477–85.
89. Argyris C. Teaching smart people how to learn. *Harv Bus Rev* 1991; 69(3):99–109.
90. Pavlov I (Anrep GV trans, ed). *Reflexes: An Investigation of the Physiological Activity of the Cerebral Cortex.* Oxford: Oxford University Press; 1927.
91. Gaba DM. Crisis resource management and teamwork training in anaesthesia. *Br J Anaesth* 2010; 105(1):3–6.
92. Kolb DA. *Experiential Learning: Experience as the Source of Learning and Development.* Englewood Cliffs, NJ: Prentice-Hall; 1984.
93. Coffield F, Moseley D, Hall E, *et al. Learning Styles and Pedagogy in Post-16 Learning. A Systematic and Critical Review.* London: Learning and Skills Research Centre; 2004.
94. Maslow A. A theory of human motivation. *Psychol Rev* 1943; 50(4):370–96.
95. Hamann S. Cognitive and neural mechanisms of emotional memory. *Trends Cogn Sci* 2001; 5(9):394–400.
96. Russell J. A circumplex model of affect. *J Pers Soc Psychol* 1980; 39(6):1161–78.
97. Issenberg SB, McGaghie WC, Petrusa ER, *et al.* Features and uses of high-fidelity medical simulations that lead to effective learning: a BEME systematic review. *Med Teach* 2005; 27(1):10–28.
98. Argyris C, Schön DA. *Theory in Practice: Increasing Professional Effectiveness.* San Francisco, CA: Jossey-Bass Publishers; 1974.
99. Rudolph JW, Simon R, Dufresne RL, *et al.* There's no such thing as "nonjudgmental" debriefing: a theory and method for debriefing with good judgment. *Simul Healthc* 2006; 1(1):49–55.
100. Boulet JR, Murray DJ. Simulation-based assessment in anesthesiology: requirements for practical implementation. *Anesthesiology* 2010; 112(4):1041–52.
101. Pratt SD. Focused review: simulation in obstetric anesthesia. *Anesth Analg* 2012; 114(1):186–90.

102. Boulet JR, Murray D. Review article: assessment in anesthesiology education. *Can J Anaesth* 2012; 59(2):182–92.
103. Murray DJ, Boulet JR, Kras JF, *et al.* Acute care skills in anesthesia practice: a simulation-based resident performance assessment. *Anesthesiology* 2004; 101(5):1084–95.
104. Bould MD, Naik VN, Hamstra SJ. Review article: New directions in medical education related to anesthesiology and perioperative medicine. *Can J Anaesth* 2012; 59(2):136–50.
105. Anderson ER, Black R, Brocklehurst P. Acute obstetric emergency drill in England and Wales: a survey of practice. *BJOG* 2005; 112(3):372–5.
106. Siassakos D, Crofts JF, Winter C, *et al.* The active components of effective training in obstetric emergencies. *BJOG* 2009; 116(8):1028–32.
107. Kirkpatrick D. *Evaluating Training Programs* (2nd ed). San Francisco, CA: Berrett-Koehler; 1998.
108. Barsuk JH, McGaghie WC, Cohen ER, *et al.* Simulation-based mastery learning reduces complications during central venous catheter insertion in a medical intensive care unit. *Crit Care Med* 2009; 37(10):2697–701.
109. Barsuk JH, Cohen ER, Feinglass J, *et al.* Use of simulation-based education to reduce catheter-related bloodstream infections. *Arch Intern Med* 2009; 169(15):1420–3.
110. Rogers GM, Oetting TA, Lee AG, *et al.* Impact of a structured surgical curriculum on ophthalmic resident cataract surgery complication rates. *J Cataract Refract Surg* 2009; 35(11):1956–60.
111. Gaba DM. Improving anesthesiologists' performance by simulating reality. *Anesthesiology* 1992; 76(4):491–4.

CHAPTER 54

Ultrasound

Sudhir Immani and John Loughrey

Introduction

The use of ultrasound in medical practice was first reported in the 1950s with one of the first descriptions of its use in clinical anaesthesia practice dating back to the late 1970s.[1] A number of reviews have recommended its usefulness in anaesthesia.[2–4] The most obvious and current application for ultrasound for obstetric anaesthetists is in the improvement of the safety, quality, and success of neuraxial anaesthesia. The description of current technique comprises the main content of this chapter. Cork and Currie both published initial reports of ultrasound application for pre-neuraxial block landmark assessment in obstetric populations in the 1980s.[5,6] However, there remains a relative paucity of good data charting the developing utility of ultrasound in obstetric anaesthesia practice and many published studies are from a small number of enthusiasts (Table 54.1). In fact, to date there is only one meta-analysis on benefits of ultrasound-guided neuraxial procedures.[7]

There are other applications of ultrasound in obstetric anaesthesia practice including vascular access, cardiac assessment, and possibly even gastric volume assessment.

Neuraxial blockade equipment

From the technical perspective, spinal ultrasound imaging is difficult, as the area of interest is protected by bone. As the ultrasound beam does not pass through bone very well, the acoustic window towards the area of interest is relatively narrow. Bony surfaces reflect most of the waves back so structures beyond bone are not 'seen' with ultrasound and a black/grey area is observed behind a thick white line on the image screen. High-frequency transducers produce high-resolution images but with poor tissue depth penetration as more sound is absorbed. Low-frequency transducers have greater tissue penetration but resolution is poorer. Most anaesthetists use a linear high-frequency ultrasound probe for superficial vascular access and brachial plexus anaesthesia. However, these probes are generally insufficient for neuraxial imaging. A curved or curvilinear array low-frequency (2–5 MHZ) probe provides depth penetration required for imaging the Ligamentum flavum(LF)–Dural (D)complex with some compromise on image quality. Linear probes can be programmed to utilize lower-frequency ultrasound, but usually down to a limit of 5–7 MHz.

Basic vertebral anatomy

A review of the anatomy of the lumbar spine is worthwhile before highlighting the sonoanatomy of the spine.

A typical vertebra can be divided into two parts (Figure 54.1): the body and the arch. The vertebral arch is made up of the following elements: pedicles, laminae, transverse processes, spinous process, and the superior and inferior articular processes[8] (Figure 54.1).

The vertebrae articulate at the facet joints (zygapophyseal joints) between the superior and inferior articular processes and at the intervertebral discs between vertebral bodies. The posterior longitudinal ligament runs along the length of the anterior wall of the vertebral canal.

The LF is a dense connective tissue ligament that bridges the interlaminar spaces. It is arch-like in cross-section and is thickest in the midline. The LF attaches to the anterior surface of the lamina above but splits to attach to both the posterior surface (superficial component) and anterior surface (deep component) of the lamina below. The spinous processes are connected at their tips by the supraspinous ligament, which is a strong fibrous cord, and along their length by the interspinous ligament, which is thin and membranous.

Within the vertebral canal lie the thecal sac (formed by the dura mater and arachnoid mater) and its contents (spinal cord, cauda equina, and cerebrospinal fluid). The epidural space is the space within the vertebral canal but outside the thecal sac.

The anatomy of the epidural space is more complex than is frequently conceptually visualized by practitioners.[9] It is divided into anterior, lateral, and posterior epidural spaces with respect to the thecal sac, with the posterior epidural space being of most interest in neuraxial blockade.

The posterior epidural space is not continuous. Instead, it is segmented into a series of fat-filled compartments in the interlaminar areas. The lateral epidural spaces are located at the level of each intervertebral foramen and contain spinal nerves, radicular vessels, and fat. The primary structure of importance in the anterior epidural space is the internal vertebral venous plexus.

The lumbar spine

The posterior surface of the laminae of the five lumbar vertebrae slopes in an anterosuperior direction (Figure 54.2). The spinous processes are broad and flat in the vertical dimension and project posteriorly, with only a slight inferior angulation.

Table 54.1 Clinical studies assessing the utility of ultrasound relevant to the obstetric population

	Study design	Methods	Findings
Sahota et al.[26]	Observational	Labouring women n = 60, BMI > 30 Ultrasound depth measured both in PSO and TM plane Another anaesthetist measured actual needle depth—midline approach	The ultrasound estimate in the PSO and TM planes, and the actual needle depth were 6.5 (1.2) cm, 6.5 (1.1) cm, and 6.6 (1.3) cm, respectively A mean difference of 0.05 cm and 95% limits of agreement of ±1 cm Good quality of images in TM plane were 68.3% where as in PSO plane were 86.7% Average BMI 39.6
Arzola et al.[28]	Observational	Labouring women (N = 61) Pre-puncture ultrasound in all	Successful identification of epidural space at pre-marked insertion point in 91.8% Agreement between ultrasound and needle depth statistically significant. 95% limits of agreement were −0.666 to 0.687 cm. Average BMI 29.7 ± 4.8. Mean needle depth to epidural space was 4.65 ± 0.72 cm
Balki et al.[16]	Observational	Labouring women with BMI >30 (N = 46) Pre-puncture ultrasound depth measured with anaesthetist performing blinded	76% epidural placement at first attempt. 95% interval correlation between ultrasound and needle depth 1.3 to −0.7 cm Mean needle depth to epidural space was 6.6 ± 1.0 cm
Currie[6]	Observational	Labouring women (N = 75)	High degree of correlation between ultrasound measurements and subsequent depth of insertion of needle
Grau T[25]	Randomized	Labouring women (N = 300) Pre-puncture ultrasound vs control All epidurals performed by a single anaesthetist	Number of puncture attempts: ultrasound 1.3 ± 0.6 vs control 2.2 ± 1.1 (P < 0.013) Effective analgesia: ultrasound 98% vs control 92% (P < 0.03)
Grau et al.[26]	Randomized	Labouring women with poorly palpable bony landmarks (N = 72)	Number of puncture attempts: ultrasound 1.5 ± 0.9 vs control 2.6 ± 1.4 (P < 0.001) Epidural failure: ultrasound 0% vs control 5.5% (P > 0.05)
Grau et al.[20]	Randomized	Women scheduled for Caesarean. 3 groups (N = 30) Pre-puncture ultrasound vs real-time ultrasound vs control	Significant reduction in the number of attempts in both ultrasound groups (P = 0.036)
Grau et al.[59]	Observational	Labouring women cohort with 9-month follow-up assessment (N = 53)	In labour, soft-tissue channel between the spinal processes was narrower and skin–epidural space distance was greater in labour
Grau et al.[60]	Observational	Labouring women (N = 100)	Strong correlation between distances measured by ultrasound and needle puncture
Grau et al.[27]	Randomized	Labouring women (N = 120) Assessment of ultrasound as teaching aid for residents performing first epidurals with pre-puncture ultrasound vs control.	Ultrasound group started with 86% ± 15% success rate and increased to 94% after 50 epidural insertions Control group started at 60% ± 16% and increased to 84% after 50 epidural insertions (P < 0.001)
Lee et al.[38]	Randomized	Postpartum women with previous dural puncture (N = 36)	Higher incidence of abnormal ligamentum flavum anatomy in dural puncture group (P < 0.0001). Sonographers were not blinded
Schlotterbeck et al.[32]	Observational	Postpartum women Accuracy of documented interspace assessment using ultrasound (N = 99)	Correct identification of puncture level in only 36.4%
Wallace et al.[29]	Observational	Obese women for caesarean (N = 36) Pre-puncture assessment	Successful anaesthesia in all patients and correlation between ultrasound assessment and needle depth. No control group was used
Shaikh et al.[7]	Meta-analysis	Randomized control trial = 14 (N = 1334) Obstetric studies = 7 Lumbar puncture = 5 studies Epidural catheterization = 9 studies	Ultrasound imaging decreased number of failed procedures (risk ratio (RR) = 0.21), traumatic procedures (RR = 0.27), insertion attempts (mean difference(MD) = −0.44), needle redirections (MD = −1.00)

Data from various sources (see references).

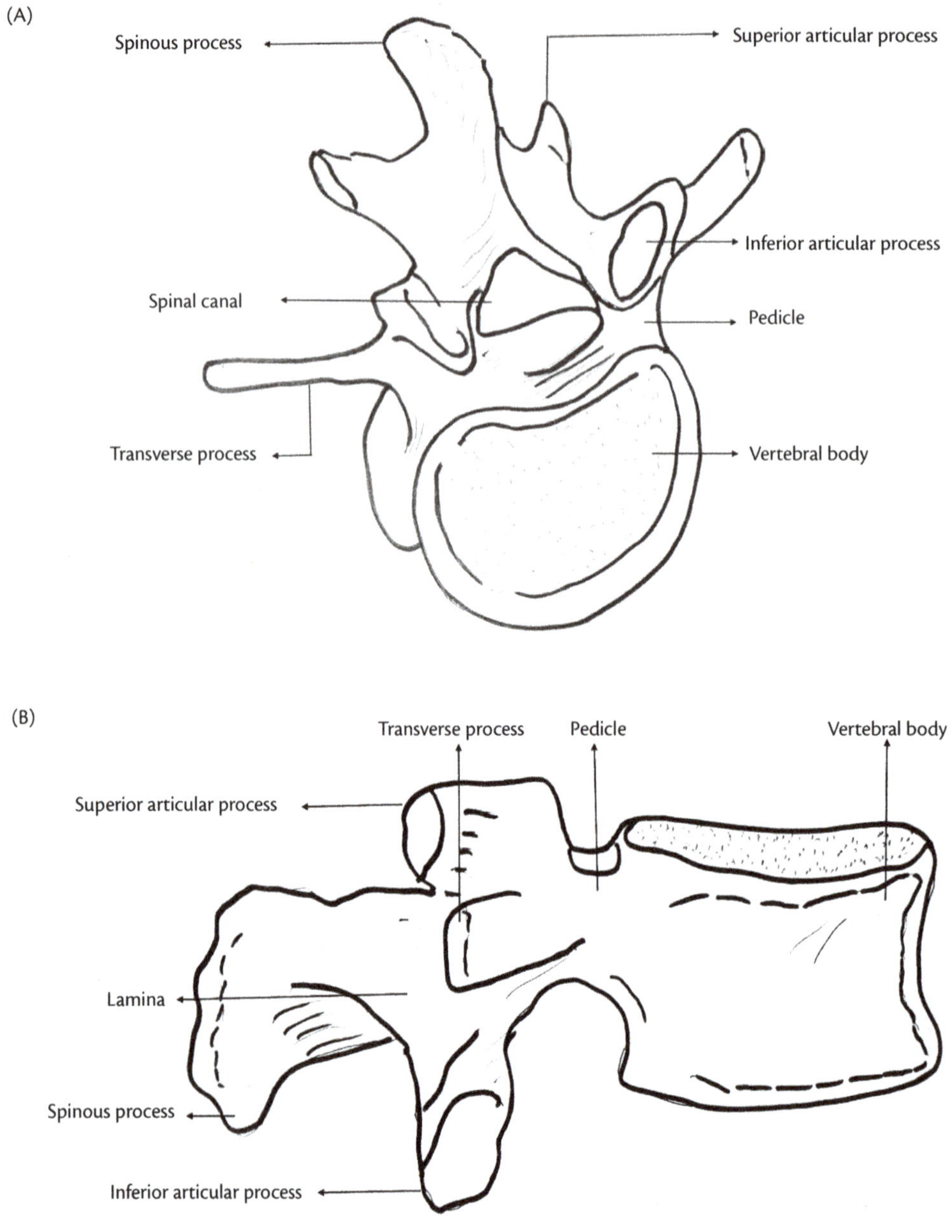

Figure 54.1 Lumbar vertebra.

Thus, accessing the vertebral canal in the midline via the interspinous and interlaminar spaces is relatively easy, with the interlaminar (paramedian) aperture being the larger. These spaces are further enlarged by forward flexion.[10] The transverse processes arise anterior to the articular processes and project posterolaterally; the L3 transverse process is characteristically the longest.[8] The facet joints and transverse processes lie in approximately the same transverse plane as the interlaminar space, and the inferior edge of the spinous process overlies the widest part of the interlaminar space.

The LF arches over the interlaminar space; deep to it lies the fat-filled compartment of the posterior epidural space. The posterior epidural space has a triangular cross-section (typically 7 mm deep in the midline anteroposterior dimension) in the lumbar region and narrows away to a virtual space anterior to the laminae.[10]. Within the thecal sac, the conus medullaris in the adult is most often located at the level of the first lumbar (L1) vertebral body; however, its location in any individual patient follows a normal distribution and may range from the middle of the 12th thoracic (T12) vertebra to the upper third of L3.[11]

The conus medullaris gives rise to the cauda equina and filum terminale. The thecal sac typically ends at the midpoint of the second sacral vertebra (S2), although in the individual patient this can range from the upper border of S1 to the lower border of S4.[12]

Sonographic assessment of the lumbar spine

Lumbar spine ultrasound scanning can be done either as a:

- 'pre-puncture' procedure to demarcate the landmarks or with
- 'real-time' scanning to provide dynamic images during epidural placement.

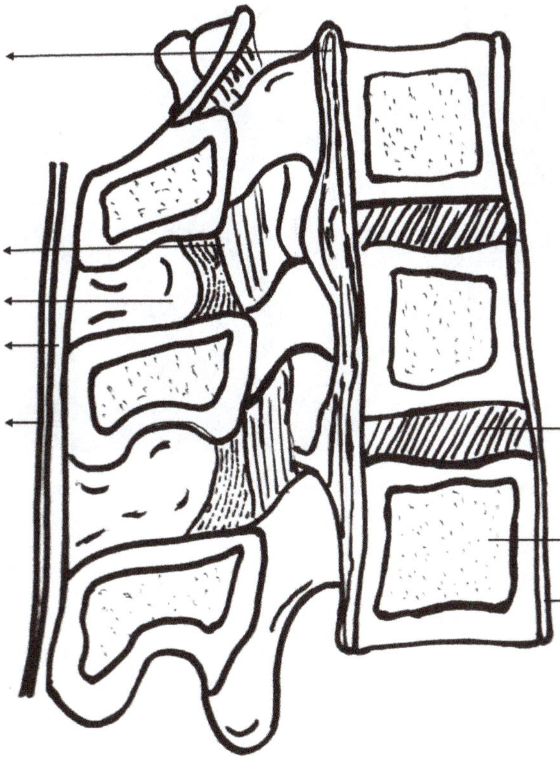

Figure 54.2 Lumbar spine.

Currently, the 'pre-puncture' method is the most widely practised, as it is relatively simple and easy to perform and provides clinically reliable information.[13] It is important to ensure that the scanning is performed with the patient in the same position as for the needle placement. The following information can be obtained during pre-puncture ultrasound scanning:

- The correct level of the interlaminar space
- The midline of the bony spine
- The skin puncture point corresponding to a good starting approach point for a needle
- The angle for needle insertion
- The depth to the epidural space
- The potentially difficult or variant anatomy.

Preparation for scanning

During pre-procedure scanning of the lumbar spine, patients should be placed in the position in which the block is to be performed. An initial screen depth setting of 7–8 cm for a normal size patient or 9–11 cm for patients with higher body mass should be set as appropriate. The depth, focus, and gain settings of the ultrasound machine should be adjusted as needed during the scanning process to produce an optimal image.

There are two basic orientations of the ultrasound probe and beam:

1. *Paramedian sagittal oblique (PSO) plane* , when the beam is oriented in the sagittal plane of the spine lateral to the median (midline) sagittal plane with a slight tilt towards the median plane (Figure 54.3)
2. *Transverse median (TM) plane*, when the beam is orientated parallel to the transverse or horizontal plane (Figure 54.4).

Paramedian sagittal oblique views

Identifying the sacrum

There are two ways of reaching the desired interlaminar space: identifying the level by noting the thoracic level above (by finding the 12th rib) and then counting caudally to the desired level; alternately the sacrum can be identified from below. The horizontal white hyperechoic line found 2–3 cm lateral to the midline in the PSO plane is the upper border of sacrum (Figure 54.5).

Counting the interlaminar spaces

Once the upper border of sacrum is identified, the probe should be advanced in the cephalad direction in the same PSO plane. The first indentation or 'dip' of the hyperechoic white line usually is the L5–S1 interlaminar space.

This image is then followed by a 'saw-tooth' pattern (Figure 54.6) wherein the teeth of the saw represent the lamina interrupted by interspaces. Hence the next dip after the L5–S1 interlaminar space is the L4–5 interlaminar space and so on. If the probe is over the midline, the spinous processes are observed instead of laminae. These appear more superficial and rounded than laminae and are more difficult to use when assessing the correct interspace.

Selecting the ideal interlaminar space

Once the interlaminar space count is established, the preferred level below L2 is chosen based on the ease of

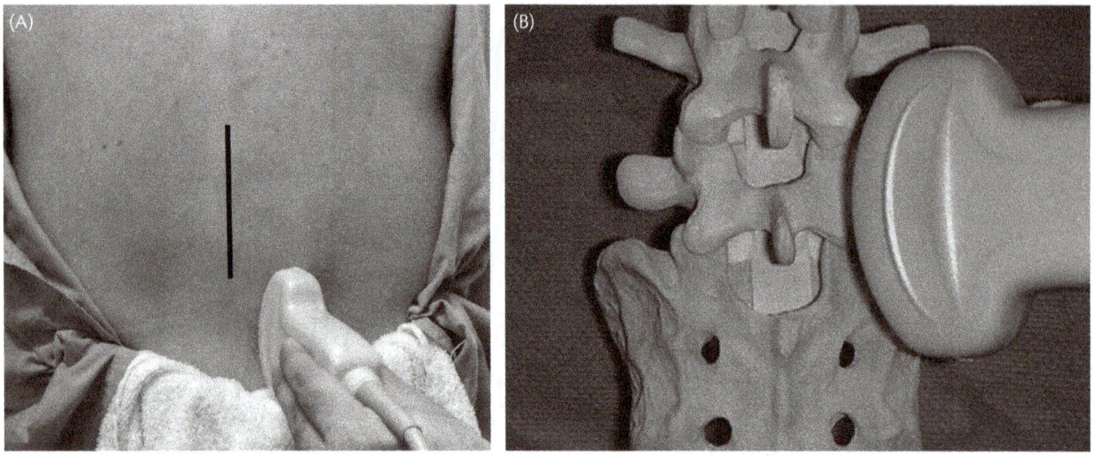

Figure 54.3 (A) Ultrasound probe orientation in paramedian saggital oblique position (PSO plane) (B) Ultrasound probe orientation in PSO plane in relation to spine.
(B) This figure was published in *Anesthesiology Clinics*, Volume 26, Jose Carlos Almeida Carvalho, Ultrasound-Facilitated Epidurals and Spinals in Obstetrics, pp. 145–158, Copyright (2008).

visualization of certain structures. These structures are seen as two parallel (dorsal and ventral) hyperechoic lines (an 'equal' sign—Figure 54.7).

The dorsal line is of more significance to the anaesthetist and consists of the LF–dura mater (D) (posterior complex). These two structures are generally seen as one line but in certain patients with a better acoustic window, they can be seen split into two hyperechoic lines with the hypoechoic epidural space in between them.

The ventral line consists of three structures namely ventral dura, posterior longitudinal ligament, and vertebral body (anterior complex). Clear visibility of the anterior complex predicts an easy neuraxial placement compared with partial or no visibility, which is associated with difficult spinal or epidural anaesthesia.[14]

Ideally, the interlaminar space with both lines visualized should be considered for neuraxial anaesthesia, but even if only the ventral line is visible the chances of success are still high.[14] The depth of LF–D from skin can be measured here and should be noted, but it is also accurately measured in the TM view.

Marking the selected interlaminar space

Once the interlaminar space is selected, it has to be carefully marked. The middle of the probe corresponds to the midpoint of the image on screen. Fixed markings on the probe help here and smaller probes in future would reduce inaccurate marking. Stabilize the probe with one hand and with the other hand mark the midpoint of the probe and draw a horizontal line lateral to it (Figure 54.8). This marking is essential because when the probe is shifted to the TM approach, it is very easy for it to drift over a space above or below.

Transverse midline views

Once the interlaminar space is chosen and marked, the ultrasound probe is rotated by 90° to lie on the same interlaminar space horizontally.

Pattern recognition in TM plane

In this plane we see the structures classically described as the 'flying bat'. This pattern recognition is of key importance as the point

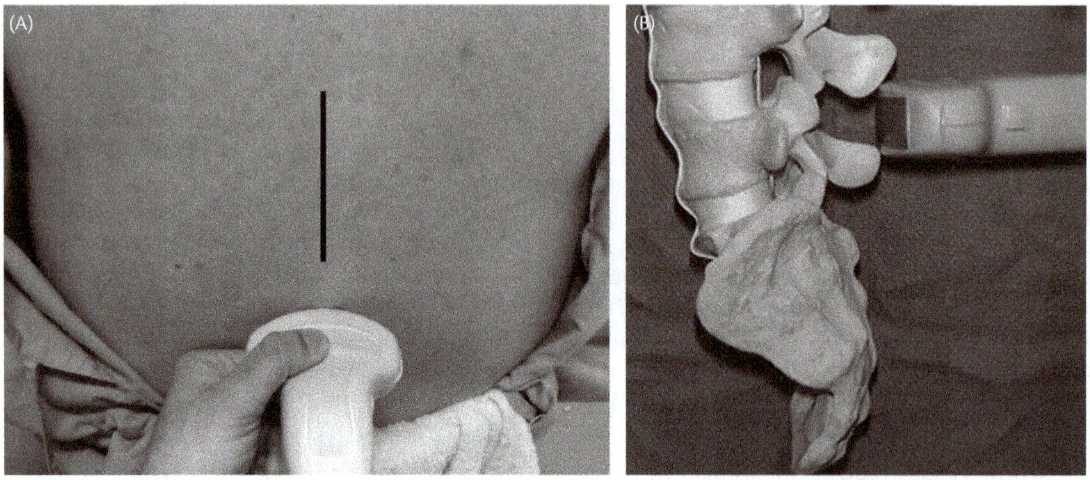

Figure 54.4 (A) Ultrasound probe orientation in transverse median plane (TM PLANE) (B) Utrasound probe orientation in transverse median plane (TM PLANE)—Lateral view in relation to Spine.
(B) This figure was published in *Anesthesiology Clinics*, Volume 26, Jose Carlos Almeida Carvalho, Ultrasound-Facilitated Epidurals and Spinals in Obstetrics, pp. 145–158, Copyright (2008).

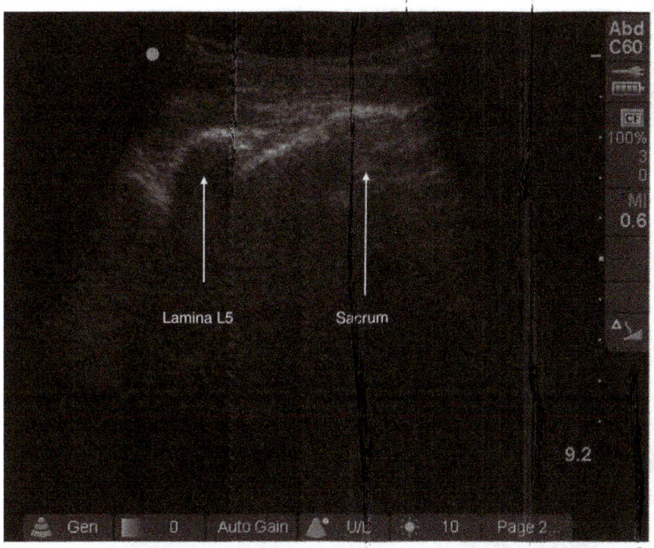

Figure 54.5 Ultraound view of Sacrum in Paramedian saggital oblique view (PSO plane).

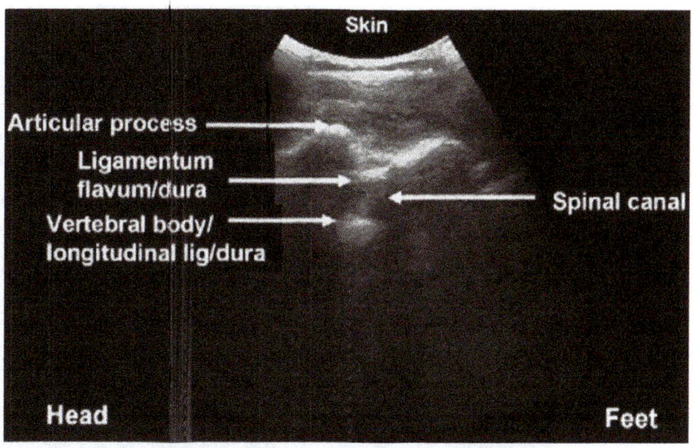

Figure 54.7 The 'equal' sign comprising the ligamentum flavum and the anterior border of the vertebral body.

of needle entry is based on this. The structures that can be visualized in this plane include the LF–D (posterior complex), the ventral dura/posterior longitudinal ligament/vertebral body (anterior complex), the articular processes comprising facet joints, and the transverse processes (Figure 54.9).

The posterior complex and the anterior complex can be visualized as midline structures, which also produce a hyperechoic 'equal' (=) sign in the middle of the interspace. The articular processes and transverse processes appear as the bilateral symmetric hyperechoic structures in a more lateral position.[15] The transverse processes appear as the lateral elongations of the LF–D unit reflections and are not seen well in thin patients where the curved probe loses contact with the skin.

Marking the midline

In the TM plane, as the transducer is moved cephalad or caudad to the interspace, the upper or lower spinous processes can be visualized. Hence, the midline of the spine can be identified as corresponding to the spinous processes, which produces a hyperechoic signal below the skin with a hypoechoic triangular shadow underneath (Figure 54.10).

Thus, scanning in this plane can determine both the midline of the spine and the middle of the interspace. In obese parturients this may be the only discernible bony structure, which helps with identifying the true midline when this is not palpable.

Estimating the depth of dura (skin to LF–D distance)

Once the best image of the interspace structures or the '=' sign is captured in the TM plane, the image is frozen on the screen. With the aid of a built-in caliper on the ultrasound machine, the depth to the epidural space can be measured as the distance from the skin to the ventral border of the LF–D complex (Figure 54.11). It is advisable to measure the depth in the TM plane and to confirm the measurement with scanning in the PSO plane. It should be noted that the depth to the epidural space continues to increase as we scan down

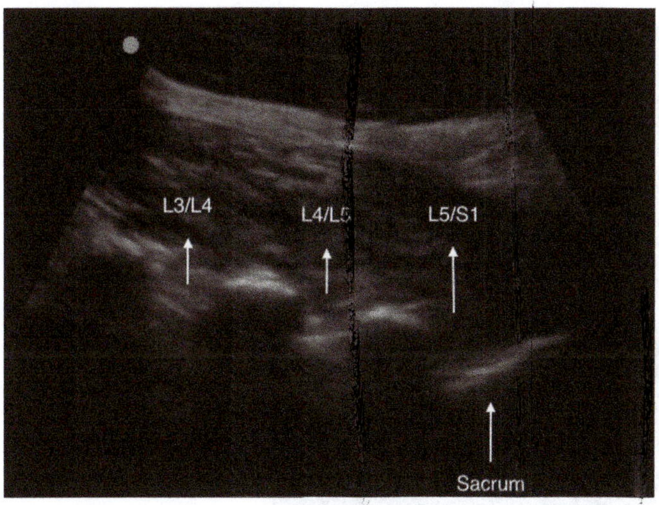

Figure 54.6 Sawtooth pattern.

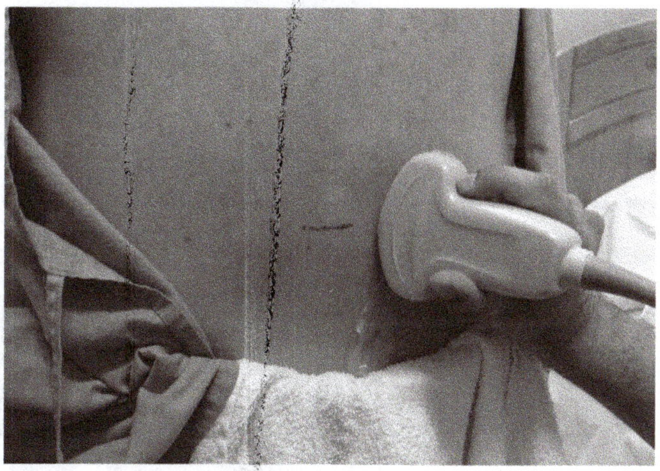

Figure 54.8 Marking the interlaminar space.

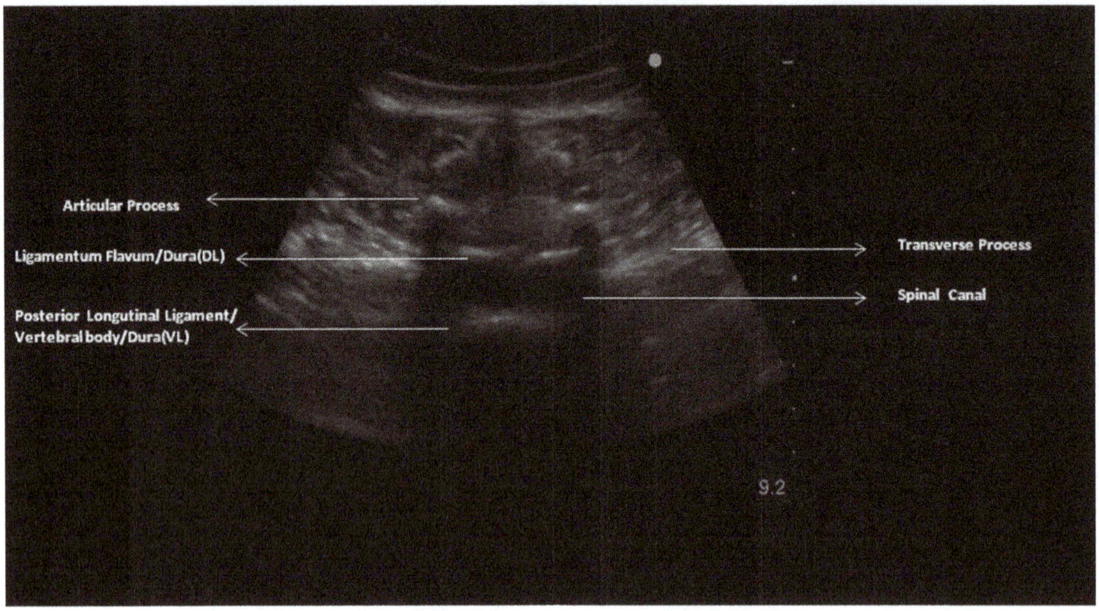

Figure 54.9 Flying bat pattern. The ears of the 'bat' comprise the articular processes comprising facet joints and the 'head' of the bat comprises the ligamentum flavum/dura line.

the lumbar intervertebral spaces. The information obtained from both the PSO and TM planes can complement each other. It has been suggested that measuring the anteroposterior diameter of the dural sac may provide information regarding dose requirements.

The compression of the skin from ultrasound probe should be taken into account while measuring the depth, and generally in a normal pregnant patient would account for 0.5 cm,[16] but in obese patients depth measurement to the epidural space may be less accurate.

Noting the angle of ultrasound probe

In addition to marking the insertion point, the angle of the transducer providing the best image of the interspace structures must be replicated by the needle trajectory. If the beam can pass through to the thecal sac, the needle will make its way through the same passage to the target if on the same trajectory and plane.

Marking the point of entry

With the transducer kept still, and making sure that the hyperechoic '=' sign is visualized, the skin is marked at the centre of both the upper and the lateral aspects of the transducer. The transducer is then removed, and lines are drawn to connect these marks. The insertion point is determined by the intersection of these two lines (Figure 54.12).

In this manner, the insertion point for both the midline and the paramedian punctures can be determined by scanning in the transverse and the paramedian sagittal planes, respectively. The needle insertion point is marked by indenting the skin as antiseptics will erase the marker. Since midline punctures are commonly performed in the obstetric population, a transverse approach is preferred to determine the insertion point.

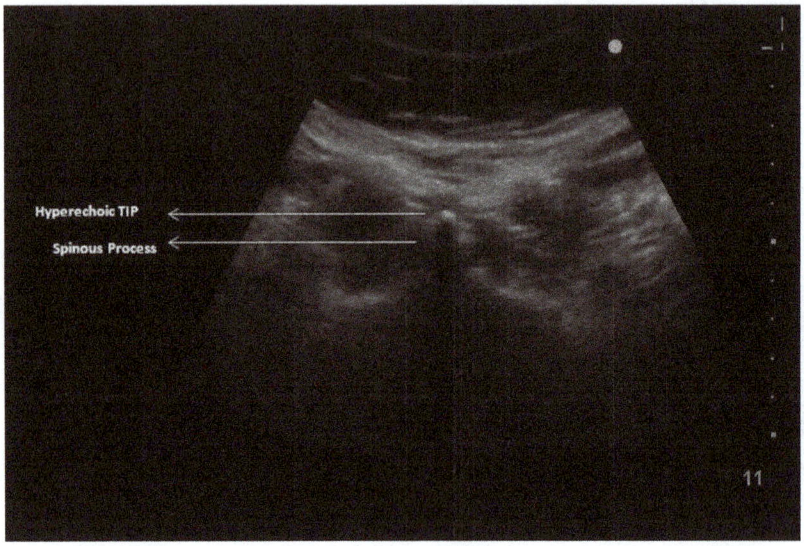

Figure 54.10 Spinous process.

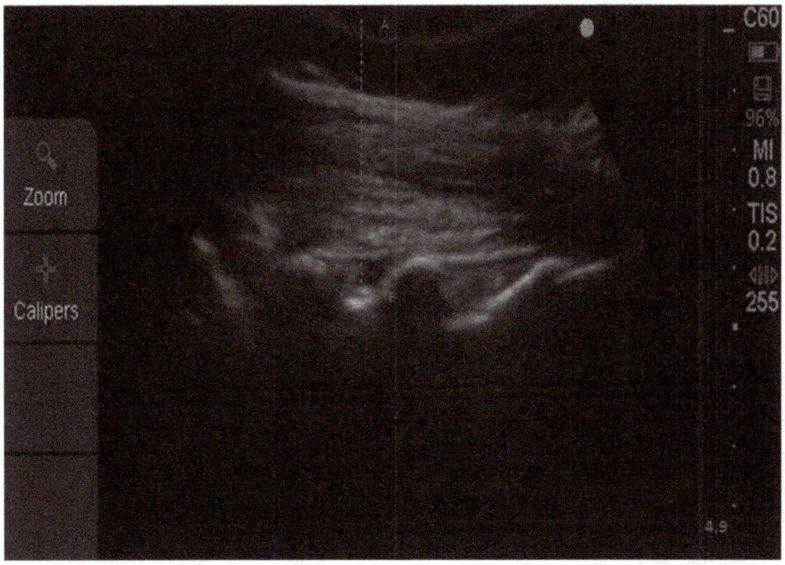

Figure 54.11 (A) Depth, PSO plane. (B) Depth, TM plane.

Variant sonoanatomy

Certain patients with abnormal sonoanatomy, patients with morbid obesity, scoliosis, and spinal instrumentation, may pose a considerable challenge for the placement of neuraxial anaesthesia. Pre-procedural ultrasound in these patients can help us to determine the presence of anatomy amenable to neuraxial anaesthesia and to choose the best intervertebral space or avoid a difficult intervertebral space.

In obese patients, subcutaneous fat makes it difficult to palpate the landmarks and hence ultrasound can be utilized to mark the midline of the intervertebral space and the appropriate intervertebral level is marked best in the PSO plane. Care should be taken not to compress the ultrasound probe too hard on to the skin as it can underestimate the depth to the LF–D complex. In most patients, the depth to the dura is less than 8 cm. If the ultrasound predicts a depth of more than 8 cm a long needle may be selected for these patients.[16]

In patients with scoliosis, there is variable degree of axial rotation of the vertebral bodies and angulation of spinous processes. The sonographic image in these patients can reveal the location of the spinous process lateral to the virtual midline of the patient, asymmetry of the articular and transverse processes, and discontinuous LF in the TM plane (Figure 54.13 and Figure 54.14).

In such situations, several interspaces should be scanned, and the interspace with normal sonoanatomy and continuous LF should be chosen for the neuraxial block.[17]

In patients with spinal instrumentation, ultrasound can help in determining the intervertebral space with preserved anatomy and thus neuraxial anaesthesia can still be contemplated in this group of patients.[18]

Learning curve

A great deal of training is required before one can be efficient in ultrasound-guided spinal and epidural anaesthesia. Margarido et al.[19] have shown that even after attending lectures and workshops, novices requires more than 20 attempts to master critical tasks necessary for locating accurate ultrasound landmarks. Common flaws included missing the L5–S1 space, not marking the skin meticulously, and inadvertently sliding the transducer to a lower segment while marking the skin insertion point. Thus, ultrasound should not be reserved for technically difficult cases because it requires experience in routine cases with easily identified palpable landmarks before it can be used effectively in difficult cases.

Real-time scanning

Real-time ultrasound scanning can be performed as an out-of-plane technique by scanning in the PSO approach and inserting the epidural needle in the midline or as part of an in-plane technique.[20,21] The obvious limitations of this technique include poor demarcation of individual structures, such as the LF and D, and the need for an assistant to perform scanning if an epidural with loss-of-resistance is used. An operator has to revert to standard blind loss-of-resistance using both hands when the needle is sent on a satisfactory path. However, the utilization of epidural syringes with an auto detect loss-of-resistance function may facilitate a single skilled operator in performing ultrasound-guided epidural placement.[22] A single operator combined spinal–epidural technique has been described in a case series which involves a modification of the ultrasound transducer with biopsy bracket and needle guide using geometrical principles.[23] A GPS needle tracking system is also described, which allows the operator to make adjustments to needle trajectory during advancement, which ensures greater precision in reaching the target.[24] At present, the role of neuraxial real-time ultrasonography is clinically restricted and advances in the transducer design and technology are required to establish its clinical relevance.

Efficacy of ultrasound-guided procedures

A 2013 meta-analysis[7] has shown that ultrasound imaging can reduce the risk of failed lumbar punctures and epidural

(A)

(B)

(C)

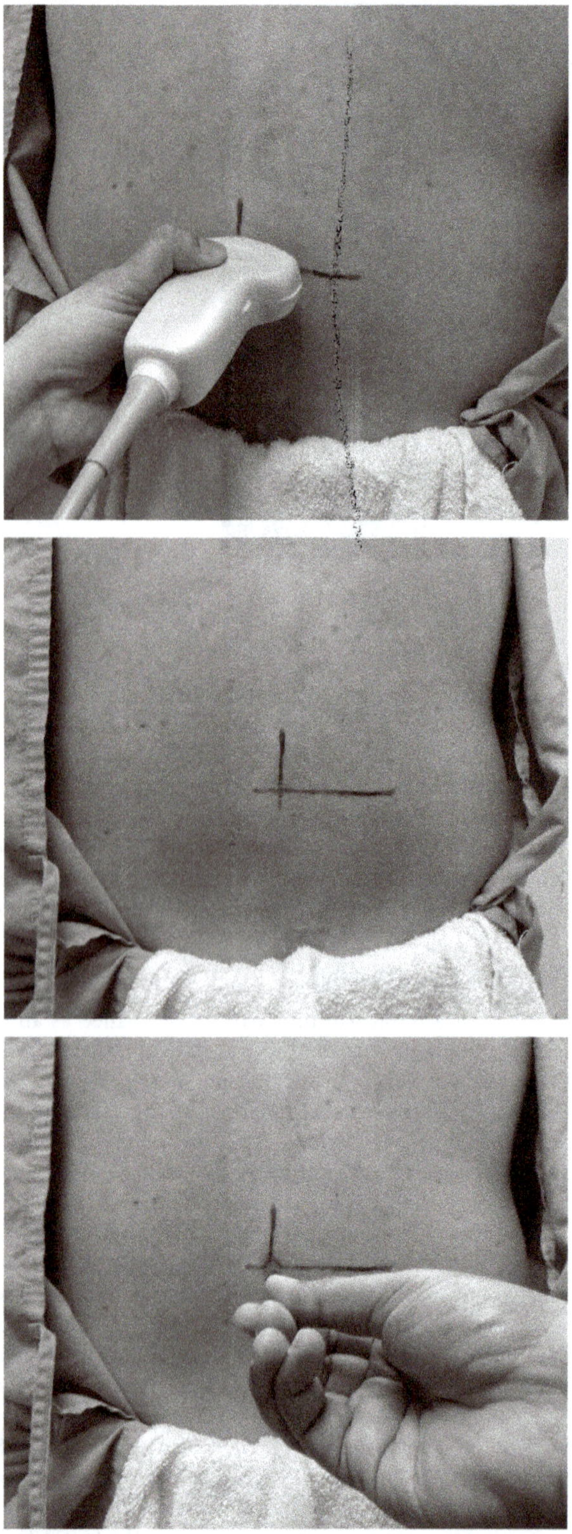

Figure 54.12 Marking point of entry.

catheterizations as well as reduce the risk of traumatic procedures and the number of needle insertions and redirections.

Grau et al. demonstrated that ultrasound guidance improved the success of blocks, minimized the complication rate, and improved overall patient satisfaction when compared with the conventional palpationmethod.[20,25–27] Such benefits were also demonstrated in many other studies.[28–30]

The inaccuracy of clinical palpation to confirm an intervertebral level is well documented, as have the risks of an inadvertently high intervertebral space selection for spinal anaesthesia.[31] Ultrasound imaging has been shown to be superior to palpation in correctly identifying lumbar intervertebral level, with traditional landmark palpation techniques erring to select a higher level than was intended or recorded in up to 50% ofcases.[32,33] As ultrasound equipment becomes more widely available, documentation of its use may become the accepted standard of care.

Several studies involving obstetric patients have shown an excellent correlation between the ultrasound-estimated depth to the epidural space and the actual needle depth. The expected depth to the epidural space can be predicted within a range of ± 0.7 cm in non-obese parturients and ±1 cm in obese parturients with a 95% confidence interval.[16,28] In obese parturients, the quality of image capture in the TM plane is generally inferior to the PSO plane and this requires excessive pressure form the ultrasound transducer which, in turn, can measure a false low value. The depth to epidural space can reasonably be estimated in the PSO plane and this corresponds well with the depth estimated from the TM plane.[34]

Ultrasound guidance has also been used for placement of an epidural blood patch,[35–37] and Lee et al. have suggested that pre-puncture imaging may identify defects in LF predisposing some parturients to unintended dural puncture at that interspace.[38] In addition to reduced skin punctures and needle redirections, enhanced analgesic success of ultrasound-guided epidural placement has also been reported.[38] Thecal sac anteroposterior diameter can be measured using ultrasound although a correlation between this and predicted height of spinal anaesthesia has not been demonstrated.[39] The length of the lumbar spine determined by ultrasound, rather than the lumbar spine volume, combined with the weight or body mass index of the subject, is of particular value in predicting the intrathecal spread of local anaesthetic during combined spinal–epidural analgesia for labour.[40]

Concerns regarding the potential for increased time required to site an epidural where ultrasound is utilized are overstated as ultrasound leads to fewer attempts at epidural space localization and is likely to reduce overall procedure time in patients with difficult anatomic landmarks.[41]

Clinical guidelines

On the basis of the available studies which included paediatric practice, in 2008 the UK National Institute for Clinical Excellence (now National Institute of Health and Care (NICE)) published a recommendation stating that ultrasound may be effective in achieving correct placement of epidural catheters.[42] Reduced needling time enhances safety and the patient experience and this appears to be the main benefit of incorporating ultrasound assessment into obstetric anaesthesia practice.

Vascular access

Ultrasound-guided central venous cannulation gained significance following a meta-analysis by Randolph et al. in 1996.[43] This showed a reduction in placement failure, decreased incidence of multiple attempts, and decreased rate of complications with ultrasound-guided cannulation compared to standard

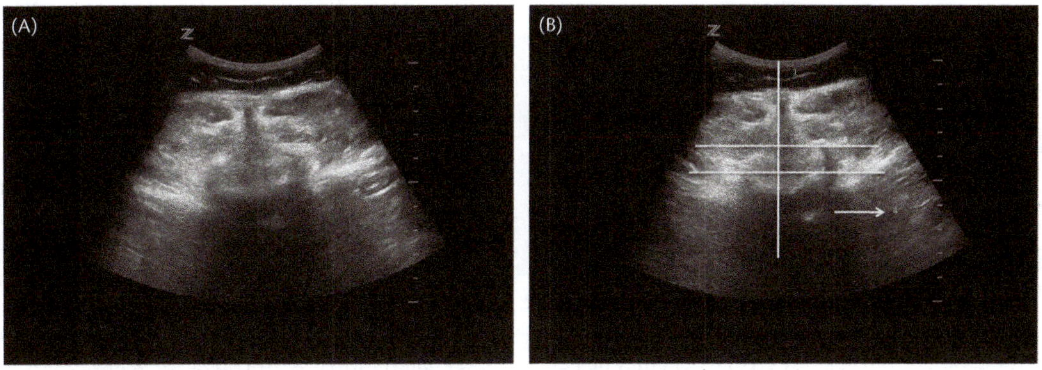

Figure 54.13 (A) Scoliosis. (B) Scoliosis—note the planes:

1. Midline plane: the spinous process is at an angle to midline
2. Plane of right articular process
3. Plane of left articular process plane
4. PLL–VB: visible only on the right side.

landmark techniques. These results were confirmed by another meta-analysis in 2003 comparing the use of two-dimensional ultrasound guidance with an anatomical landmark technique.[44] Based on these and other studies, NICE recommended that two-dimensional ultrasound guidance should be considered in most clinical circumstances where central venous cannulation is indicated.[45] Ultrasound-guided placement facilitates accurate central vascular access with more limited patient positioning for comfort. Ultrasound for central venous cannulation has proven to be most valuable in complicated cases, such as patients with coagulopathy, obese or hypovolaemic patients, those who cannot tolerate recumbent position, or who have had multiple previous cannulations.[46] For central venous catheterization, it has been shown that real-time ultrasound guidance is better than the pre-puncture imaging of anatomy.[47] The common technique for ultrasound-assisted central vein cannulation is the short-axis out-of-plane view. In addition to central venous catheters, ultrasound guidance is increasingly used for peripheral venous cannulation in patients with difficult venous access,[48] and for insertion of arterial catheters for invasive blood pressure monitoring. This has obvious potential in obese parturients although central venous line insertion has become less common.

General anaesthesia

O'Sullivan et al. have published on effects of labour and opioids on gastric emptying and residual gastric volumes in parturients. Ultrasound-based technology in many of these studies was used to assess gastric volumes.[49] Perlas et al. have shown that the gastric antral cross-sectional area, as measured by ultrasonography correlates well with gastric volume and also can provide accurate qualitative information regarding gastric content type. Bedside ultrasonography could potentially become a clinically useful non-invasive tool to stratify perioperative aspiration risk.[50] As skills among obstetric anaesthetists improve, the idea of using ultrasound technology to assess gastric volumes in a non-elective case outside a research setting is thought-provoking and may guide clinical decision-making with respect to anaesthesia technique.

Location of the cricoid cartilage for correct application of cricoid pressure during rapid sequence induction is traditionally performed by the landmark technique, but may also be identified using ultrasound. Ultrasound technology may useful to identify the cricothyroid membrane, which may lead to improved safety when considering percutaneous tracheal cannulation.[51]

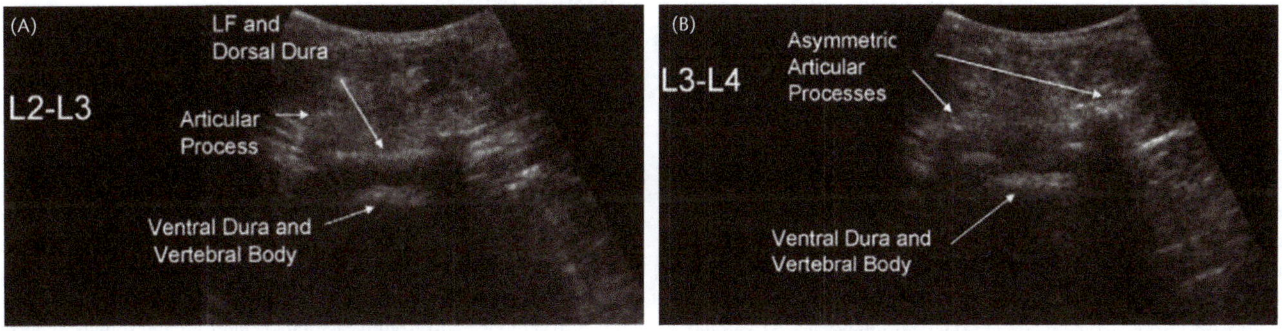

Figure 54.14 (A) Normal vertebra. (B) Scoliosis.
This figure was published in *Anesthesiology Clinics*, Volume 26, Jose Carlos Almeida Carvalho, Ultrasound-Facilitated Epidurals and Spinals in Obstetrics, pp. 145–158, Copyright (2008).

Cardiac evaluation

Transthoracic cardiac imaging is now feasible with the higher-resolution equipment now utilized in most centres for regional anaesthesia. Bedside ultrasound evaluation of the hypotensive parturient may help to differentiate non-invasively between hypovolaemia and other conditions such as cardiomyopathy or pulmonary embolism.[52]

Acute and chronic pain control

There has been some interest in the literature in abdominal wall infiltration techniques for post-caesarean analgesia.[53] Field blocks such as the transversus abdominis plane (TAP) block, may be performed with enhanced accuracy using ultrasound. Although the block was originally described without ultrasound, using a landmark technique, complications such as peritoneal injection or haematoma are possible. The sonoanatomy of the muscle planes is more clearly defined in the area between the level of the anterior superior iliac crest, the subcostal margin and the umbilicus.[54] The TAP block as originally described uses clinical landmarks at the mid-axillary line, above the iliac crest, at the lumbar triangle of Petit.[55] However, the sonoanatomy, in terms of identifying muscle and fascial planes at this point are less clear. Performance of the block in a more anterior site with ultrasound may yield comparable efficacy and studies are awaited. Though McMorrow et al.[56] have shown that TAP block using a landmark technique does not provide comparable analgesia or additional benefit to spinal morphine for post-caesarean analgesia, they have concluded that lack of ultrasound for their block could have erroneous placement of the drug either too superficially or too deep (i.e. intraperitoneal) and further studies are warranted using ultrasound. Furthermore, it is likely that clinically useful catheter-based techniques may demonstrate the most benefit in postoperative analgesia, rather than single-shot techniques. Nevertheless, ultrasound will undoubtedly have a role in the evolution and development of abdominal field anaesthesia for post-caesarean analgesia as part of a multimodal balanced analgesic plan.

Pelvic girdle pain syndromes, which involve pubic symphysis, sacroiliac, and coccygeal-related pain, are a relatively rare but disabling constellation of syndromes which have been treated with local application of anaesthetic and steroid agents. Ultrasound may be used to avoid fluoroscopy and the risks of radiation to the fetus. Obturator nerve blockade, which has been described for chronic perineal pain syndromes, has been performed using ultrasound.[57]

Cost

The cost of purchasing high-resolution equipment with at least two different probes and accessories can be substantial and in the region of EUR 50,000. More basic ultrasound technology sufficient for central venous catheterization is less expensive and justified on safety grounds. Access to devices commonly used by obstetricians may be readily available in patient areas and with appropriate specification, be sufficient to explore initial neuraxial assessment. Ultrasound has been suggested as one area with improvement potential on future reductions in anaesthesia-related maternal mortality.[58] A reduced potential for neuraxial injury from inadvertent high intervertebral space selection where spinal anaesthesia is planned may justify more widespread use. Until more data are available of the benefits to high-risk parturients, the cost of the equipment will be the main barrier to wider implementation in addition to limited technical expertise.

Conclusion

Placement of epidural catheters or spinal needles is an area where widespread use of ultrasound will potentially become more commonplace. Ultrasound may become increasingly useful in other invasive procedures such as vascular access and field blocks. The pace of development in portable ultrasound technology brings new refinements to image quality and we can expect wider availability of ultrasound technology on our delivery suites and operating theatres and further innovations in clinical application.

Acknowledgements

We are extremely grateful to the following people who have helped us throughout in making this text possible. Dr J.C. Carvalho, Dr M. Balki, Dr Amar Nandhkumar, Dr David Monks, Dr Sesha Smitha Poilimetla. We thank Elsevier for allowing us to reproduce the images (54.3B, 54.4B, Figures 54.7, 54.14A, 54.14B) which were published in Carvalho JC. Ultrasound-facilitated epidurals and spinals in obstetrics. *Anesthesiol Clin* 2008; 26:145–58. Copyright Elsevier.

References

1. Grange P, Foster P, Pretorius LK. Application of the Doppler ultrasound bloodflow detector in supraclavicular brachial plexus block. *Br J Anaesth* 1978; 50:965–7.
2. Horlocker TT, Wedel DJ. Ultrasound-guided regional anesthesia: in search of the holy grail. *Anesth Analg* 2007; 104:1009–11.
3. Liu SS, Ngeow JE, Yadeau JT. Ultrasound-guided regional anesthesia and analgesia: a qualitative systematic review. *Reg Anesth Pain Med* 2009; 34:47–59.
4. Marhofer P, Chan VW. Ultrasound-guided regional anesthesia: current concepts and future trends. *Anesth Analg* 2007; 104:1265–9.
5. Cork RC, Kryc JJ, Vaughan RW. Ultrasonic localization of the lumbar epidural space. *Anesthesiology* 1980; 52:513–16.
6. Currie JM. Measurement of the depth to the extradural space using ultrasound. *Br J Anaesth* 1984; 56:345–7.
7. Shaikh F, Brzezinski J, Alexander S, *et al.* Ultrasound imaging for lumbar punctures and epidural catheterisations: systematic review and meta-analysis. *BMJ* 2013; 346:f1720.
8. Cramer GD. The lumbar region. In Cramer GD, Darby SA (eds) *Basic and Clinical Anatomy of the Spine, Spinal Cord and ANS* (2nd ed). St. Louis, MO: Mosby; 2005: 242–307.
9. Hogan QH. Epidural anatomy: new observations. *Can J Anaesth* 1998; 45:R40–8.
10. Cousins MJ, Veering BT. Epidural neural blockade. In Cousins MJ, Bridenbaugh PO (eds) *Neural Blockade in Clinical Anesthesia and Management of Pain* (3rd ed). Philadelphia, PA: Lippincott–Raven; 1998:243–320.
11. Saifuddin A, Burnett SJ, White J. The variation of position of the conus medullaris in an adult population: a magnetic resonance imaging study. *Spine* 1998; 23:1452–6.
12. Macdonald A, Chatrath P, Spector T, *et al.* Level of termination of the spinal cord and the dural sac: a magnetic resonance study. *Clin Anat* 1999; 12:149–52.
13. Carvalho JC. Ultrasound-facilitated epidurals and spinals in obstetrics. *Anesthesiol Clin* 2008; 26:145–58.

14. Weed JT, Taenzer AH, Finkel KJ, *et al.* Evaluation of preprocedural ultrasound examination as a screening tool for difficult spinal anaesthesia. *Anaesthesia* 2011; 66(10):925–30.
15. Balki M. Locating the epidural space in obstetric patients-ultrasound a useful tool: continuing professional development. *Can J Anaesth* 2010; 57(12):1111–26.
16. Balki M, Lee Y, Halpern S, *et al.* Ultrasound imaging of the lumbar spine in the transverse plane: the correlation between estimated and actual depth to the epidural space in obese parturients. *Anesth Analg* 2009; 108:1876–81.
17. McLeod A, Roche A, Fennelly M. Case series: ultrasonography may assist epidural insertion in scoliosis patients. *Can J Anesth* 2005; 52: 717–20.
18. Costello JF, Balki M. Cesarean delivery under ultrasound guided spinal anesthesia in a parturient with poliomyelitis and Harrington instrumentation. *Can J Anesth* 2008; 55:606–11.
19. Margarido CB, Arzola C, Balki M, *et al.* Anesthesiologists' learning curves for ultrasound assessment of the lumbar spine. *Can J Anesth* 2010; 57:120–6.
20. Grau T, Leipold RW, Fatehi S, *et al.* Real-time ultrasonic observation of combined spinal-epidural anaesthesia. *Eur J Anaesthesiol* 2004; 21:25–31.
21. Karmakar MK, Li X, Ho AM, *et al.* Real-time ultrasound-guided paramedian epidural access: evaluation of a novel in-plane technique. *Br J Anaesth* 2009; 102:845–54.
22. Riley ET, Carvalho B. The Episure syringe: a novel loss of resistance syringe for locating the epidural space. *Anesth Analg* 2007; 105:1164–6.
23. Tran D, Kamani AA, Al-Attas E, *et al.* Single-operator real-time ultrasound-guidance to aim and insert a lumbar epidural needle. *Can J Anaesth* 2010; 57(4):313–21.
24. Wong SW, Niazi AU, Chin KJ, *et al.* Real-time ultrasound-guided spinal anesthesia using the SonixGPS® needle tracking system: a case report. *Can J Anaesth* 2013; 60(1):50–3.
25. Grau T, Leipold RW, Conradi R, *et al.* Efficacy of ultrasound imaging in obstetric epidural anesthesia. *J Clin Anesth* 2002; 14:169–75.
26. Grau T, Leipold RW, Conradi R, *et al.* Ultrasound control for presumed difficult epidural puncture. *Acta Anaesthesiol Scand* 2001; 45:766–71.
27. Grau T, Bartusseck E, Conradi R, *et al.* Ultrasound imaging improves learning curves in obstetric epidural epidural anesthesia: a preliminary study. *Can J Anesth* 2003; 50:1047–50.
28. Arzola C, Davies S, Rofaeel A, *et al.* Ultrasound using the transverse approach to the lumbar spine provides reliable landmarks for labor epidurals. *Anesth Analg* 2007; 104:1188–92.
29. Wallace DH, Currie JM, Gilstrap LC, *et al.* Indirect sonographic guidance for epidural anesthesia in obese pregnant patients. *Reg Anesth* 1992; 17:233–6.
30. Chin KJ, Ramlogan R, Arzola C, *et al.* The utility of ultrasound imaging in predicting ease of performance of spinal anesthesia in an orthopedic patient population. *Reg Anesth Pain Med* 2013; 38(1):34–8.
31. Reynolds F. Damage to the conus medullaris following spinal anaesthesia. *Anaesthesia* 2001; 56:238–47.
32. Schlotterbeck H, Schaeffer R, Dow WA, *et al.* Ultrasonographic control of the puncture level for lumbar neuraxial block in obstetric anaesthesia. *Br J Anaesth* 2008; 100:230–4.
33. Whitty R, Moore M, Macarthur A. Identification of the lumbar interspinous spaces: palpation versus ultrasound. *Anesth Analg* 2008; 106:538–40.
34. Sahota JS, Carvalho JC, Balki M, *et al.* Ultrasound estimates for midline epidural punctures in the obese parturient: paramedian sagittal oblique is comparable to transverse median plane. *Anesth Analg* 2013; 116(4):829–35.
35. Prasad GA, Simon G, Wijayatilake S. Ultrasound-assisted epidural blood patching. *Int J Obstet Anesth* 2008; 17:376–7.
36. Khayata I, Lance Lichtor J, *et al.* Ultrasound-guided epidural blood patch. *Anesthesiology* 2011; 114(6):1453.
37. Gnaho A, Nguyen V, des Déserts MD, *et al.* Ultrasound-guided epidural blood patch. *Eur J Anaesthesiol* 2010; 27(2):221–2.
38. Lee Y, Tanaka M, Carvalho JC. Sonoanatomy of the lumbar spine in patients with previous unintentional dural punctures during labor epidurals. *Reg Anesth Pain Med* 2008; 33:266–70.
39. Arzola C, Balki M, Carvalho JC. The antero-posterior diameter of the lumbar dural sac does not predict sensory levels of spinal anesthesia for cesarean delivery. *Can J Anesth* 2007; 54:620–5.
40. Fanning N, Arzola C, Balki M, *et al.* Lumbar dural sac dimensions determined by ultrasound helps predict sensory block extent during combined spinal-epidural analgesia for labor. *Reg Anesth Pain Med* 2012; 37(3):283–8.
41. Chin KJ, Perlas A, Chan V, *et al.* Ultrasound imaging facilitates spinal anesthesia in adults with difficult surface anatomic landmarks. *Anesthesiology* 2011; 115(1):94–101.
42. National Institute for Health and Clinical Excellence. *Ultrasound-Guided Catheterisation of the Epidural Space.* London: NICE; 2008. http://www.nice.org.uk/nicemedia/pdf/IPG249Guidance.pdf
43. Randolph AG, Cook DJ, Gonzales CA, *et al.* Ultrasound guidance for placement of central venous catheters: a meta-analysis of the literature. *Crit Care Med* 1996; 24:2053–8.
44. Hind D, Calvert N, McWilliams R, *et al.* Ultrasonic locating devices for central venous cannulation: meta-analysis. *BMJ* 2003; 327:361.
45. National Institute for Health and Clinical Excellence. *Guidance on the Use of Ultrasound Locating Devices for Placing Central Venous Catheters.* London: NICE; 2002. http://www.nice.org.uk/guidance/ta49
46. Karakitsos D, Labropoulos N, De Groot E, *et al.* Real-time ultrasound-guided catheterisation of the internal jugular vein: a prospective comparison with the landmark technique in critical care patients. *Crit Care* 2006; 10:R162.
47. Hosokawa K, Shime N, Kato Y, *et al.* A randomized trial of image-based skin surface marking versus real-time ultrasound-guided internal jugular vein catheterization in infants. *Anesthesiology* 2007; 107:720–4.
48. Bauman M, Braude D, Crandall C. Ultrasound-guidance vs. standard technique in difficult vascular access patients by ED technicians. *Am J Emerg Med* 2009; 27:135–40.
49. Kubli M, Scrutton MJ, Seed PT, *et al.* An evaluation of isotonic "sport drinks" during labor. *Anesth Analg* 2002; 94:404–8.
50. Perlas A, Chan VW, Lupu CM, *et al.* Ultrasound assessment of gastric content and volume. *Anesthesiology* 2009; 111(1):82–9.
51. Nicholls SE, Sweeney TW, Ferre RM, *et al.* Bedside sonography by emergency physicians for the rapid identification of landmarks relevant to cricothyroidotomy. *Am J Emerg Med* 2008; 26:852–6.
52. Dennis AT. Transthoracic echocardiography in obstetric anaesthesia and obstetric critical illness. *Int J Obst Anaesth* 2011; 20(2):160–8.
53. McDonnell JG, Curley G, Carney J, *et al.* The analgesic efficacy of transversus abdominis plane block after cesarean delivery: a randomized controlled trial. *Anesth Analg* 2008; 106:186–91.
54. Tran TM, Ivanusic JJ, Hebbard P, *et al.* Determination of spread of injectate after ultrasound-guided transversus abdominis plane block: a cadaveric study. *Br J Anaesth* 2009; 102:123–7.
55. McDonnell JG, O'Donnell B D, Farrell T, *et al.* Transversus abdominis plane block: a cadaveric and radiological evaluation. *Reg Anesth Pain Med* 2007; 32:399–404.
56. McMorrow RC, Ni Mhuircheartaigh RJ, Ahmed KA, *et al.* Comparison of transversus abdominis plane block vs spinal morphine for pain relief after Caesarean section.*Br J Anaesth* 2011; 106(5):706–12.
57. Fujiwara Y, Sato Y, Kitayama M, *et al.* Obturator nerve block using ultrasound guidance. *Anesth Analg* 2007; 105:888–9.
58. Arendt KW, Segal S. Present and emerging strategies for reducing anesthesia-related maternal morbidity and mortality. *Curr Opin Anaesthesiol* 2009; 22:330–5.
59. Grau T, Leipold RW, Horter J, *et al.* The lumbar epidural space in pregnancy: visualization by ultrasonography. *Br J Anaesth* 2001; 86:798–804.
60. Grau T, Leipold R, Conradi R, *et al.* Ultrasonography and peridural anesthesia. Technical possibilities and limitations of ultrasonic examination of the epidural space. *Anaesthesist* 2001; 50:94–101.

CHAPTER 55

International outreach

Gordon Yuill and Simon Millar

Maternal mortality and morbidity: a global problem

Maternal mortality

The tenth and current revision of the International Classification of Diseases, Injuries and Causes of Death (ICD-10) defines maternal mortality as 'the death of a woman while pregnant or within 42 days of termination of pregnancy, from any cause related to or aggravated by the pregnancy or its management, but not from accidental or incidental causes'.[2] Both the World Health Organization (WHO) and the Centre for Child and Maternal Health Enquiries (CMACE) further divide deaths into those that are *directly* related to pregnancy and conditions that are unique to pregnancy, and those that are *indirectly* related to pregnancy where an existing or developing disease is exacerbated by the pregnancy.

The maternal mortality ratio (MMR), the number of direct and indirect maternal deaths per 100,000 live births, is an often used health indicator when discussing national and global progress and comparisons (Figure 55.1). When the WHO determined that its Millennium Development Goal 5 (MDG 5) was to improve maternal health, the headline target it chose was to reduce the MMR by three-quarters between 1990 and 2015. This may prove to be an ambitious objective, yet by 2010 there were an estimated 287,000 deaths worldwide representing a MMR of 240 and a decline of 47% from the 1990 levels (Figure 55.2).[3] The difference between developing and developed regions is highlighted by a MMR that is 15 times higher in the former (Figure 55.3). Even this is probably an underestimate in countries with poorly developed data collection and death registration systems.[4]

Beyond the Numbers is a WHO programme that encompasses a maternal mortality review tool kit.[5] It encourages countries to review their maternal mortalities and offers a number of ways to do this allowing for varied logistical and financial circumstances. The longest running example of such a review is the *Confidential Enquiries into Maternal Deaths in the United Kingdom*, coordinated by CMACE. The most recent of its eight triennial reports was published in 2011 reviewing the years 2006–2008,[6] and calculated the MMR in the United Kingdom as 11.39 (95% confidence interval (CI) 10.09–12.86)/100,000 maternities.

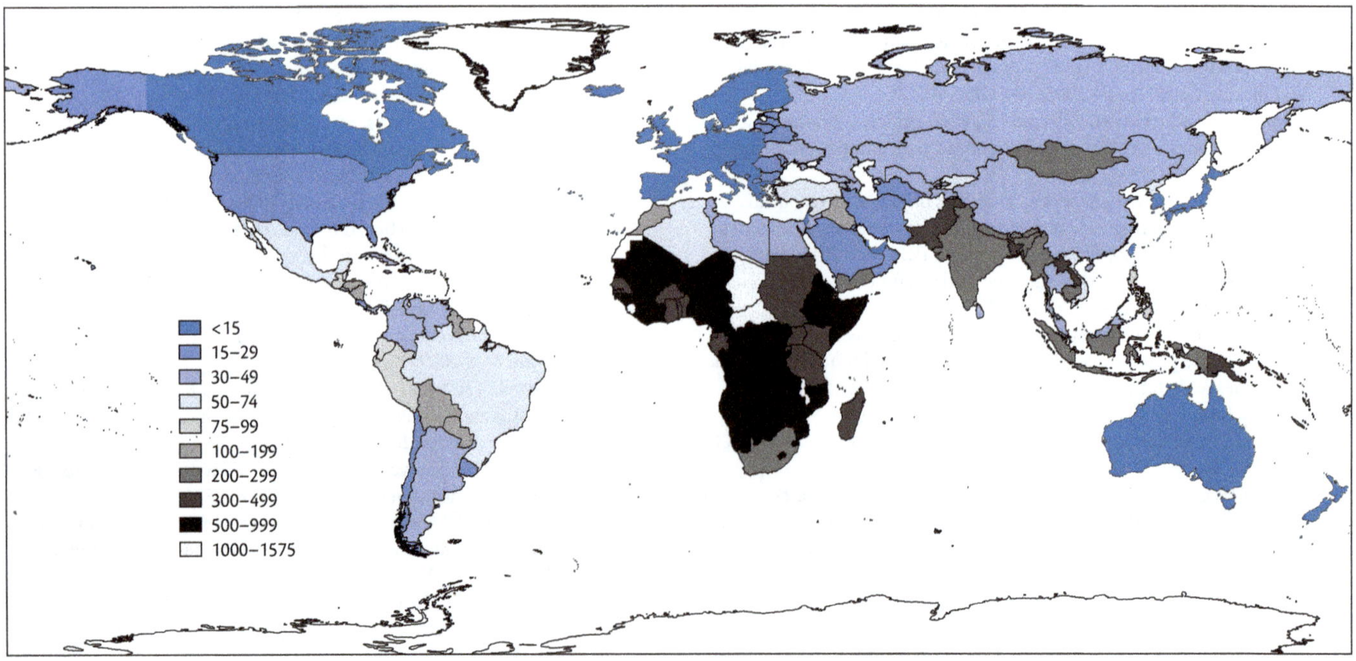

Figure 55.1 (See colour figure section). Maternal mortality ratio per 100,000 live births, 2008.

Reprinted from *The Lancet*, Volume 375, number 9726, Margaret C Hogan *et al.*, Maternal mortality for 181 countries, 1980–2008: a systematic analysis of progress towards Millennium Development Goal 5, pp. 1609–1623, Copyright (2010), with permission from Elsevier.

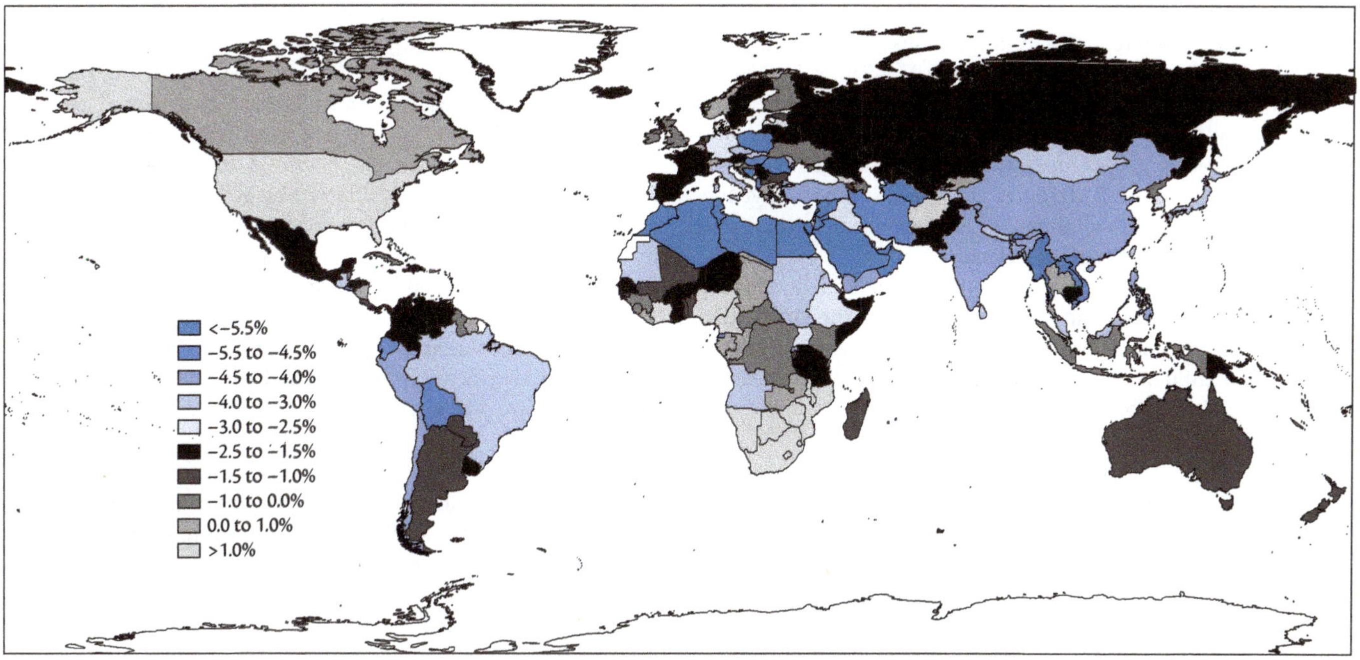

Figure 55.2 (See colour figure section). Yearly rate of decline in maternal mortality ratio, 1990–2008.

Reprinted from *The Lancet*, Volume 375, number 9726, Margaret C Hogan *et al.*, Maternal mortality for 181 countries, 1980–2008: a systematic analysis of progress towards Millennium Development Goal 5, pp. 1609–1623, Copyright (2010), with permission from Elsevier.

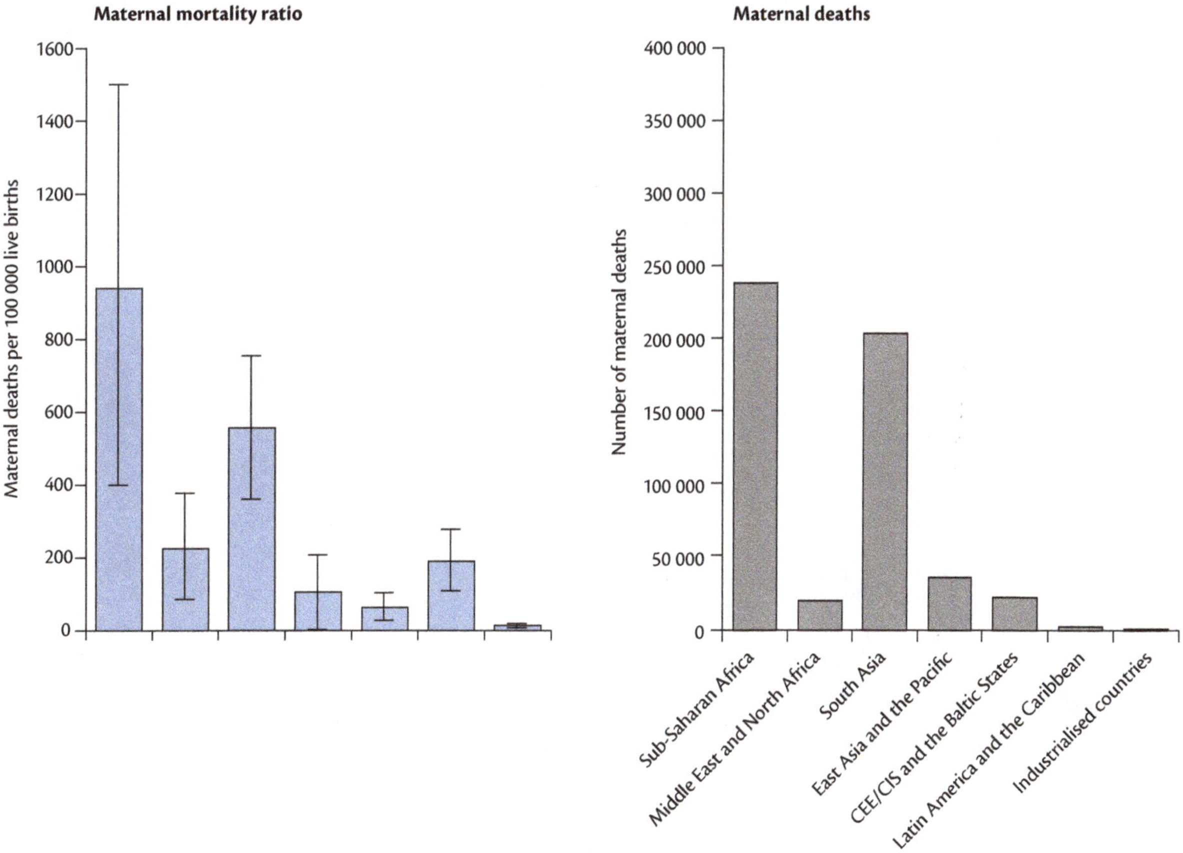

Figure 55.3 Regional variation in maternal mortality ratio and number of maternal deaths.

Reprinted from *The Lancet*, Volume 368, number 9542, Ronsmans C, Graham W, Maternal survival 1. Maternal mortality: who, when, where and why, pp. 1189–1200, Copyright (2006), with permission from Elsevier. Data from WHO, UN Children's Fund, UN Population Fund. Maternal mortality in 2000: estimates developed by WHO, UNICEF, UNFPA. Geneva: World Health Organization; 2004.

This was a statistically significant decline from 13.95 (95% CI 12.45–15.64)/100,000 reported in the previous triennium. By contrast, the WHO reported in 2010 that the MMR in sub-Saharan Africa was 500/100,000 live births.

Another way to qualify the disparity between countries is to look at the *lifetime risk* of maternal death, which estimates the probability of maternal death during a women's reproductive life. In 2010, Save the Children quoted the lifetime risk in Afghanistan as 1/6, compared to 1/47,600 in Ireland.[7]

Such discrepancies between the developed and developing countries are alarming and have been cited as 'the largest discrepancy of all public-health statistics'.[8] It is substantially greater than that for child or neonatal mortality, and some of the reasons behind it will be explored later in this chapter.

Causes of maternal death

The vast majority of maternal deaths occur around labour, delivery, and the immediate postpartum period, with a substantial number occurring in hospital.[9] Such data as demonstrated in Figure 55.4 confirms that professional and trained care should be focused on this period. In 2006, a WHO systematic review of causes of maternal death found that direct causes accounted for most of the deaths, with haemorrhage, hypertensive diseases, and infections being the main causes (Figure 55.5).[10] This is despite haemorrhage being described as the ' one major cause of maternal mortality in which women were dying needlessly for want of common skills that every midwife and practitioner should posses'.[11] Deaths due to unsafe abortion remain close to 13% of all maternal deaths, representing an actual number of 47,000.[12] The WHO estimates that 21.6 million unsafe abortions took place worldwide in 2008, with almost all of them in developing countries.

Human immunodeficiency virus (HIV), malaria, tuberculosis, and hepatitis undoubtedly contribute to the indirect causes of maternal mortality, especially in sub-Saharan Africa. The sheer prevalence of such diseases and the associated lack of available testing, under-diagnosing, and under-reporting make it difficult to assess their importance as a cause of death. However, 'in countries that are most severely affected by HIV the AIDS epidemic has thought to have reversed previous gains in maternal mortality'.[9] In Uganda, the overall MMR is around 900/100,000 but is reported as 1300/100,000 in HIV-infected mothers.[9]

Although deaths from accidents, murders, or suicides are classed as incidental and excluded from maternal mortality statistics, there is evidence from India and Bangladesh that the pregnancy may have played a role.[9]

Where women die

Many of the worldwide maternal deaths occur in hospital and fall into one of three scenarios: they arrive in a moribund state too late to benefit from emergency care; they arrive with complications and could have been saved if they had received timely and effective interventions; and those that are admitted for normal delivery who subsequently develop serious complications (natural or iatrogenic) and die with or without receiving emergency care.[9] The latter two scenarios raise concerns regarding the quality of hospital care. Numerous studies have shown that delays in recognition and treatment of life-threatening complications, as well as substandard practices, contribute directly to maternal deaths.[13,14] In cases where women arrive in a moribund state, it is likely that problems exist with referrals between facilities, or there are community barriers to accessing care, such as physical, cultural, or financial.[9,15]

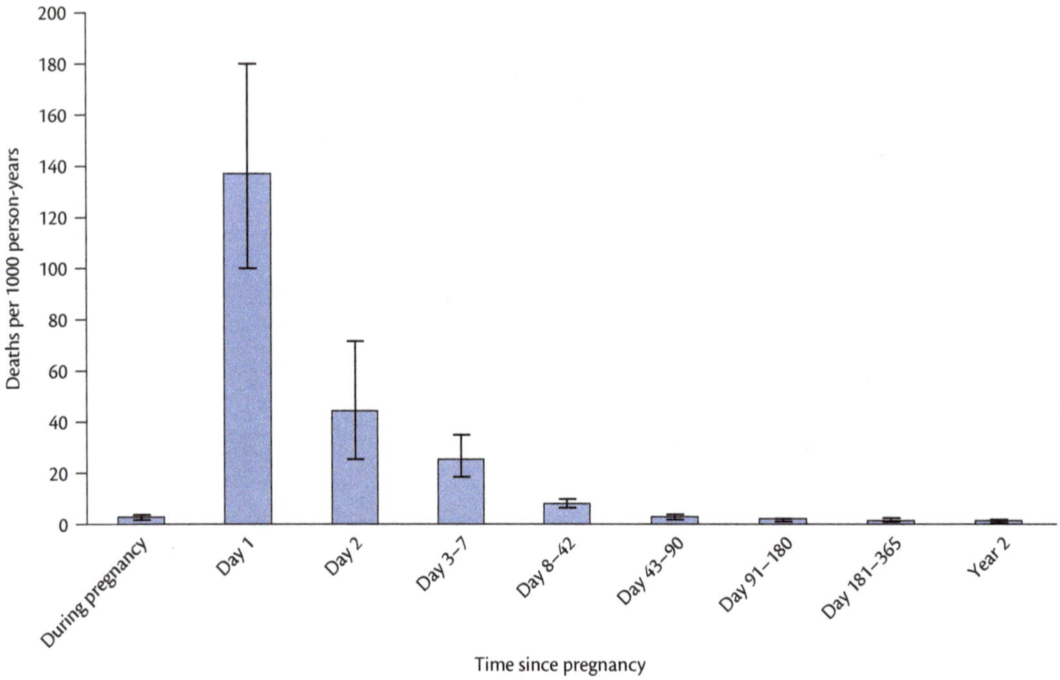

Figure 55.4 Mortality during pregnancy and by time since end of pregnancy in Matlab, Bangladesh.

Reprinted from *The Lancet*, Volume 368, number 9542, Ronsmans C, Graham W, Maternal survival 1. Maternal mortality: who, when, where and why, pp. 1189–1200, Copyright (2006), with permission from Elsevier. Data from Hurt LS, Ronsmans C. Time since pregnancy and mortality in women of reproductive age in Matlab, Bangladesh. Paper presented at the British Society for Population Studies; December 2002; London, UK.

Maternal morbidity

For every maternal death in the developing world, it is estimated that 30 women suffer morbidity during childbirth, such as chronic anaemia, infertility, stress incontinence, vaginal fistulae, chronic pelvic pain, emotional depression, and physical exhaustion.[16]

Reasons for differences between the developed and the developing world

The gap in the delivery of healthcare between the developed and developing nations is mainly caused by economic, geographical, sociobehavioural, cultural, and clinical factors.

Economic factors

Health planners face formidable challenges in the poorest countries. There are limited material and human resources, low government spending on health (often less than US$10/person/year), weak administrative and managerial support and a huge burden of disease.[17] One of the main focuses of MDG 5 is to increase the number of deliveries that are attended by skilled health personnel. The regions with the highest maternal mortality, sub-Saharan Africa and Southern Asia, are also those with the lowest coverage of births by skilled health personnel. In developing regions over all, the proportion of deliveries attended by skilled health personnel rose from 55% in 1990 to 65% in 2010.[18]

Even if obstetric services are accessed they are severely limited. Most anaesthetics are provided by non-physicians, nurses, or unqualified personnel facing erratic electrical supplies, inconsistent oxygen delivery, paucity of drugs or equipment, and even lack of running water.[17] The inadequate public spending on health has led to a poor quality of care characterized by long waiting times, lack of medication, and inappropriately trained staff. There is often an erosion of ethical values and professional conscience and a general culture of impunity. There are major problems with procurement, storage, and management. Corruption is increasingly recognized as a consequence.[19] Workforce issues such as

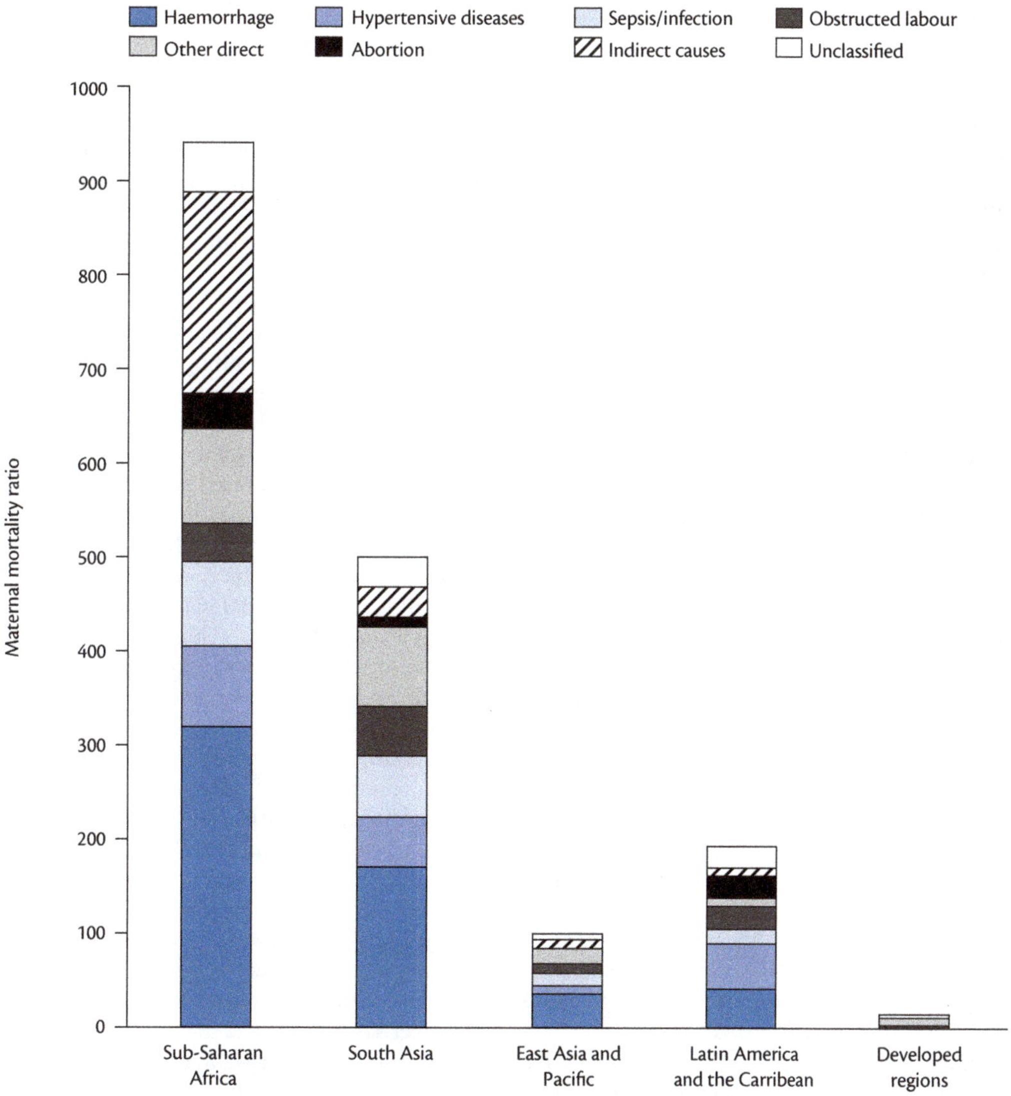

Figure 55.5 (See colour figure section). Maternal mortality ratios for 2000 by medical cause and world region.

Reprinted from *The Lancet*, Volume 368, number 9542, Ronsmans C, Graham W, Maternal survival 1. Maternal mortality: who, when, where and why, pp. 1189–1200, Copyright (2006), with permission from Elsevier. Data from WHO, UN Children's Fund, UN Population Fund. Maternal mortality in 2000: estimates developed by WHO, UNICEF, UNFPA. Geneva: World Health Organization; 2004.

emigration of skilled workers, absenteeism through illness, and migration away from the health sector due to poor working conditions leads to a further burden on the healthcare system and economies of developing countries.[20]

Geographical factors

Although one might expect that differences in maternal mortality between world regions may be explained by economic growth, it is not that simple. Despite similar gross national incomes per head, Vietnam and Sri Lanka have achieved much lower MMRs than Yemen and Ivory Coast.[9] Indeed, internal variations such as geographical, economic, and social factors, are not just confined to the developing world, and hence inequalities in the risk of maternal death are found everywhere.

Differences in maternal mortality between urban and rural areas within poor countries are also substantial. In Egypt, the MMR was more than twice as high in the nomadic Frontier region than in the Metropolitan region (120 vs 48 deaths/100,000).[21] In Afghanistan, the differences were even more striking, with mortality being 418/100,000 in the capital city of Kabul compared with 6507/100,000 in the remote district of Ragh.[22]

Sociobehavioural and cultural factors

In addition to financial and physical access to obstetric services there are sociobehavioural and cultural factors. Such barriers include late recognition by women and families of the need to seek care that is either intentional or unintentional and transportation difficulties in reaching hospitals.[15] Most women labour in their houses for several days and go to hospital only as a last resort because delivery is considered 'natural', not as an 'illness' requiring hospitalization. Unfortunately, death during labour or delivery may also be accepted as normal and inevitable.[15] Additionally, a lack of health education and/or poor reputation of healthcare facilities leave many patients unconvinced or frankly afraid of the value of modern obstetric management.[15,23] A random questionnaire administered to a group of rural women in the Akosombo district of Ghana revealed that about 70% of women associated hospital confinement with severe discomfort, especially related to caesarean delivery.[23] Others have a natural disinclination towards caesarean delivery because their peer groups insult them openly if they have been unable to deliver vaginally, considered the 'natural' way.[23] A lack of support and privacy in the hospital is a factor keeping some away and women may associate surgery with mortality.[15] Furthermore, it is a status symbol to have large families and women believe that caesarean delivery will limit the number of children that they may bear.[23] In some cultures, a pregnant woman with complications or a woman in labour cannot be taken to the hospital without the husband's consent, further delaying care.[15,23] These social issues, along with the physical impediments of travel to referral centres, put the lives of the mother and the fetus at risk.

Figure 55.6 shows the barriers to uptake of professional birthing care faced by countries with marginal exclusion and those with massive deprivation. In both settings, all of these barriers play a part in coverage. The scarcity of providers, supportive infrastructure, and policies are the primary barriers for women in sites of massive deprivation; however, reluctance to use services and poor quality care detract from use where services are available.[24]

Clinical factors

Anaesthetists are an integral part of the obstetric team in the United Kingdom, and participate in over 50% of parturients care.[25] Anaesthetists have knowledge of acute physiology and are skilled at fluid management, invasive monitoring, and the other aspects of critical care that are essential when dealing with a critically ill mother with obstetric haemorrhage, sepsis, and eclampsia. In the developing world, many women present with life-threatening complications and could be saved if the anaesthetic provider was skilled at recognizing the need for, and able to carry out, prompt and effective resuscitation.[16]

Most studies, however, identify the same issues—few medically qualified anaesthetists, lack of appropriate training and supervision for non-medical anaesthetists, limited monitoring of anaesthesia, and inadequate supplies of drugs and equipment, including blood for transfusion.[26] The lack of trained anaesthetic personnel also seems to have an impact on caesarean delivery rates. The WHO may recommend a caesarean delivery rate of between 5% and 10%, but in reality it is often below 1% for the poorest populations, often in sub-Saharan Africa.[27] In India, medical officers are discouraged from practising anaesthesia—there are few training positions, remuneration and working conditions are poor, and most doctors prefer to work in private practice in urban areas or migrate.[28] Medical migration is also rife in sub-Saharan Africa. Currently in Uganda, for example, there are 14 physician anaesthetists in a population of 30 million—approximately 1 anaesthetist per 2 million people.[29] By comparison, in the United States, the ratio is 1/4000 and in the United Kingdom, 1/5000. Most Ugandan anaesthesia providers work in cities, in conditions that would still be considered austere by Western standards. Postgraduate training programmes in Uganda remain unfilled because of difficulty recruiting and funding trainees. In 2010, there were only 12 anaesthesia residents in training although 47 positions were available.[30] The annual cost of training is approximately US$3500, nearly ten times the estimated mean annual household income in Uganda.[30] In neighbouring Kenya (population 32 million), there are 120 anaesthetists, but only 13 of these are employed in the public sector. The remainder work in private practice in the capital, Nairobi. There are several hundred surgeons at Kenyatta National Hospital, the national referral and teaching hospital, but only nine anaesthetists.[30] Thus the vast majority of anaesthetics are administered by non-physician anaesthetic providers working alone, unsupervised, and often with limited training. This should be considered when reading some reports of worryingly high perioperative mortality rates for caesarean deliveries in Africa in the region of 1–2%.[31–35] Most of these deaths were avoidable and one-third of deaths are directly attributable to anaesthesia, mainly due to airway problems. Another significant cause is the lack of access to blood transfusion.

As well as staffing concerns, health facilities are also woefully lacking. Two surveys in Uganda showed that few facilities had running water, electricity, a functional operating theatre, or midwives. Also that only 23% of anaesthetists had the facilities to deliver safe anaesthesia to an adult having major surgery, 13% to deliver safe anaesthesia to a child, and 6% had the facilities to deliver safe anaesthesia to a mother undergoing caesarean delivery (spinal needles, blood for transfusion, oxytocic agents, antihypertensive agents, or magnesium sulphate). Furthermore, ten anaesthetists were working without oxygen supplies.[29,36]

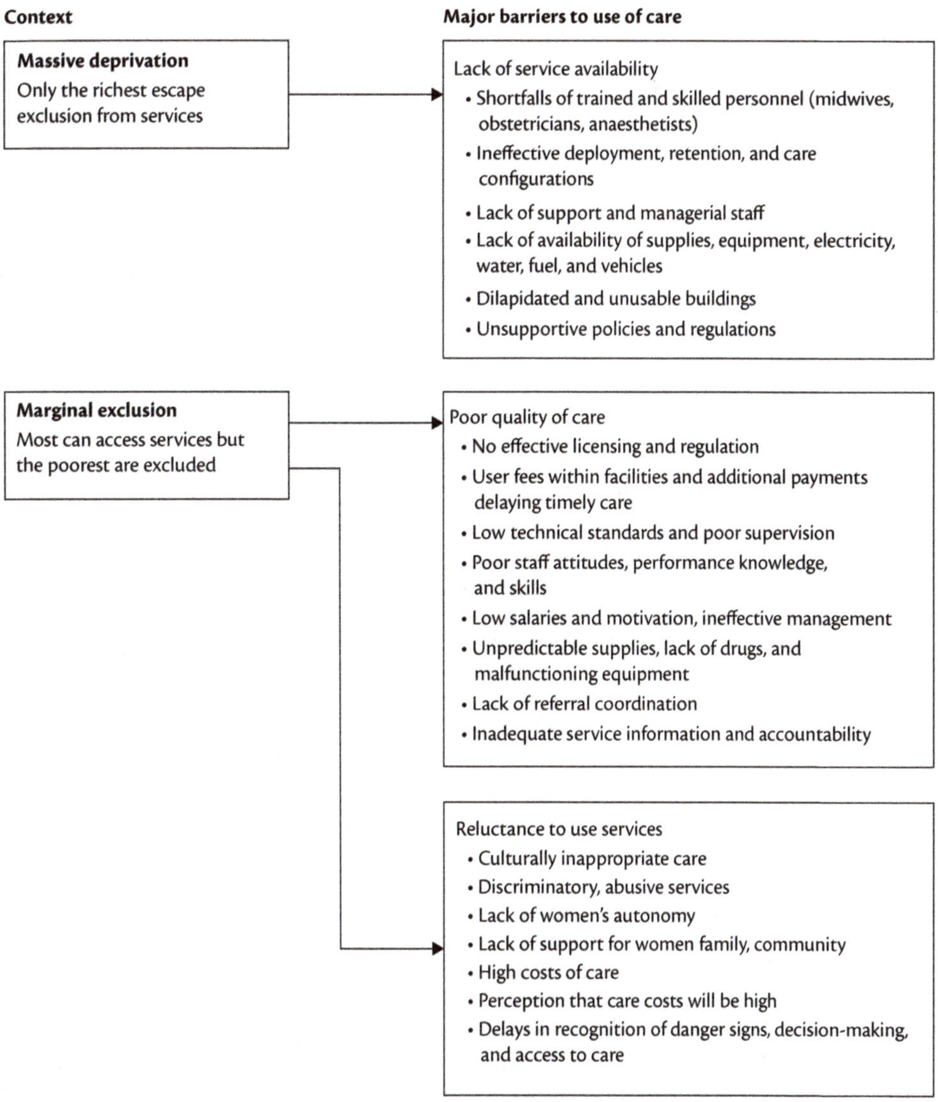

Figure 55.6 Barriers to scaling up according to context.

Reprinted from *The Lancet*, Volume 368, number 9544, Koblinsky M, Matthews Z, Hussein J *et al.*, Maternal Survival 3: Going to scale with professional skilled care, pp. 1377–1386, Copyright (2006), with permission from Elsevier.

Outcome would be better if a few common needs were met: access to a suitable facility to receive care, a sufficient number of competently trained medical staff, and a sustainable source of supplies and equipment.

International outreach: a global response

A concern for human welfare means that the developed world cannot be passive and inactive whilst such a global disparity exists. Thus aid, humanitarian and outreach organizations, and programmes have developed allowing nations and individuals to help. Some examples of an exhaustive list are discussed below.

National governmental aid

As long ago as 1970, the General Assembly of the United Nations agreed that 'each economically advanced country will progressively increase its official development assistance (ODA) to the developing countries and will exert its best efforts to reach a minimum net amount of 0.7% of its gross national product at market prices by the middle of the decade'.[37] However, in economic crises, aid to foreign countries is often the first victim of cutbacks. In 2014, only five countries (Sweden, Luxembourg, Norway, Denmark, and the United Kingdom) had met this target (see Figure 55.7).

The Department for International Development (DFID) is the UK department with responsibility for managing Britain's aid to poor countries.[38] ODA is the internationally agreed standard definition of aid, with the UK ODA in 2011 being £8,570 million or 0.56% of UK gross national income (GNI).[39] The UK government is committed to raising ODA to 0.7% of GNI by 2013.[39] However, in the current economic crisis, aid to foreign countries is often the first victim of cutbacks. The DFID contributes to the running costs of United Nations Agencies such as the WHO. It also supports the World Bank and Regional Development Banks, and the European Commission. It further supported a number of global health

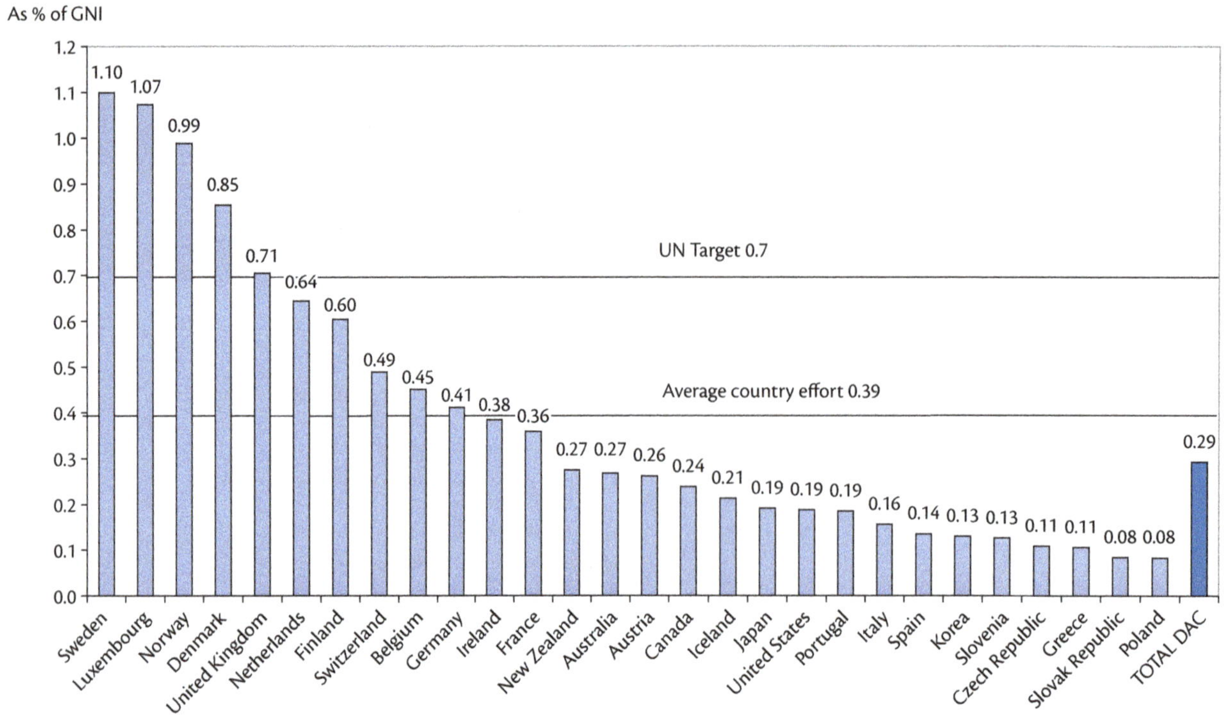

Figure 55.7 Official development assistance as per cent of gross national income (GNI) 2014.
Data taken from http://www.oecd.org/dac/stats/development-aid-stable-in-2014-but-flows-to-poorest-countries-still-falling.htm June 2015.

initiatives, and allocations directly to countries are based on need, historical relationships, the governance and policy environment, and their strategic importance for regional development.[38] The DFID works with national governments in countries where the annual health budget is nearer to £5–10 per person rather than the £1500 in the United Kingdom, to address the challenges already mentioned in this chapter and to help strengthen the systems that underpin delivery of basic health services—the trained staff, infrastructure, drug and commodity supply, and management and information systems. Where possible this is done by directly funding the national budget to support countries to implement their own health plans that reflect national priorities.[38]

World Health Organization

The WHO has been promoting safety and quality in healthcare since its inception.[40] In response to mounting attention that iatrogenic harm represented a public health problem comparable with deaths and injuries from road traffic accidents, the WHO established a programme for action called the *Global Patient Safety Challenge.* The first challenge, *Clean Care is Safer Care,* made a major impact in improving hand washing and thereby preventing the spread of infection. The aim of the second challenge, *Safe Surgery Saves Lives,* is to reduce errors in surgical care to avoid injury.

Safe surgery saves lives

The goal of the Safe Surgery Saves Lives challenge is to improve the safety of surgical care around the world by ensuring adherence to proven standards of care in all countries.[41] In 2007 and 2008, a WHO pilot study involving hospitals in eight cities around the globe demonstrated that the use of a simple surgical checklist, developed by the WHO, can lower the incidence of surgery-related deaths and complications by one-third during major operations. This has since been reproduced in the Netherlands showing that with the use of the checklist, surgery complications were reduced by more than one-third and deaths were reduced by almost half.[42] Since the release of the WHO Surgical Safety Checklist globally more than 3900 hospitals representing more than 122 countries have registered as Safe Surgery Saves Lives participating hospitals.[41] If there are an estimated 234 million operations performed globally each year then at least half a million deaths per year would be preventable with effective implementation of the WHO Surgical Safety Checklist worldwide.[41]

Safe childbirth checklist

Following the success of the Surgical Safety Checklist the WHO has developed a pilot edition of the Safe Childbirth Checklist, to support the delivery of essential maternal and perinatal care practices. It contains 29 items addressing the major causes of maternal death (haemorrhage, infection, obstructed labour and hypertensive disorders), intrapartum-related stillbirths (inadequate intrapartum care), and neonatal deaths (birth asphyxia, infection, and complications related to prematurity) in low-income countries. It was developed following a rigorous methodology and tested for usability in ten countries across Africa and Asia.[43] A collaboration was launched in November 2012 inviting organizations to study the implementation and usefulness of the checklist in diverse health-care settings. It is hoped to have as much of an impact, if not more, than that seen by the implementation of the Surgical Safety Checklist.

Anaesthesia societies

The World Federation of Societies of Anaesthesiologists

The World Federation of Societies of Anaesthesiologists (WFSA) was formed in 1955. It's objectives are 'exclusively educational, scientific, and charitable in nature and are to make available the highest standards of anaesthesia, pain medicine, trauma management, resuscitation, and preoperative/critical care medicine to all peoples of the world and to disseminate the same amongst them'.[44] This is achieved by dissemination of scientific information, recommending standards of training, encouraging research into all aspects of anaesthesia, establishing safety measures including standardization of equipment, and by providing information regarding opportunities for postgraduate training and research.[45] The WFSA is a federation of 126 national societies of anaesthesia and is part funded by an annual subscription from each national society (US$2 per member), 50% of any profit from the World Congress, and charitable funds collected by the WFSA Foundation.[45]

The 'Global Oximetry project' *Lifebox* of the Safety & Quality of Practice Committee will be discussed later in this chapter.

International Standards for the Safe Practice of Anaesthesia

In 1992, the WFSA adopted the *International Standards for the Safe Practice of Anaesthesia*, revisions of which have been ratified in 2008 and 2010.[46] These standards are recommended for anaesthesia professionals throughout the world. They are intended to provide guidance and assistance to anaesthesia professionals, their professional societies, hospital and facility administrators, and governments for improving and maintaining the quality and safety of anaesthesia care. For some, these standards will represent a future goal, while for others they may have already been implemented and be regarded as mandatory. In settings where the standards regarded as mandatory are not met, the WFSA recommend that the provision of anaesthesia should be restricted to procedures which are absolutely essential for the urgent or emergency saving of life or limb. In addition, provision of anaesthesia care at standards lower than those outlined as mandatory for elective surgical procedures cannot be construed as safe acceptable practice.[46] Table 55.1 gives a detailed outline of the integration of the practice standards with the levels of facilities/infrastructure, the goal being that all providers meet the 'Highly Recommended' standards and striving to meet as many of the 'Recommended' and 'Suggested' standards as well.[46]

The Publication Committee of the WFSA has a number of activities, including *Update in Anaesthesia*—a twice-yearly journal produced in English, French, Spanish, Chinese, and Russian distributed free of charge; and *Anaesthesia Tutorial of the Week*—an electronic peer-reviewed tutorial which is emailed out, free of charge, around the world. They have also encouraged the donation of books and journals from anaesthetists to colleagues without access to them.[45]

The Obstetric Committee of the WFSA has formed strong links with the Obstetric Anaesthetists' Association (OAA) and the Association of Anaesthetists of Great Britain and Ireland (AAGBI), successfully delivering projects such as the *Obstetric Anaesthesia for Developing Countries* textbook—specifically targeted at anaesthetic providers in resource-poor areas; *Obstetric Anaesthesia Resource Discs*—including a webcast of the 2008 OAA 3-day course with slides and abstract book, video of how spinals work, back copies of the *International Journal of Obstetric Anaesthesia* (IJOA), *Update in Anaesthesia*, and *Anaesthesia Tutorial of the Week*; and the *Safer Anaesthesia From Education (SAFE) Obstetric Anaesthesia* training course (see below).

Association of Anaesthetists of Great Britain and Ireland

The Association of Anaesthetists of Great Britain and Ireland (AAGBI) was a founder member of the WFSA in 1955 and has long assisted its members and colleagues working elsewhere in more challenging circumstances.[47]

The International Relations Committee of the AAGBI promotes education, research, and safety in international anaesthesia. Its aims are to support anaesthetists who train, work, or undertake research in low- and middle-income countries, distribute educational materials and develop high-quality anaesthesia training courses, and to promote access to safe surgery and anaesthesia as a public health priority.[48] Their many activities include offering funding for projects, individual travel grants, and long-term voluntary work. They administer the *Overseas Anaesthesia Fund* to support a book donation project, anaesthesia fellows in Uganda, the *SAFE Obstetric Anaesthesia* course and the global pulse oximetry project, *Lifebox*. The *SAFE Obstetric Anaesthesia* course is a 3-day refresher course in obstetric anaesthesia that has been developed in consultation with the WFSA. It is aimed at non-physician anaesthetists in developing countries and consists of short lectures, interactive sessions, and workshops that focus on recognition and management of the leading causes of maternal death in resource poor settings, and includes the principles of the WHO Safe Surgery Saves Lives project. It was successfully piloted in Uganda in June 2011 and with grants from the British Council and the WFSA, in conjunction with the WHO and the Director General of Maternal and Child Health, further training in Uganda, Bangladesh, and Liberia is to be rolled out.[48,49]

Many collaborations exist with government bodies, other organizations, and charities to establish educational programmes in Liberia, Zambia, and Kenya.[48]

Obstetric Anaesthetists' Association

The OAA was formed in 1969 to promote the highest standards of anaesthetic practice in the care of the mother and baby and has an international membership of over 2450. The OAA provides both education and training for anaesthetists in the United Kingdom and overseas and a resource for women seeking information about pain relief in labour and anaesthesia for caesarean delivery, translated into up to 37 languages.[50] The OAA and its membership have a long history of supporting obstetric anaesthesia around the world including nations with under-resourced healthcare systems where maternal mortality and the provision of safe obstetric anaesthesia remain challenging problems. As well as offering grants and bursaries, the OAA targets obstetric issues specifically—aiming to provide more focused educational outreach and support, mainly by running short lecture-based refresher courses.[51]

The Global Oximetry project

The Global Oximetry project is a great example of various organizations, bodies, networks and industry working together for the greater good.

Pulse oximetry is accepted as an essential part of modern anaesthesia practice and use of a pulse oximeter has been regarded as standard for many years.[52,53] Unfortunately it is either unavailable

Table 55.1 Guide to infrastructure, supplies and anaesthesia standards at three levels of healthcare facility, infrastructure, and supplies

Level 1 (Should meet at least *HIGHLY RECOMMENDED* anesthesia standards) Small hospital/health centre	Level 2 (Should meet at least *HIGHLY RECOMMENDED* and *RECOMMENDED* anesthesia standards) District/provincial hospital	Level 3 (Should meet at least *HIGHLY RECOMMENDED, RECOMMENDED* and *SUGGESTED* anesthesia standards) Referral hospital
Rural hospital or health centre with a small number of beds (or urban location in an extremely disadvantaged area); sparsely equipped operating room (OR) for 'minor' procedures Provides emergency measures in the treatment of 90–95% of trauma and obstetrics cases (excluding cesarean section) Referral of other patients (for example, obstructed labour, bowel obstruction) for further management at a higher level	District or provincial hospital (e.g. with100–300 beds) and adequately equipped major and minor operating rooms Short-term treatment of 95–99% of the major life-threatening conditions	A referral hospital of 300–1000 or more beds with basic intensive care facilities. Treatment aims are the same as for Level 2, with the addition of: Ventilation in OR and ICU Prolonged endotracheal intubation Thoracic trauma care Hemodynamic and inotropic treatment Complex neurological and cardiac surgery Basic ICU patient management and monitoring for up to 1 week: all types of cases, but possibly with limited provision for: Multi-organ system failure Hemodialysis Prolonged respiratory failure Metabolic care or monitoring
Essential procedures	**Essential procedures**	**Essential procedures**
Normal delivery Uterine evacuation Circumcision Hydrocele reduction, incision and drainage Wound suturing Control of hemorrhage with pressure dressings Debridement and dressing of wounds Temporary reduction of fractures Cleaning or stabilization of open and closed fractures Chest drainage (possibly) Abscess drainage	Same as Level 1 with the following additions: Cesarean section Laparotomy (usually not for bowel obstruction) Amputation Hernia repair Tubal ligation Closed fracture treatment and application of plaster of Paris Acute open orthopedic surgery: e.g. internal fixation of fractures Eye operations, including cataract extraction Removal of foreign bodies: e.g. in the airway Emergency ventilation and airway management for referred patients such as those with chest and head injuries	Same as Level 2 with the following additions: Facial and intracranial surgery Bowel surgery Pediatric and neonatal surgery Thoracic surgery Major eye surgery Major gynecological surgery, e.g. vesicovaginal repair
Personnel	**Personnel**	**Personnel**
Paramedical staff/anesthetic officer (including on-the-job training) who may have other duties as well Nurse-midwife	One or more trained anesthesia professionals District medical officers, senior clinical officers, nurses, midwives Visiting specialists or resident surgeon and/or obstetrician/gynecologist	Clinical officers and specialists in anesthesia and surgery
Drugs	**Drugs**	**Drugs**
Ketamine 50 mg/mL injection Lidocaine 1% or 2% Diazepam 5 mg/mL injection, 2 mL *or* midazolam 1 mg/mL injection, 5 mL Pethidine 50 mg/mL injection, 2 mL Morphine 10 mg/mL, 1 mL Epinephrine (Adrenaline) 1 mg Atropine 0.6 mg/mL Appropriate inhalation anesthetic if vaporizer available	Same as Level 1, but also: Thiopental 500 mg/L g powder or propofol. Suxamethonium bromide 500 mg powder Pancuronium Neostigmine 2.5 mg injection Ether, halothane or other inhalation anesthetics Lidocaine 5% heavy spinal solution, 2 ml Bupivacaine 0.5% heavy or plain, 4 mL Hydralazine 20 mg injection	Same as Level 2 with these additions: Propofol Nitrous oxide Various modern neuromuscular blocking agents Various modern inhalation anesthetics Various inotropic agents Various intravenous antiarrhythmic agents Nitroglycerine for infusion Calcium chloride 10% 10 IM injection

	Furosemide 20 mg injection Dextrose 50% 20 mL injection Aminophylline 250 mg injection Ephedrine 30/50 mg ampoules Hydrocortisone (?) Nitrous oxide	Potassium chloride 20% 10 mL injection for infusion
Equipment: capital outlay	**Equipment: capital outlay**	**Equipment: capital outlay**
Adult and pediatric self-inflating breathing bags with masks Foot-powered suction Stethoscope, sphygmomanometer, thermometer Pulse oximeter Oxygen concentrator or tank oxygen and a draw-over vaporizer with hoses Laryngoscopes, bougies	Complete anesthesia, resuscitation and airway management systems including: Reliable oxygen sources Vaporizer(s) Hoses and valves Bellows or bag to inflate lungs Face masks (sizes 00–5) Work surface and storage Pediatric anesthesia system Oxygen supply failure alarm; oxygen analyzer Adult and pediatric resuscitator sets Pulse oximeter, spare probes, adult and pediatric* Capnograph* Defibrillator (one per O.R. suite / ICU)* ECG (electrocardiograph) monitor* Laryngoscope, Macintosh blades 1–3(4) Oxygen concentrator[s] [cylinder] Foot or electric suction IV pressure infusor bag Adult and pediatric resuscitator sets Magill forceps (adult and child), intubation styler and/or bougie Spinal needles 25 G Nerve stimulator Automatic non-invasive blood pressure monitor	Same as Level 2 with these additions (per operating room or per ICU bed, except where stated): ECG (electrocardiograph) monitor* Anesthesia ventilator, reliable electric power source with manual override Infusion pumps (2 per bed) Pressure bag for IV infusion Electric or pneumatic suction Oxygen analyzer* Thermometer [temperature probe*] Electric warming blanket Electric overhead heater Infant incubator Laryngeal mask airways sizes 2,3, 4 (3 sets per O.R) Intubating bougies, adult and child (1 set per O.R) Anesthetic agent (gas and vapour) analyser Depth of anesthesia monitors are being increasingly recommended for cases at high risk of awareness but are not standard monitoring in many countries.
Equipment: disposable	**Equipment: disposable**	**Equipment: disposable**
Examination gloves IV infusion/drug injection equipment Suction catheters size 16 FG Airway support equipment, including airways and tracheal tubes	ECG electrodes IV equipment (minimum fluids: normal saline, Ringer's lactate and dextrose 5%) Pediatric giving sets Suction catheters size 16 FG Sterile gloves sizes 6–8	Same as Level 2 with these additions: Ventilator circuits Yankauer suckers Giving sets for IV infusion pumps Disposables for suction machines
Oral and nasal airways	Nasogastric tubes sizes 10–16 FG Oral airways sizes 000–4 Tracheal tubes sizes 3–8.5 mm Spinal needles sizes 22 G and 25G Batteries size C	Disposables for capnography, oxygen analyzer, in accordance with manufacturers' specifications: Sampling lines Water traps Connectors Filters—fuel cells

*It is preferable to combine these modalities all in one unit.

Note: drug concentrations and quantities are indicative only. All equipment should be appropriate for patients' age and size

Reproduced from Springer and the *Canadian Journal of Anaesthesia*, volume 57, 2010, pp. 1027–34, International Standards for a Safe Practice of Anesthesia 2010, Merry AF, Cooper JB, Soyannwo O, Wilson IH, Eichorn JH, With kind permission from Springer Science and Business Media.

or is only patchily available in many low- and middle-income countries, with an estimated 77,700 operating theatres worldwide currently working without pulse oximeters.[54] The Global Oximetry initiative was launched in 2004, as a partnership between AAGBI, WFSA, and GE Healthcare, promoting oximetry in low-resource countries.[53] Since then, WHO patient safety has worked with the Harvard School of Public Health, WFSA, AAGBI, and many other partners around the world to facilitate the development of pulse oximetry technical standards that led to the development of a high-standard, low-cost pulse oximeter. This had led to the development of a charity project, *Lifebox*, that addressed the pulse oximeter gap by making pulse oximeters available to low- and middle-income countries. The *Lifebox* statement of purpose is 'to preserve and protect the health of patients worldwide by providing and assisting in the provision of equipment and support services in low-resource and lower–middle-income countries at no or reduced cost; and to advance the education in healthcare of the general public and especially those in the medical or similar professions by the provision of education and training worldwide'.[55]

Anaesthesia outreach and educational mission

There is no doubt that there is a hunger for advancement in obstetric anaesthesia amongst practitioners in the developing world. This is matched by a considerable interest from individuals in the developed world in helping support a change for the better.[56] In the earlier sections in this chapter, some of the ways that governments and large global and national organizations can support, help, and influence change on a wider and more general scale have been discussed. However, significant work and change can be achieved by more focused educational outreach and support. Howell describes four key components to making a project really effective, worthwhile, sustainable, and successful:[56]

1. Local champions. The local practitioners must be enthusiastic, keen to listen, learn, and drive change forward themselves. Identifying these key people is crucial, requiring a good deal of planning, often including a reconnaissance trip or a fact-finding mission.
2. Teaching and supporting appropriate concepts, in an appropriate way. This needs intuition, sensitivity, and an ability to listen and to grasp the local needs and possibilities. It is unwise to assume to know what local practitioners need without establishing the local circumstances.
3. Team members must be flexible, able to engage with the local practitioners well, and quickly adapt to an unaccustomed environment, which may be a considerable culture shock.
4. Ongoing support and follow-up are needed to cement relationships between organizations and to provide continual reinforcement and encouragement for the local practitioners.

Kybele, Mothers of Africa, and the *Tropical Health and Education Trust (THET)* are successful examples of such focused educational outreach in obstetric anaesthesia.

Kybele

Kybele is a non-profit humanitarian organization dedicated to improving childbirth safety worldwide through educational partnerships. The role of Kybele is to bring professional medical teams into host countries, to work alongside doctors and nurses in their home hospitals, to improve healthcare standards.[57] Since 2004, Kybele has conducted medical training in Turkey, Croatia, Ghana, Georgia, Armenia, Romania, Egypt, Mongolia, and Brazil. Kybele has sponsored 16 major in-country medical conferences and has trained hundreds of doctors and nurses. It has developed an educational model to quickly implement sustainable interventions at a minimal cost, whilst being culturally sensitive and country specific.

A programme is initiated by an invitation submitted by a physician from a prospective country. A site visit is then arranged and a small team and the host observe conditions and practices within several hospitals. As already mentioned, the enthusiasm and friendship that develops between the host and the team is crucial in the development of a successful and sustainable programme. Then a project is designed with the host physician to fit the specific needs of the country for return with a full multidisciplinary team about 12 months later. A full trip generally lasts 10–14 days, comprising of a national conference and on-site training, working alongside doctors and nurses within their home hospitals. Kybele maintains collaboration with host countries and repeat visits are encouraged to sustain development, growth and change. Following this format, Kybele has shown a significant increase in the uptake of regional anaesthesia in Croatia, Armenia, and Georgia.[58–60] Kybele has also seen a reduction in the MMR of a large regional hospital in Ghana from 496/100,000 live births in 2007 to 328/100,000 in 2009, a period of sustained visits from their multidisciplinary team.[61]

Mothers of Africa

Mothers of Africa is a medical educational charity that trains medical staff in sub-Saharan Africa to care for mothers during pregnancy and childbirth. It was initially established as a link between the academic departments in Togo and Benin and the academic and NHS departments of the University Hospital of Wales in 2005. Since then educational visits to Togo, Benin, Liberia, Zambia, Ethiopia, and Tanzania have been completed, providing a mixture of seminars, lectures, workshops, and in-theatre teaching.[62,63]

Tropical Health and Educational Trust

THET is a specialist global health organization that educates, trains, and supports health workers through global health partnerships, strengthening health systems and enabling people in low- and middle-income countries to access essential healthcare. It encourages and supports links between hospitals and healthcare training institutions in the countries of the southern hemisphere and their counterparts in the United Kingdom, or indeed any economically developed country. These links can be used to equip staff with essential skills, including anaesthetic skills, to improve morale, to increase their motivation, and thus to contribute to a strengthened infrastructure.[64,65] Throughout the dialogue between the northern and southern partners it remains essential that the southern partner defines the needs of their hospital or training school, and that the northern partner remains sensitive to the southern partner's superior knowledge of the local context. Both partners have to be innovative, adaptable, and ready to adopt methods that are new and that may not yet have been tested in the context of a developing country.[65] Advantages of a link are that it can be flexible, adapt to changing needs, and provide for a wide range of healthcare workers and service development. They do have to be long-term if they are to contribute to international development, short-term interventions do not work.[65]

Anaesthesia in developing countries: the experience

This chapter has already discussed some of the problems in developing countries due to a critical shortage of staff and resources, and how stretched healthcare services are by diseases such as malaria and HIV, the loss of trained staff to developed countries, and the insecurities and economic effects of long-term conflict.[29] These factors ensure that a visiting anaesthetist from the developed world will experience a very different anaesthetic environment in the developing world.

Hodges et al. conducted a survey of Ugandan anaesthetists in 2006 to demonstrate the reality of anaesthesia in developing countries.[29] They found that only 6% of anaesthetists were able to provide a safe anaesthesia service for caesarean delivery by both general and spinal anaesthesia. The hospitals unable to provide safe anaesthesia for caesarean delivery had a total estimated caseload of 32,784 cases. Seventy-eight per cent of anaesthetists worked in hospitals where magnesium sulphate was unavailable for at least some of the time. Thirteen per cent worked without oxytocin or ergometrine for some of the time.[29] With regards to spinal anaesthesia, 59% of anaesthetists had no spinal anaesthetic solution at least some of the time, and comments included 'the surgeons do not like the technique' and 'there is no spinal anaesthesia performed since there are no spinal needles. The district cannot afford to buy such needles'.[29] Table 55.2 and Table 55.3 illustrate what drugs are available, showing that anaesthesia is largely ketamine based, with ether as the main volatile agent. Supplies of suxamethonium were unreliable and non-depolarizing neuromuscular blocking drugs were not commonly used. Very worryingly, blood for transfusion was only available to 23% of anaesthetists, and 10% of anaesthetists always worked without oxygen.[29]

Table 55.2 Availability of anaesthetic drugs. Values are number (%) of anaesthetists

n = 91	Always available	Sometimes available	Never available	Don't know
Ketamine	84 (92%)	3 (3%)	4 (4%)	0
Thiopental	54 (59%)	22 (24%)	14 (15%)	1
Suxamethonium	50 (54%)	21 (23%)	18 (19%)	2
Non-depolarizing relaxant	14 (15%)	11 (12%)	63 (69%)	3
Neostigmine	15 (16%)	6 (6%)	63 (69%)	7
Halothane	35 (38%)	15 (16%)	36 (39%)	5
Ether	62 (68%)	19 (20%)	9 (9%)	1
Pethidine/morphine	41 (45%)	28 (30%)	20 (21%)	2
Naloxone	9 (9%)	15 (16%)	55 (60%)	12
Atropine	77 (84%)	6 (6%)	6 (6%)	2

Reproduced with permission from Hodges SC, Mijumbi C, Okello M *et al.* Anaesthesia services in developing countries: defining the problems. *Anaesthesia*, volume 62, pp. 4–11, Copyright © 2007 John Wiley and Sons.

Table 55.3 Availability of other essential drugs. Values are number (%) of anaesthetists

n = 91	Always	Sometimes	Never	Don't know
Adrenaline	68 (74%)	17 (18%)	3 (3%)	3
Ephedrine/metaraminol/ phenylephrine	41 (45%)	20 (21%)	26 (28%)	4
Spinal local anaesthetic	36 (39%)	26 (28%)	28 (30%)	1
Local anaesthetics for blocks	64 (70%)	17 (18%)	7 (7%)	3
Magnesium	18 (19%)	35 (38%)	36 (39%)	2
Hydralazine	28 (30%)	31 (34%)	28 (30%)	4
Diazepam	74 (81%)	16 (17%)	0 (0%)	1
Labetalol	27 (29%)	27 (29%)	28 (30%)	9
Oxytocin	52 (57%)	29 (31%)	7 (7%)	3
Ergometrine	74 (81%)	13 (14%)	1 (1%)	3
Oxygen	58 (63%)	23 (25%)	10 (10%)	0
Intravenous fluid	62 (68%)	25 (27%)	2 (2%)	0
Nitrous oxide	0 (0%)	3 (3%)	84 (92%)	4
Blood for transfusion	21 (23%)	54 (59%)	15 (16%)	1

Reproduced with permission from Hodges SC, Mijumbi C, Okello M *et al.* Anaesthesia services in developing countries: defining the problems. *Anaesthesia*, volume 62, pp. 4–11, Copyright © 2007 John Wiley and Sons.

Equipment

The design of anaesthesia equipment for use in hospitals in the developing world must take into account the local conditions, particularly whether reliable supplies of compressed oxygen and electricity are available.[66]

Equipment for delivery of inhalational anaesthesia

The developing world often has to cope with extremes of temperature, humidity, and dust, and thus an anaesthetic machine must be physically robust, easy to understand and operate, require minimal servicing and have affordable, readily available spare parts. It should also be capable of functioning without compressed gases or electricity. In the developed world, a continuous flow plenum machine is favoured for many reasons: its accurate delivery of volatile agents, presence of a reservoir bag acting as a respiratory indicator, the use of a T-piece, nitrous oxide, and circle circuit systems. However, there are many drawbacks when considering the developing world, especially the requirement of compressed gas supplies that may well be scarce. In addition, nitrous oxide and soda lime supplies are problematic and expensive. Thus it is not unusual to come across an 'anaesthetic machine graveyard' within many hospitals in Africa.[66]

One solution to these problems is draw-over anaesthesia, consisting of a low-resistance breathing circuit with one-way valves to prevent re-breathing, a self-inflating bag or bellows to ventilate the patient, and a draw-over vaporizer such as the EMO (Epstein, Macintosh, Oxford) or the OMV (Oxford Miniature Vaporiser) vaporizers seen in Figure 55.8. This system is usually robust, portable, easy to assemble, and requires minimal maintenance.[67,68]

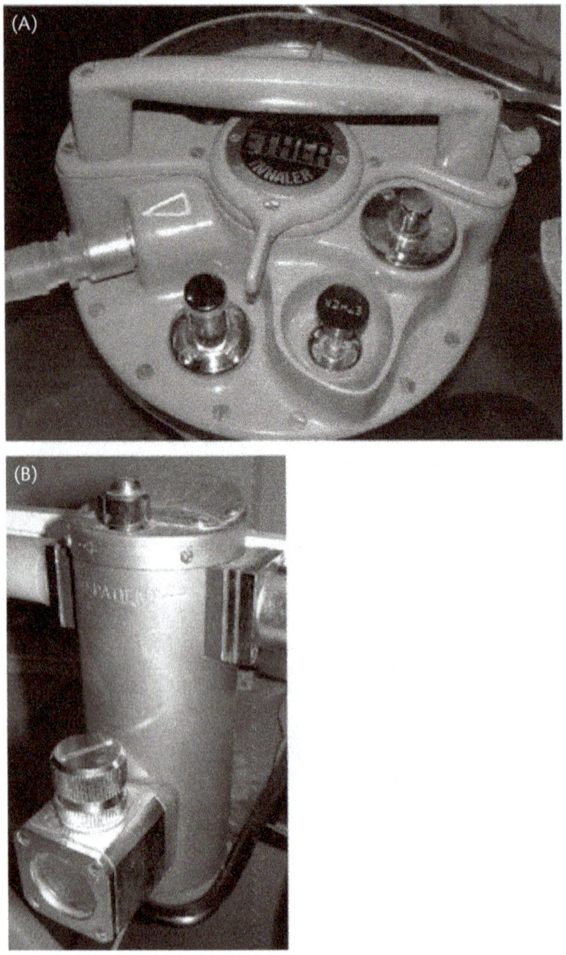

Figure 55.8 (A) An Epstein, Macintosh, Oxford (EMO) ether vaporizer. (B) An Oxford Miniature Vaporiser (OMV).
Reproduced with permission from McCormick BA, Eltringham RJ., Anaesthesia equipment for resource-poor environments, *Anaesthesia*, volume 62, Suppl1, pp. 54–60. Copyright © 2007 John Wiley and Sons.

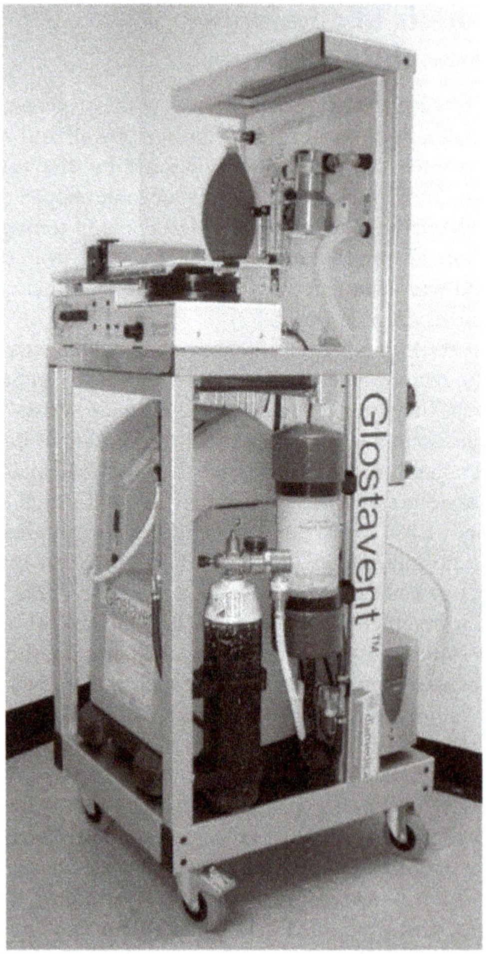

Figure 55.9 The Glostavent®.
Reproduced with permission from McCormick BA, Eltringham RJ., Anaesthesia equipment for resource-poor environments, *Anaesthesia*, volume 62, Suppl1, pp. 54–60. Copyright © 2007 John Wiley and Sons.

Oxygen concentrators

An oxygen concentrator will produce oxygen at 95% concentration by passing atmospheric air through zeolite to adsorb nitrogen, thus reducing dependence on cylinder supplies. If excessive flows are demanded, the delivered concentration is reduced. Small concentrators, which meet WHO's standards can deliver 4 L/min of oxygen (>90%) consuming approximately 350 watts (thus electricity or an AC generator are required). Concentrators are usually the cheapest source of oxygen at roughly 30–50% the cost of cylinders.[69]

The Glostavent®

The Glostavent® (Diamedica, Barnstaple, Devon, UK) is the first anaesthetic machine that meets the WFSA performance standard for anaesthetic equipment for low- and low–middle-income countries.[70] It combines an oxygen concentrator, gas-driven ventilator, low-resistance vaporizer, modified draw-over breathing circuit, uninterruptible power supply (UPS), and a reserve oxygen cylinder (see Figure 55.9).[66] It is robust, able to withstand extremes of temperature and humidity, does not require nitrous oxide or soda lime, and accidental delivery of a hypoxic mixture is impossible.[69] It can be used in either draw-over or continuous flow mode, with any breathing circuit, on any size patient using most of the commonly used inhalational agents.

Ketamine

Ketamine is a very versatile inexpensive drug and plays an invaluable role in the developing world. In regions where access and funding for a wider range of drugs is problematic, its broad range of clinical applications is ideal. Its good safety profile and ease of storage makes it ideal for use in areas where refrigerators, complex monitoring, electricity, and oxygen may all be in short supply or unreliable.[71]

Ketamine is a phencyclidine derivative that has an antagonistic action at *N*-methyl-D-aspartate receptors throughout the central nervous system. Being both water- and lipid-soluble, ketamine may be administered by a number of routes, and indeed intravenous (IV), intramuscular (IM), oral, rectal, subcutaneous, epidural, and transnasal routes have all been described.[71]

Typical doses for ketamine are induction of anaesthesia: 0.5–1.5 mg/kg IV or 4–10 mg/kg IM; maintenance of anaesthesia: 10–30 mcg/kg/min via IV infusion; sedation and analgesia: 0.2–0.75 mg/kg IV or 2–4 mg/kg IM followed continuous infusion of 5–20 mcg/kg/min with or without supplemental oxygen.[72]

Ketamine anaesthesia usually maintains the airway with some preservation of pharyngeal and laryngeal reflexes. As this is not guaranteed, airway protection must still be a priority in circumstances where aspiration is a risk, such as induction of general anaesthesia for caesarean delivery. Partial airway obstruction may be overcome by simple airway manoeuvres, and apnoea after a rapid IV bolus may require a brief period of bag–mask ventilation. Bronchodilation is a useful effect that is used in the management of moderate to severe asthma, most likely mediated by a central effect inducing catecholamine release and secondly via inhibition of vagal pathways to produce an anticholinergic effect acting directly on bronchial smooth muscle.[71]

Ketamine produces an increase in blood pressure, stroke volume, and heart rate whilst maintaining systemic vascular resistance, making it an ideal agent for the shocked patient but less appropriate for patients with severe ischaemic heart disease.[71]

It produces a dissociative anaesthesia, characterized by the patient often having their eyes open and making reflex movements during anaesthesia and surgery. Hallucinations occur during recovery in up to 30% of patients, particularly in females and after large and or rapid IV boluses. These can be reduced by premedication with benzodiazepines.

Its potent analgesic qualities mean it can be used as the sole analgesic agent intraoperatively, although a balanced technique will reduce the amount of ketamine required. Some studies have shown that its intraoperative use has led to a decreased opiate requirement postoperatively, and it is extremely useful itself as a postoperative, acute pain, and chronic pain agent.

Neuraxial anaesthesia

In modern anaesthesia practice, neuraxial techniques are preferred to general anaesthesia for many types of surgery, particularly in obstetric care. Improved outcomes have been recorded in the United Kingdom, but the techniques remain underutilized in many parts of the world. With encouragement, training, and a regular supply of appropriate needles and local anaesthetic agents, the advantages of regional techniques in the developing world could be realized.[73]

Drugs are in short supply in the developing world, funding can be erratic, and storage and stock-keeping inadequate.[73] As already discussed, Hodges et al. found that 30% of Ugandan anaesthetists stated that they never had, and 28% stated that they only sometimes had, local anaesthetic solution for spinal anaesthesia in their hospitals.[29] Unfortunately, that can lead to practitioners using multidose vials of local anaesthesia putting the patient at risk of infection. A series of 27 patients over 18 years with iatrogenic meningitis in a referral hospital in India has been reported. All cases followed spinal anaesthesia, often caesarean delivery. The mortality rate was 36%.[74]

The prevailing hot and humid climate of much of the developing world can also cause a problem with storage of drugs and equipment. This was noticed to devastating effect in Sri Lanka after the 2004 tsunami when five women contracted *Aspergillus fumigatus* meningitis following spinal anaesthesia for caesarean delivery. Unfortunately three of these women died. Subsequent examination of supplies confirmed that 43 syringes from three different manufacturers were contaminated with *Aspergillus fumigatus*. The Ministry of Health stores were found to be full of post-tsunami donations and the regular procurements were being kept in a poorly maintained humid warehouse.[75]

Lack of equipment, or inadequate or inappropriate equipment, for neuraxial anaesthesia is an ongoing problem. The most commonly used needle in Zambia is the 22 G Quincke needle, for cost reasons.[73] A study in Ghana using the same needle found an incidence of 33% postdural puncture headache in women having caesarean delivery, and the headaches were generally rated as mild to moderate.[76]

There is also a lack of training in neuraxial anaesthesia, exacerbated by the lack of access to textbooks. This is demonstrated by the poor understanding of physiological changes that occur during spinal anaesthesia for caesarean delivery. It is not uncommon for a woman to undergo this operation without any form of left lateral tilt applied.[73] It can only be hoped that this can be overcome with increased Internet access and other teaching.

What about epidural analgesia? It is argued that analgesia in labour is a fundamental human right and that an epidural may also be a medical necessity in some parturients. Once again, however, lack of equipment, drugs, and monitoring prevent the establishment of many epidural programmes. There is also resistance from many obstetricians who are unfamiliar with these techniques and are impatient to wait for onset of analgesia and anaesthesia. These challenges can be overcome, especially with the ambition, drive, and support of key team players of the health institution.[77]

Critical care

The provision of obstetric critical care in developing nations is a huge task for medical professionals and health administrators. The gap in delivery of obstetric critical care between developing and developed nations is similarly caused by economic, sociobehavioural, clinical, and cultural factors.[78] However, the value of allocating increased nurse/patient ratios, appropriate monitoring and greater medical supervision to a percentage of hospital beds is equally valid in the resource limited location as any other.[79] Eighty per cent of perioperative caesarean delivery deaths occur in the postoperative period on the general world, so it is appropriate to consider how to identify and observe these vulnerable patients at this critical time.[33] Some isolated studies from the developing world have shown very high mortality (16.8–68.4%) among obstetric patients admitted to the intensive care unit.[78] The disparity in the quality of care within developing countries is very wide though, with the practice in some private urban institutions rivalling those in the developed world.[79]

Conclusion

As we have entered the twenty-first century, the rate of globalization, technical development, and interdependence between countries and economies has increased at an incredible pace, and yet we are still faced with 'the largest discrepancy of all public-health statistics'; the lifetime risk of maternal death for some women in this world is as high as 1 in 6. This is an unacceptable scar on the world's conscience that demands a humanitarian response from us all, not just as nations but as individuals as well.

References

1. Hogan MC, Foreman KJ, Naghavi M, *et al.* Maternal mortality for 181 countries, 1980–2008: a systematic analysis of progress towards Millennium Development Goal 5. *Lancet* 2010; 375:1609–23.
2. World Health Organization. *International Classification of Diseases (ICD).* 2010. [Online] www.who.int/classifications/icd/en/
3. United Nations. *The Millennium Development Goals Report 2012.* New York: United Nations, 2012. http://www.un.org/en/development/desa/publications/mdg-report-2012.html
4. Graham W, Hussein J. The right to count. *Lancet* 2004; 363:67–8
5. World Health Organization. *Beyond the Numbers—Reviewing Maternal Deaths and Complications to Make Pregnancy Safer.* Geneva: WHO; 2004. http://www.who.int/reproductive-health
6. Centre for Maternal and Child Enquiries (CMACE). Saving Mother's Lives; reviewing maternal deaths to make motherhood safer: 2006–2008. The Eighth Report on Confidential Enquiries into Maternal Deaths in the United Kingdom. *BJOG* 2011; 118 Suppl 1:1–203.
7. Save the Children. *Women on the Front Lines of Health Care; State of the World's Mothers 2010.* [Online] http://www.savethechildren.org/site/c.8rKLIXMGIpI4E/b.6178267/k.CE3/Women_on_the_Front_Lines_of_Health_Care.htm
8. Mahler H. The safe motherhood initiative: a call to action. *Lancet* 1987; 365:668–70.
9. Ronsmans C, Graham W. Maternal survival 1. Maternal mortality: who, when, where and why. *Lancet* 2006; 368:1189–200.
10. Khan KS, Wojdyla D, Say L, *et al.* WHO systematic review of causes of maternal deaths. *Lancet* 2006; 367:1066–74.
11. Loudon I. *Death in Childbirth. An International Study of Maternal Care and Maternal Mortality 1800–1950.* Oxford: Oxford University Press; 1992.
12. World Health Organization. *Unsafe Abortion: Global and Regional Estimates of the Incidence of Unsafe Abortion and Associated Mortality in 2008* (6th ed). Geneva: WHO; 2011.
13. Van den Broek N, Graham W. Quality of care for maternal and newborn health: the neglected agenda. *BJOG* 2009; 116 Suppl 1:18–21.
14. Wagaarachchi PT, Fernando L. Trends in maternal mortality and assessment of substandard care in a tertiary care hospital. *Eur J Obstet Gynecol Reprod Biol* 2002; 101:36–40.
15. Thaddeus S, Maine D. Too far to walk: maternal mortality in context. *Soc Sci Med* 1994 38(8):1091–110.
16. Clyburn P, Morris S, Hall J. Anaesthesia and safe motherhood. *Anaesthesia* 2007; 62 Suppl 1:21–5.
17. Nambiar B, Lewycka S, Mwansambo C, *et al.* Planning health care in developing countries. *Anaesthesia* 2007; 62 Suppl 1:5–10.
18. United Nations. *The Millennium Development Goals Report 2012.* New York: United Nations; 2012.
19. Russell S. The economic burden of illness for households in developing countries. A review of studies focusing on malaria, tuberculosis and human immunodeficiency virus/acquired immunodeficiency syndrome. *Am J Trop Med Hyg* 2004; *71*:147–55.
20. Fitzhugh M. Doctors and soccer players—Africa professionals on the move. *N Engl J Med* 2007; 356:440–3.
21. Gipson R, El Mohandes A, Campbell O, *et al.* The trends of maternal mortality in Egypt from 1992–2000: an emphasis on regional differences. *Matern Child Health J* 2005; 9:71–82.
22. Bartlett LA, Mawji S, Whitehead S, *et al.* Where giving birth is a forecast of death: maternal mortality in four districts of Afghanistan, 1999–2002. *Lancet* 2005; 365:864–70.
23. Kwawukume EY. Caesarean section in developing countries. *Best Pract Res Clin Obstet Gynecol* 2001; 15:165–78.
24. Koblinsky M, Matthews Z, Hussein J, *et al.* Maternal survival 3: going to scale with professional skilled care. *Lancet* 2006; 368:1377–86.
25. The Association of Anaesthetists of Great Britain and Ireland, The Obstetric Anaesthetists Association. *Guidelines for Obstetric Anaesthesia Services.* London: AAGBI, OAA; 1998 (revised 2005).
26. Walker IA, Wilson IH. Anaesthesia in developing countries—a risk for patients. *Lancet* 2008; 371:968–9.
27. Ronsmans C, Holtz S, Stanton C. Socioeconomic differences in caesarean section rates in developing countries: a retrospective analysis. *Lancet* 2006; 368:1516–23.
28. Mavalankar D, Rosenfield A. Maternal mortality in resource-poor settings: policy barriers to care. *Am J Pub Health* 2005; 95:200–3.
29. Hodges SC, Mijumbi C, Okello M, *et al.* Anaesthesia services in developing countries: defining the problems. *Anaesthesia* 2007; 62:4–11.
30. Dubowitz G. Global health and global anesthesia. *Int Anesthesiol Clin* 2010; 48:39–46.
31. Heywood AJ, Wilson IH, Sinclair JR. Perioperative mortality in Zambia. *Ann R Coll Surg (England)* 1989; 71:354–8.
32. Hansen D, Gausi SC. Anaesthesia in Malawi: complications and deaths. *Tropical Doctor* 2000; 30:146–9.
33. Fenton PF, Whitty CJW, Reynolds F. Caesarean section in Malawi: prospective study of maternal and perinatal mortality. *BMJ* 2003; 327:587–90.
34. McKenzie AG. Operative mortality at Harare Central Hospital 1992–94: an anaesthetic view. *Int J Obstet Anaesth* 1998; 7:237–41.
35. Tomta K, Ouro-Bang'na Manan AF, Abouaangbevi S, *et al.* Deaths associated with anaesthesia in Togo, West Africa. *Trop Doct* 2005; 35:220–2.
36. Mboyne AK, Mutabazi MG, Asimwe JB, *et al.* Declining maternal mortality ratio in Uganda: priority interventions to achieve the Millennium Development Goal. *Int J Gynecol Obstet* 2007; 98:285–90.
37. International Development Strategy for the Second United Nations Development Decade. *UN General Assembly Resolution 2626 (XXV), 24 October 1970, paragraph 42.* [Online] http://www.un-documents.net/a25r2626.htm
38. Tyson S, Gordon M. United Kingdom government aid. *Anaesthesia* 2007; 62 Suppl 1:11–14.
39. Department for International Development. *Annual Report and Accounts 2011–12.* [Online] http://www.dfid.gov.uk/Documents/publications1/departmental-report/2012/Annual-report-accounts-2011-12.pdf
40. Cherian MN, Merry AF, Wilson IH. The World Health Organization and Anaesthesia. *Anaesthesia* 2007; 62 Suppl 1:65–6.
41. World Health Organization. *Safe Surgery Saves Lives.* [Online] http://www.who.int/patientsafety/safesurgery/en/index.html
42. De Vries EN, Prins HA, Crolla RMPH, *et al.* Effect of a comprehensive surgical safety system on patient outcomes. *N Engl J Med* 2010; 363:1928–37.
43. World Health Organization. *Safe Childbirth Checklist.* [Online] http://www.who.int/patientsafety/implementation/checklists/childbirth/en/index.html
44. World Federation of Societies of Anaesthesiologists. Website. [Online] http://www.anaesthesiologists.org
45. Enright A, Wilson IH, Moyers JR. The World Federation of Societies of Anaesthesiologists: supporting education in the developing world. *Anaesthesia* 2007; 62 Suppl 1:67–71.
46. Merry AF, Cooper JB, Soyannwo O, *et al.* International standards for a safe practice of anesthesia 2010. *Can J Anesth* 2010; 57:1027–34.
47. Aitken H, O'Sullivan E. The International Relations Committee of the Association of Anaesthetists of Great Britain and Ireland. *Anaesthesia* 2007; 62 Suppl 1:72–4.
48. The Association of Anaesthetists of Great Britain and Ireland. *The International Relations Committee.* [Online] http://www.aagbi.org/international/international-relations-committee
49. World Federation of Societies of Anesthesiologists. *WFSA Obstetric Committee Report (2008–2012).* [Online] http://www.anaesthesiologists.org/document-files/2012%20Obstetrics%20Report.pdf
50. Obstetric Anaesthetists' Association. Website. [Online] http://www.oaa-anaes.ac.uk
51. Howell PR. Supporting the evolution of obstetric anaesthesia through outreach programs. *Int J Obstet Anaesth* 2009; 18:1–3.

52. Eichorn J. Pulse oximetry as a standard of practice in anaesthesia. *Anaesthesiology* 1993; 78:432–6.
53. Thoms G, McHugh GA, O'Sullivan E. The Global Oximetry initiative. *Anaesthesia* 2007; 62 (Suppl 1):75–7.
54. Funk LM, Weiser TG, Berry WG, *et al.* Global operating theatre distribution and pulse oximetry supply: an estimation from reported data. *Lancet* 2010; 376:1055–61.
55. Lifebox. Website. [Online] http://www.lifebox.org
56. Howell PR. Supporting the evolution of obstetric anaesthesia through outreach programs. *Int J Obstet Anaesth* 2009; 18:1–3.
57. Kybele. Website. [Online] http://www.kybeleworldwide.org
58. Kopic D, Sedernsky M, Owen MD. The impact of a teaching program on obstetric anaesthesia practices in Croatia. *Int J Obstet Anaesth* 2009; 18:4–9.
59. Amroyan A, Millar S, Owen MD. Survey of obstetric anesthesia practices in Armenia. *Anesthesiology* 2007; 106:A60.
60. Ninidze N, Bodin S, Ivester T, *et al.* Advancing obstetric anaesthesia practices in Georgia through clinical education and quality improvement methodologies. *Int J Gynecol Obstet* 2013; 120(3):296–300.
61. Srofenyoh E, Ivester T, Engmann C, *et al.* Advancing obstetric and neonatal care in a regional hospital in Ghana via continuous quality improvement. *Int J Gynecol Obstet* 2012; 116:17–21.
62. Mothers of Africa. Website. [Online] http://www.medicine.cardiff.ac.uk/mothers-africa
63. Morris S, Clyburn, Harries S, *et al.* Mothers of Africa—an anaesthesia charity. *Anaesthesia* 2007; 62 Suppl 1:108–112.
64. Tropical Health & Education Trust (THET). Website. [Online] http://www.thet.org
65. Parry EHO, Percy DB. Anaesthesia and hospital links: strengthening healthcare through South-North hospital partnerships. *Anaesthesia* 2007; 62 Suppl 1:15–20.
66. McCormick BA, Eltringham RJ. Anaesthesia equipment for resource-poor environments. *Anaesthesia* 2007; 62 Suppl 1:54–60.
67. Kamm G, Wilson IH. Draw-over anaesthesia, part 1: theory. *Update Anaesth* 1992; 2:3–4.
68. Simpson S, Wilson IH. Draw-over anaesthesia review. *Update Anaesth* 2002; 15:13–18.
69. Dobson MB. Oxygen concentrators for district hospitals. *Update Anaesth* 1999; 10:1–4.
70. Diamedica (UK) Limited. *The Glostavent Anaesthesia Machine.* [Online] http://www.diamedica.co.uk/english/product_details.cfm?id=196
71. Craven R. Ketamine. *Anaesthesia* 2007; 62 (Suppl 1):48–53.
72. Pai A, Heining M. Ketamine. *CEACCP* 2007; 7 (2):59–63.
73. Schnitteger T. Regional anaesthesia in developing countries. *Anaesthesia* 2007; 62 (Suppl 1):44–47.
74. Pandian JD. Iatrogenic meningitis after lumbar punctures—a preventable health hazard. *J Hosp Infect* 2004; 56:119–24.
75. Gunaratne PS, Wijeyaratne CN, Chandrasiri P, *et al.* An outbreak of Aspergillus meningitis following spinal anaesthesia for caesarean section in Sri Lanka: a post-tsunami effect? *Ceylon Med J* 2006; 51(4):137–42.
76. Kodali BS, Jagannathan DK, Owen MD. Establishing an obstetric neuraxial service in low-resource areas. *Int J Obstet Anesth* 2014; 23:267–73.
77. Nafiu OO. Postdural puncture headache in obstetric patients: experience from a West African teaching hospital. *Int J Obstet Anaesth* 2007; 16:4–7.
78. Bajwa SJS, Bajwa SK. Perspectives, challenges and drawbacks of obstetric critical care in developing nations. *Int J Intensive Care* 2012; 19:123–9.
79. Towey RM, Ojara S. Intensive care in the developing world. *Anaesthesia* 2007; 62 Suppl 1:32–7.

APPENDIX 1

Guidelines

Wint Mon, York-Mui Liu, Ioanna Mavridou, and Roshan Fernando

Anaesthesia

Association of Anaesthetists of Great Britain and Ireland. *Consent for Anaesthesia*. Revised Edition, 2006

http://www.aagbi.org/sites/default/files/consent06.pdf

This guideline from the Association of Anaesthetists of Great Britain and Ireland (AAGBI) aims to address the conduct of obtaining consent for anaesthesia and the amount of information which is necessary to ensure that a patient can give fully informed consent prior to an anaesthetic intervention.

Key points

- Patients for elective surgery should be given information about their anaesthetic prior to meeting the anaesthetist on the day of surgery. The anaesthetic room is not an appropriate place to provide such information.
- Information given to a patient should be tailor made to each patient's individual needs and preferences.
- Issues discussed should be clearly document by the anaesthetist. There is presently no requirement for formal signed consent before anaesthesia.
- If a patient lacks capacity, then anaesthetists should act in accordance with the Mental Capacity Act 2005 (http://www.legislation.gov.uk/ukpga/2005/9/contents).
- Every effort should be made to minimize harm and maximize benefit to the patient, especially if a trainee is to perform a practical procedure on the patient.

The Mental Capacity Act 2005

http://www.legislation.gov.uk/ukpga/2005/9/contents

- Capacity can be defined as the ability to understand and retain any information which is given, use the information to make an informed decision, and communicate any decision made following such consideration of information.
- A person may lack capacity on either a temporary or permanent basis.
- Any decision made or performed under this act must be in the best interests of the patient. When determining what may be in the patient's best interests, it may be necessary to take into consideration any prior wishes expressed, any legal documentation signed by the patient (e.g. Lasting Power of Attorney), or carry out a consultation with the patient's friends, family, or carers.
- All efforts must be made to help the patient communicate with the medical team.
- A patient must not be deemed to lack capacity simply because they make an unwise decision. Likewise, a patient must not be considered to lack capacity simply based on their age or appearance.

AAGBI Guideline: *Pre-Operative Assessment and Patient Preparation—The Role of the Anaesthetist*, January 2010

http://www.aagbi.org/sites/default/files/preop2010.pdf

This guideline describes the role of anaesthetists in preoperative services.

Key points

- Anaesthetists should lead the preoperative assessment service to ensure that the patients are pre-assessed and optimized appropriately for their operations.
- In addition, high-risk patients should be identified at this stage and counselled about their risks for the surgery. The level of care required at the postoperative phase must also be identified at this stage.
- Skilled nurse practitioners can provide a cost-effective pre-assessment service. They should communicate effectively with anaesthetists and the rest of the perioperative team in order to prepare the patients appropriately for their surgery.
- Children and their families must be provided with suitable preoperative information. They should be admitted to the designated children ward for the perioperative period.
- Preoperative tests should be requested according to national and local guidelines.
- Anaesthetic departments should arrange one consultant whole-time equivalent to run high-risk pre-assessment clinics on a daily basis.
- High standards of perioperative care should be maintained for the patients who are admitted for emergency surgery.
- All departments should have a lead consultant for the pre-assessment service.

AAGBI Guideline: *Recommendations for Standards of Monitoring During Anaesthesia and Recovery,* March 2007

http://www.aagbi.org/sites/default/files/standardsofmonitoring07.pdf

Key Points

- The patient must be monitored and cared for continuously by an appropriately trained anaesthetist throughout the conduct of anaesthesia.
- Standard monitoring equipment and the alarm limits must be checked by the anaesthetist before use.
- The anaesthetist must document the monitoring devices used and the information they provided on the anaesthetic record.
- The following monitoring devices are essential for the safe conduct of anaesthesia:
  - Minimum monitoring for neuraxial anaesthesia or sedation for an operative procedure: electrocardiogram (ECG), pulse oximetry, and non-invasive blood pressure monitoring.
  - Minimum monitoring for induction and maintenance of general anaesthesia: ECG, pulse oximetry, non-invasive blood pressure monitoring, airway gases (O_2, CO_2 and anaesthetic volatile agent), and airway pressures.
  - Devices that should be immediately available: a nerve stimulator if a muscle relaxant is used, a device to check the temperature, capnograph, and ECG.
  - Minimum monitoring for recovery from anaesthesia: pulse oximetry and non-invasive blood pressure monitoring.

Difficult Airway Society Guideline: *Unanticipated Difficult Intubation During Rapid Sequence Induction,* 2004

http://www.das.uk.com/files/rsi-Jul04-A4.pdf

The Difficult Airway Society (DAS) has produced algorithms for the management of the difficult airway during intubation and extubation. The algorithm for the management of unanticipated difficult intubation during rapid sequence induction can be found via the above-mentioned link.

DAS Guideline: *Rescue Techniques for 'Can't Intubate, Can't Ventilate' Situation,* 2004

http://www.das.uk.com/files/cvci-Jul04-A4.pdf

DAS has produced algorithms for the management of the difficult airway during intubation and extubation. Rescue techniques for 'can't intubate, can't ventilate' situation can be found via the above link.

National Institute for Health and Care Excellence. *Inadvertent Perioperative Hypothermia: The Management of Perioperative Hypothermia in Adults.* Clinical Guideline 65, April 2008

http://guidance.nice.org.uk/cg65

The National Institute for Health and Care Excellence (NICE) has issued this guideline to prevent and manage inadvertent hypothermia in surgical patients.

Perioperative care

Patients and their carers should be informed that:

- keeping warm during the perioperative period will reduce the risk of surgical complications such as bleeding.
- they should bring additional warm clothing.

When measuring patient temperature, healthcare professionals should:

- remember that they may need to make some adjustments in certain devices to estimate core temperature.

Preoperative phase

- Patients are regarded as high risk for developing perioperative hypothermia if they have any two of the following factors:
  - ASA grade higher than II.
  - Temperature before the surgery is lower than 36.0°C.
  - Require both general and neuraxial anaesthesia.
  - Having major surgery.
  - Risk factors to develop cardiovascular complications during the perioperative period.
- If the patient's temperature is below 36.0°C, they should be actively warmed preoperatively and intraoperatively.

Intraoperative phase

- The patient's temperature should be measured preoperatively and every 30 minutes intraoperatively.
- If the patient requires intravenous fluid (500 mL or more) or blood products, a fluid warming device must be used and set at 37°C.
- If the anaesthesia and surgery is longer than 30 minutes, the patient must be actively warmed during the procedure.

Postoperative phase

- Temperature monitoring must be continued in the recovery. It should be measured every 15 minutes.
- Patients should not be discharged from the recovery if their temperature is below 36.0°C.

AAGBI Guideline: *Infection Control in Anaesthesia,* October 2008

http://www.aagbi.org/sites/default/files/infection_control_08.pdf

Also published as Association of Anaesthetists of Great Britain and Ireland. Infection control in anaesthesia. *Anaesthesia* 2008; 63:1027–36.

Key points

- Every anaesthetic department should have a named consultant to liaise with the hospital infection control team.
- Standard precautions must be applied to prevent the transmission of infection between patients and staff or between patients.
- Effective hand washing must take place immediately before every episode of direct patient contact.
- Every anaesthetist must follow the hospital infection control policy. All sharps must be discarded into an approved sharps container.

- Single-use disposable equipment should be used wherever appropriate. All reusable anaesthetic equipment must be decontaminated as per national standards.
- Anaesthetic facemasks, oral and nasal airways, and endotracheal tubes should be single use. A new, effective bacterial/viral breathing circuit filter must be placed between the anaesthetic machine and the patient. Breathing circuits should be changed on a daily basis.
- Anaesthetists must use maximum barrier precautions for certain invasive procedures. These include insertion of central venous catheters, spinals, epidurals, and caudals. Chlorhexidine or iodine-based preparations can be used to clean the procedure site.

Glahn KP, Ellis FR, Halsall PJ, *et al.* Recognizing and managing a malignant hyperthermia crisis: guidelines from the European malignant hyperthermia group. *Br J Anaesth* 2010; 105:417–20

http://bja.oxfordjournals.org/content/105/4/417.full.pdf

The authors of this article have produced consensus guidelines for the recognition and the management of malignant hyperthermia (MH). This is of particular use in countries which do not have their own guideline. The AAGBI have produced their own MH flowchart (see http://www.aagbi.org/sites/default/files/mh_guideline_for_website.pdf).

Popat M, Mitchell V, Dravid R, *et al.* Difficult airway society guidelines for the management of tracheal extubation. *Anaesthesia* 2012; 67:318–40

http://www.das.uk.com/content/das-extubation-guidelines

DAS has produced algorithms for the management of the difficult airway during intubation and extubation. The algorithm for the management of tracheal extubation can be found via the above-mentioned link.

AAGBI Safety Guideline: *Immediate Post-Anaesthesia Recovery 2013*, March 2013

http://www.aagbi.org/sites/default/files/immediate_post-anaesthesia_recovery_2013.pdf

Also published as Association of Anaesthetists of Great Britain and Ireland. Immediate post-anaesthesia recovery 2013. *Anaesthesia* 2013; 68:288–97.

Key points

- After general or neuraxial anaesthesia, patients should be transferred to a designated recovery area, compliant with national standards.
- There must be a formal handover from the anaesthetist to an appropriately trained and registered practitioner.
- All departments must have agreed, written criteria that patients should fulfil before being discharged to the ward.
- All recovery areas must have an emergency call system, which is tested on a regular basis.
- If a patient, who does not fulfil the discharge criteria, is in the recovery area, there must be at least two staff present. One of them must be a trained, registered practitioner.
- All recovery practitioners should have appropriate training to the standard set by the UK National Core Competencies for Post-Anaesthesia Care.
- An anaesthetist or a registered recovery practitioner should give one-to-one care to the patient until he or she regains control of the airway, the cardiovascular and respiratory parameters are stable, and he/she is able to communicate.
- It is the anaesthetist's responsibility to remove an endotracheal tube. Capnography must be applied if an endotracheal tube is still *in situ*.
- Recovery areas for children must be appropriately equipped and staffed.
- All the above-mentioned standards should be applied to all post-anaesthetic care areas including those in obstetric units, endoscopy, radiology, cardiology, dental units, and psychiatric units. Only registered post-anaesthesia care unit practitioners should recover the patients in those areas.
- Patient safety should be a primary concern. Patient privacy and dignity should be respected.
- If a critically ill patient is managed in the recovery area due to intensive care bed shortage, the critical care team should take the primary responsibility of that patient's care.
- There must be regular audits and incident reporting systems in all recovery units.

Royal College of Anaesthetists: *Raising the Standard: A Compendium of Audit Recipes* (Section 8.8 Technique of Anaesthesia for Caesarean Section), 2012

http://www.rcoa.ac.uk/system/files/CSQ-ARB-section8.pdf

In this audit recipe book, the Royal College of Anaesthetists recommends the proposed standard for quality improvement audits that should be carried out in individual hospitals.

Proposed standards for the technique of anaesthesia for caesarean delivery

- Greater than 95% of elective caesarean deliveries should be performed under neuraxial anaesthesia.
- Greater than 85% of emergency caesarean deliveries should be performed under neuraxial anaesthesia.
- The conversion rate from neuraxial to general anaesthesia in elective caesarean deliveries should be less than 1%.
- The conversion rate from neuraxial to general anaesthesia in emergency caesarean deliveries should be less than 3%.

The American Society of Anesthesiologists task force on obstetric anesthesia. Practice guidelines for obstetric anesthesia. *Anesthesiology* 2007; 106:843–863

http://anesthesiology.pubs.asahq.org/article.aspx?articleid=1923100

Summary of recommendations

- *Peri-anaesthetic evaluation*
  - History—maternal health, anaesthetic and obstetric history.

- Examination—airway, cardiovascular, respiratory, and examination of the back.
- A system of communication must be in place to encourage early referral to the anaesthetist from other members of the multidisciplinary team.
- A routine intrapartum platelet count is not required in a healthy parturient.
- A group and screen or cross-match must be requested, based on the maternal history and risk factors for bleeding.
- Fetal heart rate should be monitored before and after neuraxial analgesia.

◆ *Aspiration prophylaxis*

- Uncomplicated labouring women are allowed to drink clear liquids. Solid foods should be avoided in labouring patients.
- For those undergoing an elective caesarean delivery, modest amount of clear liquids can be allowed up to 2 hours before the induction of anaesthesia, and solid food is allowed up to 6–8 hours before the induction.
- Non-particulate antacids and H_2 receptor antagonists for aspiration prophylaxis are recommended before surgical procedures.

◆ *Anaesthetic care for labour and delivery*

- Resources must be available to treat complications resulting from local anaesthetic and opioid drugs.
- Intravenous fluid should be started before the neuraxial analgesia or anaesthesia and continued throughout the duration of the neuraxial block.
- Early neuraxial analgesia should be considered in the following women if there is no contraindication:
- Women who are attempting vaginal birth after previous caesarean delivery.
- Women with twin pregnancies or pre-eclampsia.
- Women with anticipated airway problems or obese women.
- When continuous infusion of epidural analgesia (CIE) is used, the lowest concentration of local anaesthetic that provides adequate analgesia should be used. An opioid may be added to improve the analgesic quality, reduce local anaesthetic concentration, and minimize motor block.
- Single injection of spinal opioid with or without local anaesthetic or combined spinal epidural (CSE) can be used for labour analgesia.
- Patient-controlled epidural analgesia (PCEA) is preferable to CIE as it is effective and flexible and causes less motor blockade.

◆ *Manual removal of retained placenta (MRP)*

- There is no preferred anaesthetic technique for the MRP. The woman should be haemodynamically stable before receiving neuraxial anaesthesia.
- Nitroglycerine may be used to relax the uterus for the removal of retained placenta.

◆ *Anaesthetic choices for caesarean delivery*

- The delivery suite should have equipment and support personnel comparable to main operating theatres.
- Neuraxial anaesthesia is preferable to general anaesthesia for most caesarean deliveries. However, in situations such as persistent fetal bradycardia, suspected ruptured uterus, severe haemorrhage, and placental abruption, general anaesthesia may be the most suitable choice.
- Left lateral tilt position should be applied in all caesarean deliveries to achieve uterine displacement.
- Both phenylephrine and ephedrine can be used to treat hypotension related to neuraxial blockade.
- Neuraxial opioids are preferred over parenteral opioids.

◆ *Postpartum tubal ligation*

- Patients should follow routine fasting guidelines prior to surgery and aspiration prophylaxis should be considered.
- Neuraxial anaesthesia is preferred to general anaesthesia.

◆ *Management of obstetric and anaesthetic emergencies*

- All institutions offering obstetric care should have facilities to manage major haemorrhage. In emergencies, O-negative or type-specific blood can be used. When blood is not available or a patient refuses blood products, cell salvage should be considered.
- The anaesthetist should be familiar with the difficult intubation drill. If an intubation attempt fails, one should continue ventilating with a face mask and cricoid pressure or with a laryngeal mask airway. If ventilation is not possible, a surgical airway should be instituted.
- Delivery suites should also have basic and advanced life support facilities. Uterine displacement should be applied during cardiopulmonary resuscitation. If spontaneous circulation is not achieved within 4 minutes, perimortem caesarean delivery should be performed.

Working Party on Obstetric Anesthesia of the Belgian Association for Regional Anaesthesia (BARA). Belgian guidelines and recommendations for safe practice in obstetric anesthesia. *Acta Anaesthesiol Belg* 2003; 54:119–125

http://www.bara2001.be/guidelines/belgian-guidelines-and-recommendations-for-safe-practice-in-obstetric-anesthesia.aspx

Guideline 1: Pre-anaesthetic evaluation

- The entire parturient file should be available to the attending anaesthetist.
- If a parturient has significant medical problems (ASA III or above), her obstetrician should inform the anaesthetic team as soon as feasible.
- A repeat platelet count is not necessary in women with uncomplicated pregnancies if the platelet counts were normal in the third trimester.
- If a woman is booked for caesarean delivery or if she has any risk factor for bleeding, group and screen should be performed.

Guideline 2: Equipment

- An operating theatre should be available 24/7 for caesarean deliveries and obstetric emergencies.
- All labour and delivery rooms should have the following facilities: oxygen supply, suction, emergency call buzzer, adequate lighting, electric power points, electronic fetal heart rate monitoring, non-invasive blood pressure and maternal heart rate monitoring. and continuous pulse oximetry.
- An operating theatre should have all standard anaesthetic equipment including those required to deal with difficult intubation.
- A well-equipped resuscitation cart and uterine displacement equipment should be available on all delivery suites.

Guideline 3: Sterile technique

- Before the neuraxial block, the parturient's back should be cleaned with an antiseptic solution and allowed to dry for 2 minutes. All injectable solutions should be aspirated from the original ampoule in a sterile manner. The anaesthetist should wear a facemask, a cap, and sterile gloves.

Guideline 4: Anaesthetic staffing and availability

- An anaesthetist must ensure maternal observations and fetal heart rate are normal, and they must be available for at least 30 minutes after the initiation of neuraxial analgesia.
- The level of the blockade and quality of the analgesia should be documented on the observation chart at least every hour.
- An anaesthetist and other appropriate staff must be readily available for an urgent caesarean delivery.

Guideline 5: Midwifery tasks

- There should be a written hospital policy for the maintenance of neuraxial analgesia.
- Midwives are responsible for the continuous care and monitoring of the mother and the fetus during the period of epidural blockade.
- Midwives should be trained to assist anaesthetists with administering neuraxial and general anaesthesia in theatre, and to care for parturients in the immediate postoperative period.

Guideline 6: Monitoring of mother and fetus during neuraxial labour analgesia

- Before the start of the neuraxial block:
- Fetal heart rate, maternal blood pressure and pulse
- After the initiation of neuraxial block:
- Maternal blood pressure and heart rate pulse every 5 minutes for 30 minutes and until the parameters are stable• Fetal heart rate continuously for at least 30 minutes

Guideline 7: Monitoring during anaesthesia for caesarean delivery

- Anaesthetists should use standard monitoring for caesarean delivery as for any surgical procedure.
- Parturients must be positioned with 30° left lateral tilt.

Guideline 8: Ambulation

- Parturients are allowed to ambulate after neuraxial analgesia if there is no contraindication. However, a parturient's ability to mobilize need to be assessed by a midwife or an anaesthetist.
- The parturient must be accompanied by a responsible adult when she ambulates.

Guideline 9: Fluid intake, nil per oral-policy and aspiration prophylaxis

- Uncomplicated parturients are allowed to drink clear fluid in labour.
- Women on the elective caesarean delivery list are allowed to eat solid food up to 6 hours before the operation and clear liquid up to 2 hours before the procedure.
- All caesarean delivery patients must have aspiration prophylaxis.

Guideline 10: Caesarean delivery

- Neuraxial anaesthesia is the recommended technique for elective caesarean delivery.
- General anaesthesia should not be started until the surgeon is scrubbed and ready to perform the procedure.
- Prophylactic antibiotics should be given as per hospital policy.
- Anaesthetic trained staff must be available throughout the procedure.

Guideline 11: Maternal and neonatal resuscitation

- The anaesthetist should direct maternal resuscitation in a shared effort with the obstetricians.
- The anaesthetist may assist in neonatal resuscitation after having considered the benefit for the newborn against the risk to the mother under his or her care.

Guideline 12: High-risk pregnancies

- Any high-risk parturient must be referred to the anaesthetist as soon as possible. An anaesthetic plan should be documented in advance of the delivery.
- Invasive monitoring facilities should be available in the delivery suites.

ACOG Practice Bulletin 36: *Obstetric Analgesia and Anaesthesia*, July 2002

http://www.acog.org/~/media/List of Titles/PBListOfTitles.pdf?dmc=1&ts=20140222T1342330971 (ACOG practice bulletins may be viewed by ACOG members or with a valid ATHENS password)

This guideline is produced to give obstetricians a better understanding of available methods of analgesia and anaesthesia.

Available methods of anaesthesia and analgesia

Parenteral

- Opioid drugs can be given as intermittent doses or as patient-controlled analgesia.
- When compared with neuraxial analgesia, parenteral agents result in higher pain scores on a visual analogue scale.

- Patients should be aware of the risks of aspiration and maternal and fetal respiratory depression.
- All parenteral drugs have significant transplacental passage.
- Norpethidine, an active metabolite of pethidine has a long neonatal half-life, and can cause prolonged neonatal sedation.

Epidural

- Indications for epidural analgesia include maternal request and medical indications.
- Medical indications are anticipated airway difficulty, malignant hyperthermia, selected forms of respiratory and cardiovascular disease, and prevention of autonomic hyperreflexia in patients with high spinal cord lesion.
- Epidural preparations usually consist of low-dose local anaesthetic with an opioid drug to decrease the risk of motor blockade and increase the chance of spontaneous vaginal delivery.
- Prospective cohort studies (see Practice Bulletin for details) have found no significant association between epidural analgesia and chronic back pain.
- The mechanism of epidural-related fever is unclear. Intrapartum fever results in a significant risk of maternal and neonatal antibiotic treatment.
- Epidural analgesia can prolong the labour by 40–90 minutes. It can also increase the need for oxytocin to augment labour.
- There is also a higher risk of prolongation of the second stage of labour. The rate of operative vaginal delivery is increased in women who use epidural analgesia.
- Most anaesthetists will perform an epidural block if platelet counts are higher than 100,000/μL.
- If patients are on a once-daily regimen of low-molecular-weight heparin (LMWH), neuraxial analgesia or anaesthesia should not be offered within 12 hours of the last dose.
- If patients are on twice-daily LMWH, a neuraxial procedure should not be performed within 24 hours of the last dose.
- Routine platelet count is, however, not necessary in uncomplicated women in labour.
- Neuraxial analgesia and anaesthesia are preferred in patients with pre-eclampsia if there is no contraindication.
- Breastfeeding success is not affected by intrapartum epidural analgesia.

Spinal

- Single-shot spinals can be used for pain relief in the second stage of labour and for procedures such as caesarean delivery and tubal ligation.

Combined spinal–epidural

- This method provides rapid-onset analgesia and ability to insert an epidural catheter to continue the analgesia. It can also be used for caesarean delivery and post-caesarean pain relief.

General anaesthesia

- Induction to delivery time should be reduced when using general anaesthesia.
- All inhaled anaesthetic agents can cause neonatal depression, uterine relaxation, and increase the risk of haemorrhage.

Local anaesthesia

- Various local anaesthetics are used for infiltration for perineal and vaginal repairs.
- Obstetricians also use local anaesthetics in pudendal nerve blocks for operative vaginal deliveries.

Maternal mortality

- Failed intubation rate in the obstetric population is tenfold higher than that of the non-obstetric population.
- In patients with a higher risk of requiring caesarean delivery, neuraxial analgesia should be recommended early during labour.

Postoperative analgesia

- Opioids are administered with local anaesthetic intrathecally or epidurally at the time of caesarean delivery. They can provide analgesia for 12–24 hours after delivery.
- Non-steroidal anti-inflammatory drugs (NSAIDs) should also be given if there is no contraindication.

Obstetric Anaesthetists' Association Clinical Guideline: *Inadequate Regional Block*, 2011

http://www.oaa-anaes.ac.uk/ui/content/content.aspx?id=173

- Inadequate neuraxial block has clinical and medicolegal consequences.
- The Obstetric Anaesthetists' Association (OAA) clinical guideline page has example guidelines on inadequate neuraxial block from three UK National Health Service (NHS) hospitals.
- In order to prevent inadequate block in the operating theatre, it is advised that the duty anaesthetist ensures labour epidurals are working effectively at the beginning of the shift and replaces any ineffective epidurals early.
- Upper block levels vary among different guidelines, ranging from 'T4 cold' to 'T4 cold and T5 touch'.
- The anaesthetist must ask the obstetrician to stop the surgery once the patient complains of pain.
- Choice of pain-relieving strategies depends on the stage of the operation. Options include Entonox®, intravenous opioids such as alfentanil, other analgesics such as ketamine, local infiltration by the obstetrician, and general anaesthesia.
- All guidelines emphasize the importance of accurate documentation.
- It is good practice to visit the mother after surgery to explain the events that occurred in theatre.

Royal College of Anaesthetists. *Report and Findings of the Third National Audit Project (Chapter 16: Complications after Obstetric CNB)*, January 2009

http://www.rcoa.ac.uk/nap3

Summarized under 'Neurology'.

Fourth National Audit Project. Major Complications of Airway Management in the UK: Results of the Fourth National Audit Project of the Royal College of Anaesthetists and the Difficult Airway Society. London: Royal College of Anaesthetists, 2011

http://www.rcoa.ac.uk/nap4

Learning points and recommendations for obstetric cases are summarized.

Learning points

1. Physiological changes in pregnancy, active labour, and isolated location increase the complexity of management of airway complications when they occur.
2. All theatre personnel (obstetricians, midwives, and operating department practitioners) should be aware of the considerable difficulty in managing airway complications in obstetric patients.
3. Three out of four parturients were obese and had complex obstetric, medical, and anaesthetic issues.
4. While preparing failed intubation strategies, it should be recognized that it is not always possible to wake the patient up.
5. Decisions regarding management of complex patients require multidisciplinary collaboration when forming initial and backup plans.

Recommendations

1. Obstetric anaesthetists should maintain airway skills which include the management of difficult and failed tracheal intubation and 'can't intubate, can't ventilate' scenario.
2. Obstetric anaesthetists should be competent in the use of second-generation supraglottic airway devices, which give better protection against aspiration and facilitate ventilation and/or intubation.
3. Anaesthetic departments should ensure airway skills and equipment are available whenever awake fibreoptic intubation is indicated.
4. Recovery staff including midwives should be trained and be competent to recover patients following an anaesthetic.

AAGBI Safety Guideline: *Management of Severe Local Anaesthetic Toxicity*, December 2010

http://www.aagbi.org/sites/default/files/la_toxicity_2010_0.pdf

Summarized under 'Critical Care and Resuscitation'.

Analgesia

Committee of Origin: Obstetrical Anaesthesia (Approved by the ASA House of Delegates). *Statement on Pain Relief During Labour*, last amended in October 2010

http://www.asahq.org/~/media/legacy/for%20members/documents/standards%20guidelines%20stmts/statement%20pain%20relief%20labor.pdf

This is a joint statement from the American Society of Anesthesiologists (ASA) and the American College of Obstetricians and Gynecologists (ACOG).

Summary of the statement

- Labour causes severe pain for many women. Maternal request should be a sufficient indication for the provision of pain relief in labour provided there is no contraindication. Pain relief should also be offered when clinically indicated.
- Neuraxial analgesia is the most effective method of analgesia and it is also the least depressing to the central nervous system.
- The American Society of Anesthesiologists (ASA) and the American College of Obstetricians and Gynecologists (ACOG) believe that women should not be deprived of labour analgesia and anaesthesia services due to the lack of health insurance or inadequate nursing participation.
- Labour nursing personnel should be able to manage epidural infusions, adjust dosage and discontinue infusions under the supervision of a physician.

NICE. *Intrapartum Care: Care of Healthy Women and their Babies During Childbirth* (Section 8: Coping with Pain in Labour: Non-Epidural). Clinical Guideline 190, December 2014

http://www.nice.org.uk/guidance/cg190/evidence/cg190-intrapartum-care-full-guideline3

Pain-relieving strategies

- Women who wish to use breathing and relaxation techniques and massage therapy in labour should be supported.
- Use of birthing pool is recommended for pain relief. Maternal and water temperatures need to be monitored hourly. The water temperature should not rise above 37.5°C. The bath or birthing pool should be cleaned as outlined in a protocol agreed with the microbiology department.
- Acupuncture, acupressure, and hypnosis should not be provided but if women wish to use them, they should not be prevented from doing so.

Non-pharmacological analgesia

- Transcutaneous electrical nerve stimulation (TENS) is not an effective analgesic technique in established labour.

Inhalational analgesia

- Entonox® should be accessible in all birthing areas. However, women should be informed about the side effects of Entonox®, which include nausea and dizziness.

Intravenous and intramuscular opioids

- All birthing units should have commonly used opioids such as diamorphine and pethidine as options for pain relief. However, women should be made aware about possible side effects associated with these drugs and that these side effects may affect both her and her unborn child. (See section 8.6.4.1.4 on page 347 of NICE guidance for a full list of side effects.)
- Women should be made aware that if they have received an opioid analgesic, they should avoid using a birthing pool within 2 hours of administration or if they feel drowsy.

American Society of Anesthesiologists task force on neuraxial opioids. practice guidelines for the prevention, detection, and management of respiratory depression associated with neuraxial opioid administration. *Anesthesiology* 2009; 110(2):218–30

http://www.guideline.gov/content.aspx?id=15133 [currently being updated] http://www.asahq.org/~/media/Sites/ASAHQ/Files/Public/Resources/standards-guidelines/practice-guidelines-for-the-prevention-detection-and-management-of-respiratory-depression.pdf

This guideline was produced to prevent and manage respiratory depression after the administration of neuraxial opioids.

Identification of patients at increased risk of respiratory depression

- Anaesthetists should carry out a focused history and examination before giving neuraxial opioids. Anaesthetists should enquire about symptoms of sleep apnoea and current medication history, including preoperative opioid use.

Prevention of respiratory depression after neuraxial opioids

- Patients with sleep apnoea, on non-invasive positive airway pressure ventilation treatment, should bring their own equipment to the hospital.
- Epidural opioids have a lower risk of respiratory depression compared to parenteral opioids.
- Neuraxial morphine should not be given to outpatient surgical patients.
- The lowest effective dose of neuraxial opioids should be given, in order to reduce the risk of respiratory depression.
- In patients who have had neuraxial opioids, parenteral opioids should be used cautiously, if necessary.

Detection of respiratory depression

- All patients receiving neuraxial opioids should be monitored for the adequacy of ventilation, oxygenation, and sedation (Table A1.1).

Table A1.1 Monitoring required for neuraxial opioids

Type of neuraxial opioid administration	Monitoring
Single-injection neuraxial lipophilic opioids (e.g. fentanyl)	Monitoring for a minimum of 2 h Continuous monitoring for first 20 min, then once per hour until 2 h have passed After 2 h, monitoring should depend on the clinical condition
Continuous infusion or patient-controlled epidural analgesia (PCEA) with neuraxial lipophilic opioids	Monitoring during the entire time of infusion Continuous monitoring for the first 20 min, then once per hour until 12 h has passed From 12 to 24 h, monitor once every 2 h After 24 h, monitor at least once every 4 h
Continuous infusion or PCEA with neuraxial hydrophilic opioids (e.g. morphine)	Monitoring during the entire time of infusion Monitoring once per hour for the first 12 h after initiation From 12 to 24 h, monitor once every 2 h After 24 h, monitor at least once every 4 h

Management and treatment

- Oxygen should be given if patients have reduced consciousness, respiratory depression, or hypoxaemia.
- Reversal agents should be available.
- If severe airway obstruction or hypoxia occurs, non-invasive positive-pressure ventilation should be commenced.

OAA clinical guideline: *Remifentanil*

http://www.oaa-anaes.ac.uk/ui/content/content.aspx?id=191

Remifentanil PCA guidelines from five NHS trusts were described on the OAA website.

- Some hospitals offer remifentanil PCA as one of the routine analgesic options while others offer it if women have any contraindications to neuraxial analgesia.
- Remifentanil PCA should be set up by an anaesthetist.
- Typical remifentanil PCA protocols consist of doses ranging from 20 mcg to 40 mcg delivered stat with a lockout of 2 minutes. Background infusions should not be used. A dedicated cannula must be used for the PCA.
- A midwife must be present in the room to provide constant one-to-one care.
- Continuous pulse oximetry should be applied. Observations including heart rate, blood pressure, respiratory rate, sedation, and pain scores should be monitored and documented every 30 minutes.
- The midwife should start oxygen supplementation if the oxygen saturation is less than 93% or the woman becomes drowsy. Criteria that warrant an anaesthetist's presence include oxygen saturation of less than 90% despite oxygen therapy, sedation score more than 2, and respiratory rate of less than 8 breaths per minute.
- *Sedation score:*
  1: Fully awake
  2: Drowsy
  3: Eyes closed but rousable by voice
  4: Eyes closed but rousable by physical stimulus
  5: Eyes closed and not rousable.
- Contraindications to remifentanil PCA include opioid allergy, opioid analgesia administration in the last 4 hours, premature labour, and ASA III and above.
- Remifentanil PCA use should be regularly audited.

Royal College of Anaesthetists: *Raising the Standard: A Compendium of Audit Recipes* (Section 8.9: Pain Relief after Caesarean Section), 2012

http://www.rcoa.ac.uk/system/files/CSQ-ARB-section8.pdf

- It is vital to provide adequate pain relief after caesarean delivery (CD) so that the mother can start mobilizing and look after the baby.
- Patients after surgery should have a pain score of 3 cm or less on a visual analogue scale (VAS) of 0–10 cm.

- Proposed standards by the Royal College of Anaesthesia are:
  - Nine out of ten women should have a pain score of 3 or less when assessed with a 10 cm VAS.
  - Regular NSAIDs should be given to all postoperative women if there is no contraindication.
  - Opioids should be given epidurally or intrathecally in all women who undergo CD under neuraxial anaesthesia.
  - The following observations should be performed every hour after an administration of opioids.
    - Respiratory rate
    - Sedation score
    - Pain score.
  - There should be adequate perioperative pain relief in over 90% of women undergoing CD.

MotherToBaby: a service of the organization of teratology information specialists

http://www.otispregnancy.org/

- The Organization of Teratology Information Specialists provides evidence-based information about drug and substance exposures in pregnancy.
- Teratology information of the drugs related to the anaesthetic practice is described as follows:
  - *Acetaminophen (paracetamol).* It is safe to take during pregnancy and during breastfeeding. There is no evidence to cause miscarriage or birth defects.
  - *Ibuprofen and other NSAIDs.* There is some evidence that NSAIDs may have a negative effect on the implantation of the early fetus. If NSAIDs are taken in the first and second trimesters, there is a possible association with certain birth defects, such as gastroschisis. During the third trimester, NSAIDs can cause premature closure of ductus arteriosus. NSAIDs are safe to use in breastfeeding mothers. NB Use of aspirin in pregnancy is not discussed in their factsheet.
  - *Opioids.* There is no strong evidence of causing miscarriage or birth defects. If a mother has been on prescription opioids, signs of withdrawal should be monitored in the baby. When opioids are used for a short period in recommended doses during breastfeeding, they are unlikely to cause harm to the baby.
  - *Benzodiazepines.* They do not significantly increase the risk of birth defects. There is some evidence that benzodiazepines can increase the risk of preterm birth and low birth weight in infants when the mother takes them during pregnancy. Signs of withdrawals should also be monitored in the neonates. During breastfeeding, long acting benzodiazepines should be avoided.

Crews KR, Gaedigk A, Dunnenberger HN, *et al.* Clinical Pharmacogenetics Implementation Consortium (CPIC) guidelines for codeine therapy in the context of cytochrome P450 2D6 (CYP2D6) genotype. *Clin Pharmacol Ther* 2012; 91:321–6

http://onlinelibrary.wiley.com/doi/10.1038/clpt.2011.287/epdf

This evidence-based guideline aims to look at the effect that individuals with different variations of the cytochrome P450 2D6 genotype have on codeine metabolism. It makes recommendations regarding the use of codeine in these individuals.

Key points

- *Ultrametabolizer phenotype*: 1–2% of the population. These individuals are more likely to produce morphine after codeine administration, so increasing their risk of toxicity. It is advisable that codeine and perhaps tramadol should be avoided in these individuals.
- *Extensive metabolizer phenotype*: 77–92% of the population. These individuals have normal codeine metabolism and can safely be given codeine according to the manufacturer's recommendations (15–60 mg every 4 hours).
- *Intermediate metabolizer phenotype*: 2–11% of the population. These individuals have reduced morphine formation after codeine. In such patients, the analgesic effect should be monitored after administration of 15–60 mg of codeine every 4 hours. If there is no benefit, then consider changing to morphine or another analgesic. Tramadol metabolism may be similarly affected.
- *Poor metabolizer phenotype*: 5–10% of the population. These individuals have severely reduced morphine formation after codeine and thus derive no analgesic benefit from codeine. Tramadol should also be avoided in these individuals.

Rigg JR, Jamrozik K, Myles PS, *et al.*; MASTER anaesthesia trial study group. epidural anaesthesia and analgesia and outcome of major surgery: a randomised trial. *Lancet* 2002; 359(9314):1276–82

http://www.thelancet.com/journals/lancet/article/PIIS0140-6736(02)08266-1/fulltext

- In this multicentre trial, 915 high-risk patients undergoing major abdominal surgery were randomized to epidural and control (alternative analgesic regimen) groups.
- Most adverse outcomes were not reduced by the use of general anaesthesia combined with an epidural or by postoperative epidural analgesia.
- However, lower pain scores and a reduction in respiratory failure were seen in the epidural group.

Cardiovascular

NICE. *Hypertension in Pregnancy: The Management of Hypertensive Disorders During Pregnancy.* Clinical Guideline 107, August 2010

http://www.nice.org.uk/guidance/cg107

Primary or secondary hypertension may present in women of childbearing age. Hypertensive disease in pregnancy is associated with significant maternal morbidity, as it increases the lifetime cardiovascular risk. Hypertensive disorders in pregnancy may also have a significant impact on neonatal outcomes: 5% of all stillbirths result from pre-eclampsia, whereas hypertension in pregnancy accounts for 8–10% of all preterm births. This guideline covers the diagnosis and management of hypertension during conception, pregnancy, labour, and the postpartum period.

Key points

- Women at high risk of pre-eclampsia should be advised to take aspirin 75 mg from 12 weeks' gestation until delivery.
- Proteinuria in pregnancy should be monitored using an automated reading-strip or a spot urea:creatinine ratio, especially if in secondary care setting.
- Women who are taking angiotensin-converting enzyme inhibitors (ACEIs) or angiotensin receptor blockers (ARBs) should be advised of the risk of teratogenicity with these drugs and efforts should be made to substitute them with safer alternatives.
- Women with uncomplicated chronic hypertension should aim to keep their blood pressure below 150/100 mmHg.
- Patients with gestational hypertension and pre-eclampsia should be offered an integrated care package, which covers monitoring and management in the community, admission to hospital for inpatient treatment, and plans for labour and delivery.
- Following consultation with an obstetric consultant, biochemical and clinical parameters to expedite delivery before 34 weeks' gestation should be documented in the notes of all women with pre-eclampsia.
- All women with pre-eclampsia should be offered a follow-up appointment 6–8 weeks postpartum.
- Women need to be warned of the risks of recurrence of gestational hypertension (13–53%) and pre-eclampsia (16–55%) in future pregnancies.

Action on Pre-eclampsia. *PRECOG: The Pre-Eclampsia Community Guideline*, 2004

http://action-on-pre-eclampsia.org.uk/wp-content/uploads/2012/07/PRECOG-Community-Guideline.pdf

This guideline has been written to assist healthcare providers in the community with the surveillance, diagnosis, and management of pregnant women, who may be at risk of or have been diagnosed with hypertensive disease of pregnancy and possible pre-eclampsia. The guideline was developed in collaboration with the Royal College of Midwives, the Royal College of General Practitioners, and the National Childbirth Trust.

Key points

- Pre-eclampsia is a major cause of maternal and fetal morbidity and mortality.
- According to the Magpie collaborative group, pre-eclampsia is associated with stillbirth, fetal growth restriction, and preterm birth.
- Most deaths associated with pre-eclampsia are secondary to substandard care, a failure to identify and act on risk factors at booking, and a failure to recognize and treat the signs and symptoms of pre-eclampsia after 20 weeks' gestation.
- *Recommendation 1*: Identifiable risk factors for pre-eclampsia at booking include primiparity, maternal age greater than 40, multiple pregnancy, maternal obesity, previous history of pre-eclampsia, family history of pre-eclampsia, or proteinuria at booking.
- *Recommendation 2*: Early referral to a centre which manages pre-eclampsia should be made for women with a multiple pregnancy, pre-existing medical conditions which predispose to pre-eclampsia, a history of pre-eclampsia, or two of the risk factors mentioned in recommendation 1.
- *Recommendation 3*: women with a higher risk of developing pre-eclampsia should be reviewed more frequently (e.g. every 3 weeks) than those with a low risk. Women should be made aware that pre-eclampsia can develop at any time after 20 weeks and that they can self-refer.
- *Recommendation 4*: At every assessment, the following five factors should be looked for: new hypertension (diastolic blood pressure (BP) > 90 mmHg), new or significant proteinuria, maternal headache or visual disturbance, epigastric pain or vomiting, and reduced fetal movements or small growth.
- *Recommendation 5*: the subsequent management of proteinuria detected on screening will depend on the presence of hypertension and other symptoms. Women with new proteinuria after 20 weeks with a diastolic BP greater than 90 mmHg or a systolic BP greater than 170 mmHg associated with visual disturbances or headaches require immediate admission for further assessment.
- *Recommendation 6*: an appropriate sized BP cuff needs to be used, with the patient in a semi-recumbent position with the arm at the level of the heart. Korotkoff sound V should be used to determine the diastolic BP and palpation to estimate the systolic BP.
- *Recommendation 7*: all staff measuring proteinuria need to be suitably trained to use and interpret a dipstick result. Using an automated dipstick reader may reduce error. Twenty-four-hour urine collection should be used to quantify the amount of excreted urine.
- *Recommendation 8*: fetal growth needs to be assessed in the community but there is no evidence to suggest which method of assessment is superior.

The task force on the management of cardiovascular diseases during pregnancy of the European Society of Cardiology (ESC). ESC guidelines on the management of cardiovascular diseases during pregnancy. *Eur Heart J* 2011; 32:3147–97.

http://www.escardio.org/static_file/Escardio/Guidelines/publications/PREGN Guidelines-Pregnancy-FT.pdf

This guidance was developed by the European Society of Cardiology and is endorsed by the European Society of Gynaecology, the Association for European Paediatric Cardiology, and the German Society for Gender Medicine.

Key points

- *Surveillance*: offer pre-pregnancy counselling in all women with known or suspected cardiovascular system disease. Echocardiography, exercise testing, and magnetic resonance imaging (MRI) without contrast may be used to assess cardiac function in pregnant women. Echocardiography to assess for fetal cardiac abnormalities should be undertaken from week 13 of gestation. Where possible, radiation, catheter techniques and surgical interventions should be avoided.

- *Congenital heart disease*: care should be individualized and the risks of pregnancy depend on the underlying disease itself. A vaginal delivery remains possible. Pregnancy should be avoided in patients with pulmonary hypertension and Eisenmenger syndrome due to the high risk of maternal mortality. Maternal cyanosis (SpO_2 < 85%) is associated with a low probability of fetal survival (<12%). Fontan circulation remains a moderate to high risk to pregnancy.
- *Aortic disease*: when aortic dissection occurs in high-risk individuals, it is more likely to occur in the last trimester (50%) or early postpartum (33%). Pregnancy should be discouraged in patients with Marfan syndrome, who have an aortic root diameter of greater than 45 mm. About 50% of patients with a bicuspid aortic valve and aortic stenosis have dilatation of the ascending aorta and remain at risk of dissection. A caesarean delivery should be considered when the aortic root diameter is greater than 45 mm.
- *Valvular heart disease*: moderate to severe mitral stenosis will need treatment prior to conception. Treatment for aortic stenosis before pregnancy is dependent on symptoms and cardiac function. Regurgitant lesions are better tolerated in pregnancy than stenotic lesions. Patients with metallic heart valves will need their oral anticoagulation modified to reduce fetal teratogenicity and to minimize the risk of bleeding.
- *Coronary artery disease*: primary percutaneous coronary intervention (PCI) with a bare metal stent is the treatment of choice in pregnant women, presenting with an acute coronary syndrome (ACS) or ST elevation myocardial infarction (STEMI). Women with coronary artery disease may consider pregnancy if there is no ongoing ischaemia and left ventricular ejection fraction (LVEF) greater than 40%.
- *Cardiomyopathies*: peripartum cardiomyopathy may develop in the last trimester or immediately postpartum. If the ejection fraction has not normalized after delivery, then a subsequent pregnancy should be discouraged due to a recurrence risk of 30–50% and the chance that left ventricular (LV) function may deteriorate by up to 50% during pregnancy. Patients with dilated cardiomyopathy have a high risk of deterioration, whilst those with hypertrophic cardiomyopathy tolerate pregnancy well.
- *Arrhythmias*: these may occur in pregnant women, though the incidence of life-threatening arrhythmias is rare. Direct cardioversion should be considered in unstable patients and pacemaker insertion is recommended in the presence of complete heart block.
- *Hypertension*: drug treatment in severe gestational hypertension is beneficial. Alpha-methyldopa is the agent of choice during pregnancy. Labetalol has comparable efficacy to alpha-methyldopa and may be used in severe hypertension. Calcium channel blockers are second choice agents.
- *Venous thromboembolism*: all pregnant women should undergo a risk assessment in pregnancy. High-risk patients should receive antenatal prophylaxis with LMWH, which should continue for 6 weeks postpartum.
- *Drug therapy during pregnancy*: no specific recommendations. In the case of an emergency, drugs which are not recommended in pregnancy and breastfeeding should not be withheld from the mother.

Table A1.2 Definition of different grades of hypertension

Grade of hypertension	Measured clinic readings	Average ambulatory or home BP readings
Stage 1	140/90 mmHg or higher	135/85 mmHg or higher
Stage 2	160/100 mmHg or higher	150/95 mmHg or higher
Severe	Systolic BP reading 180 mmHg or higher *or* diastolic BP reading 110 mmHg or higher	

NICE. *Hypertension: Clinical Management of Primary Hypertension in Adults*. Clinical Guideline 127, August 2011

http://www.nice.org.uk/guidance/cg127

This link to the updated quick reference guide replaces NICE Clinical Guideline 34 from 2006.

Key points

- Definitions (see Table A1.2):
- Patients with stage 1 hypertension should be considered for referral to specialist services for further investigation if:
    - Less than 40 years of age
    - No evidence of end-organ damage
    - No cardiovascular disease
    - No renal disease
    - No diabetes.
- Antihypertensive agents should be started in patients with stage 2 hypertension or above.
- The choice of antihypertensive agent will depend on age, race, and response to treatment.
- Lifestyle changes such as exercise and alcohol consumption should be addressed in the management of hypertension.

Chronic maternal infections

Royal College of Obstetricians and Gynaecologists. *The Prevention of Malaria in Pregnancy*. Green-Top Guideline No. 54A, April 2010

https://www.rcog.org.uk/globalassets/documents/guidelines/gtg54apreventionmalariapregnancy0410.pdf

This guideline is designed to provide evidence-based medicine for the treatment of women living in the United Kingdom who may travel to malarial regions whilst pregnant.

Key points

- Malaria infection in pregnancy may be harmful to both the mother and the fetus. Where there is low immunity to malaria (e.g. in the UK), infection is associated with maternal mortality, miscarriage, stillbirth, and premature labour. In regions where malaria is endemic, the infection may lead to babies with low birth weights and the concomitant health problems associated with it.

- It is advisable that where possible, a trip to a region where malaria is endemic should be postponed or avoided for a woman who is planning to become pregnant or who is pregnant. If travel is unavoidable, the woman should be encouraged to seek advice from a centre experienced in treating malaria regarding risks and avoidance strategies.
- Pregnant women returning from an malaria-endemic region should be advised that a fever or flu-like illness after travelling or up to a year after return may be suggestive of malaria infection.
- Malaria prevention may be divided into for components using the 'ABCD' formula:
    - **A**wareness of risk—women should be made aware of the signs and symptoms of malaria and be warned that even despite prophylaxis, they may still develop malaria.
    - **B**ite prevention—the use of 20% DEET repellent in pregnant women has not been associated with any adverse effects, even though DEET may be found in the cord blood of 8% of fetuses. Given that the consequences to the fetus may be devastating in malaria, 50% DEET should be used. Pyrethroid sprays quickly kill mosquitoes whereas permethrin sprays repel and kill mosquitoes and both may be used when pregnant. Bed nets impregnated with long-lasting pyrethroids have been recommended for use by the WHO (Level 1++ evidence). After sunset, long-sleeved clothing and long trousers should be worn. Presently, there is not enough evidence to recommend the use of any herbal remedies in the prevention of mosquito bites.
    - **C**hemoprophylaxis—there is no one drug which offers 100% protection against malaria. It is advisable to avoid travel to a malaria-endemic region whilst pregnant and not to become pregnant whilst taking chemoprophylaxis. However, chemoprophylaxis appears to be associated with a low risk of teratogenicity. In the second and third trimesters and whilst breastfeeding, mefloquine 5 mg/kg once a week is the recommended chemoprophylaxis. It may also be used in the first trimester, but specialist opinion should be sought before starting it. All other available drugs for chemoprophylaxis are not recommended for use during pregnancy.
    - **D**iagnosis and treatment—malaria should be suspected if a woman complains of a flu like illness or has a temperature of 38°C or above. Suspected malaria is a medical emergency and should be treated as soon as possible is with quinine 600 mg three times a day for 7 days and clindamycin 450 mg three times a day for 5–7 days. Once this course has been completed, mefloquine should be started 1 week after the last treatment dose of clindamycin and quinine.

Royal College of Obstetricians and Gynaecologists. *The Diagnosis and Treatment of Malaria in Pregnancy.* Green-Top Guideline No. 54B, April 2010

https://www.rcog.org.uk/globalassets/documents/guidelines/gtg-54bdiagnosistreatmentmalariapregnancy0810.pdf

This guideline offers advice regarding the drug treatment of malaria in pregnant women.

Key points

- Diagnosis of malaria may be difficult due to the lack of specific signs and symptoms. A travel history to a malaria-endemic region should be sought in all women presenting with a pyrexia of unknown origin.
- A blood film should be performed in all suspected cases to confirm the diagnosis. Rapid diagnostic tests which detect malarial antigen or enzyme in the blood may be used but are less specific than a blood film.
- A delay in diagnosis or treatment are common reasons for deaths in Europe and the United States due to malaria.
- If a patient who is febrile has had three negative malarial blood films more than 12–24 hours apart may have malaria excluded as a possible diagnosis.
- Women with uncomplicated malaria should be admitted to hospital whereas those with severe and complicated malaria should be admitted to the intensive care unit.
- The drug treatment for the different types of malaria are summarized in Table A1.3, which is from the guideline:
- Complications of malaria in pregnancy include the following:
    - Hypoglycaemia less than 2.2 mmol/L: may be profound and persistent and be a result of treatment with quinine.
    - Pulmonary oedema or acute respiratory distress syndrome (ARDS): regularly monitor jugular venous pressure or central venous pressure, and aim to keep right atrial pressure below 10 cmH_2O.
    - Severe anaemia less than 8 g/100 mL: slowly transfuse 1 unit of packed red cells with frusemide or consider exchange transfusion.
    - Secondary bacterial infection: this should be suspected especially if the patient becomes hypotensive.
- Cases of severe malaria should be managed by a multidisciplinary team which includes an obstetrician, anaesthetist, and intensive care physician to ensure the best care is provided to both the mother and the baby.
- Uncomplicated malaria is not an indication for induction of labour.
- The woman should be made aware of the possibility of vertical transmission to the baby and blood films should be performed on the placenta, cord, and baby's blood as well as sending the placenta off for histological examination.
- The risks of thromboprophylaxis should be considered in such cases and should be withheld if the platelet count is falling or below 100, which is suggestive of thrombocytopaenia.
- Babies born to mothers with a confirmed diagnosis of malaria in pregnancy should be screened with standard blood films at birth and every week for 28 days.

Guidelines for the Management of Syphilis. In James D, Steer P, Weiner C, et al. (eds) *High Risk Pregnancy: Management Options* (2nd ed). Philadelphia, PA: WB Saunders; 2003

Guidelines for treatment of syphilis are shown in Table A1.4.

Table A1.3 UK treatment guidelines for malaria in pregnancy

Severity	Indication	Drug and dosage
Severe or complicated malaria	Any species	Artesunate IV 2.4 mg/kg at 0, 12, and 24 hours, then daily thereafter. When the patient is well enough to take oral medication she can be switched to oral artesunate 2 mg/kg (or IM artesunate 2.4 mg/kg) once daily, plus clindamycin. If oral artesunate is not available, use a 3-day course of Riamet® or Malarone® or a 7-day course of quinine and clindamycin at 450 mg 3 times a day for 7 days
		Alternative: Quinine IV 20 mg/kg loading dose (no loading dose if patient already taking quinine or mefloquine) in 5% dextrose over 4 hours and then 10 mg/kg IV over 4 hours every 8 hours plus clindamycin IV 450 mg every 8 hours (maximum dose quinine 1.4 g). When the patient is well enough to take oral medication she can be switched to oral quinine 600 mg 3 times a day to complete 5–7 days and oral clindamycin 450 mg 3 times a day for 7 days (an alternative rapid quinine-loading regimen is 7 mg/kg quinine dihydrochloride IV over 30 minutes using an infusion pump followed by 10 mg/kg over 4 hours) **Note**: quinine dosing should be reduced to 12-hourly dosing if IV therapy extends more than 48 hours or if the patient has renal or hepatic dysfunction. Quinine is associated with severe and recurrent hypoglycaemia in late pregnancy
Uncomplicated malaria	*Plasmodium falciparum*	Oral quinine 600 mg 8-hourly and oral clindamycin 450 mg 8-hourly for 7 days **or** Riamet® 4 tablets/dose for weight > 35 kg, twice daily for 3 days **or** Malarone® 4 standard tablets daily for 3 days
	Vomiting but no signs of severe or complicated malaria	Quinine 10 mg/kg dose IV in 5% dextrose over 4 hours every 8 hours plus IV clindamycin 450 mg every 8 hours. When the patient is well enough to take oral medication she can be switched to oral quinine 600 mg 3 times a day to complete 5–7 days and oral clindamycin can if needed be switched to 450 mg 3 times a day 7 days
Non-falciparum malaria	*P. vivax, P. ovale, P. malariae*	Oral chloroquine (base) 600 mg followed by 300 mg 68 hours later. Then 300 mg on day 2 and again on day 3
	Resistant *P. vivax*	As for uncomplicated malaria *P. falciparum*
	Preventing relapse during pregnancy	Chloroquine oral 300 mg weekly until delivery
	Preventing relapse after delivery	Postpone until 3 months after delivery and G6PD testing
	P. ovale	Oral primaquine 15 mg single daily dose for 14 days
	P. vivax	Oral primaquine 30 mg single daily dose for 14 days
	G6PD (mild) for *P. vivax* or *P. ovale*	Primaquine oral 45–60 mg once a week for 8 weeks

Table A1.4 Recommended treatment for drug treatment of different stages of syphilis

Stage of disease	Recommended treatment
Early syphilis (primary, secondary, or latent syphilis of <1 year duration)	Benzathine penicillin G 2.4 million units IM in a single dose *Alternatives*: ◆ Tetracycline 500 mg orally 4 times daily for 2 weeks ◆ Erythromycin 500 mg orally 4 times daily for 2 weeks ◆ Ceftriaxone 1 g IM daily for 10 days
Late latent syphilis (> 1 year duration and cardiovascular syphilis)	Benzathine penicillin G 2.4 million units IM weekly for 3 consecutive weeks *Alternative*: ◆ Tetracycline 500 mg orally 4 times daily for 4 weeks
Neurosyphilis	Aqueous crystalline penicillin G, 3–4 million units IV every 4 h for 10–14 days, followed by benzathine penicillin G 2.4 million units IM weekly for 3 consecutive weeks *Alternative*: ◆ Aqueous procaine penicillin G 2.4 million units IM daily and probenecid 500 mg orally 4 times daily, both for 10–14 days

Complications or problems in reproductive medicine

Royal College of Obstetricians and Gynaecologists. *The Management of Ovarian Hyperstimulation Syndrome.* Green-Top Guideline No. 5, 2006

https://www.rcog.org.uk/en/guidelines-research-services/guidelines/gtg5/

This guideline aims to provide an evidence-based approach to managing ovarian hyperstimulation syndrome (OHSS). Healthcare workers may be unfamiliar with the presentation of OHSS as it is a disease associated with assisted conception, which may take place at sites separate to acute hospitals. This guideline includes outpatient management, admission criteria, and basic inpatient management of OHSS.

Key points

- OHSS is a systemic disease, which results from increased capillary permeability leading to leakage of fluid from the vascular compartment and accumulation in third spaces. In severe cases, the condition can lead to organ dysfunction, thrombosis, and ARDS.
- OHSS may occur in up to 33% of pregnancies in a mild form.
- Diagnosis of OHSS is usually clinical, associated with a history of taking gonadotrophins or antioestrogens.
- Any death resulting from OHSS must be reported to the Confidential Enquiries into Maternal Deaths (now MBRRACE).
- There are four grades of OHSS: mild, moderate, severe, and critical.
- Mild and moderate OHSS may be managed in the outpatient setting. Advice, antiemetics, and analgesia should be offered to these patients.
- Severe and critical OHSS require inpatient admission and management by a multidisciplinary team, which may include intensive care. Daily assessment should include measuring abdominal girth and assessing hydration state.
- Intravenous fluid replacement may be indicated if there is evidence of haemoconcentration (Hb > 14g/dL, haematocrit > 45%).
- Ultrasound-guided drainage of ascites may need to be performed if there is abdominal distension and oliguria despite adequate volume replacement.
- Thromboprophylaxis should be started on all women admitted with OHSS and may need to be continued after discharge, depending on other risk factors.

NICE. *Ectopic Pregnancy and Miscarriage.* Clinical Guideline 154, 2012

https://www.nice.org.uk/guidance/cg154/resources/guidance-ectopic-pregnancy-and-miscarriage-pdf

Fetal loss in early pregnancy accounts for over 50,000 admissions each year in the United Kingdom. The rate of ectopic pregnancy in the United Kingdom is about 11/1000 pregnancies, with a mortality rate of about 0.2/1000 pregnancies. This guideline addresses the pastoral, medical, and surgical management of ectopic pregnancy and miscarriage.

Key points

- These women must be treated sympathetically, with care and dignity. Throughout the management process, the patient and her partner must be given the opportunity to ask questions and seek advice regarding their care.
- Where an early pregnancy assessment unit exists, the woman should be able to self-refer and access the facility 7 days a week. Staff working in these units should be appropriately trained in communication with and management of such patients.
- Staff should be aware that clinical presentation in these cases may be varied. There should be access to pregnancy tests in all units.
- If ultrasound scanning is required, then a transvaginal scan should be offered. If this scan is unacceptable, then a transabdominal scan may be performed and the patient must be made aware of the limitations of the scan.
- Serum human chorionic gonadotropin (hCG) measurement should not be used to determine the viability of the pregnancy. Rather, it should be used to guide subsequent management.
- Management of miscarriage may be expectant (where no treatment is given and the patient is observed to see if the condition resolves), medical or surgical.
- Misoprostol, not mifepristone, should be offered for incomplete or missed miscarriage. This ideally should be given vaginally, but oral is an acceptable alternative. Analgesics and antiemetics should be offered concurrently.
- Surgical management of miscarriage includes manual vacuum aspiration under local anaesthetic or general anaesthetic.
- Systemic methotrexate should be offered as first-line treatment of ectopic pregnancy where appropriate.
- Surgical treatment should be first-line treatment of ectopic pregnancy in certain circumstances including the presence of severe pain and a fetal heart beat on ultrasound. The surgery should be performed laparoscopically where possible and this may include salpingectomy or salpingotomy.
- Anti-D should be offered to all Rhesus-negative women undergoing surgical management of miscarriage or ectopic pregnancy.
- A pregnancy of unknown location (PUL) is one where there is a positive serum hCG test but no embryo can be seen on ultrasound scanning. An ectopic pregnancy cannot be ruled out in these cases. Serial serum hCG testing should be taken 48 hours apart and must be used to guide subsequent management rather than try to determine the position of the embryo. If there is an increase of 63% in serum hCG after 48 hours, a viable intrauterine pregnancy is possible. A decrease of serum hCG by more than 50% after 48 hours is suggestive of a miscarriage.

Royal College of Obstetricians and Gynaecologists. *The Investigation and Treatment of Couples with Recurrent First-trimester and Second-trimester Miscarriage.* Green-Top Guideline No. 17, 2011

https://www.rcog.org.uk/en/guidelines-research-services/guidelines/gtg17/

Miscarriage is defined as 'the spontaneous loss of pregnancy before the fetus reaches viability'. Recurrent miscarriage is defined as 'the loss of three or more consecutive pregnancies' and affects 1% of couples trying to conceive.

Key points

- Increasing parental age is associated with an increased risk of miscarriage. The association with other epidemiological risk factors like caffeine intake, smoking, and anaesthetic gases is equivocal.
- Lupus anticoagulant, anticardiolipin antibodies, and anti-B_2 glycoprotein I antibodies are collectively known as antiphospholipid antibodies and are detected in 15% of women with recurrent miscarriage.
- Genetic factors include parental chromosomal rearrangements and chromosomal abnormalities of the embryo.
- Uterine malformations and cervical weakness may also cause miscarriage but the true incidence is unknown.
- Bacteraemia or viraemia resulting from a severe infection can lead to miscarriage. The organisms screened for in TORCH (toxoplasmosis, rubella, cytomegalovirus, herpes simplex, HIV) do not fulfil this criteria and such screening should be abandoned.
- Both inherited and acquired thrombophilias (e.g. factor V Leiden, deficiencies in protein C/S) have been associated with recurrent miscarriage as a result of promoting thrombosis.
- Investigations for recurrent miscarriage:
  - Test the woman for antiphospholipid antibodies and screen for thrombophilias.
  - Perform cytogenetic analysis on products of conception of the third and subsequent miscarriage.
  - Perform a pelvic ultrasound scan to assess uterine anatomy.
- Treatment options for recurrent miscarriage:
  - Refer patient to a specialist clinic.
  - Consider treatment with low-dose aspirin and heparin in women with antiphospholipid syndrome. There is no benefit from the use of corticosteroids in these patients.
  - Refer for genetic counselling should abnormal karyotyping be found.
  - Serial cervical ultrasonography to assess cervical weakness. Cerclage should only be performed if it is deemed to benefit the woman.
  - Presently, there is insufficient evidence to support the use of hormonal or metformin supplementation.

Royal College of Obstetricians and Gynaecologists. *The Management of Early Pregnancy Loss*. Green-Top Guideline No. 25, 2006

This guideline has now been superseded by NICE Clinical Guideline 154 as referenced earlier in this section.

Royal College of Obstetricians and Gynaecologists. *The Management of Tubal Pregnancy*. Green-Top Guideline No. 21, 2010

https://www.rcog.org.uk/globalassets/documents/guidelines/gtg21_230611.pdf

The annual rate of ectopic pregnancies is about 11.1/1000 pregnancies. During the triennium of 1997–1999, there were 13 maternal deaths from a tubal pregnancy. Management of such pregnancies must be provided on an individual basis, taking into account the clinical presentation and the future fertility requirements of the woman.

Key points

- Management may be surgical (laparotomy or laparoscopy), medical, or, occasionally, by observation alone.
- In the stable patient, laparoscopic surgery is preferable to the open approach.
- In the unstable patient, surgical management must be by the most expedient method. Usually this is the open approach.
- In suitable cases (serum hCG < 3000 IU/L and minimal symptoms), methotrexate may be offered as medical management of an ectopic pregnancy in an outpatient setting.
- Expectant management (observation alone) is suitable for women who are stable, with minimal symptoms and the location of the pregnancy is unknown or is identified on ultrasound and is associated with a falling serum hCG which was less than 1000 IU/L to start with.
- All Rhesus-negative women who have a suspected or confirmed ectopic pregnancy should be given anti-D immunoglobulin.

Royal College of Obstetricians and Gynaecologists. *The Management of Gestational Trophoblastic Disease*. Green-Top Guideline No. 38, 2010

https://www.rcog.org.uk/globalassets/documents/guidelines/gt38managementgestational0210.pdf

Gestational trophoblastic disease (GTD) refers to a group of conditions encompassing complete and partial molar pregnancies, as well as malignant conditions of invasive mole, choriocarcinoma, and placental site trophoblastic tumour. The incidence of GTD in the UK is 1/714 live births.

Key points

- Complete moles are diploid and are formed solely from paternal genetic tissue and usually arise when a single sperm duplicates after fertilizing an 'empty' ovum. Partial moles, on the other hand, are triploid in origin and are formed from both paternal and maternal genes.
- A molar pregnancy typically presents with erratic vaginal bleeding, severe vomiting, disproportionate uterine enlargement, and early miscarriage. Although ultrasound is useful, histological examination of the tissues of conception is required to confirm the diagnosis.
- Medical evacuation of a molar pregnancy should be avoided, as there is a theoretical risk of trophoblastic tissue embolization, and dissemination from the use of oxytocic drugs. Suction evacuation is the treatment of choice and anti-D should be given where appropriate.
- Should a woman develop persistent vaginal bleeding following a pregnancy, they should be investigated for gestational trophoblastic neoplasia (GTN).
- All women diagnosed with GTD should be given written information regarding their condition and referred to a trophoblastic

screening centre for follow-up. They should be advised not to try to conceive until their follow-up is complete.

- Women who receive chemotherapy as treatment for GTN should not try to conceive for at least a year after completion of treatment. These women are also at risk of early menopause and of developing secondary tumours.

Royal College of Obstetricians and Gynaecologists. *Cervical Cerclage*. Green-Top Guideline No. 60, 2011

https://www.rcog.org.uk/globalassets/documents/guidelines/gtg_60.pdf

Cervical cerclage is used to manage women who are at high risk of mid-trimester loss. Preterm birth is defined as delivery before 37 weeks' gestation and is the leading cause of perinatal death and disability, especially in those born before 33 weeks. The rate of preterm births continues to rise globally despite interventions aimed at preventing it.

Key points

- There are several different indications for the insertion of a cervical cerclage:
  - History-indicated cerclage—inserted at 12–14 weeks' gestation in women who have had three or more previous preterm births and/or second trimester losses.
  - Ultrasound-indicated cerclage—sonographic assessment of the cervix occurs between 14–24 weeks' gestation. A cerclage may be indicated in cases of shortened cervical length without exposed fetal membranes, associated with a previous history of preterm birth or spontaneous mid-trimester miscarriage.
  - Rescue cerclage—this is used as a salvage procedure when there is premature cervical dilatation with exposed fetal membranes in the vagina. The decision to insert one must be made by a senior obstetrician and once inserted, it may delay delivery by up to 5 weeks.
  - Transvaginal cerclage (McDonald)—a purse-string suture is placed where the cervix meets the vaginal without mobilizing the bladder.
  - High transvaginal cerclage (Shirodkar)—a transvaginal purse-string suture placed following bladder mobilization, to allow insertion above the level of the cardinal ligaments.
  - Transabdominal cerclage—a suture is performed at laparotomy or laparoscopy and is placed it at the junction of the cervix and isthmus. This method is associated with increased maternal morbidity. It needs to be inserted preconceptually or in early pregnancy and may be considered when vaginal cerclage has failed.
  - Occlusion cerclage—a continuous non-absorbable suture is placed to occlude the external os so that the mucus plug may be retained.
- There is no evidence to support the use of history or ultrasound-indicated cervical cerclage in women with multiple pregnancies, as the cerclage itself is associated with an increased risk of preterm delivery and pregnancy loss.
- There is insufficient evidence to support the routine use of a cervical cerclage to prevent preterm delivery in women with uterine anomalies.
- The use of preoperative antibiotics and the type of anaesthetic used to insert a cerclage should be made at the discretion of the theatre team.
- Routine bed rest, abstinence from sexual intercourse, and ultrasound surveillance is not recommended. Post-procedural care should be decided on an individual basis.
- A cerclage should be removed before labour, typically between 36 and 37 weeks, unless delivery is by caesarean delivery, where the suture may be removed after delivery.
- In cases of preterm premature rupture of membranes between 24 and 34 weeks' gestation where there is no evidence of infection, removal of the suture may be delayed by 48 hours.

NICE. *Fertility: Assessment and Treatment for People with Fertility Problems*. Clinical Guideline 156, February 2013

https://www.nice.org.uk/guidance/cg156/resources/guidance-fertility-pdf

Key priorities for implementation

- A woman of reproductive age who fails to conceive after unprotected sex for a year, in the absence of any cause of infertility, should be assessed along with her partner.
- Early specialist referral is recommended for those women who are over 36 years of age or those who have a known cause of (or known risk factor) for infertility.
- Oral ovarian stimulation agents should not be offered to those with unexplained infertility.
- *In vitro* fertilization (IVF) treatment should be offered to women with unexplained infertility, who have not conceived after 2 years of regular unprotected sex.
- People with unexplained infertility, mild endometriosis, or mild male factor infertility should be advised to try to conceive for a total of 2 years before IVF is offered.
- A full cycle of IVF treatment should include one episode of ovarian stimulation and the transfer of any fresh and frozen embryo(s).
- Criteria for referral for IVF are shown in Table A1.5.
- The recommended number of fresh or frozen embryos to be transferred are described in Table A1.6.

Table A1.5 Referral criteria for IVF

Age	Previous history and treatment	Recommended treatment
<40 years	2 years of regular unprotected sex or 12 cycles of artificial insemination	3 full cycles of IVF
40–42 years	2 years of regular unprotected sex or 12 cycles of artificial insemination No previous IVF No history of low ovarian reserve	1 full cycle of IVF

Table A1.6 Recommended number of embryos to be transferred

Age	First cycle	Second cycle	Third cycle
<37 years	Single	Single if top quality embryos are available Double if there is no top quality embryo	No more than 2 embryos
37–39 years	Single if top quality embryos are available Double if there is no top quality embryo	Single if top quality embryos are available Double if there is no top quality embryo	No more than 2 embryos
40–42 years	Double		

Critical care and resuscitation

AAGBI Safety Guideline: *Blood Transfusion and the Anaesthetist: Management of Massive Haemorrhage*, November 2010

http://www.aagbi.org/sites/default/files/massive_haemorrhage_2010_0.pdf

This guideline by the AAGBI covers massive haemorrhage from a variety of causes, and is not limited to just the obstetric population. The guideline was designed to address the fact that at the time of initial writing, only 16% of emergency departments had a massive haemorrhage protocol in place.

Key points

- Emphasis is made on good clinical leadership, good teamwork, and clear communication with various departments in the hospital, including the telephone operator, blood bank, and porters, in order to provide coordinated care for the critically ill patient.
- The main treatment points are to:
  - stop the bleeding
  - assess the patient
  - alert other team members of the massive haemorrhage incident
  - transfer the patient to an appropriate place for ongoing care.
- Resuscitation of the patient involves inserting wide-bore cannulae, taking baseline bloods including a cross-match sample and infusing intravenous fluids. Near-patient testing of bloods (e.g. TEG®/ROTEM®/Hemocue®) may be used if available.
- Once control of the bleeding has been achieved, resuscitation should continue to normalize blood pressure, acid–base balance, and temperature. The use of vasopressors should be avoided where possible and active warming should be started as soon as convenient.
- Patients with a massive haemorrhage almost certainly develop a coagulopathy and this must be anticipated during resuscitation. A fibrinogen less than 1 g/L or prothrombin time and activated partial thromboplastin time greater than 1.5 times normal are suggestive of coagulation problems and are predictive of microvascular bleeding. Early use of 15 mL/kg fresh frozen plasma (FFP) may address these issues. Established coagulopathy may need more than 15 mL/kg of FFP. Fibrinogen concentrate is an alternative and if fibrinogen is unavailable, cryoprecipitate may be used.
- A platelet count below 50×10^9/L is suggestive of microvascular bleeding and platelets should be kept above 75×10^9/L where possible.
- The military regimen of 1:1:1 red cell:FFP:platelet is not routinely recommended in the management of massive haemorrhage in a hospital setting, unless the patient has had coincidental severe trauma.
- Tranexamic acid, correction of hypocalcaemia and hypomagnesaemia, and recombinant factor VIIa may be considered for use in the management of massive haemorrhage.
- Venous thromboprophylaxis should be started as soon as possible after the haemorrhage has been controlled due to the fact that these patients develop a procoagulant state afterwards.
- A system for collecting blood, checking blood, and tracing transfused blood products must be in place in each hospital.

European resuscitation council. european resuscitation guidelines. *Resuscitation* 2005; 6751:51–2

The Resuscitation Council UK advocates (https://www.resus.org.uk/pages/GL2010.pdf, p. 73), that intraosseous access is now an acceptable route of drug administration and should be performed should there be two unsuccessful attempts at intravenous cannulation during resuscitation. Both the tibial and humeral routes are acceptable.

Royal College of Obstetricians and Gynaecologists. *Maternal Collapse in Pregnancy and the Puerperium.* Green-Top Guideline No. 56, January 2011

https://www.rcog.org.uk/globalassets/documents/guidelines/gtg56.pdf

This publication from the Royal College of Obstetricians and Gynaecologists provides a succinct account of the aetiology of maternal collapse and the physiological changes which occur in pregnancy. It offers practical information regarding the initial resuscitation, as well as the subsequent management and investigation of such patients, including the need for a perimortem caesarean delivery.

Key points

- Early modified warning scores should be used for all patients on the delivery suite to help early identification of the ill patient.
- There are many causes of maternal collapse. The following are discussed in the guideline:
  - Haemorrhage
  - Thromboembolism
  - Amniotic fluid embolism
  - Cardiac disease
  - Sepsis

- Drug toxicity or overdose
- Eclampsia
- Intracranial haemorrhage
- Anaphylaxis.

- All staff who may be responsible for looking after a pregnant patient should be aware of the physiological changes of pregnancy and the impact these have on resuscitation.
- Maternal resuscitation should follow the resuscitation algorithms provided by the Resuscitation Council (UK), with some modification.
- A perimortem caesarean delivery should be performed within 5 minutes of the collapse. This should not be delayed by moving the woman to theatre. The obstetrician should use the caesarean technique which they are most familiar with to deliver the baby.
- Clear documentation of the events, with timings, should be undertaken. All maternal deaths should be reported to MBRRACE-UK.
- A debriefing session should occur with the patient and their family as well as the staff involved in the management of the incident.

AAGBI Safety Guideline: *Management of Severe Local Anaesthetic Toxicity*, December 2010

http://www.aagbi.org/sites/default/files/la_toxicity_2010_0.pdf

Key points

- Recognize signs of local anaesthetic toxicity. These are usually neurological and cardiovascular.
- Immediate management: stop local anaesthetic injection and provide supportive treatment.
- Control seizures with benzodiazepines, thiopental, or propofol in incremental doses.
- In circulatory arrest, start cardiopulmonary resuscitation, treat arrhythmia as per standard advanced life support protocol, and commence lipid emulsion therapy.
- In the absence of circulatory arrest, use conventional therapies to treat hypotension and arrhythmia, and consider lipid emulsion therapy.
- Lipid emulsion therapy:
  - Give an initial intravenous bolus of 20% lipid emulsion (1.5 mL/kg over 1 minute).
  - Start an intravenous infusion of 20% lipid emulsion at 15 mL/kg/h.
  - After 5 minutes, give a maximum of two further boluses (same dose) and double the rate of infusion to 30 mL/kg/h if cardiovascular stability has not been restored or an adequate circulation deteriorates. Leave 5 minutes between boluses.
  - A cumulative dose should not exceed 12 mL/kg.
  - Continue the infusion until an adequate circulation is restored or maximum dose of lipid emulsion is given.
- Patient should be transferred to a clinical area with appropriate equipment and suitably trained staff.
- Exclude pancreatitis by regular review, including daily amylase or lipase assays for 2 days.
- Report cases in the United Kingdom to the appropriate regulatory authority.

OAA Clinical Guidelines: *Modified Early Obstetric Warning Score (MEOWS)*, 2009

http://www.oaa-anaes.ac.uk/ui/content/content.aspx?id=186

Key points

- The early warning score was introduced in order to recognize deteriorating patients early and to instigate treatment at the earliest opportunity.
- Examples of MEOWS from four NHS hospitals are described on the OAA website.
- Physiological parameters measured are pulse, blood pressure, oxygen saturation, respiratory rate, conscious level, temperature, and urine output. Some units also incorporate pain scores and partograms into the MEOWS charts.
- Colour triggers are usually used at the upper and lower limits to alert midwives to take action. (Red colour as an alert to take urgent action and amber to suggest that the patient's condition is worsening, and an escalation of treatment is required.)
- A clear algorithm of the action plan required for different levels of triggers needs to be available.
- The algorithm should include whom to call for help, how to escalate if help is not immediately available, and frequency of observations required if a patient's condition deteriorates.
- Regular audit is required to check staff compliance with the MEOWS.

Centre for Maternal and Child Enquiries (CMACE). Saving mothers' lives: reviewing maternal deaths to make motherhood safer: 2006–2008. The eighth report of the confidential enquiries into maternal deaths in the United Kingdom. *BJOG* 2011; 118(Suppl 1):1–203.

http://www.hqip.org.uk/assets/NCAPOP-Library/CMACE-Reports/6.-March-2011-Saving-Mothers-Lives-reviewing-maternal-deaths-to-make-motherhood-safer-2006-2008.pdf

The top ten overall recommendations are summarized here:

1. Women of childbearing age with a pre-existing medical condition should be made aware throughout their pregnancy that their condition may worsen and require a change in medication which may affect their unborn child. Such counselling services should be an integral part of the commissioning of community care of the pregnant woman.
2. All pregnant women who do not speak English should have access to professional interpretation services.
3. All referrals made to other specialties for a pregnant patient should be regarded as urgent and it should be clearly documented on the referral that the patient is pregnant. Such

referrals should be made following consultation with senior clinicians.

4. All women whose pregnancies are likely to be complicated by serious medical or mental health conditions, regardless of whether the condition existed prior to pregnancy, should be referred to specialist centres for expert care in a timely fashion. Those providing care of the parturient in the community should be allowed to make such referrals without prior approval from an obstetrician. However, the obstetrician should be kept informed if any such referrals are made.
5. All clinical staff must complete regular training for the identification and initial management of serious obstetric conditions or other medical emergencies, such as sepsis. Clinical staff must also take regular training for basic, intermediate, and advanced life support skills appropriate for their positions.
6. There should be a routine use of a national modified early obstetric warning score (MEOWS) chart in all pregnant or postpartum women who become unwell. MEOWS was introduced to recognize deteriorating patients early and to instigate treatments at the earliest opportunity. The management of pregnant or postpartum women with an acute severe illness requires a multidisciplinary team approach. Obstetric trainees should seek help early from senior medical, anaesthetic and critical care staff.
7. All pregnant women with pre-eclampsia and a systolic blood pressure of 150–160 mmHg or higher require urgent antihypertensive treatment in line with the guidelines from NICE. Antihypertensive treatment may be considered in women who do not fulfil the BP criteria but are otherwise high risk of becoming seriously unwell from hypertensive disease in pregnancy.
8. All pregnant and recently delivered women should be informed of the risks and signs of genital tract infection and how to prevent its transmission. All clinical staff should follow local infection control policy, and be aware of the signs and symptoms of sepsis. High-dose intravenous broad-spectrum antibiotics should be given within the first hour of recognition of septic shock or severe sepsis.
9. A high-quality local review must take place when there is a maternal death. The results of the review must be discussed with all maternity staff. The recommendations from the review process must be implemented and audited at regular intervals.
10. Specialist pathologists who perform maternal autopsies should have this agreed in their job plans. Furthermore, the provision of such services should be streamlined so fewer centres are able to perform high quality autopsies.

Key points

- All anaesthetic practitioners should have regular drills in the management of failed intubation to maintain this core skill.
- The multidisciplinary team should be involved in the management of the acutely unwell parturient with early anaesthetic and critical care involvement.
- If a woman has had a fully working epidural during labour and the decision is made for an operative delivery, then her epidural should be topped up as soon as is possible to provide surgical anaesthesia. If this is established outside the theatre environment, then appropriate monitoring and necessary precautions should be implemented.
- If a serious untoward incident occurs, all the drugs and equipment used should be kept for review until the cause of the incident has been determined.
- A woman should be fully awake before extubation if she has been given a general anaesthetic with a potentially full stomach. The insertion of an 'in and out' nasogastric tube to decompress the stomach prior to extubation may be considered in such cases.
- Parturients with severe pre-eclampsia should have BP control instigated early with regular monitoring in a high dependency unit environment. Anaesthetic and where necessary critical care input should be instituted early on.
- A parturient with sepsis should be managed with broad-spectrum antibiotics, cardiovascular support including inotropes, and appropriate fluid resuscitation to prevent circulatory collapse. Transfer to critical care and surgery should be considered in management of severe sepsis.
- Women with known risk factors for major haemorrhage should be managed in specialist maternity units. Management of major haemorrhage may require the use of cell salvage and specialist services such as interventional radiology or critical care.
- The acute anaphylaxis management algorithm should be immediately available in all clinical areas.
- There must be a clear escalation pathway to provide additional skilled assistance, if the medical staff on the delivery suite are busy and a woman with an acute, severe illness requires high-dependency care.

Confidential Enquiry into Maternal and Child Health. *Why Mothers Die 2000–2002: The Sixth Report of the Confidential Enquiries into Maternal Deaths in the United Kingdom* (Chapter 17: Trends in Intensive Care), 2004

http://www.hqip.org.uk/assets/NCAPOP-Library/CMACE-Reports/33.-2004-Why-Mothers-Die-2000-2002-The-Sixth-Report-of-the-Confidential-Enquiries-into-Maternal-Deaths-in-the-UK.pdf

This chapter discusses the importance of early recognition of the sick parturient. It also stresses the significance of the early involvement of senior help, to assist in the resuscitation and management of the acutely unwell parturient.

Key points

- As with other surgery, elective cases requiring intensive care postoperatively should be pre-arranged with the intensive care unit. This may require the cancellation of other planned surgery if bed capacity is reached.
- Aggressive resuscitation and treatment for the sick parturient should begin on the ward prior to arriving in intensive care.

Appropriate lines and invasive monitoring should be instituted on the ward where possible.

- A blood gas should be performed as soon as possible and a metabolic acidosis must be treated seriously.
- Early communication with the intensive care consultant should occur when there is a sick patient on the delivery suite.
- Appropriately modified early warning scores should be used on labour ward. Tachypnoea is an early sign of a deteriorating patient and should always be investigated.
- It is possible to provide a higher level of care in obstetric theatres if there is a delay in admission to the intensive care unit.
- Where available, intensive care outreach teams must be utilized to assist with maternal resuscitation.
- In the management of major obstetric haemorrhage, the priorities are to stop the bleeding, correct the haemoglobin and clotting, and to call for senior anaesthetic help as soon as possible.

This theme continues to be important in the global care of the sick parturient and is reiterated in Chapter 16 'Critical Care', pp.173–180 of the *Eighth Report of the Confidential Enquiries into Maternal Deaths in the UK* (http://www.oaa-anaes.ac.uk/assets/_managed/editor/File/Reports/2006-2008%20CEMD.pdf):

- Severe sepsis remains an important cause of significant morbidity and mortality and should be managed with early protocol-driven care based on the Sepsis Care Bundles prior to transfer to intensive care (see following 'Surviving Sepsis Campaign' section).
- The use of modified early warning scores for pregnant women can assist in the detection of the deteriorating parturient.
- Where available, the early involvement of critical care outreach teams would assist in maternal resuscitation.
- Maternal resuscitation in major obstetric haemorrhage should include early use of clotting factors and blood products to reduce the volume of crystalloids infused. A coordinated response from the wider multidisciplinary team ensures that appropriate products are given in a timely fashion. More information can be found from reading the Royal College of Obstetricians and Gynaecologists Green-Top Guideline No. 52 (May 2009): *Prevention and Management of Postpartum Haemorrhage* (http://www.rcog.org.uk/files/rcog-corp/GT52PostpartumHaemorrhage0411.pdf), which is summarized in Chapter 35 of this book.
- Simulation scenarios should be used to help train staff and maintain their skills in managing obstetric emergencies.

Surviving Sepsis Campaign. *Sepsis Six Care Bundle*

http://www.survivingsepsis.org/SiteCollectionDocuments/SSC_Bundle.pdf

This two-page care bundle outlines the goals, investigations, and treatment strategies that need to be established within the first hour of presentation, when managing the acutely unwell septic patient.

Key points

- Give high-flow oxygen via facemask
- Obtain blood cultures (ideally before giving antibiotics)
- Prescribe and administer broad-spectrum antibiotics
- Give intravenous fluid boluses as needed
- Take bloods including haemoglobin and serum lactate
- Measure hourly urine output.

Endocrine

Scottish Intercollegiate Guidelines Network. *Management of Diabetes: A National Clinical Guideline.* SIGN 116, March 2010

http://www.sign.ac.uk/pdf/sign116.pdf

This guideline by the Scottish Intercollegiate Guidelines Network (SIGN) encompasses the management of type 1 and type 2 diabetes in pregnant and non-pregnant patients. Good glycaemic control before conception and during pregnancy can lead to good maternal and fetal outcomes. Diabetes is associated with miscarriage, pre-eclampsia, maternal infection, fetal congenital malformation, and late intrauterine death. The following points summarize the management of diabetes in pregnancy.

Key points

- The care of a pregnant woman with diabetes should involve a multidisciplinary team, which includes an obstetrician and a physician with an interest in diabetes. There should be good communication between team members.
- The choice of contraception should be decided on an individual basis. The oral contraceptive pill (OCP) may not be suitable for all women due to the presence of diabetic vascular complications. Intrauterine devices and hormonal implants are effective alternatives.
- Pre-pregnancy care with a multidisciplinary team leads to improved maternal and fetal outcomes. Pre-pregnancy glycaemic control should aim for an HbA1c of less than 7%. The higher the HbA1c, the higher the risk of fetal malformations.
- High-dose folic acid 5 mg should be given to diabetic women prepregnancy and continued up to 12 weeks' gestation.
- The use of metformin and glibenclamide in early pregnancy is not associated with any additional risk of teratogenesis or pregnancy loss. The use of other types of sulphonylureas should be avoided due to their ability to cross the placenta.
- The use of statins and ACEIs should be avoided due to the increased risk of fetal malformations.
- Dietetic advice should be available to women pre- and during pregnancy to ensure optimum glycaemic control. Postprandial glucose monitoring should be advised in women with gestational diabetes (GDM) and may be considered in women with type 1 or 2 diabetes.
- The choice of insulin therapy should be made on an individual basis. Human insulins are licensed for use during pregnancy but oral hypoglycaemic agents are not.
- Pregnancy-induced hypertension and thromboembolism should be screened for and managed accordingly.

- Women and their partners should be educated in recognizing the signs of hypoglycaemia and ketoacidosis, as these may be associated with fetal death. Appropriate treatment advice including self-referral to hospital should be given.
- Retinopathy may deteriorate during pregnancy and monitoring is advocated prepregnancy and in each trimester in women with type 1 and 2 diabetes. Early referral to an ophthalmologist is recommended.
- Pre-existing diabetic nephropathy is associated with poorer pregnancy outcomes. Close attention should be given to monitoring and managing blood pressure in these patients.
- Both macrosomia and intrauterine growth restriction (IUGR) are more likely in women with diabetes. In cases of suspected IUGR, fetal monitoring with growth scans and umbilical artery Doppler should be carried out.
- Once diagnosed with GDM, dietary advice to lower blood glucose should be offered. Treatment with oral hypoglycaemic agents and/or insulin may be needed.
- In women with diabetes, delivery should occur within 40 weeks. These women have a higher rate of caesarean delivery compared with the normal population. An agreed plan should be made in advance regarding insulin management in labour and intravenous insulin and dextrose may be necessary to maintain blood glucose between 4 and 7 mmol/L in labour.
- There is no need to routinely admit babies born to mothers with diabetes to the neonatal unit, but they should be monitored closely for neonatal hypoglycaemia. This is defined as a blood sugar below 2.6 mmol/L and is associated with neurodevelopmental problems. In the postpartum period, women with type 1 and 2 diabetes will need to be followed up and their doses of insulin may need to be adjusted. Dietary advice, weight loss, and lifestyle changes need to be given to women with GDM postpartum as they are at risk of developing type 2 diabetes in later life. They will also need to be given good preconception counselling in subsequent pregnancies.

NICE. *Diabetes in Pregnancy.* Clinical Guideline 63, March 2008

http://www.nice.org.uk/guidance/CG063

In England and Wales, 2–5% of all pregnancies are complicated with diabetes, 87.5% of which are due to GDM. This guideline contains best practice advice regarding women with diabetes who are either planning to become pregnant, who are pregnant, or who have recently delivered. Poorly managed diabetes of any type during pregnancy can have serious implications for both the mother and fetus.

Key points

- Preconception advice needs to be offered to all diabetic women of childbearing age, with emphasis on good glycaemic control in order to minimize effects on the developing fetus. Women with diabetes should be encouraged to take folic acid 5 mg a day before conception and up to 12 weeks' gestation to minimize the risk of neural tube defects.
- Women should be encouraged to keep and maintain their HbA1c below 6.1% to minimize the likelihood of congenital malformations. . Women with an HbA1c more than 10% need to be strongly discouraged from getting pregnant.
- Metformin and fast-acting insulins (aspart and lispro) are safe to use in early pregnancy. All other oral hypoglycaemics should be stopped and substituted with insulin. Statins and ACEIs should also be discontinued before conception.
- Digital retinal assessment with tropicamide should be offered to women either preconception or at their first appointment after conception.
- An assessment of renal function should also be made early in pregnancy and referral to a nephrologist where proteinuria is greater than 2 g/day.
- Risk factors for GDM include previous history of GDM, family history of GDM, and body mass index (BMI) greater than 30 kg/m^2. Diet and exercise may reduce the likelihood of developing GDM.
- Ten to 20% of women with GDM will require treatment with metformin or insulin during pregnancy.
- Screening for GDM should be in the form of a 2-hour oral glucose tolerance test at 24–28 weeks' gestation.
- Any woman with suspected diabetic ketoacidosis should be admitted to a level 2 facility, with both medical and obstetric input.
- All women with diabetes should be offered ultrasound scanning with a four-chamber view of the fetal heart and outflow tracts between 18 and 20 weeks' gestation.
- Fetal well-being should be assessed using ultrasound to determine the rate of growth and volume of amniotic fluid every 4 weeks between 28 and 36 weeks' gestation.
- During pregnancy, the diabetic team should aim to contact the woman every 1–2 weeks to assess maternal well-being.
- Beta-mimetic drugs should not be used for tocolysis in this group.
- Delivery should be offered after 38 weeks' gestation where possible, by elective caesarean delivery or induction of labour.
- Anaesthetic assessment of women with diabetes should occur in the third trimester.
- During labour and delivery, blood glucose should be maintained between 4 and 7 mmol/L. In women treated with insulin, an intravenous insulin and dextrose infusion may be required.
- If a general anaesthetic has been given, the maternal blood glucose should be checked every 30 minutes from induction until she is fully conscious.
- Fetal blood glucose should be measured 2–4 hours after delivery. Women should be encouraged to start early feeding and at 2–3-hourly intervals until the pre-feed neonatal blood glucose is greater than 2 mmol/L.
- The baby may be looked after by the mother after birth, unless there is an indication for neonatal intensive care admission.
- Women with type 1 diabetes should reduce their insulin postpartum and be aware that they are at risk of hypoglycaemia, particularly if they are breastfeeding.

- Women with GDM should be given exercise, dietary, and lifestyle advice in the postpartum period, a fasting blood glucose check 6 weeks after delivery, and annually thereafter.

CMACE/Royal College of Obstetricians and Gynaecologists Joint Guideline: *Management of Women with Obesity in Pregnancy*, March 2010

http://www.hqip.org.uk/assets/NCAPOP-Library/CMACE-Reports/15.-March-2010-Management-of-Women-with-Obesity-in-Pregnancy-Guidance.pdf

Maternal obesity is defined as a BMI of greater than 30 kg/m^2 at the first antenatal appointment. Obesity in pregnancy is associated with serious adverse outcomes including miscarriage, GDM, pre-eclampsia, postpartum haemorrhage, and neonatal death. It is also associated with a higher caesarean delivery and lower breastfeeding rate when compared with women with a normal BMI.

Key points

- Advice on weight loss, exercise, and diet should be given in primary care to all women of childbearing age. They should also be made aware of the risks and complications associated with obesity in pregnancy.
- Women should be encouraged to take 5 mg of folic acid a day during preconception and the first trimester and 10 mcg of vitamin D daily during pregnancy and breastfeeding.
- All antenatal clinics should have provision to manage obese patients.
- Women with a BMI greater than 40 kg/m^2 should have an antenatal appointment with an obstetric anaesthetist to discuss the potential plan and anticipate any difficulties during labour and delivery.
- Antenatal thromboprophylaxis should only be given if there is a specific indication following appropriate assessment. Postpartum, these women should be encouraged to mobilize as soon as possible. All women with a BMI greater than 40 kg/m^2 should be offered thromboprophylaxis for a week postpartum, regardless of the mode of delivery.
- During antenatal assessment of blood pressure, an appropriately sized cuff needs to be used and the size of the cuff should be documented in the notes. Surveillance for pre-eclampsia should be in accordance with the PRECOG (Pre-eclampsia Community Guideline) guidelines (see earlier in the 'Cardiovascular' section).
- All women with a booking BMI of greater than 30 kg/m^2 should be screened for gestational diabetes as per NICE guidelines (see NICE Clinical Guideline 63, summarized earlier in this section).
- Women with obesity should have an antenatal appointment to discuss plans for labour and delivery and the potential complications which may occur. An individual plan should be made in each case. Delivery should occur in a consultant-led unit where there are appropriate neonatal support services.
- When admitted in labour, it is important to inform the duty anaesthetist and an experienced obstetrician early, so that they are able to assess the patient and make the necessary plans for labour and delivery.
- Midwifery care should continue throughout labour. These patients should have an intravenous line inserted early and have active management of the third stage of labour.
- The theatre team should be informed if the woman weighs more than 120 kg and is due to have an operative procedure in theatre.
- Antibiotic prophylaxis should be given before caesarean delivery due to the higher risk of poor wound healing.
- Where there is more than 2 cm of subcutaneous fat, suturing of the subcutaneous space should occur to minimize the risk of wound infection and separation.
- Postpartum, women should be encouraged to breastfeed and advice offered regarding lifestyle, weight management, and diet.

NICE. *Obesity: The Prevention, Identification, Assessment and Management of Overweight and Obesity in Adults and Children*. Clinical Guideline 43, December 2006

http://www.nice.org.uk/guidance/CG43

This guideline offers advice on the prevention, identification, assessment, and management of overweight and obesity in adults and children.

Key points

- Local authorities, schools, and nurseries should endeavour to provide facilities and activities, which promote a more healthy and less sedentary lifestyle.
- Health practitioners should be able to offer advice and support to overweight adults and children regarding diet, lifestyle changes, and weight management programmes. Referral to specialists may be needed in individuals with complex care needs.
- Drug treatment to assist with weight loss should only be started in adults following a full discussion of the risks and benefits.
- Bariatric surgery is recommended as a treatment option in the following circumstances:
  - A BMI of 40 kg/m^2 or more or a BMI between 35 and 40 kg/m^2 with other significant disease (e.g. hypertension or diabetes) which would be improved with weight loss.
  - All other appropriate weight loss measures have been tried and failed to produce or maintain weight loss for at least 6 months.
  - The person has been or will be managed by a specialist obesity service.
  - The person is generally fit for anaesthesia and surgery.
  - The person is motivated and will commit to long term follow-up.
  - Surgery may be offered as a first-line treatment in patients with a BMI of 50 kg/m^2 in whom surgery would be appropriate.

Fetal

Royal College of Obstetricians and Gynaecologists. *Management of Monochorionic Twin Pregnancy*. Green-Top Guideline No. 51, 2008

https://www.rcog.org.uk/globalassets/documents/guidelines/t51managementmonochorionictwinpregnancy2008a.pdf

This is summarized under 'Intrapartum Care'.

Royal College of Obstetricians and Gynaecologists. *The Management of Breech Presentation*. Green-Top Guideline No. 20b, 2006

https://www.rcog.org.uk/globalassets/documents/guidelines/gtg-no-20b-breech-presentation.pdf

This is summarized under 'Intrapartum Care'.

NICE. *Antenatal Care: Routine Care for Healthy Pregnant Women*. Clinical Guideline 62, March 2008

http://www.nice.org.uk/guidance/cg62

Key points on antenatal fetal assessments

- For a woman who is nulliparous with an uncomplicated pregnancy, ten antenatal appointments should be offered.
- For a woman who is multiparous with an uncomplicated pregnancy, seven appointments should be adequate.
- An early ultrasound scan should be carried out to determine the gestational age and to detect multiple pregnancies.
- An ultrasound scan to screen for structural anomalies should be offered ideally between 18 and 20 weeks' gestation. This should be done by an appropriately trained sonographer and with equipment of an appropriate standard.
- By April 2007, pregnant women should be offered screening for Down's syndrome with a test, which provides a detection rate of above 75% and a false-positive rate of less than 3%.
- Pregnant women should be offered an estimation of fetal size by measuring the symphysis–fundal distance at each antenatal appointment.
- Fetal presentation should be examined by abdominal palpation at 36 weeks or later, when presentation is likely to influence the birth plan. Suspected fetal malpresentation should be confirmed by an ultrasound.
- Routine formal fetal-movement counting is not recommended.
- Routine auscultation of the fetal heart is not recommended. However, when requested by the mother, an auscultation of the fetal heart may give reassurance.
- Routine use of antenatal electronic fetal heart rate monitoring (cardiotocography) should not be offered to women with an uncomplicated pregnancy.

NICE. *Intrapartum Care: Care of Healthy Women and their Babies During Childbirth*. Clinical Guideline 190, December 2014

http://www.nice.org.uk/guidance/CG190

Key points on intrapartum fetal monitoring

First stage of uncomplicated labour in low-risk women

- Intermittent auscultation of the fetal heart after a contraction should be carried out for at least 1 minute, at least every 15 minutes.
- Fetal heart rate (FHR) should be recorded as an average.
- Maternal pulse should be monitored hourly to differentiate the two heart rates.

Second stage of labour in low-risk women

- Intermittent auscultation of the fetal heart should be done after a contraction for at least 1 minute, at least every 5 minutes.
- The maternal pulse should be palpated if fetal bradycardia or any other FHR anomaly is suspected.

Low-risk women should be monitored using continuous electronic fetal monitoring (EFM) for the following circumstances:

- Significant meconium-stained liquor (should also be considered for light meconium-stained liquor)
- Abnormal FHR (<110 bpm, >160 bpm or any decelerations after a contraction)
- Maternal pyrexia
- Fresh bleeding in labour
- Augmentation of labour with oxytocin
- Maternal request.

Complicated labour

- Continuous EFM should be done in complicated labour.
- A systematic assessment of EFM should be undertaken every hour.
- In cases of suspected or confirmed acute fetal compromise, delivery should be done within a time appropriate for the condition.
- If fetal death is suspected, fetal viability should be confirmed with a real-time ultrasound assessment.
- Fetal blood sampling is advised in the presence of a pathological trace, unless there is acute compromise.

Fetal monitoring after epidural analgesia

- Continuous EFM should be carried out for at least 30 minutes during the establishment of neuraxial analgesia and after each bolus of 10 mL or more of a 0.1% bupivacaine solution (10 mg).

ACOG Practice Bulletin No. 88, December 2007. Invasive prenatal testing for aneuploidy. *Obstet Gynecol* 2007; 110(6):1459–67

http://www.acog.org/~/media/List of Titles/PBListOfTitles.pdf?dmc=1&ts=20140223T0705285265

Summary of recommendations

- Amniocentesis is not recommended before 15 weeks of gestation due to the high risk of miscarriage and complications.
- Pregnancy loss rate after mid-trimester amniocentesis is less than 1/300–500.
- In experienced centres, pregnancy loss rate after chorionic villus sampling is the same as that of amniocentesis.
- Risk factors for fetal aneuploidy include:
    - One major or at least two minor structural defects on the fetal ultrasound scan

- previous fetus or child with an autosomal trisomy or sex chromosome abnormality
- parental aneuploidy, chromosomal translocation, or chromosomal inversion.

◆ Invasive diagnostic testing to detect aneuploidy should be available to all women.

International Society of Ultrasound in Obstetrics and Gynecology (ISUOG) Practice Guidelines: *Performance of First-Trimester Fetal Ultrasound Scan*, January 2013

http://www.isuog.org/NR/rdonlyres/9225E408-C904-4A7F-84AE-812E456FBDDD/0/ISUOG1stTguidelines2013.pdf

Key points

◆ First-trimester fetal ultrasound scan is performed for the following reasons:
- To confirm viability
- To establish an accurate gestation age
- To determine the number of fetuses
- To assess chorionicity and amnionicity if it is a multiple pregnancy

◆ At the end of first trimester, an ultrasound scan can be used to detect gross fetal abnormalities and to measure nuchal translucency as part of aneuploidy screening.

◆ Many malformations may, however, develop later in pregnancy.

◆ The scan is offered between 11 and 13^{+6} weeks' gestation.

◆ The sonographer should have specialized training that is suitable for the practice of diagnostic ultrasound scans for pregnant women.

◆ B and M mode ultrasound scans are safe for all stages of pregnancy.

◆ The following assessments should be performed during first-trimester ultrasound scans:
- Viability—confirm the presence of an embryo with cardiac activity and the presence of an intrauterine gestational sac.
- Early pregnancy measurements—crown–rump length (CRL) provides a more accurate assessment of gestational age when compared with mean gestational sac diameter.
- First trimester measurements—CRL, biparietal diameter and head circumference are usually measured.
- Fetal anatomy assessments for first trimester are described in the appendices.
- Chromosomal anomaly assessment—Nuchal translucency measurement should be done between 11 and 13^{+6} weeks.

International Society of Ultrasound in Obstetrics and Gynecology (ISUOG) Practice Guidelines: *Performance of Routine Mid-Trimester Fetal Ultrasound Scan*, 2010.

http://www.isuog.org/NR/rdonlyres/EA865840-6CA3-45AC-9E99-FBAF775119A9/0/ISUOGGuidelinesmidtriscan20101210.pdf

Key points

◆ Mid-trimester ultrasound is performed to give accurate diagnostic information to optimize the antenatal care for the mother and fetus.

◆ The following assessments should be made during mid-trimester ultrasound scan:
- Cardiac activity
- Fetal size/age
- Number of fetuses
- Basic fetal anatomy
- Placental appearance and location.

◆ A mid-trimester ultrasound is usually performed between 18 and 22 weeks' gestation.

◆ The sonographer should have specialized training that is suitable for the practice of diagnostic ultrasound scans for pregnant women.

◆ Prenatal ultrasound scans are safe for mothers and fetuses.

◆ Biparietal diameter, head circumference, abdominal circumference, and femur diaphysis length are used to assess gestational age and fetal size.

◆ Amniotic fluid volume can be assessed subjectively or objectively using ultrasonographic measurements.

◆ In the case of multiple pregnancy, the following additional evaluations should be carried out.
- Visualization of placental cord insertion
- Chorionicity
- Distinguishing features (gender, unique markers, and position in uterus).

◆ Recommended minimum requirements for basic mid-trimester fetal anatomical survey are described in the appendices of the guidelines.

Advice from the Health Protection Agency, the Royal College of Radiologists and the College of Radiographers: *Protection of Pregnant Patients During Diagnostic Medical Exposures to Ionizing Radiation*, 2009

http://www.rcr.ac.uk/docs/radiology/pdf/HPA_Diagnostic_Pregnancy.pdf

Key points

◆ The radiation dose from any diagnostic procedure does not pose any significant risk to the mental and physical development of the fetus or death.

◆ Exposure of the fetus to radiation up to 1 milligray gives a childhood cancer risk of less than 1 in 10,000. This is considered to be an acceptable risk.

◆ The risk of childhood cancer is doubled with increasing levels of radiation exposure greater than a few milligrays. As a result, all investigations involving radiation should be avoided in pregnancy. However, if they are necessary or performed inadvertently, the childhood cancer risk remains below 1 in 200.

- Examples of high-dose procedures are barium enema, lumbar spine X-ray and computed tomography (CT), 99mTc bone scan, abdominal CT, and pelvis CT.
- There is a negligible risk of radiation-induced hereditary conditions in the offspring of an unborn child.

ACOG Practice Bulletin 106: *Intrapartum Fetal Heart Rate Monitoring: Nomenclature, Interpretation, and General Management Principles*, July 2009

http://www.acog.org/~/media/List of Titles/PBListOfTitles.pdf?dmc=1&ts=20140228T0623236788

The American College of Obstetricians and Gynecologists has published this guideline to describe the role of intrapartum fetal heart rate monitoring in the decision-making process of obstetric and gynaecology care.

Summary of recommendations

- The use of electronic fetal monitoring (EFM) is associated with an increased rate of instrumental and caesarean delivery.
- EFM has a high false-positive rate for predicting cerebral palsy (>99%) The use of EFM does not reduce the incidence of cerebral palsy.
- When EFM tracing shows recurrent variable decelerations, amnioinfusion should be performed to relieve umbilical cord compression. (Amnioinfusion is a procedure in which a needle is introduced into the uterine cavity under ultrasound guidance and saline is infused to increase the volume of amniotic fluid.)
- Pulse oximetry is not clinically useful for evaluating fetal status.
- Reinterpretation of the FHR tracing, especially if the neonatal outcome is known, may not be reliable.
- A three-tiered system for the categorization of fetal heart rate patterns is recommended. (See 'A Three-Tiered System for the Categorization of Fetal Heart Rate Patterns' in Appendix 2 in this book.)
- High-risk labouring women should be monitored with continuous EFM.

Gastrointestinal

Royal College of Obstetrician and Gynaecologists. *Obstetric Cholestasis*. Green-Top Guideline No. 43, April 2011

https://www.rcog.org.uk/globalassets/documents/guidelines/gtg_43.pdf

Obstetric cholestasis may complicate up to 1.5% of pregnancies, with an increased risk in parturients of Indian and Pakistani-Asian origin. This guideline summarizes the evidence for the fetal risks associated with obstetric cholestasis, which include preterm birth and fetal death.

Key points

- Unexplained pruritus, especially of the palms and soles of the feet, with deranged liver function tests (LFTs), which resolve after delivery, suggests obstetric cholestasis. In suspected cases, LFTs should be repeated every 1–2 weeks in pregnancy and resolution of LFTs confirmed 10 days after delivery.
- Compared with uncomplicated pregnancies, there is an increased risk of neonatal death associated with obstetric cholestasis, though this risk has not been quantified.
- A woman with obstetric cholestasis should be considered 'high risk' and her care and delivery of the baby should be conducted in a hospital by a consultant-led specialist team. Those providing intrapartum care should be aware of the risks of premature delivery, increased risks of passage of meconium, caesarean delivery, and postpartum haemorrhage.
- Continuous fetal monitoring during labour should be used. There is no one specific test or imaging modality, which can reliably predict fetal outcome.
- Regarding delivery, a discussion with the woman about both the maternal and fetal risks associated with induction of labour at 37^{+0} weeks' gestation should take place. In those with severe derangement of LFTs, there may be a stronger case in favour of an early expedited delivery.
- Women should be informed that there is no one test which is able to predict the incidence of stillbirth should the pregnancy continue beyond 37^{+0} weeks.
- There is no evidence that any one specific treatment may affect outcome. Emollient creams and chlorpheniramine may provide maternal symptomatic relief, but are not proven to improve outcome. There is insufficient evidence to recommend the use of S-adenosyl methionine (SAMe); however, ursodeoxycholic acid (UDCA) does appear to improve pruritus and LFTs in women with obstetric cholestasis, but again the maternal and fetal safety data concerning its use is lacking.
- Women with obstetric cholestasis may become deficient in vitamin K so a discussion regarding the use of oral vitamin K supplementation should take place, especially where there is a prolongation of the prothrombin time.
- Follow-up of women postnatally should take place with a liver specialist and the LFTs should be repeated.

NICE. *Antenatal Care: Routine Care for Healthy Pregnant Women*. Clinical Guideline 62, 2008

https://www.nice.org.uk/guidance/cg62/chapter/1-Guidance#management-of-common-symptoms-of-pregnancy

Section 1.4.1 in this guidance covers the symptomatic management of nausea and vomiting in pregnancy.

Key points

- Nausea and vomiting usually resolves spontaneously between 16 and 20 weeks' gestation and is not associated with poor pregnancy outcomes.
- Ginger and the acupuncture pressure point P6 on the wrist are recommended non-pharmacological symptomatic treatments.
- Antihistamines are the recommended pharmacological treatment.

Wegrzyiak LJ, Repke J, Ural SH. Treatment of hyperemesis gravidarum. *Rev Obstet Gynecol* 2012; 5(2):78–84

http://www.ncbi.nlm.nih.gov/pmc/articles/PMC3410506/pdf/RIOG005002_0078.pdf

Hyperemesis is defined as 'uncontrolled vomiting requiring hospitalization, severe dehydration, muscle wasting, electrolyte imbalance, ketonuria, and weight loss of more than 5% of body weight' and complicates between 0.3% and 2.3% of pregnancies. The symptoms are at their worst between 9 and 20 weeks of gestation and 5% of women may require hospital admission for management of hyperemesis and dehydration. Women who suffer from hyperemesis in their first pregnancy have a high risk of suffering from hyperemesis in subsequent pregnancies.

Key points

- Infants born to mothers with hyperemesis are at risk of preterm delivery, small for gestational age, low birth weights, and a 5-minute Apgar score of less than 7.
- The pathogenesis of hyperemesis is not fully understood but may be due to effects of hormones, gastrointestinal dysfunction, thyrotoxicosis, autonomic dysfunction, liver abnormalities, *Helicobacter pylori* infection, or psychosomatic reasons.
- Dietary changes to manage symptoms include reducing meal sizes, increasing protein and carbohydrate intake, drinking electrolyte beverages, and avoiding any known food triggers.
- Affected women should be advised to avoid stress and rest as much as possible. Psychological support may be necessary as the condition may be very debilitating.
- Intravenous fluids may be necessary to treat dehydration. Electrolytes should be monitored and replaced as necessary.
- Thiamine 1.5 mg/day should be given routinely to all women with prolonged vomiting.
- Antiemetics should not be used before 12–14 weeks' gestation due to the possible risk of teratogenicity. First-line treatment, as recommended by the 2004 guidelines produced by the American Congress of Obstetricians and Gynecologists, should be intravenous dimenhydrinate, metoclopramide, or promethazine.
- Droperidol, ondansetron, and methylprednisolone have also been used in the research literature.
- Ginger has also been shown to reduce nausea and vomiting, most likely by increasing gastric motility and decreasing stimuli to the chemoreceptor trigger zone.
- Supplementary feeding via a nasogastric tube or total parental nutrition may need to be considered in severe cases.
- The use of acupuncture at the pressure point P6, which is 5 cm proximal to the wrist crease, has been shown to reduce the incidence of nausea and vomiting, by presumably blocking nociceptive transmission and autonomic reflexes.
- Hypnosis to control autonomic responses has been studied to assess its possible use to manage the symptoms of nausea and vomiting in pregnancy.

NICE. *Hepatitis B (Chronic) Diagnosis and Management of Chronic Hepatitis B in Children, Young People and Adults*. Clinical Guideline 165, 2013

http://www.nice.org.uk/guidance/cg165

Chronic hepatitis B infection is characterized by detection of hepatitis B surface antigen (HBsAg) in the serum for 6 months or longer. It is a condition, which may have a variable clinical presentation which range from no symptoms to the development of liver fibrosis, cirrhosis, and hepatocellular carcinoma. Treatment with antivirals is aimed at preventing these serious complications of chronic hepatitis B infection by reducing the amount of hepatitis B virus (HBV) DNA present in the blood.

With regards to pregnancy and breastfeeding, the guideline advises that tenofovir disoproxil should be offered to women who have HBV DNA levels greater than 10^7 IU/mL in the third trimester to reduce the likelihood of HBV transmission to the fetus.

British Liver Trust Factsheet: *Acute Fatty Liver of Pregnancy*, 2012

http://www.britishlivertrust.org.uk/liver-information/liver-conditions/acute-fatty-liver-of-pregnancy/

Acute fatty liver of pregnancy (AFLP) affects 1/20,000 pregnancies and usually occurs in the third trimester. Risk factors include primiparity, male fetuses, and multiple births. The exact cause of the condition is unknown. Some experts believe it is related to pre-eclampsia whereas others have noted an association with fetal long-chain acyl-CoA dehydrogenase (LCHAD). LCHAD is a rare autosomal recessive condition where unmetabolized fetal free fatty acids are returned via the placenta to the maternal circulation and deposit in the liver.

Key points

- Symptoms of AFLP include nausea and vomiting, abdominal pain, general malaise, jaundice, and excessive thirst.
- The differential diagnosis of AFLP includes acute viral hepatitis, pre-eclampsia, HELLP syndrome, and obstetric cholestasis.
- Blood tests to investigate AFLP include taking LFTs and in particular looking for raised levels of alanine aminotransferase (ALT) and aspartate aminotransferase (AST). In some cases there may also be raised levels of alkaline phosphatase (ALP) and gamma-glutamyl transferase (GGT). Full blood count, urea and electrolytes, clotting screen, glucose, uric acid and lactate dehydrogenase should also be checked.
- Investigations include liver ultrasound, MRI, or CT scan.
- Once diagnosed, the patient should be admitted and the condition monitored with regular blood tests. The mode of delivery will need to be discussed with the patient and may include caesarean delivery.
- After delivery, the woman should continue to be monitored and this may require transfer to a high dependency unit. Complications of AFLP include infection, pancreatitis, liver failure, and death. In severe cases, a liver transplant may be necessary.
- There is a risk that AFLP may recur in future pregnancies, but again this is poorly understood.

Ko HH, Yoshida E. Acute fatty liver of pregnancy. *Can J Gastroenterol* 2006; 20(1):25–30.

http://www.ncbi.nlm.nih.gov/pmc/articles/PMC2538964/

AFLP is a condition with an incidence of 1/10,000 to 1/15,000 pregnancies and is characterized by microvesicular fatty infiltration of hepatocytes without any evidence of inflammation or necrosis. It has a maternal mortality rate of 75% and fetal mortality rate of 85%. With prompt diagnosis and treatment, these rates may be reduced to 18% and 23% respectively. The mainstay of treatment is supportive with expedited delivery of the fetus.

Key points

- The condition may present between 28 and 40 weeks of gestation, typically occurring at 35–36 weeks.
- Patients may present with a variety of vague symptoms such as anorexia, malaise, nausea, headache, and abdominal pain, which makes the diagnosis of AFLP difficult. Consistent clinical findings suggestive of the condition include fever and jaundice. In severe cases, patients may present with signs of multiorgan involvement including renal failure, pancreatitis, encephalopathy, and gastrointestinal bleeding. Women may also have concomitant pre-eclampsia and HELLP syndrome. Due to the vague symptoms, AFLP is sometimes a diagnosis of exclusion.
- A maternal metabolic acidosis may develop as a result of AFLP, which in turn could adversely affect the fetus. Correction of this acidosis will help fetal well-being but early delivery may be indicated.
- Laboratory findings of AFLP include the following:
  - Raised white blood cell count greater than 15×10^9/L
  - Normal haematocrit except in the presence of haemorrhage
  - Haemolysis
  - Thrombocytopaenia
  - Prolonged prothrombin time and partial thromboplastic time
  - Low fibrinogen level
  - Disseminated intravascular coagulation
  - Raised serum aminotransferases (ALT and AST)
  - Raised ammonia, amino acid level, lactic acidosis, uric acid, bilirubin as a sign of liver failure
  - Hypoglycaemia
  - Raised ALP—however, this may normally occur in women in the third trimester
  - Raised urea and creatinine levels as a sign of renal failure.
- Investigation of the condition using liver ultrasound and CT scanning to identify fatty infiltration of the liver has low sensitivity and specificity. However, wider availability of laboratory testing for viral hepatitis and other serum markers of AFLP have made the need for liver biopsy less critical for the diagnosis to be made.
- Once the diagnosis of AFLP has been made, the mother should be admitted and resuscitated accordingly. This may require admission to intensive care. Fetal assessment during resuscitation and correction of coagulation abnormalities needs to also take place.
- Once the mother has been stabilized, delivery of the fetus needs to be arranged. Vaginal delivery may be considered in uncomplicated cases but caesarean delivery may be needed in the more serious cases.
- Postpartum, the woman should be closely monitored as coagulation defects and haemorrhage remains a risk, as does hypoglycaemia.
- Pancreatitis may complicate AFLP, especially after hepatic and renal dysfunction.
- Liver transplantation may be needed in cases of fulminant liver failure which has failed to respond to resuscitation and delivery of the fetus.

Riely CA. Liver disease in the pregnant patient. *Am J Gastroenterol* 1999; 94(7):1728–32

http://s3.gi.org/physicians/guidelines/LiverDiseaseinPregnantPatient.pdf

These clinical guidelines have been developed in association with the American College of Gastroenterology. ALP usually rises in the third trimester, however the rest of the LFTs remain unchanged by pregnancy. Therefore any changes in LFTs other than ALP warrant further investigation.

Key points

- Liver diseases which may occur in pregnancy depend on the gestation:
  - *First trimester*—hyperemesis gravidarum which in extreme cases require intravenous fluids and resuscitation. Peptic ulcer disease and acute viral hepatitis needs to be excluded
  - *Second trimester*—pre-eclampsia, variceal bleeding in associated with portal hypertension, acute viral hepatitis, obstetric cholestasis
  - *Third trimester*—pre-eclampsia, acute viral hepatitis which tends to be worse in the third trimester, AFLP, HELLP
- Other disorders which affect the liver may occur coincidentally with pregnancy:
  - Viral or drug-induced hepatitis
  - Gallstones
  - Malignancy with metastases to the liver
  - Thrombosis of outflow tracts of the liver (e.g. Budd–Chiari syndrome)
  - Chronic hepatitis B or C—there is no increased risk to the mother, however transmission to the fetus may occur.

Alcohol intake in pregnancy

NICE guidance to the consumption of alcohol during pregnancy is contained in the NICE antenatal care guideline CG62 (https://www.nice.org.uk/guidance/cg62).

Key points

- Women who are planning to become pregnant or who may be pregnant should avoid alcohol in the first trimester due to the increased risk of miscarriage.
- Although there is uncertainty regarding the amount of alcohol which may be safely consumed during pregnancy, women who choose to continue to drink alcohol should limit the amount to 1–2 units per week.
- Pregnant women should avoid getting drunk or binge drinking (consumption of >7.5 units in one sitting) to avoid harm to the fetus.
- 1 small glass of wine = 1.5 units.
- 5 small glasses of wine = 7.5 units.

Food intake in labour

NICE. *Intrapartum Care: Care of Healthy Women and their Babies During Childbirth* (Section 4.4: Eating and Drinking in Labour). Clinical Guidance 190, December 2014

http://www.nice.org.uk/guidance/cg190/resources/guidance-intrapartum-care-care-of-healthy-women-and-their-babies-during-childbirth-pdf

- Women in established labour are allowed to drink as long as there are no complications.
- Isotonic drinks may be consumed instead of water in labour.
- If no opioids have been offered and there are no risk factors suggesting a likely operative delivery, a low-risk woman may be allowed to eat in labour.

OAA Clinical Guideline: *Oral Intake in Labour*, 2014

http://www.oaa-anaes.ac.uk/ui/content/content.aspx?id=187

- Selected guideline examples from two NHS trusts are shared on the OAA website.
- Low-risk women may take clear fluids and eat a light diet during labour.
- High-risk women may drink clear fluid in labour, but they should not eat solid food.
- Factors, which constitute high-risk pregnancy, vary marginally in the different trust (hospital) guidelines.
- Examples of high-risk factors are morbid obesity, multiple pregnancy, previous caesarean delivery or uterine scar, pre-eclampsia, diabetes mellitus, breech presentation, slow progress, oxytocin infusion, and signs of fetal distress.

American Society of Anesthesiologists task force on obstetric anesthesia. practice guidelines for obstetric anaesthesia. *Anesthesiology* 2007; 106:843–63

- Low-risk labouring women are allowed to drink clear liquids. For those undergoing an elective caesarean delivery, modest amounts of clear liquids can be allowed up to 2 hours before the induction of anaesthesia.
- Solid foods should be avoided in labouring patients. For elective surgical patients, solid food is allowed up to 6–8 hours before the induction of anaesthesia.

Aspiration prophylaxis

NICE. *Intrapartum Care: Care of Healthy Women and their Babies During Childbirth* (Section 4.4: Eating and Drinking in Labour). Clinical Guidance 190, December 2014

http://www.nice.org.uk/guidance/cg190/resources/guidance-intrapartum-care-care-of-healthy-women-and-their-babies-during-childbirth-pdf

- H_2 antagonists and antacids should only be offered to parturients who have received opioid analgesia in labour or have developed risk factors which make a general anaesthetic more likely. They should not be offered as routine to otherwise low-risk parturients.

OAA Clinical Guideline: *Antacid Prophylaxis*, 2010

http://www.oaa-anaes.ac.uk/ui/content/content.aspx?id=168

- Selected guideline examples from two NHS trusts are shared on the OAA website.
- H_2 receptor antagonists (e.g. ranitidine 150 mg to 300 mg orally or 50 mg intravenously) should be given to all elective surgery patients, emergency surgery patients and high-risk women in labour.
- Sodium citrate 30 mL 0.3M should be given orally, before induction of general anaesthesia for emergency surgery.

American Society of Anesthesiologists task force on obstetric anesthesia. practice guidelines for obstetric anaesthesia. *Anesthesiology* 2007; 106:843–63

- Administration of non-particulate antacids, H_2 receptor antagonists, and/or metoclopramide for aspiration prophylaxis is recommended before surgical procedures.

Haematological

Royal College of Obstetricians and Gynaecologists. *Antepartum Haemorrhage*. Green-Top Guideline No. 63, November 2011

https://www.rcog.org.uk/globalassets/documents/guidelines/gtg_63.pdf

Antepartum haemorrhage (APH) is one which occurs between 24 weeks of pregnancy and delivery. The most important causes of APH are placenta praevia and placental abruption. Management of APH is important, as it is responsible for 50% of maternal deaths worldwide as well as being a cause of preterm labour in 20% of cases with subsequent neonatal morbidity. This guideline is restricted to the management of antepartum haemorrhage.

Key points

- Due to multifactorial causes, APH itself cannot be reliably predicted.
- If a woman has had a placental abruption in a previous pregnancy, she is at increased risk of further abruption in subsequent pregnancies. Other risk factors for placental abruption include pre-eclampsia, increasing maternal age, intrauterine infections, multiple pregnancy, and fetal growth restriction. A comprehensive list of risk factors is included in the document.
- There is an increased risk of bleeding later in pregnancy if it has occurred in the first trimester.

- Evidence suggests that the causes of placental abruption are related to conditions, which develop during pregnancy whereas factors which lead to placenta praevia tend to exist prior to pregnancy.
- Risk factors for placenta praevia are strongly related to the number of previous caesarean deliveries and also include advanced maternal age and smoking.
- Women should report all episodes of vaginal bleeding in pregnancy to their antenatal care providers.
- APH should be suspected if the woman complains of continuous abdominal pain and the uterus feels tense on palpation. If the pain is intermittent in nature, then labour should be suspected.
- In cases of suspected placenta praevia, an ultrasound scan should be performed first to rule out the diagnosis before performing a digital examination of the vagina.
- Investigations to assess APH include Kleihauer blood test, coagulation screen, full blood count, cross match of 4 units, ultrasound scan to determine placental location and cardiotocograph monitoring of the fetus.
- Women with bleeding heavier than spotting or streaking should be admitted to hospital for observation and further management.
- If a woman presents with APH after 24 weeks of gestation and before 35 weeks, a course of antenatal steroids should be given.
- Tocolytics are not advised for use in patients who present with a major APH and are clinically unstable or there is evidence of fetal distress.
- If fetal death occurs following an APH, where possible, vaginal delivery is recommended.
- A caesarean delivery is recommended if there is evidence of fetal distress.
- Where possible, a neuraxial anaesthetic technique should be performed to facilitate operative delivery. A consultant anaesthetist should be present in the management of unstable patients. A general anaesthetic may be considered in very unstable patients for caesarean delivery.
- A woman who has suffered an APH is at risk of postpartum haemorrhage. Provisions should be made to manage and observe the woman after delivery.
- Coagulopathy needs to be managed with the replacement of clotting factors and by seeking advice from haematologists.

Royal College of Obstetricians and Gynaecologists. *Prevention and Management of Postpartum Haemorrhage*. Green-Top Guideline No. 52, April 2011

https://www.rcog.org.uk/globalassets/documents/guidelines/gt52postpartumhaemorrhage0411.pdf

Primary postpartum haemorrhage (PPH) is defined as 'the loss of 500 mL of blood or more from the genital tract within 24 hours of delivery' and is the most common form of major obstetric haemorrhage. It remains one of the major causes of maternal deaths globally. This guideline is limited to the management of PPH.

Key points

- Minor PPH—blood loss of 500–1000 mL.
- Major PPH—blood loss of greater than 1000 mL and can be further subdivided into:
  - moderate—blood loss of 1000–2000 mL
  - severe—blood loss of greater than 2000 mL.
- Once a PPH has been identified, the patient must be monitored and assessed for signs of haemodynamic instability and ongoing bleeding and appropriate protocol-driven management must begin.
- Most women suffering a PPH do not have any identifiable risk factors.
- Active management of the third stage of labour and the use of prophylactic oxytocics (e.g. oxytocin 5 or 10 IU IM), can reduce the risk of PPH.
- A multidisciplinary team including a senior obstetrician, anaesthetist, haematologist, and senior midwife will need to be involved in the management of a PPH.
- Once identified, there are four components to the management of PPH, which need to occur simultaneously: communication, resuscitation, monitoring and investigation, and arresting the bleeding. If large amounts of fluids have been used in resuscitation, a coagulopathy is likely to develop. Replacement of clotting factors and fibrinogen will need to be considered. Recombinant factor VIIa, although not widely advocated, could be considered as a potential treatment following discussion with a haematologist—there is a risk of thrombosis associated with its use.
- If anaesthesia is required, the anaesthetist will need to assess the woman for haemodynamic instability and provide the most appropriate anaesthetic as necessary. Haemodynamic instability is a relative contraindication to neuraxial anaesthesia.
- Uterine atony is the most common cause of PPH. Other causes include coagulation abnormalities, retained tissues, and trauma to the genital tract.
- Uterine atony may be managed by a variety of pharmacological methods using oxytocin, ergometrine, carboprost, and misoprostol. See guideline for full dosing regimen.
- Surgical methods to manage uterine atony include balloon tamponade, brace suturing, bilateral ligation of uterine or internal iliac arteries, and selective arterial embolization.
- Hysterectomy must be considered early on in the management of PPH and a second consultant obstetrician or gynaecologist should be consulted in the decision to proceed with one.
- Secondary PPH is usually associated with endometritis. Antibiotics (ampicillin and metronidazole with gentamicin in certain circumstances) and surgical removal of retained products of conception need to be considered in the management of secondary PPH.

Royal College of Obstetricians and Gynaecologists. *Placenta Praevia, Placenta Accreta and Vasa Praevia: Diagnosis and Management*. Green-Top Guideline No. 27, January 2011

https://www.rcog.org.uk/globalassets/documents/guidelines/gtg_27.pdf

Placenta praevia and accreta are significant causes of maternal and fetal morbidity and mortality. The rising rate of caesarean deliveries, in combination with increasing maternal age, means that the incidence of these conditions is going to increase. This guideline covers the diagnosis as well as the antepartum and peripartum management of these conditions.

Key points

- Placenta praevia is the condition where the placenta has implanted wholly or in part in the lower segment of the uterus.
- Placenta accreta, increta, and percreta are types of morbidly adherent placenta and describe the extent of the invasion of the myometrium by the placenta.
- Vasa praevia describes the condition where fetal blood vessels penetrate through the membranes and appear below the presenting part of the fetus. These vessels are fully exposed, and not protected by any placental tissue or umbilical cord. It has an incidence of about 1/2000 to 1/6000 pregnancies. The main risks are to the fetus, as these vessels are at risk of rupture and catastrophic haemorrhage following fetal membrane rupture, with a mortality rate of about 60%.
- Placenta praevia should be suspected in women presenting with vaginal bleeding after 20 weeks' gestation. This can then be confirmed with ultrasound scanning to determine the placental location. A transvaginal scan is more accurate than a transabdominal scan.
- Should the placenta be found to cover or overlap the cervical os at the 20-week scan, the patient should be followed up to determine the final location of the placenta closer to the time of delivery.
- In women who have had a previous caesarean delivery, the placental location should be determined to assess the risk of a morbidly adherent placenta developing.
- Any antenatal anaemia should be treated and women should be counselled about the risks of preterm delivery and major obstetric haemorrhage. Outpatient care may be suitable for women with minor placenta praevia or who are otherwise asymptomatic.
- If the placenta is more than 2 cm from the cervical os, then a vaginal delivery may be considered. Elective caesarean delivery may be considered after 38 weeks for placenta praevia and between 36 and 37 weeks for a suspected morbidly adherent placenta.
- Thorough preparation involving both consultant obstetric and anaesthetic care along with availability of blood products must be in place prior to delivery. The use of cell salvage may also be considered.
- The choice of anaesthetic is determined by the anaesthetist managing the case. There is insufficient evidence to recommend either anaesthetic technique (i.e. neuraxial block or general anaesthesia).
- When performing the caesarean delivery, it is worth considering making the uterine incision at a site away from the placenta to reduce the risk of bleeding and to allow further assessment of the placenta to then guide further management.
- Women must be warned of the risk of a hysterectomy following delivery of the baby.
- Should the placenta not separate after the delivery of the baby, one strategy would be to leave the placenta *in situ*. In these cases, women must be warned of the risks of infection and bleeding. Prophylactic antibiotics may be given to minimize the risk.
- At present, there are no recommendations to screen routinely for vasa praevia.
- Colour transvaginal Doppler ultrasound may be used to confirm the diagnosis in suspected cases of vasa praevia.
- A caesarean delivery should be performed to deliver the baby if bleeding occurs in a woman with known vasa praevia.

Royal College of Obstetricians and Gynaecologists. *Blood Transfusion in Obstetrics*. Green-Top Guideline No. 47, May 2015

https://www.rcog.org.uk/globalassets/documents/guidelines/gtg-47.pdf

There are many conditions in obstetrics which may require the need for a blood transfusion. Inappropriate management of haemorrhage may be associated with maternal morbidity and mortality. It is accepted that a blood transfusion itself is not without risks, therefore strict procedures and checking policies should be followed, even in an emergency.

Key points

- During antenatal screening, a haemoglobin (Hb) level less than 10.5 g/dL must be investigated and treated. Oral iron supplementation is the first-line treatment, with parenteral iron use in those patients unable to tolerate or comply with oral therapy.
- Blood loss at delivery must be minimized. One way of achieving this is to actively manage the third stage.
- Women who are at high risk of a peripartum haemorrhage, must be encouraged to deliver in hospital.
- All women should have their blood group and antibodies checked routinely at booking and at 28 weeks' gestation.
- Ensure that a parturient has a valid cross-match sample on the day of delivery.
- Elective use of cell salvage may be considered in cases where blood loss is expected to be greater than 1500 mL.
- The decision to transfuse blood must be made on both clinical and haematological grounds. Patients with Hb greater than 10 g/dL should not be transfused, whereas those with Hb less than 6 g/dL almost always require transfusion.
- FFP, platelets, and cryoprecipitate may be needed in the management of coagulopathy and their use should be given on

clinical grounds rather than waiting for formal coagulation screen results.

- Platelets should not be allowed to fall below 50×10^9/L, so it is advisable to transfuse a pool of platelets when levels fall to 75×10^9/L.
- Anti-D immunoglobulin will need to be given to a Rhesus-negative woman if the platelets are Rhesus positive.
- There is no evidence to support the prophylactic use of recombinant factor VIIa in caesarean delivery, but its use may be considered when managing major haemorrhage.
- Transfusion should be considered in the peripartum period if the Hb is about 7–8 g/dL. The decision to transfuse should be based on symptoms and clinical examination.
- In women who object to receiving a blood transfusion, their Hb must be optimized as much as possible in the antepartum period and appropriate planning for delivery should be made.

AAGBI Safety Guideline: *Blood Transfusion and the Anaesthetist: Management of Massive Haemorrhage*, November 2010

http://www.aagbi.org/sites/default/files/massive_haemorrhage_2010_0.pdf

This guideline is described under 'Critical Care and Resuscitation'.

Lee CA, Chi C, Pavord SR. The obstetric and gynaecological management of women with inherited bleeding disorders—review with guidelines produced by a taskforce of UK haemophilia centre doctors' Organisation. *Haemophilia* 2006; 12:301–36

http://onlinelibrary.wiley.com/doi/10.1111/j.1365-2516.2006.01314.x/full

This article summarizes the evidence around the obstetric and anaesthetic management of women with coagulation disorders who become pregnant. The main conditions of haemophilia, von Willebrand's disease (vWD), and factor XI deficiency are covered.

Haemophilia

- All carriers of haemophilia should be offered prepregnancy counselling in order to discuss the options regarding conception methods and prenatal diagnosis (grade C evidence, level IV).
- Chorionic villus sampling should be used to test for haemophilia in the fetus antenatally. Maternal clotting should be tested before the procedure is carried out (grade C evidence, level IV).
- It is important to determine the fetal gender as early as possible: if the fetus is female, the need for further invasive testing is avoided. If the fetus is male, then invasive fetal monitoring, forceps, and vacuum extraction should be avoided, unless the coagulation status of the fetus is known to be normal. The parents need to be informed of the need to determine fetal gender early in pregnancy (grade C evidence, level IV).
- Known carriers of haemophilia should have their clotting factors (VIII and IX) checked at booking, and 28 and 34 weeks' gestation to help determine the most appropriate mode of delivery and to anticipate any treatment which may be needed (grade C evidence, level IV).
- Recombinant factor VIII and IX is the treatment of choice in pregnant carriers of haemophilia A and B (grade C evidence, level IV).
- Neuraxial blocks for labour and delivery are permitted if the coagulation screen is normal and the relevant factor level is above 50 IU/dL. The procedure should be performed by an experienced anaesthetist and the density and duration of the anaesthetic block should be monitored. Any abnormal prolongation in anaesthetic blockade must be investigated by MRI to exclude an epidural haematoma.
- The use of NSAIDs should be avoided if the clotting factors are below normal (grade C evidence, level IV).
- The use of a fetal scalp electrode should be avoided in male fetuses known to be affected or who have an unknown coagulation status (grade C evidence, level IV).
- Factor levels should be monitored and kept above 50 IU/dL for 3 days after vaginal delivery and for 5 days after caesarean delivery.
- In neonates with known haemophilia or unknown coagulation status, IM injections and venepuncture should be avoided. Vitamin K may be given orally, with routine immunizations given subcutaneously or intradermally. Circumcision should be delayed until the coagulation status of the neonate is known and any treatment reviewed by the haematologist (grade C evidence, level IV).
- The risk of intracranial haemorrhage is estimated to be about 1–4% and is associated with significant morbidity. A cranial ultrasound or CT scan should be arranged in all neonates where labour has been premature, traumatic, or if there is any evidence of bleeding. Treatment should be given to raise plasma clotting levels to 100 IU/dL (grade C evidence, level IV).

Von Willebrand disease

- Prenatal diagnosis should be offered to and discussed with women with vWD, where there is an identifiable genetic mutation (grade C evidence, level IV).
- Patients with vWD should have the following factors checked at booking, and 28 and 32 weeks' gestation: vWF:Ag, vWF:AC and FVIII:C and the levels should be kept above 50 IU/dL for any invasive procedures or delivery (grade C evidence, level IV).
- Desmopressin increases FVIII and vWF levels and may be used in pregnancy. However repeated doses and its use in pre-eclampsia should be avoided. Women need to be monitored for the possibility of fluid retention after its administration (grade C evidence, level IV).
- Patients with vWD type 1 do not require any prophylactic treatment for delivery. Those with vWD type 2 only need treatment for operative delivery or in cases of perineal trauma. Only patients with vWD type 3 need treatment for all modes of delivery (grade C evidence, level IV).

- An epidural may be sited in patients with vWD type 1 whose vWF activity is above 50 IU/dL. It is not recommended in women with vWD types 2 and 3 (grade C evidence, level IV).
- Women with a vWF activity level below 50 IU/dL should receive prophylactic treatment before the onset of labour and planned caesarean delivery (grade C evidence, level IV).
- VWF activity and FVIII levels should be maintained above 50 IU/dL and monitored for 3 days after vaginal delivery and for 5 days after caesarean delivery. Tranexamic acid may be considered in the management of any prolonged or intermittent postpartum haemorrhage (grade C evidence, level IV).
- Invasive monitoring, vacuum extraction, and the use of rotational or mid-cavity forceps should be avoided in all fetuses at risk of vWD, except in those with mild disease. The cord blood should be sent off for analysis (grade C evidence, level IV).

Factor XI deficiency

- Factor XI deficiency is inherited in an autosomal fashion and exhibits a more variable bleeding tendency compared with haemophilia A and B. Efforts should be made to identify the individual's bleeding tendency and the existence of any confounding factors (grade C evidence, level IV).
- Factor XI levels should be checked at booking, and 28 and 32 weeks' gestation. Management may be expectant ('watch and wait'). Only patients with very low levels or a positive bleeding history should be given prophylactic treatment with FXI concentrate or virally inactivated FFP to cover any invasive procedures (grade C evidence, level IV).
- To minimize the risk of a haematoma, an epidural may be sited following consultation with a haematologist who may advocate the administration of FXI concentrate. An epidural should be avoided in women with severe disease or a significant bleeding history.
- Where given, prophylactic treatment should be continued for 3 days after vaginal delivery and for 5 days after caesarean delivery (grade C evidence, level IV).

NICE. *Sickle Cell Acute Painful Episode: Management of an Acute Painful Sickle Cell Episode in Hospital.* Clinical Guideline 143, June 2012

https://www.nice.org.uk/guidance/cg143

Sickle cell disease affects about 12,500 to 15,000 people in the United Kingdom. Acute painful sickle cell episodes (or painful crises) may be unpredictable in nature and vary in duration. They result from the blockage of small blood vessels by sickle-shaped red blood cells. The management of these painful crises are a source of complaints in hospitals, as patients may experience long delays in analgesia, inadequate analgesia, and accusations of drug-seeking behaviour. This guideline aims to detail the principles of management in hospital.

Key points

- An acute, painful sickle cell episode should be regarded as a medical emergency and analgesia should be offered within 30 minutes of arrival in hospital. The patient and their family should be involved in the management of the crisis from the outset.
- Simple analgesics such as paracetamol and NSAIDs should be offered in addition to opioids. Discussion with the patient regarding previous analgesic management should occur to help guide management. Pethidine should not be given in an acute episode.
- Other causes of acute pain should be looked for and excluded when assessing a patient presenting with an acute crisis.
- The patient should have basic observations recorded and the effectiveness of pain relief documented. A patient-controlled analgesia may be needed, especially if the patient is requiring frequent doses of strong opioids.
- Antiemetics, laxatives, and antipruritics should be offered to those patients on opioids.
- As the crisis resolves, the analgesia regimen may need to be reduced and each hospital should have local protocols to guide how this may be done.
- Corticosteroids should not be used in the treatment of uncomplicated acute painful sickle cell episodes.
- On discharge, patients and carers should be given information about how to manage the current episode, where to seek help and support, when to return to hospital, and any side effects or possible complications that may develop from any treatment they have received.

NICE. *Venous Thromboembolism in Adults Admitted to Hospital: Reducing the Risks.* Clinical Guidance 92, January 2010

https://www.nice.org.uk/guidance/cg92

Assessing the risk of venous thromboembolism and bleeding

- A venous thromboembolism (VTE) assessment must be done for all patients on admission.
- Medical patients who have reduced mobility for more than 3 days and have risk factors are at increased risk of VTE.
- Surgical and trauma patients have an increased of VTE if they have prolonged surgery, reduced mobility, intra-abdominal pathology, or risk factors.
- Risk factors for VTE include age of patient, dehydration, and medical comorbidities. See the guidelines for a full comprehensive list.
- The bleeding risk must be evaluated before the patient is offered pharmacological thromboprophylaxis.
- The bleeding and VTE risks must be reassessed within 24 hours of admission and whenever the clinical condition changes.
- The risk of VTE may be reduced through the use of pharmacological prophylaxis until the patient is no longer at risk and by encouraging mobilization when it is safe to do so.
- Patient and carer education regarding prevention and treatment of VTE should begin before discharge planning.
- Pregnant women or women who have delivered in the preceding 6 weeks should be offered VTE prophylaxis if they are at

increased risk of developing VTE. See guidelines for maternal risk factors for VTE.

AAGBI, OAA, Regional Anaesthesia UK Guidance Document: *Regional Anaesthesia and Patients with Abnormalities of Coagulation* (RAPAC), 2011

http://www.aagbi.org/sites/default/files/rapac_2013_web.pdf

This consensus document offers guidance regarding the performance of neuraxial blocks in patients who are taking medication to alter their coagulation and their recommendations are summarized in four tables within the document.

Key points

- The time needed to wait before performing a block is dependent on the anticoagulant used (see tables in guideline for further details).
- In a patient with altered coagulation, central neuraxial blocks pose a higher risk compared to a superficial nerve block.
- The more abnormal the coagulation, the higher the risk of post-procedure complications. It is advisable that an anaesthetist who has experience in performing the block undertakes the procedure in these high-risk patients.
- Coagulation may be abnormal in trauma, sepsis, uraemia, liver failure, massive transfusion, and disseminated intravascular coagulopathy. Further assessment is needed before performing a block in such situations.

Gogarten W, Vandermeulen E, Van Ake H, *et al.* Regional anaesthesia and antithrombotic agents: recommendations of the European Society of Anaesthesiology. *Eur J Anaesthesiol* 2010; 27:999–1015

http://www.csen.com/guidelines.pdf

This guideline was produced to minimize the risk of bleeding complications associated with neuraxial anaesthesia techniques.

Recommended minimum time intervals between antithrombotic drugs and neuraxial procedures are the same as the RAPAC guideline for commonly used drugs such as prophylactic unfractionated heparin (UFH), prophylactic and treatment doses of LMWH, and aspirin.

Horlocker T, Wedel DJ, Rowlingson JC, *et al.* Regional anesthesia in the patient receiving antithrombotic or thrombolytic therapy: American Society of Regional Anesthesia and Pain Medicine Evidence-Based Guidelines (Third Edition). *Reg Anesth Pain Med* 2010; 35(1):64–101

http://journals.lww.com/rapm/Fulltext/2010/01000/Regional_Anesthesia_in_the_Patient_Receiving.13.aspx

This guideline describes the neuraxial anaesthetic management of surgical patients who are receiving common antithrombotic drugs and herbal medicines such as garlic, ginkgo, and ginseng.

Key points

- In obstetric patients, oral anticoagulants should be changed to LMWH or UFH of similar dosing before 36 weeks' gestation.
- LMWH should be stopped 36 hours before the planned induction of labour or caesarean delivery. Intravenous or subcutaneous UFH can be used as a bridging therapy if necessary. UFH must be stopped 4–6 hours before the planned delivery.
- If a pregnant woman on LMWH goes into labour, she should be instructed to stop the drug until she has been assessed by the obstetric team.
- A plan must be made for restarting anticoagulation in the postpartum period when planning neuraxial analgesia or anaesthesia.
- Re-initiation of thromboprophylaxis should be withheld for 12 hours after abdominal delivery or removal of the epidural catheter, whichever is later. If the patient requires therapeutic anticoagulation, it must be started 24 hours after delivery. (NB These timings differ from THE AAGBI and OAA RAPAC guidelines discussed earlier.)

Royal College of Obstetricians and Gynaecologists. *Reducing the Risk of Venous Thromboembolism During Pregnancy and the Puerperium.* Green-Top Guideline No. 37a, April 2015

https://www.rcog.org.uk/globalassets/documents/guidelines/gtg-37a.pdf

VTE is a preventable cause of morbidity and mortality in the parturient. Effective thromboprophylaxis can markedly reduce the risk of developing VTE in this population. VTE may occur at any stage during pregnancy, but the highest risk remains in the postpartum period.

Key points

- VTE is more likely to occur following a caesarean delivery compared with a vaginal delivery, but the risk of VTE remains regardless of the mode of delivery.
- Once risk assessed, VTE prophylaxis should be started as early in the pregnancy as is practical.
- Women who are considered at very high risk of VTE will usually be on long-term oral anticoagulation prior to conception. They should be counselled about the teratogenic risks to the fetus from oral anticoagulants, such as warfarin. They require treatment with higher-dose LMWH (usually divided into two 12-hourly doses) during pregnancy and 6 weeks postpartum or until they are converted back to their oral regimen. They will also need specialized care provided by haematologists and obstetricians throughout pregnancy and delivery. In certain situations, such as mechanical heart valves, it may be necessary to continue with oral anticoagulants throughout pregnancy.
- Women at high risk of VTE require treatment with LMWH during pregnancy and for 6 weeks postpartum. This includes women who have had previous VTE (excluding VTE as a result from major surgery).
- Women with inherited thrombophilia which have resulted in the development of a VTE should be managed by specialists with knowledge of haemostasis in pregnancy, who may consider monitoring anti-Xa levels and consider antithrombin replacement prior to delivery.

- The guideline contains more details regarding management of specific inherited and acquired thrombophilias.
- Thrombophilia screening should be offered to women who have had a non-oestrogen-provoked VTE in the presence of a minor risk factor, as this will determine further antenatal management and treatment.
- Women with an asymptomatic inherited thrombophilia and no other risk factors may be monitored for VTE during pregnancy and be offered LMWH for at least 7 days postpartum.
- A neuraxial anaesthetic technique should not be performed within 12 hours of a prophylactic dose of LMWH or within 24 hours of a treatment dose of LMWH. Suitable analgesic alternatives should be offered to these women in labour.
- A prophylactic dose of LMWH may be given at least 4 hours after a central neuraxial block or removal of an epidural catheter.
- The first prophylactic dose of LMWH should be given as soon as possible after delivery as long as there is no haemorrhage and no neuraxial anaesthetic technique was used.
- LMWHs are as safe and effective as UFH. Danaparoid and fondaparinux may be considered as alternatives in women who are intolerant of LMWHs, following consultation with a haematologist.
- Low-dose aspirin may be used safely in pregnancy to manage antiphospholipid syndrome but it is not advised for use as thromboprophylaxis in pregnancy.
- Graduated compression stockings may be considered for use in women as thromboprophylaxis where treatment with LMWH or an alternative is contraindicated, after a caesarean delivery, or if they are at high risk of developing VTE.
- Each woman should be risk assessed for VTE in the postpartum period. The duration of treatment may range from 10 days to 6 weeks after delivery depending on the number of risk factors present.
- Women with a BMI greater than 40 kg/m^2 should be offered prophylactic LMWH at an appropriate dose for their weight for 10 days after delivery.
- Following caesarean delivery, all women should be risk assessed to identify those who will require prophylactic LMWH for 10 days postpartum.

Royal College of Obstetricians and Gynaecologists. *Thromboembolic Disease in Pregnancy and the Puerperium: Acute Management*. Green-Top Guideline No. 37b, April 2015

https://www.rcog.org.uk/globalassets/documents/guidelines/gtg-37b.pdf

Venous thromboembolism (VTE) continues to be the main cause of direct maternal deaths during the latest Confidential Enquiries review (2009–2012). Although it is known that pregnant women are at particularly high risk of developing VTE, especially in the puerperium, the subjective clinical assessment of these patients can be unreliable. This guideline offers an evidence-based approach to the investigation and management of women where VTE is suspected.

Key points

- If VTE is clinically suspected, all women should have investigations arranged promptly and LMWH started until the diagnosis has been excluded.
- Leg elevation and compression stockings should be advised in addition to LMWH for the treatment of VTE.
- Compression duplex ultrasound is the first-choice investigation for VTE in the lower leg. Should the scan be negative and clinical suspicion is low, then LMWH may be discontinued. If the scan is inconclusive, it should be repeated on days 3 and 7 and LMWH continued until the diagnosis has been excluded.
- If iliac vein thrombosis is suspected, magnetic resonance venography or contrast venography may be considered instead of duplex ultrasound.
- Where an acute pulmonary embolus (PE) is suspected, a chest X-ray should be performed in the first instance. Where this is normal, a duplex scan should be performed. Should both these tests be negative and the patient still has clinical signs suggestive of a PE, either a ventilation-perfusion (V/Q) scan or a computed tomography pulmonary angiography (CTPA) scan should be performed. LMWH should be continued until the diagnosis has been excluded.
- Compared with CTPA, there is a slightly increased risk of childhood cancer with V/Q scanning but a reduced maternal risk of developing breast cancer.
- Should a patient have symptoms of both PE and deep vein thrombosis, then duplex scan should initially be performed. If this scan is positive, then no further tests are necessary and appropriate treatment should be started.
- Due to physiological changes in coagulation during pregnancy, especially in the later stages and the immediate postpartum period, performing a D-dimer test to exclude a VTE is not advisable as it is likely to be raised.
- Prior to starting anticoagulation therapy, baseline bloods should be taken, including full blood count, urea and electrolytes, liver function tests, and coagulation screen. It is not necessary to perform a thrombophilia screen.
- If treatment with LMWH is required, the daily dose should be based on either the booking or the most recent body weight. LMWH does not cross the placenta nor does it increase the risk of severe bleeding in the peripartum period.
- Anti-Xa levels to monitor the effect of LMWH should only be performed in women at the extremes of weight (<50 kg or >90 kg).
- A multidisciplinary approach must be taken when managing a life-threatening PE. Treatment with intravenous UFH should be started with consideration given to thrombolysis, thoracotomy, or surgical embolectomy.
- An inferior vena cava filter should be considered for women who have either an iliac VTE, are at risk of a PE or who continue to develop a PE despite adequate anticoagulation.
- Once the diagnosis of VTE has been confirmed, treatment with LMWH should continue for the duration of pregnancy.

Presently it is not certain whether the daily dose should be given as a single dose or divided into two doses. Women should have their platelet count monitored for 14 days after starting therapeutic LMWH to monitor for thrombocytopaenia. Due to adverse effects on the fetus, it is not advisable to use oral anticoagulants in pregnancy.

- Newer agents (e.g. fondaparinux) may be considered in patients who have an adverse reaction to all forms of heparin or danaparoid.
- Once a woman is in established labour, no further doses of LMWH should be given. For planned deliveries, LMWH should be stopped 24 hours prior to delivery and neuraxial anaesthesia.
- After a caesarean delivery, LMWH should be restarted 3 hours later or more than 4 hours of epidural catheter removal. The epidural catheter should only be removed more than 12 hours after the last injection of LMWH.
- Should the activated partial thromboplastin time be prolonged close to the time of delivery following treatment with LMWH, protamine sulphate can be given to correct this.
- Due to the increased risk of bleeding, consideration should be given to leaving a wound drain *in situ* or using clips or intermittent sutures to close the skin to allow drainage of a potential haematoma. Intravenous UFH should be continued postoperatively if there is increased risk of bleeding.
- LMWH should be continued for at least 6 weeks postpartum and until 3 months of treatment in total has been given. Oral anticoagulants may be used in this period. Neither LMWH nor warfarin is contraindicated in breastfeeding.
- Oral warfarin should be restarted on day 5 postpartum. It may be necessary to delay re starting warfarin longer than 5 days in patients who are at high risk of postpartum haemorrhage.
- Using LMWH for more than 12 weeks postpartum helps prevent post-thrombotic syndrome. The evidence for prolonged postpartum use of compression stockings in preventing post-thrombotic syndrome is inconclusive.
- Women require follow-up and counselling on the need for further anticoagulation treatment in subsequent pregnancies, ideally in a joint obstetric haematology clinic.

Further advice regarding the management of the pregnant or recently pregnant patient with thromboembolic disease may be found in NICE Clinical Guideline 92 'Venous Thromboembolism: Reducing the Risk' (pp.31–33), published in January 2010 (http://www.nice.org.uk/nicemedia/pdf/CG92NICEGuidelinePDF.pdf).

Sibai BM. Diagnosis, controversies and management of the syndrome of hemolysis, elevated liver enzymes and low platelet count. *Obstet Gynecol* 2004; 103(5 Pt 1):981–91

http://www.utilis.net/Morning%20Topics/Obstetrics/HELLP,%20Sibai.pdf

This review article collates information from various expert sources to provide guidance for clinicians in the diagnosis and management options available to parturients with HELLP.

Key points

- HELLP is an acronym which stands for H = haemolysis, EL = elevated liver enzymes, LP = low platelets. It is a condition which comprises of these abnormal laboratory results and is a separate condition to pre-eclampsia.
- Haemolysis is defined as 'the presence of microangiopathic haemolysis' and is the hallmark of HELLP syndrome. Haemolysis may be detected using laboratory tests by an abnormal peripheral smear, raised serum bilirubin, raised lactate dehydrogenase or a significant fall in serum haemoglobin levels.
- Liver enzymes used to assess the severity of HELLP include serum AST, ALT, and bilirubin. However, there is no consensus regarding which liver enzymes should be used or how elevated the enzymes need to be in the diagnosis of HELLP.
- Again, there is no consensus in the literature regarding how low the platelets need to be in order to diagnosis HELLP. Low values in studies range from 75,000/mm^3 to 279,000/mm^3.
- The lack of consensus of laboratory values is partly due to the wide range of different assays available which test for liver enzymes and thrombocytopaenia. The author advises that individuals should be familiar with the normal values for these laboratory tests in their own institution.
- HELLP may be diagnosed during the expectant management of pre-eclampsia, in labour or postpartum. The maternal and fetal outcomes vary depending on when HELLP is diagnosed and how frequent blood tests are performed.
- Clinical presentation is variable and women may complain of non-specific symptoms such as malaise, a recent viral-like illness, nausea, and vomiting. More specific symptoms may include right upper quadrant or epigastric pain, headaches, visual disturbances, hypertension, and proteinuria. Some may even present with symptoms of thrombocytopaenia. There is no one symptom which has been consistently found to be present in every woman diagnosed with pre-eclampsia or HELLP.
- Acute fatty liver of pregnancy, antiphospholipid syndrome, and acute pancreatitis are some of the differential diagnoses of HELLP syndrome.
- The presence of HELLP is associated with a maternal mortality rate of 1%. It is also associated with increased maternal morbidity including pulmonary oedema (8%), acute kidney injury (3%), disseminated intravascular coagulation (15%), placental abruption (9%), and adult respiratory distress syndrome (< 1%). Pregnancies complicated by HELLP lead to an increased risk of wound haematoma and blood transfusion.
- There is an increase in perinatal mortality rates associated with HELLP, with values ranging from 7.4% to 20.4%. The higher mortality rates tend to be in pregnancies where HELLP develops at an earlier gestational age (e.g. 28 weeks or less).
- Once diagnosed, HELLP syndrome is a progressive condition with associated deterioration in the maternal condition. Experts agree that if the condition is diagnosed after 34 weeks' gestation, then prompt delivery is indicated. There is also agreement that delivery is indicated if HELLP develops before

34 weeks and there is associated multiorgan dysfunction or evidence of fetal distress.

- There is disagreement in the management of women who develop HELLP before 34 weeks' gestation, who are otherwise stable and there is no evidence of fetal distress. Some experts advocate the use of corticosteroids to assist with fetal lung maturation and delivery within 24 hours. Others advocate a more expectant approach with close monitoring of the woman and only expedite delivery when there is a deterioration in the condition or fetal distress develops. Regardless of the management, there remains an increased fetal mortality rate despite expedited delivery.
- It is accepted that corticosteroid use improves fetal outcomes in women who develop HELLP before 34 weeks' gestation. Some studies have reported improvement in platelet numbers following corticosteroid administration, allowing women to have epidural anaesthesia for delivery. However, there is good evidence to suggest that the use of corticosteroids results in a reduction in maternal morbidity.
- In all patients where HELLP is suspected, immediate admission to hospital for observation on the delivery suite is advised. Magnesium sulphate should be given as a seizure prophylaxis and hypertension treated to maintain a systolic BP below 160 mmHg or a diastolic BP below 105 mmHg. Hydralazine, labetalol, or nifedipine may be used to treat hypertension. Laboratory tests should then be taken and sent to confirm or exclude the diagnosis of HELLP.
- Regarding when to delivery, if the diagnosis is confirmed before 35 weeks' gestation, then transfer to a tertiary centre is recommended if the maternal condition is stable. The decision of when to deliver is made by determining if the maternal condition has been stabilized, fetal well-being has been assessed, and whether there is a need to delay delivery whilst corticosteroids are given to aid fetal lung maturation.
- The presence of HELLP syndrome is not an indication for immediate caesarean delivery. The decision to delivery by caesarean should be based on gestational age, presence or absence of labour, fetal well-being, and cervical Bishop score. Vaginal delivery may be indicated if the patient is in labour or there has been rupture of membranes and there are no obstetric contraindications to vaginal delivery.
- Pain relief for vaginal delivery may be provided by intermittent boluses of systemic opioids. Pudendal block is contraindicated due to the risk of haematoma formation and bleeding. Epidural analgesia is contraindicated if the platelet count is below 75,000/mm^3. For caesarean delivery, general anaesthesia may be indicated in the presence of a platelet count below 75,000/mm^3.
- Platelet transfusion is indicated either before or after delivery if there is significant bleeding or the platelet count is below 20,000/mm^3.
- After delivery, close monitoring of vital signs, fluid status, laboratory tests, and pulse oximetry should be continued for 48 hours. The majority of patients show resolution of the condition within 48 hours of delivery.
- HELLP may develop in the postpartum period within a few hours of delivery up to 7 days after birth, with the majority occurring within 48 hours. Management remains the same: the use of magnesium sulphate prophylaxis, BP management, and the use of laboratory tests to monitor the disease progression.
- The rate of recurrence of pre-eclampsia in subsequent pregnancies is 20%, whereas the rates of HELLP range between 2% and 19%. Women should be counselled about the need for close monitoring in any future pregnancies. There is presently no preventative treatment against the development of HELLP in subsequent pregnancies.

Imaging

NICE. *Ultrasound-Guided Catheterisation of the Epidural Space.* Interventional Procedure Guidance 249, 2008

https://www.nice.org.uk/guidance/ipg249

This guidance acknowledges that there is limited evidence on the use of ultrasound to assist epidural catheter placement. It does support, however, that it is a safe technique and may be a helpful way of achieving successful localization of the epidural space. This guideline covers epidural catheter placement in the obstetric and non-obstetric populations.

Key points

- Ultrasound may be used to guide the epidural needle towards the epidural space in real time. The conventional loss of resistance technique is still used as a safeguard.
- Ultrasound may also be used in a pre-puncture technique whereby the depth of the epidural space is located using the ultrasound and the ideal puncture site is marked on the back. The epidural catheter is then inserted using the conventional loss of resistance technique.
- Studies suggest that the use of both pre-puncture and real-time ultrasound-guided techniques to assist epidural catheter placement is associated with fewer attempts to locate the epidural space and with higher patient satisfaction.
- Studies in children showed that the use of ultrasound was associated with faster epidural catheter placement and with a higher success rate in terms of epidural effectiveness.
- With regards to safety, the use of the ultrasound was associated with a lower rate of dural puncture, aspiration of blood in the catheter and lower number of patients reporting 'severe' headache after an epidural.

NICE. *Guidance on the Use of Ultrasound Locating Devices for Placing Central Venous Catheters.* Technology Appraisal Guidance 49, 2002

https://www.nice.org.uk/guidance/ta49/resources/guidance-guidance-on-the-use-of-ultrasound-locating-devices-for-placing-central-venous-catheters-pdf

Central venous catheters (CVCs) are inserted by a range of medical personnel for a variety of indications. When using the landmark technique, the failure rate for the insertion of CVCs may be as high as 35%. The complications associated with the insertion of CVCs include arterial puncture, pneumothorax, arteriovenous fistula, and multiple attempts. This guidance offers advice regarding the use of ultrasound to assist the insertion of CVCs, with a view to minimizing complications.

Key points

- Ultrasound guidance should be used to assist in the insertion of CVCs in both elective and emergency situations. All those involved in inserting CVCs should undergo appropriate training in the use of ultrasound.
- The use of ultrasound allows identification of the target vein, detection of any anatomical abnormalities, and can rule out vessel thrombosis.
- Compared with the landmark technique, ultrasound-guided CVC insertion in the internal jugular vein has been associated with:
    - reduced risk of failed catheter placement
    - reduced risk of catheter placement complications
    - reduced failure on first attempt at catheter placement
    - fewer number of attempts to successfully place the catheter.
- Similar findings were found when ultrasound was used to assist CVC insertion in infants.
- Similar results were also found when ultrasound was used to assist CVC placement in the subclavian vein. However, the operators in this study were relatively inexperienced in inserting CVCs into the subclavian vein using the landmark technique.
- Ultrasound guidance significantly reduced the number of attempts needed to successfully insert a CVC into a femoral vein compared with the landmark technique.
- The use of audio-guided ultrasound technique is not recommended.

Intrapartum care

Safer Childbirth: Minimum Standards for the Organisation and Delivery of Care in Labour, October 2007

http://www.rcoa.ac.uk/system/files/PUB-Safer_Childbirth.pdf

Joint publication from the Royal College of Obstetricians and Gynaecologists, Royal College of Midwives, Royal College of Anaesthetists and Royal College of Paediatrics and Child Health.

This publication provides the minimum essential standards for staffing, training, and equipment required for providing a safe environment for the parturient and neonate.

Key points

- CMACE, along with the Confidential Enquiry into Stillbirths and Deaths in Infancy (CESDI) and the Confidential Enquiry into Maternal Deaths (CEMD) have recommended a review into the organization and provision of maternity care services.
- Through good teamwork, it is possible to provide safe and effective patient-centred care. The importance of the individual roles of the midwife, obstetrician, anaesthetist, paediatrician, and other support staff involved in the care of the pregnant patient is highlighted.
- Changes in shift patterns and recruitment shortages have resulted in inadequate numbers of midwives to provide the appropriate care to labouring women. Appropriately trained maternity care assistants can assist but not substitute midwifery care.
- 'Modernising Medical Careers' and changes to working times have reduced the availability and experience of junior medical staff on labour ward, thus requiring consultant obstetricians to be more present on labour ward.
- Maternity services are associated with higher litigation costs than other services.
- Better organization and provision of services requires good communication and strong leadership to maintain and boost staff morale.
- Clear, concise documentation should be maintained at all times. This is especially important should an incident arise.
- Due to the changing role of the anaesthetist on labour ward, a suitably trained anaesthetist should be available to manage labour analgesia and provide appropriate anaesthesia for operative delivery.
- Paediatric staff on labour ward must be competent in neonatal life support.
- Every attempt should be made to keep the mother and baby together after birth.

Royal College of Obstetricians and Gynaecologists. *Placenta Praevia, Placenta Accreta and Vasa Praevia: Diagnosis and Management*. Green-Top Guideline No. 27, January 2011

http://www.rcog.org.uk/files/rcog-corp/GTG27PlacentaPraeviaJanuary2011.pdf

This guideline is summarized under 'Haematological'.

Royal College of Obstetricians and Gynaecologists. *Preterm Premature Rupture of Membranes*. Green-Top Guideline No. 44, 2006 (Minor Amendment 2010)

https://www.rcog.org.uk/globalassets/documents/guidelines/gtg_44.pdf

This revised guideline makes recommendations regarding the diagnosis, investigation, and management of preterm premature rupture of membranes (PPROM). PPROM occurs in about 2% of pregnancies but is associated with 40% of preterm deliveries, which in turn is associated with significant neonatal morbidity and mortality.

Key points

- PPROM is known to be associated with preterm birth, neonatal sepsis, and pulmonary hypoplasia, which can lead to neonatal death.
- Women with intrauterine infections have earlier deliveries and neonates born with sepsis have a mortality rate four times higher than neonates born without sepsis.
- PPROM is best diagnosed through history and a sterile speculum examination. An ultrasound scan can be used to assist diagnosis in some cases.

- Once diagnosed, women should be observed for signs of chorioamnionitis, which include maternal pyrexia, offensive vaginal discharge, and fetal tachycardia. There is no need to carry out weekly high vaginal swabs or blood tests. Cardiotography (CTG) may be useful in assessing fetal tachycardia.
- Presently there is not enough evidence to support the use of routine amniocentesis to detect subclinical infection in women with PPROM.
- Erythromycin should be given for 10 days once PPROM has been diagnosed as this has been shown to reduce the number of deliveries occurring 48 hours after PPROM. Co-amoxiclav should be avoided as studies showed an increase in neonates born with necrotizing enterocolitis following maternal treatment with co-amoxiclav. Penicillin or clindamycin should be given if group B *Streptococcus* is isolated in PPROM.
- Corticosteroids should be given in cases of PPROM occurring between 24 and 34 weeks' gestation to reduce the incidence of neonatal respiratory distress syndrome.
- Ritodrine has been shown to delay delivery for 24 hours after PPROM but this effect does not persist beyond 24 hours. Other studies involving tocolytics did not show any benefit and their routine use is not recommended.
- Delivery of the baby should be considered after 34 weeks. If delivery is to be delayed, the woman should be warned of the increased risk of chorioamnionitis and the reduced risk of neonatal respiratory problems.
- It is advisable to admit women with PPROM for monitoring and treatment.
- Amnioinfusion during labour is not recommended in PPROM as it does not prevent umbilical cord compression. (Amnioinfusion is a procedure in which a needle is introduced into the uterine cavity under ultrasound guidance and saline is infused to increase the volume of amniotic fluid.)

Royal College of Obstetricians and Gynaecologists. *Antenatal Corticosteroids to Reduce Neonatal Morbidity and Mortality.* Green-Top Guideline No. 7, 2010

https://www.rcog.org.uk/globalassets/documents/guidelines/gtg_7.pdf

Antenatal corticosteroids have been previously shown to reduce the incidence of respiratory distress syndrome and are also beneficial in preventing other complications of prematurity, such as intraventricular haemorrhage. This guideline aims to provide up-to-date information regarding the most appropriate use of corticosteroids antenatally and in neonates. The use of corticosteroids shows no benefit for the mother.

Key points

- A single course of corticosteroids should be offered to women between 24^{+0} and 34^{+6} weeks' gestation, who are at risk of preterm delivery. Corticosteroids may be considered in women less than 24 weeks' gestation but the decision must be made by a senior clinician.
- Antenatal corticosteroids have the best chance of reducing neonatal mortality from respiratory distress syndrome between 24 hours and up to 7 days after the second dose has been given.
- A single course of antenatal corticosteroids does not appear to have any immediate or long-term adverse effects on the mother or fetus. There remains insufficient evidence regarding the adverse effects following multiple courses of antenatal corticosteroids.
- Antenatal corticosteroids should be used with caution in women with a systemic infection. Senior review should be sought when considering a delay in delivery for steroid prophylaxis in women with overt chorioamnionitis.
- Antenatal corticosteroids should be given to all women who are at risk of preterm delivery before 34^{+6} weeks' gestation and in all elective caesarean deliveries before 38^{+6} weeks' gestation.
- Diabetes mellitus is not a contraindication to giving antenatal corticosteroids. However, these patients need to be closely monitored and additional insulin may need to be given.
- The corticosteroid agent of choice to enhance lung maturation is betamethasone 12 mg in two doses or dexamethasone 6 mg in four doses. Both are given intramuscularly.

Royal College of Obstetricians and Gynaecologists. *Tocolysis for Women in Preterm Labour.* Green-Top Guideline No. 1B, 2011

https://www.rcog.org.uk/globalassets/documents/guidelines/gtg1b26072011.pdf

Preterm birth is defined as delivery before 37^{+0} weeks' gestation. Infant mortality in this age group was 42/1000 live births compared with 5/1000 live births overall. The mortality rate in the first year of infants born before 32^{+0} weeks is 144/1000 compared with 1.8/1000 live births of those born at term. Very preterm birth is defined as delivery before 32 weeks and is responsible for 51% of infant deaths. Commonly used tocolytic agents in the United Kingdom include beta-agonists, calcium channel blockers, oxytocin receptor antagonists, prostaglandin synthetase inhibitors, nitric oxide donors, and magnesium sulphate.

Key points

- The use of a tocolytic drug may prolong a pregnancy by up to 7 days. However, there is no evidence that these drugs improve neonatal outcomes. Nonetheless, it is worth considering using them if the delay in delivery facilitates care, for example, completing a course of steroids, allowing an *in utero* transfer.
- Both nifedipine and atosiban are effective in delaying delivery by up to 7 days.
- Nifedipine is associated with an improvement in neonatal outcome, when compared to beta-agonists, though the long-term effects are unknown.
- Beta-agonists can delay birth by up to 48 hours compared to placebo, but there is no evidence to suggest they are superior to other tocolytic agents. However, they have a high frequency of adverse effects.
- Nifedipine, atosiban, and cyclooxygenase inhibitors have fewer adverse effects compared to beta-agonists but it is unclear how these agents compare with each other.
- Although there is no strong evidence to support the use of magnesium sulphate to reduce the risk of preterm birth, studies have shown it to decrease the risk of cerebral palsy following

preterm delivery. For this reason, magnesium sulphate should be given to those at risk of preterm delivery.

- It is not recommended to administer more than one tocolytic agent at one time due to an increased risk of adverse side effects.

Royal College of Obstetricians and Gynaecologists. *Management of Monochorionic Twin Pregnancy*. Green-Top Guideline No. 51, 2008

https://www.rcog.org.uk/globalassets/documents/guidelines/t51managementmonochorionictwinpregnancy2008a.pdf *(Reference 45 in chapter 33)*

A monochorionic (MC) twin pregnancy is one where both twins share a single placenta. About 1/3 of twin pregnancies are monochorionic. A major risk in MC pregnancies is the development of vascular placental anastomoses between the two umbilical circulations, resulting in twin-to-twin transfusion syndrome (TTTS).

Key points

- TTTS occurs in about 10–15% of MC pregnancies and is more likely due to unidirectional flow in an artery–vein anastomosis rather than a bidirectional artery–artery anastomosis. TTTS can occur in both monochorionic, monoamniotic (MCMA) and monochorionic, diamniotic (MCDA) twin pregnancies, though it is more common in MCDA due to a high number of protective artery–artery anastomoses in MCMA.
- All women with a twin pregnancy should be offered an ultrasound examination at 10–13 weeks' gestation. Chorionicity is best assessed before 14 weeks, with a sensitivity and specificity of 89.9% and 99.5% respectively.
- The diagnosis of TTTS is made on specific ultrasound criteria: single placenta, concordant gender, oligohydramnios.
- Evidence of abnormal bladder size and haemodynamic and cardiac compromise suggest severe TTTS.
- MC twin pregnancies have a higher rate of fetal loss than dichorionic (DC) twin pregnancies.
- There is not enough evidence to suggest nuchal translucency measurements should be used routinely to predict TTTS.
- All MC twin pregnancies should have a detailed ultrasound scan assessment, which includes views of the heart. Fetal echocardiography should be considered in cases of suspected severe TTTS.
- In uncomplicated MC twin pregnancies, routine ultrasound scanning should be performed every 2–3 weeks after 16 weeks.
- The Quintero classification system can be used to grade the severity of TTTS (see Appendix 2 of this book).
- Severe TTTS should be treated with laser ablation if diagnosed before 26 weeks' gestation. Some anastomoses may be missed and TTTS can recur later in the pregnancy in up to 14% of cases treated with laser ablation.
- In severe TTTS, selective termination of one twin or complete termination of pregnancy are alternative options which need to be discussed.
- Aim to deliver uncomplicated MC pregnancy at 36–37 weeks' gestation. It is appropriate to aim for a vaginal delivery unless there are indications for a caesarean delivery.
- Should one twin die *in utero*, the surviving twin has a 12% chance of death and 18% chance of neurological abnormalities. Such women should be referred to a specialist fetal medicine centre.
- There is a high chance of cord entanglement in MCMA twin pregnancies and these are best delivered at 32 weeks by caesarean delivery following a course of antenatal corticosteroids.

Royal College of Obstetricians and Gynaecologists. *The Management of Breech Presentation*. Green-Top Guideline No. 20b, 2006

https://www.rcog.org.uk/en/guidelines-research-services/guidelines/gtg20b/

This guideline provides information regarding the route of delivery and the choice of various techniques, which may be used during delivery of a breech presentation. Breech presentation occurs in about 3–4% of term pregnancies.

Key points

- A planned caesarean delivery for a breech presentation carries a reduced perinatal mortality and early neonatal morbidity compared with planned vaginal delivery. However, there is no evidence to suggest that the long-term health of the baby is affected by the mode of delivery.
- Compared with vaginal delivery, caesarean delivery carries a small increase in serious immediate complications.
- Women should be assessed for suitability for a vaginal breech delivery. If there are any unfavourable features, then caesarean delivery should be considered.
- A vaginal breech delivery should occur in a place where there are facilities to perform an emergency caesarean delivery. If favourable, an induction of labour may take place but the labour should not be augmented.
- An epidural is not routinely advocated. The woman should have a choice regarding labour analgesia.
- Continuous CTG monitoring during labour should still occur. However, fetal blood sampling from the buttocks is not recommended.
- If there is a delayed second stage, a caesarean delivery should be considered.
- The maternal position advocated to facilitate a breech delivery is the dorsal or lithotomy position.
- There are various manoeuvres which may be performed to facilitate breech delivery: Lovset, Mauriceau–Smellie–Veit, and Burns–Marshall. (see Appendix 2 of this book).
- Routine breech extraction is not recommended.
- Routine caesarean delivery should not be performed for a preterm breech fetus or a twin pregnancy where the second twin is breech.

Royal College of Obstetricians and Gynaecologists. *Birth after Previous Caesarean Birth*. Green-Top Guideline No. 45, February 2007

https://www.rcog.org.uk/globalassets/documents/guidelines/gtg4511022011.pdf

- Women with a previous history of caesarean birth should have antenatal counselling regarding the options of a planned vaginal birth after caesarean (VBAC) and a repeat elective caesarean delivery, if they fulfil the following criteria:
  - Previous operation was an uncomplicated lower segment transverse caesarean delivery
  - There is no complication in the current pregnancy at term
  - There is no reason to suggest vaginal delivery would be unsuccessful.
- The final decision for the mode of delivery should be made ideally by 36 weeks' gestation. The management plan should be clearly documented, in case labour starts prior to the scheduled date.
- The chances of successful planned VBAC are between 72% and 76%.
- If a woman has had a classical caesarean delivery, elective repeat caesarean delivery (ERCD) should be recommended.
- Women with a previous uterine incision other than a low transverse caesarean delivery or two previous uncomplicated lower transverse caesarean deliveries should be counselled by a consultant obstetrician regarding the potential risks, if they wish to consider VBAC.
- Women considering the birth options after a previous caesarean delivery, should be aware of the risks detailed in Table A1.7.
- Planned VBAC should take place in an appropriately staffed and equipped delivery suite. Facilities for immediate caesarean delivery and advanced neonatal resuscitation must be available. Continuous electronic fetal monitoring should be applied. Continuous intrapartum care must be given so that uterine scar rupture can be promptly identified.
- It is safe to use epidural analgesia in planned VBAC.
- If labour is induced and/or augmented, there is two- to three-fold increased risk of uterine rupture and 1.5-fold increased risk of caesarean delivery when compared with spontaneous labour.

Table A1.7 Possible birth risks after a previous caesarean delivery

Complication	Planned VBAC	ERCD
Uterine rupture	22–74/10,000	No risk
Blood transfusion	1% additional risk compared to ERCD	
Birth related perinatal death	2–3/10,000 additional risk compared to ERCD	
Neonatal hypoxic ischaemic encephalopathy	8/10,000 risk	
Neonatal respiratory problems	2–3%	3–4%
Anaesthetic risk	Extremely low for both	
Serious complications for future pregnancies		Elevate the risks

- Serial cervical assessments should be performed preferably by the same person to assess if there is adequate progress.
- A consultant obstetrician should discuss with the woman the parameters of progress that would necessitate discontinuing VBAC.

Royal College of Obstetricians and Gynaecologists. *Operative Vaginal Delivery*. Green-Top Guideline No. 26, January 2011

https://www.rcog.org.uk/globalassets/documents/guidelines/gtg26.pdf

Key points

- The following factors have been shown to reduce the need for operative vaginal delivery:
  - Continuous support during labour
  - Upright or lateral positions
  - Avoiding the use of an epidural for pain relief.
- Delayed pushing should be allowed in primiparous women with an epidural in order to reduce the need for rotational and midcavity deliveries.
- A standard classification of operative vaginal delivery should be used. (outlet, low, mid and high; see Appendix 2 in this book).
- For gestations of less than 34 weeks, vacuum extraction should not be used.
- For gestations between 34 weeks and 36 weeks, vacuum extraction should be used with caution.
- All women should be given information about operative vaginal delivery during the antenatal period. A written consent should be signed before a trial of operative vaginal delivery in the operating theatre.
- An experienced obstetrician, who is competent at mid-cavity deliveries, must be present from the outset for all rotational or mid-cavity operative vaginal delivery.
- Operative vaginal deliveries, which have a higher chance of failure, should be performed in a place where a caesarean delivery can be performed immediately.
- The options for rotational delivery are Kielland forceps, manual rotation followed by direct traction forceps or rotational vacuum extraction. An experienced obstetrician should perform the rotational delivery.
- When there is no progressive descent with moderate traction during each contraction or where delivery is not imminent following three contractions of a correctly applied instrument by an experienced operator, operative vaginal delivery should be abandoned.
- An incident form must be submitted for any adverse outcomes, including unsuccessful instrumental delivery.
- Paired cord blood samples should be taken after all attempts at operative vaginal delivery.
- There is an increased neonatal morbidity with failed operative vaginal delivery. The neonatologist should be informed when this occurs to ensure appropriate management of the baby.

- There is inadequate evidence to support the routine use of prophylactic antibiotics in operative vaginal delivery.
- Venous thromboembolism risk needs to be reassessed after delivery.
- Regular paracetamol and diclofenac should be prescribed if not contraindicated.
- Women should be offered physiotherapy to prevent urinary incontinence following operative vaginal delivery.
- Individualized care should be given to all women who have sustained a third- or fourth-degree perineal tear.

NICE. *Induction of Labour.* Clinical Guideline 70, July 2008

http://www.nice.org.uk/guidance/cg70/resources/guidance-induction-of-labour-pdf

Key recommendations

- At the 38-week antenatal visit, all women should be informed of the risks associated with pregnancies that last longer than 42 weeks (e.g. placental insufficiency, meconium aspiration syndrome, fetal macrosomia, and birth injury).
- Women should be informed about membrane sweep, induction of labour between 41 and 42 weeks, and expectant management.
- Women offered an induction of labour, should be informed about:
  - the reasons for induction
  - time, place, and method of induction
  - pain relief options
  - alternative options if the woman does not choose to have an induction of labour or if an induction is not successful
  - the risks and benefits of each induction method.
- Induction of labour should be offered to the women with uncomplicated pregnancies between 41 and 42 weeks to avoid the risks associated with prolonged pregnancy.
- If a woman presents with PPROM after 34 weeks, she should be made aware of the risks to her and the baby as well as the availability of neonatal facilities, prior to a decision of induction of labour. Vaginal prostaglandin E_2 is the method of choice for induction. It is given as a gel, tablet, or controlled release pessary. Women should be informed about the risks of uterine hyperstimulation.
- If the induction fails, the woman's condition should be fully assessed, and electronic fetal monitoring should be instituted. Subsequent treatment options include a repeat attempt at induction or a caesarean delivery.

Royal College of Obstetricians and Gynaecologists. *Shoulder Dystocia.* Green-Top Guideline No. 42, March 2012

http://www.rcog.org.uk/files/rcog-corp/GTG42_25112013.pdf

Key points

- Risk assessment tools for shoulder dystocia are insufficiently predictive to prevent the majority of cases.
- Risk of shoulder dystocia can be reduced by an induction of labour at term in women with GDM. However, the induction does not prevent shoulder dystocia in non-diabetic women with a suspected fetal microsomia.
- Elective caesarean delivery should be considered in diabetic women with an estimated fetal weight of more than 4.5 kg.
- In women with previous history of should dystocia, a caesarean or vaginal delivery may be appropriate. The management decision ought to be made jointly by the woman and her medical team.
- All maternity staff should be aware of the methods for diagnosing shoulder dystocia and the manoeuvers used to facilitate delivery. The birth attendant should routinely observe for the following signs:
  - Difficulty with delivery of the face and chin
  - The head remaining tightly applied to the vulva or even retracting (turtle-neck sign)
  - Failure of restitution of the fetal head
  - Failure of the shoulders to descend.
- Routine traction in an axial direction can be applied in order to diagnose shoulder dystocia. Once shoulder dystocia is recognized, help should be called immediately.
- McRoberts' manoeuvre should be the first intervention. Suprapubic pressure can be applied to facilitate the McRoberts' manoeuvre.
- Internal manoeuvres or 'all-fours' position are both second-line manoeuvres.
- Third-line manoeuvres should be considered cautiously to avoid unnecessary morbidity and mortality.
- The team should prepare for possible postpartum haemorrhage and severe perineal tears.
- A neonatal clinician should examine the baby to rule out any injury.
- All maternity staff should take part in the shoulder dystocia training every year. High-fidelity equipment should be used in the training.

Neonatal

Nuffield Council of Bioethics and the British Association of Perinatal Medicine. *Guidelines on Giving Intensive Care to Extremely Premature Babies*, 2006

http://nuffieldbioethics.org/report/neonatal-medicine-2/guidelines-intensive-care-extremely-premature-babies/

- At 25 weeks or more of gestation: intensive care should be started unless the baby suffers from a severe abnormality which is not conducive with any meaningful duration of life.
- Between 24^{+0} and 24^{+6} weeks' gestation: intensive care treatment should be initiated apart from in circumstances where the clinicians and parents concur that such treatment in view of the neonate's current clinical condition would not be beneficial to the neonate.

- Between 23^{+0} and 23^{+6} weeks' gestation: parents should be consulted for their wishes regarding intensive care therapy. However, the clinicians should not feel duty bound to commence treatment if they feel that such treatment would cause more harm to the neonate and would not be of any further benefit.
- Between 22^{+0} and 22^{+6} weeks' gestation: due to the likelihood of a poor outcome, resuscitation of the neonate should not be attempted unless the parents repeatedly request such course of action after thorough discussion with doctors regarding the likely outcome of such actions and the doctors agree that it ought to be attempted.
- Before 22 weeks: resuscitation should only be attempted in clinical research settings.

Resuscitation Council (UK) Guideline: *Newborn Life Support*, 2010

Details of the algorithm may be found using the following link: http://www.resus.org.uk/pages/resuscitation-guidelines/

Neurological

OAA Clinical Guideline: *Postdural Puncture Headache: PDPH – Diagnosis and Management*, March 2014

http://www.oaa-anaes.ac.uk/ui/content/content.aspx?id=176

Key points

- PDPH is an important cause of morbidity following obstetric anaesthesia.
- The PDPH guidelines from three NHS hospitals in the United Kingdom can be found on the OAA clinical guideline page.
- PDPH is typically fronto-occipital. It is usually associated with neck stiffness and gets worse on sitting or standing up.
- When reviewing a patient with postpartum headache, the anaesthetist should consider differential diagnoses such as meningitis, intracranial haemorrhage, migraine, and cerebral vein thrombosis.
- Conservative treatment includes hydration, simple analgesia, and occasionally caffeine.
- If the headache is severe or if it does not improve with conservative management, an epidural blood patch (EBP) should be offered.
- An EBP should be performed under full aseptic precautions.
- Most hospitals advise women to lie flat for 2 hours after the blood patch.
- All women who have received a blood patch should be offered aftercare instructions prior to discharge.
- Patients should be informed to contact the hospital or the duty anaesthetist or attend the emergency department if their symptoms get worse or if there is any change in neurology.
- All patients with PDPH should be followed up by the anaesthetist by telephone or outpatient appointment after discharge from hospital.

Royal College of Anaesthetists. *Report and Findings of the Third National Audit Project* (Chapter 16: Complications after Obstetric CNB), January 2009

http://www.rcoa.ac.uk/nap3

- The initial census phase of this project identified that 45% of all central neuraxial blocks (CNBs) are performed for obstetric indications.
- Out of 12 cases correctly reported after obstetric CNBs, five patients made a full and rapid recovery. The remaining seven patients were considered to have a potentially disabling complication.
- There were no cases of paraplegia or death after obstetric CNB.

Key points

- Obstetric CNB is associated with fewer major complications compared to CNBs for other indications (most notably perioperatively).
- Obstetric causes should also be considered when neurological deficits occur. A neurologist's opinion and electrophysiological studies may add considerable information.
- Multiple attempts at performing neuraxial blockade, which is associated with significant bleeding, may increase the risk of neuraxial infection despite full aseptic precautions.
- Although a headache after delivery is a common occurrence and is usually benign, it is important to exclude dural puncture, meningitis, and subdural haematoma as possible causes.
- The final height of a spinal block may be difficult to predict following a recent effective epidural for labour analgesia. In such cases, a CSE may be advisable as it allows the possibility for block height adjustment.
- Clinicians should be aware that giving drugs via the wrong route is more common in obstetric practice than in other clinical areas.

Psychiatric

Oates MR, Cantwell R. Deaths from Psychiatric Causes. In Centre for Maternal and Child Enquiries (CMACE). Saving mothers' lives: reviewing maternal deaths to make motherhood safer: 2006–2008. The eighth report on confidential enquiries into maternal deaths in the United Kingdom. *BJOG* 2011; 118(Suppl. 1):132–42

http://www.oaa-anaes.ac.uk/assets/_managed/editor/File/Reports/2006-2008%20CEMD.pdf

This chapter discusses the maternal deaths resulting from suicide or accidental substance overdose and makes recommendations for their management.

Key points

- All women should have a full history taken including any previous psychiatric illnesses. Their current mental state should also be assessed. All women with a previous history of psychiatric illness should be referred to a psychiatrist, even if they are currently well. These women should be followed up for a minimum of 3 months after delivery.

- Pregnant and recently delivered women should be able to easily access psychiatric services where they may be assessed, admitted, and treated. Where possible, the same mental health team should be involved to maintain continuity of care.
- There should be specialist teams in the community who are able to treat at-risk women in the peripartum period. Facilities should be made available to admit women either late in pregnancy or early in the postpartum period where mother and baby are able to be cared for together by such teams.
- Good communication is necessary, especially when English is not the main language, when a diagnosis of a psychiatric disorder is made of physical symptoms, distress, or agitation.
- Suicides in recently delivered women were more common in white, affluent women over the age of 30. It is important not to stereotype those from lower socioeconomic backgrounds as being high risk of suicide.
- Women with a previous history of a serious affective disorder such as bipolar disease or severe depression are at increased risk of suicide. Such women should be closely followed up and monitored for signs of recurrence.
- Puerperal psychosis remains rare. Healthcare providers must remain vigilant to this condition as the clinical symptoms may have a sudden onset and deteriorate rapidly, thus endangering the life of the mother and baby.
- The welfare and safeguarding needs of the child must be considered when managing a woman with a mental illness.
- Women may conceal or hide the nature or extent of their substance abuse. Community teams should provide support including regular monitoring and prescription of relevant substitutes. Such women should be referred to specialists for management of their on-going obstetric care.

NICE. *Antenatal and Postnatal Mental Health: Clinical Management and Service Guidance.* Clinical Guideline 192, June 2015

http://www.nice.org.uk/guidance/cg192/resources/guidance-antenatal-and-postnatal-mental-health-clinical-management-and-service-guidance-pdf

This evidence-based guideline covers the management of both new and pre-existing mental health disorders in women of childbearing age. It also covers the teratogenic risk of psychotropic medication and the risks if used while breastfeeding. Individual diseases including depression, generalized anxiety disorders, panic disorder, and obsessive–compulsive disorder are discussed in more detail within the guidance.

Key points

- A woman may need to be referred for preconception counselling. In particular, the effects of any current psychotropic medication on the fetus, possible drug substitutions during pregnancy, and impact of the drugs on the ability to breastfeed should be discussed before conception. The woman should be counselled about the consequences of stopping such medication before or during pregnancy.
- Women should be asked about any current or past mental health problems they or their families have encountered. This should be asked at the booking visit and also during the postpartum review at 4–6 weeks and 3–4 months.
- If a woman is assessed to require psychological treatment, this should be arranged to occur within a month of the initial assessment.
- When starting treatment, the risks of the treatment should be clearly explained to the patient. This is particularly important when deciding which antidepressant to use, as the safety profile in pregnancy varies with each class of drug. An individualized treatment plan made in agreement with the patient should be implemented. Healthcare providers should be aware that the needs of the patient may change throughout the pregnancy and in the postpartum period and treatment should be adjusted as necessary.
- There should be a network of specialist services to provide support and advice to women with mental health problems in the perinatal period.
- Where possible, involve the patient and partner in decisions about her care and that of the baby.

Scottish Intercollegiate Guidelines Network. *Management of Perinatal Mood Disorders.* SIGN 127, March 2012

http://www.sign.ac.uk/pdf/sign127.pdf

This guideline from SIGN is an updated version of SIGN guideline 60 'Postnatal depression and puerperal psychosis'. It offers advice regarding the prevention, assessment, diagnosis, and treatment for perinatal mood disorders. The quick reference guide may be accessed by this link: http://www.sign.ac.uk/pdf/qrg127.pdf. The guideline offers advice on using various psychotropic drugs including antidepressants, lithium, antiepileptic drugs, and antipsychotics.

Key points

- Mood disorders, depression, antenatal anxiety, and postpartum psychosis are covered in this guideline.
- All women should be asked about personal and family history of postpartum psychosis and any other affective disorders. Women who are at high risk of developing a postpartum affective disorder, should have a detailed plan regarding management in late pregnancy and regarding psychiatric follow-up in the early postpartum period. There should be a multidisciplinary team input in the support and management of such patients.
- As a minimum, women should be asked about depressive symptoms at booking and during postpartum follow up at 4–6 weeks and 3–4 months.
- For the treatment of mild to moderate depression, cognitive behavioural therapy may be an option (level B evidence).
- Contraception should be discussed with women of childbearing age who are on psychotropic medication. Valproate should not be routinely prescribed to women of childbearing age due to the risk of teratogenicity and neurobehavioural toxicity.

- Electroconvulsive therapy administered during pregnancy is effective and is of low risk to the mother and fetus.

Renal

EBPG Expert Group on Renal Transplantation. European best practice guidelines for renal transplantation. Long term management of the transplant patient. Section IV: Pregnancy in renal transplant patients. *Nephrol Dial Transplant* 2002; 17(Suppl 4):50–55

http://ndt.oxfordjournals.org/content/17/suppl_4/50.full.pdf+html

This article offers evidence-based guidelines for the management of renal transplant recipients who become pregnant.

Key points

- Fertility is usually restored following a successful renal transplantation. If the kidney is functioning well prior to conception, then pregnancy has no adverse effect on kidney function or the graft survival in the long term (level B evidence).
- It is advisable to consider pregnancy 2 years after successful transplantation as long as the graft is functioning well and there are no adverse symptoms such as proteinuria or evidence of rejection (level B evidence).
- A woman who has had a renal transplant and becomes pregnant, should be treated as a high-risk patient and managed jointly by a renal physician and an obstetrician. Once the pregnancy has been confirmed, the function of the graft should be closely monitored as well as continuing to monitor for signs of infection or rejection. Such women are at risk of premature delivery. Fetal well-being should be closely monitored as there is a risk of associated low birth weight.
- Urine cultures should be performed every month throughout pregnancy to monitor for bacterial infections. If detected, then these infections should be treated to prevent further complications. There should also be monitoring for possible viral infections (level B evidence).
- There is a risk of acute graft rejection following delivery. This should be closely monitored for and immunosuppressive drugs should be adjusted accordingly to prevent this (level C evidence).
- Women with a renal transplant are at increased risk of developing pre-eclampsia, especially if they have previously suffered with arterial hypertension. Blood pressure along with markers of end-organ dysfunction must be closely monitored for every 2–4 weeks with adjustment in any antihypertensive drugs as necessary (level B evidence).
- Current evidence suggests that ciclosporin and tacrolimus, either with or without steroids, may continue to be used safely during pregnancy. However, it is not advisable to breastfeed while on these drugs due to the transfer of drugs in breast milk. There is insufficient evidence presently to safely recommend the use of other immunosuppressive agents in pregnancy (level C evidence).
- A vaginal delivery is recommended where possible but in about 50% of cases, a caesarean delivery is advised. These women should deliver in a specialist centre where both renal and obstetric teams are present. After delivery, monitoring of blood pressure, fluid balance, and graft function should continue (level C evidence).

Respiratory

Edenborough FP, Borgo G, Knoop C, *et al.* Guidelines for the management of pregnancy in women with cystic fibrosis. *J Cyst Fibros* 2008; 7 Suppl 1:S2–S32

http://www.sciencedirect.com/science/article/pii/S1569199307001294

As more women with cystic fibrosis (CF) are surviving to childbearing age, these consensus guidelines have been developed to help provide evidenced-based care for this population. The maternal outcome following pregnancy is variable and emphasis is placed on maintaining optimal CF treatment in the preconception period and maintaining it throughout pregnancy.

Key points

- Where possible, preconception counselling, including genetic testing of one or both partners, should be undertaken to fully prepare the couple for the realities of pregnancy and having a child.
- Drug treatment needs to be rationalized to minimize the potential teratogenic effects.
- Where possible, preconception lung function should be optimized and stabilized, as both maternal and fetal outcomes are related to this. Optimization may include the use of antibiotics to suppress chronic infection, physiotherapy techniques, and mucolytics. In the event of an acute lung infection, additional contraception may be required to prevent a pregnancy occurring whilst using potentially teratogenic drugs.
- Where possible, preconception assessment of the adequacy of dietary intake with a dietician needs to take place. If suboptimal, then vitamin supplementation or supplementary enteral feeding may be needed.
- Pregnant women with all forms of diabetes have been shown to have poorer outcomes than those without diabetes. In such cases, diabetes needs to be carefully controlled through diet and insulin.
- Absolute contraindications to pregnancy are pre-existing pulmonary hypertension and cor pulmonale. A forced expiratory volume in 1 second (FEV_1) greater than 60% is recommended for pregnancy, whereas FEV_1 less than 50% is an indication for termination of pregnancy.
- Termination of pregnancy in CF patients may be medical or surgical. The choice of anaesthetic for surgical termination will need to be considered on an individual case basis, but general anaesthesia is generally avoided to minimize adverse effects on the lungs.
- A coordinated, multidisciplinary approach is required to provide support for CF patients who are pregnant.

- The majority of pregnancies end with spontaneous vaginal deliveries. A caesarean delivery may be considered in women with severe CF or in those who would not tolerate a prolonged Valsalva manoeuvre.
- Labour analgesia may be effectively provided by an epidural. The use of opioids and nitrous oxide needs to be carefully considered depending on the lung function of the individual.
- A neuraxial anaesthetic technique is recommended for caesarean delivery, followed by recovery in a high dependency setting, with early physiotherapy.
- A pregnancy occurring in a patient who has received a heart–lung transplant should be considered high risk, as the babies are at risk of intrauterine growth restriction and premature delivery. Such pregnancies have typically occurred 2 years after transplant.
- Support, both physical and psychological, should be maintained for women with CF after delivery to help them cope with managing their condition and the needs of a newborn baby.
- The outcomes of mothers following delivery are variable, but appear closely related to the severity of the CF.

Service provision

AAGBI and OAA Guidelines: *OAA/AAGBI Guidelines for Obstetric Anaesthetic Services 2013*, 2013

http://www.aagbi.org/sites/default/files/obstetric_anaesthetic_services_2013.pdf

This is an updated joint guideline from the AAGBI and OAA which is designed to ensure that obstetric patients receive the same standards of care as those recommended for the general surgical population.

Key points

- A suitably trained 'duty anaesthetist' should be immediately available to look after patients on the delivery suite at all times. There must be a designated consultant in charge of the care of the patients on the delivery suite, who should be easily contactable by the duty anaesthetist at any time.
- There should be separate teams to manage elective and emergency work on the delivery suite to avoid delays in both the elective and emergency work.
- There must be an increase in the presence of a consultant anaesthetist on the delivery suite to match the increasing workload of the obstetric anaesthetist. Elective obstetric anaesthetic services must also be consultant led. This needs to be in addition to the consultant sessions required to cover emergency work on the delivery suite.
- There may need to be restructuring in the provision of maternity services, with the merger of smaller units who may not be able to meet the demands and financial implications for a consultant-led service.
- There should be planned outpatient antenatal review of high-risk parturients and anaesthetists on the delivery suite must be given adequate notice when a high-risk patient is admitted to the delivery suite.
- In units that offer a 24-hour epidural service, the waiting time for an epidural should not exceed 30 minutes. There should be local guidelines in place regarding the appropriate levels of staffing to provide care for women with neuraxial analgesia in labour.
- All women undergoing a caesarean delivery should be reviewed by an anaesthetist preoperatively.
- There should be a suitably staffed recovery area to manage postpartum women.
- Maternal critical care is a developing area and staff should be trained to recognize the sick parturient and know who to contact should the situation arise.
- There should be good communication between all members of the multidisciplinary team to promote effective team working and improve patient safety.
- There should be suitable resuscitation facilities for parturients and neonates on the delivery suite.

Safer Childbirth: Minimum Standards for the Organisation and Delivery of Care in Labour, October 2007

http://www.rcoa.ac.uk/system/files/PUB-Safer_Childbirth.pdf

This guideline is summarized under 'Intrapartum Care'.

General Medical Council. *Consent: Patients and Doctors Making Decisions Together*, 2008

http://www.gmc-uk.org/guidance/ethical_guidance/consent_guidance_contents.asp

This 2008 guideline replaces *Seeking Patients' Consent: The Ethical Considerations* (1998). The guidance is an extension of the guidance, which is issued in *Good Medical Practice (2013)* (http://www.gmc-uk.org/guidance/good_medical_practice.asp), which requires doctors to be certain to have obtained consent from the patient or an appropriate authority before performing any examination, investigation, or treatment on the patient.

Key points

- Doctors and patients must develop a partnership based on trust where all aspects of treatment, no matter how minor, may be discussed in an informed way. If the patient has capacity, the doctor must respect the decision made by the patient.
- A doctor should be able to assess whether a patient has capacity. If the patient is deemed to lack capacity, then healthcare professionals must act according to the Mental Capacity Act 2005. Further guidance may be found at: http://www.legislation.gov.uk/ukpga/2005/9/contents and http://www.justice.gov.uk/downloads/protecting-the-vulnerable/mca/mca-code-practice-0509.pdf.
- If a patient requests a treatment which the doctor believes will not benefit the patient, the reasons for this request should be explored and discussed. A doctor is not obliged to provide the patient with treatment which will not benefit them. The doctor must explain their reasons for this decision and discuss other treatment options with the patient including seeking a second opinion.

- Throughout the consultation process, patients must be given the opportunity to ask questions and seek advice regarding their treatment. At all stages, comprehension must be checked to ensure that the patient fully understands what they may or may not be agreeing to.
- Reasons for withholding information from a patient must be clearly recorded. Furthermore, if a patient does not wish to be given information about their condition or their treatment, it must be made clear to them that their consent may not be valid as a result.
- Before taking consent from a patient for a procedure, the person taking consent must be suitably trained and act in accordance with this guidance.
- A patient's consent may be implied, oral, or written. The doctor must ensure that the patient is giving their consent voluntarily and that they have been adequately informed.
- A young person's ability to give consent is based more on their ability to understand and consider options rather than their actual age. Further guidance may be found at: http://www.gmc-uk.org/guidance/ethical_guidance/consent_guidance_involving_children_and_young_people.asp.
- In an emergency situation, where it is not possible to obtain a patient's consent, treatment may be given if it is necessary to save their life or to prevent further serious deterioration in their condition. Once the patient regains capacity, they should be informed about the treatment they have received and understand it.

General Medical Council. *0–18 years – Guidance for All Doctors*, 2007

http://www.gmc-uk.org/guidance/ethical_guidance/children_guidance_index.asp

Key points

- Children and young adults should be treated as individuals who are owed a right to confidentiality and be given respect for any decisions they make.
- It is the clinician's responsibility to act in the child's or young person's best interests as well a safeguard them against all forms of harm.
- The law surrounding the provision of care for children and young adults may be complex, so help from senior colleagues should be sought where necessary.
- During discussions of treatment and care for a young patient, it is necessary to listen not only to the patient's opinions, but also to those of the parents or carers.
- A doctor must be prepared that, in some instances, a young patient may request to be seen alone, without their parents or carers present.
- A young person may be considered as having capacity to consent to a procedure if they fulfil the criteria outlined in the Mental Capacity Act 2005 outlined in the following points.
- A young person aged 16 or over may be presumed to have consent, whereas a child under 16 needs to be assessed for competency.
- The law in the United Kingdom regarding the consent to treatment in young persons aged between 16 and 17 varies according to which country you are in.
- Parents cannot override the decision of a competent young person who refuses treatment. Legal advice should be sought if a competent young person refuses a treatment which may be life-saving to them.

Parental responsibility

Parental responsibility is held by all mothers. A father may also have parental responsibility if he was married to the mother at the time of the child's birth, if they jointly registered the birth with the mother (from 1 December 2003 onwards), or if he attained parental responsibility through agreement with the child's mother or through a court order. Parental responsibility may also be held by a legally appointed guardian, the local authority in whose care a child is or a person with an emergency protection order for the child (https://www.gov.uk/parental-rights-responsibilities/who-has-parental-responsibility).

Royal College of Anaesthetists Website: *The Risks of Anaesthesia*

http://www.rcoa.ac.uk/patients-and-relatives/risks

This website provides a link to a series of articles written by anaesthetists addressing various concerns patients and their relatives may have regarding to anaesthesia. The topics listed on the website are:

- 'Feeling sick' http://www.rcoa.ac.uk/system/files/PI-Risk1_3.pdf
- 'Sore throat' http://www.rcoa.ac.uk/system/files/PI-Risk2_1.pdf
- 'Shivering' http://www.rcoa.ac.uk/system/files/PI-Risk3_1.pdf
- 'Damage to lips, teeth and tongue' http://www.rcoa.ac.uk/system/files/PI-Risk4_3.pdf
- 'Damage to the eye during general anaesthesia' http://www.rcoa.ac.uk/system/files/PI-Risk5_0.pdf
- 'Post-operative chest infection' http://www.rcoa.ac.uk/system/files/PI-Risk6_2.pdf
- 'Becoming confused after an operation' http://www.rcoa.ac.uk/system/files/PI-Risk7_1.pdf
- 'Awareness during general anaesthesia' http://www.rcoa.ac.uk/system/files/PI-Risk8_1.pdf
- 'Serious allergy during an anaesthetic (anaphylaxis)' http://www.rcoa.ac.uk/system/files/PI-Risk9_1.pdf
- Headache after a spinal or epidural injection
- 'Nerve damage associated with an operation during a general anaesthetic' http://www.rcoa.ac.uk/system/files/PI-Risk10_2.pdf
- 'Nerve damage associated with a spinal or epidural injection' http://www.rcoa.ac.uk/system/files/PI-Risk11_1.pdf
- 'Nerve damage associated with peripheral nerve block' http://www.rcoa.ac.uk/system/files/PI-Risk12_1.pdf
- 'Equipment failure' http://www.rcoa.ac.uk/system/files/PI-Risk13_1.pdf

- 'Death or brain damage' http://www.rcoa.ac.uk/system/files/PI-Risk14_2.pdf

Obstetric Anaesthetists' Association Website

http://www.oaa-anaes.ac.uk/content.asp?ContentID=221

This website has information leaflets in a variety of different languages. These may be printed out and given to the parturient and their families to help facilitate understanding and aid consent during labour and delivery. The different information leaflets are:

- 'Pain relief in labour'
- 'Caesarean section'
- 'Epidural information card'
- 'Phrase cards'
- 'High body mass index (BMI)'
- 'Headache after epidural'
- 'Regional anaesthesia for unplanned CS (caesarean section)'
- 'General anaesthesia for unplanned CS (caesarean section).'

General Medical Council Guidance for Doctors: *Confidentiality*, 2009

http://www.gmc-uk.org/guidance/ethical_guidance/confidentiality.asp

This guidance is designed to aid and assist doctors in how they may maintain respect and confidentiality when caring for patients.

Key points

- Although confidentiality is crucial to developing trust between a patient and a doctor, sometimes it may be necessary to share patient information with appropriate individuals to provide safe, effective care for both the individual patient and others in their community.
- Confidentiality is an important duty but not an absolute one. A doctor may disclose information if there is a legal requirement to do so, if the patient consents, or if it is in the public interest to do so.
- Patients have a legal right to know how their information will be used and to have access to or copies of their health records when requested. They should also be informed of any requests from external parties for disclosure of information, even if their consent is not required.
- For research purposes, unidentifiable, codified data may be disclosed without patient consent.
- When considering to disclose patient information in the public interest, it may be necessary to consult with a Caldicott Guardian or other similar advisor, who is impartial and not immediately connected with the use of the information to be disclosed. The Privacy Advisory Committee in Northern Ireland can advise on this matter. The Privacy Advisory Committee in Scotland, however, performs a different role, so the Caldicott Guardian should be consulted.
- It should be established with the patient with whom they would like their information to be shared with (e.g. parents, carers, and other family members). Although it is not a breach of confidentiality to listen to concerns from other family members regarding a patient's condition, a doctor should make it clear that they may not be able to discuss the patient's treatment or condition with that relative if the patient does not wish so.

British Medical Association Guidance: *Confidentiality and Disclosure of Information Toolkit*

http://www.bma.org.uk/practical-support-at-work/ethics/confidentiality-tool-kit

This website is made up of 16 readily downloadable cards, which cover specific areas relating to confidentiality including children, adults who lack capacity, and the deceased. The cards are designed to help assist the doctor regarding making decisions about patient confidentiality.

Surgical

Chen MM, Coakley FV, Kaimal A, *et al.* Guidelines for computed tomography and magnetic resonance imaging use during pregnancy and lactation. *Obstet Gynecol* 2008; 112(2 Pt 1):333–40

Key points

- This article describes evidence-based guidelines for the use of CT, MRI, and contrast media during pregnancy for selected indications including suspected acute appendicitis, pulmonary embolism, renal colic, trauma, and cephalopelvic disproportion.
- Risks and benefits of all imaging modalities should be discussed with patients.
- Suspected appendicitis—ultrasound is the investigation of choice. If it is negative, MRI or CT can be obtained.
- Suspected pulmonary embolism—CT is the initial diagnostic investigation.
- Suspected renal colic—ultrasound should be the initial imaging of choice.
- Trauma—ultrasound is the initial imaging evaluation for trauma. If serious injury is suspected, CT should be performed.
- Suspected cephalopelvic disproportion—pelvimetry is rarely required, but if necessary, low-dose CT pelvimetry can be performed.
- Contrast scans—iodinated contrast seems safe to use in pregnancy. Intravenous gadolinium is contraindicated, and should be used only if it is absolutely essential. It is safe to continue breastfeeding after receiving iodinated contrast or gadolinium.

Society of American Gastrointestinal and Endoscopic Surgeons. *Guidelines for Diagnosis, Treatment, and Use of Laparoscopy for Surgical Problems During Pregnancy*, 2011

http://www.sages.org/publications/guidelines/guidelines-for-diagnosis-treatment-and-use-of-laparoscopy-for-surgical-problems-during-pregnancy/

Key points on the surgical techniques

- Laparoscopy can be performed safely in any trimester of pregnancy.
- Pregnant patients should be positioned with left lateral tilt to avoid vena cava compression.
- Initial abdominal access can be performed with an open technique (Hasson), Veress needle, or an optical trocar. The location should be adjusted according to the uterine fundal height and previous incisions.
- CO_2 insufflation pressure should be maintained between 10 and 15 mmHg.
- Intraoperative and postoperative venous thromboprophylactic measures should be performed. LMWH should be given in patients undergoing extended major operations.
- Fetal heart rate monitoring should be carried out preoperatively and postoperatively in patients undergoing emergency procedures.
- The obstetric team should be consulted.
- Tocolytics should not be given routinely. However, it should be considered when there are signs of preterm labour.

NICE. *Surgical Site Infection: Prevention and Treatment of Surgical Site Infection*. Clinical Guideline 74, October 2008

http://www.nice.org.uk/guidance/CG74

Key points

- Surgical site infection is an infection which occurs in a wound after an invasive operation.
- All surgical patients and their carers should receive clear information on the risks of surgical site infections and methods of prevention and treatment.

Preoperative phase

- Routine hair removal is not recommended for clean non-prosthetic uncomplicated surgery.
- An electric clipper with a disposable head should be used on the day of surgery if hair removal is essential.
- Antibiotic prophylaxis is required for the following types of surgery:
  - Clean surgery which involves an insertion of a prosthesis or an implant
  - Clean surgery where there is a risk of contamination from other sites
  - Contaminated surgery.
- Local antibiotic guidelines should be used for the surgical prophylaxis.
- When the prophylaxis is required, a single shot of intravenous antibiotic is given at the induction of anaesthesia, or earlier if the surgery involves the use of tourniquet.

Intraoperative phase

- The surgical site should be cleaned immediately before incision using an antiseptic solution, such as povidone-iodine or chlorhexidine.

Postoperative phase

- A non-touch technique must be employed when changing surgical dressings. If the wound is left open to heal without surgical intervention, advice from a tissue viability nurse should be sought in order to choose a suitable dressing.

World Health Organization. *WHO Guidelines for Safe Surgery 2009: Safe Surgery Saves Lives*, 2009

http://whqlibdoc.who.int/publications/2009/9789241598552_eng.pdf

Ten essential objectives and recommendations

1. The theatre team should confirm the patient's identity and correct site of operation.
2. A professionally trained anaesthesia provider must be present throughout the case, and monitor the patient appropriately.
3. The team must be prepared for life-threatening loss of airway or respiratory function.
4. Risk of high blood loss should be assessed. Appropriate monitoring, adequate intravenous access, and blood products must be available if the risk of bleeding is high.
5. Allergies must be identified preoperatively.
6. The team should minimize the risk of surgical site infection by administering appropriate prophylactic antibiotics and antiseptic skin preparation.
7. A full count of swabs, instruments, and other items should be carried out by the team.
8. All surgical specimens must be correctly labelled with the patient's details, the specimen name, and the site and side from which the specimen was taken.
9. The surgeon should inform all team members of the critical steps of the operation; nursing staff and the anaesthetist should communicate any concerns clearly.
10. Regular audits of surgical capacity, and outcomes should be carried out.

NICE. *Caesarean Section*. Clinical Guideline 132, November 2011

http://publications.nice.org.uk/caesarean-section-cg132

This guideline gives evidence-based recommendations for the management of women who may require a caesarean delivery.

Woman-centred care

- Pregnant women should receive evidence-based information about caesarean delivery (CD) during the antenatal period. The information should include the indications for CD, the risks, benefits, and implications of CD on future births.

Planned CD is offered for the following indications

- Breech presentation—if external cephalic version is contraindicated or unsuccessful
- Multiple pregnancy—if the first twin is not cephalic
- Placenta praevia—both minor and major
- Morbidly adherent placenta

- Women with HIV who are not receiving antiretroviral drugs or who have a viral load of 400 copies/mL on antiretroviral drugs
- Women who are co-infected with HIV and hepatitis
- Women with primary herpes simplex infection in the third trimester of pregnancy
- Maternal request—after explaining the risks and benefits of CD and offering support including mental health support.

Factors reducing the likelihood of CD during intrapartum care

- Continuous support during labour
- A partogram with 4-hour action line to monitor labour progress
- Induction of labour beyond 41 weeks' gestation in uncomplicated pregnancies.

Eating during labour

- Isotonic drinks during labour can prevent ketosis.

Procedural aspects of CD

- Planned CD should not routinely take place before 39 weeks' gestation.
- Classification of urgency:
  1. Immediate threat to the life of woman or fetus (decision to delivery interval (DDI) 30 minutes)
  2. Maternal or fetal compromise, which is not immediately life-threatening (DDI 75 minutes in most cases)
  3. No maternal or fetal compromise but needs early delivery
  4. Delivery timed to suit woman or staff
- All women should have haemoglobin assessment before the CD. If they are at risk of blood loss of more than 1000 mL, the CD should take place at a hospital where there is an on-site blood transfusion service.
- Women should be offered neuraxial anaesthesia for CD if they do not have any contraindications. When general anaesthesia is required, it should include preoxygenation, cricoid pressure, and rapid sequence induction. Each maternity unit should have regular failed intubation drills. Antacids should be given before the CD and antiemetics should be offered during the CD. The operating table should be tilted 15°.

Surgical techniques

- Antibiotics should be given before skin incision.
- The Joel Cohen transverse incision should be used.
- After delivery, 5 units of oxytocin should be given as a slow intravenous injection. The placenta is removed by controlled umbilical cord traction. Exteriorization of the uterus is not generally recommended.
- Umbilical artery pH should be measured after all CDs with suspected fetal compromise.
- Thromboprophylaxis should be offered to all women who have had CD.

Care of the baby born by CD

- A practitioner skilled in newborn resuscitation should be present at CD if performed under general anaesthesia or if there is evidence of fetal compromise.

Care of the woman undergoing CD

Table A1.8 Monitoring requirements for women undergoing a CD

After CD	One-to-one care (until women regain airway control and cardiorespiratory stability)
After recovery from anaesthesia	Observations every half hour for 2 hours and hourly afterwards (if stable)
For women who have had intrathecal opioids	A minimum of hourly observations for 12 hours (after diamorphine), 24 hours (after morphine)
For women who have had epidural opioids or those who have patient-controlled analgesia with opioids	Hourly monitoring throughout the treatment and at least 2 hours after cessation of treatment

- Women should be offered intrathecal opioids for intra- and postoperative analgesia. NSAIDs should be offered as an adjunct provided there is no contraindication.
- If women are recovering well, they can eat and drink after the procedure. Urinary catheters should be removed 12 hours after the last neuraxial bolus.
- Monitoring requirements for women undergoing CD are described in Table A1.8.

Recovery following CD

- Women should be given appropriate wound care.
- Healthcare practitioners should be also aware of the signs and symptoms for urinary problems, endometritis, and thromboembolic disease.
- Women should be given an opportunity to discuss the indication for CD and birth options for future pregnancies.

Pregnancy and childbirth after CD

- When discussing future birth options, the following factors should be considered: maternal preferences, risks and benefits of repeat CD, and risks and benefits of planned vaginal birth after CD.

Royal College of Obstetricians and Gynaecologists and Royal College of Anaesthetists. *Classification of Urgency of Caesarean Section – A Continuum of risk*. Good Practice No. 11, April 2010

http://www.oaa-anaes.ac.uk/assets/_managed/editor/File/RCoA/Good%20Practice%2011%20CS%20FINAL.pdf

This guideline reinforces the practice of using a nationally agreed classification system for grading the urgency of caesarean delivery and formalizes the idea that the urgency of caesarean delivery represents a continuum of risk.

Summary of recommendations

- Delivery suites are encouraged to use the modified Lucas classification (see Appendix 2 in this book) of urgency of caesarean delivery. Use of the colour spectrum from green to red signifies the spectrum of risk associated with caesarean deliveries.

- There must be effective communication among the members of the multidisciplinary team in emergency cases. The team should reassess the category of urgency when the patient arrives to the theatre.
- Delivery suites should organize a formal drill for 'emergency caesarean delivery' on a regular basis.

APPENDIX 2

Scores and scales

Wint Mon, York-Mui Liu, Ioanna Mavridou, and Roshan Fernando

Analgesia

Bromage scoring system for motor block

(Chapter 1)
The Bromage scoring system is used to measure the degree of lower limb motor block (see Table A2.1).

Visual Analogue Scale (VAS)

(Chapters 14, 15, and 18)

No pain Severe pain

Figure A2.1 Visual Analogue Scale.

- VAS is usually described as a horizontal line, 100 mm in length. (See Figure A2.1)
- Word descriptors of pain severity are placed at each end.
- The patient is asked to mark on the line where they feel represents their perception of pain.
- The VAS score is obtained by measuring from the left hand of the scale to the point that the patient marked in millimetres.

Verbal rating scale (VRS)

(Chapters 14, 15, and 18)

1. No pain
2. Mild pain
3. Moderate pain
4. Severe pain.

Table A2.1 Bromage scoring system for lower limb motor block

Grade	Criteria
I	Free movement of legs and feet
II	Just able to flex knees with free movement of feet
III	Unable to flex knees, but with free movement of feet
IV	Unable to move legs or feet

Reproduced from Bromage PR. A comparison of the hydrochloride and carbon dioxide salts of lidocaine and prilocaine in epidural analgesia. *Acta Anaesthesiologica Scandinavica*, volume 9, Suppl. XVI: 55–69, Copyright © 1965 John Wiley & Sons.

- The VRS consists of a list of adjectives to describe increasing pain intensity.
- The most common words used are no pain, mild, moderate, and severe pain.
- Numbers are usually assigned to these adjectives to make the documentation easier.

Numerical rating scale (NRS)

(Chapters 14, 15, and 18)

0 1 2 3 4 5 6 7 8 9 10
No pain Severe pain

Figure A2.2 Numerical Rating Scale.

- 0 on NRS scale represents no pain and 10 is for severe pain (see Figure A2.2).
- Patient is asked to choose a number from 0 to 10 which best describes the intensity of his/her pain.

Antenatal care

(Chapter 6)
NICE guideline: *Routine Antenatal Care for Healthy Pregnant Women*, March 2008. http://www.nice.org.uk/guidance/cg62

For a summary of what should happen at antenatal appointments, see Table A2.2.

Assisted conception

(Chapter 9)
NICE Guideline: *Fertility: Assessment and Treatment for People with Fertility Problems*, February 2013. http://www.nice.org.uk/guidance/CG156

See Table A2.3 for a glossary of terms used in *in vitro* fertilization (IVF).

Critical care and resuscitation

SPOILT acronym for intrauterine resuscitation

- Syntocinon off
- Position—full left lateral

Table A2.2 Antenatal appointments and summary of what should happen at the appointments

First contact with a midwife or a doctor	◆ Advice on food hygiene and lifestyle ◆ Folic acid supplements ◆ Antenatal screening tests
Booking appointments	◆ Information on antenatal care pathway ◆ Advice on nutrition, including vitamin D supplements ◆ Information about maternity benefits and antenatal classes ◆ Calculate body mass index ◆ Measure blood pressure and test urine ◆ Offer dating scan and screening tests
16 weeks	◆ Review any screening tests ◆ Measure blood pressure and test urine
18–20 weeks	◆ Anomaly scan
25 weeks	◆ Check fundal height ◆ Measure blood pressure and test urine
28 weeks	◆ Check fundal height ◆ Measure blood pressure and test urine ◆ Offer first anti-D treatment to Rhesus D-negative mothers ◆ Further blood screening tests
31 weeks	◆ Review test results ◆ Measure fundal height ◆ Measure blood pressure and test urine
34 weeks	◆ Advice on how to prepare for labour and birth ◆ Offer second anti-D treatment to Rhesus D-negative mothers ◆ Check fundal height ◆ Measure blood pressure and check urine
36 weeks	◆ Information on breastfeeding and how to care for the newborn baby ◆ Information about vitamin K and screening tests for the newborn baby ◆ Advice on postnatal depression ◆ Measure fundal height ◆ Assess the position of the baby and discuss about an external cephalic version if the baby is breech ◆ Measure blood pressure check urine
38 weeks	◆ Give information about prolonged pregnancy ◆ Check fundal height ◆ Measure blood pressure and check urine
40 weeks	◆ Give information about prolonged pregnancy ◆ Check fundal height ◆ Measure blood pressure and check urine
41 weeks	◆ Check the size of the abdomen ◆ Measure blood pressure and check urine ◆ Offer a membrane sweep ◆ Offer an induction of labour

National Institute for Health and Clinical Excellence (2007) CG 62 *Routine antenatal care for healthy pregnant women*. London: NICE. Available from www.nice.org.uk/CG62 Reproduced with permission. NICE disclaimer: information accurate at time of press.

Table A2.3 IVF glossary

AIH	Artificial insemination using partner's sperm
ART	Assisted reproduction technology It includes intrauterine insemination (IUI), *in vitro* fertilization (IVF), intracytoplasmic sperm injection (ICSI) and donor insemination (DI).
DET	Double embryo transfer
DI	Donor insemination—the placement of donor sperm into the vagina, cervix, or womb
ET	Embryo transfer—the placement of one or more embryos in the uterus or fallopian tube
FSP	Fallopian sperm perfusion
GIFT	Gamete intrafallopian transfer—a procedure in which eggs are retrieved from a woman, mixed with sperm and immediately replaced in one of the woman's fallopian tubes so that they fertilize inside the body
ICI	Intracervical insemination—clinical delivery of sperm into the cervical os
ICSI	Intracytoplasmic sperm injection—a variation of IVF in which a single sperm is injected into the inner cellular structure of an egg
IUI	Intrauterine insemination—clinical delivery of sperm into the uterine cavity
IVF	*In vitro* fertilization—a technique in which eggs are collected from a woman and fertilized with a man's sperm outside the body
MESA	Microsurgical epididymal sperm aspiration
OHSS	Ovarian hyperstimulation syndrome
PESA	Percutaneous epididymal sperm aspiration
TEFNA	Testicular fine needle aspiration
TESA	Testicular sperm aspiration
TESE	Testicular sperm extraction
ZIFT	Zygote intrafallopian transfer

National Institute for Health and Care Excellence (2013) CG 156 *Fertility: assessment and treatment for people with fertility problems*. Manchester: NICE. www.nice.org.uk/CG156 Reproduced with permission. NICE disclaimer: information accurate at time of press.

- Oxygen
- IV—infusion of 1 L crystalloid
- Low blood pressure—consider vasopressor
- Tocolysis—e.g. terbutaline.

Reprinted from *International Journal of Obstetric Anesthesia*, Volume 11, issue 2. J.A. Thurlow, S.M. Kinsella, intrauterine resuscitation: active management of fetal distress, pp. 105–116, Copyright © 2002 with permission from Elsevier.

Adult Advanced Life Support Algorithm Resuscitation Council UK, 2010

(Chapter 22)

The algorithm and an explanation of how it should be applied in clinical practice is detailed in the following link: https://www.resus.org.uk/pages/als.pdf.

Clinical features of local anaesthetic toxicity

(Chapter 1)

Table A2.4 Neurological and cardiovascular features of local anaesthetic toxicity

Neurological features	Cardiovascular features
Sudden change in mental status	Sinus bradycardia
Loss of consciousness	Asystole
Agitation	Conduction abnormalities
Seizures—tonic clonic convulsion	Ventricular tachyarrhythmia

Data from http://www.aagbi.org/sites/default/files/la_toxicity_2010_0.pdf.

AAGBI safety guideline: *Management of Severe Local Anaesthetic Toxicity*, December 2010. http://www.aagbi.org/sites/default/files/la_toxicity_2010_0.pdf

See Table A2.4 for clinical features of local anaesthetic toxicity.

APACHE—Acute Physiology and Chronic Health Evaluation

- A scoring system applied within 24 hours of admission to intensive care to generate a morbidity score
- APACHE I contained 34 physiological variables. APACHE II and III scoring systems have further refined the data collected.

SAPS—Simplified Acute Physiology Score

- 12-point physiological scoring system applied 24 hours after admission
- Integer score generated between 0 and 163 which predicts mortality between 0% and 100%
- SAPS II now superseded by SAPS III
- Compared with APACHE II, it is much better at comparing patients with different diseases.

MPM—Mortality Prediction Model

- Scoring system to assess risk of death in intensive care
- Patients scored at 24, 48, and 72 hours after admission.

Classification of shock

See Table A2.5 for different classes of shock.

Protocol for management of minor postpartum haemorrhage

See Figure A2.3 for the protocol for management of minor postpartum haemorrhage.

Blood loss 500–1000 mL, no signs of clinical shock.

Alert midwife-in-charge

↓

Alert first-line obstetric and anaesthetic staff trained in the management of postpartum haemorrhage

↓

Insert 1 × 14 G cannula and consider taking bloods for group & screen, full blood count, coagulation screen including fibrinogen

↓

Start giving warmed crystalloids IV

↓

Record pulse and blood pressure every 15 minutes

↓

Reassess the situation and keep the patient and partner informed

↓

Identify the cause of the bleeding and manage accordingly

Figure A2.3 Protocol for management of minor postpartum haemorrhage.
Reproduced from: Royal College of Obstetricians and Gynaecologists. *Prevention and management of postpartum haemorrhage*. Green-top Guideline No. 52. London: RCOG; 2009, with the permission of the Royal College of Obstetricians and Gynaecologists.

Table A2.5 Classification of shock

	Class I	Class II	Class III	Class IV
Blood loss (mL)	Up to 750	750–1500	1500–2000	2000 or more
Blood loss (% blood volume)	Up to 15%	15–30%	30–40%	40% or more
Pulse rate (bpm)	<100	>100	>120	140 or higher
Blood pressure	Normal	Normal	Decreased	Decreased
Pulse pressure	Normal/increased	Decreased	Decreased	Decreased
Capillary refill	Normal	Decreased	Decreased	Decreased
Respiratory rate	14–20	20–30	30–40	>35
Urine output (mL/hour)	30 or more	20–30	5–15	Negligible
Central nervous system—mental status	Slightly anxious	Anxious	Anxious—confused	Confused—lethargic
Fluid replacement	Crystalloid	Crystalloid	Crystalloid and blood	Crystalloid and blood

Estimated Blood Loss Based on Patient's Initial Presentation (table 3.1) page 69 of the Ninth Edition Advance Trauma Life Support Student Manual. Reproduced with permission of American College of Surgeons.

Protocol for management of major postpartum haemorrhage

See Figure A2.4 for the protocol for management of major postpartum haemorrhage

Blood loss more than 1000 mL and continuing to bleed or clinical shock.

Alert midwife-in charge AND an experienced midwife

↓

Call obstetric middle grade and alert the consultant

Call anaesthetic middle grade and alert the consultant

Alert consultant clinical haematologist on call

Alert blood transfusion laboratory

Call porters to enable delivery to specimens and blood

Alert one team member to document all events, timings, drugs given, etc.

↓

Assess patient using 'ABC' and administer oxygen via facemask at 10–15 L/min

↓

Insert 2 × cannulae (14 G) and take bloods for cross-match (4 units minimum), full blood count, coagulation screen including fibrinogen, renal and liver function to check baseline

↓

Lie patient flat and try to keep them warm

Monitor temperature every 15 minutes. Continuously monitor pulse, blood pressure, and respiratory rate

Insert a Foley catheter to measure urine output

Consider inserting an arterial line

↓

Start giving warmed crystalloids rapidly until blood is available. Blood filters should not be used as they slow the rate of fluid administration

↓

Blood products given include red cells, fresh frozen plasma, platelets, and cryoprecipitate. Recombinant factor VIIa should only be used based on coagulation results

↓

Identify and treat the cause of the bleeding as appropriate

↓

Reassess the situation and consider transfer and admission to high dependency or intensive care units when stable

Figure A2.4 Protocol for management of major postpartum haemorrhage

Reproduced from: Royal College of Obstetricians and Gynaecologists. *Prevention and management of postpartum haemorrhage*. Green-top Guideline No. 52. London: RCOG; 2009, with the permission of the Royal College of Obstetricians and Gynaecologists.

Table A2.6 Apgar score

	Score 0	Score 1	Score 2
Activity (tone)	Limp	Some flexion	Active motion
Pulse	Absent	<100/min	>100/min
Grimace (reflex irritability)	No response	Grimace	Cry or active withdrawal
Appearance (skin colour)	Blue	Peripherally blue and centrally pink	Pink
Respiration	Absent	Weak cry or irregular respiration	Good cry

Reproduced with permission from Virginia Apgar, A Proposal for a New Method of Evaluation of the Newborn Infant, *Survey of Anesthesiology*, Volume 19, Issue 4, Copyright © 1975 Wolters Kluwer Health, Inc.

Fetal medicine and neonates

Apgar score

(Chapter 1)

The score is assessed at 1-minute and 5-minute intervals. Initial resuscitation measures should not be delayed to assess the Apgar score at 1 minute. A score of 3 is critically low; a score of 7–9 at 5 minutes is normal. See Table A2.6.

Fetal blood sampling results

(Chapter 4)

NICE guideline: *Fetal Blood Sampling*, November 2013. http://www.nice.org.uk/nicemedia/pdf/efmguidelinenice.pdf

- pH of 7.25 or more = normal
- pH of 7.21–7.24 = borderline
- pH of 7.20 or less = abnormal.

National Institute for Health and Clinical Excellence (2014) CG 190 *Intrapartum care: care of healthy women and their babies during childbirth*. London: NICE. Available from www.nice.org.uk/CG190 Reproduced with permission. NICE disclaimer: information accurate at time of press.

Normal umbilical cord gases

(Chapter 4)

See Table A2.7 for normal umbilical cord gas values. Data presented are mean values ± standard deviation.

Cardiotocography—electronic fetal monitoring

(Chapter 6)

NICE guideline: *Intrapartum Care*, September 2007. http://guidance.nice.org.uk/CG55/NICEGuidance/pdf/English

Table A2.7 Normal umbilical cord gas values

	Venous blood	Arterial blood
pH	7.35 ± 0.05	7.28 ± 0.05
pCO_2 (mmHg)	38 ± 5.6	49 ± 8.4
pO_2 (mmHg)	29 ± 5.9	18 ± 6.2
Base excess	−4 ± 2	−4 ± 2
Bicarbonate	20 ± 2.1	22 ± 2.5

Reprinted from *American Journal of Obstetrics and Gynecology*, Volume 151, issue 6, Edward R. Yeomans, John C. Hauth, Larry C. Gilstrap, Daniel M. Strickland, Umbilical cord pH, Pco2, and bicarbonate following uncomplicated term vaginal deliveries, pp. 798–800, Copyright © 1985 with permission from Elsevier.

Table A2.8 Description of cardiotocograph (CTG) features

Description	Baseline (beats/min)	Variability (beats/min)	Decelerations
Normal/Reassuring	100–160	≥5	None or early
Non-reassuring	161–180	<5 for 30–90 minutes	Variable decelerations ◆ dropping from baseline by ≤60 beats/min and taking ≤60 seconds to recover ◆ present for >90 minutes ◆ occurring with >50% of contractions Or Variable decelerations ◆ dropping from baseline by >60 beats/min or taking >60 seconds to recover ◆ present for up to 30 minutes ◆ occurring with >50% of contractions Or Late decelerations ◆ present for up to 30 minutes ◆ occurring with >50% of contractions
Abnormal	>180 or <100	<5 for >90 minutes	Non-reassuring variable decelerations ◆ still occurring 30 minutes after commencing conservative management ◆ occurring with >50% of contractions Or Late decelerations ◆ present for >30 minutes ◆ not improving with conservation management ◆ occurring with >50% of contractions Or Bradycardia or a single prolonged deceleration lasting ≥3 minutes

National Institute for Health and Clinical Excellence (2008) CG 55 Intrapartum care. London: NICE. Available from www.nice.org.uk/CG655 Reproduced with permission. NICE disclaimer: information accurate at time of press.

Typical fetal doses and risks of childhood cancer for some common imaging procedures

(Chapter 10)

Advice from the Health Protection Agency, The Royal College of Radiologists and the College of Radiographers: *Protection of Pregnant Patients during Diagnostic Medical Exposures to Ionizing Radiation*, 2009.
http://www.hpa.org.uk/webc/HPAwebFile/HPAweb_C/1238230848746

Table A2.10 shows a number of common diagnostic X-ray examinations with their typical fetal doses and associated cancer risks.

WHO: *Breastfeeding and Maternal Medications*, 2002

(Chapter 11)

World Health Organization. *Breastfeeding and Maternal Medication. Recommendations for Drugs in the Eleventh WHO Model List of Essential Drugs*. 2002. http://whqlibdoc.who.int/hq/2002/55732.pdf

See Table A2.11 for WHO recommendations for maternal medication during breastfeeding.

STAN analysis

(Chapter 12)

Amer-Wahlin I, Arulkumaran S, Hagberg H, *et al*. Fetal electrocardiogram: ST waveform analysis in intrapartum surveillance. *BJOG* 2007; 114:1191–3.

ST waveform analysis of fetal electrocardiogram (ECG) for intrapartum surveillance (STAN) is a new method of fetal monitoring, and is used in conjunction with cardiotocography (CTG) during labour. It has been used in the expert centres in Scandinavia. STAN simplified clinical guidelines recommend that if STAN events occur with suspicious or abnormal CTG (Table A2.12), an appropriate intervention should be performed within 20 minutes. During the first stage of labour, the interventions should include intrauterine resuscitation and the treatment for maternal low blood pressure. Caesarean section is recommended if there is no improvement. For the second stage of labour with active pushing, an appropriate intervention is an operative delivery, unless spontaneous vaginal delivery is imminent.

A three-tiered system for the categorization of fetal heart rate patterns

(Chapter 20)

ACOG Practice Bulletin 106: *Intrapartum Fetal Heart Rate Monitoring: Nomenclature, Interpretation, and General Management Principles*, July 2009. http://www.acog.org/~/media/List of Titles/PBListOfTitles.pdf?dmc=1&ts=20140228T0623236788 (ACOG practice bulletin may be viewed by ACOG members or with a valid ATHENS password).

The three categories of the fetal heart rate (FHR) interpretation system are shown in Table A2.13.

Gastrointestinal system

Liver function tests in pregnancy

(Chapter 2)

Table A2.9 Management for different CTG categories

Category	Definition	Interpretation	Management
Normal/reassuring	All 3 features are normal/reassuring	◆ normal CTG ◆ no non-reassuring or abnormal features ◆ healthy fetus	◆ Continue CTG and normal care ◆ If CTG was commenced due to concerns arising from intermittent auscultation, remove CTG after 20 minutes if there are no non-reassuring or abnormal features and no ongoing risk factors
Non-reassuring and CTG suggests need for conservative management	1 non-reassuring feature AND 2 normal/reassuring features	May be associated with increased risk of fetal acidosis (If accelerations are present, fetal acidosis is unlikely)	◆ Consider possible underlying causes ◆ If baseline rate is >160 beats per minute, check maternal temperature and heart rate. If either is raised, give paracetamol and fluid ◆ Start ≥ 1 conservative measures • Encourage the woman to mobilise or adopt a left lateral position and avoid being supine • Give oral or intravenous fluid • Stop oxytocin if being used and/or offer tocolysis ◆ Inform co-ordinating midwife and obstetrician
CTG is abnormal and indicates need for conservative measures and further testing	1 abnormal feature OR 2 non-reassuring features	More likely to be associated with fetal acidosis	◆ Consider possible underlying causes ◆ If baseline rate is > 180 beats per minute, check maternal temperature and heart rate. If either is raised, give paracetamol and fluid ◆ Start ≥ 1 conservative measures ◆ Inform co-ordinating midwife and obstetrician ◆ Offer to take an FBS after starting conservative measures. Or expedite birth if an FBS cannot be taken and no accelerations are seen from scalp stimulation ◆ Take action sooner than 30 minutes if late decelerations are seen with tachycardia and/or reduced variability ◆ Inform consultant obstetrician if any FBS result is abnormal ◆ Discuss with consultant obstetrician if an FBS cannot be obtained or a third FBS is thought to be necessary
CTG is abnormal and indicates need for urgent intervention	Bradycardia or a single prolonged deceleration with baseline < 100 beats per minute lasting ≥3 minutes	Very likely to be associated with current fetal acidosis or imminent rapid development of fetal acidosis	◆ Start ≥ 1 conservative measures ◆ Inform co-ordinating midwife ◆ Urgent ask for obstetric help ◆ Prepare for urgent birth ◆ Expedite birth if persists for 9 minutes ◆ If fetal heart rate recovers before 9 minutes, reassess decision to expedite birth in discussion with the woman

Table A2.10 Typical fetal doses and risks of childhood cancer for some common diagnostic medical exposures

Procedure	Fetal dose range (mGy)	Childhood cancer risk
X-ray chest	0.001–0.01	<1/1,000,000
X-ray CT pulmonary angiogram	0.01–0.1	1/1,000,000 to 1/100,000
X-ray CT chest and liver	0.1 to 1.0	1/100,000 to 1/10,000
X-ray lumbar spine X-ray CT lumbar spine X-ray CT abdomen	1.0 to 10	1/10,000 to 1/1000
X-ray CT pelvis X-ray CT pelvis and abdomen X-ray CT, pelvis, abdomen, and chest	10–50	1/1000 to 1/200

CT, computed tomography.

Adapted with permission from Public Health England. *Protection of Pregnant Patients during Diagnostic Medical Exposures to Ionising Radiation.* http://www.hpa.org.uk/webc/HPAwebFile/HPAweb_C/1238230848746

Table A2.11 WHO recommendations for drugs during breastfeeding

	Compatible with breastfeeding	Compatible but monitor infants for side effects	Avoid if possible and monitor infants for side effects	Avoid if possible. May inhibit lactation	Avoid
Thiopentone Ketamine Ether N_2O Oxygen	✓				
Bupivacaine Lignocaine	✓				
Atropine		✓			
Diazepam		Short-acting preferable			
Morphine Codeine Pethidine		✓ (Avoid repeated doses)			
Ibuprofen Paracetamol	✓				
Chlorpheniramine			✓		
Dexamethasone Hydrocortisone	In single dose				
Prednisolone	✓				
Carbamazepine Phenytoin Sodium valproate Phenobarbital		✓			
Magnesium sulphate	✓				
Beta lactam drugs	✓ (No data available for imipenem and cilastatin)				
Erythromycin	✓				
Gentamicin		✓			
Metronidazole			✓		
Clindamycin			✓		

Haematology

Changes in coagulation

(Chapter 2)

See Table A2.15 for reference ranges for thromboelastography parameters.

See Table A2.16 for ROTEM reference limits.

Intrapartum care

Bishops score

(Chapter 12)

Bishops score assesses how readily patients will go into labour after an induction (Table A2.17):

- Scores of less than 5 = unfavourable
- Score of more than 5 = favourable.

The planes of Hodge

(Chapter 12)

The planes of Hodge are used to assess the progress of labour and to ascertain the engagement of the fetal head. There are four horizontal parallel planes:

I the superior strait, high in the pelvis

II the level of the inferior aspect of symphysis pubis

III the level of ischial spines

IV the level of the tip of coccyx.

Table A2.12 STAN events and CTG findings that warrant an intervention within 20 minutes

	Intermediary CTG	Abnormal CTG	Pre-terminal CTG
Episodic T/QRS rise	>0.15	>0.1	Immediate delivery
Baseline T/QRS rise	>0.01	>0.05	
Biphasic ST	Three biphasic ST events	Two biphasic ST events	

Reproduced from Amer-Wahlin I, Arulkumaran S, Hagberg H, Maršál K, Visser G. Fetal electrocardiogram: ST waveform analysis in intrapartum surveillance. *BJOG: An International Journal of Obstetrics and Gynaecology*, volume 114, issue 10, pp. 1191–1193, Copyright © 2007 John Wiley & Sons.

Kleihauer acid elution test

- Also known as Kleihauer–Betke test or Kleihauer–Betke stain.
- This test is used to measure the amount of fetal haemoglobin in the maternal blood which has been transferred during the pregnancy in Rhesus-negative mothers.
- The percentage of fetal blood cells compared with maternal cells (FMH) is calculated from a blood slide which has been subjected to an acid bath to remove adult haemoglobin and Shephard's stain to highlight fetal haemoglobin.
- Flow cytometry is a more sensitive method to measure FMH but is not available in all hospitals.

Data from Betke K, Kleihauer E. Fetaler und bleibender Blutfarbstoff in Erythrozyten und Erythroblasten von menschlichen Feten und Neugeborenen. *Blut*, volume 4, issue 4, pp. 241–249 Copyright © 1958 Springer.

Risk factors for placental abruption

- Abruption in a previous pregnancy
- Pre-eclampsia
- Fetal growth restriction
- Non-vertex presentation
- Polyhydramnios
- Increasing maternal age
- Multiparity
- Low body mass index
- Pregnancy following assisted reproduction techniques
- Intrauterine infection
- Premature rupture of membranes
- Abdominal trauma
- Smoking
- Drug misuse—in particular, cocaine and amphetamine use in pregnancy.

Reproduced from: Royal College of Obstetricians and Gynaecologists. *Antepartum Haemorrhage*. Green-top Guideline No. 63. London: RCOG; 2011, with the permission of the Royal College of Obstetricians and Gynaecologists.

Risk factors of placenta praevia

- Previous placenta praevia
- Previous caesarean delivery—risk increases with increasing number of previous caesarean deliveries
- Previous termination of pregnancy
- Multiparity

Table A2.13 Three-tier fetal heart rate interpretation system

	Baseline rate	Baseline FHR variability	Accelerations	Decelerations
Category I	110–160 beats per minute	Moderate	Present or absent	Early deceleration—absent or present Late or variable deceleration—absent
Category II	Bradycardia—not accompanied by absent baseline variability Tachycardia	Minimal baseline variability Absent variability with no recurrent decelerations Marked baseline variability	Absence of induced acceleration after fetal stimulation	Recurrent variable decelerations accompanied by minimal or moderate baseline variability Prolonged deceleration >2 minutes but <10 minutes Recurrent late decelerations with moderate baseline variability Variable decelerations with other characteristics such as slow return to baseline, overshoots, or 'shoulders'
Category III	Absent baseline FHR variability and any of the following: Recurrent late decelerations Recurrent variable decelerations Bradycardia Sinusoidal pattern			

Reproduced with permission from George Macones, Gary Hankins, Catherine Spong, *et al.*, The 2008 National Institute of Child Health and Human Development Workshop Report on Electronic Fetal Monitoring: Update on Definitions, Interpretation, and Research Guidelines, *Obstetrics & Gynecology*, Volume 112, Issue 3, pp. 661–666, Copyright © 2008 Wolters Kluwer Health, Inc.

Table A2.14 Liver function tests in pregnancy

	Non-pregnant	Pregnant
Albumin (g/L)	33–41	24–31
AST (U/L)	1–30	1–21
ALT (U/L)	1–40	1–30
Bilirubin (micromol/L)	3–22	3–14
ALP (U/L)	25–100	125–250

- Advanced maternal age (> 40 years)
- Multiple pregnancy
- Smoking
- Endometrial deficiency secondary to:
  - uterine scar
  - endometritis
  - manual removal of placenta
  - curettage
  - submucous fibroid
- Assisted conception.

Reproduced from: Royal College of Obstetricians and Gynaecologists. *Antepartum Haemorrhage*. Green-top Guideline No. 63. London: RCOG; 2011, with the permission of the Royal College of Obstetricians and Gynaecologists.

Amnioinfusion

A technique used to increase the amount of amniotic fluid around the fetus during pregnancy. Using ultrasound guidance, a needle is inserted into the uterine cavity and either saline or Hartmann's solution is infused until the level of amniotic fluid is normal. This procedure may be repeated if oligohydramnios occurs.

Table A2.15 Preoperative and postoperative TEG thromboelastography parameters

	Pregnant (preoperative) n = 50; mean (2 standard deviations)	Pregnant (postoperative) n = 50; mean (2 standard deviations)	Non-pregnant reference range; 2 standard deviations
R time (min)	7.0 (1.0–13.0)	6.6 (2.4–10.8)	4–8
K time (min)	2.0 (0.2–3.8)	1.8 (0.4–3.2)	0–4
MA (mm)	75.4 (64.6–86.2)	76.4 (66.8–86.0)	54–72
Alpha angle (degree)	64.8 (47.6–82.0)	67.3 (53.5–81.1)	47–74
Ly30 (%)	1.6 (0–8.8)	0.7 (0–4.9)	0–8
CI	1.2 (–5.4–7.8)	1.8 (–3.4–7.0)	-3–3

Table A2.16 ROTEM® thromboelastometer 95% reference limits for third trimester parturients and non-pregnant female controls

Test		Pregnant, median (95% reference limits)	Control,median (95% reference limits)
INTEM®	CT (s)	140 (86–168)	151 (113–266)
	CFT (s)	48 (33–108)	54 (35–120)
	Alpha angle (degree)	81 (71–83)	79 (63–83)
	MCF (mm)	71 (55–79)	64 (57–73)
EXTEM®	CT (s)	47 (31–80)	48 (30–91)
	CFT (s)	50 (34–86)	61 (37–104)
	Alpha angle (degree)	80 (64–83)	78 (66–83)
	MCF (mm)	73 (66–92)	66 (53–74)
FIBTEM®	CT (s)	49 (20–95)	48 (29–92)
	CFT (s)	N/A	N/A
	Alpha angle (degree)	78 (33–86)	69 (16–81)
	MCF (mm)	25 (15–38)	17 911–37)

Atosiban

This oxytocin receptor agonist is used as a tocolytic agent to delay preterm delivery. It is licensed for use in the United Kingdom. It is significantly more expensive than nifedipine.

Nifedipine

This is a calcium channel antagonist. Although no direct comparison has been made comparing the efficacy of nifedipine with atosiban, a systematic review adjusted for indirect comparison showed that nifedipine was associated with a non-significant trend towards increased likelihood of delay in delivery by 48 hours.

Table A2.17 Bishops score

Cervical features	Scores			
	0	1	2	3
Dilatation (cm)	0	1–2	3–4	5–6
Effacement (%)	0–30	40–60	60–70	80+
Presenting part in relation to ischial spine (cm)	–3	–2	–1/0	+1/+2
Consistency	Firm	Medium	Soft	
Position	Posterior	Mid-position	Anterior	

Table A2.18 The Quintero classification system

Stage	Classification
I	There is a discrepancy in amniotic fluid volume with oligohydramnios of a maximum vertical pocket (MVP) ≤ 2 cm in one sac and polyhydramnios in other sac (MVP ≥ 8 cm). The bladder of the donor twin is visible and Doppler studies are normal
II	The bladder of the donor twin is not visible (during length of examination, usually around 1 hour) but Doppler studies are not critically abnormal
III	Doppler studies are critically abnormal in either twin and are characterized as abnormal or reversed end-diastolic velocities in the umbilical artery, reverse flow in the ductus venosus or pulsatile umbilical venous flow
IV	Ascites, pericardial or pleural effusion, scalp oedema or overt hydrops present
V	One or both babies are dead

Reproduced from: Royal College of Obstetricians and Gynaecologists. *Management of monochorionic twin pregnancies*. Green-top Guideline No. 51. London: RCOG; 2008, with the permission of the Royal College of Obstetricians and Gynaecologists. Adapted by permission from Macmillan Publishers Ltd: *Journal of Perinatology*, volume 19, pp. 550–5, Quintero RA *et al*., Staging of twin-twin transfusion syndrome, copyright (1999).

The Quintero classification system of staging twin-to-twin transfusion (TTTS)

The Quintero system of staging TTTS is shown in Table A2.18.

Lovset manoeuvre

This manoeuvre is used for a vaginal breech delivery when the arms are extended above the baby's head. Once the scapula is visible, the operator holds the baby by the hips and rotates the body up by 180° to bring the arm in front of the face. The operator is then able to sweep the arms down across the face to free it. The body is then returned to the anterior position and the procedure repeated to free the other arm as needed.

Mariceau–Smellie–Veit manoeuvre

This manoeuvre is used to help deliver the fetal head in a vaginal breech delivery. An assistant applies suprapubic pressure on the mother. The operator then inserts their left hand into the vagina and uses their index and middle fingers to palpate and press on the fetal maxilla to bring the head into flexion. The palm of the left hand should rest on the fetal chest and the right hand is placed on the shoulder of the fetus and gently pulls the fetus in the direction of the fetal pelvis.

Burns–Marshall manoeuvre

This manoeuvre is used to facilitate the delivery of the fetal head in a vaginal breech delivery. Once the trunk has been delivered and the nape of the neck is visible under the pubic arch, the baby's trunk is then gradually lifted and brought up to the mother's abdomen by the operator holding the ankles with their right hand and swinging the baby upwards. The operator's left hand should be there to guard the perineum as the head is being delivered.

Medicolegal issues

Parental responsibility

Parental responsibility is held by all mothers. A father may also have parental responsibility if he was married to the mother at the time of the child's birth, if he jointly registered the birth with the mother (from 1 December 2003 onwards), or if he attained parental responsibility through agreement with the child's mother or through a court order. Parental responsibility may also be held by a legally appointed guardian, the local authority who has care of the child, or a person with an emergency protection order for the child (https://www.gov.uk/parental-rights-responsibilities/who-has-parental-responsibility).

The following cases are discussed further within Chapter 29:

- *Bartley* v *Studd* [1995]
- *Bolam* v *Friern Hospital Management Committee* [1957]
- *Bolitho* v *City and Hackney H.A.* [1998]
- *R* v *Bateman* [1925]
- *R* v *Adomako* [1994]
- *Crawford* v *Board of Governors of Charing Cross Hospital* [1953]
- *Early* v *Newham Health Authority* [1994]
- *Wickline* v *California* [1986]
- *Kent* v *Griffiths* [2000]
- *Chester* v *Afshar* [2004]
- *Re C* [1994]
- *B* v *NHS Hospital Trust* [2002]
- *Hewer* v *Bryant* [1970]
- *Re W (A Minor) (Medical Treatment)* [1992]
- *Gillick* v *West Norfolk and Wisbech Area Health Authority* [1986]
- *Re L (medical Treatment: Gillick Competency)* [1998]
- *Burke* v *United Kingdom* [2006]
- *HE* v *NHS Trust* [2003]
- *Re MB* [1997]
- *Re S* [1992]
- *Norfolk and Norwich NHS Trust* v *W* [1996]
- *Tameside and Glossop Acute Services Trust* v *CH* (a patient) [1996]
- *St George's Healthcare NHS Trust* v *S, R V Collins and others, ex parte S* [1998]
- *R* v *Bourne* [1939]
- *Re F* [1989]
- *X* v *Y* [1988]
- *W* v *Egdell* [1990]
- *Palmer* v *Tees HA* [2000]
- *Nicholas Lewis* v *Secretary of State for Health & Michael Redfern* [2008]
- *Wilsher* v *Essex Area HA* [1988].

Neurology

Chiari malformations

These are malformations in the cerebellum and occur usually as a result of insufficient space within the posterior cranial fossa causing the cerebellum and brainstem to be pushed down through the foramen magnum and into the upper spinal canal (see http://www.ninds.nih.gov/disorders/chiari/detail_chiari.htm).

There are four different types:

- *Type 1*—there is extension of the cerebellar tonsils into the foramen magnum without brainstem involvement. This is the most common form and may be asymptomatic, with some cases found incidentally. This is the only type which may be acquired.
- *Type 2*—otherwise known as 'classic Chiari malformation', is where there is extension of both cerebellum and brainstem into the foramen magnum. In addition, the cerebellar vermis may be only partially complete or absent. This type of malformation is usually accompanied by a myelomeningocele. The term 'Arnold-Chiari malformation' specifically describes type 2 malformations.
- *Type 3*—the cerebellum, brainstem, and occasionally part of the fourth ventricle herniate through the foramen magnum and into the spinal cord. The herniated cerebellar tissue can also enter an occipital encephalocoele. This is the most serious form of Chiari malformation and is associated with severe neurological defects.
- *Type 4*—this is associated with an incomplete or underdeveloped cerebellum, otherwise known as 'cerebellar hypoplasia'. The cerebellar tonsils are found in their normal position but parts of the cerebellum are missing and there may be visible portions of the skull and spinal cord.

The International Headache Society's classification of headache disorders: diagnostic criteria for postdural (post-lumbar) puncture headache

(Chapter 27)

A. Any headache fulfilling criterion C

B. Dural puncture has been performed

C. Headache develops within 5 days of dural puncture

D. Not better accounted for by another ICHD-3 diagnosis

Reproduced with permission from The International Classification of Headache Disorders, 3rd edition (beta version), *Cephalalgia*, Volume 33, pp.629–808, Copyright © 2013 SAGE. http://cep.sagepub.com/content/33/9/629.full

Psychiatric

Risk factors for antenatal depression

- Maternal anxiety
- Life stress
- Prior depression
- Lack of social support
- Domestic violence
- Unintended pregnancy
- Relationship factors.

This guideline was produced only for NHS Scotland in 2010 by SIGN, and is due for review in 2016. The current status of SIGN guidelines in Scotland is available at http://www.sign.ac.uk. The grant of permission to any other person or body outside the UK to reprint or otherwise use the SIGN guidelines in any way is given on the strict understanding that such a person or body is not the intended user of the guidelines and the guidelines are used entirely at the person's or body's own risk. SIGN, Healthcare Improvement Scotland and NHS Scotland accept no responsibility for any adverse outcomes resulting from such use. Scottish Intercollegiate Guidelines Network (SIGN). *Management of perinatal mood disorders*. Edinburgh: SIGN; 2012. (SIGN publication no. 127). [cited 16 07 2015]. Available from URL: http://www.sign.ac.uk.

Risk factors for postnatal depression

- Past history of psychopathology and psychological disturbance during pregnancy
- Lack of social support
- Poor relationship with partner
- Recent life events
- Baby blues—an emotionally labile state experienced by the majority of women after childbirth, which commonly presents on the second or third postnatal day
- Obstetric complications
- History of abuse
- Low family income
- Lower occupational status
- Parents' perceptions of their own upbringing
- Unplanned pregnancy
- Unemployment
- Not breastfeeding
- Antenatal parental stress
- Antenatal thyroid dysfunction
- Coping style
- Longer time to conception
- Depression in fathers
- Having two or more children.

This guideline was produced only for NHS Scotland in 2010 by SIGN, and is due for review in 2016. The current status of SIGN guidelines in Scotland is available at http://www.sign.ac.uk. The grant of permission to any other person or body outside the UK to reprint or otherwise use the SIGN guidelines in any way is given on the strict understanding that such a person or body is not the intended user of the guidelines and the guidelines are used entirely at the person's or body's own risk. SIGN, Healthcare Improvement Scotland and NHS Scotland accept no responsibility for any adverse outcomes resulting from such use. Scottish Intercollegiate

Guidelines Network (SIGN). *Management of perinatal mood disorders*. Edinburgh: SIGN; 2012. (SIGN publication no. 127). [cited 16 07 2015]. Available from URL: http://www.sign.ac.uk.

Risk factors for postpartum psychosis

- Pre-existing psychotic illness (especially bipolar disorder)
- Personal history of postpartum psychosis
- Antenatal admission for psychosis or bipolar disorder
- Family history of affective psychosis
- Discontinuation of mood stabilizer prophylaxis
- Primiparity
- Delivery complications.

This guideline was produced only for NHS Scotland in 2010 by SIGN, and is due for review in 2016. The current status of SIGN guidelines in Scotland is available at http://www.sign.ac.uk. The grant of permission to any other person or body outside the UK to reprint or otherwise use the SIGN guidelines in any way is given on the strict understanding that such a person or body is not the intended user of the guidelines and the guidelines are used entirely at the person's or body's own risk. SIGN, Healthcare Improvement Scotland and NHS Scotland accept no responsibility for any adverse outcomes resulting from such use. Scottish Intercollegiate Guidelines Network (SIGN). *Management of perinatal mood disorders*. Edinburgh: SIGN; 2012. (SIGN publication no. 127). [cited 16 07 2015]. Available from URL: http://www.sign.ac.uk

Renal

Renal function values in non-pregnant and pregnant women

(Chapter 2)
See Table A2.19 for renal reference ranges.

Criteria for considering pregnancy in renal transplant recipients

1. Good general health for about 2 years after transplantation
2. Good stable allograft function [serum creatinine < 177μmol/L (2 mg/dL), preferably <133 μmol/L (<1.5 g/dL)]
3. No recent episodes of acute rejection and no evidence of ongoing rejection
4. Normal blood pressure on minimal antihypertensive regimen (only one drug)

Table A2.19 Reference ranges for renal function in non-pregnant and pregnant women

	Non-pregnant	Pregnant
Sodium (mmol/L)	135–145	132–140
Potassium (mmol/L)	3.5–5.5	3.2–4.6
Creatinine (mmol/L)	0.06–0.1	0.04–0.08
Urea (mmol/L)	2.5–6.8	1.0–3.8

This table was published in *Anesthesiology: Churchill's Ready Reference*, Michael Mythen *et al*, The Labour Ward, p. 163, Copyright Elsevier (2010).

5. Absence of, or minimal, proteinuria (< 0.50 g/day)
6. Normal allograft ultrasound (absence of pelvicalyceal distension)
7. Recommended immunosuppression:
   a. Prednisolone < 15 mg/day
   b. Azathioprine ≤ 2 mg/kg/day
   c. Cyclosporine or tacrolimus at therapeutic levels
   d. Mycophenolate mofetil (MMF) and sirolimus are contraindicated
   e. MMF and sirolimus should be stopped 6 weeks before conception is attempted.

Reproduced with permission from IV. 10 Pregnancy in renal transplant recipients, *Nephrology Dialysis Transplantation*, Volume 17, Suppl 4, Copyright © 2002 Oxford University Press.

Surgery

Classification for operative vaginal delivery

(Chapter 12)
Royal College of Obstetricians and Gynaecologists. Green-top guideline 26: *Operative Vaginal Delivery*, 2011. https://www.rcog.org.uk/globalassets/documents/guidelines/gtg26.pdf

The classification for operative vaginal delivery, as adapted from the American College of Obstetrics and Gynecology 2000, has four classes: outlet, low, mid, and high.
OutletIn this situation the fetal head is low down in the pelvis so that it is in the perineum and the scalp is visible without the need to part the labia. The reference point is the sagittal suture and without exceeding rotation of 45°, it can be visualized in one of four positions:

- Anterioposterior diameter
- Right occiput anterior
- Left occiput anterior
- Posterior position.

Low

The most palpable part of the fetal scalp per vaginum is at station 2+ cm or more and is not in contact with the pelvic floor. There are two subcategories in this class depending on whether the degree of rotation is greater or less than 45° from the occipitoanterior position.

Mid

In this category, the most palpable part of the fetal scalp per vaginum is between the ischial spines and station 2+ cm. Again, there are two subdivisions depending on whether the degree of rotation from the occipitoanterior position is greater or less than 45°. Abdominal palpation should only be able to detect up to 1/5 of the fetal head.

High

This is not included in the classification as it is not recommended that operative vaginal delivery should be attempted if more than 2/5 of the fetal head may be palpated abdominally and the fetal head is assessed to be above the ischial spines per vaginum.

Table A2.20 WHO Surgical Safety Checklist

Before induction of anaesthesia (with at least nurse and anaesthetist)	Before skin incision (with nurse, anaesthetist and surgeon)	Before patient leaves operating room (with nurse, anaesthetist and surgeon)
Has the patient confirmed his/her identity, site, procedure, and consent? • Yes **Is the site marked?** • Yes • Not applicable **Is the anaesthesia machine and medication check complete?** • Yes **Is the pulse oximeter on the patient and functioning?** • Yes **Does the patient have a:** **Known allergy?** • No • Yes **Difficult airway or aspiration risk?** • No • Yes, and equipment/assistance available **Risk of >500m1 blood loss (7m1/kg in children)?** • No • Yes, and two /Vs/central access and fluids planned	• **Confirm all team members have introduced themselves by name and role.** • **Confirm the patient's name, procedure, and where the incision will be made.** **Has antibiotic prophylaxis been given within the last 60 minutes?** • Yes • Not applicable **Anticipated Critical Events** **To Surgeon:** • What are the critical or non-routine steps? • How long will the case take? • What is the anticipated blood loss? **To Anaesthetist:** • Are there any patient-specific concerns? **To Nursing Team:** • Has sterility (including indicator results) been confirmed? • Are there equipment issues or any concerns? **Is essential imaging displayed?** • Yes • Not applicable (with nurse, anaesthetist and surgeon)	**Nurse Verbally Confirms:** • The name of the procedure • Completion of instrument, sponge and needle counts • Specimen labelling (read specimen labels aloud, including patient name) • Whether there are any equipment problems to be addressed **To Surgeon, Anaesthetist and Nurse:** • What are the key concerns for recovery and management of this patient?
This checklist is not intended to be comprehensive. Additions and modifications to fit local practice are encouraged.	Revised 1/2009	© WHO, 2009

Reprinted with permission from *WHO Surgical Safety Checklist* (first edition), 2008.

WHO surgical safety checklist

(Chapter 20)

The World Health Organization Surgical Safety Checklist is shown in Table A2.20.

WHO safer childbirth checklist

(Chapter 55)

The World Health Organization (WHO) developed the Safer Childbirth Checklist (www.who.int/patientsafety/implementation/checklists/childbirth/en/index.html) in response to the high mortality rate of pregnant women and neonates in low-resource settings, most of which were preventable. The checklist consists of 29 points, which address the major causes in low-income countries, of:

- Maternal death: haemorrhage, hypertensive disorders, obstructed labour, infection
- Intrapartum-related stillbirths: inadequate intrapartum management
- Neonatal deaths: infection, asphyxia, prematurity.

The checklist is divided into four sections and the points covered in each section are summarized in Table A2.21. This checklist is currently being trialled in over 100 hospitals and this study should be completed by 2015.

Lucas classification

(Chapter 20)

For definitions of different grades of caesarean delivery according to the Lucas classification, see Table A2.22.

Dupuis classification

(Chapter 20)

Table A2.21 Summary of the WHO Safer Childbirth Checklist

Section	Points covered
1. On admission	Patient identity, basic monitoring, need for any treatment including magnesium sulphate and antimicrobials
2. Just before pushing/ caesarean delivery	Appropriate equipment for delivery present, need for any antibiotics or magnesium sulphate
3. Soon after birth (within 1 hour)	Identify any maternal bleeding and manage appropriately, need for any further neonatal care
4. Before discharge	No further maternal bleeding, need for maternal or neonatal antibiotics, establishing feeding in neonate

Data from http://www.who.int/patientsafety/implementation/checklists/childbirth/en/index.html.

Table A2.22 The Lucas classification of caesarean delivery

Grade	Definition
1. Emergency	Immediate threat to life of woman or fetus
2. Urgent	Maternal or fetal compromise which is not immediately life-threatening
3. Scheduled	Needing early delivery but no maternal or fetal compromise
4. Elective	At a time to suit the woman and maternity team

Reprinted from Lucas DN, Yentis SM, Kinsella SM, Holdcroft A, May AE, Wee M, *et al.* Urgency of caesarean section: a new classification. *Journal of the Royal Society of Medicine*, volume 93, pp. 346–50, copyright © 2000. SAGE.

Classification for emergency caesarean delivery

- *Red*: Very urgent caesarean delivery for life-threatening maternal or fetal situation
- *Orange*: Urgent caesarean delivery
- *Green*: Non urgent intrapartum caesarean delivery

Reprinted from *European Journal of Obstetrics & Gynecology and Reproductive Biology*, Volume 140, edition 2, Olivier Dupuis *et al.*, Red, orange and green Caesarean sections: A new communication tool for on-call obstetricians, pp. 206–11, Copyright © 2008 with permission from Elsevier.

Criteria for diagnosing persistent post-surgical pain

(Chapter 25)

- Pain that develops after surgery
- Pain of at least 2 months' duration
- Other causes have been excluded.

Reproduced with permission from W. A. Macrae, Chronic post-surgical pain: 10 years on, *British Journal of Anaesthesia*, Volume 101, Issue 3, pp.77–86, Copyright © 2008 Oxford University Press.

Index

Illustrations (figures and tables) are comprehensively referred to from the text. Therefore, significant items in illustrations have only been given a page reference in the absence of their concomitant mention in the text referring to that illustration.

E

I

N

The manufacturer's authorised representative in the EU for product safety is Oxford University Press España S.A. of el Parque Empresarial San Fernando de Henares, Avenida de Castilla, 2 – 28830 Madrid (www.oup.es/en or product.safety@oup.com). OUP España S.A. also acts as importer into Spain of products made by the manufacturer.

www.ingramcontent.com/pod-product-compliance
Lightning Source LLC
Chambersburg PA
CBHW081453141225
36740CB00053B/405
9780198713333